CARDIOPULMONARY RESUSCITATION [a]

Steve C. Haskins

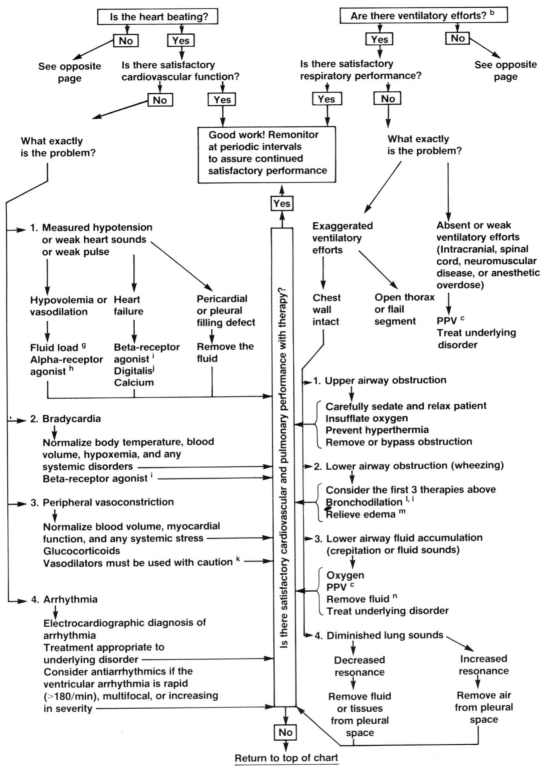

Is the heart beating?
- No → See opposite page
- Yes → Is there satisfactory cardiovascular function?
  - No → What exactly is the problem?
  - Yes → **Good work! Remonitor at periodic intervals to assure continued satisfactory performance**

Are there ventilatory efforts? [b]
- Yes → Is there satisfactory respiratory performance?
  - Yes → **Good work! Remonitor...**
  - No → What exactly is the problem?
- No → See opposite page

What exactly is the problem? (cardiovascular)

1. Measured hypotension or weak heart sounds or weak pulse

- Hypovolemia or vasodilation → Fluid load [g] / Alpha-receptor agonist [h]
- Heart failure → Beta-receptor agonist [i] / Digitalis [j] / Calcium
- Pericardial or pleural filling defect → Remove the fluid

2. Bradycardia

Normalize body temperature, blood volume, hypoxemia, and any systemic disorders
Beta-receptor agonist [i]

3. Peripheral vasoconstriction

Normalize blood volume, myocardial function, and any systemic stress
Glucocorticoids
Vasodilators must be used with caution [k]

4. Arrhythmia

Electrocardiographic diagnosis of arrhythmia
Treatment appropriate to underlying disorder
Consider antiarrhythmics if the ventricular arrhythmia is rapid (>180/min), multifocal, or increasing in severity

What exactly is the problem? (respiratory)

Exaggerated ventilatory efforts
- Chest wall intact
- Open thorax or flail segment

Absent or weak ventilatory efforts (Intracranial, spinal cord, neuromuscular disease, or anesthetic overdose)
→ PPV [c] / Treat underlying disorder

Is there satisfactory cardiovascular and pulmonary performance with therapy?
- Yes
- No → Return to top of chart

1. Upper airway obstruction

Carefully sedate and relax patient
Insufflate oxygen
Prevent hyperthermia
Remove or bypass obstruction

2. Lower airway obstruction (wheezing)

Consider the first 3 therapies above
Bronchodilation [l, i]
Relieve edema [m]

3. Lower airway fluid accumulation (crepitation or fluid sounds)

Oxygen
PPV [c]
Remove fluid [n]
Treat underlying disorder

4. Diminished lung sounds
- Decreased resonance → Remove fluid or tissues from pleural space
- Increased resonance → Remove air from pleural space

---

[n] Exudate: liquify with nebulized saline and systemic hydration; expectorant tracheal suction [o]

Transudate: minimize pulmonary hydrostatic pressure (venodilators [k], diure costeroids; treat systemic disorder; postural drainage; tracheal suction.

[o] Haskins, S.C., Management of Pulmonary Disease in the Critical Patient, in 2 and Critical Care, Lea & Febiger, Philadelphia, 1983.

D1226319

Section Editors	Section
Douglas H. Slatter	*Development of Veterinary Surgery*
Alan J. Lipowitz	*Surgical Biology*
Andreas Von Recum	*Surgical Methods*
Michael M. Pavletic	*Skin and Adnexa*
Melvin Helphrey	*Body Cavities*
Eberhard Rosin / Colin E. Harvey	*Alimentary System*
C. R. Bellenger	*Hernias*
A. Wendell Nelson	*Respiratory System*
George Eyster	*Cardiovascular System*
Anthony Schwartz	*Hemolymphatic System*
Stephen T. Simpson	*Nervous System*
Douglas H. Slatter	*Eye and Adnexa*
Dudley E. Johnston	*Male Reproductive System*
Dudley E. Johnston	*Female Reproductive System*
Bruce A. Christie	*Urinary System*
Anthony Schwartz	*Endocrine System*
Colin E. Harvey	*The Ear*
Stephen P. Arnoczky	*Musculoskeletal System*
Dennis D. Caywood	*Oncology*
Donald C. Sawyer	*Anesthetic Considerations*

TEXTBOOK OF
SMALL
ANIMAL SURGERY

Volume II

Edited by

Douglas H. Slatter,
B.V.Sc., M.S., Ph.D., F.R.C.V.S.

Diplomate, American College of Veterinary Surgeons
Diplomate, American College of Veterinary Ophthalmologists

Animal Eye and Surgical Clinic
La Habra, California

W.B. SAUNDERS COMPANY
Philadelphia   London   Toronto   Mexico City   Rio de Janeiro   Sydney   Tokyo   Hong Kong

W. B. Saunders Company: West Washington Square
                          Philadelphia, PA   19105

                          1 St. Anne's Road
                          Eastbourne, East Sussex BN21 3UN, England

                          1 Goldthorne Avenue
                          Toronto, Ontario M8Z 5T9, Canada

                          Apartado 26370—Cedro 512
                          Mexico 4, D.F., Mexico

                          Rua Coronel Cabrita, 8
                          Sao Cristovao Caixa Postal 21176
                          Rio de Janeiro, Brazil

                          9 Waltham Street
                          Artarmon, N.S.W. 2064, Australia

                          Ichibancho, Central Bldg., 22-1 Ichibancho
                          Chiyoda-Ku, Tokyo 102, Japan

Library of Congress Cataloging in Publication Data

Main entry under title:

Textbook of small animal surgery.

1. Veterinary surgery—Collected works.   I. Slatter, Douglas H.
   II. Title: Small animal surgery.   [DNLM: 1. Surgery, Operative—Veterinary. SF 911 T355]

SF911.T49   1985   636.089'7   83–14294

ISBN 0–7216–8348–7

Complete Set   ISBN   0–7216–8348–7
    Volume I   ISBN   0–7216–8349–5
   Volume II   ISBN   0–7216–8350–9

Textbook of Small Animal Surgery

Last digit is the print number: 9   8   7   6   5   4   3   2

To Our Patients

Contributors

Shehu U. Abdullahi, D.V.M., Ph.D.
Lecturer, Department of Surgery and Medicine, Faculty of Veterinary Medicine, and Director, Small Animal Medicine Section, Veterinary Teaching Hospital, Amadu Bello University, Zaria, Nigeria.

J. W. Alexander, D.V.M., M.S.
Diplomate, American College of Veterinary Surgeons. Professor and Chairman, Division of Agricultural and Urban Practice, and Director, Veterinary Medical Teaching Hospital, Virginia–Maryland Regional College of Veterinary Medicine, Blacksburg, Virginia.

Lorel K. Anderson, D.V.M.
Assistant Professor, Department of Small Animal Clinical Sciences, College of Veterinary Medicine, and Staff Veterinarian, Veterinary Clinical Center, Michigan State University, East Lansing, Michigan.

Steven Paul Arnoczky, D.V.M.
Diplomate, American College of Veterinary Surgeons. Associate Professor of Surgery, Cornell University Medical College; Associate Research Scientist, Division of Research, Director, Division of Laboratory Animal Care, and Director, Laboratory of Comparative Orthopaedics, The Hospital for Special Surgery, New York, New York.

Michael Aronsohn, V.M.D.
Clinical Assistant Professor of Surgery, School of Veterinary Medicine, Tufts University; Staff Surgeon, Angell Memorial Animal Hospital, Boston, Massachusetts.

John D. Bacher, D.V.M., M.S.
Chief, Surgery Unit, National Institutes of Health, Bethesda, Maryland.

J. E. Bartels, B.S., D.V.M., M.S.
Diplomate, American College of Veterinary Radiology. Professor of Radiology and Head, Department of Radiology, College of Veterinary Medicine, Auburn University, Auburn, Alabama.

Christopher R. Bellenger, B.V.Sc., Ph.D.
Associate Professor of Veterinary Surgery, Faculty of Veterinary Science, University of Sydney, New South Wales, Australia.

R. John Berg, D.V.M.
Resident in Surgery, Veterinary Teaching Hospital, Colorado State University, Fort Collins, Colorado.

Jeffrey L. Berzon, D.V.M.
Diplomate, American College of Veterinary Surgeons. Veterinary Specialists of Connecticut, P. C., West Hartford, Connecticut.

C. W. Betts, D.V.M.
Diplomate, American College of Veterinary Surgeons. Professor of Surgery, School of Veterinary Medicine, and Staff Surgeon, Veterinary Teaching Hospital, North Carolina State University, Raleigh, North Carolina.

A. G. Binnington, D.V.M., M.S.
Diplomate, American College of Veterinary Surgeons. Associate Professor, Department of Clinical Studies, Ontario Veterinary College, University of Guelph, Ontario, Canada.

Stephen I. Bistner, D.V.M.
Diplomate, American College of Veterinary Surgeons. Associate Professor of Comparative Ophthalmology, College of Veterinary Medicine, University of Minnesota, St. Paul, Minnesota.

Dale E. Bjorling, D.V.M., M.S.
Assistant Professor, Department of Small Animal Medicine and Surgery, College of Veterinary Medicine, University of Georgia, Athens, Georgia.

Charles E. Blass, D.V.M., M.S.
Assistant Professor of Veterinary Surgery, Department of Veterinary Clinical Sciences, College of Veterinary Medicine, Louisiana State University, Baton Rouge, Louisiana.

Mark S. Bloomberg, D.V.M., M.S.
Diplomate, American College of Veterinary Surgeons. Associate Professor and Chairman, Department of Surgical Sciences, College of Veterinary Medicine, and Associate Professor of Orthopaedic Surgery, Veterinary Medical Teaching Hospital, University of Florida, Gainesville, Florida.

Julia T. Blue, D.V.M., Ph.D.
Assistant Professor, Clinical Pathology, New York State College of Veterinary Medicine, Cornell University, Ithaca, New York.

David L. Bone, D.V.M.
Assistant Professor of Surgery, Department of Small Animal Clinics, College of Veterinary Medicine, Purdue University, West Lafayette, Indiana.

Harry W. Boothe, D.V.M., M.S.
Diplomate, American College of Veterinary Surgeons. Associate Professor, Department of Small Animal Medicine and Surgery, College of Veterinary Medicine, and Veterinary Teaching Hospital, Texas A&M University, College Station, Texas.

Adele L. Boskey, Ph.D.
Associate Professor, Biochemistry, Cornell University Medical College; Senior Scientist and Director, Laboratory of Ultrastructural Biochemistry, The Hospital For Special Surgery, New York, New York.

K. C. Bovée, D.V.M., M.Med.Sc.
Professor of Medicine, School of Veterinary Medicine, University of Pennsylvania, Philadelphia, Pennsylvania.

Gale Gilbert Bowman, D.V.M.
Practitioner, Raleigh, North Carolina.

Kyle G. Braund, D.V.M., M.S., Ph.D., F.R.C.V.S.
Diplomate, American College of Veterinary Internal Medicine. Associate Professor, School of Veterinary Medicine, and Staff Neurologist, Department of Small Animal Surgery and Medicine, School of Veterinary Medicine, Auburn University, Auburn, Alabama.

William R. Brawner, Jr., D.V.M., Ph.D.
Diplomate, American College of Veterinary Radiology. Assistant Professor, Department of Radiology, School of Veterinary Medicine, Auburn University, Auburn, Alabama.

Eugene M. Breznock, D.V.M., M.S., Ph.D.
Diplomate, American College of Veterinary Surgeons. Associate Professor, Department of Veterinary Surgery, School of Veterinary Medicine, and Chief, Small Animal Surgery Service, Veterinary Medical Teaching Hospital, University of California, Davis, California.

Ronald M. Bright, D.V.M., M.S.
Diplomate, American College of Veterinary Sur-

geons. Department of Urban Practice, College of Veterinary Medicine, University of Tennessee, Knoxville, Tennessee.

Alan H. Brightman II, D.V.M., M.S.
Diplomate, American College of Veterinary Ophthalmologists. Associate Professor, Department of Veterinary Clinical Medicine, College of Veterinary Medicine, and Ophthalmologist, Veterinary Medicine Teaching Hospital, University of Illinois, Urbana, Illinois.

Nancy O. Brown, V.M.D.
Diplomate, American College of Veterinary Surgeons. Practitioner, Hickory Veterinary Hospital, Plymouth Meeting, Pennsylvania; Consultant in Surgery, The Animal Medical Center, New York, New York.

Philip A. Bushby, B.S., D.V.M., M.S.
Diplomate, American College of Veterinary Surgeons. Associate Professor, College of Veterinary Medicine, Mississippi State University, Mississippi State, Mississippi.

Rhondda B. Canfield, B.V.Sc.
Tutor in Veterinary Anatomy, Department of Veterinary Anatomy, Faculty of Veterinary Science, The University of Sydney, New South Wales, Australia.

Joseph M. Carillo, D.V.M.
Diplomate, American College of Veterinary Internal Medicine. Staff, Internal Medicine—Neurology, The Animal Medical Center, New York, New York.

Dennis D. Caywood, D.V.M., M.S.
Diplomate, American College of Veterinary Surgeons. Associate Professor of Small Animal Surgery, Department of Small Animal Sciences, College of Veterinary Medicine, University of Minnesota, St. Paul, Minnesota.

Elizabeth D. Chambers, D.V.M., M.S.
Veterinary Ophthalmologist, Animal Eye & Surgical Associates, San Diego, California.

Bruce A. Christie, M.V.Sc.
Diplomate, American College of Veterinary Surgeons. Senior Lecturer in Veterinary Anatomy, Veterinary Preclinical Sciences, University of Melbourne, Parkville; Consultant in Soft Tissue Surgery, Veterinary Clinical Sciences, University of Melbourne, Werribee, Victoria, Australia.

William G. Connor, Ph.D.
Associate Professor, Division of Radiation Oncology,

Department of Radiology, University of Arizona Medical Center, Tucson, Arizona.

Cynthia S. Cook, D.V.M.
Resident, Ophthalmology, School of Veterinary Medicine, North Carolina State University, Raleigh, North Carolina.

Daniel M. Core, D.V.M.
Staff Surgeon, Martin Animal Hospital, Shreveport, Louisiana.

Susan M. Cotter, D.V.M.
Diplomate, American College of Veterinary Internal Medicine. Associate Professor of Medicine, School of Veterinary Medicine, Tufts University; Angell Memorial Animal Hospital; Lecturer in Cancer Biology, Harvard School of Public Health, Boston, Massachusetts.

Stephen W. Crane, D.V.M.
Diplomate, American College of Veterinary Surgeons. Professor of Surgery, School of Veterinary Medicine, North Carolina State University, Raleigh, North Carolina.

Dennis T. Crowe, Jr., D.V.M.
Diplomate, American College of Veterinary Surgeons. Assistant Professor of Surgery, Department of Small Animal Medicine, College of Veterinary Medicine, and Staff Surgeon, Small Animal Teaching Hospital, University of Georgia, Athens, Georgia.

William R. Daly, D.V.M.
Diplomate, American College of Veterinary Surgeons. Houston Veterinary Referral Surgery Service, Houston, Texas.

A. P. Davies, D.V.M., M.S.
Diplomate, American College of Veterinary Internal Medicine. Clinical Associate Professor, Department of Small Animal Clinical Sciences, College of Veterinary Medicine, and Lewis Hospital for Companion Animals, University of Minnesota, St. Paul, Minnesota.

Mark W. Dewhirst, D.V.M., Ph.D.
Assistant Professor, Division of Radiation Oncology, Duke University Medical Center, Durham, North Carolina.

Bonnie DeYoung
Surgery Research Technician, School of Veterinary Medicine, North Carolina State University, Raleigh, North Carolina.

David J. DeYoung, D.V.M.
Diplomate, American College of Veterinary Surgeons. Associate Professor of Surgery, Department of Companion Animal and Special Species Medicine, School of Veterinary Medicine, North Carolina State University, Raleigh, North Carolina.

W. Jean Dodds, D.V.M.
Chief, Laboratory of Hematology, Center for Laboratories and Research, New York State Health Department, Albany, New York.

Mary L. Dulisch, D.V.M., M.S.
Diplomate, American College of Veterinary Surgeons. Staff Surgeon, Angell Memorial Animal Hospital, Boston, Massachusetts.

Erick L. Egger, D.V.M.
Diplomate, American College of Veterinary Surgeons. Assistant Professor of Small Animal Surgery, College of Veterinary Medicine and Biomedical Sciences, and Orthopedic Surgeon, Veterinary Teaching Hospital, Colorado State University, Fort Collins, Colorado.

J. E. Eigenmann, D.V.M., Dr.Med.Vet., Ph.D.
Assistant Professor of Medicine, Department of Clinical Studies, School of Veterinary Medicine, University of Pennsylvania, Philadelphia, Pennsylvania.

Glenn S. Elliott, D.V.M.
Resident, Internal Medicine/Clinical Oncology, Purdue University, West Lafayette, Indiana.

Gary W. Ellison, D.V.M., M.S.
Diplomate, American College of Veterinary Surgeons. Assistant Professor, College of Veterinary Medicine, University of Florida, Gainesville, Florida.

T. Evans, D.V.M., M.S.
Diplomate, American College of Veterinary Anesthesiologists. Associate Professor, College of Veterinary Medicine, and Section Chief, Anesthesia, Veterinary Clinical Center, Michigan State University, East Lansing, Michigan.

George E. Eyster, V.M.D., M.S.
Diplomate, American College of Veterinary Surgeons. Professor of Thoracic and Cardiovascular Surgery, College of Veterinary Medicine, and Veterinary Clinical Center, Michigan State University, East Lansing, Michigan.

Roy T. Faulkner, D.V.M., M.S.
Staff Surgeon, Skyway Animal Hospital, St. Petersburg, Florida.

Daniel A. Feeney, D.V.M., M.S.
Diplomate, American College of Veterinary Radiology. Associate Professor of Radiology, College of Veterinary Medicine, University of Minnesota, St. Paul, Minnesota.

Beverly Ann Gilroy, D.V.M.
Diplomate, American College of Veterinary Anesthesiologists. Associate Professor of Anesthesiology, Department of Anatomy, Physiological Sciences and Radiology, School of Veterinary Medicine, and Head, Anesthesia Section, Veterinary Teaching Hospital, North Carolina State University, Raleigh, North Carolina.

Norman Gofton, B.V.Sc.
Assistant Professor, Ontario Veterinary College, University of Guelph, Ontario, Canada.

John Grandage, B.Vet.Med.
Associate Professor of Anatomy, School of Veterinary Studies, Murdoch University, Perth, Western Australia.

Jacqueline L. Grandy, D.V.M.
Diplomate, American College of Veterinary Anesthesiologists. Assistant Professor, College of Veterinary Medicine and Biomedical Sciences, and Veterinary Teaching Hospital, Colorado State University, Fort Collins, Colorado.

Kenneth M. Greenwood, D.V.M.
Private referral surgery practice, Ellenwood, Georgia.

C. R. Gregory, D.V.M.
Assistant Professor of Surgery, School of Veterinary Medicine, University of California, Davis, California.

Ronald L. Grier, D.V.M., Ph.D.
Diplomate, American College of Veterinary Surgeons. Professor, Department of Veterinary Clinical Sciences, College of Veterinary Medicine, Iowa State University, Ames, Iowa.

C. B. Grindem, D.V.M., Ph.D.
Diplomate, American College of Veterinary Pathologists. Assistant Professor, School of Veterinary Medicine, North Carolina State University, Raleigh, North Carolina.

L. R. Grono, B.V.Sc., M.Sc., Ph.D.
Associate Professor and Head, Department of Veterinary Surgery, and Surgeon, Veterinary Clinic, University of Queensland, St. Lucia, Queensland, Australia.

Nancy L. Hampel, D.V.M., M.S.
Staff Surgeon, Broadway Animal Hospital, El Cajon, California.

H. W. Hannah, B.S., J.D.
Lawyer, Texico, Illinois 62889.

Reinier P. Happé, D.V.M., Ph.D.
Lecturer in Small Animal Gastroenterology, Faculty of Veterinary Medicine, State University of Utrecht, The Netherlands.

R. M. Hardy, D.V.M., M.S.
Diplomate, American College of Veterinary Internal Medicine. Associate Professor, College of Veterinary Medicine, University of Minnesota, St. Paul, Minnesota.

David E. Harling, D.V.M.
Visiting Instructor in Ophthalmology, Department of Companion Animals and Special Species, School of Veterinary Medicine, North Carolina State University, Raleigh; Director and Clinician, Battleground Veterinary Hospital, Greensboro, North Carolina.

Benjamin L. Hart, D.V.M., Ph.D.
Professor of Neurobiology and Behavior, Department of Physiological Sciences, School of Veterinary Medicine, and Director, Behavioral Service, Veterinary Medical Teaching Hospital, University of California, Davis, California.

Sandee M. Hartsfield, D.V.M., M.S.
Diplomate, American College of Veterinary Anesthesiologists. Professor, Department of Small Animal Medicine and Surgery, College of Veterinary Medicine, and Veterinary Anesthesiologist, Veterinary Teaching Hospital, Texas A&M University, College Station, Texas.

Colin E. Harvey, B.V.Sc.
Diplomate, American College of Veterinary Surgeons. Professor of Surgery, School of Veterinary Medicine, University of Pennsylvania, Philadelphia, Pennsylvania.

Steve C. Haskins, D.V.M., M.S.
Diplomate, American College of Veterinary Anesthesiologists. Associate Professor, Department of Veterinary Surgery, School of Veterinary Medicine, and Section of Anesthesiology and Intensive Care, Veterinary Medical Teaching Hospital, University of California, Davis, California.

Joe Hauptman, D.V.M., M.S.
Diplomate, American College of Veterinary Surgeons. Assistant Professor of Surgery, Department of Small Animal Clinical Sciences and Veterinary Clinical Center, College of Veterinary Medicine, Michigan State University, East Lansing, Michigan.

Melvin L. Helphrey, D.V.M.
Diplomate, American College of Veterinary Surgeons. Private practice, Seminole, Florida.

Ralph A. Henderson, D.V.M., M.S.
Diplomate, American College of Veterinary Surgeons. Associate Professor, Department of Small Animal Surgery and Medicine, and Chief, Small Animal Surgery, School of Veterinary Medicine, Auburn University, Auburn, Alabama.

H. Philip Hobson, B.S., D.V.M., M.S.
Diplomate, American College of Veterinary Surgeons. Professor and Chief, Department of Small Animal Surgery, College of Veterinary Medicine, Texas A&M University, College Station, Texas.

Richard E. Hoffer, D.V.M., M.S.
Diplomate, American College of Veterinary Surgeons. Professor of Surgical Sciences, School of Veterinary Medicine, University of Wisconsin, Madison, Wisconsin.

David L. Holmberg, D.V.M., M.V.Sc.
Diplomate, American College of Veterinary Surgeons. Associate Professor of Surgery, Department of Veterinary Anesthesiology, Radiology and Surgery, Western College of Veterinary Medicine, University of Saskatchewan, Saskatoon, Saskatchewan, Canada.

R. D. Horne, D.V.M., M.S.
Diplomate, American College of Veterinary Surgeons. Professor of Surgery, School of Veterinary Medicine, Auburn University, Auburn, Alabama.

Don A. Hulse, B.S., D.V.M.
Diplomate, American College of Veterinary Surgeons. Professor of Surgery, College of Veterinary Medicine, Texas A&M University, College Station, Texas.

Richard J. Indrieri, M.S., D.V.M.
Diplomate, American College of Veterinary Internal Medicine (Neurology). Assistant Professor, Neurology and Neurosurgery, Department of Small Animal Clinical Sciences, College of Veterinary Medicine, Michigan State University, East Lansing, Michigan.

Wolfgang Janas
Veterinary Research Assistant, Biomedical Engineering Center, Purdue University, West Lafayette, Indiana.

K. Ann Jeglum, V.M.D.
Assistant Professor of Medical Oncology, School of Veterinary Medicine, and Head of Clinical Oncology Service, Veterinary Hospital, University of Pennsylvania, Philadelphia, Pennsylvania.

Richard G. Johnson, D.V.M.
Director of Surgery, Broadway Animal Hospital, El Cajon, California.

Dudley E. Johnston, M.V.Sc.
Professor of Surgery, School of Veterinary Medicine, University of Pennsylvania, Philadelphia, Pennsylvania.

Gary R. Johnston, D.V.M., M.S.
Diplomate, American College of Veterinary Radiology. Associate Professor of Comparative Radiology, College of Veterinary Medicine, University of Minnesota, St. Paul, Minnesota.

Shirley D. Johnston, D.V.M., Ph.D.
Diplomate, American College of Theriogenologists. Assistant Professor, Small Animal Medicine, College of Veterinary Medicine, University of Minnesota, St. Paul, Minnesota.

R. L. Jones, D.V.M., Ph.D.
Assistant Professor, Department of Microbiology and Environmental Health, and Head, Bacteriology Section, Diagnostic Laboratories, College of Veterinary Medicine and Biomedical Sciences, Colorado State University, Fort Collins, Colorado.

J. Michael Kehoe, D.V.M., Ph.D.
Professor and Chairman, Department of Microbiology/Immunology, Northeastern Ohio Universities College of Medicine, Rootstown, Ohio.

Mark D. Kittleson, D.V.M., Ph.D.
Diplomate, American College of Veterinary Internal Medicine. Assistant Professor, Department of Small Animal Clinical Sciences, College of Veterinary Medicine, and Cardiologist, Veterinary Clinical Center, Michigan State University, East Lansing, Michigan.

J. S. Klausner, D.V.M., M.S.
Diplomate, American College of Veterinary Internal Medicine. Associate Professor, Veterinary Internal Medicine, College of Veterinary Medicine, University of Minnesota, St. Paul, Minnesota.

L. Klein, V.M.D.
Diplomate, American College of Veterinary Anesthesiologists. Associate Professor of Anesthesia, School

of Veterinary Medicine, University of Pennsylvania, New Bolton Center, Kennett Square, Pennsylvania.

Alan Klide, V.M.D.
Diplomate, American College of Veterinary Anesthesiologists. Associate Professor of Anesthesia, School of Veterinary Medicine, University of Pennsylvania, Philadelphia, Pennsylvania.

Charles D. Knecht, V.M.D., M.S.
Diplomate, American College of Veterinary Surgeons and *American College of Veterinary Internal Medicine (Neurology).* Professor and Head, Department of Small Animal Surgery and Medicine, School of Veterinary Medicine, Auburn University, Auburn, Alabama.

Ronald J. Kolata, D.V.M., M.S.
Diplomate, American College of Veterinary Surgeons. Research Associate Professor, Departments of Surgery and Comparative Medicine, School of Medicine, St. Louis University, St. Louis, Missouri.

Joe N. Kornegay, D.V.M., Ph.D.
Diplomate, American College of Veterinary Internal Medicine. Associate Professor, Department of Companion Animal and Special Species Medicine, School of Veterinary Medicine, and Veterinary Teaching Hospital, North Carolina State University, Raleigh, North Carolina.

D. J. Krahwinkel, D.V.M., M.S.
Diplomate, American College of Veterinary Surgeons and *American College of Veterinary Anesthesiologists.* Head, Department of Urban Practice, College of Veterinary Medicine, and Professor of Surgery, Veterinary Teaching Hospital, University of Tennessee, Knoxville, Tennessee.

Gary C. Lantz, D.V.M.
Diplomate, American College of Veterinary Surgeons. Assistant Professor of Surgery, Department of Small Animal Clinics, College of Veterinary Medicine, Purdue University, West Lafayette, Indiana.

J. D. Lavach, D.V.M., M.S.
Diplomate, American College of Veterinary Ophthalmologists. Associate Professor of Ophthalmology, College of Veterinary Medicine and Biomedical Sciences, Colorado State University, Fort Collins, Colorado.

M. P. Lavery, R.N., B.S.N.
Surgical Nurse, Veterinary Medical Teaching Hospital, Virginia-Maryland Regional College of Veterinary Medicine, Blacksburg, Virginia.

George E. Lees, D.V.M., M.S.
Diplomate, American College of Veterinary Internal Medicine. Associate Professor, Department of Small Animal Medicine and Surgery, College of Veterinary Medicine, and Veterinary Teaching Hospital, Texas A&M University, College Station, Texas.

Arnold S. Lesser, V.M.D.
Diplomate, American College of Veterinary Surgeons. Director, Flushing Veterinary Hospital, Flushing; Staff Surgeon, Surgical Referral Service, Huntington, New York.

Stephen H. Levine, D.V.M., M.S.
Veterinary Medical Associate, Department of Small Animal Clinical Sciences, College of Veterinary Medicine, University of Minnesota, St. Paul; Director of Surgery, Minneapolis Veterinary Referral Services, Minneapolis, Minnesota.

Alan J. Lipowitz, D.V.M., M.S.
Diplomate, American College of Veterinary Surgeons. Associate Professor of Surgery and Chairman, Department of Small Animal Clinical Sciences, College of Veterinary Medicine, University of Minnesota, St. Paul, Minnesota.

William D. Liska, D.V.M.
Diplomate, American College of Veterinary Surgeons. Research Instructor in Orthopedics, Baylor College of Medicine; Staff Surgeon, Westbury Animal Hospital, Inc., Houston, Texas.

Philip Litwak, D.V.M., Ph.D.
Diplomate, American College of Veterinary Surgeons. Thoratec Laboratories Corporation, Berkeley, California.

A. A. M. E. Lubberink, D.V.M., Ph.D.
Lecturer in Soft Tissue Surgery, Small Animal Clinic, Faculty of Veterinary Medicine, State University of Utrecht, The Netherlands.

Charles L. Martin, D.V.M., M.S.
Diplomate, American College of Veterinary Ophthalmologists. Professor, Department of Small Animal Medicine, College of Veterinary Medicine, and Chief, Small Animal Medicine Service, Veterinary Teaching Hospital, University of Georgia, Athens, Georgia.

Louis McCoy
Senior Surgical Technician, Henry Bergh Memorial Animal Hospital, A.S.P.C.A., New York, New York.

D. M. McCurnin, D.V.M.
Diplomate, American College of Veterinary Surgeons. Professor of Surgery, Department of Clinical

Sciences, College of Veterinary Medicine and Biomedical Sciences, and Hospital Director, Veterinary Teaching Hospital, Colorado State University, Fort Collins, Colorado.

Wayne N. McDonell, D.V.M., Ph.D.
Diplomate, American College of Veterinary Anesthesiologists. Professor of Anesthesiology, Ontario Veterinary College, and Veterinary Medical Director, Veterinary Teaching Hospital, University of Guelph, Ontario, Canada.

H. Vince Mendenhall, D.V.M., Ph.D.
Senior Surgical Research Specialist, 3M Center, and Chief Surgeon, Veterinary Surgical Specialists, St. Paul, Minnesota.

David F. Merkley, D.V.M., M.S.
Diplomate, American College of Veterinary Surgeons. Associate Professor, Department of Veterinary Clinical Sciences, College of Veterinary Medicine, Iowa State University, Ames, Iowa.

Jennifer N. Mills, B.V.Sc., M.Sc.
Lecturer in Clinical Pathology, School of Veterinary Studies, Murdoch University, Murdoch, Western Australia.

J. L. Milton, D.V.M., M.S.
Diplomate, American College of Veterinary Surgeons. Associate Professor, School of Veterinary Medicine, Auburn University, Auburn, Alabama.

Robert W. Moore, D.V.M., M.S.
Staff Surgeon, South Shores Pet Clinic, San Pedro, California.

Robert J. Munger, D.V.M.
Diplomate, American College of Veterinary Ophthalmologists. Staff Veterinarian, Alcon Laboratories, and Veterinary Ophthalmologist, Animal Ophthalmology Clinic, Dallas, Texas.

A. Wendell Nelson, D.V.M., M.S., Ph.D.
Diplomate, American College of Veterinary Surgeons. Professor of Clinical Sciences, College of Veterinary Medicine and Biomedical Sciences, and Small Animal Surgeon, Veterinary Teaching Hospital, Colorado State University, Fort Collins, Colorado.

Teresa Nesbitt, D.V.M.
Research Associate, Duke University Medical Center, Durham, North Carolina.

M. E. Newman, D.V.M.
Resident in Surgery, Small Animal Clinic, School of Veterinary Medicine, Auburn University, Auburn, Alabama.

Alan M. Norris, D.V.M.
Diplomate, American College of Veterinary Internal Medicine. Assistant Professor, Department of Small Animal Medicine, Ontario Veterinary College, University of Guelph; Staff Internist, Veterinary Referral Clinic of Toronto, Toronto, Ontario, Canada.

Phillip N. Ogburn, D.V.M., Ph.D.
Associate Professor of Cardiology, Department of Small Animal Clinical Science, College of Veterinary Medicine, University of Minnesota, St. Paul, Minnesota.

N. Bari Olivier, D.V.M.
Instructor and Resident, Internal Medicine and Cardiology, Veterinary Clinical Center, College of Veterinary Medicine, Michigan State University, East Lansing, Michigan.

Marvin L. Olmstead, D.V.M., M.S.
Diplomate, American College of Veterinary Surgeons. Associate Professor, College of Veterinary Medicine, Ohio State University, Columbus, Ohio.

Don B. Olsen, D.V.M., Ph.D.
Research Professor of Surgery, School of Medicine, College of Medicine, University of Utah, Salt Lake City, Utah.

Patricia N. Olson, D.V.M., Ph.D.
Diplomate, American College of Theriogenologists. Assistant Professor, College of Veterinary Medicine and Biomedical Sciences, Colorado State University, Fort Collins, Colorado.

E. Christopher Orton, D.V.M., M.S.
Assistant Professor, Department of Clinical Sciences, College of Veterinary Medicine and Biomedical Sciences, and Veterinary Teaching Hospital, Colorado State University, Fort Collins, Colorado.

Carl A. Osborne, D.V.M., Ph.D.
Diplomate, American College of Veterinary Internal Medicine. Professor, Department of Small Animal Clinical Sciences, College of Veterinary Medicine, University of Minnesota, St. Paul, Minnesota.

Richard D. Park, D.V.M., Ph.D.
Diplomate, American College of Veterinary Radiology. Professor of Radiology, Department of Radiology and Radiation Biology, College of Veterinary Medicine and Biomedical Sciences, and Radiologist, Veterinary Teaching Hospital, Colorado State University, Fort Collins, Colorado.

Robert B. Parker, D.V.M.
Diplomate, American College of Veterinary Sur-

geons. Associate Professor and Chief, Small Animal Surgery, College of Veterinary Medicine, University of Florida, Gainesville, Florida.

Michael A. Pass, B.V.Sc., M.Sc., Ph.D.
Senior Lecturer in Physiology and Pharmacology, University of Queensland, St. Lucia, Queensland, Australia.

Clark S. Patton, D.V.M., M.S.
Diplomate, American College of Veterinary Pathologists. Associate Professor, Department of Pathobiology, College of Veterinary Medicine, University of Tennessee, Knoxville, Tennessee.

Michael M. Pavletic, D.V.M.
Diplomate, American College of Veterinary Surgeons. Assistant Professor of Surgery, School of Veterinary Medicine, Tufts University; Member, Surgical Staff, Angell Memorial Animal Hospital, Boston, Massachusetts.

Robert D. Pechman, Jr., D.V.M.
Diplomate, American College of Veterinary Radiology. Associate Professor, Department of Veterinary Clinical Sciences, School of Veterinary Medicine, Louisiana State University, Baton Rouge, Louisiana.

Robert L. Peiffer, Jr., D.V.M., Ph.D.
Diplomate, American College of Veterinary Ophthalmologists. Associate Professor, Departments of Ophthalmology and Pathology, School of Medicine, University of North Carolina, Chapel Hill, North Carolina.

Roger C. Penwick, V.M.D.
Assistant Professor of Small Animal Surgery, Department of Medicine and Surgery, College of Veterinary Medicine, and Clinician, Small Animal Surgery, Boren Veterinary Medical Teaching Hospital, Oklahoma State University, Stillwater, Oklahoma.

Victor Perman, D.V.M., Ph.D.
Diplomate, American College of Veterinary Pathologists. Professor and Chairman, Department of Veterinary Pathobiology, College of Veterinary Medicine, and Clinical Pathologist, Veterinary Teaching Hospital, University of Minnesota, St. Paul, Minnesota.

David J. Polzin, D.V.M., Ph.D.
Diplomate, American College of Veterinary Pathologists. Assistant Professor, Department of Small Animal Clinical Sciences, College of Veterinary Medicine, and Staff Internist, Lewis Hospital for Companion Animals, University of Minnesota, St. Paul, Minnesota.

Dennis L. Powers, D.V.M.
Assistant Professor of Bioengineering, Clemson University, Clemson, South Carolina.

Raymond G. Prata, D.V.M.
Diplomate, American College of Veterinary Surgeons. Surgeon, Neurosurgery and Orthopedics, Oradell Animal Hospital, Inc., Oradell, New Jersey.

Kenneth R. Presnell, D.V.M., M.Sc.
Diplomate, American College of Veterinary Surgeons. Professor of Small Animal Surgery, Head, Department of Veterinary Anesthesiology, Radiology and Surgery, Western College of Veterinary Medicine, University of Saskatchewan, Saskatoon, Saskatchewan, Canada.

Curtis W. Probst, D.V.M.
Assistant Professor, Small Animal Surgery, Department of Small Animal Clinical Sciences, Veterinary Clinical Center, Michigan State University, East Lansing, Michigan.

Maralyn R. Probst
Cardiology Research Technician, Department of Small Animal Clinical Sciences, Veterinary Clinical Center, Michigan State University, East Lansing, Michigan.

Peter I. Punch, B.Sc., B.V.M.S.
Practitioner, Perth, Western Australia.

Marc R. Raffe, D.V.M., M.S.
Assistant Professor of Comparative Anesthesiology, College of Veterinary Medicine, University of Minnesota, St. Paul, Minnesota.

Richard Read, B.V.Sc.
Postgraduate student, School of Veterinary Medicine, Murdoch University, Murdoch, Western Australia.

R. W. Redding, D.V.M., M.Sc., Ph.D.
Diplomate, American College of Veterinary Internal Medicine (Neurology). Professor, Departments of Veterinary Physiology and Pharmacology and Small Animal Surgery and Medicine, School of Veterinary Medicine, Auburn University Auburn, Alabama.

Daniel C. Richardson, D.V.M.
Diplomate, American College of Veterinary Surgeons. Assistant Professor of Surgery, School of Veterinary Medicine, North Carolina State University Raleigh, North Carolina.

Ken Richardson, B.Sc., B.V.Sc., Ph.D.
Lecturer, Veterinary Anatomy, School of Veterinary Studies, Murdoch University, Perth, Western Australia.

Ralph C. Richardson, D.V.M.
Diplomate, American College of Veterinary Internal Medicine. Associate Professor of Medicine, and Chief, Clinical Oncology, College of Veterinary Medicine, Purdue University, West Lafayette, Indiana.

Robert C. Rosenthal, D.V.M., M.S.
Diplomate, American College of Veterinary Internal Medicine. Assistant Professor, Department of Medical Sciences, School of Veterinary Medicine, University of Wisconsin, Madison, Wisconsin.

Anne E. Rosin, D.V.M.
Instructor, Clinical Pathology, Department of Pathobiological Sciences, School of Veterinary Medicine, University of Wisconsin, Madison, Wisconsin.

Eberhard Rosin, D.V.M., Ph.D.
Diplomate, American College of Veterinary Surgeons. Associate Professor, School of Veterinary Medicine, University of Wisconsin, Madison, Wisconsin.

Donald C. Sawyer, D.V.M., Ph.D.
Diplomate, American College of Veterinary Anesthesiologists. Professor of Anesthesia, Department of Small Animal Clinical Sciences, College of Veterinary Medicine, and Veterinary Clinical Center, Michigan State University, East Lansing, Michigan.

Anthony Schwartz, D.V.M., Ph.D.
Diplomate, American College of Veterinary Surgeons. Professor and Chairman, Department of Surgery, School of Veterinary Medicine, Tufts University; Member, Surgical Staff, Angell Memorial Animal Hospital, Boston, Massachusetts.

Peter D. Schwarz, D.V.M.
Assistant Professor, Department of Clinical Sciences, College of Veterinary Medicine and Biomedical Sciences, Colorado State University, Fort Collins, Colorado.

Kay L. Schwink, D.V.M.
Resident in Ophthalmology, College of Veterinary Medicine, Iowa State University, Ames, Iowa.

Peter K. Shires, B.V.Sc., M.S.
Diplomate, American College of Veterinary Surgeons. Associate Professor, School of Veterinary Medicine, and Surgeon, Veterinary Teaching Hospital, Louisiana State University, Baton Rouge, Louisiana.

Andy Shores, D.V.M., M.S.
Neurology/Neurosurgery Resident, Department of Small Animal Surgery and Medicine, School of Veterinary Medicine, Auburn University, Auburn, Alabama.

Stephen T. Simpson, D.V.M., M.S.
Diplomate, American College of Veterinary Internal Medicine (Neurology). Associate Professor, School of Veterinary Medicine, and Staff Neurologist, Small Animal Clinic, Auburn University, Auburn, Alabama.

Douglas H. Slatter, B.V.Sc., M.S., Ph.D., F.R.C.V.S.
Diplomate, American College of Veterinary Surgeons and *American College of Veterinary Ophthalmologists.* Veterinary Ophthalmologist and Surgeon, Animal Eye and Surgical Associates, San Diego, California.

D. D. Smeak, B.S., D.V.M.
Assistant Professor of Surgery, College of Veterinary Medicine, and Surgeon, Ohio State University, Columbus, Ohio.

C. W. Smith, D.V.M., M.S.
Diplomate, American College of Veterinary Surgeons. Professor, Department of Veterinary Clinical Medicine, College of Veterinary Medicine, and Chief, Small Animal Surgery, Veterinary Medical Teaching Hospital, Urbana, Illinois.

Donald C. Sorjonen, D.V.M.
Assistant Professor, School of Veterinary Medicine, and Staff Neurologist, Small Animal Clinic, Auburn University, Auburn, Alabama.

Eugene P. Steffey, V.M.D., Ph.D.
Diplomate, American College of Veterinary Anesthesiologists. Professor and Chairman, Department of Surgery, School of Veterinary Medicine, and Chief of Anesthesia/Critical Patient Care, Veterinary Medical Teaching Hospital, University of California, Davis, California.

Sharon Stevenson, D.V.M., M.S.
Diplomate, American College of Veterinary Surgeons. Postgraduate Research Pathologist, Department of Pathology, School of Veterinary Medicine, University of California, Davis, California.

Steven L. Stockham, B.V.M., M.S.
Diplomate, American College of Veterinary Pathologists. Assistant Professor of Veterinary Clinical Pathology, College of Veterinary Medicine, University of Missouri, Columbia, Missouri.

Elizabeth A. Stone, D.V.M., M.S.
Diplomate, American College of Veterinary Surgeons. Assistant Professor of Surgery, Department of Clinical Studies, School of Veterinary Medicine, University of Pennsylvania, Philadelphia, Pennsylvania.

Steven J. Susaneck, D.V.M., M.S.
Diplomate, American College of Veterinary Internal Medicine. Staff Oncologist, Westbury Animal Hospital, Inc., Houston, Texas.

Steven F. Swaim, D.V.M., M.S.
Professor of Surgery, Department of Small Animal Surgery and Medicine, School of Veterinary Medicine, Auburn University, Auburn, Alabama.

James Tomlinson, B.S., D.V.M., M.V.Sc.
Assistant Professor of Surgery, College of Veterinary Medicine, and Head of Orthopedic Surgery, University of Missouri, Columbia, Missouri.

James P. Toombs, D.V.M., M.S.
Assistant Professor of Surgery, Department of Small Animal Medicine, College of Veterinary Medicine, and Staff Surgeon, Small Animal Orthopedics, Veterinary Teaching Hospital, University of Georgia, Athens, Georgia.

Cynthia M. Trim, B.V.Sc.
Associate Professor and Anesthesiologist, College of Veterinary Medicine, University of Georgia, Athens, Georgia.

Alan Tucker, Ph.D.
Associate Professor, Department of Physiology and Biophysics, College of Veterinary Medicine and Biomedical Sciences, Colorado State University, Fort Collins, Colorado.

David C. Twedt, D.V.M.
Diplomate, American College of Veterinary Internal Medicine. Associate Professor, Department of Clinical Sciences, College of Veterinary Medicine and Biomedical Sciences, and Staff Gastroenterologist, Veterinary Teaching Hospital, Colorado State University, Fort Collins, Colorado.

Frederik J. Van Sluys, D.V.M.
Lecturer in Small Animal Surgery, Faculty of Veterinary Medicine, State University of Utrecht, The Netherlands.

P. B. Vasseur, D.V.M.
Diplomate, American College of Veterinary Surgeons. Assistant Professor, Department of Surgery, School of Veterinary Medicine, University of California, Davis, California.

William Ardene Vestre, D.V.M., M.S.
Diplomate, American College of Veterinary Ophthalmologists. Assistant Professor, School of Veterinary

Medicine, Purdue University, West Lafayette, Indiana.

Andreas F. von Recum, D.V.M., Dr. med.vet., Ph.D.
Professor and Head, Department of Bioengineering, College of Engineering, Clemson University, Clemson, South Carolina.

Stanley D. Wagner, D.V.M.
Instructor, College of Veterinary Medicine, Kansas State University, Manhattan, Kansas.

Tom L. Walker, B.S., D.V.M., M. S.
Diplomate, American College of Veterinary Surgeons. Associate Professor of Surgery, Department of Urban Practice, College of Veterinary Medicine, University of Tennessee, Knoxville, Tennessee.

Richard Walshaw, B.V.M.S.
Diplomate, American College of Veterinary Surgeons. Associate Professor, Department of Small Animal Clinical Sciences, College of Veterinary Medicine, and Surgeon, Veterinary Clinical Center, Michigan State University, East Lansing, Michigan.

Andy Wasilewski, M.S.
Director of Data Processing, School of Veterinary Medicine, North Carolina State University, Raleigh, North Carolina.

Joseph P. Weigel, B.S., D.V.M.
Diplomate, American College of Veterinary Surgeons. Associate Professor of Surgery, Department of Urban Practice, College of Veterinary Medicine, University of Tennessee, Knoxville, Tennessee.

Walter E. Weirich, D.V.M., Ph.D.
Diplomate, American College of Veterinary Surgeons. Professor and Head, Department of Small Animal Clinics, School of Veterinary Medicine, Purdue University, West Lafayette, Indiana.

Pamela G. Whiting, D.V.M.
Fellow, Liver Disease Research, National Institute of Arthritis, Diabetes, Digestive and Kidney Diseases, National Institutes of Health; Veterinary Medical Teaching Hospital, School of Veterinary Medicine, University of California, Davis, California.

James W. Wilson, B.S., D.V.M., M.S.
Diplomate, American College of Veterinary Surgeons. Department of Surgical Sciences, School of Veterinary Medicine, University of Wisconsin, Madison, Wisconsin.

Stephen J. Withrow, D.V.M.
Diplomate, American College of Veterinary Surgeons. Professor of Surgery, College of Veterinary Medicine and Biomedical Sciences, and Chief, Clinical Oncology Service, Veterinary Teaching Hospital, Colorado State University, Fort Collins, Colorado.

Peggy M. Wykes, D.V.M., M.S.
Private practice (surgical specialty), Reference Surgical Veterinary Practice, Englewood, Colorado.

Preface

Surgery is that fascinating and stimulating branch of therapeutic science that deals with the treatment of disease and injury by manipulative or operative methods. It requires of its practitioners not only a knowledge of diseases and their diagnosis, but also specific technical skills necessary for the operative treatment of disease. Although it is often fashionable to decry the importance of one or the other of these aspects of surgery, a surgeon's clinical results nevertheless reflect his expertise in both areas. This requirement places an additional burden on the aspiring surgeon, who must acquire both the knowledge and skills through arduous training, either by means of graduate institutional training programs or in veterinary practice.

Textbook of Small Animal Surgery is directed to the student as a text and to the veterinary practitioner and surgeon-in-training as a reference, in the hope that the rigors of training will not relegate him to the "surgical technician" category—the present-day equivalent of the barber-surgeon of previous centuries—but rather to development as a complete surgeon, whose diagnostic and treatment methods are firmly based in modern surgical science and compare favorably in results and methods with those of his colleagues. The book is also directed to the busy clinician as a source of information in routine clinical situations, when the unusual, stimulating, and challenging may become submerged in a sea of necessary but mundane procedures.

As in other specialties, the volume of new information in surgery is awesome, and the authors have attempted to distill the clinically and scientifically relevant material in one place. It is often difficult to differentiate material that will be necessary to an understanding of treatment methods currently under development from that of lesser importance. Where more than one method of treatment exists, authors have been encouraged to compare them, where possible, and the reasons for their apparent success or lack of it. The information presented is keyed to the vast literature of surgical science and published knowledge. I hope that the contents will stimulate users to read further in the literature of the subject and will assist them in the daily and effective treatment of our trusting patients.

Constructive suggestions by veterinarians, students, and other users of the text are welcome for the continued development of *Textbook of Small Animal Surgery*.

DOUGLAS H. SLATTER

Acknowledgments

I am endebted to the Section Editors, who have labored with skill and diligence in planning their sections and coordinating their respective contributing authors, and with patience when confronted with constant reminders of the task at hand. The efforts of each author are appreciated—the fruits of their intense labors are very evident. To the many veterinary and medical colleagues and farsighted teaching institutions who have allowed publication of illustrations previously published or otherwise, without charge, I extend my sincere thanks, for it is only by contributions such as this that illustration of a surgery text of this type is possible. Ray Kersey as well as the staff of the W. B. Saunders Company, especially Sandy Reinhardt, Virginia Ingaran, Amy Grodnick, and Janet Macnamara-Barnett, have been outstanding in the assistance, forbearance, and encouragement they have offered in the many phases of production of the book.

Contents

Volume I

Contents

Volume II

Section XII

Eye and Adnexa

Douglas H. Slatter
Section Editor

Principles of Ophthalmic Surgery

Douglas H. Slatter

INTRODUCTION

Attention to detail is more essential to success in opthalmic surgery than in other types of surgery, and failure to complete seemingly minute pharmacological preoperative, procedural, or postoperative details may cause unnecessary complications with intraocular or corneal surgery. Consequently, considerable discussion of apparently similar surgical techniques that differ in small details is encountered in the literature. The authors of the ophthalmic surgery section have compared techniques where sufficient information exists and have described the most appropriate techniques in their experience where information is limited. However, despite its rigors, few areas of therapeutics offer the same potential for relief of distress and improvement of quality of life and cosmetic appearance of the patient as ophthalmic surgery.

ANESTHESIA

General anesthesia is used for all but the most minor ophthalmic procedures, e.g., suture removal and superficial foreign body removal. A useful regimen follows.

1. Minimum data base, including a preoperative physical examination and a complete blood count, serum protein, urinalysis, and BUN (and blood glucose for animals with cataract) for all patients over five years of age.

2. Preoperative medication with acepromazine (0.05 mg/kg). The routine use of atropine is no longer regarded as essential by some anesthetists, evidence indicating that it may cause more arrhythmias than it prevents.[12] In ophthalmic surgery, the presence of the oculocardiac reflex probably indicates that atropine should be used.

3. Induction of anesthesia with sodium thiamylal, sodium pentothal, or alfaxalone (in cats) and immediate intubation. Some surgeons use muscle relaxants, such as pancuronium, during intraocular procedures.

4. Maintenance with methoxyflurane, or halothane and nitrous oxide. (Note: nitrous oxide should not be used if a postoperative air bubble is to be placed in the eye.)

The combination of acepromazine and methoxyflurane provides the advantages of prolonged postoperative analgesia and tranquilization and reduced dangers of inducing cardiac arrhythmias or ventricular fibrillation with intraocular epinephrine ("epinephrine syncope") during the surgical procedure compared with halothane. Most general anesthetics decrease intraocular pressure and tear production. Methods of monitoring physiological parameters during anesthesia are discussed in Chapters 186 and 197.

PREOPERATIVE PREPARATION

Pharmacological Preparation

Anti-inflammatory Agents

The canine eye (and to a much lesser degree the feline eye) rapidly becomes inflamed during or after ocular surgical procedures. Corticosteroids are frequently used both systemically and topically for several days before ophthalmic procedures or cyclocryotherapy to reduce miosis and the release of protein into the aqueous when the anterior chamber is opened, and to limit postoperative inflammation. Corticosteroids are thought to reduce the release of prostaglandins, which mediate some of the protein release through vascular walls, and the direct action of prostaglandins on the smooth muscle of the iris sphincter, the cause of intraoperative miosis.[19] In addition to preoperative topical and systemic administration of corticosteroids, an intravenous bolus may be given about 30 minutes before surgery.

Complications seen with the use of steroids are associated with slow wound healing and decreased resistance to bacterial and fungal infections.[8] To limit these complications, it is recommended that nonabsorbable sutures (nylon or polypropylene) be used in the globe and left in place until wound strength is sufficient. Prophylactic antibiotics should be bactericidal and should be changed regularly during the pre- and postoperative periods.

Prostaglandins are important mediators of ocular inflammation,[20] including protein release during intraocular surgery. Inhibitors of prostaglandin synthetase reduce vascular permeability when administered preoperatively. In the dog, acetylsalicylic acid (30 mg/kg per os every 8 hours for 40 hours before surgery) reduces aqueous protein concentrations.[2] Unfortunately, platelet numbers are depressed by acetylsalicylic acid with consequent effects on clotting time, a particularly undesirable complication in intraocular surgery.[10] Indomethacin[13] also inhibits prostaglandin synthetase in the eye but must be administered carefully and with food because of systemic toxicity in dogs. Although not approved for use in the dog, Flunixin meglumine (0.5 mg/kg) has been widely used systemically as a preoperative prostaglandin inhibitor. Antihistamines are also believed to reduce protein release and are used by some ophthalmic surgeons 30 to 60 minutes before the eye is opened.

Osmotic Agents

Intravenous mannitol causes decreased intraocular pressure and vitreous body volume[9] and has been widely used to reduce loss of vitreous during intraocular surgery. Although the necessity of this practice has been questioned,[14] I have found it to be beneficial and without complications provided the patient is normally hydrated before surgery and not hypotensive. An interaction between mannitol and methoxyflurane resulting in life-threatening pulmonary edema has been reported,[4] but is not common and has not been substantiated experimentally.

Antibacterials

Because of the normal bacterial flora of the conjunctival sac (Tables 100–1 and 100–2) and tarsal glands and the frequent use of immunosuppressive drugs, preoperative preparation with a broad spectrum bactericidal antibiotic preparation is advisable for elective procedures. Before intraocular procedures, solutions are preferable to ointments to prevent entry of oily bases into the eye and subsequent chronic inflammation.

After induction of anesthesia, the periocular area is carefully clipped and cilia on the upper lid are removed. "Clipper burn," or traumatic dermatitis, should be avoided to minimize postoperative scratching. Special care must be taken if the globe has been penetrated to prevent hair from entering the conjunctival sac during clipping and to avoid placing

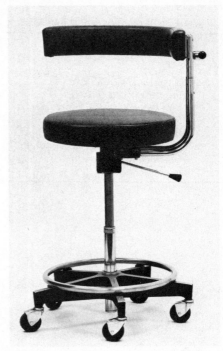

Figure 100–1. An ophthalmic operating stool with arm rest.

pressure on the eye. K-Y jelly may be placed in the sac prior to clipping and removed with the adherent hair after clipping is completed.

1. Gross contamination is first removed with gauze sponges soaked in sterile saline.

2. The periocular area is carefully scrubbed with povidone iodine solution diluted with saline. (Note:

TABLE 100–1. Normal Flora of the Canine Conjunctival Sac

	Percentage of Cases with Positive Cultures		Percentage of Cases with Positive Cultures
Western United States[1]		Eastern Australia[11]	
Staphylococcus epidermidis	46	Staphylococcus epidermidis	16
Staphylococcus aureus	24	Staphylococcus aureus	39
Streptococcus spp. (β-hemolytic)	2	Bacillus spp.	29
Streptococcus spp. (α-hemolytic)	4	Corynebacterium spp.	19
Bacillus spp.	12	Streptococcus spp. (β-hemolytic	1
Gram-negative organisms	7	Streptococcus spp. (α-hemolytic)	3
(Mima [Acinetobacter] spp., Neisseria spp., Moraxella spp., Pseudomonas spp.)	75	Streptococcus spp. (nonhemolytic)	3
Diphtheroids		Yeasts	5
	55	Micrococcus spp.	3
Mid-western United States[17]	45	Neisseria spp.	2
Staphylococcus epidermidis	7.3	Pseudomonas sp.	1
Staphylococcus aureus	34	Nocardia sp.	1
Streptococcus spp. (β-hemolytic)	26	Escherichia coli	1
Streptococcus spp. (α-hemolytic)	14	Clostridium sp.	1
Neisseria spp.	30	Enterobacter sp.	1
Pseudomonas spp.		Flavobacterium sp.	
Diphtheroids		Branhamella catarrhalis	

TABLE 100–2. Normal Flora of the Feline Conjunctival Sac in the Western United States[5]

Organism	Percentage of Cases with Positive Cultures	
	Conjunctiva	Lids
Staphylococcus aureus	10.4	8.8
Staphylococcus epidermidis	16.3	13.3
Mycoplasma spp.	5	—
Bacillus spp.	2.9	1.7
Streptococcus spp. (α-hemolytic)	2.5	1.7
Corynebacterium spp.	1.3	—
Escherichia coli	—	0.4

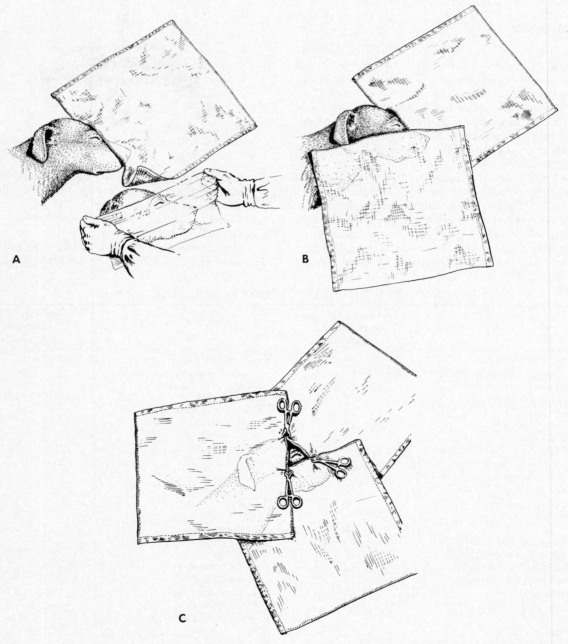

Figure 100–2. Draping for ocular surgery. *A,* The first field drape in position. *B,* The second field drape in position. *C,* The third field drape and Backhaus towel clamps in position.

povidone scrub solution, which contains detergents harmful to the cornea, should not be used.)

3. The corneal and conjunctival surfaces are irrigated with balanced salt solution,* and a drop of broad spectrum antibiotic solution may be instilled prior to surgery.

4. A final preparation of ethyl alcohol followed by povidone iodine may be used, provided the alcohol is not allowed to enter the conjunctival sac.

Positioning of Patient and Surgeon

Ophthalmic surgery is performed with the surgeon seated. An arm rest is used to steady both hands for finer movements. An adjustable stool and arm rest are commonly combined (Fig. 100–1). The patient's head is placed on an elevated soft bag, e.g., bean bag, so that the eye can be positioned as required by the surgeon.

Draping

Three field drapes are placed around the eye and fastened with small towel clamps (Fig. 100–2). A fenestrated drape with a 3-cm eccentrically placed hole is positioned over the eye. This drape should be large enough to cover the remainder of the patient. A sterile dental rubber dam with a hole in it or adhesive plastic drapes are used by some surgeons. Full aseptic precautions should be used for intraocular surgery, although some requirements may be relaxed for simple external procedures involving the lids and third eyelid. For intraocular procedures, starch powder, which may cause postoperative endophthalmitis, should be removed from surgical gloves with sterile saline. Similarly, cellulose sponges are preferable to cotton-tipped applicators which may shed fibers.

SURGICAL EQUIPMENT AND SUPPLIES

Illumination and Magnification

Ophthalmic surgery is performed in a semi-darkened room with a focal light to reduce reflections in

*Alcon Laboratories, Fort Worth, TX.

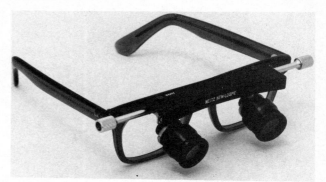

Figure 100–4. A simple magnifying loupe with interchangeable lenses of different magnification suitable for basic ophthalmic surgery. Such an instrument can be worn with the light source shown in Figure 100–3.

the transparent ocular media that make inner structures difficult or impossible to see. For adnexal surgery a standard operating light is suitable, but for finer procedures a focal or head-mounted light source that generates as little heat as possible is desirable to limit drying and heating of delicate structures (Fig. 100–3).

Surgical procedures involving the cilia, lacrimal puncta, or globe usually require magnification. A loupe of the type used in ocular examination (Fig. 100–4) with a magnification of from 2.5 to 4.0× and a focal length of 20 to 30 cm is recommended. For more intricate procedures, e.g., correction of distichiasis or intraocular procedures, an operating microscope is now considered essential. Available microscopes vary from simple table-mounted models (Fig. 100–5) with fixed magnification and illumination and no provision for viewing by an assistant to elaborate and expensive instruments, with power focusing, variable magnification, photographic outlets, assistant's eyepieces, multiple light sources, and provisions for video recording (Fig. 100–6).

Successful microsurgery requires considerable training and practice. Instruments for use with an operating microscope are considerably smaller and more delicate than those used for unmagnified surgery and have matte surfaces to prevent reflection.

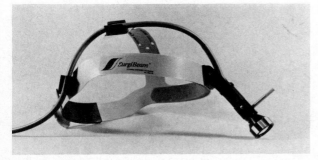

Figure 100–3. Head-mounted fiberoptic light source.

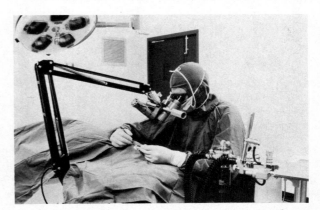

Figure 100–5. A basic operating microscope with a magnification of 10× and sterile handles to allow manipulation by the surgeon.

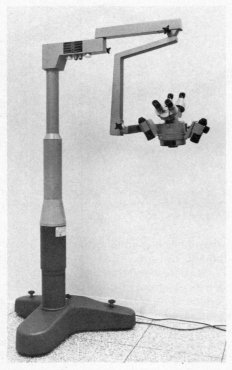

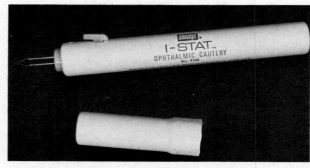

Figure 100–6   *Figure 100–7*

Figure 100–6. A Zeiss operating microscope with power-operated focus and zoom, multiple light sources, and an assistant's eye piece.

Figure 100–7. A disposable, battery-driven, hand-held electrocautery unit. The unit has a continuous operating time of 20 to 30 minutes and, although disposable, may be resterilized with ethylene oxide for repeated use.

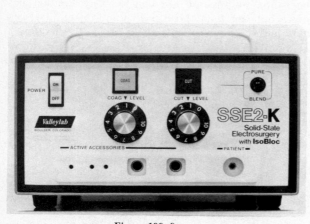

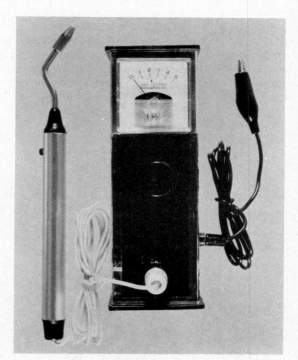

Figure 100–8   *Figure 100–9*

Figure 100–8. An electrosurgical unit capable of supplying pure or blended currents for cutting or coagulation or both. These units should not be used for electroepilation.

Figure 100–9. A battery-operated epilator that has been modified for veterinary use by the addition of a tongue electrode (alligator clip) to complete the electrical circuit. Such units supply 1 to 5 ma of direct current.

Hemostasis

Methods of hemostasis used in ophthalmic surgery include pressure with a cotton-tipped applicator; ligation of vessels, especially in lid and orbital surgery; electrocautery; electrohemostasis; and the use of 1:10000 epinephrine solution. Electrocautery may be applied by small, hand-held disposable battery-driven units (Fig. 100–7). Electrohemostasis with alternating current supplied by larger units (Fig. 100–8), which are also capable of supplying cutting or blended currents, is particularly useful when profuse hemorrhage is expected, e.g., in tumor excision, blepharoplastic procedures, and procedures involving the iris and choroid. These larger units that supply alternating current should not be used for epilation in place of the appropriate units supplying small amounts of direct current for elecrolysis (Fig. 100–9), as severe tissue necrosis may result (Fig. 100–10).

Cryotherapy

The biological usage of cryotherapy is discussed in Chapter 173. In veterinary ophthalmic surgery, cryotherapy is used for the selective destruction of neoplasms, removal of luxated lenses, treatment of distichiasis, and destruction of parts of the ciliary body in the control of glaucoma (cyclocryotherapy).[3] Cyclocryotherapy is one of the major recent advances in canine glaucoma therapy. General cryosurgical equipment may be used for periocular tumors, but for small lesions or for use on the globe, ophthalmic cryosurgical units with a probe diameter of approximately 3 mm are necessary (Fig. 100–11). These units are cooled by nitrous oxide and have a minimum temperature of approximately −89°C.

Suture Materials and Needles

The principles that apply to the selection of ophthalmic suture material are:

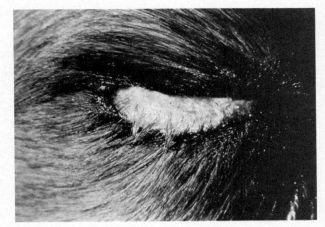

Figure 100–10. Severe necrosis of the lower lid resulting from use of an electrosurgical unit for epilation. (Courtesy of Dr. G. Severin.)

1. The suture should be as fine as is consistent with the surgeon's ability, training, and equipment and the patient's temperament.

2. Suture materials that may touch the cornea must be soft and pliable.

3. Chromic gut is not used in the cornea because of local tissue reactions. For buried sutures, e.g., beneath the conjunctiva and in subcutaneous sites, polyglycolic and polyglactic acid sutures (Dexon and Vicryl) respectively have many advantages (see Chapter 27).

4. Absorbable materials should not be used as the sole suture in a major corneal or scleral wound when nonirritant materials are available. A mixture of sutures may be used. The use of synthetic absorbable material as the sole suture in an eye immunosuppressed for intraocular surgery is inadvisable unless the sutures are removed at the normal time. In these circumstances, very acute infections (less than 12 hours) with organisms not normally pathogenic may occur around the suture and be most damaging and difficult to control. The tendency for difficult infections to occur with these sutures has been recorded in other tissues.[18]

TABLE 100–3. Suture Material Selection

Tissue	Recommended Sutures	Size
Lids	Silk—soft and pliable (do not substitute)	6/0, 4/0
	Nylon—nonirritating, but short sutures may be traumatic	4/0, 3/0
Conjunctiva (bulbar, palpebral)	Polyglycolic acid (PGA)	7/0, 6/0, 5/0
	Polydioxanone	
	Polyglactic acid (PGL)	
	Chromic gut	6/0
Third eyelid	Silk (do not substitute)	4/0
	Nylon	3/0, 4/0
Cornea	Nylon (preferred)	10/0, 8/0, 7/0, 6/0 (10/0—operating microscope)
	Silk (do not substitute)	8/0, 7/0, 6/0
	PGA, Polydioxanone (should not be used as sole suture material; should be removed after same time period as silk)	8/0, 7/0

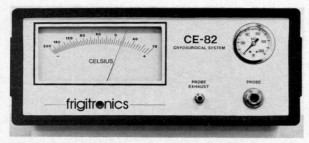

Figure 100–11. Frigitronics N20 cryosurgical unit for direct ocular use. A temperature of −89°C is reached with this equipment. A large variety of probes are available, but the glaucoma and lens probes are most suited to veterinary use.

5. Fine nonirritant suture materials limit postoperative inflammation. Fine nylon may be left in the cornea much longer than silk.

Recommended suture materials for different situations are listed in Table 100–3. Nylon also results in less inflammation around the suture in the upper lid when used for third eyelid flaps.

Surgical Needles

For corneal suturing, the micropoint spatula GS-9 (Ethicon) or cutting micropoint G-1 needle is recommended. For eyelids and third eyelid, a cutting PS-2 needle is recommended. Swaged needles cause much less trauma on passage through tissue than needles with eyes, and are strongly recommended.

Scalpel Blades

Three systems are commonly used.
1. Beaver handle with #64 or #65 blade (Fig. 100–12). Numerous other Beaver blades are available for special purposes in ophthalmic surgery (Fig. 100–24E), but the #64 and #65 are most generally useful.
2. Standard #3 handle with #11 and #15 blades (Fig. 100–13).
3. Swiss blade breaker/holder (Fig. 100–14) and

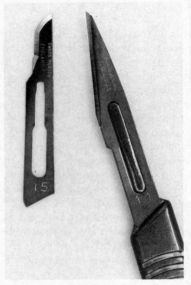

Figure 100–13. Standard #3 handle with #15 and #11 blades.

sliver of razor blade (Fig. 100–15). A fragment of a razor blade is much sharper and thinner than a standard scalpel blade and is more suitable for partial tarsal plate excision in the treatment of extensive distichiasis in very thin eyelids. For very thin eyelids in certain breeds, such a blade is almost mandatory for accurate tarsal plate excision if cryotherapy is not available.

MISCELLANEOUS SUPPLIES

Irrigating Solutions

Balanced salt solution* is preferable to saline for intraocular irrigation, as it causes less osmotic damage

---

*Alcon Laboratories; Fort Worth, TX.

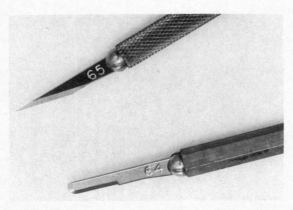

Figure 100–12. Hexagonal and circular milled Beaver handles with #64 and #65 blades, respectively.

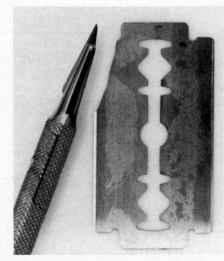

Figure 100–14. Swiss blade breaker/holder and razor blade.

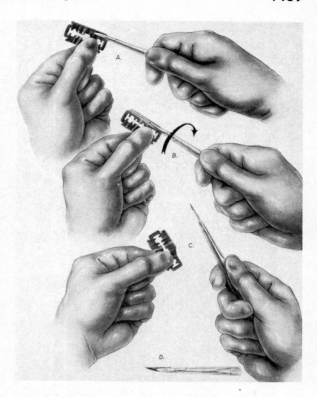

Figure 100–15. Steps in preparation of knives from razor blades. *A,* The blade is grasped by the bladeholder in such a manner that the honed edge of the blade extends slightly beyond, and is parallel to, the jaw of the bladeholder. *B,* With the blade firmly grasped between the index finger and thumb of one hand, the other hand, with the blade holder, twists it quickly in the direction of the arrow. *C* and *D,* The end of the blade breaks, leaving a triangular piece of the blade in the grip of the bladeholder. When mounted in the handle this provides the cutting edge of the knife. A longer or shorter blade can be obtained, depending on the angle at which the blade is broken. (Reprinted with permission from Castroviejo, R.: *Atlas of Keratectomy and Keratoplasty.* W. B. Saunders, Philadelphia, 1966.)

to the corneal endothelium. For preoperative preparation saline may be used. Solutions containing glutathione have been shown to cause even less endothelial damage[6] but are not yet commercially available. Sterile water should not be used near the eye, as intraocular use results in severe osmotic damage to the endothelium.

Sponges

Cellulose sponge wedges* (Fig. 100–16) are recommended for penetrating ocular wounds. Sterile cotton-tipped applicators are useful for controlling conjunctival hemorrhage but should not be placed inside the eye or near a penetrating wound because of the danger of loose cotton strands gaining entrance.

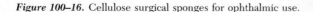

*Weck-cel, Edward Weck S Co., Long Island, NY.

Standard cotton surgical sponges should be treated with similar caution.

CARE AND STERILIZATION OF OPHTHALMIC INSTRUMENTS

Ophthalmic instruments require special care because of their delicate and fragile nature. Instruments are individually cleaned and dried, care being taken to preserve teeth, points, and cutting edges. They must not be placed in groups for washing, as damage will occur. Ultrasonic cleaning is very useful and limits damage to delicate surfaces by handling. Instruments should be inspected regularly by the surgeon for faults and repaired early. Tubular silicone cuffs may be placed over the ends of instruments to protect them during autoclaving (plastics may melt). Instruments may be protected during autoclaving or

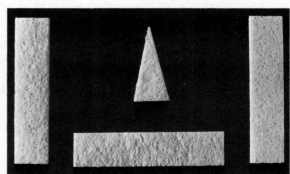

Figure 100–16. Cellulose surgical sponges for ophthalmic use.

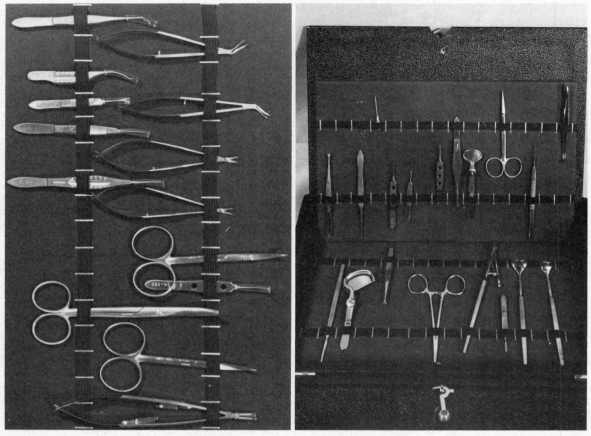

Figure 100–17. An instrument board for safe storage of instruments. Some boards of this type may be autoclaved. (Reprinted with permission from Bistner, S. I., Aguirre, G., and Batik, G.: *Atlas of Ophthalmic Surgery.* W. B. Saunders, Philadelphia, 1977.)

storage by placing them on racks or boards (Fig. 100–17) or, ideally, in a perforated instrument case (Fig. 100–18).

Three methods of sterilization are commonly used: autoclaving, ethylene oxide sterilization, and dry heat sterilization (see also Chapter 20). Ethylene oxide

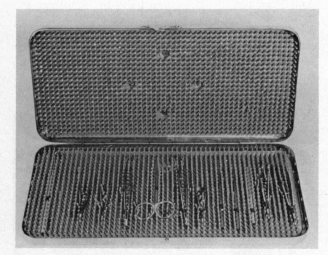

Figure 100–18. A perforated instrument case with flexible rubber fingers suitable for autoclaving or storing instruments.

sterilization is least damaging to instruments. However, ethylene oxide is very toxic to tissues, and instrument packs must be aired for 48 hours before use. Steam sterilization is commonly used, although over a long period corrosion and damage may occur to fine cutting edges, especially with poor-quality equipment. The dry heat sterilizer is useful for fine instruments, but has the disadvantage of requiring sterilization at 150°C for one and one-half hours (160°C damages fine edges).[16] Dry heat ovens should contain a fan and a thermostatic switch.

PREVENTION OF SELF-TRAUMA

The prevention of self-trauma after surgical procedures is important, especially when a cycle of scratching has been established prior to surgery and when fine sutures are used. A variety of methods are available for use, either singly or in combination.

1. An Elizabethan collar or plastic bucket (Fig. 100–19).

2. Bandaging dewclaws on the forelegs (Fig. 100–20).

3. Bandaging the eye.[15] This method is rarely necessary; the bandage is difficult to keep on and limits the frequency of observation and medication.

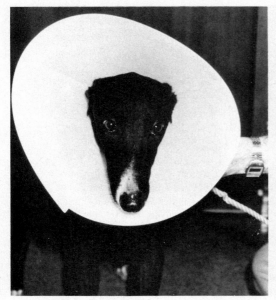

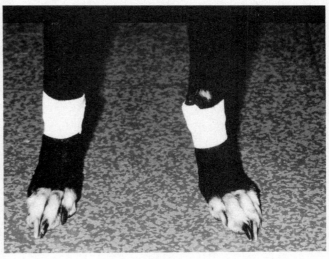

Figure 100–19   *Figure 100–20*

Figure 100–19. An Elizabethan collar to protect the eye from being rubbed or scratched. A plastic bucket with the bottom removed may be used similarly, attached to the animal's collar.

Figure 100–20. Dewclaws bandaged with adhesive tape to prevent rubbing.

Painful anterior segment lesions can be rendered much less painful with the use of appropriate cycloplegics for ciliary spasm, e.g., in uveitis, or for third eyelid flaps for painful corneal lesions.

4. Tranquilization in severe cases, e.g., diazepam or acetylpromazine as necessary.

It is often useful to leave a collar or bucket in place for several days after suture removal until all irritation has subsided, as some patients will commence rubbing or scratching soon after leaving the clinic.

EXPOSURE AND FIXATION OF THE GLOBE

Good exposure and control of the globe are primary prerequisites of successful ophthalmic surgery. The efforts required to achieve exposure in animal patients differ markedly from the simpler methods necessary in humans, primarily because the eye deviates in a inferomedial direction under general anesthesia (the "reversed Bell's phenomenon"). The third eyelid also restricts exposure.

Exposure

Numerous designs of lid retractors and speculae are available. For short procedures, especially when the animal is not under anesthesia, a lid speculum is useful (Fig. 100–21). For major ophthalmic procedures, the Castroviejo and Maumenee-Park speculae are recommended (Fig. 100–22).

Canthotomy

A lateral canthotomy greatly improves exposure of the eye (Fig. 100–23). The lateral canthus is incised with straight Mayo scissors up to but not including the orbital ligament. The area should *not* be crushed with hemostats before incision, as healing is retarded. Infiltration with dilute epinephrine solution will reduce hemorrhage. After the ophthalmic procedure is completed, the incision is closed in two layers. The first layer of simple interrupted sutures of 6/0 Vicryl or Dexon apposes the conjunctiva underlying the incision. The second layer of simple interrupted sutures of 4/0 silk closes the skin. In the second

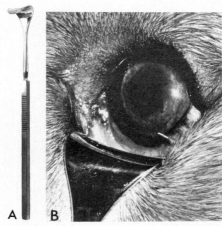

A   **B**

Figure 100–21. *A*, A lid retractor. A number of different sizes are available. *B*, Lid retractor in place.

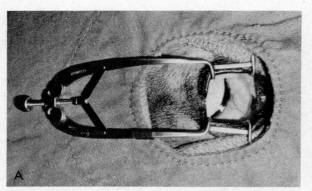
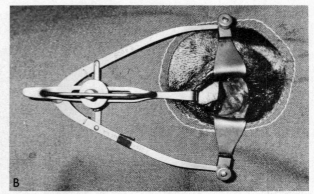

Figure 100–22. *A*, A self-retaining Castroviejo lid speculum in place. If additional exposure is needed, a lateral canthotomy may be performed. *B*, A self-retaining Maumenee-Park lid speculum in place. This speculum has the advantage of being able to retract in three directions.

layer, the first suture is placed at the former junction of the upper and lower lids and emerges from the lid margin in the same way as the suture used to close a lid laceration. Dehiscence of canthotomy incisions can usually be avoided if this procedure is followed.

Fixation

Scleral Fixation Sutures

Scleral fixation sutures are invaluable but must be placed partially through the sclera (unlike in the human eye). Passing the suture beneath the insertion of the dorsal rectus muscle is usually inadequate in animals because the muscle either cannot be identified or is too thin and flat to offer secure anchorage. A suture of 3/0 or 4/0 silk with a swaged cutting needle is placed 1 to 2 mm from the limbus and is tagged lightly with either a small hemostat or serrefines. Care must be taken not to penetrate the sclera when placing the suture. Additional sutures may be placed inferiorly, nasally, or temporally as required. When the suture is removed, one arm is cut close to the conjunctiva to reduce trauma rather than drawing

Text continued on page 1447

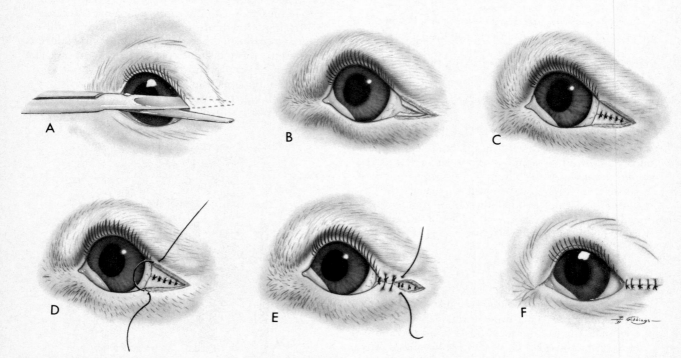

Figure 100–23. Lateral canthotomy. *A*, Position of the scissors. *B*, The canthotomy performed. *C*, Closure of the conjunctiva with simple interrupted sutures of 6-0 Vicryl or Dexon. *D*, The first suture of the second layer is placed at the lateral canthus and emerges at the lid margin. *E*, The incision is closed with simple interrupted sutures of 4-0 silk or Ethibond. *F*, The incision accurately sutured.

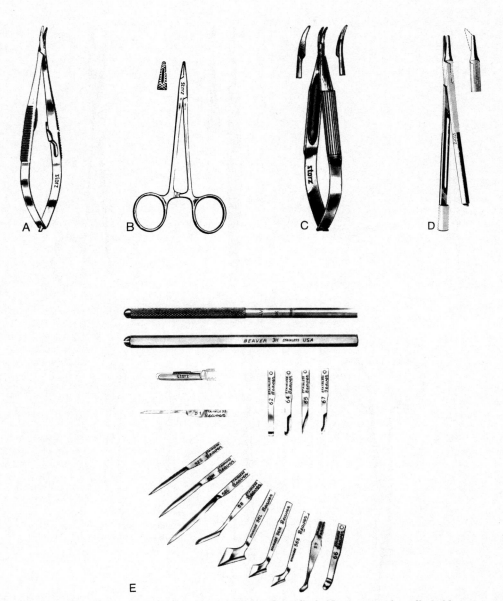

Figure 100–24. Common ophthalmic instruments. *A,* Castroviejo curved needle holders. *B,* Derf needle holders. *C,* Troutman needle holders (microsurgery). *D,* Swiss blade breaker. *E,* Selection of Beaver blades and handles.

Illustration continued on following page

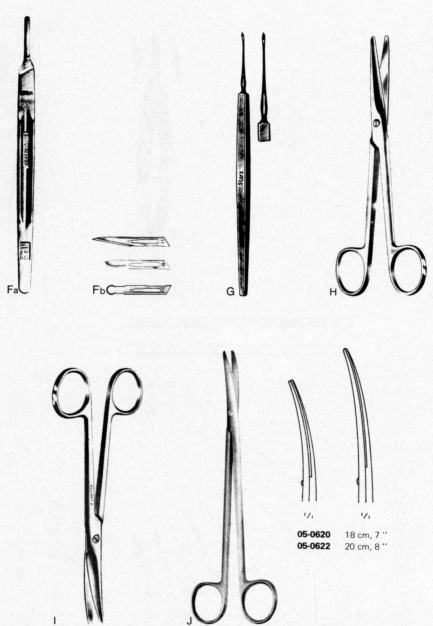

Figure 100–24 *Continued. Fa* and *Fb*, Bard-Parker blades. *G*, Foreign body spud. *H*, Straight Mayo scissors. *I*, Curved Mayo scissors. *J*, Curved Metzenbaum scissors.

Illustration continued on opposite page

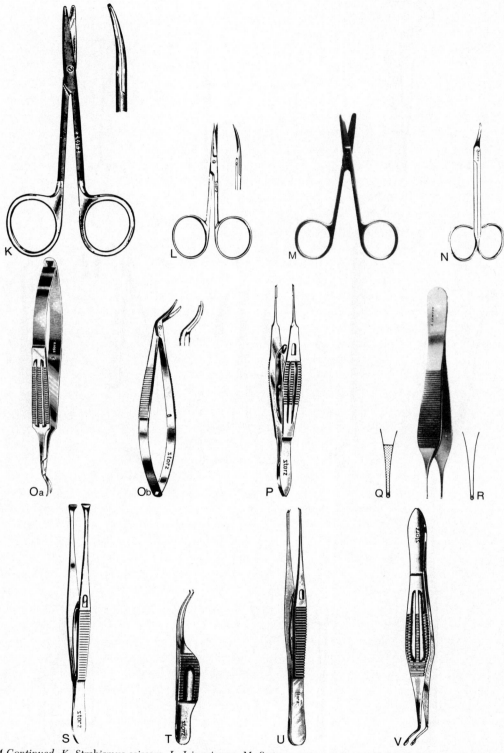

Figure 100–24 *Continued.* *K,* Strabismus scissors. *L,* Iris scissors. *M,* Spencer suture scissors. *N,* McGuire corneal scissors. *Oa* and *Ob,* Castroviejo corneal scissors (left- and right-handed). *P,* Castroviejo forceps with tying platforms. *Q,* Adson tissue forceps. *R,* Adson tissue forceps (toothed). *S,* Von Grafe fixation forceps. *T,* Colibri forceps. *U,* Elschnig-O'Brien forceps. *V,* Arruga capsule forceps.

Illustration continued on following page

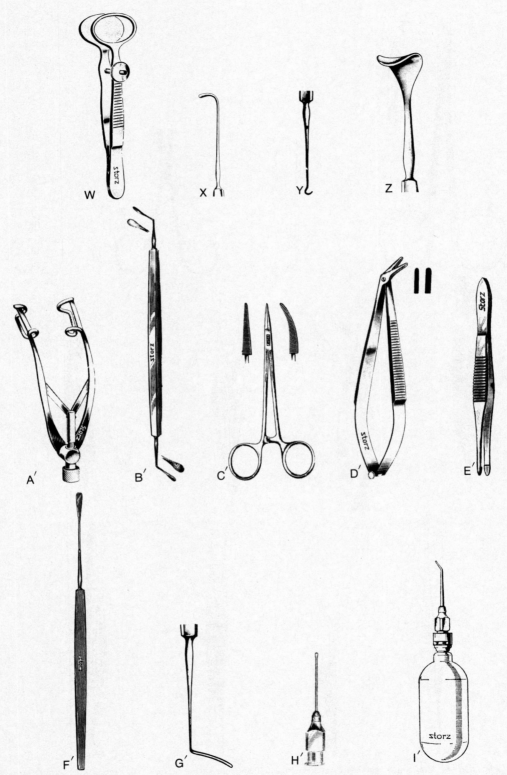

Figure 100–24 *Continued.* W, Chalazion forceps. X, Muscle hook. Y, Iris hook. Z, Lid retractor. A', Castroviejo lid speculum. B', Martinez corneal knife dissector. C', Halsted curved hemostats. D', Scleral punch. E', Cilia forceps. F', Kimura spatula. G', Cyclodialysis spatula. H', Lacrimal cannula. I', Silicone irrigating bulb and anterior chamber needles.

TABLE 100–4. Basic Ophthalmic Instrument Set

Instrument tray (35 × 25 cm)
Saline bowl (10-cm diameter)
Sponges (7 cm)
Cellulose sponges
Scalpel handle (#3), blades (#11, 15)
Castroviejo lid speculum
Castroviejo conjunctival forceps
Adson toothed (1 × 2) tissue forceps
Colibri corneal forceps
Castroviejo corneal forceps
Elschnig-O'Brien fixation forceps
Derf needle holders
Strabismus scissors
Straight Mayo scissors
Spencer suture scissors
McGuire corneal scissors
Silicone irrigating bulb
Curved Halsted mosquito hemostats
Curved Metzenbaum scissors
Curved mosquito hemostats
Irrigating cannula

the whole suture through the tissue. Subconjunctival hemorrhage is frequent with scleral fixation sutures.

Instruments

A number of instruments are available for fixation of the globe to restrict movement, but each suffers from the same disadvantage: when placed securely enough to firmly grasp the sclera, the instrument traumatizes the conjunctiva. If the conjunctiva alone is grasped, poor fixation results because it is so mobile. Fine Halsted hemostats (Fig. 100–24C') and Elschnig-O'Brien forceps (Fig. 100–24U) are used for fixation of the globe.

TABLE 100–5. Advanced Ophthalmic Instrument Set

Extraocular	Intraocular
Distichiasis clamps	Iris scissors
Swiss blade breaker/holder	Lens loupe
Castroviejo needle holders	Arruga lens capsule forceps
Troutman needle holders	McGannon lens capsule forceps
Beaver scalpel handle (blades #64, 65)	Scleral punch
Cystitome	Cystitome
Foreign body spud	Iris hook (sharp, dull)
Desmarres chalazion clamp	O'Gawa irrigation cannula
Chalazion spoon	Cyclodialysis spatula
Muscle hook	Flieringa fixation righs
Martinez corneal elevator	Jamieson calipers
Maumenee-Park lid speculum	
Tying forceps	

OPHTHALMIC SURGICAL INSTRUMENTS

Ophthalmic instruments are illustrated in Figure 100–24. A basic list of instruments suitable for procedures commonly performed in general practice is given in Table 100–4. More sophisticated extraocular and intraocular instruments are listed in Table 100–5. Eponyms applied to instruments indicate the designer, often there being many different designs of a particular instrument.

1. Bistner, S. I., Roberts, S. R., and Anderson, R. P.: Conjunctival bacteria: clinical appearances can be deceiving. Mod. Vet. Pract. 50:45, 1969.
2. Brightman, A. H., Helper, L. C., and Hoffman, W. E.: Effect of aspirin on aqueous protein values in the dog. J.Am.Vet.Med.Assoc. 178:572, 1981.
3. Brightman, A. H., Vestre, W. A., Helper, L. C., and Tomes, J. E.: Cryosurgery for the treatment of canine glaucoma. J. Am. Anim. Hosp. Assoc. 18:319, 1982.
4. Brock, K. A., and Thurmon, J. C.: Pulmonary edema associated with mannitol administration. Can. Pract. 6:31, 1979.
5. Campbell, L.: Ocular bacteria and mycoplasma of the clinically normal cat. Fel. Pract. 3:10, 1973.
6. Edelhauser, H. F., Van Horn, D. L., Schultz, R. O., and Hyndiuk, R. A.: Comparative toxicity of intraocular irrigating solutions on the corneal endothelium. Am. J. Ophthalmol. 81:473, 1976.
7. Floman, N., and Zor, U.: Mechanism of steroid action in ocular inflammation. Inhibition of prostaglandin production. Invest. Ophthalmol. 16:69, 1977.
8. Gelatt, K. N., and Rubin, L. F.: Delayed postoperative staphylomas in dogs. J. Am. Vet. Med. Assoc. 154:283, 1969.
9. Havener, W. H.: Ocular Pharmacology, 3rd Ed. C. V. Mosby, St. Louis, 1974, p. 441.
10. Magrane, W. G.,: Cataract extraction: a follow-up study (429 cases). J. Small Anim. Pract. 10:545, 1969.
11. McDonald, P. J., and Watson, A. D. J.: Microbial flora of normal canine conjunctivae. J. Small Anim. Pract. 17:809, 1976.
12. Muir, W. W.: Effects of atropine on cardiac rate and rhythm in dogs. J.Am.Vet.Med.Assoc. 172:917, 1978.
13. Nuefeld, A. H., Chavis, R. M., and Sears, M. L.: Degeneration release of norepinephrine causes transient ocular hyperemia mediated by prostaglandins. Invest. Ophthalmol. 12:167, 1973.
14. Peiffer, R. L.: Current concepts in ophthalmic surgery. Vet.Clin. North Am. 10:455, 1980.
15. Slatter, D. H.: Fundamentals of Veterinary Ophthalmology. W. B. Saunders, Philadelphia, 1981.
16. Stallard, H. B.: Eye Surgery. 5th ed. John Wright, Bristol, 1973, p. 31.
17. Urban, M., Wyman, M., Rheins, M., and Marraro, R. V.: Conjunctival flora of clinically normal dogs. J. Am. Vet. Med. Assoc. 161:201, 1972.
18. Varma, S., Lumb, W. V., Johnson, L. W., and Ferguson, H. L.: Further studies with polyglycolic acid (Dexon) and other sutures in infected experimental wounds. Am. J. Vet. Res. 42:571, 1981.
19. Waitzman, M. B., and King, C. D.: Prostaglandin influences on intraocular pressure and pupil size. Am. J.Physiol. (Lond.) 212:329, 1967.
20. Whitelocke, R. A. F., and Eakins, K. C.: Vascular changes in the anterior uvea of rabbits produced by prostsglandins. Arch. Ophthalmol. 89:495, 1973.

101 Lids

Alan H. Brightman II

ANATOMY

The eyelids are thin mobile folds of skin that normally cover the eye. In cross section, the lids are composed of the external epidermal surface, the orbicularis oculi muscle, the tarsal plate, the tarsal (meibomian) glands, and the palpebral conjunctiva (Fig. 101–1).[16] The lid margins are demarcated from the skin by a mucocutaneous border 2 to 3 mm from the lid margin. The openings of the tarsal glands (20 to 40 per lid) can be seen on the surface of the lid margins. Upon everting the lids, these glands can be seen under the conjunctiva as white cords extending ventrally 5 to 7 mm from the lid margin. The tarsal glands secrete a phospholipid-rich, sebaceous material that forms the superficial lipid layer of the tear film.

The tarsus, or tarsal plate, is a poorly defined fibrous sheet that supports the lids and is continuous with the septum orbitale, which is attached to the orbital periosteum.

The cilia (eyelashes) in the dog are found on the outer surface of the upper lid margin. The dog has no cilia on the lower lid, and the cat has no cilia at all.[8] At the base of these cilia, sweat glands (glands of Moll) and sebaceous glands (glands of Zeis) open near or into the adjacent hair follicle.[16]

Muscles of the Eyelid

The orbicularis oculi muscle lies anterior to the tarsal plate and encircles the palpebral fissure (Fig. 101–2). It is innervated by the palpebral nerve, which is a branch of the facial nerve (cranial nerve VII).[8]

The orbicularis oculi functions as a sphincter to close the lids. In most species, the muscle is anchored medially to the orbit by fascia and laterally by the retractor anguli oculi lateralis. These attachments of the orbicularis oculi preserve the elliptical shape of the palpebral fissure. The muscle that elevates the upper lid is the levator palpebrae superioris. It is innervated by the oculomotor nerve (cranial nerve III). Müller's muscle, which is indistinguishable from the levator palpebrae superioris, provides sympathetic tone to keep the upper lid elevated without conscious effort. The sensory nerve to the lids is the ophthalmic branch of the trigeminal nerve (cranial nerve V).[8]

CONGENITAL ABNORMALITIES OF THE EYELIDS REQUIRING SURGICAL CORRECTION

Ophthalmia Neonatorum

The lids in newborn puppies normally separate at 10 to 15 days. In some puppies, but rarely other species, an acute purulent conjunctivitis occurs prior to lid separation. The lids are swollen, and a purulent exudate is observed from the medial canthus or nares. In these cases, it is imperative to open the lids surgically as soon as possible to prevent corneal damage.[14] A muscle hook or tenotomy scissors is inserted medially or laterally at the canthus (Fig. 101–3). In most cases the lids separate when gentle

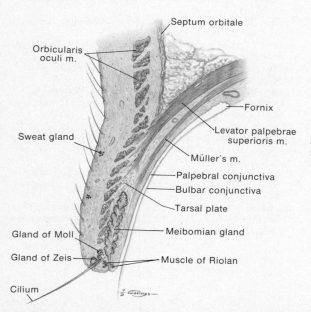

Septum orbitale

Orbicularis oculi m.

Sweat gland

Fornix

Levator palpebrae superioris m.

Müller's m.

Palpebral conjunctiva

Bulbar conjunctiva

Tarsal plate

Gland of Moll

Meibomian gland

Gland of Zeis

Muscle of Riolan

Cilium

Figure 101–1. Anatomy of the normal eyelid. (Reprinted with permission from Slatter, D.: *Fundamentals of Veterinary Ophthalmology.* W. B. Saunders, Philadelphia, 1981.)

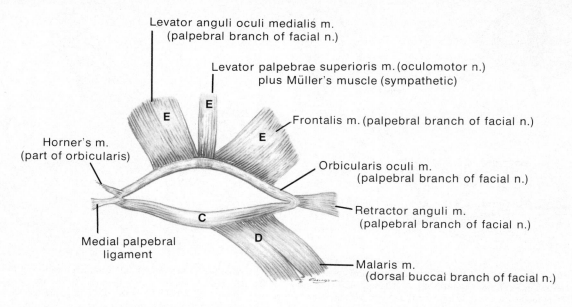

Levator anguli oculi medialis m.
(palpebral branch of facial n.)

Levator palpebrae superioris m.(oculomotor n.)
plus Müller's muscle (sympathetic)

Frontalis m.(palpebral branch of facial n.)

Horner's m.
(part of orbicularis)

Orbicularis oculi m.
(palpebral branch of facial n.)

Retractor anguli m.
(palpebral branch of facial n.)

Medial palpebral
ligament

Malaris m.
(dorsal buccai branch of facial n.)

E—Elevate upper lid
D—Depress lower lid
C—Constrict palpebral fissure

Figure 101–2. Actions and innervations of the muscles of the eyelid. (Reprinted with permission from Slatter, D.: *Fundamentals of Veterinary Ophthalmology.* W. B. Saunders, Philadelphia, 1981.)

upward pressure is applied with the instrument. Flushing the cul-de-sacs with a sterile eye wash and applying an appropriate antibiotic four to six times a day for several days usually result in rapid recovery.[14]

Colobomas

A coloboma, or agenesis of the eyelid, is a defect in the lid margin. The disease rarely occurs in the dog but has been reported in cats.[2,8,19] In cats, the defect usually involves the lateral portion of the upper lid. Depending on the severity of the defect, the condition can result in entropion, trichiasis, blepharospasm, or secondary keratitis.

Surgical correction of the defect using a horizontal

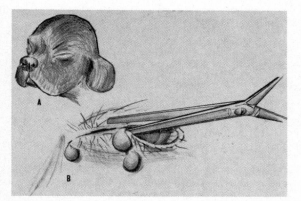

Figure 101–3. *A,* Ophthalmia neonatorum. Discharge seeping from behind closed lids. *B,* Separation of the lids with blunt tenotomy scissors. (Reprinted with permission from Magrane, W.: *Canine Ophthalmology,* 3rd ed. Lea & Febiger, Philadelphia, 1977.)

pedicle graft (Fig. 101–4) is usually required if the lesion is causing clinical signs of disease.[1] The procedure involves preparing a graft site by splitting the skin and conjunctiva. A pedicle graft is harvested from the lower lid and is sutured into the defect. Care must be taken to suture the conjunctiva to the pedicle so that hair from the skin does not rub on the cornea. The conjunctiva-to-pedicle sutures should be 6-0 or 7-0 chromic gut, and 5-0 or 6-0 silk is used for the skin sutures.

Narrow Palpebral Fissure
(Blepharophimosis, Micropalpebral Fissure)

This condition is congenital in the chow chow, Kerry blue terrier, collie, shetland sheepdog, and bull terrier.[2,14,19] If the condition is associated with concomitant microphthalmia, surgical correction may not be necessary. In a dog with a normal-sized globe, however, this condition may result in entropion (inversion of the lid margins). Enlargement of the palpebral fissure by performing a canthotomy and canthoplasty usually corrects the entropion (Fig. 101–5).[1]

The canthotomy is performed by drawing the lateral canthus laterally with the thumb and forefinger. The canthus is cut with blunt scissors to the desired length. After the canthotomy has been performed, permanent lengthening of the palpebral fissure can be achieved with a canthoplasty. The preferred canthoplasty is a modification of the technique first proposed by Smythe.[1]

In those cases requiring substantial enlargement of

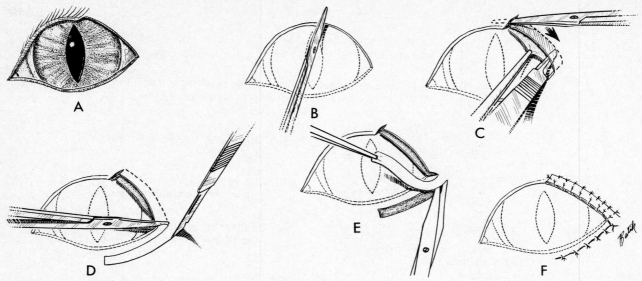

Figure 101–4. Horizontal pedicle graft for correction of eyelid coloboma. *A,* Incomplete development of the temporal aspect of the upper eyelid can result in chronic keratitis. *B,* A recipient bed is prepared in the upper lid to receive the pedicle graft. The nasal end of the lid defect is made square by trimming the defect with a Stevens tenotomy scissors. *C,* The lid is split along the length of the upper defect, separating the skin–orbicularis layer from the underlying conjunctiva. The lid splitting is continued nasally for a distance of 3 mm into the normal lid. *D,* The horizontal pedicle flap to be transposed is prepared by making two incisions through the skin and orbicularis of the lower lid. The first incision is made parallel to and 2 mm from the lid margin; the second incision is made 5 mm from the lid edge, providing a 3-mm horizontal flap. The length of the pedicle flap depends on the size of the defect to be filled. The incisions into the lower lid are parallel but diverge slightly to form a broader base as they reach the lateral canthus. The lateral canthus is cut to the uppermost edge of the pedicle, permitting the pedicle to be rotated to its new position in the upper lid. The horizontal skin–orbicularis oculi pedicle flap is bluntly dissected free. *E,* A thin strip of skin–orbicularis muscle in the recipient bed is removed from the upper lid to create a fresh wound to receive the pedicle graft. The pedicle graft is moved to its new position. *F,* The pedicle flap is sutured in place with interrupted 6–0 silk, nylon, or Dexon. The conjunctiva is sutured to the edge of the pedicle flap, creating a new lid margin. All sutures should be placed to avoid corneal irritation. Hair does not grow on the new lid margin, which consists of tarsus that becomes epithelialized and heals with a smooth border. The lower lid defect is closed with simple interrupted sutures. (Reprinted with permission from istner, S., Aguirre, G., and Batik, G.: *Atlas of Veterinary Ophthalmic Surgery*. W. B. Saunders, Philadelphia, 1977.)

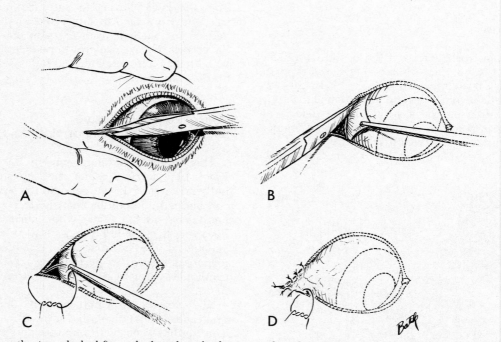

Figure 101–5. Lengthening palpebral fissure by lateral canthoplasty. *A,* A lateral canthotomy is performed. The size of the canthotomy is equivalent to the desired size of palpebral fissure. Hemorrhage is minimal and is controlled by pinpoint electrocautery. *B,* After performing the canthotomy, the palpebral conjunctiva is undermined by blunt dissection, using a Stevens tenotomy scissors. The blunt dissection, involving the conjunctiva of both the upper and lower temporal lids, is carried to the fornix. *C,* The conjunctiva is sutured to the new lateral canthus with simple interrupted 6-0 silk sutures, and the knots are tied on the outside of the lid. The canthotomy incision must be lined by conjunctiva to prevent the development of adhesions between raw lid surfaces. *D,* The palpebral fissure is lengthened. The sutures are removed in 14 to 21 days. (Reprinted with permission from Bistner, S., Aguirre, G., and Batik, G.: *Atlas of Veterinary Ophthalmic Surgery*. W. B. Saunders, Philadelphia, 1977.)

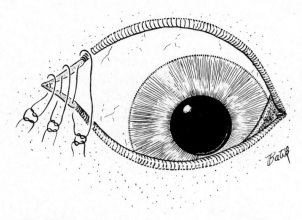

Figure 101–6. Permanent shortening of palpebral fissure.

the palpebral fissure, a wedge of lid margin can be removed above and below the lateral canthus. The edges of the conjunctiva are sutured to the debrided lid margins with 6-0 silk sutures.

Large Palpebral Fissure (Macropalpebral Fissure)

Too large a palpebral fissure, in the presence of a normal-sized globe, can result in ectropion (eversion of the lid margins). Although the condition rarely causes ocular disease, certain breeds, such as the English bulldog, spaniel, and hounds, may require shortening of the fissure.[14,19] The procedure may also be indicated in cases of phthisis bulbi or endophthalmos secondary to loss of orbital fat.

The procedure performed to shorten the palpebral fissure is a permanent tarsorrhaphy. The lateral lid margins are removed to the canthus.* The amount of tissue to be removed varies with each individual. Usually between one-quarter and one-third of the margins can be closed without causing an unacceptable cosmetic appearance. A strip of tissue 2 to 3 mm wide and parallel to the margins is removed (Fig. 101–6). The cut margins are sutured with 5-0 silk in an interrupted pattern. The sutures should be left in place for about 14 days to ensure that the wound will heal.

CONGENITAL AND ACQUIRED EYELID DISEASES

Entropion

Entropion is defined as an inversion of the eyelid margin in which the eyelashes rub the cornea. This condition often results in a superficial irritation of the

conjunctiva and cornea. Chronic ocular discharge and blepharospasm are commonly seen (Fig. 101–7). If not surgically treated, the condition can lead to vascularization, pigmentation, and possible ulceration of the cornea. There are three commonly accepted etiologies: congenital, spastic, and acquired.

Congenital Entropion

Congenital entropion is usually a bilateral condition that is commonly seen in dogs. The lower lateral lid is most frequently affected, followed by the upper lid, and, infrequently, the medial lower lid. The chow chow, bloodhound, Labrador retriever, English bulldog, Doberman pinscher, Chesapeake Bay retriever, St. Bernard, rottweiler, poodle, Irish setter, and Shar Pei are predisposed to entropion.[14,19]

Diagnosis of this disease is usually easy. Surgical correction is satisfactory in most cases. Whenever possible, it is wise to postpone entropion correction until the dog is four to six months of age and its facial features have matured. Application of a topical antibiotic ointment three to four times a day coats the eyelashes and hairs rubbing on the cornea and should be used until surgery is performed.

Surgical Correction

Many techniques have been suggested for the correction of simple entropion. The technique that provides the most consistent result is a modified Holtz-Celus procedure (Fig. 101–8)[8,19] involving excision of a half-moon-shaped flap of skin 2 to 3 mm from the lid margin. The skin excision should be 3 to 4 mm wider than the affected area of lid. The area of skin to be removed is crushed with Halsted or Crile forceps by grasping the fold of skin with the edge of the instrument. After initially placing the forceps on the skin fold, fine adjustments in the size of the fold can be made by releasing skin or pulling more skin into the jaws of the forceps before crushing. The hemostats are clamped tightly and left in place for about 30 seconds before being removed. The fold of skin is removed with blunt scissors. Some surgeons prefer to make a free-hand incision with a scalpel to reduce most operative scarring. This method has the advantage of causing slightly less tissue trauma, but more hemorrhage is encountered. In severe cases of entropion, a small strip of orbicularis muscle may be removed in an effort to create greater internal scarring and reduce the amount of postoperative skin stretching. This is accomplished by grasping the exposed muscle with small Bishop-Harmon forceps and cutting a strip of muscle with tenotomy scissors. Care must be taken not to cut through the palpebral conjunctiva. The skin is closed with 5-0 or 6-0 silk sutures placed about 2 mm apart in a simple interrupted pattern. Subcutaneous suturing is not necessary.

Immediately postoperatively, the lids should be in a normal position. During the first few days of

---

*Editor's note: In brachycephalic breeds, corneal exposure may be reduced by medial tarsorrhaphy.

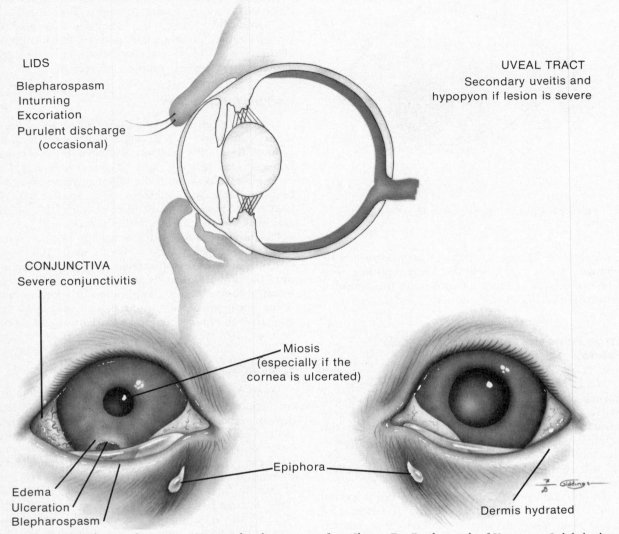

LIDS

Blepharospasm
Inturning
Excoriation
Purulent discharge
(occasional)

UVEAL TRACT
Secondary uveitis and
hypopyon if lesion is severe

CONJUNCTIVA
Severe conjunctivitis

Miosis
(especially if the
cornea is ulcerated)

Epiphora

Edema
Ulceration
Blepharospasm

Dermis hydrated

Figure 101–7. Clinical signs of entropion. (Reprinted with permission from Slatter, D.: *Fundamentals of Veterinary Ophthalmology.* W. B. Saunders, Philadelphia, 1981.)

recovery, the lids appear to be slightly overcorrected, but as the swelling subsides they return to normal. When in doubt it is better to slightly undercorrect than to overcorrect and create an ectropion. Postoperative treatment consists of placing an antibiotic ointment in the eye and on the wound twice a day. No wound adhesions or infections have been observed following antibiotic application. A plastic Elizabethan collar should be placed on the animal to prevent self-injury. Sutures are removed 10 to 14 days postoperatively.

The two major reasons for failure to achieve a good cosmetic result are (1) not making the incision close enough to the lid margin, and (2) placing the sutures too far apart.

Spastic Entropion

This disease is usually unilateral and can occur at any age. The cause of the lid inversion is spasm of the orbicularis oculi muscle secondary to ocular irritation. The etiology includes conjunctivitis, foreign bodies, keratoconjunctivitis sicca, trichiasis, distichiasis, ectopic cilia, and corneal ulceration. A de-

Figure 101–8. Pinch technique for entropion. *A,* Preoperative appearance of the entropion. *B,* The "rolled-in" area is everted and the necessary amount of skin is placed between the forceps. *C,* The second pair of forceps is applied and final adjustments are made before clamping. *D,* The forceps are removed. *E,* The strip of skin is excised, starting at the temporal canthus and including all of the clamped area. The strip is kept taut throughout the excision. *F,* The excised area with orbicularis oculi undisturbed. *G,* The incision is sutured with simple interrupted sutures of 6-0 silk, 1.5 to 2.0 mm apart. A generous bite of tissue should be taken to prevent premature pulling out as the wound heals, but the sutures should not be tied tight, as postoperative edema may cause tearing of the surrounding tissue. (Redrawn after Severin, 1976.) (Reprinted with permission from Slatter, D.: *Fundamentals of Veterinary Ophthalmology.* W. B. Saunders, Philadelphia, 1981.)

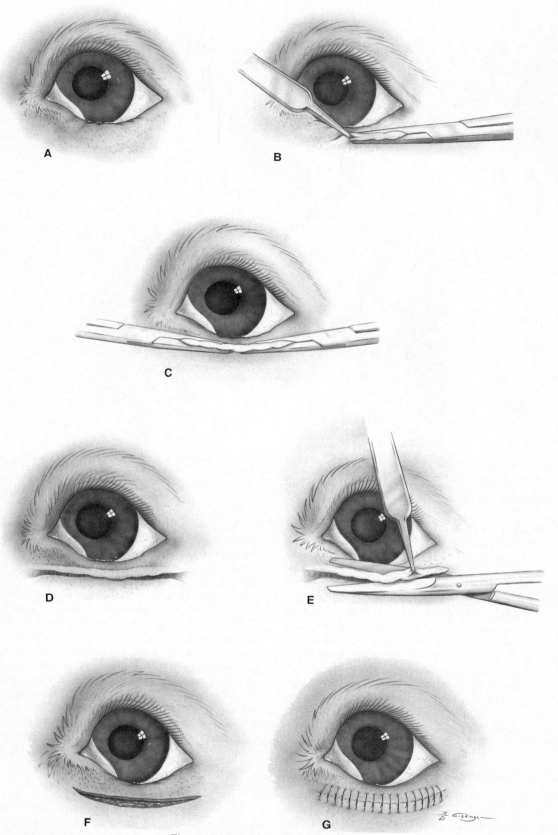

Figure 101-8. See legend on opposite page

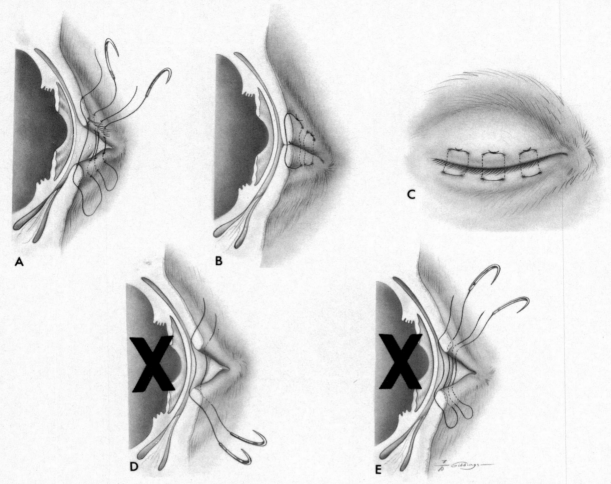

Figure 101–9. A, B, and C, Placement of interrupted intermarginal horizontal mattress sutures in temporary tarsorrhaphy. D and E, Incorrect suture placement, which results in corneal abrasions from the sutures. (After Severin, G. A.: *Veterinary Ophthalmology Notes.* Fort Collins, CO, 1976. Reprinted with permission from Slatter, D.: *Fundamentals of Veterinary Ophthalmology.* W. B. Saunders, Philadelphia, 1981.)

tailed ocular examination should be performed to determine the underlying cause. Initial therapy should be directed at correcting the original problem. Many cases of spastic entropion resolve after the inciting irritant is removed. One diagnostic method to help differentiate spastic from congenital or acquired entropion is to place several drops of topical anesthetic on the eye. If the entropion resolves spontaneously it was most likely spastic in nature.

If the entropion persists once the underlying cause has been corrected, one can use a third eyelid flap or a temporary tarsorrhaphy (Fig. 101–9) to reduce further irritation. Sutures for both of these procedures are removed in two to three weeks. If all else has failed, a standard entropion correction will cure the condition.

Acquired Entropion

Entropion is a common sequela to endophthalmos from loss of the orbital fat or temporalis muscle atrophy. Endophthalmos caused by retraction of the globe by the retractor oculi muscle secondary to

ocular pain will generally not cause entropion. An abnormally small globe with normal lid structure as seen with phthisis bulbi or microphthalmos can also result in entropion. The surgical correction of this type of entropion is best accomplished by performing a lateral canthoplasty to shorten the palpebral fissure (Fig. 101–10). This is accomplished by separating the skin from the orbicularis oculi muscle at the lateral canthus with a small scalpel (Beaver #64 blade). A triangular flap of skin is removed from the upper lid proportional to the amount of closure required. A flap from the lower lid is sutured into the defect in the upper lid. Suturing is completed with 6-0 silk in an interrupted pattern. This procedure has the advantage of providing a palpebral fissure proportionate to the globe size while correcting the acquired entropion.

Medial Entropion and Facial Folds

In poodles, Pekingese, and pugs the lid margins at the medial canthus may be slightly inverted. This condition is occasionally seen in Persian cats. The

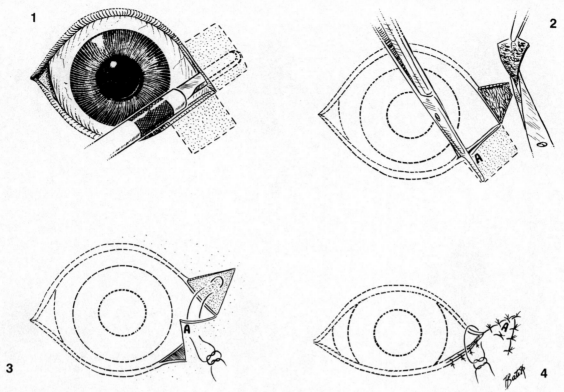

Figure 101–10. *1,* The amount of palpebral fissure to be closed is estimated by pinching the lids closed at the lateral canthus. The upper and lower lids are then split over an area that encompasses the amount of closure desired. The lid-splitting technique separates skin–orbicularis muscle from the underlying conjunctiva. *2,* A cut *(A)* is made at the nasal end of the lid split in the lower lid, and the tarsal (ciliary) margin of this undermined lower lid flap is removed. A similar cut at the nasal end of the upper lid split is made, and the incision is extended outward and downward to end at the lateral canthus. This triangular piece of skin–orbicularis muscle is removed from the upper lid. *3,* A double-armed 4-0 silk suture is used to place a mattress suture in the upper eyelid tarsoconjunctiva and then through the lower lid skin-muscle flap. The lower lid is then drawn upward to fit into the defect created in the upper lid, and the mattress suture is tied. *4,* Additional 6-0 silk sutures are used to secure the flap and recreate the lateral canthus. Care must be taken to close the lid-splitting defect in the lower lid. (Reprinted with permission from Bistner, S. I., Aguirre, G., and Batik, G.: *Atlas of Veterinary Ophthalmic Surgery.* W. B. Saunders, Philadelphia, 1977.)

lacrimal puncta may be slightly compressed, and epiphora may be the only presenting sign. Those cats and dogs having only minor epiphora may not benefit from surgical intervention because the defect may be so slight that the problems associated with overcorrection outweigh the potential benefit of surgery. Medical therapy using 5 mg of oral tetracycline once a day often eliminates the staining of the tears on the facial fur of these patients and further negates surgical intervention. The brachiocephalic breeds such as the Pekingese and pug often have a combination of medial entropion and prominent facial folds.[8,14,19] One or both of these conditions can cause keratitis and eventually pigment infiltration of the cornea from the medial limbus. Once this pigmentary keratitis is diagnosed, it is necessary to determine if and what surgery is necessary. In older dogs (seven to eight years and older) in which the pigment has infiltrated only one-fourth or less of the cornea and no visual loss is observed, surgery is generally not necessary.

In younger dogs with progressive pigmentary keratitis, close examination usually reveals the cause of the irritation, which may require surgical intervention.

Repair of medial entropion is accomplished by the same technique as that outlined for congenital entropion (see Fig. 101–8). Care must be taken not to cut or suture the lacrimal puncta. Removal or reduction of the nasal folds is indicated when the hairs on the folds rub on the cornea. This can be accomplished by crushing the tissue to be removed with forceps and excising it with blunt scissors (Fig. 101–11). A better cosmetic result is obtained if the incision is made on the posterior aspect of the folds. Usually, the nasal folds must be reduced to at least one-half their original height. The sutures are placed in an interrupted pattern with 6-0 or 5-0 silk and are removed 10 to 14 days postoperatively. Concurrent superficial keratectomy for pigmentary keratitis is unnecessary, since correction of the medial entropion

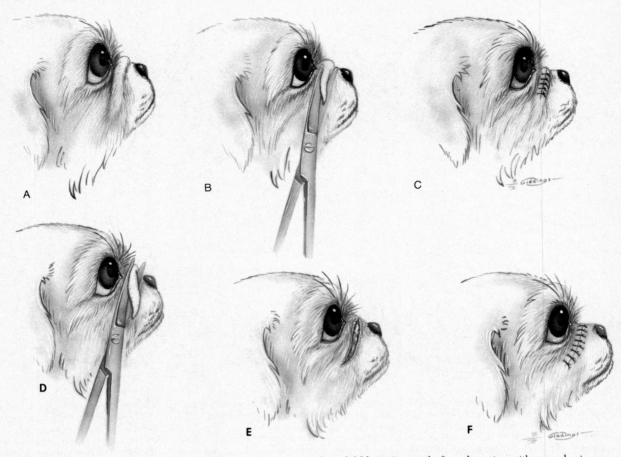

Figure 101–11. A–C, Partial removal of the nasal fold. A, Lateral view of nasal fold. B, Removal of nasal portion with curved scissors. Note that the anterior portion of the fold is removed. C, The sutured wound with a small fold remaining that is more prominent laterally. The knots are placed on the anterior side of the incision to limit corneal contact. D–F, Total removal of the nasal fold. D, Removal of the fold starting laterally. E, The fold removed. F, The fold sutured. The knots are placed on the anterior side of the incision to reduce the chance of corneal contact. (Redrawn after Severin, 1976.) (Reprinted with permission from Slatter, D.: *Fundamentals of Veterinary Ophthalmology.* W. B. Saunders, Philadelphia, 1981.)

or nasal folds stops the physical irritation to the cornea. Pigmentation decreases with time and the judicious use of corticosteroids. In addition, many superficial keratectomies performed on Pekingese and pugs for pigmentary keratitis often result in severe corneal scarring with no improvement in vision; therefore, I strongly recommend against it.

Combined Entropion-Ectropion

Certain breeds, such as the St. Bernard, Doberman pinscher, English bulldog, and cocker spaniel, may exhibit a lid deformity that involves both an inversion and eversion of one or both lids.[2,19] Typically, these dogs have a lateral entropion and a central ectropion of both the upper and lower lids. They are usually presented prior to six months of age with a profound mucopurulent discharge and severe keratoconjunctivitis.

There are several theories regarding the cause of this disease. It has been proposed that there may be an absent or poorly functioning retractor anguli oculi muscle, which is responsible for providing lateral tension on the lid.[21] This muscle is thought to perform the function of the lateral canthal ligament in man. The possibility that the underlying cause is simply excessive facial skin in breeds such as the St. Bernard must also be considered.

The condition requires a surgical procedure that not only corrects the entropion but also provides lateral traction on the canthus to correct the ectropion. Wyman has outlined a lateral canthoplasty recommended for this lid abnormality (Fig. 101–12).[21] This technique involves making either a free-hand incision or a crush-and-cut incision on both the upper and lower lids, extending around the lateral canthus. After the skin is removed, two strips of upper and lower orbicularis oculi muscle are freed laterally from the lid to the lateral canthus. The skin is undermined over the zygomatic arch, and a cruciate-type suture pattern with 3-0 Dexon or nylon is used to join the strips of orbicularis. This "artificial" lateral ligament is pulled as far laterally as possible and sutured into the periosteum of the zygomatic arch. The skin is closed with 5-0 silk suture in an interrupted pattern.

The major problems encountered with this proce-

dure are (1) cutting the orbicularis strips so far past the lateral canthus that they provide little or no traction, (2) failure to suture the orbicularis strips to the periosteum or other ligamentous tissue, resulting

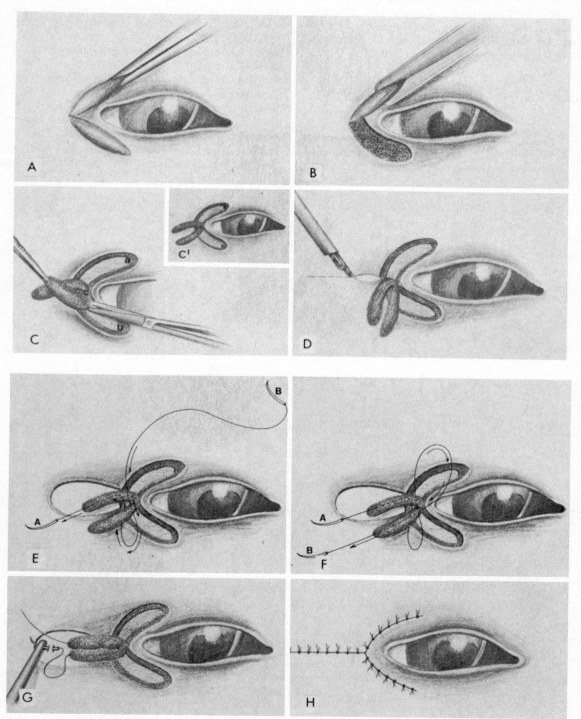

Figure 101–12. Lateral blepharoplasty for correction of combined entropion-ectropion. *A,* Folds of upper and lower lids are made to meet opposite the lateral canthus. *B,* Excision of folds. *C,* Commencing at *(a)* and *(b),* tongues of orbicularis muscle are dissected to terminate in a single bundle base. Step completed *(C').* *D,* Skin incision is made from the base of the muscle bundle to an area over the temporal bone. *E,* Tongues are brought together at the base. One needle *(A)* traverses the base and is turned and brought up through the opposite tongue. *F,* The second needle *(B)* is brought up the length of the other tongue. *G,* The bundle is "tacked" to the periosteum over the inferior process of the temporal bone. *H,* Skin closure. (Reprinted with permission from Magrane, W. G.: *Canine Ophthalmology.* 3rd ed. Lea & Febiger, Philadelphia, 1977.)

in a loss of tension on the lateral canthus, and (3) making the skin incisions too far from the lid margins to correct the entropion.

In most cases there is more postoperative swelling than is encountered with a standard entropion correction. Hot packing twice a day for two or three days while the animal is still hospitalized is recommended. An Elizabethan collar should be placed on the animal, and sutures are removed after 14 days.

Ectropion

Ectropion, or eversion of the lid margin, is a common finding in many breeds of dogs. It is particularly common in the St. Bernard, bloodhound, American cocker spaniel, basset hound, and bull-

dog.[8,14,19] The condition is usually congenital and generally involves the lower eyelids but can result from scarring.

Most dogs with congenital ectropion do not require surgical correction. Only those animals experiencing chronic keratitis or conjunctivitis that is unresponsive to medical therapy should be considered for surgery (Fig. 101–13).

Of the numerous techniques available for correcting both congenital and acquired ectropion, the Warton-Jones blepharoplasty (V-Y technique) is the simplest and most commonly used (Fig. 101–14).[19] This procedure involves making a V-shaped incision through the skin ventral to and slightly wider than the everted area. The flap is undermined to within 2 to 3 mm of the eyelid margin. The incision is closed from the base dorsally. The amount of closure can be

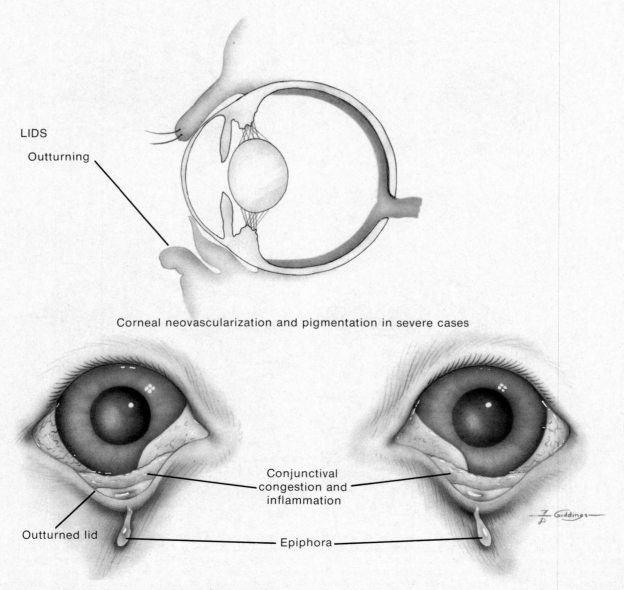

LIDS
Outturning

Corneal neovascularization and pigmentation in severe cases

Conjunctival congestion and inflammation

Outturned lid

Epiphora

Figure 101–13. Clinical signs of ectropion. (Reprinted with permission from Slatter, D.: *Fundamentals of Veterinary Ophthalmology.* W. B. Saunders, Philadelphia, 1981.)

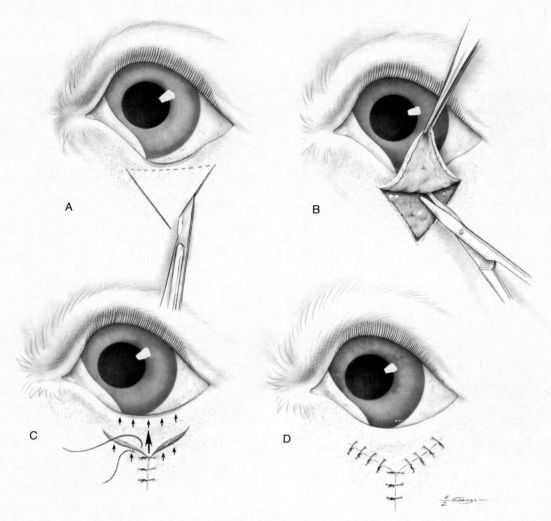

Figure 101–14. Wharton-Jones blepharoplasty. *A,* Skin triangle outlined and incisions made. *B,* Skin flap elevated and dissected beneath. *C,* Vertical portion formed (defect + 3 mm). *D,* Completed Y incision sutured with 6-0 or 4-0 silk. (Reprinted with permission from Slatter, D.: *Fundamentals of Veterinary Ophthalmology.* W. B. Saunders, Philadelphia, 1981.)

gauged by moving the flap up until the eversion is corrected. The remaining sides of the incision are closed. Subcutaneous suturing is neither indicated nor needed in this procedure. The incision is closed with 5-0 or 6-0 silk in an interrupted pattern.

On rare occasions, after successfully correcting the eyelid abnormality, excessive conjunctiva, which is not cosmetically acceptable, is present in the ventral fornix. In such cases, the conjunctiva may be excised by grasping a fold of conjunctiva with a straight hemostat and clamping it. The newly formed ridge is cut with scissors and the wound closed with 6-0 chromic gut or Vicryl in a continuous pattern.

In severe cases in which the V-Y technique will not correct the ectropion, a modification of the Kuhnt-Szymonowski technique can be used (Fig. 101–15).[8,19] This procedure involves removing a wedge of lid margin of appropriate width to shorten the margin adequately. The crush-and-cut technique can be used to outline the area to be excised. Once the tissue is removed, the conjunctiva and tarsal

tissues are closed in a continuous pattern to assure good apposition. The skin is closed with 5-0 or 6-0 silk in an interrupted pattern.

EYELID TUMORS

Eyelid tumors are common in the dog. The tarsal gland adenoma is the most frequently diagnosed eyelid tumor in the dog.[12] Less commonly found are adenocarcinomas, melanomas, and papillomas. The tarsal gland adenoma, as with most tumors of the canine eyelid, is clinically benign, and surgical excision is usually curative. Cryosurgery using liquid nitrogen at −20°C can also be used to treat these tumors (see Cryosurgery hereafter).

Excision of Eyelid Tumors

A full thickness eyelid resection is the simplest procedure for removal of tarsal gland adenomas in

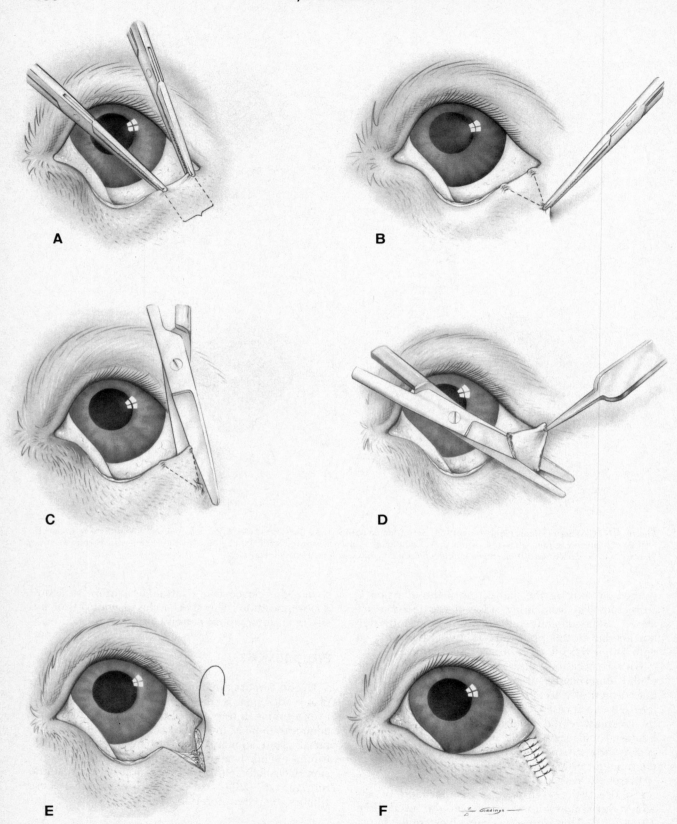

Figure 101–15. Modified Kuhnt-Szymonowski procedure. *A,* The lid margin is marked laterally. *B,* An estimate of the amount of margin to be removed is made, and the lid is marked. The ventral end of the triangle is marked 10 to 14 mm below. *C,* The first incision is made with straight Mayo scissors. *D,* The second incision is made. *E,* The triangular piece removed. Note that the conjunctival defect is smaller, justifying one layer of sutures in the skin in some cases. *F,* The wound sutured with 6-0 silk. (Reprinted with permission from Slatter, D.: *Fundamentals of Veterinary Ophthalmology.* W. B. Saunders, Philadelphia, 1981.)

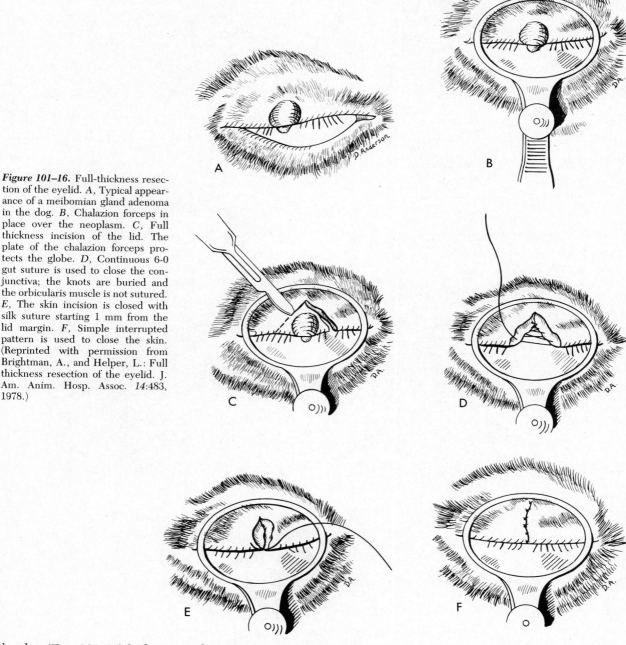

Figure 101–16. Full-thickness resection of the eyelid. *A,* Typical appearance of a meibomian gland adenoma in the dog. *B,* Chalazion forceps in place over the neoplasm. *C,* Full thickness incision of the lid. The plate of the chalazion forceps protects the globe. *D,* Continuous 6-0 gut suture is used to close the conjunctiva; the knots are buried and the orbicularis muscle is not sutured. *E,* The skin incision is closed with silk suture starting 1 mm from the lid margin. *F,* Simple interrupted pattern is used to close the skin. (Reprinted with permission from Brightman, A., and Helper, L.: Full thickness resection of the eyelid. J. Am. Anim. Hosp. Assoc. *14*:483, 1978.)

the dog (Fig. 101–16).[3] This procedure can be used in lesions that involve up to one-third of the lid margin on either the upper or lower lid. Immobilizing the lesion with a Desmarres chalazion clamp or using hemostats to crush along the proposed incisions decreases bleeding. A V incision is made with blunt scissors including a 2 to 3 mm strip of normal tissue on each side of the tumor. If a chalazion clamp is used, the tissue edges can be moved closer together and the clamp retightened prior to suturing. The wound is closed by suturing only the conjunctiva and skin. This allows the lid to stretch and return to a near normal appearance postoperatively. The con-

junctiva is closed using 5-0 or 6-0 chromic gut in a continuous pattern, starting at the bottom of the V and working toward the margin. The skin is closed with 5-0 or 6-0 silk in an interrupted pattern starting at the lid margin.

Tumors that require excision of one-third or more of the eyelid require more extensive restoration techniques. For lesions that do not involve the full thickness of the eyelid, partial thickness tissue advancement may be used (Fig. 101–17).[2,19] This technique preserves the palpebral conjunctiva. If, however, the majority of the lower lid is removed, a mucocutaneous flap from the lower lip can be used

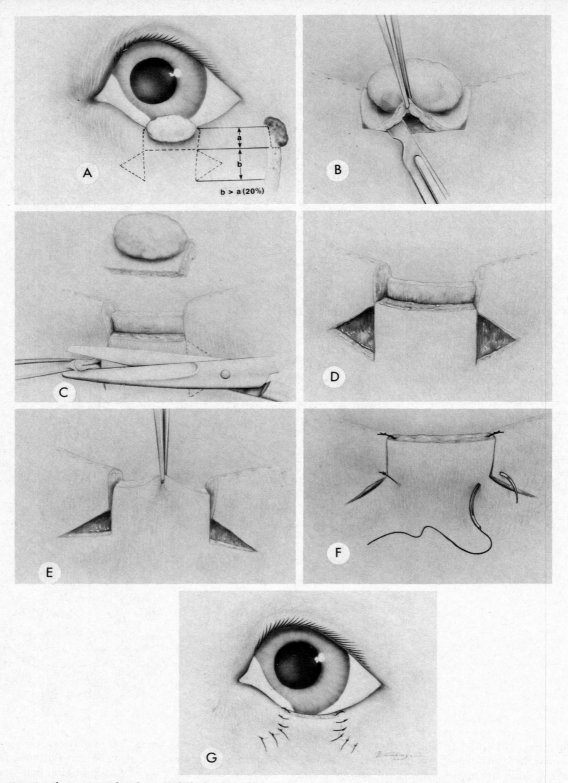

Figure 101–17. Advancement flap for partial thickness lesions. *A,* The tumor (or defect) before excision. As the conjunctiva is not involved, it is not removed. Incisions are outlined by dotted lines. The incisions are marked on the patient with a plastic surgery marking pen. The vertical sides of the triangles are 20 per cent longer than the vertical incisions adjacent to the tumor to allow for wound contraction. *B,* A square or rectangular incision is made around the tumor. The tumor is dissected off from the base toward the lid margin. *C,* The tumor is removed and placed in fixative. The tumor is pinned to a piece of cardboard to allow the ophthalmic pathologist to examine the margins for evidence of tumor. Note: If tumor is present in any margin, excision has been incomplete. The previously marked triangle is elevated and excised. *D,* The triangles have been removed and all incisions completed. *E,* To prevent tension on the wound, the tissues surrounding the triangles and the flap are undermined. The flap is advanced to the margin with no tension on it. *F,* Simple marginal sutures of 6–0 silk are placed. Sutures are placed at the corners of the incision to assist in accurate placement of subsequent sutures. *G,* Remaining sutures in place 2 mm apart. If the conjunctiva is mobile it is sutured to the skin edge, filling the defect with a simple continuous suture. This helps prevent retraction of the advancement flap. (Reprinted with permission from Slatter, D.: *Fundamentals of Veterinary Ophthalmology.* W. B. Saunders, Philadelphia, 1981.)

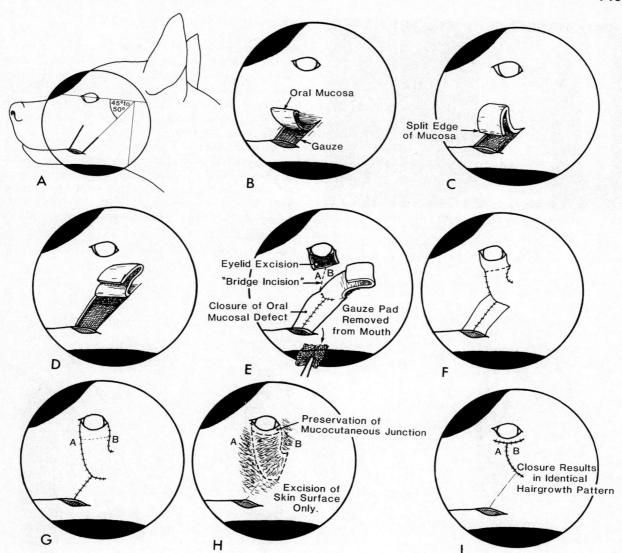

Figure 101–18. Mucocutaneous subdermal plexus flap. *A,* Proposed full thickness lip incisions are drawn with a marking pen at a 45° to 50° angle to a line passing through the medial and lateral canthi. Reference incision lines slightly diverge to avoid accidental narrowing of the cutaneous pedicle. Gauze pads beneath the lip will support it when incising the lip margin. *B,* Elevation of the full-thickness lip flap to expose the mucosal surface. *C,* Oral mucosa is carefully split at a level sufficient to replace the missing lower lid conjunctiva. *D,* The cutaneous pedicle is carefully dissected from the oral mucosa and underlying structures. Care must be exercised to avoid traumatizing the pedicle's vital subdermal plexus, to avoid severing any underlying facial structures, and to avoid the development of an unnecessarily long cutaneous transfer pedicle. *E,* Oral mucosal defect is apposed with a buried suture pattern. A "bridge incision" is used to connect the donor and recipient beds for suture placement of the transfer pedicle. Undermining of edge B should be avoided to prevent circulatory compromise to the graft. *F,* Graft is sutured into place by apposing the oral mucosa to the remaining conjunctival edges with a buried interrupted suture pattern. The cutaneous surface is sutured with a simple interrupted pattern. *G,* Completion of the closure of the recipient bed. Folds and skin puckers should be left alone to avoid vascular compromise to the graft in this first stage. *H,* In four to six weeks, the surgeon has the option of removing the cutaneous transfer pedicle and closing the defect by simple apposition of skin edges A and B. *I,* Completion of optional second-stage revision procedure to improve cosmetic results. Apposition of edges A and B will give a normal hair growth pattern. Second stage revision can be used to re-establish a more normal graft edge in the event of partial necrosis of the outer lip margin. (Reprinted with permission from Pavletic, M. M., Nafer, L. A., and Confer, A. W.: Mucocutaneous subdermal plexus flap from the lip for lower lid restoration in the dog. J. Am. Vet. Med. Assoc. *180*:921, 1982.)

for restoring the lid.[15] The use of a mucocutaneous subdermal plexus flap has several advantages over other procedures (Fig. 101-18). It can replace extensive areas of eyelid and provides a new mucous membrane to replace the palpebral conjunctiva. Good cosmetic results have been obtained in the dog with this procedure.

Alternate methods for removing small tumors of the eyelid include electrocautery and cryosurgery. A loop attached to a surgical electrocautery unit aids in removal of papillomas, melanomas, and small basal cell carcinomas. The cornea must be protected, since heat cautery wounds of the cornea are very slow to heal. Also, electrocautery may be contraindicated if microscopic examination of the excised tissue is desired, since it coagulates small tumors and alters their histological architecture.

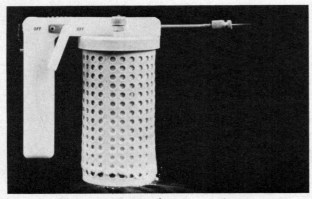

Figure 101–19. Liquid nitrogen applicator.

Cryosurgery (See also Chapter 173)

Cryosurgery is an alternative to excision of eyelid tumors.[6] Only liquid nitrogen should be used as the cooling agent because other substances, such as nitrous oxide, may not yield temperatures low enough to destroy neoplastic tissues. Although cryosurgery is not a painful procedure, general anesthesia is usually recommended.

The most commonly used cryosurgical technique for the removal of eyelid tumors is the freeze-thaw-refreeze method.[6] Thermocouples should be placed under and at the edges of the lesion prior to freezing. Liquid nitrogen* is sprayed (Fig. 101–19) on the center of the mass until thermocouples indicate

---

*Kryospray, Brymill Corp., Vernon, CT.

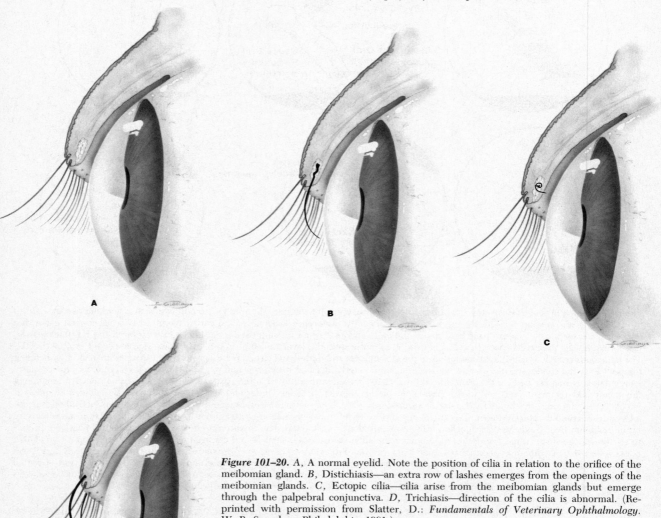

Figure 101–20. *A,* A normal eyelid. Note the position of cilia in relation to the orifice of the meibomian gland. *B,* Distichiasis—an extra row of lashes emerges from the openings of the meibomian glands. *C,* Ectopic cilia—cilia arise from the meibomian glands but emerge through the palpebral conjunctiva. *D,* Trichiasis—direction of the cilia is abnormal. (Reprinted with permission from Slatter, D.: *Fundamentals of Veterinary Ophthalmology.* W. B. Saunders, Philadelphia, 1981.)

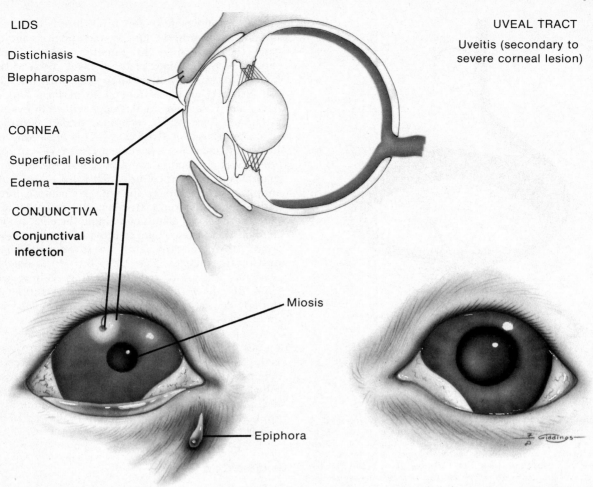

LIDS

Distichiasis

Blepharospasm

CORNEA

Superficial lesion

Edema

CONJUNCTIVA

Conjunctival infection

UVEAL TRACT

Uveitis (secondary to severe corneal lesion)

Miosis

Epiphora

Figure 101–21. Clinical signs of distichiasis. (Reprinted with permission from Slatter, D.: *Fundamentals of Veterinary Ophthalmology.* W. B. Saunders, Philadelphia, 1981.)

$-20°C$. The tissue is allowed to thaw to $0°C$ and is then refrozen to $-20°C$. Lesions can be expected to slough in five to seven days. Bleeding and postoperative infections are of little concern with cryosurgery. One drawback to the use of cryosurgery in dogs is that hair that grows into the previously frozen area is depigmented and the resulting white spot may be objectionable in black or dark-colored animals.

EYELASH-RELATED DISEASES

Distichiasis, districhiasis, trichiasis, and ectopic cilia all result in corneal irritation or ulceration (Fig. 101–20). These cilia-related diseases are most frequently encountered in dogs. In some breeds, such as the cocker spaniel, distichiasis (cilia emerging from the tarsal [meibomian] gland openings) and districhiasis (more than one cilium emerging from the gland opening) are common findings.[14] Many of these dogs have little or no adverse effects from the presence of these cilia and therefore do not require surgical treatment. In other dogs, however, chronic keratitis or ulceration may result and surgery is indicated (Fig. 101–21).

Surgical Correction

There are several methods described to treat distichiasis or districhiasis. Manual epilation can be accomplished using either cilia forceps or jeweler's forceps. This method may be useful when a corneal ulcer has developed in a dog who has had distichiasis without complications for years. Once the cornea becomes ulcerated, the distichiasis may prevent healing by mechanically rubbing the loosely adhered, healing epithelium. Manual epilation yields only temporary results but often relieves the irritation long enough for the cornea to heal before the cilia grows back.

Electroepilation can be used to treat distichiasis permanently when only five or six cilia are present on each lid. To permanently destroy the hair follicle in the tarsal gland, a thin wire (25 gauge or less) is passed down the hair shaft and current is applied until the cilia can be removed with little tension.

When the number of cilia on each eyelid exceeds that which can be easily removed with electroepilation, surgical excision is indicated. Various techniques have been described for resecting the cilia at the lid margin.[8,19] The classic method for removal of

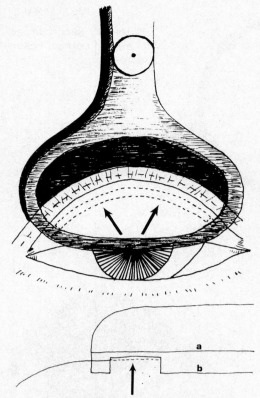

Figure 101–22. Conjunctival resection for distichiasis removal. *A*, Incision lines (arrows) on the conjunctival surface of the everted eyelid. *B*, Cross section of the eyelid, demonstrating the cilia and excised tissue (arrow), tarsus (*a*), and palpebral conjunctiva (*b*). (Reprinted with permission from Campbell, L. H., and McCree, A. V.: Conjunctival resection for the surgical management of canine distichiasis. J. Am. Vet. Med. Assoc. *171*:275, 1977.)

cilia is the partial tarsal plate excision. This can be accomplished by making an incision on each side of the tarsal gland opening and removing a V-shaped section of the tarsal plate containing the hair folli-

cles.[8,19] An alternate to this procedure is to make an incision anterior to the tarsal gland openings and then carry the incision to the palpebral side of the lid, thus removing a block of tarsal plate. Both of these techniques work well on large dogs with thick lids. These procedures are difficult to perform and may have poor results in smaller dogs with thin eyelids.

The most acceptable technique to date is conjunctival resection (Fig. 101–22).[4,20] This technique minimizes the chances of secondary cicatricial entropion, which was a common complication of the earlier lid margin splitting procedures. The procedure entails simply everting the eyelid with a chalazion forceps and doing a transconjunctival en bloc resection of the bases of the tarsal glands containing the cilia. Another method that also appears to provide excellent results is the use of electrocautery to sever the cilia and destroy the follicles (Fig. 101–23).[17] It has not been necessary to suture or use grafting techniques to close the defect in the conjunctiva. Postoperative therapy consists of applications of an antibiotic ointment twice daily.

An alternative to the previously mentioned techniques for the treatment of distichiasis and trichiasis is the use of cryosurgery.[7] Nitrous oxide is the cooling agent of choice in the procedure, since it freezes the follicle but does not cause as much tissue destruction as liquid nitrogen. A cryoprobe is transconjunctivally applied for 60 seconds. The tissue is allowed to thaw and is then refrozen for 45 seconds.

Ectopic Cilia

Ectopic cilia originate from the tarsal gland and penetrate the conjunctiva (see Fig. 101–20). Superficial corneal ulceration is a common finding associated with ectopic cilia, and the disease should be suspected with any small ulcer that fails to heal with medical therapy.[10] Most ectopic cilia occur at the base of the tarsal glands on the upper lid. Unlike

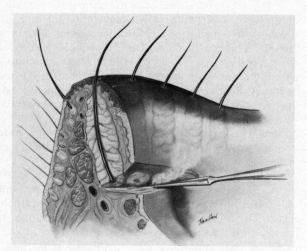

Figure 101–23. Basal meibomian gland cautery. An electrocautery unit with a medium coagulation setting is used to sever the distichia and destroy the follicle. (Reprinted with permission from Riis, R.: Basal meibomian gland cautery, a surgical technique for distichiasis. Proc. Am. Soc. Vet. Ophthal., Las Vegas, 1982, pp. 88–93.)

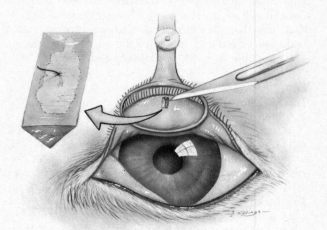

Figure 101–24. Ectopic cilium resection. The offending area of the lid is clamped with a Desmarre's chalazion clamp for hemostasis, and the lid is everted. The wedge for resection is outlined. (Reprinted with permission from Slatter, D.: *Fundamentals of Veterinary Ophthalmology.* W. B. Saunders, Philadelphia, 1981.)

distichiasis, ectopic cilia usually involve one individual cilium rather than a row. They may be very difficult to locate, and occasionally careful examination, under anesthesia, with high magnification may be necessary to make the diagnosis. Simple en bloc excision is the preferred treatment (Fig. 101–24). Suturing the defect in the conjunctiva is not necessary.

CHALAZION

A chalazion is an accumulation of secretory products in a blocked tarsal gland. It is a relatively common disease in the dog but rare in other species and is usually recognized as a painless swelling 4 to 6 mm from the lid margin. It appears as a thickened yellow-white swelling seen through the palpebral conjunctiva when the eyelid is everted. A chalazion

must be differentiated from a tarsal gland adenoma, which becomes more invasive, and a hordeolum, which contains purulent material. The treatment of choice for chalazion is incision and curettage of the lesion (Fig. 101–25). This may be done under either manual restraint or general anesthesia, depending on the patient. If general anesthesia is used, a chalazion clamp can be used to stabilize the lid. Attempts to manually express a chalazion should be avoided, because a rupture of the gland may lead to lipid granulomas in the surrounding tissue due to the release of inspissated material.

HORDEOLUM

A hordeolum is a bacterial (usually *Staphylococcus aureus*) infection of either the lash follicle and associated gland of Zeis (external hordeolum) or the tarsal gland (internal hordeolum). Unlike a chalazion or a

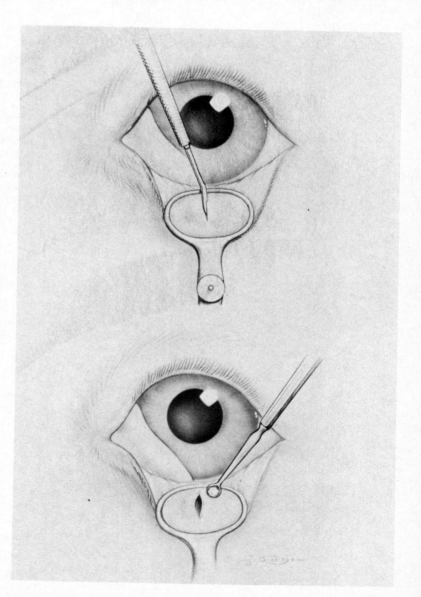

Figure 101–25. Treatment of chalazion. *A*, A chalazion clamp has been applied, and the lesion is incised through the palpebral conjunctiva with a #11 blade. *B*, Removal of granulomatous material and secretion with a chalazion spoon or curette. (Reprinted with permission from Slatter, D.: *Fundamentals of Veterinary Ophthalmology*. W. B. Saunders, Philadelphia, 1981.)

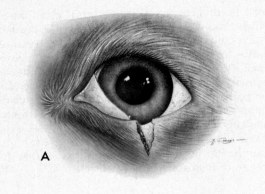

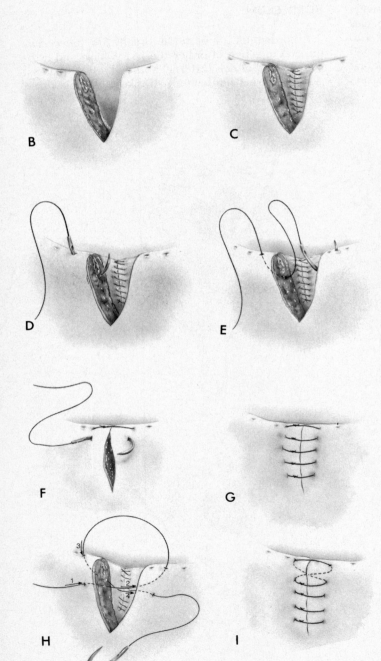

Figure 101–26. Simple two-layer repair. *A,* Initial injury before debridement. *B,* Wound after debridement and ready for suturing. *C,* The conjunctiva is sutured with 6-0 Vicryl in a simple, continuous pattern. *D,* The marginal suture is placed first, in two separate bites. *E,* The second bite. *F,* The marginal suture is carefully tied to ensure apposition of the margins. The knot lies along the margin. The wound is sutured with simple interrupted suture of 6-0 silk 2 mm apart. The first suture beneath the margin relieves tension on the marginal suture. *G,* The wound sutured. *H,* A figure-eight suture pattern may be used in place of the first two sutures. *I,* The wound sutured using a figure-eight technique. (Redrawn after Severin, 1976.) (Reprinted with permission from Slatter, D.: *Fundamentals of Veterinary Ophthalmology.* W. B. Saunders, Philadelphia, 1981.)

lid tumor, a hordeolum is characterized by marked inflammation of the surrounding tissue. External hordeolums are usually raised, painful pustules on the external lid margin. Internal hordeolums are not raised as much as the external lesions. They appear as small white pustules along the base of the tarsal glands. Treatment consists of lancing the lesions with the tip of a scalpel or the point of an 18-gauge needle. The purulent material is expressed from the lids. Hot packing and topical and systemic antibiotics may also be used depending on the severity of the disease.

LACERATIONS

A full thickness laceration of the eyelid is best repaired using a simple two-layer technique. If the wound is near the medial canthus, the nasolacrimal puncta and canaliculi should be checked to assure they are not involved in the wound. Should the nasolacrimal system be involved, the canaliculi should be cannulated with a large monofilament suture or polyethylene tube to maintain patency during healing.

The two-layer closure is accomplished after debridement of the wound edges. The conjunctiva is sutured in a simple continuous pattern with 6-0 Vicryl or gut. The lid margins are carefully apposed using the suture pattern described in Figure 101–26. No subcutaneous sutures are used in this technique. This has the advantage of allowing the natural elasticity of the skin and conjunctiva to stretch back to a near normal eyelid shape. If the tarsal plate is sutured, the resultant scarring may prevent the eyelid from healing with the excellent cosmetic result obtained by the two-layer closure.

1. Bistner, S. I., Aquirre, G., and Batik, G.: *Atlas of Veterinary Ophthalmic Surgery.* W. B. Saunders, Philadelphia, 1977.
2. Blogg, J. R.: *The Eye in Veterinary Practice.* W. B. Saunders, Philadelphia, 1980.
3. Brightman, A. H., and Helper, L. C.: Full thickness resection of the eyelid. J. Am. Anim. Hosp. Assoc. *14*:483, 1978.
4. Campbell, L. H., and McCree, A. V.: Conjunctival resection for the surgical management of canine distichiasis. J. Am. Vet. Med. Assoc. *171*:275, 1977.
5. Crowley, J. P., and McGloughlin, P.: Hereditary entropion in lambs. Vet. Rec. 75:1104, 1963.
6. Farris, H. E., and Fraunfelder, F. T.: Cryosurgical treatment of ocular squamous cell carcinoma of cattle. J. Am. Vet. Med. Assoc. *168*:213, 1976.
7. Frueh, B. R.: Treatment of distichiasis with cryotherapy. Ophthalmic Surg. *12*:100, 1981.
8. Gelatt, K. N.: *Textbook of Veterinary Ophthalmology.* Lea & Febiger, Philadelphia, 1981.
9. Grier, R. L., Brewer, W. G., Paul, S. R., and Theilen, G. H: Treatment of bovine and equine ocular squamous cell carcinoma by radiofrequency hyperthermia. J. Am. Vet. Med. Assoc. *177*:55; 1980.
10. Helper, L. C., and Magrane, W. G.: Ectopic cilia of the canine eyelid. J. Small Anim. Pract. *11*:185, 1970.
11. Hilbert, B. J., Farrell, R. K., and Grant, B. D.: Cryotherapy of periocular squamous cell carcinoma in the horse. J. Am. Vet. Med. Assoc. *170*:1305, 1977.
12. Krehbiel, J. D., and Langham, R. F.: Eyelid neoplasms of dogs. Am. J. Vet. Res. *36*:115, 1975.
13. Lavach, J. D., and Severin, G. A.: Neoplasia of the equine eye, adnexa and orbit—a review of 68 cases. J. Am. Vet. Med. Assoc. *170*:202, 1977.
14. Magrane, W. G.: *Canine Ophthalmology*, 3rd ed. Lea & Febiger, Philadelphia, 1977.
15. Pavletic, M. M., Nafe, L. A., and Confer, A. W.: Mucocutaneous subdermal plexus flap from the lip for lower eyelid restoration in the dog. J. Am. Vet. Med. Assoc. *180*:921, 1982.
16. Prince, J. H., Diesem, C. D., Eglitis, I., et al.: *Anatomy and Histology of the Eye and Orbit in Domestic Animals.* Charles C Thomas, Springfield, 1960.
17. Riis, R.: Basal Meibomian gland cautery, a surgical technique for distichiasis. Proc. Am. Soc. Vet. Ophthalmol. 1982, pp. 88–93.
18. Severin, G. A.: *Veterinary Ophthalmology Notes.* 2nd ed. Colorado State University Bookstore, Fort Collins, CO, 1976.
19. Slatter, D. H.: *Fundamentals of Veterinary Ophthalmology.* W. B. Saunders, Philadelphia, 1981.
20. White, J. H.: Correction of distichiasis by tarsal resection and mucous membrane grafting. Am. J. Ophthalmol. *80*:507, 1975.
21. Wyman, M.: Lateral canthoplasty. J. Am. Anim. Hosp. Assoc. 7:196, 1971.
22. Wyman, M., Rings, M. D., Tarr, M. J., and Aldon, C. L.: Immunotherapy in equine sarcoid. J. Am. Vet. Med. Assoc. *171*:449, 1977.

Chapter **102**

The Conjunctiva

Robert J. Munger

EMBRYOLOGY

The conjunctival epithelium develops from surface ectoderm, whereas the underlying connective tissue develops primarily from neural crest–derived mesenchyme (mesectoderm). The surface ectoderm differentiates to form nonkeratinizing stratified squamous-to-columnar epithelium containing goblet cells as well as the major and minor lacrimal glands. The lacrimal glands represent end-stage differentiations of conjunctival buds that grow into the mesenchyme. During development, embryonic conjunctiva can become sequestered to form dermoid cysts, which are lined by mucus-producing conjunctival-type epithelium and which may involve the lids or orbit.[26,29,38,47,56]

GROSS AND MICROSCOPIC ANATOMY

The conjunctiva is a mucous membrane consisting of two layers, the epithelium and the substantia propria. (The tear film is sometimes referred to as a third layer because of its intimate association with the conjunctiva and its importance in preserving the health and function of the conjunctiva and cornea. See Chapter 103.) It has three distinct areas: the palpebral conjunctiva, the bulbar conjunctiva, and the forniceal conjunctiva. The palpebral conjunctiva lines the inner surfaces of the upper and lower lids and both surfaces of the third eyelid. It originates at the mucocutaneous junction of the upper and lower lid margins and extends to the fornices. The substantia propria of the palpebral conjunctiva is firmly bound to the lids near the margins but becomes more movable toward the fornices. The lacrimal caruncle, a modified portion of the palpebral conjunctiva, is a small, fleshy mass at the medial canthus containing hairs and should not be mistaken for a dermoid. It should be removed with the lids whenever an enucleation with permanent tarsorrhaphy is performed. The bulbar conjunctiva covers the anterior sclera and extends from the limbus to the fornices. The substantia propria of the bulbar conjunctiva has a delicate, areolar structure and is freely movable over the sclera except near the limbus, where it is firmly bound by its fusion with Tenon's capsule. The conjunctival fornices are formed by the reflection of the bulbar and palpebral conjunctivae upon each other, thus creating the dorsal and ventral conjunctival sacs. The substantia propria of the conjunctiva becomes redundant at the fornices. It is augmented dorsally by the fibrous expansion of the levator aponeurosis and Müller's muscle and ventrally by the fibrous expansion of the ventral rectus muscle sheath and ventral tarsal muscle. These facial attachments hold the fornices in place and prevent the conjunctiva from displacing anteriorly over the cornea (especially during upward gaze).[26,29,36,38,47,52,56]

The conjunctival epithelium is a nonkeratinized stratified columnar epithelium that becomes stratified squamous epithelium near the limbus and lid margins. Near the fornices the epithelium contains numerous goblet cells, but few (if any) are present near the limbus and lid margins. These goblet cells as well as small crypts (simple invaginations) in the bulbar and palpebral conjunctiva produce the mucinous layer of the tear film.[12,26,35] Melanophores are often found in the conjunctival epithelium, and melanin granules in the cytoplasm of these cells should not be mistaken for pathological inclusions during cytological examination.[26,29,36,38,46,47,56]

The substantia propria of the conjunctiva can be divided into two layers, an adenoid or glandular layer and a deep fibrous layer. The adenoid layer is composed of a connective tissue network enclosing lymphocytes and plasma cells, and active lymphoid follicles (formed in response to antigenic stimulation) may be found throughout this layer. Such follicles are particularly numerous in the fornices and on the bulbar surface of the third eyelid.[19,26,29,38,47,48,52,56,63]

The blood supply for the conjunctiva is derived from the anterior ciliary arteries via the vascular arcades of the lids and the superficial branches of the ciliary arteries themselves. Because the bulbar conjunctiva is nearly transparent, the superficial vessels of the conjunctiva, which are light pink and tortuous, may be seen overlying the deeper, straighter, dark red branches of the anterior ciliary arteries that anastomose with the conjunctival vessels at the limbus.[26,29,36,38,47,52,56] Sensory innervation of the conjunctiva is by the ophthalmic branch of the trigeminal nerve.[26,38,47,56]

CONJUNCTIVAL PHYSIOLOGY

Conjunctival Healing

The conjunctiva responds rapidly to injury and has great regenerative capacity.[26,36,39,52,54–56] Because of the extensive vascular and lymphatic network in the conjunctiva, intracellular and intercellular edema occurs rapidly following injury.[26,39,52,56] Epithelialization of conjunctival and corneal wounds occurs, with sliding and mitosis of epithelial cells covering the defect soon after the wound edges adhere to the episcleral tissues.[26,54,56] Indeed, it is the conjunctival epithelium that is responsible for re-epithelialization of the cornea in lesions in which the corneal epithelium is completely denuded.[55] Subepithelial conjunctival healing begins within hours of injury, with infiltration of inflammatory cells and proliferation of fibroblasts and capillaries.[26,52,56] Healing of simple conjunctival lacerations generally occurs within 24 to 48 hours, so that suturing of such wounds is not required. Suturing of more extensive wounds with 5-0 or 6-0 absorbable suture is generally recommended to minimize scarring, although even large wounds with baring of the sclera are generally re-epithelialized quickly.[5,26,52,54,55]

Physiological Responses in Disease

The responses of the conjunctiva to disease are many and include vascular changes, cellular infiltrates and exudates, edema (chemosis), emphysema, follicle and papule formation, and swelling. Of all the responses, changes in the conjunctival vasculature are probably the most obvious owing to the semitransparent nature of the tissue. Hyperemia of the conjunctiva may be active, such as that produced with irritation, allergic conditions, and local or systemic disease; or it may be passive owing to venous obstruction or congestion resulting from glaucoma, uveitis, or intraocular neoplasia. Pallor of the conjunctival vessels is commonly associated with anemia. Conjunctival hemorrhages, especially large subconjunctival hemorrhages, are usually caused by trauma, but ecchymoses may occur in association with clotting disorders, blood dyscrasias, and severe systemic inflammatory diseases.[26,36,52,54,56]

Because the episcleral (ciliary) vessels and conjunctival vessels can be affected by intraocular and systemic diseases, differentiating the conjunctival vessels from episcleral vessels can be extremely important in distinguishing between diseases involving only the conjunctiva and more severe diseases affecting other ocular structures. Conjunctival vessels branch profusely and are bright red, movable, and more numerous at the fornices and in the palpebral conjunctiva than near the limbus. Ciliary vessels remain stationary and are a deeper red, relatively straight, and most prominent at the limbus. The direction of blood flow is also unique, with blood flowing from fornix to limbus in conjunctival vessels and from limbus to fornices in the ciliary vasculature.[26,52,56] Conjunctival vessels, which extend into the cornea, are superficial and easily distinguishable as separate branching vessels, whereas ciliary vessels are deeper and straighter. Topical application of 1:100,000 epinephrine to the eye results in blanching of the conjunctival vessels, whereas the deeper ciliary vessels remain injected. When the deep ciliary vessels are injected, intraocular disease is probable and a thorough ophthalmic examination is indicated.[26,52,56]

Cellular infiltrates and exudates present in conjunctival disease provide a means of classifying the stage of the disease and probable etiology. Conjunctival smears in which the predominant cells are neutrophils are usually indicative of bacterial or acute conjunctivitis, whereas lymphocytes and monocytes are more often associated with viral, chlamydial, or chronic conjunctivitis. The lymphocytes associated with chronic conjunctivitis arise from lymphoid follicles that proliferate in the conjunctiva after antigenic stimulation. Epithelial hypertrophy and goblet cell proliferation also occur with chronic conjunctivitis, so that keratinized epithelial cells and goblet cells are seen in conjunctival smears. Keratinization of epithelial cells is particularly common in conjunctivitis associated with tear film deficiencies. The rare presence of basophils and eosinophils is indicative of a parasitic or allergic etiology, and a diagnosis of conjunctival neoplasia can be made when neoplastic cells are observed in the smears.[34,45,56]

Swelling of the conjunctiva may be due to chemosis, conjunctival emphysema, or solid tissue masses. Chemosis of the conjunctiva (escape of intravascular fluids into the loose subepithelial tissues) occurs readily with manipulation or other irritation of the conjunctiva. It may be a result of direct injury to the conjunctival vasculature as well as indirect injury through the release of vasoactive chemical mediators of inflammation.[39] Conjunctival emphysema usually occurs when air escapes into the orbit through fractures in the bony walls of the paranasal sinuses. Solid tissue masses are usually associated with proliferative keratoconjunctivitis, episcleritis, scleritis, or neoplasia.[26,34,52,54,56]

TABLE 102–1. Criteria for Diagnosis of Antibody-Mediated Disease*

Antibody-antigen ratio (Ab/Ag) in ocular fluids greater than Ab/Ag in serum
Abnormal accumulations of plasma cells in ocular lesions
Abnormal immunoglobulin accumulations at site of injury
Complement fixed by immunoglobulins at site
Accumulation of eosinophils at site
Association with antibody-mediated disease elsewhere in the body

*At least one criterion should be fulfilled.

Immune Responses

The conjunctiva is subject to normal as well as abnormal immune reactions, which may be manifested as resistance to infections, immune deficiencies, and hypersensitivity. Locally acting factors, primarily secretory IgA antibodies and cell-mediated immunity, are the primary determinants in conferring conjunctival resistance to infection.[19,43,48] Circulating (humoral) antibodies act mainly to neutralize agents before they reach target cells in the tissue and hence contribute less to protection from infectious diseases that primarily affect the conjunctiva. Immune deficiencies and hypersensitivities may initiate primary conjunctival disease, predispose the conjunctiva to infection, or exacerbate pre-existing infectious disease. Table 102–1 contains criteria of immune-mediated diseases. More complete discussions on immune-related diseases are available but are beyond the scope of this chapter.[19,43,48]

DIAGNOSTIC METHODS

Bacterial and viral cultures, conjunctival smears, and conjunctival biopsies may be easily performed and are particularly indicated in refractory or progressive conjunctival diseases. The techniques and diagnostic indications for microbiological cultures and conjunctival smears have been extensively discussed in existing literature, and readers are referred to those sources for detailed discussions.[26,30,45,56] Table 102–2 lists the typical cytological features of specific conjunctivitides.[34,56]

Small snip biopsies of conjunctiva (especially bulbar conjunctiva) are easily obtained after instillation of a local anesthetic such as proparacaine in the conjunctival sac. The conjunctiva is grasped with a fine-toothed forcep, and the "tented" conjunctiva is excised quickly with tenotomy or iris scissors. As long as the biopsy is small the site heals rapidly, and suturing is not required. Occasionally, highly-strung or aggressive animals must be heavily sedated or briefly anesthetized for biopsy. For biopsy of larger conjunctival masses or conjunctival and episcleral tissues, a short-acting general anesthetic is advisable, and suturing of the conjunctiva may be necessary.

TABLE 102–2. Cellular Response Associated with Specific Conjunctivitides

Disease	Cellular Response
Acute bacterial conjunctivitis	Predominantly neutrophils, few mononuclear cells, many bacteria, degenerating epithelial cells
Chronic bacterial conjunctivitis	Predominantly neutrophils, many mononuclear cells, degenerate or keratinized epithelial cells, goblet cells, bacteria may or may not be seen, mucus, fibrin
Feline herpesvirus conjunctivitis	Pseudomembrane formation, giant cells, fibrin, erythrocyte, neutrophils, and mononuclear cell numbers depend on stage of infection
Feline mycoplasmal conjunctivitis	Predominantly neutrophils, fewer mononuclear cells, basophilic coccoid or pleomorphic organisms on cell membrane.
Feline chlamydial conjunctivitis	Predominantly neutrophils, mononuclear cells in subacute cases are increased in numbers, plasma cells, giant cells, basophilic cytoplasmic inclusions early in the disease
Keratoconjunctivitis sicca	Epithelial cells keratinized, goblet cells, mucus, neutrophilic response marked if there is much infection, bacteria
Canine distemper	Varies with stage of disease: early, giant cells and mononuclear cells; later, neutrophils, goblet cells, and mucus; infrequent intracellular inclusions
Allergic conjunctivitis	Eosinophils, neutrophils may be marked, basophils possible

(Reprinted with permission from Lavach, J. D., et al.: Cytology of normal and inflamed conjunctivas in dogs and cats. J. Am. Vet. Med. Assoc. *170*:722, 1977.)

GENERAL SURGICAL PRINCIPLES

Most discussions of veterinary ophthalmic surgery describe techniques and neglect the basic physical forces that act on the ocular tissues. Because these forces affect the sectioning and manipulation of the tissues (and thus the success of the procedure), it is extremely important that they be considered. Eisner (1980) and Troutman (1974) should be consulted for more detailed discussions of these basic techniques.[14,63]

Levels of Surgical Dissection

Three layers are encountered during surgical dissection of the conjunctiva. The first two layers are the closely adhered epithelial lamella and the subepithelial fibrous layer. The third layer is actually a space, the episcleral space, that contains sparsely distributed fibers of connective tissue that loosely attach the fibrous layer to the sclera. The episcleral space extends to within 2 mm of the limbus, where it is obliterated by firm adhesion of the subepithelial fibrous layer to the sclera in the "perilimbic zone."[14]

Tissue Mobility and Sectility

The ease with which a tissue can be smoothly cut, i.e., its sectility, decreases as its elasticity and mo-

bility increase. Because the conjunctiva is highly mobile and elastic, it tends to shift ahead of cutting instruments toward areas where it is firmly anchored or under greater tension. As a result, incisions started parallel to the limbus deviate toward the fornix unless countertraction is exerted against the tension created by the perilimbal attachments of the conjunctiva. In addition, the sectility of the conjunctiva is greater where it is more firmly anchored, and limbal and scleral attachments increase the risk of conjunctival perforation ("buttonholing") by shifting the conjunctiva into the path of the cutting instrument. The risk of perforation is directly proportional to the distance travelled by the cutting instrument (Fig. 102–1).[14]

Deviation of incisions and perforation of the conjunctiva may be avoided by proper regulation of traction on the conjunctiva, cutting in small steps near the scleral attachments of conjunctival fibers, and careful guidance of cutting instruments. Gentle traction on the conjunctiva using delicate forceps to equally counter tension created by tissue attachments and adhesions prevents tissue displacement and deviation of the incision. Avoiding folds in the conjunctiva and stretching the conjunctiva so it is flat further minimize the risk of perforation. Limbal-based conjunctival flaps may be reflected onto the cornea and tensed during perilimbal dissection. This increases tension on fibers at the dissection margin (increasing their sectility) while decreasing tension on fibers near the conjunctival surface (decreasing their sectility).

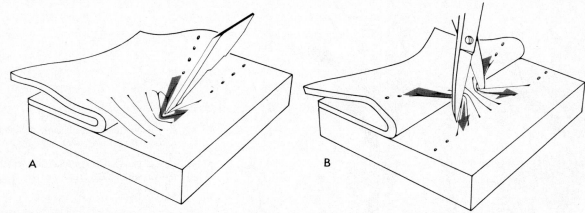

Figure 102–1. Effect of lateral shifting tendency during dissection at the limbus. The fibers of a reflected limbus-based conjunctival flap are shifted toward their scleral attachments in front of a blade moving parallel to the limbus. The greater the distance travelled by the blade, the more tissue is shifted toward the sclera. Ultimately, the conjunctival surface may enter the cutting path and be sectioned. *A,* Lateral shifting tendency when cutting with a razor blade tip. *B,* Shifting tendency when cutting with scissors. Tissue is pulled between the blades during closure. Since the danger of perforation depends on the distance travelled by the cutting point, it varies with the aperture angle and can be reduced by dissection with a small aperture (i.e., in many small snips). (Reprinted with permission from Eyster, G.: *Eye Surgery—An Introduction to Operative Technique.* Springer-Verlag, New York, 1980.)

The tensed fibers may be sectioned parallel to the limbus near their scleral attachments with minimal tissue shifting (Fig. 102–2).[14]

Deep dissection of the conjunctiva with access to the episcleral space is necessary for surgery on the

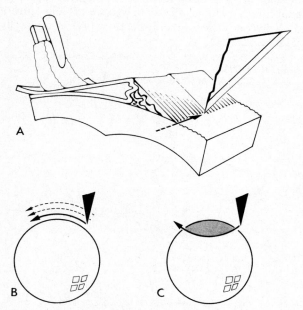

Figure 102–2. Prevention of perforations. *A,* Selective fiber tension at the margin of fixation zones. If the dissected conjunctival flap is reflected onto the globe, selective tension is exerted on the peripheral fibers exposed directly to the cutting edge. Meanwhile, the more central fibers and vulnerable epithelial layer are relaxed and, therefore, less sectile. *B* and *C,* Guidance direction during dissection near the limbus. To avoid injury to the conjunctival flap, no vectors should be directed toward the cornea. *B,* The cutting point is directed parallel to the limbus to avoid vectors in the corneal direction. *C,* "Slewing movements" produce vectors in the corneal direction and thus endanger the conjunctival flap. (Reprinted with permission from Eyster, G.: *Eye Surgery—An Introduction to Operative Techniques.* Springer-Verlag, New York, 1980.)

extraocular muscles or sclera and as a preliminary step for certain intraocular procedures. The space may be opened by incising the conjunctiva either parallel to the globe at the limbus, creating a fornix-based conjunctival flap, or perpendicular to the globe at a point caudal to the limbus, creating a limbus-based flap (Fig. 102–3). Dissection is continued bluntly, adjacent to the sclera where sectility of interstitial fibers is greatest. Sharp dissection is required where the tissues are firmly fixed (around scars and in the perilimbal zone), and care is required to avoid perforation of the flap.

Superficial dissection of the conjunctiva—separation of the epithelial lamella from the subepithelial fibrous layer—is more demanding than deep dissection. Dissection may be facilitated by tensing the subepithelial fibers with instruments or by infiltrating the area with sterile saline (with or without epinephrine added).[14] When fluid infiltration is used, the fluid must be injected just below the conjunctival surface. The injection cannula preferably should be advanced during injection, forming numerous fluid-filled chambers. As dissection progresses, each chamber collapses individually, thus maintaining adequate tension in the undissected tissues; a single, large chamber would collapse immediately, resulting in a complete loss of tension on the surrounding subepithelial fibers. If the episcleral space is inadvertently entered or if natural deep fixation is lost as dissection progresses toward the fornix, traction sutures or forceps may be used to artificially fix the deep tissues, thus exploiting lamellar deflection to keep the dissection superficial (Fig. 102–4). The requirements of superficial dissection are best summarized by Eisner, "Superficial dissection therefore requires a skillful blending of tension and countertension, a continual adjustment to ever-changing tensions, and a close monitoring of the 'danger zone' between the scissor blades."[14]

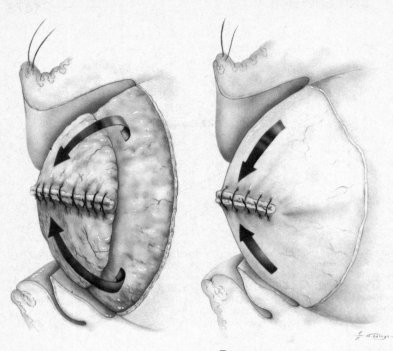

A   **B**

Figure 102–3. Conjunctival flaps. *A*, Limbus-based flap. *B*, Fornix-based flap. (Reprinted with permission from Slatter, D. H.: *Fundamentals of Veterinary Ophthalmology.* W. B. Saunders, Philadelphia, 1981.)

Suturing the Conjunctiva

The conjunctiva of dogs and cats is extremely delicate, and successful placement of sutures in the conjunctiva requires careful handling with proper instrumentation. Delicate-toothed forceps, such as extra-delicate Bishop-Harmon or Colibri forceps (see Chapter 100), are highly desirable during dissection and suturing, since larger forceps may shred the tissue. Appropriately delicate suture and needles are also essential, and no suture larger than 5-0 should be used for the conjunctiva. Small, swaged-on, taper-point, or spatula needles are best, but small cutting needles are also acceptable. A simple interrupted or continuous pattern of 6-0 to 7-0 absorbable suture (polyglycolic acid* or polyglactin 910†) is generally

---

*Dexon, Davis & Geck, Div. of American Cyanamid Co., Pearl River, NY 10965.

†Vicryl, Ethicon Inc., Somerville, NJ 08876.

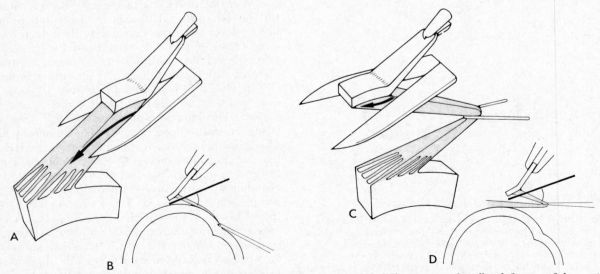

Figure 102–4. Inversion of the angle of attack for the cutting point. The subepithelial fibers cause a lamellar deflection of the cutting point when under tension. The angle of attack determines the direction of deflection. *A*, If the subepithelial fibers *above* the scissors are pulled toward the scissors joint, as by traction on the epithelial lamella, they deflect the cutting point downward (toward the sclera), and the resulting superficial layer increases in thickness. *B*, Inversion of the direction of attack by traction on the globe (traction suture through the *sclera*) during the dissection of fibers fixed at the sclera. *C*, If the subepithelial fibers *below* the scissors are pulled in the direction of the scissor joint, the angle of attack is inverted, the cutting point is driven upward, and the lamella becomes thinner. *D*, Inversion of the direction of attack by traction sutures through the *subepithelial fibers* in areas lacking adequate deep fixation (e.g., the conjunctiva of the fornix). (Reprinted with permission from Eyster, G.: *Eye Surgery—An Introduction to Operative Techniques.* Springer-Verlag, New York, 1980.)

preferred for most closures. If a nonabsorbable suture is used, 6-0 to 7-0 silk or 8-0 monofilament nylon may be used, depending on the circumstances. For the best apposition of tissues during closure of the conjunctiva, the needle and suture must pass through both the epithelial lamellae and the subepithelial fibrous layer (including Tenon's capsule) on both sides of the wound.

Postoperative Therapy

In general, treatment with topical antibiotic solutions or ointments administered four to six times daily for three to ten days following surgery is sufficient. If severe infection of the conjunctiva or surrounding tissues is present, appropriate systemic antibiotics are indicated.[5,26,52,54,55] Topical corticosteroids may be used in combination with the antibiotics unless contraindicated by resistant infectious disease or the presence of corneal ulceration.

CONGENITAL CONJUNCTIVAL DISEASE

Dermoids

Conjunctival dermoids (dermolipomas) are relatively uncommon choristomas arising in the conjunctiva and consisting of dermal elements such as epidermis, dermis, fat, sebaceous glands, and hair follicles. Dermoids are light tan or brown to black in color. Their size is variable, and they may extend across the limbus to involve the cornea. Occasionally they may involve the eyelids or orbit. Enlargement of the tumor is uncommon and usually negligible when it occurs. Small dermoids cause relatively little irritation, but larger dermoids, particularly those containing hair, may be irritating enough to cause blepharospasm and epiphora. They must be differentiated from the lacrimal caruncle and subconjunctival lacrimal cysts.[13,26,36,54,56]

Treatment of dermoids is by surgical excision. Some animals (especially those with small dermoids) show no evidence of irritation and may tolerate them without treatment. When only the conjunctiva is involved, the dermoid can be removed by simple conjunctivectomy and dissection down to bare sclera. When the dermoid extends into the cornea, superficial lamellar keratectomy (see Chapter 105) must be performed. Dissection of the superficial lesions may be continued from the episcleral space across the limbus. This results in removal of approximately the superficial third of the cornea, and healing with minimal scarring may be expected. With deeper lesions, more severe disorganization of the corneal stroma is present, and corneal scarring is much more likely. After excision of the dermoid, the surrounding conjunctiva may be mobilized and closed with a simple interrupted or simple continuous suture pattern utilizing 6-0 or 7-0 absorbable suture. If a keratectomy is performed, the conjunctiva may be similarly sutured to the sclera adjacent to the limbus.[5,13,26,36,54,56]

The Lacrimal Caruncle

The lacrimal caruncle is a normal structure in the medial canthus that contains hair follicles. In dogs

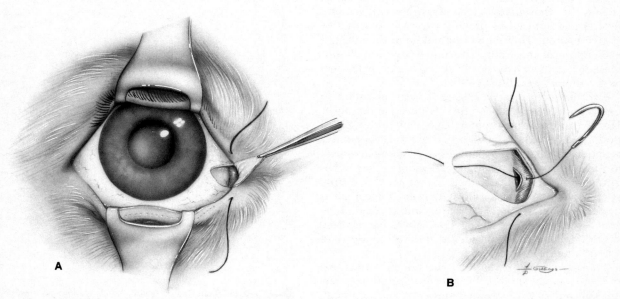

Figure 102–5. Sliding conjunctival flap for excision of the lacrimal caruncle. *A,* The dermis is dissected off and a conjunctival flap is created. *B,* The sliding flap is sutured to the edge of the medial palpebral ligament with one or two simple interrupted sutures of absorbable suture. NOTE: The lacrimal canaliculi have been cannulated with 3-0 monofilament suture to aid identification of and prevent inadvertent damage to these structures. (Reprinted with permission from Slatter, D. H.: *Fundamentals of Veterinary Ophthalmology.* W. B. Saunders, Philadelphia, 1981.)

with exophthalmos and occasionally in poodles, the hairs are long enough to cause mild superficial keratitis, medial corneal pigmentation, irritation of the adjacent conjunctiva, and persistent epiphora. Excision of the tissue resolves the problem, but care must be exercised to avoid the adjacent lacrimal canaliculi, which may be identified by cannulation through the lacrimal puncta with 3-0 monofilament nylon. The tissue defect is closed by mobilizing bulbar conjunctiva and suturing it to the medial palpebral ligament (Fig. 102–5).[56]

Subconjunctival Lacrimal Cysts

Infrequently, subconjunctival lacrimal cysts occur with congenital misplacement of lacrimal tissue. The conjunctiva bulges over the cyst, which may contain serous fluid, and can usually be transilluminated. Differential diagnoses include conjunctival neoplasia, subconjunctival foreign bodies, dermoids, orbital or global neoplasia with subconjunctival extension, and dacryoadenitis. Treatment consists of excisional biopsy of the cyst, duct, and associated glandular tissue. Usually this can be accomplished by incision of the conjunctiva and careful subconjunctival dissection, but occasionally a lateral canthotomy and subcutaneous dissection may be necessary.[46]

ACQUIRED CONJUNCTIVAL DISORDERS

Traumatic Disorders

Abrasions and small lacerations of the conjunctiva heal rapidly and usually require only short-term topical antibiotic therapy. More severe lacerations should be thoroughly cleaned with gentle saline flushes and sutured to prevent excessive scarring or symblepharon. Thorough examination of the eye and exploration of the wound are imperative to rule out foreign bodies or damage to other ocular structures (e.g., scleral lacerations).

Subconjunctival hemorrhage is very alarming to owners but is usually of little clinical importance. However, extensive hemorrhage may hide scleral perforations, and thorough ocular examination (under sedation or anesthesia if necessary) should be performed. Subconjunctival hemorrhage usually resorbs gradually over 10 to 14 days. Treatment is mainly supportive with topical antibiotics and topical corticosteroids unless the latter are contraindicated by concurrent ocular disease. Evaluation for clotting disorders should be considered in severe cases and when hemorrhage persists.

Subconjunctival emphysema occurs after fractures of the paranasal sinus walls, and the presenting signs are subconjunctival swelling and crepitus. Thorough ocular examination to rule out intraocular damage, and skull radiographs with thorough evaluation of the sinuses are indicated. The air usually resorbs within two weeks, and systemic broad spectrum antibiotics

should be administered to inhibit orbital infection with organisms from the sinuses.[26,45,53,55]

Symblepharon

A symblepharon is an adhesion of the palpebral conjunctiva to the bulbar conjunctiva that may also involve the cornea. Infrequently it may be a congenital anomaly, but more often it arises as a sequela to trauma, surgery, severe acute keratoconjunctivitis (e.g., chemical burns, neonatal conjunctivitis), or chronic recurrent keratoconjunctivitis (e.g., feline herpetic keratoconjunctivitis). The more severe or chronic the disease, the greater the risk of symblepharon formation. A symblepharon can markedly contract the conjunctival sac and can even limit ocular and lid motility when it is severe.[26,33,36,40,45,54,56,60]

Prevention of symblepharon should be a major goal in the treatment of the previously mentioned types of conjunctivitis. Daily use of a glass rod or blunt stainless steel spatula to separate adhesions of the conjunctiva along with removal of necrotic debris and exudates and use of appropriate topical antibiotics, artificial tears, and lubricants is helpful. Judicious use of topical corticosteroids unless contraindicated by corneal ulceration or the risk of exacerbation of herpetic infection will provide faster resolution of inflammation.[25,26,45,50,52,56] Soft therapeutic contact lenses may be used in some corneal injuries to reduce the risk of symblepharon formation.[13]

Once a symblepharon has formed, it can only be resolved surgically. A partial symblepharon that does not involve the cornea or interfere with ocular motility or lid and tear dynamics need not be repaired. If correction is desired, small adhesions may be severed

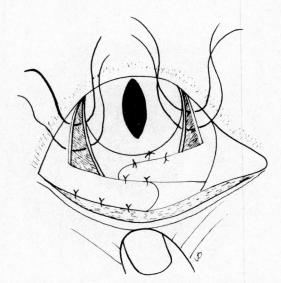

Figure 102–6. Teale-Knapp technique of symblepharon repair. Following mobilization of the symblepharon, the fornix is reconstructed using rotating conjunctival pedicle flaps from each side of the cornea. (Reprinted with permission from Peiffer, R. L.: Feline ophthalmology. *In* Gelatt, K. N. (ed.): *Textbook of Veterinary Ophthalmology.* Lea & Febiger, Philadelphia, 1981.)

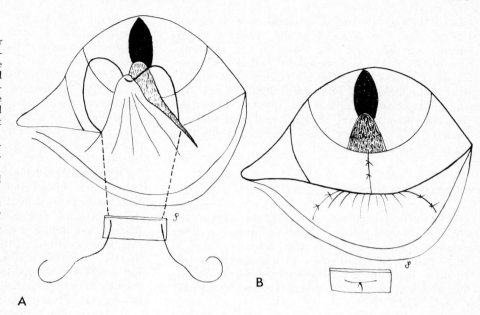

Figure 102–7. Arlt technique for symblepharon repair. *A,* The adherent conjunctiva is shaved off the cornea and the incision continued onto the palpebral surface. A double-armed 4-0 (or 5-0) silk suture is passed through the mobilized flap and the eyelid to emerge at the edge of the lower orbital rim. *B,* The bulbar conjunctiva is mobilized by blunt dissection and sutured with 6-0 absorbable material. The flap of conjunctiva is sutured to the fornix with similar material. The knots may be buried. The skin sutures are tightened and tied over a tension device. (Reprinted with permission from Peiffer, R. L.: Feline ophthalmology. *In* Gelatt, K. N.: *Textbook of Veterinary Ophthalmology.* Lea & Febiger, Philadelphia, 1981.)

and the eye treated with an antibiotic/corticosteroid ointment several times daily. The bulbar and palpebral conjunctival surfaces should be separated several times daily until they are re-epithelialized to prevent re-adhesion.[26,45,52,56,57] A more extensive adhesion that does not involve a wide area may be resolved by dissecting it away from the globe and mobilizing the surrounding conjunctiva to allow primary closure of the defect in the bulbar conjunctiva.[16,45,50,60]

When the symblepharon is so large that simple closure is not possible, resection combined with conjunctival flaps or free grafts is required (Fig. 102–

6). When the cornea is involved the adhesion is freed by lamellar dissection (superficial keratectomy), and dissection is continued bluntly over the sclera and almost to the lid margin, thus freeing the adhesion as a mobile flap, which is used to reline the palpebral surface. Scar tissue in the fornix and on the lid beneath the flap is dissected and removed, creating a pocket as deep as the normal fornix. Two double-armed, 5-0 silk mattress sutures are placed (from without to within) in each outer third of the flap to aid in retraction of the flap during dissection. When dissection is complete, each double-armed suture is

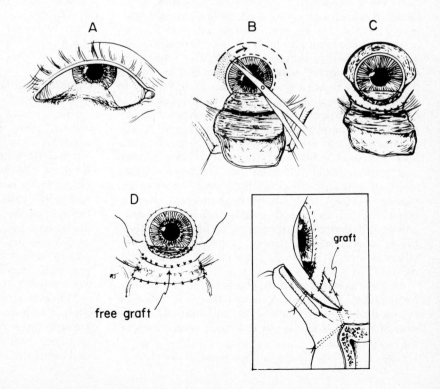

Figure 102–8. Variation of the Arlt technique for repair of symblepharon involving the cornea. *A, B,* and *C,* After freeing the conjunctiva from the cornea and sclera, a strip of bulbar conjunctiva is dissected 180° from the defect and mobilized across the cornea as a bridge flap to cover the sclera adjacent to the limbus. *D,* The conjunctiva dissected from the cornea is used to reline the palpebral surface, and a free graft has been used to reconstruct the fornix. Note deep sutures anchoring the forniceal portion of the graft to the orbital rim and passing through the skin. (Reprinted with permission from Tenzel, R. R.: Statement of the problem and treatment of chemical injuries. *In* Guibor, P., and Gougleman, H. (eds.): *Problems and Treatments of Contracted Sockets, Exenterated Orbits and Alkali Burns.* Intercontinental Medical Book Co., New York, 1973.)

passed through the freed forniceal area to emerge through the skin adjacent to the orbital rim. The sutures are then tied over small buttons or stents. The scleral defect is covered by pedicle, advancement, or bridge flaps from adjacent bulbar conjunctiva. If the fornix still has a large defect, a free graft can be placed in this area as described in subsequent sections (Conjunctival Flaps, and Conjunctival Grafts).[16,45,50,60] Figures 102–7 and 102–8 illustrate variations of this technique.

Inflammatory Tumors

Inflammatory tumors involving the conjunctiva are rare in cats and are more common in dogs, although the incidence is still relatively low. In dogs, three distinct diseases are recognized: granulomatous reactions to subconjunctival injections, proliferative keratoconjunctivitis, and ocular nodular fasciitis.[4,7,13,21,26,54,56,57]

Inflammation following subconjunctival drug injection is usually transient and subsides as the drug is resorbed, provided the drug is acceptable for subconjunctival use. The subconjunctival injection of some repository corticosteroids (methylprednisolone*) commonly results in a creamy white plaque, which can persist beneath the conjunctiva for months. Occasionally these plaques elicit painful granulomatous inflammation and should be excised under short-acting general anesthesia.[56]

Proliferative keratoconjunctivitis may be unilateral or bilateral and is most commonly seen in young to middle-aged collies. The cause is unknown, but hypopigmentation and exposure to intense sunlight have been suggested as contributory factors.[7,54,56,57] Characteristic lesions are raised, yellow to red masses involving the bulbar conjunctiva, adjacent cornea (usually at the temporal limbus), and the margin and anterior surface of the third eyelid. The lesions are closely incorporated with the conjunctiva and move with it. Growth is rapid, and blindness secondary to corneal involvement may occur if the disease is untreated. Corneal opacities (usually cholesterol deposits) are common in the cornea adjacent to the advancing edge of the lesion. Histologically, the lesions resemble fibrous histiocytomas seen in man and contain proliferating fibrous connective tissue and histiocytes as well as infiltrations of lymphocytes, plasma cells, and polymorphonuclear leukocytes.[7,26,54,56,57] In the dog, the term *proliferative keratoconjunctivitis* is preferred to *fibrous histiocytoma*, since the latter tumor is neoplastic in man, whereas lesions in the dog are considered nonneoplastic.[56,57]

Ocular nodular fasciitis is characterized by benign, firm, raised, flesh-colored masses that may be single or multiple and unilateral or bilateral. Distribution of lesions is similar to that seen with prolifera-

tive keratoconjunctivitis, except that the eyelids and sclera may also be involved. On the globe the masses arise from episcleral tissue and are often firmly adhered to the sclera. Usually the conjunctiva is freely movable over the nodule. Histologically, the lesions are highly vascularized, solid, nonencapsulated, inflammatory nodules in which the predominant cells are proliferating fibroblasts arranged haphazardly or in bundles. Lymphocytes and plasma cells are usually present, and occasional accumulations of histiocytes may be noted.[4,21,26,54,56]

Differential diagnoses for inflammatory conjunctival tumors should include the diseases previously mentioned as well as neoplasia and exuberant granulation tissue. The history and presence of drug plaques will define granulomas secondary to subconjunctival injections. Although movement of the conjunctiva over the nodular mass and involvement of the eyelids is more suggestive of ocular nodular fasciitis than proliferative keratoconjunctivitis, biopsy is necessary for a definitive diagnosis.

Early treatment of both ocular nodular fasciitis and proliferative keratoconjunctivitis with topical, subconjunctival (intralesional), and systemic steroids may be attempted. Proliferative keratoconjunctivitis responds better to corticosteroid therapy, but long-term topical and subconjunctival therapy is usually necessary.[7,26,54,56,57] Large, protuberant masses should be excised, and when this requires a superficial keratectomy, topical and subconjunctival corticosteroids should be withheld until the corneal site has re-epithelialized. Beta irradiation of lesions using a strontium-90 applicator followed by topical corticosteroids is the treatment of choice for early lesions or as an adjunct to surgical excision. A dosage of 4000 to 5000 rads per site is best.[7,54,56] Ocular nodular fasciitis responds poorly to corticosteroids, but recurrence after excision is uncommon even when excision of a lesion is incomplete.[21,26,54,56]

Conjunctival Neoplasms (see also Chapter 180)

Conjunctival neoplasia is uncommon in the dog and even rarer in the cat. In one long-term study of a beagle colony of 1,680 dogs, only 14 dogs (19 lesions) exhibited proliferative or neoplastic lesions.[24] In dogs, the most frequent neoplasms of the conjunctiva are benign hemangiomas, viral papillomas, and histiocytomas. Other tumors reported involving the conjunctiva are squamous cell carcinomas, hemangiosarcomas, melanomas, fibrosarcomas, and angiokeratomas.[2–4,6,8,9,22–24,26,37,44,45] The appearance and biological behavior of most conjunctival tumors are quite typical and allow the clinician to make a presumptive diagnosis of the type of neoplasia.

Whenever tumors involve the bulbar conjunctiva, limbus, or cornea, careful examination of all intraocular structures for transcleral extension is imperative, and such examinations should utilize biomicroscopy and ophthalmoscopy (direct and indirect). Evaluation

---

*Depo-Medrol, The Upjohn Co., Kalamazoo, MI 49001.

of the iridocorneal angle should also be performed using gonioscopy. Early excisional biopsy for histopathological evaluation should be obtained to properly identify the neoplasm and plan therapy. Epibulbar melanomas are possible exceptions to this rule, since the results of a small study involving six dogs with epibulbar melanomas suggested that these tumors in older dogs (8 to 11 years) may remain noninvasive and nonprogressive. The study concluded that surgical removal could be postponed in dogs in that age range as long as the tumors are stationary. However, epibulbar tumors in younger dogs in the study were more aggressive and required surgical removal (see Chapter 105).[33]

Because of the loose attachment of the bulbar conjunctiva to the globe, neoplasms involving only the bulbar conjunctiva can be easily removed. Small tumors may be resected after applying a topical anesthetic. The tumor is grasped and snipped off, leaving the wound to heal rapidly by second intention. Good restraint or sedation is advisable, as some deep sensation may remain and the patient may move its head as the conjunctiva is resected. Resection of larger tumors may require closure of the conjunctiva with a continuous pattern of 6-0 absorbable suture. If necessary, advancement conjunctival flaps may be mobilized from adjacent bulbar conjunctiva for closure. Free grafts from the buccal mucosa are rarely necessary.

Tumors that involve the palpebral conjunctiva, limbus, or cornea require more careful dissection and wound closure. Lid involvement usually accompanies tumors of the palpebral conjunctiva, and resection of the lids may be necessary (see Chapter 101). Tumors involving the superficial cornea and limbus as well as bulbar conjunctiva may be dissected via superficial keratectomy, which is carried past the limbus and beneath the involved conjunctiva. Healing of the wound progresses faster if the bulbar conjunctiva is sutured to the sclera adjacent to the limbus. This technique has been utilized with melanomas, histiocytomas, papillomas, and squamous cell carcinomas, and the prognosis for nonrecurrence is fair to good as long as excision is complete.[3,5,8,11,22,26,37,44,45,54] Beta irradiation of the area of excision with a strontium-90 applicator (5000 to 9500 rads/site) before closure of the conjunctiva is beneficial for squamous cell carcinomas, histiocytomas, and hemangiomas.[1,2,9,10,16,18,22,48,50,60,63]

Cryosurgery and low-current radiofrequency-induced hyperthermia are alternatives to surgical excision of selected conjunctival tumors.[2,20,22,26,28,53,54,56] Although these techniques have not been evaluated extensively for conjunctival tumors in small animals, both have been used in large animals, especially for squamous cell carcinomas.[14,27,31,32,42,49,61,64] Cryotherapy has been used for skin and lid neoplasms in small animals, and hyperthermia has been used successfully for the treatment of squamous cell carcinomas in cats and dogs.[2,20,22,28,45,54,61] Vascular tumors such as hemangiomas and hemangiosarcomas may be more re-sistant to these treatments owing to the temperature-dispersing tendencies of their blood-filled spaces.[53] The relative paucity of conjunctival tumors has hampered evaluation of the susceptibility of different conjunctival tumors to cryotherapy and hyperthermia, and further studies are warranted.

Because most conjunctival tumors can be easily managed by one of the previously mentioned surgical techniques alone or in combination with irradiation, chemotherapy and immunotherapy have not been used extensively in the treatment of primary conjunctival tumors. Bacillus Calmette Guérin (BCG) has been used in large animals for ocular squamous cell carcinomas and sarcoids and in experimental conjunctival malignant melanomas in hamsters.[41,51,54,58,65] Several excellent references are available for a more complete consideration of these modes of therapy.[51,58,61]

Irradiation of conjunctival neoplasms is best accomplished with beta irradiation utilizing a strontium-90 applicator. Surgical removal or reduction of the tumor is necessary, and radiation is applied to the tumor bed. The use of radioactive implants is not suitable for use in the conjunctiva because of its delicate structure and high mobility and because of the levels of radiation subsequently delivered to intraocular structures.[1,10,11,17,18,54,59,64]

CONJUNCTIVAL FLAPS

Conjunctival flaps may be broadly classified into four types: (1) hood flaps, (2) bridge flaps, (3) complete flaps, and (4) pedicle flaps (Figs. 102–9 to 102–11). They are indicated for repair of large defects in adjacent areas of conjunctiva (when simple apposition of the wound edges is not possible), for covering recurrent corneal erosions, and for treatment of deep or progressive ulcers. Such flaps over corneal ulcers protect the weakened area of the cornea while providing direct access of vascular and fibrous connective tissues to the ulcer. This direct blood supply to the wound is beneficial, since serum contains collagenase inhibitors, which counteract collagenase produced in necrotic and infected corneal tissues.[13,25,56] In addition, antibiotics administered systemically have direct access to the cornea. Direct contact of the fibrovascular tissue of the flap with the corneal ulcer allows more rapid healing through migration and proliferation of the fibroblasts and blood vessels to fill the wound. Flaps also raise the temperature of the cornea and thus theoretically facilitate healing by increasing corneal cellular metabolism.[26,56]

Hood Flaps. Hood flaps prepared from the bulbar conjunctiva are useful for covering peripheral corneal lesions. A 180° incision is made in the conjunctiva at the limbus, and the conjunctiva is superficially dissected for 1.0 to 1.5 cm toward the fornix. The flap is pulled centrally and sutured directly to the cornea with four to six interrupted sutures of 7-0 or 8-0 nylon or silk (Fig. 102–9). A penetrating groove may

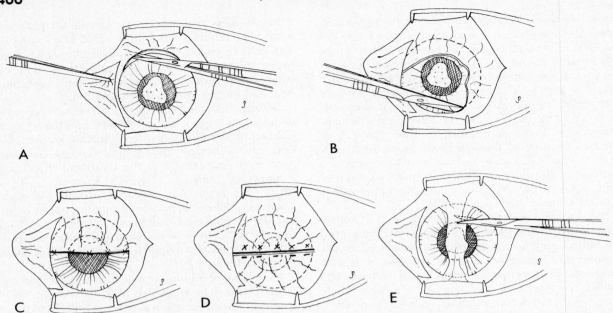

Figure 102–9. Preparation of hood (180°) and complete (360°) bulbar conjunctival flaps. *A* and *B,* The conjunctiva is incised at the limbus and dissected from the episcleral tissues. *C,* For the hood (180°) flap, four to six 6-0, nonabsorbable, simple interrupted sutures anchor the leading margin of the conjunctiva directly to the cornea. *D,* Five to six interrupted mattress sutures of 5-0 or 6-0 nonabsorbable suture are used to appose the dorsal and ventral bulbar conjunctiva for the complete bulbar conjunctival flap. *E,* After removal of the sutures from the complete bulbar conjunctival flap, the conjunctiva is adherent to the corneal ulcer site. The remaining conjunctiva is transected, leaving a small graft in the corneal defect. (Reprinted with pemission from Helper, L. C.: The canine nictitating membrane and conjunctiva. *In* Gelatt, K. N. (ed.): *Textbook of Veterinary Ophthalmology.* Lea & Febiger, Philadelphia, 1981.)

be prepared in the cornea to facilitate anchoring of the flap. Anchoring the flap only at the limbus or in the conjunctiva adjacent to the advanced flap has been advocated, but the flap is usually less stable and may shift prematurely. Sutures are removed when the flap has been in place for 10 to 21 days. Thereafter, the conjunctival flap will gradually retract and re-attach at the limbus except where it has adhered to the corneal defect. The adhesion may break down spontaneously within seven to ten days following suture removal. If not, the remaining pedicle of conjunctiva is severed just proximal to its adhesion to the cornea, allowing the freed conjunctiva to retract to the limbus. Both suture removal and severance of the conjunctival pedicle can usually be performed after administration of a topical anesthetic. The "island" of conjunctiva on the cornea gradually re-organizes and is incorporated into the corneal scar. Topical antibiotic/corticosteroid therapy is utilized to reduce corneal vascularization and scarring.

Complete (360°) Flaps. Complete bulbar conjunctival flaps (sometimes referred to as double hood flaps) are prepared by continuing the limbal conjunctival incision 360° around the limbus. Superficial dissection of the conjunctiva is performed toward the fornices for 1.0 to 1.5 cm, thus mobilizing the bulbar conjunctiva and creating dorsal and ventral flaps, which are advanced over the cornea to meet centrally. The flaps are apposed with five or six horizontal mattress sutures of 5-0 silk (see Fig. 102–9). As with the hood flap, the sutures are left in place for 10 to 21 days. Occasionally sutures may pull loose prematurely. The resulting gap in the flap can usually be

resutured utilizing moderate to heavy sedation and a topical local anesthetic. Sutures are removed and adhesions managed as discussed for hood flaps.

Bridge (Bucket Handle) Flaps. Bridge flaps may be used to cover part or all of the cornea (depending on its width) or to fill defects in the bulbar conjunctiva on the opposite side of the cornea during symblepharon correction. The degree of conjunctival dissection necessary is proportional to the width and distance of the defect from the flap. The conjunctiva is first superficially dissected from the limbus as for the

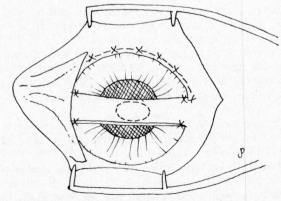

Figure 102–10. The bridge or strip bulbar conjunctival flap, usually a band of conjunctiva, is connected at both ends for treatment of corneal ulcers. This flap is predominantly a graft and does not provide as much support to the weakened cornea as other types of bulbar flaps. (Reprinted with permission from Helper, L. C.: The canine nictitating membrane and conjunctiva. *In* Gelatt, K. N. (ed.): *Textbook of Veterinary Ophthalmology.* Lea & Febiger, Philadelphia, 1981.)

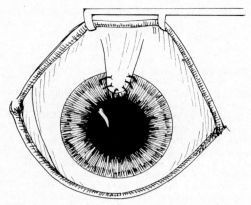

Figure 102–11. Pedicle flap of fornix-based bulbar conjunctiva is advanced over the cornea after freeing it at the limbus. The flap is sutured directly to the corneal defect with interrupted 7-0 or 8-0 nonabsorbable sutures.

complete conjunctival flap, and the flap is created via a second incision in the conjunctiva 1.0 to 1.5 cm from and parallel to the limbal incision. Once the flap is freed it can be shifted over the cornea or into a conjunctival defect and sutured with 7-0 to 8-0 silk or 8-0 nylon sutures in a simple interrupted or continuous pattern (Fig. 102–10; see Fig. 102–8). When the flap is used to cover the cornea, it may be anchored in scleral grooves parallel to the limbus for wide flaps or in parallel grooves in the cornea on each side of narrower flaps. Bridge flaps that totally cover the cornea are more difficult to prepare than complete (360°) flaps and offer no advantage over the latter. Thin bridge flaps that partially cover the cornea offer less support and are more fragile than complete flaps but do permit limited vision.

Pedicle Flaps. Pedicle flaps may be constructed from either bulbar or palpebral conjunctiva. Flaps from the latter are much more difficult to dissect, are more subject to disruption due to combined eyelid and globe movements, and have no advantage over similar flaps constructed of bulbar conjunctiva. Flaps may be dissected and advanced from the limbus and sutured to the cornea (Fig. 102–11) or advanced or rotated to close adjacent conjunctival defects (see Fig. 102–6). Nonabsorbable sutures (7-0 or 8-0) are used to secure the flap to the cornea, and 5-0 or 6-0 absorbable sutures may be used to close conjunctival defects. Suture removal is as previously described, and adhesions to the cornea are managed as discussed with hood and complete flaps. Pedicle flaps to the cornea have a distinct advantage over complete flaps in that they are directly sutured into the corneal defect and permit minimally restricted vision. However, they are technically more difficult to prepare.

CONJUNCTIVAL GRAFTS

Free conjunctival grafts are rarely necessary in small animals, and the techniques are adapted from those used in man. Whenever possible conjunctiva should be used to replace conjunctiva. Donor conjunctiva can be obtained from the fornices of the same or fellow eye and placed in the recipient site. Silk or absorbable sutures (7-0) may be used to close the donor site and secure the graft. The size of the attainable graft is limited, and buccal mucosa can be used as an acceptable alternative. Because contracture of grafts occurs postsurgically, the donor tissue should be considerably larger than the defect to be covered. When buccal mucosal grafts are used, they must be well trimmed of fat and submucosal tissue for the best healing and postoperative appearance. When the defect involves the conjunctival fornix, the graft must be anchored in the fornix. A Silastic tube or small rubber catheter is cut to a sufficient length to overlap the graft edges. Three or four double-armed 4-0 silk sutures can then be passed through or over the tube, through the fornix, out through the skin and tied over buttons or stents. When possible, the suture should be anchored to the periosteum of the orbital rim before passing through the skin (Fig. 102–8).

1. Banks, W. C., and England R. B.: Radioactive gold in the treatment of ocular squamous cell carcinoma of cattle. J. Am. Vet. Med. Assoc. 163:745, 1973.
2. Barrie, K. P., Gelatt, K. N., and Parshall, C. P.: Eyelid squamous cell carcinoma in four dogs. J. Am. Anim. Hosp. Assoc. 18:123, 1982.
3. Belkin, P. V.: Malignant melanoma of the bulbar conjunctiva in a dog. Vet. Med./Sm. Anim. Clin. 70:957, 1975.
4. Belhorn, R. W., and Henkind, P.: Ocular nodular fasciitis in a dog. J. Am. Vet. Med. Assoc. 150:212, 1967.
5. Bistner, S. I., Aguirre, G., and Batik, G.: Atlas of Veterinary Ophthalmic Surgery. W. B. Saunders, Philadelphia, 1977, pp. 139–146.
6. Blodi, F. C., and Ramsey, F. K.: Ocular tumors in domestic animals. Am. J. Ophthalmol. 64:627, 1967.
7. Blogg, J. R.: Proliferative keratoconjunctivitis in the collie. Pro. Am. Coll. Vet. Ophthalmol. 8:89, 1977.
8. Bonney, C. H., Koch, S. A., Confer, A. W., and Dice, P. F.: A case report: A conjunctivocorneal papilloma with evidence of viral etiology. J. Sm. Anim. Pract. 21:183, 1980.
9. Buyukmihic, N., and Stannard, A. A.: Canine conjunctival angiokeratomas. J. Am. Vet. Med. Assoc. 178:1279, 1981.
10. Candlin, F. T., and Levine, M. H.: The use of beta radiation on corneal lesions in the dog. North Am. Vet. 33:632, 1952.
11. Catcott, E. J., Tharp, V. L., and Johnson, L. E.: Beta ray therapy in ocular diseases of animals. J. Am. Vet. Med. Assoc. 122:172, 1953.
12. Cotchin, E.: Melanotic tumors of dogs. J. Comp. Pathol. 65:115, 1955.
13. Dice, P. F.: The canine cornea. In Gelatt, K. N. (ed.): Textbook of Veterinary Ophthalmology. Lea & Febiger, Philadelphia, 1981, pp. 343–373.
14. Eisner, G.: Eye Surgery—An Introduction to Operative Techniques. Springer-Verlag, New York, 1980.
15. Farris, H. E., and Fraunfelder, F. T.: Cryosurgical treatment of ocular squamous cell carcinoma of cattle. J. Am. Vet. Med. Assoc. 168:213, 1976.
16. Fox, S. A.: Ophthalmic Plastic Surgery, 5th ed. Grune and Stratton, New York, 1976.
17. Frauenfelder, H. C., Blevins, W. E., and Page, E. H.: 90Sr for treatment of periocular squamous cell carcinoma in the horse. J. Am. Vet. Med. Assoc. 180:307, 1982.
18. Friedell, H. L., Thomas, C. I., and Krohmer, J. S.: An evaluation of the clinical use of a strontium 90 beta-ray applicator with a review of the underlying principles. Am. J. Roentgenol. 71:25, 1954.
19. Friedlander, M. H.: Allergy and Immunology of the Eye. Harper and Row, New York, 1979.
20. Grier, R. L., Brawer, W. G., Jr., and Theilen, G. H.:

Hyperthermic treatment of superficial tumors in cats and dogs. J. Am. Vet. Med. Assoc. *177*:227, 1980.

21. Gwin, R. M., Gelatt, K. N., and Peiffer, R. L.: Ocular nodular fasciitis in the dog. J. Am. Vet. Med. Assoc. *170*:611, 1977.

22. Gwin, R. M., Gelatt, K. N., and Williams, L. W.: Ophthalmic neoplasms in the dog. J. Am. Anim. Hosp. Assoc. *18*:853, 1982.

23. Hare, C. L., and Howard, E. B.: Canine conjunctivocorneal papillomatosis: A case report. J. Am. Anim. Hosp. Assoc. *13*:688, 1977.

24. Hargis, A. M., Lee, A. C., and Thomassen, R. W.: Tumor and tumor-like lesions of perilimbal conjunctiva in laboratory dogs. J. Am. Vet. Med. Assoc. *173*:1185, 1978.

25. Havener, W. H.: *Ocular Pharmacology*, 4th ed. C. V. Mosby, St. Louis, 1978, pp. 572–575.

26. Helper, L. C.: The canine nictitating membrane and conjunctiva. In Gelatt, K. N. (ed.): *Textbook of Veterinary Ophthalmology*. Lea & Febiger, Philadelphia, 1981, pp. 330–342.

27. Hilbert, B. J., Farrell, R. K., and Grant, B. D.: Cryotherapy of periocular squamous cell carcinoma in the horse. J. Am. Vet. Med. Assoc. *170*:1305, 1977.

28. Holmberg, D. L.: Cryosurgical treatment of canine eyelid tumors Vet. Clin. North Am. *10*:831, 1980.

29. Jakobiec, F. A., and Iwamoto, T.: The ocular adnexa: Lids, conjunctiva and orbit. In Fine, B. S., and Yanoff, M. (eds.): *Ocular Histology*. Harper and Row, New York, 1979, pp. 290–342.

30. Joseph, J. M.: Tissue culture and chick embryo techniques. In Sonnenwirth, A. C., and Jarrett, L. (eds.): *Gradwohl's Clinical Laboratory Methods and Diagnosis*, Vol. II. C. V. Mosby, St. Louis, 1980, pp. 2002–2010.

31. Joyce, J. R.: Cryosurgical treatment of tumors of horses and cattle. J. Am. Vet. Med. Assoc. *168*:226, 1976.

32. Kainer, R. A., Stringer, J. M., and Lueker, D. C.: Hyperthermia for treatment of ocular squamous cell tumors in cattle. J. Am. Vet. Med. Assoc. *176*:356, 1980.

33. King, J. H., Jr., and Wadsworth, J. A. C.: *An Atlas of Ophthalmic Surgery*, 3rd ed., J. B. Lippincott, Philadelphia, 1981, pp. 211–242.

34. Lavach, J. D., Thrall, M. A., Benjamin, M. M., and Severin, G. A.: Cytology of normal and inflamed conjunctivas in dogs and cats. J. Am. Vet. Med. Assoc. *170*:722, 1977.

35. Lindmark, R. C.: Alkali burns-prosthetic fittings. In Guibor, R., and Gougleman, H. (eds.): *Problems and Treatments of Contracted Sockets, Exenterated Orbits and Alkali Burns*. Intercontinental Medical Book Co., New York, 1973, pp. 139–142.

36. Magrane, W. G.: *Canine Ophthalmology*, 3rd ed. Lea and Febiger, Philadelphia, 1977, pp. 101–102.

37. Martin, C. L.: Canine epibulbar melanomas and their management. J. Am. Anim. Hosp. Assoc. *17*:83, 1981.

38. Martin, C. L., and Anderson, B. G.: Ocular anatomy. In Gelatt, K. N. (ed.); *Textbook of Veterinary Ophthalmology*. Lea and Febiger, Philadelphia, 1981, pp. 17–18.

39. McDonald, T. O., et al.: Eye irritation. In Marzulli, F. N., and Maibach, H. I. (eds.): *Dermatotoxicology*, 2nd ed. Hemisphere Publishing Corp., New York, 1983, pp. 555–610.

40. Mulberger, R. D.: Trauma with lid deformities. In Guibor, P., and Gougleman, H. (eds.): *Problems and Treatments of Contracted Sockets Exenterated Orbits and Alkali Burns*. Intercontinental Medical Book Co., New York, 1973, pp. 859–867.

41. Murphy, J. M., Severin, G. A., Lavach, J. D., Helper, D. I., and Lueker, D. C.: Immunotherapy in ocular equine sarcoid. J. Am. Vet. Med. Assoc. *174*:269, 1979.

42. Neuman, S. M., Kainer, R. A., and Severin, G. A.: Reaction of normal equine eyes to radiofrequency current-induced hyperthermia. Am. J. Vet. Res. *43*:1938, 1982.

43. O'Connor, G. R.: Eye diseases. In Fudenberg, H. H., Stites, D. P., Caldwell, J. L., and Wells, J. V. (eds.): *Basic and Clinical Immunology*. Lange Medical Publications, Los Altos, 1976, pp. 579–586.

44. Peiffer, R. L.: Hemangioma of the nictitating membrane in a dog. J. Am. Vet. Med. Assoc. *172*:832, 1978.

45. Peiffer, R. L.: Feline ophthalmology. In Gelatt, K. N. (ed.): *Textbook of Veterinary Ophthalmology*. Lea and Febiger, Philadelphia, 1981, pp. 521–568.

46. Playter, R. F., and Adams, L. G.: Lacrimal cyst (dacryops) in two dogs. J. Am. Vet. Med. Assoc. *171*:736, 1977.

47. Prince, J. H., Diesem, C. D., Eglitis, I., and Ruskell, G. L.: *Anatomy and Histology of the Eye and Orbit in Domestic Animals*. Charles C Thomas, Springfield, 1960, pp. 45–51.

48. Rahi, A. H. S., and Gainer, A.: *Immunopathology of the Eye*. Blackwell Scientific Publications, London, 1976.

49. Riis, R. C.: Equine ophthalmology. In Gelatt, K. N. (ed.): *Textbook of Veterinary Ophthalmology*. Lea and Febiger, Philadelphia, 1981, pp. 601–604.

50. Roper-Hall, M. J. (ed.): *Stallard's Eye Surgery*, 6th ed. John Wright and Sons Ltd., Bristol, 1980, pp. 377–392.

51. Rutgard, J., et al.: Calmette-Guerin bacillus treatment of experimental conjunctival malignant melanoma. Arch. Ophthalmol. *95*:2214, 1977.

52. Scheie, H. G., and Albert, D. M.: *Textbook of Ophthalmology*, 9th ed. W. B. Saunders, Philadelphia, 1977, pp. 554–565.

53. Seim, H. B. III: Mechanisms of cold-induced cellular death. Vet. Clin. North Am. *10*:755, 1980.

54. Severin, G. A.: *Veterinary Ophthalmology Notes*, 2nd ed. Colorado State University Press, Fort Collins, 1976, pp. 137–151.

55. Shapiro, M. S., Friend, J., and Thoft, R. A.: Corneal re-epithelialization from the conjunctiva. Invest. Ophthalmol. Visual Sci. *21*:135, 1981.

56. Slatter, D. H.: *Fundamentals of Veterinary Ophthalmology*, W. B. Saunders, Philadelphia, 1981.

57. Smith, J. S., Bistner, S., and Riis, R.: Infiltrative corneal lesions resembling fibrous histiocytoma: Clinical and pathological findings in six dogs and one cat. J. Am. Vet. Med. Assoc. *169*:722, 1976.

58. Spradbrow, P. B., Wilsonk, B. E., Hoffmann, D., and Kelly, W. R.: Immunotherapy of bovine ocular squamous cell carcinomas. Vet. Rec. *100*: 376, 1977.

59. *Strontium-90 Radiation, Technical Information and Instruction Manual for Users of the Model NB-1 Eye Therapy Source*. New England Nuclear, Boston.

60. Tenzel, R. R.: Statement of the problem and treatment of chemical injuries. In Guibor, P., and Gougleman, H. (eds.): *Problems and Treatments of Contracted Sockets, Exenterated Orbits and Alkali Burns*. Intercontinental Medical Book Co., New York, 1973, pp. 143–145.

61. Theilen, G. H., and Madewell, B. R. (eds.): *Veterinary Cancer Medicine*. Lea & Febiger, Philadelphia, 1978.

62. Troutman, R. C.: *Microsurgery of the Anterior Segment of the Eye*, Vol. I: Introduction and Basic Techniques. C. V. Mosby, St. Louis, 1974.

63. Vaughn, B., and Asbury, T.: *General Ophthalmology*. Lange Medical Publications, Los Altos, 1980, pp. 59–88.

64. Williams, L., and Gelatt, K. N.: Food animal ophthalmology. In Gelatt, K. N. (ed.): *Textbook of Ophthalmology*. Lea and Febiger, Philadelphia, 1981, pp. 622–632.

65. Wyman, M., Rings, M. D., Tarr, M. J., and Alden, C. L.: Immunotherapy in equine sarcoid: A report of two cases. J. Am. Vet. Med. Assoc. *171*:449, 1977.

Chapter **103** # The Lacrimal System

J. D. Lavach

The lacrimal system produces and removes tears. In the normal animal there is coordinated secretion of glandular products, which combine to form the precorneal tear film. This film is distributed across the cornea and performs several important functions. A substantial portion of tear volume is lost through evaporation, and the remainder drains away (Fig. 103–1).

The initial part of this chapter provides a working knowledge of the anatomy of the nasolacrimal system. A limited discussion has been directed toward methods of evaluating and testing the function of the nasolacrimal system. Finally, congenital and acquired diseases of the lacrimal system and their contemporary surgical treatments are illustrated and described.

ANATOMY OF THE LACRIMAL SYSTEM

The lacrimal gland produces most of the tears.[15] Histologically, it is similar to the serosalivary gland.[30,60] Being a modified skin gland, it has a tubuloalveolar arrangement, containing both serous and mucous acini.[60] The lacrimal gland is located in the superotemporal region of the orbit between the globe nasally and the orbital ligament and zygomatic process of the frontal bone temporally.[18] It is enclosed within a fold of periorbita but is isolated from the rectus muscles by a fascial plane. The size in dogs varies: 0.5 to 2.0 cm long, 3.0 to 1.5 cm wide, and 0.7 to 1.5 cm thick.[18] The emptying ducts are continuous from the deeper lobe through the superficial lobe; hence damage to the superficial portions of the ducts or their openings renders the gland nonfunctional. The ducts in dogs (3 to 5 or 15 to 20) are not grossly visible but open through the conjunctiva in the superior temporal fornix.[18,74]

The gland of the third eyelid is an accessory lacrimal gland. The gland encompasses the stem of the hyaline cartilaginous shaft in the third eyelid and is heart-shaped with the apex pointing ventrally. The secretions are mixed and seromucoid in the dog and serous in the cat.[49,60] In the dog, 29 to 57 per cent of the aqueous phase of the precorneal film may be produced by this gland.[15,37] The secretions pass through two to four invisible[18] ducts that open into the inferior cul-de-sac between the globe and third eyelid.

The tarsal (meibomian) glands are grossly visible through the thin palpebral conjunctiva and have a palisade appearance, perpendicular to the margin of the eyelid (Fig. 103–2). The gland openings are visible and line the margin of the eyelid. In dogs approximately 40 openings are found in the upper eyelid and fewer (usually 28 to 34) in the lower eyelid. Each opening is about 80 microns (0.08 mm) in diameter.[60] The secretion is a lipid-laden sebaceous material, which can be manually expressed on the margin of the eyelid as a cream-colored exudate.

The intraepithelial goblet cells are the primary source of the mucoid layer of the tears. The cells are scattered throughout the palpebral conjunctiva, including the reflections on the third eyelid, but are most prevalent in the fornices. Goblet cells are not normally found in the bulbar conjunctiva.

Modified sebaceous sweat glands, the glands of Moll (ciliary glands), are usually found near and parallel with the eyelash follicles. The sebaceous glands of Zeis are usually paired and attached to a follicle, supplying it with sebum.[59]

The upper and lower eyelids each have a small opening, the punctum lacrimale, which is the beginning of the lacrimal drainage system. The puncta are 2 to 5 mm from the nasal canthus at the site where the eyelid margin becomes much thicker and more rigid, and are situated just nasal to the most nasally located tarsal gland. The punctal openings are oval or slit-like and may be 0.2 to 0.5 mm wide and 0.5 to 1.0 mm long.[18,30] The long axis is parallel to the eyelid margin. Occasionally the puncta lack pigment, but usually the rim of the punctum is pigmented in comparison to adjacent palpebral tissues.

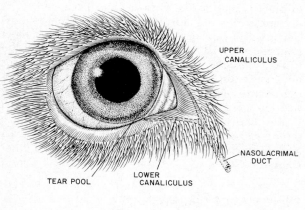

UPPER CANALICULUS

NASOLACRIMAL DUCT

TEAR POOL

LOWER CANALICULUS

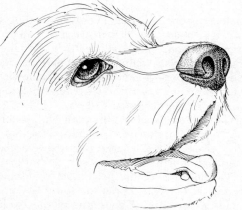

Figure 103–1. The nasolacrimal system.

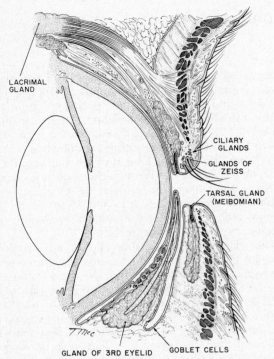

LACRIMAL
GLAND

CILIARY
GLANDS

GLANDS OF
ZEISS

TARSAL GLAND
(MEIBOMIAN)

GLAND OF 3RD EYELID   GOBLET CELLS

Figure 103–2. A cross-section of the globe and eyelids showing sources of the precorneal tear film.

After entering a punctum, the tears pass into the upper or lower canaliculus. The upper canaliculus lies just beneath the palpebral conjunctiva and parallels the eyelid margin for a short distance before making an abrupt turn and entering the nasolacrimal sac. The lower canaliculus turns into the sac just below the site where the upper canaliculus enters.[18,30] The total length of each canaliculus is between 4.0 and 7.0 mm, and the diameter varies in dogs from 0.5 to 1.0 mm.[18,26,30] The canaliculi are lined with stratified squamous epithelium.[30]

The lacrimal sac is not always a distinct structure in animals, as it is in man. In some animals it is vestigial and visible only at the confluence of the upper and lower canaliculi and the beginning of the nasolacrimal duct. The lining of the outflow channel changes from stratified squamous epithelium in the canaliculi to columnar epithelium in the lacrimal sac and nasolacrimal duct.[30] The lacrimal sac (2.0 to 5.0 × 0.5 to 2.0 mm)[18] occupies the fossa in the lacrimal and frontal bones just posterior to the lacrimal crest.

The nasolacrimal duct begins caudally at the lacrimal sac. The duct continues rostrad through the bony channel of the lacrimal bone and into the lacrimal sulcus of the maxilla. This section is the narrowest portion of the nasolacrimal duct. The duct emerges from the bony capsule at the conchal crest, which is adjacent to the second premolar tooth, or at the infraorbital canal.[18,30] This is about one-fourth of the total length of the duct. It then curves rostrad in a gentle ventral arch.[18] After leaving the bony canal, the duct continues in the medial wall of the maxilla, deep to the nasal mucosa. This middle portion is about one-half the length of the duct.[18] An accessory opening is present in approximately 50 per cent of dogs at the root of the upper canine tooth.[51, 83] When present, this auxiliary opening is a slit on the medial wall of the duct and is 2 to 5 mm in length. The rostral fourth of the duct passes through the cartilages that form the ventral and lateral walls of the external nares.[18] The duct makes an abrupt 90° turn 2 mm from the orifice and proceeds to open onto the floor of the nasal cavity at the junction of the ventral and lateral walls, approximately 1 cm inside the opening of the external nares. The orifice may be surrounded by pigmented tissue and may be visible as a slight indentation in the mucosal surface. A nasal speculum or forceps must be used to retract the alar cartilage laterally to see the opening in the nasal vestibule. A small malar artery follows the nasolacrimal duct to its opening in the nose.[30]

TEAR MOVEMENT

Tears pass from the lacrimal gland across the cornea, blend with other secretory components, and pool in the lacrimal lake. The pool is not always evident owing to eyelid and globe relations but exists inferiorly in the nasal canthus. The heavy, oily secretions from the tarsal glands help to prevent spillage of tears onto the face and direct the tears toward the lacrimal lake. Several theories have evolved to explain the passage of tears from the palpebral fissure to the lacrimal lake and down into the nose.[52,74,78,82] A combination of contraction of the orbicularis muscle, gravity, capillary action, and a syphoning effect from the lacrimal sac may be required to propel the tears. Consequently, patent outflow apparatus does not ensure removal of tears unless physiological function is present. Little tear secretion occurs during sleep in man, and approximately one-half of the total tear volume is lost through evaporation.[78] For a discussion of the composition and function of tears and mucous threads, the reader is referred to other sources.[38,50]

PRINCIPLES OF DIAGNOSIS

A detailed history of ocular events, including duration of abnormality, ocular discharge, pain, and previous medications, may be useful in arriving at the correct diagnosis. A complete ophthalmic examination should be performed on all patients; however, this discussion is limited to the specific evaluation of the tears and the nasolacrimal system.

An initial, direct visual examination with magnification and focal illumination provides essential information. Any ocular discharge is noted and classified as mucoid, purulent, serous, or a combination thereof. The location of the accumulated discharge may be important (i.e., upper or lower eyelid or inferior cul-de-sac only). The status of the eyelids, conjunctiva, and cornea may be related to tears or outflow abnormalities. The size, shape, and position of each punctum and the relationship of the globe to the eyelids and the lacrimal lake should be evaluated.

SPECIAL DIAGNOSTIC METHODS

Cytology

Exudate from the eye is collected from the apparent source (e.g., the conjunctiva, eyelids, or punctum) for culturing and sensitivity testing. Cytological evaluation from impression smears or scrapings may yield additional information. Any exudate obtained from the nasolacrimal system should be cultured. Any foreign body expelled during flushing should be cultured to obtain the best therapeutic results.

Tear Production

The use and value of the Schirmer tear test have been well documented in small animals.[1,10,15,29,36,37,64,80] Patients presented with abnormal ocular discharge should have the tear volume measured. Repeated tests may be necessary to determine the presence or absence of normal tear volume and response to treatment.

Lacrimal Patency

Vital dyes such as fluorescein and rose bengal may be instilled into the conjunctival sac; the external nares are observed for appearance of the dye, indicating physiological function as well as patency. The time it takes for the solution to pass to the nostril is variable, but it should pass within five minutes.

The nasolacrimal drainage apparatus may be flushed to evaluate patency. A combination of topical anesthesia and firm restraint facilitates flushing and prevents iatrogenic damage to the drainage system. The nares are tilted downward while flushing. If the nares are elevated during flushing and an accessory opening is present in the lacrimal canal, the retrograde flow may stimulate swallowing and gagging as the fluid enters the pharynx. Magnification may be used to assist in viewing the puncta. The technique for flushing requires a small (3-ml) syringe filled with saline and a lacrimal needle. A 20- to 25-gauge lacrimal needle with a 90-degree bend at the tip is sufficient for the upper punctum. The examiner should gently roll the upper eyelid up, apply slight lateral traction to stabilize the eyelid, and expose the punctum. The tip of the lacrimal needle is held parallel to the eyelid margin and directed toward the nasal canthus. Once the punctum is entered, the lacrimal needle should not be inserted more than 2 mm into the canaliculus. Gentle irrigation produces leakage around the needle and lower punctum simultaneously. If patent, saline should flow out the external nares. In some dogs a few drops of seromucoid material may precede the flow of saline from the nostril. In cats, the procedure may require chemical restraint in addition to the topical anesthetic used in dogs. If resistance to flow is encountered, the needle should be withdrawn slightly.

Insertion of the needle into the nasolacrimal sac and bony canal is contraindicated in conscious patients. Sudden head movements may cause the needle to damage the sac or duct. The lower punctum and canaliculus are important outflow channels. Inadvertent damage caused by insertion of the lacrimal needle and flushing may lead to poor tear outflow and permanent epiphora.

The upper portion of the lacrimal outflow system may be examined by use of a blunt probe of malleable stainless steel or silver. A variety of diameters are available down to 0000. Probing the nasolacrimal system is restricted to anesthetized patients and allows the examiner to physically explore from the canaliculi to the lacrimal sac and into the proximal bony canal. It is useful in detecting concretions or other firm debris in the canaliculi or sac. The probe is inserted into the upper punctum parallel to the eyelid margin while the upper eyelid is held under lateral tension. At this point, the probe is rotated upward 90° and immediately slides into the bony canal. This is the extent of maximum insertion of a semirigid probe. The same procedure may be used when probing the lower canaliculus; however, it may be more difficult to enter the bony portion of the canal. The probe should not be forced into the canaliculus or canal, since severe damage may result.

Monofilament nylon suture material (size 0 to 2) may be used as a soft stent to probe the outflow system.[66] The end of the suture should be smooth and the tip flamed to round off the sharp edge. The upper punctum is entered and the suture passes with minimal resistance until the sac is entered. At the exit from the sac some initial resistance may be encountered until the tip "finds" the entrance to the bony canal. This bony entrance may be the narrowest portion of the canal, and if passage is not possible, a smaller diameter suture should be used. After entering the canal the suture should pass easily with minimal resistance. In 50 per cent of dogs the suture exits at the accessory opening near the root of the upper canine tooth and continues out the nostril. In the remainder of patients the suture passes down to the nasal orifice and may lodge just inside the opening, requiring elevation of the alar flap of cartilage to allow passage onto the floor of the nasal vestibulum.

Dacryocystorhinography

Radiographic evaluation of the nasolacrimal system requires plain films of the skull and contrast studies

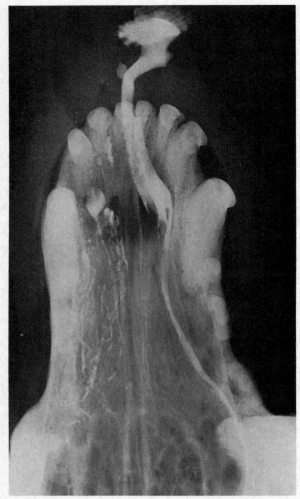

Figure 103–3. Dacryocystorhinogram in a normal dog.

TABLE 103–1.   Etiology of Epiphora[55]

A. Eyelid abnormalities
B. Congenital anomalies of the nasolacrimal system
   1. Atresia
   2. Hypoplasia
C. Acquired anomalies
   1. Trauma
   2. Infection
D. Foreign bodies
E. Neoplasia
F. Parasympathetic stimulation
   1. Cholinergic drugs (pilocarpine)
   2. Anticholinesterase drugs (demecarium bromide)
G. Lacrimal gland inflammation
   1. Traumatic lesions
   2. Infectious process
H. Trigeminal irritation
   1. Lesions of the eyelids, conjunctiva, cornea, and iris
   2. Glaucoma
I. Retinal stimulation by glare and excessive light
J. Tear staining syndrome

exceeds the capacity for drainage and evaporation.[19] Lacrimation caused by psychic stimulation does not occur in lower animals, but lacrimation may be stimulated by external stimuli or as a response to pain (Table 103–1).

CONGENITAL ANOMALIES OF DRAINAGE

Congenital anomalies of the drainage apparatus are occasionally seen in small animals. Some anomalies are insignificant and epiphora is not present. In others, a constant state of increased moisture is noticed during the first three to four months of life. The discharge is clear and free of copious amounts of mucoid or purulent material. The chief owner complaint is altered appearance and not patient discomfort or disability. A few patients have scalding of the skin and secondary dermatitis.

Congenital anomalies of drainage are: (1) absence of punctum, (2) conjunctival membrane, (3) stenotic punctum, (4) misplaced punctum, (5) atresia of canaliculi or lacrimal duct, and (6) eyelid abnormalities.

Absence of punctum. Several dog breeds,[5, 25] including cocker spaniels, golden retrievers, Samoyeds, toy poodles, miniature poodles, and Bedlington terriers, and the Persian cat may lack one or more puncta.

If either the upper or lower punctum is present, epiphora may not exist. If only the lower is absent, epiphora will more likely be present than if only the upper is absent, because the lower punctum is more important in removing tears. A thorough examination with magnification is necessary to establish the absence of a punctum. If the upper and lower puncta are absent, a slight depression in the conjunctiva may be identified where the opening would normally be located. If only one punctum is absent, the site of

(Fig. 103–3) under general anesthesia. Several commercial contrast media are available, including a 37% iodized poppyseed oil and a 37% organically bound iodine solution. The lower punctum is occluded and the contrast material flushed gently through the upper punctum until several drops appear at the nasal opening. Flushing with normal saline prior to using contrast medium removes mucoid debris and reduces air bubbles which may alter interpretation. Routine lateral, oblique, and dorsoventral exposures are made. In addition, a nonscreen, open mouth exposure may provide greater detail of the duct. A complete discussion of the techniques and results of dacryocystorhinography has been published.[26,81]

Epiphora and Lacrimation

Epiphora is defined as overflow of tears onto the face as the result of an impaired outflow apparatus. Lacrimation is an increased production of tears that may result in tear overflow when the production

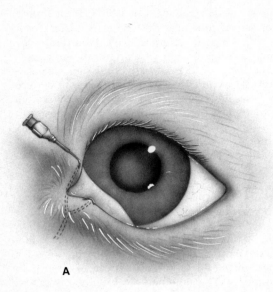

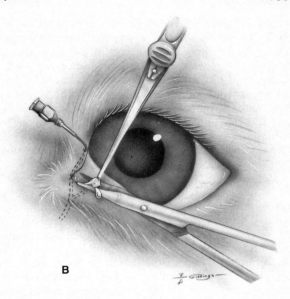

A

B

Figure 103–4. Repair of imperforate punctum using pressurized fluid. *A,* The opposing punctum is cannulated, and pressure is applied via a saline-filled syringe to elevate the obstructing conjunctiva over the other punctum. The use of methylene blue solution aids in locating the bleb. Some loss of saline occurs down the nasolacrimal duct. *B,* The tissue is grasped with fine forceps and incised with strabismus scissors. Antibiotic and corticosteroid preparations are applied to prevent scarring and obstruction for seven to ten days. Daily dilation may be necessary for a few days to prevent closure. (Reprinted with permission from Slatter, D. H.: *Fundamentals of Veterinary Ophthalmology.* W. B. Saunders, Philadelphia, 1981.)

the atretic punctum may bulge, since the canaliculus may be filled with mucus or inflammatory debris from a low-grade dacryocystitis and canaliculitis. The site may be surrounded by a pigmented rim of conjunctiva with a nonpigmented center. If one punctum is present, it may be cannulated, and gentle flushing may permit a tenting up or slight ballooning of the conjunctiva at the site of the atretic punctum (Fig. 103–4). Retrograde catheterization from the nasal orifice may allow the catheter to push up against the conjunctiva as a landmark for incision. If the exact site cannot be determined, a 25-gauge hypodermic needle may be used.

A stab incision is made by sliding the needle parallel to the lid margin and penetrating the conjunctiva at the anticipated site of the punctum. Slight resistance is met going into the conjunctiva. If properly placed and if the canaliculus is present, the needle slides into the canaliculus. The needle should not be advanced more than the length of the point or the canaliculus may be lacerated. A surgical blade (e.g., #15 Bard-Parker) may be used to cut down onto the needle, or the needle may be used as a knife to slightly enlarge the opening. An alternative technique is to pick up the conjunctiva over the anticipated site of the opening and excise a 1 × 2 mm piece of conjunctiva with scissors. Minimal bleeding occurs with either of these techniques.

After establishing the punctal opening, the nasolacrimal system is flushed to expel any debris and confirm patency. Postoperative treatment consists of the use of a topical antibiotic corticosteroid solution three to four times daily for five to seven days. Tears should continue to flow through the new punctum, and patency should be maintained without further

surgery. In a small number of patients, two complications may occur: (1) the punctal opening may close with granulation tissue or cicatrix, necessitating reoperation; this is more likely if a concurrent infectious conjunctivitis is present or if infection is present in the canaliculus; or (2) epiphora may still be present when the drainage system does not have adequate functional capacity, even though the punctum is open and patency is established.[19]

If a new punctal opening is established and is not satisfactory (i.e., does not give the clinical impression of probable drainage), a monofilament nylon suture may be passed as previously described. A larger, polyethylene catheter is threaded over the monofilament nylon and pulled through the nasolacrimal system.[66,70] The nylon guide is removed and the

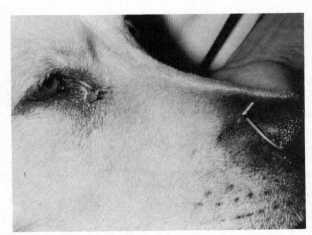

Figure 103–5. Polyethylene tubing sutured in place for treatment of dacryocystitis.

tubing is sutured in place at the nasal canthus and on the haired skin just posterior to the planum nasale (Fig. 103–5). This drainage tube remains in place for three to four weeks until the wounds have epithelialized and postsurgical inflammation has subsided.

Conjunctival membrane. A condition similar to congenital absence of the punctum occurs when a conjunctival membrane or flap is present over the punctum, providing a partial or complete obstruction. The treatment is similar to that previously described for establishing a punctal opening.

Stenotic punctum. Stenotic puncta are occasionally found in the Manx and Persian cat. Small, apparently hypoplastic or incomplete openings are seen in some dogs.[5] This may represent incomplete atresia of punctal openings. A lacrimal dilator, a blunt, taper-pointed instrument, may be introduced through the small punctum and gradually advanced into the canaliculus. The procedure may be repeated until the orifice is sufficiently dilated. Additionally, the punctum may be enlarged by excision. A one-, two-, or three-snip technique may be used immediately following dilation.[5,53,74] A canaliculus knife or scissors is gently inserted into the punctum while the eyelid is stretched laterally. The blade edge is parallel to the lid margin, and the incision is made horizontally through the posterior portion of the canaliculus for 1 to 2 mm (one-snip). The second (two-snip) and third (three-snip) cuts, if made, are performed with scissors and result in the removal of a triangular flap of conjunctiva (Fig. 103–6).

An alternative technique, utilizing juxtapunctal cautery, has been described in humans.[20] The aim is to create strictures that will contract and open the puncta. Follow-up care may not be necessary if an adequate opening is created; however, a nasolacrimal tube may be placed and sutured as previously described.

Misplaced punctum. Misplaced puncta are seen most commonly in brachycephalic breeds of dogs and less frequently in cats. Usually the misplaced punc-

tum is near the normal site but is 1 to 2 mm more medial or lateral and may be further from or closer to the eyelid margin. Animals with Waardenburg's syndrome or congenital blepharophimosis may have puncta that open more laterally than normal. Enlargement of the punctum by a three-snip procedure may increase the efficiency of the drainage system enough to eliminate the epiphora. Surgical repositioning of the punctum and proximal canaliculus may be accomplished after catheterization of the canal.[27] Alternatively, a blepharoplasty may be performed to increase the efficiency of the puncta in collecting tears. In most patients treatment is not necessary.

Supernumerary puncta are rare and incidental and usually do not have any associated functional alterations.

Atresia of canaliculi or lacrimal duct. The canaliculi or nasolacrimal duct may be obstructed by a membrane owing to failure of the facial fissure to close properly. This anomaly is usually associated with lethal defects. Rarely a dog is presented with a normal punctum and canaliculus but an obstruction of the bony canal. This condition requires surgery to establish communication between the nasolacrimal sac and the nasal cavity.

Eyelid abnormalities. Eyelid abnormalities include notching, entropion, ectropion, nasal folds, inferior medial entropion, and eyelid cicatrix. Malpositioned or misshapen eyelids are seen in many breeds of dogs. Irish setters, golden retrievers, and bloodhounds often have a slight to marked notch in the upper eyelid 3 to 4 mm from the nasal canthus. This notch may interfere with the function of the upper punctum and canaliculus. Eyelids that are notched are difficult to correct. Fortunately, in most cases the lower punctum is normal and epiphora is not present. Entropion and ectropion may alter the position of the lacrimal lake and puncta and may produce epiphora. Facial hairs touching the cornea produce increased lacrimation, which is exaggerated by faulty tear drainage. Standard surgical procedures (see Chapter 101) usually correct the defect and allow the punctum to return to normal position and function.

Inferior medial entropion is described as a specific disease process that causes epiphora.[57] Treatment calls for removal of a small, triangular wedge of skin just beneath the nasal portion of the lower eyelid. The most common error seen with this procedure is failure to remove enough skin to correct the entropion adequately.

TEAR STAINING SYNDROME

The tear staining syndrome is a clinical entity affecting several breeds of dogs and some cats. The characteristic appearance is chronic facial moisture and secondary staining of facial hairs. The nasolacrimal system is patent when flushed, but a functional blockage exists. The absence of obvious abnormalities or obstructions to drainage makes this condition a

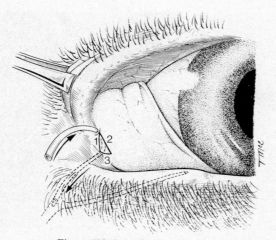

Figure 103–6. 1,2,3-snip procedure.

diagnostic enigma. Previous treatments of epiphora have included medical and surgical techniques.[6,10,11,21,32–39,42,62,76]

Medical treatment of tear staining. Epiphora has been palliatively managed with topical creams and pastes to protect the facial hair and skin but without success. One medical approach is based on a theory that tetracyclines may bind with circulating porphyrins[32,68] or lactoferrin-like pigments[70] and prevent hair staining. The face remains wet but the hair is not stained; therefore the tear staining is less noticeable. Another medical treatment is based on the concept that affected dogs have a chronic low-grade inflammation of the nasal or pharyngeal area and tonsils.[10, 11] This inflammation could produce edema of the nasolacrimal system and lead to functional blockage. Systemic and topical treatment with antibiotics and corticosteroids for two weeks is required to improve most patients. Recurrences may be expected, and some consideration may be given to tonsillectomy.

Surgical treatment of tear staining. A histological study of 91 glands of the third eyelid was performed on glands obtained from 47 dogs with epiphora.[46] The results were not correlated with clinical signs, suggesting that the gland of the third eyelid is not responsible for epiphora and that the benefit derived by removing the gland is a reduction of the total tear volume. Surgical removal of the gland of the third eyelid effectively reduces the tear volume by up to 50 per cent. This relatively simple procedure should not be attempted unless the Schirmer tear values are known to exceed 20 mm in 60 seconds.* The potential for keratoconjunctivitis sicca and its consequences

---

*Editor's note: Some authors recommend 14 mm.

should be thoroughly discussed and explained prior to using this approach to control epiphora.

In small breeds of dogs and cats with epiphora, the orbits are shallow and the globes are prominent. Close examination reveals an absence of a lacrimal lake and poor eyelid closure during blinking. Hence, the tears may not be propelled to the puncta and into the canaliculi. Surgery has been suggested to reduce the tautness of the eyelids and allow the formation of a lacrimal lake.[16] The technique involves grasping the nasal canthus and applying gentle anterior and lateral traction. At the same time, a small stab incision is made through the conjunctiva near the mucocutaneous junction of the nasal canthus. Small tenotomy scissors are advanced into the conjunctival incision, and the nasal canthal ligamentous support is transected. The conjunctival wound is closed with a 6-0 absorbable suture. Care must be used to avoid the canaliculi; catheterization prior to surgery will help identify them. If the large vessels that cross the nasal rim of the orbit are damaged, hemorrhage may result and produce subconjunctival and retrobulbar accumulations of blood.

Hair may grow from the nasal canthus when a plaque of skin extends beyond the normal limits of the mucocutaneous junction of the nasal canthus. The hairs cause corneal irritation and serve as wicks for the tears. If facial staining and constant moisture persist on the face, the offending tissue may be excised. Sutures are not usually necessary, but if they are placed, care should be used to avoid excessive tension that would alter the position or function of the punctum and canaliculi. In a similar procedure, the dermal tissue is dissected from the conjunctiva and the margins are bluntly undermined, exposing the medial palpebral ligament (Fig. 103–7).[13] The

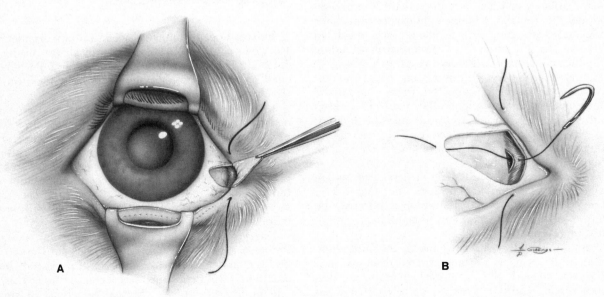

A **B**

Figure 103–7. Sliding conjunctival flap for treatment of dermoid. *A*, The dermis is dissected off and a conjunctival flap is created. *B*, The sliding flap is sutured to the edge of the medial palpebral ligament with one or two simple interrupted sutures of 5-0 Vicryl. (Reprinted with permission from Slatter, D. H.: *Fundamentals of Veterinary Ophthalmology.* W. B. Saunders, Philadelphia, 1981.)

exposed margin of the ligament is freed from the nasal bone. A 6-0 absorbable suture attaches the cut edge of the conjunctiva to the margin of the medial palpebral ligament. This procedure may have the additional benefit of increasing the size of the lacrimal lake.

As previously described, several types of congenital anomalies may be responsible for altered drainage of tears. Often, more than one defect is present and multiple procedures may be required to correct the epiphora. In a few patients, it may be impossible to establish a consistent balance between tear production and tear removal, and some epiphora is permanent.

ACQUIRED ANOMALIES OF TEAR OUTFLOW

Spastic entropion. Proper eyelid position and function are essential for even distribution and removal of tears. Inward rolling of the eyelid stimulates lacrimation, alters the position of the puncta, and inhibits normal function. Surgical correction of entropion is necessary to restore eyelid function and normal tear outflow.

Cicatricial entropion. Old wounds or infected tissues around the eyelid may lead to scar formation and may inhibit eyelid movement. The scar tissue must be freed and the eyelid function restored to regain normal function of the lacrimal system.

Blepharitis. Swelling of the eyelids may result from systemic or localized disease processes. Insect bites and local injury may produce enough hemorrhage and edema to alter eyelid and lacrimal function. Each condition must be treated appropriately to restore normal function of the lacrimal outflow apparatus.

Conjunctivitis. Acquired occlusion of the punctum may result in epiphora. Conjunctival infections or inflammation may cause edema and thickening and occlude the puncta. Chemical injury or infections associated with conjunctival ulcers may result in scarring of the punctum or a symblepharon occluding the punctum. In cats with upper respiratory diseases, e.g., herpesvirus, the symblepharon may be extensive. If the third eyelid is affected, there is additional interference with the proper movement of the tears to the punctum. These adhesions may be incised, but often reform postoperatively. This permanent alteration often results in epiphora, even though patency may be established.

Folliculosis. Extensive follicle or papule formation may inhibit tear flow and occlude the punctum in young dogs. The etiology is unknown but may be allergic. Appropriate treatment of the follicles eliminates the epiphora.

Autoimmune disease. Erosions of the mucocutaneous junction, as in the pemphigoid diseases, may be associated with closure of the punctum and epiphora. Each condition must be correctly diagnosed and treated specifically. Once under control, the patency of the nasolacrimal system may be established as previously described with stents and tubing.

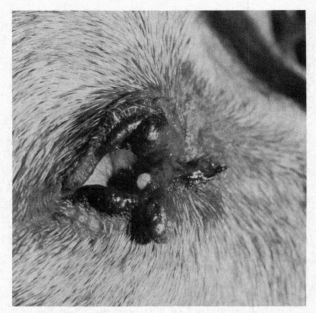

Figure 103–8. Multiple melanomas of the eyelids in a Vizsla.

The creation of a new drainage pathway may be considered if patency cannot be established.

Neoplasia. Neoplastic tissue involving the eyelids may interfere with normal eyelid function or may obstruct the punctum and create epiphora. The result is a thick eyelid margin, alteration of eyelid function, and punctal occlusion (Fig. 103–8). Techniques for the treatment of medial canthal tumors have been described.[13] The goal of treatment is to remove the tumor and maintain lacrimal drainage.

ACQUIRED OCCLUSION OF THE CANALICULI, SAC, OR NASOLACRIMAL DUCT

Idoxuridine. In humans, occlusion of a canaliculus has been caused by prolonged topical use of idoxuridine.[53] This side effect has not been reported in small animals but should be considered if idoxuridine therapy is used over long periods.

Upper respiratory infections. In small animals, occlusion of the nasolacrimal system may follow several disease processes. Upper respiratory infections in cats and chronic bacterial infections can extend into the canaliculus and nasolacrimal sac. Often the primary disease responds to appropriate treatment, but organisms may remain in the isolated sac, and reinfection is possible. Repeated flushing with antibiotic/steroid combinations is indicated.

Dacryocystitis. Dacryocystitis is inflammation of the nasolacrimal sac. Chronic, low-grade dacryocystitis is characterized by epiphora and persistent conjunctivitis. In man, this has been described as a "silent dacryocystitis."[75] Typical infections in small animals result in epiphora with a mucoid to mucopurulent discharge from the lower punctum. The discharge has a stringy nature and often contains bubbles. Digital pressure over the nasal canthus may result in extrusion of material from the upper and lower puncta. Chronic infections have an associated canaliculitis. The punctum may be elevated and hyperemic, with the appearance of granulating tissue. The most severe signs are usually evident in the lower punctum and canaliculus. Pain may be present over the sac, but rarely can a detectable swelling of the sac be seen. Dacryocystitis usually results from single or multiple foreign bodies lodging in the canaliculus, sac, or duct.

The treatment for dacryocystitis is establishment of patency by mechanical flushing and removal of foreign material and debris.[54] Long-standing cases are difficult to catheterize, and a complete evaluation, including culturing of the exudate and dacryocystorhinography, is necessary. Localized bony involvement of the sac may be encountered. Periosteal reaction may narrow or occlude the lumen and prevent catheterization. If a catheter cannot be passed, repeated efforts using a smaller diameter monofilament nylon suture are indicated. Once the catheter is in place, a larger polyethylene tube is threaded and passed (see previous discussion). As the polyethylene tube is passed over the suture, resistance may be encountered at the sac and considerable effort may be required to force a channel through obstructing fibrous tissue. Some hemorrhage is expected and is self-limiting. Once the polyethylene catheter is placed, it is not removed until the disease is controlled. Inadvertent or premature removal may lead to re-obstruction or considerable difficulty in recatheterization. Follow-up care consists of appropriate topical antibiotic solutions, but systemic antibiotics may be warranted.

Dacryolith. Dacryoliths in humans are often associated with mycotic infections, but this is rarely encountered in small animals.[53] Most concretions are semirigid and can be broken up by catheterization and flushing. If a solid concretion is encountered, a dacryocystotomy may be indicated (see Dacryocystorhinostomy).

Mucocele. Mucocele of the lacrimal sac is rare but may be either congenital or acquired. Facial swelling by a fluctuating mass over the lacrimal sac with minimal pain and an absence of signs of infection suggest a mucocele. Radiographs may assist in the diagnosis. I have treated such a mucocele by needle aspiration of the sac and catheterization with tubing. There was no recurrence during the subsequent two years.

Neoplasia. Primary neoplasia of the canaliculus, sac, or duct is rare. Local involvement may occur from extension of primary nasal tumors.[28] Metastatic tumors have been located in the sac (Fig. 103–9), orbit, sinuses, or nasal passages. Palpation of the rim of the orbit and the region of the lacrimal sac reveals a firm mass that is not usually painful and that must be differentiated from a mucocele. Clinically, the neoplastic tissue mass is hard and not fluctuant, as is a mucocele. Treatment involves appropriate therapy

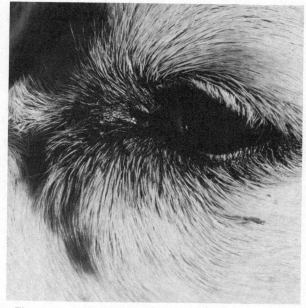

Figure 103–9. Metastatic adenocarcinoma of the lacrimal sac.

directed at the primary tumor. Local dissection and removal are possible and are indicated for histopathological evaluation and prognosis. It may be possible to remove the mass from the area of the sac and observe the opening in the lacrimal bone for the nasolacrimal duct. If the punctum is catheterized, the catheter can be pulled through the cut end of the canaliculus, threaded into the bony canal, and sutured in place. If the bony canal is not visible, a dacryocystorhinostomy may be performed to enhance drainage.

Lacerations. Superficial lacerations of the conjunctiva may involve the punctum or canaliculus. If only the punctum is damaged, it is unlikely that sufficient scarring will occur to produce epiphora. If the canaliculus is lacerated, however, surgical repair is indicated. Passage of a monofilament nylon suture from the punctum into the lacerated end is possible by visual inspection in some patients. In others, the distal portion is not visible until nasal (retrograde) passage is accomplished. Since about 50 per cent of dogs have an accessory opening, it may be impossible for the suture to follow the nasolacrimal duct out through the cut end. If the suture does pass, it is usually easy to thread the previously identified proximal end out through the punctum. If it cannot be catheterized, retrograde flushing may permit a stream of fluid to identify the cut end. Boiled milk has been suggested as a good flushing solution, as it is colored and will not stain tissues.[79] Pigtail probes (Worst) are available with hook ends or eyeholes and may assist in identifying the cut ends of the canaliculus and passing catheters (Fig. 103–10).[9,70] The use of pigtail probes is controversial in man, since some canalicular damage may result from the manipulations. Once the canaliculus is catheterized, a single,

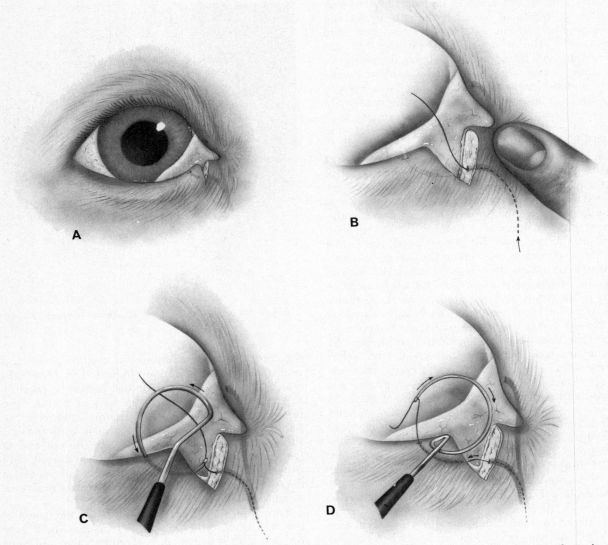

Figure 103–10. Nasolacrimal catheterization for canalicular laceration. *A*, Laceration of lid margin and canaliculus. *B*, A fine nylon (e.g., 2-0) thread is passed up the nasolacrimal duct from the nose. The superior punctum from which it normally emerges is occluded by finger pressure, and the thread is manipulated to emerge from the severed inferior canaliculus. *C*, A Worst probe is passed, and the suture is tied to it and pulled through the punctum *(D)*. (Reprinted with permission from Slatter, D. H.: *Fundamentals of Veterinary Ophthalmology.* W. B. Saunders, Philadelphia, 1981.)

simple interrupted suture of a 7-0 absorbable material is placed through the deep tissue below the canaliculus (Fig. 103–11). A second suture is placed above the canaliculus in a similar fashion, and a 4-0 suture is placed full thickness from skin to conjunctiva and back out to skin to complete the closure. Sutures are not placed directly through the canaliculus.[61] The tube should be left in place for 12 weeks in dogs to assure healing without stricture.[73]

SURGICAL CREATION OF A NEW DRAINAGE APPARATUS

Dacryocystorhinostomy. A dacryocystorhinostomy may be used in patients with an obstructed sac or canal. A skin incision is made parallel to the nose

and 2 to 3 mm medial to the nasal canthus. The incision continues ventrally 2 cm over the sac. The exact position of the sac is determined by palpation of the inferior rim of the orbit. The incision should be full thickness through the skin but not so deep as to injure the large vessels. The skin and vessels are retracted, and the sac is identified. If the sac is redundant and not readily visible, palpation of the maxillary bone and lacrimal bones may reveal the lacrimal crest and fossa; catheterization of the canaliculi may "point" to the junction of the upper and lower canaliculi. A bone drill or trephine is used to enter the bone at the level of the sac.

At this point in human patients, an attempt is made to suture the nasal mucosa to the sac and thereby create a continuous epithelium-lined channel for outflow.[82] Failure to do so results in uncontrolled

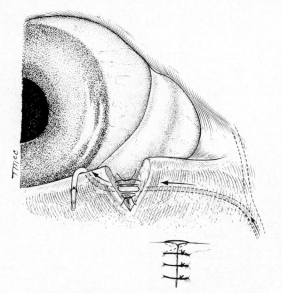

Figure 103–11. Closure of canalicular laceration.

granulation and eventual closure of the duct. In small animals this procedure has not been described. It is difficult to identify the sac, and it would be extremely difficult to suture it to the nasal mucosa. Therefore, in dogs and cats, the largest size polyethylene tubing that will pass through the punctum and canaliculus should be threaded through the new bony canal and sutured in place as described for dacryocystitis. The catheter should be left in place for at least four months to ensure continued patency. Continued evaluation of the tubing is necessary. In the event of loss, it should be replaced immediately.

Conjunctivorhinostomy. Conjunctivorhinostomy has been used for the treatment of obstruction of the lacrimal duct in dogs.[47] A skin incision is made 1 cm from the nasal canthus and beneath the medial palpebral ligament (Fig. 103–12). The incision is extended to 3 cm parallel to the inferior orbital rim and is continued down through the orbicularis muscle, exposing the periosteum of the maxilla. The lacrimal crest is palpated, and the periosteum is incised and elevated for 1.5 cm anterior to the crest. An 8- to 10-mm diameter trephine is placed over the bone after the periosteum is retracted and the maxillary sinus is entered. I prefer to use a bone drill to enter the sinus. Part of the lacrimal crest is removed using small rongeurs. This ensures a smooth channel with a straight entrance from the nasal canthus. A rectangular block of buccal mucosa is removed from the mouth and sutured around a polyethylene tube with the mucosal surface in contact with the tube. The tube is then guided over a Bowman's lacrimal probe for support. A #11 scalpel blade is used to make a stab incision from the nasal canthal conjunctiva down to the trephined opening. The mucosal graft with polyethylene tube is threaded from the conjunctival wound down to the trephined portal. The mucosal graft should lie in the new bony canal without bend-

ing or strictures. The mucosal graft should be firmly sutured to the periosteum with absorbable sutures and flushed with saline to ensure patency. The skin wound is closed, but the tubing should be left in place as long as possible to increase the chances of a mucosa-lined fistula resulting.

Method of Covitz. In the technique described by Covitz, Hunziker, and Koch, a small Steinmann pin is directed ventromedially into the orbital rim toward the nasal cavity (Fig. 103–13).[17] The pin is aimed at the ipsilateral external nares, with the shaft of the pin and handle lying on the dorsolateral orbital rim. The globe is slightly depressed by the shaft of the pin. A series of larger pins is used until one larger than the outside diameter of the catheter to be placed is used. The tract should be flushed with saline prior to catheterization. Either polyethylene or Silastic tubing may be used in lengths of 2.5 to 3.8 cm. A flanged end or rim should be applied to the tubing and is used to suture the tubing in place at the mucocutaneous junction of the nasal canthus. If the tubing does not slide easily into place, nasal mucosal folds may be obstructing the bony opening and can be flushed out of the way. The tube can be guided into place if it is threaded onto a malleable probe, which adds some rigidity.

A topical antibiotic/steroid ointment is applied three times daily for three to four days and then once daily until the tubing is removed. The tube should be flushed at least once weekly. The sutures are removed two weeks after surgery; however, the tubing is left in place for at least eight weeks. Premature removal results in overgrowth of the canal with granulating tissue. If the tube is accidentally lost it should be replaced immediately. The actual relief of epiphora is usually not noticed until after the final tube is removed. If tubing with a flange or collar is not available, the surgeon may suture polyethylene tubing to the skin of the face and at the exit of the nares as described previously for other conditions.

Conjunctivobuccostomy. Conjunctivobuccostomy has been described as an alternative surgical procedure for the treatment of epiphora due to obstructed canaliculi (Fig. 103–14).[27] The technique is much simpler than dacryocystorhinostomy, conjunctivorhinostomy, or the method of Covitz because bone is not involved. A stab incision is made through the conjunctiva of the lower fornix, and a tunnel is bluntly created downward until the oral mucosa can be entered between the lip and the upper dental arcade. Care should be taken to avoid injuring the opening of the parotid duct near the upper fourth premolar tooth. Polyethylene tubing is placed into the canal and sutured at the conjunctival and oral ends. The tube should be left in place for a minimum of two months to ensure epithelialization of the tract and permanent fistulization. Postoperative care includes daily administration of topical antibiotics and steroids.

The previously described procedures are commonly complicated by closure of the newly created outflow channel, and the client must be informed of the care and potential complications. Only an expe-

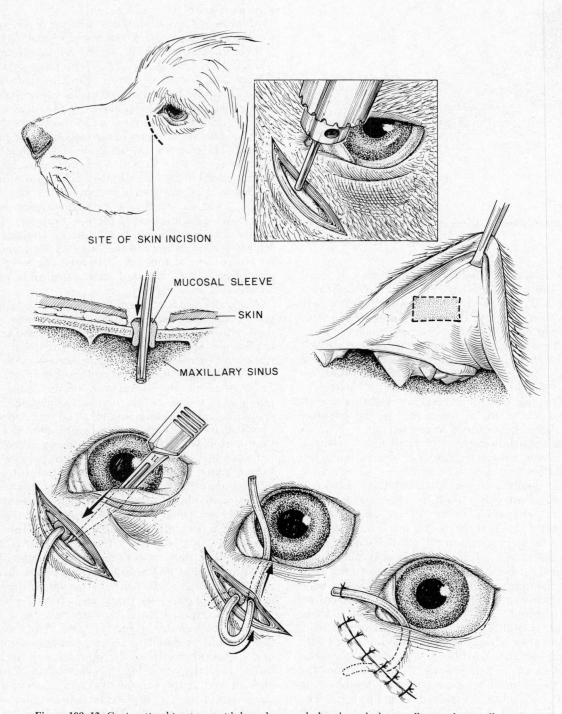

SITE OF SKIN INCISION

MUCOSAL SLEEVE

SKIN

MAXILLARY SINUS

Figure 103–12. Conjunctivorhinostomy with buccal mucosal plug through the maxilla into the maxillary sinus.

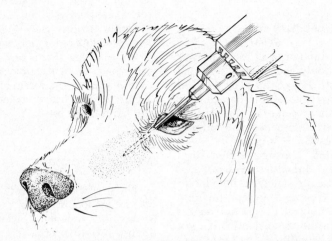

Figure 103–13. Position of pin and chuck to create a new outflow channel.

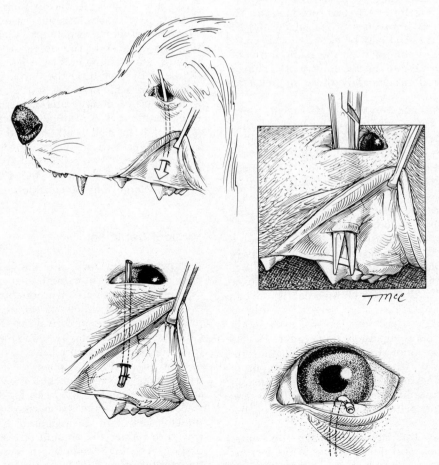

Figure 103–14. Conjunctivobuccostomy.

rienced ophthalmic surgeon should attempt any of these procedures.

DEFICIENCY OF PRECORNEAL TEAR FILM

Diseases resulting in reduction or absence of precorneal tear film are commonly encountered in small animals. Fortunately, most cases of dry eyes respond to medical treatment and are transient in nature. The following discussion presents some of the known causes of keratoconjunctivitis sicca in small animals and the surgical approaches for treatment.

Premature eyelid opening. During the first 10 to 14 days of neonatal life the immature eyes of small animals are protected by a physiological ankyloblepharon. After the eyelids separate, lacrimal function is evident. Premature opening of the eyelid results in keratoconjunctivitis sicca, since lacrimation has not begun. Fortunately, this condition is rarely reported.[3,22,25]

Infectious conjunctivitis. Several disease processes may result in damage to the tear-producing glands and cells. Chronic infection of the conjunctiva by any microorganism may result in changes in the epithelium and may interfere with tear production. The emptying channels from the lacrimal gland and the gland of the third eyelid may be closed or obliterated by scarring of the conjunctiva. Local disease processes such as an abscess or a cellulitis may damage the lacrimal gland. Fortunately these sequelae are uncommon.

Systemic disease. Systemic diseases such as canine distemper may cause adenitis of the lacrimal gland and gland of the third eyelid, which may result in transient or permanent disability. Feline upper respiratory diseases characterized by conjunctival ulcers and symblepharon may occlude the ducts from the glands.

Drug-induced deficiency. Many systemic pharmacological agents, including urinary analgesics, sulfonamides, and parasympatholytic drugs, reduce tear production.[1,3,12,48,69,71,72,77] Permanent damage may result following long-term treatment with these drugs. Some dogs maintained on sulfonamides (e.g., boxers treated with sulfasalazine for chronic colitis) develop keratoconjunctivitis sicca after several months or years without signs of previous lacrimal dysfunction.

Antidiarrheal parasympatholytic (neomycin sulfate and methylscopolamine bromide) combinations reduce tear volume. In most patients treatment for diarrhea is short-term and tear reduction is transient. The reduced tear volume may not be clinically manifested unless the patient already has reduced tear production.

Trauma. Head trauma may damage the central nervous system or local nerve supply to the lacrimal gland and reduce tear production. Parasympathomimetic stimulation with topical or oral pilocarpine may result in a marked increase in tear production in such cases.[63,67]

Neoplasia. Any neoplasm of the central nervous system or orbit may decrease tear production. Usually, other signs of disease are present, such as head tilt, facial paralysis, and ataxia.

Senile atrophy. Senile atrophy of the lacrimal gland may occur in older pets with chronic keratoconjunctivitis and low Schirmer values in the absence of other primary ocular or systemic disease. Microscopic examination of the lacrimal glands from old dogs with hyposecretion has revealed a nonspecific atrophy of the lacrimal gland.

Medical Treatment

The medical treatment of keratoconjunctivitis sicca has been documented.[63,67] Topical antibiotics, corticosteroids, mucolytic agents, and parasympathomimetics are all useful. The usual recommendation is topical treatment for two to three weeks, followed by re-evaluation. If the Schirmer tear values have not improved, oral pilocarpine therapy is instigated. One drop of a 2 per cent pilocarpine solution for each 5 kg of body weight is applied to food twice daily. Every three days the dose is increased by one drop until signs of gastrointestinal stimulation, including excessive drooling, eructation, diarrhea, and vomiting, are produced. The dosage is adjusted for each patient, maintaining oral treatment for a minimum of 30 days. By that time the cumulative action of the pilocarpine will have elicited a response from the lacrimal glands if any functional gland remains. Topical treatment is continued throughout this course. The initial topical treatment and combined topical and systemic treatment are continued for a total of six to eight weeks. If sequential Schirmer tear values have not indicated improvement by this time, surgical treatment may be considered.

Surgical Treatment

Punctal occlusion.* The simplest surgical procedure is performed in patients that are not completely dry and have limited tear production. The puncta are occluded, and as much of the tears as possible is preserved in the conjunctival sac. The puncta can be closed with sutures or by touching a heated spatula to the orifice. Diathermy has also been reported as a method of closing the puncta.[74] In my experience with punctal closure, the clinical benefits are minimal and do not eliminate the need for other treatments.

Permanent partial tarsorrhaphy. In addition to punctal occlusion, the palpebral fissure can be narrowed to reduce the amount of tears lost from evaporation. The best technique is a canthoplasty at the temporal canthus.[40] The conjunctival flap is prepared

---

*Editor's note: The use of punctal occlusion is of controversial effectiveness in animals.

from the upper tarsal conjunctiva and is pulled into an opening created at the lower eyelid margin. The upper and lower eyelid margins are excised adjacent to this flap, and the skin edges are sutured together. The flap supplies the additional support, which, if not utilized, may result in wound dehiscence.

Parotid duct transposition. For dogs and cats with no measurable tear volume and chronic keratocon-junctivitis that has not responded to medical treatment, parotid duct transposition may be used.[7,31,44,66,67] Prior to surgery, medical treatment is necessary to ensure complete loss of lacrimal function. Presurgical culturing and sensitivity testing and proper antibiotic therapy are mandatory. The client must be well informed of the disease process, the alternative use of topical therapy instead of surgery,

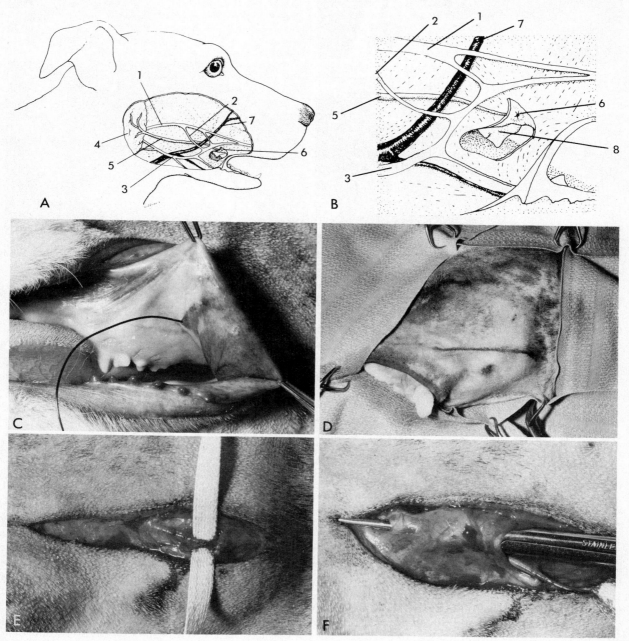

Figure 103–15. Parotid duct transposition. *A* and *B*, Cutaway diagram of the face *(A)* and enlargement of area where duct enters mouth *(B)*. Dorsal buccal nerve *(1)*; anastomosis of dorsal and ventral buccal nerves *(2)*; ventral buccal nerve *(3)*; parotid salivary gland *(4)*; parotid duct *(5)*; papilla of parotid duct *(6)*; facial vein *(7)*; upper carnassial tooth *(8)*. *C*, Monofilament nylon suture marker in place in the parotid duct. *D*, Pledget of cotton soaked with 1:750 aqueous benzalkonium chloride placed over the parotid duct papilla. The course of the duct is marked on the skin. *E*, Umbilical tape passed beneath parotid duct so that the duct can be manipulated without damaging it with forceps. *F*, Completed dissection beneath the facial vein and branches of buccal nerve with blunt scissors.

Illustration continued on following page

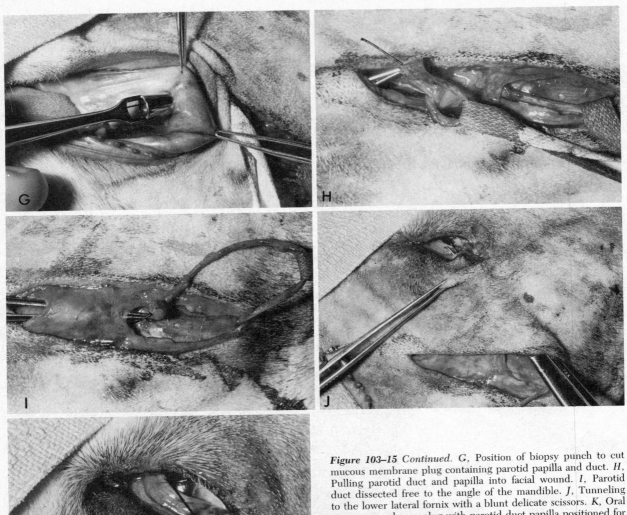

Figure 103–15 Continued. *G,* Position of biopsy punch to cut mucous membrane plug containing parotid papilla and duct. *H,* Pulling parotid duct and papilla into facial wound. *I,* Parotid duct dissected free to the angle of the mandible. *J,* Tunneling to the lower lateral fornix with a blunt delicate scissors. *K,* Oral mucous membrane plug with parotid duct papilla positioned for suturing to the conjunctiva. (Reprinted with permission from Severin, G. A.: Keratoconjunctivitis sicca. Vet. Clin. North Am. 3:407, 1973.)

and what to expect following surgery. Only an experienced surgeon should perform this procedure. Two approaches to the transposition have been used.

Open approach. The open technique was described first and is preferred by some ophthalmic surgeons because the structures are completely visible (Fig. 103–15).[31,44,67,70] Following catheterization, the duct is palpated through the skin over the masseter muscles. A skin incision is made directly over the duct for 2 to 5 cm, depending on the size of the dog. The incision is carefully continued down to the duct, and the duct is isolated and retracted by applying a loop of umbilical tape around the duct. The loop allows manipulation of the duct without forceps, which may damage the duct. The duct is freed from the tissues posterior to the parotid gland. The overlying tissues

are dissected from the duct with care and patience. The surgeon should avoid transecting the branches of the buccal nerves when possible. The duct passes beneath the superficial facial vein, which is also avoided. Accidental incision of the vein produces hemorrhage and necessitates ligation. The deep side of the duct is not freed from its attachments at this point. Careful dissection is continued until the duct enters the oral mucosa. The last centimeter prior to the duct's entrance into the oral cavity is difficult to dissect, as the duct lies tightly adherent to the oral mucosa. The lip is retracted and a 6-mm Keyes skin biopsy punch is used to outline the oral mucosa around the papilla. The punch is rotated gently, with its greatest pressure anteriorly as the duct lies just under the mucosa posteriorly. Too much pressure will transect the duct. The papilla is cut free from the remaining mucosal attachments with small scissors. Once the papilla is completely freed, it is passed back through the canal under the superficial facial vein and into the skin incision. Some additional dissecting may be performed from the deeper side of the duct to free it from muscular fascia. Scissors are directed from the skin incision to the lower conjunctival cul-de-sac, and the conjunctiva is entered between the lateral margin of the third and lower eyelids. This pathway lies on the fascia of the masseter muscle and should not be placed at other levels. The papilla and free duct are carried through the canal, and the papilla is sutured in place with six to eight 7-0 absorbable sutures. The skin and oral wounds are closed in a routine fashion.

Closed approach. The closed technique involves working through an oral incision only and is not described further here.[41]

Immediate postoperative care consists of systemic and topical antibiotic therapy for five days. Several small meals during each day stimulate parotid flow (a small blood clot can be milked from the duct through the skin the first postoperative day). Proper flow must be ascertained immediately to correct any complications (see hereafter). The major postoperative complication is failure of the duct to function.[4,8,33,65] This is usually due to a twisting of the duct during surgery. Preoperative catheterization and careful placement of the transposed duct reduce this complication. Postsurgical stricture may impede the flow of saliva at any time after surgery. Strictures probably result from poor dissection of the duct or rough handling of the tissues, which stimulates more fibrosis. Uncontrolled conjunctival infections may also lead to fibrosis and closure of the duct.[65] If a duct fails to function, it should be catheterized and evaluated for patency. If a stricture is found, the duct is surgically exposed and examined. When a stricture is near the papilla, the duct may be transected below the stricture and the cut end of the duct sutured into the conjunctival sac. If a stricture occurs further from the papilla, the duct may not be of sufficient length to reach the conjunctival sac and a surgical solution may be impossible.

Complications of parotid duct transposition. Immediate complications of parotid duct transposition include nonfunctioning parotid gland, twisting or kinking of the duct, bending around a vessel or nerve, and suturing through the duct. Delayed complications include slippage of papilla into subcutaneous tissues, stricture formation, skin maceration, and solid deposits on the cornea and eyelids.

Skin infections resulting from maceration by saliva are a potential problem, and it may be necessary to apply petrolatum or other ointment around the eyelids to protect the skin. When maceration occurs, it is usually transient, since the volume of saliva seems to decrease with time. The hair should be kept short around the eyelids to reduce the amount of retained moisture. A few dogs have a continuous large volume of saliva accumulation on the eyelids and face. In two dogs the owners requested reversal or ligation of the parotid duct, since the facial dermatitis and treatment were considered more objectionable than the medical treatment for the dry eyes. Another potential complication is the appearance of chalklike deposits on the eyelid margins and on and in the cornea.[67] The material in the deposits may be irritating and may require a superficial corneal abrasion and the use of EDTA to remove them. Periodic use of mucolytic agents (Acetylcysteine) prevents the accumulation of deposits.

1. Aguirre, G.: Keratoconjunctivitis sicca caused by sulfadiazine. J. Am. Vet. Med. Assoc. *162*:8, 1973.
2. Aguirre, G., and Rubin, L. F.: Ophthalmitis secondary to congenitally open eyelids in a dog. J. Am. Vet. Med. Assoc. *156*:70, 1970.
3. Aguirre, G. D., Rubin, L. F., and Harvey, C. E.: Keratoconjunctivitis sicca in dogs. J. Am. Vet. Med. Assoc. *158*:1566, 1971.
4. Baker, G. J., and Formston, C.: An evaluation of transplantation of the parotid duct in the treatment of keratoconjunctivitis sicca in the dog. J. Small Anim. Pract. *9*:261, 1968.
5. Barnett, K. C.: Imperforate and microlachrymal puncta in the dog. J. Small Anim. Pract. *20*:481, 1979.
6. Deleted in press.
7. Bennett, J. E.: The management of total xerophthalmia. Trans. Am. Ophthalmol. Soc. *66*:503, 1968.
8. Betts, D. M., and Helper, L. C.: The surgical correction of parotid duct transposition failures. J. Am. Anim. Hosp. Assoc. *13*:695, 1977.
9. Billson, F. A., Taylor, H. R., and Hoyt, C. S.: Trauma to the lacrimal system in children. Am. J. Ophthalmol. *86*:828, 1978.
10. Bryan, G. M.: Diseases of the nasolacrimal system. *In* Kirk, R. W. (ed.); *Current Veterinary Therapy VI*. W. B. Saunders, Philadelphia, 1977, pp. 618–624.
11. Bryan, G. M., and Michelson, E.: Epiphora in the poodle. West. Vet. *16*:13, 1978.
12. Bryan, G. M., and Slatter, D. H.: Keratoconjunctivitis sicca induced by phenazopyridine in dogs. Arch. Ophthalmol. *90*:310, 1973.
13. Carter, J. D.: Reconstructive surgery for juxtapunctal neoplasms of the lower eyelid. J. Am. Vet. Med. Assoc. *157*:199, 1970.
14. Carter, J. D.: Medial conjunctivoplasty for aberrant dermis of the Lhasa Apso. J. Am. Anim. Hosp. Assoc. *9*:242, 1973.
15. Chang, S. H., and Lin, A. C.: Effects of main lacrimal gland and third eyelid gland removal on the eye of dogs. J. Chinese Soc. Vet. Sci. *6*:13, 1970.
16. Covitz, D.: Diseases of the lacrimal apparatus. *In* Kirk, R. W. (ed.): *Current Veterinary Therapy VII*, W. B. Saunders, Philadelphia, 1980, pp. 553–558.
17. Covitz, D., Hunziker, J., and Koch, S. A.: Conjunctivorhinostomy: a surgical method for the control of epiphora in the dog and cat. J. Am. Vet. Med. Assoc. *171*:251, 1977.
18. Diesem, C.: Organ of vision. *In* Getty, R. (ed.): *Sisson and Grossman's The Anatomy of Domestic Animals*, 5th ed. W. B. Saunders, Philadelphia, 1975.
19. Duke-Elder, S., and MacFaul, P. A.: The ocular adnexa. *In: System of Ophthalmology*, Vol. 13. H. Kimpton, London, 1974.
20. Fein W.: Cautery applications to relieve punctal stenosis. Arch. Ophthalmol. *95*:145, 1977.
21. Filipek, M. E., and Rubin, L. F.: Effect of metronidazole on lacrimation in the dog: a negative report. J. Am. Anim. Hosp. Assoc. *13*:339, 1977.
22. Fox, M. W.: Congenitally opened eyelids in the dog. Mod. Vet. Pract. *46*:88, 1965.

23. Fried, J. J., and Goldzieher, M. A.: The endocrine treatment of keratoconjunctivitis sicca. Am. J. Ophthalmol. 27:1003, 1944.

24. Gelatt, K. N.: Pediatric ophthalmology. Vet. Clin. North Am. 3:321, 1973.

25. Gelatt, K. N.: Premature eyelid opening and exposure keratitis in a puppy. Vet. Med./Sm. Anim. Clin. 69:863, 1974.

26. Gelatt, K. N., Cure, T. H., Guffy, M. M., and Jessen, C.: Dacryocystorhinography in the dog and cat. J. Small Anim. Pract. 13:381, 1972.

27. Gelatt, K. N., and Gwin, R. M.: Canine lacrimal and nasolacrimal systems. In Gelatt, K. N. (ed.): Veterinary Ophthalmology. Lea and Febiger, Philadelphia, 1981, pp. 309–329.

28. Gelatt, K. N., Ladds, P. W., and Guffy, M. M.: Nasal adenocarcinoma with orbital extension and ocular metastasis in a dog. J. Am. Anim. Hosp. Assoc. 6:132, 1970.

29. Gelatt, K. N., Peiffer, R. L., Erickson, J. L., and Gum, G. G.: Evaluation of tear formation in the dog, using a modification of the Schirmer tear test. J. Am. Vet. Med. Assoc. 166:368, 1975.

30. Getty, R.: The eye, orbit, and adnexa. In Miller, M. E., Christensen, G. C., and Evans, H. E. (eds.): Anatomy of the Dog. W. B. Saunders, Philadelphia, 1964.

31. Gwin, R. M., Gelatt, K. N., and Peiffer, R. L.: Parotid duct transposition in a cat with keratoconjunctivitis sicca. J. Am. Anim. Hosp. Assoc. 13:42, 1977.

32. Harrison, V. A.: Letter to the editor. Vet. Rec. 76:437, 1964.

33. Harvey, C. E., and Koch, S. A.: Surgical complications of parotid transposition in the dog. J. Am. Anim. Hosp. Assoc. 7:122, 1971.

34. Harvey, C. E., Koch, S. A., and Rubin, L. F.: Orbital cyst with conjunctival fistula in a dog. J. Am. Vet. Med. Assoc. 153:1432, 1968.

35. Hayes, K. C.: Vitamin A. In: Nutritional Management of Dogs and Cats. Ralston-Purina Company, St. Louis, 1975.

36. Helper, L. C.: The effect of lacrimal gland removal on the conjunctiva and cornea of the dog. J. Am. Vet. Med. Assoc. 157:72, 1970.

37. Helper, L. C., Magrane, W. G., Koehm, J., and Johnson, R.: Surgical induction of keratoconjunctivitis sicca in the dog. J. Am. Vet. Med. Assoc. 165:172, 1974.

38. Holly, F. J., and Lemp, M. A.: Tear physiology and dry eyes. Surv. Ophthalmol. 22:69, 1977.

39. Howard, D. R.: The surgical correction of epiphora. Vet. Med./Sm. Anim. Clin. 1969.

40. Jenssen, H. E.: Canthus closure. Comp. Cont. Ed. 1:735, 1979.

41. Jenssen, H. E.: Keratitis sicca and parotid duct transposition. Comp. Cont. Ed. 1:721, 1979.

42. Kerpsack, R. W., and Kerpsack, W. R.: The orbital gland and tear staining in the dog. Vet. Med./Sm. Anim. Clin. 61:121, 1966.

43. Kuhns, E. L., and Keller, W. F.: Effects of postsurgical ligation of the transposed parotid duct. Vet. Med./Sm. Anim. Clin. 74:515, 1979.

44. Lavignette, A. M.: Keratoconjunctivitis sicca in a dog treated by transposition of a parotid salivary duct. J. Am. Vet. Med. Assoc. 148:778, 1966.

45. Leopold, I. H. (ed.): The Lacrimal Apparatus, Monograph I, The Dry Eye, Tear Film and Dry Eye Syndromes. Office Seminars in Ophthalmology, Allergan Pharmaceuticals, Irvine, 1978.

46. Loeffler, V. K., Branscheid, W., Rodenbeck, H., and Ficus, H. J.: Histologische Untersuchungen an Nickhautdrüsen von Hunden mit vermehrtem Tränenfluss. Kleintierpraxis 23:215, 1978.

47. Long, R. D.: Relief of epiphora by conjunctivorhinostomy. J. Small Anim. Pract. 16:381, 1975.

48. Ludders, J. W., and Heavner, J. E.: Effect of atropine on tear formation in anesthetized dogs. J. Am. Vet. Med. Assoc. 175:585, 1979.

49. Martin, C. L., and Anderson, P. G.: Ocular anatomy. In Gelatt, K. N. (ed.): Veterinary Ophthalmology. Lea and Febiger, Philadelphia, 1981, pp. 12–121.

50. McDonald, J. E.: Surface phenomena of tear films. Trans. Am. Ophthalmol. Soc. 66:905, 1968.

51. Michel, G.: Anatomy of the lachrymal glands and ducts in the dog and cat. Deutsch. Tier. Wochenschr. 62:347, 1955.

52. Milder, B.: The lacrimal apparatus. In Moses, R. A. (ed.): Adler's Physiology of the Eye, 7th ed. C. V. Mosby, St. Louis, 1981.

53. Miller, S. J. H.: Diseases of the lacrimal apparatus. In: Parson's Diseases of the Eye, 16th ed. Churchill-Livingston, New York, 1978.

54. Murphy, J. M., Severin, G. A., and Lavach, J. D.: Nasolacrimal catheterization for treating chronic dacryocystitis. Vet. Med./Sm. Anim. Clin. 72:883, 1977.

55. Newell, F. W.: Ophthalmology, Principles and Concepts, 4th ed. C. V. Mosby, St. Louis, 1978.

56. Patwardhan, V. N.: Hypovitaminosis A in the epidemiology of xerophthalmia. Am. J. Clin. Nutr. 22:1106, 1969.

57. Peiffer, R. L., Gelatt, K. N., Gwin, R. M., and Williams, L. W.: Correction of inferior medial entropion as a cause of epiphora. Canine Pract. 5:27, 1978.

58. Playter, R. F., and Adams, L. G.: Lacrimal cyst (dacryops) in two dogs. J. Am. Vet. Med. Assoc. 171:736, 1977.

59. Pollock, R. V. H.: The eye. In Evans, H. E., and Christensen, G. C. (eds.): Miller's Anatomy of the Dog, 2nd ed. W. B. Saunders, Philadelphia, 1979.

60. Prince, J. H., Diesem, C. D., Eglitis, I., and Ruskell, G. L.: Anatomy and Histology of the Eye and Orbit in Domestic Animals. Charles C Thomas, Springfield, 1960.

61. Putterman, A. M.: In Peyman, G. A., Sanders, D. R., and Goldberg, M. F. (eds.): Principles and Practice of Ophthalmology, Vol. 3. W. B. Saunders, Philadelphia, 1980.

62. Roberts, S. R.: Abnormal tear secretion in the dog. Mod. Vet. Pract. 43:37, 1962.

63. Rubin, L. F., and Aguirre, G.: Clinical use of pilocarpine for keratoconjunctivitis sicca in dogs and cats. J. Am. Vet. Med. Assoc. 151:313, 1967.

64. Rubin, L. F., Lynch, R. K., and Stockman, W. S.: Clinical estimation of lacrimal function in dogs. J. Am. Vet. Med. Assoc. 147:946, 1965.

65. Schmidt, G., Magrane, W. G., and Helper, L. C.: Parotid duct transposition: a followup study of 60 eyes. J. Am. Anim. Hosp. Assoc. 6:235, 1970.

66. Severin, G. A.: Nasolacrimal duct catheterization in the dog. J. Am. Anim. Hosp. Assoc. 8:13, 1972.

67. Severin, G. A.: Keratoconjunctivitis sicca. Vet. Clin. North Am. 3:407, 1973.

68. Severin, G. A.: Veterinary Ophthalmology Notes, 2nd ed. Colorado State University, Ft. Collins, 1976.

69. Slatter, D. H.: Keratoconjunctivitis sicca in the dog produced by oral phenazopyridine hydrochloride. J. Small Anim. Pract. 14:749, 1973.

70. Slatter, D. H.: Fundamentals of Veterinary Ophthalmology. W. B. Saunders, Philadelphia, 1981.

71. Slatter, D. H.: Disorders of the lacrimal system, part 1. Deficiency of precorneal tear film. Comp. Cont. Ed. 2:801, 1980.

72. Slatter, D. H., and Davis, W. C.: The toxicity of phenazopyridine. Arch. Ophthalmol. 91:484, 1974.

73. Snead, J. W., Rathbun, J. E., and Crawford, J. B.: The effects of silicone tube on the canaliculus: an animal experiment. Ophthalmology 87:1031, 1980.

74. Startup, F. G.: Diseases of the Canine Eye. Williams & Wilkins, Baltimore, 1969.

75. Theodore, F. K.: Silent dacryocystitis. Arch. Ophthalmol. 40:157, 1948.

76. Thun, R., Abraham, R. S., and Helper, L. C.: Effect of tetracycline on tear production in the dog. J. Am. Anim. Hosp. Assoc. 11:802, 1975.

77. Todenhofer, V. H.: Toxische Nebenwirkungen von Sulfadiazin

(Debenal, Sulfatidin) bei der Anwendung als Geriatrikum für Hunde. Deutsch. Tier. Wochenschr. 76:14, 1969.

78. Veirs, E. R. (ed.): *The Lacrimal System, Clinical Application.* Grune & Stratton, New York, 1955.

79. Veirs, E. R. (ed.): *The Lacrimal System, Proceedings of the 1st International Symposium.* C. V. Mosby, St. Louis, 1971.

80. Veith, L. A., Cure, T. H., and Gelatt, K. N.: The Schirmer tear test in cats. Mod. Vet. Pract. *51*:48, 1970.

81. Yakely, W. L., and Alexander, J. E.: Dacryocystorhinography in the dog. J. Am. Vet. Med. Assoc. *159*:1417, 1971.

82. Yamaguchi, M. (ed.): *Recent Advances on the Lacrimal System.* 3rd International Lacrimal Symposium, Kyoto, 1978.

83. Zictzschmann, O., Ackernecht, E., and Grau, H.: *In* Ellenberger, W., and Baum, H.: *Handbuch der vergleichenden Anatomie der Haustiere,* 18th ed. Springer-Verlag, Berlin, 1943.

Chapter 104

Third Eyelid

Robert L. Peiffer, Jr., and David E. Harling*

SURGICAL ANATOMY

The nictitating membrane, or third eyelid,† is a modified fold of conjunctiva located at the medial canthus. The membrane follows the curvature of the globe, its bulbar (inner) surface being concave and the palpebral (outer) surface convex. It is covered with mucosal epithelium, contiguous with the conjunctival epithelium of the fornices, on both the bulbar and palpebral surfaces. The leading margin of the membrane may be pigmented.

The third eyelid is supported by a flat, T-shaped hyaline cartilage, the arms of which are parallel to the leading edge, whereas the shaft is embedded in the gland of the third eyelid at its base. The gland is surrounded by adipose tissue and is classified as seromucoid in the dog and serous in the cat.[15] Secretions of the gland reach the bulbar conjunctival surface via multiple ducts[11,15,17] and contribute approximately 30 per cent of the aqueous portion of the tear film.[5–7] Fibrous attachments between the gland of the third eyelid and the periorbital tissue limit the gland's movement and prevent it from prolapsing.[17]

Diffuse, slightly elevated lymphoid follicles are located beneath the bulbar conjunctival surface of the third eyelid and may become chronically inflamed and hypertrophied, with a cobblestone-like appearance.

Blood is supplied to the third eyelid by branches of the ophthalmic artery.[15] The third eyelid is innervated by sympathetic fibers via the cranial cervical ganglion (efferent) and the infraorbital nerve of the ophthalmic nerve (afferent).[15]

Movement of the third eyelid is primarily passive;[17] retraction of the globe by the retractor bulbi muscle (abducens nerve) results in superotemporal elevation. The position of the third eyelid is partially determined by sympathetic tone; smooth muscle fibers can be demonstrated histologically, and their function is suggested clinically by elevation of the third eyelid with the sympathetic denervation in Horner's syndrome.[15,18,19]

In the cat there are two sheets of smooth muscle arising medially and ventrally from the fascia of the medial and ventral rectus muscles, which retract the membrane; these muscles are supplied by sympathetic fibers. Active elevation may also be associated with contraction of the lateral rectus muscle, supplied by the sixth cranial nerve.[18,19]

FUNCTION

The four primary functions of the third eyelid include (1) protection of the cornea and removal of foreign bodies, (2) secretion of precorneal tear film, (3) dispersion of the tear film, and (4) immunological activity. Because of these functions, removal of the third eyelid is rarely indicated; histologically confirmed malignancy and irreparable trauma are the only exceptions. If the membrane is removed the eye becomes predisposed to exposure keratoconjunctivitis and keratoconjunctivitis sicca.[5–7]

CONGENITAL ABNORMALITIES

An incomplete, dorsally encircling third eyelid remnant may be seen as an incidental finding, especially in American cocker spaniels and beagles.[17]

In both dogs and cats, lack of marginal pigmentation may increase sensitivity to solar radiation.[17] In cases of solar sensitivity, topical corticosteroid preparations or tattooing may be of benefit.

Dermoids of the third eyelid occur in the dog and cat. Surgical excision with plastic repair if necessary is the treatment of choice.

ACQUIRED DISORDERS

Cartilage Abnormalities

Inversion or eversion of the third eyelid may occur spontaneously as a congenital, but more frequently as a spontaneous, defect or secondary to improper suture placement for a third eyelid flap. Eversion is

---

*Medical illustrator for this chapter was Thomas Waldrop.

†Nomina Anatomica Veterinaria now describes the nictitating membrane as the "palpebra tertia" or third eyelid.

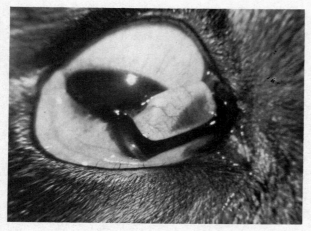

more common in German shepherds, German short-haired pointers, Weimaraners, St. Bernards, New-foundlands, Chesapeake Bay retrievers, English bull-dogs, and Great Danes, and the condition may be inherited.[10] The spontaneous condition is usually seen before six months of age[2] (Fig. 104–1). The cartilage of the membrane develops a curl, usually outward, and the third eyelid develops a scroll-like appearance on the leading edge. The curl may occur anywhere from the vertical stem of the T to the eyelid edge or to the ends of the horizontal arm. The condition causes little discomfort unless secondary keratitis or conjunctivitis occurs. Chronic low-grade irritation and unsightly appearance warrant excision of the involved cartilage in most cases.[4,16]

The membrane is fixed and everted with forceps and stabilized nasally and temporally; two pairs of small Babcock forceps are ideal. The conjunctiva is

Figure 104–1. Eversion of the cartilage of the third eyelid in the right eye of a six-month-old Great Dane.

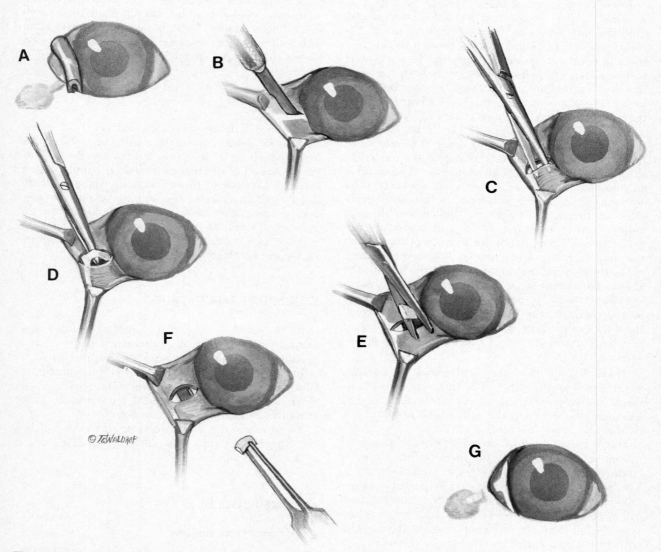

Figure 104–2. Repair of everted cartilage of the third eyelid. *A,* Appearance prior to surgery. *B,* Incision of mucosa on the bulbar surface of the nictitating membrane over the deformed cartilage. *C,* Blunt dissection with strabismus scissors to free the cartilage from the bulbar and palpebral mucosa. The cartilage is dissected free *(D)* and the deformed cartilage is resected *(E). F,* Mucosa may be sutured with knots buried, or the incision may be left to heal by secondary intention. *G,* Immediately postoperatively the membrane should lie flat on the globe.

incised on the posterior surface of the membrane parallel to and over the curled cartilage. The deformed cartilage is isolated from the bulbar and palpebral conjunctiva using blunt dissection with strabismus scissors, taking care to avoid puncturing the palpebral surface. The exposed distorted cartilage is excised and the mucosa is apposed. Absorbable sutures (6-0 to 8-0) may be used to pull the conjunctiva over the exposed edge of the cartilage. Knots should be buried to avoid corneal irritation (Fig. 104–2).

If the horizontal portion of the T is involved, the dissection is more difficult but can be completed with care. Aftercare consists of treatment with a topical antibiotic ophthalmic ointment three times daily for five to seven days.

Protrusion of the Gland of the Third Eyelid

Protrusion of the gland of the third eyelid results from prolapse of the gland up and over the free edge of the membrane (Fig. 104–3). This condition may result from a congenital, possibly inherited, aplasia or hypoplasia of the connective tissue attachments between the base of the gland and the periorbital tissue.[17] The gland everts while remaining attached to the cartilage. The condition may be unilateral or bilateral and occurs in all breeds but is most commonly seen in the American cocker spaniel, English bulldog, basset hound, and the beagle between 3 and 12 months of age. Since the gland supplies part of the aqueous phase of the tear film, removal predisposes to keratoconjunctivitis sicca, especially if lacrimal function is otherwise compromised; of 160 dogs presented with keratoconjunctivitis sicca, 38 had previous resection of the third eyelid or its gland. Although not conclusive, these data strongly suggest that removal of the gland is contraindicated. The treatment of choice is repositioning of the gland by suturing it to the episclera[1] (Fig. 104–4A). The membrane is fixed in an everted position with Babcock forceps nasally and temporally to provide support (Fig. 104–4B). The conjunctival epithelium is excised over the gland from its most superior aspect to the fornix of the conjunctiva and across the bulbar conjunctiva to the limbus. The conjunctiva is bluntly dissected free from the gland (Fig. 104–4C). The inferior limbus is grasped at the 6 o'clock position with fine-toothed forceps, and the globe is rotated superiorly. A 4-0 absorbable mattress suture is passed through the exposed inferior nasal bulbar fascia and episclera and placed through the glandular tissue at the apex of the gland (Fig. 104–4D). When the suture is tied, the gland returns to a position inferior to the globe (Fig. 104–4E). Complications include penetration of the globe at the time of placement of the episcleral suture. Use of a small spatulate needle and adequate exposure and stabilization of the globe prevent this. With adequate placement of sutures, the success rate approaches 100 per cent, although an occasional gland reprolapses.

Alternatively, the prolapsed gland may be partially excised.[8,16] A Schirmer tear test should be performed prior to surgical removal of the gland; a value of less than 10 mm is a contraindication to excision. Excision of the prolapsed gland is performed by clamping the tissue with straight mosquito forceps and excising the distal part with scissors or a surgical scalpel (Fig. 104–4 F and G). To maintain partial secretion, only two-thirds of the gland is excised. Additionally, only a minimal amount of cartilage from the vertical portion of the T should be removed, as radical removal may affect the ability of the lid to sweep across the cornea.

Aftercare for either procedure consists of application of an ophthalmic antibiotic ointment two to three times daily for five to seven days.

Lacerations

The third eyelid is often lacerated in cat fights. If the free edge is only slightly torn it may be trimmed under topical anesthesia to remove any trailing flap of tissue.

If the membrane is extensively torn, primary repair of acute tears or secondary repair of more chronic tears is performed under general anesthesia. The wound edges are debrided if necessary, and, with care and magnification, the torn membrane can usually be reconstructed to its original shape. The knots of full thickness sutures should be placed on the palpebral surface to avoid corneal irritation.

Prominence of the Third Eyelid

Unpigmented third eyelids may appear more prominent than normal, especially if unilateral. Usually it is only necessary to assess the condition and explain its nature to the owner to relieve anxiety.

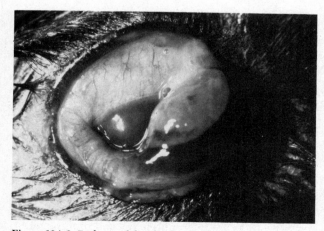

Figure 104–3. Prolapse of the gland of the third eyelid in the right eye of a young American cocker spaniel. Note the relationship of the prolapsed gland to the pigmented margin of the nictitating membrane and the accompanying conjunctivitis.

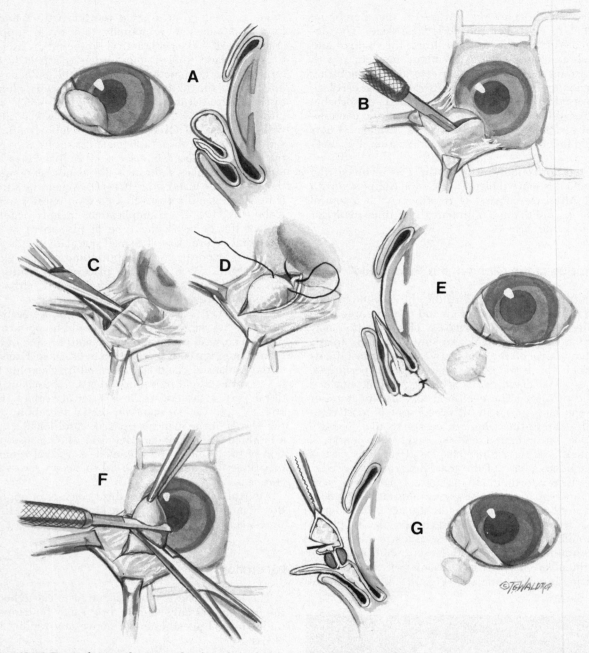

Figure 104–4. Two techniques for repair of prolapsed gland of the third eyelid. *A,* Prolapse of the gland of the nictitating membrane up and over the free edge. *B,* Incision through the bulbar mucosa of the membrane. *C,* Dissection of the mucosa overlying the gland. *D,* The globe is rotated dorsally and 4-0 absorbable mattress suture placed in the inferior nasal bulbar fascia and the prolapsed base of the gland. *E,* The gland is positioned ventral to the globe as the suture is tied. *F,* An alternate technique involves placing a hemostat proximal to the portion of gland to be excised. *G,* Resection of gland distal to crushed area.

In cats the third eyelids may become prominent following transient upper respiratory infections or gastroenteritis. Although the etiology is unknown, the condition is proposed to be related to decreased sympathetic tone.[19] The condition is symmetrical and bilateral, usually self-limiting with a two- to eight-week course, and is not a surgical disease. Topical 1.0% phenylephrine administered twice daily usually produces at least a partial symptomatic improvement.[13]

Speculative and demonstrated causes of bilateral protrusion of the third eyelid include parasites such as *Dipylidium caninum* and *Spirometra* spp., dehydration, ocular inflammation, rapid weight loss, wasting associated with severe systemic disease, senility, and tranquilization with acetylpromazine. Horner's syndrome, space-occupying orbital lesions, and foreign bodies[3] are associated with unilateral third eyelid protrusion, as are microphthalmia and phthisis bulbi. Systemic diseases that may cause endophthalmos or protrusion of the membrane include tetanus, rabies, canine distemper, and meningitis. If the third eyelid covers the pupillary axis and impairs vision, it may be desirable to conservatively resect the free edge of the membrane including the stem of the cartilage. Remove no more tissue than is needed to clear the optic axis, preserving the glandular tissue. The free edge may be oversewn with absorbable 6-0 suture in a continuous fashion to speed healing and reduce scarring. An alternative procedure is to leave the edge of the membrane intact and excise a full thickness ellipse of tissue from the mid portion of the nictitans and suture in a manner that allows the shortened membrane to lie flat on the globe.[12] This produces a more cosmetic appearance and preserves the functional edge to distribute the tear film.

Proliferative Diseases of the Third Eyelid

Follicular Conjunctivitis (Lymphoid Hyperplasia of the Bulbar Surface of the Third Eyelid)

On the bulbar surface of the third eyelid are lymphoid follicles that are part of the local ocular immune system. Chronic irritation and immunological stimulation initiate proliferation of these follicles. If the stimulus persists, follicles may also develop on the palpebral surface and conjunctiva, resulting in follicular conjunctivitis. Once the follicles have hypertrophied to a certain point, the condition becomes self-sustaining even when the original insult has resolved. Mucoid discharge may become prominent.

Causes of follicular hyperplasia in the dog include any chronic ophthalmic inflammation associated with bacterial infection, mechanical irritation from distichiasis, entropion, ectropion, parasites, and dust and pollen allergens. This disease is uncommon in cats, and when seen is often related to chlamydial conjunctivitis.[13]

Pulling the topically anesthetized membrane upward and forward with smooth forceps reveals the hyperplastic follicles, red and roughened in appearance. If the conjunctiva is affected one will see follicles on the palpebral and bulbar conjunctiva as well.

Although mild cases may respond to topical antibiotic-corticosteroid preparations, severe, chronic, or recurrent cases require the removal of the follicles. The follicles may be vigorously abraded with gauze, scraped from the surface with a scalpel blade, or (authors' preference)* shaved off with sharp scissors. Hemorrhage is controlled with gentle pressure. Chemical cautery is difficult to control and is not recommended. Postoperative topical antibiotic-corticosteroid ointments are prescribed for seven to ten days.

Inflammatory Hyperplasia

The third eyelid may become diffusely and markedly thickened in association with chronic inflammatory disease. Diffuse inflammation may be associated with chronic superficial keratitis in the German shepherd (Überreiter's disease) characterized by plasma cell infiltration (Fig. 104–5) and focal proliferative lesions seen with proliferative keratoconjunctivitis in the rough- and smooth-coated collie (Fig. 104–6). Excisional biopsy may be indicated to rule out neoplasia and confirm the clinical diagnosis. Although the primary therapy of either condition is medical, excisional biopsy is of therapeutic value in proliferative keratoconjunctivitis.

---

*Editor's note: The treatment of this condition is controversial. Some ophthalmologists prefer intense local immunosuppression with corticosteroids.

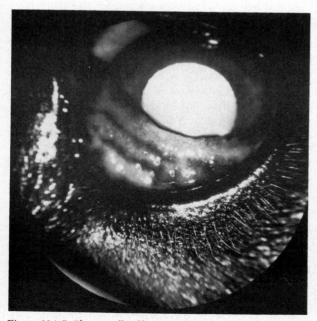

Figure 104–5. Plasma cell infiltration of the third eyelid in the left eye of a six-year-old female German shepherd. The disease is bilateral and may or may not be associated with corneal lesions of chronic superficial keratitis.

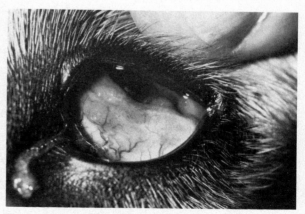

Figure 104–6. Nodular involvement of the third eyelid in a four-year-old female collie with bilateral proliferative keratoconjunctivitis.

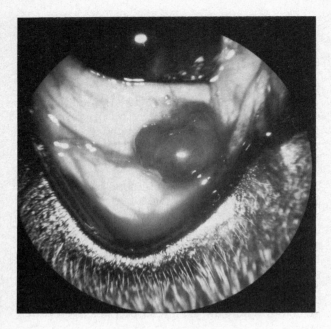

Figure 104–7. Hemangiosarcoma of the third eyelid in a Samoyed.

Neoplasms of the Third Eyelid

Neoplasia of this structure in the dog is uncommon. Reported tumors include fibrosarcoma,[2] lymphosarcoma, mastocytoma, hemangioma and hemangiosarcoma,[14] squamous cell carcinoma, and adenocarcinoma of the nictitating gland (Fig. 104–7). If possible, excisional biopsy without removal of the entire membrane and gland is preferable; the affected tissue is simply excised full or partial thickness as required. The margin of the membrane is supported with forceps and the neoplastic tissue is defined and excised, using sharp and blunt dissection as necessary. Surgical defects are closed following the principles described for repair of lacerations. Alternatively, neoplasms can be treated with cryosurgery, which often results in minimal destruction to the third eyelid, even when extensively frozen. Radiation may be effective in squamous cell carcinomas, lymphosarcomas, and mastocytomas.

Surgical Procedures

Reconstruction of Previously Excised Third Eyelid

In chronic keratoconjunctivitis in which the third eyelid has been surgically removed, temporary corneal protection can be afforded by tarsorrhaphy or conjunctival flaps. For more permanent control of exposure keratitis, the use of autografts of oral mucosa transplanted to the conjunctiva has been described.[9] The procedure includes elevation of an appropriate-sized flap (20 × 7 mm) of buccal mucosa and underlying connective tissue and suturing it in place in a prepared bed in the medial canthus, with the mucosal epithelial side placed as the palpebral surface. Silk suture material (4-0) is removed in 18 to 28 days. Although variably notched or partially depigmented, the function of the missing membrane is preserved, and, in spite of shrinkage by about one-third, the grafts remained viable in three out of four procedures.

Third Eyelid Flaps

The third eyelid provides a readily available protective bandage for the cornea. Ulceration, laceration, keratoconjunctivitis sicca, seventh nerve paralysis, reduction of proptosis of the globe, or any condition in which corneal coverage, support, or protection is needed is an indication for a third eyelid flap. General anesthesia is preferable, although sedation and topical and local anesthetic may be considered. The upper eyelid is grasped with forceps and a suture is placed from the superior temporal skin surface into the fornix (Fig. 104–8A), through the third eyelid in an anterior to posterior direction (Fig. 104–8B), back through 5 to 6 mm from the first bite (Fig. 104–8C), and back through the fornix and skin (Fig. 104–8D). A second suture is placed in a similar pattern, and in large animals a third suture may be used (Fig. 104–8E). Sutures should be placed just below the T arms of the cartilage and may be passed through the base of the cartilage near the midpoint of the membrane. Stents, such as plastic or rubber tubing, buttons, or a heavy rubber band may be used to control tension; sutures are tied gently but not so tightly that they tear the membrane (Fig. 104–8F and G).

In an alternative method the suture is placed from

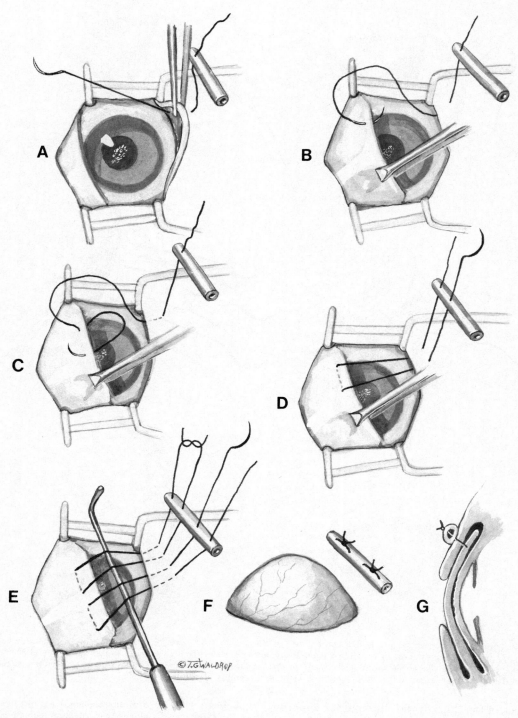

Figure 104–8. Third eyelid flap to the upper eyelid. *A*, The upper lid is grasped and a suture is placed through the superior temporal lid into the fornix. *B*, The suture is passed beneath the arms of the cartilage or through the base of the cartilage at the midpoint. *C*, Note direction of the needle in placing the mattress suture. *D*, The first suture is placed. *E*, The second suture is placed in a similar fashion; sutures may be placed through or over a stent to minimize tension. *F*, Completion of nictitating membrane flap. Three sutures may be used in large breeds. *G*, Cross section demonstrates proper positioning of sutures and third eyelid.

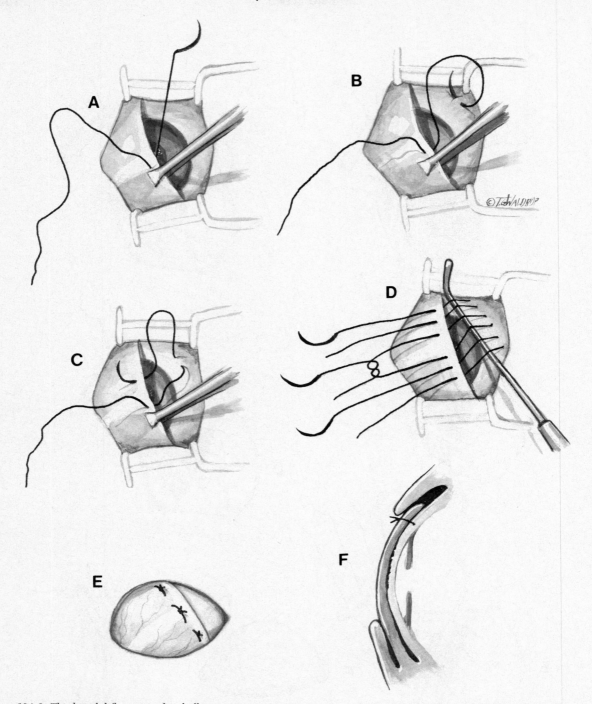

Figure 104–9. Third eyelid flap sutured to bulbar conjunctiva. *A*, Suture is passed anterior to posterior through the membrane beneath the cartilage. *B*, Suture is placed through the bulbar conjunctiva and underlying Tenon's capsule and episclera. *C*, The suture is passed back through the membrane. *D*, Three sutures usually are placed and are tied gently snug. *E*, Note positioning of knots and suture. *F*, Cross section demonstrating proper suture placement and nictitating membrane position.

front to back of the third eyelid; through the superior temporal conjunctiva, Tenon's capsule, and episclera; and back through the third eyelid (Fig. 104–9). The advantage of this technique is that the membrane moves with the eye and is perhaps more closely apposed. It is especially useful in brachycephalic breeds, in which the prominent globe makes a flap to the upper eyelid difficult to place without marked tension.

1. Blogg, J. R.: Surgical replacement of a prolapsed gland of the third eyelid ("cherry eye"), a new technique. Aust. Vet. Pract. 9:75, 1979.
2. Buykmichi, N.: Fibrosarcoma of the nictitating membrane in a cat. J. Am. Vet. Med. Assoc. 167:934, 1975.
3. Gelatt, K. N.: Foreign body beneath the nictitating membrane. Vet. Med./Sm. Anim. Clin. 66:468, 1971.
4. Gelatt, K. N.: Surgical correction of everted membrane in the dog. Vet. Med./Sm. Anim. Clin. 67:291, 1972.
5. Gelatt, K. N., Peiffer, R. L., Jr., Erickson, J. L., and Gum, G. G.: Evaluation of tear formation in the dog, using a

modification of the Schirmer tear test. J. Am. Vet. Med. Assoc. *106*:368, 1975.

6. Helper, L. C.: The effect of lacrimal gland removal on the conjunctiva and cornea of the dog. J. Am. Vet. Med. Assoc. *157*:72, 1970.

7. Helper, L. C., Magrane, W. G., et al.: Surgical induction of keratoconjunctivitis sicca in the dog. J. Am. Vet. Med. Assoc. *164*:172, 1974.

8. Howard, D. R.: Hypertrophy of the nictitans gland. Vet. Med./Sm. Anim. Clin. *64*:304, 1969.

9. Kuhns, E. L.: Oral mucosa grafts for membrana nictitans replacement. Mod. Vet. Pract. *58*:768, 1977.

10. Martin, C. L.: Everted membrane nictitans in German short-haired pointers. J. Am. Vet. Med. Assoc. *157*:1229, 1970.

11. Miller, M. E. L., Christensen, G. C., and Evans, H. E. (eds.): *Anatomy of the Dog*. W. B. Saunders, Philadelphia, 1964, pp. 838–840.

12. Ojay, E., and Milinsky, H. L.: Surgical correction of unpigmented prominent membrane nictitans. J. Am. Vet. Med. Assoc. *144*:857, 1969.

13. Peiffer, R. L., Jr.: Feline ophthalmology. *In* Gelatt, K. N. (ed.): *Veterinary Ophthalmology*. Lea and Febiger, Philadelphia, 1981, pp. 521–568.

14. Peiffer, R. L., Jr., Duncan, J., and Terell, T. G.: Hemangioma of the nictitating membrane in a dog. J. Am. Vet. Med. Assoc. *172*:832, 1978.

15. Prince, J. H., Diesem, C. D., Eglitis, I., and Ruskell, G. L.: Anatomy and histology of the eye and orbit of domestic animals. Charles C Thomas, Springfield, 1960, pp. 86–88.

16. Richards, D. S.: Removal of hypertrophied nictitans gland. Vet. Med./Sm. Anim. Clin. *68*:1107, 1973.

17. Severin, G. S.: *Veterinary Ophthalmology Notes*, 2nd ed. Fort Collins, 1976, pp. 101–110.

18. Thompson, J. W.: The nerve supply to the nictitating membrane of the cat. J. Anat. *95*:371, 1967.

19. Wyman, M.: The nictitating membrane. *In* Bojrab, H. J. (ed): *Pathophysiology in Small Animal Surgery*. Lea and Febiger, Philadelphia, 1981, p. 66.

Cornea and Sclera

Chapter **105**

Douglas H. Slatter

INTRODUCTION

The structure and function of the cornea are uniquely specialized, and a knowledge of these features and the normal reactions of the tissue to disease is necessary to achieve acceptable surgical results. For a more detailed discussion, the reader is referred to standard texts.[13,18,39]

ANATOMY[28]

The transparent cornea is the anterior window in the fibrous coat of the eye. The sclera is the posterior opaque part, and the limbus is the zone of transition between the two.

The cornea has five layers (Fig. 105–1): the precorneal tear film, epithelium and basement membrane, stroma, Descemet's membrane (basement membrane of the endothelium), and endothelium.

The precorneal tear film covers the cornea and conjunctiva to a depth of 7μ. Each of its three layers is different in composition and function (Fig. 105–2).[18] The outer superficial layer is composed of oily materials and phospholipids from the tarsal (meibomian) glands and serves two functions: (1) to increase the surface tension and bind the precorneal tear film to the corneal surface, and (2) to limit evaporation of the aqueous layer beneath. The middle, or aqueous, layer is mostly water derived from the lacrimal and nictitans glands and serves the following functions:

1. Flushing of foreign material from the conjunctival sac.

2. Lubrication of the passage of lids and third eyelid over the epithelial surface.

3. A conduit for the passage of oxygen, inflammatory cells, and immunoglobulins (IgA and IgG) to the cornea.

4. A smooth corneal surface for greatest optical efficiency.

The inner mucoid layer consists of mucoproteins derived from the conjunctival goblet cells. Its primary function is to bind the hydrophilic, lipophobic aqueous layer to the hydrophobic, lipophilic corneal epithelium with bipolar mucoprotein molecules.

The corneal epithelium is composed of simple stratified squamous and nonkeratinized cells and is attached to its basement membrane by hemidesmosomes. As the basal cells near the basement membrane undergo mitosis, daughter cells are forced toward the surface and gradually lose their organelles. Fibrocytes, keratocytes, collagen, and ground substance comprise about 90 per cent of the corneal stromal substance.[18] Collagen fibrils within it are arranged in a parallel fashion to form interlacing sheets or lamellae. The regular spacing of stromal collagen fibrils is important in maintaining corneal transparency and distinguishes the stroma from the collagen in scar tissue and sclera (Figs. 105–3 and 105–4). Stromal keratocytes are capable of synthesizing collagen, glycosaminoglycans, and mucoprotein of the ground substance.

Descemet's membrane (see Fig. 105–1) is the basement membrane of the endothelium and is continuously laid down by the endothelium throughout life. It is composed of fine collagen fibrils and is

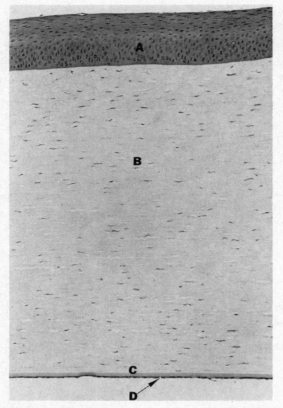

Figure 105–1. Microscopic structure of the cornea. *A*, Epithelium; *B*, stroma; *C*, Descemet's membrane; *D*, endothelium.

elastic in nature. If ruptured, the ends tend to curl because of this elasticity (Fig. 105–5). In a descemetocele in which the overlying stroma has been destroyed, Descemet's membrane often protrudes dramatically because of this elasticity. After rupture, the endothelium secretes a new membrane to fill small defects. Descemet's membrane does not stain with fluorescein, and its presence as a dark, transparent bulge in the center of a corneal ulcer or wound is a grave sign indicating impending rupture.

The endothelium is one cell thick and lies posterior and adjacent to Descemet's membrane (see Fig. 105–1). It has a limited ability to replicate depending on age and species,[16] and when endothelium is lost the defect is replaced by the migration of existing adjacent cells. With advancing age, the number of endothelial cells (which can be determined in the living

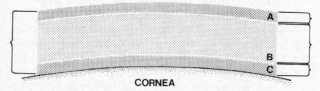

Figure 105–2. Precorneal tear film. *A*, Superficial lipid layer; *B*, aqueous layer; *C*, inner mucoid layer.

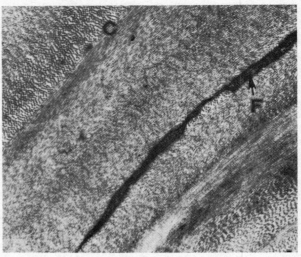

Figure 105–3. Interlacing lamellae cross at right angles in a dog cornea. The lamellae consist of regularly spaced collagen fibrils *(C)* separated by ground substance. A process of a keratocyte *(F)* is present between lamellae. (Reprinted with permission from Shively, J. N., and Epling, G. P.: Fine structure of the canine eye: cornea. Am. J. Vet. Res. *31:*713, 1970.)

animal by specular microscopy) decreases.[16] The endothelium is of particular relevance to the surgeon because it is extremely susceptible to osmotic and traumatic damage during surgical procedures. Loss of corneal endothelium beyond the ability of adjacent cells to compensate or replicate results in permanent corneal edema and opacity.

The sclera is the largest part of the fibrous outer coat of the globe and has three layers: the episclera, sclera proper, and the lamina fusca, which lies adjacent to the choroid (Fig. 105–6).

The episclera is composed of a dense, highly vascular layer that binds Tenon's capsule (fascia bulbi) to the sclera. Collagenous fibers within the episclera blend into the superficial sclera stroma. Anteriorly, the episclera thickens and blends with Tenon's capsule and subconjunctival connective tissue near the limbus.

The sclera is composed of collagen fibers and fibroblasts. The collagen fibers vary in diameter and orientation in different parts of the globe. The scleral collagen fibrils differ from corneal fibrils in their considerable variation in diameter and the absence of regular fixed spacing between them.

The lamina fusca is the zone of transition between the sclera and the uvea (the middle or vascular coat of the eye). The lamina fusca contains scleral collagen bundles that separate and intermingle with widely separated bundles in the choroid and ciliary body. The sclera is perforated posteriorly by the optic nerve at the lamina cribrosa, a sieve-like opening through which the fibers of the optic nerve pass. The short posterior ciliary nerves and arteries pierce the sclera around the nerve and enter the choroid. The long posterior ciliary arteries and nerves pierce the sclera near the optic nerve and pass forward horizontally to

Figure 105–4. Summary diagram of the corneal stroma. *A,* Fibroblasts. This diagram shows six fibroblasts lying between the stromal lamellae. The cells are thin and flat, with long processes that contact fibroblast processes of other cells lying in the same plane. These cells were once believed to form a true syncytium, but electron microscopy has disproved this idea. There is almost always a 200 Å wide intercellular space separating the cells. Unlike fibroblasts elsewhere, these cells occasionally join each other at a macula occludens.

B, Lamellae. The cornea is composed of a very orderly, dense, fibrous connective tissue. Its collagen, which is a very stable protein having a half-life estimated at 100 days, forms many lamellae. The collagen fibrils within a lamella are parallel to each other and run the full length of the cornea. Successive lamellae run across the cornea at an angle to each other. Three fibroblasts are seen between the lamellae.

C, Diagram to show the theoretical orientation of the corneal collagen fibrils. Each of the fibrils is separated from its fellows by an equal distance. Maurice has explained the transparency of the cornea on the basis of this very exact equidistant separation. As a result of this arrangement the stromal lamellae form a three-dimensional array of diffraction gratings. Scattered rays of light passing through such a system interact with each other in an organized way, resulting in the elimination of scattered light by destructive interference. The mucoproteins, glycoproteins, and other components of the ground substance are responsible for maintaining the proper position of the fibrils.

D, Orientation of the collagen fibrils in an opaque cornea. The diagram shows the orderly positions of the fibrils to have been disturbed. Because of this disarrangement, scattered light is not eliminated by destructive interference and the cornea becomes hazy. Edema fluid in the ground substance also produces clouding of the cornea by disturbing the interfibrillar distance.

(Reprinted with permission from Hogan, M. J., Alvarado, J. A., and Weddell, J. E.: *Histology of the Human Eye.* W. B. Saunders, Philadelphia, 1971.)

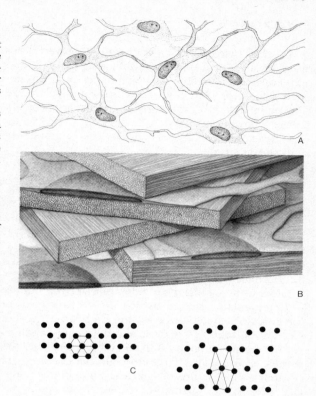

the ciliary body within the sclera. In the dog these arteries carry most of the arterial supply to the anterior segment,[20] a feature of considerable importance in the prognosis following ocular prolapse when the anterior ciliary arteries have been torn from their insertions with the extraocular muscles. The anterior ciliary arteries and vortex veins enter and leave the sclera, respectively, in the area overlying the ciliary body.

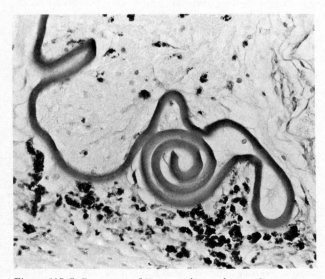

Figure 105–5. Retraction of Descemet's membrane after rupture. PAS stain.

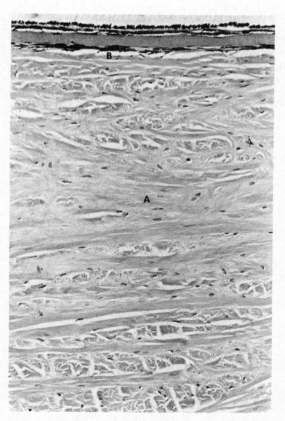

Figure 105–6. Layers of the canine sclera. *A,* Scleral stroma; *B,* lamina fusca.

PHYSIOLOGY

The transparent cornea is the most powerful refracting surface in the eye. Both transparency and curvature are maintained by anatomical and physiological features. Although the cornea and sclera are similar in structure, the cornea is transparent owing to the following features:

1. Lack of blood vessels and reduced numbers of cells in the stroma.
2. Lack of pigment.
3. Control of water content.
4. A smooth optical surface provided by the precorneal tear film.
5. A higher mucopolysaccharide content.
6. A regular, highly organized arrangement of collagen fibrils of very uniform diameter and spacing, which eliminates the scattering of light by destructive interference.

Glucose metabolism provides most of the energy requirements of corneal tissues. About two-thirds of the glucose is metabolized via the Embden-Meyerhof pathway and the Krebs' cycle and the remaining third via the hexose monophosphate shunt.[29] Because the cornea is avascular, it requires alternate sources of oxygen: aqueous, precorneal tear film, limbal capillary plexus, and palpebral conjunctival capillaries (Fig. 105–7). The endothelium receives most of its oxygen from the aqueous, but atmospheric oxygen is the major source for the remainder of the cornea.

Water enters the cornea under the influence of intraocular pressure,[29] is attracted by stromal collagen and mucopolysaccharides, and leaves by evaporation from the corneal surface. The control of water entry and the maintenance of the state of relative dehydration ("detergescence") are both important to transparency and are energy dependent. The endothelium

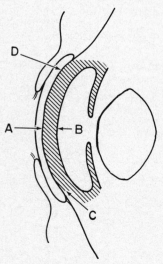

Figure 105–7. Sources of oxygen available to cornea. *A,* Precorneal film; *B,* aqueous humor; *C,* limbal capillaries; *D,* palpebral conjunctival capillaries. (Reprinted with permission from Scheie, H. G., and Albert, D. M.: *Textbook of Ophthalmology.* 9th ed. W. B. Saunders, Philadelphia, 1977.)

functions as a "fluid pump," moving water from the stroma back to the aqueous against the intraocular pressure.[26] The epithelium also controls water content by preventing entry from the precorneal tear film. Interference with the oxygen supply of the epithelium (e.g., by an impermeable contact lens) increases anaerobic glycolysis and causes the accumulation of lactic acid and water and corneal edema. Both endothelium and epithelium contain large amounts of Na^+- and K^+-activated ATPase associated with the sodium pump. If the corneal epithelium is removed, water enters the stroma from the precorneal film and gross swelling occurs until a new layer of epithelium covers the denuded area and fluid balance is restored. The recognition of this swollen edematous stroma is important after keratectomy.

Corneal transparency is affected by variations in the amount of water in the corneal stroma (corneal edema, which causes swelling and separation of the collagen fibril lattice), the arrangement of the collagen fibrils (irregular arrangement or diameter in scar tissue), the presence of blood vessels, and alterations to the optical surface (removal of epithelium or precorneal film). The effect of altered spacing between collagen fibrils can be demonstrated by pressing on the globe (this increases intraocular pressure and distorts the lattice). This causes corneal opacity by scattering light. As soon as the pressure is released, transparency returns. This mechanism differs from that seen in corneal edema due to elevated intraocular pressure (glaucoma), in which endothelial damage and elevated pressure result in an increase in stromal water.

PATHOLOGICAL RESPONSES[9]

Several properties affect the corneal response to pathological processes. Because of its avascularity, which limits cellular and humoral access, and compact construction, which limits the penetration of new blood vessels and cells, pathological reactions tend to be sluggish, chronic, and intractable. Unstable factors, such as fluid balance and state of dehydration, together with the regular arrangement of collagen fibrils are responsible for the precarious state of transparency. Changes that would be very mild in other tissues, e.g., edema, slight scar formation, or change in tissue tension, may greatly alter transparency and are of greater significance in the cornea.

Exogenous disorders must first pass the corneal epithelium, a very effective barrier to bacteria and bacterial toxins because of its unique sensitivity and impervious superficial cells. Bacteria rarely cause primary keratitis in dogs and cats. Once the integrity of the epithelium has been breached, microorganisms establish themselves within the avascular stroma.

The spread of disease processes from other ocular tissues is a common cause of corneal disorders. Examples include the entry of infectious canine hepatitis virus into the cornea from the aqueous, the effects of uveitis (including corneal edema), infiltration of corneal stroma by inflammatory cells and blood vessels in canine chronic superficial keratitis (Überreiter's syndrome), and the trauma of misplaced cilia in distichiasis.

Endogenous disorders apparently arising within the cornea include lipid deposition in hyperlipoproteinemia, endothelial dystrophy in dogs, and corneal bullae formation in corneal dystrophy of Manx cats.

NORMAL CORNEAL HEALING[19]

Epithelium

The regenerative capacity of corneal epithelium is very great. Within a very short time, cells surrounding the margin of a lesion slide over the affected area (Fig. 105–8). An entirely denuded cornea can be covered in four to seven days.[32] Once cells have covered the defect, mitosis occurs and the multilayered epithelial surface is reconstituted. During the sliding process, melanocytes from the limbus may be carried into formerly transparent areas. Small deficiencies in underlying stroma may be filled with epithelial cells, forming an epithelial facet (Fig. 105–9).

Stroma

Superficial stromal defects are filled by epithelial facets. Deeper defects are covered initially by epi-

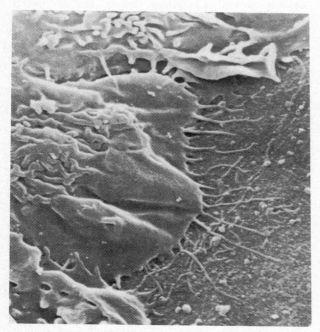

Figure 105–8. Filopodia extending from an epithelial cell over bare basement membrane at the edge of an epithelial defect. (Reprinted with permission from Pfister, R. R.: The healing of corneal epithelial abrasions in the rabbit: a scanning electron microscope study. Invest. Ophthalmol. *14*:648, 1975.)

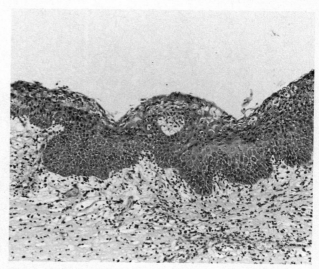

Figure 105–9. Epithelial facet and associated subepithelial inflammatory cell infiltration after a superficial corneal injury in a canine cornea.

thelium, with regeneration of stroma following from beneath. Because regeneration is often incomplete, overall corneal thickness may be reduced. Uncomplicated stromal wounds heal in an avascular fashion (see hereafter), but infected or destructive lesions heal in a vascularized fashion.

Avascular Healing

Several events take place during avascular healing. (1) Neutrophils infiltrate and surround the lesion under chemotactic influences. These cells reach the lesion from the precorneal tear film and stroma via limbal conjunctival vessels. (2) Keratocytes in the immediate area die. In surrounding areas, keratocytes transform to fibrocytes and migrate to the damaged area, where they synthesize collagen and mucopolysaccharides of the ground substance. An epithelial covering facilitates these processes, and if it is not present, healing is delayed. (3) From about 48 hours following injury, macrophages invade the lesion, remove cellular debris, and subsequently transform into keratocytes. The collagen fibrils laid down by the regenerating stroma are irregular and opaque. Within the ensuing weeks, the density of the scar decreases but it does not disappear altogether. Scar resolution is greater in feline than canine corneas.

Vascular Healing

In vascular healing of destructive lesions, cellular infiltration is more extensive than that in avascular healing, and the area is invaded by blood vessels originating from the limbal plexus (Fig. 105–10). Granulation tissue is laid down and forms a more dense scar than that laid down in avascular healing. Eventually the blood vessels collapse but do not disappear; they remain as "ghost vessels" and are

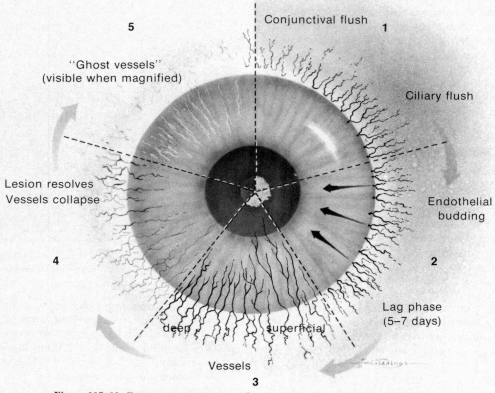

5

"Ghost vessels"
(visible when magnified)

Conjunctival flush   **1**

Ciliary flush

Lesion resolves
Vessels collapse

Endothelial
budding

4

2

deep   superficial

Lag phase
(5–7 days)

Vessels

3

Figure 105–10. Diagrammatic sequence of corneal vascularization in a simple injury.

visible with a slit lamp. Irregularities in the corneal surface are filled by the epithelial process mentioned previously. Corneal nerves damaged by the lesion gradually regenerate, and sensation slowly returns to the affected area.

Endothelium

Because of its elasticity, Descemet's membrane retracts when damaged and curls toward the anterior chamber, exposing a small area of stroma. Neighboring endothelial cells slide in to cover the area, and a new Descemet's membrane is laid down. In extensive lesions, endothelium may not cover the area, and an area of swollen and edematous stroma persists. The endothelium itself is a very delicate tissue, and, if widely damaged, permanent opacity results. Endothelial regeneration occurs in dogs[3] and rabbits[44] and to a lesser extent in cats,[44] primates, and humans.[43]

Corticosteroids and Corneal Healing

Corticosteroids inhibit epithelial regeneration, infiltration with inflammatory cells, fibroblastic activity,

and endothelial regeneration.[9,39] The strength of the resulting wound is lessened, collagenases are potentiated many times,[6] and the risk of infection is greatly increased (Fig. 105–11). Alternatively, corticosteroids are particularly useful after an epithelial cover has been achieved to control the production of irregularly sized or oriented collagen fibrils, which reduce transparency.

INTERPRETATION OF CORNEAL PATHOLOGICAL REACTIONS

Although there are numerous specific keratopathies, the majority of clinically important lesions exhibit one of the following reactions: edema, vascularization, scar formation, pigmentation, or accumulation of an abnormal substance within the cornea.

Edema

Corneal edema results when excess fluid accumulates within the stroma and forces the collagen lamellae apart, causing loss of transparency. Fluid accumulates when regulating functions of the epithe-

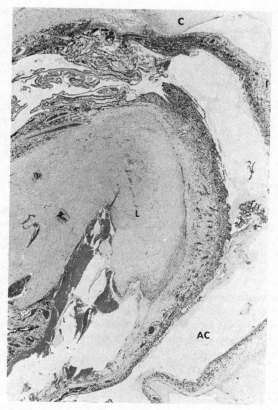

Figure 105–11. Ruptured descemetocele, endophthalmitis, and disorganization due to infection by *Pseudomonas* spp. after treatment of a minor corneal wound with subconjunctival corticosteroids in a dog. *C*, Cornea; *I*, iris; *L*, lens; *AC*, anterior chamber.

lium and endothelium are disturbed, by either removal or functional alteration. On examination, the cornea is hazy blue either in localized areas around an injury or throughout, as in glaucoma or endothelial dysfunction. Corneal edema is usually reversible if fluid balance is re-established and the underlying cause removed. Chronic corneal edema may result in vascularization or, less commonly, bullous keratopathy. In bullous keratopathy, fluid-containing vesicles form in or beneath the epithelium.

Corneal edema may be cleared temporarily for examination by hyperosmotic solutions, e.g., 5% NaCl solution or ointment, 40% glucose solution, 50% glycerin, or 5% polyvinylpyrrollidone solution.*

Vascularization

There are no blood vessels in the normal cornea. Vessels invade the corneal stroma in response to various pathological processes and during vascularized stroma healing. Corneal vascularization may be either superficial or deep.

Superficial vessels occur in the anterior third of the stroma and are continuous with the conjunctival circulation at the limbus. These superficial vessels branch (arborize) more than deep vessels, although in central corneal lesions the part of the vessel nearest the limbus may be straight. Superficial vessels are a brighter red than deep vessels, which branch less and are usually short, straight, and darker red in color. Deep vessels are continuous with the ciliary circulation and disappear from view at the limbus. The depth of invading vessels gives some indication of the depth of the inciting lesion. The sequence and timing of corneal vascularization is shown in Figure 105–10. A knowledge of this sequence is important both for diagnostic evaluation of corneal lesions and during postoperative assessment.

In complicated stromal lesions, especially when the stimulus in the cornea remains, vessels may not collapse and further vascularization and formation of granulation tissue occur. In general, vascularization is a beneficial response (e.g., during stromal repair after prolapse of the globe in the dog), but vessels result in decreased transparency, ingrowth of pigment, and, in some cases, transport of antibodies and inflammatory cells that are not desirable if a transparent cornea is to be maintained. Thus, control of vascularization is often attempted by the application of corticosteroids and beta radiation, e.g., after superficial keratectomy for superficial erosion when an epithelial covering is present. Beta radiation can be used prior to re-establishment of the epithelium.

*Adsorbonac, Burton Parsons Co., Washington, DC.

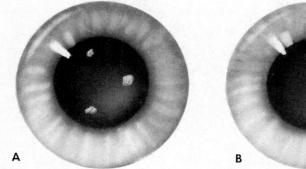
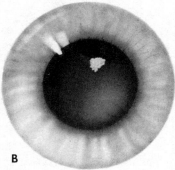
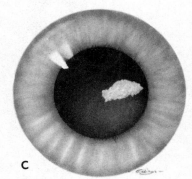

A B C

Figure 105–12. Types of corneal scars. *A*, Nebula. *B*, Macula. *C*, Leukoma. If the iris attaches to the leukoma it is called an "adherent leukoma."

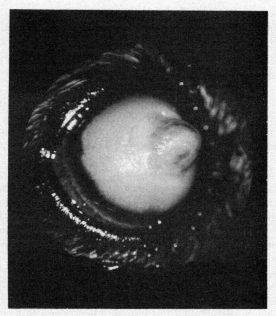

Figure 105–13. A descemetocele with corneal edema and vascularization in a Pekingese.

Scar Formation

Repair of destroyed corneal stroma has been previously described and results in disorganized collagen fibrils of differing diameters—an area of decreased transparency. With time, corneal scars in cats tend to increase in transparency, but in dogs pigmentation and, less frequently, lipid deposition may occur. The deeper the initial injury, the more dense and permanent the resulting scar and the less the tendency for clearing. Very superficial stromal injuries are filled in by epithelial facets. With increasing size and density, corneal opacities are termed nebula, macula, and leukoma (Fig. 105–12). Extensive loss of substance with subsequent cicatrization may result in a thin cornea that bulges (corneal ectasia or kerectasia).

If the stroma is entirely destroyed and Descemet's membrane is forced outward by the intraocular pressure, the lesion is termed a *descemetocele* (Fig. 105–13). Descemetoceles frequently form after unremitting ulceration, and, if untreated, the membrane either ruptures, with loss of aqueous and collapse of the anterior chamber, or becomes surrounded by scar tissue. Descemetoceles do not stain with fluorescein (Fig. 105–14). If the cornea does rupture, the escaping aqueous carries the iris forward into the rupture. If the iris is incorporated into the healing wound, an anterior synechia is formed. If the iris is carried out of the wound, a prolapse of the iris exists (Fig. 105–15).

Opacity resulting from uncomplicated corneal stromal wounds may be limited by the judicious use of corticosteroids provided that: (1) infection has been controlled, (2) an epithelial covering can be demonstrated with fluorescein, and (3) the structural integrity of the cornea is not compromised. Under these circumstances, topically applied corticosteroids (e.g, 0.1% dexamethasone or 1% prednisolone drops, three to four times daily) decrease vascularization, reduce pigmentation, and improve final transparency.

Pigmentation

Corneal pigmentation ("pigmentary keratitis") is a nonspecific response to corneal inflammation, either severe or mild, and not a primary disease. Melanin may be deposited in the stroma or epithelium. Stromal pigment originates from proliferation of normal limbal melanoblasts that migrate into the stroma with blood vessels during vascularization and in response to the same stimulus that caused the ingrowth of blood vessels.

Pigment in the corneal epithelium arises from the basal layer, which is of the same embryological origin as the layer containing pigment in the conjunctiva.

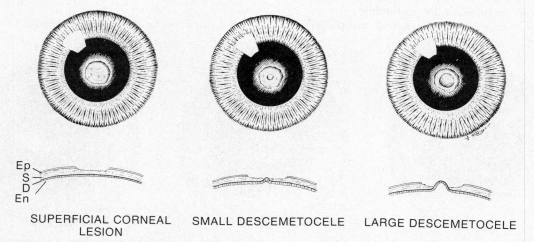

Ep
S
D
En

SUPERFICIAL CORNEAL   SMALL DESCEMETOCELE   LARGE DESCEMETOCELE
LESION

Figure 105–14. Staining characteristics of corneal lesions. *Ep,* epithelium; *S,* stroma; *D,* Descemet's membrane; *En,* endothelium.

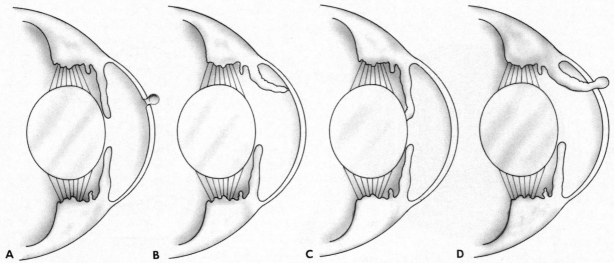

Figure 105–15. Corneal lesions. *A*, Descemetocele. *B*, Anterior synechia. *C*, Posterior synechia. *D*, Iris prolapse.

Epithelial pigmentation is more common in chronic corneal diseases, especially when continuous exposure or irritation is present, e.g., distichiasis, irritation from nasal folds, or chronic exposure in Pekingese and pugs. In these disorders, removal of the stimulus usually prevents the progression of pigmentation. Stromal pigmentation is usually associated with more severe corneal pigmentation and vascularization. In chronic exposure or lack of precorneal tear film, the corneal epithelium may revert to a simple skin pattern with thickening, rete peg formation, keratinization, and pigmentation. Pigmentation with melanin must be distinguished in cats from feline focal corneal necrosis in which the brownish black is believed to be keratin and necrotic stroma.[10]

Pigmentation itself is not normally treated unless vision is threatened. The underlying cause should be removed when possible, e.g., removal of cilia or nasal folds, reduction of the lid aperture in brachycephalic breeds, and control of inflammation in chronic superficial keratitis.[39] Methods used in the treatment of conditions causing pigmentation include superficial keratectomy, β irradiation,[39] and treatment of underlying inflammation with topical corticosteroids.

SURGICAL PROCEDURES

Treatment of Corneal Injuries

In the presence of a penetrating wound of the globe, pressure on the globe may result in further intraocular damage. Initially, a third eyelid flap should be placed over the eye to protect it from further damage until skilled assistance is available. A careful examination is required to evaluate the extent of intraocular injuries. One of the most common causes of severe endophthalmitis and secondary glaucoma leading to enucleation in dogs is unsuspected damage to the lens and its capsule following a perforating corneal injury. If no other intraocular damage is evident, the wound is sutured after routine exposure and fixation of the globe.

Equipment

Magnifying loupe ($\times 2$ to $\times 4$) or operating microscope
   Lid retractors
   Ophthalmic needle holders
   Corneal scissors
   Iris scissors
   Corneal forceps
   Cyclodialysis spatula
   Anterior chamber irrigating bulb and needle
   Fine suture (7-0 or 8-0 silk or 8-0–10-0 nylon with swaged needle)
   Cellulose sponge ("Weckcel")

Balanced salt solution (Alcon) for irrigation. (Epinephrine [1:10,000] and dilute heparin may be added to control hemorrhage and fibrin, respectively.)

Closure of a Corneal Wound

1. The corneal endothelium is exquisitely sensitive to trauma. It should not be touched with instruments or flushed vigorously with irrigating solutions. When the edges of a corneal wound are held, the stroma and the epithelium only are touched with the forceps.

2. The edges of corneal wounds are not debrided; as much tissue as possible is left in place to complete closure.

3. If the wound is fresh, an attempt is made to replace any protruding iris with an iris repositor. This process may be assisted if the anterior chamber is reconstituted with sodium hyaluronate. If the tissue is damaged, the protruding iris is excised with iris scissors. Hemorrhage may be severe if the excision

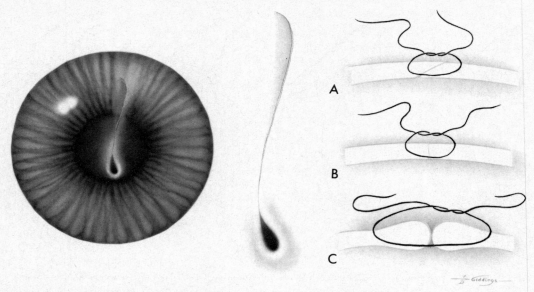

Figure 105–16. Repair of corneal laceration. The diagram illustrates suggested placement of nylon suture material for shelved laceration (A), vertical laceration (B), and laceration with edematous margins (C). (Redrawn after Paton, D., and Goldberg, M. F.: *Management of Ocular Injuries*. W. B. Saunders, Philadelphia, 1976.)

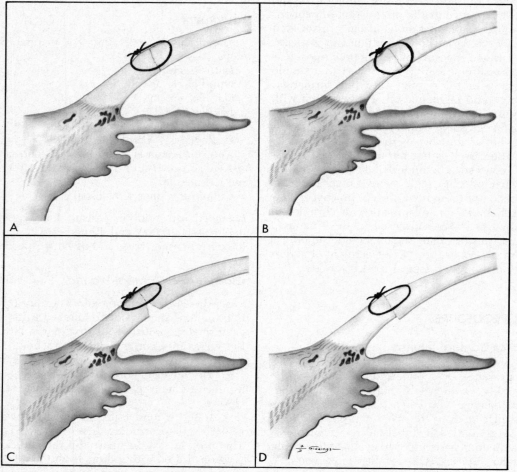

Figure 105–17. A, A correctly placed corneal suture. B, Suture incorrectly penetrates the anterior chamber. C, Suture is too superficial, resulting in poor endothelial closure and persistent edema. D, Bites of the suture are uneven, resulting in poor apposition of the wound edges. (Redrawn after Severin, G.: *Veterinary Ophthalmology Notes*. 2nd ed. Colorado State University Bookstore, Ft. Collins, CO, 1976.)

is near the major arterial circle of the iris; electrocautery is advised.

4. Blood and fibrin clots in the anterior chamber are carefully removed with a cyclodialysis spatula before the wound is closed.

5. Partial thickness sutures are used in the cornea rather than full thickness penetrating sutures (Figs. 105–16 and 105–17).

6. The cornea is sutured with simple interrupted sutures placed about 1 mm apart.

7. After partial closure of the corneal wound, the anterior chamber is carefully irrigated to remove loose debris.

8. The wound is closed and the anterior chamber is reconstituted with balanced salt solution or a small air bubble (Fig. 105–18). In uncomplicated corneal

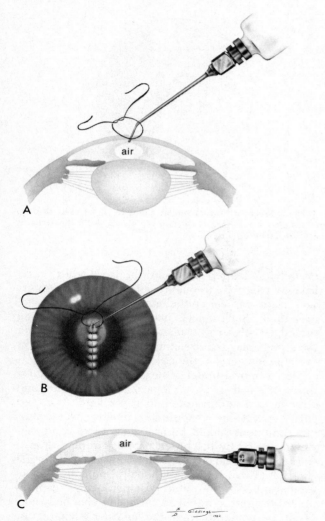

Figure 105–18. Reconstruction of the anterior chamber with a sterile air bubble or balanced salt solution. *A* and *B*, A cannula may be placed between the wound edges or (*C*) via a 25-gauge needle from the limbus. With the sterile air bubble method, care must be taken to use as little air as possible, since, if air gets behind the iris, "air block" glaucoma can occur. Balanced salt solution is preferable to air. (Redrawn after Severin, G.: *Veterinary Ophthalmology Notes.* 2nd ed. Colorado State University Bookstore, Ft. Collins, CO, 1976.)

wounds, some sutures may be removed after seven days.

The prognosis for a corneal wound depends on its initial depth and severity. Lacerations usually have a good prognosis, as do wounds that penetrate the superficial layers only rather than perforating the entire thickness of the cornea. Perforating wounds heal more frequently by vascularization with more scar tissue and opacity. Ruptures of the cornea have a poorer prognosis than do simple lacerations or perforating wounds owing to the greater disruption of tissues adjacent to the wound edge.

Therapy of Descemetocele

A descemetocele is a protrusion of Descemet's membrane through a defect in the corneal epithelium and stroma (see Figs. 105–13 and 105–15) and requires urgent repair because of the risk of corneal rupture. The cause of the initial corneal lesion must be treated and the cornea given structural support to prevent rupture. Direct suturing is often possible in small descemetoceles but produces corneal distortion (astigmatism), which is of little visual significance in dogs and cats. A limiting factor in direct suturing is that the surrounding cornea may not be strong enough to retain sutures.

Therapy

Infected or severely damaged ulcer margins are debrided.

The defect is closed with direct suturing (Fig. 105–19). As the edges are often edematous or lack strength, horizontal mattress sutures may be useful. The anterior chamber is reconstituted with an air bubble or balanced salt solution. For simple lacerations and penetrating wounds, direct suturing is usually the best treatment. If direct closure is not possible, several alternatives are available.

1. Insertion of an allograft of cornea into the defect to add support. The lesion will eventually vascularize, and the button will be rejected, but the cornea may be saved. Because of the availability of donor tissue when required and other therapeutic techniques this method is not often used.

2. Corneoscleral transposition from an adjacent area of normal cornea. Donor tissue is always available for this method, but it is time-consuming to perform. Even though it may result in opacity in the donor bed, the result is often preferable to a dense scar in the area of the original central lesion.

3. Use of a conjunctival flap (see Chapter 102) to support the lesion and aid in vascularization. Of the numerous kinds available, a 360° flap is the easiest to perform. Further support may be given with a third eyelid flap or temporary tarsorrhaphy. Whether to use a third eyelid flap or a conjunctival flap is a matter of personal preference, but in general third eyelid flaps are easier to perform and for many

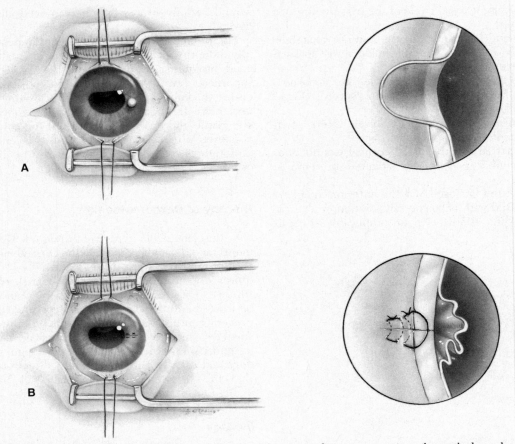

Figure 105–19. Direct suturing of a descemetocele. A, Descemetocele prior to direct suturing. A similar method may be used for deep ulcers in danger of rupture. B, A number of horizontal mattress sutures are placed as necessary to close the defect (7-0 or 8-0 nylon is ideal). Descemet's membrane is not penetrated by the suture. The cornea heals with vascularization.

surgeons give excellent results. For more severe lesions, the conjunctival flap has the theoretical advantage in that it may supply fibroblasts to the stroma in an area of severe corneal destruction.

Topical and systemic antibiotics (e.g., chloramphenicol), atropine (1%), and antiproteases (acetylcysteine) are used postoperatively. Tissue adhesives have been used in such wounds[22] but cannot be recommended until the results of their use are further evaluated in controlled studies.

Severe penetrating wounds of a cornea chronically affected with ulcerative or inflammatory lesions and loss of tissue (e.g., in brachycephalic breeds) often lead to a healed and scarred cornea with loss of the anterior chamber. Iris bombé and secondary glaucoma are frequent sequelae.

Removal of Corneal Foreign Bodies

Corneal foreign bodies are removed to limit pain, reduce the risk of infection, and prevent vascularization and scar formation. Small embedded foreign bodies are removed with an instrument known as a foreign body spud (see Fig. 100–23G). In an emergency, a 25- or 26-gauge needle may be used with a

magnifying loupe. Adherent foreign bodies, e.g., flakes of paint, are frequently found lying in a depression in the corneal epithelium, with the lids passing over them. Such objects may be removed by lifting the edge with an instrument. Objects embedded in the stroma may require an incision in the epithelium over the long axis of the object.

After removal under either local or general anesthesia, a broad spectrum topical antibiotic q.i.d. and atropine are administered to control infection and ciliary spasm due to secondary uveitis. (Note: atropine ointment should be used in cats to avoid salivation caused by the bitter taste of atropine drops.) Corneal epithelial healing is normally rapid, and local anesthetics that inhibit epithelial healing are unnecessary and contraindicated postoperatively. Inappropriate attempts to remove a corneal foreign body may result in penetration of the anterior chamber or corneal damage with more severe vascularization and scar formation.

Superficial Keratectomy

Keratectomy is removal of the corneal epithelium or stroma. Because the corneal stroma does not regenerate, the number of successive keratectomies that can be performed on the same site is limited to two or three, depending on how much tissue is removed with each procedure. Therefore, keratectomy is of limited use in a pathological process that is likely to continue postoperatively. Use of an op-

erating microscope greatly improves the results in this procedure.

Superficial keratectomy is indicated in several situations.

1. Removal of neoplasms encroaching from the limbus.

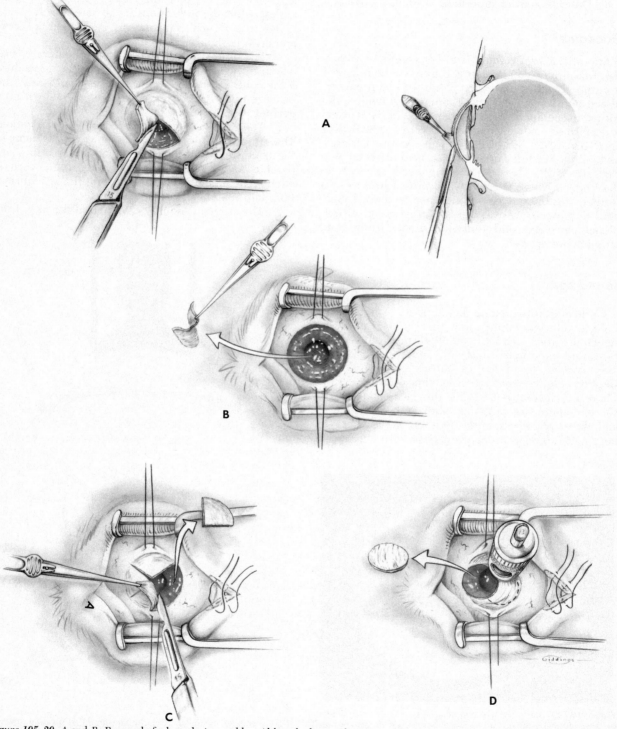

Figure 105–20. *A* and *B,* Removal of a large lesion *en bloc.* Although clear at this stage, the cornea soon becomes edematous. *C,* Division of the cornea into quadrants. *D,* Outline of the area to be removed with a corneal trephine. The canthotomy is closed. (Redrawn after Severin, G.: *Veterinary Ophthalmology Notes.* 2nd ed. Colorado State University Bookstore, Ft. Collins, CO, 1976.)

2. Removal of superficial opaque tissue in specific keratopathies to improve vision, e.g., chronic superficial keratitis (Überreiter's syndrome).

3. Treatment of specific keratopathies, e.g., superficial corneal erosion syndrome in corgis and boxers and focal corneal necrosis (mummification/sequestration) in cats.

4. Debridement of superficial epithelial wounds.

Procedure

Superficial keratectomy is either complete or partial. In complete keratectomy, the area to be removed is outlined with a corneal trephine set to a predetermined depth (e.g., 0.3 to 0.4 mm) or by dividing the cornea in segments (Fig. 105–20). The initial incision is performed under magnification with a #64 Beaver or #15 Bard-Parker blade, and dissection is continued with a Martinez or similar corneal dissector (see Fig. 100–23B). The stroma is removed in sheets to the limbus, where it is cut with corneal scissors or a scalpel. Postoperatively, the cornea is stained daily with fluorescein to evaluate the progression of epithelial coverage, and topical antibiotic drops and atropine are applied.

Keratoplasty

Corneal transplantation (keratoplasty) is not widely used in veterinary ophthalmic surgery. It is useful in selected cases, such as bilateral corneal edema due to canine endothelial dystrophy, in which it is the only specific treatment of choice[17] (Fig. 105–21). Reports of long-term success in clinical cases are few. There are several reasons for this lack of long-term success: there are problems with graft rejection,[8,24] and there are fewer indications for keratoplasty in dogs and cats than in man, in whom visual performance as distinct from relative decreased vision is more critical than in dogs and cats. The importance of microsurgical technique and immunosuppression with corticosteroids to the success of canine keratoplasty has been reported[27] and results contrasted with those of studies in which they were not used.[8] In general, the feline cornea has a higher degree of long-term success than the canine cornea after keratoplasty, but the indications in cats are fewer.

Before a corneal transplant is recommended, several criteria should be fulfilled.

1. The animal must have a severe bilateral visual handicap, as the benefit gained with the procedure if the contralateral eye has vision does not justify the expense to the owner and risk to the animal with the current rate of success.

2. The cornea should be free of vascularization. This condition is often not met, however, as many of the conditions that reduce corneal transparency are chronic and eventually vascularize, e.g., chronic edema, pigmentation, chronic keratitis, scar formation, and feline focal corneal necrosis.

3. The surgeon should be trained in the use of the

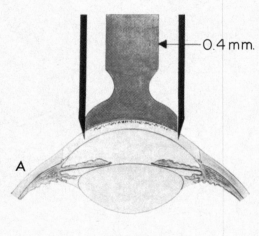

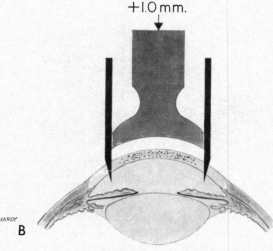

Figure 105–22. Lamellar (A) and penetrating (B) keratoplasty with a corneal trephine. (Reprinted with permission from Castroviejo, R.: Atlas of Keratectomy and Keratoplasty. W. B. Saunders, Philadelphia, 1966.)

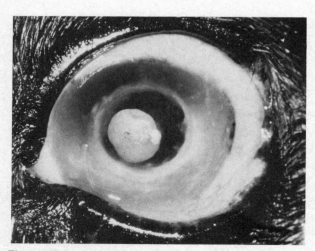

Figure 105–21. Postoperative appearance 16 months after a penetrating corneal graft in a 12-year-old Boston terrier with corneal edema due to corneal dystrophy. The clear donor button contains an area of opacity, probably calcification. (Courtesy of Dr. G. L. Gwin.)

operating microscope[42] and should be familiar with keratoplasty techniques.

Corneal grafts are of two main types: penetrating and lamellar (Fig. 105–22).

Penetrating Keratoplasty

Penetrating keratoplasty is used to replace scarred or diseased cornea. Affected tissue is removed full thickness and is replaced with a donor button lined with viable endothelium. Major problems encountered with penetrating keratoplasty in dogs are formation of protein-rich ("plasmoid") aqueous, shrinkage of the donor button after harvesting and before insertion in the recipient, and postoperative vascularization. Formation of plasmoid aqueous may be minimized by pretreatment with: (1) systemic corticosteroids, e.g., prednisolone 1 to 2 mg/kg orally, daily for three days; (2) antiprostaglandins for 24 to 48 hours, e.g., 300 mg acetylsalicylic acid orally two to three times daily; (3) systemic antihistamines, e.g., chlorpheniramine 0.5 mg/kg intramuscularly 45 minutes before the recipient eye is opened; and (4) heparin (1000 units/ml), 0.1 to 0.2 ml instilled into the anterior chamber of the recipient when it is opened.

Technique (Figure 105–23)

1. With the trephine depth set to 1.0 mm the lesion is removed (Fig. 105–23A) and the trephine is withdrawn as soon as the anterior chamber is penetrated (Fig. 105–23B).

2. If the corneal disc is not completely removed, corneal scissors are used to complete removal (Fig. 105–23C and D).

3. Any bevel or tags of tissue are trimmed from the edge of the incision with the same scissors and either fine corneal forceps or jeweler's forceps (Fig. 105–23E and F).

4. The surface of the donor button is washed with Neosporin solution, and the graft is removed from the donor eye (Fig. 105–23G and H). Alternatively, the cornea and a rim of sclera 4 to 5 mm in width may be removed from the donor eye and placed epithelium down onto an excavated Teflon block. The donor disc may then be cut from the endothelial surface, taking care not to allow the trephine to contact the endothelial surface. Whichever method is used, the endothelial surface should be preserved and not touched. Note that the donor button must be 0.5 mm larger than the recipient bed to allow for shrinkage.[27]

5. The donor button is removed (Fig. 105–23I and J).

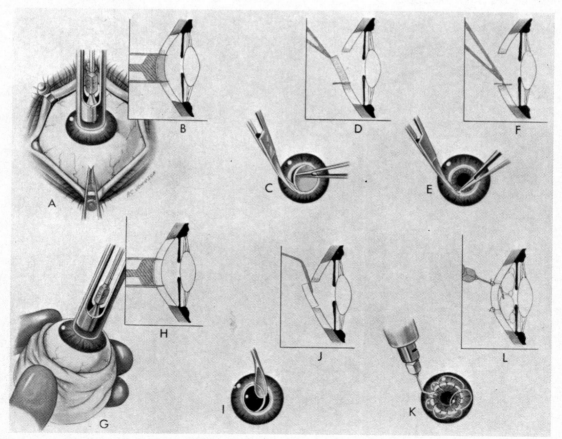

Figure 105–23. Penetrating keratoplasty. (Reprinted with permission from Castroviejo, R.: *Atlas of Keratectomy and Keratoplasty.* W. B. Saunders, Philadelphia, 1966.)

6. The button is placed into the recipient bed and sutured in place with four cardinal sutures, one in each quadrant. The suturing is completed with either multiple interrupted sutures or a continuous suture with buried knot. The cardinal sutures may be removed.[42] The anterior chamber is reconstituted with balanced salt solution and air (Fig. 105–23K and L).

7. Postoperatively, antibiotic and corticosteroid solutions are applied three to four times daily.

Postoperative vascularization is minimized by using fine sutures (e.g., 8-0 to 10-0 nylon), careful technique, and topical corticosteroids (e.g., 0.1% dexamethasone three to four times daily). Sutures are removed after 8 to 18 days.[27]

Lamellar Keratoplasty

In this type of graft,[21] epithelium and superficial layers of the stroma are dissected free and replaced with donor tissue, usually as an aid to structural support during the healing phase of a corneal wound, e.g., as in descemetocele or after removal of an opacity or scar.

Technique (Figure 105–24)

1. The area to be removed is outlined with the blade of the trephine set at 0.4 mm (Fig. 105–24A).

2. The lesion is removed with a corneal dissector or corneal scissors (Fig. 105–23B).

3. The donor eye is washed with antibiotic solution. The donor lamellar graft is removed from the donor eye (the graft is 0.5 mm larger than the recipient bed (Fig. 15–24D). A corneal dissector may be used in place of an electrokeratome.

4. The donor tissue is sutured into the recipient bed with either a continuous running suture with buried knot[42] or multiple interrupted sutures (Fig. 105–24E).

5. Postoperatively, topical antibiotic and corticosteroid solutions are applied three to four times daily.

Penetrating Corneoscleral Allograft

Replacement of continuous cornea and sclera from a donor of the same species is the treatment of choice for canine epibulbar melanoma when the tumor infiltrates the cornea or sclera. Canine epibulbar melanoma (Fig. 105–25) is a distinct tumor entity[25] and must be distinguished from melanosis of the conjunctiva and extension of intraocular melanoma through the cornea and sclera. In intraocular melanoma the intraocular mass or its sequelae are visible during examination of the anterior chamber. Melanosis of the conjunctiva has the potential for malignant transformation in the dogs, and local resection with β irradiation is the treatment of choice rather than cornea scleral resection and allografting.[40]

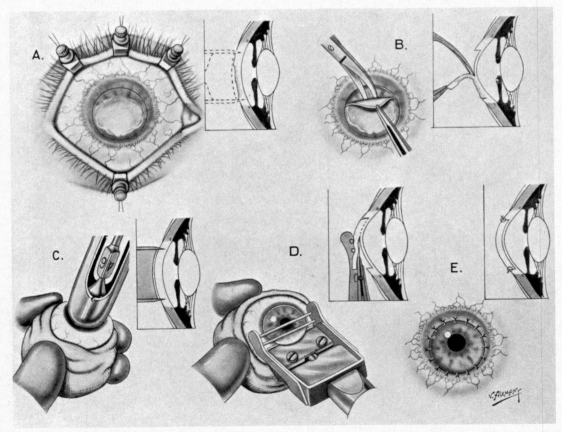

Figure 105–24. The technique of lamellar keratoplasty. A Martinez corneal dissector may be used in place of an electrokeratome (D). (Reprinted with permission from Castroviejo, R.: *Atlas of Keratectomy and Keratoplasty.* W. B. Saunders, Philadelphia, 1966.)

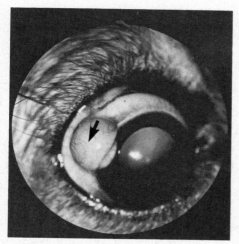

Figure 105–25. Amelanotic epibulbar melanoma (arrow) in a two-year-old American cocker spaniel. Note the typical dorsolateral limbal position. (Reprinted with permission from Martin, C. L.: Canine epibulbar melanomas and their management. J. Am. Anim. Hosp. Assoc. *17*:83, 1981.)

Donor tissue is collected aseptically as soon as possible before resection of the lesion and is kept on a sterile gauze pad moistened with balanced salt solution. All traces of uveal tissue are removed from the inner surface of the graft to reduce the severity of postoperative immune reactions. The technique for resection and placement of the graft is illustrated (Fig. 105–26). The graft is sutured with 8-0 to 10-0 monofilament nylon, and the eye is treated topically with a broad spectrum antibiotic, e.g., gentamicin four to six times daily, and a corticosteroid solution,

e.g., 1% prednisolone at the same frequency, for seven to ten days. The graft slowly vascularizes around its margins, sutures are removed, and therapy is discontinued.

Corneoscleral Transposition

Corneoscleral transposition[30] is replacement of part of the cornea by adjacent sclera, which is mobilized to fill a defect when a lesion is removed (Fig. 105–27). The technique is indicated when insufficient tissue remains to fill a defect after removal of a large lesion. Alternatives to this technique include penetrating keratoplasty and penetrating corneoscleral allograft.[12, 25]

ADVANCES IN CORNEAL SURGERY AND THERAPEUTICS

Sodium Hyaluronate

Sodium hyaluronate (Healon) is a viscous disaccharide polymer that is widely used during intraocular procedures in man. It is inserted into the anterior chamber during surgery to facilitate dissection and prevent adhesion of tissues; this decreases handling of the cornea and loss of endothelial cells.

Keratoprosthesis

Prosthokeratoplasty is replacement of part of the cornea with a prosthesis. The technique is applicable

Figure 105–26. Penetrating corneoscleral allograft. *A*, The conjunctiva is incised and retracted. *B*, The affected cornea and sclera are excised full thickness with scissors or scalpel after initial use of an electroscalpel to reduce hemorrhage. *C*, Oversized donor tissue is sutured along one scleral edge. *D–G*, Remaining edges of the graft are trimmed and sutured. *H*, Adjacent conjunctiva is mobilized and sutured to the graft. (Reprinted with permission from Martin, C. L.: Canine epibulbar melanomas and their management. J. Am. Anim. Hosp. Assoc. *17*:83, 1981.)

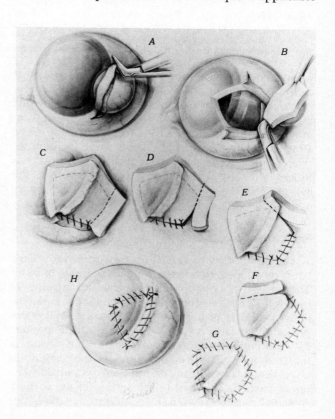

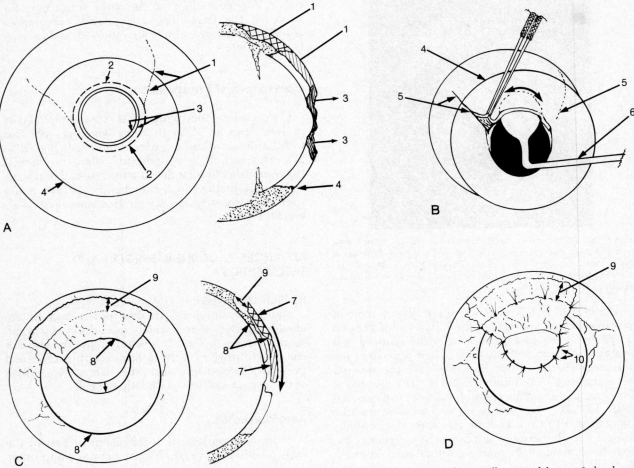

Figure 105–27. Corneoscleral transposition. *A*, Step 1. *1*, Line of graft excision; *2*, borders of surgically excised lesion; *3*, border of necrotic tissue; *4*, limbus. *B*, Step 2. *5*, Borders of graft tissue; *6*, corneal dissector. *C*, Step 3. *7*, Scleral and corneal parts of grafts; *8*, limbus of graft and globe; *9*, gap created in sclera by sliding the graft toward the cornea. *D*, Step 4. *10*, Placement of sutures. (Reprinted with permission from Parshall, C. J.: Lamellar corneal-scleral transposition. J. Am. Anim. Hosp. Assoc. 9:270, 1973.)

when penetrating keratoplasty has a poor prognosis owing to severe corneal scarring or vascularization. A variety of corneal prostheses have been developed experimentally, but methylmethacrylate is most commonly used in man.[35] The prostheses have been attached to the cornea by silicone, bone, or methacrylate screw devices incorporated in the prosthesis to help prevent extrusion of the prosthesis from the cornea. None are commonly used in veterinary ophthalmic surgery.

Refractive Keratoplasty[2, 35]

A number of controversial surgical procedures have been developed to correct refractive errors in man. They have in common the mechanical turning of frozen tissue either the patient's own tissue (keratomileusis) or that of a donor (keratophakia, epikeratophakia) on a lathe to the desired optical parameter. In keratomileusis and keratophakia, the tissue is inserted into the corneal stroma of the patient to alter the refractive power. In epikeratophakia the donor tissue is attached to the surface of the cornea. Radial keratotomy[11] is a technique in which nu-

merous radial incisions are made in the cornea to reduce its refractive power in severe myopia (nearsightedness). These techniques are not currently used in veterinary ophthalmology.

Tissue Adhesives

Tissue adhesives can be used to close corneal wounds but are used more in veterinary ophthalmic surgery for the treatment of superficial corneal ulceration, especially in brachycephalic breeds susceptible to recurrent ulceration.[22] The glue is applied to the dried lesion with a sterile toothpick and remains in place for two to three days, providing additional support to the cornea. When used in this manner, the glue supports the cornea while normal vascularized healing takes place beneath. The technique has not been shown to have significant advantages over coverage of the lesion with a third eyelid flap.

Hydrophilic Contact Lenses

Hydrophilic contact lenses are occasionally used to cover corneas with severe bullous keratopathy and can also be used to administer drugs to the cornea in high concentrations.[39] A lens that fits the eye properly is placed in an antibiotic solution until saturated with the drug and then is applied to the eye. The antibiotic diffuses from the lens and enters the cornea in high concentrations. The lens must be recharged with drugs several times daily, the frequency depending on the properties of the individual drug and the composition of the lens.

Corneal Preservation

Corneas can be preserved by a variety of techniques for subsequent keratoplasty, although a shortage of donor tissues has not stimulated their use in veterinary surgery. Culture of endothelial cells and replacement of damaged endothelium have recently been achieved in animals[1] and await application to clinical problems such as endothelial dystrophy.

CORNEAL DISORDERS OF SURGICAL IMPORTANCE
Ulcerative Keratitis[39]

A corneal ulcer occurs when corneal epithelium and a variable amount of stroma are missing. Small acute ulcers heal rapidly, but chronic lesions may heal slowly if at all.

Progression. Corneal ulcers may progress to involve deeper layers, as shown in the box at the bottom of the page. In treating corneal ulceration, the most important step is to determine and remove the cause of the ulceration, then to try to create an ideal environment for healing of the lesion and prevention of progression, with surgical treatment to prevent rupture. Regardless of the initial cause, all corneal ulcers have the potential to progress to endophthalmitis if not treated. The most common causes of ulceration in the dog and cat are listed (Table 105–1).

Normal corneal epithelium is a very effective barrier against invading bacteria. In simple traumatic injuries with a small epithelial defect, healing is rapid. If the ulcer becomes infected or if the epithelium is unable to attach to the underlying stroma, healing is delayed, and progression to a deep ulcer and beyond may occur. Progression of the lesion may be limited to a small area of the cornea, or the whole cornea may become affected.

In chronic or infected ulcers, proteases may speed the progression ("melting") of a simple ulcer to rupture and iris prolapse (within 24 hours in some cases). Proteases are produced by healing epithelium, bacteria (*Pseudomonas* spp. especially), neutrophils, and possibly stroma.[3, 15, 38] Their action is potentiated by

TABLE 105–1. Etiology of Corneal Ulceration

Dog	Cat
Trauma	Trauma
Foreign body	Foreign body
Distichiasis	Herpetic keratitis
Keratitis sicca	Entropion
Entropion	
Superficial corneal erosion	
Chronic corneal edema	
Tumors of lid margin	

corticosteroids. Proteases are not important in the pathogenesis of all corneal ulcers, but those in which they are active have a grayish, gelatinous appearance around the margin, which must be distinguished from the uncomplicated corneal edema found around any penetrating corneal wound to which tear fluid has access. Corneal ulceration causes secondary uveitis, which may result in hypopyon.

Diagnosis. Clinical signs of corneal ulceration are illustrated (Fig. 105–28).

Corneal ulcers are frequently invisible even with good lighting. For this reason, all red and painful eyes must be stained with fluorescein and the intraocular pressure measured. Ancillary diagnostic tests (bacterial culture, corneal scraping for Gram and Giemsa staining) are also useful depending on the stage of the ulcer (see box at bottom of page 1528).

The clinical handling of a corneal ulcer is summarized in Table 105–2. Occasionally it is necessary to institute treatment phases 1 and 2 without knowing the cause, either because it is obscure or because the structural integrity of the eye must be preserved while awaiting laboratory results. The stage reached by the ulcer determines which methods are chosen in phases 2 and 3. In addition to the measures outlined, topical atropine therapy (1% t.i.d.) is instituted to relieve ciliary spasm and pain due to secondary anterior uveitis and decrease the formation of anterior synechiae between a miotic pupil and the cornea.

In most cases no attempt is made to inhibit this secondary uveitis or to remove purulent exudate and inflammatory cells from the anterior chamber, as the immunoglobulins and macrophages aid in resolution of the ulcer. The use of vitamin A, estrogens, or chemical cautery (liquid phenol, iodine) is not recommended in the treatment of indolent ulceration. Careful surgical debridement, use of antibiotics, and physical coverage of the lesion are more consistent with the principles of corneal wound healing and yield excellent results when properly applied. The following combination of antibiotics, atropine, antiprotease agents, and base is commonly and effectively used.[39]

Superficial ulceration	→	Deep ulceration	→	Descemetocele	→	Iris prolapse	→	Endophthalmitis

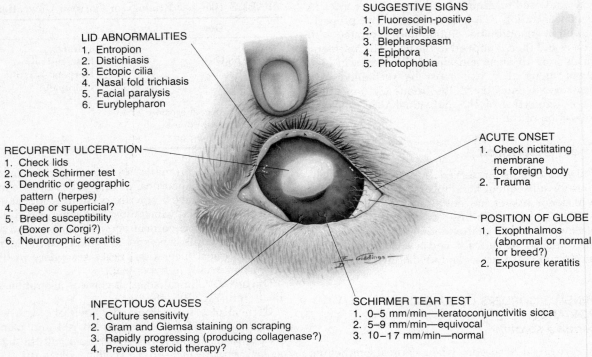

LID ABNORMALITIES
1. Entropion
2. Distichiasis
3. Ectopic cilia
4. Nasal fold trichiasis
5. Facial paralysis
6. Euryblepharon

SUGGESTIVE SIGNS
1. Fluorescein-positive
2. Ulcer visible
3. Blepharospasm
4. Epiphora
5. Photophobia

RECURRENT ULCERATION
1. Check lids
2. Check Schirmer test
3. Dendritic or geographic pattern (herpes)
4. Deep or superficial?
5. Breed susceptibility (Boxer or Corgi?)
6. Neurotrophic keratitis

ACUTE ONSET
1. Check nictitating membrane for foreign body
2. Trauma

POSITION OF GLOBE
1. Exophthalmos (abnormal or normal for breed?)
2. Exposure keratitis

INFECTIOUS CAUSES
1. Culture sensitivity
2. Gram and Giemsa staining on scraping
3. Rapidly progressing (producing collagenase?)
4. Previous steroid therapy?

SCHIRMER TEAR TEST
1. 0–5 mm/min—keratoconjunctivitis sicca
2. 5–9 mm/min—equivocal
3. 10–17 mm/min—normal

Figure 105–28. Clinical signs of corneal ulceration.

Acetylcysteine 20% ("Mucomyst")	6.0 ml
Atropine ophthalmic solution 1%	6.0 ml
Chloramphenicol succinate 20%	1.2 ml
(or gentamicin 5%)	(1.5 ml)
Artificial tear solution	q.s. to 25.0 ml

Acetylcysteine has been shown to retain its potency at room temperature,[7] thus reducing the handling problems formerly associated with refrigeration of this medication.[39] For details of other protease inhibitors, readers are referred to general veterinary ophthalmology texts.[39] In uncomplicated ulcers coverage with a third eyelid flap (see Chapter 104) or a conjunctival flap (see Chapter 102) should be maintained for seven to ten days. During this time medications are placed on top of the flap. If any of the following signs appear, the flap is removed and the cornea examined for:

1. Purulent discharge.
2. Sudden voluminous watery discharge, which may indicate corneal rupture and escape of aqueous.

3. Hemorrhagic discharge.
4. Sudden, painful blepharospasm.

A small amount of discharge from an eye with a third eyelid is normal. Flaps usually relieve much of the discomfort of painful corneal lesions.

During the healing phase, deep and superficial vascularization occurs, with formation of granulation tissue in the wound bed. Residual scar formation is lessened if corticosteroids are used with care (after an epithelial cover has been demonstrated with fluorescein). At this stage the lesion should be checked frequently and any steroids administered in a topical form that can be quickly discontinued if infection or poor healing occurs, e.g., 1% prednisolone (Prednefrin Forte) or 0.1% dexamethasone (Maxidex). Combined antibiotic steroids may be used provided no infection is present.

Neoplasia

Corneal neoplasms in dogs and cats are uncommon. Squamous cell carcinomas are the most common,

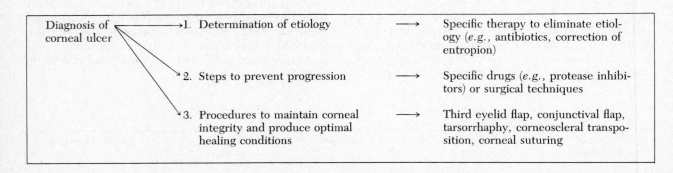

Diagnosis of corneal ulcer	→ 1. Determination of etiology	⟶	Specific therapy to eliminate etiology (*e.g.*, antibiotics, correction of entropion)
	→ 2. Steps to prevent progression	⟶	Specific drugs (*e.g.*, protease inhibitors) or surgical techniques
	→ 3. Procedures to maintain corneal integrity and produce optimal healing conditions	⟶	Third eyelid flap, conjunctival flap, tarsorrhaphy, corneoscleral transposition, corneal suturing

TABLE 105–2. Treatment of Corneal Ulceration

Type of Ulcer	Phase 1	Phase 2	Phase 3
Simple superficial ulcer	Topical antibiotics Correction of lid defects (*e.g.*, entropion, cilia) Topical atropine	Rarely necessary	Rarely necessary
Uncomplicated deep ulcer	Topical antibiotics Topical atropine	Antiprotease agents Debridement	Third eyelid flap Tear replacement
Complicated deep ulcer	Topical, subconjunctival, and systemic antibiotics (subpalpebral lavage) Topical atropine	Antiprotease agents Debridement (surgical, chemical)	Conjunctival or third eyelid flap Tear replacement
Descemetocele	Topical, subconjunctival, and systemic antibiotics (subpalpebral lavage) Topical atropine	Antiprotease agents	Conjunctival or third eyelid flap Tear replacement or corneoscleral transposition
Iris prolapse	Topical, subconjunctival, and systemic antibiotics (subpalpebral lavage) Topical atropine	Antiprotease agents	Resection or replacement of prolapsed iris Conjunctival or third eyelid flap Suture lacerations Reconstitution of anterior chamber

especially in lightly pigmented animals, in which they may involve the conjunctiva, cornea, and lids. Depending on the extent of invasion, they are treated by surgical excision (superficial keratectomy, corneoscleral transposition, corneoscleral allografting) or cryotherapy and β radiation therapy[39] (see Chapters 169, 170 and 180). Although chemotherapy and immunotherapy are used in ocular squamous cell carcinomas in cattle and horses, their use has not been described extensively in dogs and cats (see Chapters 171 and 172).

Dermoids (Dermolipoma)

Dermoids (see Chapter 102) usually involve both conjunctiva and cornea. Those involving the cornea are removed by superficial keratectomy with local conjunctivectomy. Dermoids may extend to deeper corneal layers, and even after uneventful keratectomy corneal scarring occasionally occurs.

Bullous Keratopathy

Bullous keratopathy is a nonspecific response to chronic corneal disease. It begins as formation of small vesicles in the epithelium that coalesce to form larger bullae. The surrounding epithelium and stroma are edematous and often vascularized, because of either the bullae or the underlying corneal disease.

Differential Diagnosis. Bullous keratopathy must be distinguished from descemetocele, iris prolapse, and epithelial inclusion cysts.[39]

Treatment. Bullous keratopathy should be managed as follows:

1. Treatment of the underlying disorder, if known, e.g., herpetic keratitis.
2. Surgical removal of the bullae by superficial keratectomy.
3. Initial coverage with a third eyelid flap and routine administration of topical antibiotics, atropine, and protease inhibitors.[39]
4. Continued protection of the cornea with a hydrophilic contact lens and artificial tear solutions, e.g., Adsorbotear.* Although the use of hypertonic preparations (e.g., 5% sodium chloride, 5% Adsorbonac*) has been advocated to remove fluid from the vesicles, I have found them to be of limited use for long-term treatment. In the long term, bullous keratopathy has a guarded prognosis.

Feline Focal Corneal Necrosis[10]

Focal corneal necrosis (corneal mummification,[45] sequestration,[39] keratitis nigrum[5]) occurs most commonly in Persian cats and less frequently in the Siamese and domestic short-haired breeds. The etiology is unknown, but the disease usually occurs after previous ulceration or keratitis and consists of dark necrotic corneal stroma tightly attached to the cornea. The lesion may extend down to Descemet's membrane in severe cases.

Clinical Signs. The clinical signs of feline focal corneal necrosis are (1) slowly progressive focal, brownish black corneal lesion (often of several months duration), (2) corneal vascularization, (3) epiphora, and (4) pain and blepharospasm.

---

*Burton Parsons and Co., Washington, D.C.

Treatment. Before treatment is attempted, the lesion should have ceased to enlarge, as a nonprogressive lesion is less likely to recur postoperatively. The necrotic material must be removed by superficial keratectomy before the cornea will heal. The use of an operating microscope is recommended because the lesion is often deep, and extreme care must be exercised during keratectomy to avoid corneal penetration. Postoperatively, the site is covered with a third eyelid flap and treated with topical antibiotics and atropine as for an ulcer (see Table 105–2). Topical corticosteroids may be used in the healing phase to reduce corneal opacity, provided herpesfelis is not the cause of the initial lesion. Prolonged corneal coverage is occasionally necessary, and the condition does recur.

Superficial Corneal Erosion

Superficial corneal erosion is seen most commonly in the boxer[34] and corgi[39] although other breeds are affected. Affected dogs usually have a history of blepharospasm and epiphora that have been resistant to treatment with topical antibiotics, sometimes for several months.

Clinical Signs. The clinical signs of superficial corneal erosion are unilateral chronic blepharospasm, epiphora, and photophobia.

The lesions may be due to separation of the corneal epithelium from the basal lamina because of a defect in the hemidesmosomes,[14, 37, 39] although abnormalities of the basal epithelial cells and anterior stroma have been noted.[41] Affected areas are usually 3 to 4 mm in diameter, have a ragged outline, cause intense pain, and stain with fluorescein. Epithelium often accumulates at the periphery, causing a "rolled-up" appearance, as it does not attach to the underlying stroma. Superficial corneal erosions usually do not stimulate vascularization unless very chronic; this is a useful feature in differential diagnosis.

Treatment. Superficial keratectomy is the treatment of choice.[31, 39] The lesion and a margin of 2 to 2.5 mm of normal surrounding tissue are removed superficially, preferably using an operating microscope. The cornea is covered and treated as for a superficial ulcer (see Table 105–2). The eye is medicated with topical broad spectrum antibiotics and atropine, t.i.d. for two days before and seven days after surgery. After removal of the flap, topical corticosteroid therapy (prednisolone 1%, dexamethasone 0.1% t.i.d.) is used to reduce scar formation. The lesions rarely recur in the same eye after treatment.

Epithelial Inclusion Cysts

Epithelial inclusion cysts[23] are a rare corneal lesion in which a fluid-filled sac lined with epithelium is present in the corneal stroma. The cyst appears as an elevation 3 to 4 mm in diameter on the corneal surface. It has been proposed that they are caused by traumatic inclusion of epithelium into the stroma. The cyst is removed by superficial keratectomy.

Superficial Pigmentary Keratitis

Superficial pigmentary keratitis occurs most frequently in the Pekingese, pug, and Boston terrier. It is a nonspecific, chronic, low-grade keratitis with pigmentation of the superficial stroma and epithelium[39] due to one or more of the following: (1) chronic exposure of the cornea with prominent globes and a large palpebral fissue (euryblepharon) (see Chapter 101), (2) distichiasis (see Chapter 101), and (3) nasal fold trichiasis (see Chapter 101).

Pigmentation frequently advances to occlude the central cornea and interfere with vision before the owner is aware of its presence. The condition is treated by correction of the causative factors to prevent progression of pigmentation rather than removal of pigment.

Pseudopterygium

Pseudopterygium is an adhesion of conjunctiva to a superficial corneal lesion preventing passage of light and is named because of its similarity to the human condition—pterygium—which does not occur in dogs or cats. Its most common cause is herpesfelis infection in young cats (see Chapter 102). In severe cases the whole cornea may be affected. The conjunctival epithelium may be removed by keratectomy, but regrowth is not uncommon.

1. Bahn, C. F., MacCallum, D. K., Lillie, J. H., Meyer, R. F., and Martoni, C. L.: Complications associated with bovine corneal endothelial cell-lined homografts in the cat. Invest. Ophthalmol. Vis. Sci. 22:73, 1982.
2. Barraquer, J. I.: Corneoplastic surgery. Proc. 2nd Int. Corneoplastic Conf., London, 1967.
3. Befanis, P. J., Peiffer, R. L., and Brown, D.: Endothelial repair of the canine cornea. Am. J. Vet. Res. 21:113, 1981.
4. Berman, M. B., Dohlman, C. H., Davison, P. F., et al.: Characterization of collagenolytic activity in the ulcerating cornea. Exp. Eye Res. 11:225, 1971.
5. Blogg, J. R.: The Eye in Veterinary Practice. W. B. Saunders, Philadelphia, 1980.
6. Brown, S. I.: Collagenase and corneal ulcers. Invest. Ophthalmol. 10:203, 1971.
7. Costa, N. D., and Slatter, D. H.: The potency of acetylcysteine in pharmaceutical preparations—effects of temperature and storage. Aust. Vet. J. 60:195, 1983.
8. Dice, P. F., Severin, G. E., and Lumb, W. V.: Experimental autogenous and homologous corneal transplantation in the dog. J. Am. Anim. Hosp. Assoc. 9:245, 1973.
9. Duke-Elder, S., and Leigh, A. G.: System of Ophthalmology, Vol. VIII., Diseases of the Outer Eye, Part 2. Henry Kimpton, London, 1965.
10. Formston, C., Bedford, P. G. C., Staton, J. F., and Tripathi, R. C.: Corneal necrosis in the cat. J. Small Anim. Pract. 15:19, 1974.
11. Fyodorov, S. N., and Durnev, V. V.: Operation of dosaged dissection of corneal circular ligament in cases of myopia of mild degree. Ann. Ophthal. 11:1885, 1979.
12. Gelatt, K. N.: Excision of adenocarcinoma of iris and ciliary body. J. Am. Anim. Hosp. Assoc. 6:59, 1970.

13. Gelatt, K. N.: *Veterinary Ophthalmology*. Lea & Febiger, Philadelphia, 1981.
14. Gelatt, K. N., and Samuelson, D. A.: Recurrent corneal erosions and epithelial dystrophy in the boxer dog. J. Am. Anim. Hosp. Assoc. *18*:453, 1982.
15. Gordon, J. M., Bauer, E. A., and Eisen, A. Z.: Collagenase in human cornea—immunologic localization. Arch. Ophthalmol. *98*:341, 1980.
16. Gwin, R. L., Lerner, I., Warren, J. K., and Gum, G.: Decrease in canine corneal endothelial cell density and increase in corneal thickness as functions of age. Invest. Ophthal. Vis. Sci. *22*:267, 1982.
17. Gwin, R. M., Polack, F. M., Warren, J. K., Samuelson, D. A., and Gelatt, K. N.: Primary canine corneal endothelial cell dystrophy: Specular microscopic evaluation and therapy. J. Am. Anim. Hosp. Assoc. *18*:471, 1982.
18. Hogan, M. J., Alvarado, J. A., and Weddell, J. E.: *Histology of the Human Eye*. W. B. Saunders, Philadelphia, 1971.
19. Hogan, M. J., and Zimmerman, L. E.: *Ophthalmic Pathology — A Text and Atlas*. W. B. Saunders, Philadelphia, 1962.
20. Keough, E. M., Wilcox, L. M., Connally, R. J., and Hotte, C. E.: The effect of complete tenotomy on blood flow to the anterior segment of the canine eye. Invest. Ophthalmol. Vis. Sci. *19*:1355, 1980.
21. Khodadoust, A. A.: Lamellar corneal transplantation in the rabbit. Am. J. Ophthalmol. *66*:1111, 1968.
22. Koch, S. A.: Paper presented at 12th Ann. Sci. Meeting, Am. Coll. Vet. Ophthalmol., Lake Tahoe, Nevada, 1982.
23. Koch, S. A., Langloss, J. H., and Schmidt, G.: Corneal epithelial inclusion cysts in four dogs. J. Small Anim. Pract. *164*:1192, 1974.
24. Kuhns, E. L., Keller, W. F., and Blanchard, G. L.: The treatment of pannus in dogs by use of a corneal scleral graft. J. Am. Vet. Med. Assoc. *162*:950, 1973.
25. Martin, C. L.: Canine epibulbar melanomas and their management. J. Am. Anim. Hosp. Assoc. *17*:83, 1981.
26. Maurice, D. M.: The location of the fluid pump in the cornea. J. Physiol. (London) *221*:43, 1972.
27. McEntyre, J.: Experimental penetrating keratoplasty in the dog. Arch. Ophthalmol. *80*:372, 1968.
28. Morrin, L. A., Waring, G. O., and Spangler, W.: Oval lipid opacities in beagles: Ultrastructure of normal beagle cornea. Am. J. Vet. Res. *43*:443, 1982.
29. Moses, R. A.: *Adler's Physiology of the Eye*, 6th ed. C. V. Mosby, St. Louis, 1975.
30. Parshall, C. J.: Lamellar corneal-scleral transposition. J. Am. Anim. Hosp. Assoc. *9*:270, 1973.
31. Peiffer, R. L., Gelatt, K. N., and Gwin, R. M.: Superficial keratectomy in the management of indolent ulcers of the boxer cornea. Canine Pract. *3*:31, 1976.
32. Pfister, R. R.: The healing of corneal epithelial abrasions in the rabbit: a scanning electron microscope study. Invest. Ophthalmol. *14*:648, 1975.
33. Refojo, M. F., Dohlmann, C. H., Ahmad, B., Carroll, J. M., and Allen, J. C.: Evaluation of adhesives for corneal surgery. Arch. Ophthalmol. *80*:645, 1968.
34. Roberts, S. R.: Superficial indolent ulcer of the cornea in boxer dogs. J. Small Anim. Pract. *6*:111, 1966.
35. Roper-Hall, M. J.: *Stallard's Eye Surgery*, 6th ed. John Wright and Son, Bristol, 1980.
36. Rosenthal, J. J.: Bullous keratopathy: a latent complication of chronic corneal disease. Vet. Med./Sm. Anim. Clin. *69*:181, 1974.
37. Shively, J. N., and Epling, G. P.: Fine structure of the canine eye: cornea. Am. J. Vet. Res. *31*:713, 1970.
38. Slansky, H. H., and Dohlman, C. H.: Collagenase and the cornea. Surv. Ophthal. *14*:402, 1970.
39. Slatter, D. H.: *Fundamentals of Veterinary Ophthalmology*. W. B. Saunders, Philadelphia, 1981.
40. Slatter, D. H.: Unpublished data. 1981.
41. Slatter, D. H., and Rockey, J. D.: Superficial corneal erosion in dogs. Light and electron microscopic studies, in preparation, 1983.
42. Troutman, R. C.: *Microsurgery of the Anterior Segment of the Eye*. C. V. Mosby, St. Louis, 1974.
43. Van Horn, D. L., and Hyndiuk, R. A.: Endothelial wound repair in primate cornea. Exp. Eye Res. *21*:113, 1975.
44. Van Horn, D. L., Sendele, D. D., and Seidman, S.: Regenerative capacity of the corneal endothelium in the rabbit. Invest. Ophthalmol. *16*:597, 1977.
45. Verwer, M. A.: Partial mummification of the cornea in cats—the corneal sequestrum. Proc. 32nd Mtg. Am. Anim. Hosp. Assoc., 1965, pp. 112–118.

Iris and Ciliary Body

Chapter **106**

Robert L. Peiffer, Jr., and Cynthia S. Cook

Surgery on the iris and ciliary body is infrequently indicated. Surgical procedures for glaucoma involve manipulation of these tissues; however, these techniques are discussed in Chapter 110. This chapter examines iridotomy as a means of controlling pupillary aperture; iridectomy for removing localized tumors of the iris; iridocyclectomy for excision of anterior segment neoplasms; pupillary membranectomy to manage one of the most common complications of cataract surgery; and aspiration of iris and ciliary body epithelial cysts.

SURGICAL ANATOMY AND PHYSIOLOGY

The iris and ciliary body consist of connective tissue of mesodermal origin, lined posteriorly by a two-layered epithelium of neuroectodermal origin. The iris epithelium is heavily pigmented with melanin in both layers; the basilar portion of the anterior layer is made up of smooth muscle, which forms the dilator muscle of the iris, an alpha-adrenergic smooth muscle. This layer continues posteriorly over the ciliary body as a densely pigmented sheet of cuboidal cells continuous with the retinal pigment epithelium. The posterior pigmented iris epithelium lines the pupil as the pupillary ruff and continues as a nonpigmented epithelial layer over the surface of the ciliary body. The iris epithelium is pigmented even in blue-eyed individuals; only in true albinos is it devoid of melanin granules. It is the amount of stromal melanin that gives the iris its characteristic color. The iris is divided grossly into a peripheral ciliary zone and a thinner, central pupillary zone by the collarette.

The pupillary zone contains the sphincter muscle, formed by a 1.5 mm ring of smooth muscle encircling the pupil within the posterior stroma. It is a cholinergic smooth muscle that constricts to produce miosis. This phenomenon can be induced with parasympathomimetic drugs and also occurs in response to the release of prostaglandins[6] and other mediators of inflammation.

The iris and ciliary body receive a vascular supply from the long posterior ciliary arteries, which originate from the ophthalmic artery near the posterior pole and follow a transcleral and intrachoroidal route to the anterior segment. The anterior ciliary arteries, which are continuations of the muscular branches of the ophthalmic artery, enter the globe at the insertions of the extraocular muscles. They contribute less significantly to anterior uveal perfusion in the dog than in primates.[5] Each long posterior ciliary artery terminates as a medial and lateral branch entering the iris at the 9 and 3 o'clock positions. These branch dorsally and ventrally along the peripheral half of the ciliary zone to form the major arterial circle, which is incomplete at the 12 and 6 o'clock positions. Radial vessels emanate from this circle, travelling toward the pupil as well as retrograde into the ciliary body, where they anastomose with the short posterior ciliary arteries. These vessels lack perivascular connective tissue sheaths, which minimize surgical hemorrhage in primates.[5] Significant bleeding is usually avoided, however, if the major arterial circle is not transected. Fibrinous exudation from the iris vasculature and miosis are frequent surgical complications that can be minimized by preoperative treatment with systemic antiprostaglandins (aspirin 32.5 mg/kg) and topical mydriatics and antibiotic/steroids for three days. Epinephrine (0.5 ml of a 1:10,000 solution), instilled intraocularly at the time of surgery, can be employed to enlarge the pupil, and judicious use of intracameral heparin may be used to inhibit fibrin clotting. Topical, subconjunctival, and systemic corticosteroids and topical mydriatics are used postoperatively to reduce surgically induced inflammation, thereby decreasing the incidence of complications.[3]

Ciliary body landmarks include the ora ciliaris retinae, or junction between the pars plana of the ciliary body and the peripheral retina; this area in the dog is located 8 mm posterior to the limbus superiorly and temporally but only 4 mm inferiorly and nasally.[1] Iridocyclectomy extending posterior to the ora may cause peripheral retinal dialysis and detachment. The ciliary epithelium produces aqueous humor; although it is not clear to what extent this tissue can be excised without impairing aqueous humor dynamics, it is probably less than one-fourth. The zonules arise from both the pars plana and the pars plicata of the ciliary body. Manipulations that cause extensive zonular disruption may lead to lens dislocation or ciliary body hemorrhage.

IRIDOTOMY

The most common indication for sphincter iridotomy is enlargement of the pupillary aperture during cataract surgery. If the pupil constricts prior to lens extraction or is less than 3 mm following extraction, a one- to four-quadrant sphincterotomy is performed as necessary to enhance exposure or achieve at least a 5-mm pupil.

The technique is described and illustrated in Figure 106–1. Incision with scissors is preferable to grasping and tearing, as it is less traumatic and more readily controlled. Significant hemorrhage can almost always be prevented if the major arterial circle in the base of the ciliary zone is avoided. An incision can safely be made to a depth of 2 to 3 mm. If the iris must be incised further, hemorrhage can be prevented by incising with wet-field cautery. If hemorrhage does occur, closing the incision and re-establishing the anterior chamber and intraocular pressure hasten clotting. After several minutes, blood and clots are gently irrigated or extracted from the anterior chamber.

As in all anterior segment surgery, care must be taken to avoid corneal endothelial damage; gentle irrigation should be minimal and should be directed away from the endothelium, and instruments within the anterior chamber must not come in contact with the endothelium.

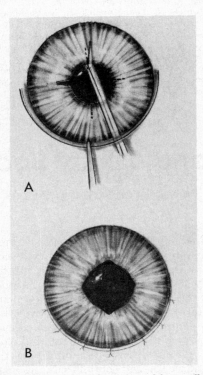

Figure 106–1. Iridotomy. *A,* Enlargement of the pupillary aperture may be achieved by incising the sphincter muscle of the iris. The procedure is best performed with sharp scissors and a formed anterior chamber in the superior and lateral quadrants; gentle retraction of the cornea and an "open sky" technique are necessary to incise the iris at the 12 o'clock position. Minimizing the incision to a depth of 2 mm prevents significant hemorrhage. *B,* The resultant pupil appears diamond-shaped rather than round if four-quadrant sphincterotomy is performed.

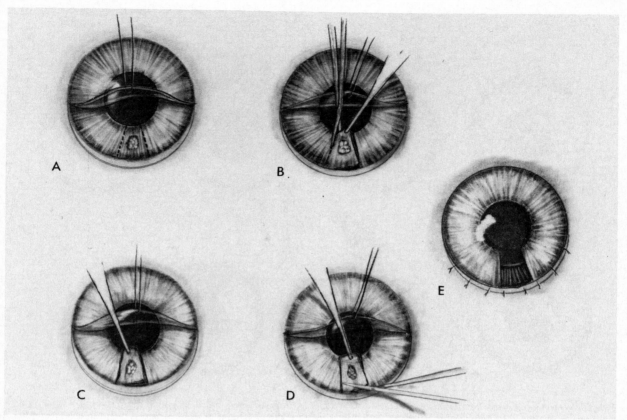

Figure 106–2. Sector iridectomy for excisional biopsy of an inferior iris lesion. *A*, Following an inferior 180° corneoscleral incision, the cornea is gently retracted. Lesions in the superior quadrants are excised with a similar incision and a formed anterior chamber. Dotted lines indicate area of planned excision. Note that liberal margins of grossly normal tissue are allowed. *B*, While exerting gentle traction on the pupillary margin, the lateral iris margins are incised with scissors or cautery. If hemorrhage does occur, the corneal flap is replaced, the anterior chamber is formed, and the bleeding vessels are allowed to clot before irrigating the anterior chamber and proceeding. *C* and *D*, The base of the iris can be transected by tearing (*C*) or by incision (*D*). *E*, Postoperative appearance. The corneoscleral incision is closed with interrupted sutures of 7-0 polyglactin 910 (Vicryl), and the anterior chamber is reformed with lactated Ringer's or a similar solution. The lens equator, zonules, and ciliary processes will be seen through the keyhole pupil.

IRIDECTOMY

Sector iridectomy is indicated for excisional biopsy of iris lesions, creation of a pupillary aperture following formation of extensive posterior synechia or pupillary membranes, and management of acute inflammatory posterior synechia with iris bombé and secondary glaucoma. In the last-named situation, a combined posterior sclerectomy-cyclodialysis-transscleral iridencleisis, which not only restores normal pathways of aqueous flow[3,4] but provides a filtering procedure to alleviate the possibility of persistent glaucoma from peripheral anterior synechiae secondary to iris bombé, is preferred. If simple iridectomy is used, the technique illustrated in Figure 106–2 for excisional biopsy is modified by initially freeing the adherent pupillary margin with a blunt iris hook or a cyclodialysis spatula.

IRIDOCYCLECTOMY

Excision of the iris and ciliary body is used infrequently for tumors of the anterior uvea. This technique may be used to remove ciliary body adenomas, which usually involve only the ciliary processes. Anterior uveal malignant melanomas and ciliary body adenocarcinomas are usually diagnosed only when they have been present for some time and have extended into the outflow pathways or posteriorly into the choroid, retina, or deep sclera. The ideal surgical candidate has an uninvolved iridocorneal angle on gonioscopic examination, a discrete, well-defined lesion confined to the iris or ciliary body, and no secondary uveitis or glaucoma. A thorough clinical examination, including indirect ophthalmoscopy with scleral depression under general anesthesia, critical transillumination, and ultrasonography, facilitates this challenging clinical diagnosis. In most cases, 45 to 60° is the maximum tolerable extent of uveal excision. Although invasive melanomas and adenocarcinomas may be removed with this technique,[2] involvement of the angle structures and deep sclera may make it difficult to define the extent of such tumors. The possibility of residual neoplasm with the potential for metastasis is high. In addition, manipulation during the surgical procedure may enhance seeding or metastasis of the tumor. We believe

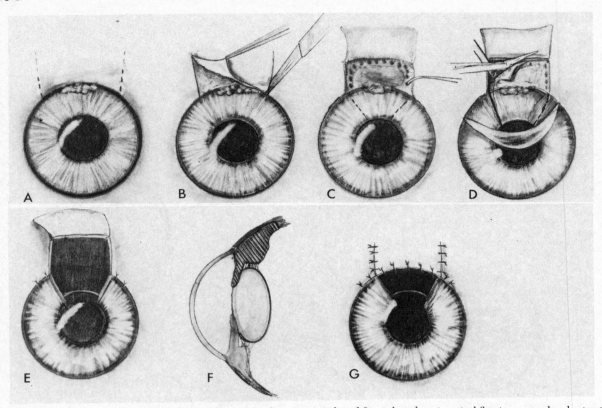

Figure 106–3. Iridocyclectomy for excision of an anterior uveal tumor. *A,* A broad fornix-based conjunctival flap is prepared and retracted; conjunctiva is not shown to simplify the drawings. Dotted lines indicate lateral margins of planned scleral flap and deeper excision. *B,* With sharp dissection, a half-thickness posterior-based scleral flap is prepared. *C,* Cautery is applied around the margins of the excised flap to minimize hemorrhage when the underlying ciliary body is excised. Dotted lines indicate extent of planned iris excision. *D and E,* A corneoscleral incision is made beyond the extent of planned excision to allow mobility of the corneal flap. Scissors are used to excise the iris, the deep cornea and sclera, and the ciliary body along the area made by the flap. A suction cutter is utilized to remove vitreous if it appears in the wound. *F,* The hatched area indicates the tissues excised, which include the deep sclera and peripheral cornea, the iridocorneal angle structures, the iris, and the ciliary body. *G,* The flap and corneoscleral incision are closed with interrupted sutures of 7-0 polyglactin 910 (Vicryl), and the anterior chamber is reformed with lactated Ringer's or a similar solution. The conjunctival flap may be sutured in place or allowed to reposition and heal without sutures.

that, unless the fellow eye is blind, enucleation is the procedure of choice in such cases. Iridocyclectomy is illustrated in Figure 106–3.

PUPILLARY MEMBRANECTOMY

The formation of pupillary iridocapsular membranes is a common sequela to cataract surgery in the dog and may also occur following anterior uveitis, especially lens-induced uveitis. If extensive, these membranes may impair vision or block the flow of aqueous, precipitating secondary glaucoma. When the lens is present, a sector iridectomy is indicated. However, in an aphakic animal, membranectomy is a simple, effective secondary procedure that frequently allows the patient to see, salvaging an otherwise unsuccessful cataract surgery. The technique

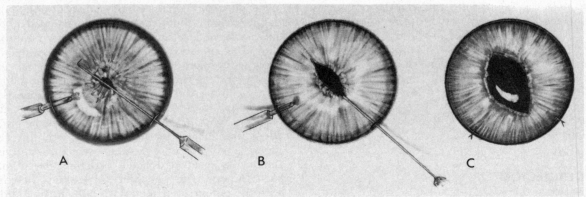

Figure 106–4. Pupillary membranectomy. *A,* Two 2- to 3-mm limbal incisions are made at the 4 and 8 o'clock positions. An infusion port or needle is placed through one incision, and a 27-gauge needle with its tip bent 90° is placed through the other. *B,* The needle is rotated and its tip manipulated to engage the iris. The needle is gently depressed and drawn across the membrane. *C,* The instruments are withdrawn, and the incisions are closed with interrupted sutures of 7-0 polyglactin 910 (Vicryl).

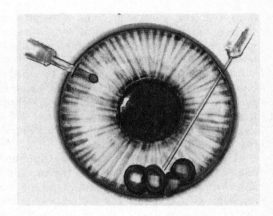

Figure 106–5. Aspiration of pupillary cysts. Incisions identical to those described for membranectomy are made at the 10 and 2 o'clock positions, and the infusion port is inserted. A straight 25-gauge needle is used to aspirate the cysts.

is illustrated in Figure 106–4, using one needle for infusion and one for transection of the membrane.

The ideal surgical candidate for a pupillary membranectomy has a formed anterior chamber and near-normal intraocular pressure. Generally, the longer after the initial cataract surgery the membranectomy is performed the better, allowing surgically induced inflammation to resolve. In our experience, the procedure as described carries approximately a 50 per cent success rate; failures result from reformation of pupillary membranes. The procedure can be repeated but is less likely to produce a satisfactory result, and sector iridectomy should be considered if a single membranectomy is unsuccessful.

ASPIRATION OF EPITHELIAL CYSTS

Cysts of the iris and ciliary body epithelium may develop spontaneously or subsequent to trauma or inflammation. They may be attached to the ciliary processes or pupillary margin or may be observed free-floating in the anterior chamber. These cysts are distinguished clinically by their regular margins and transparency when transilluminated. Although benign, they may be aspirated if they become excessively large or if they contact the corneal endothelium or to differentiate them from malignant melanomas or cystic ciliary body adenomas when clinical distinction is not possible.*

The surgical technique is identical to that used for membranectomy, except that a straight 20-gauge needle is used for aspiration (Fig. 106–5). As the cyst is aspirated, the bevel of the needle is used to transect the base of the cyst if it is attached to uveal tissue. Aspirated tissue should be submitted for histopathological examination.

1. Donovan, R. J., et al.: Histology of the normal collie eye. II. Uvea. Ophthalmology 6:1175, 1974.
2. Gelatt, K. N., Henry, J. D., and Straffus, A. C.: Excision of an adenocarcinoma of the iris and ciliary body in a dog. J. Am. Anim. Hosp. Assoc. 6:59, 1970.
3. Peiffer, R. L.: Current concepts in ophthalmic surgery. Vet. Clin. North Am. 10:455, 1980.
4. Peiffer, R. L., et al.: Combined posterior sclerectomy, cyclodialysis and trans-scleral iridencleisis in the management of primary glaucoma. Canine Pract. 6:54, 1977.
5. Van Buskirk, E. M.: The canine eye: the vessels of aqueous drainage. Invest. Ophthalmol. Visual Sci. 18:223, 1979.
6. Waitzman, M. B., and King, C. D.: Prostaglandin influences on intraocular pressure and pupil size. Am. J. Physiol. 212:329, 1967.

*Editor's note: This technique may also be used when large numbers of cysts in the posterior chamber cause angle closure glaucoma—an unusual complication seen in Great Danes.

Chapter **107**

Lens

Robert L. Peiffer, Jr., and Gale Bowman

Surgery of the lens is limited to extraction, which is indicated when visual impairment is due to opacification, when the lens is dislocated, and when lens-induced uveitis does not respond to medical therapy.

Medical illustrator for this chapter was Mr. Thomas Waldrop.

EMBRYOLOGY

The lens develops from a lens placode, which develops from surface ectoderm by induction by the underlying optic vesicle between days 15 and 17 of gestation in the dog. The modified surface ectoderm (lens placode) invaginates and separates from the surface to form the spherical lens vesicle by the nineteenth gestational day. The cells lining the posterior of the sphere elongate anteriorly, resulting in a solid structure totally enclosed by epithelial cell basement membrane (lens capsule) and lined anteriorly by cuboidal epithelial cells. The obliteration of the lens vesicle cavity is completed by 30 days gestation. These fibers remain at the central core of the lens as the embryonic nucleus.

The cells along the equator elongate in an anterior and posterior direction between the capsule, with its anterior monolayer of epithelium, and the embryonic nucleus; this occurs by the 25th day of gestation. As the fibers meet fibers from the opposite side, they are sealed together by an amorphous cement substance. Because the fibers are the same length, their terminal junctions collectively form a Y pattern called the anterior and posterior suture lines; the posterior Y is inverted as compared with the upright, anterior Y. The fibers formed prior to birth comprise the embryonic and fetal nuclei. Cell division and elongation continue after birth and throughout life, resulting in compaction of central lens fibers, forming the adult nucleus. The zone of "young" lens fibers between capsule and nucleus is the cortex.

Although the lens is an avascular tissue in the adult, **in utero** it is enveloped posteriorly by the tunica vasculosa lentis and anteriorly by the developing anterior uveal vasculature and pupillary membrane, both of which are fully developed in the dog by 30 days gestation and which may persist in the neonate.[1,3] Persistent tunica vasculosa lentis can be associated with posterior lenticonus and posterior axial capsular cataracts,[20,29] and adherent persistent pupillary membranes may cause anterior capsular cataract.

Development of the zonular fibers, which suspend the lens, is the result of secretion of the tertiary vitreous by the ciliary neuroepithelium. These fibers extend from the equatorial lens capsule to the pars plicata and pars plana of the ciliary body.[2,23]

ANATOMY

The adult lens is composed of anterior and posterior capsules, anterior epithelium, fibers, and amorphous cement. It is an optically transparent structure located between the iris and vitreous and suspended by the zonular fibers, which join the lens to the ciliary body. The lens is bounded by the anterior and posterior chamber and iris anteriorly and the vitreous posteriorly. Firm vitreolenticular adhesions, hyaloideocapsular ligaments, are present.

The anterior lens capsule is thicker than the posterior capsule, which is formed by the posterior lens epithelium during lens development. The capsule is composed of a collagen framework with interstices of mucopolysaccharide and has elastic properties that permit alteration in the shape of the lens owing to

the effect of the ciliary muscle, which exerts traction on the lens capsule via the zonular fibers in the process of accommodation. As a general rule, the ciliary muscle is poorly developed in subprimates, and accommodation is not as active nor as important a process in subprimates as in the higher species. The lens capsule also acts as a semipermeable membrane between the ocular fluids and the lens.

The anterior lens epithelium is a monolayer of cuboidal cells, which divide equatorially, elongate, and migrate centrally, forming the lens bow of the lens cortex.

The cortex is the zone of developing lens fibers, the nuclei of which are arranged at the lens bow. As the cells elongate, they extend anteriorly and posteriorly as lens fibers and take a more central position, increasing in length with loss of the nucleus. Opposing fibers meet to form the suture lines. The cortex is less dense than the nucleus and often is difficult to remove completely during extracapsular lens extraction.

The center of the lens consists of the innermost embryonic nucleus, the fetal nucleus, and the adult nucleus. The embryonic nucleus has no Y sutures, since the fibers are formed by the anterior elongation of the posterior lens epithelium. The fetal nucleus is the next layer of the lens to form and surrounds the embryonic nucleus. The adult nucleus is continuously formed throughout life. As the cortical fibers are compressed concentrically, they become relatively dehydrated. In the older animal this frequently results in nuclear sclerosis.[6,8,22,23]

PHYSIOLOGY AND BIOCHEMISTRY

The lens is involved in the refraction of light, controlled to some extent by the process of accommodation. The ability of a medium to refract light requires (1) optical clarity for the transmission of light, and (2) an interface between tissues of different optical density and thus a difference in velocity of the light passing through the medium (refractive index). The greatest degree of refraction in the eye takes place at the cornea and, to a lesser degree, at the lens. This results in light focused on the retina.

The lens in man and some animals has the ability to change shape, thus allowing focus adjustments for objects at varying distances. This process is called accommodation and requires a pliable lens and capsule, intact zonular fibers, and a functional ciliary muscle. The process involves a complex, poorly defined reflex pathway. To accommodate for near vision, the ciliary muscle contracts, releasing tension on the zonular fibers, which allows the lens capsule to relax and the lens to assume a more spherical shape. As the lens ages, it loses its elasticity owing to compaction and dehydration of lens fibers with an associated decrease in ability to accommodate.

Maintaining lens transparency is a primary function of the anterior lens epithelium and intact lens capsule. The anterior lens epithelium has a high metabolic rate and actively transports carbohydrates, electrolytes, and amino acids into the lens. Glucose is the primary energy source for lens epithelial metabolism, and abnormal sugar metabolism may result in lens opacification, as seen with diabetic and galactose cataracts.

The lens substance is composed primarily of intracellular protein (60 per cent) and water (40 per cent). Potassium is sequestered intracellularly, and sodium is extruded.[6]

IMMUNOLOGY

The lens is an immunologically unique tissue. If lens protein is exposed to the immune system it is recognized as a foreign substance. Lens protein is sequestered and potentially antigenic for the following reasons: (1) the lens capsule is formed before the immune system develops; lens protein is thus never recognized as "self"; (2) the lens is avascular; and (3) the lens is enclosed by a capsule that is impermeable to cells and large molecules.

An animal immunized by injection of lens protein develops serum antibodies against lens protein regardless of the animal species from which it came, demonstrating that lens protein is organ- rather than species-specific.[6]

Lens protein may be exposed to the body as a result of leakage through the lens capsule during liquefaction of a cataract, traumatic lens rupture, or extracapsular lens extraction. The characteristics of the antigen, including potency, quantity, and duration, govern the severity of the inflammatory reaction. Leakage of soluble lens protein from a hypermature cataract may result in mild to moderate anterior uveitis, which usually responds to topical cortico-steroid therapy. Acute traumatic lens rupture may result in severe intraocular inflammation. Planned extracapsular lens extraction exposes residual lens material to the immune system; if most of the lens material is successfully removed, the resultant inflammation is mild and responsive to anti-inflammatory therapy. Intracapsular lens extraction results in minimal inflammation relative to the surgical invasion of the globe.

ROLE OF THE LENS IN ANIMAL VISION

Accommodation is poorly developed in domestic animals: the dog and cat possess one to two diopters of accommodative power compared with ten diopters in man. Although mature cataracts may permit light and dark perception, they result in functional blindness. Although many dogs and cats adjust remarkably well to vision loss, successful cataract extraction allows restoration of functional vision—the ability to recognize people and objects. Dogs and cats compensate adequately for the loss of accommodation and

the surgically induced hyperopia, and although occasional errors in visual function occur, they are insignificant compared with the improvement that surgery affords.

CONGENITAL ANOMALIES

Lens development is intimately related to the optic vesicle and, therefore, the overall development of the eye, and congenital lens abnormalities may occur either as isolated lesions or in association with multiple abnormalities.

Congenital anomalies of the lens include the following:

1. *Microphakia*—a smaller than normal lens that may or may not be associated with cataract.

2. *Spherophakia*—a spherically shaped lens that is frequently microphakic.

3. *Lenticonus*—protrusion of lens capsule anteriorly or posteriorly; this condition may be associated with persistent hyaloid and hyperplastic primary vitreous. The lens capsule may rupture, releasing lens material into the vitreous.[1,5,14]

4. *Coloboma*—notching of the lens equator in typical or atypical position, usually associated with similar defects in the iris, ciliary body, and zonules.

5. *Cataract*—opacification of the lens fibers or capsule.

Cataract

Cataract is a nonspecific disease that results in opacification of the lens fibers or capsule. Cataracts may be characterized clinically according to stage of development, location within the lens, age of the animal at the time of development, and etiology.

The stages of development of a cataract include the initial opacity and, if the cataract is progressive, subsequent degeneration of the lens. The stages of development are incipient, immature, mature, and hypermature.[3,21]

Incipient. Focal opacification of the lens or its capsule. The animal can still see. This stage may or may not be progressive.

Immature. Opacity is more or less diffuse, although there may be areas of variable density. The fundic reflex is present, and the animal may experience some visual impairment.

Mature. Total dense opacification of the lens with absence of the fundic reflex. Visual function is significantly impaired. Cataract surgery is recommended at this stage.

Hypermature. Lens protein liquifies and may leak through the capsule. If leakage is extensive with significant resorption of protein, the lens capsule becomes wrinkled, initially at the equator. The nucleus, which is insoluble albuminoid protein, may migrate inferiorly within the lens capsule to form a morgagnian cataract. Uveitis may result from leakage of lens protein. The fundic reflex may be present peripherally, and the animal may see if resorption is extensive.

Intumescence

If a cataract becomes hydrated, the lens swells and increases in size. Resultant shallowing of the anterior chamber or pupillary block may cause secondary glaucoma.

Classification

Location is an aid in defining etiology, and cataracts may be capsular, subcapsular, cortical, or nuclear. These are further described as axial or equatorial, anterior or posterior, and according to the position of the hands on a clock (e.g., 3 o'clock position).

Age of the animal when the cataract first appears may be used to classify the cataract as one of the following:

Congenital. The cataract is present at birth. Congenital cataracts may be inherited or noninherited.[9, 13, 28]

Developmental. An inherited bilateral cataract that occurs after birth, usually in young animals, but in such breeds as the American cocker spaniel, miniature poodle, and Boston terrier, may not appear until later in life.[4, 10–12, 24, 26, 27, 31, 32]

Senile. Occurring in aged animals, preceded or accompanied by nuclear sclerosis.

Etiology may be difficult to determine; cataracts may occur secondary to ocular diseases, including uveitis, retinal degeneration, and glaucoma; in association with systemic metabolic disease, including diabetes mellitus[19] and Cushing's disease; or secondary to blunt or penetrating trauma; or they may represent a congenital developmental disorder. The majority of canine cataracts are inherited.

Cataracts are a surgical disease; there is no reliable topical, systemic, or intraocular medication that will prevent progression or induce resorption of cataracts. Lens extraction is performed by either intracapsular or extracapsular techniques, depending on whether the lens capsule remains intact.

Extracapsular lens extraction is routinely performed for the majority of cataract extractions owing to the strong hyaloideocapsular ligament; intracapsular extraction almost invariably results in disruption of the hyaloid membrane with increased incidence of vitreous presentation and associated complications, including corneal edema, glaucoma, and retinal detachments. With the extracapsular technique, the posterior lens capsule and vitreous face are not disturbed.

Extracapsular Lens Extraction

Cataracts are among the most common ocular diseases seen in our practice; one out of five animals are presented with cataracts or suspicion of cataracts. Although not all of these patients are candidates for surgery, cataract extraction is among the most successful and most rewarding procedures the veterinary ophthalmologist can perform.

Selection of Patients

The objective of cataract surgery is to restore functional vision. Because of the ability of the dog and cat to adjust and compensate for incomplete lens opacity or monocular blindness, functional vision is not significantly impaired until bilateral cataracts approach maturity. The owner of the pet is the best judge of when surgery should be contemplated. When the animal is bumping into objects constantly and is unable to maintain its normal lifestyle and personality, cataract extraction should be considered.

Of prime importance is the establishment of integrity of the retina and the central visual pathways. It is discouraging to both client and surgeon to have a technically successful procedure fail to restore vision because of disease of the retina or optic nerve. To evaluate the neural visual components, history, ophthalmoscopy, visual function tests, and electrophysiology should be used in combination.

Inherited retinal degenerations are increasing in incidence and are the primary cause of failure in technically successful cataract surgery. Owing to mechanisms that are poorly understood, animals with inherited or inflammatory retinal degeneration are likely to develop associated cataracts. The problem is complicated by the fact that breeds with a high incidence of inherited retinal degeneration, such as the miniature and toy poodle and the Irish setter, also have primary genetic cataracts unassociated with retinal disease.

Pupillary responses are unreliable as the sole method of assessing peripheral and central vision potential. The majority of cataract patients should demonstrate complete, brisk direct and consensual responses to a bright focal light source in a darkened room in the presence of even the densest cataract. With some variability, these responses persist in the presence of well-advanced retinal degeneration. The ganglion cell fibers that mediate this reflex are distinct from the visual fibers that extend to the lateral geniculate body and thus provide no information as to the status of the optic radiation and visual cortex. Iris atrophy is not infrequently observed in miniature poodles, and lesions involving the third cranial nerve may also result in absence of pupillary reflexes in the presence of intact visual components. Thus, although it is always reassuring to observe normal pupillary reflexes, they provide minimal definitive information.

History is helpful in addition to the owner's observations of changes in the animal's appearance or behavior. Without exception, visual and ophthalmoscopic changes in inherited retinal degeneration always precede associated cataract development. Thus, a reliable history suggesting visual impairment accompanied or followed by rather than preceded by noticeable cataract development indicates an intact visual system. If inherited retinal degeneration is present, a history of initial nyctalopia (night blindness) may be elicited. Critical ophthalmoscopy performed while the cataracts are still immature, rather than waiting until the fundus cannot be critically examined, is of benefit to all involved. Ophthalmoscopy prior to maturity of the cataract approaches 100 per cent reliability. The rare dog with genetic tendencies to develop both retinal degeneration and primary cataracts will provide an occasional disappointment if the retinal degeneration develops subsequent to the primary cataract.

The ability to negotiate an obstacle course under photopic and scotopic conditions may be of value in those cases in which the fundus reflex can be obtained although lens changes prohibit a critical fundic examination. As a general rule of thumb, if a fundic reflex can be obtained, some vision should be present and should change minimally with alterations in ambient light if the retina is healthy.

Electrophysiology provides the most reliable criterion for critical evaluation. Ideally, an electroretinogram should be performed on all patients with cataracts; in those breeds with predisposition to inherited retinal degeneration, electroretinography is a prerequisite to cataract surgery. In a retrospective study of 54 miniature poodles presented with cataracts at the University of Minnesota from 1975 to 1976, 42 (78 per cent) had associated progressive retinal atrophy as determined by ophthalmoscopy (23 dogs) or electroretinography (19). The surgeon who attempts cataract surgery without an electroretinogram will have fewer successes than will a surgeon who utilizes the test. If history, pupillary responses, or neurological findings suggest the possibility of a defect in the central visual system, evaluation of visually evoked responses may be considered in addition to electroretinography. Ultrasonography may be of value in the detection of retinal detachment.

A large percentage of young dogs (between one and three years of age) with inherited developmental cataracts (seen most frequently in the Afghan hound, American cocker spaniel, Irish setter, and miniature and toy poodle) undergo spontaneous resorption of their cataracts. Active resorption, demonstrated by mild lens-induced uveitis and an irregular lens capsule, is an indication to delay surgery. Although these liquified cataracts may be aspirated, approximately 40 per cent resorb such that cataract surgery is unnecessary. We prefer to manage these animals with topical application of 1.0% atropine sulfate to enhance peripheral vision and corticosteroids to temper the uveitis. The animal should be examined monthly, and cataract surgery should be recommended only when active resorption has subsided without restoration of visual function.

Cataract surgery is an elective procedure; thorough multisystem evaluation should be performed prior to surgery. Concurrent related diseases (such as diabetes mellitus or Cushing's disease) or unrelated diseases (such as renal decompensation or heartworm disease) should be identified and adequately controlled. In older patients with systemic disease who have adjusted reasonably well to their visual impairment, the complications of anesthesia should be weighed against the benefits of improved vision.

Philosophies of Cataract Surgery

With rare exceptions, we perform cataract surgery on one eye only because of the ability of an animal to function well with monocular vision, lower cost to the owner, and the reduced insult to the patient in terms of anesthesia time and postoperative discomfort. Also it is reassuring to know that, in case of failure, one can offer the client an alternative—an operation on the fellow eye. Of course, both cataracts may be removed at one or two sittings at the owner's insistence or if acute visual function is necessary, as in hunting or obedience dogs.

The procedure for cataract removal, when performed with appropriate preoperative treatment and instrumentation, is not difficult. However, the incidence of intraoperative or postoperative complications is high compared with that of other procedures, and these complications frequently have disastrous effects on the visual outcome. With experience and greater understanding of ocular anatomy, physiology, and pathology, recognition and management of complications are facilitated, with improved success. The results of 470 cataract extractions performed between 1979 and 1981 reflect a progressive increase in success rate commensurate with experience and refinement of technique that levels off at approximately 90 per cent. In regard to technical refinement, the routine use of microsurgical technique and anterior vitrectomy has likewise significantly improved our results. These data support the theory that results are most likely to be rewarding in the hands of an experienced cataract surgeon, using an operating microscope and the instrumentation and experience necessary to perform anterior vitrectomy.

Routine Procedures and Techniques

Adequate preoperative preparation minimizes intraoperative and postoperative complications. The canine eye responds to even meticulous surgery with intraoperative constriction of the pupil, which hampers exposure, necessitates increased intraocular manipulation, and intensifies postoperative inflammation. Treatment with oral aspirin and topical antibiotic-corticosteroids and 1% atropine sulfate solutions for three days prior to surgery minimizes these problems. Prostaglandins play a role in both pupillary constriction and inflammation, and aspirin, which inhibits synthesis of prostaglandin, provides results superior to those seen with the use of corticosteroids alone.[18]

Planned extracapsular extraction is the

rule.[11, 18, 25, 30] The posterior capsule and the hyaloid membrane of the anterior vitreous are intimately associated, and intracapsular extraction or tearing of the posterior capsule is invariably associated with vitreous presentation. Although not always disastrous, vitreous presentation adds an undesirable challenge that frequently precipitates other complications. In addition, enzymatic dissolution of the zonules is unreliable in the dog, and intracapsular extraction results in excessive traction on the ciliary processes.

Stable, deep anesthesia is important. Under light anesthesia, the animal may move when the iris is touched and intraocular pressure may increase owing to extraocular muscle contraction. The stability of anesthesia induced with methoxyflurane is preferred over that induced with halothane, but the usually quieter recovery from halothane reduces the likelihood of trauma during a stormy recovery.

The positioning of the patient is crucial to the success of the procedure. The muzzle should be elevated to enable the surgeon to see the iris and lens surface in a horizontal plane. Lateral canthotomy is routinely performed. A traction suture of 4-0 silk placed through the conjunctiva under the insertion of the superior rectus muscle may be necessary. A similar suture is placed through and is used to retract the third eyelid if necessary. The incision should be a minimum of 180°; it is difficult to accurately predict lens size prior to surgery, and attempting to deliver an intumescent lens through a small incision results in undue trauma and residual lens material in the anterior chamber. A corneoscleral incision under a limbal-based conjunctival flap or a clear corneal incision without a flap may be used. A corneoscleral incision heals more rapidly than a clear corneal incision; corneal scarring at the incision site is minimized; accurate apposition of the surgical wound margin is facilitated; if corneal dehiscence occurs, the intraocular contents are not exposed to the environment; and absorbable suture knots may be covered by the flap so that postoperative irritation does not occur. These advantages offset the additional three to five minutes it takes to dissect the flap and control the minimal hemorrhage associated with a corneoscleral incision. A clear corneal incision is more efficient in terms of time and provides slightly better exposure, without obstruction by the flap. Preplaced sutures hinder exposure and maneuverability, and we prefer to have unobstructed access to the anterior segment should complications arise.

Capsulectomy is performed with a cryoprobe or capsule forceps. Although it is easier to obtain a good equatorial capsular tear with a cryoprobe, the incidence of posterior capsule disruption is increased. The capsule is grasped as superficially and as widely as the dilated pupil allows without compromising a view of the forceps teeth. The forceps are closed, elevated minutely, and gently rotated. The lens cortex and nucleus are removed *in toto*; liquified or residual cortex may be gently irrigated or aspirated with a blunt needle. If a pupil of less than 3 mm

results, sphincter iridectomy is performed. This is exceptional, however. Closure is with 7-0 polyglactin 910 in a simple interrupted pattern or 9-0 nylon in a continuous interlocking pattern (Figs. 107–1 and 107–2).

Postoperative care is critical and is aimed at reducing inflammation and maintaining pupil size. Triamcinolone acetonide (0.5 ml) is administered subconjunctivally in the inferior quadrants. Oral corticosteroids are continued for seven days. Topical 1.0% atropine sulfate, 2.5% phenylephrine, and antibiotic-corticosteroid solutions are applied every two hours daily for the first three days, which is the critical period for control of pupillary size. Bandages are not used as the surgery is tolerated remarkably well. Atropine and topical corticosteroids are continued until the inflammation has subsided, usually at four weeks. The patient is re-examined 1, 2, 4, 12, and 24 weeks and 1 year after surgery.

Complications

Intraoperative complications include miosis, which can be largely prevented by adequate premedication and minimal intraocular manipulations; hemorrhage from the ciliary processes while performing the capsulectomy or from the sphincterotomy incision if one is necessary; vitreous presentation; corneal edema; and posterior capsular opacity. A small pupil is managed by sphincterotomy and postoperative medication. Ciliary process hemorrhage occurs in approximately 2 per cent of cases, and iris hemorrhage occurs in approximately 20 per cent of animals subjected to three- or four-quadrant sphincterotomy. In both instances, bleeding is minimal and self-limited. The vessels are encouraged to clot by reforming the anterior chamber and delaying manipulations for three to five minutes. The blood can be irrigated or gently teased from the anterior chamber. A small amount of residual hyphema, although not desirable, is resorbed over two to three weeks without adverse consequences.

Vitreous presentation occurs in about 15 per cent of planned extracapsular extractions, with a higher incidence in animals with incomplete cataract resorption. Vitreous presentation is managed by an anterior chamber air bubble if the hyaloid membrane is intact. Unfortunately, the hyaloid membrane usually ruptures and the vitreous must be removed from the anterior chamber to reduce the likelihood of disastrous sequelae. Anterior vitrectomy may be performed with cellulose sponges, excising the gel vitreous as close to the plane of the iris as possible, or with a disposable vitreophage.*[17] The vitreophage is preferred because it minimizes intraocular manipulation and traction to the retina. Vitrectomy is performed until the anterior chamber is completely free of vitreous and the iris plane assumes a concave appearance.

Administration of preoperative mannitol does not

---

*Kaufman Vitrector II, Concept, Clearwater, FL.

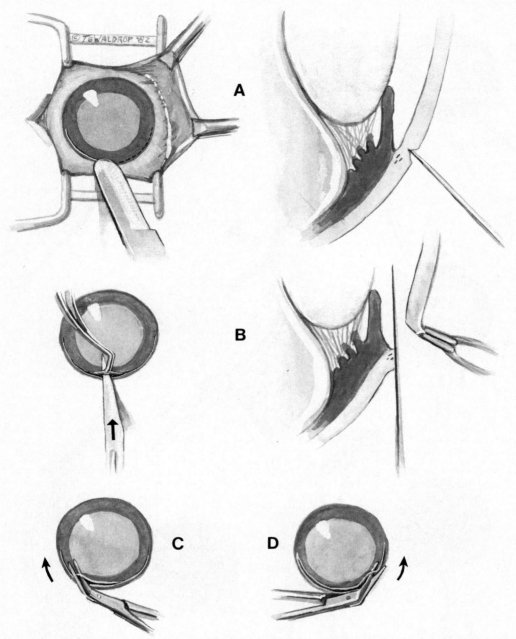

Figure 107–1. Extracapsular cataract extraction via a clear corneal incision. *A*, Using a #64 Beaver blade 1 mm anterior to the limbus, a 180°, 3/4-depth corneal incision is made. *B*, The anterior chamber is entered with a #65 Beaver blade at the 12 o'clock position. *C* and *D*, The corneal incision is completed with left- and right-handed corneoscleral scissors, following the previously made corneal groove.

appear to influence the incidence of vitreous presentation in the normotensive dog, with 1 of 12 dogs in each group developing this complication in a prospective study comparing treated and nontreated patients.[18]

Mild transient corneal edema is a common postoperative feature that occurs proportional to (1) mechanical trauma from intraocular irrigation or lens-endothelial contact during extraction, and (2) postoperative inflammation. In our series, severe persistent corneal edema was not seen without associated glaucoma or vitreous touch.

In approximately 2 per cent of patients with cata-

racts, the posterior capsule is translucent or opaque at the time of surgery. If the fundus cannot be seen during surgery, the capsule should be incised or removed. Except for a 3 mm superior opening, the corneal incision is closed and the anterior chamber reformed with saline; the posterior capsule is then incised with a hooked 23-gauge needle. The linear incision will usually widen to prevent unimpaired observation of the posterior pole. If it does not, the incised margins are grasped and the capsule teased away from the hyaloid membrane. Vitrectomy is performed if necessary.

Postoperative complications include (1) pupillary

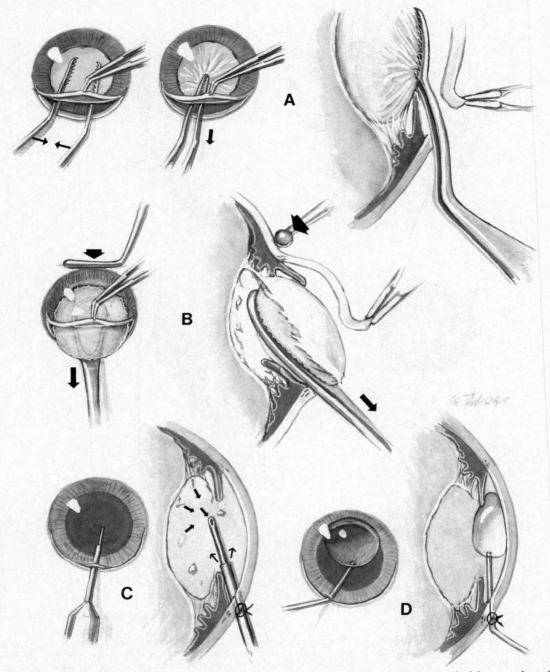

Figure 107–2. Extracapsular cataract extraction (continued). *A,* The corneal flap is grasped with a fine-toothed forcep and gently elevated to allow entrance of the toothed capsulotomy forceps. The capsulotomy forceps are inserted into the anterior chamber with closed jaws. As the forceps are positioned over the anterior lens capsule, the jaws are opened, gently depressed, and closed to grasp the anterior lens capsule. With gentle elevation and rotation of the capsulotomy forceps, the anterior lens capsule tears at the equator. *B,* A lens loop is positioned to gently depress the superior iris. An extraocular muscle hook is placed opposite the lens loop on the outside of the globe 2 mm posterior to the limbus; gentle pressure is exerted to deliver the lens. *C,* Following anterior chamber irrigation, the corneal incision is closed with simple interrupted sutures; the anterior chamber is re-established with saline solution. Residual lens debris may be aspirated. *D,* An air bubble one-third the volume of the anterior chamber reconstitutes the anterior chamber and closure is completed. Balanced salt solution may be used in preference to air.

membrane with or without pupillary occlusion and secondary glaucoma; (2) glaucoma without pupillary obstruction; and (3) retinal detachment. The first complication is almost invariably associated with in-tense postoperative inflammation related to residual lens material or excessive intraocular manipulation and the third to unplanned intracapsular extraction and anterior vitrectomy. Although focal opacification of the posterior capsule and synechiae of iris to posterior capsule are not uncommon, good functional vision persists around the secondary cataract if a pupil is maintained. Scarring of the limbal cornea in the area of incision is expected and is of no consequence, even if associated with peripheral anterior synechiae.

Corneoplasty may be performed as a salvage procedure in dogs with pupillary membrane with or without iris bombé. Vision was restored in 5 of 11 eyes that we operated on. Presently available suction-cutting machines manipulated through the pars plana offer promise in the management of this common complication.

Our experiences are similar to those of Startup,[30] Magrane,[16] and Roobs and coworkers[25]; the increased success rate may be the result of improved technology and the relatively short-term follow-up for the described series. For example, retinal detachment may occur several months to years following surgery.

Phakoemulsification

Because of the tendency of the canine iris to constrict during surgery and the density of the majority of canine cataracts, especially the nucleus, sonication and aspiration of cataractous lenses with the instruments currently available is less rewarding than the extracapsular technique described previously.

Intraocular Lenses

The use of intraocular plastic lenses has achieved widespread acceptance in human ophthalmology. These lenses may be clipped or sutured to the iris or inserted into the anterior chamber or lens capsule bag. Because of the marked inflammatory response of the canine eye, significant differences in anterior chamber and pupil size, and the ability of our patients to function well without optical correction, their routine use in veterinary ophthalmology is not recommended.

Lens Dislocation

Lens dislocation can be complete (luxation) or partial (subluxation, some intact zonules remaining). The lens may dislocate into the anterior chamber (anterior luxation) or the vitreous (posterior luxation) or may remain within the retropupillary space (subluxation). The condition may occur after blunt trauma but is most frequently seen as a spontaneous bilateral problem in the terrier breeds, most likely related to inherited zonular weakness.[15] Obstruction of aqueous flow from the posterior to anterior chamber by the dislocated lens or displaced vitreous frequently causes secondary glaucoma. Primary lens dislocation must be distinguished from secondary pathology associated with chronic glaucoma, in which buphthalmos and zonular stretching lead to this condition.

Lens extraction is rarely indicated in cases of lens dislocation associated with chronic glaucoma.

Prevention or effective management of glaucoma secondary to primary lens luxation demands lens extraction. Lens extraction is recommended in all cases of anterior lens luxation, subluxation associated with clinical disease (glaucoma or anterior uveitis), and posterior luxation associated with glaucoma that cannot be controlled medically.

Intracapsular cryoextraction is the technique of choice for a primary dislocated lens. Although the zonular attachments are damaged, the hyaloideocapsular ligament is usually intact, and the surgeon who operates on a dislocated lens must be prepared to perform a vitrectomy prior to or subsequent to removal of the lens.

Preoperative preparation of the eye varies with the location of the dislocated lens. Anterior lens luxation is considered a nonelective surgical procedure owing to the potential for damage to the corneal endothelium or glaucoma as a result of pupillary block. Preoperative topical pilocarpine may maintain a small pupil, which traps the lens in the anterior chamber and facilitates extraction; however, miosis may precipitate vitreous pupillary block, and topical pilocarpine should be used only immediately prior to surgery. If the intraocular pressure is significantly elevated (greater than 40 mm Hg), intravenous mannitol should be given at a dosage of 1 mg/kg one hour before surgery to minimize vitreous presentation and spontaneous choroidal hemorrhage.

Subluxation of the lens should be treated surgically if associated with uveitis, glaucoma, or cataract. Subluxated lenses are allowed to remain, in the absence of other clinical signs, in patients with a functional fellow eye; one-eyed patients should be managed more conservatively. Dilation of the pupil with topical 1.0% atropine sulfate and 2.5% phenylephrine is performed prior to surgery.

Posterior luxation ("couching") of the lens may cause intermittent glaucoma and the risk of anterior luxation of the lens. The procedure is elective and is indicated in the presence of glaucoma.

Exposure of and approach to the anterior chamber are identical to those used during extracapsular lens extraction. An *ab externo* incision may be used to avoid puncture of the lens capsule if the lens is luxated anteriorly. If vitreous protrudes during the corneoscleral incision, it is ignored until the incision is complete. Once exposure of the anterior chamber is achieved, the technique for the intracapsular extraction varies with the position of the lens.

With anterior luxation or subluxation of the lens, the cornea is retracted and vitrectomy performed, if necessary, to allow direct access to the lens. Posterior lens luxation involves a more extensive vitrectomy to remove the vitreous between the surgeon and the lens. The lens capsule is dried with a cellulose sponge, and the tip of the cryoprobe is applied to the lens capsule superiorly. Once the cryoprobe is firmly adherent, the lens is carefully extracted as the surgeon separates the posterior vitreal attachments with a cyclodialysis spatula in a gentle sweeping movement in the plane of the iris. Anterior vitrectomy is performed if vitreous is present within the anterior chamber following extraction. Three interrupted 7-0 vicryl sutures close the corneal incision, and the anterior chamber is preformed with saline and an air bubble to allow optimal apposition of the corneal wound. Once the closure is completed, an air bubble one third the size of the anterior chamber is injected and routine closure of the canthotomy is performed (Fig. 107–3). Postoperative therapy is similar to that following extracapsular lens extraction. Intraocular inflammation is less than with extracapsular extraction, as lens protein is never exposed and is completely removed.

Postoperative complications include corneal edema, pupillary membrane, persistent glaucoma, and retinal detachment.[18] Significant corneal edema may be associated with preoperative mechanical trauma from an anteriorly luxated lens or postoperative vitreous in the anterior chamber in direct contact with the endothelium. The former complication may be managed by thin conjunctival flaps or corneal

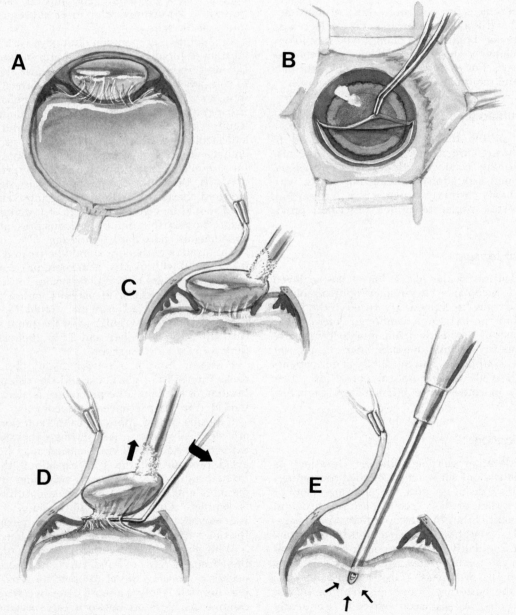

Figure 107–3. Intracapsular cryoextraction of dislocated lenses. *A,* Anterior dislocation of the lens with the vitreal attachments to the posterior lens capsule intact. *B,* The approach to the anterior chamber is the same as that used in Figure 107–1. *C,* The corneal flap is retracted with a corneal forcep, and a cryoprobe is applied to the lens. *D,* Once the cryopexy to the lens is achieved, the lens is removed while relieving vitreal attachment with a spatula. *E,* Intracapsular lens extraction is followed by an anterior vitrectomy as demonstrated with a Kaufman vitrector.

transplantation if time and topical hyperosmotic agents fail to restore vision. The latter complication is preventable with good surgical technique; if it does occur, re-operation and vitrectomy are indicated.

Pupillary membranes are uncommon compared with extracapsular cataract extraction and are usually associated with intra- or postoperative intraocular hemorrhage; if significant, surgical management as discussed previously may be considered.

Postoperative intraocular pressure should be monitored closely and regularly. Continued elevation uncontrollable by medication is an indication for further surgical intervention. Such circumstances are unusual, and removal of the dislocated lens generally cures glaucoma.

Retinal detachment is the most common and perhaps most discouraging of complications; its incidence is 15 to 20 per cent in animals that require vitrectomy. The majority of detachments occur two to four weeks postoperatively and are associated with peripheral tears of the retina. If the detachment is recent (within two weeks), surgical correction may be indicated, with drainage of the subretinal fluid and cryopexy followed by scleral buckling.

1. Aguirre, G., and Bistner, S.: Posterior lenticonus in the dog. Cornell Vet. 63:455, 1973.
2. Aguirre, G. D., Rubin, L. F., and Bistner, S.: Development of the canine eye. Am. J. Vet. Res. 33:2399, 1972.
3. Barnett, K. C.: Types of cataract in the dog. J. Am. Anim. Hosp. Assoc. 8:2, 1972.
4. Barnett, K. C.: Hereditary cataract in the dog. J. Small Anim. Pract. 19:109, 1978.
5. Barrie, K. P., et al.: Posterior lenticonus, microphthalmia, congenital cataracts and retinal folds in an Old English Sheepdog. J. Am. Anim. Hosp. Assoc. 15:715, 1979.
6. Bistner, S., Rathbun, W., Peiffer, R., Jr., Hammer, R. and Shaw, D.: The lens of the dog—basic ultrastructural anatomy and biochemistry. Proc. Am. Coll. Vet. Ophthalmol. 11:129, 1980.
7. Donovan, R. H., et al.: Histology of the normal collie eye. III. Lens, retina and optic nerve. Ann. Ophthalmol. 6:1299, 1974.
8. Formstron, C.: Observation on subluxation and luxation of the crystalline lens in the dog. J. Comp. Pathol. 55:168, 1945.
9. Gelatt, K. N.: Cataracts in the Golden Retriever dog. Vet. Med./Sm. Anim. Clin. 67:113, 1972.
10. Gelatt, K. N., et al.: Cataracts in Chesapeake Bay retrievers. J. Am. Vet. Med. Assoc. 175:1176, 1979.
11. Heywood, R.: Juvenile cataracts in the Beagle dog. J. Small Anim. Pract. 12:171, 1971.
12. Hirth, R. S., Greenstein, E. T., and Peer, R. L.: Anterior capsular opacities (spurious cataracts) in Beagle dogs. Vet. Pathol. 18:181, 1974.
13. Koch, S. A.: Cataracts in interrelated Old English Sheepdogs. J. Am. Vet. Med. Assoc. 160:299, 1972.
14. Lavach, J. D., and Severin, G. A.: Posterior lenticonus and lenticonus interum in the dog. J. Am. Anim. Hosp. Assoc. 13:685, 1977.
15. Lawson, D. D.: Luxation of the crystalline lens in the dog. Trans. Ophthalmol. Soc. U.K. 59:259, 1969.
16. Magrane, W. G.: Cataract extraction: A follow-up study (429 cases). J. Small Anim. Pract. 10:545, 1969.
17. Peiffer, R. L., Jr.: Surgical management of dislocated lenses with vitrectomy using a disposable vitreophage. Vet. Med./Sm. Anim. Clin. 75:1299, 1980.
18. Peiffer, R. L., Jr.: Current concepts in ophthalmic surgery. Vet. Clin. North Am. 10:455, 1980.
19. Peiffer, R. L., Jr., Gelatt, K. N., and Gwin, R. M.: Diabetic cataracts in the dog. Can. Pract. 4:18, 1977.
20. Peiffer, R. L., Jr., Gelatt, K. N., and Gwin, R. M.: Persistent primary vitreous and a pigmented cataract in a dog. J. Am. Anim. Hosp. Assoc. 13:478, 1977.
21. Playter, R. F.: The development and maturation of a cataract. J. Am. Anim. Hosp. Assoc. 13:317, 1977.
22. Prince, J. H., et al.: Anatomy and Histology of the Eye and Orbit in Domestic Animals. Charles C Thomas, Springfield, 1960.
23. Quinn, A. J.: Embryology, anatomy and physiology of the lens. Canine Pract. 8:6, 1981.
24. Roberts, S. R., and Helper, L. C.: Cataracts in the Afghan hound. J. Am. Vet. Med. Assoc. 160:427, 1972.
25. Roobs, R. L., Brightman, A. H., Helper, L. C., and Magrane, W. G.: Extracapsular cataract extraction: A review of 283 operations. Proc. Am. Coll. Vet. Ophthalmol. 11:239, 1980.
26. Rubin, L. F.: Cataracts in Golden Retrievers. J. Am. Vet. Med. Assoc. 165:457, 1974.
27. Rubin, L. F., and Flowers, R. D.: Inherited cataracts in a family of standard Poodles. J. Am. Vet. Med. Assoc. 161:207, 1972.
28. Rubin, L. F., Koch, S. A., and Huber, R. J.: Hereditary cataracts in miniature Schnauzers. J. Am. Vet. Med. Assoc. 154:1456, 1969.
29. Stades, F. C.: Persistent hyperplastic tunica vasculosa lentis and persistent hyperplastic primary vitreous (PHTVL/PHPV) in 90 closely related Doberman Pinschers: Clinical aspects. J. Am. Anim. Hosp. Assoc. 16:739, 1980.
30. Startup, F. C.: Cataract surgery in the dog. J. Small Anim. Pract. 8:667, 1967.
31. Yakely, W. L.: A study of heritability of cataracts in the American Cocker Spaniel. J. Am. Vet. Med. Assoc. 172:814, 1978.
32. Yakely, W. L., Hegreberg, G. A., and Padgett, G. A.: Familial cataracts in the American Cocker Spaniel. J. Am. Anim. Hosp. Assoc. 7:127, 1971.

Chapter 108

Vitreous

Robert L. Peiffer, Jr., and Cynthia S. Cook

Indications for surgical manipulation of the vitreous in veterinary ophthalmic surgery are uncommon and are usually encountered secondary to other intraocular procedures. Anterior presentation of the vitreous during removal of the dislocated or cataractous lens is a frequent complication in dogs. Removal of posterior segment foreign bodies, organized hemorrhage, and opaque vitreous due to asteroid hyalosis are less frequent indications for vitreous surgery. In the past, a wide range of potentially disastrous complications resulted in a conservative approach to vitreous surgery. However, improvements in techniques and instrumentation have extended the scope of vitreous surgery beyond frantic attempts to remove an unwelcome and unanticipated tissue from an undesirable location.

SURGICAL ANATOMY AND PHYSIOLOGY

The vitreous is a transparent connective tissue consisting of collagen and mucopolysaccharides, primarily hyaluronic acid, that fills the posterior segment of the globe. The definitive (secondary) vitreous is of neuroectodermal origin and is formed around the fetal hyaloid artery system (primary vitreous) by gestational day 45 in the dog.[1] The volume of this tissue is approximately 3 ml in the dog and cat.[7] In adults, the vitreous is avascular, atrophy of the hyaloid artery occurring during the first two postnatal months. The zonular fibers attaching the lens to the ciliary body constitute the tertiary vitreous.

Collagen fibrils within the vitreous are continuous with Müller cell processes, which form the internal limiting membrane of the retina.[8] Firm areas of attachment to adjacent structures occur at three locations: the peripheral posterior lens capsule (ligamentum hyaloid capsulare), the ora ciliaris retinae (vitreous base), and at the margin of the optic nerve. The main body of the vitreous is divided into a peripheral cortical portion; an intermediate zone; and the central primary vitreal remnant, Cloquet's canal (Fig. 108–1). The cortical vitreous is loosely attached to the retina and, contrary to that of man, is less dense than the central zone.[19] Cellular components of the vitreous are scarce, consisting primarily of macrophages called hyalocytes. These cells are most numerous near the vitreal base. At its boundaries, the vitreous condenses to form the hyaloid membrane.

HISTORICAL ASPECTS

Removal of opaque vitreous was first described in man in 1890 using an approach through the pars

plana of the ciliary body.[9] Modifications of this technique have been used extensively to clear vitreal opacities (hemorrhage, amyloidosis), to manage retinal detachment by reducing traction and removing vitreous sequestered behind the detachment, to remove posterior segment foreign bodies, and to prevent anterior vitreal prolapse in the aphakic eye.[4, 10, 14, 16–18, 20, 26] An anterior approach to vitrectomy through a limbal incision was introduced in the late 1960s and was subsequently applied to treatment of persistent hyperplastic vitreous, certain types of glaucoma, removal of vitreous opacities, and management of vitreal incarceration in corneal wounds.[3, 4, 11, 13, 15, 20, 25, 27]

Techniques of vitreous removal have involved the use of cellulose sponges, which readily adhere to and absorb liquified vitreous, with transection of fibrils using scissors.[2, 12, 13] A mechanized suction cutter was developed for use with the pars plana approach.[16, 18] Several years later, a simple, disposable vitreophage, which has veterinary applications, was introduced for use in the anterior approach.[3, 15, 22]

Early in the development of vitrectomy techniques, controversy existed over proper replacement of vitreous with a substance of similar properties in order to maintain normal anatomical relationships, tamponade the retina against the pigmented epithelium, and reduce traction. Absorbable and nonabsorbable materials that have been used include saline; gases (air, O_2, N_2, NO_2); body fluids (cerebrospinal fluid, aqueous humor, vitreous grafts); hyaluronic acid; and silicone oil.[20,24] No substance is completely satisfactory, and currently a balanced salt solution, which is rapidly replaced by aqueous humor, is the most practical for use in veterinary ophthalmology.[13,14]

PATHOPHYSIOLOGY AND INDICATIONS

Owing to intimate anatomical relationships between the vitreous and the retina, any process altering the volume or structure of the vitreous may cause retinal detachment. Syneresis, or liquefaction, of the vitreous can occur as a result of senile changes or inflammation. Postinflammatory scarring, or cicatrization, can result in the formation of traction bands that separate the inner retina from the underlying pigmented epithelium.

Lack of vascular supply to the vitreous results in slow clearing of hemorrhage and response to infection. Abnormal vascularization can occur by ingrowth of retinal blood vessels (neovascularization) and is a challenging problem in persons with diabetic retinopathy. These neovascular proliferations are fragile and can bleed into the vitreous. Fortunately, this is unusual in animals.[23]

Vitreal surgery in animals is rarely a primary or elective procedure. However, removal of opaque vitreous owing to asteroid hyalosis has been successfully performed, and similar techniques may be uti-

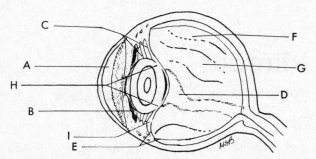

Figure 108–1. Zones within the vitreous. *A,* Anterior chamber; *B,* posterior chamber; *C,* zonules (tertiary vitreous); *D,* Cloquet's canal (remnant of primary vitreous); *E,* vitreous base; *F,* cortical vitreous; *G,* intermediate zone of vitreous; *H,* hyaloideocapsular ligament; *I,* anterior hyaloid membrane.

lized to remove posterior segment foreign bodies. Veterinary applications in the management of retinal detachment have not been described. The most frequent indication for vitrectomy for the veterinary ophthalmic surgeon is found during intracapsular extraction of a dislocated lens in which some degree of vitreal prolapse is expected owing to the firm attachment of the posterior lens capsule to the anterior hyaloid membrane. Inadvertent tearing of the posterior lens capsule during extracapsular cataract extraction may also result in the appearance of vitreous through the pupil.

The surgeon may be faced with signs of imminent rupture of the hyaloid face, such as iris prolapse through the initial limbal incision, ballooning forward of the iris and narrowing of the anterior chamber, and the actual appearance of the vitreous face. In such cases, it may be possible to sweep the anterior hyaloid behind the iris with a cyclodialysis spatula or prevent anterior vitreal prolapse by aspiration of liquified vitreous through the pupil by a pars plana approach. Rupture of the anterior hyaloid with vitreous presentation into the anterior chamber is an indication for anterior vitrectomy.

TECHNIQUES

Pars Plana Vitrectomy

This approach is useful in the prevention of anterior vitreal prolapse. The globe is stabilized using a scleral support ring and is entered with a 1-inch, 20- to 22-gauge needle over the pars plana ciliaris, located 6 to 8 mm behind the limbus. Anatomical relationships are critical (Fig. 108–2); an anterior approach may result in ciliary trauma and hemorrhage or damage to the lens. If the retina is penetrated by the needle posterior to the pars plana, the resulting retinal hole may lead to detachment. Overzealous aspiration can also result in retinal traction. Liquified vitreous can be gently aspirated (0.25 to 2.00 cc), accompanied by posterior displacement of the vitreous face and deepening of the anterior chamber. Liquified vitreous may be minimal in the young animal or may lie in pockets beyond safe penetration of the needle, leading to discouraging results from attempted aspiration. Small amounts of vitreous removed in this fashion need not be replaced. Modifications of this technique may be utilized in combination with indirect ophthalmoscopy to remove small vitreous opacities or to obtain vitreous biopsies.

Use of the vitreous suction cutter, with or without infusion, in combination with the operating microscope and fiberoptic illumination represents a significant improvement over the earlier pars plana procedure. The procedure can be done in the eye with lens intact with a small incision, maintaining a normal globe and leaving the anterior chamber intact.

Anterior Vitrectomy

Once formed vitreous is present within the anterior chamber, anterior vitrectomy is necessary. This technique, which requires minimal instrumentation, involves the use of cellulose sponges to absorb the liquid components and readily adhere to formed vitreous, facilitating gentle elevation (Fig. 108–3). Vitreous is excised, a little at a time, at the level of the iris until the anterior chamber deepens and no further vitreous appears. Great care is taken to avoid contact with the corneal endothelium as the cellulose swells; a broad, 180° corneoscleral incision facilitates

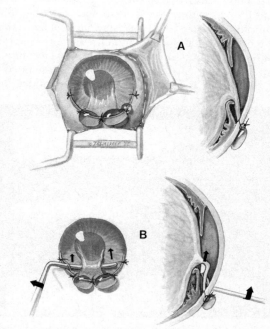

Figure 108–3. *A*, Vitreous incarcerated in a corneoscleral wound. *B*, Sweeping vitreous from incision using a cyclodialysis spatula, with replacement of vitreous behind the iris.

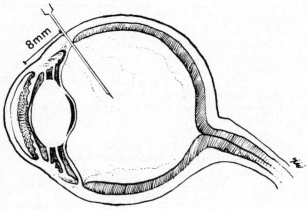

Figure 108–2. Anatomical relationships in a pars plana vitrectomy. Similar techniques are used to aspirate vitreous for diagnostic purposes.

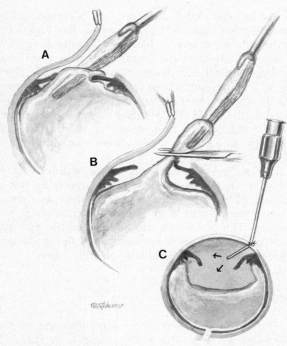

Figure 108–4. Anterior vitrectomy using a cellulose sponge. *A,* Vitreous is allowed to adhere to the sponge. *B,* The sponge is gently retracted, and vitreous fibrils are transected at the level of the iris. *C,* After closure of the corneal incision, an infusion of balanced salt solution is used to reform the anterior chamber and re-establish normal anatomical relationships.

the procedure. Small particles of cellulose left within the eye cause granulomas and chronic inflammation in man.[13]

If vitreous is incarcerated into a corneoscleral wound once closure has started, it may be swept behind the iris with a cyclodialysis spatula[5] (Fig. 108–4). Simple, disposable vitreophages are available that combine controlled suction by an assistant-operated syringe with atraumatic tissue resection via a rotating or guillotine-like blade within an aspirating needle (Fig. 108–5). These instruments markedly reduce the

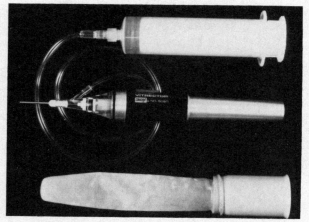

Figure 108–5. The disposable vitreophage consists of a battery-powered motor, an assistant-operated syringe to provide suction, and a rotary cutting blade. The power source is enclosed in a sterile latex sleeve and coupled to the cutting unit during the procedure.

time required for vitrectomy and minimize traction on the retina and are particularly applicable when more than a small amount of vitreous must be removed, as with a lens dislocation, posterior segment foreign body, or vitreous opacification. In these situations, a large "open sky" exposure is indicated, involving up to a 200° corneal incision and multiple sphincterotomies if necessary to maintain an enlarged pupil. The excised vitreous is replaced with saline, and an air bubble is used to reform the anterior chamber. The technique is most frequently used in cryoextraction of a dislocated lens. If vitreous appears as the globe is entered, the incision is extended and vitreous is excised until the cryoprobe can be applied directly to the lens capsule. If vitreous does not appear, the cryoprobe is used to elevate the lens through the incision. Vitreous attachments are separated from the posterior lens capsule in the plane of the pupil with a lens loop or cyclodialysis spatula. Vitreous is excised until the anterior chamber is empty and the iris is concave.

COMPLICATIONS

Complications associated with vitrectomy may occur at surgery or in the postoperative period. In humans, these include cystic macular edema, persistent uveitis, retinal detachment, vitreous hemorrhage, keratopathy, peaked pupil, and glaucoma.[6,11] The radical anterior approach can lead to corneal dehydration due to exposure. However, the canine cornea seems to be more resistant, with a lower incidence of corneal complications.[21]

Complications of anterior vitrectomy associated with canine lens removal are summarized in Table 108–1. Incomplete removal of vitreous from the anterior chamber can lead to glaucoma due to blockage of outflow pathways and pupillary and cyclitic mem-

TABLE 108–1. Complications Following Canine Anterior Vitrectomy*

Anteriorly displaced lens (n = 42)	
Retinal detachment	4 (9.5%)
Persistent corneal edema	2 (4.8%)
(without vitreous touch)	
Glaucoma	4 (9.5%)
Posteriorly displaced lens (n = 15)	
Retinal detachment	3 (20.0%)
Glaucoma	2 (13.3%)
Vitreous presentation during planned extracapsular cataract extraction (n = 364)	
Vitreous presentations requiring anterior vitrectomy	48 (13.2%)
Retinal detachment	8 (16.7%)
Glaucoma	2 (4.2%)

*Associated with lens removal performed with a disposable vitreophage between 1978 and 1982.

branes and endothelial damage due to vitreocorneal contact. Excessive manipulation and traction on the vitreous can lead to the most serious complications of vitrectomy. During pars plana vitrectomy, failure to cut through the vitreous base cleanly may push the vitreous ahead of the needle, the resulting traction producing retinal dialysis and detachment. Excessive traction or removal of vitreous can also lead to retinal detachment. Hemorrhage may result from cutting vitreous proliferations containing vessels.

1. Aguirre, G. D., Rubin, L. F., and Bistner, S. J.: Development of the canine eye. Am. J. Vet. Res. 33:2399, 1972.
2. Barraquer, F.: Surgery of the dislocated lens. Trans. Am. Acad. Ophthalmol. Otolaryngol. 76:44, 1972.
3. Binder, P. S.: Anterior vitrectomy in cataract surgery, aphakic keratoplasty, and patients with vitreous pathology using a simple vitreophage. Ann. Ophthalmol. 6:947, 1974.
4. Binder, P. S.: Present surgical approaches to vitrectomy. Ann. Ophthalmol. 7:1377, 1975.
5. Castroviejo, R.: Handling of eyes with vitreous prolapse. Am. J. Ophthalmol. 48:397, 1959.
6. Cerasoli, J. R., and Kasner, D.: A follow-up study of vitreous loss during cataract surgery managed by anterior vitrectomy. Am. J. Ophthalmol. 71:1040, 1971.
7. Cole, D. F.: Comparative aspects of the intraocular fluids. In Dawson, H., and Graham, L. T. (eds.): Comparative Physiology, Vol. 1, Academic Press, New York, 1974.
8. Foos, R. Y.: Vitreoretinal juncture; topographical variations. Invest. Ophthalmol. 12:801, 1972.
9. Ford, V.: Proposed surgical treatment of opaque vitreous. Lancet. 1:462, 1890.
10. Freeman, H.: Recent advances in vitreous surgery. Invest. Ophthalmol. 12:549, 1973.
11. Gardner, R. C.: Anterior vitrectomy. Ann. Ophthalmol. 7:723, 1975.
12. Iliff, C. E.: Management of vitreous loss after cataract extraction. Arch. Ophthalmol. 83:319, 1970.
13. Kasner, D.: Vitrectomy: A new approach to the management of vitreous. Highlights Ophthalmol. 11:304, 1969.
14. Kasner, D., Miller, G. R., Taylor, W. H., Sever, R. J., and Norton, E.: Surgical treatment of amyloidosis of the vitreous. Trans. Am. Acad. Ophthalmol. Otolaryngol. 72:410, 1968.
15. Kaufman, H. E.: Vitrectomy from the anterior approach. Vitrectomy for the anterior segment surgeon. Ophthalmic Surg. 6:58, 1975.
16. Machemer, R.: A new concept for vitreous surgery. 2. Surgical technique and complication. Am. J. Ophthalmol. 74:1022, 1972.
17. Machemer, R., and Norton, E.: A new concept for vitreous surgery. 3. Indications and results. Am. J. Ophthalmol. 74:1034, 1972.
18. Machemer, R., Parel, J. M., and Buettner, H.: A new concept for vitreous surgery. 1. Instrumentation. Am. J. Ophthalmol. 73:1, 1972.
19. Martin, C. L., and Anderson, B. G.: Ocular anatomy. In Gelatt, K. (ed.): Veterinary Ophthalmology. Lea & Febiger, Philadelphia, 1981, pp. 80–84.
20. Michaels, R. G., Machemer, R., and Mueller-Jensen, K.: Vitreous surgery: History and current concepts. Ophthalmic Surg. 5:13, 1974.
21. Peiffer, R. L., Jr.: Clinical and histopathologic effects of lensectomy and anterior vitrectomy in the canine eye. J. Am. Anim. Hosp. Assoc. 15:421, 1979.
22. Peiffer, R. L., Jr.: Removal of a luxated lens and anterior vitrectomy using a disposable vitreophage. Vet. Med./Sm. Anim. Clin. 75:1249, 1980.
23. Peiffer, R. L., Jr., Armstrong, J. R., and Johnson, P. T.: Animals in ophthalmic research: Concepts and methodologies. In Gay, W. I. (ed.): Methods of Animal Experimentation. Academic Press, New York, 1981, pp. 140–235.
24. Peyman, G. A., Ericson, E. S., and May, D. R.: A review of substances and techniques of vitreous replacement. Surv. Ophthalmol. 17:41, 1972.
25. Peyman, G. A., May, D. R., and Ericson, E. S.: Techniques of vitreous removal. Surv. Ophthalmol. 17:29, 1972.
26. Tolentino, F. I., Donovan, R. H., and Freeman, H. M.: Biomicroscopy of the vitreous in collie dogs with fundus abnormalities. Arch. Ophthalmol. 73:700, 1965.
27. Turtz, A. I.: Anterior vitrectomy. Ophthalmic Surg. 1:14, 1970.

Chapter 109

Orbit

Douglas H. Slatter and Elizabeth D. Chambers

INTRODUCTION

The orbit is the bony cavity surrounding the eye. Many orbital disorders are treated surgically, and manipulative procedures are frequently used in the diagnosis of orbital disease. Major features of orbital anatomy and pathophysiology are discussed before the diseases themselves. For a more detailed discussion of the diagnosis of orbital disease, readers are referred to veterinary ophthalmology texts.[7, 15]

The orbit of the dog and cat[5] separates the eye from the cranial cavity but allows blood vessels and nerves to pass through numerous foramina joining the two (Figs. 109–1 through 109–7). The length of the optic nerve is greater than the distance from the eye to the optic foramen (Fig. 109–8).

The dorsolateral wall of the orbit is not composed of bone but is formed by the dense, collagenous orbital ligament between the zygomatic process of the frontal bone and the frontal process of the zygomatic bone (see Fig. 109–1).[6] The orbit is completely enclosed by the periorbita, connective tissue that lies next to the bony walls and is thickened laterally as the orbital ligament (see Fig. 109–8).

The periorbita also surrounds the extraocular muscles and forms Tenon's capsule, which blends with the sclera and conjunctiva near the limbus. It is continuous with the periosteum of the facial bones around the orbital rim, the orbital septum, and the dura of the optic nerve at the optic foramen. The orbital fat pad lies between the periorbita and the orbital wall posteriorly. The extraocular muscles arise

Text continued on page 1554

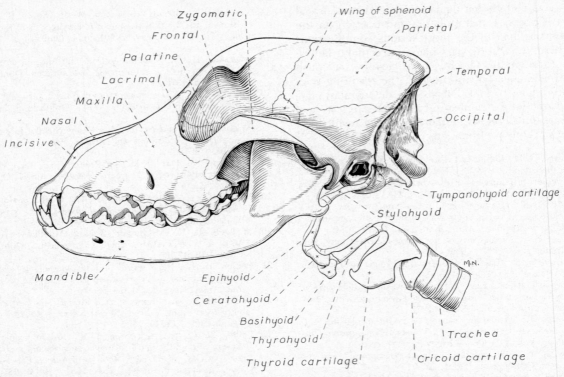

Figure 109–1. Bones of the skull, hyoid apparatus, and laryngeal cartilages. (Reprinted with permission from Evans, H. E., and Christensen, G. C. (eds.): *Miller's Anatomy of the Dog*. 2nd ed. W. B. Saunders, Philadelphia, 1979.)

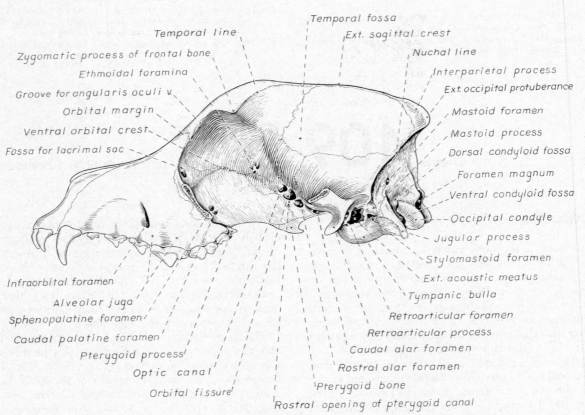

Figure 109–2. Skull, lateral aspect (zygomatic arch removed). (Reprinted with permission from Evans, H. E., and Christensen, G. C. (eds.): *Miller's Anatomy of the Dog*. 2nd ed. W. B. Saunders, Philadelphia, 1979.)

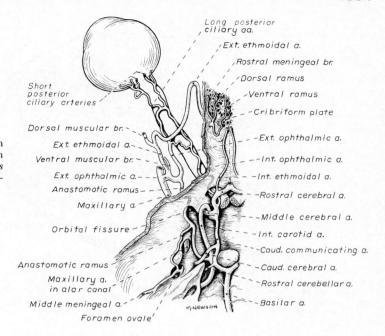

Figure 109–3. Arteries of the orbit and base of the cranium in the dog, dorsal aspect. (Reprinted with permission from Evans, H. E., and Christensen, G. C. (eds.): *Miller's Anatomy of the Dog.* 2nd ed. W. B. Saunders, Philadelphia, 1979.)

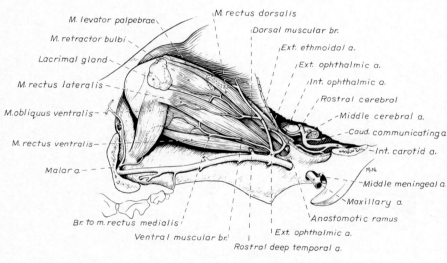

Figure 109–4. Arteries of the orbit and extrinsic ocular muscles in the dog, lateral aspect. (Reprinted with permission from Evans, H. E., and Christensen, G. C. (eds.): *Miller's Anatomy of the Dog.* 2nd ed. W. B. Saunders, Philadelphia, 1979.)

Figure 109–5. Scheme of the terminal branches of the maxillary artery in the dog, lateral aspect. (Reprinted with permission from Evans, H. E., and Christensen, G. C. (eds.): *Miller's Anatomy of the Dog.* 2nd ed. W. B. Saunders, Philadelphia, 1979.)

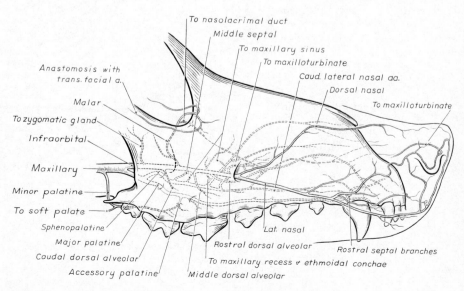

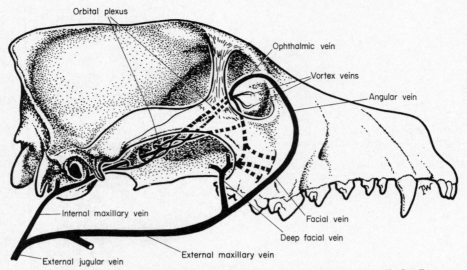

Figure 109–6. The venous drainage of the eye and orbit. (Reprinted with permission from Startup, F. G.: *Diseases of the Canine Eye.* Williams & Wilkins, Baltimore, 1969.)

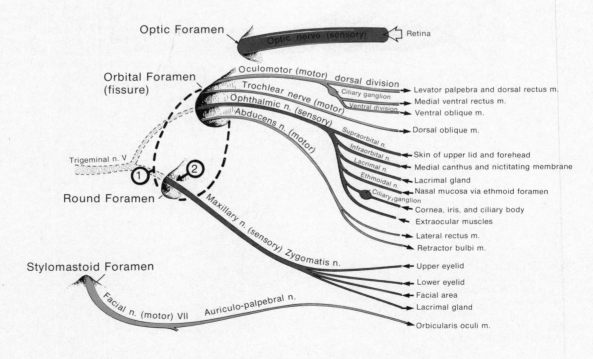

① Round and orbital foramina fuse in the pig and ruminants, forming the <u>foramen orbitorotundum</u>

② Only orbital branches shown here

Figure 109–7. Nerve supply to the eye.

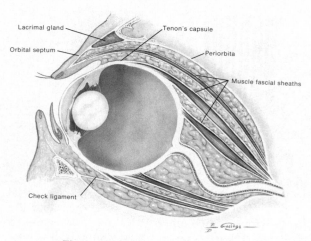

Figure 109–8. Division of the periorbita.

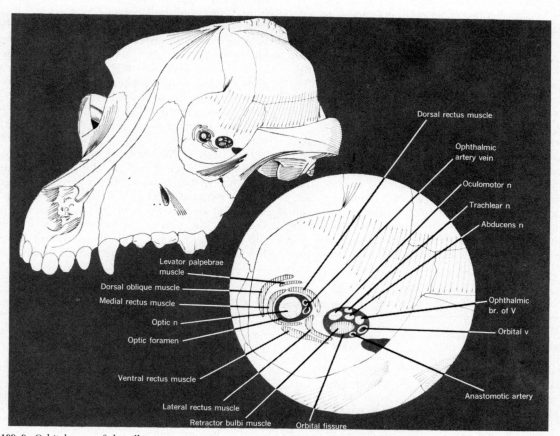

Figure 109–9. Orbital apex of dog illustrating structures passing through the optic foramen and orbital fissure as well as extraocular muscle attachments. (Reprinted with permission from Gelatt, K. N.: *Textbook of Veterinary Ophthalmology*. Lea & Febiger, Philadelphia, 1981.)

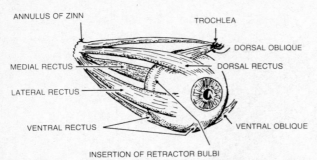

Figure 109–10. General arrangement of the orbital muscles. (After Prince, J. H., et al.: *Anatomy and Histology of the Eye and Orbit in Domestic Animals.* Charles C Thomas, Springfield, 1960.)

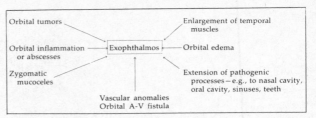

Figure 109–11. Mechanisms of exophthalmos.

from the annulus of Zinn, which surrounds the optic foramen and fissure (Figs. 109–9 and 109–10).

Innervation and function of the extraocular muscles are listed in Table 109–1.

The lacrimal gland lies beneath the orbital ligament on the dorsolateral surface of the globe and is surrounded by the periorbita (see Fig. 109–8).

PATHOLOGICAL MECHANISMS

The orbit is a confined space. Increases and decreases in the volume of its contents move the eye in relation to the orbital rim, the face, and the other eye. The periorbita and extraocular muscles provide three possible compartments for disease processes to occupy (see Fig. 109–8): (1) within the muscle cone, (2) outside the muscle cone but within the periorbita, or (3) within the orbit but outside the periorbita, i.e., beneath the periosteum (periorbita) or behind the periorbita laterally.

Space-occupying lesions, e.g., tumors, zygomatic mucocele, and abscesses, push the eye rostrally, causing exophthalmos, and often cause protrusion of the mucous membrane behind the last upper molar (Fig. 109–11), where the periorbita is unrestrained by a bony wall. Reduction in the volume of orbital contents causes the eye to recede into the orbit (enophthalmos) and the third eyelid to protrude.

The position of space-occupying lesions alters the direction in which the globe is displaced and is useful in localizing a mass for biopsy or excision (Fig. 109–12). Exophthalmos leads to increased evaporation of the precorneal tear film with exposure keratitis, ulceration, and conjunctivitis. Because the orbit and subconjunctival tissues are connected, pathological orbital edema is often seen clinically as chemosis, e.g., orbital cellulitis/abscess. Obstruction of posterior venous drainage may exacerbate this chemosis.

The proximity of the paranasal sinuses (Fig. 109–13), teeth, zygomatic gland, and vertical ramus of the mandible to the orbit influences the extension of disease processes in these structures by affecting the orbital tissues. Infections and neoplasms in the sinuses or nasal cavity may invade the orbit, usually through the thin medial wall[6] of the orbit where the frontal, lacrimal, and palatine bones join. Fractures in the walls of the sinuses after trauma may allow air to escape into the orbit, causing orbital or subconjunctival emphysema.[3] Air may also enter the orbit from the nasolacrimal duct after enucleation of the globe.[1, 12] Although uncommon, such passage of air may be caused by increased pressure within the nasal cavity during expiration in brachycephalic dogs with collapsed external nares and elevated intranasal pressure.

Infections of the roots of molar teeth may cause orbital infections as well as the more common discharging fistula beneath the eye. Sialocele of the canine zygomatic gland with enlargement can cause the gland to protrude into the ventral orbit and be visible in the ventral conjunctival fornix or behind the last upper molar. When the mouth is opened, the vertical ramus of the mandible moves forward,

TABLE 109–1. Innervation of the Extraocular Muscles

Muscle	Innervation	Action
Dorsal rectus m.	Oculomotor III	Elevates globe
Ventral rectus m.	Oculomotor III	Depresses globe
Medial rectus m.	Oculomotor III	Turns globe nasally (medially)
Lateral rectus m.	Abducens VI	Turns globe temporally (laterally)
Dorsal oblique m.	Trochlear IV	Intorts globe (rotates 12 o'clock position nasally)
Ventral oblique m.	Oculomotor III	Extorts globe (rotates 12 o'clock position temporally)
M. retractor bulbi	Abducens VI	Retracts globe
M. levator superioris	Oculomotor III	Elevates upper lid

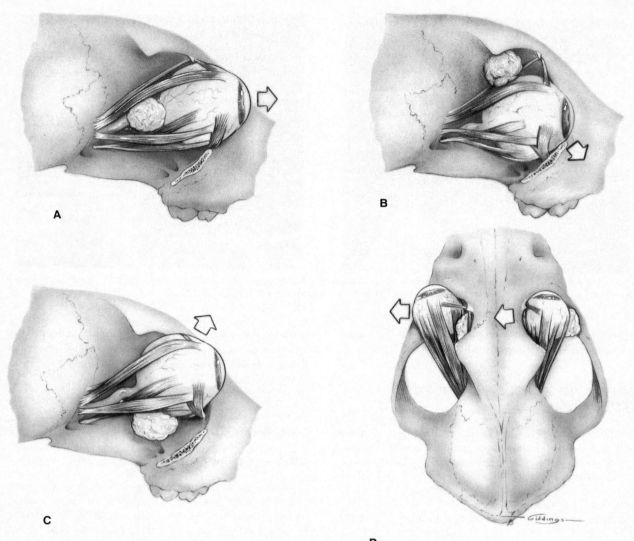

Figure 109–12. Effects of position of space-occupying lesions on the direction of globe displacement. *A*, Within muscle cone. *B*, Dorsal mass. *C*, Ventral mass. *D*, Nasal and temporal masses.

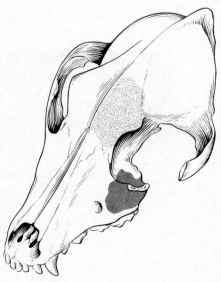

Figure 109–13. Relationship of the paranasal sinuses to the orbital walls in the dog. (Reprinted with permission from Evans, H. E., and Christensen, G. C. (eds.): *Miller's Anatomy of the Dog.* 2nd ed. W. B. Saunders, Philadelphia, 1979.)

Mesaticephalic

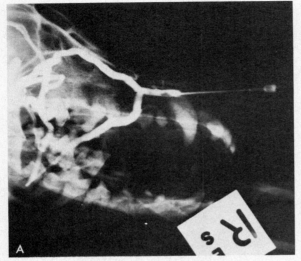 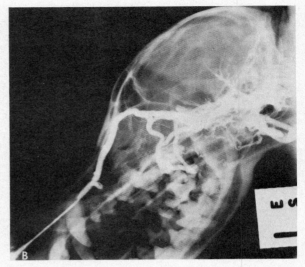

Figure 109–14. *A*, Lateral orbital venogram (right eye). *B*, Venogram of left orbit in a five-year-old poodle with a lymphoid pseudotumor in the inferonasal orbit. The inferior ophthalmic vein has been obliterated. (Courtesy of Dr. R. Dixon.)

pressing on the orbital contents and causing pain if cellulitis or abscess is present.

DIAGNOSTIC METHODS AND SIGNS OF ORBITAL DISEASE

Methods of diagnosis and localization especially useful for orbital disorders include orbital contrast venography (Fig. 109–14),[4] contrast orbitography,[13] ultrasonography, orbital arteriography,[18] and aspiration and cytology. Contrast venography and aspiration and cytology are the most readily available methods. Computer-assisted tomography, thecography of the optic nerve,[10] and radiographic imaging of the optic foramen are available in radiological referral centers. Signs associated with orbital lesions include exophthalmos, displacement of the globe (see Fig. 109–12), chemosis, protrusion of the third eyelid, conjunctival erythema, periorbital swelling, pain on opening the mouth if inflammation is present, indentation of the globe from the posterior with folding of the overlying retina, interference with vision if the optic nerve is affected, and alteration of direct and consensual reflexes.

ORBITAL DISORDERS

Orbital Inflammation

Orbital inflammation occurs in both dogs and cats, either as a diffuse orbital cellulitis or, in advanced cases, as an orbital or retrobulbar abscess. It is usually assumed to be caused by penetration of foreign bodies from the mouth (Fig. 109–15) or by hematogenous bacteria.

The clinical signs of orbital inflammation include pyrexia, chemosis, protrusion of the third eyelid, pain on opening the mouth, variable exophthalmos,

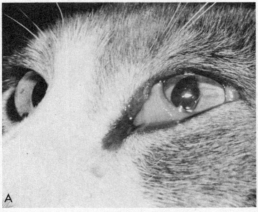 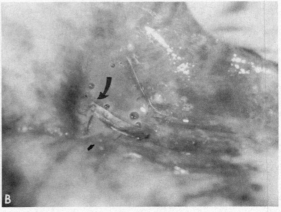

Figure 109–15. *A*, Acute retrobulbar abscess in a cat with exophthalmos, protrusion of the third eyelid, chemosis, and pain on opening the mouth. *B*, Foreign body behind the last molar tooth of a dog with acute retrobulbar abscess. The foreign body was 6 cm in length. (Courtesy of Dr. Stephen Bistner.)

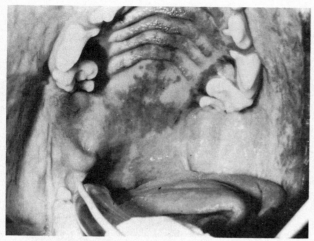

Figure 109–16. Fluctuant reddened mucous membrane behind the last upper molar.

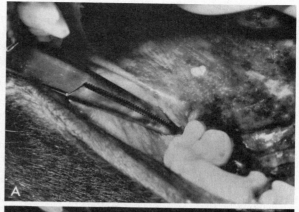

fluctuating red swelling in the oral mucous membrane behind the last upper molar (Fig. 109–16), periorbital swelling, and anorexia. The clinical signs are usually acute.

Based on clinical signs alone it is often impossible to distinguish orbital cellulitis from abscess. However, in cellulitis pain is less evident and pyrexia and anorexia are less severe. The two diseases can usually be differentiated by the lack of discharge when the orbit is drained to the oral cavity. Orbital inflammation is distinguished from other causes of exophthalmos by its acute onset, pain, pyrexia, and the frequent occurrence of leukocytosis with neutrophilia.

Treatment

Cellulitis and abscesses are treated by ventral drainage to the oral cavity and systemic and local antibiotics. Drainage is through an incision behind the last upper molar (Fig. 109–17). The mucous membrane is incised and a pair of curved Crile hemostats or a blunt probe is inserted (Fig. 109–18) and gradually advanced and opened in small steps until the orbit is reached. Dependent drainage to the

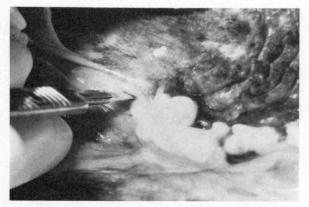

Figure 109–17. Site of incision for drainage of retrobulbar abscess.

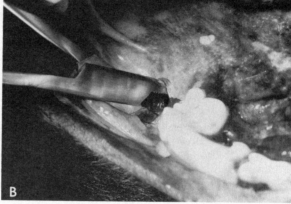

Figure 109–18. Gradual insertion of hemostats to establish drainage from the orbit to the oral cavity.

orbit is established, and small pockets of exudate (sometimes under pressure) may be released.

The orbit is flushed with sterile saline or crystalline penicillin solution via the oral incision with a blunt needle or lacrimal cannula. Systemic antibiotics are administered for five to seven days, and soft foods are fed during the recovery period, which is usually short (one to two days). Topical antibiotics may be used if severe conjunctivitis was present prior to drainage. Exploratory orbitotomy may occasionally be required if response to therapy is poor or to locate foreign bodies.

Zygomatic Mucocele[11, 14]

A mucocele is a leakage of saliva from a gland or duct with inflammation and fibrosis. Mucocele of the zygomatic salivary gland beneath the eye occurs in dogs spontaneously and after trauma to the head. Although not common, it must be considered in the differential diagnosis of exophthalmos, space-occupying orbital lesions, and posterior oropharyngeal masses.

The clinical signs include protrusion of the oral mucous membrane behind the last upper molar, the presence of a mass in the ventral conjunctival fornix, protrusion of the third eyelid, exophthalmos, and painless orbital swelling. The clinical signs vary with the position of the mucocele in the orbit. Aspiration of fluid from within the mucocele reveals tenacious, straw-colored fluid. A zygomatic sialogram may be useful in outlining the extent of the mucocele for therapy.

The treatment of choice is resection of the gland and mucocele via a local orbitotomy. Any of the following approaches may be used: (1) posterior to the orbital ligament, (2) dorsal to the zygomatic arch, (3) through the ventral conjunctival fornix, or (4) if an oral lesion is visible behind the last upper molar.

Orbital Emphysema[1, 12]

Air may enter the orbit from the paranasal sinuses after trauma (Fig. 109–19) or from the nasolacrimal duct after enucleation (Fig. 109–20). The air is palpable as crepitus beneath the conjunctiva or periocular skin.

If emphysema is present, a radiographic study may indicate the source of the air. Systemic antibiotics are used to prevent infection of the orbit from the sinuses. In the few cases reported, spontaneous resolution has occurred. If emphysema occurs after enucleation, the nasolacrimal duct may be cannulated, exposed at its upper end, and ligated.

Orbital emphysema after enucleation is more common in brachycephalic breeds. This may be due to higher pressure in the nasal cavity near the exit of

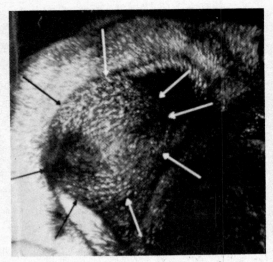

Figure 109–20. Orbital emphysema following enucleation in a pug. (Reprinted with permission from Martin, C. L.: Orbital mucocele in a dog. Vet. Med/Small Anim. Clin. 66:986, 1971.)

the nasolacrimal duct during expiration, to collapsed nares, or to a narrowed airway. Ligation of the dorsal end of the duct during enucleation in these breeds should prevent the development of emphysema.

Orbital Cyst[8]

Orbital cysts rarely occur because either the lacrimal gland or the gland of the third eyelid has been left in the orbit during enucleation. Care must be taken to remove these glands during enucleation. If the cyst ruptures, a fistula may form. Because of its position within the periorbita, the cyst is often difficult to see and remove. If a cyst has formed, the orbit is opened and the tissue is located and removed.

Other Orbital Disorders[5, 17]

The differential diagnoses of other orbital conditions are considered in Table 109–2.

SURGICAL PROCEDURES

Orbital Drainage

Ventral orbital drainage to the oral cavity was discussed previously.

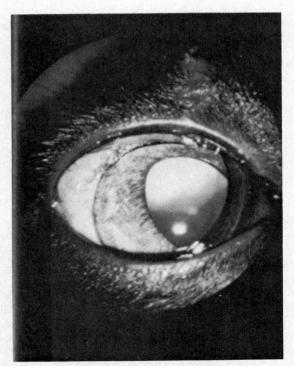

Figure 109–19. Subconjunctival emphysema following orbital trauma in a cat. (Reprinted with permission from Bryan, G.: Subconjunctival emphysema in a cat. Vet. Med./Small Anim. Clin. 72:1087, 1977.)

Enucleation

Enucleation is removal of the globe and the third eyelid (Fig. 109–21) and is indicated for intraocular neoplasia, severe perforating ocular trauma, intract-

TABLE 109–2. Summary of Orbital Diseases*

Type of Disorder	Condition	Clinical Signs
Developmental abnormalities	1. Shallow orbit (brachycephalic breeds)	1. Exophthalmos, exposure keratitis, corneal ulceration, pigmentation
	2. Microphthalmos, anophthalmos	2. Small or absent globe, narrow palpebral fissure, prominent third eyelid, epiphora, blindness
	3. Hydrocephalus with orbital malformation	3. Exotropia, hypotropia, poor vision
	4. Euryblepharon	4. Long palpebral fissure resulting in apparent exophthalmos
	5. Orbital arteriovenous fistula	5. Exophthalmos, fremitus, pulse detectable ("exophthalmos pulsans")
Trauma	1. Hemorrhages	1. Subconjunctival and episcleral hemorrhages; retrobulbar hemorrhage with exophthalmos or proptosis
	2. Penetrating foreign bodies (grass awns, needles, etc., from mouth)	2. Discharging sinus fluid through the conjunctiva, periocular skin, buccal mucosa; pain on opening mouth
	3. Orbital fractures	3. Pain, crepitus; skin abrasions, displacement of globe
Infections	1. Bacterial, fungal	1. Ocular discharge usually secondary to penetrating foreign bodies from conjunctiva or oral cavity; sinusitis, rhinitis, or infections of roots of teeth
	2. Parasites (*Dirofilaria immitis; Pneumonyssus caninum*)	2. Granulomatous lesions due to wandering larvae, *e.g.*, *Dirofilaria* (rare), or extension of infection from nasal cavity (*Pneumonyssus*)
Neoplasia	1. Primary orbital neoplasms—sarcoma, meningioma, adenocarcinoma from nasal cavity, lymphosarcoma in cattle	1. Exophthalmos, exposure keratitis, strabismus, displacement of globe
	2. As for (1), plus nasal or neurologic signs	
Miscellaneous conditions	1. Zygomatic mucocele	1. Exophthalmos, strabismus, swelling in any part of orbit, or behind upper last molar tooth
	2. Infections of roots of teeth (especially carnassial)	2. Discharging fistula beneath eye in dogs
	3. Dehydration	3. Enophthalmos, protrusion of third eyelid
	4. Eosinophilic myositis	4. Exophthalmos, pain with dysphagia in acute stage; enophthalmos potentiated by opening mouth in chronic stage when temporal muscles have atrophied
	5. Horner's syndrome	5. Enophthalmos, miosis, ptosis, protrusion of nictitating membrane, ipsilateral sweating in horses, dermal vasodilation, and hypothermia

*Reprinted with permission from Slatter, D.H.: *Textbook of Veterinary Ophthamology*. W. B. Saunders, Philadelphia, 1981.

Modified from Smith, J.S.: Diseases of the orbit. *In* Kirk, R.W. (ed.): *Current Veterinary Therapy VI*. W. B. Saunders, Philadelphia, 1977.

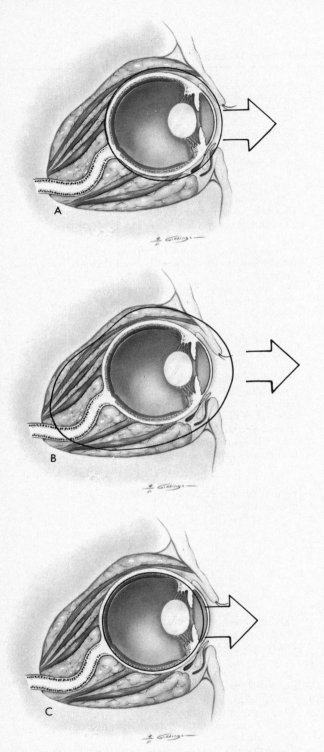

Figure 109–21. Diagram of (A) enucleation, (B) exenteration, and (C) evisceration.

able glaucoma when other treatment methods have failed, and uncontrollable enophthalmitis or panophthalmitis. In dogs and cats the lateral subconjunctival technique gives excellent results. The use of cryotherapy, intrascleral prostheses, and intraocular gentamicin injections has reduced the need for enucleation in glaucoma therapy.

Lateral Subconjunctival Enucleation[2]

A lateral canthotomy is performed for 1 to 2 cm to improve exposure. The conjunctiva is grasped near the limbus with toothed forceps, and a 360° perilimbal incision is made (Fig. 109–22A). The conjunctiva and extraocular muscles are elevated from the sclera with curved Metzenbaum or Mayo scissors to the optic nerve (Fig. 109–22B). If possible, the lacrimal gland, which is found dorsolaterally over the globe, should be left attached to it.

The optic nerve is severed with either scissors or an electrosurgical tonsil snare (Fig. 109–22C). Excess traction on the optic nerve, especially in cats, may damage the optic chiasm and impair vision in the other eye. A ligature may be placed around the optic nerve and nearby long and short posterior ciliary vessels. Hemorrhage in the orbit is controlled by either ligation or pressure from surgical sponges. The third eyelid is grasped and removed (Fig. 109–22D), and the orbit is *temporarily* packed with sponges. The eyelids are removed entirely (Fig. 109–22E) at this later stage to prevent blood from obscuring the earlier dissection during removal of the globe.

Surgical sponges are removed, and the conjunctiva and Tenon's capsule are closed with simple interrupted sutures of 4-0 absorbable material. Any further hemorrhage is contained by the sutured conjunctiva (Fig. 109–22F). The lid incisions are closed with simple interrupted sutures of 4-0 silk, nylon, or Vicryl (Fig 109–22G).

Postoperative swelling is common, especially if hemorrhage has continued, but usually resolves in three to four days. The owner may observe a drop of red fluid on the nose from the nasal end of the nasolacrimal duct during the postoperative period as clots within the orbit break down. With enucleation, orbital fat and extraocular muscles are retained, making the defect after healing more cosmetic than after evisceration. A number of techniques have been used to reduce the orbital defect. Silicone prostheses are the latest to gain acceptance.

The size of the orbital implant (see Fig. 109–29) (16 to 22 mm) is determined by the depth and diameter of the orbital defect. The silicone sphere is prepared by removing one-third of the circumference

---

Figure 109–22. Enucleation. *A,* A lateral canthotomy is performed. *B,* The globe is dissected free from the conjunctiva via a perilimbal incision. Extraocular muscle insertions and periorbita are dissected from the globe back to the optic nerve. *C,* The optic nerve is transected and the eye removed. *D,* The cavity is packed with sponges for *temporary* hemostasis, and the third eyelid is removed completely. *E,* The lid margins are removed. *F,* The sponges are removed, and the conjunctiva is sutured with 3-0 Vicryl or chromic gut. *G,* The entire lid incision is sutured with 3-0 silk.

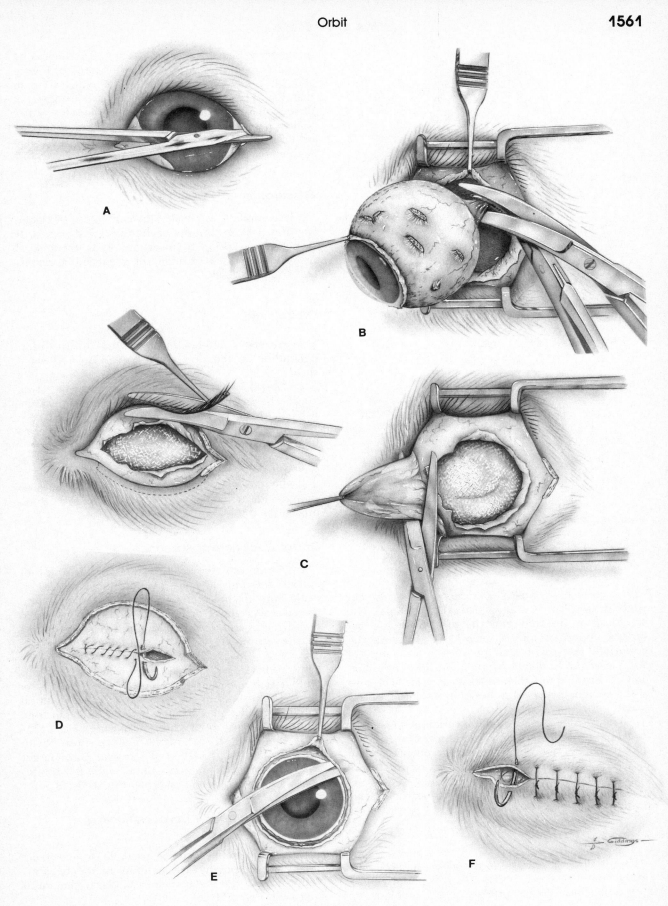

Figure 109–22. *See legend on opposite page*

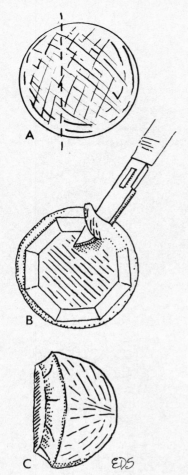

Figure 109–23. Preparation of the orbital prosthesis. *A,* One-third of the silicone sphere is removed. *B* and *C,* The cut edge is contoured to resemble a watch glass.

with a clean horizontal slice and contouring the cut edges using a No. 10 scalpel blade (Fig. 109–23). The prosthesis is inserted into the orbit with the flat surface uppermost. It is secured by suturing the periorbital fascia with a simple continuous suture of 4-0 Vicryl. Crystalline sodium penicillin (1 million units) is instilled into the orbital space prior to closure of the conjunctiva and also before the skin incision is closed.

All enucleated globes should be examined histologically, as the clinical reason for enucleation is frequently inaccurate, e.g., intraocular neoplasia may masquerade as endophthalmitis or glaucoma.[15] Foreign materials, e.g., antibiotic powders, setons, or irritating antiseptic solutions, should not be placed in the orbit before closure.

Exenteration

Exenteration is removal of the globe, adnexa, and orbital contents (see Fig. 109–21). It is performed to stop a noxious disease process, e.g., neoplasia or fulminating, uncontrollable infection. The technique of transpalpebral exenteration is illustrated in Figure 109–24. The technique differs from enucleation in that the lids are incised initially and the plane of dissection is outside the extraocular muscles rather than adjacent to the sclera. Because more of the orbital contents are removed with this method than with enucleation, the postoperative defect is greater.

Evisceration

Evisceration is removal of the contents of the globe (see Fig. 109–21) but not of the sclera and cornea. It is performed prior to insertion of an intrascleral prosthesis in the treatment of advanced glaucoma (see Chapter 110).

Orbitotomy

There are a number of approaches to the orbit, depending on the site and degree of desired exposure.

1. Dorsal, nasal, and temporal transconjunctival approach, for lesions anterior to the equator of the globe.

2. Limited orbitotomy with transection of the orbital ligament for lesions posterior to the globe.

3. Complete orbitotomy with zygomatic arch resection for extensive orbital exposure.

Preliminary examination and diagnostic techniques should indicate which is the most appropriate approach for the lesion being treated.

Dorsal Conjunctival Approach

This approach is used for lesions either inside or outside the muscle cone. A perilimbal incision is made through the conjunctiva, and dissection is continued either above or beneath the insertions of the dorsal rectus and dorsal oblique muscles, depending on the site of the lesion in relation to the muscle cone (Fig. 109–25A). The use of electrocautery aids hemostasis. Dorsally, a vortex vein may be encountered 4 to 6 mm back from the limbus. If the lesion is inside the muscle cone, dorsal rectus and dorsal oblique muscles may be transected 3 to 4 mm from their scleral insertions to aid exposure (Fig. 109–25B). In closing, these muscles may be sutured with mattress sutures of 4-0 to 6-0 Vicryl or chromic gut and the conjunctiva closed with a simple 6-0 continuous suture of the same material (Fig. 109–25C).

Nasal and Temporal Transconjunctival Approaches

These approaches may be used for lesions lying nasally or temporally and anterior to the equator. They are performed in a manner similar to the dorsal approach (Fig. 109–26).

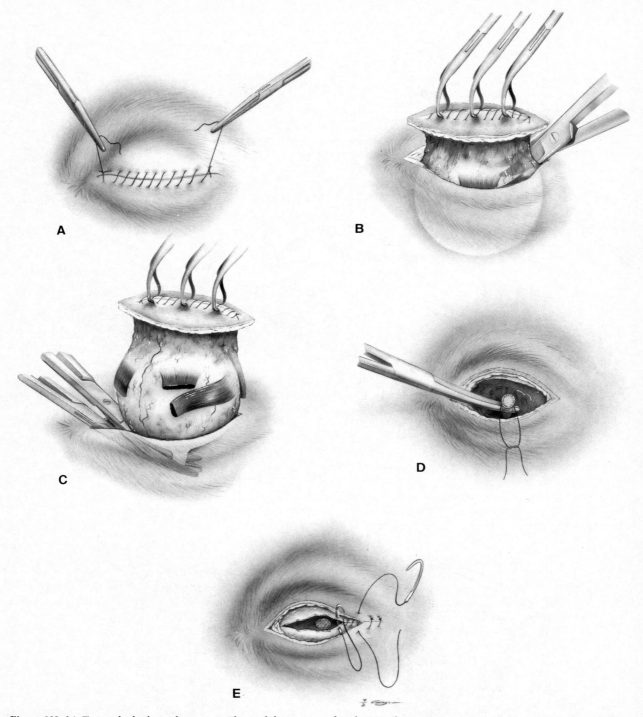

Figure 109–24. Transpalpebral enucleation. *A*, The eyelids are sutured with a simple continuous suture tied at either end and are held with hemostats. *B*, A periocular incision is made and dissection carried down outside the extraocular muscles to the apex of the orbit. *C* and *D*, The optic nerve and associated vessels are clamped and ligated and transected. *E*, Conjunctiva and Tenon's capsule are sutured with 3-0 chromic gut or Vicryl, and the skin is closed with simple interrupted sutures of a nonabsorbable material appropriate for the size and environment of the patient (e.g., 4-0 silk or nylon for cats and dogs).

Partial Orbitotomy with Orbital Ligament Transection

This technique is useful for removal of zygomatic mucoceles and lesions in the lateral orbit (Fig. 109–27). The dense collagenous orbital ligament may be transected above or slightly below the lateral canthus. It should be resutured with nonabsorbable monofilament nylon, e.g., 2-0, to prevent disruption during the slow healing process.

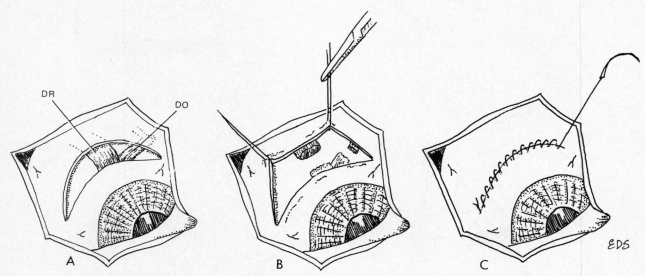

Figure 109–25. Dorsal conjunctival approach to the orbit. *A,* The dorsal rectus (*DR*) and dorsal oblique (*DO*) muscles are exposed. *B,* The muscles are transected to increase surgical exposure. *C,* The conjunctiva is closed with a simple continuous suture of 4-0 Vicryl or silk.

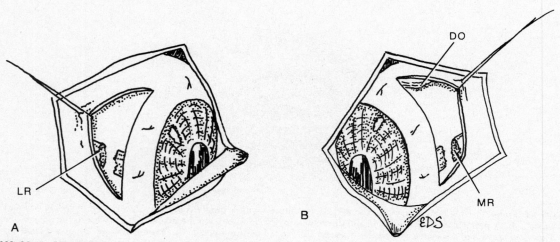

Figure 109–26. *A,* Temporal (lateral) conjunctival approach to the right eye with exposure and transection of the lateral rectus (*LR*) muscle. *B,* Nasal (medial) conjunctival approach to the right eye with exposure of the medial rectus (*MR*) and dorsal oblique (*DO*) muscles and transection of the medial rectus muscle.

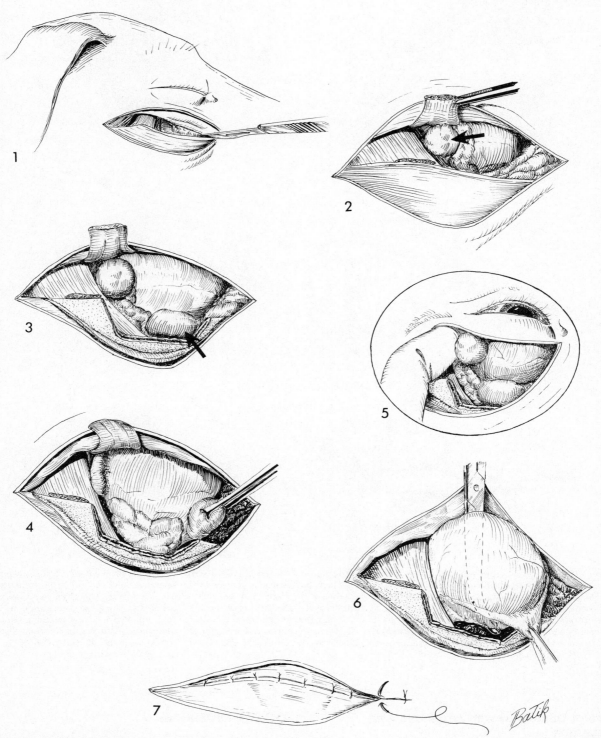

Figure 109–27. Exposure of the interior lateral orbit by limited orbitotomy. The globe, zygomatic salivary gland, and transected orbital ligament are visible. (Reprinted with permission from Bistner, S. I., Aguirre, G., and Batik, G.: *Atlas of Veterinary Ophthalmic Surgery*. W. B. Saunders, Philadelphia, 1977.)

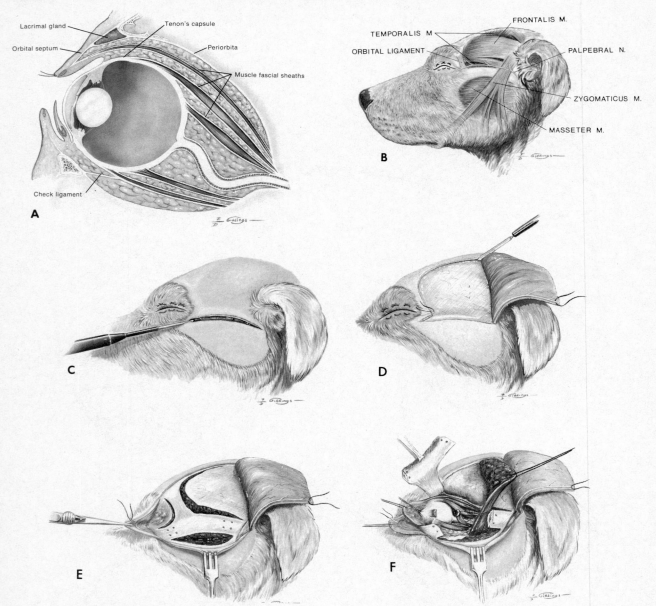

Figure 109–28. Lateral orbitotomy with zygomatic arch resection. *A,* Diagram of the three divisions of the orbital fascia: Tenon's capsule, periorbita, and fascial sheaths of extraocular muscles. *B,* Major anatomical structures in the operative field. *C,* Initial horizontal skin incision over the zygomatic arch. *D,* Outline of skin incisions, with reference to palpable surface landmarks. The initial skin flap with adherent frontalis muscle is reflected posteriorly. *E,* Incision of the aponeurosis of the temporal muscle along the external frontal and sagittal crests and the dorsal margin of the zygomatic arch. Temporal muscle attachment to periosteum of parietal and temporal bones is broken down, and the muscle is reflected posteriorly. *F,* Zygomatic arch is reflected dorsally. (Reprinted with permission from Slatter, D. H., and Abdelbaki, Y.: Lateral orbitotomy by zygomatic arch resection in the dog. J. Am. Vet. Med. Assoc. *175:*1179, 1979.)

Lateral Orbitotomy with Zygomatic Arch Resection[16]

This extensive and time-consuming approach affords excellent exposure of deeper orbital structures and is indicated for removal of neoplasms and foreign bodies and for diagnostic and experimental procedures. The technique is illustrated in Figure 109–28, and further details have been published.[16]

OCULAR PROSTHESES

Prostheses for ocular use in animals are of three types: intraorbital, intrascleral, and extrascleral.

Intraorbital Prosthesis

Implantation of a silicone prosthesis after enucleation or exenteration reduces the facial distortion.

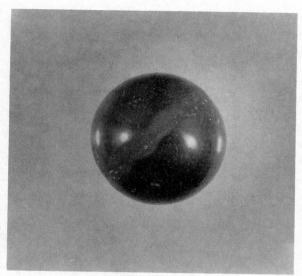

Figure 109–29. Silicone prosthesis.

caused by removal of orbital contents. The major complication is dislodgment of the prosthesis and rotation within the orbit. The contour of the skin is pushed outward and the desired cosmetic effect is lost. Preoperative bacterial invasion is minimized by the prophylactic use of bactericidal antibiotics. Extrusion of the prosthesis is rare.

Intrascleral Prosthesis (See also Chapter 110)

The intrascleral silicone prosthesis is used in dogs and to a lesser extent in cats in the treatment of chronic intractable glaucoma in blind, painful eyes. It provides the clinician and owner with an acceptable alternative to enucleation. The prosthesis (Fig. 109–29) is inserted in the eye with a prosthesis inserter after evisceration. In buphthalmic eyes the sclera and cornea shrink to conform to the size of the prosthesis. A complication rate of about 10 per cent has been reported.[9]

Extrascleral Prosthesis

The extrascleral prosthesis is a porcelain hemisphere that is manufactured to fit over the surface of a phthitic or deformed eye. An eye is painted on the surface of the porcelain after it has been accurately fitted. These prostheses are rarely used in small animals but are more commonly fitted to horses.

1. Bedford, P. G. C.: Orbital Pneumatosis as an unusual complication to enucleation. J. Small Anim. Pract. *20*:551, 1979.
2. Bellhorn, R. W.: Enucleation technique. A lateral approach. J. Am. Anim. Hosp. Assoc. *8*:59, 1972.
3. Bryan, G. M.: Subconjunctival emphysema in a cat. Vet. Med./Sm. Anim. Clin. 72:1087, 1973.
4. Dixon, R. T., and Carter, J. D.: Canine orbital venography. J. Am. Vet. Rad. Soc. *13*:43, 1973.
5. Duke-Elder, S.: *System of Ophthalmology*, Vol. I: The Eye in Evolution. H. Kimpton, London, 1958.
6. Evans, H. E., and Christensen, G. C.: *Miller's Anatomy of the Dog*, 2nd ed. W. B. Saunders, Philadelphia, 1981.
7. Gelatt, K. N. (ed.): *Veterinary Ophthalmology*. Lea & Febiger, Philadelphia, 1981.
8. Harvey, C. E., Koch, S. A., and Rubin, L. F.: Orbital cyst with conjunctival fistula in a dog. J. Am. Vet. Med. Assoc. *153*:1432, 1968.
9. Koch, S. A.: Intraocular prosthesis in the dog and cat—the failures. J. Am. Vet. Med. Assoc. *179*:883, 1981.
10. Le Couteur, R. A., Scagliotti, R. H., Beck, K. A., and Holliday, T. A.: Indirect imaging of the canine optic nerve using metrizamide (optic thecography). J. Am. Vet. Med. Assoc. *43*:1424, 1982.
11. Martin, C. L.: Orbital mucocele in a dog. Vet. Med./Sm. Anim. Clin. 66:36, 1971.
12. Martin, C. L.: Orbital emphysema. Vet. Med./Sm. Anim. Clin. 66:986, 1971.
13. Munger, R. T., and Ackerman, N.: Retroorbital injections in the dog: a comparison of three techniques. J. Am. Anim. Hosp. Assoc. *14*:490, 1978.
14. Schmidt, G. M., and Betts, C. W.: Zygomatic salivary mucoceles in the dog. J. Am. Vet. Med. Assoc. *172*:940, 1978.
15. Slatter, D. H.: *Fundamentals of Veterinary Ophthalmology*. W. B. Saunders, Philadelphia, 1981.
16. Slatter, D. H., and Abdelbaki, Y.: Lateral orbitotomy by zygomatic arch resection in the dog. J. Am. Vet. Med. Assoc. *175*:1179, 1979.
17. Smith, J. S.: Diseases of the orbit. *In* Kirk, R. W. (ed.): *Current Veterinary Therapy VI*. W. B. Saunders, Philadelphia, 1977.
18. Ticer, J. W.: *Radiographic Technique in Small Animal Practice*. W. B. Saunders, Philadelphia, 1975.

Chapter **110**

Glaucoma

Charles L. Martin and William A. Vestre

INTRODUCTION

Glaucoma can occur in all domestic species, but it is an important therapeutic enigma in the dog because of its relatively high incidence in certain breeds (Table 110–1). Glaucoma is a sign, rather than a disease, as many diversified etiologies may result in the "final common pathway" leading to increased intraocular pressure (IOP). Owing to the variety of conditions that may precipitate glaucoma, particular emphasis is placed on a thorough examination of the normal as well as the affected eye for prognosis and

TABLE 110–1. Breed Predisposition and Types of Glaucoma

American cocker spaniel	Closed angle
Basset hound	Closed angle
Samoyed	Closed angle
Siberian husky	Closed angle
Norwegian elkhound	Closed and open angle
Brittany spaniel	Closed angle
Beagle	Open angle
Miniature toy poodle	Open and closed angle
Wire- and smooth-haired fox terrier	Lens displacement ± closed angle
Sealyham terrier	Lens displacement

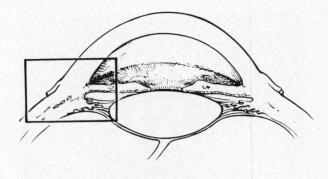

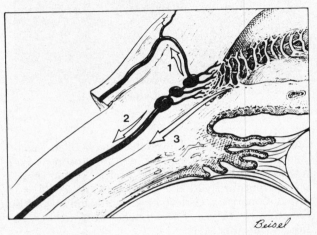

Figure 110–1. The routes of aqueous drainage from the canine iridocorneal angle. Aqueous taken up by the venous system in the angle may drain anteriorly to the episceral and conjunctival veins (1), posteriorly into the vortex venous system (2), or through the ciliary muscle interstitium to the suprachoroid and diffuse through the sclera (uveoscleral flow, 3).

therapy. Theoretically, therapy should be specific for the etiology.

Glaucoma may be defined as an elevation in intraocular pressure that results in impaired ocular function. Ocular hypertension is the presence of increased IOP without optic nerve changes or visual deficits. The latter condition poses a dilemma to the veterinary ophthalmologist as to whether therapy should be initiated. In man, up to 35 per cent of the optic nerve fibers are lost before visual field defects are present, 50 per cent of the fibers are lost before the milder visual field disturbances are detected, and 90 per cent of the fibers are lost in patients with severe glaucomatous field losses.[56,58] In view of the disparity between clinical detection of dysfunction and histopathological lesions, it is prudent to treat all animals with persistent ocular hypertension.

The reported upper limit of normal intraocular pressure is 27 to 30 mm Hg as measured with the Schiøtz tonometer and using the human conversion tables.[8,27,33] Peiffer and associates have calculated a Schiøtz tonometer conversion table for the dog that results in significantly higher IOP readings (i.e., the scale reading that converts to 24 mm Hg in the human table converts to 38 mm Hg in the dog table).[53] Thus, the two tables create confusion in interpreting the upper limits of normal IOP for the dog, and veterinarians should be aware of this. Furthermore, values from applanation tonometers in clinical use appear to agree more closely with those on the human calibration table. The IOP should not vary more than 5 mm Hg between eyes of the same dog.[33]

ANATOMY AND PHYSIOLOGY

Aqueous humor is produced continuously by the ciliary processes and leaves the eye mainly via the iridocorneal angle.[64] Alterations in production or outflow or both may be responsible for variations in intraocular pressure. Aqueous is produced by a combination of passive ultrafiltration, diffusion, and dialysis and active secretion. Secretion is usually given the dominant role (65 to 70 per cent), but Pederson and Green reported that only 35 per cent of the total amount of aqueous was formed by secretion.[51]

The ciliary body is divided into the anterior pars plicata (ciliary processes) and the posterior pars plana. Grossly, the ciliary processes are 60 to 70 triangular blades separated by deep valleys (Fig. 110–1). The zonules originate posteriorly in the pars plana and sweep forward, ensheathing the sides and ridge of the process to the tips before passing to their insertion on the lens equator.[47,66] In relation to external landmarks, the ciliary processes are 3 to 5 mm posterior to the limbus, depending on the region. The dorsal region has a wider scleral shelf at the limbus, placing the ciliary processes at a greater distance from the limbus.

Aqueous produced in the posterior chamber flows through the pupil and leaves mainly through the iridocorneal angle. The iridocorneal angle is that region where the base of the iris attaches to the peripheral cornea and sclera (Figs. 110–2 and 110–3; see Fig. 110–1). In viewing the angle from the anterior chamber, the main structure observed is the pectinate ligament, which originates from the anterior extremity of the iris base and inserts in the peripheral cornea. The pectinate ligament consists of numerous strands that may branch and interconnect but, in general, are single strands with relatively

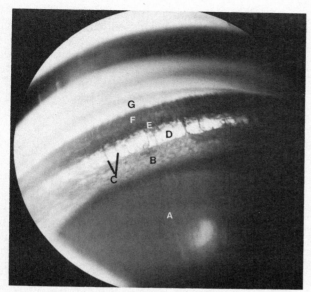

Figure 110–2. Goniophotograph of a normal dog. *A*, Pupil; *B*, iris; *C*, pectinate ligament strands; *D*, bluish-white zone of the uveal trabeculae; *E*, deep pigmented zone; *F*, superficial pigmented zone; *G*, cornea.

wide spaces between them. An accessory row of strands arises slightly deeper in the angle. Clinically, a bluish-white zone denotes the ciliary or uveal trabeculae that loosely fill the ciliary cleft between the base of the ciliary body and iris and the sclera (see Fig. 110–2). The degree of pigmentation in the angle varies in the same eye as well as between eyes. The pigmentation of the pectinate ligament is the same as that of the adjacent iris. The insertion of the pectinate ligament strands may have a dark, narrow zone of pigmentation (deep zone) that may continue

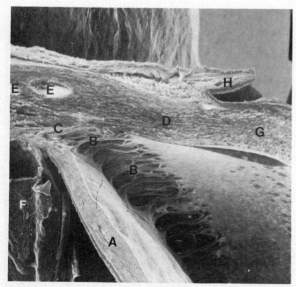

Figure 110–3. Combined frontal and sagittal scanning electron micrograph of the canine iridocorneal angle (× 32). *A*, Iris; *B*, primary row of pectinate ligament fibers; *C*, uveal trabeculae; *D*, limbus; *E*, scleral venous plexus; *F*, ciliary process; *G*, corner; *H*, conjunctiva.

obliquely and superficially to line the scleral shelf and may be visible as a grayer, wider zone of pigmentation that extends beyond the deep zone.[3,30,42,43,45,67]

In addition to the previously described angle structures, compact corneoscleral trabeculae (cribriform ligament)— meridional ciliary muscles that extend anteriorly to insert near the termination of Descemet's membrane—are found on sagittal section. Numerous small vascular channels, trabecular "veins," in the deep sclera drain aqueous from the corneoscleral trabeculae. They drain into larger collecting veins and then into the large channels of the scleral venous plexus in the midsclera. The scleral venous plexus consists of 2 to 4 interwoven large channels in the midsclera that communicate posteriorly with the vortex venous system and anteriorly with the episcleral and conjunctival veins (see Fig. 110–1).[42,43,67,69]

In addition to vascular uptake in the trabecular meshwork, aqueous drainage has been demonstrated in the dog via a posterior uveoscleral route.[12,18] The uveoscleral flow of aqueous is through the angle into the ciliary muscle interstitium to the suprachoroidal space, where aqueous is probably absorbed by choroidal vessels and orbital lymphatics (see Fig. 110–1).

CLINICAL SIGNS AND DIAGNOSTIC TECHNIQUES

The signs of glaucoma are pressure dependent and range from completely occult with elevated intraocular pressure only, to florid with all signs present. Intraocular pressure in the mid 40s to 50 mm Hg begins to produce typical external signs of vascular injection, pupillary dilation, and corneal edema.

Increased Intraocular Pressure

All signs of glaucoma are nonspecific for the presence of *active* glaucoma, so an objective measurement of intraocular pressure is necessary. Although objective measurement may not be necessary for the initial diagnosis, it is required when following the response to therapy in those cases that do not develop obvious hypotony.

Tonometry is the measurement of intraocular tension. Digital tonometry, using two fingers (not thumbs) to palpate the firmness of the eye through the closed upper lid, is a crude technique and differentiates only soft, medium, and hard eyes. The most practical instrument for tonometry in the dog is the Schiøtz tonometer, which measures the amount of corneal indentation that a plunger with a given weight produces. The higher the intraocular pressure, the less the indentation. The amount of indentation is measured on a scale that is usually converted to mm Hg on a table (Fig. 110–4). The tonometer must be vertical to avoid plunger friction, the plunger should be freely movable, and the instrument should be

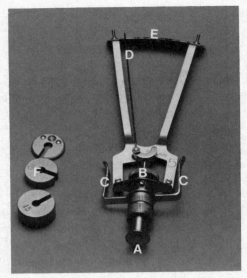

Figure 110–4. Schiøtz tonometer with additional weights. *A,* Footplate with protruding plunger; *B,* weight on proximal portion of plunger; *C,* tabs used to hold tonometer; *D,* pointer that plunger pushes, indicating scale reading; *E,* scale of tonometer (out of view); *F,* additional weights used on glaucomatous eyes.

near the central cornea to conform to the curved footplate. After applying a topical anesthetic, the entire weight of the instrument is rested on the globe for 1 to 2 seconds, and two to four readings are taken to determine consistency. The lids are held open by distant pressure near the orbital rim to avoid transferring pressure to the globe. Additional sources of error with Schiøtz tonometry are deviations in corneal curvature (buphthalmos or microphthalmos), corneal scars and irregularities, and severe corneal edema.

Dilated Pupil

In uncomplicated glaucoma without iris adhesions, the pupil dilates at about 45 to 50 mm Hg. Thus, mydriasis is neither a sensitive nor specific sign of glaucoma, although it is frequent. The pathogenesis of pupillary dilation with increased intraocular pressure is uncertain but is associated with sphincter ischemia as it correlates with diastolic blood pressure, above which there is a demonstrated lack of vascular perfusion of the iris.[9,62] Direct and consensual reflexes are absent, and miotics are ineffective until IOP is lowered.

Conjunctival Vascular Injection

Various degrees of conjunctival injection are present in most cases of canine glaucoma, depending on cause, chronicity, abruptness of onset, and degree of pressure elevation. Vascular injection occurs before pupil dilation and is similar to that seen in intraocular inflammation. Large conjunctival veins that bend near the limbus and drain the episcleral and scleral plexus are selectively injected. With acute high IOP, capillary engorgement as well as large vessel engorgement may be present. The presumed cause of the conjunctival injection is collapse of the posterior intrascleral veins in the thin equatorial sclera and increased venous drainage via the anterior routes (see Fig. 110–1).[37]

Corneal Pathology

Corneal opacification occurs with increased intraocular pressure by disruption of normal corneal lamellar arrangement resulting in light scattering and corneal edema.[74] Corneal edema may be mild or so severe as to make it difficult to evaluate intraocular structures. Although corneal edema is pressure dependent, considerable individual susceptibility exists. Chronic edema usually results in corneal vascularization. Epithelial edema combined with the cellular toxicity of topical anesthetics and perhaps mechanical trauma of tonometry or lagophthalmos may result in epithelial erosions and ulcer complications, i.e., iris prolapse. Severe edema may interfere with accurate tonometry by altering the corneal indentability (rigidity).

Marked stretching of the globe frequently results in breaks in Descemet's membrane (Descemet's streaks) that are permanent and specific for glaucoma. Descemet's streaks appear as curvilinear lines that may branch and can be localized with the slit lamp to the posterior cornea (Fig. 110–5).

Chronic corneal edema combined with lagophthalmos and decreased corneal sensation usually results in a degenerative pannus or a superficially scarred cornea. In those individuals or breeds with marked limbal pigmentation, the cornea may become com-

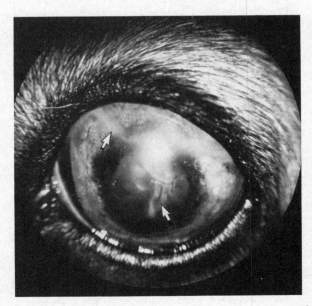

Figure 110–5. Breaks in Descemet's membrane *(arrows)* associated with glaucoma.

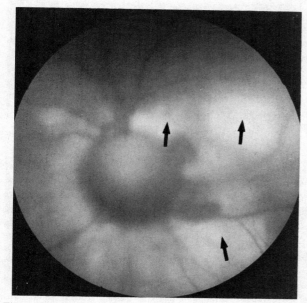

Figure 110–6. Optic nerve cupping, peripapillary hemorrhages, and retinal infarcts (*arrows*) in a Siberian husky with acute onset of high intraocular pressure.

pletely pigmented. Corneal scarring may significantly alter Schiøtz tonometer readings.

Fundus Abnormalities

The fundus may appear normal in acute, modest pressure elevations, but with higher pressure, retinal vascular attenuation, optic disc hemorrhages, and papilledema may be visible (Fig. 110–6). In chronic IOP elevations, peripapillary or diffuse hyperreflectivity of the tapetum and attenuation of the retinal

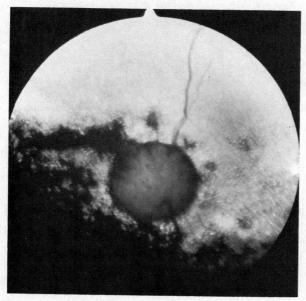

Figure 110–7. Optic disc atrophy with mild cupping, retinal vascular attenuation, loss of vessels, and diffuse tapetal hyperreflectivity from chronic glaucoma.

vessels may be seen. Various degrees of optic nerve atrophy with cupping, loss of myelin, and change in color to grayish-white are present in chronic cases (Fig. 110–7). Advanced changes may appear similar to those seen in progressive retinal atrophy, with attenuated retinal vessels, hyperreflectivity of the tapetum, and atrophy of the optic disc.[37] Glaucomatous posterior segment changes may be differentiated from progressive retinal atrophy by the lack of bilateral symmetry and the presence of optic disc cupping.

Ocular Pain

Most animals with primary glaucoma have epiphora but lack blepharospasm or ocular pain that is recognized by the owner. Once the intraocular pressure is reduced to normal, it is common for owners to comment on how playful the animal appears. Pain with glaucoma is usually manifested as sleepiness, depression, irritability, and reduced playfulness. The relief of ocular pain is one of the main goals in the therapy of chronic glaucoma. Pain should be considered present even if the owner is not aware of it.

Decreased Vision or Blindness

Increased IOP for two to four hours to a few days may cause loss of vision in acute high pressure glaucoma,[26,57,60] or an insidious loss may occur with modest elevations of IOP. One of the frustrations of treating glaucoma is late presentation for therapy of the involved eye. Client education and experience usually result in earlier presentation of the second eye with primary glaucoma.

There are two main theories of glaucoma-induced optic nerve and retinal damage: vascular and mechanical.[50] The vascular theory states that tissue damage results from ischemia when intraocular pressure interferes with tissue perfusion.[25] The retina can only sustain 100 minutes of complete anoxia before irreversible damage occurs.[26] The cat retina suffers complete ischemia at an IOP of 100 mm Hg.[78] In the mechanical theory, increased IOP causes the lamina cribrosa to bow outward, distorting and disregistering its pores or passages. The resulting distortion pinches the axon bundles, thus interfering with axoplasmic flow and causing axonal death.[15, 31, 57] Interference in axoplasmic flow has been demonstrated in beagles with glaucoma.[77] Both of these mechanisms are probably involved in the usual case of acute canine glaucoma with high intraocular pressure.

Buphthalmos

Enlargement of the globe is a typical and specific, but not a sensitive, sign of canine glaucoma. Once significantly stretched, the globe remains large even if IOP returns to normal. The young eye is most susceptible to stretching, and extreme buphthalmos may cause lagophthalmos and a grotesque appearance. In the buphthalmic eye, accurate Schiøtz tonometer readings may not be obtainable because the corneal curvature does not fit the tonometer footplate or because of corneal scarring and altered scleral rigidity.

Luxated Lenses

Various degrees of lens luxation are commonly associated with glaucoma, and it is often difficult to interpret their role in the pathogenesis. Buphthalmos frequently results in rupture of part of the zonular circumference with consequent subluxation that usually does not progress to complete luxation. The signs of subluxation are an aphakic crescent, iridodonesis, and alterations in depth of the anterior chamber (either deepening or local shallowing). How a subluxated lens induces glaucoma is unclear, and the usual theories of pupil block and angle closure are often questioned.

Lens luxation into the anterior chamber may precipitate glaucoma or may turn chronic glaucoma into an acute syndrome. Anterior lens luxation with a normal iridocorneal angle may not precipitate pressure elevations or may do so intermittently. The lens may be clear or cataractous. Anterior lens displacements are usually obvious but may be hidden by corneal edema. Posterior luxations may be overlooked if the pupil is not dilated or if the lens is transparent. A deep anterior chamber, iridodonesis, and vitreous herniation through the pupil indicate possible lens displacement.

Aqueous Flare

Increased aqueous protein and pigment clumps may be observed in many forms of glaucoma. Increased protein in the aqueous is caused by increased vascular permeability, e.g., with anterior uveitis. The protein content is often as high as 4.5 to 5.0 gm/dl, and it is suspected that the protein may precipitate pressure elevations by obstructing trabecular spaces.

CLASSIFICATION AND PATHOGENESIS OF GLAUCOMA (Table 110–2)

The classification of glaucoma in animals is similar to that in man, although species differences exist in the anatomy and physiology, e.g., signs and relative incidence of types.[75] Glaucoma is divided into two broad categories, primary and secondary, and these in turn are each subdivided according to the gonioscopic findings of an open, narrow, or closed angle.

Primary glaucoma is that not caused solely by acquired intraocular lesions. Primary glaucoma is potentially bilateral, although the onset is usually asynchronous (often by years), and a genetic inheri-

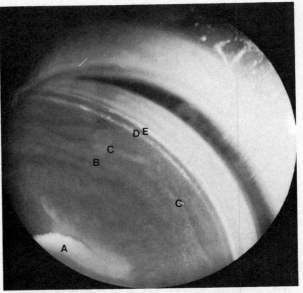

Figure 110–8. Goniophotograph of a basset hound's angle with severe goniodysgenesis. The opposite eye had glaucoma and a similar-appearing angle, but IOP in this eye was normal. Note the absence of an obvious pectinate ligament. *A*, Pupil; *B*, iris in a deep anterior chamber; *C*, major arterial circle of the iris; *D*, angle covered with lightly pigmented mesoderm; *E*, deep pigmented zone. The thin white zone with pigment streaks simulates a narrow angle with a short pectinate ligament at low magnification but with high magnification can be identified as a sheet continuous with the iris.

tance is suspected in most cases as reflected in the breed predisposition (see Table 110–1).[2,34,38] The definition of primary glaucoma is not clear-cut; detailed examinations reveal that in many instances of appar-

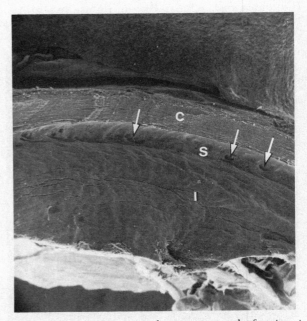

Figure 110–9. Frontal scanning electron micrograph of an American cocker spaniel with moderate goniodysgenesis (× 21). Arrows indicate holes in sheet that allows aqueous passage. *I*, Iris; *S*, sheet covering angle; *C*, cut cornea. (Reprinted with permission from Martin, C. L., and Wyman, M.: Primary glaucoma in the dog. Vet. Clin. North Am. 8:257, 1978.)

TABLE 110–2. Classification of Canine Glaucoma

I. Open angle glaucoma: Normal, wide angle on gonioscopy
   A. Primary: no observable predisposing factors, angle normal on gonioscopy, bilateral, breed predisposition (see Fig. 110–2)
   B. Secondary: normal angle obstructed by aqueous contents or elevated episcleral venous pressure interferes with aqueous drainage
      1. Inflammation—WBC and fibrin obstruct outflow
      2. Hyphema—erythrocytes and fibrin obstruct outflow
      3. Pigment—Deposition or proliferation obstructs outflow
      4. Lipids in anterior chamber obstruct outflow
      5. Anterior luxated lens—may obstruct angle or create pupil block
      6. Elevated episcleral venous pressure—arteriovenous fistula, orbital lesion, or increased blood pressure (rare)
II. Closed angle glaucoma: Angle is collapsed or covered with peripheral iris or connective tissue
   A. Primary
      1. Congenital: goniodysgenesis—maldeveloped angle covered with mesodermal tissue; usually bilateral; age of glaucoma onset varies (see Figs. 110–8 to 110–10)
      2. Acquired: closure associated with abnormal anterior chamber conformation
         a. Forward displacement of lens presumably due to slack zonules; creates a relative pupillary blockage from increased adhesive forces between lens and iris (see Fig. 110–11)
         b. Shallow anterior chamber with small anterior segment; pupillary block may occur that results in peripheral anterior synechia
         c. Plateau iris—iris plane is flat, but peripheral iris has a recess adjacent to angle, which is susceptible to angle closure with pupillary blockage
   B. Secondary closed angle: Acquired lesions precipitate closure of previously normal angle; also, angle conformations under II A. have an increased susceptibility to pupillary blockage
      1. Associated with pupillary block
         a. Intumescent lens
         b. Posterior synechia, iris bombé
         c. Subluxated lens, luxated lens
         d. Aphakic vitreous herniation
         e. Increased volume in vitreous compartment, i.e., accumulation of aqueous, swelling of vitreous
      2. No pupillary block
         a. Neoplasia with invasion of angle and/or pushing iris forward or thickening of iris
         b. Inflammation with peripheral anterior synechia
         c. Subluxated lens pushing iris base forward
         d. Epithelial downgrowth—perforating corneal wound with epithelium proliferating over angle

ent "secondary" glaucoma the acquired lesion may have been an initiating event in an eye predisposed by an abnormal angle or anterior chamber conformation. When two or more conditions produce ocular decompensation, it is difficult to determine the relative importance of each condition. The genetics of most types of glaucoma has proved elusive, possibly indicating the influence of environmental or compound factors.[1,35,79]

Congenital glaucoma is rare, and classification by age of onset overlaps other methods of classification, serving little purpose.

Most primary glaucoma in the dog is associated with bilateral closed angles even though it is seen initially as a unilateral glaucoma (Fig. 110–8).[4,21,34,48] The cause for closure cannot be determined in many cases, but it is present in the absence of inflammation, is often tolerated for years without decompensation, and can be seen at any age.[49] In many of these eyes, a severe form of goniodysgenesis or an arrest in angle development is present, but in aged dogs one may question the likelihood of a congenital lesion.[44] Closed angles in normotensive eyes have flow holes near their corneal insertion (Fig. 110–9).[46,49] These holes are presumably more prone to obstruction than the normal open space between the pectinate liga-

ment. If obstruction occurs suddenly, an acute syndrome may develop. If slowly progressive closure occurs, an insidious onset of glaucoma results. Acquired intraocular lesions may obstruct these pores and be misdiagnosed, or normal covert intraocular changes may precipitate obstruction, i.e., lens growth, pupil size, and endothelial proliferation. Obstruction of the sheet creates a pressure differential, pushing it outward to collapse the ciliary cleft and causing it to adhere to the inner sclera (Fig. 110–10). The latter finding is usually interpreted histopathologically as a peripheral anterior synechium.[34,48]

A closed angle is usually seen gonioscopically as a thin, lighter circumferential zone that may have some radial pigment streaks but no distinct pectinate ligament.[4,48,49] The latter appearance is often misinterpreted as a narrowed filtering cleft and is called a "narrow angle" (see Fig. 110–8).

Primary open angle glaucoma is rare in the dog but has been studied in detail in the beagle, in which it is a simple recessive trait.[19] Many beagles with open angle glaucoma later develop a closed angle, but this differs from the primary closed angle glaucoma in the sequence of events, i.e., in the latter instance closed angle is present prior to pressure elevation.[22,52]

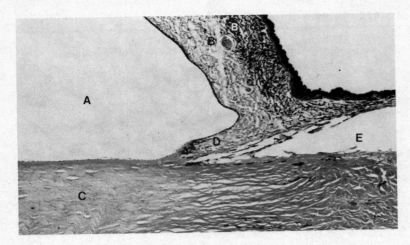

Figure 110–10. Sagittal histologic section of the angle of a basset hound with goniodysgenesis. The pressure in this eye was normal, but the opposite eye was glaucomatous. *A,* Anterior chamber; *B,* iris; *C,* cornea; *D,* mesodermal sheet covering the angle and pulling the iris base forward; *E,* ciliary cleft. If the sheet becomes occluded, obstructing aqueous flow, the sheet and iris base are pushed against the inner sclera, obliterating the ciliary cleft.

Secondary glaucoma is caused by acquired intraocular abnormalities and, depending on the etiology, may be unilateral or bilateral (Fig. 110–11). Secondary glaucoma is associated with acquired diseases that alter fluid dynamics at the pupil or angle and may vary from inflammation to neoplasia.[39]

EMERGENCY THERAPY

All recently functional eyes should be treated with emergency medical therapy to reduce intraocular pressure whether surgery is planned or not. A delay of several hours may be critical considering the high intraocular pressures that are often present. Surgical patients should have normal pressures, if possible, to minimize the internal shock to homeostasis that occurs when decompressing the eye from a high intraocular pressure to 0 mm Hg.

Systemic Therapy

The first line of emergency therapy is osmotic diuresis. The osmotic diuretics create a hyperosmolar vascular space, which withdraws extravascular fluid into the vessels. The ocular effect is to withdraw fluid from the vitreous as well as the aqueous.[63,73] Osmotic agents that remain in the vascular system without leaking into the eye produce a longer hypotony with less rebound of water into the eye. The effect is dose- and rate-dependent. Thirst is stimulated with the hyperosmotic blood; therefore, water should be restricted for two to three hours so that the drug effect is not neutralized. In addition to the ocular hypotonic effect, mannitol increases the ocular perfusion and retinal oxygen tension, benefiting the glaucomatous eye.[13]

Many agents, such as mannitol, glycerol, urea, sorbitol, lactate, ascorbate, ethyl alcohol, dextrose, sucrose, and isosorbide, have potential as osmotic agents, but in veterinary practice mannitol and glycerol are routinely used. Mannitol, 1 to 2 gm/kg, is given slowly intravenously for three to five minutes or by intravenous drip. The hypotensive effect occurs in about 15 to 30 minutes and usually lasts for four to six hours, although some eyes have low pressure for 48 hours after emergency therapy before the pressure rises again. Repeat injections of mannitol can be given, but dehydration of the patient may reach critical levels and the response to subsequent injections is greatly diminished after the second dose. Caution should be used in animals with cardiac disease, as the rapid infusion of mannitol may overload the circulatory system and create pulmonary edema.

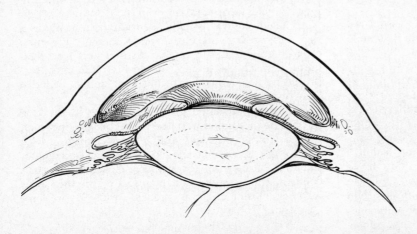

Figure 110–11. Anterior chamber conformation with forward displacement of the lens creating a convex iris plane. Conformation predisposes to pupillary blockage and secondary angle closure.

TABLE 110–3.   Carbonic Anhydrase Inhibitors for Glaucoma Therapy

Drug	Dose (mg/kg)	Frequency of Administration
Acetazolamide	10–30	b.i.d. to t.i.d.
Dichlorphenamide	2–4	b.i.d. to t.i.d.
Methazolamide	2–4	b.i.d. to t.i.d.

Orally administered glycerol (glycerin), although not as effective as mannitol, lowers the intraocular pressure within 15 to 30 minutes.[16] The dosage of 1 to 2 gm/kg orally may cause gastric irritation and vomiting, but it is nontoxic and does not induce the diuresis that mannitol does.

Carbonic anhydrase inhibitors (CAI) are the second type of drug used. The hypotensive effect of CAI is independent of the diuretic effect, as the ocular effect occurs in a nephrectomized patient and other potent non-CAI diuretics have minimal ocular effect.[14] Although the exact ocular mechanism is unknown, CAIs decrease aqueous secretion by about 40 to 50 per cent and have a minimal effect on the facility of outflow.[24, 36, 41] The intraocular pressure was decreased with a single administration of CAI by 24 per cent in normal and 29 per cent in glaucomatous beagles.[20] In general, the decrease in pressure begins within one hour and lasts for about eight hours, with minor variations with drug and dosage. An intravenous form of acetazolamide is available and may produce a recognizable reduction in pressure after ten minutes. Three CAI preparations are available, and the recommended dosages are given in Table 110–3. Acetazolamide is the best known and most available of the group. Side effects are similar with all the preparations, but individual tolerance to side effects and to individual products is quite variable. Some patients do not tolerate any of the products at therapeutic doses, but intolerance to one does not ensure intolerance to all. The primary side effects noted are panting, vomiting, anorexia, and acidosis.[23] Vestibular signs of nystagmus and circling have also been noted on several occasions.

Topical Therapy

Epinephrine decreases aqueous formation as well as increases the outflow facility.[28,65] Decreased aqueous formation with epinephrine is independent of the effect of the CAI decrease, and together they have an additive effect. As epinephrine dilates the pupil it may create or aggravate angle closure. The main indication for use of epinephrine is open angle glaucoma. Epinephrine is available as hydrochloride, borate, and bitartrate in concentrations of 0.5 to 2.0%. Dipivalyl epinephrine is available as a proform of epinephrine. The addition of two pivalyl groups makes epinephrine more lipophilic, and the resultant (eight to ten times) better corneal penetration allows lower drug concentrations to be used, avoiding many of the deleterious side effects. Once in the cornea and anterior chamber, hydrolysis of the pivalyl groups occurs.[40]

The use of miotics in emergency therapy should be restricted to direct-acting agents such as pilocarpine. The more potent cholinesterase inhibitors should be avoided because of their systemic toxicity if used frequently as well as their potentiation of bleeding and inflammation if surgery is performed.[24] The mydriasis of glaucoma is not overcome with miotics until the pressure is lowered.

Pilocarpine is available in concentrations of 0.25 to 10.0%, but 2.0% was the most efficient concentration in a study in beagles, with no additional benefits resulting from the higher concentrations.[76] Although minimal ocular effects are noted while the intraocular pressure is elevated, pilocarpine should be given to be present when the pressure is lowered. Administration at 30-minute intervals for two treatments and then at six-hour intervals should deliver adequate drug concentration without complicating systemic side effects. Some individuals are very sensitive to pilocarpine-induced ciliary spasms, and if a tolerance does not develop, therapy may have to be discontinued. Miotic therapy is contraindicated with secondary glaucomas due to inflammation.

Timolol maleate is a β-adrenergic blocker that decreases aqueous production up to 48 per cent in man and has little effect on the pupil.[10] Although laboratory evidence in the cat indicates some effect with the commercial concentrations of 0.25 and 0.5%, a significant lowering of pressure has not been noted clinically in veterinary ophthalmology, and timolol maleate is not routinely used.[32]

In summary, emergency medical therapy consists of an osmotic diuretic, a CAI (oral or IV), and topical pilocarpine. Once the intraocular pressure is lowered, maintenance therapy with a CAI and pilocarpine is continued to determine the chronic response to therapy. Most acute high pressure glaucomas are associated with closed angles or mechanical obstructive phenomena and respond poorly to chronic medical therapy. Persistence with medical therapy often simply prolongs the inevitable surgical procedure, and more ocular damage occurs owing to the erratic control. The owner should be warned of this initially, so that the decision for surgery can be made early in the course of therapy.

SURGICAL THERAPY

Before any surgical procedures are attempted on a glaucomatous eye, a thorough ophthalmic examination must be performed to determine the cause of the glaucoma and select the most rational therapy and prognosis. Retinal and optic nerve damage must be accurately defined, as the selection of therapy may depend on restoration of vision as opposed to cosmetic appearance and pain relief alone. If CAIs have been administered, blood gas determinations may be important, as acidosis may persist for up to 36 hours after their withdrawal.[23] Acid-base imbalances are corrected prior to induction of general anesthesia.

Surgical therapy is divided into those procedures that increase aqueous outflow, e.g., filtering procedures; those that decrease aqueous production, e.g., cyclocryotherapy[17]; and salvage procedures used to relieve pain and provide a cosmetically acceptable eye, e.g., intraocular prosthesis or induction of hypotony. The last-named procedures destroy the retina and are not acceptable for a potentially functional eye.

Various procedures increase the outflow of aqueous humor with success rates ranging from 30 to 50 per cent.[5, 17] Procedures designed to increase aqueous outflow include iridencleisis, corneoscleral trephination, cyclodialysis, sclerectomy, and anterior chamber implantation. Combinations of these procedures are often used, with the best success rates reported for corneoscleral trephination with peripheral iridectomy[5] and combined posterior sclerectomy-cyclodialysis-transscleral iridencleisis.[54]

Procedures That Increase Aqueous Outflow

Combined Sclerectomy-Cyclodialysis-Iridencleisis

The combination of sclerectomy, cyclodialysis, and iridencleisis creates a direct pathway from the anterior chamber into the subconjunctival space. The iris pillars are positioned through the scleral defect into the subconjunctival space to create a filtering wick.

Technique

The animal is positioned and prepared in a routine fashion for intraocular surgery. An 8-mm wide limbus-based conjunctival flap is prepared, including both conjunctival and Tenon's capsules. The flap is at least 10 mm long. The underlying sclera is bared (Fig. 110–12A–K), and a block of sclera 2 × 5 mm is outlined. The anterior border of this block is 3 to 5 mm posterior to the limbus (see Fig. 110–12D) and is incised until black uveal tissue is visible. Bleeding is usually profuse owing to the scleral venous plexus, and hemostasis is effected with low-temperature elec-

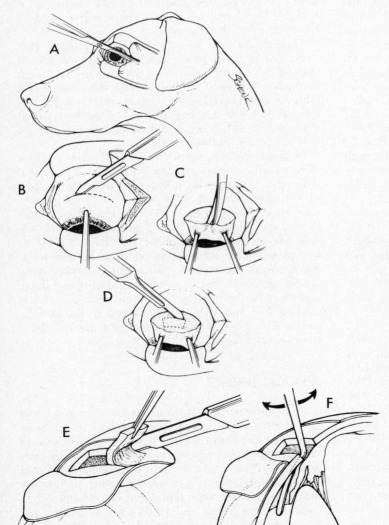

Figure 110–12. Procedure for combined cyclodialysis, sclerectomy, and iridencleisis. (Reprinted with permission from Peiffer, R. L., Gwin, R. M., Gelatt, K. N., and Schenk, M.: Combined posterior sclerectomy, cyclodialysis and trans-scleral iridencleisis in the management of primary glaucoma. Canine Pract. 4:54, 1977.)

Illustration continued on opposite page

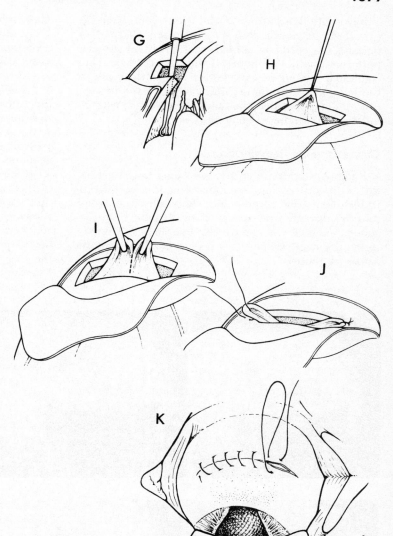

Figure 110–12 Continued

trocautery and dilute epinephrine. The scleral block is gently separated from the uveal tissue and removed (see Fig. 110–12C). A cyclodialysis spatula is inserted into the suprachoroidal space and passed into the anterior chamber, allowing aqueous to escape via the newly created stoma (see Fig. 110–12F). A broad cyclodialysis (separation of ciliary body from suprachoidal space) is performed by gently sweeping with the spatula. A blunt iris hook is passed through the cyclodialysis space into the anterior chamber, and the pupillary margin of the iris is hooked and the iris gently withdrawn (see Fig. 110–12G and H). The iris is grasped with fine forceps at the pupillary margin and torn to its base or split by electrocautery. Cautery minimizes hemorrhage, which can be extensive as the arterial circle of the iris is torn (see Fig. 110–12I). The iris pillars are retained in the scleral defect by a simple interrupted absorbable suture to the sclera (see Fig. 110–12J). Large fibrin and blood clots are removed from the anterior chamber by flushing

and forceps manipulation. To decrease hemorrhage and fibrin accumulation, the irrigating solution may include dilute epinephrine (1/10,000) and dilute heparin (1 to 2 I.U./ml of solution), respectively. If possible, the anterior chamber is reformed with air or a balanced salt solution. The conjunctiva is closed with a simple or continuous pattern of absorbable suture material, e.g., 6-0 Vicryl* (see Fig. 110–12K).

Postoperative therapy consists of topical antibiotic-corticosteroid drops and, if inflammation is severe, subconjunctival or systemic anti-inflammatory doses of corticosteroids. The pupil is maintained in a mid-dilated state by the use of topical pilocarpine and epinephrine. Anti-inflammatory medication is discontinued in one to two weeks. Intraocular pressure is measured at one, three, and eight weeks and then every three months after surgery. If IOP begins to rise, standard medical therapy for glaucoma is begun.

*Ethicon, Somerville, NJ.

Favorable long-term control (one year) can be expected in approximately 40 per cent of cases.[54] The prognosis is better in animals that have had surgery performed within 48 hours of the initial attack. This combined technique gave better results than any of the individual techniques and was applicable to narrow angle, closed angle, and, to a lesser extent, inflammation-induced glaucomas.

Corneoscleral Trephination

Bedford reported a 44 per cent long-term success rate with corneoscleral trephination and a peripheral iridectomy.[5] The corneoscleral hole allows aqueous to drain directly from the anterior chamber into the subconjunctival vasculature and lymphatics. The peripheral iridectomy prevents occlusion of the surgical fistula by the iris.

Technique

The animal is positioned and prepared in a routine fashion for intraocular surgery. A 6-mm wide limbus-based conjunctival and Tenon's capsule flap is dissected to bare the sclera. The flap is 10 mm long and is dissected forward to the limbus (Fig. 110–13A). Electrocautery is used for point hemostasis. The anterior edge of a trephine 2 mm or greater is placed at the scleral margin at the 12 o'clock position to prevent corneal and conjunctival flap damage. The trephine passes through the scleral shelf and underlying cornea to enter the anterior chamber anterior to the pectinate ligament insertion at the iris root (Fig. 110–13B). The trephine is tilted anteriorly, allowing part of the corneoscleral disc to remain attached and preventing loss into the anterior chamber. The initial outflow of aqueous usually pushes the disc outward where it can be grasped and re-

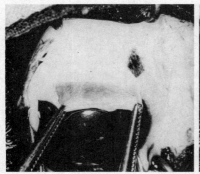
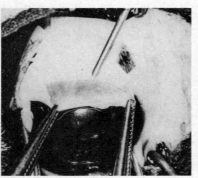
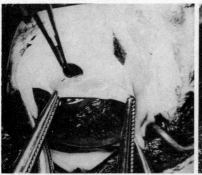
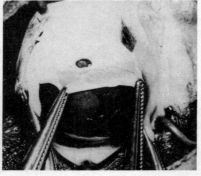
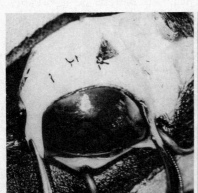
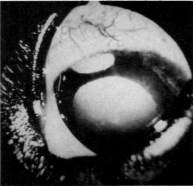

Figure 110–13. Procedure for corneoscleral trephination and peripheral iridectomy. (Reprinted with permission from Bedford, P. G.: The surgical treatment of canine glaucoma. J. Small Anim. Pract. *18*:713, 1977.)

moved. The adjacent peripheral iris usually bulges into the trephine hole and is further withdrawn for a peripheral iridectomy performed with scissors or electrocautery (Fig. 110–13C). The iris is repositioned into the anterior chamber. Minor hemorrhage may be controlled with 1:10,000 epinephrine. After fibrin and blood clots are removed by flushing or aspirating through the trephine hole, the anterior chamber is reformed with air or a balanced salt solution (Fig. 110–13D). The conjunctival flap is replaced and sutured with 6-0 absorbable suture material (Fig. 110–13E). Postoperative therapy is the same as for combined sclerectomy-cyclodialysis-iridencleisis. Postoperative complications leading to surgical failure include occlusion of the trephine hole by iris and fibrosis of the conjunctiva occluding the drainage site. A conjunctival bleb may not be present postoperatively and is not a criterion of success. A late complication is vitreous prolapse through the iridectomy leading to occlusion of the trephine hole.

The success rate for this procedure was about 40 to 50 percent, with the best results seen in those animals operated on before excessive adhesions had formed. This procedure is applicable to narrow angle, closed angle, and open angle glaucoma.

Other filtering procedures that have been advocated for canine glaucoma include combined sclerectomy with cyclodialysis and iridocyclectomy, iridectomy, cyclodialysis, and iridencleisis.

Additional procedures used in human glaucoma therapy to increase outflow, such as gonipuncture, goniotomy, and trabeculectomy, have not been critically evaluated in the dog.

Strips or tubes of silicone have been inserted into the anterior chamber to communicate with the subconjunctival spaces and have been somewhat successful in the dog.[55] After a limbal-based conjunctival flap is dissected, the implant is inserted into the anterior chamber through a small limbal stab incision and secured with sutures to the sclera to prevent migration. Topical anti-inflammatory drugs and antibiotics are administered postoperatively. Loss of function of the implant is due initially to obstruction of the tube by inflammatory debris or later to fibrosis of the filtering bleb. Implants with a valve mechanism to maintain pressure are available and deserve critical evaluation.

Luxated Lens Removal

The role of lens displacement and lens luxation in canine glaucoma is not totally understood. The presence of a luxated lens with glaucoma does not imply that the luxation was the cause of the glaucoma but does markedly complicate medical management. Removal of a luxated lens may simplify medical management if the drainage angle remains partially open. In some breeds in which primary lens luxation is suspected as a primary disease, e.g., wire-haired and smooth fox terriers and Sealyham terriers, removal of a luxated lens may control glaucoma without long-term medical management.

Anteriorly luxated lens in eyes that can see should be removed, as they may precipitate acute glaucoma and inflammation and may cause corneal endothelial damage. Anteriorly luxated lenses in chronically blind eyes with glaucoma pose a therapeutic dilemma. Removal of the lens in this case may not control the pressure, and a more pragmatic and less expensive mode of therapy is perhaps indicated (e.g., salvage surgical procedure). A posteriorly luxated lens with no pressure elevation is not usually removed. Lens extraction is covered elsewhere (Chapter 107), but several points are crucial in the removal of the anterior luxated lens. Preoperative treatment consists of medically controlling the IOP and constricting the pupil with the anteriorly luxated lens. In anticipation of vitreous loss, intravenous mannitol and complete muscle relaxation with pancuronium are valuable adjuncts. Prostaglandin inhibitors are routinely given prior to intraocular surgery. The pupil should be constricted with anterior lens luxation, as many of the lenses are quite mobile and may fall into the vitreous cavity if the patient is moved. If necessary, the lens may be fixed in place by small (25-gauge) hypodermic needles at right angles to each other placed through the limbus behind the lens.

Entrance into the eye can be via either a clear corneal incision or a limbal incision under a conjunctival flap. Removal of a luxated lens is intracapsular, usually with the aid of a cryoextractor to grasp the lens. Vitreous remains attached to the posterior lens and is gently teased away with a cyclodialysis spatula as the lens is elevated. Vitreous that remains herniated through the pupil is excised using scissors and cellulose sponges. All solid vitreous should be behind the pupil at the end of surgery. Postoperative management is similar to routine cataract extraction, but postoperative inflammation is usually much less than with extracapsular extraction. The IOP should be gently monitored in the immediate postoperative period as well as in the follow-up period of one to two years. Retinal detachments are relatively common after intracapsular extractions with vitreous loss.

Procedures that Decrease Aqueous Production

The second method of surgical management of glaucoma involves decreasing aqueous production by ciliary body destruction to the level at which the reduced outflow can keep IOP at the normal or subnormal range. Two methods for damaging the ciliary body are cyclodiathermy and cyclocryotherapy.

Cyclodiathermy is the application of intense heat within the ciliary body. A limbus-based conjunctival flap is prepared to expose the sclera. A diathermy needle is inserted 5 to 6 mm posterior to the limbus directly into the ciliary body at six to ten different sites. This technique causes necrosis of the sclera and severe postoperative inflammation, requiring intense postoperative therapy. Cyclodiathermy tends to be unpredictable and results in significant phthisis bulbi. The technique is not widely used.

In cyclocryotherapy, cold is used to destroy the ciliary epithelium and decrease aqueous production. Cyclocryotherapy has been used in glaucoma therapy in humans since 1950 and has proved highly effective in treating several forms of glaucoma. The treatment may have to be repeated at a later date if IOP begins to rise as the ciliary epithelium begins to regenerate. The technique is highly effective in canine glaucoma therapy, with success rates up to 90 per cent reported.[7]

The cryogen used for freezing the ciliary epithelium can be liquid nitrogen, carbon dioxide, or nitrous oxide. Nitrous oxide cryosurgical units are preferred because of ease of handling, reproducibility of results, ease of storage, and availability of the cryogen and a wide variety of instruments. A cryoprobe with a thermocouple incorporated to monitor tip temperature is preferred.

With a cryoprobe tip frozen to -60 to $-80°C$ applied to the surface of the globe, a predictable cooling curve is obtained (Fig. 110–14). The temperature decreases rapidly during the first minute, with only gradual cooling from one to three minutes of freezing. Freezing of the ciliary processes to $-10°C$ is reached in 135 seconds using a 2.5-mm diameter cryoprobe at -60 to $-80°C$ with nitrous oxide as the cryogen. With nitrous oxide as a cryogen, the ciliary body temperature does not reach the $-20°C$ previously thought necessary for destruction of cells. The ciliary epithelium appears to be sensitive to cold, and a temperature of $-10°C$ is adequate to cause hypotony in dogs.[70] A wide range of cryotherapy techniques produce the desired decrease in IOP.[71]

Cyclocryotherapy may be applied with the animal under heavy sedation, but general anesthesia is preferred for better manipulation of the globe. The eyelids are retracted with a speculum. A lateral canthotomy is required. The cryoprobe tip is placed firmly on the conjunctiva 5 mm posterior the limbus, and each site is frozen for two minutes (Fig. 110–15). The process is repeated at six to eight approximately equally spaced locations around the globe. In cats and in dogs with a small palpebral fissure, it is difficult to correctly place the cryoprobe over 360°. The freezing site under the third eyelid is the most difficult to expose without freezing excessive adjacent conjunctiva. This region is exposed by rolling the globe upward with forceps placed adjacent to the limbus near the freezing site, not by pulling on the third eyelid; this shortens the cul-de-sac and the probe cannot be positioned. Once freezing is begun, cryoadhesion allows easy manipulation of the globe. There is no advantage to specifically trying to overlap the freeze locations; in fact, the subsequent chemosis

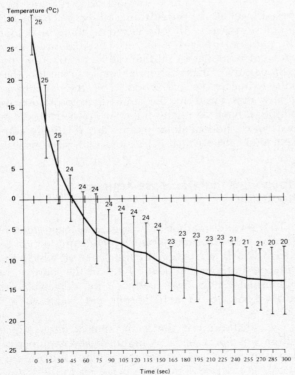

Figure 110–14. Typical cooling curve of average ciliary body temperature (°C ± 1 S. D.) for 25 eyes cannulated with a 24-gauge thermocouple and frozen using a 2.5-mm diameter cryoprobe tip with nitrous oxide as the cryogen. Numbers above each point indicate total number of eyes measured.

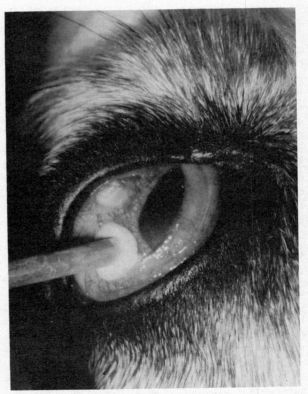

Figure 110–15. Cyclocryotherapy with formation of ice ball at cryoprobe tip placed 5 mm posterior to limbus. A previously frozen area is thawing, and the conjunctiva is chemotic and inflamed.

may make freezing at the earlier location slightly less effective. Repeat freeze-thaw cycles in a given location are no more effective than single freezes and result in more severe postoperative chemosis. Overzealous cryotherapy may result in phthisis bulbi.

After cryotherapy, marked conjunctivitis, chemosis, and uveitis occur. A subconjunctival injection of 1 mg dexamethasone is administered at the end of the cryotherapy and topical antibiotic-steroids are administered for 10 to 14 days. In functional and recently functional eyes, the IOP is monitored postoperatively, as one-fourth to one-third of eyes have a transient increase in IOP following cryotherapy. Objective measurements of IOP may be impossible for two to three days after freezing owing to excessive chemosis and edema of the eyelids. Thus, animals whose vision may return are maintained on their preoperative carbonic anhydrase inhibitors until pressures have returned to normal and are then challenged by withdrawal of the drug.

The patient is re-evaluated at two to three weeks and two months postoperatively and then at three-month intervals. The IOP may gradually increase as ciliary epithelium regenerates. If IOP increases, medical management may control the pressure or cyclocryotherapy may be repeated.

Cyclocryotherapy has advantages over filtering procedures because it is noninvasive, easily repeatable, less expensive, technically easier, and more successful.

Complications of cyclocryotherapy include phthisis bulbi, hyphema, and choroidal and retinal detachments. Owing to a high incidence of retinal detachments produced by cryotherapy in normal eyes, prophylactic cryotherapy on an eye with ocular hypertension but no clinical signs of glaucoma is not recommended.[71]

Cyclocryotherapy is useful for narrow, closed, and open angle glaucoma. Glaucoma secondary to uveal inflammation responds but with a lower success rate than primary glaucoma. The procedure was originally designed for pain relief in blind eyes but has been used on glaucomatous globes with preservation of vision in many.

Salvage Surgical Procedures for Glaucoma

Ocular Prosthesis[6,72]

Ocular evisceration and insertion of a prosthesis is indicated in chronically blind, painful eyes that do not have an ocular tumor, infection, or deep corneal ulcer. The preservation of a nearly normal eye is very desirable to most owners, who invariably elect the prosthesis over enucleation.

The prosthesis selected is 1 to 2 mm larger than the horizontal corneal diameter. If the globe is greatly enlarged, the contralateral normal eye is measured for the size of implant. Most canine eyes take a sphere of 17 to 22 mm in diameter.[6]

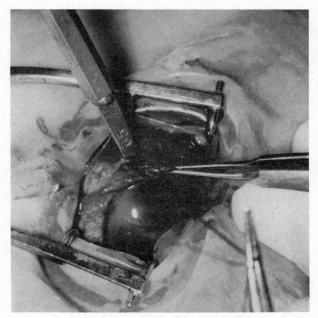

Figure 110–16. Evisceration of a globe prior to prosthesis implantation. A limbus-based conjunctival flap has been prepared, and the eye is stabilized with preplaced sutures. The globe is entered by a stab incision with a sharp blade.

A limbus-based conjunctival and Tenon's flap is made beginning 5 mm posterior to the limbus and extending approximately 150°. Two preplaced stay sutures are positioned in the sclera, 3 and 5 mm posterior to the limbus to retract the globe, and a stab incision 2 mm posterior to the limbus is made into the eye with a #11 Bard-Parker blade (Fig. 110–16). The incision is lengthened around the limbus for 150 to 160° with scissors. The iris root may be swept with a cyclodialysis spatula or the ciliary body simply

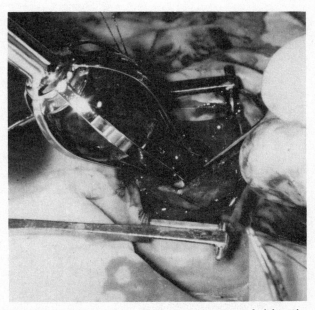

Figure 110–17. Introduction of sphere into eviscerated globe. The procedure is accompanied by marked hemorrhage.

grasped and removed with forceps. Hemorrhage is excessive and suction is useful to keep the field free of blood. The uvea, retina, lens, and vitreous are removed, leaving only the fibrous tunic. The corneal endothelium is protected during the intraocular manipulations. Once all intraocular contents are removed, the black sphere* is positioned with a sphere introducer (Fig. 110–17). The scleral incision is closed with either simple interrupted absorbable sutures, e.g., 5-0 Vicryl, or, if there is no tension on the incision, e.g., with a buphthalmic globe, by a continuous pattern. A small amount of air or balanced salt solution is injected between the implant and cornea. The conjunctiva is closed with a simple continuous suture. In buphthalmic eyes a temporary tarsorrhaphy may be performed to protect the cornea during postoperative swelling.

Postoperative complications include extrusion of the implant through a central corneal ulceration, recurrence of an unsuspected ocular tumor around the implant, and extrusion due to intraocular infection.[29] Despite the occasional failure, the prosthesis is a viable alternative to enucleation for the painful glaucomatous globe nonresponsive to less radical therapy.

Vitreal Injections

An inexpensive alternative to surgery in blind, painful glaucomatous eyes is intravitreal injection of gentamicin. Under narcoleptic sedation, .50 to 1.0 ml of vitreous is aspirated with a 22-gauge needle

---

*Jardon Plastic Research Corp., Southfield, MI.

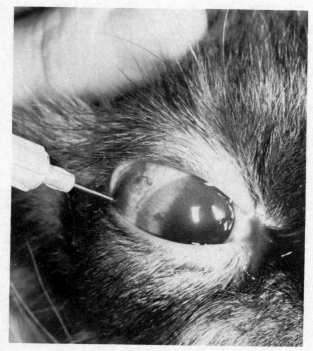

Figure 110–18. Site for vitreous aspiration and injection.

inserted through the pars plana (8 to 10 mm posterior to the limbus) in the dorsolateral quadrant (Fig. 110–18), and 25 mg of gentamicin* is injected. Gentamicin is toxic to the ciliary epithelium (and retina), and causes a marked reduction in aqueous production and hypotony. The technique is useful only as an inexpensive salvage procedure, as phthisis bulbi may occur.

Enucleation (see Chapter 109)

Although once considered standard surgical therapy for chronic canine glaucoma, enucleation is indicated mainly in glaucoma associated with an intraocular tumor, overwhelming infection, or a pragmatic owner. The low cost and high efficacy of cyclocryosurgery, intraocular implants, and vitreal injections make enucleation the last choice of all the surgical procedures available in treating canine glaucoma.

SUMMARY

Most cases of canine glaucoma cannot be controlled medically and require surgery. The type of surgical procedure selected depends on the equipment available, whether return of vision is a goal, the cause of glaucoma, and the surgeon's preference. Currently, cyclocryotherapy gives the most consistent response but is not without complications.

1. Alsbirk, P. H.: Anterior chamber depth and primary angle closure glaucoma II. A genetic study. Acta Ophthalmol. *53*:436, 1975.
2. Barnett, K. C.: Glaucoma in the dog. J. Small Anim. Pract. *11*:113, 1970.
3. Bedford, P. G.: Gonioscopy in the dog. J. Small Anim. Pract. *18*:615, 1977.
4. Bedford, P. G.: A gonioscopic study of the iridocorneal angle in the English and American breeds of Cocker Spaniel and the Basset Hound. J. Small Anim. Pract. *13*:631, 1977.
5. Bedford, P. G.: The surgical treatment of canine glaucoma. J. Small Anim. Pract. *18*:713,1977.
6. Brightman, A. H., Magrane, W. G., Huff, R. W., and Helper, L. C.: Intraocular prosthesis in the dog. J. Am. Anim. Hosp. Assoc. *13*:481, 1977.
7. Brightman, A. H., Vestre, W. A., Helper, L. C., and Tomes, J. E.: Cryosurgery for the treatment of canine glaucoma. J. Am. Anim. Hosp. Assoc. *18*:319, 1982.
8. Bryan, G.: Tonometry in the dog and cat. J. Small Anim. Pract. 6:117, 1965.
9. Charles, S. T., and Hamasaki, D. I.: The effect of intraocular pressure on the pupil size. Arch. Ophthalmol. *83*:729, 1970.
10. Coakes, R. L., and Brubaker, R. F.: The mechanism of timolol in lowering intraocular pressure. Arch. Ophthalmol. *96*:2045, 1978.
11. Cole, D. F.: Aqueous humour formation. Doc. Ophthalmol. *21*:116, 1966.
12. Cruise, L., and McClure, R.: Posterior pathway for aqueous humor drainage in the dog. Am. J. Vet. Res. *42*:992, 1981.
13. Ernest, J. T., Stern, W. H., and Trimble, J. L.: The effect of mannitol infusion on retinal function and oxygen tension. Invest. Ophthalmol. Vis. Sci. *16*:670, 1977.
14. Friedman, Z., Krupin, T., and Becker, B.: Ocular and systemic effects of acetazolamide in nephrectomized rabbits. Invest. Ophthalmol. Vis. Sci. *23*:209, 1982.

*Gentocin, Schering Corp., Kenilworth, NJ.

15. Gaasterland, D., Tanishima, T., and Kuwabara, T.: Axoplasmic flow during chronic experimental glaucoma. Invest. Ophthalmol. Vis. Sci. 17:838, 1978.

16. Galin, M. A., Davidson, R., and Schacter, N.: Ophthalmological use of osmotic therapy. Am. J. Ophthalmol. 62:629, 1966.

17. Gelatt, K. N.: The canine glaucomas. In Gelatt, K. N.(ed.): Veterinary Ophthalmology. Lea & Febiger, Philadelphia, 1981, pp. 390–434.

18. Gelatt, K. N., Glenwood, G., Williams, L. and Barrie, K.: Uveoscleral flow of aqueous humor in the normal dog. Am. J. Vet. Res. 40:845, 1979.

19. Gelatt, K. N., and Gum, G. G.: Inheritance of primary glaucoma in the Beagle. Am. J. Vet. Res. 42:1691, 1981.

20. Gelatt, K. N., Gum, G. G., Williams, L. W., et al.: Ocular hypotensive effects of carbonic anhydrase inhibitors in normotensive and glaucomatous Beagles. Am. J. Vet. Res. 40:334, 1979.

21. Gelatt, K. N., and Ladds, P. W.: Gonioscopy in dogs and cats with glaucoma and ocular tumors. J. Small Anim. Pract. 12:105, 1971.

22. Gelatt, K. N., Peiffer, R. L., Gwin, R. M., et al.: Clinical manifestations of inherited glaucoma in the Beagle. Invest. Ophthalmol. Vis. Sci. 16:1135, 1977.

23. Haskins, S. C., Munger, R. J., Helphrey, M. G., et al.: Effect of acetozolamide on blood acid-base and electrolyte values in dogs. J. Am. Vet. Med. Assoc. 179:792, 1981.

24. Havener, W.: Ocular Pharmacology, 4th ed. C. V. Mosby, St. Louis, 1978.

25. Hayreh, S. S.: Pathogenesis of cupping of the optic disc. Br. J. Ophthalmol. 58:863, 1974.

26. Hayreh, S. S., and Weingeist, T. A.: Experimental occlusion of the central artery of the retina IV: Retinal tolerance time to acute ischemia. Br. J. Ophthalmol. 64:818, 1980.

27. Heywood, R.: Intraocular pressures in the Beagle dog. J. Small Anim. Pract. 12:119, 1971.

28. Kaufman, P. L., and Barany, E. H.: Adrenergic drug effects on aqueous outflow facility following ciliary muscle retrodisplacement in the cynomolgus monkey. Invest. Ophthalmol. Vis. Sci. 20:644, 1981.

29. Koch, S. A.: Intraocular prosthesis in the dog and cat: The failures. J. Am. Vet. Med. Assoc. 179:883, 1981.

30. Lescure, F.: L'angle camerulaire du chien étude goniophotographique. Proc. World Vet. Congr. 17:1001, 1963.

31. Levy, N. S.: The effect of elevated intraocular pressure on axoplasmic transport in the optic nerve of the Rhesus monkey. Doc. Ophthalmol. 43:181, 1977.

32. Liu, H. K., and Chiou, C. Y.: Ocular hypotensive effects of timolol in cat eyes. Arch. Ophthalmol. 98:1467, 1980.

33. Lovekin, L.: Primary glaucoma in dogs. J. Am. Vet. Med. Assoc. 145:1081, 1964.

34. Lovekin, L., and Bellhorn, R. W.: Clincopathologic changes in primary glaucoma in the Cocker Spaniel. Am. J. Vet. Res. 29:379, 1968.

35. Lowe, R. F.: Primary angle-closure glaucoma inheritance and environment. Br. J. Ophthalmol. 56:13, 1972.

36. Macri, F. J., and Cevario, S. J.: A possible vascular mechanism for the inhibition of aqueous humor formation by ouabain and acetazolamide. Exp. Eye Res. 20:563, 1975.

37. Magrane, W. G.: Canine glaucoma. I. Method of diagnosis. J. Am. Vet. Med. Assoc. 131:311, 1957.

38. Magrane, W. G.: Canine glaucoma. II. Primary classification. J. Am. Vet. Med. Assoc. 131:372, 1957.

39. Magrane, W. G.: Canine glaucoma. III. Secondary classification. J. Am. Vet. Med. Assoc. 131:374, 1957.

40. Mandell, A. I., and Podos, S. M.: Dipivalylepinephrine (DPE): A new pro-drug in the treatment of glaucoma. In Leopold, I. H., and Burns, R. P. (eds.): Symposium on Ocular Therapy, Vol. 10. John Wiley & Sons, New York, 1977.

41. Maren, T. H.: The rates of movement on Na$^+$, Cl$^-$, and HCO$^-$ from plasma to posterior chamber: Effect of acetazolamide and relation to the treatment of glaucoma. Invest. Ophthalmol. Vis. Sci. 15:356, 1976.

42. Martin, C. L.: Biomicroscopic examination of the normal canine anterior segment. Master's Thesis, The Ohio State University, 1968.

43. Martin, C. L.: Gonioscopy and anatomical correlations of the drainage angle of the dog. J. Small Anim. Pract. 10:171, 1969.

44. Martin, C. L.: Development of pectinate ligament structure of the dog: Study by scanning electron microscopy. Am. J. Vet. Res. 35:1433, 1974.

45. Martin, C. L.: The normal canine iridocorneal angle as viewed with the scanning electron microscope. J. Am. Anim. Hosp. Assoc. 11:180, 1975.

46. Martin, C. L.: Scanning electron microscopic examination of selected canine iridocorneal angle abnormalities. J. Am. Anim. Hosp. Assoc. 11:301, 1975.

47. Martin, C. L., and Anderson, B. G.: Ocular anatomy. In Gelatt, K. N. (ed.): Veterinary Ophthalmology. Lea & Febiger, Philadelphia, 1981, pp.12–121.

48. Martin, C. L., and Wyman, M.: Glaucoma in the Basset Hound. J. Am. Vet. Med. Assoc. 53:1320, 1968.

49. Martin, C. L., and Wyman, M.: Primary glaucoma in the dog. Vet. Clin. North Am. 8:257, 1978.

50. Minckler, D. S., and Spaeth, G. L.: Optic nerve damage in glaucoma. Surv. Ophthalmol. 26:128, 1981.

51. Pederson, J. E., and Green, K.: Aqueous humor dynamics: Experimental studies. Exp. Eye Res. 15:277, 1973.

52. Peiffer, R. L., and Gelatt, K. N.: Aqueous humor outflow in Beagles with inherited glaucoma: Gross and light microscopic observations of the iridocorneal angle. Am. J. Vet. Res. 41:861, 1980.

53. Peiffer, R. L., Gelatt, K. N., Jessen, C. R., et al.: Calibration of the Schiotz tonometer for the normal canine eye. Am. J. Vet. Res. 38:1881, 1977.

54. Peiffer, R. L., Gwin, R. M., Gelatt, K. N., and Schenek, M.: Combined posterior sclerectomy, cyclodialysis and transscleral iridencleisis in the management of primary glaucoma. Can. Pract. 4:54, 1977.

55. Pritchard, D. L., and Hamlet, M. P.: A silastic-dacron implant for the treatment of glaucoma. Vet. Med. Sm./Anim. Clin. 65:1191, 1970.

56. Quigley, H. A.: Glaucoma's optic nerve damage: Changing clinical perspectives. Ann. Ophthalmol. 14:611, 1982.

57. Quigley, H. A., and Addicks, E. M.: Chronic experimental glaucoma in primates. II. Effect of extended intraocular pressure elevation on optic nerve head and axonal transport. Invest. Ophthalmol. Vis. Sci. 19:137, 1980.

58. Quigley, H. A., Addicks, E. M., and Green, W. R.: Optic nerve damage in human glaucoma. III. Quantitative correlation of nerve fiber loss and visual field defect in glaucoma, ischemic neuropathy, papilledema, and toxic neuropathy. Arch. Ophthalmol. 100:135, 1982.

59. Quigley, H. A., Flower, R. W., Addicks, E. M., and McLeod, D. S.: The mechanism of optic nerve damage in experimental acute intraocular pressure elevation. Invest. Ophthalmol. Vis. Sci. 19:505, 1980.

60. Radius, R. L., and Anderson, D. F.: Reversibility of optic nerve damage in primate eyes subjected to intraocular pressure above systolic blood pressure. Br. J. Ophthalmol. 65:661, 1981.

61. Rutkowski, P. C., and Thompson, H. S.: Mydriasis and increased intraocular pressure. I. Pupillographic studies. Arch. Ophthalmol. 87:21, 1972.

62. Rutkowski, P. C., and Thompson, H. S.: Mydriasis and increased intraocular pressure, II. Iris fluorescein studies. Arch. Ophthalmol. 87:25, 1972.

63. Robbins, R., and Galin, M. A.: Effect of osmotic agents on the vitreous body. Arch. Ophthalmol. 82:694, 1969.

64. Sears, M. L.: The aqueous. In Moses, R. A. (ed.): Adler's Physiology of the Eye, 7th ed. C. V. Mosby, St. Louis, 1981, pp. 204–226.

65. Townsend, D. J. and Brubaker, R. F.: Immediate effect of epinephrine on aqueous formation in the normal human eye as measured by fluorophotometry. Invest. Ophthalmol. Vis. Sci. 19:256, 1980.

66. Troncoso, M. U.: Microanatomy of the eye with the slitlamp microscope. II. Comparative anatomy of the ciliary body, zonula and related structures in mammallia. Am. J. Ophthalmol. 25:1, 1942.
67. Troncoso, M. U.: The intrascleral vascular plexus and its relations to the aqueous outflow. Am. J. Ophthalmol. 25:1153, 1942.
68. Troncoso, M. U., and Castroveijo, R.: Microanatomy of the eye with the slitlamp microscope. I. Comparative anatomy of the angle of the anterior chamber in living and sectioned eyes of mammalia. Am. J. Ophthalmol. 19:481, 1936.
69. VanBuskirk, M. E.: The canine eye: The vessels of aqueous drainage. Invest. Ophthalmol. Vis. Sci. 18:223, 1979.
70. Vestre, W. A., and Brightman, A. H.: Ciliary body temperatures during cyclocryotherapy in the clinically normal dog. Am. J. Vet. Res. 44:135, 1983.
71. Vestre, W. A., and Brightman, A. H.: The effects of cyclocryotherapy on the clinically normal canine eye. Am. J. Vet. Res. 44:187, 1983.
72. Vestre, W. A., Brightman, A. H., and Helper, L. C.: Use of an intraocular prosthesis in the cat. Fel. Pract. 8:23, 1978.
73. Vucicevic, Z. M., Tark, E., and Ahmad, S.: Echographic studies of osmotic agents. Ann. Ophthalmol. 11:1331, 1979.
74. Waltman, S. R.: The cornea. In Moses, R. A. (ed.): Adler's Physiology of the Eye, 7th ed., C. V. Mosby, St. Louis, 1981, pp. 38–62.
75. Watson, P.: Comparative aspects of glaucoma. J. Small Anim. Pract. 11:129, 1970.
76. Whitley, R. D., Gelatt, K. N., and Gum, G. G.: Dose response of topical pilocarpine in the normotensive and glaucomatous Beagle. Am. J. Vet. Res. 41:417, 1980.
77. Williams, L. W., Gelatt, K. N., Gum, D. A., et al.: Orthograde rapid axoplasmic transport and ultrastructural changes of the optic nerve of normotensive, acute ocular hypertensives and glaucomatous Beagles. Proc. Am. Coll. Vet. Ophthalmol. 11:172, 1980.
78. Wündsch L.: Experimentall-kritische Studie zum Problem der retinalen Ischämie. Albrecht von Graefes Arch. Klin. Ophthalmol. 197:241, 1975.
79. Wyman, M., and Ketring, K.: Congenital glaucoma in the Basset Hound: A biologic model. Trans. Am. Acad. Ophthalmol. Otolaryngol. 81:645, 1976.

Chapter **111**

Ocular Emergencies and Trauma

Steven I. Bistner

EVALUATION OF THE TRAUMATIZED EYE

Ocular emergencies include the following: corneal abrasion or chemical irritation; lid laceration; corneal foreign body; acute infectious keratitis; corneal or scleral laceration; contusion and penetrating intraocular injury; proptosis of the globe; endophalmitis; and acute glaucoma. When an animal is presented with an ocular emergency, the following procedures should be performed to obtain a diagnosis and institute effective therapy:

1. Obtain an adequate history from the owner. This may reveal previous ocular disease, the instillation of some chemical irritant, or trauma. Determine when the injury occurred and if any medication or eye wash has been used.

2. Examine the eye for any discharge, blepharospasm, or photophobia. Note the type of any discharge present. If the animal is in extreme discomfort and the eye is completely closed, *do not* try to force open the lids. This may extrude intraocular contents if a corneal laceration is present. If a severe corneal ulcer, laceration, or penetrating wound is present, the animal should be anesthetized and preparations made for surgery prior to examination.

3. Note the position of the globe within the orbit and the presence of exophthalmos or proptosis. If the eye is exophthalmic, there is frequently strabismus and protrusion of the third eyelid, exposure keratitis, and, in cases of retrobulbar or zygomatic salivary gland inflammation, pain on opening the mouth. Note any displacement of the globe medially or temporally.

4. Note any swelling, contusions, or lacerations of the lids and whether the lids cover the cornea. Determine the depth of any lid lacerations. Penetrating lid lacerations may be associated with secondary injury to the globe.

5. Palpate the orbital margins for fractures, crepitus, air, and cellulitis.

6. Examine the conjunctiva for hemorrhage, chemosis, lacerations, or foreign bodies and the superior and inferior conjunctival cul-de-sacs for foreign bodies. With the animal under topical anesthesia, a sterile cotton swab can be used to "sweep" the conjunctival fornix free of foreign bodies. Elevate the third eyelid with small, fine-toothed forceps and examine its bulbar aspect for foreign bodies.

7. Examine the cornea for opacities, ulcers, foreign bodies, abrasions, or lacerations. A loupe and a good focal source of illumination are important in this examination. A Finoff transilluminator with halogen illumination (3.5 volt) is an excellent source of focal illumination.

8. Record pupil size; shape; and response to light, both direct and consensual; and the presence of anisocoria.

9. Examine the anterior chamber and note its depth and the presence of hyphema, iridodonesis, or iridodialysis.

10. If indicated and if the cornea is undamaged, measure intraocular pressure.

11. Dilate the eye with 1% tropicamide drops and examine the fundus with a direct or indirect ophthalmoscope, noting intraocular or retinal hemorrhage, edema, or retinal detachment.

OCULAR EMERGENCIES

Differential Diagnoses

Acute Vision Loss

Sudden loss of vision or marked visual impairment may involve one or both eyes. The following differential diagnoses should be considered:

1. Massive vitreous or retinal hemorrhage from any cause (no pain).
2. Bilateral optic neuritis or retrobulbar optic neuritis (painful).
3. Retinal detachment (no pain).
4. Severe anterior and/or posterior uveitis (painful).
5. Severe keratitis with blepharospasm (painful).
6. Acute congestive glaucoma (painful).

Asymmetry of Pupils

Pupillary asymmetry may be caused by any of the following:

1. Traumatic uveitis with miosis of the pupil.
2. Horner's syndrome—miosis of the ipsilateral side.
3. Intraorbital trauma to ciliary nerves or ganglia—mydriasis.
4. Optic neuritis or optic nerve avulsion—mydriasis with acute vision loss.
5. Iridodialysis and rupture of iris sphincter—mydriasis.
6. Unilateral use of topical mydriatic or miotic drugs.
7. Diffuse central neurological disease—increased CSF pressure.

Chemical Burns

Chemical irritation of the eye may result from accidental contact with a noxious agent, such as a cleaning solution containing soap or lye (sodium hydroxide), or from intentional discharge of chemical agents, such as mace, lye, or other noxious gases, into the face of an animal.

Immediate first aid is aimed at removing the offending chemical from the eye with irrigation using large amounts of water or saline. Particles of solid material that adhere to the cornea or remain in the conjunctival cul-de-sacs are removed.

In general, acidic compounds are less dangerous than lye compounds.[20] Acidic compounds denature surface proteins and stop their penetration, whereas basic compounds destroy protein and penetrate deeper ocular structures.[29]

Highes' classification[29] of chemical ocular irritation indicates the extent of ocular injury following chemical irritation:

1. Mild
   a. Erosion of corneal epithelium
   b. Faint haziness of cornea
   c. No ischemic necrosis of conjunctiva and sclera
2. Moderately severe
   a. Corneal opacity blurs iris details
   b. Minimal ischemic necrosis of conjunctiva and sclera
3. Very severe
   a. Blurring of pupillary outline
   b. Blanching of conjunctiva and sclera

With mild chemical irritation, epithelial tags and remnants are carefully removed using a fine cotton swab, with the animal under topical anesthesia. The pupil is dilated with atropine and, if necessary, 10% phenylephrine. A synergistic affect is obtained when indirect-acting atropine and the direct-acting phenylephrine are combined. Infection, especially with gram-negative organisms, may be prevented by the topical application of gentamicin ointment five times daily.

The animal should be prevented from rubbing the eye by placing a collar or bucket over the head. If pain is severe, hospitalization and the systemic administration of pethidine (Demerol), 3 to 6 mg/kg every six to eight hours, may be indicated. Once reepithelialization has taken place and if interstitial keratitis, vascularization, or granulation tissue remain, topical corticosteroids such as 0.1% dexamethasone can be used topically.

If there is stromal necrosis of the cornea in moderately severe anterior ocular segment injury, additional steps may be necessary. Antiprotease agents,[6] such as acetylcysteine 10%, may be administered, using two drops five to seven times daily topically. Thin conjunctival flaps in combination with topical acetylcysteine 10%, antibiotics, and atropine aid in controlling secondary uveitis.

Lid Injuries

Lid contusions and lacerations are most commonly associated with bite wounds or vehicular trauma. Surgical treatment of lid lacerations is similar to that of other areas of the body, except that very careful primary repair must be undertaken to ensure adequate physiological and cosmetic results. An accurate understanding of lid anatomy is necessary before attempting lid surgery (see Chapter 101).

The lids are a two-layered structure; the anterior layer is composed of skin and orbicularis muscle, and the posterior layer is composed of tarsal glands, connective tissue, and conjunctiva. Meticulous repair

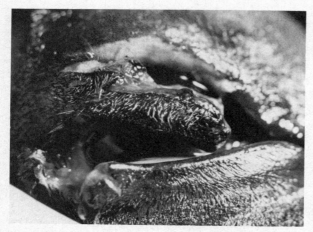

Figure 111–1. Severe lacerations of the lid with avulsion of the lid from the lateral canthus. Very careful debridement, cleansing, and re-apposition of lid was required using a two-layered closure.

of lid lacerations is important if good cosmetic and physiological results are to be obtained. The age and type of injury are important considerations. Lacerations of the lid margin *without* lid avulsion that are presented 24 to 48 hours after injury and are grossly contaminated should not be immediately operated on but rather carefully cleaned, the eye evaluated for further injury, the lids treated with topical antibiotics, and any systemic infections controlled. The animal can undergo careful surgical repair to the lid in five to seven days.

When the lid is torn away from its lateral or medial attachments, blood supply to the lid may be compromised and atrophy of the damaged piece of lid may occur (Fig. 111–1). Although avulsions may be grossly contaminated and 24 to 48 hours old, they should be carefully cleaned, minimally debrided, and resutured in an attempt to restore adequate circulation.

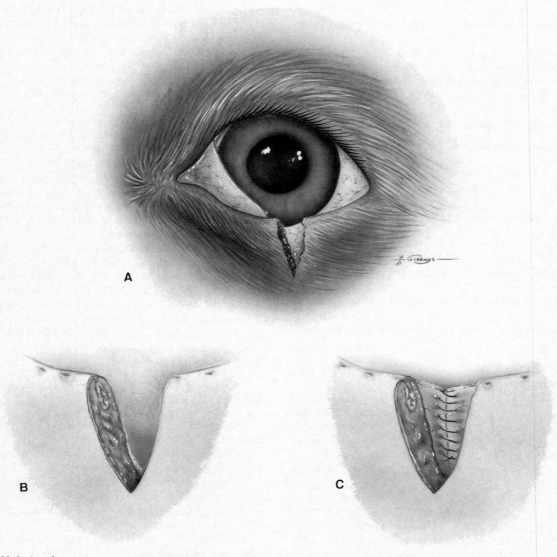

Figure 111–2. Simple two-layer repair. *A,* Initial injury before debridement. *B,* Wound after debridement and ready for suturing. *C,* The conjunctiva is sutured with 6-0 Vicryl in a simple, continuous pattern.

Illustration continued on opposite page.

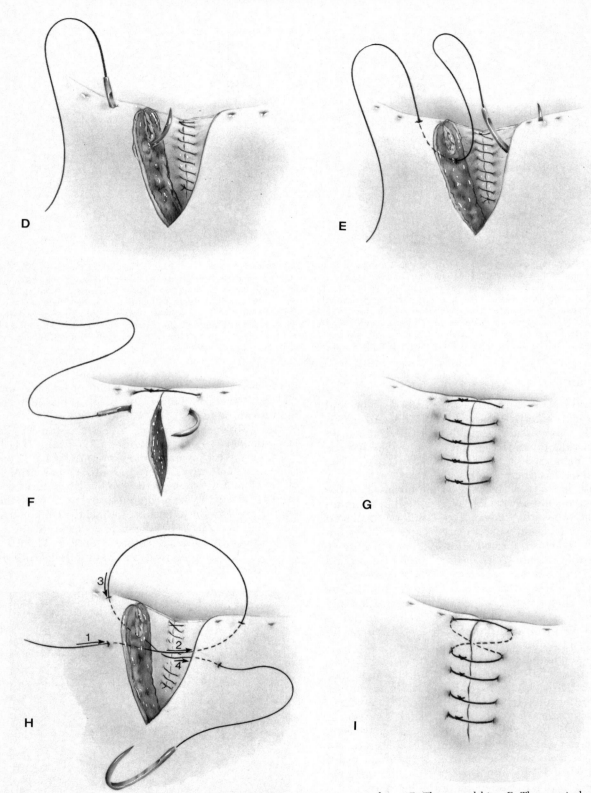

Figure 111–2 Continued. D, The marginal suture is placed first, in two separate bites. *E*, The second bite. *F*, The marginal suture is carefully tied to ensure apposition of the margins. The knot lies along the margin. The wound is sutured with simple interrupted suture of 6-0 silk, 2 mm apart. The first suture beneath the margin relieves tension on the marginal suture. *G*, The wound sutured. *H*, A figure-eight suture pattern may be used in place of the first two sutures. *I*, The wound sutured using a figure-eight technique. (Reprinted with permission from Slatter, D. H.: *Fundamentals of Veterinary Ophthalmology.* W. B. Saunders, Philadelphia, 1981.)

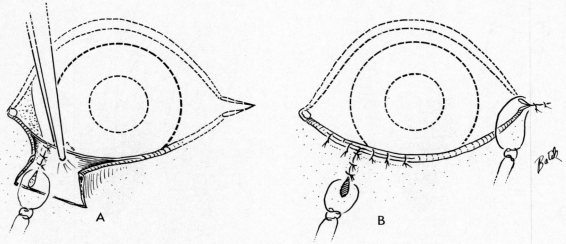

Figure 111–3. Marginal lid wound repair by lid splitting and conjunctival resection. *A*, The lower lid in the area of the lower punctum has been split into skin-orbicularis muscle and conjunctiva. The punctum is not incised. The tumor-containing portions of the epidermal and conjunctival tissues have been removed as wedge resections. The edges of the skin-orbicularis portion are undermined. If mobilization of the skin is difficult, a lateral canthotomy should be performed. The conjunctiva is closed with 6–0 chromic gut tied, with the knots lying between the conjunctiva and the skin. *B*, The undermined skin-orbicularis area is closed with simple interrupted 6–0 silk sutures. The lateral canthotomy permits the lid to be moved nasally to facilitate closure. The split lid margin is closed with 6–0 silk sutures, with the knots tied on the outside of the lid margin. Sutures are removed in 10 to 14 days. (Reprinted with permission from Bistner, S. I., Aguirre, G., and Batik, G.: *Atlas of Veterinary Ophthalmic Surgery.* W. B. Saunders, Philadelphia, 1977.)

Treatment

The lid laceration is lavaged with sterile saline and any foreign material removed aseptically. All hair is carefully clipped and irrigated from the wound, and a 1% povidone iodine solution is applied around the wound margins but not in the wound itself. The surgical field is draped aseptically.

A full thickness lid wound laceration involves the conjunctiva, muscle-fascial layer, and skin. A minimum of two suture layers gives well-approximated lid closure. Ragged wound margins are trimmed and necrotic tissue is debrided. However, *as much tissue as possible should be saved* to minimize wound contracture and lid deformity. When correcting a ragged lid margin, the tarsus is trimmed in a slightly curved fashion, permitting slight overcorrection and "pouting" of the suture incision when the lid is sutured vertically. This helps to ensure tight lid closure and reduces scarring.[14]

The conjunctiva is closed with interrupted absorbable sutures (5/0 to 7/0) of collagen, chromic gut, polyglycolic or polyglactic acid. All knots are buried beneath the conjunctiva to prevent corneal abrasion. The lid margins must be made parallel. The skin is closed with nylon, silk, polyglycolic or polyglactic acid, and small sutures (5/0 to 7/0) are used. An everting effect should be achieved at the skin closure line. It is especially important to close the marginal lid defect to prevent notching of the lid margin.

Closure of lid margin defects not involving more than one-fourth to one-third of the lid margin can usually be accomplished without placing abnormal tension on the lid margin. If more than one-fourth of the lid margin has been lost, blepharoplasty must be performed to close the defect while preserving normal lid structure. Numerous blepharoplastic techniques can be used.[4, 14, 15, 20, 27, 28]

The two-layer technique to close extensive lid lacerations is shown in Figures 111–2 and 111–3. Splitting the lid separates the skin-muscle layer from the tarsoconjunctival layer, permitting mobilization of the skin. Interrupted 6-0 chromic gut sutures are used to close the tarsoconjunctival layer, with the knots buried on the anterior surface of the conjunctiva (see Fig. 111–2D). The skin-muscle layer is closed with interrupted 6-0 silk sutures (see Fig. 111–2 F–I). Thus, the conjunctival and skin-muscle sutures are in two different planes.

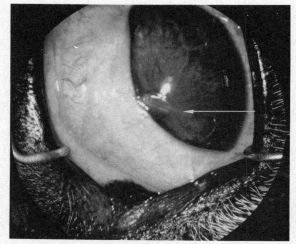

Figure 111–4. Corneal foreign body. A grass awn, partially hidden by the prolapsed third eyelid, is embedded in the corneal stroma. Note the miotic pupil resulting from secondary uveitis.

Lacerations of the lids near the medial canthus can present difficult problems if a canalicular laceration is also present. For repair of canalicular defects, see Chapter 103.

Corneal Foreign Bodies

Foreign bodies are frequently seen in dogs and occasionally in cats. In working dogs, awns, grass seeds, and oat hulls may enter the anterior segment of the eye and become embedded in the conjunctival fornices or cornea (Figs. 111–4 and 111–5). Blepharospasm, photophobia, pain, keratitis, and secondary uveitis may develop. The foreign body may penetrate the corneal stroma and enter the anterior chamber.

Paint chips frequently fall on the canine cornea when the dog is in the area while the owner is removing paint from a wall. Animals are presented with an active keratitis caused by this foreign body.

In all cases of corneal foreign bodies, removal of the foreign body is the most effective treatment. Removal usually has to be done with the animal under topical or general anesthesia. If a foreign body is embedded in the cornea, the epithelium may have to be carefully incised to remove it. Following removal, the active keratitis is treated with topical antibiotics and atropine, and interstitial keratitis and granulation tissue are controlled with topical corticosteroids, e.g., 0.1% dexamethasone ointment or drops.

Acute Infectious Keratitis

Infectious keratitis is an ocular emergency because of the rapidity with which certain forms of infection spread, destroy the corneal stroma, and result in corneal perforation, endophthalmitis, and loss of the affected eye.

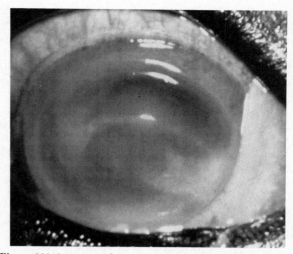

Figure 111–6. Acute infectious keratitis with rapid development of corneal edema, corneal stromal cellular infiltrates, mucopurulent stromal necrosis, and secondary anterior uveitis with possible hypopyon formation. The infectious organism was a *Pseudomonas* spp.

Clinical Diagnosis

The following signs may be significant in considering whether an active keratitis is associated with microbial infection: (1) rapidly developing keratitis in a previously normal eye (signs appear and within 24 to 48 hours become much more severe); (2) loss of corneal epithelium accompanied by stromal cellular infiltrates and stromal edema; (3) mucopurulent stromal necrosis; and (4) secondary anterior uveitis with possible hypopyon (Figs. 111–6 and 111–7).

Confirmation of Infectious Keratitis

Corneal and conjunctival cultures are easy to perform and can quickly confirm a diagnosis of infectious keratitis. The following materials are needed to perform a corneal or conjunctival culture: (1) sterile

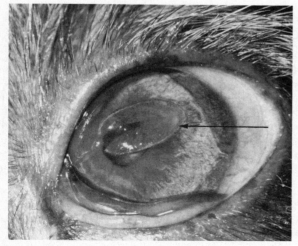

Figure 111–5. An oat hull (arrow) is attached to the cornea and must be surgically removed.

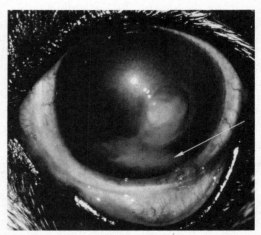

Figure 111–7. Intrastromal corneal abscess in a Boston terrier. There is secondary uveitis with hypopyon formation (*arrow*). Care must be practiced in handling these dogs, as the stromal abscesses are often very deep and descemetoceles are present (see management of complicated corneal stromal loss).

cotton-tipped applicators or calcium alginate swabs; (2) bacterial culture media including blood agar plate, thioglycollate broth, and Sabouraud dextrose agar plates; (3) Kimura platinum spatula or other spatula that can be sterilized in the heat of an open flame; (4) alcohol lamp; (5) glass slides with etched ends; (6) Gram's stain; and (7) Giemsa stain.

To obtain viable corneal cultures, a wet swab should be used. Topical anesthetics should not be placed in the eye prior to culturing, because anesthetics contain antiseptics that may alter bacterial growth. A sterile swab is moistened in thioglycollate broth, the excess fluid is wiped off, and the moistened swab is gently wiped over the cornea. The swab is immediately plated onto culture media.

Corneal scrapings are made with the Kimura platinum spatula. A topical anesthetic, e.g., 0.5% proparacaine hydrochloride,* is used on the cornea. The glass slides are dipped in 95% methanol and wiped clean, and the margins and base of the ulcer are carefully scraped. Mucus or mucopurulent discharge should be disregarded; corneal cellular infiltrate is spread onto the surface of two slides. The slides are stained with Gram's and Giemsa stains. New methylene blue stain can be used for immediate evaluation of cytological detail.

Treatment

The initial selection of antibiotics is based on the results of Gram staining. Until culture results prove otherwise, it can generally be assumed that gram-positive infections are caused by penicillin-resistant *Staphylococcus* spp. and gram-negative rod infections are caused by *Pseudomonas* spp.

The treatment for gram-positive infections includes subconjunctival therapy with methicillin, 100 mg/0.5 ml, and gentamicin, 20 mg; topical treatment with a concentrated solution of gentamicin and cefazolin if it can be applied frequently (requires hospitalization) or gentamicin ointment; and, in severe cases, systemic therapy with intravenous methicillin or ampicillin.

Infection with gram-negative rods can be treated subconjunctivally with gentamicin, 20 mg, and carbenicillin, 125 mg/0.5 ml; topically with fortified gentamicin drops or gentamicin ointment; and, in severe cases, systemically with gentamicin, 2 mg/kg every eight hours.

Pseudomonas Infections

Keratitis produced by *Pseudomonas aeruginosa* is a rapidly spreading and destructive corneal disease. In *Pseudomonas*-induced keratitis, the cornea becomes very edematous and necrotic and there is frequently an associated uveitis with hypopyon (see Fig. 111–6). *Pseudomonas* produces proteolytic enzymes[6,18,19] and additionally may stimulate collag-

enase production,[3,6] which causes the rapid spread of infection and the destruction of corneal stroma with perforation.

The drug of choice for *Pseudomonas* infections is gentamicin. Additionally, tobramycin, polymyxin B, and colistin have been effective in treating *Pseudomonas* ulcers.

Additionally, disodium EDTA* is used to inhibit the proteoglycan enzyme produced by *Pseudomonas*. A solution is made by adding 0.4 ml of EDTA (150 mg/ml) to a 15-ml bottle of Adapt† drops. Two drops are administered five times daily.

Additional Treatment

Additional treatment measures include the following:

1. The animal is hospitalized whenever possible to provide intensive treatment.

2. Pain associated with secondary uveal inflammation is controlled with a mydriatic-cycloplegic agent such as atropine (1 to 4%).

3. If the cornea appears very soft, collagenase may be present and an antiprotease agent such as 10% acetylcysteine drops‡ may be used (two drops every two hours for the first 24 to 48 hours).

4. Careful cleaning to remove necrotic corneal tissue may be helpful. A sterile swab and a small amount of 2% iodine solution may be used to remove necrotic tissue. The eye is washed carefully with a sterile collyrium.§

5. Self-mutilation is prevented by placing collars around the neck or buckets over the head of the animal.

6. Pain is relieved with systemic agents. ||

7. When extensive loss of corneal stroma may result in imminent perforation, a conjunctival or nictitating membrane flap may be surgically placed over the cornea. In severe corneal infections I prefer not to cover the cornea; however, good results have been obtained with covered corneas and the previously mentioned treatment measures.

Corneal Lacerations (Tables 111–1 to 111–3)

Corneal lacerations may be penetrating or perforating (passing through the cornea). Perforating corneal lacerations may cause prolapse of intraocular contents. Frequently, pieces of uveal tissue or fibrin effectively but temporarily seal the wound and permit the anterior chamber to re-form. Manipulation of these wounds should be avoided until the animal has been anesthetized. Care is used in anesthetizing an

---

*Ophthaine, E. R. Squibb & Sons Inc., Princeton, NJ.

*Endrate, Abbott Laboratories, North Chicago, IL.
†Burton, Parsons & Co., Inc., Washington, DC.
‡Mucomyst, Mead Johnson Pharmaceutical Division, Evansville, IN.
§Dacriose, CooperVision Pharmaceuticals, Inc., San German, PR.
|| Demerol, Winthrop Laboratories, New York, NY.

TABLE 111–1.   Preparation of Fortified Antibiotic Eye Drops*

Penicillin G
1. Remove 5 ml "tears" from 15-ml tear substitute squeeze bottle.
2. Add 5 ml "tears" to 1 vial penicillin G (5 million units).
3. Replace 5 ml reconstituted penicillin into tear squeeze bottle (10 ml + 5 ml = 15 ml).
4. Final concentration of penicillin = 333,000 U/ml.

Oxacillin
1. Remove 7 ml "tears" from a 15-ml tear substitute squeeze bottle.
2. Add 7 ml "tears" to ampoule oxacillin (1 gm).
3. Replace 7.2 ml reconstituted oxacillin into tear squeeze bottle (8 ml + 7.2 ml = 15.2 ml).
4. Final concentration of oxacillin = 66 mg/ml.

Carbenicillin
1. Reconstitute 1 vial carbenicillin (1 gm) with 9.5 ml sterile water.
2. Add 1.0 ml reconstituted carbenicillin into 16-ml tear substitute squeeze bottle (15 ml + 1 ml = 16 ml).
3. Final concentration of carbenicillin = 6.2 mg/ml.

Ticarcillin
1. Reconstitute 1 vial ticarcillin (1 gm) with 10 ml sterile water.
2. Add 1.0 ml reconstituted ticarcillin into 15-ml tear substitute squeeze bottle.
3. Final concentration of ticarcillin = 6.3 mg/ml.

Cephaloridine
1. Remove 2 ml "tears" from a 15-ml tear substitute squeeze bottle and discard.
2. Add 2 ml sterile saline to 1 ampoule cephaloridine (500 mg).
3. Replace 2.4 ml reconstituted cephaloridine into tear squeeze bottle (13 ml + 2.4 ml = 15.4 ml).
4. Final concentration of cephaloridine = 32 mg/ml.

Cefazolin
1. Remove 2 ml "tears" from a 15-ml tear substitute squeeze bottle and discard.
2. Add 2 ml sterile saline to 1 ampoule cefazolin (500 mg).
3. Replace 2.2 ml reconstituted cefazolin into tear squeeze bottle (13 ml + 2.2 ml = 15.2 ml).
4. Final concentration of cefazolin = 33 mg/ml.

Vancomyin
1. Remove 9 ml "tears" from a 15-ml tear substitute squeeze bottle and discard.
2. Add 10 ml sterile water to 1 vial vancomycin (500 mg).
3. Replace 10.2 ml reconstituted vancomycin into tear substitute squeeze bottle.
4. Final concentration of vancomycin = 31 mg/ml.

Gentamicin
1. Add 2.0 ml parenteral gentamicin to the 5-ml dropper bottle of commercial ophthalmic gentamicin.
2. Final concentration of gentamicin = 14 mg/ml.

Tobramycin
1. Remove 2 ml "tears" from a 15-ml tear substitute squeeze bottle and discard.
2. Add 2 ml parenteral tobramycin (80 mg) to tear substitute squeeze bottle (13 ml + 2 ml = 15 ml).
3. Final concentration of tobramycin = 5 mg/ml.

Amikacin
1. Remove 2 ml "tears" from a 15-ml tear substitute squeeze bottle and discard.
2. Add 2 ml parenteral amikacin (100 mg) to tear substitute squeeze bottle (13 ml + 2 ml = 15 ml).
3. Final concentration of amikacin = 6.7 mg/ml.

Bacitracin
1. Remove 9 ml "tears" from a 15-ml tear substitute squeeze bottle.
2. Add 3 ml "tears" to each of 3 commercial vials of bacitracin (50,000 U each).
3. Replace 9.6 ml reconstituted bacitracin into tear squeeze bottle (9.6 ml + 6 ml = 15.6 ml).
4. Final concentration of bacitracin = 9600 U/ml.

Neomycin
1. Remove 2 ml "tears" from a 15-ml tear substitute squeeze bottle.
2. Add 2 ml "tears" to 1 vial neomycin (500 mg).
3. Replace 2 ml reconstituted neomycin into tear squeeze bottle (13 ml + 2 ml = 15 ml).
4. Final concentration of neomycin = 33 mg/ml.

*Adapted from Baum, I.: Antibiotic use in ophthalmology. *In* Duane, T.D. (ed.): *Clinical Ophthalmology*, Vol. 4. Harper and Row, Hagerstown, 1980, Chapter 26.

TABLE 111–2.   Preparation of Antibiotics for Subconjunctival Injection*

Process	Ampi-cillin	Baci-tracin	Carbe-nicillin	Cepha-loridin	Colistin†	Genta-micin	Methi-cillin	Neo-mycin	Peni-cillin G	Vanco-mycin
Amount in commercially prepared vial	1000 mg	50,000 U	1000 mg	500 mg	150 mg	80 mg/ 2.0 ml	1000 mg	500 mg	5.0 megaU	500 mg
Number of vials needed	1	1	1	1	1	1	1	1	1	1
Diluent volume to be added to the vial	5.0 ml	2.5 ml	5.0 ml	2.5 ml	2.0 ml		5.0 ml	1.0 ml	2.5 ml	5.0 ml
Volume to remove for injection	0.5 ml	0.5 ml	0.5 ml	0.5 ml	0.3 ml	0.5 ml	0.5 ml	0.5 ml	0.5 ml	0.25 ml
Antibiotic dose in injection volume	100 mg	10,000 U	100 mg	100 mg	25 mg	20 mg	100 mg	250 mg	1.0 megaU	25 mg

*Adapted from Jones, D. B.: Initial therapy of suspected microbial corneal ulcers II. Specific antibiotic therapy based on corneal smears. Surv. Ophthalmol. *24:97*, 1980.

†Sodium colistimethate, Coly-Mycin, parenteral, Parke-Davis, Morris Plains, NJ.

**TABLE 111–3. Subconjunctival Antibiotic
Dosages for Treatment of Keratitis***

Antibiotic	Dosage
Ampicillin	50 to 250 mg
Bacitracin	10,000 U
Carbenicillin	100 mg
Cephaloridine	100 mg
Cephalothin	100 mg
Chloramphenicol, sodium succinate suspension	50 to 100 mg
Colistin	15 to 30 mg
Erythromycin (lactobionate or gluceptate)	50 to 100 mg
Gentamicin	10 to 20 mg
Kanamycin	10 to 20 mg
Lincomycin	50 to 150 mg
Methicillin	100 to 200 mg
Neomycin	100 to 500 mg
Penicillin G	300,000 to 1,000,000 U
Polymyxin B	10 mg
Streptomycin	50 to 100 mg
Tobramycin	40 mg
Vancomycin	25 mg

*Reprinted with permission from Bistner, S.I.: Clinical diagnosis and treatment of infectious keratitis. Comp. Cont. Ed. 3:1056, 1981.

animal with a corneal laceration, because struggling or excitement during administration of anesthetic may result in loss of the temporary seal in the corneal laceration and extrusion of intraocular contents. In addition, an intraocular foreign body may be present concurrently with a perforating corneal laceration. The globe should be examined carefully and radiographs of the globe and orbit taken if necessary.

Complicated Corneal Lacerations

This refers to corneal injuries accompanied by one or a combination of the following: iris prolapse, hyphema, cataract formation, luxation of the lens, or loss of vitreous (Figs. 111–8 and 111–9).

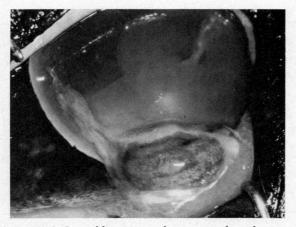

Figure 111–8. Corneal laceration with incarcerated uveal tissue in the wound and severe secondary uveitis (see management of complicated corneal lacerations).

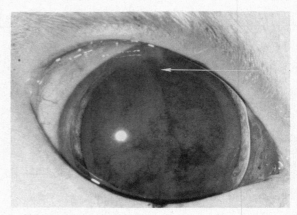

Figure 111–9. Corneal laceration (*arrow*) in a cat caused by a cat's claw. Note that the aqueous is plasmoid and that hyphema is present. Immediate treatment for traumatic uveitis is indicated, and the corneal laceration must be sutured. The pupil is widely dilated because the cat had already been given topical atropine as part of the uveitis treatment.

If examination of the eye reveals a damaged lens with rupture of the anterior lens capsule, extraction of the lens via an extracapsular approach may be indicated. If the corneal wound is small, the wound is first closed and a limbal or corneal section made to extract the lens. I have found damage to the lens to be a frequent problem with cat claw injuries to the eyes of dogs or cats. The claws are long and penetrate the cornea and anterior chamber, lacerating the anterior lens capsule. The lens becomes intumescent (swollen), and cataractous changes occur. The anterior chamber narrows as the lens swells. These lenses have been removed by phacofragmentation and suction as well as with a standard planned extracapsular approach following repair of the corneal laceration. If the lens is not removed, phacolytic uveitis and secondary glaucoma will develop.

Incarceration or prolapse of uveal tissue in corneal wounds presents a difficult surgical problem. The tendency for iris prolapse depends on the size of the wound. If the wound is small and there is a small iris prolapse of short duration, it may be repositioned with an iris spatula. The spatula is introduced into the anterior chamber through the corneal wound to sweep free possible anterior synechiae. If hyphema is present, the anterior chamber is irrigated with BSS* and the blood clots are removed. The wound is closed with 7-0 or 8-0 silk, nylon, or 7-0 collagen sutures, and the anterior chamber is re-formed (Fig. 111–10). Mydriatics are used postoperatively to correct the associated traumatic uveitis and to prevent anterior synechia formation if the wound is in the central cornea.

If at the time of surgical repair the surgeon cannot effectively replace prolapsed iris or if the iris is excessively contaminated and necrotic, it should be excised.

The uveal tissue can be trimmed from the corneal

---

*Balanced Salt Solution, Alcon Laboratories, Fort Worth, TX.

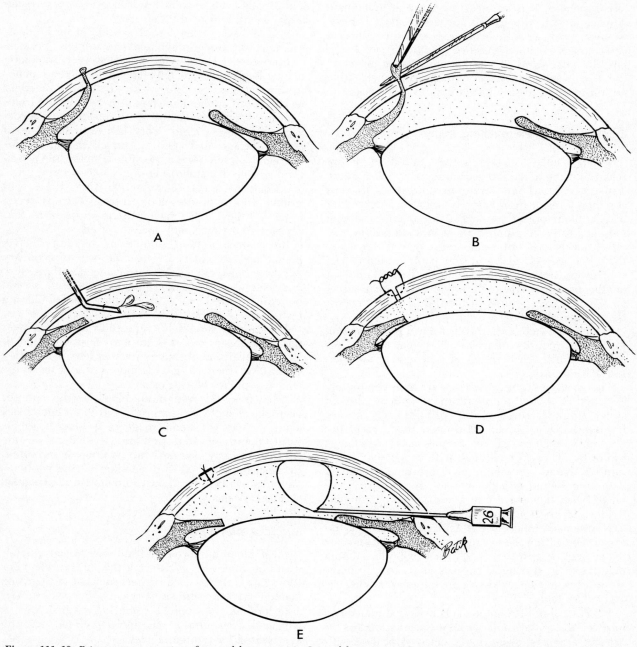

Figure 111–10. Primary reconstruction of corneal laceration. *A,* Corneal laceration with incarcerated iris and secondary hyphema and uveitis. *B,* Incarcerated viable iris should be repositioned whenever possible. The corneal wound may have to be enlarged to replace the iris with either a cyclodialysis spatula or an iris spatula. If extensive anterior synechiae have already occurred, incarcerated iris may be removed using an electroscalpel or scissors. *C,* If possible, the iris is swept free from its adhesion to the cornea with an anterior chamber irrigating needle or iris spatula. If the lens capsule appears ruptured or the lens dislocated, a limbal incision is made and the lens extracted. *D,* In repairing corneal wounds, a 4.5-mm atraumatic needle is used if adequate magnification is available. I prefer 8–0 silk or nylon or 7–0 collagen. The sutures are placed in the deeper two-thirds of the cornea to ensure coaptation of Descemet's membrane and to prevent posterior gaping of the wound. If possible, the needle bite is approximately 1 mm on either side of the wound margin. *E,* Once the anterior chamber has been closed, it is reformed with balanced salt solution via a limbal injection using a 26-gauge needle. (Reprinted with permission from Bistner, S. I., Aguirre, G., and Batik, G.: *Atlas of Veterinary Ophthalmic Surgery.* W. B. Saunders, Philadelphia, 1977.)

wound using an electroscalpel or scissors and the wound swept with a blunt cyclodialysis spatula to free additional adhesions. An electroscalpel is preferred, as it minimizes the profuse hemorrhage that accompanies iridectomies in domestic animals. The

corneal wound is then repaired as previously described.

When a corneal laceration is presented with prolapse of the iris, lens, vitreous, and ciliary processes, a decision must be made whether, under these circumstances, it is better to perform an immediate enucleation. If the eye is very soft and there is extensive damage, enucleation is the procedure of choice once the animal has been medically stabilized. On the other hand, if there is any chance of saving the eye, repair can be attempted and enucleation performed if necessary in ten days to two weeks.

Contusion and Penetrating Injury

Severe ocular contusions are caused by injury resulting from a sudden acceleration or deceleration imparted by a blunt force. In animals contusions commonly result from being hit by a car, kicked, hit with a blunt object, or kicked by a larger animal, e.g., a horse. A number of factors determine the effect of this form of trauma on the eye: (1) impact of the force on the globe at the point of injury, (2) contrecoup impact in direct line with the force but on the opposite side of the globe, and (3) indirect force when the globe is pushed or "hurled" against the orbital contents.[8, 15, 20, 24, 30]

Ocular damage can result from disturbance of functional integrity of tissues; vascular damage resulting in either hemorrhage or ischemia; or mechanical tearing of tissue.

The orbits of dogs and cats are not completely enclosed in bone; therefore these animals do not suffer from fractures of the orbital floor, as are frequently seen in man. However, fractures of the zygomatic arch or maxillary, frontal, or lacrimal bones can occur. Therefore, animals with concussive ocular injuries should be radiographed to evaluate damage. Attention should also be paid to the maxillary and mandibular bones for any evidence of mandibular fracture or luxation of the temporomandibular joint.

Hyphema is blood in the anterior chamber of the eye. Blood within the eye may come from the anterior uveal tract or posterior uveal tract or both. Trauma may result in tearing of the iris at its root (iridodialysis), permitting excessive bleeding from the iris and ciliary body.

Usually, simple hyphema resolves spontaneously in seven to ten days and does not cause vision loss.[7, 21] Loss of vision following hyphema is associated with secondary ocular injuries, including glaucoma, traumatic iritis, cataract, retinal detachment, endophthalmitis, and corneal scarring.

Severe trauma to the globe or a direct blow to the head can result in retinal or vitreous hemorrhage, with a distinctive ophthalmoscopic appearance.[27] Retinal and vitreous hemorrhage associated with trauma usually resorbs spontaneously over a two- to three-week period.[24] Unfortunately, vitreous hemorrhage can produce vitreous traction bands as it organizes, eventually producing retinal detachment. Extensive retinal hemorrhage may be associated with scarring and glial proliferation as the blood resorbs. Expulsive choroidal hemorrhage can occur at the time of injury

and usually leads to retinal detachment, severe visual impairment, and total vision loss.

Several basic principles are significant in the management of traumatic hyphemas in animals. Because of the vascular anatomy of the uveal tract, traumatic uveitis is also present following concussive or penetrating intraocular injury with hyphema. Bleeding usually stops spontaneously unless a traumatic iridodialysis or retinal detachment and posterior choroidal rupture have occurred. Very little can be done to control intraocular bleeding. Animals should be confined and kept as quiet as possible. Rebleeding within the first five days following injury may occur.

Secondary uveal inflammation should be controlled. Topical prednisolone acetate 1% drops, seven to nine times daily, and atropine drops 1 to 2%, three to four times daily, may be used.

Intraocular pressure should be monitored. Hyphema and secondary uveitis can lead to secondary pupillary block or angle closure glaucoma. If pressure increases, an oral carbonic anhydrase inhibitor should be administered, e.g., dichlorphenamide 125 mg t.i.d. for a 15-kg dog.

The animal should be repeatedly observed over the initial five to ten days during resorption of blood. If intraocular complications such as lens subluxation or luxation occur, surgery is indicated to remove the lens if pupillary block exists.

After five to seven days, blood in the anterior chamber changes from a bright red to a bluish-black color ("eight-ball hemorrhage"). If total hyphema persists and elevated pressure is evident despite medical therapy, surgical intervention is indicated. Surgical therapy varies, depending on the hyphema and the availability of instrumentation and skilled surgical assistance.

Surgical Intervention

If the blood has formed a firm, well-organized clot, it can be removed by entering the anterior chamber through a limbus-based corneal incision in the same manner as for cataract surgery.[4, 7, 9, 20, 21, 25, 27] The anterior chamber may be gently irrigated with a balanced salt solution,* the incision closed, and the eye treated for traumatic uveitis.

If the hyphema is still partially liquified, anterior chamber irrigation and suction can be carefully carried out. Many techniques are available to do this, but, in general (unless very sophisticated automatic irrigators with hand pieces are available), two surgeons are needed, one to irrigate, and the other to aspirate, even when a double-walled needle is used.

Sophisticated anterior chamber irrigating and vitreous cutting units using microsurgical handles and needles are available. They work well in hyphemas of both the anterior and posterior chamber. Unfortunately, they are expensive for the limited use they

---

*BSS, Alcon Laboratories, Fort Worth, TX.

would receive in private practice. The only unit that might be economically feasible is the Concept Portable Vitreophage Unit (Kaufman Vitrector II* vitreous suction cutter with reciprocating cutting action).

The use of medications such as vitamin C, vitamin K, calcium, rutin, or estrogenic substances does not appear to accelerate a normal clotting mechanism.[21,23] There is some evidence that the use of aminocaproic acid† may minimize rebleeding by inhibiting fibrinolysis in the damaged blood vessels.[11]

It is important to emphasize that surgical intervention and blind probing of the anterior chamber in an attempt to remove blood or blood clots may cause serious surgical complications, such as rebleeding, luxated lens, extensive iris damage, and damage to the corneal endothelium.

Ocular Foreign Bodies

Periorbital, scleral, or corneal punctures or lacerations may be due to penetrating foreign bodies. The most common foreign bodies associated with ocular injuries in small animals are birdshot, air gun pellets, and glass. The site of intraocular penetration may be obscured by the eyelids (Figs. 111–11 and 111–12).

A foreign body entering the eye may take several trajectories, depending on its velocity and angle of entry. It may penetrate the cornea and fall into the anterior chamber or become lodged in the iris, or it may penetrate the anterior capsule of the lens, producing a cataract. Some metallic, high-speed foreign bodies may perforate the cornea, iris, and lens to lodge in the posterior wall of the eye or in the vitreous or may pass entirely through the eye and remain within the orbit.

There are numerous techniques available to determine the presence and location of ocular foreign bodies.[5,10,12,15,16] Direct observation is the best means

---

*Concept Inc., Clearwater, FL.
†Amicar, Lederle Laboratories, Pearl River, NY.

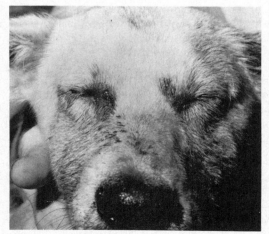

Figure 111–11. This dog was shot in the head with a shotgun. Severe blepharospasm is evident because of traumatic uveitis from the wounds in and around the eye.

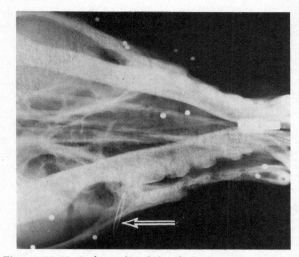

Figure 111–12. Radiographs of the skull of the dog in Figure 111–11 were taken, and a Flieringa metallic ring was placed under the lids *(arrow)* to help outline the location of the orbit. Penetrating wounds of the globe such as this must be sutured and the eyes treated for traumatic uveitis. Pieces of "shot" should not be recovered from the eye unless they are easily retrievable.

of locating a foreign body. Examination with the biomicroscope or indirect ophthalmoscope may prove invaluable in locating foreign bodies. The anterior chamber and anterior drainage angle can be directly viewed with the aid of a gonioprism. Careful ocular examination should be performed as early as possible before secondary ocular inflammation or cataract formation opacifies the ocular media. Indirect demonstration of an intraocular foreign body may be achieved by radiographic techniques.[15,16]

In addition to radiography, the more refined technique of ultrasonography may be employed to locate foreign bodies. This technique is most valuable in evaluating the extent of intraocular damage when there is extensive corneal edema or secondary cataract formation. Ultrasonic evaluation of the traumatized globe may be helpful in evaluating the presence of hyphema, lens luxation, lens rupture, vitreous hemorrhage, retinal detachment, and foreign bodies.

Intraocular penetration by a foreign body always results in a guarded prognosis, and the outcome depends on the foreign body's chemical nature and its position within the eye. Foreign bodies made of iron or copper can produce extensive ocular inflammation.[12,15,22]

Chalcosis[22] is produced by retention of copper or its alloys of bronze or brass and results in rapid inflammation, hypopyon, and localized abscess formation. Slow release of copper results in deposition of copper on limiting membranes within the eye, especially Descemet's membrane and the anterior lens capsule.

Retained foreign bodies of iron and steel may lead to repeated episodes of ocular inflammation and siderosis.[12] In siderosis, iron pigments are deposited in the cornea, iris, and lens, and degenerative changes occur in these areas as well as in the retina. Other metals besides copper and iron may produce ocular inflammatory reactions.[12] Precious metals, stone, carbon, glass, building plaster, and rubber are usually inert in the eye; however, the mechanical trauma produced by these objects may produce serious sequelae.

When considering removing any foreign body from an eye, the dangers of leaving the foreign body in the eye must be weighed against the dangers of surgical removal. Foreign objects in the anterior chamber are much easier to remove than objects at the posterior pole. Removal of foreign bodies from the vitreous has consistently produced poor results.

Proptosis of the Globe

Proptosis of the globe secondary to trauma is common in brachycephalic breeds. A greater degree of initiating contusion is required in the doliocephalic breeds than in the brachycephalic breeds. Therefore, secondary damage to the eye and central nervous system associated with proptosis of the globe may be far greater in the collie than in the Pekingese.

One should not disregard the general physical condition of the animal presented with a proptosed globe, despite the urgency of globe replacement. Careful evaluation of the cardiovascular system for evidence of shock and examination of the respiratory and nervous systems should be carried out. Treatment to establish an adequate airway and control shock, overt bleeding, and so on should be carried out before any attempt is made to replace the eye. While this initial examination and treatment are being carried out, the proptosed globe must be protected against further exposure and drying. This can be accomplished by using sponges soaked in cold, hypertonic 10% dextrose to reduce ocular edema and prevent corneal drying.

Proptosis of the globe results in several pathological phenomena that must be considered in establishing treatment and prognosis. (1) Occlusion of the vortex and ciliary veins of the eye by the lids produces venous stasis and a form of congestive glaucoma. The resulting venous stasis also limits accessibility of intravenous medication to the eye. Venous stasis is relieved once the eye is replaced in the orbit. (2) Proptosis results in marked exposure keratitis and corneal necrosis. Initial protection of the eye with moist gauze soaked in a hypertonic solution will prevent excessive drying. (3) Proptosis of the globe can be associated with iritis, chorioretinitis, retinal detachment, luxation of the lens, and avulsion of the optic nerve.

An attempt should be made to replace most proptosed globes. Exceptions are eyes in which the intraocular contents have been extruded or in which massive destruction of the intraocular contents has taken place or when the owner wishes to have the eye removed because of cosmetic or economic considerations.

Treatment

Surgical replacement of the proptosed globe should be carried out with the animal under general anesthesia. A lateral canthotomy extending from the canthus to the orbital ligament (Fig. 111–13) is made to widen the palpebral fissure. The orbital ligament should not be cut; however, if the globe cannot be replaced by enlarging the palpebral fissure with a canthotomy, it can be partially severed. To facilitate identification, 5-0 silk sutures may be placed at the ends of the severed ligament. Following replacement of the globe, the ligament is sutured with 5.0 to 6.0 nylon.

Using gentle pressure to the globe with a moistened, sterile sponge, an attempt is made to replace the globe.[27] Swelling of the globe and retro-orbital hemorrhage or edema may make this difficult. Paracentesis of the globe should be avoided, since sudden release of intraocular pressure combined with tension on the globe by the lids can result in choroidal hemorrhage, retinal detachment, luxation of the lens, and a general displacement of all intraocular structures. In addition, probing of the retro-orbital space with a needle in an attempt to aspirate blood or fluid should be avoided because further damage to the globe and optic nerve may result. Nylon sutures (5.0) are preplaced for a third eyelid flap. The third eyelid flap helps keep the globe in the orbit and protects the cornea if the lid sutures become loose and the lids part too early. Three nonpenetrating mattress sutures of 4.0 to 5.0 nylon are preplaced in the lid margins. The eye is gently replaced in the orbit, and the third eyelid and lid sutures are tightened. Other techniques for replacement of the globe have been described.[27] Small pieces of plastic tubing are used under the sutures to prevent pressure necrosis of the skin overlying the lids. After replacing the eye in the orbit, 2 to 4 mg of methylprednisolone acetate are injected into the retrobulbar space to reduce inflammation.

Postoperative treatment is designed to control traumatic iritis and the extensive corneal damage that is associated with proptosis and exposure. Systemic broad spectrum antibiotics are indicated. Atropine ointment (1%) is used topically, and topical steroids* and antibiotics are used five to six times daily. Although steroids are a "two-edged sword," the extensive vascularization, inflammation, and scar tissue that can form after ocular injury make them a very valuable aid in treating traumatic proptosis. The topical medication can be delivered as either an ointment or drops (in the case of prednisolone acetate, 1% placed through the eyelid margins directly on the cornea). If trauma to an eye has been extensive, topical steroids are supplemented with systemic steroids for a one-week period.

---

*Editor's Note: The use of *topical* steroids in the control of corneal vascularization after proptosis is controversial and is regarded as contraindicated by some veterinary ophthalmologists.

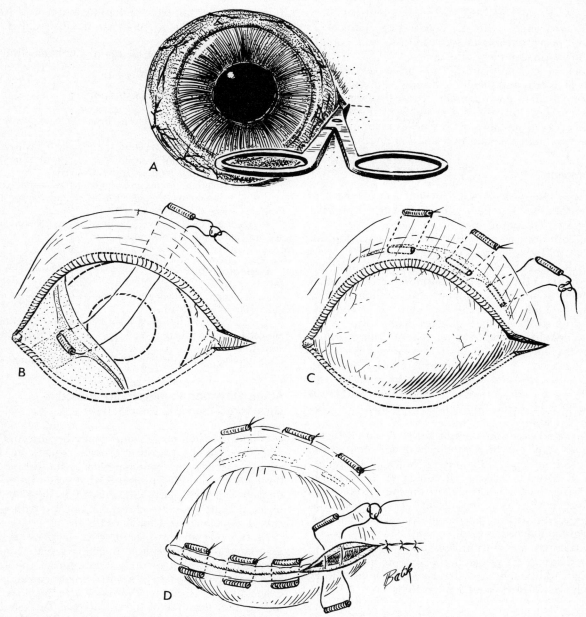

Figure 111–13. Repair of proptosis of the globe. *A,* An acutely proptosed eye is presented, showing congestion and chemosis. The lateral canthus is incised with blunt-tipped scissors to reduce compression of the eyelids on the globe. *B,* Sutures are preplaced for a third eyelid flap (see Chapter 104). *C,* The third eyelid is brought over the globe, and the sutures are tied. *D,* The lateral canthotomy has been closed. A temporary tarsorrhaphy is created, making sure that the sutures emerge in the middle of the eyelid margin. (Reprinted with permission from Bistner, S. I., Aguirre, G., and Batik, G.: *Atlas of Veterinary Ophthalmic Surgery.* W. B. Saunders, Philadelphia, 1977.)

Sutures are left in place until intraorbital swelling is markedly reduced, usually ten days to three weeks. The sutures are removed and the globe is inspected. If proptosis recurs, the sutures are replaced and removed after an additional two weeks.

Extraocular muscle injury and the resultant strabismus are very common following proptosis. The most frequent deviation observed is upward and outward, indicating possible paralysis or rupture of the medial rectus, dorsal oblique, and ventral rectus muscles or an overaction of the lateral or dorsal rectus muscle. Strabismus is most noticeable imme-

diately following removal of the lid sutures. In most cases, a relatively normal visual axis returns in three to four months following the initial injury. Keratitis sicca and optic nerve atrophy are also common sequelae to proptosis of the globe.

Endophthalmitis

Endophthalmitis (inflammation of the eye and its contents) is more severe than uveitis, and often an infectious agent is associated with this inflammatory reaction. In dogs and cats, endophthalmitis is most often associated with a penetrating intraocular wound, postsurgical infections, and ruptured corneal wounds with secondary infections.

Signs of endophthalmitis are more severe than those of uveitis and include extreme pain, very deep scleral vascular engorgement, corneal edema with large numbers of cells and proteins in the anterior chamber, large amounts of vitreous exudate, systemic signs, e.g., anorexia and pyrexia, and neutrophilia.

Treatment

If very severe structural damage is not evident and the cornea has not been ruptured with intraocular tissue loss, treatment may be attempted.

An anterior or vitreous chamber aspiration for culture and cytological examination should be performed. This requires either a short-acting anesthetic or sedation of the patient. Endophthalmitis in animals produces a plasmoid aqueous, and although small gauge needles (25- or 26-gauge) are less traumatic, they frequently become plugged with fibrin. A 20-gauge needle is used to enter the anterior chamber at the limbus, and the aspirate is examined by culture and cytology.[1,4,13] Large numbers of polymorphonuclear leukocytes and gram-negative or gram-positive bacteria are indicative of active infection, and treatment should begin immediately without awaiting culture results.

The rapid determination of glucose content in the vitreous may aid in distinguishing infectious from noninfectious endophthalmitis.[31] Material is applied to a Dextrostix from a vitreous tap. In bacterial infections, bacteria use glucose in the vitreous and glucose is reduced or absent. In noninfectious endophthalmitis the vitreous glucose content is normal (greater than 10 mg/dl).

Antibiotics and anti-inflammatory agents at prescribed dosage are placed in the aqueous and vitreous cavity.[1] Additionally, in vitreal disease, a vitrectomy may be performed (see Chapter 108).

Initial Therapy

The intraocular antibiotic regimen for the treatment of endophthalmitis is as follows:

1. Intraocular gentamicin, 0.1 mg, and cephaloridine (Loridine), 0.25 mg.
2. Subconjunctival gentamicin, 25 mg, and cephaloridine, 1 mg, or methicillin, 100 mg.
3. Topical gentamicin ophthalmic ointment.
4. Systemic cephaloridine intravenously.

Intraocular aspiration should be repeated at 48 hours, and if bacteria are still evident and culture positive, the intraocular antibiotic regimen should be repeated.

Because infections associated with endophthalmitis can spread via the optic nerve and meninges to the central nervous system, resulting in meningitis, it is important to either treat endophthalmitis or, if treatment is not successful, enucleate the diseased globe.

Preparation of Gentamicin and Cephaloridine for Intraocular Injection

Intraocular Gentamicin, 0.1 mg

1. Withdraw 0.1 ml (4 mg) from the vial (40 mg/dl gentamicin).
2. Add to 9.9 ml of nonbacteriostatic saline if final volume of 0.25 ml for injection is desired *or* to 3.9 ml of nonbacteriostatic saline if 0.1 ml volume is desired.
3. 10 ml contains 4 mg gentamicin; 1 ml contains 0.4 mg; 0.25 ml contains 0.1 mg; *or* 4 ml contains 4 mg; 1 ml contains 1 mg; 0.1 ml contains 0.1 mg.
4. Inject either 0.25 ml containing 0.1 mg gentamicin *or* 0.1 ml containing 0.1 mg gentamicin.

Cephaloridine

1. Reconstitute powder with 10 ml sterile sodium chloride (1000 mg in 10 ml).
2. Add 0.1 ml (10 mg) of suspension to 3.9 ml nonbacteriostatic saline; 10 mg in 4 ml contains 1 mg cephaloridine in 0.4 ml.
3. Inject 0.1 ml containing 0.25 mg cephaloridine.

Acute Elevation in Intraocular Pressure— Glaucoma (See also Chapter 110)

Glaucoma is an ocular emergency because uncontrolled elevated intraocular pressure causes irreversible damage to the ganglion cells of the retina and optic nerve, resulting in irreversible vision loss. This damage can take place within 24 to 48 hours of the onset of acute pressure elevation. For the pathogenesis of glaucoma see Chapter 110.

In the dog and cat, acute rises in pressure are associated with preceding intraocular disease (secondary glaucoma) that severely compromises the anterior drainage angle. In the initial treatment of acute congestive glaucoma it is important to consider the differential diagnosis of the major problems producing secondary narrow angle glaucoma.

Anterior Uveitis

Uveitis is one of the most common causes of glaucoma. It rapidly produces a plasmoid aqueous, which can lead to a blockage of the trabecular meshwork with fibrin and cells, secondary broad-based anterior synechia, and elevations in intraocular pressure. Cyclytis is, in my experience, a diagnosis that often goes undetected until the zonular ligaments supporting the lens are broken and the lens subluxates or luxates through the pupil or into the anterior chamber (Fig. 111–14). Careful examination with a biomicroscope in many early lens luxation cases has shown protein in the anterior chamber and vitreous; inflammatory cells, especially in the vitreous; and

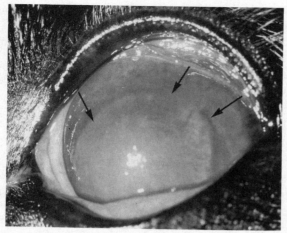

Figure 111–14. Acute congestive glaucoma in a dog. Subluxated lens in a dog with cyclitis (inflammation of the ciliary body). The zonular ligaments ruptured secondary to inflammation and the lens moved forward, becoming trapped in the pupillary space. The outline of the lens is indicated by the arrows. Severe uveitis as well as elevated intraocular pressure is evident. Treatment involved treating the uveitis and surgically removing the subluxated lens.

active cyclytis. Cyclytis and lens luxations are primarily seen in terriers and smaller breeds of dogs.

Basset hounds with acute congestive unilateral glaucoma (Fig. 111–15) have active severe uveitis that has caused decompensation of a poorly formed anterior drainage angle and secondary glaucoma. When the normal eye is gonioscopically evaluated, the angle is usually very poorly developed and narrowed and appears as if it, too, could develop increased pressure if anything caused "decompensation."

The animal presented with acute lens subluxation or luxation into the anterior chamber and secondary anterior uveitis and cyclytis can be improved by surgical removal of the lens and control of underlying intraocular inflammation. Early diagnosis of pupillary block glaucoma *is essential* if a good prognosis is to be established.

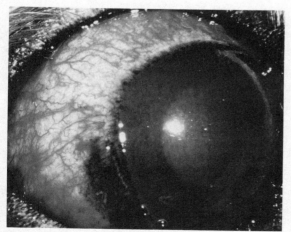

Figure 111–15. Acute glaucoma with episcleral engorgement and corneal edema.

Lens Intumescence

This term means enlargement or swelling of the lens.[27] Intumescence leads to pupillary block, a narrowing of the anterior drainage angle because fluid in the posterior chamber pushes the iris forward with resultant peripheral anterior synechia.

Treatment (see also Chapter 110)

Initial treatment in acute elevations of intraocular pressure is directed at the reduction of pressure using osmotic agents such as mannitol, 1 gm/kg given IV slowly. The effect of the drug develops over a 30- to 60-minute period and lasts three to four hours. Oral osmotic agents (glycerin 50 to 75%) can also be given (8 to 12 cc to a 15-kg dog every eight hours).

Carbonic anhydrase inhibitors can be used to decrease the production of aqueous fluid. Numerous drugs are available. However, an initial loading dose can be achieved with acetazolamide, 250 to 500 mg by intravenous bolus to a 15- to 20-kg dog. The initial loading dose can be followed with oral dichlorphenamide, 50 mg/20 kg every eight hours. Dichlorphenamide produces less serious side effects, including vomiting, diarrhea, panting, and weakness, than other carbonic anhydrase inhibitors.

Once the initial, acutely elevated intraocular pressure is controlled, careful examination may indicate the underlying cause of the glaucoma, and further appropriate therapy, such as treatment for uveitis, lens removal, cyclocryotherapy, or filtration, can be undertaken.[1]

1. Baum, J. L.: Bacterial endophthalmitis. *In* Fraunfelder, F. T., and Roy, T. H. (eds.): *Current Ocular Therapy.* W. B. Saunders, Philadelphia, 1980, pp. 439–440.
2. Baum, J. L.: Antibiotic use in ophthalmology. *In* Duane, T. D. (ed.): *Clinical Ophthalmology,* Vol. 4. Harper and Row, New York, 1980, Chapter 26.
3. Bistner, S. I.: Clinical diagnosis and treatment of infectious keratitis. Comp. Cont. Ed. 3:1056, 1981.
4. Bistner, S. I., Aguirre, G., and Batik, G.: *Atlas of Veterinary Ophthalmic Surgery.* W. B. Saunders, Philadelphia, 1977.
5. Bronson, N. R. II: Management of magnetic foreign bodies. *In* Freeman, H. M. (ed.): *Ocular Trauma.* Appleton-Century-Crofts, New York, 1979, pp. 179–186.
6. Brown, S. I., and Weller, C. A.: The pathogenesis and treatment of collagenase induced disease of the cornea. Trans. Am. Acad. Ophthalmol. Otolaryngol. 74:375, 1970.
7. Byron, H. M.: The contused globe: Management of traumatic hyphema and secondary glaucoma. Instruction course, Am. Acad. Ophthalmol., 1975.
8. Cherry, P. M. H.: Indirect traumatic rupture of the globe. Arch. Ophthalmol. 96:252, 1978.
9. Coleman, J. D.: Surgical management of traumatic lens injuries. *In* Freeman, H. M. (ed.): *Ocular Trauma.* Appleton-Century-Crofts, New York, 1979, pp. 205–214.
10. Coleman, J. D., and Smith, M. E.: Ultrasound in the preoperative evaluation of trauma. *In* Freeman, H. H.: *Ocular Trauma.* Appleton-Century-Crofts, New York, 1979, pp. 23–30.
11. Crouch, E. R., Jr., and Frenkel, M.: Aminocaproic acid in

the treatment of traumatic hyphema. Am. J. Ophthalmol. *81*:355, 1976.

12. Ellis, P. P.: Intraocular foreign body—steel or iron. *In* Fraunfelder, F. T., and Hampton, R. (eds.): *Current Ocular Therapy.* W. B. Saunders, Philadelphia, 1980, pp. 286–288.

13. Forster, R, K.: Endophthalmitis. *In* Duane, T. D. (ed.): *Clinical Ophthalmology*, Vol. 4. Harper and Row, New York, 1980, Chapter 24.

14. Fox, S. A.: *Ophthalmic Plastic Surgery*, 4th ed. Grune and Stratton, New York, 1970.

15. Freeman, H. M. (ed.): *Ocular Trauma.* Appleton-Century-Crofts, New York, 1979.

16. Hanafee, W. N. (ed.): Symposium on radiology of the orbit. Radiol. Clin. North Am. *10*:1, 1972.

17. Hogan, M. J., and Zimmerman, L. E. (eds.): *Ophthalmic Pathology*, 2nd ed. W. B. Saunders, Philadelphia, 1962.

18. Jones, D. B.: Initial therapy of suspected microbial corneal ulcers. II. Specific antibiotic therapy based on corneal smears. Surv. Ophthalmol. *24*:97, 1979.

19. Jones, D. B., Liesegang, T. J., and Robinson, N. M.: *Laboratory Diagnosis of Ocular Infections*, Cumitech 13. American Society for Microbiology, Washington, D.C., 1981.

20. Paton, D., and Goldberg, M. F.: *Management of Ocular Injuries.* W. B. Saunders, Philadelphia, 1976.

21. Read, J. E.: Trauma: ruptures and bleeding. *In* Duane, T. D. (ed.): *Clinical Ophthalmology, External Diseases*, Vol. 4. Harper and Row, New York, 1980, pp. 5–12.

22. Rosenthal, A. R., Appleton, B., and Hopkins, J. L.: Intraocular copper foreign bodies. Am. J. Ophthalmol. 78:671, 1974.

23. Rynne, M. V., and Romano, P.: Systemic corticosteroids in the treatment of traumatic hyphema. J. Ped. Ophthalmol. 17:141, 1980.

24. Sarin, L. K., and Reinert, C. G.: Retinopathy in ocular trauma. *In* Duane, T. D. (ed.): *Clinical Ophthalmology*, Vol. 3. Harper and Row, Hagerstown, 1976. Chapter 31.

25. Sholiton, D. B., and Solomon, O. D.: Surgical management of black ball hyphema with sodium hyaluronate. Ophthalmic Surg. *12*:820, 1981.

26. Slansky, H. H., Berman, M. B., Dohlman, C. H., and Rose, J.: Cysteine and acetyl cysteine in the prevention of corneal ulcerations. Ann. Ophthalmol. 2:488, 1970.

27. Slatter, D. H.: *Fundamentals of Veterinary Ophthalmology.* W. B. Saunders, Philadelphia, 1981.

28. Smith, B.: Eyelid reconstruction. *In* Soll, D. B., and Asbell, R. L. (eds.): *Management of Complications in Ophthalmic Plastic Surgery.* Aesculapius Publishing Co., Birmingham, 1976, pp. 221–243.

29. Thoft, R. A., and Dohlman, C. H.: Chemical and thermal burns of the eye. *In* Freeman, H. M. (ed.): *Ocular Trauma.* Appleton-Century-Crofts, New York, 1979, Chapter 14.

30. Wilson, F. M. II: Traumatic hyphema, pathogenesis and management. Ophthalmology 87:910, 1980.

31. Wong, R.: Endophthalmitis. An exhibit at Am. Acad. Ophthalmol. Meeting, Atlanta, Georgia, 1981.

Section XIII

Male Reproductive System

Dudley E. Johnston
Section Editor

Chapter 112

Anatomy of the Male Genital Organs

Harry W. Boothe and Dudley E. Johnston

TESTIS

The testes are positioned obliquely within the scrotum, with their long axis directed dorsocaudally. Each testis is oval and thicker in its dorsoventral measurement than its lateral measurement. The testis of a 12-kg dog has the following average dimensions: length, 3 cm; width, 2 cm; and thickness, 2 cm. The fresh organ weighs approximately 8 gm.[1]

Because they originate in the body cavity, the testes have a serosal covering.[6] The vaginal tunics, parietal and visceral, envelop the testis and structures of the spermatic cord (Figs. 112–1 to 112–3). The parietal vaginal tunic is the outer layer, whereas the visceral vaginal tunic is continuous with the parietal peritoneum of the abdominal cavity.[1] The visceral vaginal tunic leaves the caudal epididymis at an acute angle and becomes the parietal vaginal tunic. This results in a small circumscribed area on the epididymis that is not covered by peritoneum.[2] Deep to the vaginal tunic is the tunica albuginea, a dense, white, fibrous capsule.[1] The tunica albuginea, which is not elastic, contains the superficial branches of the testicular artery and vein. It joins the mediastinum testis at the epididymal attachment to the dorsomedial border of the testis. Connective tissue lamellae, septula testis, from the deep surface of the tunica albuginea converge centrally to form the mediastinum testis. These connective tissue septa contain blood vessels, lymphatics, and nerves and divide the testis into many lobules.[6] The mediastinum testis is a mass of fibrous tissue that runs lengthwise through the middle of the testis.

The testis and epididymis are connected to the parietal vaginal tunic at the caudal extremity of the epididymis by the caudal ligament of the epididymis,

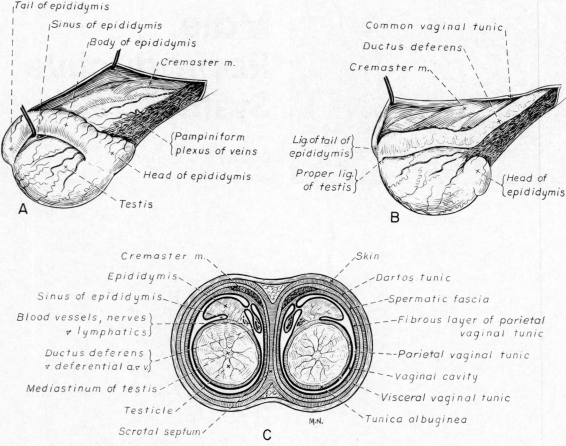

Figure 112–1. Structures of testes and scrotum. *A*, Right testis, lateral aspect. *B*, Left testis, medial aspect. *C*, Schematic cross-section through scrotum and testes. (Reprinted with permission from Evans, H. E., and Christensen, G. C. (eds.): *Miller's Anatomy of the Dog*. 2nd ed. W. B. Saunders, Philadelphia, 1979.)

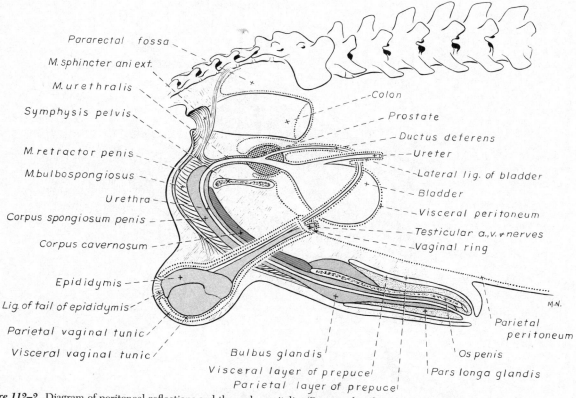

Figure 112–2. Diagram of peritoneal reflections and the male genitalia. (Reprinted with permission from Evans, H. E., and Christensen, G. C. (eds.): *Miller's Anatomy of the Dog.* 2nd ed. W. B. Saunders, Philadelphia, 1979.)

stabilizing the testis. The testis is also indirectly stabilized by the spermatic cord and its reflected vaginal tunics.

The testicular artery is tortuous and arises from the aorta at the level of the fourth lumbar vertebra (Fig. 112–4).[1] The right testicular artery originates cranial to the left. The testicular vein follows the arterial pattern but forms an extensive pampiniform plexus in the spermatic cord. The right testicular vein empties into the caudal vena cava at the level of the origin of its arterial counterpart.[1] The left testicular vein terminates in the left renal vein.

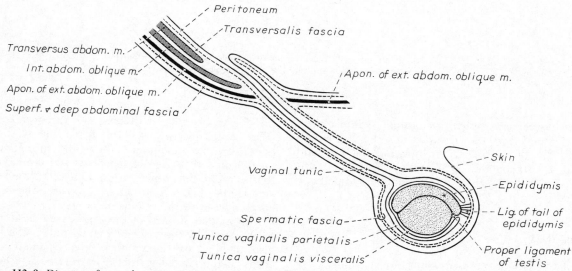

Figure 112–3. Diagram of sagittal section of inguinal canal and vaginal process of the male. (Reprinted with permission from Evans, H. E., and Christensen, G. C. (eds.): *Miller's Anatomy of the Dog.* 2nd ed. W. B. Saunders, Philadelphia, 1979.)

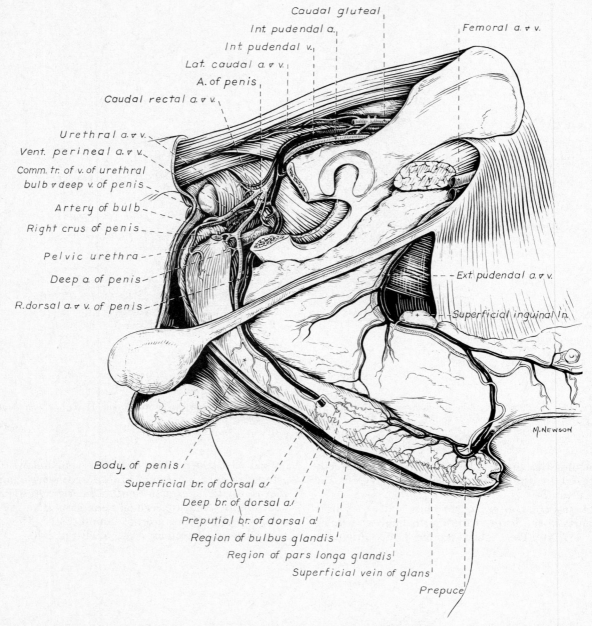

Caudal gluteal
Int. pudendal a.
Int. pudendal v.
Lat. caudal a. & v.
A. of penis
Caudal rectal a. & v.
Femoral a. & v.

Urethral a. & v.
Vent. perineal a. & v.
Comm. tr. of v. of urethral
bulb & deep v. of penis
Artery of bulb
Right crus of penis
Pelvic urethra
Deep a. of penis
R. dorsal a. & v. of penis
Ext. pudendal a. & v.
Superficial inguinal l.n.

M. NEWSON

Body of penis
Superficial br. of dorsal a.
Deep br. of dorsal a.
Preputial br. of dorsal a.
Region of bulbus glandis
Region of pars longa glandis
Superficial vein of glans
Prepuce

Figure 112–4. Topographic relations of the penis and other pelvic structures. (The right ischium is removed.) (Reprinted with permission from Christensen, G. C.: Angioarchitecture of the canine penis and the process of erection. Am. J. Anat. 95:227, 1954.)

The testicular lymphatics anastomose into a variable number of trunks that drain into the iliac lymph nodes. The testicular nerve supply is autonomic and contains postganglionic sympathetic fibers. These fibers arise from the third to fifth lumbar sympathetic ganglia.[2]

EPIDIDYMIS

The epididymis is relatively large in the dog. It lies along the dorsolateral border of the testis in both the dog and cat and is divided into three parts: The head communicates with the testis and is slightly larger than the remainder of the epididymis. It begins on the medial surface of the testis but immediately twists around the cranial extremity to reach the lateral side.[1] The body is the middle part. The tail is continuous with the ductus deferens.

The medial surface of the epididymis is attached to the testis by the visceral vaginal tunic. The tail is also attached by the tough proper ligament of the testis to the caudal testicular extremity. The artery of the ductus deferens, a branch of the prostatic artery, supplies the epididymis and anastomoses with the testicular artery.[1] Epididymal lymphatics drain into the iliac lymph nodes.

SPERMATIC CORD

The spermatic cord begins at the deep inguinal ring (Fig. 112–3), the point at which its component parts converge to leave the abdominal cavity.[1] The spermatic cord is contained within the parietal and visceral vaginal tunics. Its constituents are the ductus deferens, the small artery and veins of the ductus deferens, the testicular artery, the pampiniform plexus, the plexus of testicular nerves, and the testicular lymphatics. The ductus deferens and its vessels are enveloped by one fold of visceral vaginal tunic, the mesoductus deferens. The testicular vessels, nerves, and lymphatics are covered by another fold, the mesorchium. The mesoductus deferens is attached to the mesorchium, which is continuous with the parietal vaginal tunic.

The ductus deferens, the continuation of the duct of the epididymis connects the epididymis with the pelvic urethra. The ductus deferens begins at the tail of the epididymis, runs along the dorsomedial border of the testis, and ascends in the spermatic cord. It averages 18 cm in length and 2.3 cm in diameter in a 12-kg dog. The artery and vein of the ductus deferens accompany it to the epididymis. The artery anastomoses with the testicular artery in the spermatic cord.[1] The vein empties into the internal iliac vein. Parasympathetic fibers from the pelvic plexus are distributed to the smooth muscle of the ductus deferens.

The cremaster muscle accompanies the spermatic cord through the superficial inguinal ring. This muscle arises from the caudal free border of the internal abdominal oblique muscle and attaches to the parietal vaginal tunic near the testis. The cremaster muscle is surrounded by the spermatic fascia, a continuation of the abdominal fascia.

PENIS

The penis is composed of three principal divisions: root, body, and distal portion (Fig. 112–5). The distal portion, the glans, is subdivided into a bulbus glandis and a pars longa glandis. The root is attached to the tuber ischii by the left and right crura. Each crus is composed of the proximal part of the corpus cavernosum and the ischiocavernosus muscle covering it (Figs. 112–6 to 112–8).[1] The corpus spongiosum contains the penile urethra and is situated ventrally. The bulb of the penis is a bilobed expansion of the corpus spongiosum, located between the crura at the ischial arch.

The body of the penis begins at the blending of the crura and extends just beyond the proximal end of the os penis. The body is directly continuous with the root. The corpus cavernosum and the corpus spongiosum constitute the main substance of the penile body.

The glans of the canine penis is located immediately cranial to the scrotum. The proximal portion of the glans is composed of the bulbus glandis. The distal three-fourths of the glans is made up primarily of the pars longa glandis. The distal half of the bulbus glandis is overlapped by the caudal third of the pars longa glandis.

The corpora of the penis contain enlarged venous spaces. The corpora cavernosa arise from the ischial tuberosity and continue distally in the dorsolateral part of the body of the penis as far as the os penis. The right and left cavernous bodies are separated by a fibrous median septum. Each corpus cavernosum is covered by a thick layer of collagenous and elastic fibers, the tunica albuginea. The corpus spongiosum originates within the pelvic cavity and surrounds the penile urethra throughout its course. It is located in a groove on the urethral side of the penis. The corpus spongiosum narrows in diameter until it enters the glans penis, where it gives off numerous shunts that supply the bulbus glandis with blood. The corpus spongiosum continues in the pars longa glandis to the external urethral orifice.

The bulbus glandis surrounds the proximal part of the os penis. Its thickest dimension, and greatest potential for expansion, is located dorsally. The bulbus glandis is separated from the pars longa glandis by a fibrous septum. The pars longa glandis is similar to the bulbus glandis in structure but has erectile tissue dorsally and laterally only. The pars longa glandis is not capable of expansion comparable to that of the bulbus glandis.

The os penis begins caudal to the bulbus glandis and extends almost to the tip of the glans. The distal end is extended by a slightly curved fibrocartilaginous projection. The proximal two-thirds of the os penis is indented ventrally by a distinct groove, which is occupied by the penile urethra and surrounding corpus spongiosum. The os penis is attached to the bulbus glandis, pars longa glandis, and tunica albuginea.

There are four paired extrinsic penile muscles in the dog: retractor penis, ischiocavernosus, bulbospongiosus, and ischiourethralis muscles (see Figs. 112–6 and 112–7). The retractor penis muscles are composed principally of smooth muscle fibers. They arise from the first two caudal vertebrae, blend with the external anal sphincter, run along the ventral surface of the penis, and insert in the penis at the fornix of the prepuce. The ischiocavernosus muscles originate from the ischial tuberosity and insert on the corpus cavernosum. The bulbospongiosus muscles arise from the external anal sphincter, cover the superficial surface of the bulb of the penis, and fuse with the retractor penis muscles at the proximal third of the penile body. The ischiourethralis muscles

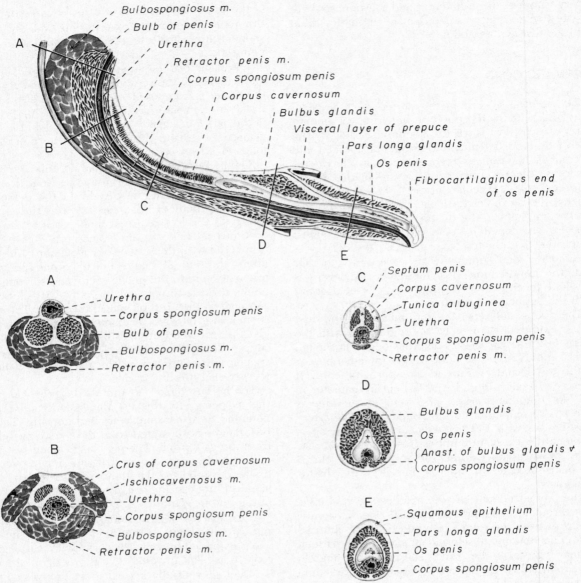

Labels in upper drawing:
- A
- B
- C
- D
- E
- Bulbospongiosus m.
- Bulb of penis
- Urethra
- Retractor penis m.
- Corpus spongiosum penis
- Corpus cavernosum
- Bulbus glandis
- Visceral layer of prepuce
- Pars longa glandis
- Os penis
- Fibrocartilaginous end of os penis

A:
- Urethra
- Corpus spongiosum penis
- Bulb of penis
- Bulbospongiosus m.
- Retractor penis m.

B:
- Crus of corpus cavernosum
- Ischiocavernosus m.
- Urethra
- Corpus spongiosum penis
- Bulbospongiosus m.
- Retractor penis m.

C:
- Septum penis
- Corpus cavernosum
- Tunica albuginea
- Urethra
- Corpus spongiosum penis
- Retractor penis m.

D:
- Bulbus glandis
- Os penis
- Anast. of bulbus glandis ∀ corpus spongiosum penis

E:
- Squamous epithelium
- Pars longa glandis
- Os penis
- Corpus spongiosum penis

Figure 112–5. Internal morphology of the penis. *Upper drawing,* A parasagittal section. *Lower drawing,* Cross-sections made at five levels indicated by corresponding letters on upper drawing. (Reprinted with permission from Christensen, G. C.: Angioarchitecture of the canine penis and the process of erection. Am. J. Anat. 95:227, 1954.)

originate from the dorsal aspect of the ischial tuberosity and insert into a fibrous ring at the urethral bulb.

The principal source of blood to the penis is derived from three branches of the artery of the penis, the continuation of the internal pudendal artery.[1] All three branches—artery of the bulb, deep artery of the penis, and dorsal artery of the penis—anastomose with one another. The paired arteries of the bulb enter the corpus spongiosum to supply the corpus spongiosum, penile urethra, and pars longa glandis. The deep artery of the penis passes through the tunica albuginea to enter the corpus cavernosum. The dorsal artery of the penis, the continuation of the main trunk, is located on the dorsolateral surface of the os penis beneath the erectile tissue. The dorsal artery of the penis supplies the corpus spongiosum, bulbus glandis, and pars longa glandis.

The venous drainage of the penis occurs via the internal and external pudendal veins. The pars longa glandis is drained by both the deep vein of the glans to the bulbus glandis and the superficial vein of the glans to the external pudendal vein. The dorsal veins of the penis run along the dorsolateral surface of the penile body and drain the bulbus glandis. The deep vein of the penis and the vein of the urethral bulb drain the corpus cavernosum and corpus spongiosum, respectively.

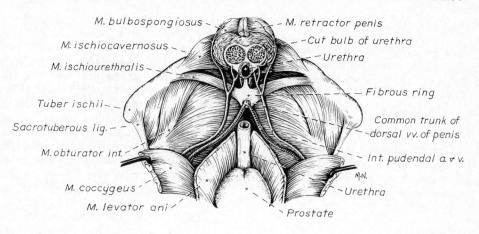

Figure 112–6. Dorsal view of ischiourethral muscles. (The pelvic urethra is cut off at the urethral bulb and removed.) (Reprinted with permission from Evans, H. E., and Christensen, G. C.: (eds.): *Miller's Anatomy of the Dog.* 2nd ed. W. B. Saunders, Philadelphia, 1979.)

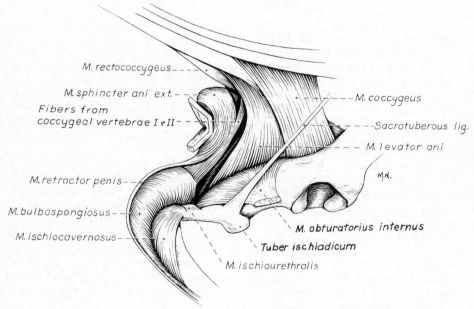

Figure 112–7. Root of penis with superficial muscles, lateral aspect. (Reprinted with permission from Evans, H. E., and Christensen, G. C. (eds.): *Miller's Anatomy of the Dog.* 2nd ed. W. B. Saunders, Philadelphia, 1979.)

Figure 112–8. Superficial muscles of male perineum, caudal aspect. (Reprinted with permission from Evans, H. E., and Christensen, G. C. (eds.): *Miller's Anatomy of the Dog.* 2nd ed. W. B. Saunders, Philadelphia, 1979.)

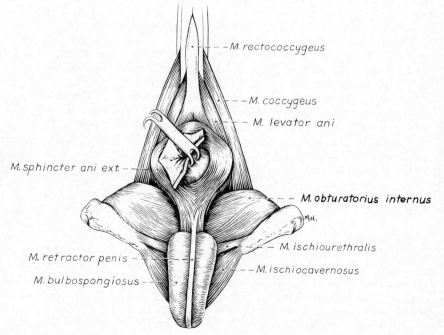

The penis is supplied by nerves from the pelvic and sacral plexuses. The dorsal nerve of the penis passes on the dorsolateral surface of the penis and is the chief sensory nerve to the penis. Penile lymphatics drain into the superficial inguinal lymph nodes.

The feline penis is shorter and directed caudally. Its urethral surface faces caudodorsally and its dorsum faces cranioventrally.[6] Like that of the dog, the penis of the cat consists of a proximal cavernous and a distal osseous part. The free part of the penis of a sexually mature cat is studded with small cornified papillae, penile spines.[6]

PREPUCE

The canine prepuce is a complete tubular sheath that covers the pars longa glandis and part of the bulbus glandis in the nonerect penis. It is firmly attached and continuous with the skin of the ventral abdominal wall.[1] The dorsal prepuce is composed of two layers of integument. On its ventral, lateral, and the cranial aspects of its dorsal surface, the prepuce is composed of three layers of integument. The outer layer is skin, and the inner layers, parietal and visceral, are made up of thin, stratified squamous epithelium. The parietal layer is a continuation of the outer skin layer onto the wall of the preputial cavity. It extends to the fornix, which is located at the level of the middle of the bulbus glandis. The parietal layer is stippled with many lymph nodules and nodes, particularly along the fornix. The visceral, or inner, layer extends from the preputial fornix to the external urethral orifice. It is continuous with the cavernous urethra. The paired preputial muscle, which extends from the xiphoid cartilage to the dorsal wall of the prepuce is derived from the cutaneous trunci muscle.[1]

The blood supply to the visceral and parietal layers of the prepuce is derived primarily from the dorsal artery of the penis and the external pudendal artery. The artery of the bulb of the penis contributes some to the blood supply of the visceral layer. The caudal superficial epigastric artery supplies the preputial skin. The principal venous drainage of the visceral and parietal layers is the superficial and deep veins of the glans, the dorsal vein of the penis, and the external pudendal veins. Preputial lymphatics drain to the superficial inguinal lymph nodes.

SCROTUM

The canine scrotum is a membranous pouch located approximately two-thirds of the distance from the preputial orifice to the anus. It is spherical, divided into two cavities by a median septum, and located between the thighs. The scrotal wall consists of two layers. The outer skin is thin, pigmented, and covered with fine scattered hairs. The deeper layer is the dartos, composed of smooth muscle mixed with collagenous and elastic fibers. The dartos forms a common lining for both halves of the scrotum and contributes to the scrotal septum. The septum is continuous with the abdominal fascia dorsally. The scrotum contains the testes, epididymides, the distal part of the spermatic cord with its associated spermatic fascia and vaginal tunics, and the distal cremaster muscle. The external spermatic fascia attaches to the caudal aspect of the scrotum as the scrotal ligament. The external pudendal artery is the principal blood vessel to the scrotum. The draining veins parallel the arteries. Lymphatic drainage is to the superficial inguinal lymph nodes.

The feline scrotum is located just ventral to the anus. It is densely covered with hair.

PROSTATE

The prostate gland surrounds the proximal portion of the urethra at the neck of the bladder (Fig. 112–9). The gland is semioval in transverse section, and the dorsal surface is flattened with a mid-dorsal groove that can be palpated rectally. The urethra traverses the prostate gland slightly dorsal to the midpoint of the gland.

The prostate gland has a thick capsule, and a prominent median septum divides the gland into right and left lobes. Each lobe is further divided into lobules by capsular trabeculae. The lobules consist of numerous compound tubuloalveolar glands lined by columnar epithelium. Ducts arise from these glands and enter the prostatic urethra at multiple sites. Smooth muscle fibers are present in the capsule of the prostate gland. Muscle fibers from the wall of the urinary bladder extend onto the dorsal surface of the gland.

The blood supply of the prostate gland is mainly via the prostatic artery,[3,5] which usually arises from the internal pudendal artery at the level of the second or third sacral vertebra. The prostatic artery gives rise to the artery of the ductus deferens and the middle rectal artery before ramifying on the surface of the gland. Anastomoses occur between the prostatic vessels and those from the urethra and the rectum. Prostatic blood drains by the prostatic and urethral veins into the internal iliac vein. Prostatic lymph drains into the iliac lymph nodes. The prostate receives parasympathetic nerve fibers from the pelvic plexus (which is formed by the pelvic nerve) and sympathetic nerve fibers from the hypogastric nerve following the artery of the deferent duct.

The two deferent ducts enter the craniodorsal surface of the prostate. They are in close contact with each other and pass caudoventrally through the gland to open into the urethra by two slits on each side of the colliculus seminalis.[2]

The size and weight of the prostate varies with age, breed, and body weight.[7,8] The growth of the prostate has been divided into three phases, normal

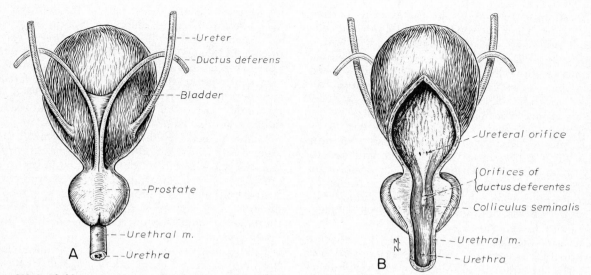

Figure 112–9. Bladder and prostate. *A*, Dorsal aspect. *B*, Ventral aspect, partially opened on midline. (Reprinted with permission from Evans, H. E., and Christensen, G. C. (eds.): *Miller's Anatomy of the Dog.* 2nd ed. W. B. Saunders, Philadelphia, 1979.)

growth in young adults, hyperplasia during middle to adult life, and senile involution.[7]

The anatomical relations and the position of the prostate vary with the age of the dog. The prostate is entirely situated within the abdominal cavity at birth and moves caudally into the pelvis when the urachal remnant breaks down at about two months of age.[4] The gland remains within the pelvic canal until sexual maturity, when it increases in size and its cranial border extends into the abdomen. Usually, at four years of age one-half of the gland is cranial to the pelvic inlet, and by 10 years of age the entire gland is outside the pelvis. The external relations of the gland change with age. Dorsally, the prostate is separated from the rectum by the two layers of peritoneum that form the rectogenital space. The ventral surface of the prostate is retroperitoneal and is covered by large masses of fat, which obscure the gland, its blood vessels, and the neck of the bladder.

1. Evans, H. E., and Christensen, G. C. (eds.): *Miller's Anatomy of the Dog*, 2nd ed. W. B. Saunders Co., Philadelphia, 1979.
2. Evans, H. E., and deLahunta, A.: *Miller's Guide to the Dissection of the Dog.* W. B. Saunders Co., Philadelphia, 1971.
3. Gordon, N.: Surgical anatomy of the bladder, prostate gland and urethra in the male dog. J. Am. Vet. Med. Assoc. *136*:215, 1960.
4. Gordon, N.: The position of the canine prostate gland. Am. J. Vet. Res. *22*:142, 1961.
5. Hodson, N.: On the intrinsic blood supply to the prostate and pelvic urethra in the dog. Res. Vet. Sci. *9*:274, 1968.
6. Nickel, R., Schummer, A., Seiferle, E., and Sack, W. O.: *The Viscera of the Domestic Mammals.* Springer-Verlag, New York, 1973.
7. O'Shea, J. D.: Studies on the canine prostate gland. 1. Factors influencing its size and weight. J. Comp. Pathol. *72*:321, 1962.
8. Schlotthauer, C. F., and Bollman, J. L.: The prostate gland of the dog. Cornell Vet. *26*:342, 1936.
9. Vlahos L., Karatzas, G., Giannopoulos, A., et al.: Visualization of the lymphatics of the vulva and scrotum by direct intratissue injection of the dye. Br. J. Urol. *50*:205, 1978.

Chapter **113** Physiology of the Male Genital Organs

Harry W. Boothe and Dudley E. Johnston

The male reproductive tract is designed to produce mature spermatozoa, to store them until they are needed, and to discharge them in a convenient fluid into the female so that they can ascend the female tract. Androgens, also produced by the male genital tract, are vital to male reproductive activity. The production and release of androgens are regulated by feedback mechanisms.[10]

TESTES

The testes release spermatozoa and fluid into the seminiferous tubules and elaborate male sex hormones.[10] Both testicular functions are regulated by gonadotrophins. The testes require precise thermoregulation to maintain normal function (see "Spermatic Cord" and "Scrotum").

The seminiferous tubules are the exocrine portion of the testis. They are composed of supporting cells (Sertoli cells) and spermatogenic cells.[1] In addition to providing support, Sertoli cells are involved in spermiation (the release of spermatozoa) and estrogen production. Spermiation is mediated by gonadotrophins.[12] Sertoli cells are more resistant to many noxious agents than other cells of the testis.[17]

Spermatogenesis is the sequence of events by which spermatogonia are transformed into spermatozoa.[1] This process consists of mitotic and meiotic activity, as well as a maturation phase.[17] Spermatogenesis is a continuous process that is controlled by gonadotrophins from the pituitary. It is decreased by elevated testicular temperatures, nutritive deficiencies, and many noxious agents.

The interstitial cells of the testis (Leydig cells) are the principal constituent of the endocrine portion of the testis. Sertoli cells also have an endocrine function. Leydig cells produce androgens in response to interstitial cell–stimulating hormone (ICSH) in synergy with follicle-stimulating hormone (FSH) and probably prolactin.[17] Androgens are involved with spermatogenesis, maintenance of the accessory glands and secondary sex characteristics, and changes associated with sexual maturity. Interstitial cell function is not severely reduced in ectopic testes, in contrast to the severe damaging effect of the intra-abdominal or other ectopic position of the testis on the germinal epithelium.[17] Estrogens have been isolated from the testes of dogs and other species. The Sertoli cells are the most probable source of testicular estrogens.[17]

A blood-testis barrier comparable to the blood-brain barrier has been described.[10] The seminiferous tubules are segregated from the interstitium by two barriers: the myoid layer and the tight junctions between Sertoli cells. This barrier is influenced by gonadotrophins and temperature.[10] The significance of the blood-testis barrier is not yet fully understood. The barrier appears to be responsible for the gradient between androgen levels in the blood and in the seminiferous tubules. The antigenic properties of spermatozoa are also, in part, associated with the blood-testis barrier.

EPIDIDYMIS

The epididymis functions in the storage, maturation, and transport of spermatozoa. Functionally, the epididymis has three main regions: an initial segment (head), and a middle segment (body), and a terminal segment (tail). These functional regions do not necessarily correspond to the anatomic regions· (see Chapter 112).[10]

Spermatozoa are stored primarily in the tail of the epididymis, which is capable of preserving them for fairly long periods. Ejaculated spermatozoa in the dog and other species originate mainly from the epididymis. The location of the tail of the epididymis

in the most distal, coolest part of the scrotum may be related to its storage function. Sperm maturation also occurs in the epididymis. Maturation is characterized by changes in both structure and function: Spermatozoa acquire the progressive forward motility of mature sperm, develop the capacity for fertility, and become less resistant to thermal stress. The metabolic pattern of epididymal spermatozoa also differs from that of testicular spermatozoa.[17]

Maintenance of epididymal functions and cellular integrity depends on androgenic hormones.[22] Androgen receptors have been demonstrated in the canine epididymis.[21,22] Circulating androgen as well as testicular fluid androgen probably regulates epididymal function. One example of androgenic regulation is the effect of androgen on contractile activity in the epididymis.[10]

Epididymal resorption of whole spermatozoa has been demonstrated in the rabbit and bull.[4,12] Resorption of spermatozoa has not been shown to occur in the dog. In fact, one examination of the canine epididymal ultrastructure did not support the theory of sperm cell resorption.[4]

SPERMATIC CORD

The spermatic cord is a conduit for the transport of spermatozoa, an important part of the thermoregulation mechanism of the testes, and a contributor to sperm maturation and survival.[8] The ductus deferens is capable of secretion, absorption, and synthesis of cholesterol and sex steroids.[7,8] It is also an androgen target organ.[8]

Parasympathetic nerve fibers influence the passage of spermatozoa through the ductus deferens.[12] Stimulation of these fibers leads to contraction of both the tail of the epididymis and the ductus deferens, leading to seminal emission.[10] Semen is conveyed by peristaltic contractions of the ductus deferens into the pelvic urethra. Androgens and estrogens also influence the smooth muscle of the ductus deferens—androgens inhibit and estrogens stimulate.[12]

The vascular architecture of the spermatic cord helps maintain the scrotal temperature below general body temperature. The coiling of the testicular artery and its close proximity to the pampiniform plexus pre-cool blood flowing to the testis by a countercurrent heat exchange mechanism.[10] The cremaster muscle, which accompanies the spermatic cord, is also an important part of testicular thermoregulation. This muscle regulates the distance of the testis from the body. Contraction properties of the cremaster muscle indicate that it is a "slow" muscle. It depends upon the testis for normal tonus, because orchidectomy produces cremaster muscle atrophy.[18]

The ductus deferens metabolizes androgens and estrogens. Androgen levels in the ductus deferens are significantly higher than in peripheral plasma. These higher levels could be explained by high levels of androgen in the epididymis, by active fluid resorption in the ductus deferens, or by the presence of an androgen binder to the ductus deferens.[2] The ductus deferens may be involved in the transfer of high concentrations of androgens and estrogens into the prostatic circulation.[7,8]

PROSTATE

The prostate gland has no endocrine function and does not seem to be essential for fertility. Prostatectomized dogs are fertile; however, it has been suggested that in normal mating, prostatic fluid assists in transporting out of the urethra the small volume of spermatozoa that are stored in the ductus deferens.[14] Other than this simple technical function, the function of prostatic fluid is unknown. Semen is ejaculated in three visually distinguishable fractions. The first is clear and is followed by the sperm-bearing fraction. The third fraction, consisting of clear prostatic fluid, is ejaculated after the dog dismounts and during the "tie" or genital lock.

Forty to 50 lobules are present in the prostate, each formed by densely packed acini and all separated by fibromuscular stromas. The acini are lined by tall columnar epithelium, which is densely granulated in the apical cytoplasm.[13] These prostatic acinar epithelial cells have an extensive exocrine secretory activity and can transplant a variety of substances derived from the blood into the glandular lumen. These secretory and transport activities are constant, without the need for ejaculation. Interestingly, these activities have been studied in more detail in dogs than in humans.[16] Under basal conditions in the dog, the prostate produces 0.3 ml per 30 minutes.[20] This output is low in total protein and is hypotonic, with the major electrolytes being sodium and chloride.[19,16] During ejaculation, the active prostatic output increases 83-fold, being high in protein and isotonic.[14] During basal conditions, prostatic alveolar cells have a dynamic ability to modify the composition of the prostatic fluid in the glandular lumen by means of reabsorption of sodium and chloride. This could explain the change in osmolality of the prostatic fluid under basal conditions and during ejaculation.[20,3]

Among the secretory products of the canine prostate are many hydrolytic enzymes. Three of these, arginine esterase, acid sulfatase, and acid phosphatase, are the most sensitive markers of testicular hormones, because they are decreased 18-fold, fivefold, and five-fold, respectively, after one month of castration. Normal levels can return after two weeks of androstanediol administration.[9]

In general, activities of all enzymes except alkaline phosphatase are increased by testosterone and decreased by estrogen or hypophysectomy.[12] Measurement of certain prostatic enzyme levels in blood is an important diagnostic and prognostic test in humans, but it has not been studied adequately in dogs. The secretion of prostatic fluid is increased by stimulation of parasympathetic and sympathetic nerves.

PENIS

Erection is essential for the penis to function during copulation in all species except the dog.[17] The canine os penis facilitates vaginal entry without full erection. The basis for erection of the penis is a profound increase in blood supply. Parasympathetic stimulation increases blood flow through the internal pudendal artery, the principal source of blood to the penis.[6] Erection is accomplished by synergy of two mechanisms. First, engorgement of the cavernous bodies of the penis occurs through expansion of the arteries and contraction of the veins. Second, the dorsal penile vein is compressed against the ischial arch by the contraction of ischiocavernosus and bulbospongiosus muscles.[5,17] The extent to which the cavernous spaces expand during erection depends on development and composition of the connective tissue tunics of the penis. Erection involves primarily the glans penis in the dog and cat.[17] Enlargement of the bulbus glandis in the dog is an important part of the "tie" that occurs during copulation. The cornified spines of the feline penis stimulate ovulation.

PREPUCE

The prepuce covers the non-erect penis. At birth, the epithelial surfaces of the prepuce and penis adhere. Separation of the prepuce from the penis is under androgenic influence and usually occurs at puberty. The preputial muscles keep the prepuce over the penis. They are classified as "slow" muscles and are similar to the cremaster muscle in their contraction properties.[18]

SCROTUM

The scrotum functions in the thermoregulation of the testes.[10] The scrotal skin is thin, sparsely covered with hair, and richly supplied with sweat glands. This structure favors the dissipation of heat from the testes. The dartos, a layer of smooth muscle and connective tissue, also regulates the distance of the testis from the body. Contraction of the dartos helps bring the testis closer to the abdomen, whereas relaxation does the opposite.

1. Bloom, W., and Fawcett, D. W. (eds.): *A Textbook of Histology.* 9th ed. W. B. Saunders Co., Philadelphia, 1968.
2. Boulanger, P., Desaulniers, M., Dupuy, G. M., et al.: Androgen levels in the liquid of the canine vas deferens and peripheral plasma. J. Endocrinol. 93:109, 1982.
3. Brandes, D.: Fine structure and cytochemistry of male sex accessory organ. *In* Brandes, D. (ed.): *Male Accessory Sex Organ: Structure and Function in Mammals.* Academic Press, New York, 1974.
4. Chandler, J. A., Sinowatz, F., and Pierrepoint, C. G.: The ultrastructure of dog epididymis. Urol. Res. 9:33, 1981.
5. Christensen, G. C.: Angioarchitecture of the canine penis and the process of erection. Am. J. Anat. 95:227, 1954.
6. Colleen, S., Holmquist, B., and Olin, T.: An angiographic study of erection in the dog. Urol. Res. 9:297, 1981.

7. Dupuy, G. M., Boulanger, P., Roberts, K. D., et al.: Metabolism of sex steroids in the human and canine vas deferens. Endocrinology 104:1553, 1979.

8. Dupuy, G. M., Boulanger, P., Roberts, K. D., et al.: Detection of an androgen receptor in the canine vas deferens. J. Steroid Biochem. 13:305, 1980.

9. Frenette, G., Dube, J. Y., and Tremblay, R. R.: Effect of castration and steroid treatments on the activity of some hydrolytic enzymes in dog prostate. Prostate 4:383, 1983.

10. Glover, T. D.: Recent progress in the study of male reproductive physiology: testis stimulation; sperm formation, transport and maturation (epididymal physiology); semen analysis, storage and artificial insemination, In Greep, R. O. (ed.): Reproductive Physiology I. University Park Press, Baltimore, 1975.

11. Gouvelis, A., Baker, J. R., and Rosenkrantz, H.: Histochemistry of the canine prostate. Invest. Urol. 84:426, 1971.

12. Hansel, W., and McEntee, K.: Male reproductive processes. In Swenson, M. J. (ed.): Dukes' Physiology of Domestic Animals. 9th ed. Cornell University Press, Cornell, 1977.

13. Hohbach, C., Ueberberg, H., and Deutsch, H.: The functional cytomorphology of canine prostatic epithelium. Prog. Clin. Biol. Res. 75B:231, 1981.

14. Huggins, C.: The physiology of the prostate gland. Physiol. Rev. 25:281, 1945.

15. Isaacs, J. T.: Prostatic structure and function in relation to the etiology of prostatic cancer. Prostate 4:351, 1983.

16. Isaacs, J. T., Isaacs, W. B., Wheaton, L. G., and Coffey, D. S.: Differential effect of estrogen treatment on canine seminal plasma components. Invest. Urol. 17:495, 1980.

17. McDonald, L. E. (ed.): Veterinary Endocrinology and Reproduction. 3rd ed. Lea & Febiger, Philadelphia, 1980.

18. Spurgeon, T. L., Kitchell, R. L., and Lohse, C. L.: Physiologic properties of contraction of the canine cremaster and cranial preputial muscles. Am. J. Vet. Res. 39:1884, 1978.

19. Smith, E. R.: The canine prostate and its secretion. Adv. Sex Horm. Res. 1:168, 1975.

20. Smith, E. R.: The secretion of electrolytes by pilocarpine-stimulated canine prostate gland. Proc. Soc. Exp. Biol. Med. 132:223, 1969.

21. Younes, M., Evans, B. A. J. Chaisiri, N., et al.: Steroid receptors in the canine epididymis. J. Reprod. Fertil. 56:45, 1979.

22. Younes, M. A. and Pierrepoint, C. G.: Androgen steroid-receptor binding in the canine epididymis. Prostate 2:133, 1981.

Chapter 114

Pathophysiology of the Male Genital Organs

Harry W. Boothe and Dudley E. Johnston

Diseases of the male genital system can be classified as congenital, acquired traumatic, acquired non-traumatic, and degenerative. Pathophysiological mechanisms of the more common diseases of the male genital system are described in this chapter. Neoplastic disorders are covered in Chapter 181.

TESTIS, EPIDIDYMIS, AND SPERMATIC CORD

Cryptorchidism is probably the most common congenital defect of the testes. Cryptorchidism is a failure of one or both testes to descend into the scrotum at the usual time.[9]

Cryptorchidism may be an hereditary condition involving a single recessive autosomal gene.[5] Because of its atypical environment, the ectopic testis is exposed to normal body temperatures. Long-term exposure to normal body temperatures results in degeneration of the germinal epithelium. The interstitial cells (Leydig cells) and Sertoli cells, however, continue to function in the ectopic testis. Endocrine function of the ectopic testis is near normal, but exocrine function is absent.

Ectopic testes, particularly intra-abdominal testes, are more susceptible to torsion and neoplasia than descended testes.[21, 23] Presumably, the ectopic position allows greater movement of the testis than is possible in the scrotum.[21] The abnormal environment of the ectopic testis may partially explain why neoplasia, particularly Sertoli cell tumor and seminoma, is more commonly observed in the ectopic testis.[22] Neoplasms of ectopic testes are also observed at a younger age than neoplasms of descended testes.

The testis, epididymis, and spermatic cord are relatively accessible to injury. Any trauma to the testis, epididymis, or spermatic cord is potentially dangerous. Because of their well-developed blood supply, hemorrhage frequently accompanies trauma to these tissues. The expansile nature of the scrotum permits development of large hematomas following the rupture of even a small blood vessel.[5] Damage to testicular tissue can lead to leakage of sperm into the interstitial tissue and eventually the formation of sperm granulomas, which develop because of the antigenic properties of sperm. Antibodies and sensitized cells respond as they would to any foreign material and in some cases may influence spermatogenesis throughout both testes.[19] Local hyperthermia of the testes following trauma can result in temporarily or permanently reduced fertility. The traumatized testis is predisposed to infectious orchiepididymitis because of the accompanying edema and congestion.[19] Persistent licking of the traumatized scrotum and testes by the animal can aggravate the original injury.

Infection of the testis, epididymis, and spermatic cord may be acute or chronic, and unilateral or bilateral. Infection may occur by the hematogenous route, by local extension from penetrating wounds of the scrotum, by extension from infection of the intact scrotal skin, or by extension from the peritoneal cavity, urinary bladder, or prostate.[5, 17, 18] Infectious agents that have been incriminated as causal organisms include: *Brucella canis*, *Entamoeba coli*, *Proteus* sp., *streptococci*, *staphylococci*, *Mycoplasma* sp., *Norcardia* sp., *Mycobacterium tuberculosis* var. *hominis*, and canine distemper virus.[5, 20] Because of the accompanying inflammation and autoimmune reactions, testicular infection relatively rapidly results in reduced fertility or infertility.[4, 17, 20] Atrophy and fibrosis of the testes as well as fibrotic stenosis of the epididymis are possible sequelae of infection.[5]

Partial obstruction to the venous drainage of the testis can lead to the formation of a varicocele. Although uncommon in the dog, varicocele is a cause of reduced fertility.[1, 7, 17] The decreased semen quality may result from an increase in testicular temperature because of increased blood flow.[23]

PENIS

Inability to protrude the penis from the prepuce may be due to either congenital or acquired causes. Among those conditions that prevent normal penile protrusion are congenital phimosis, persistent penile frenulum, and acquired phimosis following preputial injury or neoplasia. Congenital phimosis is not common in the dog. Persistent penile frenulum may be due to hormonal imbalances, because the penile frenulum normally ruptures at puberty under androgenic influences.[2, 6] Mating is not possible if the penis cannot protrude beyond the prepuce. Pain and irritation, as well as balanoposthitis, are also seen.[6]

Inability to retract the penis completely into the prepuce also has both congenital and acquired causes. Congenital causes include a narrowed preputial orifice and an abnormally shortened prepuce. Acquired causes include trauma, infection, and priapism.[6, 17] The last is usually secondary to spinal cord injury or genitourinary infections.[17] The exteriorized penis becomes dry and congested. Licking of the exposed penis by the animal accentuates the inflammation. Severe penile damage can occur relatively quickly, particularly if the reduced size of the preputial orifice has a constrictive effect on the penis. Strangulation of the penis with necrosis due to interruption of blood supply can occur.

Because of its exposed position, the penis is relatively accessible to injury. The canine mating behavior is such that the erect penis is particularly prone to injury during the tie.[12] Injury to the cavernous tissue frequently results in profuse hemorrhage. Damage to the penile urethra can result in extrava-

sation of urine with accompanying edema and necrosis of tissue.[12] Fracture of the os penis and strangulation of the penis can also be seen following penile trauma. Licking of the penis by the animal often aggravates the injury.

Prolapse of the penile urethra is usually seen in young English bulldogs.[13, 24] Prolapse can follow genitourinary infection or excessive sexual excitement.[13] Swelling, hemorrhage, and drying of the prolapsed tissue occur relatively early, making nonsurgical management frequently unsuccessful. The patient frequently licks at the penis, perpetuating the inflammation.

PREPUCE

Traumatic and nontraumatic conditions of the prepuce usually result in clinical signs relating to exposure of the distal penis. Lack of adequate coverage of the distal penis leads to penile inflammation, drying, trauma, and even necrosis.

SCROTUM

Injury to the scrotum is possible because of its exposed location. Scrotal injury frequently stimulates licking by the animal, which results in further inflammation and possible infection. The delicacy of the scrotal skin makes it susceptible to irritants, including many disinfectants. Scrotal dermatitis results from irritation by both the disinfectant and the frequent licking by the animal. Scrotal dermatitis is also a prominent feature of *Brucella canis* infection.[11]

Non-neoplastic degenerative conditions of the scrotum are common in older dogs.[17, 18, 27] Chronic hyperplasia of the scrotum, particularly the heavily pigmented ventral aspect, probably results from chronic scrotal irritation. Fertility can be reduced because of the insulating effect of the thickened scrotum. Secondary infection may also occur. Varicosities of the scrotal veins also occur in older dogs. These varicosities are subepithelial in location, and scrotal trauma may lead to ulceration and repeated episodes of profuse hemorrhage.[17]

PROSTATE

The three pathological processes that affect the prostate gland with any frequency are benign enlargement, inflammation, and tumors. The most significant aspect of the pathophysiology of prostatic disease is the effect of hormones on the normal gland and particularly on the development of benign enlargement.

Benign enlargement of the prostate, by far the most common process, occurs so often in dogs over six years of age that it can almost be regarded as a normal aging process. There is no general agreement on the pathogenesis of prostatic enlargement. That the prostate in sexually immature dogs is small and has virtually no secretion is not in doubt. It increases rapidly in size and activity with sexual development, probably as a result of androgenic stimulation. The metabolites, 5α-reduced androgens, are probably responsible for this stimulation. The natural growth of the gland seems to be followed by a process of hyperplasia in the middle of adult life, so that the process of hyperplasia is superimposed on a gland that is already showing a steady rate of growth. When this process of hyperplasia remains within the normal limits of growth and when it produces an abnormal prostate are not known, and certainly the mechanism of stimulation is not understood.

Several terms are used to denote the clinical syndrome of benign enlargement of the prostate. The term "benign prostatic hyperplasia" is redundant, because all hyperplasias are benign, and the same comment can be made regarding "benign prostatic hypertrophy." The most acceptable term seems to be "hyperplasia of the prostate." It is an age-related disease.[28]

Although the cause of hyperplasia of the prostate is uncertain, the available evidence suggests that both androgens and estrogens are involved in its genesis.[25] The important role of the testis in the development of spontaneously occurring prostatic hyperplasia in the dog can be demonstrated by the fact that castration causes remission of the disease.[15] It is unclear whether the testis secretes a substance such as a hormone that induces hyperplasia, or whether testicular steroids simply permit the abnormal growth of prostatic cells associated with prostatic hyperplasia.

Prostatic hyperplasia has been induced by treating castrated dogs simultaneously with 5α-reduced androgens and 17β-estrodiol, which in the dog are derived from direct testicular secretion or peripheral conversion of testosterone that was produced in the testicles.[8, 9, 16, 26]

The prostate in the beagle enlarges for at least six years after birth whether normal or hyperplastic. In contrast, prostatic secretory function determined by ejaculate volume, as well as total ejaculate protein, declines markedly after four years of age. These reciprocal growth and functional changes in the prostate are closely associated with a progressive increase in the incidence of prostatic hyperplasia that is already apparent in some dogs by two years of age. With age there is a modest decrease in serum androgen levels with no apparent change in serum 17β-estrodiol levels. This finding suggests that the growth and functional changes that are associated with the development of prostatic hyperplasia and are initiated very early in life reflect an altered sensitivity of the prostate to serum androgens or a response to the relative decrease in the ratio of serum androgen to estrogen.[3]

More recent work has indicated that the natural history of prostatic hyperplasia in the dog is characterized by slow progression through two phases. The early phase of the disease, consisting of glandular hyperplasia, occurs as early as two and a half years of age. The later phase of the disease, consisting of cystic hyperplasia, occurs after four years. The testis of the beagle may secrete a potent estrogen that can eventually cause the prostate to grow permissively in response to endogenous androgens, resulting in prostatic hyperplasia.[10] Thus, many details are still unknown, but it seems reasonable to conclude that with advancing age an imbalance between the male and female sex hormones must be involved in the genesis of prostatic hyperplasia.

An additional pathological change in the canine prostate is the development of squamous metaplasia. This disorder is invariably associated with excess estrogen, which is due to a Sertoli cell tumor of the testis or is iatrogenically induced by excessive administration of estrogens. Squamous metaplasia can lead to enlargement of the prostate and in some cases to cyst production owing to obstruction of ducts by the metaplastic process.

Spontaneous prostatic hyperplasia in the dog has often been used as a model for study of nodular hyperplasia of the prostate in humans. Canine prostatic hyperplasia is characterized by diffuse epithelial or glandular proliferation throughout the prostate,[5] whereas human prostatic hyperplasia may arise specifically within the periurethral tissue and is characterized primarily by stromal hyperplasia. Although the cause and pathogenesis of the disorder in both dogs and humans are uncertain, it seems clear that hormonal factors are involved. In both humans and dogs, prostatic hyperplasia is an age-related disease,[28] and its development requires the presence of functioning testes.[15]

1. Al-Juburi, A., Pranikoff, K., Dougherty, K. A., et al.: Alteration of semen quality in dogs after creation of varicocele. Urology 13:535, 1979.
2. Balke, J.: Persistent penile frenulum in a cocker spaniel. Vet. Med. Small Anim. Clin. 76:988, 1981.
3. Brendler, C. B., Berry S. J., Ewing, L. L., et al.: Spontaneous benign prostatic hyperplasia in the beagle. Age-associated changes in serum hormone levels, and the morphology and secretory function of the canine prostate. J. Clin. Invest. 71:1114, 1983.
4. Burke, T. J.: Reproductive disorders. In Ettinger, S. J. (ed.): Textbook of Veterinary Internal Medicine. 2nd ed. W. B. Saunders, Philadelphia, 1983.
5. Burke, T. J., and Reynolds, H. A.: The testis. In Bojrab, M. J. (ed.): Pathophysiology in Small Animal Surgery. Lea & Febiger, Philadelphia, 1981.
6. Christie, T. R.: Phimosis and paraphimosis. In Bojrab, M. J. (ed.): Pathophysiology in Small Animal Surgery. Lea & Febiger, Philadelphia, 1981.
7. Dandia, S. D., Bagree, M. M., Vyas, C. P., et al.: Experimental production of varicocele and its effects on testes. Jpn. J. Surg. 9:372, 1979.
8. DeKlerk, D. P., Coffey, D. S., Ewing, L. L., et al.: Comparison of spontaneous and experimentally induced canine prostatic hyperplasia. J. Clin. Invest. 64:842, 1979.
9. Dunn, M. L., Foster, W. J., and Goddard, K. M.: Cryptorchidism in dogs: a clinical survey. J. Am. Anim. Hosp. Assoc. 4:180, 1968

10. Ewing, L. L., Thompson, D. J., Jr., Cochran, R. C., et al.: Testicular androgen and estrogen secretion and benign prostatic hyperplasia in the beagle. Endocrinology *114*:1308, 1984.

11. George, L. W., Duncan, J. R., and Carmichael, L. E.: Semen examination in dogs with canine brucellosis. Am. J. Vet. Res. *40*:1589, 1979.

12. Hall, M. A., and Swenberg, L. N.: Genital emergencies. *In* Kirk, R. W. (ed.): *Current Veterinary Therapy VI: Small Animal Practice.* W. B. Saunders, Philadelphia, 1977.

13. Hobson, H. P., and Heller, R. A.: Surgical correction of prolapse of the male urethra. Vet. Med. Small Anim. Clin. *66*:1177, 1971.

14. Huggins, C.: The etiology of benign prostatic hypertrophy. Bull. N.Y. Acad. Med. *23*:696, 1947.

15. Huggins, C., and Clark, P. J.: Quantitative studies of the prostatic secretion. II. The effect of castration and of estrogen injection on the normal and on the hyperplastic prostate glands of dogs. J. Exp. Med. *72*:747, 1940.

16. Jacobi, G. H., Moore, R. J., and Wilson, J. D.: Studies on the mechanism of 3α-androstanediol-induced growth of the dog prostate. Endocrinology *102*:1748, 1978.

17. Johnston, D. E., and Archibald, J.: Male genital system. *In* Archibald, J. (ed.): *Canine Surgery.* 2nd ed. American Veterinary Publications Inc., Santa Barbara, 1974.

18. Jubb, K. V. F., and Kennedy, P. C. (eds.): *Pathology of Domestic Animals.* Academic Press, New York, 1970.

19. Larsen, R. E.: Evaluation of fertility problems in the male dog. Vet. Clin. North Am. Small Anim. Pract. 7:735, 1977.

20. Lein, D. H.: Canine orchitis. *In* Kirk, R. W. (ed.): *Current Veterinary Therapy VI: Small Animal Practice.* W. B. Saunders, Philadelphia, 1977.

21. Pearson, H., and Kelly, D. F.: Testicular torsion in the dog: a review of 13 cases. Vet. Rec. *97*:200, 1975.

22. Reif, J. S., and Brodey, R. S.: The relationship between cryptorchidism and canine testicular neoplasia. J. Am. Vet. Med. Assoc. *155*:2005, 1969.

23. Saypol, D. C., Howards, S. S., Turner, T. T., and Miller, E. D., Jr.: Influence of surgically induced varicocele on testicular blood flow, temperature, and histology in adult rats and dogs. J. Clin. Invest. *68*:39, 1981.

24. Sinibaldi, K. R., and Green, R. W.: Surgical correction of prolapse of the male urethra in three English bulldogs. J. Am. Anim. Hosp. Assoc. *9*:450, 1973.

25. Tveter, K. J.: Some aspects of the pathogenesis of prostatic hyperplasia. Acta Pathol. Microbiol. Scand. *248*:167, 1974.

26. Walsh, P. C., and Wilson, J. D.: The induction of prostatic hypertrophy in the dog with androstanediol. J. Clin. Invest. *57*:1093, 1976.

27. Werpers, W. L., and Jarrett, W. F. H.: Haemangioma of the scrotum of dogs. Vet. Rec. *66*:106, 1954.

28. Zuckerman, S., and McKeown, T.: The canine prostate in relation to normal and abnormal testicular changes. J. Pathol. Bacteriol. *46*:7, 1938.

Chapter 115

Diagnostic and Biopsy Techniques—Male Genital Organs

Dudley E. Johnston and Harry W. Boothe

Many of the diagnostic techniques employed in the investigation of the male genital system are identical to techniques used in other body systems. Specific techniques for the male genital system are discussed in more detail.

History and Physical Examination

A complete history should be obtained for most problems of the male genital system. If infertility is the presenting complaint, attention should be given to the breeding history of the patient.[2, 3] The history should enable one to distinguish between secondary sterility, resulting from inability to copulate, and primary sterility.[2] A complete physical examination to detect other systemic diseases should be performed. The scrotum, testes, epididymides, spermatic cords, and prostate are carefully palpated. Prostatic palpation is not usually performed in the cat. The size, shape, and consistency of each structure and swellings, tenderness, or varicosities are noted.

The penis is withdrawn from the prepuce and examined. Inspection of the preputial reflection may require sedation.

Radiography and Laboratory Studies

Radiographic examination of the male genital system is utilized for conditions of the urethra, os penis, and prostate. Hormonal assays, including progesterone, estrogen, and testosterone assays, may be useful in the investigation of infertility. Thyroid function testing should also be performed in males with subnormal sexual function. Serologic testing for *Brucella canis* is widely available and should be included as part of the evaluation of the male genital system.

Semen Evaluation

Semen evaluation is an important part of fertility evaluation. Semen may be collected by manual manipulation or by electroejaculation. Electroejaculation techniques have been developed for the cat.[14] Manual collection in the dog may require the presence of a teaser bitch.[3, 11] Semen should be collected in a sterile container that is free of any chemical agents. Motility, numbers, and morphology of sperm should be determined. Morphology should be evaluated for primary, secondary, and tertiary abnormalities.[14] Bacterial culture and antibiotic susceptibility testing of the semen is also recommended.

Testicular Biopsy

Testicular biopsy provides the most precise information on the condition of the seminiferous epithelium.[11] In humans, quantitative testicular biopsy correlates closely with sperm count in the absence of obstruction.[17] Usually, only one testis is sampled. Although biopsy of only one testis carries the inherent risk that a localized lesion will be missed, unilateral testicular biopsy in man provides diagnostic information equal to that yielded by bilateral biopsy in the majority of cases.[11] A number of biopsy techniques are available, including incisional, needle punch, and aspiration biopsy.[5, 9, 12]

Incisional techniques are less likely to result in architectural disruption than the other biopsy methods.[3, 5, 12] Incisional biopsy is performed under anesthesia and after preparation of the antescrotal area for aseptic surgery. An antescrotal skin incision is used. The testis is positioned with the epididymis away from the incision. The parietal vaginal tunic is incised with a scalpel blade. The tunica albuginea is incised with a sterile, thin razor blade, with care taken to avoid blood vessels. The razor blade is used to excise the bulging testicular tissue (Fig. 115–1). If bulging of the testicular tissue does not occur, a wedge of tissue should be taken by more deeply incising the parenchyma. The tunica albuginea and parietal vaginal tunic should be closed separately with fine synthetic absorbable sutures. The skin is closed with fine nonabsorbable sutures.

Percutaneous needle punch biopsy of the testis provides adequate tissue for diagnostic histological examination of the seminiferous epithelium.[5, 9, 20] The amount of tissue obtained is inferior to that obtained by incisional techniques and is insufficient for detailed assessment of spermatogenesis.[9] General anesthesia is usually required for testicular punch biopsy. Franklin-modified Vim-Silverman needles and Menghini needles have been used successfully.[5, 9] A small scrotal incision is made and the needle is inserted into the body of the testis. Aspiration with a syringe may be necessary to obtain the biopsy specimen. Digital pressure is applied to the testis over the biopsy site for one to two minutes. The wound is not sutured.

Aspiration biopsy of the testis is easier to perform than the other methods and does not usually require general or local anesthesia. Sufficient biopsy material

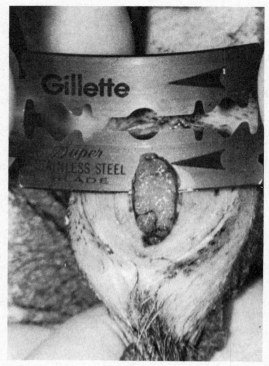

Figure 115–1. The scoop method of testicular biopsy using a razor blade. (Reprinted with permission from Burke, T. J.: Reproductive disorders. *In* Ettinger, S. J. (ed.): *Textbook of Veterinary Internal Medicine.* 2nd ed. W. B. Saunders, Philadelphia, 1983.)

is obtained to differentiate inflammatory from noninflammatory disease.[5] A 5-ml syringe and 22- or 23-gauge needle are used. After gentle surgical preparation of the scrotum, the needle is introduced into the body of the testis. Two or three passes may be necessary while the plunger is retracted. The syringe plunger is carefully released prior to withdrawal of the needle from the testis. Digital pressure is applied to the biopsy site for one to two minutes.

Testicular tissue specimens should not be placed in formalin solution, because it causes tubular shrinkage and poor nuclear detail. Bouin's, Stieve's, or Zenker's fixative should be used.[12] Possible complications of testicular biopsy include hemorrhage, infection, local hyperthermia, scarring, adhesions, and atrophy.[9, 12] A temporary, slight decrease in sperm count may be associated with biopsy of the testes.[9] This decrease may be due to local hyperthermia or an antigen-antibody reaction initiated by liberation of sperm antigen at biopsy.[5]

Epididymal biopsy is usually not performed because of the likelihood of postoperative obstruction. Epididymal obstruction in humans is treated by anastomosing the ductus (vas) deferens to the epididymis (vasoepididymostomy) proximal to the obstruction. A microscopic technique for anastomosing the ductus (vas) deferens directly to the epididymal tubule has been described.[15, 16] Such a technique could be utilized in the dog; however, it is not known what portions of the canine epididymis are necessary for sperm maturation.[11] With the possible exception of the ductus deferens, the spermatic cord is usually not sampled for biopsy. Following biopsy of the ductus deferens, microsurgical anastomosis (vasovasotomy) using a single-layer penetrating suture is recommended.[4, 10] Improved results of vasovasotomy in dogs have been demonstrated if the nerves of the ductus deferens are spared during vasectomy.[5]

Because of their accessible location, biopsy of the penis, prepuce, and scrotum is usually performed by fine-needle aspiration or impression smear. Excisional biopsy techniques can also be employed. Hemorrhage following penile biopsy is controlled by ligation and suturing of the tunica albuginea and penile mucosa separately with fine absorbable material. Full-thickness preputial biopsy sites are closed in two layers. Excisional biopsies of the scrotum should not traumatize the parietal vaginal tunic of the testes.

PROSTATE

When evaluating prostatic disease in the dog, the clinician first determines whether the prostate gland is diseased and is the cause of the clinical syndrome, and secondly differentiates between the various pathological processes that can occur within the gland. On the one hand, the prostate gland can be innocently incriminated as the cause of clinical signs in dogs, and on the other hand, it can be overlooked when it is diseased. The term "prostatitis" is frequently used to denote any enlargement of the prostate, and no attempt is made to distinguish among the various causes of enlargement. In general, a diseased prostate gland in the dog is seen as an enlarged gland, and therefore the clinician's responsibility is to differentiate between the various causes of prostatic enlargement. O'Shea[13a] in 1962 examined 240 unselected adult dogs and showed a wide range of variation in the relative weight of the prostate gland in different individuals. In each year of life there is a wide variation, even among prostates of similar structure. It must be presumed that these glands are within normal limits, and yet the clinician is faced with the problem of determining whether a gland is normal in size when it can show such wide variation. For example, in German shepherds, the relative weight of the prostate in grams per kilogram of body weight varies from 0.18 to 5.6. The weight of the prostate is of little assistance to the clinician in evaluating the prostate; the dimensions of the gland are more important. Unfortunately, little work has been done on the dimensions of the normal gland, and in certain breeds, notably the Scottish terrier, the relative prostate weight is significantly different from that in other breeds. The mean relative weight of the prostate in seven Scottish terriers in O'Shea's series was approximately four times as great as the mean of all other adult dogs.

Palpation of the Prostate

The prostate gland is originally an abdominal organ, becomes a pelvic organ in young puppies, and assumes a position at the rim of the pelvis or in the abdomen in adult dogs. Therefore, it assumes an abdominal location as enlargement occurs, whether this enlargement is due to the normal hypertrophy of the gland or to a disease entity. The prostate should be examined by rectal and abdominal palpation. When it is within the pelvic canal, the gland can usually be examined by inserting a finger into the pelvic canal per rectum. However, it may be necessary to use the other hand to push upwards on the caudal abdomen, in order to displace its contents towards the pelvic inlet and displace the gland caudally to the examining finger in the rectum.

The size, shape, surface texture, position, and consistency of the gland should be evaluated with the finger. The prostate gland is normally symmetrical, with right and left lobes separated by a shallow dorsal groove. The surface should be smooth, and the consistency uniform and slightly spongy.

Palpation of the normal prostate is not painful, but the dog can experience pain because of the presence of the examining finger distending the anus and anal sphincter. The examining finger should come to rest on the surface of the prostate, and the clinician should delay further evaluation of pain response until the dog accepts the presence of the examining finger. Then, careful digital pressure is applied directly to the gland to evaluate pain. A pain response is commonly seen with prostatitis and prostatic neoplasia.

Radiography

The normal prostate usually cannot be seen on survey radiographs because of the overlying pelvic bone and muscle mass of the thigh. With advancing age or disease, the gland becomes larger and advances cranially into the abdomen. In these cases, a mass of soft tissue density can be seen between the pelvic inlet and the urinary bladder, and one should assume that this mass is the prostate gland unless proven otherwise.

In many cases, radiography indicates only that the prostate is enlarged and is not helpful in distinguishing between the various disease processes. However, in selected instances, useful information can be obtained concerning the differential diagnosis of the prostatic enlargement. Calcification of the prostate that is seen occasionally in inflammatory and neoplastic diseases can be seen radiographically. Prostatic calculi, a rare phenomenon, can usually be seen on survey radiographs. The size of the gland as determined radiographically can occasionally be of value. The mean normalized area values for hyperplastic and inflammatory prostatic disease do not differ. Also, the mean normalized area values for cystic and neoplastic prostates are similar. However, the mean normalized area values for prostatic cysts and neoplasms can be significantly larger than for hyperplastic and inflammatory prostatic disease. In addition, the prostate is more symmetrical in circumference in hyperplastic and inflammatory disease than in cystic and neoplastic prostatic disease. Prostatic cysts and neoplasms also tend to be asymmetrical not only in circumference but also in relation to the prostatic urethra.[11]

Urethrograms, cystograms, and cystourethrograms can be useful in evaluating the presence and cause of prostatic enlargement. In some cases there is a large, vaguely defined soft tissue mass in the caudal abdomen, and it is not possible in survey radiographs to differentiate the urinary bladder from the prostate. Injection of contrast material can outline the urinary bladder, show the position of the urethra in relation to the prostatic mass, and reveal the presence or absence of reflux of contrast material into the prostate. Reflux into the prostate probably does not occur in most normal dogs. However, all four prostatic disease processes can be associated with reflux of contrast material into the parenchyma. Therefore prostatic reflux of contrast material is not helpful in distinguishing among the various prostatic disease processes.[11]

Prostatic neoplasms can invade the pubis and vertebral bodies, and osseous destructive or productive lesions can be seen radiographically.

Evaluation of Prostatic Fluids

Examination of fluid from the prostate is generally regarded as a valuable means of evaluating prostatic pathology. Prostatic massage is a common method of obtaining prostatic fluid in humans, but it has limited application in the dog because of technical difficulties. The small volume of fluid in the dog is difficult to obtain as well as to differentiate from urethral and bladder debris.

In dogs, the usual technique for prostatic massage begins with tranquilization. With aseptic technique, a urethral catheter is inserted into the bladder. Aseptic technique involves using a sterile catheter after cleaning the exteriorized penis with soap and water. It is probably preferable to avoid antiseptic agents that could be carried in with the catheter and inhibit growth of microorganisms in the sample. After the catheter is passed into the bladder, all urine is removed. The bladder can be flushed with 5 ml of sterile saline solution, and this fluid can be aspirated to be compared with a later sample obtained by prostatic massage. The catheter is retracted until rectal palpation indicates that the tip is immediately caudal to the prostate gland. The prostate is then massaged rectally. Another 5 ml of sterile saline solution is injected into the catheter while the urethra is gently occluded around the catheter to prevent retrograde loss of the sample. The catheter is slowly advanced into the bladder as aspiration is done.

It is probably necessary in this test to compare the pre- and post-massage samples bacteriologically and cytologically, to differentiate disease of the prostate from disease of other areas of the urinary tract. More accurate results from prostatic massage may be possible through use of an alternative technique. Prior to taking of a sample, the dog should be allowed to urinate to clear the urethra of debris. The tip of the penis is removed from the prepuce and gently washed with soap and water; however, a catheter is not used. While the penis is protruding, the prostate is massaged rectally, and fluid dripping from the urethral orifice is collected in a sterile container. Unfortunately, it is not always possible to obtain samples of prostatic fluid by this means.[3, 4]

Ejaculation of the dog may be a more reliable method of obtaining prostatic fluid than prostatic massage. The ejaculate should be obtained as cleanly as possible after exteriorizing and washing the exposed penis. The ejaculate is collected in a sterile container. It may be partially fractionated if desired. In normal dogs the clear fluid obtained during the terminal part of ejaculation has a higher content of prostatic fluid. However, complete separation of testicular and prostatic components of the semen is not possible.

Cytological examination and bacterial cultures are usually done on the prostatic massage fluids or the ejaculate. Abnormalities in the fluid can originate from the urethra, prostate, ductus deferens, epididymis, or testicle, and contamination from the prepuce can occur. Standard bacteriological culture methods are used. In one evaluation of clinically normal aging dogs, bacteria of several species, primarily gram-positive cocci, were isolated from ejaculates in 11 of 18 dogs.[1] The concentration of bacteria varied from 550/ml to more than 100,000/ml. The large numbers of organisms isolated from a few dogs indicate that one must interpret the results of culture of ejaculates cautiously when trying to determine whether prostatic infection is present. It is likely that bacteriological culture is useful only to verify the presence of prostatitis that has been diagnosed by other means and also to indicate the type of bacteria and their antibiotic susceptibility. In the same 18 dogs, massaging the prostate was not associated with recovery of bacteria.[1]

The ejaculate or prostatic fluid may be examined cytologically. In general, the procedure involves air-drying the slides, staining with new methylene blue or Wright's stain, and examining for evidence of inflammation or presence of bacteria. Generally, only a few white blood cells per high-power field are present and bacteria are not seen. In addition, examination of semen or prostatic fluid for neoplastic cells of prostatic origin can also be done, although negative results do not rule out prostatic neoplasia.

Prostatic Biopsy

Both percutaneous fine-needle aspiration biopsy and needle punch biopsy can be done on the enlarged canine prostate. In addition, incisional biopsy can be done during a laparotomy. Techniques for prostatic aspiration and biopsy in dogs have been described, and some complications have been reported. [4, 5, 9, 10, 19]

Fine-needle aspiration biopsy is the simplest and safest of the three biopsy techniques. However, the specimen obtained is not adequate for tissue section. The aspirate can be examined cytologically and cultured for bacteria. The enlarged prostate gland must be adequately immobilized for a transperineal or transabdominal approach, depending on the location of the gland. For transperineal biopsy, an assistant forces the prostate caudally by abdominal palpation while the operator performs the rectal examination and the aspiration biopsy. The area lateral to the anus is surgically prepared, and a 22-gauge spinal needle of appropriate length is inserted through the skin and parallel to the rectum. The needle is guided to the prostate gland, the stylus is removed, a syringe is attached, and aspiration is performed as the needle is advanced into the gland. If fluid is not obtained, aspiration is continued as the needle is retracted and advanced through the tissue of the prostate three or four times. For transabdominal aspiration biopsy, the dog is placed in lateral recumbency, and the enlarged prostate gland is fixed by abdominal manipulation and brought as close to the body wall as possible. The aspirate is obtained in the same manner as for transperineal biopsy.

Punch biopsy of the prostate is done using a Trucut disposable biopsy needle.* The biopsy is obtained either transperineally or transabdominally as described for aspiration biopsy. Generally, sufficient material is obtained for histological section. [2, 3, 10, 19]

Potential complications of biopsy include dissemination of infection, hemorrhage, and urethral fistula formation. Complications from the procedure have been few and have included hematuria and mild periprostatic hemorrhage. Urethral fistulae have not been seen in spite of penetration of the urethra during the biopsy procedure. If prostatitis or prostatic abscess is suspected, fine-needle aspiration should be done instead of punch biopsy.

Biopsy after exposure of the gland at laparotomy has the advantage of thorough examination of the prostate and selection of the biopsy site. The urethra should not be penetrated during the incisional biopsy, and the opening in the prostate should not be closed with nonabsorbable sutures, which could act as a nidus for infection.

Other Tests for Prostatic Disease

In humans, several tests have been evaluated for preliminary screening and for definitive diagnosis of prostate disease, especially carcinomas. These tests fall into two main categories: first, measurement of enzymes, including acid phosphatase and lactic de-

hydrogenase V/1 ratio, and second, imaging procedures such as ultrasonography and nuclear magnetic resonance. In 1980, a survey of the results of screening tests for prostatic carcinoma in humans indicated that rectal examination was more accurate than nine other more sophisticated and more costly procedures. [8]

The new physical imaging procedures will probably prove to be more accurate and useful than present tests, including radiography. In particular, it should be possible to detect early the presence of a nodule, which could be neoplastic, or a cyst, either of which could be deep within the gland and undetectable by present means.

1. Barsanti, J. A.: Evaluation of diagnostic techniques for canine prostatic diseases. J. Am. Vet. Med. Assoc. 177:160, 1980.
2. Burke, T. J.: Sterility in the male. In Bojrab, M. J. (ed.): Pathophysiology in Small Animal Surgery. Lea & Febiger, Philadelphia, 1981.
3. Burke, T. J.: Reproductive disorders. In Ettinger, S. J. (ed.): Textbook of Veterinary Internal Medicine. 2nd ed. W. B. Saunders, Philadelphia, 1983.
4. Esk, P. C., and Pabst, R.: Improved results of vasovasostomy after sparing of nerves during vasectomy. Fertil. Steril. 35:363, 1981.
5. Finco, D. R.: Biopsy of the testicle. Vet. Clin. North Am. 4:377, 1974.
6. Finco, D. R.: Diseases of the prostate gland of the dog. In Morrow, D. A. (ed.): Current Therapy in Theriogenology. W. B. Saunders, Philadelphia, 1980.
7. Finco, D. R.: Prostate gland biopsy. Vet. Clin. North Am. 4:367, 1974.
8. Guinan, P., and Bush, I.: The accuracy of the rectal examination in the diagnosis of prostate carcinoma. N. Engl. J. Med. 303:499, 1980.
9. James, R. W., Heywood, R., and Fowler, D. J.: Serial percutaneous testicular biopsy in the beagle dog. J. Small Anim. Pract. 20:219, 1979.
10. Lamesch, A. J., and Doctu, N.: Microsurgical vasovasostomy. Eur. Surg. Res. 13:299, 1981.
11. Larsen, R. E.: Evaluation of fertility problems in the male dog. Vet. Clin. North Am. 7:735, 1977.
12. Larsen, R. E.: Testicular biopsy in the dog. Vet. Clin. North Am. 7:747, 1977.
13. Leeds, E. B., and Leav, I.: Perineal punch biopsy of the canine prostate gland. J. Am. Vet. Med. Assoc. 154:925, 1969.
13a. O'Shea, J. D.: Studies on the canine prostate gland. J. Comp. Pathol. Ther. 72:321, 1962.
14. Platz, C. C., Jr., and Seager, S. W. J.: Semen collection by electroejaculation in the domestic cat. J. Am. Vet. Med. Assoc. 173:1353, 1978.
15. Silber, S. J.: Microscopic vasoepididymostomy: specific microanastomosis to the epididymal tubule. Fertil. Steril. 30:566, 1978.
16. Silber, S. J.: Reversal of vasectomy and the treatment of male fertility; role of microsurgery, vasoepididymostomy, and pressure-induced changes of vasectomy. Urol. Clin. North Am. 8:53, 1981.
17. Silber, S. J., and Rodriguez-Rigau, L. J.: Quantitative analysis of testicle biopsy: determination of partial obstruction and prediction of sperm count after surgery for obstruction. Fertil. Steril. 36:480, 1981.
18. Stone, E. A.: Radiographic interpretation of prostatic disease in the dog. J. Am. Anim. Hosp. Assoc. 14:115, 1978.
19. Weaver, A. D.: Transperineal punch biopsy of the canine prostate gland. J. Small Anim. Pract. 18:573, 1977.
20. Wilson, G. P.: Surgery of the male reproductive tract. Vet. Clin. North Am. 5:537, 1975.

*Travenol Laboratories, Inc., Deerfield, IL.

Chapter 116 Testis, Epididymis, and Spermatic Cord

Harry W. Boothe

TESTIS

Anorchism and Monorchism

Congenital absence of both testes in small animals is rare.[2] Monorchism is reported, usually the left testis being absent.[17] Diagnosis of these conditions is made by careful palpation of the scrotum and inguinal region and exploratory celiotomy. A thorough search of the abdomen should be performed to establish the lack of one or both testes, epididymides, and ductus deferentes.

Testicular Hypoplasia

Testicular hypoplasia may be present unilaterally or bilaterally. Hypoplastic testes are usually freely movable within the scrotum and may be difficult to palpate, particularly in the obese patient. The testes are usually of normal or soft consistency. When accompanied by excessive connective tissue, however, the hypoplastic testis is firmer than normal.[18] Testicular hypoplasia with normal Leydig (interstitial) cell function probably occurs in the dog. However, hypoplasia of both the interstitial cells and the germinal epithelium may also be seen. Some dogs with testicular hypoplasia exhibit signs of feminization.

Cryptorchidism

Cryptorchidism is a failure of one or both testes to descend into the scrotum at the usual time.[10] The usual time of testicular descent is at birth, although descent may occur normally at any time up to six months of age. This condition may be unilateral or bilateral, and the position of the ectopic testis may be prescrotal, inguinal, or abdominal.[10] Unilateral cryptorchidism is more common, with the right testis being more commonly undescended.[10, 30] The ectopic testis is probably more commonly located in the abdomen than in the inguinal region.[8, 29] The reported incidence of canine cryptorchidism varies widely from 0.8 per cent for a large study of dogs of all ages to 10 per cent for a smaller study of dogs at least six months of age.[8]

Diagnosis of cryptorchidism, particularly in a young pup, may be difficult. Testes may be located in the scrotum but be difficult to palpate because of their small size, especially in the obese pup. Testes may also be freely movable between the scrotum and inguinal canal. A final diagnosis of cryptorchidism should not be made until the dog is approximately six months of age.[3, 10] Ectopic testes, unless tumorous or diseased, are uniformly smaller than descended testes. Locating an extra-abdominal ectopic testis by palpation is usually possible, although often difficult. Intra-abdominal ectopic testes are usually palpable only when enlarged.

Cryptorchidism is more common in the chihuahua, miniature schnauzer, Pomeranian, poodle, Shetland sheepdog, Siberian husky, and Yorkshire terrier.[27] Small breeds have a 2.7 times greater risk of cryptorchidism than other breeds.[27] The genetic basis of canine cryptorchidism is unclear. The hereditary nature of this problem in the miniature schnauzer has been discussed.[8]

Undescended testes fail to develop a germinal epithelium. The interstitial cells, however, continue to function. Androgen is produced by the ectopic testis in near-normal amounts. No spermatozoa are produced because of the elevated temperature of the abnormal testicular environment.[18] Secondary characteristics develop normally, even in the bilateral cryptorchid.

Both torsion and neoplasia are more commonly observed in the undescended testis, particularly the intra-abdominal testis.[11, 24, 26, 29, 34] Torsion occurs because the intra-abdominal site presumably allows greater movement of the testis than is possible in the scrotum (see "Spermatic Cord Torsion").[26] There is also a strong association between cryptorchidism and testicular neoplasia in the dog. Cryptorchid dogs have a risk of testicular tumors 13.6 times that of normal dogs.[15] Approximately 50 per cent of the Sertoli cell tumors (58 of 108) and 33 per cent of the seminomas (23 of 68) occurred in cryptorchid testes in one study of canine testicular neoplasia, compared with 10.2 per cent and 11.8 per cent, respectively, in breed-matched noncryptorchid control dogs.[29] Dogs developed neoplasms in cryptorchid testes at a younger age than dogs with descended testes. Signs of feminization have also been more commonly observed with Sertoli cell tumors of cryptorchid testes than of scrotal testes.[23, 29]

Treatment

Medical and surgical attempts to move the ectopic testes into the scrotum have been largely unsuccessful in the dog.[34] Orchiopexy is not condoned in veterinary medicine because of the heritable nature of cryptorchidism.[6] Although the incidence of testicular neoplasia in dogs is unknown, the higher risk of neoplasia in cryptorchid testes may justify the prophylactic removal of the undescended testis. The high incidence of multiple tumors of more than one histological type in the same or opposite testis justifies bilateral orchidectomy.[6] Another advantage of performing early bilateral orchidectomy in the unilaterally cryptorchid dog is to decrease the possibility of perpetuating the defect.

The surgical technique for removal of the cryptorchid testis varies with its location. The extra-abdominal ectopic testis is removed by the usual technique. The intra-abdominal testis is generally approached from a ventral median abdominal incision. The location of the retained testis can be determined by tracing (1) the ductus deferens from its prostatic termination to the testis, (2) the testicular artery from its aortic origin to the testis, (3) the testicular vein from its termination in the caudal vena cava (or left renal vein) to the testis, or (4) the gubernaculum testis to the testis. Once located, the vessels and ductus deferens are doubly ligated and divided. Histological evaluation of the testes should be performed.

Prognosis following castration of the cryptorchid dog is generally good even with testicular neoplasia. Testicular neoplasms are generally benign, and the incidence of observed metastases is low (see Chapter 181).[6, 23]

Orchitis

Orchitis in the dog is not uncommon and is frequently accompanied by epididymitis. Infection reaches the testis most commonly by reflux along the vas deferens from the urinary bladder, urethra, or prostate.[17, 18] Bacterial organisms frequently found are *Escherichia coli, Proteus vulgaris,* staphylococci, and streptococci.[22] Although not a common feature, orchitis may be seen in *Brucella canis* infection.[12] Penetrating wounds of the scrotum may also result in orchitis.

Acute orchitis is usually suppurative, with the formation of one or more abscesses in the testis and epididymis. Involvement of the parietal vaginal tunic in the inflammatory process may result in formation of a fistula through the scrotal skin to the exterior.[18] In chronic orchitis, the testis may be completely atrophied or firm and fibrotic. The scrotal contents usually adhere to the tunics and cannot be moved freely.[22]

Clinical signs of acute orchitis include testicular pain and tenseness and scrotal edema. Abscess of the testis and scrotum may be noted. Systemic signs of infection, including leukocytosis, pyrexia, and listlessness, may be present. Signs of chronic orchitis are usually limited to the finding of a small, firm, irregular testis with an enlarged epididymis.[18] Adhesions between the parietal and visceral vaginal tunics may occur. Fibrosis of the epididymis can result in spermatocele formation. Fertility is reduced in both acute and chronic orchitis because of thermal degeneration and autoimmune reactions.[5, 22] Bilateral involvement eventually leads to sterility.[17] Diagnosis is made by physical examination, cytological and bacteriological examination of the semen, and, possibly, serologic examination.[22]

Treatment

Treatment of orchitis depends on the extent of involvement and the breeding usefulness of the dog. Severely traumatized or abscessed testes are surgically removed. Removal of chronically inflamed testes is justified to prevent continuing episodes of acute inflammation.[6] Antibacterial drugs, local hypothermia, and, possibly, anti-inflammatory drugs are used to treat less severe orchitis.[5] Primary foci of infection elsewhere in the urogenital tract should be eliminated. Local treatment of sinus tracts in the parietal tunic and scrotum involves excision, drainage, and flushing with an appropriate antibiotic. Prognosis for maintaining fertility is guarded. Orchitis is quite resistant to antibiotic or chemotherapeutic treatment. Orchidectomy is usually the treatment of choice, particularly if the patient is not a valuable breeding dog.[22]

Testicular Trauma

Despite their exposed location, testes are not commonly traumatized in small animals. They may be injured by either blunt trauma or penetrating wounds. Minor blunt testicular trauma is accompanied by temporary pain, mild swelling, and bruising of the testis and scrotum. More severe blunt trauma may result in local hemorrhage and rupture of the tunica albuginea, and massive scrotal hematoma may occur because of the expansile nature of the tissue.[6] Penetrating wounds frequently cause hemorrhage and may lead to local infection. Leakage of sperm following a penetrating wound may lead to spermatic granulomas after the original injury has healed.

Diagnosis of testicular trauma is made on physical examination. Scrotal lesions are not consistently present in mild testicular trauma. Local pain and swelling of the testis with possible hindlimb lameness are usually seen. More severe lesions of the testes are usually accompanied by swelling and bruising of the scrotum. Rupture of the tunica albuginea may be difficult to detect because of swelling of the scrotum and testis. Careful palpation often reveals an abnormal testicular contour.[B] Swelling, local hypothermia, loss of sensation, and blue discoloration of the scrotum are grave signs indicating irreversible damage from ischemia.[6]

Treatment

Medical treatment is indicated for minor testicular trauma. Local hypothermia, possibly supportive bandaging, and the administration of antibiotics and corticosteroids are often used. Analgesics and diuretics may also be indicated. Fluid accumulations should be aseptically aspirated. If blood refills the scrotum, surgical exploration should be considered for hemostasis.[6] Rupture of the tunica albuginea should be surgically corrected if unaccompanied by infection. Severe testicular trauma often requires unilateral or bilateral orchidectomy. Scrotal ablation may also be necessary. Orchidectomy should be delayed until the injury can be assessed.[17]

Surgical exploration of the scrotum is performed by longitudinally incising the cranial aspect of the scrotum. Following removal of the fluid accumulations, a systematic search of the scrotum and testes is performed. The parietal vaginal tunic may be incised to repair wounds of the tunica albuginea. If orchidectomy is not indicated, bleeding vessels should be ligated with fine synthetic absorbable sutures. Tears in the tunica albuginea are sutured with fine synthetic absorbable sutures following excision of the protruding testicular tissue and thorough lavage with physiological saline. The parietal vaginal tunic and scrotum are closed separately with fine sutures. Appropriate antibiotics should be continued postoperatively.

Orchidectomy should be performed when pain, swelling, or local hyperthermia persists following trauma.[6] A midline skin incision is made just cranial to the scrotum. The affected testis is exteriorized through this incision by exerting digital pressure on the caudal scrotum.

Testicular Tumors

Testicular tumors occur commonly, particularly in the older dog (see also Chapter 181).[18] After skin tumors, testicular tumors are the second most frequently reported tumor in the male dog.[15] The three common neoplasms are seminoma, interstitial cell tumor, and Sertoli cell tumor, with about equal frequency.[15] They can occur individually, although a combination of two or more tumors in a testis is common.[17]

Palpation may be helpful in diagnosing tumors of the testes. The finding of a firm, nodular, and possibly enlarged scrotal testis is suspicious for neoplasia. An enlarged intra-abdominal testis may also be neoplastic. Some testicular tumors cannot be detected by palpation,[17] and others cause pain or signs of feminization.[4] Differential diagnoses include torsion of the spermatic cord, testicular and spermatic cord trauma, orchitis, epididymitis, spermatocele, scrotal hernia, and scrotal neoplasia.

Biopsy of the testis, or unilateral orchidectomy with biopsy, is the method of definitive diagnosis. Excisional wedge biopsy of the testis away from the epididymis is preferred to percutaneous needle techniques.[5] The chance of adhesions following testicular wedge biopsy can be reduced by slightly rotating the testis after incision through the parietal vaginal tunic but before opening the tunica albuginea.[21] Control of hemorrhage is usually accomplished with digital pressure and closure of the tunica albuginea. Less hemorrhage is encountered if a prescrotal incision rather than a scrotal incision is made.[5]

Orchidectomy

Orchidectomy in the Dog

Canine orchidectomy can be performed by either open or closed methods. Both methods use a midline prescrotal skin incision (Fig. 116–1A). The testis is pushed cranially to the skin incision, and the subcutaneous tissue is incised over the testis (Fig. 116–1B).

The first (open) method involves incision through the parietal vaginal tunic (Fig. 116–2A). Once the testis is exteriorized, the tunics are separated from the rest of the spermatic cord (Fig. 116–2B). Each is double-ligated with absorbable suture. Transfixation ligation is recommended (Fig. 116–2C).

The second (closed) method involves incision to the parietal vaginal tunic.[28] The testis is exteriorized (Fig. 116–3A) and freed from its scrotal attachment by incising the ligament of the tail of the epididymis

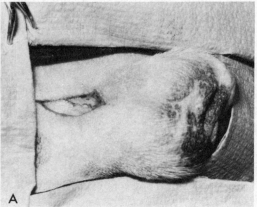
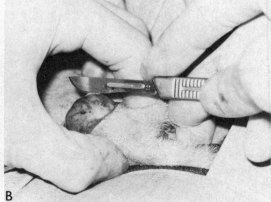

Figure 116–1. Canine orchidectomy. *A*, A prescrotal skin incision is made. *B*, The testis is pushed cranially to the skin incision. The subcutaneous tissue is incised over the testis.

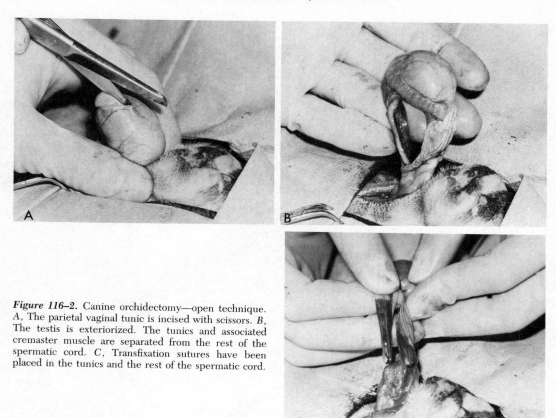

Figure 116–2. Canine orchidectomy—open technique. *A,* The parietal vaginal tunic is incised with scissors. *B,* The testis is exteriorized. The tunics and associated cremaster muscle are separated from the rest of the spermatic cord. *C,* Transfixation sutures have been placed in the tunics and the rest of the spermatic cord.

close to the testis (Fig. 116–3*B*). Fat and fascia surrounding the parietal vaginal tunic are reflected using a gauze sponge (Fig. 116–3*C*), enabling maximal exteriorization of the testis and spermatic cord (Fig. 116–3*D*). The spermatic cord with its vaginal tunics is double-ligated using two transfixation ligatures. The needle can be safely inserted through the spermatic cord between the cremaster muscle and the ductus deferens (Fig. 116–3*E* to *G*). The spermatic cord is transected distal to the ligature and returned to the inguinal region (Fig. 116–3*H*).

The other testis is removed in the same manner and through the same skin incision, if indicated. The subcutaneous tissues are closed with 3-0 absorbable suture material. The skin may be closed with nonabsorbable, interrupted sutures or by a subcuticular pattern of 3-0 absorbable suture material.

Orchidectomy in the Cat

Feline orchidectomy is usually performed by making a separate longitudinal scrotal incision over each testis (Fig. 116–4*A*). The testis is pushed caudally to the skin incision, and the subcutaneous tissue and parietal vaginal tunic are incised. The parietal vaginal tunic is grasped with hematostats, separated from the testis (Fig. 116–4*B*), and excised (Fig. 116–4*C*). The ductus deferens is transected with scissors near the testis (Fig. 116–4*D*). Four throws are placed in the spermatic cord using the ductus deferens and sper-

matic vessels (Fig. 116–4*E*). This maneuver effectively controls hemorrhage. The spermatic cord is transected distal to these square knots (Fig. 116–4*F*). The scrotal incision is left unsutured (Fig. 116–4*G*).

Complications

Complications following orchidectomy include scrotal bruising and swelling, hemorrhage, and infection. Bruising and swelling of the scrotum is relatively common following canine orchidectomy. A lower incidence of scrotal swelling is reported with the closed technique of canine orchidectomy.[28] Hemorrhage following orchidectomy may be serious, particularly if it occurs within the abdomen. Serious hemorrhage necessitates ligation of the bleeding spermatic cord, intravenous fluid therapy, and possibly a blood transfusion. A ventral median abdominal approach is often necessary to locate and ligate the spermatic cord. Infection following orchidectomy usually necessitates both local and parenteral treatment (see "Funiculitis").

Scrotal Ablation

Scrotal ablation is recommended at the time of orchidectomy whenever trauma to the scrotum is severe and suggestive of ischemia. Ablation of the scrotum may be preferred in old dogs at orchidec-

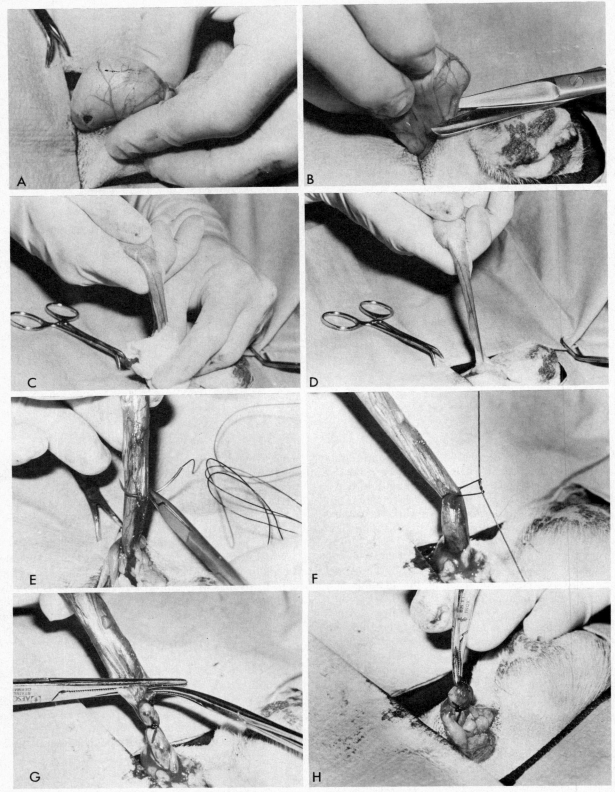

Figure 116–3. Canine orchidectomy—closed technique. *A,* The testis is exteriorized without incising the parietal vaginal tunic. *B,* The ligament of the tail of the epididymis is incised close to the testis with scissors. *C,* The fat and fascia that surround the spermatic cord are reflected proximally with a gauze sponge. *D,* The spermatic cord has been maximally exteriorized and is ready for ligation. *E,* The suture needle is inserted between the cremaster muscle *(right)* and the ductus deferens in preparation for transfixation ligation. *F,* A figure-eight transfixation ligature is being tied. The entire spermatic cord is enclosed in the ligature. *G,* Two transfixation ligatures have been placed. The spermatic cord will be transected between the two hemostats. *H,* The ligated spermatic cord is returned to the inguinal region.

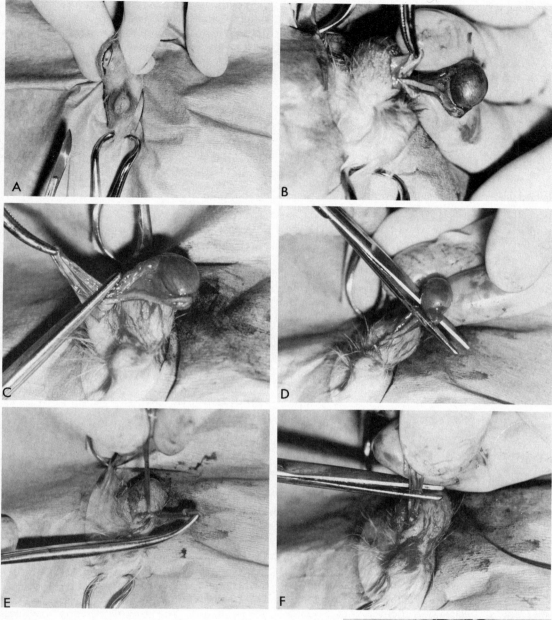

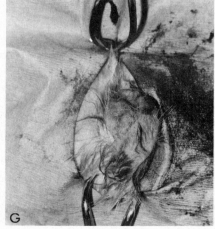

Figure 116–4. Feline orchidectomy—open technique. *A,* A separate longitudinal scrotal incision is made over each testis. *B,* The parietal vaginal tunic is grasped with hemostats and separated from the testis. *C,* The parietal vaginal tunic is excised with scissors. *D,* The ductus deferens is transected with scissors near the testis. *E,* The ductus deferens and spermatic vessels are used to tie two square knots in the spermatic cord. *F,* The spermatic cord is transected distal to the square knots. *G,* The scrotal incision is left unsutured.

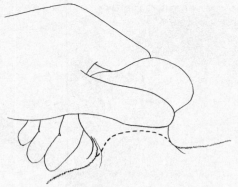

Figure 116–5. Ablation of the scrotum in the dog. The scrotum is retracted ventrally. The curved scrotal skin incision is shown as a dotted line. (Reprinted with permission from Harvey, C. E.: Scrotal ablation and castration in the dog. J. Am. Anim. Hosp. Assoc. 9:170, 1973.)

tomy to avoid postoperative problems.[14] The scrotum may also need to be ablated in scrotal neoplasia (see Chapter 120). Curvilinear incisions are made on both sides of the scrotum at its base. The incisions should curve toward the scrotum to provide adequate skin for closure (Figure 116–5).[14] Bleeders are controlled by ligation, and both testes are removed. Following transection of the scrotal septum, the skin is closed in the usual manner.

EPIDIDYMIS

Aplasia and Occlusion of the Epididymis

Segmental aplasia of the epididymis has been reported in dogs.[7, 18, 20, 25] Epididymal aplasia is due to failure of development of a portion of the mesonephric duct.[7] Bilateral epididymal aplasia results in obstruction to flow of spermatozoa and infertility. Spermatoceles and spermatic granulomas develop immediately proximal to the obstructed segment.[18]

Although biopsy is necessary to establish a diagnosis, careful palpation of the scrotal contents assists in the diagnosis of aplasia of the epididymis.[7] Repair of epididymal aplasia and occlusion is usually not attempted in small animals. Orchidectomy is generally performed.

Epididymitis

This condition usually accompanies orchitis. Epididymitis can result from an ascending infection of the genital tract, canine distemper virus, or a hematogenous infection. Canine distemper virus produces cytoplasmic and intranuclear inclusions in the epididymal epithelial cells.[18] Hematogenous infection, particularly *Brucella canis*, can result in epididymitis without signs of orchitis.[12] A secondary scrotal dermatitis frequently results from excessive licking in *B. canis* infection (see Chapter 120).

Epididymitis may produce only clinical signs of slight pain associated with epididymal enlargement.[12] More severe inflammation results in fluid accumulations between the parietal and visceral vaginal tunics, fibrosis of the epididymis, spermatocele, spermatic granuloma, and possibly abscess formation. Pyrexia and anorexia can accompany acute cases of epididymitis. Diagnosis of the causative organism often requires culture and susceptibility of fluid within the vaginal tunics, semen, urine, and possibly blood. Diagnosis of canine brucellosis involves both serological and bacteriological testing.[5] Canine distemper–induced epididymitis is diagnosed by histopathology.

Treatment

Treatment of acute suppurative epididymitis is by orchidectomy. The cavity of the vaginal tunics should be drained and allowed to heal by second intention.[17] Antibacterial drugs are used to control infection. There is no uniformly successful treatment for canine brucellosis.[5]

Prognosis for maintaining fertility following epididymitis is guarded. Testicular atrophy and chronic epididymitis are common sequelae of *B. canis* infections.[5, 12]

Epididymal Tumors

Primary epididymal tumors are rarely reported in small animals (see also Chapter 181). Local invasion of the epididymis by testicular tumors can occur.[18] Fibromas of the epididymis have been observed.[4, 17] Orchidectomy with excision of as much of the spermatic cord and vaginal tunics as necessary is the method of diagnosis and treatment.

SPERMATIC CORD

Spermatic Cord Trauma

Trauma to the spermatic cord may accompany blunt testicular trauma or penetrating wounds. The pampiniform plexus is the portion of spermatic cord most susceptible to injury.[17] Persistent hemorrhage occurs following rupture of the venous plexus. Swelling and bruising of the scrotum and spermatic cord are seen.

Definitive diagnosis is made on exploration of the scrotum and spermatic cord. An attempt should be made to preserve the testis if possible. The scrotum and parietal vaginal tunic are incised over the swelling. The hematoma is removed and as much of the pampiniform plexus as necessary is ligated. The cavity of the parietal vaginal tunic is flushed with saline. The tunic is closed with fine absorbable sutures, and the skin is closed with fine nonabsorbable sutures. Damage to the testicular artery or ductus deferens usually requires orchidectomy.

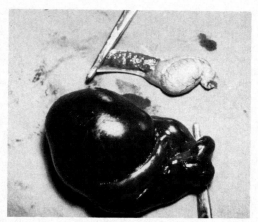

Figure 116–6. Torsion of an abdominally situated testis in a dog. The normal scrotal testis is shown at the top. (Courtesy of D. E. Johnston.)

Spermatic Cord Torsion

Torsion of the spermatic cord is uncommon in the dog (Fig. 116–6). It is reported more frequently in intra-abdominal than in scrotal testes.[11, 16, 24, 26, 33, 35, 36] Torsion occurs in both neoplastic and non-neoplastic testes. Spermatic cord torsion usually occurs as an acute illness characterized by anorexia and vomiting.[35] Other common signs include distress, lethargy, diarrhea, stiffness of the hindquarters, a palpable caudal abdominal mass, and urinary dysfunction.[26, 35] Most spermatic cord torsions in intra-abdominal testes are associated with abdominal pain.[36] Swelling and edema of the scrotum are also usually seen in spermatic cord torsion of intrascrotal testes, although pain is not consistently observed.[16, 26, 35, 36] Spermatic cord torsion in ectopic or intrascrotal testes is unknown.

Treatment

Treatment of spermatic cord torsion in the dog is orchidectomy. The testis should be examined histologically for evidence of neoplasia. There are no reports of preservation of an intrascrotal testis following derotation in the dog. Correction of spermatic cord torsion in man is performed within 12 hours of the onset of clinical signs.[19] In humans, untwisting of the spermatic cord and fixation of an intrascrotal testis within the first 72 hours results in a progressively decreased residual testicular mass. Further delay in treatment almost invariably results in complete testicular atrophy.[19]

Funiculitis

Inflammation of the spermatic cord is rare and usually reflects infection following orchidectomy.[17] Funiculitis can also occur following trauma to the cord. Inflammation of the ductus deferens rarely occurs separately; it usually accompanies other infections such as orchitis, epididymitis, and prostatitis.[17]

Clinical signs can be limited to local pain and swelling with pyrexia and stiffness in the hindlimbs. Chronic infections result in development of a scirrhous cord.[17]

Both local and parenteral treatment of funiculitis is usually indicated. Dependent drainage should be established when the condition is seen following orchidectomy. Local irrigation with a saline-antibiotic solution should be considered.[17] Appropriate parenteral antibiotics should be administered. Chronic infections following orchidectomy require resection of the involved spermatic cord and establishing drainage. Prognosis of funiculitis in the intact male is guarded for continued fertility. In humans, because of the rich blood supply and ample lymphatic drainage, funiculitis usually resolves with no permanent abnormality.[13]

Varicocele

Dilation, elongation, and tortuosity of the veins of the pampiniform plexus is referred to as varicocele.[13, 17] It is uncommon in the dog but can develop at any age. Any obstruction to the venous return from the testis can produce a varicocele. This condition can be produced experimentally by partial occlusion of the left testicular vein.[1, 9, 31] Mechanical obstruction to the blood flow through the inguinal canal by a neoplasm or hernia is the usual cause of varicocele in the dog.[17]

Clinical signs of varicocele are usually only an enlarged, soft spermatic cord and reduced fertility.[1, 9, 17] Decreased semen quality may result from an increase in bilateral testicular temperature because of increased blood flow.[31] Thrombosis of the p-ampiniform plexus following varicocele formation is occasionally observed.[18]

Asymptomatic varicoceles are not treated. Careful dissection and double ligation of the multiple abnormal venous channels of the spermatic cord may be indicated in the breeding animal. Preservation of the normal venous channels, testicular artery, and ductus deferens is imperative. Painful or traumatized varicoceles should be treated by orchidectomy.

1. Al-Juburi, A., Pranikoff, K., Dougherty, K. A., et al.: Alteration of semen quality in dogs after creation of a varicocele. Urology 13:535, 1979.
2. Arey, L. B.: *Developmental Anatomy.* W. B. Saunders, Philadelphia, 1965.
3. Ashdown, R. R.: The diagnosis of cryptorchidism in young dogs: a review of the problem. J. Small Anim. Pract. 4:261, 1963.
4. Barrett, R. E., and Theilen, G. H.: Neoplasms of the canine and feline reproductive tracts. *In* Kirk, R. W. (ed.): *Current Veterinary Therapy VI: Small Animal Practice.* W. B. Saunders, Philadelphia, 1977.
5. Burke, T. J.: Reproductive disorders. *In* Ettinger, S. J. (ed.): *Textbook of Veterinary Internal Medicine.* 2nd ed. W. B. Saunders, Philadelphia, 1983.
6. Burke, T. J., and Reynolds, H. A.: The testis. *In* Bojrab, M.

J. (ed.): *Pathophysiology in Small Animal Surgery.* Lea & Febiger, Philadelphia, 1981.

7. Copland, M. D., and Maclachlan, N. J.: Aplasia of the epididymis and vas deferens in the dog. J. Small Anim. Pract. *17*:443, 1976.

8. Cox, V. S., Wallace, L. J., and Jessen, C. R.: An anatomic and genetic study of canine cryptorchidism. Teratology *18*:233, 1978.

9. Dandia, S. D., Bagree, M. M., Vyas, C. P., et al.: Experimental production of varicocele and its effects on testes. Jpn. J. Surg. *9*:372, 1979.

10. Dunn, M. L., Foster, W. J., and Goddard, K. M.: Cryptorchidism in dogs: a clinical study. J. Am. Anim. Hosp. Assoc. *4*:180, 1968.

11. Eskew, N. E., and Kuhn, E. F.: Abdominal pain due to torsion of a retained testicle. Vet. Med. *56*:212, 1961.

12. George, L. W., Duncan, J. R., and Carmichael, L. E.: Semen examination in dogs with canine brucellosis. Am. J. Vet Res. *40*:1589, 1979.

13. Glenn, J. F.: The male genital system. *In* Sabiston, D. C., Jr. (ed.): *Davis-Christopher Textbook of Surgery.* W. B. Saunders, Philadelphia, 1977.

14. Harvey, C. E.: Scrotal ablation and castration in the dog. J. Am. Anim. Hosp. Assoc. *9*:170, 1973.

15. Hayes, H. M., Jr., and Pendergrass, T. W.: Canine testicular tumors: epidemiologic features of 410 dogs. Int. J. Cancer *18*:482, 1976.

16. Hulse, D. A.: Intrascrotal torsion of the testicle in a dog. Vet. Med. Small Anim. Clin. *68*:658, 1973.

17. Johnston, D. E., and Archibald, J.: Male genital system. *In* Archibald, J. (ed.): *Canine Surgery.* 2nd ed. American Veterinary Publications, Santa Barbara, 1974.

18. Jubb, K. U. F., and Kennedy, P. C. (eds.): *Pathology of Domestic Animals.* Academic Press, New York, 1970.

19. King, L. M., Sekaran, S. K., Sauer, D., and Schwentker, F. N.: Untwisting in delayed treatment of torsion of the spermatic cord. J. Urol. *112*:217, 1974.

20. Kirk, R. W., McEntee, K., and Bentinck-Smith, J.: Diseases of the urogenital system. *In* Catcoff, E. J. (ed.): *Canine Medicine.* American Veterinary Publications, Wheaton, Ill., 1968.

21. Larsen, R. E.: Testicular biopsy in the dog. Vet. Clin. North Am. *7*:747, 1977.

22. Lein, D. H.: Canine orchitis. *In* Kirk, R. W. (ed.): *Current Veterinary Therapy VI: Small Animal Practice.* W. B. Saunders, Philadelphia, 1977.

23. Lipowitz, A. J., Schwartz, A., Wilson, G. P., and Ebert, J. W.: Testicular neoplasms and concomitant clinical changes in the dog. J. Am. Vet. Med. Assoc. *163*:1364, 1973.

24. MacDonald, D. S., Devereux, R. J., and Bartolf, F.: Torsion of an ectopic testicle simulating a foreign body in the intestine. Can. Vet. J. *2*:117, 1961.

25. Majeed, Z. Z.: Segmental aplasia of the Wolffian duct; report of a case in a poodle. J. Small Anim. Pract. *15*:263, 1974.

26. Pearson, H., and Kelly, D. F.: Testicular torsion in the dog: a review of 13 cases. Vet. Rec. *97*:200, 1975.

27. Pendergrass, T. W., and Hayes, H. M., Jr.: Cryptorchidism and related defects in dogs: epidemiologic comparisons with man. Teratology *12*:51, 1975.

28. Phillips, J. T., and Leeds, E. B.: A closed technique for canine orchidectomy. Canine Pract. *3*:23, 1976.

29. Reif, J. S., and Brodey, R. S.: The relationship between cryptorchidism and canine testicular neoplasia. J. Am. Vet. Med. Assoc. *155*:2005, 1969.

30. Reif, J. S., Maguire, T. G., Kenney, R. M., and Brodey, R. S.: A cohort study of canine testicular neoplasia. J. Am. Vet. Med. Assoc. *175*:719, 1979.

31. Sampol, D. C., Howards, S. S., Turner, T. T., and Miller, E. D., Jr.: Influence of surgically induced varicocele on testicular blood-flow, temperature, and histology in adult rats and dogs. J. Clin. Invest. *68*:39, 1981.

32. Stansbury, R. L.: A castration technique. Feline Pract. *1*:20, 1971.

33. White, P. T., and Johnson, P., Jr.: Strangulated testicle of a cryptorchid (dog). J. Am. Vet. Med. Assoc. *126*:312, 1955.

34. Wilson, G. P.: Surgery of the male reproductive tract. Vet. Clin. North Am. *5*:537, 1975.

35. Young, A. C. B.: Two cases of intrascrotal torsion of a normal testicle. J. Small Anim. Pract. *20*:229, 1979.

36. Zymet, C. L.: Intrascrotal testicular torsion in a sexually aggressive dog. Vet. Med. Small Anim. Clin. *70*:133, 1975.

Chapter **117**

Penis

Harry W. Boothe

HYPOSPADIAS

Hypospadias, the most common developmental anomaly of the male external genitalia, is most frequently encountered in Boston terriers.[12] There is failure of fusion of the urogenital folds and incomplete formation of the penile urethra.[18] The external urethral orifice can occur anywhere on the ventral aspect of the penis from the normal opening to the perineal region (Fig. 117–1). Hypospadias is usually associated with failure of fusion of the prepuce and underdevelopment of the penis (see Chapter 118).[18]

Clinical signs may be absent if the prepuce is normal and the external urethral orifice is near the end of the penis. Occasionally, the skin and hair around the urethral orifice are urine-soaked and irritated.[18] Diagnosis of hypospadias is made by close inspection of the penis.

Surgical correction is not usually attempted in the dog, because the urethra cranial to the abnormal orifice is deficient.[12] Excision of the remnants of the prepuce and penis as well as bilateral orchidectomy may be indicated in severe cases. The urethral orifice is maintained in the perineal region.[18]

DEFORMITY OF THE OS PENIS (CURVATURE)

The os penis may rarely develop with a pronounced curvature.[12] Because of the curvature, the dog may not be able to retract the distal penis into the prepuce. The exposed part becomes dry and fissured, resulting in infection and necrosis.[12]

Treatment depends on the condition of the penis. Local treatment of the exposed penis is usually not effective without treatment of the bony curvature. It

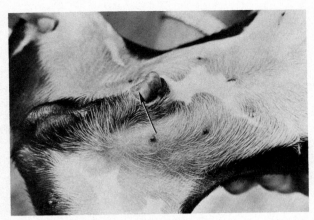

Figure 117–1. Hypospadias. The urethral orifice is located on the ventral aspect of the penis *(arrow).* The prepuce is also not fully developed.

may be possible to fracture and straighten the os penis, if infection and necrosis are not present. Partial penile amputation may be necessary in severe cases (see "Strangulation of the Penis").

PERSISTENT PENILE FRENULUM

In most domestic animals, the epithelial surfaces of the penis and prepuce are fused at birth and remain so until the onset of puberty.[4, 14] In the immature dog, the penis and prepuce are joined ventrally by a fine band of connective tissue, the frenulum. The frenulum normally ruptures by puberty.[1] Occasionally this separation is incomplete and the frenulum persists. Persistence of the frenulum has been seen in Cocker spaniels, miniature poodles, and the Pekingese (Fig. 117–2).[1, 3, 11, 13]

Pain may be evident during sexual excitement or when an attempt is made to extrude the penis. A ventral deviation of the glans is usually noted when extrusion is attempted. The patient may also continually lick the area. Surgical severing of the avascular

connective tissue is readily performed after administration of a short-acting anesthetic. The prognosis is good following surgery.

PENILE WOUNDS

Wounds to the penis may occur during mating, dog fights, and fence jumping, or from automobile accidents or gunshot.[8, 12, 15] Penile lacerations and gunshot wounds may involve the urethra. Severe penile trauma may produce a fracture of the os penis (see "Fracture of the Os Penis").

The most common clinical sign of penile wounds is hemorrhage. Hemorrhage is frequently intermittent but often profuse. Repeated hemorrhage is associated with penile erection, which in turn is caused by irritation from injury. Rupture of the penile urethra is usually accompanied by fluctuant subcutaneous swelling associated with urine extravasation.[8]

Minor injuries to the penis can be cleaned and treated with a topical antibiotic ointment. These wounds are usually allowed to heal by second intention. If significant hemorrhage occurs, the wound is debrided and sutured. Arterial bleeding is controlled by ligation, and cavernous bleeding is controlled by suturing the tunica albuginea with fine absorbable material. The penile mucosa is closed with fine absorbable material. Parenteral and local antibiotics are used postoperatively. Erection of the penis should be prevented by sedating the animal.[12]

Wounds of the penile urethra are usually treated by catheterization, provided that the urethra has not been transected. A transected urethra should be sutured with fine absorbable material and then catheterized. Catheters should remain in place for 5 to 7 days with minor penile urethral tears and up to 21 days after urethral anastomosis. Severe wounds may require partial penile amputation (see "Strangulation of the Penis").

The prognosis for penile wounds is generally good, provided that the urethra has not been transected. Some urethral narrowing is possible, especially following transection and anastomosis.

STRANGULATION OF THE PENIS

Malicious application of a rubber band around the penis or constriction of a ring of preputial hairs can cause strangulation of the penis. The penile mucosa becomes swollen with a necrotic circle, or the entire penis distal to the constriction may be necrotic.[12] The dog usually exhibits pain and may frequently lick the prepuce. Dysuria can also be seen. This condition must be distinguished from paraphimosis, because the treatments differ (see "Paraphimosis"). When damage to the penis is minor, removal of the cause and topical application of an antibiotic ointment results in prompt healing. Licking should be controlled. More severe cases accompanied by urethral swelling

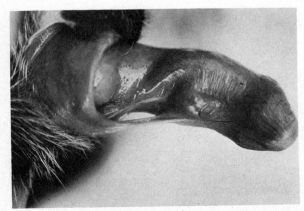

Figure 117–2. The persistent penile frenulum is evident, connecting the ventral aspect of the penis and the prepuce.

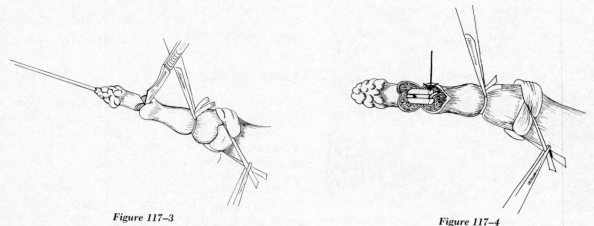

Figure 117–3

Figure 117–4

Figure 117–3. Partial penile amputation: Creation of bilateral flaps in the pars longa glandis. The penis is extruded and the prepuce is retracted with umbilical tape. Following urethral catheterization, a tourniquet is placed around the penis. The pars longa glandis is incised to create two flaps.

Figure 117–4. Partial penile amputation: Transection site in the os penis following dissection of the urethra. The urethra is transected distal to the proposed ostectomy site *(arrow)* and dissected from the groove of the os penis. (Both figures reprinted with permission from Bojrab, M. J.: Current Techniques in Small Animal Surgery. Philadelphia, Lea & Febiger, 1975.)

and constriction require an indwelling urethral catheter as well as local antibiotics. Partial amputation of the penis is indicated when the distal portion is gangrenous or when the urethra is severely damaged.

The surgical area, including the preputial cavity, is prepared in the usual manner, following induction of general anesthesia. The urethra is catheterized. The penis is withdrawn from the prepuce and kept exteriorized with a rubber tourniquet placed around the penis as far caudally as possible. The prepuce may also be retracted caudally with umbilical tape. If the penis cannot be adequately exteriorized, the prepuce is incised on the ventral midline. Bilateral flaps are created proximal to the os penis and urethra (Fig. 117–3). The urethra is dissected from the groove in the os penis. The catheter is removed, and the urethra is transected just distal to the proposed amputation site. The os penis is transected with bone-cutting forceps at the base of the flap (Fig. 117–4). The tourniquet is loosened to identify and ligate blood vessels in the erectile tissue. The flaps of erectile tissue and tunica albuginea are apposed with simple interrupted sutures of 4–0 absorbable material. The urethra is incised along its dorsal midline. The urethral edges are sutured to penile mucosa over the ventral portion of the end of the penile stump.

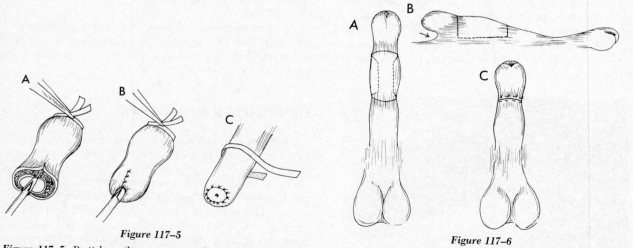

Figure 117–5

Figure 117–6

Figure 117–5. Partial penile amputation: closure of the distal end of the penis. *A,* The distal urethra is incised longitudinally on its dorsum. *B,* The cavernous tissue is closed on the dorsal aspect of the penis with fine absorbable sutures placed in the tunica albuginea. *C,* The urethral margin is sutured to the epithelium of the penis with simple interrupted absorbable sutures.

Figure 117–6. Technique for shortening of the prepuce in conjunction with partial penile amputation. *A,* A rectangular portion of prepuce is excised. *B,* A sliding skin flap will facilitate retraction of the cranial prepuce *(arrow). C,* The segments are apposed with three layers of suture. (Both figures reprinted with permission from Bojrab, M. J.: Current Techniques in Small Animal Surgery. Philadelphia, Lea & Febiger, 1975.)

Penile mucosa is sutured to penile mucosa on the dorsal portion of the penile stump (Fig. 117–5), to prevent creating too large a urethral orifice.

Shortening of the prepuce may be necessary when a large part of the glans penis has been removed.[9] A rectangular full-thickness segment of the ventral wall of the prepuce is excised (Fig. 117–6). The preputial mucous membrane is sutured with fine absorbable material in an everting pattern. The subcutaneous tissue is closed with simple interrupted absorbable sutures. The skin is apposed with simple interrupted or horizontal mattress sutures.

FRACTURE OF THE OS PENIS

This condition occurs rarely.[15, 19] Fractures usually are transverse with limited soft tissue damage, although they may be comminuted.[12]

Clinical signs depend upon the degree of soft tissue damage and fracture displacement. Dysuria and hematuria are often present. Crepitus is apparent, and urethral obstruction may be present. Urethral obstruction may also be observed in association with callus formation.[19] Radiography determines the amount of damage to the os penis.

Conservative management of this fracture is often successful.[12, 15, 19] Minimally displaced simple fractures do not require immobilization.[12] More severe fractures can be adequately immobilized with a urethral catheter. The catheter is positioned beyond the fracture site and maintained for seven days. If a catheter cannot be passed because of urethral damage, or if the fracture is unstable following urethral catheterization, open reduction and fixation with a finger plate has been successful.[19] Fractures accompanied by severe penile trauma may necessitate partial penile amputation (see "Strangulation of the Penis"). If urethral obstruction occurs because of callus formation, a prescrotal urethrostomy can be performed.

PARAPHIMOSIS

This condition occurs when the penis protrudes from the preputial sheath and cannot be replaced to its normal position. Paraphimosis is usually seen following coitus, trauma, or masturbation, particularly in young male dogs.[12] A narrow preputial orifice or hairs surrounding the preputial orifice may prevent full penile retraction.[6, 12]

Clinical signs depend upon the duration of paraphimosis. The exteriorized glans penis becomes congested and discolored owing to the constricting band of retracted prepuce. The dog frequently licks at the exposed penis, exacerbating the inflammation. Severe penile damage can result from prolonged paraphimosis. Necrosis of the exposed penis and urethral obstruction can occur quickly.

Treatment is directed at replacement of the penis into the prepuce. Lubricants, hyperosmolar solutions, and local heat or cold may be adequate to reduce the size of the penis and permit replacement. The penis is pushed caudally as the prepuce is drawn cranially. If replacement cannot be accomplished within a few hours, an indwelling urethral catheter should be sutured in place. Temporary or permanent surgical enlargement of the preputial orifice may be necessary (see Chapter 118). Long-standing cases of paraphimosis accompanied by necrosis can require partial penile amputation (see "Strangulation of the Penis").

Prognosis following repair is guarded. Recurrence is not uncommon.[6] Paraphimosis accompanied by a deficient prepuce usually requires partial penile amputation to be effective.

PRIAPISM

Defined as persistent erection not associated with sexual excitement, priapism is not commonly seen in small animals. It is usually associated with spinal cord lesions, but it may accompany constipation or genitourinary infection.[12] Priapism is distinguished from paraphimosis because the penis can be manually replaced into the prepuce. As penile congestion and swelling increase because of drying and licking, this distinguishing feature is lost.

Treatment is directed at eliminating the primary cause. Some cases will subside spontaneously.[12] The exposed penis is kept clean and moist by applying a soothing ointment. Licking should also be controlled.

PROLAPSE OF THE URETHRA

Prolapse of the urethra occurs uncommonly in the male dog. This condition is seen mainly in young English bulldogs, although it has been reported in a Boston terrier.[7, 10, 17] Prolapse may follow genitourinary infection or excessive sexual excitement.[10] Intermittent hemorrhage from the penis unassociated

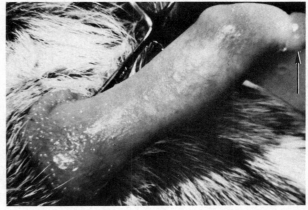

Figure 117–7. Prolapsed urethra in the canine. The exposed, hemorrhagic urethral mucosa is evident at the end of the penis (*arrow*).

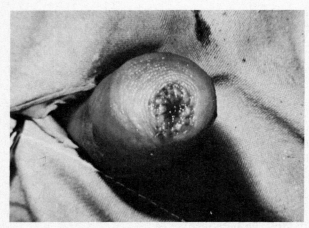

Figure 117–8. Amputation of prolapsed urethra. The urethra is sutured to the epithelium of the penis following amputation of the prolapsed portion.

with urination is often noted. The affected dog frequently licks the preputial orifice.

Diagnosis is made by finding a small, red, pea-shaped mass at the end of the penis (Fig. 117–7). Treatment should be surgical, because no spontaneous recovery has been reported.[17] The primary cause should be identified and treated. The prolapse can be reduced by inserting a lubricated catheter in the urethra or by gentle manipulation with a moistened gauze sponge. A purse-string suture of fine, nonreactive, nonabsorbable material is inserted around the exterior of the urethral orifice and tied sufficiently tight to prevent recurrence. The suture is removed in five days. Amputation of the prolapse and anastomosis of urethral and penile mucosa should be performed when the prolapse is irreducible, necrotic, or recurrent after the purse-string suture has been removed. A circular incision is made in the penile mucosa, proximal to the prolapse. An incision is then made on the ventral surface of the urethral mucosa halfway around its circumference.[17] The urethral mucosa is sutured to penile mucosa with simple interrupted sutures of 4–0 absorbable material, to prevent retraction of the urethral mucosa and to eliminate the need for stay sutures. The dorsal surface of the urethral mucosa is incised and sutured (Fig. 117–8).

Urinary antibiotics should be continued postoperatively. The dog should be prevented from licking the area. Smooth-muscle relaxants and tranquilizers may be helpful in controlling postoperative hemorrhage. Prognosis following surgical repair is good, and prolapse usually does not recur.

BALANOPOSTHITIS

This condition can be seen following penile injury or accompanying phimosis, preputial foreign bodies, or neoplasia (see Chapter 118). A slight purulent preputial discharge is regarded as normal in mature dogs, as it is not associated with inflammation of the

penile or preputial mucosa. A copious or possibly blood-tinged preputial discharge indicates balanoposthitis. The affected dog frequently licks at the prepuce. Examination reveals an inflamed, thickened mucosa of the penis and prepuce. Enlarged lymphoid nodules are noted, particularly near the fornix of the preputial cavity. Adhesions may develop between the prepuce and penis in severe cases.

Treatment is directed at eliminating the primary cause. The patient is usually anesthetized to allow complete examination. Thorough irrigation of the penis and preputial cavity should be performed with warm saline solution. Superficial curettage of the lymphoid nodules with a gauze sponge is often necessary. Adhesions between the penis and prepuce are severed. Local instillation of povidone-iodine solution is also helpful. An antibiotic ointment is instilled into the preputial cavity for a few days following curettage. The prognosis following treatment is guarded, because balanoposthitis tends to recur.

PENILE TUMORS (see also Section XIX)

Tumors of the canine penis are not uncommonly seen. There are almost no reports of genital neoplasia in male cats. Tumors involving the penis in dogs include transmissible venereal tumor, papilloma, and squamous cell carcinoma.[2] Licking and a serosanguineous preputial discharge are common clinical signs of penile transmissible venereal tumors.[5] Diagnosis is frequently made by cytological evaluation of fine-needle aspirates or impression smears from the mass. The transmissible venereal tumor responds to many modes of treatment, including radiation therapy, chemotherapy, and surgery.[2, 5, 16] Tumors involving the distal aspect of the penis may require partial

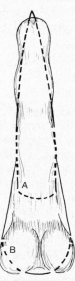

Figure 117–9. Incision sites for amputation of the prepuce *(A)* and combined amputation of the prepuce and scrotum *(B)* are shown. (Reprinted with permission from Bojrab, M. J.: Current Techniques in Small Animal Surgery. Philadelphia, Lea & Febiger, 1975.)

penile amputation (see "Strangulation of the Penis"). Tumors involving more of the penis may require a more extensive penile amputation and perineal urethrostomy. Bilateral orchidectomy and scrotal ablation may also be necessary. An elliptical incision is made along each side of the prepuce and scrotum from the cranial end of the prepuce to an appropriate level on the perineal midline (Fig. 117–9). Branches from the caudal superficial epigastric vessels are ligated in the subcutaneous tissue. The testes and scrotum are removed in a standard fashion (see Chapter 116). The penis is isolated cranial to the scrotum and is temporarily encircled with a heavy ligature proximal to the site of initial transection. The penis is transected and removed. The proximal portion of the penis is exteriorized through a separate midline perineal incision. The ventral abdominal incision is closed in a routine manner.

The temporary ligature is removed, and the penis is cut at a 45-degree angle dorsoventrally in preparation for perineal urethrostomy. Approximately 0.5 to 1 cm of the urethra is preserved distal to the point of transection. Severed arteries are ligated with 4–0 absorbable material. The urethra is incised along its dorsal midline and sutured to the penile mucosa. Simple interrupted sutures of nonabsorbable material are placed through the skin, penile mucosa, tunica albuginea, and urethral mucosa to complete the urethrostomy.[9]

1. Balke, J.: Persistent penile frenulum in a Cocker Spaniel. Vet. Med. Small Anim. Clin. 76:988, 1981.
2. Barrett, R. E., and Theilen, G. H.: Neoplasms of the canine and feline reproductive tracts. In Kirk, R. W. (ed.): Current Veterinary Therapy VI: Small Animal Practice. W. B. Saunders, Philadelphia, 1977.
3. Begg, T. B.: Persistent penile frenulum in the dog. Vet. Rec. 75:930, 1963.
4. Bharadwaj, M. B., and Calhoun, M. L.: Mode of formation of the preputial cavity in domesticated animals. Am. J. Vet. Res. 22:764, 1961.
5. Brown, N. O., Calvert, C., nd MacEwen, E. G.: Chemotherapeutic management of transmissible venereal tumors in 30 dogs. J. Am. Vet. Med. Assoc. 176:983, 1980.
6. Christie, T. R.: Phimosis and paraphimosis. In Bojrab, M. J. (ed.): Pathophysiology in Small Animal Surgery. Lea & Febiger, Philadelphia, 1981.
7. Firestone, W. M.: Prolapse of the male urethra. J. Am. Vet. Med. Assoc. 99:135, 1941.
8. Hall, M. A., and Swenberg, L. N.: Genital emergencies. In Kirk, R. W. (ed.): Current Veterinary Therapy VI: Small Animal Practice. W. B. Saunders Co., Philadelphia, 1977.
9. Henry, J. D., Jr.: The penis. In Bojrab, M. J. (ed.): Current Techniques in Small Animal Surgery I. Lea & Febiger, Philadelphia, 1975.
10. Hobson, H. P., and Heller, R. A.: Surgical correction of prolapse of the male urethra. Vet. Med. Small Anim. Clin. 66:1177, 1971.
11. Hutchison, J. A.: Persistence of the penile frenulum in dogs. Can. Vet. J. 14:71, 1973.
12. Johnston, D. E., and Archibald, J.: Male genital system. In Archibald, J. (ed.): Canine Surgery. 2nd ed. American Veterinary Publications, Inc., Santa Barbara, 1974.
13. Joshua, J.: Persistence of the penile frenulum in a dog. Vet. Rec. 74:1550, 1962.
14. Jubb, K. V. F., and Kennedy, P. C. (eds.): Pathology of Domestic Animals. Academic Press, New York, 1970.
15. Ndiritu, C. G.: Lesions of the canine penis and prepuce. Mod. Vet. Pract. 60:712, 1979.
16. Richardson, R. C.: Canine transmissible venereal tumor. Comp. Cont. Ed. Pract. Vet. 3:951, 1981.
17. Sinibaldi, K. R., and Green, R. W.: Surgical correction of prolapse of the male urethra in three English Bulldogs. J. Am. Anim. Hosp. Assoc. 9:450, 1973.
18. Smith, C. W.: Developmental anomalies. In Bojrab, M. J. (ed.): Pathophysiology in Small Animal Surgery. Lea & Febiger, Philadelphia, 1981.
19. Stead, A. C.: Fracture of the os penis in the dog—two case reports. J. Small Anim. Pract. 13:19, 1972.

Chapter **118** **Prepuce**

Harry W. Boothe

PHIMOSIS

Phimosis is the inability to protrude the penis beyond the preputial orifice. It is caused by absence of or an abnormally small preputial orifice. Congenital stenosis of the preputial orifice occurs in the dog.[4] More commonly, the orifice is narrowed because of scarring following preputial trauma or preputial neoplasia.

Congenital phimosis is usually accompanied by a distended prepuce and inability to urinate normally. Urine can often be passed only in drops or a thin stream.[5] Despite these signs, the puppy is rarely distressed. Retention of urine in the prepuce results in balanoposthitis, and the infected area may ulcerate.[9] Ulceration or sloughing of tissue at the preputial orifice can result in a spontaneous recovery.

Acquired phimosis is often accompanied by inflammation and edema of the prepuce. The dog frequently licks the area. A neoplasm or healing wound can also be present. Retention of urine within the prepuce can also be seen in severe cases.

Surgical enlargement of the preputial orifice and correction of the primary condition result in successful alleviation of the problem. A triangular incision is made over the preputial orifice after the induction of general anesthesia and appropriate preparation of the site. The skin, subcutaneous tissue, and preputial mucosa are excised, usually on the dorsal surface of the prepuce. As much tissue as possible is removed, although one ensures that the penis remains covered by prepuce. Neoplasms are excised or treated appropriately, care being taken to avoid stenosis of the preputial orifice (see "Preputial Tumors"). Bleeding vessels are ligated or cauterized, and the preputial mucosa is sutured to the skin. Simple interrupted, fine, nonabsorbable sutures are used.

Prognosis following repair of congenital phimosis is generally good. Acquired phimosis caused by neoplasia may be complicated by recurrence of the tumor. A larger-than-normal preputial orifice should be created, because postoperative fibrosis can be significant. If too much tissue is removed, particularly from the ventral prepuce, paraphimosis may result (see Chapter 117).

ABNORMALITIES OF THE PREPUCE

The prepuce may be hypoplastic or absent or may fail to fuse normally. The normal embryological closure of the genital folds over the penis does not occur, resulting in a deficient prepuce. Failure of preputial fusion usually accompanies hypospadias and underdevelopment or absence of the penis.[3, 10] A deficiency in the length of the prepuce is seen occasionally in the dog. The end of the penis is exposed, subjecting it to trauma and drying. This condition may also be a source of annoyance to the owner.[7]

Clinical signs of congenital preputial abnormalities usually are due to exposure of the distal penis. The dog frequently licks at the penis, causing inflammation. Trauma results in hemorrhage. Surgical management of congenital preputial abnormalities other than phimosis is difficult. Failure of preputial fusion is usually treated by removal of the open prepuce, partial penile amputation, and prescrotal or perineal urethrostomy.[3, 10] An elliptical incision is made along each side of the exposed preputial mucosa. The mucosa is dissected to the level of the glans penis. Hemorrhage is controlled with fine absorbable material. A partial penile amputation is performed to excise the exposed distal penis (see Chapter 117). The preputial mucosa and distal penis are excised, and the urethra is sutured to the ventral abdominal skin with fine, nonabsorbable material. Bilateral orchidectomy, scrotal ablation, and perineal urethrostomy may be necessary if the preputial defect is severe.

A deficiency in the length of the prepuce is corrected by advancing the prepuce cranially along the abdominal wall or by partial penile amputation (see Chapter 117). Simple cranial advancement of the prepuce is not often successful if much of the distal penis is exposed. After routine preparation of the area, a U-shaped incision is made in the abdominal skin immediately cranial to the prepuce. This part of the prepuce is freed from the abdominal skin and advanced cranially until the penis is covered. This point is marked. A second U-shaped skin incision is made at this level. The skin between the two incisions is excised. The prepuce is sutured in its new position using fine absorbable sutures in the subcutaneous tissue and fine nonabsorbable sutures in the skin.[5, 7]

Prognosis following repair of congenital preputial defects is guarded. Even if adequate coverage of the penis has been achieved following cranial preputial advancement with the dog anesthetized, the distal penis may remain exposed postoperatively. Partial penile amputation usually corrects this problem. Urethral stricture may occur following partial penile amputation if healing is complicated.

PREPUTIAL FOREIGN BODIES

Foreign bodies such as grass awns, plant seeds, pieces of straw, and urinary calculi can lodge in the preputial cavity. These may cause irritation, ulceration, infection, and abscess formation.[5]

Clinical signs are often mild and may be overlooked. A purulent, blood-tinged preputial discharge may be present, and the animal frequently licks the prepuce. Migration of the foreign body through the preputial mucosa at the fornix results in swelling and abscess of the tissues surrounding the penis. The animal usually is in pain, listless, and mildly pyrexic, and walks stiffly. A draining tract may be present ventral or lateral to the penis.

Removal of the foreign body from the preputial cavity usually corrects the associated balanoposthitis. Irrigation of the preputial cavity may be necessary. Draining tracts should be opened and explored for foreign bodies. Following removal of the foreign body, the tract should be flushed with antiseptic solution and drained. Systemic antibiotics may be indicated. The prognosis is usually good, provided that the foreign body is removed.

PREPUTIAL TUMORS (see also Section XIX)

The prepuce is affected by the same tumors as the skin.[1, 5] Mast cell tumors are the most frequently reported tumors of the external genitalia.[1] Transmissible venereal tumors, melanomas, and perianal gland tumors have also been reported.[1, 6, 10] Clinical signs are often minimal, unless the tumor ulcerates or involves the preputial orifice. Phimosis and balanoposthitis can result.

Diagnosis is made by incisional, excisional, or cytological biopsy. Surgical removal of the tumor with closure of the prepuce in two layers is the treatment. Care needs to be taken to assure that the penis remains covered by the prepuce. A partial penile amputation may be necessary following removal of large tumors (see Chapter 117). Orchidectomy is recommended following removal of a perianal gland tumor.

1. Barrett, R. E., and Theilen, G. H.: Neoplasms of the canine and feline reproductive tracts. *In* Kirk, R. W. (ed.): *Current Veterinary Therapy VI: Small Animal Practice.* W. B. Saunders, Philadelphia, 1977.
2. Christie, T. R.: Phimosis and paraphimosis. *In* Bojrab, M. J. (ed.): *Pathophysiology in Small Animal Surgery.* Lea & Febiger, Philadelphia, 1981.
3. Croshaw, J. E., Jr., and Brodey, R. S.: Failure of preputial closure in a dog. J. Am. Vet. Med. Assoc. *136:*450, 1960.
4. Elam, C. W., and Randle, P. O.: Peculiar preputial condition in a five-week-old puppy. Vet. Rec. *64:*98, 1952.
5. Johnston, D. E., and Archibald, J.: Male genital system. *In* Archibald, J. (ed.): *Canine Surgery.* 2nd ed. American Veterinary Publications, Inc., Santa Barbara, 1974.
6. Jubb, K. V. F., and Kennedy, P. C. (eds.): *Pathology of Domestic Animals.* Academic Press, New York, 1970.
7. Leighton, R. L.: A simple surgical correction for chronic penile protrusion. J. Am. Anim. Hosp. Assoc. *12:*667, 1976.
8. Ndiritu, C. G.: Lesions of the canine penis and prepuce. Mod. Vet. Pract. *60:*712, 1979.
9. Proescholdt, T. A., DeYoung, D. W., and Evans, L. E.: Preputial reconstruction for phimosis and infantile penis. J. Am. Anim. Hosp. Assoc. *13:*725, 1977.
10. Smith, C. W.: Developmental anomalies. *In* Bojrab, M. J. (ed.): *Pathophysiology in Small Animal Surgery.* Lea & Febiger, Philadelphia, 1981.
11. Smith, C. W.: Neoplasia of the male reproductive system. *In* Bojrab, M. J. (ed.): *Pathophysiology in Small Animal Surgery.* Lea & Febiger, Philadelphia, 1981.

Chapter **119**

Prostate

Dudley E. Johnston

HYPERPLASIA OF THE PROSTATE

Also known as benign hypertrophy of the prostate, prostatic hyperplasia is the most common disease of the prostate, occurring in approximately 60 per cent of all dogs over five years of age. Although many old dogs have hyperplastic prostates, only a few show clinical effects of the enlarged gland. The condition occurs rarely in dogs younger than five years of age.[40]

The cause of prostatic hyperplasia is poorly understood. An imbalance between estrogens and androgens is the most widely accepted cause. Hyperplasia may be a consequence of normal aging; however, a combination of estrogens and androgens is more effective in producing hyperplastic changes than androgens alone (see Chapter 114).[11, 36] A high incidence of testicular tumors has been reported in dogs with prostatic hyperplasia.[7, 33] As discussed later, squamous metaplasia of the prostate occurs with Sertoli cell tumors because of prolonged estrogenic stimulation.

Clinical Signs

Prostatic hyperplasia develops slowly, with gradual loss of weight and decline in general health. These signs can be associated with other diseases that occur in older dogs, such as chronic nephritis. Because some of these diseases and prostatic disease have signs in common, prostatic diseases can be overlooked and their treatment delayed. The major signs of prostatic enlargement are constipation and tenesmus. The enlarged prostate obstructs the pelvic canal, either because it is within the pelvic canal or because it is forced caudally into the pelvic canal from the abdomen, with increased abdominal pressure from straining. A mass within the pelvic canal simulates fullness within the bowel and results in frequent attempts at defecation. In addition, the pressure on the rectum impinges on the lumen of the bowel, resulting in constipation. As the dog strains to defecate, the enlarged gland is pushed upward and backward, thus further obstructing the pelvic canal, and fecal impaction occurs. In some cases of fecal impaction, the hard part of the feces is retained, and only liquid is passed. Unless a careful examination is carried out, the animal can be treated for diarrhea, and the treatment can aggravate the straining and discomfort.

Urinary retention is a constant feature of prostatic hyperplasia in humans. However, it is seen in only advanced cases in the dog. Urinary retention can be the result of narrowing of the lumen of the prostatic urethra, but it is more commonly associated with cranial displacement of the enlarged prostate gland into the abdomen with mechanical kinking of the urethra. During chronic retention of urine, the bladder is distended and atonic, and urinary incontinence is seen. A small amount of urine frequently spills from the grossly distended bladder. With urinary retention, cystitis and hematuria can be seen.

The possibility of prostatic disease should be investigated in all cases of perineal hernia. Although no evidence exists that prostatic enlargement and perineal hernia are associated, a dog with prostatic enlargement should be castrated after perineal hernia repair in order to reduce the chance of recurrence.[20] Other prostatic diseases such as prostatic cysts can be associated with perineal hernias.

Diagnosis

The first consideration in diagnosis is to detect an enlarged prostate gland. The second consideration is to distinguish the four common causes of prostatic enlargement and arrive at a diagnosis of prostatic hyperplasia. The clinical history of the presence of tenesmus in a dog more than five years of age, constipation, urinary incontinence or hematuria, very rarely abdominal distension, and change in gait or lameness can suggest prostatic disease.

Blood and urine examinations generally reveal no abnormalities unless there is concurrent cystitis. In most instances the enlarged prostate gland is detected by rectal palpation or a combination of rectal and abdominal palpation (see Chapter 115). In prostatic hyperplasia, the prostate gland is considerably enlarged, but the basic shape is still present. The gland is symmetrical and bilobed, with the normal dorsal groove. The surface is smooth, and the texture is homogenous and spongy. The animal should feel no pain on palpation of the gland. The prostatic enlargement can be seen on survey radiographs or by using contrast material in the urethra and bladder.

In most cases, examination of prostatic fluid and biopsy procedures are not indicated in making a diagnosis of prostatic hyperplasia.

Treatment

The treatment of prostatic hyperplasia is to reduce the size of the enlarged gland and correct constipation and urinary obstruction. Two to three weeks are usually necessary to reduce the size of the prostate gland enough to alleviate clinical signs. Therefore, two problems in nursing arise, relieving immediate problems of obstruction and allowing the animal to function for two to three weeks until prostatic enlargement is removed. It may be necessary to give enemas to empty the colon and rectum. In addition, a bulk laxative such as Metamucil (psyllium hydrophylic mucilloid) is given orally. It is often helpful to give the dog a low-residue diet such as hamburger and white rice. Because this diet is not balanced for minerals and vitamins, a mineral and vitamin supplement is generally recommended. In the presence of urinary retention, the bladder is emptied at least three times daily, by exertion of manual pressure on the abdominal wall. However, in many dogs this maneuver is not successful and catheterization is required. If repeated catheterization is necessary, it is usually preferable to place an indwelling catheter for several days. Because of urinary retention, bladder infection is usually present, and antibiotics should be given systemically. A distended bladder is likely to become atonic. It may be possible to stimulate contraction by administering a parasympathomimetic drug such as bethanecol or phenylpropanolamine.

The size of the prostate gland can be reduced by prostatectomy, castration, or administration of estrogens. Prostatectomy is rarely, if ever, indicated in treatment of prostatic hyperplasia because of the effectiveness of other methods. Other surgical procedures, such as capsulotomy and ligation of the prostatic blood supply, are not effective procedures. Partial prostatectomy is not necessary.

Castration provides effective and long-lasting relief from hyperplasia without the potentially serious side effects of hormone therapy. Following castration, the prostate atrophies, and in general, an improvement in clinical signs can be expected in two to three weeks. There is no doubt that castration is the preferred specific therapy for prostatic hyperplasia.

Hormone therapy can be used in place of castration when castration is not permitted by the owner or anesthesia and surgery are contraindicated. Large amounts of estrogenic hormones can lead to squamous metaplastic changes in the prostate and bone marrow depression with thrombocytopenia. There is little information on the optimal dose or duration of hormones in dogs. However, most clinicians recommend a dose of 0.2 to 1 mg of diethylstilbesterol orally every two to three days for approximately three to four weeks. After several weeks without therapy, the dosage can be repeated if necessary. Signs of estrogen toxicity in the dog include prostatic enlargement with cyst formation, signs of feminization, hemorrhage due to thrombocytopenia, and loss of hair.

In Europe the use of estrogen has been banned for many years, and considerable study has been done in the use of antiandrogen compounds such as cyproterone acetate (SH 714). This drug can cause a reduction in prostatic size in dogs with prostatic hyperplasia.[11] There is little information on its use in the United States.

Owners are often concerned about the effects of castration of their adult male dog. It can be expected that objectionable male behavior patterns such as roaming, fighting with other males, urine marking in the house, and mounting of other dogs or people will be altered by castration in 50 to 90 per cent of adult dogs. Other behavior patterns and characteristics such as playfulness, ability to learn, and function as a guard dog are not affected.[24]

PROSTATITIS AND PROSTATIC ABSCESS

There is confusion in the veterinary literature concerning the classification of prostatitis, prostatic abscess, and prostatic cysts. In many discussions, prostatitis is presented as an entity separate from prostatic abscess. In other discussions, prostatic abscess and prostatic cysts are regarded as similar or related entities. It seems more logical to discuss prostatitis and prostatic abscess as related entities distinguished from prostatic cysts. However, one problem with this classification is that prostatic cysts can become secondarily infected, with abscess formation.

Prostatitis in the dog can be acute, chronic, and complicated by abscess formation. Prostatitis is usually suppurative, and there is a tendency for abscess formation. It is commonly associated with prostatic hyperplasia and is probably secondary to it. Like prostatic hyperplasia, prostatitis has a high incidence in older dogs. Most prostatic infections are probably part of ascending urinary disease, and the organisms found in the prostate are those commonly isolated from urinary tract infections—including gram-negative organisms such as *Escherichia coli* and occasionally other organisms such as *Proteus* spp., staphylococci, and streptococci. Predisposing causes of prostatitis in the dog include estrogen administration and Sertoli cell tumors.

Clinical Signs

Acute prostatitis is usually suppurative, and the purulent foci either are multiple and small or coalesce to form one or several large cavities. The contour of the gland depends on the size and distribution of suppurative foci. Consequently, the prostatic lobes can be unequal in size and shape. Large abscesses can project from the gland as soft fluctuating masses that adhere to adjacent structures. The reaction in the gland is predominantly neutrophilic, and extensive scarring can follow episodes of acute prostatitis.

In acute prostatitis, the clinical signs resemble those of prostatic hyperplasia; however, the dog is generally sicker and in more pain. There can be constipation, urinary retention, urinary incontinence, tenesmus, and an increase in the size of the abdomen. A mass can generally be palpated in the caudal abdomen or can be palpated rectally. The prostate gland is increased in size, and the contour of the gland depends on the size and shape of abscess cavities. In acute prostatitis, the gland is generally softer and more spongy than normal. Fluctuating abscesses may be present (Figs. 119–1 and 119–2). In general, there is considerable pain on palpation of the enlarged prostate, whether it is palpated through the body wall or rectally. Pain is also manifested by the abnormal gait and stance of the dog. The dog walks with short, painful steps in the hind legs and generally stands with the hind legs tucked under the

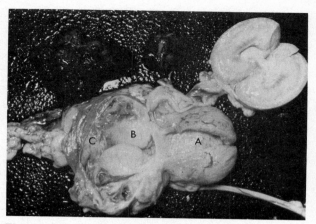

Figure 119–2. The abscess in the dog shown in Figure 119–1 has been opened to show the enlarged prostate gland. *A*, Bladder; *B*, prostate gland; *C*, abscess cavity.

abdomen to reduce pressure on the abdomen (Fig. 119–3). Systemic signs include anorexia and fever. Hematuria is a common sign, and there can be bloodstained and purulent discharge from the urethra. If a prostatic abscess ruptures into the peritoneal cavity, acute diffuse peritonitis, shock, and death can occur within one to two days.

Acute prostatitis can generally be diagnosed on the basis of clinical signs and palpation of the prostate gland. Prostatic secretions can be examined for inflammatory cells and bacteria. Cultures and sensitivity testing can be done on prostatic secretions or urine. Leukocytosis is usually present. Needle aspiration of the prostate gland is usually not required for diagnosis, although it can be done in doubtful

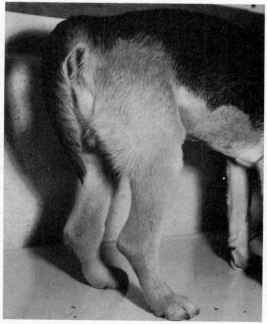

Figure 119–3. Typical appearance of a dog with a painful prostatic abscess. The tail is raised. The hind legs are advanced under the abdomen to relax the abdominal muscles and are edematous.

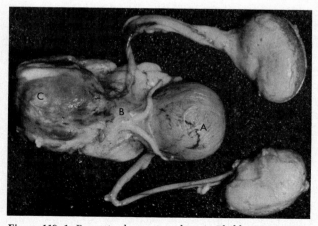

Figure 119–1. Prostatic abscess in a dog. *A*, Bladder; *B*, prostate gland; *C*, abscess.

cases. Fluid obtained by aspiration can be examined cytologically and by culture techniques. No reported complications have been reported following aspiration of prostatic abscesses (see Chapter 115).

Radiography can be used in diagnosis of acute prostatitis. However, usually it indicates only the presence of a large prostate gland and is not helpful in distinguishing among the various causes of prostatic enlargement. The expected radiographic changes in prostatitis include enlargement of the gland with cranial displacement (see Chapter 115).

Acute prostatitis is recurrent without appropriate therapy, and chronic prostatitis can be a sequel. In chronic prostatitis either there are acute episodes resembling those described previously for acute prostatitis or the condition remains chronic with a low-grade infection and many periods in which the dog is normal and afebrile. Therefore the dog is presented with signs resembling those of acute prostatitis or with a history of blood or pus at the urethral opening. With more severe infection, exudate drips from the penis constantly. The hemogram may reveal a normal or elevated white blood cell count, depending on the degree of prostatic involvement. Microscopic examination of an ejaculate or prostatic secretion reveals an inflammatory exudate. Findings of examination of prostatic aspirate are similar. On rectal palpation, the prostate gland is generally enlarged and symmetrical or asymmetrical, and there is usually some pain on palpation. The consistency of the gland varies widely. It may be soft and fluctuant in the presence of abscesses or firmer than normal with irregular areas of fibrosis. In many cases, the gland adheres to surrounding structures, as with prostatic carcinoma. Prostatic biopsy, either percutaneous or incisional at laparotomy, may be necessary to distinguish chronic fibrosis from prostatic carcinoma. In any adult male dog with a history of dripping of blood or purulent material from the urethra, chronic bacterial prostatitis should be ruled out by cytological examination and culture of the exudate, semen, or prostatic aspirate. In general, a quantitative culture that yields a greater number of organisms in semen than in midstream voided urine is evidence of primary genital infection, usually in the prostate gland.

With chronic drainage of purulent material from a prostatic abscess, massive adhesions can be seen within the peritoneal cavity. They can cause severe intestinal obstruction. Severe prostatic infections, usually with large abscess formation, can lead to an acute clinical situation in which the dog is lethargic, septicemia is present, and death can occur within a few days. Such an animal requires vigorous corrective therapy.

Treatment

Treatment of prostatitis in the dog includes correction of complications such as constipation and urinary obstruction as well as specific treatment for the infection. The complicating processes are treated as in prostatic hyperplasia.

Antibiotics are essential in treatment of prostatitis. Experimental results in normal dogs indicate that numerous antibacterial drugs are unable to diffuse readily into prostatic fluids in dogs.[21, 35, 37, 44-47, 50, 56] In these animals, negligible concentrations of ampicillin, penicillin G, cephalosporins, tetracycline, kanamycin, nitrofurantoin, and all sulfa drugs are found in prostatic fluid a few hours after intravenous administration. Differences among drugs in the diffusion in prostatic fluid are probably due to several factors, including lipid solubility, degree of ionization, plasma protein binding, and acidic or basic character of the drug. Prostatic fluid in the dog normally is more acidic than plasma, and basic antibiotics that diffuse in the fluid can be trapped there, exceeding plasma levels. Conversely, acidic drugs are excluded from prostatic fluid, depending on the degree of ionization. Weakly ionized acids can diffuse in prostatic fluid and can approach but cannot exceed plasma concentration. There are two major problems in trying to relate this experimental information to clinical prostatitis. First, there is some experimental information to show that if antibiotics are administered for prolonged periods, for example seven days, the drugs can attain effective levels in the prostatic fluid, although they did not attain effective levels immediately after administration. Secondly, the prostate-blood barrier that is undoubtedly present in normal glands is probably disrupted by inflammation. However, the clinician is advised to heed the results of these experiments, and if any of the limited range of drugs is effective on culture and sensitivity testing, it should be used. Trimethoprim and chloramphenicol are probably good choices in treatment of prostatitis in the dog.

In the treatment of chronic bacterial prostatitis, the duration of therapy and evaluation of the dog for persistent recurrent infection should be considered. Antibacterial therapy should be given for at least two weeks and in most cases for four to six weeks. Castration is generally recommended for treatment of prostatitis in the dog.[6] Controlled clinical studies of the effects of castration in prostatitis have not been done. However, prostatitis is likely to be associated with hyperplasia of the prostate. The most common procedure seems to be to castrate the dog to prevent a recurrence of the prostatitis. The operation is not always indicated during the acute phase of the inflammation. If surgery is necessary to drain a prostatic abscess, castration is certainly indicated. It leads to atrophy of the prostate gland and a significant decrease in the recurrence rate.

Prostatic abscesses can be associated with prostatitis and rarely respond to antibiotic therapy. Treatment is either drainage of the prostatic abscess or prostatectomy.[15, 23, 43] In one report, ten dogs with prostatic abscesses and four dogs with diffuse suppurative prostatitis were treated by procedures such as marsupialization, drainage, ligation of the prostatic artery, and prostatectomy.[17] The authors conclude that overall complications were more frequent with marsupialization and drainage procedures than with prostatectomy. However, they stated that to maintain urinary continence, it is critical that these former procedures should be used instead of prostatectomy. When the owner is willing to accept the risk of incontinence, prostatectomy is more reliable treatment for more severe prostatic disease. In my experience, urinary incontinence is a common complication of prostatectomy. Owners will not accept this complication, and the operation is rarely indicated. On the other hand, complications following drainage of prostatic abscesses are rare.

In 1978, Zolton described a surgical approach for treatment of prostatic abscesses in the dog.[58] In this report two to four one-centimeter rubber drains were passed from ventral to dorsal through the gland and fixed in place with one suture of chromic gut. In addition, drains were placed in the periprostatic area. Because drains are foreign bodies and irritants, this method constitutes an excessive amount of foreign material in the wound. I have used a simpler approach for many years: The animal is placed in dorsal recumbency and the abdomen is entered via a standard ventral midline incision, which should extend caudally to the pubis. The abdominal incision is held open by Balfour abdominal retractors. The region of the prostate gland is carefully examined; however, care is taken not to break down tissue, particularly adipose tissue in the periprostatic area. The prostate gland is carefully palpated and the prostatic abscess is delineated. The caudal abdomen and the prostatic abscess are packed off from the rest of the abdomen with saline-soaked laparotomy sponges (Fig. 119–4). The prostatic abscess is entered bluntly with a closed hemostat, and emerging purulent material is immediately aspirated to prevent contamination of the abdomen and surrounding tissues. The suction nozzle is inserted into the abscess cavity, and all purulent material is removed. The opening into the abscess is then enlarged. The surgeon's finger is inserted to

explore all cavities and break down loculi to encourage drainage. Because it is important to avoid the urethra in this procedure, the opening is made bluntly and lateral to the midline.

The surgeon's examining finger is inserted deep into the abscess cavity and across the midline to a point corresponding to the entry point on the other side of the abscess. A second blunt opening is made into the abscessed prostate gland at this point, and a five-millimeter Penrose drain is passed through the abscess cavity (Fig. 119–5A). There are no loose ends of drain within the abscess, and therefore there is no need to fix the end of the drain at this point. Both ends of the drain emerge from the abscess. The ends of the drain are exteriorized through the body wall, each one approximately two centimeters lateral to the prepuce (Fig. 119–5B). The drain must not be pulled tight as it passes over the urethra, because a tightly placed drain may lead to urethral obstruction. Both ends of the drain are secured firmly to the skin (Fig. 119–5C).

The advantages of this technique are (1) the drain is securely placed within the abscess because both ends are fixed to the skin and (2) because there has been minimal dissection of periprostatic tissue, infected material draining from the prostatic abscess cannot extend into the periprostatic tissue but instead follows the drain to the outside.

The drain in the abscess is left in place for three weeks. In most cases the dog must be prevented from removing the drain, by means of a bandage, an elizabethan collar, or a side brace. The dog is always castrated at operation. Purulent material is sampled for culture and sensitivity testing, and appropriate antibiotics are administered for two to three weeks.

In a series of 35 prostatic abscesses I treated in this manner, one dog had significant hemorrhage from the drain sites for several days after surgery. Bleeding stopped spontaneously and no further problems occurred. In another dog there was chronic fibrosis and residual small abscess formation in the prostate gland after removal of the drain. The other 33 dogs recovered completely from the prostatic infection, and there were no postoperative complications, including urinary incontinence. In my opinion, prostatectomy is definitely contraindicated in the treatment of prostatic abscess with one exception, as described later.

A distinction must be made at operation between a prostatic abscess and an infected prostatic cyst. If an infected prostatic cyst containing purulent material is treated by prostatic drainage as previously described, it is unlikely that the cavity of the cyst will be obliterated, and the infection probably will recur. Many reports of unsuccessful treatment of prostatic abscesses by drainage may refer to treatment of infected prostatic cysts. In these cases, the treatment of choice is marsupialization of the infected prostatic cyst, not drainage with a Penrose drain. The distinguishing surgical features of a prostatic abscess and an infected prostatic cyst are that in the latter case,

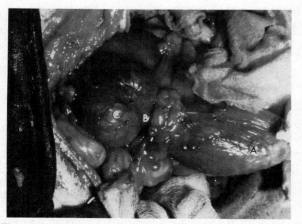

Figure 119–4. Prostatic abscess in a dog at surgical drainage. A, Bladder; B, prostate gland; C, abscess.

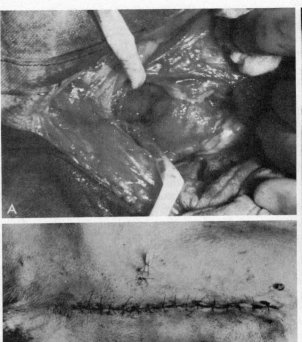

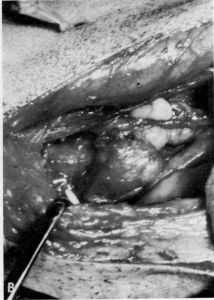

Figure 119–5. Surgical drainage of a prostatic abscess. *A,* A 5-mm Penrose drain has been passed through the abscess cavity without disturbing periprostate tissues. *B,* One end of the Penrose drain emerges through the body wall. The other end of the drain is brought out through the body wall on the opposite side of the incision. *C,* Completed prostatic abscess drainage. This drain is removed in approximately three weeks.

the wall of the abscess cavity is thickened and smooth and is lined by a smooth membrane, unlike the swollen inflamed wall of an abscess cavity. Future studies in the literature of treatment of prostatic abscess should be specific and should differentiate between the typical prostatic abscess and an infected prostatic cyst.

Prostatectomy or partial prostatectomy can be indicated in the treatment of prostatitis when the infection is chronic, there is considerable scar tissue in and around the prostate gland, and several small prostatic abscesses are present. In these cases it is difficult to remove the infection by drainage, and antibiotics and prostatectomy may be required. The owner must be informed that the dog is likely to be incontinent after this operation.

PROSTATIC CYSTS

Classification

Several classifications have been suggested for prostatic cysts in the dog, and considerable lack of agreement exists among authors.[23, 53] Prostatic hyperplasia in the dog is associated with cyst formation, although the cysts are generally microscopic. The name *cystic prostatic hyperplasia* has been given to this common prostatic enlargement in the dog. This condition has been discussed previously under the name *prostatic hyperplasia*, and it bears no relationship to the large prostatic cysts that can occur in the dog.

A second type of prostatic cyst in the dog is the cystic condition associated with squamous metaplasia. The cysts are related to exogenous estrogen administration or endogenous estrogen release by a functional Sertoli cell tumor. Prolonged administration of estrogens can produce squamous metaplasia of the prostate, which can lead to obstruction of prostatic ducts and cyst formation. This condition is discussed under "Squamous Metaplasia."

There are two main types of the classic large prostatic cyst in the dog and they are discussed here.

Prostatic Retention Cysts

There is no doubt that some large cysts are the result of the formation of large fluid-filled cavities within the parenchyma of the prostate gland. These cavities increase in size and eventually project from the wall of the prostate into the surrounding tissues. Retention cysts may be the result of obstruction of the prostatic ducts due to tissue proliferation from hyperplasia, chronic prostatitis, or neoplasia. Almost the entire parenchyma of the prostate gland may be destroyed, leaving only a thin cortex of prostatic tissue.

Paraprostatic Cysts

The second type of cyst in the dog is the paraprostatic cyst. It does not communicate with the prostate gland and does not arise from its parenchyma. In almost all cases, the prostate gland is normal or slightly enlarged. The cyst occurs in the tissue surrounding the prostate gland. Many forms of these cysts are seen in the dog, and they have two anatomical sites—in the abdomen lateral and cranial to the prostate gland, and in the pelvis caudal to the prostate gland. Some cysts occupy both sites, the main mass being in the abdomen with an extension into the pelvis, usually as far caudally as the perineum lateral to the anus. Paraprostatic cysts can also assume different forms. They can have a very thin, soft wall, usually with a smooth lining membrane, or the wall is thickened with a smooth lining membrane (Fig. 119–6). Affected animals often have masses of calcified material within the wall and projecting into the lumen in irregular stalagtite formations.

The origin of the large paraprostatic cysts has often been suggested as embryonal. Proof for this assertion is lacking.[19] Pinegger[42] in 1975 reported a case of a paraprostatic cyst arising from a uterus masculinus in a 7-year-old Hungarian Puli working dog. The dog had a grossly dilated and complete uterus masculinus causing a massive discrete swelling in the midabdomen. The mass originated from the dorsal aspect of the bladder neck and had a direct communication with the bladder lumen. It contained about 400 ml of yellow aqueous fluid with an odor of urine. This condition has been referred to recently as pyometra in the uterus masculinus.

In the dog, the prostate gland develops from the cranial portion of the urogenital sinus where the müllerian and wolffian ducts open into it. The blind sac known as the uterus masculinus is derived from the fused terminal portions of the müllerian ducts and becomes surrounded by the growing prostatic cord and eventually incorporated into the substance of the prostate.[39, 56] In the dog, the uterus masculinus

in the adult usually opens on the apex called the seminal hillock and is a short tube extending a few millimeters cranial to the substance of the prostate gland.[8] It is not possible from descriptions of recorded cases of paraprostatic cyst (except that by Pinegger[42]) to establish whether the origin was in the dorsal midline at the site of the uterus masculinus.

Clinical Signs

Few surveys have been done on prostatic cysts in the dog. A report by Weaver[53] in 1978 described discrete prostatic cysts in 12 dogs ranging in age from five to 12 years. Various breeds, including five border collies and three German shepherds, were included. There was only one small dog, a dachshund. The initial clinical signs were urinary in six cases, alimentary in five, and both urinary and alimentary in one. The duration of signs varied from two days to two years. All dogs were afebrile, and on palpation there was evidence of a smooth and painless mass in the caudal abdomen in 11 of the 12 dogs. The prostate was usually enlarged, and the caudal abdominal mass was separate from the prostate gland. An examination of blood was done in all dogs; five dogs had elevated serum urea nitrogen, four had elevated alkaline phosphatase, and three had elevated transaminase levels. All electrolyte and protein determinations were within normal limits. Four dogs had leukokytosis with neutrophilia.

The volume of the cysts varied from 90 ml to 800 ml. The cysts were in the abdomens in nine dogs, intrapelvic or both intrapelvic and intraperineal in two, and both intra-abdominal and intrapelvic in one. The degree of attachment of the cyst to the prostate varied considerably from a relatively limited pedicle to an extensive adhesion. The origin of the cyst varied, originating from the dorsal, ventral, or caudal surface of the gland. The contents of the cyst varied: colorless, pink or red/serous fluid, a gray or cloudy fluid, or a dark brown viscous material containing necrotic debris. In all instances, bacteriological culture result was negative. The specific gravity of the fluid in the cyst varied from 1.010 to 1.034. Many of the samples contained a high proportion of red cells and some contained epithelial cells.

The proportion of cases of prostatic disease that are caused by solitary prostatic cysts is generally low, varying from 2.6 to 5.3 per cent.[23, 53] Affected breeds are usually medium or large; few cases are seen in smaller breeds. There is no obvious breed preponderance among the larger dogs.

Most prostatic cysts cause no pain and can attain a very large size before becoming obvious. Interference with urination and defecation occurs only late in development, when the cysts have become large. Usually a cyst is more likely to lead to urinary than to alimentary disturbance, probably as a result of cranial displacement of the bladder neck or excessive pressure on the bladder wall. The lack of a febrile

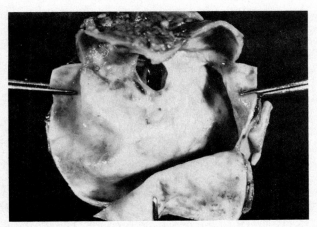

Figure 119–6. The typical smooth lining membrane in a paraprostatic cyst.

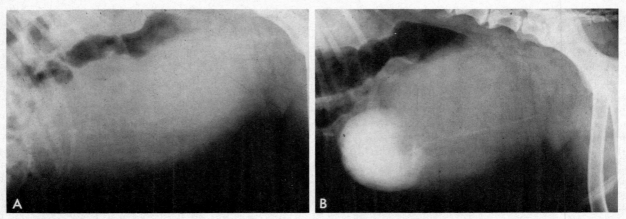

Figure 119–7. A large prostatic cyst in a dog. *A*, The cyst and the urinary bladder are indistinguishable in a survey radiograph. *B*, The urinary bladder and the urethra are seen in a cystogram.

reaction and pain on palpation are features that differentiate prostatic cysts from prostatic abscesses.

In Weaver's[53] series of twelve cases, the radiographic features of prostatic cysts on survey films were large spherical smooth masses of soft-tissue density (Fig. 119–7). In only one cyst, large calcified masses were present. In all cases, contrast radiography was used, and the contrast material did not reflux into the prostatic cyst from the urethra. Weaver[53] concluded that the striking radiographic features and the absence of fever and pain permit a firm diagnosis of prostatic cyst in most cases. He stated that the majority of prostatic abscesses have an obvious communication with the urethra, so that pneumocystography or positive-contrast cystography has usually resulted in passing of contrast material into the prostatic spaces. He stated that this reflux is not seen in prostatic cysts. In general, the prostatic cyst is seen radiographically as a large, fluid-filled mass of smooth outline occupying much of the caudal abdomen and either dorsolateral or lateral to the bladder shadow. The prostate gland itself may be obviously enlarged. Radiographic evidence of calcification can be seen in many cases.[53]

Stone and Thrall[51] in 1978 stated that infectious conditions of the prostate were thought to be the main cause of reflux of contrast material from the urethra into the prostate gland.[51] However, data from nine cases in their survey showed that all four categories of prostatic disease can have reflux of contrast material into the prostatic parenchyma, in disagreement with the findings of Weaver.[53] However, in Stone and Thrall's series of 24 dogs, only three dogs had cyst formation and these also had bacterial prostatitis. None of these cases resembled the typical prostatic cysts described by Weaver.[53] It seems likely that reflux of contrast material from the urethra is not likely to occur with paraprostatic cyst but could occur in prostatic retention cysts and in prostatic abscesses.

Treatment

Weaver[53] stated that surgery in the majority of his 12 cases proved difficult because of the extensive attachments of the cysts to the prostate and to the bladder neck. Accidental injury to the bladder neck or to the urethra can occur.[53]

Some prostatic cysts, particularly paraprostatic cysts, can be excised totally. At laparotomy the surgeon first determines that the attachment of the cyst in the region of the bladder and prostate is by a relatively narrow pedicle and that excision is possible. Extensive dissection in this area is contraindicated, because damage to the blood and nerve supply of the bladder is likely. In addition, no attempt at dissection and excision of the prostatic cyst should be undertaken if total excision of the portion near the bladder and prostate is not possible. In this situation, marsupialization is no longer possible because insufficient cyst wall remains to carry out a marsupialization procedure. I have seen severe peritoneal irritation and adhesions leading to intestinal obstruction and death in three cases of inadequate removal of a prostatic cyst. Most reports stress the benefits of marsupialization in the treatment of prostatic cysts in the dog. This procedure overcomes the problem of refilling of the cyst following other methods of drainage and the dangers associated with the resection of cysts that can be intimately associated with the bladder neck, ureters, and prostate gland. In marsupialization of a prostatic cyst, a laparotomy is done through a caudal ventral midline incision to expose the urinary bladder, prostatic cyst, and prostate gland. The diagnosis of prostatic cyst is confirmed by palpation, and a stab incision is made into the cyst with aspiration of its contents. The surgeon's finger thoroughly explores the cavity of the cyst, which has a smooth lining membrane. A site is selected for the stoma lateral to the penis and prepuce. The position depends on the size of the cyst, and the site is selected so that the cyst wall can be exteriorized at this point. The stoma should be placed as far cranially as possible. A small oval stoma is made in the skin, and the muscle fascia and muscle fibers are separated by blunt dissection into the peritoneum. Forceps are passed through the opening in the body wall to grasp the cyst wall and pull it through the opening in the body wall and the skin. The entire opening that was made previously in the cyst wall must be exteriorized. The cyst capsule is sutured to the musculature of the body wall with simple interrupted sutures of 2-0 or 0 absorbable material. Excess cyst wall is excised, and the cut edge is sutured to the skin with simple interrupted nonabsorbable suture. The excised portion of cyst wall is retained for histological examination. The lining of the prostatic cyst is treated with a cauterizing or irritating material such as tincture of iodine or silver nitrate solution, which is removed at the end of the procedure.

At operation, the cavity of the cyst is explored to determine that the cyst is entirely abdominal. If it is, the marsupialization just described is adequate therapy. If the cyst extends into the pelvis to the perineal skin, it may be necessary to pass a Penrose drain through the stoma at the site of marsupialization, through the main body of the cyst along the extension in the pelvis, and out through an opening in the perineum. In other cases it is possible to create a second marsupialization of a pelvic cyst in the perineum lateral or ventral to the anus. Every dog should be castrated to reduce the size and activity of the prostate.

Drainage from the marsupialization stoma decreases gradually and in most cases ceases completely after eight weeks, although it can persist indefinitely. In most cases the stoma eventually closes, and further surgery is not necessary. In a few cases, drainage persists and further surgery is needed to remove a small draining stalk from the prostate gland to the stoma and to close the stoma in the skin. There is some evidence that neoplasia is associated with paraprostatic cysts and prostatic retention cysts in the dog.[19, 23]

PROSTATIC NEOPLASIA

Prostatic neoplasms are rare in the dog, whereas prostatic carcinoma is the second most common cancer and the fourth leading cause of cancer-related death in humans. In dogs, prostatic neoplasia is probably the least common of the four prostatic disorders. The average age of most dogs developing prostatic carcinoma is nine to ten years, and no breed predisposition is seen.[6, 25, 32, 52, 55] Although most reports indicate that dogs that develop prostatic carcinoma are not castrated, this could be misleading information, because in any population, most dogs are probably not castrated.

Histologically, most neoplasms of the prostate gland are adenocarcinomas.[25, 32] Undifferentiated carcinomas, transitional cell carcinomas, leiomyosarcomas, and hemangiosarcomas have been reported.[31, 32, 41] The remainder of this discussion concerns prostatic adenocarcinomas.

Pathology

The pathological features of prostatic carcinomas in dogs have been described.[18] Carcinomas of the prostate gland are usually large and irregular.[32, 55] Leav and Ling[32] reported little change in gross size between hyperplastic prostate glands and neoplastic glands. The neoplastic prostate gland is generally more adherent to surrounding tissues than non-neoplastic glands, but some glands with inflammation adhere to surrounding structures. Prostatic adenocarcinomas are usually composed of variably sized and shaped alveoli lined by multiple layers of epithelial cells. In canine prostate glands that are not diffusely replaced by neoplastic cells, there are areas of hyperplasia, atrophy, and fibrosis.[32] Metastasis occurs most frequently to the iliac, lumbar, and pelvic lymph nodes, periprostatic tissue, lung, and bladder.[32, 55] Bone, mesentery, colon, rectum, and pelvic muscle may also be involved. In one report of nine prostatic adenocarcinomas, three metastasized to bone.[14] In humans, bone metastasis from prostatic carcinomas is commonly widespread and may develop before the primary prostatic carcinomas have caused clinical signs.[3] The vertebral venous system may be an important means of neoplastic spread to bone in humans, and neoplastic cells have been found in the vertebral venous plexus and basivertebral veins of two dogs.[5, 32] Radiographic changes in vertebral bodies are commonly present in prostatic carcinoma in the dog.

Cause of Prostatic Adenocarcinoma

The cause of prostatic carcinoma is not known. The effect of androgens and estrogens on prostatic volume and prostatic activity has been discussed previously.[12, 48] These hormones are probably highly significant in the development of prostatic hyperplasia in old dogs. However, because prostatic hyperplasia is common and carcinomas are uncommon, it is suggested that hyperplasia itself is not associated with neoplastic transformation.[1, 16, 24, 38, 52] In addition, testicular tumors are not associated with prostatic carcinoma.[55] The effects of previous castration on the incidence of prostatic carcinoma is also unknown, and any association is difficult to prove because there are fewer neutered than intact male dogs and because prostatic tumors are uncommon. In one study of prostatic carcinoma all 15 dogs were intact, whereas in another study 16 of 20 dogs were intact.[32, 55] In other studies, castrated dogs developed prostatic carcinoma.[18, 25] The influence of castration and the age at castration remain to be fully evaluated. In one series of 14 cases, seven of 14 dogs were castrated.[18] Unfortunately, time of castration was not known in four of the dogs; in the remaining three the length of time between castration and diagnosis of prostatic carcinoma was nine months, three years, and five years.

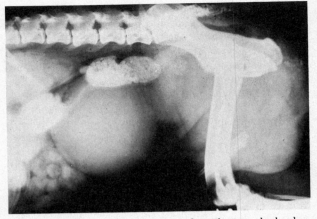

Figure 119–8. Prostatic carcinoma in a dog. The irregular borders of the prostatic mass and the area of calcification suggest a diagnosis of carcinoma, not hyperplasia; however, other tests are necessary.

Clinical Signs

The most common clinical signs of prostatic carcinoma, in order of frequency, are emaciation, rear leg lameness, lumbar pain, straining to defecate, straining to urinate, polydypsia, polyuria, and urethral bleeding.[9, 18, 32, 52, 55] In the dog, early diagnosis of prostatic carcinoma is usually not made. If the urethral lumen is invaded, dysuria, urinary retention and hematuria can occur. Clinical diagnosis of prostatic carcinoma is often difficult because this disorder is not easy to differentiate in some cases from prostatic hyperplasia, prostatic cysts, and prostatitis. The main problem occurs in the differentiation of prostatic carcinoma from prostatic hyperplasia and from chronic prostatitis in which abscess formation is not a prominent feature.

On physical examination of the prostate per rectum, the carcinomatous glands are usually large, firm, and irregularly nodular.[32, 55] This is different from prostatic hyperplasia, in which the enlargement is symmetrical and the glands have normal consistency. Prostatic carcinoma can resemble chronic prostatitis with fibrosis. Carcinomatous glands are occasionally more firmly attached to periprostatic tissues than in other diseases of the prostate, with the possible exception of prostatitis. The only two prostatic diseases in which pain can be elicited on prostatic palpation are prostatitis and prostatic carcinoma. In general, the presence of pain distinguishes prostatic neoplasia from hyperplasia and prostatic cysts. Prostatic carcinoma is usually the only prostatic disease in which surrounding bone and structures such as the rectum can be involved. Therefore, signs of rectal bleeding or obstruction, and of hind leg weakness associated with prostatic enlargement, generally point to a diagnosis of prostatic neoplasia.

Radiography can assist in diagnosis of prostatic disease, and some generalizations can be made concerning the radiographic appearance of prostatic neoplasia. In general, radiographic signs are not diagnostic (Fig. 119–8). Cystic and neoplastic prostates have a significantly greater normalized area than prostates with benign and inflammatory disease. Also, cystic and neoplastic prostate glands show both a circumferential asymmetry and an asymmetrical shape around the urethra compared with the prostate in benign and inflammatory disease.[51] The bones of the pelvis and vertebrae are examined for proliferative or lytic change, which can indicate direct or metastatic extension of prostatic neoplasia (Fig. 119–9).[25]

Urinalysis is not generally helpful in differentiating types of prostatic disease—abnormal urinalysis results can be obtained in all four prostatic disorders. Neoplastic cells have been found in the blood of dogs with prostatic adenocarcinoma.[1, 25, 32]

Evaluation of an ejaculate and fluid obtained by prostatic massage can be performed in the diagnosis of prostatic neoplasia, but in general the examination is not helpful. However, the presence of bacteria and inflammatory cells can suggest prostatitis. The finding of neoplastic prostatic cells would aid in the diagnosis of neoplasia, but a negative result is not helpful. Little information is available in the literature on the cytological examination of ejaculate and the fluid from prostatic massage in evaluation of prostatic disease.[4]

Needle aspiration and percutaneous biopsy can be diagnostic for prostatic neoplasia. It has been suggested that these techniques should not be used when acute prostatitis or prostatic abscess is likely to be present, because of the risk of introducing bacteria through the needle tract. This risk is probably more a theoretical than a real problem.[4] Percutaneous perirectal or transabdominal needle biopsy can be performed rapidly, and only light anesthesia or sedation is required. Disadvantages include the inability to see the prostate, to select diseased tissue, and to avoid puncturing blood vessels, abscesses, or the urethra. If neoplastic tissue is localized, it could be missed by a needle biopsy technique. In most reports, complications arising as a result of bleeding or entering the urethra did not occur, and the main problem with needle biopsy is missing localized tissue.[4, 32, 54] Because most prostatic carcinomas are large and can be localized by rectal or abdominal palpation, percutaneous needle biopsy is a valuable diagnostic test.

Incisional biopsy done during exploratory laparotomy is obviously a very accurate test that avoids most of the disadvantages of needle biopsy. Diseased prostatic tissue can be identified and sampled specifically.

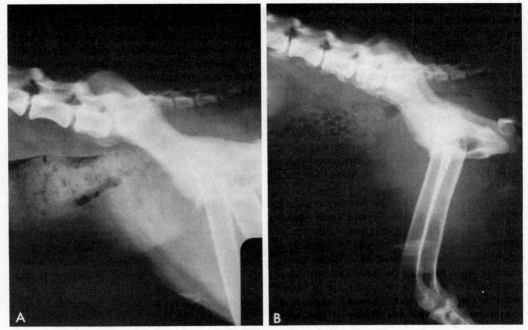

Figure 119–9. A, Bone proliferation on the pelvic bones and L7 in a dog with prostatic-carcinoma. *B*, A radiograph taken three weeks later shows marked progression of the bone lesions.

Sublumbar lymph nodes, the bladder, and periprostatic tissue can be evaluated. The disadvantages of incisional biopsy are the cost of the laparotomy and general anesthesia, and the trauma to the animal.

Transitional-cell carcinomas of the bladder and urethra can secondarily invade the prostate gland, and tumors of the prostatic urethra, usually transitional cell carcinomas, can easily be confused with primary prostatic tumors.[55]

Treatment

Prostatectomy should be done if a diagnosis is made early, when the prostate gland is relatively small and mobile. Because the diagnosis is usually made after local invasion or metastasis has occurred, prostatectomy is rarely effective in the dog. In humans, some prostatic tumors are initially androgen-sensitive and respond to castration or estrogen therapy. However, as the tumors regrow after a period of suppression they may become androgen-insensitive.[3] Other prostatic tumors are androgen-insensitive from the outset, and therefore castration is ineffective even for palliation. Castration and estrogen therapy have been reported to control temporarily the growth of canine prostatic carcinoma; however, no controlled clinical trials have been reported. In general, treatment of prostatic carcinoma in the dog is not successful. Most cases in the dog are seen only after local invasion and metastasis have occurred. The growth of the tumor is amazingly rapid, and the dog is generally euthanized in a few weeks.

SQUAMOUS METAPLASIA OF THE PROSTATE GLAND

Squamous metaplasia of the prostate gland is seen with excess estrogen, either administered orally or produced by a Sertoli cell tumor of the testicle. No reliable information exists concerning the amount of oral estrogen that can lead to metaplastic changes in the prostate.

Clinically, squamous metaplasia of the prostate produces signs identical to those of prostatic hyperplasia or prostatic cyst. Severe enlargement of previously unrecognized prostatic cysts can occur, leading to a serious clinical problem. In general, there are systemic signs of excess estrogen production or administration, including skin changes, hair loss, and bone marrow suppression. The diagnosis of squamous metaplasia of the prostate can be made by detecting the source of excess estrogen, noting the systemic signs of estrogen toxicity, and performing percutaneous needle or incisional biopsy of the prostate gland. Treatment involves removal of the source of excess estrogens, treatment of a prostatic cyst if present, and, occasionally, treatment of other prostatic conditions such as prostatitis.

PROSTATIC CALCULI

Prostatic calculi have been reported rarely in the dog. However, calcification of the prostate in association with chronic prostatitis, cysts, and prostatic neoplasia is not uncommon.[34] Prostatic calculi are found within the parenchyma or in prostatic ducts and are usually small and multiple. They are commonly composed of cholesterol, and calcium salts can be deposited on the surfaces of the stones.

Clinical signs of prostatic calculi are not characteristic and resemble those seen in other prostatic diseases and infection of the urinary tract. Prostatitis is commonly present. The prostatic calculi can occasionally be felt by rectal palpation, and if the stones are multiple, crepitus can be detected.

The diagnosis of prostatic calculi is confirmed by radiography, and the stones appear in dense, calcified masses within the parenchyma of the prostate gland. It is difficult to differentiate prostatic calculi from calcification of the prostate gland. Urethrography may be needed to differentiate urethral calculi in the prostatic urethra from prostatic calculi.

Little information is available on the treatment of prostatic calculi. It is likely that other conditions of the prostate such as prostatitis and prostatic neoplasia will be present, and they may require more urgent therapy than the calculi. Surgical removal of the calculi by incision of the prostate gland or prostatectomy is the usual treatment, if special treatment for the calculi is necessary.

TRAUMA TO THE PROSTATE

The prostate can be injured when a stiff urethral catheter pierces the wall of the prostatic urethra. This usually produces only hematuria and is probably not usually recognized. The prostate can be severely damaged with fracture of the pubis, during which the gland can be crushed between the mobile pubis and the sacrum. In most cases the prostate is fragmented, and the prostatic urethra is destroyed (Fig. 119–10).

The clinical sign is inability to urinate or the passage of blood in the urine. The diagnosis is easily confirmed by urethrography, and treatment involves removal by debridement of the fragmented prostate

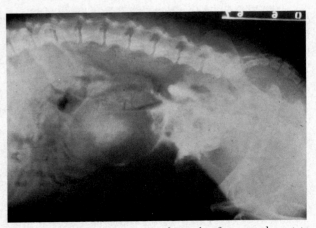

Figure 119–10. Urethrogram in a dog with a fragmented prostate gland. The femur and pubis are fractured. The dog recovered completely following prostatectomy and urethral anastomosis.

and anastomosis of the urethra. One dog in my practice with total fragmentation of the prostate and prostatic urethra in association with a pubic fracture was clinically normal after anastomosis of the urethra. In most cases the urethral anastomosis is difficult because the ends of the urethra are severely traumatized and do not hold sutures well. The concepts of suturing should be: (1) absorbable material is needed, (2) simple interrupted sutures are used, (3) the sutures should not be pulled tightly because blood supply to the cut edge can be disrupted, and (4) a watertight seal at the anastomotic site cannot be obtained. A Penrose drain is placed close to but not touching the anastomotic site, so that any urine that leaks through the anastomosis is drained to the exterior. Excellent healing of the canine urethra can occur under these circumstances.

PROSTATECTOMY IN THE DOG

Many procedures have been used to reduce the size of the prostate gland and to remove the contents of cysts and abscesses. The drainage of cysts and abscesses has been described previously. Capsulotomy, partial prostatectomy, and ligation of the prostatic vessels have been described in the dog. However, the rationale for these three procedures is unclear.

Partial prostatectomy (removing a portion of the prostatic parenchyma) has been recommended to relieve or correct prostatic hyperplasia and was described in 1931 and 1954 and, more recently, in 1984.[13, 30, 47a] In my opinion, the only indication for partial prostatectomy is the removal of infected prostatic tissue that does not respond to drainage, antibiotic administration, and castration. It may be preferable to remove diseased portions of the gland instead of the whole gland in order to avoid the urinary incontinence associated with total prostatectomy. After partial prostatectomy, castration is almost certainly indicated to produce further atrophy of the gland.

Ligation of the blood supply in the treatment of canine prostatic hyperplasia has been reported.[29] A later study failed to detect atrophy of the prostate following ligation of the blood supply.[22] Accordingly, it seems that this procedure has no place in veterinary surgery.

Complete prostatectomy in the dog has been recommended for treatment of all prostatic disease, and the incidence of its use varies among veterinary surgeons. In one report, it was stated that the complications associated with prostatectomy were fewer than those seen following drainage procedures for prostatic cysts and abscesses, and prostatectomy was recommended for treatment of many of these conditions.[17] Other reports have recommended prostatectomy for treatment of prostatic hyperplasia and prostatic neoplasia. In my opinion, prostatectomy should be performed only in the dog in early cases of prostatic neoplasia, in treatment of some intractable cases of chronic prostatitis in which the infection cannot be removed by use of drainage, antibiotics, and castration, and in some cases of prostatic trauma. Prostatectomy is rarely successful in treatment of prostatic neoplasia. In treatment of chronic prostatitis, successful results can usually be obtained by means of antibiotics and castration, and in chronic prostatitis with scarring, partial prostatectomy may be more appropriate than total prostatectomy. Unfortunately, total prostatectomy in the dog is associated with an extremely high incidence of postoperative urinary incontinence. Other complications that have been associated with the operation include perforation of the bladder or intestine, hemorrhage, infection, and urinary fistula formation.

Complete prostatectomy in the dog can be done by a perineal or prepubic approach. The perineal approach should be used only for removal of a retroflexed prostate gland that is part of a perineal hernia.[2] This approach is unsuitable for removal of an enlarged gland situated in the abdominal cavity. In perineal hernia, enlargement of the prostate is usually due to prostatic hyperplasia or congestion and hyperemia of the gland, and prostatectomy is not indicated. Therefore, the perineal approach for complete prostatectomy is rarely indicated in the dog. In most cases a prepubic laparotomy gives adequate exposure for removing an enlarged prostate gland, and only rarely does the surgeon have to enter the pelvic canal by osteotomy of the pubis. Prostatectomy in the dog by incision of the pelvic symphysis has been described, but the method involving partial reflection of the pubic bones and subsequent replacement of the bones as described by Howard in 1969 gives much better exposure of the gland.[26-28] In my technique,

the osteotomy of the pubis differs slightly from that described by Howard, in that the lateral incisions in the pubis are more lateral and the caudal incision is placed at the caudal limit of the obturator foramen. In addition, it is rarely necessary to place wire sutures in the caudal osteotomy site; fixation of the two cranial osteotomies is generally successful. As stated previously, osteotomy of the pubis is rarely needed in prostatectomy in the dog.

Preoperatively, the colon and rectum are emptied by a few days of a low-residue diet such as hamburger and white rice. Preoperative enemas are rarely needed. Infection in the urinary tract should be diagnosed, and treatment should commence before prostatectomy is done. Dogs needing prostatectomy often have chronic urinary tract disease, including interstitial nephritis with elevated serum creatinine level. Therefore preoperative and operative fluid therapy is needed.

For the prepubic approach to prostatectomy, the dog is placed in dorsal recumbency and a catheter is passed into the bladder. A skin incision is made from cranial to the umbilicus in the midline, caudally to the prepuce, and is extended to the pubis lateral to the prepuce. A large vein, the superficial epigastric vein, lies across the incision and is divided between ligatures. The penis and prepuce are retracted laterally so that the abdomen can be entered via a midline incision from the umbilicus to the pubis. The abdominal incision is held open by a Balfour abdominal retractor. Laparotomy sponges moistened with warm saline are used to isolate the bladder and prostate. The prostate is exposed by careful dissection through the periprostatic fat. Dissection then proceeds as close to the prostate as possible to avoid interfering with blood supply to the urethra and

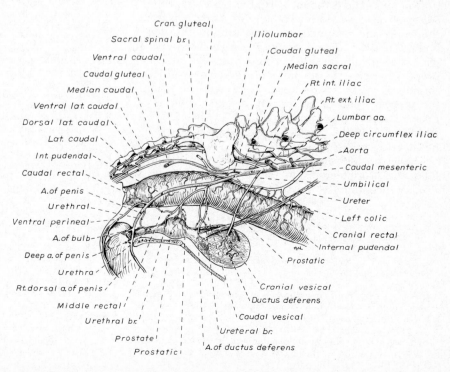

Figure 119–11. Blood supply to the prostate gland, urinary bladder, and rectum in a dog. (Reprinted with permission from Evans, H. E., and Christensen, G. C. (eds.): *Miller's Anatomy of the Dog.* 2nd ed. W. B. Saunders, Philadelphia, 1979.)

Cran. gluteal
Sacral spinal br.
Ventral caudal
Caudal gluteal
Median caudal
Ventral lat. caudal
Dorsal lat. caudal
Lat. caudal
Int. pudendal
Caudal rectal
A. of penis
Urethral
Ventral perineal
A. of bulb
Deep a. of penis
Urethra
Rt. dorsal a. of penis
Middle rectal
Urethral br.
Prostate
Prostatic

Iliolumbar
Caudal gluteal
Median sacral
Rt. int. iliac
Rt. ext. iliac
Lumbar aa.
Deep circumflex iliac
Aorta
Caudal mesenteric
Umbilical
Ureter
Left colic
Cranial rectal
Internal pudendal
Prostatic
Cranial vesical
Ductus deferens
Caudal vesical
Ureteral br.
A. of ductus deferens
Prostate
Prostatic
Cranial vesical

urinary bladder (Fig. 119–11). The prostatic arteries are clamped, divided, and ligated close to the gland. The vas deferens, which passes through the prostate gland dorsally to empty into the prostatic urethra, is divided and ligated. Considerable care is needed during this dissection to isolate completely the prostate from the periprostatic tissue without damaging blood and nerve supply to neighboring structures and to avoid injury to the colon and rectum.

Cranially, the prostatic tissue is carefully dissected away from the urinary bladder and urethra to expose some of the prostatic urethra. Generally this dissection can be done for only a short distance before it is necessary to transect the urethra as close to the prostate gland and as far away from the bladder neck as possible. This exposes the urethral catheter that was preplaced in the urinary bladder. Caudally, the urethra is transected as close to the prostate gland as possible, and the freed prostate gland is removed by slipping it off the catheter. The catheter is reinserted into the urinary bladder and the two ends of the urethra are approximated for anastomosis. The anastomosis is done using simple interrupted sutures of 3-0 absorbable suture material. Each suture is placed so that the ends of the urethra are approximated without tension and blood supply is not interrupted. It is usually preferable to insert first the sutures furthest from the surgeon, that is, on the dorsal aspect of the urethra, and to proceed in both directions around the circumference of the urethra. If any difficulty is encountered with the suturing, some urine leakage should be anticipated, and a Penrose drain is inserted close to, but not touching, the anastomotic site. The abdomen is closed routinely after irrigation with sterile saline.

Postoperatively, the catheter is left in place for one to two days. The catheter is fixed in place by passing adhesive tape around the catheter as it emerges from the penis and wrapping the tape around the dog's body. An alternative and more secure means is to pass a skin suture through the prepuce into the preputial cavity, to tie this suture securely to the catheter, to pass the suture again through the wall of the prepuce, and to tie the suture outside the prepuce. The catheter can be cut off so that its end remains within the preputial cavity and the dog does not have access to the catheter to remove it.

There is a high incidence of urinary incontinence following prostatectomy in the dog. In one survey, urinary incontinence was seen in six of seven dogs.[17]

1. Alsaker, R. D.: Neoplastic cells in the blood of a dog with prostatic adenocarcinoma. J. Am. Anim. Hosp. Assoc. 13:486, 1977.
2. Archibald, J., and Cawley, A. J.: Complete perineal prostatectomy and repair of perineal hernia. Sm. Anim. Clin. 1:73, 1961.
3. Ashley, D. J. B.: *Evan's Histological Appearances of Tumors.* 3rd ed. Churchill Livingstone, New York, 1978.
4. Barsanti, J. A., and Finco, D. R.: Canine bacterial prostatitis. Vet. Clin. North Am. 9:679, 1979.
5. Batson, O. V.: The function of the vertebral veins and their role in the spread of metastasis. Ann. Surg. 112:138, 1940.
6. Borthwick, R., and MacKenzie, C. P.: The signs and results of treatment of prostatic diseases in dogs. Vet. Rec. 89:374, 1971.
7. Campbell, J. R., and Lawson, D. D.: The signs of prostatic disease in dogs. Vet. Rec. 75:4, 1963.
8. Christensen, G. C.: The urogenital apparatus. *In* Evans, H. E., and Christensen, G. C. (eds.): *Miller's Anatomy of the Dog.* 2nd ed. W. B. Saunders, Philadelphia, 1979.
9. Clark, L., and English, P. P.: Carcinoma of the prostate gland in a dog. Aust. Vet. J. 42:214, 1966.
10. Ehrlichman, R. J., Isaacs, J. T., and Coffey, D. S.: Differences in the effects of an anti-androgen, SH 714 (6-Chlor 6–1, 2d-methylene-17-hydroxyprogesterone acetate, cyproterone acetate) on canine prostatic hyperplasia. Endocrinology 82:311, 1968.
11. Ehrlichman, R. J., Isaacs, J. T., and Coffey, D. S.: Differences in the effects of estradiol on dihydrotestosterone induced prostatic growth of the castrate dog and rat. Inv. Urol. 18:466, 1981.
12. El Etreby, M. F., and Mahrous, A. T.: Immunocytochemical technique for detection of prolactin (PRL) and growth hormone (GH) in hyperplastic and neoplastic lesions of the dog prostate and mammary gland. Histochemistry 64:279, 1976.
13. Frey, L.: Beitrag zur Prostatahypertrophie des Hundes. Tierartzl Umchav 17:297, 1954.
14. Goedegeburre, S. A.: Secondary bone tumors in the dog. Vet. Pathol. 16:520, 1979.
15. Gourley, I. M. G., and Osborne, C. A.: Marsupialization—a treatment for prostatic abscess in the dog. Anim. Hosp. 2:100, 1966.
16. Greiner, T. P., and Johnson, R. G.: Diseases of the prostate gland. *In* Ettinger, S. J. (ed.): *Textbook of Veterinary Internal Medicine.* W. B. Saunders, Philadelphia, 1983.
17. Hardie, E. M., Barsanti, J. A., and Rawlings, C. A.: Complications of prostatic surgery. J. Am. Anim. Hosp. Assoc. 20:50, 1984.
18. Hargis, A. M., and Miller, L. M.: Prostatic carcinoma in dogs. Comp. Cont. Ed. 5:647, 1983.
19. Harvey, C. E., Nunamaker, D. M., and Weber, W. T. (eds.): Clinico-Pathologic Conference from the School of Veterinary Medicine, University of Pennsylvania. Am. Vet. Med. Assoc. 155:928, 1969.
20. Hayes, H. M., Wilson, G. P., and Tarone, R. E.: The epidemiologic features of perineal hernias in 771 dogs. J. Am. Anim. Hosp. Assoc. 14:703, 1978.
21. Hessl, J. M., and Stamey, T. A.: The passage of tetracyclines across epithelial membranes with special reference to prostatic epithelium. J. Urol. 196:253, 1971.
22. Hodson, N.: On the intrinsic blood supply to the prostate and pelvic urethra in the dog. Res. Vet. Sci. 9:274, 1968.
23. Hoffer, R. E., Dykes, N. L., and Greiner, T. P.: Marsupialization as a treatment for prostatic disease: J. Am. Anim. Hosp. Assoc. 13:98, 1977.
24. Hopkins, S. G., Schubert, T. A., and Hart, B. L.: Castration of adult male dogs. Effects on roaming, aggression, urine marking and mounting. J. Am. Vet. Med. Assoc. 168:1108, 1976.
25. Hornbuckle, W. E., MacCoy, D. M., Allan, G. S., and Gunther, R.: Prostatic disease in the dog. Cornell Vet. 68(Suppl. 7):284, 1978.
26. Howard, D. R.: Surgical approach to the canine prostate. J. Am. Vet. Med. Assoc. 155:2026, 1969.
27. Knecht, C. D.: A symphyseal approach to pelvic surgery in the dog. J. Am. Vet. Med. Assoc. 149:1729, 1966.
28. Knecht, C. D., and Schiller, A. G.: Prostatectomy in the dog by incision of the pelvic symphysis. J. Am. Vet. Med. Assoc. 149;1186, 1966.
29. Kopp, H., and Stockton, N.: Ligation of blood supply in the treatment of canine prostatic hyperplasia. J. Am. Vet. Med. Assoc. 136:327, 1960.
30. Lamy, E.: Anatomie et chirurgie de la prostate du chien. Doctors Thesis, Faculty de Medicine de Paris, L'Ecole Veterinaire D'Alfort, 1931.
31. Leav, I., and Cavazos, L. F.: Some morphologic features of

normal and pathologic canine prostate. *In* Goland, M. (ed.): *Normal and Abnormal Growth of the Prostate.* Charles C Thomas, Springfield, 1975.

32. Leav, I., and Ling, G. V.: Adenocarcinoma of the canine prostate. Cancer 22:1329, 1968.

33. Lipowitz, A. J., Schwartz, A., Wilson, G. P., and Ebert, J. W.: Testicular neoplasms and concomitant clinical changes in the dog. J. Am. Vet. Med. Assoc. 163:1364, 1973.

34. Lumb, W. V.: Prostatic calculi in a dog. J. Am. Vet. Med. Assoc. 121:14, 1952.

35. Madsen, P. O., Wolf, H., Barquin, O. P., et al.: The nitrofurantoin concentration in prostatic fluid of humans and dogs. J. Urol. 100:54, 1968.

36. Merk, F. B., Leav, I., Kwan, P. W. L., and Ofner, P.: Effects of estrogen and androgens on the ultrastructure of secretory granules and intercellular junctions in regressed canine prostate. Anat. Rec. 197:111, 1980.

37. Mobley, D. F.: Erythromycin plus sodium bicarbonate in chronic bacterial prostatitis. Urology 3:60, 1974.

38. Moulton, J. E.: Tumors of the genital system. *In* Moulton, J. E. (ed.): *Tumors in Domestic Animals.* University of California Press, Berkeley, 1978.

39. Narbaitz, R.: Male sex organs. *In* Brandes, D. (ed.): *Structure and Function in Mammals.* Academic Press, New York, 1974.

40. O'Shea, J. D.: Studies on the canine prostate gland. J. Comp. Pathol. Ther. 72:321, 1962.

41. O'Shea, J. D.: Studies on the canine prostate gland. II: Prostatic neoplasms. J. Comp. Pathol. Ther. 73:244, 1963.

42. Pinegger, H.: Kleintierpraxis 20:231, 1975.

43. Pollock, S.: Prostatic abscess in the dog. J. Am. Vet. Med. Assoc. 129:274, 1956.

44. Reeves, D. S., and Chilchik, M.: Secretion of the antibacterial substance trimethoprim in the prostate fluid of dogs. Br. J. Urol. 42:66, 1970.

45. Reeves, D. S., Rowe, R. C. G., Snell, M. E., et al.: 23 further studies on the secretion of antibiotics in the prostate fluid of the dog. *In: Proceedings, Second National Symposium on Urinary Tract Infection,* London, 1972.

46. Robb, C. A., Carroll, P. T., Tippett, L. O., and Langston, J. B.: The diffusion of selected sulfonamides, trimethroprim, and diaveridine into prostatic fluid of dogs. Invest. Urol. 8:679, 1971.

47. Robb, C. A., Langston, J. B., Poe, R. D., and Bach, F. C.: Evidence against the diffusion of sulfisoxazole and sulfamethizole into the prostatic fluid of dogs. Invest. Urol. 8:37, 1970.

47a. Robertson, J. J., and Bojrab, M. J.: Subtotal intracapsular prostatectomy. Results in normal dogs. Vet. Surg. 13:6, 1984.

48. Rohr, H. P., Coffey, D. S., DeKlerk, D. P., et al.: The dog prostate under defined hormonal influences: an approach to experimental induced prostatic growth. Pathol. Res. Pract. 166:347, 1980.

49. Stamey, T. A.: *Urinary Infections.* Williams & Wilkins, Baltimore, 1972.

50. Stamey, T. A., Meares, E. M., and Winningham, D. G.: Chronic bacterial prostatitis and the diffusion of drugs into prostatic fluid. J. Urol. 103:187, 1970.

51. Stone, E. A., Thrall, D. E., and Barber, D. L.: Radiographic interpretation of prostatic disease in the dog. J. Am. Anim. Hosp. Assoc. 14:115, 1978.

52. Taylor, P. A.: Prostatic adenocarcinoma in a dog and a summary of ten cases. Can. Vet. J. 14:162, 1973.

53. Weaver, A. D.: Discrete prostatic (paraprostatic) cysts in the dog. Vet. Rec. 102:435, 1978.

54. Weaver, A. D.: Transperineal punch biopsy of the canine prostate gland. J. Small Anim. Pract. 18:573, 1977.

55. Weaver, A. D.: Fifteen cases of prostatic carcinoma in the dog. Vet. Rec. 109:71, 1981.

56. Willis, R. A.: *The Borderland of Embryology and Pathology.* Butterworth, London, 1958.

57. Winningham, D. G., Nemoy, N. J., and Stamey, T. A.: Diffusion of antibiotics from plasma into prostatic fluid. Nature 219:139, 1968.

58. Zolton, G. M., and Greiner, T. P.: Prostatic abscesses—a surgical approach. J. Am. Anim. Hosp. Assoc. 14:698, 1978.

Chapter **120** # Scrotum

Harry W. Boothe

SCROTAL INJURY

Scrotal injury is not common despite the exposed location of the scrotum.[4] Clinical signs depend upon the severity of the injury. Minor abrasions and lacerations may be initially undetected because of the paucity of clinical signs. Inflammation with or without signs of infection are seen, and the scrotum is sensitive to palpation. The animal frequently licks at scrotal wounds, causing further inflammation and possible infection. A stiff gait may be noted, and the dog often prefers to sit. More significant wounds are more likely to become infected if treatment is delayed. Trauma to the parietal vaginal tunic of the testis can result in infection within the cavity of the vaginal tunic and even orchitis.

Minor abrasions and lacerations are treated by gentle cleaning of the wound with saline, application of topical antibiotics, and prevention of self-inflicted trauma. The use of antiseptics on the scrotum is usually avoided because of the irritation they produce. More extensive wounds require suturing with fine, nonreactive skin sutures following cleaning, debridement, and local antibiotic irrigation. Severely contaminated wounds may require unilateral or bilateral castration with scrotal ablation (see Chapter 116).

The prognosis following scrotal injury is good, provided that contamination has been minimal and the parietal vaginal tunic has not been traumatized. Prevention of self-mutilation of the scrotum is the usual aftercare required. Systemic antibiotics may be indicated in extensive scrotal wounds.

INFECTION OF THE SCROTAL SKIN

The exposed location and delicacy of the scrotal skin make it relatively susceptible to irritants. A disinfectant such as iodine is frequently the cause of scrotal irritation and subsequent infection, particularly in surgical procedures and in kennels. Scrotal dermatitis is a prominent feature of *Brucella canis* infection of male dogs.[3] Infection can also be secondary to scrotal laceration. The scrotal skin is inflamed, edematous, exudative, and sensitive to palpation. Culture and susceptibility testing of the exudate determines appropriate antibiotic therapy. Management is usually directed at avoidance of further scrotal irritation and local treatment with emollients and antibiotics. Systemic antibiotics are indicated in severe cases. The prognosis is generally good; however, severe cases may require castration and scrotal ablation (see Chapter 116).

CHRONIC HYPERPLASIA OF THE SCROTUM

Hyperplasia of the scrotum is common in older dogs.[4] A thickened, wrinkled, and usually heavily pigmented ventral scrotum is seen. This condition presumably results from chronic irritation of the scrotum. Because of the insulating effect of the thickened scrotum, fertility may be reduced. Scrotal hyperplasia usually, however, is not clinically significant unless secondary infection occurs. Simple cases of scrotal hyperplasia are usually not treated. Resistant infections are treated by excision of the involved tissue and closure of the scrotum with fine sutures. It is important to avoid incising the parietal vaginal tunic. Extensive hyperplasia with infection may require castration and scrotal ablation (see Chapter 116).

VARICOSITIES OF THE SCROTAL BLOOD VESSELS

Varicose dilation of scrotal veins occurs in older dogs.[5, 6] The varicosities are seen as flattened and irregular thickenings of the scrotal skin.[5] They are subepithelial, with the overlying epithelium normal or ulcerated. Trauma leads to ulceration and repeated episodes of profuse bleeding.

Treatment involves either stimulating thrombosis of the varicose vessels with styptics or surgically removing the involved scrotal skin and blood vessels. Surgical removal is generally more effective, because recurrence following use of styptics or chemical cautery is common. All involved scrotal skin should be excised without incision of the parietal vaginal tunic. Blood vessels are ligated, and the incision is closed with fine nonabsorbable skin sutures. A support bandage and prevention of self-injury are indicated postoperatively. Extensive lesions may require excision of the majority of the scrotum. The testes can be transposed to the subcutaneous tissues lateral to the penis; however, castration is generally indicated. Prognosis depends upon the severity of the lesion. The less significant lesions require no treatment, whereas extensive lesions are treated by castration and scrotal ablation.

SCROTAL NEOPLASMS

Many cutaneous neoplasms involve the scrotum.[1, 2, 4, 6] Mastocytomas are relatively commonly reported. Because of their accessible location, scrotal neoplasms can often be differentiated by fine-needle aspiration or impression smears (see Section 19). Wide excision of a scrotal neoplasm may necessitate castration and scrotal ablation (see Chapter 116). Closure of scrotal skin following removal of a neoplasm should be performed with fine nonabsorbable sutures.

1. Barron, C. N.: Scrotal neoplasms—a report of two cases in the dog. J. Am. Vet. Med. Assoc. *115*:13, 1949.
2. Brodey, R. S.: Multiple genital neoplasia (mast cell sarcoma, seminoma, and sertoli cell tumor) in a dog. J. Am. Vet. Med. Assoc. *128*:450, 1956.
3. George, L. W., Duncan, J. R., and Carmichael, L. E.: Semen examination in dogs with canine brucellosis. Am. J. Vet. Res. *40*:1589, 1979.
4. Johnston, D. E., and Archibald, J.: Male genital system. *In* Archibald, J. (ed.): *Canine Surgery.* American Veterinary Publications, Inc., Santa Barbara, 1974.
5. Jubb, K. V. F., and Kennedy, P. C. (eds.): *Pathology of Domestic Animals.* Academic Press, New York, 1970.
6. Weipers, W. L., and Jarrett, W. F. H.: Haemangioma of the scrotum of dogs. Vet. Rec. *66*:106, 1954.

Section **XIV**

Female Reproductive System

Dudley E. Johnston
Section Editor

121 Anatomy

Elizabeth A. Stone, Peggy M. Wykes, and Patricia N. Olson

OVARY

The ovaries are oval and flattened. The ovary has a smooth surface in the prepubertal animal, but after several estrous cycles it becomes rough and nodular. The ovaries in a 10-kg dog are about 1.5 cm in length, 0.7 cm in width, 0.5 cm in thickness, and 0.3 gm in weight.[2] The feline ovary is about 1 cm in diameter.[8]

The ovaries are located 1 to 3 cm caudal to the kidneys near the abdominal wall. In multiparous animals, the ovaries are located more caudally and ventrally.[2] Canine ovaries are completely concealed within a peritoneal pouch, the *ovarian bursa*, which is formed from the mesosalpinx, a double fold of peritoneum. The bursa measures 2.5 cm to 5 cm dorsoventrally and 0.5 to 3.5 cm craniocaudally.[6] The bursa is completely closed, except for a narrow slit-like opening ventrally, and in the dog usually contains fat.[8] On the lateral surface of the ovarian bursa there is a round, fat-free area through which the ovary can usually be seen.[6] The ovarian bursa in the cat is much smaller, contains no fat, and covers only the lateral surface of the ovary. The medial surface of the feline ovary is covered ventrally and cranially by the infundibulum of the uterine tube.[4]

The ovary is attached to the dorsolateral region of the abdominal wall by the mesovarium, which is a part of the broad ligament (Fig. 121–1). The suspensory ligament of the ovary extends between the middle and ventral thirds of the last two ribs and the ventral surface of the ovary and mesosalpinx and forms the cranial portion of the free border of the broad ligament. The proper ligament of the ovary is a continuation of the suspensory ligament. It connects the caudal end of the ovary to the cranial end of the uterine horn.[2]

The ovary is divided into a medulla and a cortex. The medulla contains blood vessels, nerves, lymphatics, smooth muscle fibers, and connective tissue. The cortex contains connective tissue stroma and a large number of follicles.[2] A follicle is made up of an oocyte and its surrounding granulosa cells. A basement membrane separates the follicle from the ovarian stroma.[2] A connective tissue capsule, the *tunica albuginea,* surrounds the ovary. The peritoneal covering over the tunica albuginea is called the *superficial epithelium of the ovary.*[2]

The blood supply of the ovary is from the ovarian artery, a branch of the aorta. Branches of the uterine artery may also supply the ovary.[4] The right ovarian vein drains into the caudal vena cava. The left ovarian vein enters the left renal vein. The ovarian lymphatics drain into the lumbar lymph nodes.[2] The ovarian blood vessels are innervated by sympathetic nerves from the renal and aortic plexuses. The ovarian follicles and interstitial secretory tissues may not have sympathetic innervation.[2]

UTERINE TUBE

The uterine tube, or oviduct, of the bitch is 6 to 10 cm long.[6] The infundibulum forms the cranial end of the uterine tube. Multiple fingerlike processes, fimbriae, project from the end of the funnel-shaped infundibulum. The opening of the infundibulum into the ovarian bursa is called the abdominal ostium. The uterine tube extends cranially away from the ovary

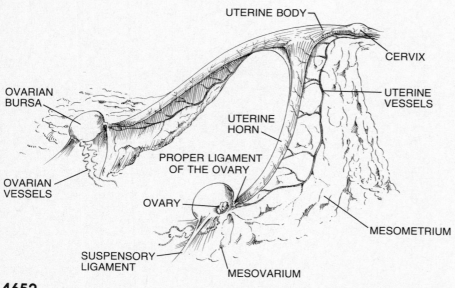

UTERINE BODY

CERVIX

OVARIAN BURSA

UTERINE VESSELS

UTERINE HORN

OVARIAN VESSELS

PROPER LIGAMENT OF THE OVARY

OVARY

MESOMETRIUM

SUSPENSORY LIGAMENT

MESOVARIUM

Figure 121–1. Anatomy of the uterus and ovary.

and then bends sharply back toward the cranial uterine horn. The opening of the uterine tube into the uterine horn is called the uterine ostium.[2]

The uterine tube is covered by a peritoneal covering, the tunica serosa. The muscular layer consists mainly of circular muscle but also contains some longitudinal and oblique fibers. The mucosal layer consists of partially ciliated columnar epithelium.[2]

The ovarian and uterine arteries supply the uterine tube. The corresponding veins drain the uterine tube. The lymphatics drain into the lumbar lymph nodes. Innervation is by the aortic and renal plexuses (sympathetic) and pelvic plexus (parasympathetic).

UTERUS

The uterus consists of a cervix, a body, and two uterine horns that connect with the uterine tubes.

The *uterine horns* in a 10-kg dog average 10 to 14 cm in length and 0.5 to 1 cm in diameter.[2] In the cat, they are about 9 to 10 cm long.[6] They lie completely within the abdominal cavity. They extend from the uterine tubes to the uterine body. At their caudal end they are united by peritoneum for a short distance, but they enter the uterine body separately.

The *uterine body* is about 1.4 cm long and 0.8 to 1 cm wide in the dog and 2 cm long in the cat[2,6] and is located in both the abdominal and pelvic cavities. In multiparous animals the entire uterine body may be located within the abdominal cavity.[2] It lies between the descending colon and the urinary bladder. An internal musculomembranous projection, not visible externally, extends 1 cm into the body of the uterus, separating the horns.[2]

The *cervix* in the dog is about 1 cm long. The *internal orifice* of the cervix faces almost dorsally; the *external orifice* is directed ventrally toward the vaginal floor.[3] The feline cervix feels like a hard oval knot at the uterovaginal junction.

The *mesometrium* is part of the broad ligament and attaches the uterus to the dorsolateral body wall. The *round ligament of the uterus* extends between the tip of the uterine horn and the deep inguinal ring. It may pass through the inguinal canal within the vaginal process and subcutaneously near the vulva.[2]

The outer layer of the uterus is termed the *tunica serosa*. It is a peritoneal covering that is continuous with the mesometrium. The muscular layer, *tunica muscularis* or *myometrium*, consists of an outer thin layer of longitudinal smooth muscle and an inner thick layer of circular smooth muscle. Within the circular layer is a vascular layer containing blood vessels, nerves, and circular and oblique muscle fibers. The innermost layer of the uterus is the *tunica mucosa*, or *endometrium*. It has a lamina propria with simple branched tubular uterine glands that open into the uterine lumen. Low columnar epithelium, which is temporarily ciliated, faces the uterine lumen.[2,6]

The ovarian and uterine arteries supply blood to the uterus. The uterine branch of the ovarian artery supplies the cranial uterine horns. The uterine artery is the main artery to the uterus. It arises from the umbilical artery, which is a branch of the internal iliac artery. The uterine branch of the urogenital artery (from the internal pudendal artery) supplies the caudal uterus, the cervix, and parts of the vagina.[6] The uterine veins follow the course of the arteries except, as mentioned above, the left ovarian vein enters the left renal artery.[2]

The uterine lymphatics drain into the hypogastric and lumbar lymph nodes. Innervation of the uterus is via the hypogastric plexus (sympathetic and visceral afferent fibers) and the pelvic nerves (parasympathetic and visceral afferent fibers).[2]

VAGINA AND VULVA

The vagina is a highly distensible musculomembranous structure that extends from the uterus to the vulva. The external genitalia, or vulva, consists of the vestibule, clitoris, and labia (see Fig. 123–1). The vestibule (derived from the urogenital sinus) joins the vagina (derived from the müllerian ducts) just cranial to the urethral opening.[5] Although no hymen is normally located at this vestibulovaginal junction, such a vestige is retained in some bitches (see hereafter).

Evaluation of the vagina via vaginoscopy is difficult owing to the unique anatomical features of the canine vagina. The vagina is an extremely long structure (10.5 to 23.5 cm) in bitches weighing 6.5 to 27 kg.[1] Unfortunately, this length prevents complete examination of the entire vagina in many dogs when otoscopic or standard vaginal speculae are used. A dorsal median postcervical fold extends from the edge of the vaginal portion of the cervix and terminates caudally by blending with smaller longitudinal folds of vaginal mucosa. Although the function of the postcervical fold is unknown, the fold can be mistaken for the cervical os during vaginoscopy.[7]

The vaginal wall consists of an inner mucosal layer, a middle smooth muscle layer, and an external coat of connective tissue. The tunica mucosa is a nonglandular, stratified squamous epithelium that undergoes histological changes during the various stages of the estrous cycle. The tunica muscularis is composed of a very thin inner layer of longitudinal muscle, a thick circular layer, and a thin outer longitudinal layer.

The vaginal artery, a branch of the urogenital artery, supplies blood to the vagina and vestibule. The vaginal veins empty into the internal pudendal veins. Vaginal lymphatics drain into the internal iliac lymph nodes. Both sympathetic and parasympathetic nerves from the pelvic plexus innervate the vagina as well as sensory afferent fibers via the pudendal nerve.

The vestibule connects the vagina with the vulvar labia, which open to form the vulvar cleft. The urethral tubercle arises from the floor of the vestibule, just caudal to the vestibulovaginal junction. Since vestibular mucosa is smooth, unlike vaginal mucosa, which contains distinct ridges, the vestibulovaginal junction can be grossly identified. The mucosal surface of the vestibule is covered by stratified squamous epithelium and contains small lobular glands located deep to the constrictor vestibuli muscles. The constrictor vestibuli and the constrictor vulvae muscles facilitate copulation by maintaining the "tie" and elevating the labia for intromission of the penis.[5]

The labia, or lips of the vulva, are derived from the embryonic genital swellings. Homologous to the scrotum of the male, the labia form the external boundary of the vulva. The labia are composed of smooth muscle, fat, and fibrous and elastic connective tissue.

The clitoris is derived from the genital tubercle in the embryo. It is a homologous structure to the penis and projects into the clitoral fossa. The clitoris is normally very small (a few mm in diameter) and does not normally contain any structure comparable to the os penis unless the bitch is exposed to anabolic steroids (i.e., intersex, drug therapy, Cushing's syndrome, and so on). The clitoris and clitoral fossa are readily seen when the lips of the vulva are spread laterally. The body of the clitoris consists of fat,

elastic connective tissue, and a tunica albuginea. The glandula clitoridis consists of erectile tissue and numerous sensory nerve endings.

Blood is carried to the vestibule, the labia, and the clitoris by branches of the left and right urogenital arteries and internal and external pudendal arteries. Satellite veins accompany these arteries. Motor innervation is supplied by branches of the pudendal, hypogastric, and pelvic nerves. Sensory fibers arise from the pudendal and genital nerves.[5]

1. Burke, T. J., and Reynold, H. A.: The female genital system. In Bojrab, M. J. (ed.): *Pathophysiology in Small Animal Surgery*. Lea & Febiger, Philadelphia, 1981, pp. 425.
2. Evans, H. E., and Christensen, G. C.: *Miller's Anatomy of the Dog*. W. B. Saunders, Philadelphia, 1979.
3. Getty, R.: *Sisson and Grossman's The Anatomy of the Domestic Animals*. W. B. Saunders, Philadelphia, 1975.
4. Ginther, O. J.: Comparative anatomy of the uteroovarian vasculature. Scope *20*:3, 1976.
5. Miller, M. E., Christensen, G. C., and Evans, H. E.: *Anatomy of the Dog*. W. B. Saunders, Philadelphia, 1964, pp. 790.
6. Nickel, R., Schummer, A., Seiferle, E., and Sack, W. O.: *The Viscera of the Domestic Mammals*. Verlag Paul Parey, New York, 1973.
7. Pineda, M. H., Kainer, R. A., and Faulkner, L. C.: Dorsal median postcervical fold in the canine vagina. Am. J. Vet. Res. *34*:1487, 1973.
8. Roberts, S. J.: *Veterinary Obstetrics and Genital Diseases (Theriogenology)*. Published by the author, Ithaca, 1971.

Chapter **122** Physiology of the Estrous Cycle and Gestation

Elizabeth A. Stone

ESTROUS CYCLE IN THE BITCH

The estrous cycle in the bitch is monoestrous with one period of receptivity during each breeding season.[25] Cycle length varies among dog breeds. Small breeds have a cycle length of four to seven months and larger breeds 6 to 12 months.[3, 23] Dogs may enter estrus (the period of receptivity) at any time of the year. As one author has stated, "the popular opinion that the dog has a regular six-month estrous period, estrus occurring twice annually with a definite seasonal trend, is in reality a misconception."[15]

Puberty begins in most dogs at six to nine months of age. Larger breeds may not have their first estrus until two years of age.[25] The estrous cycle in the bitch is divided into four stages: proestrus, estrus, diestrus, and anestrus (Table 122–1).

The onset of *proestrus* is characterized by vulvar and vaginal enlargement due to congestion, the accumulation of interstitial fluid, and the growth of

stratified squamous epithelium under the influence of estrogen.[2, 23] The mucosal lining of the cervix becomes folded and the lumen dilates.[15] A bloody discharge from red blood cells lost into the lumen of the uterus by diapedesis starts within two to four days.[6] In late proestrus the walls of enlarged ovarian follicles develop elaborate, lacelike folds consisting of vascular theca interna, basement membrane, and an avascular mural granulosa.[6] Granulosa cells lining the antrum become spherical as intracellular and intercellular secretory products accumulate. These preovulatory follicles are in a preluteinized state.[15]

The proestral bitch may become restless and start to roam. Most bitches avoid or attack all males during this period.[4]

Luteinizing hormone (LH) concentrations rise slowly for three to five days during proestrus. Peak values may occur 24 to 48 hours before ovulation[15] and about eight days before the onset of diestrus.[13] Concentrations of FSH decline during proestrus and

TABLE 122–1. Estrous Cycle in the Dog*

	Proestrus (5–15 days)	Estrus (5–15 days)	Diestrus (60–80 days)	Anestrus (variable length)
Clinical	Vulva enlarged Bloody discharge Restlessness, roaming behavior	Vulva enlarged Breeding stance Sexual receptivity Reduced vaginal discharge	No signs or Pseudopregnancy	No signs
Morphological	Congested genitalia Follicles enlarge rapidly	Congested genitalia Ovulation Corpus luteum develops Endometrial proliferation	Corpus luteum active Endometrial proliferation	Follicles slowly develop Endometrium sloughs and repairs
Hormonal	Estrogens rise and peak LH peaks 24–48 hours Progestins rise slightly	Estrogens decrease before ovulation Progestins rise	Progestins plateau and decline	No changes except near proestrus, when estrogens rise slightly

*Data from Jochie, W., and Andersen, A. C.: The estrous cycle in the dog: A review. Theriogenology 7:113, 1977; Shille, V. M., and Andersen, A. C.: The estrous cycle of the bitch. Canine Pract. Jul.–Aug:29, 1974; and Siegel, E. T.: *Endocrine Diseases of the Dog.* Lea & Febiger, Philadelphia, 1979.

increase coincidentally with or one or two days after the LH peak.[17a] Estrogen concentrations rise during proestrus and reach highest levels before the LH peak. Plasma estrogen levels are lower in the dog than in other species.[15] There is a slow preovulatory rise in progesterone levels during late proestrus.[8]

Proestrus lasts from 5 to 15 days and ends with the onset of estrus.[15]

Estrus is the period of sexual receptivity. First acceptance of the male is used as zero time in the estrous cycle of the dog. The next 24 hours are considered day 1. If the dog is not bred, day 1 of the cycle begins when the bitch assumes the breeding stance.[15]

Ovulation is spontaneous in the dog. The younger adult bitch may ovulate as early as the first day of estrus. Older bitches may ovulate later in estrus (days 1 to 5).[23] Oocytes remain in the bursal cavity for a few hours and then pass through the oviduct. Meiosis is completed in the middle and uterine portions of the oviduct. Ova cannot be fertilized until the first reduction-division step of meiosis has been completed (first polar body formation).[6, 15, 23] Oocytes remain viable for at least six days.[6]

Ovarian follicles secrete small amounts of progesterone before ovulation and before becoming luteinized. Plasma progesterone levels rise rapidly soon after the LH peak. Estrogen and LH levels return to baseline levels following ovulation.[15, 17]

Estrus continues until the bitch is no longer sexually receptive. The length of estrus averages 9 days, varying from 5 to 15 days.[6] The exact end of estrus is difficult to determine because a bitch may reject a male one day and be receptive the following day.

Diestrus is defined as "the period during which the reproductive organs are mainly under the influ-

ence of progesterone."[12] The term *metestrus* is restricted to the three- to five-day period during which the corpora lutea are becoming functional and progesterone concentrations are increasing. Since the bitch may accept the male during this period, metestrus occurs within the period of estrus.[15]

Persistence of the corpus luteum is normal in the bitch. Progesterone levels peak at about 20 to 25 days after ovulation. There is then a prolonged decline in activity until the level returns to baseline at about 70 to 80 days after ovulation.[23] Progesterone increases the number and secretory activity of the uterine glands, inhibits myometrial contractions, and maintains closure of the cervix. The presence of the uterus is not necessary for corpus luteum activity or regression, since hysterectomy does not disrupt normal cyclic ovarian activity.[23]

Nonpregnant bitches may show clinical signs of pseudocyesis (pseudopregnancy), including gradual deposition of abdominal fat, development of mammary glands, nesting, and lactation.[23] The progesterone levels in pseudopregnant dogs are no different from those in nonpregnant dogs that are at the same stage of diestrus and showing no clinical signs.[26] Some investigators consider pseudopregnancy as the normal condition in a diestral bitch.[15, 25]

Anestrus is the period between diestrus and proestrus. Concentrations of FSH during anestrus are similar to those occurring coincidentally with the preovulatory LH surge. Concentrations of LH appear to increase prior to the onset of proestrus, possibly inducing a new follicular phase.[17a] The termination of diestrus and the beginning of anestrus are not clinically obvious. There is no vaginal drainage and the vulva is small. The bitch may gain weight and have an improved physical appearance.[15]

After the influence of progesterone is over, the uterine endometrium exfoliates and regenerates. During anestrus some follicles slowly enlarge but most undergo atresia.[15] The entire genital tract is at rest until the signs of proestrus begin again. The length of anestrus is quite variable even within the same breed.[25]

GESTATION IN THE BITCH

Normally 3 to 15 ova are released at each ovulatory period. Fertilization of the canine ovum occurs in the distal portion of the oviduct. A 16- to 32-cell morula enters the uterus between 8 and 20 days postcoitus.[11, 25] Implantation occurs 18 to 22 days after the beginning of estrus.[15] The zonary placentas become established at the beginning of the second trimester of gestation.[25] Transformation of granulosa cells into lutein cells is similar in the pregnant and nonpregnant bitch.[15] Morphology and function of the corpora lutea are maintained until the end of gestation. Hypophysectomy at any stage of gestation in the dog results in abortion.

Blood supply to the placenta in the pregnant bitch comes essentially from the uterine artery. Blood supply from the ovarian artery is minimal.[1]

The gravid uterine horn is tubular and about the same diameter throughout its entire length. The fetuses are nearly equally distributed between each horn. Embryonic mortality of 20 to 40 per cent commonly occurs during gestation; there are usually more than two fetuses present in the uterus. The average number of fetuses varies among breeds: large dogs 6 to 10, medium-sized dogs 4 to 7, and small dogs 2 to 4 fetuses.[19]

The level of circulating progesterone is the same in the pregnant and diestral bitch.[26] A pregnancy specific hormone, such as pregnant mare's gonadotropin, has not been found in the bitch. Pregnancy can be diagnosed by abdominal palpation after approximately 21 days. Following implantation there is a progressive decrease in packed red blood cell volume from about 45 to 31 per cent. Body weight increases about 36 per cent during gestation.[5]

ESTROUS CYCLE IN THE QUEEN

Most female cats have seasonal polyestrous cycles.[14, 16] Cats can be induced to come into estrus by artificially increasing the length of the day.[22] Seasonality may be associated with breed, since 90 per cent of long-haired cats have a nonbreeding period during the year. Sixty per cent of short-haired cats have a nonbreeding season in Europe.[14]

The average age of puberty in one study was 9 to 10 months, with a range of 4 to 18 months. Color points reached puberty later than other breeds (13 months); Burmese cats reached puberty earlier than other breeds (7 to 8 months).[14]

The estrous cycle in the unbred cat is divided into three stages: proestrus, estrus, and anestrus. If the cat is stimulated to ovulate, the term *diestrus* describes the period of corpus luteum function. The duration of the estrous cycle is most frequently within a range of 8 to 30 days. Estrus is most often repeated at 14- to 19-day intervals.[16]

Proestrus is difficult to determine in the cat because there is no vaginal discharge or enlargement. As estrus approaches, the number of small follicles decreases and the number of large follicles increases.[16, 21] Proestrus lasts for 12 to 48 hours.[24] During proestrus the cat may cry and posture as if in estrus but will not accept the male.[19]

Estrus is characterized in the female cat by crouching accompanied by treading with the hind feet and tail displacement to one side.[19] Estrus can be induced by single or multiple injections of follicle-stimulating hormone or pregnant mare's serum gonadotropin.[7]

Cats do not ovulate spontaneously. Ovulation usually occurs 24 to 30 hours after copulation.[19] Laparoscopic studies have shown that the mean ovulation rate in queens mated daily is 3.7 ovulations during each estrus.[7] Ovulation can be induced by vaginal stimulation with a glass rod.[19] Ova reach the uterus four to five days after coitus.[9] The queen may remain receptive to the male for several days after ovulation. The average length of estrus in one study of queens mated daily was 6.5 days.[7] If coitus does not occur estrus lasts five to ten days.[19]

Peak levels of estradiol-17B correlate with vaginal cornification and estrous behavior.[16] Luteinizing hormone levels peak after vaginal stimulation.

Anestrus is the period of ovarian quiescence following estrus when ovulation has not occurred. The follicles regress to a nondetectable state within one week after estrus.[28] Some authors refer to the period following follicle regression as metestrus or postestrus.[22, 28] The term *anestrus* also denotes the quiescent period of the ovaries during the nonbreeding season.

Diestrus begins 24 to 36 hours after ovulation when the corpora lutea are formed and are secreting progesterone.[7, 16, 28] Peak levels of progesterone are reached at about 21 days after ovulation.[28]

Progesterone levels in the pseudopregnant cat are similar to those in the pregnant cat for 12 days following coitus. The levels gradually drop and reach basal levels by 40 days after coitus.[18] In the pregnant cat progesterone levels reach basal levels 63 days after coitus.[27] This is different from the dog, in which progesterone levels remain elevated longer in the pseudopregnant dog than in the pregnant dog. Clinically the pseudopregnant cat, i.e., a cat that has corpora lutea and is not pregnant, does not show signs of nesting or mammary gland development.

GESTATION IN THE QUEEN

Implantation occurs 13 days after ovulation.[17] The placenta is zonary, as in the dog.[19]

Circulating levels of estradiol-17B decline following copulation and remain low until just before parturition. Progesterone levels rise after ovulation and reach a plateau about ten days after copulation. A second peak is reached at about day 20. Progesterone levels gradually decline and return to baseline just before parturition.[27]

Pregnancy can be diagnosed in the cat by abdominal palpation after about 24 days of pregnancy. Abdominal radiographs may reveal fetal skeletons during the third trimester of pregnancy.[19]

1. Abitbol, M. M., Demeter, E., and Benaroch, T.: Uterine and ovarian blood flow in the pregnant dog. Am. J. Obstet. Gynecol. *136*:780, 1980.
2. Andersen, A. C., and Wooten, E.: The estrous cycle of the dog. *In* Cole, H. H., and Cupps, P. T. (eds.): *Reproduction in Domestic Animals*. Academic Press, New York, 1959.
3. Christie, D. W., and Bell, E. T.: Some observations on the seasonal incidence and frequency of oestrus in breeding bitches in Britain. J. Small Anim. Pract. *12*:159, 1971.
4. Christie, D. W., and Bell, E. T.: Endocrinology of the oestrous cycle in the bitch. J. Small Anim. Pract. *12*:383, 1971.
5. Concannon, P. W., Powers, M. E., Holder, W., et al.: Pregnancy and parturition in the bitch. Biol. Reprod. *16*:517, 1977.
6. Evans, H. M., and Cole, H. H.: An introduction to the study of the oestrous cycle in the dog. Mem. Univ. Calif. *9*:65, 1931.
7. Foster, M. A., and Hislaw, F. L.: Experimental ovulation and resultant pseudopregnancy in anestrous cats. Anat. Rec. *62*:75, 1935.
8. Hadley, J. C.: Total unconjugated estrogen and progesterone concentration in peripheral blood during the oestrous cycle of the dog. J. Reprod. Fert. *44*:445, 1975.
9. Herron, M. A., and Sis, R. F.: Ovum transport in the cat and the effect of estrogen administration. Am. J. Vet. Res. *35*:1277, 1974.
10. Hill, J. P., and Tribe, M.: The early development of the cat (*Felis domestica*). Q. J. Microscop. Sci. *68*:513, 1924.
11. Holst, P. A., and Phemister, R. D.: The prenatal development of the dog: preimplantation events. Biol. Reprod. *5*:194, 1971.
12. Holst, P. A., and Phemister, R. D.: Onset of diestrus in the beagle bitch: Definition and significance. Am. J. Vet. Res. *135*:401, 1974.
13. Holst, P. A., and Phemister, R. D.: Temporal sequence of events in the estrous cycle of the bitch. Am. J. Vet. Res. *36*:705, 1975.
14. Jemmet, J. E., and Evans, J. M.: A survey of sexual behaviour and reproduction of the female cat. J. Small Anim. Pract. *18*:31, 1977.
15. Jochle, W., and Andersen, A. C.: The estrous cycle in the dog: A review. Theriogenology *7*:113, 1977.
16. Lofstedt, R. M.: The estrous cycle of the domestic cat. Comp. Cont. Ed. *4*:52, 1982.
17. Nalbandov, A. V.: *Reproductive Physiology of Mammals and Birds;* 3rd ed. W. H. Freeman and Co., San Francisco, 1976.
17a. Olson, P. N., Bowen, R. A., Behrendt, M. D., et al.: Concentrations of reproductive hormones in canine serum throughout late anestrus, proestrus and estrus. Biol. Repro. *27*:1196, 1982.
18. Paape, S. R., Shille, V. M., Seto, H., et al.: Luteal activity in the pseudopregnant cat. Biol. Reprod. *13*:470, 1975.
19. Roberts, S. J.: *Obstetrics and Genital Diseases (Theriogenology)*. Published by the author, Ithaca, 1971.
20. Roszell, J. F.: Genital cytology of the bitch. Vet. Scope *19*:2, 1975.
21. Scott, P. P.: Cats. *In* Hafez, E. S. E. (ed.): *Reproduction and Breeding Techniques for Laboratory Animals*. Lea & Febiger, Philadelphia, 1970.
22. Scott, P. P., and Lloyd Jacob, M. A.: Reduction in the anoestrous period of laboratory cats by increased illumination. Nature *26*:2022, 1959.
23. Shille, V. M., and Andersen, A. C.: The estrous cycle of the bitch. Canine Pract. *Jul.–Aug.*:29, 1974.
24. Shille, V. M., Lundstrom, K. E., and Stabenfeldt, G. H.: Follicular function in the domestic cat as determined by estradiol-17B concentrations in plasma: Relation to estrous behavior and cornification of exfoliated vaginal epithelium. Biol. Reprod. *21*:953, 1979.
25. Siegel, E. T.: *Endocrine Diseases of the Dog*. Lea & Febiger, Philadelphia, 1979.
26. Smith, M. S., and McDonald, L. E.: Serum levels of luteinizing hormone and progesterone during the estrous cycle, pseudopregnancy, and pregnancy in the dog. Endocrinology *94*:404, 1974.
27. Verhage, H. G., Beamer, N. B., and Brenner, R. M.: Plasma levels of estradiol and progesterone in the cat during polyestrus, pregnancy and pseudopregnancy. Biol. Reprod. *14*:459, 1976.
28. Wildt, D. E., and Seager, S. W. J.: Laparoscopic determination of ovarian and uterine morphology during the reproductive cycle. *In* Morrow, D. A. (ed.): *Current Therapy in Theriogenology*. W. B. Saunders, Philadelphia, 1980.

Chapter **123**

Embryology

Elizabeth A. Stone, Peggy M. Wykes, and Patricia N. Olson

OVARY AND UTERUS

During early fetal life the embryonic intermediate cell mass divides into urinary (nephric) and genital regions. The gonads develop from the ventromedial portion of the intermediate cell mass, also known as the genital ridge. Although the sex of the embryo is genetically determined at fertilization, morphological evidence is not detectable until the 30th day of gestation. In the female the mesonephric tubules persist as the vestigial epoophoron and paroophoron. The mesonephric ducts also degenerate. (In the male the mesonephric tubules become the epididymis and ductus deferens.)

During fetal development the ovaries migrate caudally, but they remain within the abdominal cavity suspended by the broad ligaments. The vaginal processes that contain the round ligament migrate toward the labia. Paired müllerian ducts open cranially into the peritoneal cavity as the abdominal ostia of the uterine tubes. They form the uterine horns and unite caudally to form the uterine body.[1]

VAGINA

The canine vagina and vulva are embryologically derived from the müllerian ducts and urogenital sinus. Cranially the müllerian ducts form the uterine horns; caudally, they fuse, in part, to form the uterine body, cervix, and vagina. The cranial portion of the vestibule originates from the urogenital sinus and initially develops independent of the vagina. The urogenital sinus results from the division of the primitive cloaca. The cloaca partitions to form the rectum dorsally and the urogenital sinus ventrally. The caudally fused müllerian ducts (vagina) unite with the urogenital sinus to form the vestibulovaginal junction (Fig. 123–1).[1] A membranous partition, the hymen, marks this junction in the fetus but is normally absent by birth.

VULVA

During fetal life the external genitalia begin as an undifferentiated phallic tubercle. Labioscrotal swell-

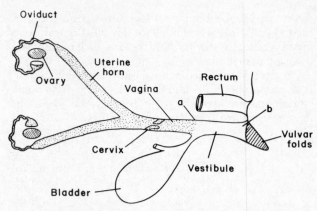

Figure 123–1. Embryological development of the female reproductive tract. Dotted area indicates structures derived from müllerian ducts. White area indicates structures derived from urogenital sinus. Lined area indicates structures derived from genital swellings. *a*, Location of hymen (vestibulovaginal junction); *b*, vestibulovulvar junction.

ings surround the phallus. The ventral portion of the phallus contains the urethral groove, which later forms the caudal vestibule. The clitoris also arises from the phallus, and the genital tubercles become the labia of the vulva.[1]

1. Evans, H. E., and Christensen, G. C.: *Miller's Anatomy of the Dog.* W. B. Saunders, Philadelphia, 1979.

Chapter 124 — Diagnostic Techniques

Elizabeth A. Stone, Peggy M. Wykes, and Patricia N. Olson

OVARY AND UTERUS

Abdominal Palpation

Examination of the ovaries by abdominal palpation is not possible unless they are grossly enlarged. It is sometimes difficult to identify the anestral or early estral uterus in a dog by abdominal palpation. It is easier to palpate the uterus in cats. The descending colon should be identified in the caudal abdomen. The tubular uterus is palpated directly ventral to the descending colon.

Pregnancy Determination

Abdominal palpation is frequently used to diagnose pregnancy in the dog and cat. In a dog at 17 to 18

days gestation, the uterus is about the same size as that of a pseudopregnant bitch. It may be possible to palpate round swellings, approximately 1.25 cm in diameter, in the uterine horns at 18 to 21 days gestation. From 24 to 32 days the spherical swellings are about 2.5 cm to 4.0 cm in diameter and are readily palpable. From 35 to 45 days gestation the swellings increase in size, elongate, lose their tenseness, and lie in the ventral abdomen. The uterus may be bent upon itself to conform to the available space in the abdomen. By day 50, it is no longer possible to palpate individual swellings of the uterus. From 55 to 63 days gestation, the fetuses should be easily palpable. Rectal palpation with the forequarters elevated may reveal the size of the fetuses.[1, 5]

Cats are usually easier to palpate than dogs. At 21 days gestation, pea-sized swellings can be felt in the uterus. By 28 days, the swellings are firm and are about 2 to 2.5 cm in diameter. The uterus is evenly distended during days 35 to 50 and may be difficult to differentiate from a pyometra.[5] Fetal heads are palpable in the bitch and queen after 50 days of gestation.[5]

Radiography can be used to diagnose pregnancy after fetal skeletal ossification during the last 15 days of gestation. Radiographs taken following pneumoperitoneum may delineate uterine swellings as early as 30 to 35 days of pregnancy.[5] The ultrasonic Doppler has been used to diagnose pregnancy at 32 to 35 days.[2]

Exploratory Laparotomy

The diagnosis of some ovarian or uterine diseases may require exploratory laparotomy and biopsy. If the ovaries are not grossly enlarged, the ovarian bursa is first incised to expose the ovaries. The presence of follicles, cysts, and corpora lutea should be noted. The bursal incision is closed with synthetic absorbable suture material. The uterine tubes can be examined, but patency cannot be determined because of the natural uterotubal valve.[6]

A uterine biopsy and bacteriological culture are taken. A 2- to 3-mm skin biopsy punch instrument can be used to take a punch biopsy. A sterile swab is inserted into the uterine lumen through the hole to obtain a sample of uterine contents for bacterial culture. The small hole in the uterus is closed with 3-0 synthetic absorbable suture.

VAGINA AND VULVA

The perineal region and vulvar labia are examined first for discharges, skin irritation, or swelling. Adequate examination of the labia often necessitates stretching the perivulvar skin folds. Prior to extensive examination of the vestibule and vagina the perivulvar area should be cleaned and rinsed and clipped of hair in some instances. Samples for microbiological or cytological examination should be obtained prior to digital examination or the insertion of nonsterile instruments into the vagina and vestibule. Short vaginal or otoscopic specula can be used to aid in the insertion of a dry sterile swab or biopsy instrument into the vagina for obtaining a sample. The use of a speculum assures sampling from the vaginal and not the vestibular epithelium. Specimens from the vagina for culture and sensitivity should be obtained with a guarded culturette to minimize contamination from the vulva.[3] Uterine biopsy forceps provide adequate tissue for histological examination. Biopsies can also be obtained through some fiberoptic units.

Vaginal specula are usually adequate for examination of the vestibular region and vestibulovaginal junction, but inspection of the vagina requires the use of a longer instrument such as a pediatric proctoscope or a custom-made tubular device that can be fitted onto an otoscopic handle.[4] The scope should be sterile and well lubricated for comfortable insertion. Prepubertal bitches or dogs with small vaginal openings may require sedation to minimize discomfort during the examination.

The cervix is rarely visible with these instruments because of the tendency of the vagina to stretch longitudinally while the scope is advanced and because the dorsal longitudinal fold (pseudocervix) prevents adequate exposure.

Endoscopic examination of the caudal reproductive tract has also been used and found to be a relatively accurate method of detecting the sexual status of a bitch. This investigative technique also has some potential for diagnosing reproductive disorders.[3]

The vagina and vestibule should always be examined by digital palpation as well as direct observation. Congenital anomalies such as vestibulovaginal bands or ring strictures (persistent hymen) are more readily detected by palpation than by direct visualization.[7]

The caudal vagina and pelvic region can be examined by placing a gloved finger into the vagina while manipulating the abdomen with the other hand. Likewise, the dorsal vaginal and vestibular walls can be evaluated by inserting a finger in the vagina while one finger of the opposite hand is inserted into the rectum.

The vagina is rarely visible by plain radiography unless this structure is greatly distended with fluid, such as is seen with vaginal segmental aplasia or traumatically induced closure of the vaginal entrance. Contrast vaginography can be helpful to demonstrate vaginal strictures, double vagina, tumors, or rectovaginal fistulas. A Foley catheter is inserted into the vestibule and secured by inflating the large bulb (30 cc). Enough Hypaque* (diluted 50:50 with saline) is injected to distend the vagina.[7] Both dorsoventral and lateral views are important for evaluation of pathological conditions.

1. Evans, H. E., and Christensen, G. C.: *Miller's Anatomy of the Dog.* W. B. Saunders, Philadelphia, 1979.
2. Helper, L. C.: Diagnosis of pregnancy in the bitch with an ultrasonic Doppler instrument. J. Am. Vet. Med. Assoc. 156:60, 1970.
3. Lindsay, F. E. F.: The normal endoscopic appearance of the caudal reproductive tract of the cyclic and noncyclic bitch: post-uterine endoscopy. J. Small Anim. Pract. 24:1, 1983.
4. Morrow, D. A.: *Current Therapy in Theriogenology.* W. B. Saunders, Philadelphia, 1980.
5. Roberts, S. J.: *Veterinary Obstetrics and Genital Diseases (Theriogenology).* Published by the author, Ithaca, 1971.
6. Senior, D. F.: Infertility in the cycling bitch. Comp. Cont. Ed. 1:17, 1979.
7. Wykes, P. M., and Soderberg, S. F.: Congenital abnormalities of the canine vagina and vulva. J. Am. Anim. Hosp. Assoc. 19:995, 1983.

*Winthrop Laboratories, New York, NY.

Chapter 125

The Ovary

Elizabeth A. Stone

CONGENITAL ANOMALIES

Agenesis of one or both ovaries has been reported in dogs.[4, 5] If both ovaries are congenitally absent, the uterus may also be absent or underdeveloped. Hypoplastic ovaries are rarely reported.[5] Supernumerary and accessory ovaries are very rare. A supernumerary ovary is a third gonad that is separate from the normally positioned ovaries. An accessory ovary is located near a normally positioned ovary, is usually connected to it, and appears to develop after a splitting of the embryonic gonad.[4]

Congenital ovarian anomalies are usually found incidentally during elective ovariohysterectomy. Occasionally, an exploratory laparotomy to determine a cause for sterility may reveal agenesis of both ovaries.

ACQUIRED OVARIAN LESIONS

Ovarian Cysts

Follicular cysts develop from the graafian follicle. Smaller cysts are lined with several layers of granulosa cells within a capsule composed of regressing theca and compressed ovarian stroma.[1] Solitary follicular cysts range in size from 1 to 5 cm. Multiple follicular cysts can form masses up to 10 cm in diameter. The component cysts are small and monolocular with no communication between individual cysts. Both ovaries may have follicular cysts.[1] Follicular cysts may result from incomplete oophorectomy when the viable remnants of ovarian tissue develop follicles that become cystic.[4] They can be produced experimentally by the injection of pregnant mare's serum gonadotropin or follicle-stimulating hormone.[4, 9]

In one postmortem study follicular cysts were found in 16 per cent of 400 unselected canine ovaries examined. They were more prevalent in nulliparous bitches and in bitches over five years of age. There was no histological evidence of estrogenic activity in the endometrium or vagina of any of the dogs studied.[1] However, clinical signs associated with follicular cysts have been reported as prolonged estrus with bloody vaginal discharge, nymphomania, cystic endometrial hyperplasia, cystic mammary hyperplasia, and genital fibroleiomyomas (fibroids).[4, 6, 8] In cats, cysts from atretic follicles can be functional. Excessive estrogen can cause prolonged estrus and even nymphomania. Behavior changes such as aggressiveness and viciousness can occur. The pathogenesis of these cysts is unknown. Cats may be predisposed to follicular cysts because ovulation and the subsequent luteinizing hormone release are not spontaneous.[7]

Lutein cysts form from the corpus luteum following ovulation. In the postmortem study previously mentioned, 2 per cent of the ovaries had lutein cysts 1.5 to 3 cm in diameter. They were thicker and more opaque than those of the follicular type. The ovaries in all the animals also contained normal corpora lutea. Histological examination of the uterus and vagina revealed changes consistent with the progesterone phase of the estrous cycle.[1] They may be associated with cystic endometrial hyperplasia or pyometra. They are found incidentally during a routine ovariohysterectomy or during an exploratory laparotomy for pyometra.

Parovarian cysts originate from the remnants of either mesonephric (wolffian) or paramesonephric tubules and ducts. They are seen more frequently in the dog than in the cat[5] and are located between the ovary and uterine horn. They are found incidentally during elective ovariohysterectomy.

Inflammatory Disease

Inflammatory disease of the ovary and oviduct is not recognized in the dog as a distinct disease. Ovaritis or pyosalpinx may occur secondary to pyometra.[4, 5]

Ovarian Tumors

See also Chapter 182.

Ovarian tumors are reported more frequently in older, nulliparous bitches. Ovarian tumors irrespective of type may occasionally stimulate the luteinization of theca cells with concomitant production of progesterone. Signs associated with prolonged progesterone stimulation include cystic endometrial hyperplasia and pyometra. Larger tumors may be palpable in the cranial right or left abdominal quadrant. They can produce signs, such as vomiting, which are consistent with a cranial abdominal space-occupying mass. Radiographic evaluation may reveal a soft tissue density mass in the same area.[2]

Granulosa cell tumors are the most common tumors of the ovary in dogs.[1, 4, 5] Bitches with granulosa cell tumors may show signs of prolonged estrogen treatment, e.g., hyperplasia and cornification of the vaginal epithelium.[1] Surgical therapy is ovariohysterectomy. It may be necessary to dissect the ovarian tumor from the body wall. Unilateral nephrectomy may be necessary if the tumor has invaded the kidney.

Papillary cystadenomas and cystadenocarcinomas occur only in the bitch. Cystadenomas are either unilocular, varying in size from 0.8 to 1.5 cm, or multilocular, varying in size from 6 to 8 cm. They are thin-walled and usually cause no derangement of the estrus cycle.[1, 4] Bitches with cystadenocarcinomas may have irregular estrous cycles, cystic endometrial hyperplasia, or ascites.[1, 5] One author states that papillary adenocarcinomas should always be considered in the differential diagnosis of ascites in adult intact bitches. The ascites develops from the obstruction of diaphragmatic lymphatic vessels by tumor fragments and from fluid secreted by tumor epithelium.[4] The tumors vary from microscopic to 10 cm or more in size.[4] When the tumor is confined within the ovarian bursa, the papillae are compressed and have a cauliflowerlike appearance. Once the papillae outgrow the bursa, their papillary nature becomes apparent and peritoneal implantation occurs readily.[4] The presence of papillae indicates malignancy. Cysts of varying size are usually scattered throughout the neoplastic mass.[4]

Surgical treatment of a confined papillary cystadenocarcinoma is ovariohysterectomy. Since confined papillary cystadenocarcinomas frequently have peritoneal implants and lung metastasis, the prognosis is poor with surgical therapy alone.

1. Dow, C.: Ovarian abnormalities in the bitch. J. Comp. Pathol. 70:59, 1960.
2. Faulkner, R. T.: Removal of a thecoma in a poodle. Vet. Med./Small Anim. Clin. 73:451, 1978.
3. Faulkner, R. T., and Johnson, S. E.: An ovarian cyst in a West Highland White Terrier. Vet. Med./Small Anim. Clin. 75:1375, 1980.
4. Jubb, K. V. F., and Kennedy, P. C.: *Pathology of Domestic Animals.* Academic Press, New York, 1970.
5. Roberts, S. J.: *Veterinary Obstetrics and Genital Diseases (Theriogenology).* Published by the author, Ithaca, 1971.
6. Rowley, J.: Cystic ovary. Vet. Med./Small Anim. Clin. 75:1888, 1980.
7. Stein, B. S.: The genital system. *In* Catcott, E. J. (ed.): *Feline Medicine and Surgery.* American Veterinary Publications Inc., Santa Barbara, 1975, pp. 303–354.
8. Vaden, P.: Surgical treatment of cystic ovaries in the dog (a case report). Vet. Med./Small Anim. Clin. 73:1160, 1978.
9. Wildt, D. E., Kinney, G. M., and Seager, S. W.: Gonadotropin induced reproductive cyclicity in the domestic cat. Lab. Anim. Sci. 28:301, 1978.

Chapter **126**

The Uterus

Elizabeth A. Stone

CONGENITAL ANOMALIES

Congenital anomalies of the canine or feline uterus are rare. The incidence of uterus unicornis is 1 of 5,000 to 10,000 necropsies.[103] Uterus unicornis complicates ovariohysterectomy, since the absence of one uterine horn is unexpected. The ovary on the side of the undeveloped uterus may be small but should be removed.[39, 59, 117] Agenesis of one uterine horn may be accompanied by unilateral renal agenesis.[103] Other congenital abnormalities of the uterus include hypoplasia, agenesis, atresia, septate uterine body, double cervix, and cornual fusion.[20, 86, 117] Most anomalies are found incidentally during elective ovariohysterectomy. Some may cause infertility or dystocia.

ACQUIRED DISEASES

Pyometra

The term *pyometra* describes the clinical condition of a pus-filled uterus, ovarian changes, and extragenital lesions occurring secondary to the uterine changes. It occurs in the mature bitch or queen and is unrelated to parturition.

After examining uteri from dogs during necropsy and after ovariohysterectomies, Dow concluded that pyometra was one stage in a series of pathological changes in the uterus. He used the term *cystic hyperplasia-pyometra complex.* Dow divided the changes into four types.[42, 43] Type I, cystic endometrial hyperplasia, occurs in middle-aged dogs and is not related to a particular stage of the estrous cycle. The thickened endometrium is lined by numerous thin-walled, translucent cysts. In type II there is a diffuse plasma cell infiltration of the endometrium in addition to the cystic endometrial hyperplasia. It only occurs during diestrus. The cervix is relaxed and patent. In type III, cystic endometrial hyperplasia is accompanied by an acute inflammatory reaction of the endometrium. Bitches that present with pyometra usually have type III uterine changes. The size of the uterus is proportional to the patency of the cervix. In Dow's study, 78 per cent of bitches with type III uteri were within the first 40 days of diestrus. In chronic endometritis, type IV, the cervix can be either open or closed. If the cervix is open, there is a chronic vaginal discharge. The horns are not greatly enlarged, the walls are thickened, and there is little pus. There is myometrial hypertrophy and fibrosis. If the cervix is closed, the uterus is greatly distended and the uterine walls may be very thin. The endometrium is atrophied and infiltrated with lymphocytes and plasma cells.[42–44]

Diffuse cystic endometrial hyperplasia occurs in cats, but focal areas of polypoid proliferation are more common. Localized cysts are interspersed with normal endometrial tissue. Larger cysts attached by slender pedicles can be found. These are usually asymptomatic unless torsion of a pedunculated cyst causes hemorrhage.[71]

Pyometra is a disease of the diestral phase of the estrous cycle, when the corpus luteum is actively secreting progesterone. Progesterone increases the number and secretory activity of the uterine glands, inhibits myometrial contractions, and maintains closure of the cervix.[63] Since pyometra can be cured by ovariectomy, the presence of the ovaries for maintenance of pyometra is essential.[43] Pyometra was induced in ovariectomized dogs by the administration of high levels of progesterone. Once the progesterone administration was stopped, the signs stopped. Estrogen alone given to ovariectomized dogs caused a mild, chronic endometrial hyperplasia. Previous treatment with estrogen decreased the dose of progesterone needed to produce pyometra.[126] Chronic progesterone administration to ovariectomized dogs produced chronic endometrial hyperplasia.[42, 43]

Long-acting progestational compounds in intact bitches cause endometrial hyperplasia with progression to pyometra in some animals.[29, 55, 74, 99, 115, 120, 139] The biological activity of medroxyprogesterone in dogs is about 24 to 48 times the activity of naturally occurring progesterone.[5] Short-term progestational compounds administered when endogenous estrogens are high may also cause pyometra.[115]

Endogenous progesterone and estrogen levels in relation to the time of estrus are similar to the corresponding patterns in normally cycling or pregnant bitches.[17, 35, 57, 58] Luteolysis may occur normally about 60 days after ovulation even when the pyometra persists.[33]

Since progesterone levels are not abnormally elevated, it has been postulated that there is a modification of the affinity of progesterone to the receptors of the endometrial cells or that there are changes in the receptors that maintain abnormally long progesterone influences on the uterine endometrium.[115]

Because cats do not ovulate spontaneously, a progesterone-dependent disease such as pyometra should occur only with sterile matings. However, pyometra is seen in unbred housecats. Dow speculates that the pet female cat may respond sexually to mild stimulation, which is sufficient to cause a cessation of estrus, ovulation, and the production of a corpus luteum.[46]

Infection is usually present in the pyometra uterus, even though it is not considered the primary cause. In the progesterone-primed uterus, an inhibition of the leukocyte response to infection[64] may predispose the uterus to infection. The epithelium from the metestral uterus binds *Escherichia coli* antigens to a greater degree than do uteri from other stages of the estrous cycle.[109] The uterus may be infected during early metestrus when the receptors for *E. coli* are developed in the endometrium and myometrium.[109] *E. coli* antigens can be precipitated from the sera of some animals with pyometra.[109]

The most common bacterium cultured from the uterine contents of dogs with pyometra is *E. coli*.[23, 35, 57, 73, 101] Other bacteria cultured include streptococcus, staphylococcus, *Klebsiella*,[35] *Proteus*, *Pseudomonas*, and *Aerobacter*.[73] A mycoplasma has been cultured from the vagina of a bitch with an open cervix pyometra.[1] Some uteri with pyometra are sterile.[23]

Bacteria have been isolated from about 85 per cent of the uteri of cats with pyometra.[46] Organisms cultured include *E. coli*, staphylococcus, and streptococcus.[35] Attempts to produce pyometra in cats by intrauterine injection of bacteria have been unsuccessful. After the simultaneous administration of progesterone and intrauterine bacteria, 25 per cent of cats showed signs of pyometra. None of the cats receiving estrogen and intrauterine bacteria became infected.[45]

Pyometra is a polysystemic disease. In one study, approximately 62 per cent of dogs with pyometra were anemic, 41 per cent had liver disease, and 48 per cent had kidney disease.[22] The nonregenerative anemia is due to a loss of red cells by diapedesis into the uterine lumen and to toxic depression of erythropoiesis.[111] The bone marrow changes are primarily hyperplasia of the myeloid elements.[19]

Minimal hepatocellular injury or necrosis is associated with pyometra. The liver signs are caused by intrahepatic cholestasis and retention of bile pigments without lobular damage. Extramedullary myelopoiesis also occurs in the liver.[24]

Asheim conducted the classic studies on the functional relationship between pyometra and renal function.[7-16] Renal dysfunction in dogs with pyometra can be attributed to the following causes:

1. Prerenal uremia can be caused by decreased renal blood flow for a variety of reasons. Dehydration (from vomiting, diarrhea, and inadequate water intake) and hypotensive shock (from toxemia, septicemia, anesthesia, or surgery) can reduce blood flow to the kidney. Prolonged reduction of renal blood flow can cause primary renal failure.

2. Primary glomerular disease has been described in animals severely ill with pyometra.[12, 15] Measurements of glomerular filtration rate (GFR) showed a normal or decreased rate. The degree of proteinuria has not been determined. The glomerular filtration rate improved in 12 to 16 days after ovariohysterectomy. A membranous or mixed membranous proliferative glomerulonephritis was seen with light microscopy. A thickened basement membrane and swollen glomerular endothelial cells were found on electron microscopy.[91] A good correlation was found between the degree of glomerular changes and the decrease in glomerular filtration rate.[15, 91]

The changes in the glomerulus may have an immune basis. The renal changes may develop in association with infection and heal after the infection is gone. Dogs that have been tested serologically usually have specific antibodies against strains of bacteria isolated from the uterus. The placenta may be antigenetically similar to glomerular structures. Damaged uterine tissue may stimulate formation of antibodies that can crossreact with glomerular structures.[26, 112] Immunofluorescent examination of the glomeruli or localization of specific bacterial antigens in glomerular deposits has not been reported. Similar renal lesions have been seen in various chronic purulent conditions[38] and in congestive heart failure, splenomegaly, and pseudopregnancy.[135] The clinical significance and specificity of the reported changes in the glomeruli are unclear. Severe loss of protein in the urine has not been reported.

3. There is a decreased tubular capacity to concentrate the glomerular filtrate in dogs with pyometra. Polydipsia occurs secondary to the inability to conserve water. The ability to dilute the urine is normal.[8] Early observations suggested that the hypothalamic-hypophyseal system contained decreased amounts of neurosecretory material.[124] Since injection of antidiuretic hormone did not restore the ability to concentrate, the possibility of a primary hypothalamic-hypophyseal lesion was eliminated.[1] No changes in concentrating ability were seen in bitches that were given progesterone and that did not develop pyometra.[8]

No correlation has been shown between decreased concentrating ability and decreased GFR. The ability to concentrate improves after ovariohysterectomy to a greater extent than does the GFR. Normal concentrating ability has been seen two to eight weeks after ovariohysterectomy.[8-10] No obvious morphological changes correlate with the dysfunction in concentrating ability.

4. Since pyometra usually occurs in older dogs, concomitant renal disease or immunological changes in the kidney may be present that are unrelated to the pyometra. Kidneys that look grossly abnormal at the time of ovariohysterectomy should be biopsied to determine the type and degree of renal disease.[61]

5. Combinations of prerenal uremia and primary acute and chronic disease may be present.

Diagnosis

Pyometra can occur in a bitch of any age after the first estrus. It occurs most frequently in bitches over six years of age within 12 weeks of the last estrus.[21, 44, 62, 122] No breed predisposition has been recognized. The reproductive history of dogs with pyometra is varied. No difference exists in the incidence of pyometra in dogs with a history of irregular heat cycle, abnormal estrus, or pregnancies. The occurrence is less frequent in dogs with a history of pseudopregnancy.[50]

Pyometra occurs much less frequently in the cat. It has been reported in spayed cats following treatment with megestrol acetate for dermatological disease. During surgical exploration, a pus-filled uterine stump and no vestigial ovarian tissue or uterine horns were found in each cat.[69, 80]

The type and severity of clinical signs with pyometra depend on the patency of the cervix, the duration of the illness, and the associated extragenital disease. Signs most frequently reported in dogs by owners include anorexia, polydipsia, depression, and vaginal discharge.[21, 62, 122, 132] Other signs noted include polyuria, nocturia, vomiting, and diarrhea. On physical examination, vaginal discharge is frequently apparent. Digital examination of the vagina should differentiate vaginal tumors as a cause of vaginal discharge. A vaginoscopic examination may be done to identify vaginitis. The majority of dogs with pyometra have normal body temperatures; about 40 per cent are febrile.[21, 122] Toxemic dogs may have subnormal body temperatures.

Signs of pyometra in cats are more subtle than in dogs. Cats may show mild anorexia and depression until the disease is well advanced. A copious vaginal discharge is not seen because of the grooming habits of the cat. Physical examination may disclose soiling of the perineal hair.[121] Abdominal distension is more apparent in the cat than in the dog.

An enlarged uterus may be palpable in the dog upon abdominal or rectal palpation. Care must be taken to avoid rupturing a distended uterus. Many dogs with pyometra are also obese,[21, 75] which makes them difficult to palpate. Abdominal palpation is easier in cats.

There are no pathognomonic laboratory findings for pyometra. The total white cell count is usually between 15,000 and 100,000,[62, 73, 109, 122] although some dogs may have a normal count.[114] A left shift that may be degenerative, with toxic neutrophils,[19] is usual. A leukopenia may also indicate a systemic toxemia. The purulent material retained within the uterus is chemotactic for neutrophils. If the uterus can drain, there is a decrease in chemotaxis, and the total number of neutrophils may be within normal limits.[111] The lymphocyte count is within normal range unless there is severe stress. The monocyte number can be elevated because of the chronicity of the suppurative process.[122]

The total red cell concentration (PCV) may be less than 36 per cent because of a normocytic normochromic anemia. However, the severity of the decreased PCV may be masked by dehydration.[111, 122] The total protein concentration is elevated because of an elevation of the globulin component.[22, 73, 109] Albumin levels may be lower than normal. Cholesterol, bilirubin, alkaline phosphatase, and lactate dehydrogenase levels may be increased, but glutamic pyruvic transaminase (SGPT) values are usually within normal limits.[22]

The status of the kidneys should be carefully evaluated in every dog with pyometra. A midstream urine sample is collected for evaluation of specific gravity. If a dehydrated or azotemic dog has a urine specific gravity value indicating lack of concentrating ability (< 1.030), primary renal dysfunction is present. Creatinine and serum urea nitrogen (SUN) elevations may reflect primary renal disease or may be secondary to prerenal decreases in renal blood flow. In one study, 70 per cent of dogs with pyometra had a normal SUN; 18 per cent had a SUN greater than 35 mg/dl.[101]

Urine for bacterial culture and urinalysis should be obtained by cystocentesis at the time of surgery to check for associated urinary tract infection. Urinary tract infection was diagnosed in 23 of 32 bitches with pyometra. The strain of *E. coli* identified was identical to the strain cultured from the uterine contents.[101] Examination of vaginal smears reveals large numbers of bacteria and neutrophils, many of which are degenerative.

The diagnosis of pyometra often can be made from the clinical history, physical examination, and laboratory values. If radiographic examination is necessary, abdominal preparation (no food, enemas) is not recommended. On survey abdominal radiographs, homologous tubular structures of fluid density may be seen in the caudal abdomen. The uterus has a similar appearance during early pregnancy and immediately post partum.[62, 101]

Animals with pyometra and a closed cervix may be a diagnostic challenge. Careful examination of the animal and laboratory values should help differentiate pyometra from other diseases causing polyuria and polydipsia, including diabetes mellitus, hyperadrenocorticism, and generalized hepatic disease.[122]

In cats, signs associated with pyometra must be differentiated from feline infectious peritonitis (FIP). Cats with either pyometra or FIP may have elevated gamma globulins. The diffuse thickening of the bowel wall in FIP must be differentiated from an enlarged uterus. An FIP titer may give a definitive diagnosis.[121]

In summary, the minimum data base for pyometra should include the following: PCV, total protein concentration, creatinine (or SUN), urine specific gravity from a midstream sample, and urine culture and urinalysis from cystocentesis taken during surgery. If surgery is not done, a urine sample should be obtained by percutaneous cystocentesis after the uterine disease has resolved. Other tests that may be needed include additional blood chemistry evaluations, abdominal radiographs, and vaginal cytological studies.

Treatment

The most common treatment for pyometra is ovariohysterectomy.[118, 121, 122] The procedure as described later needs little modification for the removal of an enlarged uterus. Special precaution is taken to avoid lacerating an enlarged, friable uterus. The recommended method for handling the uterine body is the classic triple clamp method with individual ligation of the uterine arteries. The ligatures are placed at the cranial end of the cervix to avoid leaving any uterine body, which is packed off from the rest of the abdomen before it is severed to prevent abdominal contamination. The small amount of exposed uterus is lavaged and suctioned to remove residual pus. Some descriptions of pyometra surgery have included a Parker-Kerr oversew of the uterine stump.[118] This procedure is not necessary unless the cervix is greatly distended. The disadvantages of oversewing the uterine stump include (1) the cavity that remains between the oversewn area and the cervix may continue to act as an abscess; (2) the oversewn stump contains more tissue and suture material that can contribute to a stump granuloma; and (3) the oversew technique increases operative time.

If the uterus has ruptured or is torn during surgery, the abdomen should be copiously washed with large amounts of warm, multiple electrolyte solution. Antibiotics should be administered if there has been abdominal contamination.

Corrective therapy for fluid deficits and acidosis should be started before surgery. It may be necessary to perform ovariohysterectomy before the animal can be completely stabilized. Supportive therapy should continue during and after the surgery.

Removal of corpora lutea and surgical drainage without ovariohysterectomy has been described to treat pyometra in valuable breeding bitches.[48, 54, 65] This procedure is not recommended for use in a sick, toxic animal.

After a midline abdominal incision, the ovary is exposed by carefully elongating the opening of the ovarian bursa. The oviducts must not be damaged. The corpora lutea are excised. Hemorrhage is controlled by pressure on the ovary and ligation if necessary. The bursal incision is closed with 4-0 synthetic absorbable suture material. The uterus is isolated from the abdominal cavity. A small incision is made in the body, and the contents of each horn are removed by suction. If the cervix was not open before surgery, drainage is provided by passing a catheter from the uterine lumen, through the cervix, and into the vagina. If the cervix was open before surgery, no catheter is needed. The uterine incision is closed with synthetic absorbable suture material. The uterine exudate is cultured for bacteria and appropriate antibiotics administered.[48, 54, 65] Results using this protocol have not been reported.

Medical therapy for pyometra is directed toward lowering the progesterone levels, eliminating bacteria, and opening the cervix.[89] Several investigators have reported the use of prostaglandin $F_{2\alpha}$.[20, 32, 37, 86, 88, 95, 123] Various dosage regimens have been suggested, and there is not yet an accepted protocol of treatment. At this time the drug has not been approved by the United States Food and Drug Administration for use in dogs.[86] One case of a ruptured uterus following administration of prostaglandin $F_{2\alpha}$ to a bitch with an open pyometra has been reported.[68]

Surgical therapy for pyometra in cats is similar to that performed on dogs. One case report suggests that prostaglandin $F_{2\alpha}$ can also be used in cats.[136]

Hydrometra and Mucometra

Hydrometra and mucometra are sterile accumulations of fluid within the uterus caused by the secretion of endometrial glands under the stimulation of progesterone. The type of accumulation is determined by the amount of mucin present. Drainage is impeded by a closed cervix or a polypoid cyst from cystic endometrial hyperplasia. The fluid may extend into the oviducts, causing hydrosalpinx or mucosalpinx. Hydrometra and mucometra are uncommon and are usually found incidentally during elective ovariohysterectomy.[71, 83, 84]

Diseases of the Postparturient Uterus

Subinvolution of Placental Sites

Normal involution of the uterus is complete by 12 weeks following parturition. During the first week the uterine horns are dilated and edematous. Decidual cells are found throughout the lamina propria. The placental sites are 1.5 to 3 cm in width and are rough, granular, and covered with mucus and a few blood clots. By the fourth week the dilated uterine glands are degenerating and the placental sites are thick and nodular. The uterine horns are contracted and the placental sites are narrow with few nodules by the seventh week. The endometrial glands have a normal shape by this time. By nine weeks after parturition, the uterine horns are uniform in shape and have a narrow lumen. The placental sites are a narrow brown band.[3]

With subinvolution of the placental sites, a disturbance in the normal postparturient placental degeneration and endometrial reconstruction takes place. During pregnancy, fetal trophoblastic cells invade the myometrium. These cells should die promptly and spontaneously after an abortion or full-term pregnancy. If they do not regress or degenerate, they can continue to invade the deep glandular layer and the myometrium. The retention of these cells for a prolonged time after parturition interferes with normal involution.[2]

The clinical sign of subinvolution of the placental sites is persistent serosanguineous vaginal discharge 7 to 12 weeks following parturition. It usually occurs in bitches less than two and one-half years of age after the first or second whelping. Severe anemia may develop. Abdominal palpation may reveal discrete, firm spherical enlargements of the uterine horns.[52, 110] Subinvolution of placental sites must be differentiated from cystitis, urinary bladder tumors, metritis, and vaginitis.[18] The cause of the hemorrhage may be failure of the vessels of the exposed placental bed to occlude, failure of endometrial blood vessels to thrombose, or damage to vessels by trophoblastlike cells.[2]

Treatment of choice for most animals without breeding value is ovariohysterectomy, since eroded areas could possibly rupture and result in peritonitis.[2, 18] Hysterolaparotomy and curettage of individual sites may be considered in selected animals. Documented series of cases have not been reported. This technique might be less useful if the sites were widely separated, necessitating an incision in the entire length of each horn.[18, 52] A single case of spontaneous recovery after subinvolution of the placental sites has been reported.[110] Another investigator questioned the histopathological diagnosis in this animal and stated that it was merely delayed normal involution that spontaneously resolved.[2] Spontaneous remission usually occurs, and bitches with subinvolution of placental sites rarely require medical or surgical therapy.[134a]

Metritis

Acute metritis occurs most commonly in the immediate postpartum period and is usually associated with dystocia, obstetrical manipulations, or retained placentas or fetuses. Acute metritis also may be seen after a normal whelping or following nonsterile artificial insemination.[77, 79]

Clinical signs begin within a few days of parturition. They include a malodorous, mucopurulent vaginal discharge and signs of systemic illness, such as fever, anorexia, and vomiting. The enlarged uterus may be palpable. Mastitis may also be present.[18, 77, 79, 121]

A complete blood count may reveal a neutrophilia and a degenerative left shift. If the animal is dehydrated, the PCV and the total proteins are increased. Vaginal cytology shows degenerative neutrophils and bacteria. In one study, *Escherichia* species were cultured from the uterine contents of 65 per cent of dogs and cats with postparturient metritis.[130]

Ovariohysterectomy is recommended if the owners do not want to breed the animal again or if the animal has severe systemic signs. Supportive therapy may be necessary before surgery. The puppies or kittens should be weaned and hand fed.

Medical treatment consists of uterine drainage, administration of antibiotics, and supportive therapy. A soft rubber catheter with a stylet is manipulated through the external opening of the cervix. Care is taken to avoid contacting the uterine wall. The uterus is evacuated and an antibiotic solution instilled. Broad spectrum antibiotics are used until the antibiotic sensitivity of the uterine bacteria is known. Antibiotics are instilled into the uterus daily until there is no uterine discharge, the white blood cell count is normal, and there is no fever.[77, 79]

In animals that do not respond to this treatment or in animals in which an intrauterine catheter cannot be placed through the cervix, a laparotomy can be done. If the uterus has discolored, swollen, or eroded areas, ovariohysterectomy is performed. If the uterine wall looks healthy, a hysterotomy incision is made at the uterine bifurcation to remove the uterine contents. Gentle massage of the uterus may help break down adhesions and debris. A catheter is passed from the uterus through the cervix. Antibiotics are placed into the uterus and the uterine incision is closed. The abdominal incision is closed routinely. The catheter can be used to instill antibiotics after surgery.[47, 77, 79]

Uterine Torsion

Uterine torsion is an uncommon condition in dogs and cats. One or both uterine horns can twist along the long axis or around the opposite horn, or the entire uterine body can rotate. The uterine horns or body can twist clockwise or counterclockwise from 90 to over 200 degrees of rotation.[27, 31, 67, 100, 108, 116, 121, 128, 131, 140] Torsions of gravid and nongravid uteri have been reported in dogs.[27, 31, 67, 100, 108, 116, 128, 131] Reported uterine torsions in cats have all involved one horn of a gravid uterus.[131, 140] The following causes for uterine torsion have been suggested: (1) jumping or running late in pregnancy, (2) active fetal movement, (3) premature uterine contraction, (4) partial abortion, (5) variations in the length and mobility of the proper ovarian ligament, and (5) abnormalities of the uterus.[121]

Signs of uterine torsion are not specific and usually reflect abdominal pain. The onset is often acute. The bitch or queen may crouch and strain as if in labor and may attempt to defecate. Prior delivery of a healthy or dead puppy or kitten may have occurred. There may be a vaginal discharge. The abdomen can be tense and distended. On vaginal examination, the caudal aspect of the rotated uterus occasionally may be felt. Radiographic examination often discloses a large air- or fluid-filled tubular structure.[100, 121]

The treatment of choice is ovariohysterectomy. If there are viable fetuses in the normal horn, a cesarean section can be performed first. Since there can be massive sequestration of fluid within the uterus and vascular obstruction, supportive therapy may be necessary before surgery.

Uterine Prolapse

Prolapse of the uterus occurs infrequently in dogs and cats. It has been reported in a primiparous queen and in queens and bitches that have had several normal litters without complication.[6, 82, 85, 98, 90] One horn or the entire uterus can prolapse during prolonged labor or up to 48 hours after parturition, when the cervix is extremely dilated.[6, 118] The fetuses may be expelled from one horn, which subsequently prolapses while the other horn is still gravid. Usually, however, both horns have emptied before the prolapse.[121]

Possible mechanisms of uterine prolapse include (1) overrelaxation and stretching of pelvic musculature, (2) uterine atony due to metritis, (3) incomplete separation of placental membranes, (4) severe tenesmus, and (5) postpartum contractions intensified by oxytocin release during lactation.[85, 121]

An animal with a prolapsed uterus has one or two tubular masses protruding from the vulva. If there is no visible mass at the time of presentation, digital examination reveals a uterine horn in the vagina. The uterus may be hemorrhagic, ulcerated, and encrusted with litter, hair, feces, or placental membranes. Tenesmus may continue.[121]

If the animal is in good physical condition and the uterus is healthy, manual reduction can be attempted.[82, 85, 89, 90, 121, 138] Sterile gauze sponges are soaked in warm, sterile saline and placed around the uterus. General anesthesia or epidural anesthesia is usually necessary. The uterus is cleaned with warm saline followed by an antibiotic wash and lubricated with a water-soluble jelly. Gentle manipulation with gloved fingers, a sterile smooth syringe plunger, or a long glass tube may assist reduction. After reduction the uterus can be palpated abdominally to determine its position. If partial reduction is achieved, further reduction and positioning can be done through a celiotomy. Uterine prolapse seldom recurs following proper replacement.[103] A successful pregnancy in a queen six months after the reduction of a uterine prolapse has been reported.[85]

Extensive devitalization of the uterus necessitates ovariohysterectomy after reduction of the prolapse. If reduction of the uterus is impossible, the uterus is amputated and the stump is reduced.[6, 89, 90, 121, 138] It may be necessary to stabilize a shocked, toxic animal before anesthesia and surgery. To amputate the prolapsed uterus, an incision is made into the cranial part of the uterine body near the vulva. The cranial ends of the uterine horns are visible. Gentle traction on the uterine horns may expose the ovaries. If possible, the ovarian artery should be ligated proximal to the ovary. If the ovary cannot be seen, the uterine horn is divided between two ligatures. The uterine arteries are ligated and severed. The uterus is severed and closed with simple interrupted absorbable sutures. The uterine stump is reduced through the vagina. If the ovaries remain, they should be removed through an abdominal incision.[82, 118, 121, 133]

Uterine Rupture

In dogs and cats, rupture of a gravid uterus is rare.[4, 34, 102, 103, 107, 134] The gravid uterus may rupture spontaneously during parturition or as a result of severe trauma. Fetuses expelled into the peritoneal cavity may die immediately and may resorb or cause peritonitis. If the fetal circulation remains intact, the fetuses may live to term. The extrauterine location may not be recognized until whelping, when the fetus is not delivered. An exploratory laparotomy reveals one or more fetuses within the peritoneal cavity, surrounded by adhesions. Removal of the puppies and fetal membranes is difficult if not impossible, so a poor prognosis must be given for the bitch or queen.[118]

Acute rupture of the uterus is usually treated by ovariohysterectomy. A unilateral ovariohysterectomy may preserve breeding ability. A small clean laceration may be sutured, but a repaired area may be more likely to rupture during subsequent pregnancies. Fibrotic and constricted areas predispose to infertility.[121]

An enlarged uterus secondary to pyometra may rupture before or during surgery.[72] Extensive peritoneal contamination can result. Copious lavage and careful suctioning during laparotomy are necessary to minimize contamination and the potential for peritonitis.

Uterine Intussusception

Uterine intussusception has been reported in a chow chow dog with a vaginal discharge for four weeks. At celiotomy, the left uterine horn was telescoped into itself near its junction with the uterine tube. Ovariohysterectomy was performed.[53]

Uterine Neoplasia

See also Chapter 182.

The incidence of uterine tumors in dogs is 0.3 to 0.4 per cent of canine tumors.[127] Comparable data are not available for cats. Leiomyomas are the most frequent uterine tumor; leiomyosarcomas occur much less frequently.[127]

The clinical signs may be abdominal enlargement or a palpable abdominal mass. If the tumor obstructs the lumen, a hydrometra or mucometra may develop. The tumor may be found incidentally during ovariohysterectomy or during an exploratory laparotomy. The surgical treatment is ovariohysterectomy.

Ovariohysterectomy

Indications

The most common reason for an ovariohysterectomy is elective sterilization. Ovariohysterectomy is the usual treatment for many of the uterine diseases discussed previously, e.g., pyometra, uterine torsion, uterine prolapse, and uterine rupture. Ovariohysterectomy is also indicated to prevent the recurrence of vaginal hyperplasia. Animals with diabetes or epilepsy may be spayed to prevent hormonal changes that can interfere with medication. Ovariohysterectomy before the first estrous cycle decreases the incidence of mammary gland tumors to less than 0.5 per cent compared with intact bitches. If ovariohysterectomy is performed after the first estrous cycle, the risk of mammary gland tumors increases to 8 per cent; after two estrous cycles, the risk increases to 26 per cent. Ovariohysterectomy after two and one-half years has no preventive effect on mammary gland

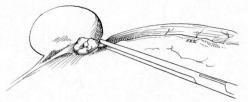

Figure 126–1. After the ovary is identified, a clamp is placed on the proper ligament of the ovary.

tumors in the bitch.[49] Similar data are not available for cats.

The minimum data base before elective ovariohysterectomy in a young dog (younger than five years of age) is a packed red cell volume (PCV) and a total plasma protein concentration determination. In an older dog, a serum urea nitrogen or creatinine level should also be determined. Other laboratory tests may be indicated before ovariohysterectomy for a diseased uterus or ovaries.

Procedure

Many variations in techniques are described.[54, 66, 76, 118] A midline abdominal incision is made extending from the umbilicus approximately 5 cm caudally in the dog. In the cat, the incision is started approximately 1 cm caudal to the umbilicus and extended caudally for 3 cm. If the uterus is distended or enlarged, the length of the abdominal incision is increased. A flank incision is occasionally used in cats.[76] The right uterine horn is located by means of an ovariohysterectomy hook or the index finger. The spleen should be avoided. A clamp is placed on the proper ligament of the ovary (Fig. 126–1) and is used to retract the ovary while the suspensory ligament is stretched or broken with the index finger (Fig. 126–2). A window is made in the mesoovarium caudal to the ovarian vessels. The ovarian pedicle is triple clamped, and the pedicle is severed between the clamp closest to the ovary and the middle clamp (Fig. 126–3). The clamp most distant from the ovary is removed so that the pedicle ligature can be placed in its groove (Fig. 126–4).

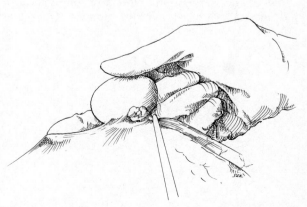

Figure 126–2. The suspensory ligament is stretched or broken.

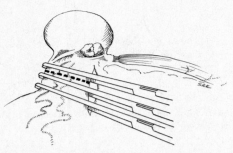

Figure 126–3. A window is made in the mesoovarium caudal to the ovarian vessels. The ovarian pedicle is triple clamped. The ovarian pedicle is severed between the clamp closest to the ovary and the middle clamp.

Absorbable suture material is used for the ligature. The pedicle is grasped with small hemostats, the remaining clamp is removed, and the pedicle is inspected for bleeding. The pedicle is gently replaced into the abdomen and the hemostat is released. The procedure is repeated on the opposite ovarian pedicle. In young dogs or cats, two clamps can be used, since it is not necessary to groove the pedicle. The broad ligament is severed or torn. If the broad ligament is vascular, it should be ligated with one or two ligatures before it is cut (Fig. 126–5).

Three clamps are placed on the uterine body just cranial to the cervix. The uterine body is severed between the proximal and middle clamps (Fig. 126–6). The uterine arteries are individually ligated caudal to the most caudal clamp. The caudal clamp is removed, and the uterus is ligated in the groove that remains (Fig. 126–7). The uterine pedicle is grasped with a small hemostat above the clamp, the clamp is removed, and the pedicle is inspected for bleeding. The pedicle is gently replaced into the abdomen and the hemostat is removed.

Complications

Ovariohysterectomy can have the same complications as any abdominal procedure, e.g., anesthesia complications, delayed wound healing, suture abscesses and infection, and self-inflicted trauma to the wound.[41, 70, 118]

Hemorrhage is reported as the most common cause of death following ovariohysterectomy.[97] Operative

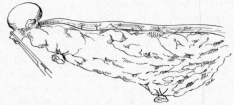

Figure 126–5. The broad ligament is ligated in one or two places and then severed.

hemorrhage may be caused by rupture of the ovarian vessels when the suspensory ligament is stretched or by tearing the vessels in the broad ligament. The uterine vessels may be torn by excessive traction on the uterine body. This can be avoided by lengthening the abdominal incision so that the uterine body near the cervix can be easily exposed. Improperly placed ligatures or defective suture material may result in hemorrhage during or after surgery. Transfixation sutures around the ovarian pedicle or the uterine arteries keep the ligature from dislodging but will not prevent bleeding if the ligature loosens. Coagulation defects may also cause hemorrhage.[97, 118]

To determine the source of the bleeding, each ligature is inspected and replaced if necessary. The abdominal incision is enlarged. The right ovarian pedicle ligature is located by using the mesoduodenum to retract the jejunum and expose the right paravertebral space. The left ovarian pedicle ligature is located by using the descending colon to retract the jejunum and expose the left paravertebral space. The ovarian pedicles are found just caudal to the kidneys. The urinary bladder is retracted ventrally and caudally to reveal the uterine pedicle between the neck of the urinary bladder and the rectum. The broad ligament is also examined for bleeding vessels.

Erosion of the uterine vessels or infection around the uterine vessel ligatures can cause intermittent bleeding from the vagina 4 to 16 days after ovariohysterectomy.[97] Erosion of the uterine vessels occurs

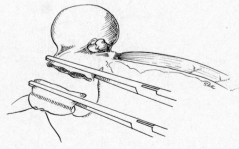

Figure 126–4. A ligature is placed in the groove left by the clamp most distant from the ovary.

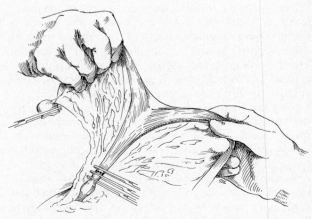

Figure 126–6. The uterus is exteriorized and three clamps are placed on the uterine body just cranial to the cervix. The uterine body is severed between the proximal and middle clamps.

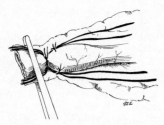

Figure 126–7. The uterine vessels are ligated on each side of the uterine body. The uterine body is ligated in the groove left by the most distal clamp.

most frequently when a single ligature is placed around the uterine body and the uterine vessels. Localized infection can occur when a transfixation suture is passed through the lumen of the uterus. An exploratory laparotomy is indicated because the bleeding may quickly become severe. The vessels may not be bleeding into the peritoneal cavity. The uterine vessels should be individually ligated at the cranial cervix. The cervix is also ligated.[97]

Recurrent estrus following ovariohysterectomy is due to residual ovarian tissue.[30, 92, 97, 118] The right ovary is incompletely removed more often than the left.[92, 97] Ovarian remnants may be more common in cats that have been spayed through a flank incision.[121] Vulval swelling, proestral bleeding, and behavioral changes may occur. Uterine stump pyometra can develop if a uterine horn or the uterine body is also present.[51, 70, 80, 93, 97, 125, 137] *Brucella canis* has been reported in a uterine stump abscess in a bitch with both ovaries.[39]

The diagnosis and treatment of recurrent estrus require an exploratory laparotomy through a midline abdominal incision and removal of all remaining ovarian tissue. It may be easier to find residual ovarian tissue if the exploratory surgery is done during estrus. Even if the ovarian remnant cannot be seen because it is hidden in fat, there may be an enlarged ovarian pedicle on the functional side. The pedicle is clamped, ligated, and severed closer to the aorta. The excised tissue should be examined histologically.

Active ovarian tissue separate from the ovarian vessels has not been documented in clinical cases. In an experimental study in cats, the ovarian cortex was completely separated from its vascular supply and sutured to the lateral abdominal wall. Estrus occurred in two of the four cats. The other two cats had cystic follicles. This demonstrated that after several months collateral circulation may activate ovarian cortical tissue even though the ovarian vessels are ligated and severed.[113] It is not known whether pieces of ovary left in the abdomen without attachment to the peritoneum will become revascularized.

Uterine stump pyometra can occur in dogs and cats after incomplete ovariohysterectomy. The source of progesterone may be endogenous from residual ovarian tissue or exogenous from progestational compounds used to treat dermatitis.[80, 93, 125, 137] Uterine

stump pyometra is prevented by the complete removal of the uterine horns and body. The uterine body ligature should be just cranial to the cervix. In cats it may be necessary to extend the abdominal incision caudally in order to excise the entire uterine body.

Fistulous tracts can develop from tissue reaction to ligature material.[96] The tract extends from an ovarian or uterine body ligature through muscle planes to the skin. A sinus develops beneath the skin as a soft, painful swelling. Blood-tinged fluid or pus intermittently discharges from the flank area (ovarian ligature) or the precrural fold, the medial thigh region, or the inguinal region (uterine ligature). Antibiotic administration may stop the drainage, but it recurs once the antibiotic ceases. In one report of 20 cases of ovariohysterectomy-related fistulous tracts, the tract originated unilaterally from an ovarian ligature in 12 animals and from the uterine ligature in 4 animals. In all these animals, braided nonabsorbable suture material (silk, multifilament nylon, linen) was used for the ligatures.[96]

Local exploration of fistulous tracts originating from the ovarian or uterine stump is of little value. A midline exploratory laparotomy should be done and all stumps examined. If the ligature is deeply imbedded in reactive tissue, the entire mass is removed. When the ovarian stump inflammatory tissue is closely associated with the renal capsule and renal parenchyma, a nephrectomy is required. If the ureter is involved, hydronephrosis can develop, necessitating nephrectomy. Uterine stump fistulous tracts can involve extensive adhesions to the bladder, uterus, mesentery, omentum, and intestines. The ureters must be protected during dissection of the fistulas to prevent further damage.[25]

Accidental *ligation of a ureter* during ovariohysterectomy causes hydronephrosis.[70, 118, 129] This can be prevented by careful identification of the uterine horns and body before ligating the uterine body. It is most likely to occur when the urinary bladder is distended and the trigone and ureterovesical junction are positioned more cranially. The ureters have more slack at this time and are more easily included in the uterine body ligature.

Urinary incontinence following ovariohysterectomy can be caused by adhesions or granulomas of the uterine stump that interfere with urinary bladder sphincter function.[106] A common ligature around the vagina and ureter can cause vaginoureteral fistulation and urinary incontinence.[98]

Estrogen-responsive incontinence can occur in older, spayed bitches.[94, 105] The recommended therapy is either oral administration of diethylstilbestrol at 0.1 to 1.0 mg per day for three to five days, followed by a maintenance dose of 1.0 mg per week, or parenteral administration of estradiol cypionate, 0.1 to 1.0 mg, at intervals of weeks to months, as needed.[105]

Body weight gains of 26 to 38 per cent have been reported following ovariohysterectomy.[28, 41] Inactivity and increased food intake contribute to the weight gain.

Ovariectomy is thought by some investigators to produce a *eunuchoid syndrome* in working dogs, i.e., decreased aggression, interest in working, and stamina.[78] A procedure has been described to prevent this syndrome. After an ovariohysterectomy, ovarian tissue is transferred to an area on the stomach that is drained exclusively by the portal vein. The graft continues to produce estradiol and progesterone, which are partially metabolized by the liver. Estrus is abolished, but brief, occasional periods of proestrus occur. The levels of estradiol in the systemic circulation are high enough to prevent the eunuchoid state.[78]

1. Adegboye, D. S.: Mycoplasmas from vagina of a bitch with open cervix pyometra. Vet. Rec. *102*:62, 1978.
2. Al-Bassam, M. A., Thomson, R. G., and O'Donnell, L.: Involution abnormalities in the postpartum uterus of the bitch. Vet. Pathol. *18*:208, 1981.
3. Al-Bassam, M. A., Thomson, R. G., and O'Donnell, L.: Normal postpartum involution of the uterus in the dog. Can. J. Comp. Med. *45*:217, 1981.
4. Allcock, J., and Penhale, B. M.: Rupture of the uterus in a bitch. Vet. Rec. *64*:353, 1952.
5. Anderson, R. K., Gilmore, C. E., and Schnelle, G. B.: Utero-ovarian disorders associated with use of medroxyprogesterone in dogs. J. Am. Vet. Med. Assoc. *146*:1311, 1965.
6. Arnall, L.: Prolapse of the uterus. Vet. Rec. *73*:750, 1961.
7. Asheim, A.: Renal function in dogs with pyometra. 1. Studies of the hypothalamic-neurohypophyseal system. Acta Vet. Scand. *4*:281, 1963.
8. Asheim, A.: Renal function in dogs with pyometra. 2. Concentrating and diluting ability. Acta Vet. Scand. *4*:293, 1963.
9. Asheim, A.: Renal function in dogs with pyometra. 3. Glomerular filtration rate, effective renal plasma flow, and the relation between solute excretion rate and maximum urine osmolarity during dehydration. Acta Vet. Scand. *5*:26, 1964.
10. Asheim, A.: Renal function in dogs with pyometra. 4. Maximum concentrating capacity during osmotic diuresis. Acta Vet. Scand. *5*:44, 1964.
11. Asheim, A.: Renal function in dogs with pyometra. 5. Sodium content of the renal medulla in relation to concentrating ability. Acta Vet. Scand. *5*:58, 1964.
12. Asheim, A.: Renal function in dogs with pyometra. 6. Sodium excretion during osmotic diuresis and its relation to the renal dysfunction. Acta Vet. Scand. *5*:69, 1964.
13. Asheim, A.: Renal function in dogs with pyometra. 7. Calcium and potassium levels in dogs with pyometra and polyuria. Acta Vet. Scand. *5*:85, 1964.
14. Asheim, A.: Renal function in dogs with pyometra. 8. Uterine infection and the pathogenesis of the renal dysfunction. Acta Pathol. Microbiol. Scand. *60*:119, 1964.
15. Asheim, A.: Renal function in dogs with pyometra. 9. Comparative pathophysiological aspects of the glomerulonephritis associated with pyometra in dogs. Acta Vet. Scand. *5*:125, 1964.
16. Asheim, A.: Pathogenesis of renal damage and polydypsia in dogs with pyometra. J. Am. Vet. Med. Assoc. *147*:736, 1965.
17. Austad, R., Blom, A. K., and Borresen, B.: Pyometra in the dog—A pathophysiological investigation. III. Plasma progesterone levels and ovarian morphology. Nord. Vet. Med. *31*:258, 1979.
18. Beck, A. M., and McEntee, K.: Subinvolution of placental sites in a postpartum bitch. A case report. Cornell Vet. *56*:269, 1966.
19. Bloom, F.: The blood and bone marrow in pyometra. North Am. Vet. *25*:483, 1944.
20. Bloom, F.: *Pathology of the Dog and Cat*. American Veterinary Publications, Inc., Santa Barbara, CA, 1954.
21. Borresen, B.: Pyometra in the dog—A pathophysiological investigation. II. Anamnestic, clinical and reproductive aspects. Nord. Vet. Med. *31*:251, 1979.
22. Borresen B.: Pyometra in the dog—A pathophysiological investigation. IV. Functional derangement of extragenital organs. Nord. Vet. Med. *32*:255, 1980.
23. Borresen, B., and Naess, B.: Microbial, immunological and toxicological aspects of canine pyometra. Acta Vet. Scand. *18*:569, 1977.
24. Borresen, B., and Skrede, S.: Pyometra in the dog—A pathophysiological investigation. V. The presence of intrahepatic cholestasis and an "acute phase reaction." Nord. Vet. Med. *32*:378, 1980.
25. Borthwick, R.: Unilateral hydronephrosis in a spayed bitch. Vet. Rec. *90*:244, 1972.
26. Boss, J. H.: The antigen distribution pattern of the human placenta. An immunofluorescent microscopic study using the kidney as an experimental model. Am. J. Pathol. *12*:332, 1963.
27. Brear, N.: Torsion of the uterus with tubal gestation in the bitch. Vet. Rec. *51*:422, 1939.
28. British Small Animal Vet. Assoc. Congress Report: Sequelae to bitch sterilization: Regional survey. Vet. Rec. *96*:371, 1975.
29. Brodey, R. S., and Fidler, I. J.: Clinical and pathologic findings in bitches treated with progestational compounds. J. Am. Vet. Med. Assoc. *149*:1406, 1966.
30. Brodey, R. S., and Harvey, C.: Excision of ovarian remnant for post ovariohysterectomy estrus (letter to the editor). J. Small Anim. Pract. *12*:699, 1971.
31. Brown, A. J.: Torsion of the gravid uterus in a bitch. Vet. Rec. *94*:202, 1974.
32. Burke, T. J.: Prostaglandin F2 alpha in the treatment of pyometra-metritis. Vet. Clin. North Am. (Small Anim. Pract.) *12*:107, 1982.
33. Chaffaux, S., and Thibier, M.: Peripheral plasma concentrations of progesterone in the bitch with pyometra. Ann. Rech. Vet. *9*:587, 1978.
34. Chivers, A. W.: An unusual finding in a cat (letter to the editor). Vet. Rec. *88*:560, 1971.
35. Choi, W.-P., and Kawata, K.: O group of *Escherichia coli* from canine and feline pyometra. Jpn. J. Vet. Res. *23*:141, 1975.
36. Christie, D. W., Bell, E. T., and Parkes, M. F.: Plasma progesterone levels in canine uterine disease. Vet. Rec. *90*:704, 1972.
37. Coulson, A.: Dinoprost in pyometritis in the bitch (letter to the editor). Vet. Rec. *105*:151, 1979.
38. Dahme, E.: The morphology of nephrosis in the dog in relation to clinical findings. Dtsch. Tierarztl. Wschr. *63*:49, 1956.
39. Dillon, A. R., and Henderson, R. A.: *Brucella canis* in a uterine stump abscess in a bitch. J. Am. Vet. Med. Assoc. *178*:987, 1981.
40. Doley, P. B.: Instances of reproduction with uterus unicornis and uterus didelphys. Vet. Med. *46*:60, 1951.
41. Dorn, A. S., and Swist, R. A.: Complications of canine ovariohysterectomy. J. Am. Anim. Hosp. Assoc. *13*:720, 1977.
42. Dow, C.: The cystic hyperplasia–pyometra complex in the bitch. Vet. Rec. *69*:1409, 1957.
43. Dow, C.: The cystic hyperplasia–pyometra complex in the bitch. Vet. Rec. *70*:1102, 1958.
44. Dow, C.: The cystic hyperplasia–pyometra complex in the bitch. J. Comp. Pathol. *69*:237, 1959.
45. Dow, C.: Experimental uterine infection in the domestic cat. J. Comp. Pathol. *72*:303, 1962.
46. Dow, C.: The cystic hyperplasia–pyometra complex in the cat. Vet. Rec. *74*:141, 1962.
47. Durfee, P. T.: Surgical treatment of postparturient metritis in the bitch. J. Am. Vet. Med. Assoc. *153*:40, 1968.

48. Ewing, G. O., Schechter, R. D., Whitney, R. C., et al.: The therapy of canine pyometra. J. Am. Anim. Hosp. Assoc. 6:218, 1970.

49. Fanton, J. W., and Withrow, S. J.: Canine mammary neoplasia. Calif. Vet. 35:12, 1981.

50. Fidler, I. J., Brodey, R. S., Howson, A. E., et al.: Relationship of estrous irregularity, pseudopregnancy and pregnancy to canine pyometra. J. Am. Vet. Med. Assoc. 149:1043, 1966.

51. Fitts, R. H.: Pyometra following incomplete oophorectomy in a bitch. J. Am. Vet. Med. Assoc. 128:449, 1956.

52. Glenn, B. L.: Subinvolution of placental sites in the bitch. 18th Gaines Veterinary Symposium, 1968, pp. 7–10.

53. Gorham, M. F., and Spink, R. R.: Uterine intussusception in a Chow Chow. Mod. Vet. Pract. 56:35, 1975.

54. Gourley, I. M.: Treatment of canine pyometra without ovariohysterectomy. In Bojrab, M. J. (ed.): Current Techniques in Small Animal Surgery. Lea & Febiger, Philadelphia, 1975, pp. 244–245.

55. Goyings, L. S., Sokolowski, J. H., Zimbelmen, R. G., and Geng, S.: Clinical, morphologic, and clinicopathologic findings in beagles treated for two years with melengestrol acetate. Am. J. Vet. Res. 38:1923, 1977.

56. Greene, J. A.: An alternative method for transfixation of the uterine stump. Can. Pract. 6:26, 1979.

57. Grindlay, M., Renton, J. P., and Ramsey, D. H.: O-groups of Escherichia coli associated with canine pyometra. Res. Vet. Sci. 14:75, 1973.

58. Hadley, J. C.: Variations in peripheral blood concentrations of progesterone and total free oestrogens in the nonpregnant bitch. Vet. Rec. 93:77, 1973.

59. Hadley, J. C.: Unconjugated oestrogen and progesterone concentrations in the blood of bitches with false pregnancy and pyometra. Vet. Rec. 96:545, 1975.

60. Hansen, J. S.: Ectopic pregnancy in a queen with one uterine horn and a urachal remnant. Vet. Med./Small Anim. Clin. 69:1135, 1974.

61. Hardy, R. M., and Osborne, C. A.: Canine pyometra: Pathophysiology, diagnosis and treatment of uterine and extra-uterine lesions. J. Am. Anim. Hosp. Assoc. 10:245, 1974.

62. Hardy, R. M., and Osborne, C. A.: Canine pyometra—a polysystemic disorder. In Kirk, R. W. (ed.): Current Veterinary Therapy VI. W. B. Saunders, Philadelphia, 1977, pp. 1229–1233.

63. Hardy, R. M., and Senior, D. F.: Canine pyometra. In Kirk, R. W. (ed.): Current Veterinary Therapy VII. W. B. Saunders, Philadelphia, 1980, pp. 1216–1219.

64. Hawk, H. W., Turner, G. D., and Sykes, J. F.: The effect of ovarian hormones on the uterine defense mechanism during the early stages of induced infection. Am. J. Vet. Res. 21:644, 1960.

65. Herron, M. R., and Herron, M. A.: Surgery of the uterus. Vet. Clin. North Am. 5:471, 1975.

66. Hess, J. L.: Use of a simultaneous ligating-dividing stapling instrument for ovariohysterectomy. Vet. Med./Small Anim. Clin. 74:1480, 1979.

67. Homer, B. L., Altman, N. H., and Tenzer, N. B.: Left horn uterine torsion in a nongravid nulliparous bitch. J. Am. Vet. Med. Assoc. 176:634, 1980.

68. Jackson, P. G. G.: Treatment of canine pyometra with dinoprost. Vet. Rec. 105:131, 1979.

69. Jones, A. K.: Pyometra in the cat (letter to the editor). Vet. Rec. 97:100, 1975.

70. Joshua, J. O.: The spaying of bitches. Vet. Rec. 77:642, 1965.

71. Jubb, K. V., and Kennedy, P. C.: Pathology of Domestic Animals, 2nd ed. Academic Press, New York, 1970.

72. Kitzman, L. M.: Endometritis and uterine rupture in a bitch. Mod. Vet. Pract. 59:535, 1978.

73. Kivisto, A.-K., Vasenius, H., and Sandholm, M.: Laboratory diagnosis of canine pyometra. Acta Vet. Scand. 18:308, 1977.

74. Knecht, C. D.: A brief survey of progestogen involvement in utero-ovarian disorders. Ill. Vet. 9:3, 1966.

75. Krook, L., Larsson, S., and Rooney, J. R.: The interrelationship of diabetes mellitus, obesity and pyometra in the dog. Am. J. Vet. Res. 21:120, 1960.

76. Krzaczynski, J.: The flank approach to feline ovariohysterectomy. Vet. Med./Small Anim. Clin. 69:572, 1974.

77. Larsen, R. E., and Wilson, J. W.: Acute metritis. In Kirk, R. W. (ed.): Current Veterinary Therapy VI. W. B. Saunders, Philadelphia, 1977, pp. 1277–1299.

78. LeRoux, P. H., and Van Der Walt, L. A.: Ovarian autograft as an alternative to ovariectomy in bitches. J. South Afr. Vet. Assoc. 48:117, 1977.

79. Lipowitz, A. J., and Larsen, R. E.: Acute metritis. In Kirk, R. W. (ed.): Current Veterinary Therapy VII. W. B. Saunders, Philadelphia, 1980, pp. 1214–1215.

80. Long, R. D.: Pyometritis in spayed cats (letter to the editor). Vet. Rec. 91:105, 1972.

81. Luckhurst, J.: Prolapse of the uterus in the cat. Vet. Rec. 73:728, 1961.

82. Maxson, F. B., and Krausnick, K. E.: Dystocia with uterine prolapse in a Siamese cat. Vet. Med./Small Anim. Clin. 64:1065, 1969.

83. McAfee, L. T.: Hydrouterus and hydrovarium in a beagle bitch. Can. Pract. Aug:46, 1977.

84. McAfee, L. T., and McAfee, J. T.: Hydrometra in a bitch. Mod. Vet. Pract. 57:829, 1976.

85. McCaig, J.: Prolapse of the uterus in the bitch. Vet. Rec. 73:628, 1961.

86. Meyer, V. N.: Medical treatment of canine pyometra. Am. Ken. Club Gazette May:48, 1982.

87. Morrow, L. L., and Howard, D. R.: Genital tract anomaly. Vet. Med./Small Anim. Clin. 67:1313, 1972.

88. Nelson, M.: Dinoprost in small animals (letter to the editor). Vet. Rec. 105:261, 1979.

89. Nelson, R. W., and Feldman, E. C.: Treatment of canine pyometra with prostaglandin F2 alpha. 31st Gaines Veterinary Symposium, 1981, pp. 10–16.

90. Newman, M. A. H.: Prolapse of the uterus in the bitch and the cat (letter to the editor). Vet. Rec. 73:680, 1961.

91. Obel, A. L., Nicander, L., and Asheim, A.: Light and electron microscopical studies of the renal lesions in dogs with pyometra. Acta Vet. Scand. 5:93, 1964.

92. Okkens, A. C., Dieleman, S. J., and Gaag, I.: Gynaecological complications following ovariohysterectomy in dogs, due to (1) partial removal of the ovaries, (2) inflammation of the uterocervical stump. Tijdschr. Diergeneesk. 106:1142, 1981.

93. Orhan, U. A.: Pyometritis in spayed cats (letter to the editor). Vet. Rec. 90:77, 1972.

94. Osborne, C. A., and Polzin, D. J.: Canine estrogen-responsive incontinence: An enigma. D.V.M. 10:42, 1979.

95. Ott, R. S., and Gustafsson, B. K.: Therapeutic application of prostaglandins for postpartum infections. Acta Vet. Scand. 77:363, 1981.

96. Pearson, H.: Ovariohysterectomy in the bitch. Vet. Rec. 87:646, 1970.

97. Pearson, H.: The complications of ovariohysterectomy in the bitch. J. Small Anim. Pract. 14:257, 1973.

98. Pearson, H., and Gibbs, C.: Urinary incontinence in the dog due to accidental vagino-ureteral fistulation during hysterectomy. J. Small Anim. Pract. 21:287, 1980.

99. Petit, G. D.: Progesterone-induced pyometra in the bitch. Anim. Hosp. 1:151, 1968.

100. Rendano, V. T., Juck, F. A., and Binnington, A. G.: Hematometra associated with pseudocyesis and uterine torsion in a dog. J. Am. Anim. Hosp. Assoc. 10:577, 1974.

101. Renton, J. P., Douglas, T. A., and Watts, C.: Pyometra in the bitch. J. Small Anim. Pract. 12:249, 1971.

102. Roberts, E.: What is your diagnosis? J. Am. Vet. Med. Assoc. 147:269, 1965.

103. Roberts, S. J.: Obstetrics and Genital Diseases (Theriogenology). Published by the author, Ithaca, 1971.

104. Robinson, G.: Uterus unicornis and unilateral renal agenesis in a cat. J. Am. Vet. Med. Assoc. 147:516, 1965.

105. Rosin, A. H., and Ross, L.: Diagnosis and pharmacological management of disorders of urinary continence in the dog. Comp. Cont. Ed. 3:601, 1981.

106. Ruckstuhl, B.: Urinary incontinence in the bitch as a complication of spaying. Schweiz. Arch. Tierheilk. *120*:143, 1978.

107. Rudolph, L.: Clinical rupture of the uterus in a dog. North Am. Vet. *12*:46, 1931.

108. Salzmann, G. B.: Torsion of the canine uterus. Mod. Vet. Pract. *55*:250, 1974.

109. Sandholm, S. M., Vasenium, H., and Kivisto, A.-K.: Pathogenesis of canine pyometra. J. Am. Vet. Med. Assoc. *167*:1006, 1975.

110. Schall, W. D., Duncan, J. R., Finco, D. R., et al.: Spontaneous recovery after subinvolution of placental sites in a bitch. J. Am. Vet. Med. Assoc. *159*:1780, 1971.

111. Schalm, O. W.: Pyometra in the dog. Calif. Vet., Oct., 1973, pp. 18–21.

112. Seegal, B. C., Hasson, M. W., Gaynor, E. C., et al.: Glomerulonephritis produced in dogs by specific antisera. I. The course of the disease resulting from injection of rabbit antidog-placenta serum or rabbit antidog-kidney serum. J. Exp. Med. *102*:789, 1955.

113. Shemwell, R. E., and Weed, J. C.: Ovarian remnant syndrome. Obstet. Gynecol. *36*:299, 1970.

114. Sheridan, V.: Unusual case of pyometra (letter to the editor). Vet. Rec. *104*:417, 1979.

115. Shille, V. M.: Canine pyometra. Vet. Med. Newsletter (Univ. Florida), Aug., 1980, p. 6.

116. Shull, R. M., Johnston, S. D., Johnston, G. R., et al.: Bilateral torsion of uterine horns in a nongravid bitch. J. Am. Vet. Med. Assoc. *172*:601, 1978.

117. Slauson, D. O., and Lewis, R. M.: Comparative pathology of glomerulonephritis in animals. Vet. Pathol. *16*:135, 1979.

118. Smith, K. W.: Female genital system. *In* Archibald, J. (ed.): *Canine Surgery*. American Veterinary Publications, Inc., Santa Barbara, 1974, pp. 762–782.

119. Sokolowski, J. H.: Prostaglandin F2 alpha-THAM for medical treatment of endometritis, metritis and pyometritis in the bitch. J. Am. Anim. Hosp. Assoc. *16*:119, 1980.

120. Sokolowski, J. H., and Zimbelmen, R. G.: Canine reproduction: Effects of multiple treatments of medroxyprogesterone acetate on reproductive organs of the bitch. Am. J. Vet. Res. *35*:1285, 1974.

121. Stein, B. S.: The genital system. *In* Catcott, E. J. (ed.): *Feline Medicine and Surgery*. American Veterinary Publications, Inc., Santa Barbara, 1975, pp. 303–354.

122. Sumner-Smith, G.: The diagnosis of "open" and "closed" pyometra in the dog and cat—I. Clinical aspects and differential diagnosis. J. Small Anim. Pract. *6*:429, 1965.

123. Swift, G. A., Brown, R. H., and Nuttall, J. E.: Dinoprost in pyometritis in the bitch (letter to the editor). Vet. Rec. *105*:64, 1979.

124. Talanti, S.: Observations on pyometra in dogs, with reference to the hypothalamic-hypophyseal neurosecretory system. Am. J. Vet. Res. *20*:41, 1959.

125. Teale, M. L.: Pyometritis in spayed cats (letter to the editor). Vet. Rec. *90*:129, 1972.

126. Teunissen, G. H. B.: The development of endometritis in the dog and the effect of oestradiol and progesterone on the uterus. Acta Endocrinol. *9*:407, 1952.

127. Theilen, G. H., and Madewell, B. R.: *Veterinary Cancer Medicine*. Lea & Febiger, Philadelphia, 1979.

128. Tompsett, J. W., and Bezner, G. A.: Torsion of the dog's uterine horn. Mod. Vet. Pract. *52*:52, 1971.

129. Turner, T.: An unusual case of hydronephrosis in a spayed Alsatian bitch. Vet. Rec. *91*:588, 1972.

130. Valle, A., and Delrieu, A.: Étude bactériologique des métrites de la chienne et de la chatte. Rec. Med. Vet. *135*:195, 1959.

131. Vlcek, Z., and Kozumplik, J.: Uterine torsion. Veterinarstvi *12*:334, 1962.

132. Walker, R. G.: The diagnosis of "open" and "closed" pyometra in the dog and cat—II. Diagnosis and clinical assessment of closed pyometritis in the bitch. J. Small Anim. Pract. *6*:437, 1965.

133. Wallace, L. J., Henry, J. D., and Clifford, J. H.: Manual reduction of uterine prolapse in a domestic cat. Vet. Med./Small Anim. Clin. *65*:595, 1970.

134. Webb, A. I.: Ventral hernia and ruptured uterus in a cat. Aust. Vet. J. *48*:212, 1972.

134a. Wheeler, S. L., Magne, M. L., Kaufman, J. L., et al.: Postpartum disorders in the bitch: A review. Comp. Cont. Ed. *6* June 1984.

135. Whitney, J. C.: Polydipsia in the dog—Symposium: 2. Polydypsia and its relationship to pyometra. J. Small Anim. Pract. *10*:485, 1969.

136. Wiessing, J., and Thomson, K. S.: Treatment of feline pyometra with dinoprost. N.Z. Vet. J. *28*:112, 1980.

137. Wilkins, D. B.: Pyometritis in spayed cats. Vet. Rec. *90*:24, 1972.

138. Wilkinson, G. T.: Prolapse of the uterus in the bitch. Vet. Rec. *73*:679, 1961.

139. Withers, A. R., and Whitney, J. C.: The response of the bitch to treatment with medroxyprogesterone acetate. J. Small Anim. Pract. *8*:265, 1967.

140. Young, R. C., and Hiscock, R.: Torsion of the uterus in the cat. Vet. Rec. *75*:872, 1963.

Chapter **127** The Vagina

Peggy M. Wykes and Patricia N. Olson

CONGENITAL ANOMALIES

Congenital abnormalities of the vagina probably occur commonly in the bitch and are occasionally associated with clinical disease. They result from abnormal development of the müllerian ducts or urogenital sinus. In most cases, congenital abnormalities of the canine reproductive tract are caused by either developmental inhibition of portions of the müllerian ducts or aberrations in the pattern of their fusion to each other or to the urogenital sinus.

Segmental Vaginal Aplasia; Hypoplasia

Segmental aplasia of the müllerian duct system is commonly reported in humans and cattle but is uncommonly found in dogs.[4, 11] The defect can occur anywhere along the vaginal wall. The occlusion may be partial (hypoplasia) and interfere with breeding or parturition, or complete (aplasia) and cause retention of uterine fluids during estrus. The latter can simulate a closed pyometra radiographically.

The method of treatment for complete or partial

vaginal occlusion depends on its location within the vagina, the breeding potential of the dog, and the degree of obstruction. In breeding bitches, caudal and midvaginal strictures have been successfully resected and the vaginal segments anastomosed.[4] No treatment may be necessary for nonbreeding, asymptomatic female dogs with partial obstruction. However, nonbreeding, symptomatic animals may require ovariohysterectomy or vaginectomy.

Whether some of the developmental defects to be described should be surgically corrected in the breeding animal is ethically debatable. The cause of segmental aplasia of the müllerian duct system in cattle may be a sex-linked trait, but a genetic etiology has not been established in the dog.[4]

Persistent Hymen

Various forms of persistent hymen are seen as the müllerian ducts fail to unite with each other or fail to fuse or cannulate with the urogenital sinus. Incomplete perforation of the hymen, taking the form of a vertical septum or annular fibrous stricture, results in stenosis at the vestibulovaginal junction (Fig. 127–1A and C).[5, 12] The latter may be confused with hypoplasia of the genital canal at the vaginal entrance, which also has a lumen but lacks a fibrous ring seen with hymen remnants (Fig. 127–1D). Contraction of the constrictor vestibularis muscle may falsely rep-

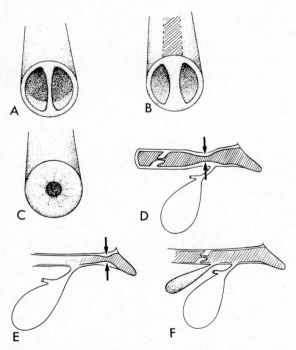

Figure 127–1. Congenital anomalies of the vagina and vulva. A, Vertical septum at vestibulovaginal junction. B, Incomplete fusion of müllerian ducts resulting in partitioning of the vagina. C, Annular stricture at vestibulovaginal orifice. D, Hypoplasia of vestibulovaginal junction. E, Stenosis at vestibulovulvar junction. F, Secondary vaginal pouch (double vagina).

resent stenosis in this location. In addition, incomplete fusion of the caudal müllerian ducts, with retention of a medial partition, results in an elongated vertical band or, rarely, a double vagina (bifid vagina) (Fig. 127–1B and F).[3, 12]

Clinical Signs

Annular fibrous strictures or vertical septa in dogs may contribute to breeding or whelping difficulties, chronic vaginitis, and urine pooling. A significant number of cases are asymptomatic. Affected female dogs have normal cycles and exhibit normal mating behavior by flagging and allowing the male to mount, but they experience pain on intromission and are unable to complete the "tie." The male may experience pain also, may dismount, or may refuse further breeding.

A history of intermittent vaginal discharge with intense licking at the vulva also has been seen in dogs with chronic vaginitis associated with vaginal obstruction.[12] The persistent vaginitis results from inadequate drainage of vaginal or uterine fluids or urine from the cranial vagina because of incomplete partitioning of the vagina and vestibule. Abnormal sloping of the vagina in a cranioventral direction ("up-and-over" vagina) also may contribute to retention of fluids. This vaginal position may be due to the cranioventral angulation of the pelvis or the degree of concavity of the symphysis pubis[6] and results in signs of urinary incontinence.[5] Urine collects in the vagina cranial to the vestibulovaginal stenosis and overflows intermittently as the dog changes position.

Diagnosis

History and clinical signs indicate the anomalies described. A digital vaginal examination is the most informative and least expensive method of diagnosis. Vaginal bands, elongated vaginal septa, or double vagina is considered when a small stoma is palpated on either side of a central partition. Bitches with annular strictures and hypoplastic lesions have a single, small vaginal opening that prevents digital penetration. Failure of the constrictor vestibularis muscle to relax may simulate a stricture. Questionable cases should be examined with the patient relaxed under general anesthesia, or during estrus when the diameter of the vestibulovaginal junction is maximal. These defects are often missed during vaginal examination with vaginal specula or otoscopic cones that bypass the anomaly. Likewise, vaginal bands and strictures are not readily appreciated with fiberoptic equipment, although it is helpful for examination and biopsy of the vaginal mucosa.

Vaginograms are performed by injection of diluted Hypaque* (50:50 with saline) into the vagina using a

---

*Winthrop Laboratories, 90 Park Ave., New York, NY.

Foley catheter. This study can demonstrate the location and expandability of a vaginal or vestibulovaginal stricture but will not differentiate the types.[13]

Treatment

Surgical correction of annular strictures and thick hymen bands is necessary in many cases to eliminate the clinical signs. Some bands can be resected per vaginam with the aid of a speculum. However, most vaginal anomalies are located at or near the vestibulovaginal junction and cannot be adequately exposed without an episiotomy.

An episiotomy incision is made that extends from the dorsal vulvar commissure toward the anus along the median raphe. Fascia and constrictor vestibularis and vulvar muscles are incised, followed by separation of the deeper vestibular bulb tissue and vaginal mucosa. The incisional edges are retracted laterally to allow exposure of the vestibulovaginal junction. A urethral catheter should be placed prior to resection of ring strictures or septa to avoid incising the urethral papilla. A curved instrument placed cranial to the band assists exposure and subsequent resection at the dorsal and ventral attachment (Fig. 127–2). Closure of the vaginal mucosa may be necessary for hemostasis if broad-based bands are removed (Fig. 127–3).

Annular strictures located at the vestibulovaginal junction require resection of submucosal fibrous tissue through a circular incision in the mucosa. Only the ventral 180° of the stricture is removed in mild cases. The mucosa is closed with an absorbable suture perpendicular to the initial incision to maximize the lumen diameter. When this procedure is not possible, the fibrous edge of the annular stricture is simply incised in several places and the stenosis expanded digitally. Expansion of these strictures by digital dilation alone is unsuccessful.

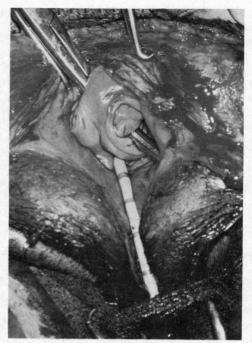

Figure 127–3. Episiotomy exposure of a broad vaginal band that partially partitions the caudal vagina.

A vestibulovaginoplasty can be attempted for hypoplasia of the vagina. The episiotomy is extended through the dorsal vaginal wall beyond the stenotic region. The vaginal wall is closed in a T fashion, using a single layer of 3-0 Vicryl in an interrupted pattern[5] (Fig. 127–4), to increase the diameter of the vaginal lumen.

Some animals may possess both types of perforate hymen (annular stricture and vertical bands). Consequently, the diameter of the vaginal opening should

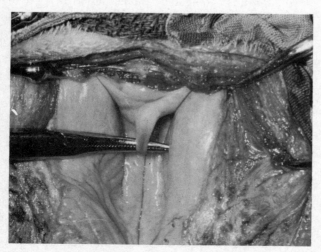

Figure 127–2. Episiotomy to expose vestibulovaginal junction. Curved hemostat is used to isolate a vertical band prior to resection at its dorsal and ventral attachments.

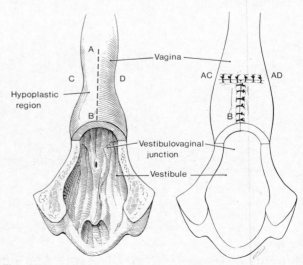

Figure 127–4. Vaginoplasty. *A,* Dorsal view of the vestibule and vagina, demonstrating a hypoplastic region (C-D). A longitudinal incision is made beyond the limits of the stenotic area (A-B). *B,* The vaginal incision is closed in a T fashion to increase the diameter of the vaginal lumen.

be carefully evaluated after septum removal. Likewise, a short, intact vertical band may flatten the vaginal entrance to suggest a stricture, but the vaginal opening expands normally after band excision.

After correction of the previously mentioned abnormalities, the episiotomy incision is closed in three layers, consisting of interrupted absorbable sutures in the vaginal mucosa, a continuous layer in the submucosa, and a subcuticular row in the skin. Postoperative management is usually not necessary when only vertical septa are removed. Permanent relief of signs can be expected after septum removal if no other genital abnormalities exist. However, some ring strictures require intermittent digital dilation after surgery to prevent cicatricial narrowing of the vaginal canal. Prognosis is more guarded for these animals.

Strictures that are located more than 2 cm cranial to the vaginal opening cannot be adequately exposed with a standard episiotomy. An abdominal approach and possible pubic osteotomy may be necessary to expose the stricture surgically. When the vagina is to be preserved, an en bloc resection of the stricture can be performed, followed by anastomosis of the vaginal components.

Abdominal exposure of the vagina is necessary when treatment by vaginectomy is considered.[5] Vaginectomy is indicated for cranial vaginal strictures, if urine pooling persists after septum removal, or when surgical removal of the occlusive tissue at the vestibulovaginal junction is unsuccessful. An ovariohysterectomy is performed, along with removal of the entire vagina in intact females. For vaginectomy, the vagina is isolated from its peritoneal support, followed by ligation of the vaginal branches of the urogenital arteries and veins. The vagina is transfixed just cranial to the urethral papilla. Extreme care should be taken to avoid interruption of the nerve and blood supply to the urethra and bladder, as well as to avoid compression or distortion of the urethral opening.

The incidence of vaginal abnormalities in animals without clinical signs is unknown. Many of these animals are spayed early in life, making hereditary predisposition difficult to evaluate.[13]

Rectovaginal Fistula

This congenital condition is often associated with imperforate anus. The rectum opens into the vagina, and the vulva functions as a common orifice for both the urogenital and gastrointestinal tracts (Fig. 127–5). A barium sulfate enema can be given via the vagina (if atresia ani is present) to demonstrate the fistula.

The severity of clinical signs varies with the size of the fistula and the dog's diet. An animal with a large fistula and on a liquid diet evacuates enough soft feces through the fistula to decompress the colon. Megacolon is a complicating factor when excessive feces collects in the colon after the diet is changed to solid food, especially if atresia ani is also present.[8]

A fistula extending from the rectum can also communicate with the vulvar vestibule (caudal to the urethral papilla) and demonstrate similar signs.

Treatment

Treatment is to restore the lumen of both the rectum and the vagina. A linear incision is made along the median raphe from just ventral to the anal sphincter to the vulva. The fistula is located and isolated by blunt dissection. The dorsal communication with the rectum is ligated with absorbable sutures placed around the fistula, and the fistula is incised. Oversewing the rectal ligature ensures a tight seal. If the tract is very short, the stoma must be oversewn primarily. The tract is also divided where it joins the vaginal (or vestibular) wall, and

Figure 127–5. Rectovaginal fistula. *A,* Rectum communicates directly with the vagina but terminates in a normal anus. *B,* Rectum terminates at the vagina. Atresia ani is present.

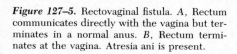
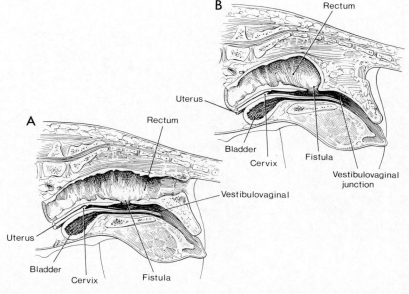

the resulting vaginal defect is closed with a double line of absorbable sutures.

Cellulitis is a complicating factor if the operative site is contaminated with feces or if the rectal incision continues to leak. Fecal incontinence often persists when this condition occurs with imperforate anus. These animals frequently lack an anal sphincter and remain incontinent even after surgical reconstruction of the anal opening.

ACQUIRED ABNORMALITIES

Vaginal Hyperplasia

During the follicular phase of the estrous cycle, the vaginal and vestibular mucosa normally become edematous and thickened. Exaggeration of this estrogenic response occasionally results in excessive mucosal folding of the vaginal floor cranial to the urethral papilla.[12] This redundant mucosa begins to protrude through the vulvar labia as a red, fleshy mass (Fig. 127–6A). The exposed tissue is subject to trauma, inflammation, and ulceration. The urethra does not become exteriorized and can be easily catheterized. Vaginal hyperplasia is most frequently seen during the first estrous period and usually regresses spontaneously during the luteal phase. Recurrence is common during succeeding estrous periods. Because the hyperplastic tissue may prevent natural breeding, affected bitches may be artificially inseminated; however, owners should be cautioned that the hyperplastic tissue occasionally recurs at parturition and may result in dystocia.

Since English bulldogs, boxers, and other brachycephalic breeds are the most commonly afflicted, owners should be informed that the condition may be hereditary.[2]

Megestrol acetate (2.0 mg/kg PO daily for seven days) can be given in early proestrus in an attempt to prevent the development of vaginal hyperplasia in bitches with a previous history of vaginal hyperplasia. Megestrol acetate is a synthetic progestogen and may be antagonistic to estrogens in the target tissue. Owners wishing to breed their bitches during the current cycle should be warned that this treatment prevents ovulation.

Gonadotropin-releasing hormone (GnRH) has also been used to treat vaginal hyperplasia in the bitch (50 μg GnRH IV once). Although administering GnRH to a bitch in estrus should assure a luteinizing hormone (LH) surge and subsequent increases in serum progesterone, most bitches with vaginal hyperplasia are already in estrus (i.e., the LH surge has already occurred). Administration of GnRH in early proestrus, or when ovarian follicles are still immature and not capable of ovulating, could result in preovulatory luteinization of follicles or ovarian cysts.

Temporary relief can be provided by application of K-Y jelly to minimize drying of the exposed mucosa. In addition to interfering with coitus, the hyperplastic tissue is esthetically displeasing to many owners, and surgical resection becomes the treatment of choice. Owners should be cautioned that vaginal hyperplasia occasionally recurs following surgical correction; since the defect appears to be in the vagina it can occur during a subsequent estrus. Ovariohysterectomy prevents further recurrence.

Surgical Treatment

The patient is placed in sternal recumbency and positioned and prepared for episiotomy, which exposes the posterior vaginal floor and allows delineation of the prolapsed tissue margins. The mass must be lifted off the vestibular floor to identify the urethra for catheterization (Fig. 127–6B). Redundant vaginal

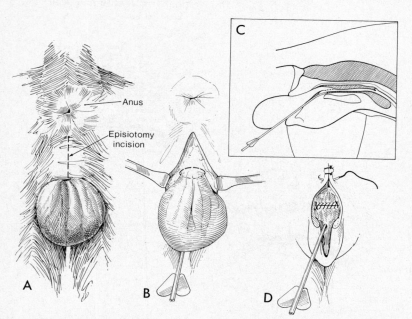

Figure 127–6. Vaginal hyperplasia. *A,* Protrusion of hyperplastic tissue through the vulvar labia. An episiotomy is necessary for better exposure. *B,* The mass is lifted off the vestibular floor to catheterize the urethra. Note that the mass originates from the vaginal floor just caudal to the urethral papilla. *C,* A transverse elliptical incision is made at the base of the mass, avoiding the urethral papilla. *D,* Vaginal wall defect is closed with a continuous suture followed by closure of the episiotomy incision.

tissue is amputated by making a transverse elliptical incision around its base (Fig. 127–6C). Closure of the vaginal defect is with a simple continuous suture of 2-0 Vicryl, avoiding the urethral orifice (Fig. 127–6D). The episiotomy incision is closed in three layers.

Vaginal Prolapse

Vaginal prolapse is much less common than vaginal hyperplasia in dogs. Prolapse of the vagina can be either partial or complete. In contrast to partial vaginal prolapse, the cervix is exteriorized with complete prolapses. In either case, a doughnut-shaped eversion of the complete vaginal circumference (including the urethral papillae) protrudes through the labia (Fig. 127–7). This is in contrast to vaginal hyperplasia, in which redundant mucosa arises primarily from the vaginal floor. The everted tissue often becomes discolored from venous congestion, ulcerates, and is easily traumatized. Displacement of abdominal or pelvic organs into the prolapse is rare, although vaginal prolapse may precede prolapse of the uterus.[10]

Brachycephalic breeds such as boxers and Boston terriers appear predisposed to vaginal prolapse. The cause of this condition is complex, but hereditary weakness of the perivaginal tissue is a proposed factor.[10] Constipation, forced separation during coitus, and size discrepancy between breeding partners may play a role in vaginal prolapse.[1] This condition

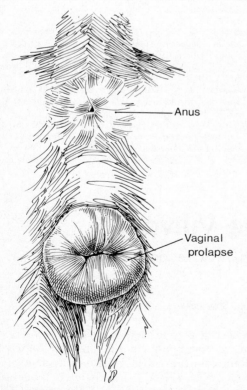

Figure 127–7. Vaginal prolapse. Eversion of the complete vaginal circumference through the vulvar labia, demonstrating the typical donut-shaped appearance.

occurs when estrogen production predominates (e.g., estrus) and with pathological hyperestrogenism (e.g., cystic ovaries). Vaginal displacement during pregnancy is very rare in the bitch, but a few cases have been reported in late gestation.[10]

Both vaginal prolapse and vaginal hyperplasia must be differentiated from tumors that arise from the vagina and vestibule (leiomyomas, fibromas, polyps, and so on). The presenting signs are very similar, and biopsy should be considered even though the majority of vaginal tumors are benign (see Chapter 182).

Treatment

With mild prolapse, no treatment may be necessary, as spontaneous regression occurs during diestrus. More severe prolapses require protection of exposed tissues until estrus passes. Attempts to replace the vaginal mucosa usually require general anesthesia. The everted tissue is first cleaned with saline or a dilute antiseptic solution (povidone-iodine*). Tissue edema can be reduced by manual compression or by application of 50% dextrose to the mucosal surface. The solution is later rinsed off to minimize mucosal irritation. A lubricated plastic syringe case can be used to push the everted tissue back into place. An episiotomy provides additional exposure for easier reduction. Once the vagina is repositioned, a urinary catheter is placed until the swelling resolves, and the reduction is maintained by placing nonabsorbable sutures across the labia. If repositioning is unsuccessful with the vulvar approach, reduction can be assisted by traction on the uterus through a ventral abdominal incision. After vaginal repositioning, recurrent prolapse can be minimized in some cases by suturing the uterine body or the broad ligaments to the abdominal wall.[1]

In severe acute or longstanding vaginal prolapse, severe hemorrhage, infection, or necrosis may exist. These animals may become dehydrated and hypotensive and should be treated accordingly. Surgical resection of the devitalized tissue is necessary to prevent further sepsis and self-mutilation and to restore the vaginal lumen. Repair is often preceded by an episiotomy for exposure and a urinary catheter is inserted to identify and protect the urethra (Fig. 127–8A). A circumferential incision is carried out in relays through the vaginal wall. One to two centimeters of the outer mucosal layer are incised, followed by resection of the inner, noninverted mucosal layer (Fig. 127–8B).[1] Hemorrhage is controlled by electrocautery, ligation, and suturing the incision edges with a series of horizontal mattress sutures. The ring-shaped incision is extended, and the next section is sutured until the entire circumference of the prolapsed vaginal tissue is resected.

A bitch with a vaginal prolapse during late preg-

---

*Prepodyne Solution, West Chemical Products, Inc., New York, NY.

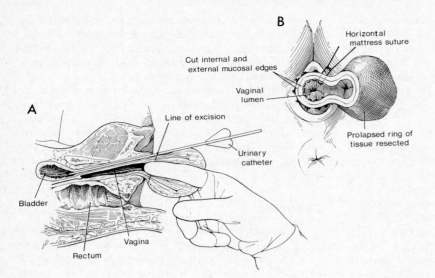

Figure 127–8. Surgical correction of vaginal prolapse. *A*, Dog is placed in dorsal recumbency. Urethral catheter is placed to identify urethral papilla; a finger can be inserted into the center of the prolapsed tissue. Note the intended line of resection. *B*, A stepwise full-thickness circumferential incision is made in the vaginal wall. Horizontal mattress sutures are placed to close the incisional edges.

nancy will probably have difficulty during parturition.[10] Therefore, surgical resection of the prolapsed tissue is preferred. Future breeding is seldom impaired following surgical resection. However, breeding is undesirable for bitches that have a tendency to prolapse, as the condition may have an hereditary component. Ovariohysterectomy causes permanent regression of vaginal prolapse and is recommended.[10]

Vaginal Trauma

Injury to the vagina most often occurs with the use of obstetrical equipment during assisted parturition. Other causes include forceful separation of dogs during mating, accidents, and malicious injuries.[9] Hemorrhage may be profuse. An episiotomy may be necessary to visualize and suture the injury. No treatment is necessary for simple contusions, but large hematomas often require removal (after one to two days) to prevent interference with future breeding or whelping.

1. Alexander, J. E., and Lennok, W. J.: Vaginal prolapse in the bitch. Can. Vet. J. 2:428, 1961.
2. Burke, T. J., and Reynold, H. A.: The female genital system. *In* Bojrab, M. J. (ed.): *Pathophysiology in Small Animal Surgery.* Lea & Febiger, Philadelphia, 1981, pp. 425.
3. Capel-Edwards, K.: Double vagina with perineal agenesis in a bitch. Vet. Rec. 101:57, 1977.
4. Gee, B. R., Pharr, J. W., and Furneaux, R. W.: Segmental aplasia of the müllerian duct system in a dog. Can. Vet. J. 18:281, 1977.
5. Holt, P. E., and Sayle, B.: Congenital vestibulovaginal stenosis in the bitch. J. Small Anim. Pract. 22:67, 1981.
6. Jones, D. E., and Joshua, J. O.: *Reproductive Clinical Problems in the Dog.* Wright PSG, Boston, 1982.
7. McConnell, D. A.: Correction of vaginovestibular strictures in the bitch. J. Am. Anim. Hosp. Assoc. 13:92, 1977.
8. Rawlings, C. A., and Capps, W. F.: Rectovaginal fistula and imperforate anus in a dog. J. Am. Vet. Med. Assoc. 159:320, 1971.
9. Smith, K. W.: Female genital system. *In* Archibald, J. (ed.): *Canine Surgery.* American Veterinary Publications Inc., Santa Barbara, 1974, p. 751.
10. Troger, C. P.: Vaginal prolapse in the bitch. Mod. Vet. Pract. 53:73, 1972.
11. Wadsworth, P. F., Hall, J. C., and Prentice, D. E.: Segmental aplasia of the vagina in a beagle bitch. Lab. Anim. 12:65, 1978.
12. Welser, J. R.: The vagina and vulva. *In* Bojrab, M. J. (ed.): *Current Techniques in Small Animal Surgery.* Lea & Febiger, Philadelphia, 1981, p. 249.
13. Wykes, P. M., and Soderberg, S. F.: Congenital abnormalities of the canine vagina and vulva. In press.

Chapter **128**

The Vulva

Peggy M. Wykes and Patricia N. Olson

CONGENITAL ABNORMALITIES

Congenital abnormalities of the canine vulva are not common; however, they may contribute to the development of vaginitis, cystitis, and difficulty with natural breeding. Some of these anomalies include vestibulovulvar stenosis, anovulvar cleft, vulvar atresia, and clitoral hypertrophy. Double vulvar formation and total vulvar agenesis are much less common.

Vulvar Stenosis

Stenosis may occur within the body of the vestibule or, more commonly, at the junction between the vestibule and the vulvar labia (vestibulovulvar junction) (see Fig. 127–1E). The latter is thought to be due to an imperfect joining of the genital folds or genital swellings. Affected female dogs experience pain when coitus is attempted and often require artificial insemination. We have seen this condition in several collie dogs. An episiotomy can be performed to permanently enlarge the vestibulovulvar opening to prevent dyspareunia (difficult mating) and potential dystocia. This procedure is performed as for episiotomy; however, the ventral third of the incision is closed in a mucocutaneous fashion, resulting in an elongated vulvar cleft.[2] As a result of increased vestibular exposure to microorganisms in the environment, the flora of the vestibule and vagina may change and predispose to urinary tract infection.[4]

Anovulvar Cleft (Vulvovaginal Cleft)

This condition is incomplete closure of the skin from the dorsal vulvar commissure to the anus (Fig. 128–1A).[1, 5] The failure of the urogenital folds to fuse dorsally allows the vestibular floor and clitoris to be directly seen. Clitoritis and hyperemia of the vestibular mucosa occur frequently subsequent to exposure and fecal contamination. This anomaly may occur in sexually normal female dogs or in conjunction with intersex states. The rarity of this defect suggests it is not hereditary.[1]

Treatment

Surgical repair is performed to reduce infection and abrasion of exposed mucous membranes and to provide a more cosmetic appearance to the perineal region. The cleft is repaired by making an inverted

V perineoplasty incision along the mucocutaneous junction between the anus and vulva (Fig. 128–1B).[1] Enough tissue should be removed to create a gap between the mucosal vaginal edge and skin edge of about 1 centimeter. Interrupted 2-0 Vicryl sutures are used in the vaginal submucosa to close the dorsal defect. This is followed by placement of interrupted nonabsorbable sutures in the skin (Fig. 128–1C and D).

Atresia of the Vulva

Vulvar hypoplasia or atrophy is most frequently recognized in spayed female dogs.[3] The vulva appears small (infantile) and is often retracted into the perineal skin folds. This results in a moist dermatitis that may be accentuated by retention of urine within the folds of skin.

Estrogens may be used to treat this condition, but because continual administration is necessary for retained vulvar size, hormonal therapy is not the treatment of choice. Prolonged use of estrogens also can result in fatal bone marrow suppression. Episioplasty improves exteriorization of the vulva and is the preferred treatment (see episioplasty procedure).

Clitoral Hypertrophy

Dogs with enlarged clitorides are often presented by owners for esthetic reasons. These animals may

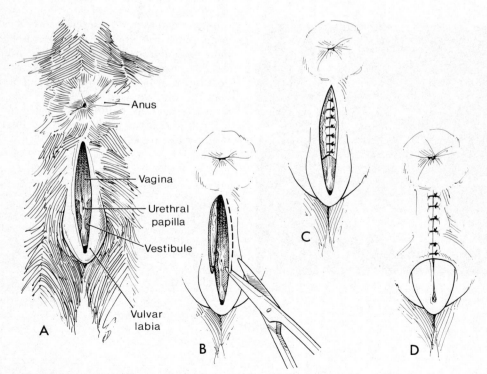

Figure 128–1. Anovulvar cleft. *A,* Incomplete closure of skin from the anus to the dorsal vulvar commissure. *B,* A V-shaped incision is made along the mucocutaneous junction between the anus and vulvar labia. *C,* Simple interrupted sutures are used to close the vaginal wall. *D,* Skin closure with simple interrupted sutures.

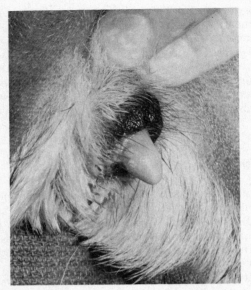

Figure 128–2. Hypertrophied clitoris protruding through the vulvar cleft.

be hermaphrodites, pseudohermaphrodites, bitches receiving anabolic steroids, or bitches with hyperadrenocorticism. Occasionally the condition is found in normal females.[3] The clitoris may protrude through the vulvar cleft if hypertrophy is severe (Fig. 128–2). The clitoris sometimes resembles a small penis and may even possess an os (baculum). Protrusion of the hypertrophied clitoris through the vulvar labia may result in clitoritis. Similarly, the mechanical irritation

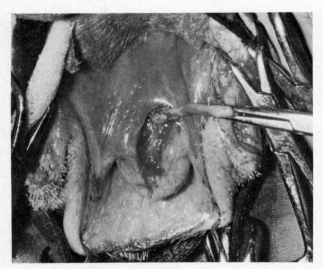

Figure 128–3. An os being surgically dissected from the clitoris through an episiotomy incision.

of an enlarged clitoris can result in vaginitis. When an os is present, clitoral enlargement may persist even after removal of the gonads; consequently, the os is surgically removed by simple dissection followed by resection of the surrounding clitoral tissues (Fig. 128–3). Large "phalluses" in dogs with intersex disorders bleed profusely when removed, and episiotomy may be needed.

ACQUIRED VULVAR ABNORMALITIES

Vulvar Hypertrophy

The vulva normally becomes swollen and edematous during the follicular stages of the estrous cycle in response to estrogen stimulation. Occasionally this vulvar enlargement becomes excessive. This swelling should dissipate with the conclusion of normal estrus. In animals experiencing prolonged estrogen stimulation from cystic ovaries or granulosa cell tumor, vulvar hypertrophy may persist. In chronic cases, the labia become thickened, pigmented, and hairless.[3] Ovariohysterectomy is an effective treatment.

Vulvar Trauma

Vulvar trauma is uncommon but usually results from dog fights, sadistic acts, injury during breeding, attempts to disrupt mating during a "tie," or difficult parturition. The wounds are usually lacerations, contusions, or puncture wounds.[4] Determination of the extent of the injury and subsequent treatment may require vaginoscopy or episiotomy. Lacerations and large puncture wounds are debrided and sutured; Penrose drains are placed if needed. Bitches in estrus should be separated from other dogs to prevent the possibility of mating and reinjury. Large vulvar hematomas are allowed to organize one to two days prior to resection. Failure to remove these may result in vestibulovulvar obstruction. Antibiotics are used to minimize infection.[3]

1. Burk, T. J., and Smith, C. W.: Vulvovaginal cleft in a dog. J. Am. Anim. Hosp. Assoc. *11*:774, 1975.
2. McConnell, D. A.: Correction of vaginovestibular strictures in the bitch. J. Am. Anim. Hosp. Assoc. *13*:92, 1977.
3. Smith, K. W.: Female genital system. *In* Archibald, J. (ed.): *Canine Surgery.* American Veterinary Publications, Inc., Santa Barbara, 1974, p. 751.
4. Welser, J. R.: The vagina and vulva. *In* Bojrab, M. J. (ed.): *Current Techniques in Small Animal Surgery.* Lea & Febiger, Philadelphia, 1981, p. 249.
5. Wilson, C. F., and Clifford, D. H.: Perineoplasty for anovaginal cleft in the dog. J. Am. Vet. Med. Assoc. *159*:871, 1971.

Chapter 129

Normal and Abnormal Parturition

Peggy Wykes and Patricia N. Olson

A thorough understanding of the physiology and endocrinology of normal parturition (eutocia) is vital for diagnosing and treating abnormal parturition (dystocia). Although the exact mechanisms that allow parturition to begin and proceed normally in the bitch are still unknown, extrapolations from other species, along with recent studies on canine parturition, provide information on the physiological and endocrinological changes that are important for normal parturition.

ENDOCRINOLOGY OF PARTURITION

Dramatic changes occur in the concentrations of some hormones in serum preceding and following whelping (Fig. 129–1). A decrease in plasma progesterone occurs in bitches 24 to 48 hours before parturition. In one study, whelping did not occur until concentrations of progesterone in the plasma fell to less than 2 ng/ml.[6] Similarly, parturition was prevented in bitches receiving progesterone implants during the week of expected whelping. Bitches either died with pups in utero or were relieved by cesarean section following periods of severe stress. These data strongly suggest that the prepartum decline in progesterone plays an important role in normal parturition.

Concentrations of corticoids increase in the serum of some pregnant bitches near the time that progesterone declines. Although the increases in corticoids observed prepartum are somewhat erratic and fail to consistently parallel the decline in progesterone in all bitches, it is possible that the prepartum elevations observed in the maternal circulation of some bitches reflect larger increases locally at the fetoplacental-uterine level. The local increase may be what is necessary for normal whelping (see "Fetal Factors").

Concentrations of prolactin also increase in the serum of pregnant bitches near whelping. The prepartum surge of prolactin is dramatic and is observed concomitantly with or immediately after the prepartum decline in progesterone. This finding supports the suggestion that prolactin release in the bitch follows abrupt decreases in concentrations of progesterone in serum and may explain why bitches spayed during diestrus occasionally begin to lactate a few days following surgery.[7, 16]

Although concentrations of estrogens increase in the serum of many species prior to parturition, it is still unclear whether or not similar increases occur in the bitch. Concannon and associates[8] reported concentrations of "total immunoreactive estrogens" in plasma to be elevated prepartum in the bitch, whereas Edquist and colleagues[10] found no elevations in estradiol during diestrus in either pregnant or nonpregnant bitches.

PHYSIOLOGY OF PARTURITION

Fetal Factors

The fetus is important in determining its own time of delivery in many species. A normal adrenal-pituitary-hypothalamic axis is necessary for eutocia in many animals. Prolonged gestation occurs in both the cow and ewe carrying a fetus with abnormal adrenal or pituitary glands. It has been speculated that fetal stress near parturition results in increased release of corticotropin-releasing hormone (CRH), which stimulates the release of adrenocorticotropic hormone (ACTH) and subsequently of cortisol. However, concentrations of ACTH decline in human fetal blood as gestation advances, with the rate of adrenal growth in the fetus increasing at a time when concentrations of ACTH are falling.[20] Although other tropic agents produced by the pituitary or placenta may stimulate fetal adrenal glands in some species, no such tropic agent has been identified for the bitch.

The increase in corticoids produced by the fetal adrenal gland is believed to stimulate the release of prostaglandins from the placenta in some species. These prostaglandins can either directly stimulate uterine contractions or enter the maternal circulation

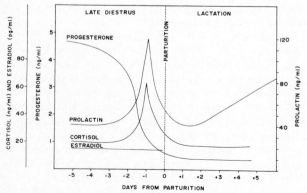

Figure 129–1. Concentrations of hormones in canine serum during late diestrus and lactation.

to stimulate the release of oxytocin from the pituitary gland, which also results in uterine contractions. However, concentrations of $PGF_{2\alpha}$ do not increase in the canine uterus prior to parturition and may not be physiologically involved in whelping.[15]

Corticoids can induce an enzyme in the pregnant ewe that is capable of hydroxylating placental progesterone to a less active progestogen that is rapidly metabolized.[12] Because progesterone inhibits myometrial cell contractility, parturition does not occur in many species until concentrations of progesterone in the serum or placenta decline. However, the canine placenta does not produce progesterone in any appreciable quantity.[21] Therefore, it is uncertain whether fetal corticoids could be responsible for lowering concentrations of progesterone in serum, because the ovaries and not the placenta produce progesterone throughout pregnancy in the bitch. However, there is some evidence for fetal participation in determining the onset of whelping. For example, gestational length is often increased in the bitch carrying a single fetus and decreased when multiple fetuses are present. A single fetus may require more time than multiple fetuses to produce sufficient corticoids for the initiation of parturition. Similarly, puppies born with head defects also have prolonged gestation periods, possibly owing to an abnormality of the adrenal-pituitary-hypothalamic axis that interferes with fetal steroid production.[2]

Maternal Factors

A decrease in the progesterone-estrogen ratio at the myometrium is generally accepted as being important for initiating normal parturition in many species. The decrease can occur through either increasing concentrations of estradiol or decreasing concentrations of progesterone. As progesterone declines (or estradiol increases) in the serum, oxytocin can initiate and maintain uterine contractions. As the fetus enters the birth canal and causes mechanical distension, nerve impulses pass to the hypothalamus and cause the release of more oxytocin into the systemic circulation. Mechanical distension of the birth canal also stimulates the sensory part of a spinal reflex arc, resulting in efferent stimulation and contractions of the abdominal muscles.

Relaxin, a polypeptide hormone isolated from the ovary or placenta in several species, causes relaxation of pelvic ligaments and increased diameter of the birth canal. In addition, relaxin may be important in allowing the uterus to expand during late gestation to accommodate growing fetuses. Although relaxin has been isolated from many species, its exact role in the pregnant bitch is undetermined.

Corticoids are elevated in the serum of bitches prior to whelping, but their contribution to lowering concentrations of serum progesterone, and hence initiating labor, is unclear. It is also uncertain whether the corticoids are of fetal or maternal origin. Administration of dexamethasone (5 mg b.i.d. for 10 days) reportedly results in intrauterine death followed by fetal resorption (when initiated at day 30 of pregnancy) or abortion (when initiated at day 45 of pregnancy).[1] Because the exact role of corticoids in inducing parturition in the bitch is still unknown, it seems prudent to avoid treating pregnant dogs with glucocorticoids.

HEMATOLOGIC CHANGES DURING PREGNANCY

The packed cell volume (PCV) declines in pregnant bitches, with an observed anemia reportedly occurring between seven and nine weeks following estrus. Similar decreases of lesser magnitude also occur in nonpregnant bitches during diestrus. Conversely, concentrations of cholesterol and protein in serum increase during diestrus in pregnant and nonpregnant bitches.[19] Increases in the circulating activity of coagulation factors VII, VIII, IX, and XI occur in pregnat but not in nonpregnant diestrous bitches.[14]

ONSET OF PARTURITION

The rectal temperature drops to less than 100°F (and frequently to less than 99°F) approximately eight to 24 hours prior to parturition and ten to 14 hours after concentrations of progesterone in the serum decline to less than 2 ng/ml.[9] Although the mechanism for hypothermia is poorly understood, the temperature drop appears to be associated with declining concentrations of progesterone, since it is also observed after concentrations of progesterone decline in the serum of diestrous bitches receiving injections of $PGF_{2\alpha}$. Anestrous bitches receiving $PGF_{2\alpha}$ do not show similar decreases in rectal temperatures.[9] A transient hypothermia has also been observed for one to two days following ovariohysterectomy in bitches relieved of pyometra, presumably again owing to a rapid decrease in concentrations of progesterone following removal of ovaries.[4]

If parturition does not follow the decline in progesterone (i.e., dystocia) the bitch soon becomes euthermic as the thermoregulatory mechanisms readjust. Therefore, the return of a normal rectal temperature does not preclude the possibility of dystocia. We have observed transient fluctuations in body temperatures with occasional drops in rectal temperatures to 99°F during the last two weeks of gestation in eutocic bitches. This pattern may be caused by fluctuations in concentrations of progesterone in the serum of some pregnant bitches. Although a brief period of hypothermia could be observed in a normal pregnancy without impending parturition, the term bitch with hypothermia must be carefully monitored for dystocia.

STAGE OF PARTURITION

Stage I

The first stage of labor is characterized by uterine contractions and dilation of the cervix. Although the uterine contractions are not externally visible to the owner, the bitch may appear restless, pant, tremble, and become anorectic. Occasionally the bitch vomits, and respiratory and heart rates may be elevated. The bitch may seek seclusion and establish a nest. This first stage of labor usually lasts for six to 12 hours, but it may persist up to 36 hours in the primiparous bitch.

Stage II

During the second stage of labor each fetus passes through the birth canal and is expelled. Although the average duration of this stage is six to 12 hours, it may continue up to 24 hours in some normal bitches. Abdominal straining is apparent and coincides with uterine contractions. As the fetus enters the birth canal, the neuroendocrine reflex (Ferguson's reflex) results in oxytocin release, which enhances uterine contractions. Distension of the birth canal also leads to stimulation of the sensory component of a spinal reflex arc, resulting in efferent stimulation and contraction of the abdominal muscles. The bitch usually lies down during the second stage of labor. Stage II can be inhibited if the bitch is disturbed or distressed. The allantois usually ruptures as the fetus enters the birth canal. The owners may notice a clear, water-like fluid pass from the vulva. Occasionally the allantoic membranes may cover the newborn, but more likely the fetus is covered by only the amnionic membranes at birth. The bitch usually licks each puppy at birth to remove the amnion. This cleaning action also aids in stimulating cardiovascular and respiratory function in the puppies. The bitch frequently eats the fetal membranes, and may sometimes therefore vomit.

Approximately 60 per cent of the puppies are born in an anterior presentation with the remaining presented in breech. The breech birth (posterior presentation) does not predispose the bitch to dystocia. Although puppies are usually delivered every one-half to one hour until whelping is finished, the interval between puppies can be variable, with up to four hours occurring between eutocic births.

Stage III

Stage III of labor is defined for monotocous species as the stage when fetal membranes are expelled. In the bitch, fetal membranes are actually passed during Stage II. Puppies can be alternately delivered from each horn, so that two puppies may be born before the placentas are passed. A thick, greenish discharge (lochia) accompanies placental separation and may be observed in all three stages of labor. This pigment is due to uteroverdin, the product of red blood cell breakdown in the canine placenta.

Uterine Involution

Uterine involution occurs over several weeks following whelping, with complete endometrial repair by three months postpartum. Lochia may be observed passing from the vulva of normal bitches for up to three weeks postpartum and must be differentiated from abnormal uterine discharges. The bitch with postpartum metritis is often systemically ill and has a malodorous discharge from the uterus that is frequently brown or brownish-red rather than green. Degenerative neutrophils are present on vaginal smears from bitches with metritis, in contrast to healthy neutrophils frequently observed in vaginal smears from normal bitches following whelping. A bright red, bloody discharge may be observed for several weeks or months following parturition in bitches with subinvolution of placental sites (SIPS). These animals are frequently less than three years of age and are often primiparous. These females are not systemically ill unless the retained placental tags of tissue, characteristic of SIPS, become secondarily infected. Generally, the hemorrhagic discharge resolves by the next estrus and no therapy is required. Rarely, the hemorrhage is so severe that ovariohysterectomy is necessary to save the bitch. Although retention of placental tags is a fairly common problem in the young bitch, retention of a whole placenta is rare in bitches of any age. Individuals retaining entire placentas are frequently systemically ill, with metritis occurring as a sequela.

ABNORMAL PARTURITION

Diagnosis

A thorough history is important in attempting to establish whether a bitch is suffering from dystocia. Although breeding dates are helpful in determining whether gestation is prolonged, they may be of limited value, since a normal bitch may be in estrus (and hence be mated) for up to 21 days. This variation in the length of estrus results in variable gestation lengths based on breeding dates. The owner should be questioned about past whelpings and previous dystocias, because some causes of dystocia (e.g., uterine inertia, vaginal anomalies, pelvic fractures) may result in subsequent whelping difficulties. Obtaining such information from an owner allows the veterinarian to decide whether medical or surgical assistance should be considered.

A complete physical examination should be performed on any bitch presented for dystocia. Assessment of the animal's general health should be performed as well as a thorough evaluation of the genital system. A digital examination of the vagina should be done to determine whether (1) a fetus is lodged in the birth canal, (2) vaginal anomalies that might result in dystocia are present, or (3) firm pressure placed on the ventral or dorsal vaginal wall results in abdominal straining (Ferguson's reflex). Absence of Ferguson's reflex suggests either that the bitch is not yet ready to deliver puppies or that uterine inertia is present and the bitch is incapable of responding to vaginal pressure. A vaginal examination is also helpful in characterizing the presence and nature of uterine discharges. The presence of lochia indicates that placental separation has begun and that whelping must quickly follow or else the fetus will die.

Rectal palpation is beneficial in evaluating pelvic diameter and identifying the presence of old pelvic fractures that may result in obstructive dystocia. Abdominal palpation is performed to determine whether fetuses are present. Occasionally a bitch that is not pregnant or has completed delivery may be presented for dystocia. Fetal heartbeats are difficult to auscultate through the abdominal wall in most bitches. Therefore, the absence of fetal heartbeats does not always correlate with fetal death, nor does the presence of fetal heartbeats guarantee the viability of each puppy. Real-time ultrasonographic equipment is now available that can accurately evaluate the heart rate and viability of individual fetuses. If fetal heart rates are absent or decreased (normal rate 200–240 beats/min) or if fetal motion is absent on real-time ultrasonographic evaluation, a dystocia is likely and the owners must be cautioned that the likelihood that all puppies will survive is small.

Survey radiographs can also be taken to evaluate fetal viability; however, radiographic changes indicative of fetal death usually do not occur until puppies have been dead for several hours (Fig. 129–2). The presence of intravascular fetal gas, usually found in the fetal heart, is not apparent radiographically until six hours following death. Overlap of the cranial bones is a less reliable sign and results from calvarial

collapse around a shrunken brain. Calvarial collapse usually occurs two days postmortem. Another sign of fetal death is an alteration in the spatial relationships between the bones of the fetal skeleton. This is especially seen in the vertebral column as a collapse of the spinal column following loss of axial muscle tone. The fetus may appear radiographically like a "bag of bones."[11] Survey radiographs are probably most valuable in determining the number of fetuses yet to be delivered.

Several criteria can suggest that dystocia is present. These are offered as guidelines and are not absolute parameters.

Signs of Toxicity in a Pregnant Bitch. Any toxic bitch in late pregnancy should be critically evaluated for dystocia. If lochia is present in the vagina, placental separation has begun for at least one puppy and perhaps more. The entire litter of puppies is usually dead by 24 hours after the onset of dystocia. The bitch usually shows signs of toxemia by 48 to 72 hours and requires vigorous care for survival.

Strong and Frequent Abdominal Straining With Failure to Produce a Puppy Within 20 Minutes. This usually suggests that a puppy is present in the birth canal but cannot pass. A puppy lodged in the birth canal will become asphyxiated if complete placental separation occurs prior to birth. Prolonged straining eventually results in uterine inertia.

Weak Straining That Fails to Produce a Puppy Within Two to Three Hours. Weak straining without delivery of a puppy suggests that the uterine contractions are incapable of bringing the fetus into the birth canal.

More Than Four Hours Since the Birth of the Last Puppy. If more than four hours have lapsed since the birth of the last puppy, parturition may be completed. If not, uterine inertia should be considered, especially if the delivery has been prolonged and the myometrium is fatigued. Although some bitches can deliver a live puppy after four or more hours have elapsed since the last born, the incidence of stillbirths dramatically rises as the time between delivered puppies increases. If inertia develops, the bitch is no longer able to deliver the remaining pups naturally.

Prolonged Gestation. The average length of estrus (or time when a bitch is receptive to mating) can range from three days to three weeks. Therefore, giving a due date for whelping based on 63 to 65 days from breeding can be erroneous for some bitches. Although whelping usually occurs 57 ± 1 days from the onset of diestrus as determined by vaginal cytology,[17] the date for the onset of the cytologic diestrus is usually not available for the bitch presented for prolonged gestation. Because breeding dates are frequently all that an owner has, a bitch should be evaluated for dystocia if 68 days have elapsed since the last mating. With this parameter some normal bitches may be included, but dogs with uterine inertia may also be identified (see "Uterine Inertia"). Because a nonpregnant diestrous bitch de-

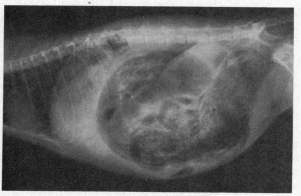

Figure 129–2. Free intrauterine gas or fetal gas is evidence of fetal death.

velops mammary gland tissue and occasionally lactates, owners may present a nonpregnant animal for prolonged gestation. Radiographic evaluation can be performed to determine whether fetuses are present (skeletons are usually visible by the 45th to 50th day of gestation), to evaluate fetuses for maturity, to measure fetal and pelvic canal size, and to detect signs of fetal death. Real-time ultrasonographic evaluation can aid in evaluating fetal motion and heart rates. Although this tool is extremely valuable, the cost limits its use for most veterinarians.

An Obvious Cause of Dystocia. An owner may say that a puppy is observed between the vulvar lips and cannot pass.

The Presence of an Abnormal Discharge at the Vulva. The presence of lochia (a greenish discharge) suggests placental separation has occurred and is a reliable sign that whelping must occur within a few hours if puppies are to survive. Rarely, a single fetus may die *in utero* several days before term and lochia is passed, with the remaining puppies being born normally at term. Because this occurrence is rare, any bitch near term that passes a greenish discharge should be critically evaluated for dystocia. A copious amount of a clear, water-like discharge suggests that the allantoic and/or amnionic fluids have passed. As with lochia, whelping should soon follow the appearance of allantoic or amnionic fluids. A bloody discharge can be observed near term in bitches experiencing a traumatic birth or suffering from uterine torsion. Severe hemorrhage can also be observed at whelping in animals that have inadequate or faulty clotting factors. Hemorrhagic discharges observed earlier in gestation are frequently associated with abortion.

TYPES OF DYSTOCIA AND BREED INCIDENCE

Several excellent reviews on canine dystocia have been published.[2, 3, 13] Both maternal and fetal factors can contribute to an abnormal parturition. Some of the factors have been categorized by Bennett (Fig. 129–3).[2] Maternal factors most frequently resulting in dystocia include decreased pelvic canal size (from immaturity, fractures, breed predisposition); abnormalities of the vagina (persistent hymen, vaginal bands, vestibulovaginal strictures, vaginal hypoplasia, tumors); abnormalities of the vestibule (vestibular strictures); and uterine malfunction (uterine inertia, uterine rupture, uterine torsion). The most common fetal factors leading to dystocia are absolute oversize of a fetus (single puppy or puppy of a breed predisposed to large head or shoulder widths); developmental defects (fetal monsters, ascites, anasarca, hydrocephalus or hydropic conditions, hypothalamic-pituitary-adrenal axis abnormalities); and faulty presentations, positions, or postures at birth. The brachycephalic breeds frequently have obstructive dystocias owing to large fetal head sizes in relation to small maternal pelvic diameters. Bulldogs, in addition, may experience inadequate contraction of the abdominal muscles, making it difficult to introduce the fetus into the pelvic canal. Dachshunds and Scottish terriers appear to have a higher incidence of primary uterine inertia, whereas St. Bernard bitches frequently develop secondary uterine inertia as a sequela to large litter size. Greyhounds have a relatively high incidence of arrested fetal development and fetal death resulting in dystocia.[2, 3, 13]

UTERINE INERTIA

Uterine inertia has been classified as primary (defect in uterine contractions not due to some other inciting cause) or secondary (due to an inciting cause). Secondary uterine inertia can occur from fatigue following an obstructive dystocia or overstretching of the myometrium due to a large litter or oversized puppy. In primary uterine inertia, the fetuses are of normal size but initiation of parturition does not occur (complete primary uterine inertia) or parturition begins normally but uterine contractions soon fail with insufficient activity to expel the remaining puppies (incomplete primary uterine inertia). This is in contrast to secondary uterine inertia, in which the uterine muscles become exhausted after prolonged contraction against an obstructed fetus or fail to contract owing to overstretching. In both types of inertia, the uterine musculature fails to respond to administration of oxytocin and the bitch fails to strain when pressure is applied *per vagina* to the pelvic canal (i.e., lack of Ferguson's reflex). Lochia is frequently observed in the vagina of bitches with complete uterine inertia, suggesting that parturition should be occurring but cannot. Normal bitches not yet ready to whelp likewise have no Ferguson's reflex when pressure is manually applied to the pelvic canal. These bitches do not have lochia present in the vagina and lack other signs of dystocia (decreased fetal heart rate, viability, or motion).

NONSURGICAL TREATMENT OF DYSTOCIA

Whether to use nonsurgical or surgical treatment to alleviate dystocia depends on several factors. If a single fetus remains, medical therapy might be considered prior to cesarean section. However, if several puppies are still to be delivered in an already fatigued bitch, surgical intervention may be more appropriate. Surgery may also be indicated when the entire litter consists of a single fetus. Because single fetuses are generally large, obstructive dystocia is more likely to occur with medical management. If a bitch is toxic, surgical intervention is beneficial to remove necrotic debris as well as the diseased uterus. On the other hand, a toxic bitch is a greater anesthetic risk, and certain precautions must be employed (see Chapter 193).

Medical therapy is frequently successful in alle-

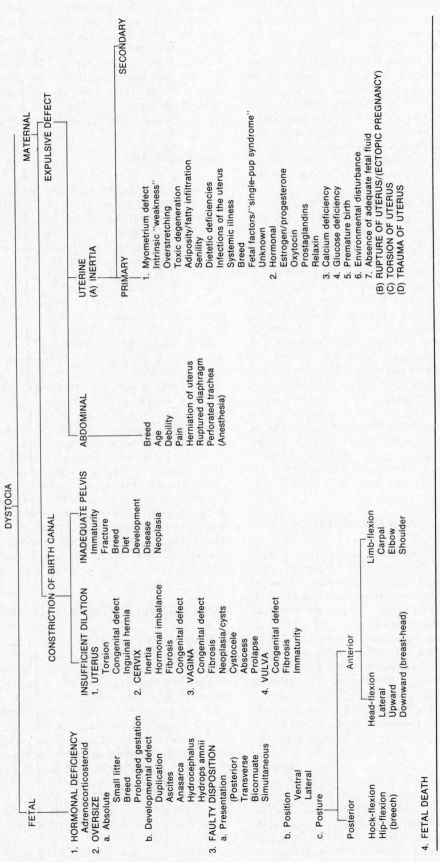

Figure 129–3. Causes of canine dystocia. (Reprinted with permission from Bennett, D.: Normal and abnormal parturition. *In* Morrow, D. A. (ed.): *Current Therapy in Theriogenology.* W. B. Saunders Co., Philadelphia, 1980.)

viating dystocias and can be used initially. If it is unsuccessful, surgery should be considered before the bitch and veterinarian are fatigued.

Ecbolics can be administered to bitches with *non-obstructive* dystocias. Ecbolics act by enhancing uterine contractions and are therefore contraindicated in dogs with obstructive dystocias. The most commonly used ecbolic is oxytocin, which has a short duration of action. It can be given intramuscularly at a dose of 5 to 20 units every 30 minutes or added to a balanced electrolyte solution so that a constant intravenous infusion delivers 5 to 20 units every 30 minutes. Oxytocin enhances placental separation. Therefore, if the bitch fails to respond to therapy during the first hour, or delivers only a single puppy every two or three hours, surgical intervention should be considered. Ergot drugs are also ecbolics but have a much longer duration of action than oxytocin. They are more likely to cause uterine rupture and will also interfere with lactation by inhibiting prolactin release from the pituitary gland.

Calcium solutions are frequently given to bitches with dystocias, because calcium is required for myometrial contractions. However, since most bitches presented for dystocia have normal concentrations of calcium in the serum, it is probably safer to use a balanced electrolyte solution that contains calcium unless the bitch is showing clinical signs of hypocalcemia (prepartum eclampsia).

Glucose solutions can be given to hypoglycemic dogs presented for dystocia. Although hypoglycemia is not common in bitches presented with dystocia, it has been reported, along with ketonuria, in three pregnant bitches with clinical signs indistinguishable from signs observed with hypocalcemia (nervousness, panting, pyrexia, trembling, tetany, seizures, or coma).[18]

Although some authors have suggested tranquilizing apprehensive bitches to promote a normal delivery, many sedatives cross the placenta and affect the fetus. Barbiturates and promazine derivatives both traverse the placenta and result in fetal depression. In addition, the immature fetal liver cannot readily metabolize these drugs.

OBSTETRICAL MANAGEMENT OF DYSTOCIA: VAGINAL DELIVERY BY DIGITAL AND FORCEPS MANIPULATION

Delivery *per vaginum* by digital or forceps manipulation can be attempted for a fetus lodged within the birth canal. The indications for assisted delivery per vagina are: (1) to correct abnormal fetal positions (breast-head, lateral head deviation, etc.); (2) to relieve obstruction due to slight fetal oversize, in order to allow normal progression of parturition (assuming secondary uterine inertia is not apparent); and (3) to extract the last remaining fetus in cases of secondary uterine inertia or to relieve obstruction by extracting a dead fetus.

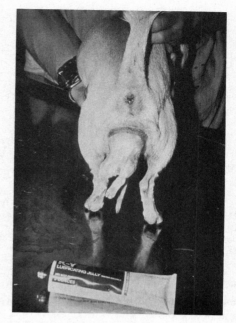

Figure 129–4. Bitch in dystocia with a puppy lodged in the birth canal. Use of a lubricant during fetal extraction minimizes trauma to both the bitch and puppy.

Manipulation of a fetus within the vagina should be done carefully to avoid trauma to either the fetus or the vaginal wall. Vaginal infection and injury can be avoided if an aseptic technique is maintained and if sufficient lubrication (K-Y Jelly)* is used during fetal extraction (Fig. 129–4). With the bitch in a standing position, simple digital manipulation should

*K-Y Jelly, Johnson & Johnson, New Brunswick, NJ 08903.

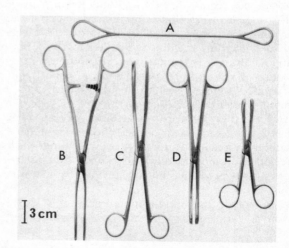

Figure 129–5. Obstetrical instruments for assisted vaginal delivery of puppies. *A*, Vestis; *B*, Rampley-type forceps; *C* and *D*, Hobday-type forceps (dog); *E*, Hobday-type forceps (cat). (Reprinted with permission from Bennett, D.: Normal and abnormal parturition. *In* Morrow, D. A. (ed.): *Current Therapy in Theriogenology.* W. B. Saunders, Philadelphia, 1980.)

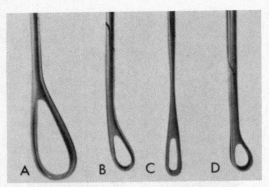

Figure 129–6. Obstetrical forceps as in Figure 129–5, showing different types of jaws. *A* and *B*, Hobday-type (dog): *C*, Rampley-type; *D*, Hobday-type (cat). (Reprinted with permission from Bennett, D.: Normal and abnormal parturition. *In* Morrow, D. A. (ed.): *Current Therapy in Theriogenology.* W. B. Saunders, Philadelphia, 1980.)

be attempted prior to manipulation with obstetrical instruments. Correction of abnormal fetal disposition is often necessary to allow fetal extraction. If the obstructed fetus is beyond digital reach, vaginal delivery of the fetus is discouraged.

Several types of instruments are used for fetal extraction. Among these are Rampley's sponge-holding forceps and Hobday's forceps (Figs. 129–5 and 129–6). The former has the advantage of maintaining a secure grasp of the fetus without significantly adding to the effective width of the fetus.[2] For a fetus in an anterior presentation, the grip is taken on the upper or lower jaw or the muzzle. Gentle traction on the fetal mandible can also be applied with an obstetrical hook (spay hook) placed in the intermandibular space.[5] Hobday's forceps are used to grasp the sides of the skull. When a fetus has already entered the vaginal vault, an obstetrical vestis is sometimes used for assistance (see Fig. 129–5). It is often helpful to elevate and secure the fetus by abdominal palpation with one hand, as digital or forceps manipulations are done *per vaginum.* After the fetus has cleared the pelvic brim, traction is applied to the fetus in caudoventral direction during periods of uterine contraction. Extreme care must be taken when traction is applied to the fetus to avoid disarticulation or amputation of tails or limbs.

A fetus in a posterior presentation can be manipulated using forceps to engage the hocks or pelvis. Slight rotational movement as well as caudoventral tension is applied to the fetus, taking care to avoid entrapment of vaginal mucosa in the obstetrical forceps.

In some cases, fetal membranes can also be removed *per vaginum.* A pair of obstetrical forceps padded with gauze is inserted into the uterus and then twisted to "wind up" the membranes prior to withdrawal.[2]

1. Austad, R., Lunde, A., and Sjaestad, O. V.: Peripheral plasma levels of estradiol 17B and progesterone in the bitch during the estrous cycle, in normal pregnancy, and after dexamethasone treatment. J. Reprod. Fertil. *46*:129, 1976.
2. Bennett, D.: Normal and abnormal parturition. *In* Morrow, D. A. (ed.): *Current Therapy in Theriogenology.* W. B. Saunders Co., Philadelphia, 1980.
3. Bennett, D.: Canine dystocia—a review of the literature. J. Small Anim. Pract. *15*:101, 1974.
4. Blevins, M.: Personal communication, 1982.
5. Collins, D. R.: A simple obstetrical technique for assisting with fetal delivery. Vet. Med. Small Anim. Clin. May:455, 1966.
6. Concannon, P. W., Powers, M. E., Holder, W., and Hansel, W.: Pregnancy and parturition in the bitch. Biol. Reprod. *16*:517, 1977.
7. Concannon, P. W., Butler, W. R., Hansel, W., et al.: Parturition and lactation in the bitch: serum progesterone, cortisol and prolactin. Biol. Reprod. *19*:1113, 1978.
8. Concannon, P. W., Hansel, W., and Visek, W. J.: The ovarian cycle of the bitch: plasma estrogen, LH and progesterone. Biol. Reprod. *13*:112, 1975.
9. Concannon, P. W., and Hansel, W.: Prostaglandin $F_{2\,alpha}$-induced luteolysis, hypothermia, and abortions in beagle bitches. Prostaglandins *13*:533, 1977.
10. Edquist, L. E., Johansson, E. D. B., Kastrom, H., et al.: Blood plasma levels of progesterone and estradiol in the dog during the estrous cycle and pregnancy. Acta Endocrinol. *78*:554, 1975.
11. Farrow, C. W., Morgan, J. P., and Story, E. C.: Late term fetal death in the dog: early radiographic diagnosis. J. Am. Vet. Radiol. *17*:11, 1976.
12. Fitzpatrick, R. J.: Pregnancy and parturition. *In* Morrow, D. A. (ed.): *Current Therapy in Theriogenology.* W. B. Saunders Co., Philadelphia, 1980.
13. Freak, M. J.: Practitioners'-breeders' approach to canine parturition. Vet. Rec. 96-303, 1975.
14. Gentry, P. A., and Fiptrap, R. M.: Plasma levels of specific coagulation factors and estrogens in the bitch during pregnancy. J. Small Anim. Pract. *18*:267, 1977.
15. Gerber, J. G., Hubbard, W. C., and Nies, A. S.: Uterine vein prostaglandin levels in late pregnant dogs. Prostaglandins *17*:623, 1979.
16. Graft, K. J., and El Etreby, M. F.: Endocrinology of reproduction in the female beagle dog and its significance in mammary gland tumorigenesis. Acta Endocrinology. *90*:1, 1979.
17. Holst, P. A., and Phemister, R. D.: Onset of diestrus in the beagle bitch: definition and significance. Am. J. Vet. Res. *35*:401, 1974.
18. Irvine, C. H. G.: Hypoglycemia in the bitch. N. Z. Vet. J. *12*:140, 1964.
19. Tietz, W. J., Benjamin, M. M., and Angleton, G. M.: Anemia and cholesterolemia during estrus and pregnancy in the beagle. Am. J. Physiol. *212*:693, 1967.
20. Winters, A. J.: Plasma ACTH levels in the human fetus and neonate as related to age and parturition. J. Clin. Endocrinol. Metab. *39*:269, 1974.
21. Zander, J.: Gestogens in human pregnancy. *In* Lloyd, C. W. (ed.): *Recent Progress in Endocrinology and Reproduction.* Academic Press, New York, 1959.

Chapter 130

Surgical Management of Dystocia

Peggy M. Wykes and Patricia N. Olson

EPISIOTOMY

Episiotomy is a procedure rarely necessary for the relief of canine dystocia. The primary indications are to relieve vestibular or vestibulovulvar strictures and to remove hymen remnants that impede the passage of a fetus.

CESAREAN SECTION (HYSTEROTOMY)

Indications

Delivery of puppies by hysterotomy is indicated when dystocia cannot be satisfactorily relieved with medical management or manipulation of a fetus by vagina. The operation is relatively safe for both the bitch and puppies when performed at the appropriate time. Ideally, surgery should be done when the dog is in relatively good health and should not be used as a treatment of last resort. When fetal death, uterine torsion, or uterine rupture occurs, the bitch can rapidly become toxic. In these conditions, following shock therapy, emergency surgery may be required to save the animal's life.

The following are guidelines for the use of cesarean section:[1, 2]

1. For prolonged gestation; normal parturition is not likely to occur after 70 days gestation.
2. For complete primary uterine inertia.
3. For incomplete primary uterine inertia, especially if several puppies remain and ecbolic agents have failed.
4. For secondary uterine inertia when several fetuses remain.
5. When abnormalities of the maternal pelvis or soft tissues exist that may impede the passage of a fetus (pelvic fractures, vaginal tumors, or imperforate hymen).
6. For relative and absolute fetal oversize.
7. For fetal monstrosities.
8. For fetal malpositioning (transverse, head-flexion, and so on) that cannot be corrected to allow delivery through the vagina.
9. For fetal death with putrefaction.

Surgical Procedure

Two surgical approaches are used for cesarean section: the ventral midline abdominal approach and the flank approach. Only the abdominal approach is described here in detail. Both procedures have advantages and disadvantages. The ventral abdominal procedure provides better exposure of the uterus, generally requires less hemostasis, results in less scarring, and is more familiar to most surgeons than the flank approach. However, the flank approach is preferred by some because it does not interfere with lactation and because it reduces the chance of wound dehiscence.

Dehydrated or toxic bitches suffering from dystocia should be stabilized with fluids, corticosteroids, and antibiotics prior to anesthesia (see anesthesia for cesarean section). The surgical patient is routinely shaved and prepared for surgery.

For the ventral abdominal approach, the animal is placed in dorsal recumbency and tilted 10 to 20° to the right. This positioning shifts the weight of the uterus away from the caudal vena cava in an effort to prevent the weight of the uterus from significantly compromising venous return to the heart and decreasing subsequent cardiac output (supine hypotensive syndrome).[3] After preparing the surgical site for aseptic surgery, the surgical field is draped and a ventral midline abdominal incision of sufficient length is made to expose the uterus. Care must be taken to avoid injury to underlying viscera as the abdomen is opened. The uterus is extracted, and moistened laparotomy sponges are used to pack the uterus from surrounding viscera to prevent contamination of the peritoneum by fetal fluids. A longitudinal incision is made on the dorsal midline of the uterine body long enough to allow removal of the fetuses (Fig. 130–1). Gentle squeezing of the uterine horn advances each individual fetus into the uterine body for extraction. The amnionic sac is opened prior to separation of the placenta from the uterus. The puppies, with attached placentas, are immediately handed to an assistant, who removes the oral and nasal secretions and towel dries the infants. The fetus often can obtain several more milliliters of blood if the placental attachment to the puppy remains intact for several minutes after uterine separation. Whether this improves fetal viability is still unknown. The umbilical cord is clamped with hemostats and cut approximately 2 cm from the fetal abdomen. The hemostats can be removed after several minutes and the umbilical stump examined for hemorrhage.

Vigorous rubbing of the puppy usually stimulates respiration. However, if the puppy fails to breathe gentle thoracic massage and artificial respiration

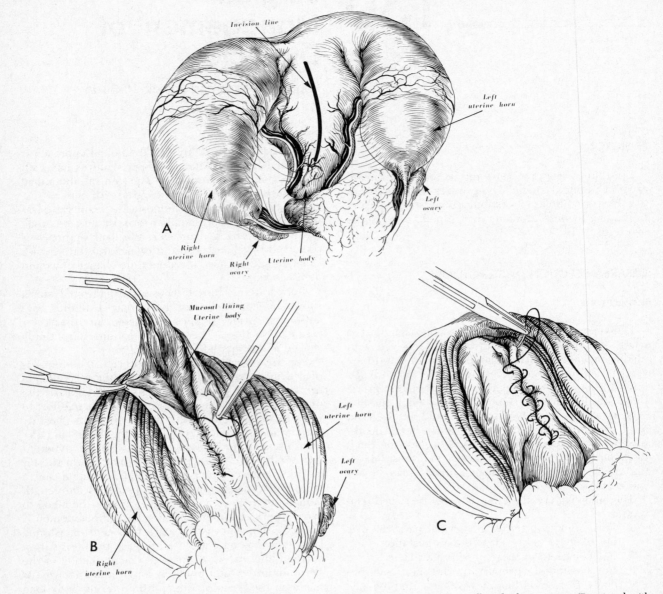

Figure 130–1. A long enough longitudinal incision is made in the dorsal body of the uterus to allow fetal extraction. (Reprinted with permission from Chambers, J. N.: Cesarean section. *In* Wingfield, W. E., and Rawlings, C. A.: *Small Animal Surgery.* W. B. Saunders, Philadelphia, 1979.)

should be attempted. Respiratory stimulants (dopamine,* one to two drops orally) also help initiate breathing. Oxygen supplementation should be administered to puppies with depressed respiration (e.g., cyanosis). One to two drops of naloxone† injected into the fetal umbilical vein or placed on the tongue will reverse the effect of narcotics used for anesthetic induction of the bitch. Some infants may take up to an hour of resuscitation before spontaneous breathing occurs. An environmental temperature (32.5°C, or 90°F) should be provided to ensure that the core temperature of the neonate is maintained after delivery.

To ensure that all fetuses are removed, the vaginal canal should be inspected, and the entire length of both uterine horns should be palpated prior to closure of the uterine incision.

Uterine involution normally begins rapidly after removal of the fetuses, especially if oxytocin is injected into the uterine wall or dripped onto the uterine surface. Complete uterine involution may take up to three months. Removal of all fetal membranes prior to uterine closure is desirable, although it is better to leave the placentas to minimize severe postoperative uterine hemorrhage if placental separation is difficult.

The uterine incision is closed with one or two layers of a continuous absorbable suture. An inverting Lembert or Cushing pattern is commonly used to

---

*Dopram, A. H. Robins Co., Richmond, VA.
†Narcon, Endo Laboratories, Inc.. Manatz, PR.

ensure an adequate seal (see Fig. 130–1). Pulling the strand tight after each suture and burying the knots tends to minimize postoperative peritoneal adhesions.

Prior to returning the uterus to the peritoneal cavity, the uterine surface should be cleaned with warm saline. Bacterial culture and sensitivity testing of peritoneal fluid resulting from uterine spillage assists selection of appropriate antibacterial drugs if peritonitis is potential. The laparotomy incision is routinely closed with simple interrupted sutures in the ventral rectus sheath, followed by placement of subcutaneous and skin sutures.

The number of cesarean sections that can be performed on the same patient is variable. Peritoneal adhesions often prevent adequate exposure of the uterus after the third cesarean section.

In cases of dystocia where the uterus is devitalized (uterine torsion or rupture) or distended with dead, emphysematous puppies, hysterectomy may be necessary to save the life of the bitch. The uterus often appears discolored (reddish-green or dark purple) and lacks normal muscle tone. An ovariohysterectomy can also be performed as an elective procedure to terminate a pregnancy or following fetal extraction to prevent further conception. For either emergency (toxic dystocia) or elective (postcesarean section) ovariohysterectomies, supportive intravenous fluid therapy is extremely important to counteract hypovolemia and shock. The surgical procedure for ovariohysterectomy of a gravid uterus is basically the same as that for a routine spay. If a cesarean section precedes an ovariohysterectomy, the uterine body incision should be closed prior to removal of the uterus to avoid spillage of uterine fluid.

Ovariohysterectomy should not interfere with the bitch's ability to mother puppies or produce milk, since ovarian hormones are necessary only for ductal and glandular development of mammary tissue, whereas prolactin and cortisol are more important in maintaining lactation.

Complications

Peritoneal infection, excessive hemorrhage, or wound dehiscence can occur as with any abdominal surgery. Peritoneal adhesions become more abundant with each cesarean section and make further abdominal surgery difficult. Incisions into the uterine horns, rather than the uterine body, can result in a uterine scar that may prevent future placentation or cause abnormal fetal development.[2]

PREVENTION

A thorough examination of the bitch for congenital abnormalities or pelvic deformities prior to mating may prevent potential breeding or parturition difficulties. A subsequent examination of the bitch is important to determine whether pregnancy has occurred and is progressing normally. The owner should be informed about proper nutrition and management of the bitch throughout the gestation and lactation periods.

1. Bennett, D.: Canine dystocia—a review of the literature. J. Small Anim. Pract. 15:101, 1974.
2. Bennett, D.: Normal and abnormal parturition. In Morrow, D. A. (ed.): Current Therapy in Theriogenology. W. B. Saunders, Philadelphia, 1980, p. 595.
3. Smith, K. W.: Female genital system. In Archibald, J. (ed.): Canine Surgery. American Veterinary Publications Inc., Santa Barbara, 1974, p. 751.

Chapter **131** # Fetal Surgery in the Dog

John D. Bacher

Fetal surgery has become an important means of investigating fetal growth, development, and physiology.[9, 71, 117] A number of investigators have used the fetal dog as a model for intestinal physiology,[11, 25, 70] urinary physiology,[18, 20, 65, 101] cardiovascular physiology,[35, 71, 72, 75, 76, 80, 134, 135] intestinal atresia,[10, 11, 86] biliary atresia,[67] hemolytic disease,[71, 74] immunological development,[36, 39, 43] and metabolic activity of the uterine-placental-fetal preparation.[16]

Recent advances in surgical technology permit virtually any operative procedure on a fetus during its intrauterine existence that can be performed postnatally.[13, 82, 105, 119] Such advances include techniques for minimizing loss of amniotic fluid by marsupialization of the fetus to the uterine wall,[73] partial[22, 99] or total extraction[82] of the fetus from the uterine cavity, and multiple uterotomies.[98, 108] Because of the umbilical attachment to the anesthetized mother, the fetus does not need to be anesthetized, nor does artificial respiration need to be provided during thoracotomies. The main problems encountered in intrauterine fetal surgery are related to the size of young fetuses and the extreme delicacy of their tissues and membranes.

The human fetus and its environment are also becoming more accessible to those concerned in ascertaining its well-being. Traditionally, guides to the status of the fetus have been auscultation of its heart rate and later the electrocardiogram. It is now possible to detect stress by the presence of meconium seen in the amniotic fluid with the aid of the amnioscope and to sample the scalp capillary blood and determine its acid-base parameters and the concentration of electrolytes and glucose. Samples of amniotic fluid can be removed by amniocentesis and examined; a high bilirubin concentration is associated with hemolytic disease whereas a low concentration of lecithin indicates the probability of breathing difficulties of the respiratory distress syndrome type at birth[48] and elevated levels of α-fetoprotein indicate an open neural tube defect.[66] Studies on cells in the amniotic fluid may reveal not only the sex of the fetus but also chromosomal abnormalities. Radiopaque contrast medium in the amniotic sac is used to delineate structures bathed by the amniotic fluid. By radiography, this technique has been used to visualize the alimentary tract and detect soft tissue abnormalities.[92–94] Timing of the passage of dye along the gastrointestinal tract is used to evaluate the chronic fetal distress syndrome.[8]

Human fetal therapy began in 1963 with the first intrauterine blood transfusion by Liley into the peritoneal cavity of a fetus with hemolytic disease.[85] Since that time a variety of medications have been administered to pregnant women because of the transplacental effects: glucocorticoids have been given to accelerate lung maturation;[84] digoxin, to treat congestive heart failure;[55] vitamin B_{12}, for fetal methylmalonic acidemia;[6] biotin, for biotin-dependent multiple carboxylase deficiency;[60] thyroxine, to accelerate pulmonary maturation[88] and to treat fetal goiter;[130] and amino acids, to reverse intrauterine growth retardation.[113]

Improved ultrasonographic assessment of the fetus early in gestation has resulted in the diagnosis of a number of fetal anomalies that may be amenable to surgical therapy *in utero*.[27, 62] If these abnormalities are diagnosed and treated early in gestation, fetal growth and development may then continue until term. Specific examples of such fetal conditions include urinary tract obstruction caused by posterior urethral valves[17, 49, 59, 61, 77] and specific cases of hydrocephalus associated with aqueductal stenosis (Fig. 131–1).[21, 29, 44, 100] In these cases, overcoming the mechanical obstruction may allow normal or nearly normal development to proceed *in utero*.

Another fetal malformation that may require correction before birth is congenital diaphragmatic hernia. Although this defect is easily correctable after birth, 50 to 90 per cent of these infants die of pulmonary insufficiency in the first three hours of life because the lung compressed by the herniated viscera is hypoplastic.[54, 58] To allow the lung to grow and develop enough to support life at birth, pulmonary compression must be relieved before birth.[57, 63] A technique for successful surgical correction *in utero* has been developed experimentally.[64]

The advantages of intrauterine repair of fetal defects include:

1. Early intervention before irreversible damage has occurred is the paramount benefit.

2. The fetal immune surveillance system is not yet intact, thus facilitating transplantation of organs and bone grafts.

3. Rapid healing is fostered by fetal growth factors.

4. The umbilicus services both respiratory and nutritional needs without extracorporeal support.

5. In some cases, infections are combated by transplacental passage of immune factors.

6. The postoperative period is technically simplified with a fetal patient.

7. Medicinal agents administered directly to the fetus have greater efficacy at reduced doses than do comparable treatments routed through the mother,

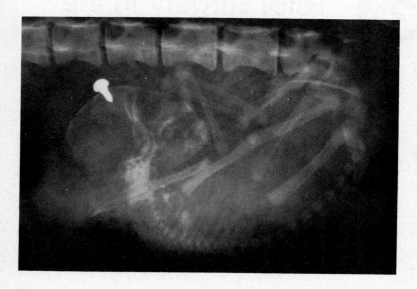

Figure 131–1. Radiograph of fetal monkey *in utero* following placement of antenatal shunt in lateral ventricle for treatment of hydrocephalus.

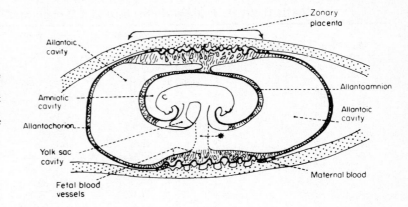

Figure 131–2. Illustration of fetal membranes in the bitch. (Reprinted with permission from Eckstein, P., and Kelly, W. A.: Implantation and development of the conceptus. *In* Cole, H. H., and Cupps, P. T. (eds.): Reproduction in Domestic Animals. Academic Press, New York, 1977.)

in which metabolism of the medication might make fetal therapy complicated.[66]

FETAL DEVELOPMENT

The time during which fetal surgery is possible depends on the organ development and size of the fetus. Accurate conception dates provide fetuses of relatively the same size and weight for comparison and surgery. Ovulation in the bitch is spontaneous and is thought to occur within 24 hours after the day of first acceptance. All ovulatory follicles rupture at almost the same time, and fertilization occurs in the oviduct.[124] The ovum enters the uterus as morulae of 16 cells or more, 8 to 12 days after mating, and they become blastocysts shortly thereafter. Free-floating blastocysts exist in the uterine horn for about seven days. At some time during this stage, probably when the conceptus measures about 1200 μm in diameter, they migrate from one uterine horn to the other and become established in approximately equal numbers in each horn regardless of the number of corpora lutea in each ovary.[68] Implantation occurs over a period of time, with edema of the endometrium being the first indication that the blastocyst has taken up a definite position along the horn. The grouping of villi around the equator of the chorioallantoic sac, beginning about days 17 to 21, forms the zonary placenta of the dog. By day 23 after insemination there is a structural attachment of the endometrium and trophoblast, and implantation is complete. From this time on, removal of consecutive embryos does not result in either repositioning of embryos or abortion of the remaining embryos.[87, 124] The stages of placentation have been illustrated by Andersen and Goldman.[7]

Implantation in the uterine wall is followed by progressive elaboration of the extraembryonic membranes that protect and nourish the embryo. As these membranes expand, they fold to form three cavities: the amniotic, the allantoic, and the yolk sac. The formation of extraembryonic membranes in the dog is illustrated in Figure 131–2. The first amniotic fold appears on day 19 or 20, and the amniotic cavity is completed on day 21.[47] The amniotic cavity provides the embryo with a free space that is cushioned with liquid. Early in development the yolk sac type of placenta is functional in the dog; however, it regresses in size while the allantoic membrane combines with the chorion to form the placenta through which nutrients, gases, and metabolic wastes are exchanged.[40]

Fetal development progresses to a grossly visible stage by about day 20, when embryos of 4 to 7 mm in length from crown to rump (C-R) can be recovered.

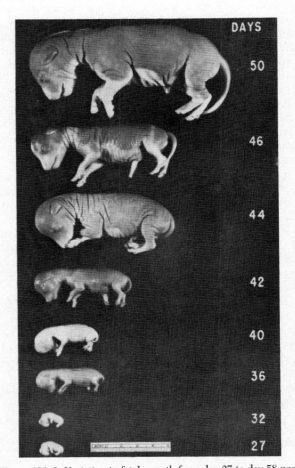

Figure 131–3. Variation in fetal growth from day 27 to day 58 post conception. (Reprinted with permission from Andersen, A. C., and Goldman, M.: Growth and development. *In* Andersen, A. C. (eds.): *The Beagle as an Experimental Dog.* Iowa State University Press, Ames, 1970.)

TABLE 131–1. Embryo-Fetus Size and Weight at Different Stages of Gestation*

| Day Post-breeding | Number | Crown-Rump Length (mm) | | Weight (gm) | |
		Average	Range	Average	Range
20	1	7.0	—	—	—
26	1	8.0	—	0.074	—
28	2	12.0	(11–13)	0.244	(0.191–0.258)
30	2	15.5	(15–16)	0.426	(0.420–0.432)
32	1	19.0	—	0.794	—
33	9	32.2	(29–38)	3.50	(2.5–4.5)
35	5	42.2	(36–45)	6.10	(5.5–7.0)
36	1	33.0	—	3.3	—
37	1	46.0	—	7.0	—
38	8	54.5	(50–58)	10.6	(9–13)
40	13	71.6	(63.0–78.1)	23.9	(20.0–28.0)
52	5	114.0	(110.0–119.0)	114.0	(100.0–138.0)
54	5	138.0	(131.0–143.0)	202.4	(176.0–222.0)
57	11	132.1	(120.0–150.0)	218.0	(190.0–260.0)
Term		160.3	(147.0–170.0)	273.6	(207.0–327.0)

*Bitches of similar prebreeding size. (Reprinted with permission from Sokolowski, J. H.: Normal events of gestation in the bitch and methods of pregnancy diagnosis. *In* Morrow, D. A. (ed.): *Current Therapy in Theriogenology.* W. B. Saunders, Philadelphia, 1980.)

The morphology of canine fetuses from days 27 to 50 is shown in Figure 131–3. Extreme variations can occur in embryo size (both C-R measurement and weight) within and between litters at a given time after breeding (Table 131–1). Competition for food with others in the litter appears to be one of the most important factors, and an increase in litter size is associated with a decrease in fetal and birth weights. Fetuses of larger bitches are generally larger at a given stage of development. In the beagle bitch, increases in fetal C-R length are linear from midgestation to about day 58 and progress at a rate of about 6 mm per day.[124]

Organogenesis advances rapidly in the embryo, so that by days 20 to 23 after breeding the aorta and mesonephric tubule are present. By days 26 to 28 the major organs, including the undifferentiated gonad, can be observed. Microscopic identification of gonadal differentiation can be accomplished about days 30 to 34, whereas sex determination by appearance of the external genitalia is not possible until after 35 days gestation.[124]

Estimation of the period of gestation is possible through serial radiographs. The fetal skeleton, however, is not visible until day 45 of gestation.[126] The 50-day fetus shows calcification of the proximal tail vertebrae. At about 55 days, six to eight tail vertebrae are visible. After that, little change is discernible.[67] The size of the fetal head is also a good guide: the larger the head, the nearer to term.

PLACENTAL PHYSIOLOGY

A basic characteristic of mammalian development is the formation of the placenta, across which nutrients for growth and waste products of metabolism are exchanged.

Hemodynamics

The uteroplacental circulation is a low-resistance system for the maternal organism. It is responsible for, or at least contributes to, marked changes in maternal cardiovascular physiology. Uterine arterial blood flow in the nonpregnant state represents about 1 per cent of maternal cardiac output. During pregnancy it rises markedly until uterine blood flow at term requires 17 per cent of the maternal cardiac output to handle the increased load imposed by the fetus and placenta.[38] Renal plasma flow and glomerular filtration rate similarly are elevated in pregnancy for the increased load imposed by the fetus and placenta.

The placenta receives approximately 50 per cent of the fetal cardiac output.[119] This high flow rate is important in the transport of oxygen and nutrients between mother and fetus and is maintained by a number of autonomic and physiological differences in the fetal circulation. Since the fetal lungs are practically useless as respiratory organs, a high vascular resistance is maintained in these organs by the mechanical effects of the unexpanded alveoli on the vessel walls and the vasoconstrictive effect of the low oxygen tension in the fetal blood. These two factors combine to shunt approximately two-thirds of the right ventricular output away from the lungs. The shunted blood is diverted toward the systemic circulation through the ductus arteriosus, which is maintained patent by the same low oxygen tension that keeps the pulmonary vessels constricted. With the large right-to-left shunt through the ductus arteriosus, a high cardiac output (almost twice that of the mother) is created; this compensates for the low oxygen tension of the fetal blood and provides a high blood flow across the placental membranes.[111]

Some blood flow is necessary on each side of the

intervillous space for myometrial and placental metabolism. It also is likely that some fetal and maternal blood never reaches any exchange area but is in effect shunted. For these reasons there is frequently a gradient in transfer, so that fetal blood levels of a given substance are either higher or lower than maternal blood levels, depending on whether it is an excretory or input product. In the case of gases such as oxygen and carbon dioxide, fetal levels remain quite different from maternal levels.

Most biological systems have considerable reserve capacity for times of stress. It is reasonable to assume that this is also true of the placenta. Radiographic studies indicate that not all spiral arterioles function simultaneously and that function may be influenced by myometrial contractions and tone. During uterine contractions, venous outflow is markedly reduced, and, because of the increase in outflow pressure, there is temporary stasis or slowing of intervillous flow and arterial input.[112] Fetal flow apparently is unaffected by myometrial contractions.

Transfer

Throughout pregnancy the placenta retains the primary role of selective permeability of materials. With particulate matter, such as blood cells, transfer is severely restricted, a function described as the "placental barrier." At the other end of the spectrum, the transfer of many essential nutrients is accelerated by a variety of transport mechanisms. As an organ for gas exchange, the placenta is far less efficient than the lung. The diffusion rate for gases per unit weight of placenta is approximately one-fiftieth that of the lung. Consequently, fetal and maternal levels of oxygen and carbon dioxide are different (Table 131–2). Gases cross the placenta by simple diffusion, the driving force being the concentration difference on both sides of the membrane. The fetus compensates for low oxygen levels by increasing its flow rates, increasing its binding power and the number of binding sites for oxygen, and shunting within the fetal body. The difference between carbon dioxide

tensions in the two circulations is less than the difference between their oxygen tensions, but it is sufficiently large to favor diffusion of carbon dioxide from the fetal to the maternal circulation since the diffusion constant of carbon dioxide is greater than that of oxygen. However, the blood of the fetus contains an increased amount of carbon dioxide when carbon dioxide tension of the mother's blood is increased.[37, 125]

Glucose is the principal source of energy for the fetus, crossing the placenta by facilitated transport. The level in the fetal blood varies with the maternal level but is always lower. There is normally a considerable excess of glucose over the supply of oxygen for its metabolism. The fetus is able to store glycogen, particularly in the liver, in higher concentration than is found in the adult.[129]

Amino acids are delivered to the fetus for protein synthesis and apparently contribute to requirements for fetal energy. They are transferred by active transport, which requires the expenditure of energy, and transport can occur against the concentration gradient. Fetal levels of most amino acids are consistently higher than are maternal levels. The natural L-amino acids are transferred more rapidly than are the D form, indicating stereospecificity. Many individual differences exist among the amino acids, suggesting different transport systems.[37]

Sodium, potassium, and chloride probably cross by simple diffusion. Calcium, iron, and phosphorus are present in higher levels in fetal than in maternal blood, suggesting active transport. Unbound iodine crosses very rapidly and is taken up in the fetal thyroid more readily than in the maternal thyroid.

The water-soluble vitamins are found in high concentrations in fetal blood, whereas fat-soluble ones are in low concentration. Phospholipids and cholesterol do not cross intact, but the placenta is readily permeable to acetate and many free fatty acids.[129]

MATERNAL PHYSIOLOGICAL CHANGES DURING PREGNANCY

Pregnancy produces physiological alterations that change the patient's responses to anesthesia. Of the many physiological alterations produced, ventilatory, cardiovascular, and gastrointestinal changes are the most important.

Ventilation Physiology

The maternal rate (including the fetal rate) of oxygen consumption rises progressively during pregnancy, reaching a peak of 20 per cent above nonpregnant levels. Some of the increment is attributed to the increased work and metabolic needs of the mother (cardiac and respiratory muscles), but the major portion of the increase is probably due to the metabolic needs of the fetus.[46] Because of elevation

TABLE 131–2. P_{CO_2} Gradient Between Mother and Fetus

Parameter (Carotid Arterial)	Maternal (Range)	Fetal (Range)
P_{O_2} (mmHg)	105 ± 1.2 (94–112)	29.7 ± 0.8 (23–35)
P_{CO_2} (mmHg)	32.6 ± 0.9 (22–39)	42.8 ± 1.3 (29–53)
pH	7.42 ± 0.007 (7.38–7.50)	7.37 ± 0.004 (7.34–7.42)

Means ± S.E. of 22 observations: range in brackets. (Reprinted with permission from Dawes, G. S.: P_{CO_2} gradient between mother and fetus. *In* Hodari, A. A., and Mariona, F. (eds.): *Physiological Biochemistry of the Fetus, Proceedings of the International Symposium.* Charles C Thomas, Springfield, Ill., 1972.)

of the diaphragm caused by the cephalad displacement of the enlarging uterus during pregnancy, the functional residual capacity and residual volume of air in the lungs are decreased by 15 to 20 per cent at term.[52] Studies available from humans during pregnancy indicate that a progressive increase in minute ventilation is effected through a modest (15 per cent) increase in respiratory rate and a significant (40 per cent) increase in tidal volume. This hyperventilation is not caused through a change in the mechanics of breathing but is stimulated by the ovarian hormones as a continuation of the luteal phase of the menstrual cycle. The respiratory alkalosis produced is compensated for by renal excretion of bicarbonate.[50]

The decrease in functional residual capacity combined with the hyperventilation that occurs normally in pregnancy permits a more rapid change in alveolar concentration of anesthetic gases. Thus anesthetic depth is achieved more rapidly, and the danger of overdosage of inhalant agents is greater with pregnant than with nonpregnant patients. In addition, anesthetic requirements for inhalation agents are decreased up to 40 per cent during pregnancy.[107] The mechanism for this decrease in anesthetic agent required is uncertain, but hormonal changes during pregnancy may be responsible. For example, progesterone levels increase 10- to 20-fold during late pregnancy.[13, 137] Progesterone has a sedative activity[122] and in large doses induces loss of consciousness in humans.[96] In addition, hypocapnia and alkalosis from hyperventilation may be associated with a fall in uterine and hence placental blood flow and a change in placental permeability. Decreases in uterine and placental blood flow may result in fetal acidosis.[15]

The decrease in functional residual capacity also lowers the oxygen reserve. Apnea of even 60 seconds produces a reduction of oxygen tension significantly greater in pregnancy than in the nonpregnant state. This rapid hypoxia indicates the importance of preoxygenation before and prompt reoxygenation following endotracheal intubation.

Cardiovascular Physiology

Pregnancy is normally characterized by significant cardiovascular developments. Maternal blood volume increases approximately 40 per cent during pregnancy.[46] This rise is due to an increase in both the plasma volume and the red cell volume.[116] The latter increases at a slower rate than the former, thus accounting for the relative anemia of pregnancy.[123] Maternal blood volume increase begins early in the first trimester and continues throughout pregnancy, but the most rapid expansion occurs during the second trimester and coincides with the period of accelerated placental vascular expansion. In humans, about 750 ml of blood flows through the maternal circulation of the placenta each minute during the latter phases of gestation. This high flow rate through the placenta decreases the total peripheral resistance of the maternal circulatory system, allowing increased venous return to the heart. Consequently, stroke volume and heart rate are increased, with a resulting 40 per cent increase in cardiac output during pregnancy.[23]

The steroid hormones of pregnancy, particularly estrogen, not only affect vascular resistance but also appear to have a direct effect on myocardial muscle. Csapo has postulated that estrogens may alter the actinomyosin-adenosine triphosphatase (ATPase) relationship in the myocardium, thereby increasing myocardial contractility.[32] More recently, it has been shown that the pre-ejection period of left ventricular systole is reduced, particularly in the second trimester.[26]

Venous pressure is not significantly changed unless the patient is in the supine position. In this situation the inferior vena cava and aorta are partially or completely compressed by the enlarging uterus. Obstruction of the vena cava not only impedes venous return to the heart, causing hypotension, but also increases uterine venous pressure, which further decreases uterine blood flow. Compression of the aorta is not associated with maternal signs but does cause arterial hypotension in the rear extremities and uterine arteries, which can further decrease uterine blood flow and cause fetal asphyxia and distress.[123]

Drugs causing vasodilation, such as halothane and thiopental sodium, or anesthetic techniques causing sympathetic block, such as epidural anesthesia, will further decrease venous return to the heart when the vena cava is obstructed. Prevention of aorta caval compression consists of left uterine displacement, either manually during surgery or by tilting the operating table 15° laterally to the left.[56, 123]

Circulatory changes within the vertebral column during pregnancy have profound effects on epidural anesthesia. Owing to increased intra-abdominal pressure, epidural veins become engorged, making inadvertent intravascular injections during lumbar epidural or caudal epidural anesthesia common. This engorgement decreases the size of the epidural space. In addition, each spinal nerve root as it passes out of its intervertebral foramen is accompanied by an epidural vein that is swollen, thus decreasing the size of the opening.[24] The decrease in size of the epidural space consequent to venous obstruction is conducive to abnormally high anesthesia following epidural injection. This complication can be avoided by small doses and careful technique.[50]

Gastrointestinal System

Pregnancy is associated with a shift in the position of the stomach due to the gravid uterus that changes the angle of the gastroesophageal junction. This makes the parturient prone to silent regurgitation and aspiration during general anesthesia. Gastric motility and emptying time are slowed, further increasing the risk of pulmonary aspiration. The hormone gastrin produced by the placenta raises the acid, chloride, and enzyme content of the stomach to levels above normal.[52]

AMNIOTIC FLUID

Function

Amniotic fluid protects the fetus from external trauma by pressure equalization. Since the intrauterine fetus is totally bathed by this medium, any sudden force applied to the reservoir is transmitted in all directions, and no localized area of the fetus receives the full impact of the blow. The watery environment provides constant lubrication between the fetus and its enveloping membranes, assuring unimpeded fetal mobility. Amniotic fluid may also play a role in the metabolic functions of the fetus. Nutritive elements may be provided through fetal swallowing of amniotic fluid. Electrolytes, carbohydrates, lipids, and protein may be derived from this supplemental source, thereby enhancing fetal metabolic growth.[106, 114] The amniotic fluid and membranes aid in dilating the cervix at parturition when, because of its slippery, mucous consistency, the fluid is an excellent lubricant for the fetus and birth canal.[115]

Origin and Fate

Many theories have been proposed to explain the formation of amniotic fluid. Few have stood the test of time, and the origin of amniotic fluid remains unclear. Amniotic fluid is present soon after the space forms by splitting of the cytotrophoblast on the dorsal surface of the embryo. At that time no vessels are supplying the chorion or amnion, and there is no fetus with functioning kidneys excreting into the amniotic sac. Therefore, some of the cells lining the amniotic cavity must have secretory function to account for the origin of the fluid. In the dog, the amnion grows to cover the entire umbilical cord and, along with the allantois, forms the allantoamnion junction (see Fig. 131–2). Fetal function also develops so that the kidney, trachea, or other sources within the fetus may be available for amniotic fluid formation.

A decrease in or absence of swallowing by the fetus is almost universally associated with hydramnios or excessive amounts of amniotic fluid. This has led to the apparently correct deduction that fetal swallowing is necessary for removal of amniotic fluid. Anomalies preventing fetal urination, such as renal agenesis, lead to oligohydramnios or decreased amounts of amniotic fluid. Fetal urine forms at least some of the amniotic fluid;[28, 114, 121] however, spontaneous discharge of urine from the dog occurs only rarely, but the ability of the urinary bladder to contract in response to stimuli increases as term approaches.[18]

The fetal trachea secretes or excretes fluid similar to amniotic fluid.[3] It also is possible that fetal alveoli are capable of resorbing water or electrolytes from the amniotic fluid. However, since fetal respiration *in utero* is spasmodic and infrequent, it is unlikely that this is a major factor in the formation or removal of amniotic fluid.[51] There is no reason to think that fetal skin serves as a diffusing membrane. Squamous epithelium does not behave this way in the adult and is not likely to do so in the fetus. The fetus is covered with vernix caseosa, which is produced by sebaceous glands and is oily. This tends to prevent any water loss through the skin.

In humans, the rate of water exchange within the amniotic cavity approaches 500 ml/hr at term.[110] Since fetal gut and kidneys cannot accommodate this rapid turnover, the major portion of it must occur across the membranes, either on the fetal surface of the placenta or, more likely, directly across amnion, allantochorion, and decidua to maternal vessels. The membranes become thin as term approaches; thus there may be less of a diffusion barrier. Diffusion studies indicate that a considerable amount of exchange takes place across both the membranes and the umbilical cord itself. Obviously, all the water, electrolytes, and other constituents within the amniotic fluid eventually must come from the mother. However, it cannot be said that amniotic fluid is an ultrafiltrate of maternal serum; the differences in composition are too great.

Amniotic fluid apparently originates from both mother and fetus. There is exchange in both directions across the fetal membranes to the cord, to the placenta, and directly to maternal vessels. Changes in any of these functions can result in dramatic changes in amniotic fluid volume.[37]

Biochemistry

In recent years, the biochemistry of amniotic fluid has been a subject of increasing interest, but much of the information gained has no clinical application, since the normal values and trends of many constituents of potential practical value have yet to be established. In addition to the cytology and the cytogenetic and biochemical testing of cultured amniotic fluid cells, electrolytes and gas tensions, proteins and amino acids, hormones and enzymes, prostaglandins and other lipids, and the products of both hemoglobin breakdown and of fibrin degradation have all been studied in the amniotic fluid itself.[45, 133]

ANESTHESIA

The ideal anesthetic agent for operative procedures on the fetus should provide adequate pain relief and skeletal as well as uterine muscular relaxation without adversely affecting the mother or fetus. Operations performed under local or spinal anesthesia may cause apprehension and excitement, which lead to impaired placental perfusion and gas exchange, most likely produced by stimulation of the sympathoadrenal system. Narcotics, hypnotics, and tranquilizing agents given in doses sufficient to cause uterine relaxation are likely to affect the cardiovascular systems of both the mother and the fetus. Pentobarbital anesthesia causes a fall in maternal Pa_{O_2} and a rise in Pa_{CO_2}. These changes are reflected in the fetus. Neuromuscular blocking agents such as curare and succinylcholine chloride have no relaxing effect on the uterus but may be used for tracheal intubation and to relax the abdominal muscles.[102]

Induction with intravenous thiopental sodium has been recommended.[33] This anesthetic crosses the placenta almost immediately and reaches peak fetal levels within two to three minutes. Ten minutes after intravenous administration of this thiobarbiturate (6 mg/kg), the fetal blood level is one-half the peak fetal blood level. Repeat intravenous injections of only one-third of the induction dose of thiopental sodium quickly induce peak fetal blood levels similar to those following the initial induction dose. Large induction doses (12 mg/kg) yield more than double the fetal blood level compared with a 6 mg/kg dose and result in perinatal depression.[5]

The potent inhalation anesthetics are the best agents to produce relaxation of uterine muscles. Of these, halothane produces the promptest relaxation needed for intrauterine manipulation.[42] A mixture of halothane with a 2:1 ratio of nitrous oxide with oxygen produces excellent uterine relaxation and depth of anesthesia.[30, 41, 97, 102] Emergence from anesthesia is also rapid and free of excitement. In most cases, it is desirable to anesthetize the fetus simultaneously with the mother. Halothane rapidly crosses the placenta. In 20 to 30 minutes, the tissue levels of halothane reach equilibrium between the mother and the fetus.

Disadvantages of halothane include its respiratory and circulatory depressant effect at high concentrations. Assisted or continuous mechanical respiration must be used throughout the procedure to ensure adequate fetal oxygenation. Hypotension is treated by reducing or discontinuing the concentration of halothane, infusing additional fluids, changing maternal position or displacing the uterus laterally to prevent compression on the aorta and vena cava, or by administration of vasopressors.

GENERAL CONSIDERATIONS IN FETAL SURGERY

Fetal surgery in dogs is most successful if performed during the last trimester of pregnancy. Prior to day 45 of gestation the tissues are too friable for any extensive manipulation or suturing.[36, 71] The optimum time appears to be at about 53 days; at this time tissues are firm enough to allow manipulation, the fetus is of adequate size, and the 10 remaining days of gestation allow adequate time for the fetus

and mother to recover from the operation.[43, 67] Sampling of umbilical cord blood, intrafetal injections, amputations, and intra-allantoic sampling or injections can be done at any stage of pregnancy.[33]

As much of the uterus as possible should be left in the maternal abdominal cavity, as the more it is pulled out the greater is the tension on the uterine vessels and the interference with the blood flow through the uterine veins. The exposed uterus is also very susceptible to dehydration and heat loss. It is important to check that the firm edge of the ventral fascia of the body wall is not compressing the uterine veins when the uterus is pulled out of the abdomen. If this occurs, the abdominal incision should be enlarged. The fetal pups near the cervix should not be used for surgery. Manipulation of these fetuses initiates labor in over 50 per cent of cases.[19, 65] Progesterone, isoxsuprine, indomethacin, fenoprofen, acetylsalicylic acid, and flufenamic acid have been used to reduce myometrial contractions in various species of animals. However, their use in dogs generally has not been needed.[71, 105]

The uterine incision can be made longitudinally along the uterine horn, at or near the antimesometrial pole or horizontally midway on the uterine wall between the prominent uterine vessels coming from the mesometrial attachment. Using the latter site results in less bleeding. If the fetal head is delivered for surgery in late gestation, the membranes should be left intact over the mouth and nose to prevent the fetus from inflating its lungs if respiratory activity is initiated.[19] An alternative to this approach is to enclose the head in a rubber glove filled with warm physiologic saline.[105]

Great care must be exercised in suturing or ligating fetal tissues. The decreased amount of connective tissue in the fetus results in increased friability. There is less tendency for sutures to cut through tissues when larger sizes are used (i.e., 3-0 versus 5-0). All fetal incisions are closed with interrupted suture patterns to prevent restricted fetal growth in the area of surgery that occurs when continuous sutures are used.[19] If the identity of the operated fetus is to be ensured at whelping, a nonabsorbable suture such as silk may be used as a marker.

Manipulation of the fetus results in varying degrees of stimulation of the autonomic nervous system and of increased hormonal activity. The fetal plasma ACTH and vasopressin concentrations may be elevated for several days after fetal surgery. These hormones, and possibly others such as catecholamines, may affect the circulation and influence responses of the cardiovascular system.[118]

The importance of lost amniotic fluid has been debated for years. Although some replacement of lost amniotic fluid has been stated to take place between midterm fetal surgery and birth in monkeys,[127] and although some investigators have made no attempt to conserve the amniotic fluid,[30, 69, 103, 117] there is suggestive evidence that loss of amniotic fluid alters the growth and development of the fetus,[79, 132] predisposes the mother to dystocia,[36, 120] and can result in fetal death.[2, 138] Dennis and colleagues reported that near-term pups survived without surrounding amniotic fluid, but that fluid was vital for the survival of more immature fetuses.[36] Hanks' balanced salt solution,[36] Ringer's lactate,[53] and warmed saline[1, 104] have been used successfully to replace lost amniotic fluid.

The fetus and uterus tolerate infection poorly; the fetus dies, the uterus aborts.[82, 91] The placenta in many species of animals provides an efficient barrier to the entrance of maternal antibodies and phagocytes into the fetal circulation. This phenomenon, coupled with the assumption that the fetus provides a fertile medium for the growth of many organisms, makes it advisable to use strict aseptic technique. Fetal[12] or maternal antibiotics, as well as the instillation of antibiotics and antifungal agents into the amniotic fluid, have been used to prevent fetal infections.[1, 83] However, antibiotics should be used cautiously when studying allantoic fluids, as alterations in amino acid, potassium, and sodium concentrations, as well as near complete disappearance of the allantoic fluid, have been reported following their use.[95]

If the protocol or special instrumentation precludes natural delivery, a cesarean section should be performed. Generally, the pups will be healthy and viable when delivered by cesarean section two or three days before the expected delivery date.

The major causes of fetal death following fetal surgery include amniotic fluid loss or leak;[4, 36] amniotic infection;[83] metabolic acidosis in the fetus from exteriorization, hemorrhage, trauma, or spasm of the umbilical vessels;[1, 36] placental damage;[36] interference with blood flow through main uterine vessels;[119] abortion;[41, 43, 56, 105, 135] and fetal breathing.[117]

Maternal Preparation

The bitch is fasted for 12 to 18 hours prior to surgery. No premedication is given. Ideally, anesthesia is induced with intravenous thiopental sodium, followed by tracheal intubation and maintenance with halothane–nitrous oxide–oxygen or methoxyflurane–nitrous oxide–oxygen. Injections of thiopental sodium supplemented with nitrous oxide and oxygen and local infiltration of lidocaine may be used. If it is not desired to anesthetize the fetus, epidural anesthesia can be used for the dam.

Oblique flank incisions, both muscle-splitting and muscle-cutting, and midline incisions may be used. If both uterine horns are to be operated on, the left dorsal lateral position with a midabdominal incision is best. In late pregnancy care should be exercised to avoid cutting into the enlarged mammary glands. Assisted or continuous mechanical respiration must be used throughout the procedure to ensure adequate fetal oxygenation. Five per cent dextrose solution should be administered to the dam during surgery. Maternal temperature should be monitored by a rectal probe, and heating pads or heat lamps should be used to maintain normal body temperature.

SURGICAL APPROACHES TO THE FETUS

Three approaches have been used to operate on fetuses *in utero*. In the first, the fetus has been completely exteriorized from the uterus, an operation performed, and the fetus left to develop in the abdominal cavity of the mother as an extrauterine pregnancy,[78, 89, 90, 131, 132, 136] or, after completion of the procedure, the fetus has been replaced in the uterus.[30, 82] A second method consists of delivering only a portion of the fetus from the uterus with return to the *in utero* position after operation.[36, 79, 81, 99, 128] In the third type, the fetus is left undisturbed *in utero*, and the operation is performed through a window in the uterine wall and the fetal membranes. The loss of amniotic fluid is kept to a minimum by pressing the fetus against the opening in the membranes and the uterine wall,[10, 43] by clamping the edges of the fetal membranes to the edges of the uterine incision,[120] by suturing the uterine wall around the uterine window to the skin of the fetus[73, 109] or by using the well technique.[70]

Certain experimental procedures, while not technically involving surgery on the fetus, are generally included in the category of intrauterine fetal surgery. These include injections into the fetus or fetal circulation. In many animals, it is possible, by hypodermic injection, to accurately place materials intravenously, intraperitoneally, or subcutaneously in the fetus during the last third of gestation without opening the uterus. Intracardial punctures can be safely made in dogs during the final third or quarter of gestation in this manner.[82] As an alternative, small uterine and membrane incisions can be made to expose the inoculation site. In fetal pups over 45 days of age, the jugular veins provide a site for intravenous inoculation and collection of blood. In younger fetuses, the umbilical vessels prove less likely to contract after trauma and are suitable sites for inoculation.[36]

Complete Exteriorization of the Fetus

For many intrauterine surgical procedures, it is desirable to take the fetal animal completely out of the uterus.[54] This is particularly true during the first one-half to two-thirds of gestation, when the fetus is most delicate and small relative to the amount of amniotic fluid. In addition, it is very difficult to get a secure atraumatic hold on the fetus through the uterine wall and membranes. The advantage of complete exteriorization of the fetus is that the operative procedure is more easily accomplished;[82] however, it may be complicated by marked contraction of the uterus following loss of its contents.[105]

Following laparotomy, the segment of uterus containing the fetus upon which surgery is to be performed is exteriorized. The position of the zonary placenta is denoted by its increased resistance to touch and by identifying the course of the uterine vessels. Orientation of the fetus is determined by palpation through the uterine wall cranial and caudal to the zonary placenta. Accurate palpation of fetal puppies less than 40 days of age is prevented by their small size and greater amount of fluid.[36]

The uterine muscle is incised above the chorioallantoic membrane as far from the zonary placenta as possible to prevent retroplacental hemorrhage or separation. Prior to cutting the fetal membranes, the amniotic fluid should be removed when fully exteriorizing the fetus.[82] This is done by inserting a 20-gauge needle into the amniotic cavity and aspirating the fluid into a graduated syringe. The amniotic fluid is placed in a sterile container, incubated at body temperature, and returned just prior to closure of the uterus. The removal of all or most of the fluid in this manner permits greater freedom for manipulating the fetus. It also avoids the problem of fluid flowing into the surgical field.

Next, the fetal membranes are incised and the fetus is gently lifted out of the uterus. Great care must be taken when handling the fetus, as the skin and subcutaneous tissues are extremely fragile and hemorrhage follows even the most gentle manipulations.[1] Care should be exercised to avoid obstructing the flow of blood in the umbilical cord. The umbilical cord of the fetal dog is sensitive to manipulation. In late-term fetal puppies, complete constriction of the umbilical arteries and veins may result from tension on the umbilical cord or the insertion of a hypodermic needle.[82] At this stage, it is necessary to moisten the skin of the fetus frequently with warmed (37°C) saline solution as the fetal temperature rapidly drops and the skin dries rapidly when exposed to the air. Keeping the operating room warm and shortening operative time are also helpful.

Fetal incisions are closed with 3-0 or 4-0 absorbable sutures in an interrupted pattern. Tissue apposition should be accomplished with the least number of sutures, including as many layers of tissue as possible. For example, abdommal incisions are closed by including all muscle layers and the peritoneum in one layer, and thoracic incisions are closed by apposing the ribs on each side of the incision with pericostal sutures including the pleura. The ribs will usually fuse but without serious impairment of function. Though fetal tissue heals well and rapidly, thoracic surgery on a fetus frequently results in adhesions of the lungs to the external pleura, resulting in pneumothorax at birth.[33]

After the surgical procedure has been completed, the edges of the uterine incision and fetal membranes are clamped together with Babcock forceps to prevent tearing or separation of the chorioallantoic membranes. The fetus is replaced by simultaneously lifting and spreading the incised edges of the uterus with Babcock forceps, while gently pushing on the fetus. This procedure generally requires an increase in the halothane concentration to provide relaxation of the myometrium. Maternal hypotension and fetal bradycardia frequently accompany this maneuver.[105] If patience is observed, this procedure can be completed with minimal difficulty or stress to either the fetus or mother. It is usually best to return the fetus to the same position from which it was taken.[82]

The uterus is sutured with 3-0 absorbable sutures on an atraumatic needle; the sutures are placed through the full thickness of the muscle and chorioallantoic membrane on each side. A continuous locking suture is used, as this helps to prevent the sutures from cutting through the muscle. Closure of the fragile amniotic membrane is unnecessary for the further development of the fetus.[36] Prior to closure of the uterus, the warmed amniotic fluid collected earlier is returned to the uterus. A second continuous suture is placed in the uterine muscle to invert the incision; this helps to prevent leakage of fluid and also relieves tension on the wound, thereby reducing the risk of rupture. When this technique is used, uterine rupture does not occur even when labor occurs soon after surgery.[105]

The gravid uterus should be carefully returned to its normal position in the abdomen. Lifting the sides of the incised abdominal wall while tilting the animal slightly head down facilitates this procedure. The abdominal incision is closed in a conventional manner. The fascial layers, which provide the main support of the abdomen, should be closed with interrupted sutures.

Partial Exteriorization

During the last third of gestation, when the fetus is larger, it is often simpler to perform surgical procedures with the fetus only partially exteriorized.[82] This procedure is feasible for operations on the extremities or the head. However, the exteriorizing of only part of the trunk may lead to compromise of the umbilical circulation or to complete extrusion of the fetus. For procedures of this kind, the uterus and placental membranes are opened in the same manner as for complete exteriorization except that a smaller incision may be desired. Often it is not necessary to remove the fluid, since the fetus can be positioned to block the opening.

The usual approach for partial exteriorization is to locate by palpation the part of the fetus to be exteriorized and position it against the site selected for incision of the uterus. If the fetus is held against the membranes and uterus in a slightly elevated position, it is possible to make the opening with little or no fluid loss. The part to be exteriorized is then gently lifted through the incision and held by moist gauze pads so that it continues to block the opening. After the operation has been completed, the edges of the incision are grasped and lifted as the fetal extremity is returned, to avoid spilling the amniotic or allantoic fluid. The membranes and the uterine wall are closed as in complete exteriorization.

Marsupialization

Marsupialization of the fetus permits extensive surgical manipulation without significantly disturbing the fetal-maternal relationship.[104] It is used in older fetuses (over 45 days of gestation), in which the fetal skin is tough enough to hold sutures. It is of particular value in lengthy procedures requiring continual access to the fetus for several hours and is used to prevent amniotic fluid loss and exposure of the sensitive umbilical vessels.[82]

The proper anatomical area of the fetus for the proposed operation is located by palpation, and it is moved outside the boundaries of the placental girdle and held against the uterine wall. A 3-0 suture on an atraumatic needle is passed through the uterine wall and fetal skin at one end of the anticipated incision. This suture is tied and a purse-string suture (3-mm bites) is placed through the uterine wall to include the chorionic membrane, amnion, and the fetal skin; it is then carried in a gentle curve lateral to the line of the proposed incision. The suture is carried back in a similar manner to the original starting point so that an elliptical area is circumscribed. This suture is pulled up snugly to prevent loss of amniotic fluid (Fig. 131–4).[33, 73]

An incision is made within the area of the ellipse through the uterine wall, fetal membranes, and skin. The cut edges of the fetal skin and uterus may be sutured together with a row of continuous 4-0 sutures to protect further against the possibility of losing amniotic fluid at the operative site. The specific operation can now be performed through the initial incision, using standard techniques.

At the conclusion of the surgical operation, the edges of the uterus and fetal skin are separated by cutting and removing the suture binding them. The fetal skin is closed with interrupted 3-0 or 4-0 absorbable suture. The uterus is closed as described previously and the purse-string is cut in several places, allowing the fetus to separate from the uterine wall.

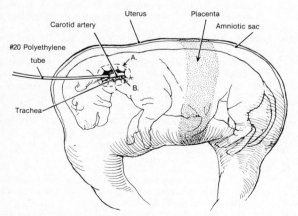

Figure 131–4. Schematic representation of catheterization of the carotid artery through a marsupialized opening in the uterine wall. Continuous mattress suture (*a*); fetal skin and uterus sutured together (*b*).

Catheterization of Carotid Artery and Jugular Vein

The practicality of catheterizing fetal vessels is determined not only by their size but also by their fragility and reactivity. In general, the earlier the gestational age, the more fragile are the vessels. In younger fetuses, the vessel walls have a high water content and tear easily with minor tension. Most vessels undergo some degree of constriction when manipulated; arteries constrict more than veins, and the degree of constriction varies in different vessels. Umbilical arteries and veins constrict actively, and this constriction may extend some distance proximally and distally from the site of manipulation. Lower limb arteries also have a marked propensity for spasm, but the carotid and jugular veins are much less reactive.[118]

Access to the fetus is gained by one of the methods previously described. An incision is made from the angle of the mandible to the shoulder. If the chin is held in extension, this places the carotid artery under tension and renders it more accessible. A small mosquito forceps is used to dissect out the artery and vein. Number 2-0 silk ties are used for cut-downs, as finer silk severs the artery. Number 20 polyethylene catheters (ID, 0.015 inches) can be used to cannulate vessels in 56-day-old fetal pups. This tubing should have a silicon lining to eliminate clotting that may occur because of high fetal hemoconcentration. Perforation of the artery is less likely if blunt catheters are used.

In adult animals, intravascular pressures are referenced to atmospheric pressure at the level of the heart as zero, and external pressure transducers are positioned at this level. In the fetus, the chest is surrounded by pressure within the uterine cavity; it is customary to reference fetal intravascular pressures to amniotic cavity pressure as the zero reference. Thus, amniotic pressure is recorded simultaneously with vascular pressures and is subtracted from them to obtain a pressure above the intrauterine level. Arterial blood pressure *in utero* is 20 to 40 mm Hg in fetal pups between 56 and 58 days of gestation.[65]

Catheterization of Umbilical Vessels

Catheterization of the umbilical vessels offers two advantages. These vessels are larger than the carotid artery and jugular vein and therefore less susceptible to rupture. Moreover, a catheter from the umbilical vessels can more easily be brought outside the uterus for serial collection of fetal blood samples. In dogs, the umbilical vessels undergo marked ramification; therefore, one branch can be catheterized without danger of obstructing the fetal circulation. The uterine tissue is incised and retracted carefully until the amniotic sac lies immediately below the incision. The sac is manipulated until the placenta is exposed with the vessels lying apposed to it. A catheter is inserted and tied to the vessels. The primary disadvantage in using this technique is that the loss of amniotic fluid tends to be greater because the amniotic sac is more vulnerable in this procedure.[65]

Other Fetal Operations

Various fetal operations have been performed successfully in dogs. Examples include cannulation of femoral vein,[65] bilateral nephrectomy,[65] catheterization and ligation of the trachea,[65] monitoring of fetal heart sounds[65] or electrocardiograms,[71, 135] thymectomy,[36, 39, 43] skin grafting,[71] inoculations,[71, 82] catheterization of urinary bladder[19, 20] and ureter,[19] abdominal laparotomies,[10, 19] thoracotomies,[71] and catheterization of the inferior vena cava[22] and stomach.[70]

1. Abrams, J. S.: Fetal surgery in sheep: Technique and results of 53 intrauterine procedures. J. Surg. Res. 13:249, 1972.
2. Adams, C. E.: Embryonic mortality induced experimentally in the rabbit. Nature 188:332, 1960.
3. Adams, F. H., Fujiwara, T., and Rowshan, G.: The nature and origin of the fluid in the fetal lamb lung. J. Pediatr. 63:881, 1963.
4. Adamsons, K., Jr.: Fetal surgery. N. Engl. J. Med. 275:204, 1966.
5. Albright, G. A.: Anesthesia in Obstetrics: Maternal, Fetal, and Neonatal Aspects. Addison-Wesley Publishing Co., Menlo Park, CA, 1978.
6. Ampola, M. G., Mahoney, M. J., Nakamura, E., and Tunaka, K.: Prenatal therapy of a patient with vitamin B$_{12}$–responsive methylmalonic acidemia. N. Engl. J. Med. 293:313, 1975.
7. Andersen, A. C., and Goldman, M.: Growth and Development. In Andersen, A. C. (ed.): The Beagle as an Experimental Dog. Iowa State University Press, Ames, 1970.
8. Asensio, S. H.: Human fetal surgery. Clin. Obstet. Gynecol. 17:153, 1974.
9. Barcroft, J., and Barron, D. H.: Movements in midfoetal life in the sheep embryo. J. Physiol. 91:329, 1937.
10. Barnard, C. N.: A method of operating on fetal dogs in utero. Surgery 41:805, 1957.
11. Barnard, C. N., and Louw, J. H.: The genesis of intestinal atresia. Minnesota Med. 39:745, 1956.
12. Bassett, J. M., and Madell, D.: The influence of maternal nutrition on plasma hormone and metabolite concentrations of foetal lambs. J. Endocrinol. 61:465, 1974.
13. Bassett, J. M., and Thorburn, G. D.: Foetal plasma corticosteroids and the initiation of parturition in sheep. J. Endocrinol. 44:285, 1969.
14. Bassett, J. M., and Thorburn, G. D.: Circulating levels of progesterone and corticosteroids in the pregnant ewe and its foetus. In Pierrepoint, C. G. (ed.): The Endocrinology of Pregnancy and Parturition: Experimental Studies in Sheep. Alpha Omega Alpha, Cardiff, 1973.
15. Battaglia, F.: Dangers of maternal hyperventilation. J. Pediatr. 70:313, 1967.
16. Benzi, G., Berte, F., Crema, A., and Arrigoni, E.: Uterine-placental-fetal preparation in situ on the dog. Investigation of metabolizing activity and tissue distribution. J. Pharm. Sci. 57:1031, 1968.
17. Berkowitz, R. L., Glickman, M. G., Walker Smith, G. J., Siegel, N. J., Weiss, R. M., Mahoney, M. J., and Hobbins, J. C.: Fetal urinary tract obstruction: What is the role of surgical intervention in utero? Am. J. Obstet. Gynecol. 144:367, 1982.
18. Bernstine, R. L.: Activity of the urinary bladder in the dog fetus. Am. J. Obstet. Gynecol. 105:431, 1969.
19. Bernstine, R. L., and Coran, A. G.: Surgical techniques in

the study of canine fetal physiology. J. Pediatr. Surg. 6:466, 1971.
20. Bernstine, R. L., Rice, F., and Homer, L. D.: Isolation and characterization of a green pigment from fetal urine. Biochem. Med. 3:422, 1970.
21. Birnholz, J. C., and Frigoletto, F. D.: Antenatal treatment of hydrocephalus. N. Engl. J. Med. 304:1021, 1981.
22. Bissonnette, J. M., Hohimer, A. R., and Richardson, B. S.: Ventriculocisternal cerebrospinal perfusion in unanesthetized fetal lambs. J. Appl. Physiol. 50:880, 1981.
23. Brinkman, C. R., III, and Woods, J. R., Jr.: Effects of cardiovascular drugs during pregnancy. Cardiovasc. Med. 1:231, 1976.
24. Bromage, P. L.: Continuous lumbar epidural analgesia for obstetrics. Can. Med. Assoc. J. 85:1136, 1961.
25. Bueno, L., and Ruckelbusch, Y.: Perinatal development of intestinal myoelectrical activity in dogs and sheep. Am. J. Physiol. 237:E61, 1979.
26. Burg, J. R., Dodek, A., Kloster, F. E., and Metcalfe, J.: Alterations of systolic time intervals during pregnancy. Circulation 49:560, 1974.
27. Canty, T. G., Leopold, G. R., and Wolf, D. A.: Maternal ultrasonography for the antenatal diagnosis of surgically significant neonatal anomalies. Ann. Surg. 194:353, 1981.
28. Chez, R. A., Smith, F. G., and Hutchinson, D. L.: Renal function in the intrauterine primate fetus. Am. J. Obstet. Gynecol. 90:128, 1964.
29. Clewell, W. H., Johnson, M. L., Meier, P. R., Newkirk, J. B., et al.: A surgical approach to the treatment of fetal hydrocephalus. N. Engl. J. Med. 306:1320, 1982.
30. Cowen, R. H., and Laurenson, R. D.: A technique of operating upon the fetus of the rabbit. Surgery 45:321, 1959.
31. Creighton, R. E., et al.: Experimental congenital diaphragmatic hernia. Proc. Can. Fed. Biol. Soc. 13:22, 1970.
32. Csapo, A.: Actomyosin formation by estrogen action. Am. J. Physiol. 162:406, 1950.
33. Cummings, J. N.: Fetal Surgery. In Archibald, J. (ed.): Canine Surgery. 2nd ed. American Veterinary Publications, Inc., Santa Barbara, 1974.
34. Cummings, J. N., and Bellville, T. P.: Transplacental passage of antibiotics and techniques for repeated sampling of the fetal lamb in situ. Am. J. Obstet. Gynecol. 86:504, 1963.
35. De Luca, F. G., Frates, R., and Corwin, R.: Intrauterine angiographic investigation of the cardiovascular and pulmonary systems of the dog fetus. J. Pediatr. Surg. 2:41, 1967.
36. Dennis, R. A., Jacoby, R. O., and Griesmer, R. A.: Intrauterine techniques for studying development of the immune response of the fetal dog. Lab. Anim. Care 18:561, 1968.
37. Dilts, P. V., and Ahokas, R. A.: Development and physiology of the placenta and membranes. In Sciarra, J. J. (ed.): Gynecology and Obstetrics. Harper and Row, Hagerstown, 1980.
38. Dilts, P. V., Brinkman, C. R., Kirschbaum, T. H., and Assali, N. S.: Uterine and systemic hemodynamic interrelationships and their response to hypoxia. Am. J. Obstet. Gynecol. 103:138, 1969.
39. Dixit, S. P., and Coppola, E. D.: Experimental surgery—Intrauterine thymectomy in the canine fetus. Can. J. Surg. 13:170, 1970.
40. Eckstein, P., and Kelly, W. A.: Implantation and development of the conceptus. In Cole, H. H., and Cupps, P. T. (eds.): Reproduction in Domestic Animals. Academic Press, New York, 1977.
41. Eng, M., Berges, P. U., Yuen, D. D., Bonica, J. J., and Ueland, K.: A comparison of the effects on the inhalation of 4% and 8% fluroxene in the pregnant primate. Acta Anaesth. Scand. 20:183, 1976.
42. Eng, M., Bonica, J. J., Akamatsu, T. J., Berges, P. U., Der Yuen, D., and Ueland, K.: Maternal and fetal responses to halothane in pregnant monkeys. Acta Anaesth. Scand. 19:154, 1975.

43. Fisher, J. H., deAlmeida, M., Nettelblad, S. A. C., and DeLuca, F. G.: Technique of thymectomy in newborn puppies and intrauterine thymectomy in dog fetuses. Trans. Am. Soc. Artif. Intern. Organs 10:244, 1964.

44. Frigoletto, F. D., Birnholz, J. C., and Greene, M. F.: Antenatal treatment of hydrocephalus by ventriculoamniotic shunting. J. Am. Med. Assoc. 248:2496, 1982.

45. Fukuda, S., and Matsuoka, O.: Placenta weight, umbilical cord length, and amniotic fluid characteristics in beagle dogs. Exp. Anim. 28:69, 1979.

46. Garden, J. M., Askenazi, J., and Lesch, M.: Assessment of cardiovascular function. In Sciarra, J. J. (ed.): Gynecology and Obstetrics. Harper and Row, Hagerstown, 1980.

47. Gier, H. T.: Early embryology of the dog. Anat. Rec. 108:561, 1950.

48. Gluck, L., Kulovich, M. V., Borer, R. G., Brenner, P. H., Anderson, G. G., and Spellacy, W. N.: Diagnosis of the respiratory distress syndrome by amniocentesis. Am. J. Obstet. Gynecol. 109:440, 1971.

49. Golbus, M. S., Harrison, M. R., Filly, R. A., Callen, P. W., and Katz, M.: In utero treatment of urinary tract obstruction. Am. J. Obstet. Gynecol. 142:383, 1982.

50. Goodger, W. J., and Levy, W.: Anesthetic management of the cesarean section. Vet. Clin. North Am. 3:85, 1973.

51. Goodlin, R. C., and Rudolph, A. M.: Tracheal fluid flow and function in fetuses in utero. Am. J. Obstet. Gynecol. 106:597, 1970.

52. Gutsche, B. B.: Maternal physiologic alterations during pregnancy. In Shnider, S. M., and Levinson, G. (eds.): Anesthesia for Obstetrics. Williams & Wilkins, Baltimore, 1979.

53. Haller, J. A., Golladay, E. S., Tepas, J. J., Inon, A. E., Mostofi, I., and Shermeta, D. W.: Fetal surgery: General management and operative technique for creating anomalies in sheep. Prog. Pediat. Surg. 12:41, 1978.

54. Hardy, K. J., Auldist, A. W., and Shulkes, A.: Congenital diaphragmatic hernia—Intrauterine repair in fetal sheep. Med. J. Aust. 2:223, 1982.

55. Harrigan, J. T., Kangos, J. J., Sikka, A., Spisso, K. R., Natarajan, N., Rosenfeld, D., Leiman, S., and Korn, S.: Successful treatment of fetal congestive heart failure secondary to tachycardia. N. Engl. J. Med. 304:1527, 1981.

56. Harrison, M. R., Anderson, J., Rosen, M. A., Ross, N. A., and Hendrickx, A. G.: Fetal surgery in the primate. I. Anesthetic, surgical, and tocolytic management to maximize fetal-neonatal survival. J. Pediatr. Surg. 17:115, 1982.

57. Harrison, M. R., Bressack, M. A., Churg, A. M., et al.: Correction of congenital diaphragmatic hernia in utero. II. Simulated correction permits fetal lung growth with survival at birth. Surgery 88:260, 1980.

58. Harrison, M. R., and DeLorimier, A. A.: Congenital diaphragmatic hernia. Surg. Clin. North Am. 61:1023, 1981.

59. Harrison, M. R., Filly, R. A., Parer, J. T., et al.: Management of the fetus with a urinary tract malformation. J. Am. Med. Assoc. 246:635, 1981.

60. Harrison, M. R., Golbus, M. S., and Filly, R. A.: Management of the fetus with correctable defect. J. Am. Med. Assoc. 246:774, 1981.

61. Harrison, M. R., Golbus, M. S., Filly, R. A., Callen, R. W., Katz, M., DeLorimier, A. A., Rosen, M., and Jensen, A. R.: Fetal surgery for congenital hydronephrosis. N. Engl. J. Med. 306:591, 1982.

62. Harrison, M. R., Golbus, M. S., Filly, R. A., Nakayama, D. K., and DeLorimier, A. A.: Fetal surgical treatment. Pediatr. Ann. 11:896, 1982.

63. Harrison, M. R., Jester, J. A., and Ross, N. A.: Correction of congenital diaphragmatic hernia in utero. I. The model: Intrathoracic balloon produces fatal pulmonary hypoplasia. Surgery 88:174, 1980.

64. Harrison, M. R., Ross, N. A., and DeLorimier, A. A.: Correction of congenital diaphragmatic hernia in utero. III. Development of a successful surgical technique using abdominoplasty to avoid compromise of umbilical blood flow. J. Pediatr. Surg. 16:934, 1981.

65. Hodari, A. A., and Thomas, L.: Experimental surgical procedures upon the fetus in obstetric research. Obstet. Gynecol. 34:204, 1969.

66. Hodgen, G. D.: Antenatal diagnosis and treatment of fetal skeletal malformations with emphasis on in utero surgery for neural tube defects and limb bud regeneration. J. Am. Med. Assoc. 246:1079, 1981.

67. Holder, T. M., and Ashcroft, K. W.: The effects of bile duct ligation and inflammation in the fetus. J. Pediatr. Surg. 2:35, 1967.

68. Holst, P., and Phemister, R. D.: The prenatal development of the dog: Preimplantation events. Biol. Reprod. 5:194, 1971.

69. Hooker, D., and Nicholas, J. S.: Spinal cord section in rat fetuses. J. Comp. Neurol. 50:413, 1930.

70. Idriss, F. S., and Nikaidoh, H.: Radiographic studies of the gastrointestinal tract of the fetus in utero. J. Pediatr. Surg. 2:29, 1967.

71. Jackson, B. T.: Approach to fetal research—Present and future. Am. J. Dis. Child. 118:812, 1969.

72. Jackson, B. T., Clarke, J. P., and Egdahl, R. H.: Direct lead fetal electrocardiography with undisturbed fetal-maternal relationships. Surg. Gynecol. Obstet. 110:687, 1960.

73. Jackson, B. T., and Egdahl, R. H.: The performance of complex fetal operations in utero without amniotic fluid loss or other disturbances of fetal-maternal relationship. Surgery 48:564, 1960.

74. Jackson, B. T., Novy, M. J., and Piasecki, G. J.: Experimental in utero hemolytic disease in dog fetuses. Surg. Forum. 17:388, 1966.

75. Jackson, B. T., Piasecki, G. J., and Egdahl, R. H.: Electrocardiographic response to experimental coarctation of the aorta in the fetus in utero. Surg. Forum 11:270, 1960.

76. Jackson, B. T., Piasecki, G. J., and Egdahl, R. H.: Experimental production of coarctation of the aorta in utero with prolonged postnatal survival. Surg. Forum 14:290, 1963.

77. Jancin, B.: Successful operations boost concept of fetus as patient. Obstet. Gynecol. News, Vol. 20, Oct. 15, 1981.

78. Jones, D. B., and Hooker, C. W.: A technique that permits manipulations of the mouse embryo. Anat. Rec. 112:417, 1952.

79. Jost, A.: On the sexual differentiation of the rabbit embryo. Remarks on the subject of certain surgical operations on the embryo. Compt. Rend. Soc. Biol. 140:461, 1946.

80. Kaneoka, T.: Electrocardiographic and polargraphic observations in the canine fetus. J. Jpn. Obstet. Gynecol. Soc. 108:19, 1963.

81. Kisken, W. A., and Swensen, N. A.: A technique of intrauterine thymectomy in the rabbit. Surgery 63:546, 1968.

82. Kraner, K. L.: Intrauterine fetal surgery. Adv. Vet. Sci. 10:1, 1965.

83. Leash, A., Sachs, L., Abrams, J., and Limber, R.: Control of Aspergillus fumigatus infection in fetal sheep. Lab. Anim. Care 18:407, 1968.

84. Liggins, G. C., and Howie, R. N.: A controlled trial of antepartum glucocorticoid treatment for prevention of respiratory distress syndrome in premature infants. Pediatrics 50:515, 1972.

85. Liley, A. W.: Intrauterine transfusion of the fetus in hemolytic disease. Br. J. Med. 2:1107, 1963.

86. Louw, J. H., and Barnard, C. N.: Congenital intestinal atresia. Observations on its origin. Lancet 269:1065, 1955.

87. Lowrey, J. C.: Surgical procedures for selective removal of canine fetuses at mid-term and beyond without effecting abortion (application in deafness research). Vet. Med. Small Anim. Clin. 70:439, 1975.

88. Mashiach, S., Barkai, G., Sack, J., Stern, E., Brish, M., Goldman, D. M., and Serr, D. M.: The effect of intraamniotic thyroxine administration on fetal lung maturity in man. J. Perinat. Med. 7:161, 1979.

89. Mayer, A.: Über den Einfluss des Eierstocks auf das Wachstum des Uterus in der Fötalzeit und in der Kindheit und über die Bedeutung des Lebensalters zur Zeit der Kastration. Ztschr. f. d. ges. Gynak. u. Geburtsh. 77:279, 1915.

90. Mayer, A.: Über die Möglichkeit operativer Eingriffe beim lebenden Saugetierfötus. Zentralbl. Gynak. 42:773, 1918.

91. McFadyen, I. R., Boonyaprakob, U., and Hutchinson, D. L.: Experimental production of anemia in fetal lambs. Am. J. Obstet. Gynecol. 100:686, 1968.

92. McLain, C. R., Jr.: Amniography studies of the gastrointestinal motility of the human fetus. Am. J. Obstet. Gynecol. 86:1079, 1963.

93. McLain, C. R., Jr.: Amniography, a versatile diagnostic procedure in obstetrics. Obstet. Gynecol. 23:45, 1964.

94. McLain, C. R., Jr.: Amniography for the diagnosis of fetal death in utero. Obstet. Gynecol. 26:233, 1965.

95. Mellor, D. J., and Slater, J. S.: Effects of antibiotic treatment on the composition of sheep fluids. Res. Vet. Sci. 12:521, 1971.

96. Merryman, W.: Progesterone anesthesia in human subjects. J. Clin. Endocrinol. Metab. 14:1567, 1954.

97. Michejda, M., Bacher, J., Hayes, N., Johnson, D., Killens, R., and Watson, W.: Estimation of gestational and skeletal age in Macaca mulatta. J. Med. Primatol. 8:143, 1979.

98. Michejda, M., Bacher, J., and Johnson, D.: Surgical approaches in fetal radiography and the study of skeletal age in Macaca mulatta. J. Med. Primatol. 9:50, 1980.

99. Michejda, M., Bacher, J., Kuwabora, T., and Hodgen, G. D.: In utero allogeneic bone transplantation in primates. Transplantation 32:96, 1981.

100. Michejda, M., and Hodgen, G. D.: In utero diagnosis and diagnosis and treatment of nonhuman primate fetal skeletal anomalies. J. Am. Med. Assoc. 246:1093, 1981.

101. Montoya, A., and Quiroga, P. J.: Direct evidence of renal function in the intrauterine canine fetus. Texas Rep. Biol. Med. 33:596, 1975.

102. Morishima, H. O., Hyman, A. I., Adamsons, K., and James, L. S.: Anesthetic management for fetal operation in the subhuman primate. Am. J. Obstet. Gynecol. 110:926, 1971.

103. Nicholas, J. S.: Notes on the application of experimental methods upon mammalian embryos. Anat. Rec. 31:385, 1925.

104. Niederhuber, J. E., Shermeta, D., Turcotte, J. G., and Gikas, P. W.: Kidney transplantation in the fetal lamb. Transplantation 12:161, 1971.

105. Novy, J. M., Walsh, S. W., and Cook, M. J.: Chronic implantation of catheters and electrodes in pregnant non-human primates. In Nathanielsz, P. W. (ed.): Animals Models in Fetal Medicine. Elsevier/North-Holland Biomedical Press, New York, 1980.

106. Ostergard, D. R.: The physiology and clinical importance of amniotic fluid. A review. Obstet. Gynecol. Surv. 25:297, 1970.

107. Palahniuk, R. J., Shnider, S. M., and Eger, E. I., II: Pregnancy decreases the requirements for inhaled anesthetic agents. Anesthesiology 41:82, 1974.

108. Parshall, C. J., and Silverstein, A. M.: Surgical approaches to the study of fetal immunology in primate animals. Ann. N.Y. Acad. Sci. 162:254, 1969.

109. Picket, L. K., and Briggs, H. C.: Biliary obstruction secondary to hepatic vascular ligation in fetal sheep. J. Pediatr. Surg. 4:95, 1969.

110. Plentl, A. A., and Gray, M. J.: Physiology of the amniotic fluid and the management of hydramnios. Surg. Clin. North Am. 37:405, 1957.

111. Pritchard, J. A., and MacDonald, P. C.: Williams Obstetrics, 16th ed., Appleton-Century-Crofts, New York, 1980.

112. Ramsey, E. M., and Donner, M. W.: Placental Vasculature and Circulation. W. B. Saunders, Philadelphia, 1980.

113. Renaud, R., Vincendon, G., Boog, G., Brettes, J. P., Schumacher, J. C., Koehl, C., Kirchstetter, L., and Gandar, R.: Injections intra-amniotiques d'acides amines dans les cas de malnutrition foetale. J. Gynecol. Obstet. Biol. Reprod. 1:231, 1972.

114. Reynolds, W. A.: Fetal sources of amniotic fluid: An enigma. In Hodari, A. A., and Mariona, F. (eds.): Physiological

Biochemistry of the Fetus. Charles C Thomas, Springfield, 1972.

115. Roberts, S. J.: Veterinary Obstetrics and Genital Diseases, 1st ed. Edwards Brothers, Inc., Michigan, 1956.

116. Roddick, J. W.: Surgical complication of pregnancy. In Sciarra, J. J. (ed.): Gynecology and Obstetrics. Harper and Row, New York, 1980.

117. Rosenkrantz, J. G., Simon, R. C., and Carlisle, J. H.: Fetal surgery in the pig with a review of other mammalian fetal technics. J. Pediatr. Surg. 3:392, 1968.

118. Rudolph, A. M., and Heymann, M. A.: The fetal circulation. Ann. Rev. Med. 19:195, 1968.

119. Rudolph, A. M., and Heymann, M. A.: Methods for studying the circulation of the fetus in utero. In Nathanielsz, P. W. (ed.): Animal Models in Fetal Medicine. Elsevier/North-Holland Biomedical Press, New York, 1980.

120. Schinekel, P. G., and Ferguson, K. A.: Skin transplantation in the fetal lamb. Aust. J. Biol. Sci. 6:533, 1953.

121. Schulman, H.: Amniotic fluid. Clin. Obstet. Gynecol. 13:542, 1970.

122. Selye, H.: Studies concerning the anesthetic action of steroid hormones. J. Pharmacol. Exp. Ther. 73:127, 1941.

123. Shnider, S. M., and Livinson, G.: Obstetric anesthesia. In Miller, R. D. (ed.): Anesthesia. Churchill Livingstone, New York, 1981.

124. Sokolowski, J. H.: Normal events of gestation in the bitch and methods of pregnancy diagnosis. In Morrow, D. A. (ed.): Current Therapy in Theriogenology: Diagnosis, Treatment, and Prevention of Reproductive Diseases in Animals. W. B. Saunders, Philadelphia, 1980.

125. Taylor, E. S.: Beck's Obstetrical Practice and Fetal Medicine, 10th ed. Williams & Wilkins, Baltimore, 1976.

126. The Quaker Oats Co.: Pregnancy Diagnosis in the Canine with Radiography. Radiographic Aids for the Veterinary Practitioner, Series 3, Summer, 1962.

127. Thomasson, B. H., and Rivitch, M. M.: Fetal surgery in the rabbit. Surgery 66:1092, 1969.

128. Turley, K., Vlahakes, G. J., Harrison, M. R., Messina, L., Hanley, F., Uhlig, P. N., and Ebert, P. A.: Intrauterine cardiothoracic surgery: The fetal lamb model. Ann. Thorac. Surg. 34:422, 1982.

129. Walker, J., MacGillinray, I., and Macnaughton, M. (eds.): Combined Textbook of Obstetrics and Gynecology, 9th ed. Churchill Livingstone, New York, 1976.

130. Weiner, S., Scharf, J. I., Bolognese, R. J., and Librizzi, R. J.: Antenatal diagnosis and treatment of a fetal goiter. J. Reprod. Med. 24:39, 1980.

131. Wells, L. J.: A method for subjecting fetal rats to laparotomy and repeated subcutaneous injections. Anat. Rec. 94:530, 1946.

132. Wells, L. J.: Subjection of fetal rats to surgery and repeated subcutaneous injections: Method and survival. Anat. Rec. 108:309, 1951.

133. Whitfield, C. R.: Amniotic fluid. In MacDonald, R. R. (ed.): Scientific Basis of Obstetrics and Gynaecology. Churchill Livingstone, New York, 1978.

134. Williams, H. B., Powers, J. D., and Hamlin, R. L.: Ventricular wall thickness in the fetal dog. Am. J. Vet. Res. 40:696, 1979.

135. Williams, H. B., Rankin, J. S., and Hamlin, R. L.: An invasive procedure for in utero fetal electrocardiology: Recording of fetal electrocardiograms by applying electrodes through the uterus. Am. J. Vet. Res. 39:183, 1978.

136. Wolf, B.: Experimentelle Untersuchungen über die Entstehung extrauteriner Schwangerschaften und über die Möglichkeit operativer Eingriffe beim lebenden Saugetierfoetus. Beitr. Path. Anat. 65:423, 1919.

137. Yannone, M. E., McCurdy, J. R., and Goldfein, A.: Plasma progesterone levels in normal pregnancy, labor and puerperium. II. Clinical data. Am. J. Obstet. Gynecol. 101:1058, 1968.

138. Zuntz, N.: Über die Respiration des Saugethier-Foetus. Pfluger's Arch. Physiol. 14:605, 1877.

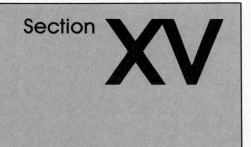

Section **XV**

Urinary System

Bruce A. Christie
Section Editor

Chapter 132

Anatomy of the Urinary Tract

Bruce A. Christie

DEVELOPMENT OF THE URINARY SYSTEM

The urinary and genital systems share a common mesodermal origin and pursue an integrated development. Much of this chapter's content is drawn from several textbooks.[1, 19, 37]

Normal Development

Kidneys and Ureters

Kidneys are compound tubular glands composed of uriniferous tubules. They arise in the embryo in a mesodermal plate called the nephrotome, which lies between the somatic and splanchnic mesoderm (Fig. 132–1A). From the nephrotome, three classes of organs develop sequentially (Fig. 132–1B and C). The first to form is the pronephros. This is the functional kidney of primitive vertebrates such as cyclostomes and the provisional kidney of larval fishes and amphibians. Pronephric tubules arise as buds from the nephrotome plate. The growing extremities of the buds unite to produce a pronephric duct. The caudal blind end of the duct grows toward and penetrates the cloaca. Pronephric tubules degenerate, but the duct is retained and used by tubules of the mesonephros, the second nephrogenic organ to develop. The duct is now known as the mesonephric or wolffian duct. The mesonephros is the permanent kidney of fishes and amphibians. In mammals, some portions of the mesonephric duct and some tubules are salvaged for use in the genital system of the male. The metanephric kidney, the third class in the sequence, is the functional kidney of reptiles, birds,

and mammals. It has a dual origin. Secretory units, or nephrons, consist of Bowman's capsule, proximal and distal convoluted tubules, and the loop of Henle. These units arise in the caudalmost portion of the nephrogenic cord, the metanephros.

The drainage duct system of the metanephros is derived from a bud growing off the mesonephric duct close to the cloaca. This bud pushes into the metanephrogenic mesoderm and, by a process of repeated dichotomous branching and absorption, differentiates into ureter, pelvis, calyces, papillary ducts, and straight collecting tubules (Fig. 132–2).

Microdissection studies have shown that in the human kidney there are 25 to 30 generations of buds.[27] The renal pelvis is formed from the first 5 generations, major calyces generations 10 through 15, and collecting tubules from succeeding generations. Each bud consists of an interstitial, or tubular, segment and the advancing end, or ampulla. Up to 25 papillary ducts, or ducts of Bellini, open into each minor calyx via the fenestrated papillary tip known as the area cribrosa. All papillary ducts that drain into the same minor calyx form the medullary pyramid. Straight collecting tubules are abundant in the medulla and project into the cortex as medullary rays (Fig. 132–3). The metanephrogenic mesoderm, which caps the medullary pyramid, is the cortex. This tissue also divides and increases in volume as the collecting tubules divide. Renal columns are regions where the cortex extends between individual pyramids. The terminal ampulla of the last generation of buds induces nephron formation. The tiny masses of metanephrogenic tissue around each terminal collecting tubule hollow into vesicles, elongate, and become tortuous. A Bowman's capsule and glomer-

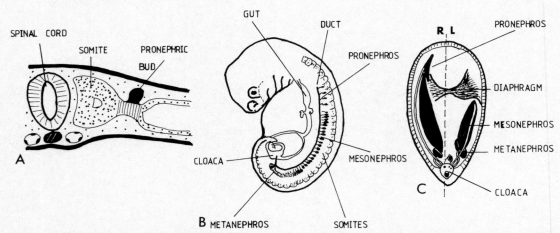

Figure 132–1. Development of the kidney and ureter. *A*, Transverse section. *B*, Sequential development of the three kidney types in mammals. *C*, Ventral dissection. The left side is drawn at a later stage than the right. (Reproduced with permission from Arey, L. B.: *Developmental Anatomy.* W. B. Saunders, Philadelphia, 1965.)

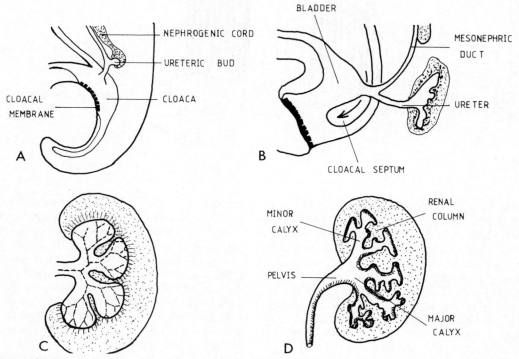

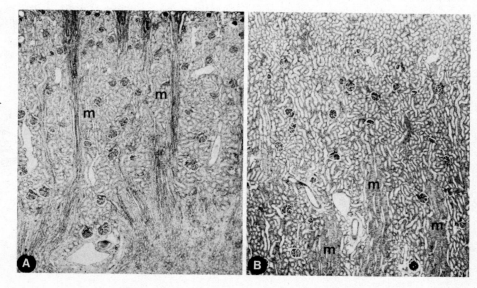

Figure 132–2. Development of the metanephros and drainage duct system. *A,* Ureteric bud from the mesonephric duct pushing into metanephrogenic cord. The cloacal membrane is the fused ectodermal/endodermal plate. *B,* A septum divides the cloaca into dorsal rectum and ventral urogenital sinus. *C* and *D,* The duct system is formed from repeated dichotomous branching. Absorption of the first 15 generations forms the pelvis and calyces. (*A, B,* and *D* reproduced with permission from Arey, L. B.: *Developmental Anatomy.* W. B. Saunders, Philadelphia, 1965.)

ulus differentiate at one end, whereas the other end becomes continuous with a nearby collecting duct.

Newer generations of nephrons develop centrifugally as the terminal ampulla grows toward the kidney capsule. From 12 to 15 nephrons ultimately attach to each of the terminal branches. It follows, therefore, that the subcapsular glomeruli are youngest. Nephron formation in each human kidney is finished at birth. Each kidney contains approximately 1,000,000 nephrons. Enlargement of the kidney after birth is due to maturation of nephrons already present. In the dog,[2] and presumably the cat, induction of more nephrons continues into the postnatal period.

Ascent of the Kidneys. The metanephros originates near the bifurcation of the aorta, but its definitive position is closer to the thoracolumbar junction. The cranial movement is brought about mostly by growth of the lumbosacral region as the marked curvature of the body of the embryo straightens out. As the kidneys ascend out of the pelvis, they rotate through

Figure 132–3. Photomicrograph of a dog's kidney to show the under-development of the outer cortex in a one-week-old pup (*A*) compared with a mature dog (*B*). The medullary rays (m) are prominent. H and E ×10.

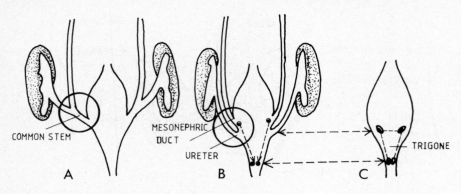

Figure 132–4. Differentiation of the cloaca. *A* and *B*, Growth and absorption of the ureter and mesonephric duct so that they acquire separate openings. These openings outline the bladder trigone (*C*).

90° so that the hilus faces medially rather than dorsally. In addition, the blood supply to the kidneys sequentially shifts from iliac arteries to the final point of origin off the aorta level with lumbar vertebral segments 2 and 3.

Lobation, Pyramids, and Lobules. As the cortex organizes over a primary pyramid, the boundary of the cortical cap is indicated by a deep groove on the surface of the kidney. Each primary pyramid, but not its papilla, subsequently divides into two or more secondary pyramids. The site of the secondary pyramids is also indicated on the surface of the kidney, giving it a lobed appearance. Fetal lobation in human kidneys progressively disappears in infancy and childhood as kidney growth causes the cortical cap on the pyramids to fuse. In the dog, the cortex and medullary pyramids fuse completely. The composite broad-based papilla is called the renal crest. Such kidneys are known as unipyramidal or unilobar kidneys even though they consist of several fused lobes. The feline kidney is a true unilobar kidney, as it contains only one lobe.

Within the lobes are found lobules. These are the functional units of the kidney containing all the uriniferous tubules whose collecting ducts course in a particular medullary (cortical) ray.

Cloacal Differentiation. The cloaca is the common endodermal chamber into which fecal, urinary, and reproductive products pass. Reptiles, birds, and non-placental mammals retain this organ. In placental mammals the cloaca is further subdivided into dorsal rectum, ventral bladder, and urogenital sinus by the growth of a wedge-shaped mesenchymal mass called the cloacal septum (see Fig. 132–2B). When this reaches the cloacal membrane (the fused ectodermal/endodermal plate), the membrane ruptures, exposing the projecting wedge, which is now called the perineal body. The perineal body merges with the lateral folds flanking the fissure that was left when the cloacal membrane was resorbed. This area becomes covered by advancing ectoderm and fuses at the median raphe. When the bladder is first formed, it still receives on either side the common stem of a mesonephric duct and ureter (Fig. 132–4A). Growth now occurs with absorption of these stems so that the four ducts acquire individual openings (Fig. 132–4B). The mesonephric ducts are displaced caudally and open close together on an elevation in the future urethra known as Müller's tubercle, or seminal colliculus. The triangular area on the dorsal wall of the bladder and urethra demarcated by these ducts is the trigone (Fig. 132–4C).

With further growth the bladder expands into an elongated sac. It has a tapering cranial extremity leading to the urachus, which is continuous at the umbilicus with the allantois. The caudal extremity, the neck, is continuous with the urethra.

The urogenital sinus (Fig. 132–5A) has pelvic and phallic portions. In the female, the short neck connecting the bladder and urogenital sinus elongates

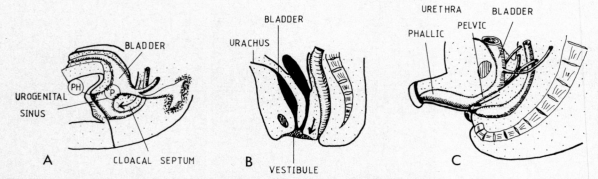

Figure 132–5. A, Development of the urogenital sinus with its pelvic (P) and phallic (PH) portions. *B,* In the female, the pelvic and phallic portions merge to create the vestibule. *C,* In the male, the phallic portion of the sinus forms the penile urethra. (Reproduced with permission from Arey, L. B.: *Developmental Anatomy.* W. B. Saunders, Philadelphia, 1965.)

into the permanent urethra (Fig. 132–5*B*), and the pelvic and phallic portions of the sinus merge to create the slitlike vestibule. The female urethra does not extend into the clitoris. In the male, the prostatic urethra between the bladder neck and Müller's tubercle is equivalent to the entire female urethra. The pelvic portion of the urogenital sinus completes the prostatic and all the membranous urethra (Fig. 132–5*C*). The phallic portion of the sinus contributes the penile urethra, which extends through the penis to the exterior.

Abnormal Development

Renal Agenesis. This can occur if the mesonephric ducts fail to develop or if no ureteric bud forms. It is primarily the branching ureteric bud penetrating into the metanephrogenic tissue that stimulates the development of nephrons. That is, in true renal agenesis, there is no ureter.

Supernumerary Kidneys. If two ureteric buds grow from the same mesonephric duct, supernumerary kidneys will result. Separate renal development is induced around each duct system. In this situation, the upper metanephric duct drains the upper (cranial) part of the kidney and the lower drains the caudal region. The upper duct is usually ectopic, since it migrates with the mesonephric duct into the urethra.[7]

Renal Hypoplasia. This is a deficiency in the total nephron population. A defect in the "inducer capability" of the ureteric bud or in the nephrogenic cord can produce renal abnormalities.[31] With extreme sites of ureteral ectopia, the abnormally placed bud unites with defective involuting nephrogenic or stromagenic mesenchymal tissue leading to hypoplasia and dysplasia. Dysplasia refers to the presence of abnormal nephrons. Normal renal parenchymal development is also impaired by complete obstruction of the urinary tract but not by incomplete obstruction.[31]

Nonascent of the Kidneys. This can affect one or both kidneys. The kidney remains in its primary pelvic position.

High Renal Ectopia. This can result in an intrathoracic kidney.[24] The diaphragm does not form completely until about eight weeks of gestation in human beings. Continued ascent of the kidney exerts pressure on the incompletely formed diaphragm, displacing it anteriorly and producing a thin membrane covering the cranial pole of the kidney.

Fused Kidneys. If during development the ureteric buds take a converging course, fused kidneys may result. The fused kidneys might or might not ascend properly.

Renal Polycystic Disease. The traditional anatomical explanation attributes renal cysts to nonunion of secretory and collecting tubules.[18] The blind secretory tubules dilate and become cysts. It is now known as a result of microdissection studies that polycystic disease can be due to dilatation and hyperplasia of collecting ducts, inhibited ampullary activity with failure to induce nephrons, or multiple abnormalities

in the ureteric bud derivatives and the nephrons.[28] The developing cysts apply pressure to surrounding normal tubules and compromise their function.

Ureteral ectopia. In the male, the bladder neck, prostatic urethra, seminal vesicles, and vas deferens all develop from the mesonephric duct and urogenital sinus. If the ureter buds off the mesonephric duct too far cranially, then with growth and absorption the metanephric duct (ureter) might not open separately into the bladder. It can be carried caudally to open into the vas deferens, seminal vesicles, or urethra.[30] The same explanation accounts for ureters that open into the bladder neck or urethra in females and also accounts for the upper (cranial) ureter being ectopic when the ureters are duplicated, as the lower (caudal) metanephric duct is absorbed normally into the bladder wall. It is less certain how ureters can open into the vagina, cervix, or uterus, as these structures are Müllerian duct derivatives. One explanation is that part of the vagina is derived from the mesonephric system and urogenital sinus.[6] However, embryological connection through Gartner's duct, a wolffian derivative that normally atrophies and disappears, is the most common explanation of an ectopic opening into the cervix and uterus.[14] In man, rare cases of an ectopic ureteral opening into the rectum have been reported.[23] Such an abnormality could be accounted for by faulty division of the cloaca by the cloacal septum.

Ureterocele. A ureterocele is a cystic dilatation of the intravesicular portion of the ureter. It may be related to a congenitally small ("pinpoint") ureteral meatus due to faulty mesonephric duct development. Urine pressure builds up, and the bladder mucosa over the region of the submucosal ureter bulges. Ureteroceles can also occur when the ureteral orifice or meatus is large. This usually occurs in an ectopic ureter. The distal portion of the ureter expands in response to the same stimulus that causes the fetal bladder to expand.[33]

Faulty Differentiation of the Cloaca. This can result in incomplete separation of the rectum and urogenital sinus. The outcome is a rectovestibular fistula in the female or a rectovesicular or rectourethral fistula in the male (Fig. 132–6). If invasion by

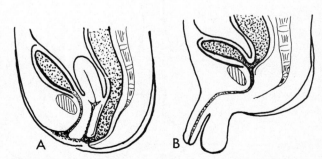

Figure 132–6. Faulty separation of the rectum and urogenital sinus can lead to rectovestibular fistula in the female (*A*) and rectourethral fistula in the male (*B*). (Reproduced with permission from Arey, L. B.: *Developmental Anatomy.* W. B. Saunders, Philadelphia, 1965.)

somatic mesoderm fails to reduce the extensive cranial extent of the early cloacal membrane (see Fig. 132–2), subsequent rupture of the membrane exposes the lining of the bladder. This condition is known as exstrophy of the bladder.

GROSS ANATOMY OF THE URINARY SYSTEM

Overview[9, 15, 36]

When the abdomen of a dog is opened and explored, most of the "within-body" urinary apparatus can be seen (Fig. 132–7). For a more complete view, the floor of the pelvis has to be removed. The renal artery, vein, and ureter enter the medial border of the kidney through a fissure called the hilus. The hilus leads to a central recess, the renal sinus, which is lined by a continuation of the kidney capsule and contains much fat. Lymph vessels and renal nerves are closely related to the renal vein and artery,

respectively. Because the aorta and vena cava lie side by side with the aorta to the left of the cava, the left kidney has a relatively long renal vein and the right kidney a relatively long renal artery.

The ureters, like the kidneys, are retroperitoneal structures. They run caudomedially along the sublumbar muscles toward the bladder. As they approach the pelvic inlet, they leave the sublumbar position and gain access to the bladder between the two layers of peritoneum that form the lateral ligaments of the bladder. The spermatic or ovarian vessels cross the cranial ureter ventrally, but the deep circumflex iliac vessels cross the caudal ureter dorsally.

Radiographic Anatomy

Contrast agents infused into the lower urinary tract or excreted into the upper urinary tract outline the urinary apparatus (Fig. 132–8). An intravenous pyelogram opacifies the entire kidney parenchyma, renal pelvis, and ureters. A pneumocystogram highlights

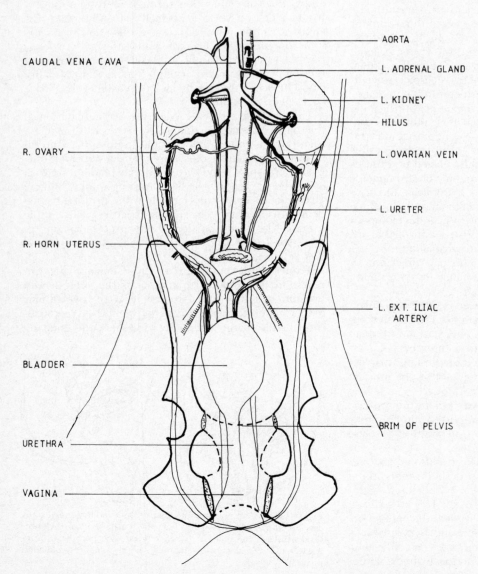

Figure 132–7. The relationships of the urinary and genital apparatus to each other and to the bony pelvis in the female dog.

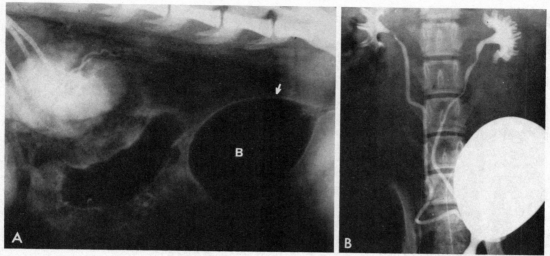

Figure 132–8. *A,* Intravenous urogram in a cat to show the point of entry of the ureters (arrow) into the bladder (B). *B,* Cystogram and retrograde pyelogram outlining the urinary apparatus in a young male dog.

the thin-walled bladder and provides negative contrast against which the ureterovesical junction can be seen. A retrograde pyelogram outlines the renal pelvis and ureters. Finally, a positive contrast voiding cystogram indicates bladder volume and shape and also the capacity of the bladder neck and proximal urethra to dilate.

Kidneys

Topography

The topographical anatomy of the kidneys is well illustrated in canine whole-body longitudinal, horizontal, and transverse sections (Fig. 132–9). The kidneys are retroperitoneal. The cranial pole of each kidney is covered with peritoneum on both dorsal and ventral surfaces, but only the ventral surface of the caudal pole is covered. The kidneys are embedded in adipose tissue and are held in the sublumbar position by subperitoneal fibroareolar tissue or renal fascia. Ventrally, this renal fascia is continuous with the connective tissue around the aorta and caudal vena cava. Medially and dorsally, it is attached to the thoracolumbar fascia. The fixation is not rigid. Both kidneys are displaced by movement of the diaphragm during respiration. The right kidney is related to the liver and is firmly attached. The left kidney is less firmly attached and can be displaced caudally by a full stomach. In cats, both kidneys are equally mobile.

Characteristics

The characteristic features of the kidneys of dogs and cats are summarized in Table 132–1. Both cat and dog have bean-shaped, unipyramidal or unilobar kidneys. The feline kidney has only one lobe, but the canine kidney contains a number of fused lobes.[12]

Canine kidneys are brown-red to brown-blue in color, depending on the degree of oxygenation of the blood they contain. Feline kidneys are red to yellow-red in color because of a large amount of intracellular fat stored in the proximal convoluted tubules.[16] Lipid content is greatest in mature cats, castrated males, and pregnant females. Feline kidneys are comparatively large, representing 0.6 to 1.0 per cent of body weight, compared with 0.6 per cent of body weight for dogs.[29] Many investigators have measured the size of normal kidneys of dogs and cats from radiographs.[11, 22, 34] The most recent study[22] recorded measurements from lateral radiographs on 167 dogs and 33 cats. Length varied between 2.5 and 3.2

TABLE 132–1. Characteristic Features of the Kidneys

Feature	Dog	Cat
Type	Unipyramidal (fused pyramids)	Unipyramidal (single pyramid)
Weight per kidney (gm)	50 to 60	7.5 to 15
Color	Brown-red to red-blue	Red to yellow-red
Kidney mass as a percentage of body weight	0.6	0.6 to 1.0
Total nephrons per kidney	415,000	190,000
Kidney length in proportion to length of lumbar vertebra (L_2)	2.9	2.7
Kidney width in proportion to length of L_2	1.6	1.7
Ventral displacement in proportion to length of L_2	L 0.7 R 0.3	0.7 0.7

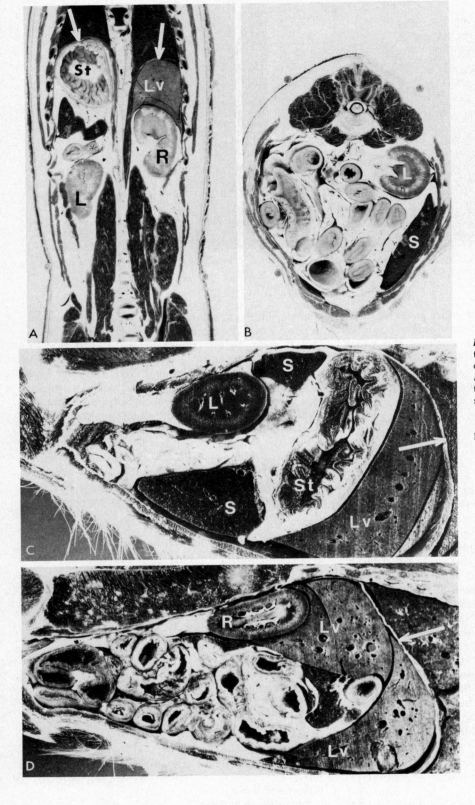

Figure 132–9. Frozen whole body sections of dogs to show the topography of the kidneys. *A*, Horizontal section. *B*, Transverse section. *C*, Left longitudinal section. *D*, Right longitudinal section. St = stomach; s = spleen; L = left kidney; R = right kidney; Lv = liver; arrows = line of the diaphragm.

lumbar vertebrae in dogs and 2.5 to 3.0 in cats. Width ranged from 1.4 to 1.8 for dogs and 1.6 to 1.9 for cats. That is, feline kidneys are shorter and broader than canine kidneys. This study also showed that kidneys from male dogs were proportionally larger than those from female dogs and that the kidneys from immature dogs were proportionally larger than those from mature dogs.

The measured ventral displacement of the kidney from the line of the lumbar vertebrae indicates that the right kidney of the dog is less likely to be displaced that the left, whereas both kidneys of the cat are equally mobile.

Structure

The adipose capsule that envelopes the kidney (see Fig. 132–9) varies in thickness with the nutritional state of the animal. The surface of the canine kidney is smooth, but that of the cat is grooved owing to the presence of large subcapsular veins that join the renal vein at the hilus (Fig. 132–10A and B).

Longitudinal midsagittal sections of canine and feline kidneys demonstrate their gross internal structure (Fig. 132–10C). The outer region, the cortex, is granular owing to the presence of glomeruli. The cortex also contains many radially directed striations of medullary substance called medullary rays. The inner region, the medulla, is paler than the cortex and divides into outer and inner zones at the point where the ascending thin loop of Henle gives way to the thick loop of Henle. The inner zone, the papilla in the cat or renal crest in the dog, projects into the renal pelvis. This region contains only thin loops of Henle, collecting ducts, and blood vessels. The renal crest is wedge shaped with a long craniocaudal axis. Clay models of the renal crest of a dog show transversely oriented fingerlike ridges that project from each side of the renal crest into the pelvic cavity.[5]

Kidney sections dorsal or ventral to the longitudinal axis of the crest (Fig. 132–10D) cut the transverse ridges and expose the recesses (diverticulae) of the renal pelvis, simulating a multipyramidal kidney with calyces. The feline kidney also has recesses in its medullary pyramid. These recesses are related more to the presence of "interlobar" blood vessels than to well-developed medullary transverse ridges. The renal pelvis is shaped like an everted umbrella and is adapted to the configuration of the ridged renal crest. The perimeter of attachment of the pelvis to the medulla courses over each ridge, thus creating a scalloped configuration and simulating a calyceal pattern on pyelography (see Fig. 132–8).

Figure 132–10. Dog and cat kidneys. *A*, With capsule in place. Capsular vessels and capsular fat are prominent features. *B*, With capsule removed, the surface of the dog kidney is smooth, whereas that of the cat shows prominent subcapsular veins. *C*, Midsagittal sections illustrate the renal crest (RC) in the dog and papilla (P) in the cat. The arrows point to the arcuate vessels. *D*, Sagittal sections to one side of the midline cut through the transverse ridges on the renal crest of the dog, simulating a multipyramidal kidney. The arrows point to the interlobar arteries, which in the cat also groove the medulla and simulate a multipyramidal kidney.

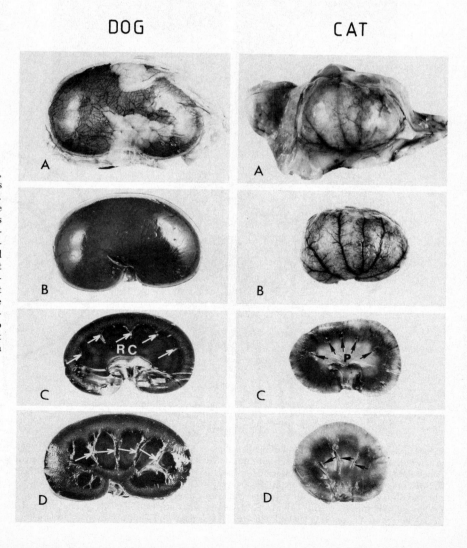

DOG   CAT

Vasculature

Arterial Circulation. After the renal artery leaves the aorta, it bifurcates into dorsal and ventral branches (Fig. 132–11A and B). Each branch gives rise to five to seven interlobar arteries. These travel between the medullary ridges outside the pelvic diverticulae and branch into arcuate arteries at the corticomedullary junction. The arcuate arteries radiate toward the periphery of the cortex, giving rise to radially directed interlobular arteries, the smallest arteries that can be readily identified by renal angiography. These arteries supply the afferent arterioles of the glomerulus.

Multiple renal arteries (Fig. 132–11D) have been

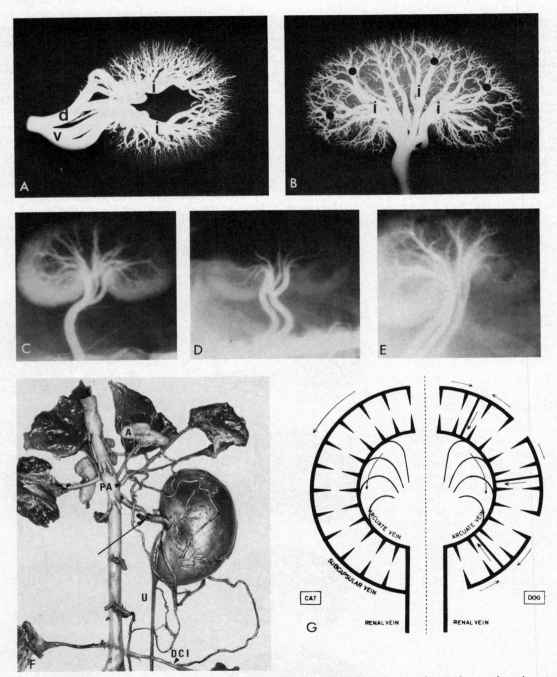

Figure 132–11. Vasculature of the kidney of a dog. *A*, Angiogram in the transverse plane showing the renal artery branching into dorsal (d) and ventral (v) branches and then into interlobar branches (i). *B*, Angiogram in the lateral plane indicating where the arcuate vessels (black dots) arise from from the interlobar vessels (i). *C–E*, Angiograms indicating single (*C*), double (*D*), and triple (*E*) renal arteries. *F*, Specimen from a dog. The right renal artery was gradually occluded, and the left kidney excised. *A* = Adrenal gland; *PA* = phrenicoabdominal trunk; *arrow* = ligated right renal artery; *U* = ureter; *DCI* = deep circumflex iliac artery. Note prominent collateral vessels on the surface of the kidney. *G*, Diagram showing the different vein systems of dog and cat kidneys. (*G* reproduced with permission from Nissen. O. I.: *The Function of Superficial and Deep Areas of Cat Kidney.* Costers Bogtrykkeri, Virum, 1969.)

observed in the left kidney in 13 per cent of dogs[29, 32] but are uncommon in cats. A single renal artery to the right kidney occurs in most dogs.

Although the renal arteries are usually described as "end arteries," a significant number of interlobar and arcuate arteries in dogs perforate the renal substance and make vascular connections with the adrenal gland, phrenicoabdominal trunk, deep circumflex iliac artery, caudal mesenteric artery, spermatic artery, and ureteral artery.[9] These vessels form an arterial circle around the kidney. They can hypertrophy (see Fig. 132–11F) and provide an alternative blood supply if renal artery flow is gradually obstructed.

Venous Drainage. Venous drainage of the kidney has deep and superficial components.[26] Capillary beds in the outer cortex drain toward the surface by superficial cortical veins, which join stellate veins beneath and within the capsule in the dog and cat. Interlobular veins drain the stellate veins into the arcuate and major renal veins in the dog, but in the cat they converge and drain via a second route into the renal vein at the hilus (Fig. 132–11G). The deeper cortical capillaries drain into deep cortical veins and from there to the renal vein. In dogs, the left renal vein also receives the left ovarian vein.[15]

Lymphatics. Renal capsular and parenchymal lymphatics are connected to interlobular plexes, which converge and leave the kidney at the hilus to terminate in the lumbar lymph nodes.[15, 35]

Innervation

Autonomic sympathetic innervation to the kidney comes from ganglia in the region of the celiac and phrenicoabdominal arteries and lumbar splanchnic nerves to form a plexus around the renal arteries. Branches of the dorsal vagal trunk (parasympathetic) also join the renal plexus.[15]

Microstructure

Medullary rays (see Fig. 132–3) form the core of the kidney lobule.[17] The core of the medullary ray is the branched collecting tubule, which receives filtrate from the many nephrons that surround it (Fig. 132–12). The medullary ray also contains descending and ascending limbs of the *loops of Henle*. Mammals have long and short loops of Henle named according to whether the U-bend occurs in the outer or inner medulla, respectively. The relative proportion of each loop depends on the species (see Chapter 133). The loops of Henle in dogs and cats are all long loops.[26] After the *efferent arteriole* leaves the vascular pole of Bowman's capsule, it forms a peritubular plexus around the uriniferous tubules of the cortex. The efferent network has many anastomotic links. Single nephron perfusion depends on the efferents of many glomeruli. The efferent arterioles of the juxtamedullary glomeruli descend into the medulla along straight paths to form a network around the medullary urin-

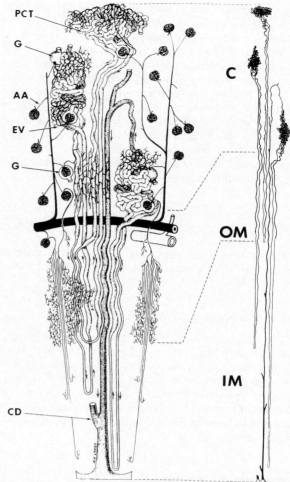

Figure 132–12. Arrangement of nephrons and collecting ducts in the kidney. C = Cortex; OM = outer medulla; IM = inner medulla; PCT = proximal convoluted tubules; G = glomeruli; AA = afferent arteriole; EV = efferent vessel; CD = collecting duct. (Reproduced with permission from Beeuwkes, R. III: The vascular organization of the kidney. Ann. Rev. Physiol., 42:531, 1980.)

iferous tubules. Venules from this capillary network return blood to the interlobular veins and arcuate veins and from there to the renal vein.[3] When a glomerular tuft invaginates into the expanded proximal end of the nephron, a *renal corpuscle* is formed. A renal corpuscle consists of the glomerular capillaries plus the parietal and visceral layers of Bowman's capsule.

The glomerular capillary is lined by fenestrated endothelial cells that lie on a basement membrane. The visceral layer of Bowman's capsule consists of highly specialized epithelial cells called podocytes. Foot processes on the podocytes interdigitate with each other and are separated by filtration slits, or pores. The site where the afferent and efferent arterioles enter and leave glomeruli is the vascular pole. At this site, the ascending limb of the loop of Henle of each nephron returns to the glomerulus of that nephron before it continues on as the distal convoluted tubule. There is a concentration of nuclei where the tubule touches the root of the glomerulus and the afferent arteriole. This group of cells is the macula densa. Between it and the glomerulus is an aggregation of smaller cells termed the *polar cushion*, or laser cells. In some parts of the glomerulus, the basement membrane derived from epithelial cells does not completely surround each capillary. Support is provided by mesangial cells, which also have phagocytic and contractile properties. The cells of the media of the afferent arteriole in the region of the glomerular root have rounded nuclei and contain granules. They are called juxtaglomerular cells and, together with the cells of the macula densa, form the juxtaglomerular complex.

Ureter

The ureters are retroperitoneal urine conduits that pursue a relatively tortuous route to the bladder (see Fig. 132–8).

The Ureteropelvic Junction

The ureter expands within the renal sinus in the dog and cat to form the renal pelvis. The periphery of the renal pelvis is adapted to the configuration of the ridged renal crest, giving it a scalloped appearance on pyelography (see Fig. 132–8). The pelvic diverticulae simulate calyces radiographically, but since the kidneys of the dog and cat are unipyramidal, calyces are not found.

Ureterovesical Junction

Ureters must be long enough to reach their point of attachment to an empty bladder retracted within the bony pelvis. As the bladder fills with urine it becomes an intra-abdominal organ. The angle of approach of the ureter to the bladder must pass beyond 90° and may even strongly recurve (Fig. 132–13). When the ureter pierces the bladder wall, it loses its outer layer of circular muscle and is surrounded by a connective tissue sheath into which detrusor muscle fasicles insert. This is the principle means by which the ureter is connected to the bladder.[8] The ureter reaches a submucosal position and runs obliquely toward the bladder neck.

The ureteral orifices are characteristically horseshoe shaped and form the base limits of the bladder trigone. The long, narrow submucosal ureter acts as a flap valve to prevent vesicoureteral reflux as bladder hydrostatic pressure is raised above ureteral peristaltic pressure.

Vessels and Nerves

The ureter has a cranial blood supply from the renal artery and a caudal blood supply from the prostatic or vaginal arteries. Cranial and caudal ureteral arteries anastomose on the ureter in the outer

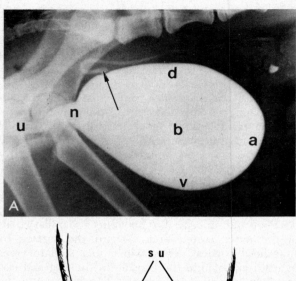

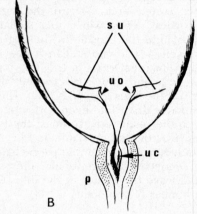

Figure 132–13. Ureterovesicular junction. *A,* Cystogram and ureterogram showing the ureter entering the bladder on its dorsal surface *(d)*, near the bladder neck *(n)*. Other regions of the bladder are identified as body *(b)*, apex *(a)*, ventral surface *(v)*, and proximal urethra *(u)*. *B,* Mucosal view of the dorsal half of the bladder of a young male dog, showing submucosal ureters *(su)*, ureteral orifices *(uo)*, urethral colliculus *(uc)*, and prostate gland *(p)*.

layers of adventitia.[25] Additional supply from surrounding vessels frequently joins the ureteral artery.[9]

Autonomic nerves supply the ureter, but their function is not clear, since ureteral peristalsis is not propagated by nervous impulses as it is in the gut but is myogenic in origin.[20]

Bladder

The bladder is a urine reservoir that varies in form, size, and position, depending on the volume of urine it contains. The bladder (see Fig. 132–13A) has a neck (vesicourethral junction), a body, and a vertex (apex). The body has dorsal (roof) and ventral (floor) surfaces. The fundus (base), used as a descriptive term in human anatomy, is equivalent to the dorsocaudal region of the body of the bladder of a dog. This term is appropriate for man, since it relates to an erect posture, but it is an inappropriate term for quadrupeds. The distended bladder lies on the floor of the abdomen and occupies a considerable volume of the abdominal cavity (Fig. 132–14A). The bladder of dogs and cats has a peritoneal covering over the entire bladder and bladder neck (Fig. 132–14*B* and *C*). Peritoneal reflections (lateral ligaments) attach the bladder to the lateral abdominal wall and ventral abdominal wall (median ligament). Obliquely ori-

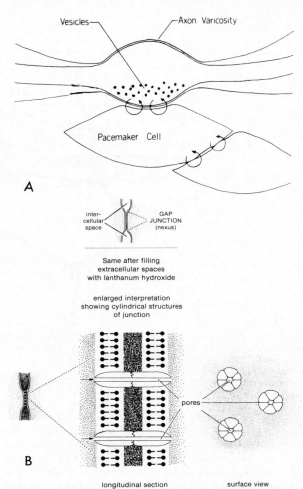

Figure 132–15. Electrical conduction in the bladder. *A,* Electrical impulses are generated at axon varicosities. *B,* The pacemaker cell depolarizes, and impulses pass to adjacent smooth muscle cells through areas of close contact called gap junctions. (*A* reproduced with permission from Bradley, W. E., Timm, G. W., and Scott, F. B.: Innervation of the detrusor muscle and urethra. Urol. Clin. North Am. *1*:3, 1974. *B* reproduced with permission from Ham, A. W., and Cormack, D. H.: *Histology*, 8th ed. J. B. Lippincott, Philadelphia, 1979.)

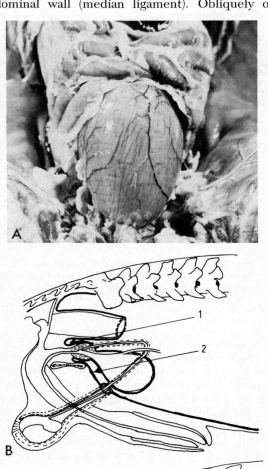

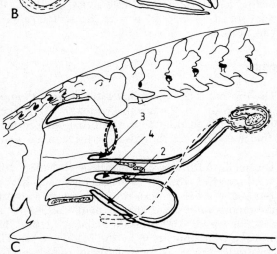

Figure 132–14. Location of the bladder in a dog. *A,* The ventral body wall has been removed to show the position of a full bladder. *B* and *C,* Longitudinal sections of male *(B)* and female *(C)* dogs showing the peritoneal covering of the bladder. Peritoneal reflections form the rectovesicular pouch *(1)* and the pubovesicular pouch *(2)*. In the female, the presence of the uterus divides the rectovesical pouch into the rectogenital pouch *(3)* and vesicogenital pouch *(4)*. (*B* and *C* modified from Evans, H. E., and Christensen, G. C.: *Miller's Anatomy of the Dog*, 2nd ed. W. B. Saunders, Philadelphia, 1979.)

ented detrusor muscle fascicles are continuous with urethral smooth muscle at the bladder neck.[21, 38] When the detrusor muscle is relaxed, the deployment of fibers at the vesicourethral junction constricts the bladder neck. This action is assisted by a concentration of submucosal elastic tissue in the region. Thus, the internal urinary sphincter is formed. It should be noted, however, that although a constriction is present at the bladder neck, the region is not an anatomical sphincter. Alpha-adrenergic receptors are found in the bladder neck and proximal urethra. These receptors are active during the late phase of bladder filling, indicating that sympathetic stimulation of the smooth muscle of this region contributes to urine continence. (Refer to Chapters 133 and 134 for physiology and pathophysiology of bladder function.)

Electrical conduction within the bladder is along each smooth muscle fiber.[4] There are few neuromuscular junctions in visceral smooth muscle. Those that are present are of the axon varicosity type rather than

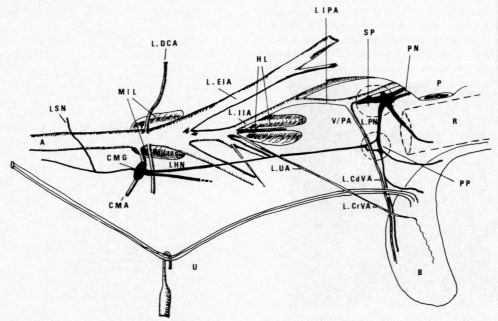

Figure 132–16. Blood and nerve supply to the bladder of a dog, viewed from the ventral surface with the bladder and left ureter displaced to the right. The prefix L stands for left. The suffix A stands for artery and N for nerve. *Arteries:* A = aorta; *CM* = caudal mesenteric; *CdV* = caudal vesical; *CrV* = cranial vesical; *DC* = deep circumflex iliac; *EI* = external iliac; *II* = internal iliac; *IP* = internal pudendal; *UA* = umbilical; *V/P* = vaginal or prostatic. *Nerves:* H = hypogastric; *SN* = lumbar splanchnic; *LPN* = pelvic; *PN* = pudendal. *Plexus: PP* = pelvic; *SP* = sacral. *Ganglion = CMG* = caudal mesenteric. *Lymph nodes: HL* = hypogastric; *MIL* = middle iliac.

the motor end-plate of skeletal muscle. When depolarization occurs in a "pacemaker" cell, impulses cross from one fiber to the next at areas of close apposition of their cell membranes (Fig. 132–15). These junctions (nexuses) are areas of low electrical resistance and are probably of the "gap junction type"[17] rather than the "tight junction type," as stated by others.[4]

Vessels and Nerves

The blood supply and innervation to the bladder of a female dog are shown in Figure 132–16. Close to its origin, the internal iliac artery gives rise to the umbilical artery. The lumen of this artery is obliterated in 50 per cent of adult dogs, forming the lateral umbilical ligament. In the remaining 50 per cent of adult dogs, the artery continues patent and supplies the cranial end of the bladder as the cranial vesical artery. The internal iliac artery branches into caudal gluteal and internal pudendal arteries. The vaginal (or prostatic) branch of the internal pudendal artery lies in the pelvic fascia with the pelvic plexus of nerves approximately level with the brim of the pelvis. Arising from this vessel is the major supply to the bladder, the caudal vesical artery, which also gives rise to the caudal ureteral artery.

The plexus of veins drain into the vaginal (or prostatic) vein, a satellite of the artery, and then into the internal iliac vein.

The bladder lymphatics drain into the hypogastric nodes, which lie in the angle between the internal iliac and median sacral arteries, and the lumbar lymph nodes, which are variably located along the aorta and caudal vena cava.[15]

The nerve supply of the urinary bladder[4] is via the pelvic parasympathetic nerves, which stimulate contraction of the detrusor muscle, and the hypogastric sympathetic nerves, which help maintain bladder neck tone. Nerve trunks from the pelvic plexus pass into the bladder adventitia near the ureters. They follow a tortuous course, pass into smooth muscle fascicles, and terminate as free nerve endings. Pudendal somatic innervation is to the striated muscle of the external urethral sphincter.

Urethra

The urethra is the canal that extends from the neck of the bladder to the urethral meatus. It conveys urine from the bladder to the external environment. In the male, the urethra also carries seminal secretions.

The male urethra is shown for the dog (Fig. 132–17) and cat (Fig. 132–18). The bladder neck is short in the dog and the urethra is divisible into prostatic, membranous, and cavernous or penile segments. In the cat, however, the prostate gland is located 3 or 4 cm from what appears to be the bladder neck. This preprostatic region has been variably called an elongated bladder neck[13] or a preprostatic portion of the membranous urethra.[10] Histological examination of these two regions shows no striated muscle surrounding the preprostatic "membranous urethra," but striated muscle is present around the true membranous urethra. Anatomically, therefore, the region is bladder neck, and the term *elongated bladder neck* is quite appropriate.

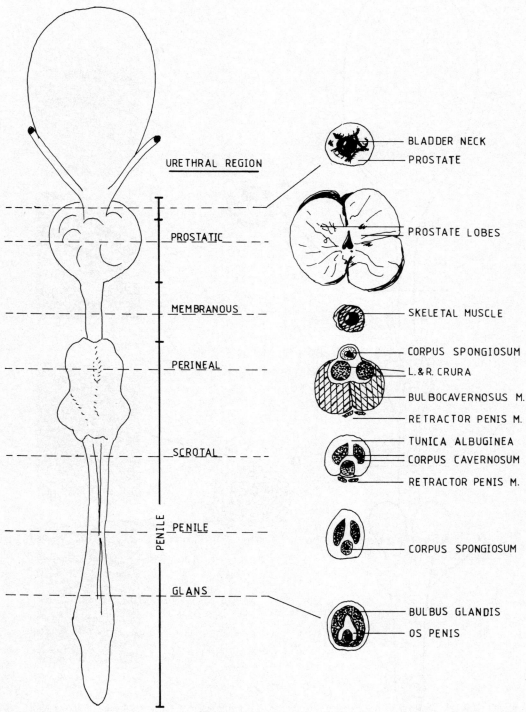

Figure 132–17. Structure of the urethra in the male dog. Transverse sections are drawn from the levels indicated in the diagram. Note that the membranous urethra has a large, transversely oriented skeletal muscle component.

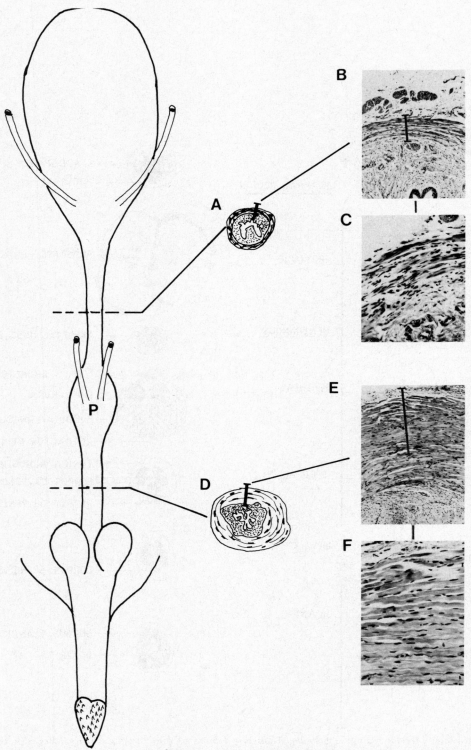

Figure 132–18. Urinary apparatus of a male cat. *A*, Transverse section of the elongated bladder neck. *B* and *C*, Photomicrographs indicate that the major component of the wall is smooth muscle. *B* H and E ×40, *C* H and E ×100. *D*, Transverse section of the membranous urethra shows a dense outer skeletal muscle layer. *E* and *F*, Photomicrographs. *E* H and E ×40, *F* H and E ×100.

1. Arey, L. B.: *Developmental Anatomy*, 7th ed. W. B. Saunders, Philadelphia, 1965, p. 295.
2. Banks, W. J.: *Applied Veterinary Histology*. Williams & Wilkins, Baltimore, 1981, p. 424.
3. Beeuwkes, R. III: The vascular organization of the kidney. Ann. Rev. Physiol. 42:531, 1980.
4. Bradley, W. E., Timm, G. W., and Scott, F. B.: Innervation of the detrusor muscle and urethra. Urol. Clin. North Am. 1:3, 1974.
5. Brodsky, S. L., Dure-Smith, P., and Zimskind, P. D.: Gross and radiological anatomy of the canine kidney. Invest. Urol. 14:356, 1977.
6. Bulmer, D.: The development of the human vagina. J. Anat. 91:490, 1957.
7. Campbell, M. F.: Anomalies of the ureter. *In* Campbell, M. F., and Harrison, J. H. (eds.): *Urology*, Vol. 2, 3rd ed. W. B. Saunders, Philadelphia, 1970, p. 1493.
8. Christie, B. A.: The ureterovesical junction in dogs. Invest. Urol. 9:10, 1971.
9. Christie, B. A.: Collateral arterial blood supply to the normal and ischemic canine kidney. Am. J. Vet. Res. 41:519, 1980.
10. Crouch, J. E.: *Text-Atlas of Cat Anatomy*. Lea & Febiger, Philadelphia, 1969, p. 167.
11. Douglas, S. W., and Williamson, H. D.: *Principles of Veterinary Radiography*, 2nd ed. Williams & Wilkins, Baltimore, 1972.
12. Ellenport, C. R.: Carnivore urogenital apparatus. *In* Getty, R. (ed.): *Sisson and Grossman's The Anatomy of the Domestic Animals*, Vol. 2. W. B. Saunders, Philadelphia, 1975, p. 1576.
13. Elliot, R.: *Reighard and Jennings Anatomy of the Cat*, 3rd ed. Holt, Rinehart and Winston, New York, 1935.
14. Emmett, J. L.: *Clinical Urography*, 2nd ed. W. B. Saunders, Philadelphia, 1964.
15. Evans, H. E., and Christensen, G. C.: *Miller's Anatomy of the Dog*, 2nd ed. W. B. Saunders, Philadelphia, 1979, pp. 544, 551, 554.
16. Finco, D. R., Kneller, S. K., and Crowell, W. A.: Diseases of the urinary system. *In* Catcott, E. J. (ed.): *Feline Medicine and Surgery*, 2nd ed. American Veterinary Publications Inc., Santa Barbara, 1975, p. 251.
17. Ham, A. W., and Cormack, D. H.: *Histology*, 8th ed. J. B. Lippincott, Philadelphia, 1979, pp. 200, 757.
18. Hildebrant, A.: Weiterer Beitrag zur pathologischen Anatomie der Nierengeschwülste. Arch. Klin. Chir. 48:343, 1894.
19. Hilderbrand, M.: Analysis of vertebrate structure. John Wiley and Sons, New York, 1974, p. 303.
20. Kiil, F.: Physiology of the renal pelvis and ureter. *In* Campbell, M. F., and Harrison, J. H. (eds.): *Urology*, Vol. 1, 3rd ed. W. B. Saunders, Philadelphia, 1970, p. 72.
21. Kirulata, H. G., Downie, J. W., and Awad, S. A.: The continence mechanisms. The effect of bladder filling on the urethra. Invest. Urol. 18:460, 1981.
22. Lee, R., and Leowijuk, C.: Normal parameters in abdominal radiology of the dog and cat. J. Small Anim. Pract. 23:251, 1982.
23. Lepoutre, M. C.: Sur un cas d'absence congenitale de la vessie. J. Urol. Méd. Chir. 48:334, 1939.
24. Malter, I. J., and Stanley, R. J.: The intrathoracic kidney. J. Urol. 107:538, 1972.
25. Mingledorff, W. E., Rinker, J. R., and Owen, G.: Experimental study of the blood supply of the distal ureter with reference to cutaneous ureterostomy. J. Urol. 92:424, 1964.
26. Nissen, O. I.: *The Function of Superficial and Deep Areas of the Cat Kidney*. Costers Bogtrykkeri, Virum, 1969.
27. Osathanondh, V., and Potter, E. L.: Development of human kidney as shown by microdissection. Arch. Pathol. 76:271, 1963.
28. Osathanondh, V., and Potter, E. L.: Pathogenesis of polycystic kidneys. Arch. Pathol. 77:459, 1964.
29. Osborne, C. A., Low, D. G., and Finco, D. R.: *Canine and Feline Urology*. W. B. Saunders, Philadelphia, 1972, p. 3.
30. Owen, R. R.: Canine ureteral ectopia—a review. 1. Embryology and aetiology. J. Small Anim. Pract. 14:407, 1973.
31. Schwartz, R. D., Stephens, F. D., and Cussen, L. J.: The pathogenesis of renal dysplasia, II and III. Invest. Urol. 19:97, 101, 1981.
32. Shively, M. J.: Origin and branching of renal arteries in the dog. J. Am. Vet. Med. Assoc. 173:986, 1978.
33. Stephens, F. D.: Caecoureterocele and concepts on the embryology and aetiology of ureteroceles. Aust. N.Z. J. Surg. 40:239, 1971.
34. Suter, P. F.: Portal vein anomalies in the dog. Their angiographic diagnosis. J. Am. Vet. Radiol. Soc. 16:84, 1975.
35. Trautmann, A., and Fiebiger, J.: *Fundamentals of the Histology of Domestic Animals* (translated and revised from the 8th and 9th German editions, 1949, by Habel, R. E., and Biberstein, E. L.). Comstock Publishing Assoc., Ithaca, 1952.
36. Warwick, R., and Williams, P. L.: *Gray's Anatomy*, 35th ed. Longman Group Ltd., Edinburgh, 1973.
37. Webster, D., and Webster, M.: *Comparative Vertebrate Morphology*. Academic Press, New York, 1974, p. 427.
38. Woodburne, R. T.: Anatomy of the bladder and bladder outlet. J. Urol. 100:474, 1968.

Chapter **133**

Physiology of the Urinary Tract

Bruce A. Christie and Anne Rosin

Markowitz once said that "ultimately, physiology may become an account of biological reactions in terms of physics and chemistry."[25] The aim of this chapter is to examine the basic anatomical and biological aspects of physiology and to correlate structure (Chapter 132) with function.[16, 36]

BASIC RENAL PROCESSES

In the kidneys, blood is pumped through the glomerular capillaries and a fluid resembling plasma is filtered. As the filtrate passes down the tubules, its composition is altered. Water and solutes are re-absorbed and solutes are added by tubular secretion. The processes of filtration, tubular re-absorption, and tubular secretion are under physiological control. The final product excreted into the renal pelvis is urine.

Renal Circulation

Blood Flow

In man, blood flow to the kidney is 1.2 to 1.3 L/min, or approximately 25 per cent of the cardiac output.

The kidney filters plasma. Renal plasma flow (RPF) can be measured using any substance that is excreted but not metabolized, stored, or produced by the kidney and that does not affect renal blood flow, e.g., para-aminohippuric acid (PAH), which is filtered and secreted. When infused at low doses, 90 per cent is removed in a single circulation through the kidney. If the amount not removed is ignored, the effective renal plasma flow (ERPF) can be calculated by measuring the concentration of PAH in the volume of urine produced during a timed period and dividing the result by the plasma PAH concentration as follows:

$$\frac{U_{PAH}V/t}{P_{PAH}} = ERPF$$

This measurement is called the PAH clearance. For humans, the ERPF is approximately 625 ml/min. If the kidney extraction rate of 90 per cent is taken into account, the actual RPF is

$$\frac{625}{0.9} = 694 \text{ ml/min.}$$

Assuming the hematocrit to be 45%, renal blood flow equals

$$\frac{694}{55} \times \frac{100}{1} = 1262 \text{ ml/min.}$$

Regional Blood Flow

The radioactive inert gases krypton[38] and xenon[3] have been used in dogs to show how renal blood flow is partitioned. Four flow regions have been detected by autoradiography: cortex, outer medulla, inner medulla, and adipose capsule (Fig. 133–1). Blood flow through the renal cortex is much greater than flow through the medulla. In anesthetized dogs, blood flows were 4.59 ml/gm of kidney tissue per minute in the cortex, 0.7 ml/gm/min in the outer medulla, and 0.1 ml/gm/min in the inner medulla.[3] Thus, the renal medulla is relatively ischemic. However, normal blood flow to the brain is only 0.5 ml/gm/min, so even in the renal medulla total blood flow is not too impoverished.[16]

Pressure in Renal Vessels

Glomerular capillary pressure in rats is approximately 50 per cent of systemic arterial pressure, or about 50 mm Hg.[6] Peritubular capillary pressure is close to 15 mm Hg. The glomerular pressure is affected by cardiac output and resistance in the afferent and efferent arterioles. A drop in blood pressure, or hypoxia, stimulates the vasomotor center in the brain and causes renal vasoconstriction. Circulating catecholamines cause a similar response. Vasoconstriction is seen first in the efferent arterioles; therefore, despite decreased renal blood flow, the glomerular filtration rate (GFR) can be maintained. If the mean systemic arterial pressure drops below

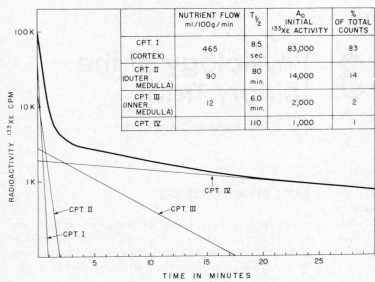

	NUTRIENT FLOW ml/100g/min	$T_{1/2}$	A_0 INITIAL [133]XE ACTIVITY	% OF TOTAL COUNTS
CPT. I (CORTEX)	465	8.5 sec.	83,000	83
CPT. II (OUTER MEDULLA)	90	.80 min.	14,000	14
CPT. III (INNER MEDULLA)	12	6.0 min.	2,000	2
CPT. IV		110.	1,000	1

Figure 133–1. Distribution of renal blood flow in a normal dog. The exponential curve was obtained by external monitoring after a single injection of xenon-133 in the renal artery. Analysis of the curve gives the four components. (Reproduced with permission from Bovee, K. C., and Webster, M. D.: Values for intrarenal distribution of blood flow using xenon 133 in the anesthetized dog. Am. J. Vet. Res. 33:501, 1972.)

90 mm Hg or if the catecholamine stimulus is large enough, GFR falls because the afferent as well as efferent arterioles constrict and perfusion pressure cannot be maintained. Vasodilation increases renal blood flow. Factors known to produce vasodilation include bacterial pyrogens, high-protein diets, and certain drugs including dopamine, acetylcholine, prostaglandin E, and bradykinin.[22]

The ability to maintain a constant renal blood flow (autoregulation) by adjusting renal vascular resistance as blood pressure changes is retained even in transplanted kidneys. Autoregulation is probably, therefore, the result of direct contraction of the smooth muscle of the afferent arteriole in response to stretch.[33]

Glomerular Filtration

Glomerular filtration rate (GFR) can be determined by measuring the urine and plasma concentration of a substance freely filtered by the kidneys but neither secreted nor absorbed. Inulin, a polysaccharide polymer of fructose, has a molecular weight of 5,200 and is extensively used to measure GFR. Inulin clearance is the concentration of inulin in a volume of urine collected during a known period of time divided by the plasma level of inulin as follows.

$$\frac{U_{In} \times V/t}{P_{In}} = GFR$$

In dogs and cats, creatinine clearance can also be used to measure GFR. Creatinine clearance is not an accurate measure of GFR in humans, since some creatinine is absorbed and some is secreted. However, as these two processes tend to cancel each other out and since endogenous creatinine clearance is easy to measure, it is still regarded as a useful index of human renal function.

Normal GFR

In man, GFR is approximately 125 ml/min, or 180 L/day. Normal urine volume is about 1 L/day; therefore, 99 per cent of the filtered plasma is re-absorbed.

The average total plasma volume in man is 3 liters; therefore, the entire plasma volume is filtered 60 times each day. GFR for other animals varies from 4 ml/min in chickens to 800 ml/min in the ox (Table 133–1).

Control of GFR

The capacity to vary GFR is related to the size of the capillary bed, the permeability of the capillaries, and the pressure gradient across the capillary wall.

Permeability. Glomerular capillaries are 50 times more permeable than capillaries in skeletal muscle and have a special structure (see Chapter 132). The endothelium of glomerular capillaries is fenestrated with pores approximately 100 nm in diameter. The pseudopodia of the epithelial cells, or podocytes, form slits approximately 25 nm wide. The basal lamina, which separates these two layers, is a hydrated gel with limited permeability, restricting the passage of plasma proteins and lipids.[13] Functionally, the "filtration barrier" permits free passage of neutral substances up to 4 nm in diameter, delays the passage of substances up to 8 nm in diameter, and excludes those over 8 nm in diameter. However, the charge as well as diameter influences the rate of passage of molecules into Bowman's space.[5] Sialoproteins in the endothelium and basement membrane are negatively charged. Therefore, negatively charged molecules in the plasma are retarded and the passage of positively charged molecules is facilitated. Albumin carries a negative charge and has an effective molecular radius of about 7.2 nm. Normally only 0.2 per cent of plasma albumin is filtered, but in nephritis the negative charge on the glomerular membrane dissipates. The result is enhanced filtration of albumin and albuminuria.

Pressure Gradients. Pressure gradients across the glomerular capillary wall have been directly measured in rats (Table 133–2). The net filtration pressure at the afferent end of the glomerulus is 15 mm Hg, but this pressure gradient falls to 0 (filtration equilibrium) toward the efferent end as fluid leaves the capillary and the osmotic pressure of the plasma rises. It is apparent that some parts of the glomerulus do not normally contribute to the production of the

TABLE 133–1. Glomerular Structure and Function*

Animal	Glomerular Filtration Rate (ml/min)	Total Glomeruli (× 10⁵)	Glomerular Diameter (μm)
Chicken	3–4	8	85
Cat	15–20	4	140
Dog	40–50	8	180
Pig	80–100	22	165
Ox	700–800	80	240

*Modified from Phillis, J. W.: *Veterinary Physiology.* W. B. Saunders, Philadelphia, 1976.

TABLE 133–2. Pressure Gradients Across Rat Glomerulus (mm Hg)*

	Afferent End	Efferent End
Glomerular capillary	45	45
Bowman's capsule hydrostatic pressure	10	10
Osmotic pressure gradient	20	35
Net filtration pressure	15	0

*Modified from Mercer, P. F., Maddox, D. A., and Brenner, B. M.: Current concepts of sodium chloride and water transport by the mammalian nephron. West. J. Med. 120:33, 1974.

glomerular ultrafiltrate.[5] The hydrostatic pressure in Bowman's capsule is about 10 mm Hg. Since the protein level in tubular fluid is very low, the osmotic gradient is equal to the colloidal osmotic pressure (oncotic pressure) of the plasma proteins (20 mm Hg). If the mean systemic arterial pressure were to drop below 60 mm Hg, glomerular pressure would be approximately 30 mm Hg and filtration would cease.

The ratio $\dfrac{\text{GFR}}{\text{RPF}}$ is called the filtration fraction. This rises when systemic blood pressure falls within physiological limits, because although RPF has decreased, GFR is maintained as a result of efferent arteriolar constriction, which maintains glomerular capillary pressure.

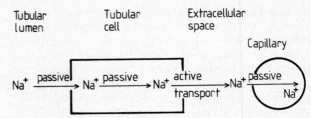

Figure 133–2. Diagrammatical representation of transepithelial transport of sodium from tubular fluid to capillary. The key component is an active process; the other three components are passive.

Tubular Function

The renal tubules handle the plasma components in the filtrate in different ways. The tubular cells can add more substance to the filtrate (tubular secretion) or may remove some or all of the substance from the filtrate (tubular re-absorption). The amount of substance excreted equals the amount filtered plus the net amount transferred by the tubules (Table 133–3). This transfer can be passive (diffusion) along a chemical or electrical gradient or active, in which case substances are transported against these gradients (transepithelial transport).

Active Re-absorption

Using re-absorption of sodium as an example (Fig. 133–2), sodium diffuses into and across the tubular cell and is actively transported into the interstitial fluid, and sodium and water flow by a bulk flow process to the capillaries. Although three of these four steps are passive, transepithelial transport is an active process. The active phase of this process can be saturated, since tubules can only handle a limited amount of any particular solute in a given time. The capacity to re-absorb glucose (Fig. 133–3) is high. If glucose is administered intravenously, none is excreted in the urine until the maximal tubular capacity (T_m) to transport glucose has been reached. When T_m is reached, any increase in plasma glucose produces a proportional increase in excreted glucose. This situation occurs in patients with diabetes mellitus. When the T_m for glucose is exceeded, very high glucose levels appear in the urine. If the T_m for the solute being re-absorbed is close to the filtered load, as it is for the phosphate ion, even a slight increase in plasma phosphate produces a large increase in excreted phosphate. In this way, the amount of phosphate ingested is balanced by the amount excreted.

Passive Re-absorption

Urea re-absorption is a passive process. As fluid passes along the tubule, water is absorbed. The urea concentration rises and so diffuses out of the tubule along the concentration gradient into the peritubular capillary.

TABLE 133–3. Renal Handling of Various Plasma Constituents in a Normal Adult Human on an Average Diet*

Substance	24 Hours				Percentage Re-absorbed	Location†
	Filtered	*Re-absorbed*	*Secreted*	*Excreted*		
Na+ (mEq)	26,000	25,850		150	99.4	P,L,D,C
K+ (mEq)	900	900‡	100	100	100.0‡	P,D,‡
Cl− (mEq)	18,000	17,850		150	99.2	P,L,D,C
HCO− (mEq)	4,900	4,900		0	100.0	P,D
Urea (mmol)	870	460§		410	53.0	P,L,D,C
Creatinine (mmol)	12	1 ‖	1 ‖	12		
Uric acid (mmol)	50	49	4	5	98.0	P
Glucose (mmol)	800	800		0	100.0	P
Total solute (mOsm)	54,000	53,400	100	700	87.0	P,L,D,C
Water (ml)	180,000	179,000		1000	99.4	P,L,D,C

*Reproduced with permission from Ganong, W. F.: *Review of Medical Physiology*. Lange Medical Publications, Los Altos, CA, 1979, p. 559.
†P = proximal tubules; L = loops of Henle; D = distal tubules; C = collecting ducts.
‡K+ is re-absorbed proximally and secreted distally. It is not certain that all of the filtered K+ is re-absorbed proximally.
§Urea diffuses into as well as out of some portions of the nephron.
‖Variable secretion and probable re-absorption of creatinine in humans.

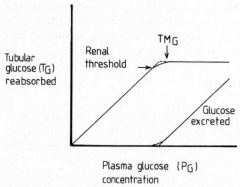

Figure 133–3. Glucose re-absorption curve. As plasma glucose rises, glucose starts to appear in the urine at the renal threshold. When tubular transport is maximum for glucose (T_{MG}), all additional filtered plasma glucose (P_G) is excreted.

Tubular Secretion

This transport process is the opposite of re-absorption and, like re-absorption, can be active or passive. Most excreted hydrogen ions (H^+) and potassium ions (K^+) enter the tubules by secretion. Many foreign chemicals, for example, penicillin, are also excreted by tubular secretion.

Regulation of Salt and Water Balance

Output

Most renal energy production is used to absorb 99 per cent of the filtered sodium (Na^+), chloride (Cl^-), and water. Sodium re-absorption is the key. It is an active process and requires expenditure of much energy. Sodium absorption produces a charge separation and results in passive re-absorption of chloride along an electrical gradient. Re-absorption of solute induces passive re-absorption of water by osmosis. However, re-absorption of water depends on the permeability of tubular epithelium, and this can vary. Tubular permeability to water is regulated in the distal tubules and collecting ducts by the hormone vasopressin or antidiuretic hormone (ADH). In the absence of ADH, permeability to water is very low. Since ADH has no effect on sodium transport, sodium continues to move out of the tubule. Since the water cannot follow, it remains in the tubule, and a large volume of urine is excreted. When ADH is present, the permeability of the distal tubules and collecting ducts to water is very high. Water re-absorption therefore follows sodium and chloride re-absorption, and urine volume is small. The action of ADH on kidney tubules is inhibited by calcium, potassium, and glucocorticoids, accounting for the polyuria seen in hypercalcemia, hyperkalemia, and steroid excess.

Control of Sodium Excretion

This depends on control of glomerular filtration rate, tubular re-absorption, and possibly a third factor.

Control of Glomerular Filtration Rate

GFR is controlled primarily by the glomerular capillary blood pressure. The reflexes that maintain total body sodium are those that also are mediated by pressure, distension, and flow receptors in the cardiovascular system. If plasma volume is decreased, for example, owing to diarrhea or hemorrhage, arterial blood pressure drops as cardiac output decreases. In addition, activation of baroreceptors in the carotid sinus, aortic arch, veins, and atria results in arteriolar vasoconstriction. These two effects decrease glomerular capillary pressure and GFR; therefore, the amount of sodium excreted is decreased.

Control of Tubular Sodium Re-absorption

This is more important than control of GFR in long-term regulation of sodium excretion. Aldosterone, a hormone produced in the adrenal cortex, stimulates sodium re-absorption by the distal tubules. If the adrenal glands are diseased or absent, loss of salt and water occurs and the patient can die of shock. The renin/angiotensin system controls production of aldosterone.

Renin/Angiotensin/Aldosterone System. The juxtaglomerular cells in the media of the afferent arterioles produce renin. Renin acts on renin substrate (angiotensinogen), a plasma protein produced by the liver, to produce angiotensin I. Converting enzyme present in the lungs and probably in all endothelial cells converts inactive angiotensin I into angiotensin II. Angiotensin II is the most potent vasoconstrictor known and, if produced in excess, will certainly result in hypertension. Angiotensin II acts directly on the adrenal cortex to increase the secretion of aldosterone. Renin release[31] is stimulated by a fall in blood pressure or by an increase in sympathetic nervous system activity. Prostaglandins generated in the renal cortex probably mediate renin release.[1] The macula densa can sense sodium and chloride concentration in the distal tubule. If the concentration is low owing to excretion of a large volume of dilute urine, renin is released and angiotensin II is produced. This results in constriction of the afferent arterioles, decreased GFR, and decreased urine production.

Third Factor

In some instances, GFR can be low and aldosterone levels high but sodium excretion is normal or increased. A third factor influencing sodium re-absorption has been postulated but not identified.[36]

Sodium Retention in Congestive Heart Failure

Deranged sodium balance can occur when kidney function is normal but heart action is defective. For example, in congestive heart failure the decreased cardiac output results in reduced glomerular filtration rate and increased aldosterone secretion. Therefore, little or no salt is excreted. There is expanded plasma volume and increased capillary pressure with increased interstitial fluid, producing edema. Obviously the primary aim of treatment of this condition is to improve the pumping action of the heart, but in support, edema fluid can be mobilized by inhibiting tubular sodium re-absorption with diuretic agents. (A further consideration of diuretic agents can be found later in this chapter.)

ADH Secretion and Extracellular Volume

Whether or not water re-absorption follows sodium re-absorption in the renal tubules depends on the presence of ADH. For changes in sodium excretion to be effective in altering extracellular volume, there must be equivalent changes in water excretion. Therefore, decreased extracellular volume must reflexly produce increased ADH production as well as stimulate aldosterone secretion. ADH is produced by hypothalamic neurons, the axons of which terminate in the posterior pituitary gland, from which ADH is released. The hypothalamic cells receive signals from baroreceptors in the left atrium.[36] These receptors are stimulated by increased arterial blood pressure, and the result of the stimulation is inhibition of ADH production. Decreased atrial pressure has the opposite effect and stimulates ADH synthesis.

Pure Water Loss and Gain

If excessive pure water is ingested, it is excreted without producing a corresponding loss of sodium. Plasma volume is expanded, therefore circulating volume increases. This results in increased left atrial pressure; ADH production is reflexly inhibited and water is excreted. This phenomenon is called *water diuresis*. The maximum urine flow for man in water diuresis is 16 ml/min. Urine flow is limited because water re-absorption in the proximal tubule is normal. If water is ingested at a faster rate than this, the extracellular fluid becomes hypotonic and body cells swell. This phenomenon is called *water intoxication*. Swelling in brain cells causes convulsions, coma, and death. If the hypothalamus is damaged and ADH production is impaired, diabetes insipidus is produced. The result is constant production of a large volume of dilute urine.

When pure water is lost from the body by dehydration, the kidneys compensate to conserve water by producing concentrated urine. For this to occur, water absorption must move ahead of sodium absorption. This is achieved by the countercurrent concentrating system, discussed later in this chapter. Dogs and cats have little capacity to adapt to water lack.[32]

Thirst

Thirst is stimulated by increased osmotic pressure of body fluids acting on osmoreceptors found in the hypothalamus. It is also stimulated by decreased extracellular volume. Hemorrhage lowers extracellular volume but does not change plasma osmolality. In this case, thirst is stimulated by the renin angiotensin system. Angiotensin II acts on receptors in the diencephalon, which in turn stimulate the hypothalamic nuclei. A dry oral mucosa strongly stimulates thirst, but this can be relieved by simply moistening the mouth and throat.

Salt Excess

There is a limit to the concentration gradient against which sodium can be pumped out of the proximal tubules. When this concentration is exceeded, an increased volume of isotonic fluid reaches Henle's loop because solutes that are not re-absorbed in the proximal tubules exert a considerable osmotic effect. Of more importance, water and solute re-absorption in Henle's loop and distal tubules decreases. This happens because the medullary hypertonicity decreases owing to an increase in medullary blood flow.[17] The resulting increased urine flow is called *osmotic diuresis*, and flows are much greater than those in water diuresis because there is decreased water re-absorption in the proximal tubules. Osmotic diuresis can be induced by infusing mannitol, a substance filtered but not absorbed, or glucose, sodium chloride, or urea at a rate that exceeds the T_m for that solute.

Urine Concentration

The capacity of the kidney to produce hyperosmotic urine determines an animal's ability to survive without water. The measure of urine concentrating capacity is osmolality or specific gravity. Osmolality is a measure of the osmotic activity of the dissolved solute and depends on the ratio of the total number of solute particles to the number of moles of solvent. For example, a protein molecule of molecular weight 100,000 has the same effect as a sodium ion, weight 23. Also, a mole of sodium chloride, since it dissociates into two particles, has twice the effect of a mole of urea or glucose, neither of which dissociates. One mole of solute dissolved in 1 kilogram of water depresses its freezing point by 1.86°C. Since most biological fluids are more dilute, the unit milliosmole is used. Therefore, the milliosmolality of a solution is defined as its freezing point depression in degrees Centigrade divided by 0.00186.

The specific gravity is a measure of the weight of solute dissolved in a given volume of water. It indicates concentration, which is tied to molecular weight but not necessarily concentrating capacity, which is related to the number of molecules of the solution. The maximum urine concentrating capacity for various animals and for humans is shown in Table 133–4.

The concentrating mechanism is known as the countercurrent system. Its action depends on the maintenance of an increasing osmolality along the medullary pyramids but with the same concentration gradient at any horizontal level. This gradient exists because the loops of Henle act as countercurrent multipliers and the vasa recta as countercurrent ex-

TABLE 133–4. Mammalian Kidney Concentrating Capacity*

Animal	Long-looped Nephrons (% of Total)	Relative Medullary Thickness	Maximum Urine Concentration (mOsm/L)
Beaver	0	1.3	516
Pig	3	1.6	1,075
Human	14	3.0	1,398
Dog	100	4.3	2,607
Cat	100	4.8	3,118
Kangaroo rat	27	8.5	5,591
Jerboa	33	9.3	6,451
Psammomys	100	10.7	4,946

*Modified from Schmidt-Nielsen, B., and O'Dell, R.: Structure and concentrating mechanism in the mammalian kidney. Am. J. Physiol. *200*:1119, 1961.

changers. The function of this system is to absorb salt in excess of water and thus concentrate the medullary interstitium and also to deliver a large volume of free water to the cortical distal tubule (Fig. 133–4). Fluid flows in opposite directions ("countercurrent") in each limb of Henle's loop. The thin descending limb is relatively impermeable to solute but highly permeable to water. Therefore, water moves into the interstitium and sodium concentration in the tubule rises. The thin ascending limb is relatively impermeable to water but relatively permeable to sodium and, to a lesser extent, urea. Therefore, sodium moves into the interstitium along a concentration gradient and takes chloride with it. The thick ascending limb is relatively impermeable

to both solute and water, but chloride is actively transported out of the tubular fluid, with sodium following along the electrical gradient. The distal tubule and outer collecting ducts are relatively impermeable to urea but permeable to water in the presence of ADH. Water leaves the lumen and urea concentration increases markedly. The inner medullary portion of the collecting duct is permeable to urea and, in the presence of ADH, also water. The sodium and urea remain in the pyramids because the vasa recta act as countercurrent exchangers. Solutes diffuse out of the ascending vessels and into the descending vessels; conversely, water diffuses out of the descending vessels and into the ascending vessels. Solutes tend to recirculate in the medulla and water tends to bypass it, therefore maintaining hypertonicity. Water removed by the collecting ducts is also returned to the general circulation by the vasa recta. The amount of urea in the medullary interstitium and urine varies with the amount filtered, and this depends on intake. Consequently, a high-protein diet increases the ability of the kidney to concentrate urine.[16]

Regulation of Potassium, Calcium, and Hydrogen Ions

Potassium. Extracellular levels of potassium are closely regulated, since it is involved in excitability of nerve and muscle. The resting membrane potential is directly related to the ratio of intracellular to extracellular potassium. An increase in extracellular potassium lowers resting potential and increases excitability. A decrease in extracellular potassium hy-

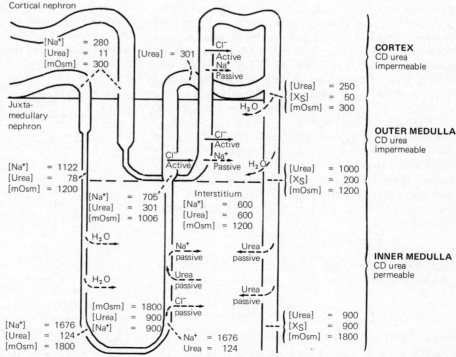

Figure 133–4. Schematic summary of the countercurrent mechanism in the renal medulla. All concentrations are in mOsm/1. CO = collecting duct; X = nonre-absorbable solute. (Modified and reproduced with permission from Ganong, W. F.: *Review of Medical Physiology.* Lange Medical Publications, Los Altos, CA, 1977, p. 538.)

perpolarizes the cell membrane and decreases excitability. The intake of dietary potassium varies. Output is regulated by the kidneys. One hundred per cent is filtered, and 100 per cent is re-absorbed, so changes in excretion are due to changes in tubular secretion. Aldosterone enhances tubular potassium secretion by the distal tubules as well as tubular sodium absorption by the proximal tubules.

Calcium. Calcium has profound effects on neuromuscular excitability. Hypocalcemia produces tetany. Therefore, extracellular levels must be kept constant. The bones, kidneys, and the gastrointestinal tract feature in calcium homeostasis. Three principal hormones regulate plasma calcium. The first is parathyroid hormone, which increases plasma calcium by stimulating osteoclasts to break down bone, liberating calcium phosphate. It also increases calcium absorption in the renal tubules and decreases tubular re-absorption of phosphate, leading to phosphaturia.

The second is 1,25-dihydroxycholicalciferol, a metabolite of vitamin D produced in inactive form by the liver and activated by the kidney. It increases intestinal re-absorption of calcium and promotes mobilization of calcium from the bone. Chronically diseased kidneys lose their ability to form 1,25-dihydroxycholicalciferol. Plasma calcium is therefore low, stimulating the parathyroid glands and producing hyperparathyroidism.

The third hormone is calcitonin, produced by the thyroid gland. It acts to decrease plasma calcium by inhibiting bone re-absorption. Its secretion is related to the calcium concentration in the blood supplying the thyroid gland.

Hydrogen Ions. Hydrogen ion concentration is very closely regulated because even small variations in pH can adversely affect enzyme function. Hydrogen ions are generated in the body by metabolic processes. Many proteins contain phosphorus and sulphur, which are metabolized to phosphoric and sulphuric acids. These acids dissociate completely, generating much hydrogen ion. They are therefore strong acids. Organic acids such as fatty acids and lactic acid are end products of metabolism. They weakly dissociate to produce some hydrogen ions and are therefore called weak acids. The major source of hydrogen ion is from metabolically produced carbon dioxide. This reacts with water to produce carbonic acid, which dissociates into hydrogen ions and bicarbonate ions. During the period between generation and excretion, the majority of hydrogen ions are buffered. Buffers act by reversibly binding hydrogen ions (H^+).

$$\text{Buffer} + H^+ \rightleftharpoons H - \text{Buffer}$$

Important buffers are bicarbonate/carbon dioxide, plasma proteins, intracellular phosphate, and hemoglobin.

$$H^+ + HCO_3^- \rightleftharpoons H_2CO_3 \rightleftharpoons H_2O + CO_2$$

Increased production of hydrogen ion drives the reaction to the right. This continues as long as the lungs can generate and remove CO_2. Increased hydrogen ion concentration stimulates the respiratory center of the brain to increase ventilation rate. The hydrogen ions generated in metabolically active tissues from CO_2 and water are buffered by hemoglobin in the red blood cells. Reduced hemoglobin has a greater affinity for hydrogen ions than oxyhemoglobin. In the lungs, reduced hemoglobin becomes oxyhemoglobin. It loses its affinity for hydrogen ions, which are released. The hydrogen ions react with plasma bicarbonate to produce carbon dioxide and water. This reaction is catalyzed by carbonic anhydrase. The carbon dioxide and water diffuse into the alveoli and are expired.

Acidification of the Urine

The kidneys can also excrete hydrogen ion. Hydrogen ion is generated in the renal tubular cell in the presence of carbonic anhydrase (Fig. 133–5). For each H^+ excreted, one Na^+ enters the cell. Na^+ is pumped into the interstitial fluid in exchange for potassium (K^+). If there were no buffers in the urine, the secreted H^+ would diffuse back into the interstitial fluid. The urine buffers are bicarbonate (HCO_3^-), phosphate (HPO_4^{--}), and ammonia (NH_3) (Fig. 133–6).

In the proximal tubule, most of the secreted H^+ reacts with HCO_3^- to produce H_2CO_3, which breaks down to yield CO_2 and water. The CO_2 diffuses into the cell and can repeat the cycle. In this way, HCO_3^- is re-absorbed. Thus, for each H^+ excreted, one Na^+ and one HCO_3^- enter the interstitial fluid and diffuse into the blood. If a chloride load is given, e.g., ammonium chloride or calcium chloride, some is re-absorbed by the kidney tubules, but much is excreted, taking with it an equivalent amount of sodium and the appropriate amount of water. Excretion of Na^+ means that the alkali reserve (HCO_3^-) is depleted; therefore, the amount of urine titratable acid

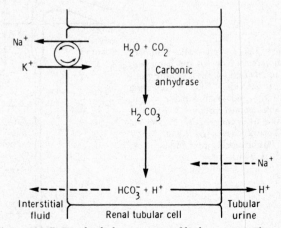

Figure 133–5. Renal tubular secretion of hydrogen ion. The solid arrows crossing cell boundaries indicate an active transport system, and the broken arrow indicate diffusion. (Reproduced with permission from Ganong, W. F.: *Review of Medical Physiology*. Lange Medical Publications, Los Altos, CA, 1977, p. 538.)

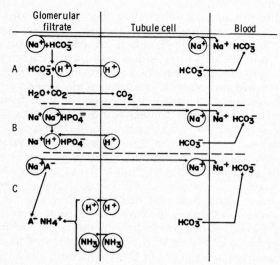

Figure 133–6. Urinary buffers for secreted H^+ contribute to (A) reabsorption of filtered bicarbonate by CO_2 movement, (B) formation of titratable acid from phosphate ion, and (C) ammonium ion formation from NH_3. Note that for each H^+ excreted, one Na^+ and one HCO_3^- enter the blood stream. (Reproduced with permission from Ganong, W. F.: *Review of Medical Physiology.* Lange Medical Publications, Los Altos, CA, 1977, p. 538.)

increases and the ammonium ion concentration rises. That is, the urine becomes acid. In the distal tubules and collecting ducts, phosphate concentration is high. The reaction is as follows.

$$H^+ + HPO_4^{--} \rightleftharpoons H_2PO_4^{--}$$

This reaction produces urine titratable acid. This is measured by the amount of alkali that has to be added to return the pH to 7.4. Titratable acid is only a fraction of secreted acid, since it does not measure the H^+ that combines with HCO_3^- or ammonia (NH_3).

If the amount of H^+ generated exceeds the capacity of HCO_3^- and HPO_4^{--} to handle it, ammonia can be generated in the tubules and collecting ducts by the deamination of glutamine. The NH_3 diffuses into the lumen and combines with H^+ to yield NH_4^+. Although the cell membrane is permeable to NH_3, it is not permeable to NH_4^+. In chronic acidosis, ammonia production gradually increases as hydrogen ion concentration in the tubular fluid remains elevated for more than a few days. This is called adaptation.

Diuretics

Previously in this chapter, the consideration of water and electrolyte balance and urine concentration laid the physiological foundation for the action of the diuretic agents. The mechanisms of action of commonly used diuretics are summarized in Table 133–5.

The major purpose of diuretic therapy is to rid the body of excess sodium and water and thereby eliminate edema and hypertension. Most of the clinically used diuretic drugs exert their effect by interfering with sodium chloride re-absorption in the renal tubules. Electrolyte depletion, particularly of potassium, can accompany prolonged use of the potent diuretics furosemide and ethacrynic acid. Potassium depletion is not seen when the organomercurials or

TABLE 133–5. Mechanism of Action of Various Diuretics*

Agent	Mechanism of Action
Water	Inhibits vasopressin secretion
Ethyl alcohol	Inhibits vasopressin secretion
Large quantities of osmotically active substances such as mannitol and glucose	Produce osmotic diuresis
Xanthines such as caffeine and theophylline	Probably decrease tubular re-absorption of Na^+ and increase GFR
Acidifying salts such as $CaCl_2$ and NH_4Cl	Supply acid load; H^+ is buffered, and anion is excreted with Na^+ when the ability of the kidney to replace Na^+ with H^+ is exceeded
Organic salts of mercury such as mercaptomerin (Thiomerin) and meralluride (Mercuhydrin)	Inhibit Cl^- re-absorption in the medullary thick ascending limb of the loop of Henle; inhibit K^+ secretion
Carbonic anhydrase inhibitors such as acetazolamide (Diamox)	Decrease H^+ secretion throughout nephron, with resultant increase in Na^+ and K^+ excretion
Metolazone (Zaroxolyn), thiazides such as chlorothiazide (Diuril)	Inhibit Cl^- re-absorption in the distal cortical portion of the loop of Henle and proximal portion of the distal tubule
Furosemide (Lasix), ethacrynic acid (Edecrin), and bumetanide	Inhibit Cl^- re-absorption in the medullary thick ascending limb of the loop of Henle
K^+-retaining natriuretics such as spironolactone (Aldactone), triamterene (Dyrenium), and amiloride (Colectril)	Inhibit Na^+-K^+ "exchange" in the distal portion of the distal tubule by inhibiting the action of aldosterone (spironolactone) or by inhibiting K^+ secretion (triamterene, amiloride)

*Reproduced with permission from Ganong, W. F.: *Review of Medical Physiology.* Lange Medical Publications, Los Altos, CA, 1979, p. 560.

the potassium-retaining natriuretics such as the steroid lactone spironolactone, or triamterene are used.

Erythropoietin and the Kidney

Hemorrhage or hypoxia enhances erythropoiesis. This is mediated by the hormone erythropoietin, a glycoprotein with an approximate molecular weight of 46,000.[14] The kidneys are the primary site of production of this hormone. Humans can maintain a low basal level of erythropoiesis after bilateral nephrectomy,[28] but dogs cannot.[27]

The production of erythropoietin occurs in two stages. A renal erythropoietic factor (REF), or erythrogenin, has been isolated from the mitochondria of the renal cortex and medulla.[18] It is postulated that REF acts as an enzyme on a globulin substrate in the plasma, probably produced in the liver, to produce erythropoietin.[24]

Benign renal lesions such as cysts and malignant renal lesions can cause increased erythropoietin production with polycythemia. It is suggested that the lesions cause compression and relative anoxia of the surrounding renal tissue, which stimulates erythropoietin production.[30]

Prostaglandins and the Kidney

Prostaglandins are oxygenated, cyclic, 20–carbon chain fatty acids. Prostaglandins are present in most biological tissues and fluids and have a role in vasodilation and constriction, regulation of body temperature, platelet aggregation, reproduction, inflammation, gastrointestinal function, autonomic neurotransmission, and cardiovascular and renal function.[20]

The prostaglandin precursor is arachidonic acid. This is converted by the microsomal enzyme prostaglandin endoperoxide synthetase (cyclooxygenase) to unstable prostaglandin endoperoxides. Aspirin and the nonsteroidal anti-inflammatory agents indomethacin and phenylbutazone inhibit this metabolic step.[20] The endoperoxides are transformed by specific enzymes in the presence of cofactors and oxygen into a series of biologically active lipids, including prostaglandins, thromboxanes, and prostacyclins.

The renal prostaglandins are synthesized primarily by the interstitial cells and the collecting duct cells of the renal papilla. Some synthesis also occurs in the renal cortex in glomeruli and collecting tubules. The major prostaglandin produced is PGE_2, and this is metabolized by prostaglandin dehydrogenase, mainly in the renal cortex and lungs.[1]

The prostaglandins react with other intrarenal systems. They play a part in sodium excretion by producing changes in renal hemodynamics. Their presence produces an increase in renal blood flow associated with redistribution of blood to the inner cortex and papilla.[1] Diuretics that act on the loop of Henle produce a similar effect. The diuresis can be blocked by indomethacin, an antiprostaglandin, suggesting that the diuretic action is mediated by prostaglandin.[8] The prostaglandins act in water excretion by inhibiting the action of vasopressin.[11] The interaction of prostaglandins with the renin/angiotensin/aldosterone axis has been extensively studied. Exogenous prostaglandin stimulates renal cortical renin release by a direct effect on the macula densa cells.[38] They also play a part in the sympathetic[7] and baroreceptor-mediated[29] renin release.

In anesthetized animals, inhibition of endogenous prostaglandin synthesis produces significant changes in renal blood flow and distribution.[29] In ureteral obstruction, there is increased production of PGE_2 and thromboxane, particularly in the cortex, which probably contributes to the afferent glomerular vasoconstriction observed in this condition.[37]

Urine Storage and Neurology of Micturition

In the nonvoiding state, the urinary bladder is a reservoir with flaccid walls that generate little pressure, whereas the urethra is a high-resistance valve designed to prevent the passage of urine. This state is dominated by sympathetic autonomic nervous activity with beta-adrenergic stimulation facilitating relaxation of the detrusor smooth muscle and alpha-adrenergic stimulation of the bladder neck and proximal urethra providing muscle tone and allowing continence to be maintained. In voiding, the bladder becomes a pump that expels urine under high pressure while the urethra opens into a minimum resistance conduit. As the detrusor contracts and urine is forced into the urethra, urethral resistance drops to a level equal to or less than intravesicular pressure.[15, 34] Parasympathetic stimulation of the urinary bladder with inhibition of alpha-adrenergic sympathetic stimulation to the urethra allows micturition to occur. The normal urethra should maintain continence under resting conditions as well as under physiological stresses. It should assist or at least not hinder voiding until the bladder is empty.

The bladder and urethra are continuous structures and function interdependently. The autonomic centers of the spinal cord that control micturition are normally regulated by the cerebral cortex, the micturition center of the pons, and the cerebellum, all of which modify the spinal reflex arc that results in bladder emptying.[4] Without the cerebral cortex, micturition can still occur but cannot be voluntarily controlled. The cerebellum provides an inhibiting influence on micturition via the brain stem.[4]

Critical to the proper functioning of the bladder and urethra is the normal integration of their neural and muscular components. A complex network of parasympathetic, sympathetic, and somatic nerves supply the lower urinary tract. The detrusor smooth muscle of the bladder is richly innervated by excitatory parasympathetic cholinergic nerves, which are uniformly distributed throughout the muscle.[19] These nerve fibers compose the pelvic nerve, which originates in the sacral spinal cord. As the bladder fills with urine, these sensory fibers detect changes in the stretch of the detrusor muscle. When the bladder is filled to capacity, a "desire to void" reflex is initiated. The parasympathetic afferent fibers discharge impulses to the sacral spinal cord, from where signals of bladder capacity are relayed to the brain stem.[4] Here reflex integration occurs, resulting in efferent signals to the sacral spinal cord, activation of pre- and postganglionic parasympathetic neurons, and excitation of detrusor muscle fibers. This wave of excitation spreads through the detrusor muscle via areas of fusion of the outer components of adjacent cell membranes (gap junctions), resulting in contraction.[4, 21]

Urethral smooth muscle is continuous with the detrusor muscle at the vesicourethral junction.[12] Although there is no specific anatomical sphincter in that area, the proximal urethral smooth muscle acts like a sphincter and provides the major resistance to urine flow in the resting state.[2] Urethral smooth muscle is sympathetically innervated via fibers of the hypogastric nerves originating from the thoracolumbar spinal cord and caudal mesenteric ganglion. Sympathetic innervation is more important to the resting tone of the urethra than is parasympathetic innervation.[10]

Striated muscle forms a well-developed encircling sleeve distal to the midpoint of the urethra in the female and in the postprostatic membraneous urethra in the male.[12, 21] This muscle is the external urethral sphincter and is innervated by sympathetic fibers of the hypogastric nerves and somatic fibers of the pudendal nerves.[15] The external urethral sphincter maintains a low tone in the nonvoiding state, but its major function is rapid contraction to prevent urine leakage should a sudden increase in intravesical or intra-abdominal pressure occur.[9]

As the detrusor muscle contracts, the neck of the bladder is pulled open and urine is forced into the proximal urethra. Simultaneously, there is reflex inhibition of sympathetic and somatic spinal neurons, resulting in relaxation of the urethral smooth and striated muscle.[15] When the bladder is empty, parasympathetic neurons cease discharging, and the detrusor muscle relaxes. Sympathetic and somatic neurons are no longer inhibited and the urethral sphincters return to a normal state of contraction.[4]

1. Attalah, A. A., and Lee, J. B.: Prostaglandins renal function and blood pressure regulation. *In* Lee, J. B. (ed.): *Prostaglandins (Current Endocrinology)*. Elsevier Inc., New York, 1982, pp. 251–301.
2. Awad, S. A., and Downie, J. W.: Relative contributions of smooth and striated muscles to the canine urethral pressure profile. Br. J. Urol. 48:347, 1976.
3. Bovee, K. C., and Webster, G. D.: Values for intrarenal distribution of blood flow using xenon 133 in the anesthetized dog. Am. J. Vet. Res. 33:501, 1972.
4. Bradley, W. E., Timm, G. W., and Scott, F. B.: Innervation of the detrusor muscle and urethra. Urol. Clin. North Am. 1:3, 1974.
5. Brenner, B. M., Baylis, C., and Deen, W. M.: Transport of molecules across renal glomerular capillaries. Physiol. Rev. 56:502, 1976.
6. Brenner, B. M., Troy, J. L., and Daugharty, T. M.: The dynamics of glomerular filtration in the rat. J. Clin. Invest. 50:1776, 1971.
7. Campbell, W. B., Graham, R. M., and Jackson, E. K.: Role of renal prostaglandins in sympathetically mediated renin release in the rat. J. Clin. Invest. 65:448, 1979.
8. Data, J. L., Rane, A., Gerkens, J., Wilkinson, G. R., Nies, A. S., and Branch, R. A.: The influence of indomethacin on the pharmacokinetics, diuretic response, and hemodynamics of furosemide in the dog. J. Phamacol. Exp. Ther. 206:431, 1978.
9. De Groat, W. C., and Booth, A. M.: Physiology of the urinary bladder and urethra. Ann. Intern. Med. 92:312, 1980.
10. Downie, J. W., and Awad, S. A.: Role of the neurogenic factors in canine urethral wall tension and urinary incontinence. Invest. Urol. 14:143, 1976.
11. Dunn, M. J., Greely, H. P., Valtin, H., Kinter, L. B., and Beevwkes, R. III: Renal excretion of prostaglandins E_2 and $F_2 \alpha$ in diabetes insipidus rats. Am. J. Physiol. 235:F624, 1978.
12. Evans, H. E., and Christensen, G. C.: *Miller's Anatomy of the Dog*, 2nd ed. W. B. Saunders, Philadelphia, 1979, pp. 578, 594.
13. Farquhar, M. G., Wissig, S. L., and Palade, G. E.: Glomerular permeability. J. Exp. Med. 113:47, 1961.
14. Fisher, J. W.: Erythropoietin: Pharmacology, biogenesis and control of production. Pharmacol. Rev. 24:459, 1972.
15. Fletcher, T. E., and Bradley, W. E.: Neuroanatomy of the bladder-urethra. J. Urol. 119:153, 1978.
16. Ganong, W. F.: *Review of Medical Physiology*, 9th ed. Lange Medical Publications, Los Altos, CA, 1979, pp. 467, 538–564.
17. Gennari, F. J., and Kassirer, J. P.: Osmotic diuresis. N. Engl. J. Med. 291:714, 1974.
18. Gordon, A. S., Cooper, G. W., and Zanjani, E. D.: The kidney and erythropoiesis. Sem. Hematol. 4:337, 1967.
19. Gosling, J.: The structure of the bladder and urethra in relation to function. Urol. Clin. North Am. 6:31, 1979.
20. Hall, A. K., and Behrman, H. R.: Prostaglandins, biosynthesis, metabolism, and mechanism of cellular action. *In* Lee, J. B. (ed.): *Prostaglandins (Current Endocrinology)*. Elsevier Inc., New York, 1982, p. 1.
21. Ham, A. W., and Cormack, D. H.: *Histology*, 8th ed. J. B. Lippincott, Philadelphia, 1979, pp. 200, 779, 899.
22. Hollenberg, N. K., Adams, D. F., Mendell, P., Abrams, H. L., and Merrill, J. P.: Renal vascular response to dopamine. Clin. Sci. Mol. Med. 45:733, 1973.
23. Jacobson, L. O., Goldwasser, E., Fried, W., and Plzak, L.: Role of the kidney in erythropoiesis. Nature 179:633, 1957.
24. Kuratowska, Z.: The renal mechanism of the formation and inactivation of erythropoietin. Ann. N.Y. Acad. Sci. 147:128, 1968.
25. Markowitz, J., Archibald, J., and Downie, H. G.: *Experimental Surgery*, 4th ed. Bailliere, Tindall, and Cox Ltd., London, 1959, p. 9.
26. Morrison, A. R.: Prostaglandins and the kidney. Am. J. Med. 69:171, 1980.
27. Naets, J. P.: The role of the kidney in erythropoiesis. J. Clin. Invest. 39:102, 1960.
28. Nathan, D. G., Beck, L. G., Hampers, C. L., and Merrill, J. P.: Erythropoiesis in anephric man. J. Clin. Invest. 43:2158, 1964.
29. Oates, J. A., Whorton, R., Gerkens, J. F., Branch, R. A., Hollifield, J. W., and Frolich, J. C.: The participation of prostaglandins in the control of renin release. Fed. Proc. 38:72, 1979.
30. Peterson, M. E., and Zanjani, E. D.: Inappropriate erythropoietin production from a renal carcinoma in a dog with polycythemia. J. Am. Vet. Med. Assoc. 179:995, 1981.

31. Reid, I. A., Morris, B. J., and Ganong, W. F.: The renin-angiotensin system. Ann. Rev. Physiol. *40*:377, 1978.
32. Schmidt-Nielsen, K.: *Desert Animals. Physiological Problems of Heat and Water.* Oxford University Press, London, 1964.
33. Shipley, R. E., and Study, R. S.: Changes in renal blood flow. Am. J. Physiol. *167*:676, 1951.
34. Tanagho, E. A., Meyers, F., and Smith, D.: Urethral resistance: Its components and implications. II. Striated muscle component. Invest. Urol. 7:195, 1969.
35. Thornburn, G. D., Kopald, H. H., Herd, J. A., Hollenberg, M., O'Morchoe, C. C. C., and Barger, A. C.: Intrarenal

distribution of nutrient blood flow determined with Krypton[85] in the unanesthetized dog. Circ. Res. *13*:290, 1963.
36. Vander, A. J., Sherman, J. H., and Luciano, D. S.: *Human Physiology, The Mechanisms of Body Function,* 2nd ed. McGraw-Hill, New York, 1975, p. 319.
37. Yarger, W. E., Schocken, D. D., and Harris, R. H.: Obstructive nephropathy in the rat. J. Clin. Invest. 65:400, 1980.
38. Yun, J., Kelly, C. H., Bartter, F. C., and Smith, H., Jr.: The role of prostaglandins in the control of renin secretion in the dog. Life Sci. *23*:945, 1978.

======================= Chapter **134**

Pathophysiology and Therapeutics of Urinary Tract Disorders

Kenneth C. Bovée, Anne Rosin, and Benjamin L. Hart

RENAL INSUFFICIENCY AND RENAL FAILURE

This section deals with reduced renal function in three characterized syndromes. Although these syndromes may not include all possible renal diseases, they provide a useful focus for the evaluation of clinical and laboratory tests for the surgeon. The syndromes include urinary tract obstruction, acute renal failure, and chronic renal failure. The detection of these syndromes requires clinical and laboratory data from a routine examination. After confirmation, the syndrome should be analyzed to determine severity, causal factors, and therapeutic approaches. The most common questions for a surgeon concerning an animal with renal failure are: Is the animal safe for surgery? What is the rationale for surgery? Is renal failure reversible? What are the relative benefits and risks of surgery?

The three syndromes have significant pragmatic value, because each is easily recognized and requires different medical and surgical treatment. Each syndrome is caused by a large number of abnormalities that affect renal function. After the diagnosis is confirmed, natural distinctive characteristics, categories of pathophysiology, and specific etiologies become apparent.

Renal insufficiency is defined as reduction in renal function in the absence of dramatic clinical signs. Renal insufficiency may be transient or permanent and may occur in any of these three syndromes. Overt clinical signs or significant azotemia may not be recognized until renal function has been reduced by 70 per cent of normal. The term *renal failure* refers to more significant loss of renal function with

dramatic clinical signs. Failure usually implies the loss of a major portion of renal tissue on a permanent basis. Renal failure is associated with a group of metabolic abnormalities termed *uremia*.

Urinary Tract Obstruction

Obstruction of urine outflow is a common and potentially reversible cause of renal failure. Urinary tract obstruction is generally divided into two forms, acute and chronic. When acute obstruction is complete and bilateral, it threatens life. Death results within 65 to 70 hours if the obstruction is not relieved. After relief of the obstruction, renal function may return to normal in several days. Acute incomplete or acute unilateral obstruction might not be clinically obvious.

Chronic urinary tract obstruction is commonly unilateral or incomplete and may go unrecognized for long periods. If obstruction persists, the kidney may be irreversibly damaged. The presence of chronic obstruction may be obvious or silent. It may be recognized readily with anuria, dysuria, or abdominal pain or may be undetected for long periods with manifestations of pyuria, fever, or vague abdominal pain. Urinary tract obstruction is secondary to other diseases of the urinary tract, abdomen, or pelvis.

Causes

The incidence of acute obstruction is generally thought to be higher than that of chronic obstruction, but many cases of chronic obstruction are undetected.

Males have a higher incidence than females owing to different anatomy of the urethra. A combination of factors, including diameter of the urethra, predisposition to metabolic urinary calculi in males, and obstruction due to prostatic disease, contributes to the higher incidence in males. Obstruction may be mechanical or functional. The most common mechanical cause of obstruction is urinary calculi (Chapter 140). The most common cause of functional obstruction is neurogenic or atonic bladder, and this is discussed later in this chapter under Urine Incontinence. Acute obstruction is usually not associated with anatomical defects of the urinary tract. In contrast, chronic obstruction is commonly associated with neoplasia, strictures, urolithiasis, atonic bladder, and prostatic diseases.

Clinical Signs and Laboratory Findings

The clinical signs of acute complete obstruction are straining upon urination, frequency of urination, dysuria with oliguria or anuria, and abdominal pain. Table 134–1 outlines the clinical and laboratory data commonly used to identify urinary tract obstruction and distinguish it from acute or chronic renal failure. Pain due to urinary tract obstruction is secondary to stretching of the collecting system or renal capsule. The severity of pain appears to correlate with the rate of distention rather than the degree of dilation. Pain is usually associated with anorexia, restlessness, and stranguria.

Clinical signs of chronic obstruction may include moderate polydypsia and polyuria, which might not be associated with azotemia. It should be emphasized

TABLE 134–1. Clinical and Laboratory Data Base

Finding	Urinary Tract Obstruction	Acute Renal Failure	Chronic Renal Failure
Azotemia	X	X	X
Uremic symptoms		X	X
Urinary retention	X		
Edema/ascites		X	X
Anuria/oliguria	X	X	
Tender bladder	X		
Distended bladder after voiding	X		
Gross polyuria			X
Blood chemistry			
↑ BUN/creatinine	X	X	X
↑ or ↓ sodium			
↑ potassium	X	X	
↑ chloride or ↓ CO_2		X	X
↑ phosphorus	X	X	X
↑ or ↓ calcium			X
Blood count			
anemia			X
Urinalysis			
proteinuria		X	X
glycosuria	X	X	
casts		X	X

that large volumes of urine suggest rather than rule against chronic obstructive disease. Animals with chronic obstruction may not show symptoms of azotemia until renal failure is far advanced.

Animals with acute obstruction have a tense painful abdomen, distended urinary bladder, engorged external genitalia, and enlarged and sensitive kidneys. If azotemia is present, vomiting, "uremia breath," dehydration, and hypothermia may be present. Labored respiration may be present owing to metabolic acidosis. A sterile catheter should be passed into the urethra to determine its patency. A careful rectal examination and abdominal palpation are essential to evaluate pelvic or abdominal masses.

Physical findings associated with chronic obstruction are more discrete, and such animals may require special diagnostic tests including a radiographic examination. An abdominal examination may reveal an enlarged kidney bladder, or other abdominal masses such as a tumor or cystic calculus. Observation of the voiding pattern and force of the urine stream may suggest bladder atony. Hematuria is commonly noted by owners. This finding suggests calculi, infection, inflammatory disease, or neoplasia.

The laboratory evaluation should include a urinalysis, urine culture, complete blood count, plasma creatinine concentration, and sodium, potassium, calcium, chloride, and phosphorus measurements if azotemia is present. Obstruction is usually associated with microscopic and gross hematuria. A careful examination of the urine sediment is particularly important during chronic obstruction to determine the presence of inflammatory or infectious disease.

Urine is commonly dilute in all forms of obstruction. Glycosuria is transiently seen during and after acute obstruction. Azotemia due to acute obstruction is marked by elevated plasma creatinine and urea nitrogen levels, hyperphosphatemia, hyperkalemia, and metabolic acidosis. Acute obstruction is always life-threatening, death resulting from hyperkalemia and metabolic acidosis.

Animals with chronic obstruction may have azotemia after a variable period of time associated with chronic renal failure. There are no specific blood chemistry tests to distinguish urinary tract obstruction from other causes of chronic failure.

Pathophysiology

The effects of urinary tract obstruction on renal function must be considered during and after relief of obstruction. Dramatic changes in renal function occur during the first 24 hours of complete bilateral obstruction. After relief of obstruction, there is a marked increase in sodium and water excretion in the urine despite a severe reduction in GFR, a natriuretic state referred to as postobstructive diuresis. After relief of unilateral obstruction or incomplete obstruction, there may be no dramatic increase in sodium and water excretion, even though fractional excretion of these substances is increased from the postobstructive kidney. During unilateral obstruction, the nonobstructed kidney undergoes changes, which may mask the presence of obstruction in the opposite kidney. Relief of chronic obstruction usually leads to less dramatic changes in renal function.

The loss of urine concentrating capacity is the first function lost after any form of urinary tract obstruction.[82] Glomerular filtration rate (GFR) and renal plasma flow are decreased during acute obstruction.[11, 30] Loss of the ability to excrete acid occurs when urine is not excreted.

After complete obstruction in dogs, renal blood flow decreases to approximately 50 per cent of normal.[81] This reduction occurs in both unilateral and bilateral complete obstruction. During chronic unilateral obstruction, decreases in renal blood flow progressively occur so that after two months flow is about 10 per cent of normal.[74]

After relief of complete obstruction of 24 hours duration, renal blood flow returns to approximately 60 per cent of normal in dogs.[81] It appears that renal blood flow gradually returns to normal over a period of days after relief of obstruction.

During acute bilateral urinary tract obstruction, GFR is markedly reduced, and is approximately 20 per cent of normal immediately after relief of 24 hours obstruction.[80] Although GFR returns toward normal, as does renal blood flow, after relief of obstruction, it remains reduced for several days. During chronic obstruction GFR is variably decreased from 20 to 70 per cent of normal.[79] After relief of unilateral obstruction, recovery of GFR to between 50 and 75 per cent occurs within six weeks in dogs.[55] These results suggest that after the relief of chronic obstruction a return of renal function may be seen and may be greater if the more severely obstructed kidney is released first.

The postobstructive diuresis that occurs immediately after relief of obstruction is an important phenomenon related to renal function. This diuresis is marked by a transient increase in urine volume and excessive loss of solutes in the urine. Urine is usually dilute and contains large quantities of sodium, which leads to inappropriate losses after the relief of bilateral obstruction. The phenomenon of postobstructive diuresis has been described in cats with complete urethral obstruction.[16] Excessive urinary loss of sodium may lead to negative sodium balance persisting for two days after the relief of obstruction. A concomitant loss of excessive water in the urine may persist for three to four days. Although the animal may have dramatic polyuria and may suffer from dehydration, serum sodium concentration remains normal during the diuresis.

During acute bilateral obstruction, plasma potassium concentration increases. After relief of obstruction, potassium loss in the urine increases.[11] Excessive urinary potassium loss during the postobstructive diuresis may lead to a negative potassium balance three to five days after relief of the obstruction. Although the functional defect is self-limiting, it may lead to significant hypokalemia during the diuretic phase.

Reduced ability to concentrate the urine is a feature of almost all types of obstruction. After relief of bilateral obstruction, many factors may influence urine concentration, including decreased re-absorption of filtrate resulting in increased delivery in collecting ducts, increased osmotic load per nephron due to azotemia, and direct effect on collecting duct transport due to sustained increase in intrapelvic hydrostatic pressure. The clinical significance of the concentrating defect lies in the potential dehydration that may occur for several days after the relief of obstruction.

During acute obstruction, metabolic acidosis occurs in both cats and dogs.[16, 77] After relief of 24 hours of unilateral obstruction, urine pH and plasma bicarbonate are decreased, which may lead to acidosis for a short interval.

Treatment

Animals with complete acute obstruction have a potentially lethal disease that must be relieved and treated immediately. The site of blockage must be determined and the obstruction removed as soon as possible. The most direct measure is to bypass the obstruction with a catheter that decompresses the fluid column behind the obstruction. Surgical correction of the primary disease is advisable as soon as the patient is stabilized for surgery. Severe acidosis, hyperkalemia, and azotemia may preclude immediate surgery. Animals with azotemia, hypothermia, and dehydration should be hospitalized for intensive treatment.

An intravenous catheter should be placed in a peripheral vein for administration of warmed fluids (2.5% dextrose in 0.5% saline) to replace the estimated fluid deficit, which ranges between 5 and 15 per cent. Rate of administration should be 5 to 15 ml/kg/hr. Expansion of the extracellular fluid volume may partially correct the reduced GFR associated with obstruction.[18] The urinary obstruction should be mechanically relieved or the bladder decompressed per urethra or by cystocentesis with a urinary catheter that can be maintained in the bladder. Based on the severity of clinical signs or on specific measurement of the severity of acidosis, sodium bicarbonate should be administered intravenously. The rate varies between 3 and 9 mEq/kg body weight, depending on the severity of clinical signs. One-half of the calculated dose is given as a slow intravenous bolus and the rest administered intravenously with the rehydrating fluids over the next few hours. When the fluid deficit has been replaced, administration of fluid is slowed to the maintenance rate of 60 to 80 ml/kg/day. When serum potassium is normal, a balanced electrolyte solution is substituted for the dextrose/saline solution. Although potassium-containing solutions are contraindicated initially because of hyperkalemia, reduced potassium intake combined with increased urinary potassium loss tends to cause hypokalemia during recovery, which may result in anorexia, muscle weakness, ileus, and bladder atony. This may be corrected by adding 10 to 20 mEq of potassium to each liter of maintenance fluids or by giving oral potassium supplementation.

Using these measures, azotemia should be corrected within 24 to 48 hours after the initiation of treatment. In some animals fluid administration must be dramatically increased to match urinary output. Potassium supplementation is usually not necessary once animals begin to eat voluntarily. Permanent surgical correction of the mechanical obstruction may take place as soon as hyperkalemia, acidosis, and severe azotemia are corrected. The timing of surgery is highly variable, depending on the severity of these metabolic abnormalities; it may require from 6 to 48 hours to make the patient stable for surgery.

Chronic incomplete obstruction usually requires extensive radiographic studies to confirm the diagnosis and then surgical correction. Complications of obstruction, such as renal failure, anemia, calculi, and infection, require specific management prior to or after surgery. Surgical correction need not be hastily entered into in the majority of cases.

Finally, all animals that have had recurrent obstruction with or without infection require careful long-term surveillance. A periodic evaluation should include a complete physical examination, urinalysis, urine culture, and renal function tests as well as a radiographic examination.

Acute Renal Failure

Acute renal failure is defined as recent loss of renal function owing to potentially reversible damage of the renal parenchyma. It may be difficult to distinguish from chronic renal failure. Anuria or oliguria may be present during the early stages of the disease but may change to polyuria, which may be confusing. Additional evidence is the occurrence of renal failure without anemia, a finding that is less common in chronic renal failure. Rapid increases in BUN, serum creatinine, potassium, and phosphate levels and metabolic acidosis are consistent findings. It is particularly helpful to know if the serum creatinine level and GFR were normal within a reasonable time before the illness. Hence, these measurements should be part of the data base in all "at risk" patients.

Causes

Reduced renal hemodynamics represent a major predisposing factor to acute renal failure. Reduced renal perfusion, hypotension, hypovolemia, and sudden circulatory collapse are the most common initiating factors. These may result from a large number of disease processes including hemorrhage, trauma, prolonged anesthesia, extensive surgery, and reduced cardiovascular function.

A variety of nephrotoxins may also cause acute renal failure including heavy metals, organic compounds, antimicrobial agents, pigments, acute infectious agents, and hypercalcemia. Antimicrobials are important nephrotoxins, particularly the aminoglycosides and amphotericin B. The aminoglycoside gentamicin disrupts renal tubular cell function and causes ultrastructural changes in the glomerulus.[2, 10] The onset of acute renal failure due to aminoglycosides ranges from a few days to two weeks. Therefore, the onset of clinical signs is much later than that found with primary reduction of renal hemodynamics. Hypercalcemic nephropathy as a result of malignancy may also cause acute renal failure. Serum calcium concentrations in excess of 13 mg/dl may result in a renal concentrating defect, tubular necrosis, and calcification of the kidney.[19] Hypervitaminosis D may cause a similar nephropathy.[70]

Clinical Signs and Laboratory Findings

Animals with acute renal failure are generally depressed, hypovolemic, and hypothermic and have acute and severe gastrointestinal signs. Kidneys are usually normal in size or enlarged. Oliguria with concentrated urine suggests acute rather than chronic renal failure. Laboratory studies should include a complete blood count; BUN; serum creatinine, sodium, potassium, phosphorus, and calcium; acid-base evaluation; and urinalysis (see Table 134–1). The complete blood count is usually nonspecific unless there is an infectious cause. Animals with acute renal failure usually have a normal hematocrit, whereas those with chronic renal failure tend to have anemia. Moderate to severe azotemia is usually present. Serum inorganic phosphorus is elevated as in chronic failure. Hyperkalemia and acidosis are commonly present in acute failure but would not be expected until the terminal stages of chronic failure. Serum potassium concentration may range from 6 to 10 mEq/L. Acidosis is commonly accompanied by deep and labored respiratory motions. Bicarbonate deficits are frequently 5 to 15 mEq/L.

Urinalysis may be helpful in differentiating acute failure from other forms of renal failure. Urinary concentrating capacity is lost in the early stages of this disease, but urine specific gravity in the absence of fluid deprivation is highly variable. Proteinuria and glycosuria are commonly present. Glycosuria is usually transient and is due to reduced tubular reabsorption of glucose. A urine sediment examination is helpful to confirm acute failure, as the sediment may contain many casts that suggest an acute inflammatory or ischemic process.

Radiographic studies to confirm acute failure are of limited practical value. Normal or enlarged kidneys suggest acute failure, in contrast to small, shrunken kidneys, which suggest chronic disease. Conventional intravenous urograms are seldom helpful in differentiating the two forms of disease because reduced blood flow to the kidneys occurs in both. A renal arteriogram may confirm the presence of the normal vascular pattern and suggest acute failure. However, this procedure is not practical and may not be safe in many cases of acute failure during the early stages of the disease. Whether contrast radiography further decreases renal function in this situation is controversial.

Confirmation of the diagnosis may be by renal biopsy. A biopsy may be helpful to exclude chronic renal disease, but it seldom provides a specific etiology or prognosis in acute failure. A wedge biopsy or even a percutaneous needle biopsy may be contraindicated owing to the dangers of anesthesia and bleeding tendencies associated with renal failure.

Pathophysiology

Acute renal failure occurs in four stages: (1) onset, (2) oliguric or maintenance stage, (3) diuretic stage, and (4) recovery. During the initial stage the renal insult occurs with a reduction in glomerular filtration and urine volume. The time period varies from one day to a few days. The oliguric or maintenance stage may persist for several days or weeks with continued reduction in GFR and oliguria. During this time the initiating factors of failure persist or trigger additional factors that maintain the disease. The diuretic phase is recognized by a progressive increase in urine output that may or may not be associated with improved renal function. Urine volume may increase dramatically for one to two weeks while healing and repair continue or while the disease process is maintained. If azotemia subsides during the diuretic phase, a recovery phase begins and may last for days or weeks. Complete stabilization of renal function may require one or two months, and the animal may be left with a subclinical stage of chronic renal failure.

Four major mechanisms participate in the production and maintenance of acute failure. No single event or sequence of events uniformly represents the pathophysiological sequence.[22] After an ischemic or nephrotoxic insult, alterations in renal hemodynamics, cellular injury to the glomerulus, arteriolar vasoconstriction, tubular ischemia, tubular leakage, intratubular obstruction, and decreased glomerular permeability occur. The exact sequence of these events is unclear. If nephrotoxins are the initial insult, it is presumed that altered function and structure of tubules and glomeruli are primary with hemodynamic changes occurring as a secondary event. When ischemia is the initial insult, vasoconstriction appears to initiate reduced renal blood flow, filtration formation, and urine output. In the maintenance stages, many of these factors appear to be interrelated to maintain vasoconstriction, tubular back leak, and altered glomerular permeability.

Treatment

Surgery is seldom indicated in the treatment of acute renal failure. In fact, surgery is likely to be contraindicated in most animals owing to hyperkalemia, acidosis, and prolonged bleeding time. Treatment is divided into conservative measures and dialysis. Conservative measures are directed toward correction of major metabolic disturbances such as reduced extracellular fluid volume, hyperkalemia, acidosis, and azotemia. The first priority is correction of renal hemodynamic disorders and alleviation of biochemical abnormalities until renal repair can take place.

Conservative measures can only be pursued when an indwelling intravenous catheter is maintained for repeated sampling of plasma and administration of fluid and electrolytes. A catheter should be implanted that will remain secure and sterile for several days. The animal should be given a reduced dose of antibiotics (owing to renal failure) to prevent vascular infection. A urinary catheter attached to a closed sterile drainage system is placed in the urinary bladder for continual measurement of urine volume.

Diuretic agents have been advocated in the treatment of oliguric acute renal failure when volume replacement alone fails to initiate urine production. The protective effects of diuretics are related to reduced vascular resistance, increased renal blood flow, and increased solute excretion.[24] These agents are of little benefit during the maintenance stage and later than 12 to 24 hours after initiation of acute failure. Mannitol has been extensively used and reported to improve renal function and survival secondary to traumatic injury, surgery, and shock. In dogs mannitol increases GFR, renal blood flow, urine output, and survival when administered prior to or shortly after the induction of several models of acute failure.[8, 15, 56, 66]

After surgery, trauma, or nephrotoxic exposure resulting in oliguria, mannitol administration may be of considerable benefit in protecting renal function. Infusion of 0.25 to 0.5 gm/kg body weight given with fluid replacement to dogs is beneficial. If a diuresis results, a maintenance infusion of 5 to 10% mannitol in normal saline or a balanced electrolyte solution can be continued to promote diuresis for 12 to 24 hours. If a diuresis does not occur within one hour of the first dose, additional doses should not be given.

Extension of extracellular fluid volume using isotonic saline or hypertonic saline is of little benefit compared with mannitol.[56] Although hypertonic glucose has been suggested in place of mannitol, there are no clinical or experimental studies to support its efficacy in acute failure. If osmolar excretion is the major factor in protecting renal function in acute renal failure, mannitol is likely to be more effective than glucose owing to its limited volume of distribution and specific influence on renal hemodynamics and tubular re-absorption.

The use of diuretics that work on the loop of Henle has been suggested for use in acute failure. These agents have been inconsistently effective compared with mannitol in improving renal function experimentally. The efficacy of these agents in clinical medicine remains controversial. The use of dopamine or dopamine in conjunction with mannitol enhances renal blood flow in dogs with acute renal failure.[52]

Metabolic acidosis is treated in a manner similar to that described for urinary obstruction. Repeated bicarbonate administration every 6 to 12 hours may be necessary for several days to combat acidosis.

The management of persistent hyperkalemia and severe azotemia requires more aggressive therapy during the second and third days of acute failure if conservative management is not adequate. Peritoneal dialysis and hemodialysis may be considered and applied for a period of 3 to 14 days until it is clear whether renal function will return and is adequate to support the animal. Peritoneal dialysis and hemodialysis are discussed in Chapter 136 and elsewhere.[61, 72]

Chronic Renal Failure

In chronic renal failure, GFR has been reduced for a long interval, and there is little likelihood of rapid deterioration or hope of significant improvement. This term includes all degrees of azotemia including renal insufficiency, which may be detected before the uremic symptoms appear. The time scale is months to years.

Causes

The causes of chronic failure are multiple, varied, and commonly unknown. A detailed list of causes will not be discussed here. The causes of chronic failure are usually not surgical diseases and cannot be corrected by surgical intervention. The exceptions include diseases resulting in chronic urinary tract obstruction and pyelonephritis. When animals are presented with clinical signs of chronic renal failure, etiology cannot be determined with certainty at the end stage. A renal biopsy with tissue diagnosis of chronic interstitial nephritis tells little about the pathogenesis or time course of the disease.

Clinical Signs and Laboratory Findings

The common clinical and laboratory findings seen with chronic failure are outlined in Table 134–1. Evidence of chronicity includes stable azotemia and stable reduced GFR for more than three months and a gradual decline of function over years. Most animals have some degree of polyuria, anorexia, or osteodystrophy or small kidneys as seen on routine x-ray films. The presence of nonresponsive anemia indicates chronic rather than acute failure.

The presence of hyperphosphatemia or abnormalities in serum calcium concentration are indicators of chronicity but are seldom helpful, since serum phosphorus alterations may also be present in acute failure. Chronic failure may also include the coexistence of acute renal failure, which may obscure their differences. Chronic failure includes irreversible nephron loss with a permanent reduction in renal function, whereas acute failure includes reductions in GFR resulting from reversible causes such as volume depletion, heart failure, and urinary tract obstruction. Although these factors are generally minor and their correction will usually not return GFR to an improved state, they should be recognized and corrected. The value of the search for reversible factors contributing to chronic failure is often determined by judgment of the severity and duration of azotemia.

Metabolic Abnormalities in Uremia

As chronic failure progresses, a number of complex alterations in renal function occur to maintain metabolic balance until the later stages of renal failure. These functional responses to nephron loss have recently been described for the dog.[12] Three basic patterns of adaptation occur during progressive renal failure in regard to specific types of solutes. For example, one group of solutes has a pattern of no regulation by surviving nephrons. These solutes, including urea and creatinine, are characterized by a rise in plasma concentration as GFR is reduced. A second group of solutes has limited regulation during renal failure, e.g., phosphate ion. Phosphate is excreted in higher quantities into the urine during the early stages of renal failure, resulting in normal plasma phosphate concentration. However, adaptive ability fails when GRF falls below 25 per cent of normal, and then plasma concentration progressively rises as GFR falls. A third pattern of solutes is associated with complete regulation, as in the case of sodium and potassium. These solutes are regulated by renal tubular mechanisms that maintain normal plasma concentrations throughout the course of renal disease and failure.

The pattern of metabolic abnormalities in uremia is irregular. In some animals, regulatory failure for sodium and water may occur first. This may lead to inability to regulate extracellular fluid volume. Alternatively, inadequate production of erythropoietin may result in anemia as the first sign. Certain endocrinopathies may result in, for example, excess production of parathyroid hormone associated with malabsorption of calcium and impaired release of calcium ions from bone. Or, a group of vague gastrointestinal symptoms, malnutrition, anorexia, poor energy utilization, and abnormal metabolism of carbohydrates may lead to clinical signs. Therefore, during the early course of chronic failure the presenting signs may be highly variable and confusing.

A typical animal with progressive chronic failure may pass through four stages.

Stage 1. During this stage there is only a reduction in renal reserve. Until at least 50 per cent of normal nephrons have been lost, there is no evidence of chemical abnormalities or azotemia. The excretory and regulatory functions of the kidney are preserved in this stage, and clinical signs are absent. This stage is commonly missed in clinical evaluation unless renal clearance studies are performed.

Stage 2. This stage may be termed *renal insufficiency*. Manifestations include mild azotemia, impaired ability to concentrate urine, nocturia, and polyuria. Anorexia may be intermittently seen, but body weight and physical appearance are relatively normal. A mild anemia may be present. The animal is in a precarious state, which may be revealed by reduced fluid intake, vomiting, or diarrhea leading to more pronounced azotemia.

Stage 3. This stage is associated with persistent and frank renal failure with anemia, hyperphosphatemia, isosthenuria, and marked polyuria. Intermittent anorexia, weakness, listlessness, and intermittent vomiting with debilitation are found.

Stage 4. The final stage is uremia when all the consequences of metabolic abnormalities become obvious. Clinical signs are more advanced than in stage 3 and include severe gastrointestinal disturbances, nervous signs, and severe anemia.

Consideration of these four stages is helpful to determine if animals are safe candidates for surgery. Those in stages 1 and 2 are generally considered safe for mandatory surgery but should be carefully evaluated for elective procedures, particularly if prolonged general anesthesia is required. Animals in stage 3 are poor candidates for general surgery. If surgery is necessary, renal function and the degree of metabolic abnormalities must be evaluated. During and after surgery special care must be given to maintain extracellular fluid volume, renal blood flow, hematopoietic function, and electrolyte and acid-base balance.

The major metabolic abnormalities of uremia are listed in Table 134–2. All these abnormalities are discussed in a recent review.[13] Three important and newly elucidated disturbances (endocrine disturbances, anemia, and renal osteodystrophy) are discussed here.

Uremia is associated with a variety of endocrine abnormalities, including excessive production of hormones, inadequate production of hormones, reduced metabolic or renal clearance of hormones, and abnormal metabolism of hormones. In some cases, as

TABLE 134–2. Metabolic Disturbances of Uremia

Uremic toxins
Cellular function and composition
Biochemical disturbances
Nitrogen metabolism
Fat metabolism
Endocrine alterations
Gastrointestinal changes
Fluid, electrolyte, and acid-base changes
Hematological abnormalities
Renal osteodystrophy
Neurological changes
Cardiovascular abnormalities

TABLE 134–3. Alterations in Plasma Concentration of Some Hormones in Uremia

Increased	*Decreased*
Parathyroid hormone	Somatomedin
Growth hormone	Erythropoietin
Prolactin	Triiodothyronine
Insulin	Testosterone
Glucagon	
Calcitonin	
Gastrin	
Follicle-stimulating hormone	
Luteinizing hormone	

with parathyroid hormone, clinical disturbances have been identified and the role of the hormone has been clarified. The important polypeptide hormones that are not removed from the circulation in adequate quantities during renal failure include parathyroid hormone, glucagon, insulin, and pituitary hormones. Therefore, increased plasma concentrations of these hormones occur during renal failure (Table 134–3). Parathyroid hormone is a key element in renal osteodystrophy and is discussed later.

The significance of elevations in plasma concentration of other polypeptide hormones such as growth hormone, prolactin, calcitonin, gastrin, and the sex hormone precursors is unclear. Elevated plasma insulin concentration is associated with peripheral insensitivity to the action of insulin caused by a uremic toxin and reduced renal clearance of insulin during renal failure. Elevated glucagon concentrations are related to carbohydrate metabolism but may also play a role in the regulation of blood flow to specific tissues during renal failure. Decreased production of hormones such as erythropoietin and thyroid hormone may play a role in the uremic syndrome.

It is clear that reduced erythropoietin production during renal failure leads to reduced production of red blood cells. Reduced thyroid function may be partly due to a defect in the peripheral conversion of thyroxin to T_3 (triiodothyronine). Although some uremic subjects have reduced plasma thyroid hormone concentration, it is not clear whether this reflects the metabolic state of subjects with renal failure. A reduced thyroid hormone level may be appropriate for subjects with reduced metabolism due to renal failure. The side effects of these multiple endocrinopathies and their interrelationships may explain many of the mechanisms of metabolic disturbances in uremia.

The anemia of chronic renal failure may be a major limiting factor in survival of these animals. Fatigue, listlessness, weakness, and anorexia are clinical signs contributed to by the presence of anemia. The pathogenesis of anemia includes deficiency of erythropoietin. Experiments in animals indicate that reduction in the availability of this hormone is the central factor in reduced erythropoiesis, and replacement of the hormone increases bone marrow production.[73] Reduced red cell life span may also be a factor contributing to anemia. The hemostatic mechanism is abnormal during uremia, leading to insidious loss of red blood cells. The major hemostatic defect in uremia appears to be related to abnormal platelet function. The result may be prolonged bleeding time although the number of circulating platelets is normal. This qualitative platelet defect has been described in dogs with acute renal failure.[51] It is likely that the most significant blood loss during uremia is through insidious gastrointestinal bleeding.

Renal osteodystrophy is a major metabolic abnormality with widespread secondary effects. Although the bony changes may be associated with rubber jaw, a fractured mandible, or bowed long bones, the most devastating lesions may occur in soft tissues and may lead to a progression of renal failure. The pathogenesis of renal osteodystrophy involves three main abnormalities: malabsorption of calcium, altered vitamin D metabolism, and hyperparathyroidism. Their interrelationships are shown in a simplified schematic fashion in Figure 134–1. Chronic failure is characterized by marked impairment in the intestinal absorption of calcium. This intestinal defect appears restricted to the vitamin D–dependent active or carrier-mediated calcium transport sites in the duodenum and jejunum. The defect appears to be a derangement of vitamin D metabolism. Since 1,25-$(OH)_2D3$ functions principally to regulate calcium absorption, acquired alterations in its production by renal disease could play a major role in altering the intestinal absorption of calcium.

Secondary hyperparathyroidism in uremic patients represents the cellular and biochemical adaptations of the parathyroid gland to sustained reduction in calcium intake or slight hypocalcemia. As a result of excessive parathyroid hormone release, serum calcium concentration remains normal during renal failure owing to a release of calcium from bone stores. In this situation the parathyroid gland enters an autonomous secretory state. The control of phosphate balance is achieved primarily by renal excretion of filtered phosphate with parathyroid hormone playing a significant role. The subsequent rise in circulating parathyroid hormone promotes a greater degree of phosphaturia by the remaining nephrons and normalizes circulating phosphate concentration. Hyperphosphatemia was initially caused by reduced GFR but is now corrected by altered tubular excretion of phosphate due to parathyroid hormone. The importance of phosphate balance in the control of hyperparathyroidism has been confirmed in studies using uremic dogs, in which it was found that dietary phosphate restriction controls hyperparathyroidism.[46] The longstanding elevations in circulating parathyroid hormone have several effects in addition to remodelling bone.

Several toxic effects have been attributed to excessive parathyroid hormone, and this substance may now be considered as a uremic toxin. The possible relationship of excessive parathyroid hormone, calcium, and phosphorus abnormalities in uremia include soft tissue calcification, bone pain, fractures, retarded growth, neuropathy, altered mental state, and sodium and bicarbonate renal reabsorption. The most significant of these is probably soft tissue calcification. Both metastatic and dystrophic calcification occur during chronic failure. Metastatic calcification is a reflection of an abnormal chemical balance resulting in mineral deposition in normal tissues. Hyperphosphatemia or an elevated [calcium] × [phosphate] product probably is an important component in this complication. It is generally believed that when the [calcium] × [phosphate] product is greater than 60, soft tissue calcification occurs. Although the tissue sites of calcification have not been carefully quantitated in uremic animals, mineralization is common in lungs, kidneys, arteries, stomach, and myocardium. The significance of soft tissue calcification is that it may cause serious injury to renal tissues and further advance renal failure. This leads to the therapeutic approach of dietary phosphate restriction or other medical management of phosphate levels.

METABOLIC CONSEQUENCES AND ALTERED RENAL FUNCTION AFTER URINARY DIVERSION

Urinary diversion procedures include ureteroileostomy, ureterosigmoidostomy, trigonal-colonic anastomosis, transureteroureterostomy, and cutaneous end ureterostomy. Experience with these procedures is primarily in dogs. The objectives of urinary diversion are to provide for adequate urinary drainage, to preserve renal function, and to minimize secondary effects of diversion. Untoward consequences are not expected when a technically competent transureteroureterostomy is performed.[23] Problems associated with the use of bowel as a urinary conduit include ascending infection resulting in pyelonephritis and

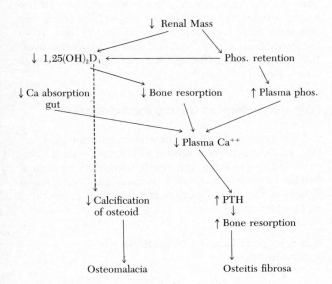

Figure 134–1. Pathogenesis of renal osteodystrophy.

reduced renal function, electrolyte imbalances secondary to absorption of urinary solutes, and stenosis at the site of intestinal anastomosis causing impaired ureteral function, leakage of urine, or progressive hydronephrosis. The problems of cutaneous end ureterostomy in domestic animals have not been studied, since this procedure is considered impractical in domestic animals.

Infection of the upper urinary tract is a major concern when using any urinary diversion technique.[83] Infections include pyelonephritis, pyelitis, and ureteritis. Pyelonephritis is the most serious infection, as it may lead to reduced renal function or permanent loss of renal mass. Ureteritis may also be important in that it leads to altered function of the submucosal ureter, which may allow vesicoureteral reflux and renal infection.[20] Bacterial cultures from the ureters, renal pelvis, and renal parenchyma usually contain the same organisms as those found in the gastrointestinal contents; i.e., *E. coli*, *Proteus* spp., and *Klebsiella*. The incidence of pyelonephritis in dogs with trigonal-colonic anastomosis was 30 per cent regardless of duration of anastomosis.[14] Similar results were found with trigonal-ileal anastomosis in dogs.[62] The rate of pyelonephritis in ureteroileostomy varied from 25 to 80 per cent.[64, 68] In similar studies the incidence of pyelonephritis ranged from 7 to 67 per cent for ureterosigmoidostomy.[64, 68] The lower incidence of pyelonephritis after diversion to the large bowel seemed to be related to the preservation of a normal ureterovesicular junction, as in trigonal-colonic anastomosis, or to the creation of a long submucosal tunnel, as in ureterocolonic anastomosis. The valvelike function of these structures is thought to protect against ascending infection.[54] This so-called antireflux anastomosis prevents pressure waves within the lumen of the bowel ascending the ureter to the renal pelvis, whereas end-to-side, mucosa-to-mucosa anastomosis allows transmission of pressure from the lumen of the bowel to the ureter.[45] Pyelonephritis was also found in 50 per cent of dogs with an ileal conduit to the skin.[71] Pyelonephritis may lead to rapid deterioration of renal function or it may persist as a minor infection that smolders along for years without causing major renal insufficiency.

Abnormal levels of plasma electrolytes and other solutes are less likely with urine diversion into the colon compared with diversion into the small intestine.[45, 53] Electrolytes are more readily absorbed from the small intestine than the colon. In studies using isolated intestinal loops, it was found that chloride, urea, and phosphate are absorbed more readily than sodium or potassium. Bicarbonate is readily lost in an intestinal loop.[53] Serum inorganic phosphorus and blood urea are the most frequently elevated constituents in the plasma as a result of absorption from the colon.[14] The increases in concentration may be minor, and values may remain in the high-normal range. It should be understood that these changes may have no relation to renal function in this situation.

Changes in glomerular filtration rate have been studied in dogs after trigonal-colonic anastomosis.[14] In dogs from which bacteria were not cultured from the kidneys, the mean reduction in GFR was only 12 per cent. In dogs from which bacteria were cultured from the kidneys, the mean decrease was 40 per cent. Although renal function as measured by filtration rate was reduced after the surgical procedure, serum creatinine values remained within normal limits. The decrease in GFR in dogs that did not have a kidney infection suggests that the mild pyelitis present in these dogs, or perhaps increased ureteral pressure, may have been responsible for the reduced renal hemodynamics.

These problems associated with urinary diversion are usually obvious within a few days after surgery. Their presence must be sought out along with other postsurgical problems such as stenosis at the site of anastomosis, hydronephrosis, abnormal gastrointestinal motility, and urinary obstruction. The metabolic complications previously mentioned are usually minor. They must be separated from deterioration of renal function, which is monitored by a long-term surveillance plan. Once the postsurgical period is passed without complications, serum creatinine measurements, intravenous urogram, or radioisotope imaging should be used to monitor renal function.

PATHOPHYSIOLOGY AND PHARMACOLOGICAL MANAGEMENT OF URINARY INCONTINENCE

Urinary incontinence is the failure of voluntary control of the urinary bladder and urethral sphincters, resulting in inability to control urination. Dysfunction of any of the various components that control micturition or the storage and voiding of urine can result in incontinence. This disorder is more common in dogs than in cats and more frequent in females than males. An understanding of the anatomy of the lower urinary tract and of the physiology of normal urination and continence is essential if one is to establish the cause of urinary incontinence or institute proper drug therapy for the specific disorder (see Chapters 132 and 133).

Pathophysiology of Urinary Incontinence

Urinary incontinence and urinary outflow obstruction are frequently encountered in small animal practice. These problems can occur secondary to neurological lesions, hormonal imbalances, congenital abnormalities, and diseases of the bladder, urethra, or prostate gland.

Neurological Causes of Urinary Incontinence

Neurological lesions that affect micturition can usually be divided into upper motor neuron lesions and lower motor neuron lesions. Abnormalities of the cerebral cortex, brainstem, cerebellum, or spinal cord above the L_7 spinal cord segment (L_5 vertebral body) may result in incontinence and are considered upper motor neuron lesions with respect to micturition. Abnormalities of the sacral spinal cord segments or sacral nerve roots or branches may result in lower motor neuron incontinence.

Upper Motor Neuron Lesions

Lesions from the pons to the L_7 spinal cord segments may result in detrusor areflexia, with hyperreflexia and increased tone of the external urethral sphincter. Thus, there is loss of voluntary control of urination, and manual expression of the bladder is difficult. One to two weeks following the injury, spinal reflexes usually initiate a sequence of bladder filling, contraction, and emptying, which is incomplete and involuntary. The bladder is referred to as spastic, hyperreflexic, or automatic. The external urethral sphincter remains hypertonic. The combination of incomplete bladder emptying with increased urethral resistance to urine flow results in residual urine.

Abnormalities of the cerebellum or partial long tract lesions may result in detrusor hyperreflexia with little or no residual urine. In these cases, urination is frequent and inappropriate. Partial long tract lesions may also result in detrusor urethral dyssynergia or reflex dyssynergia, a condition in which bladder contraction and urethral relaxation are not synchronous.[28] Interruption of the reflex pathways from the pelvic and pudendal nerve origin in the caudal spinal cord to the sympathetic origin in the thoracolumbar spinal cord may result in increased smooth muscle tone of the urethra. Additionally, decreased inhibition to the skeletal muscle of the external urethral sphincter may contribute to increased outflow resistance. Reflex dyssynergia creates functional urethral obstruction, characterized by sudden cessation of voiding with continued straining to urinate and a residual urine volume. This condition mimics mechanical urethral obstruction.

Lower Motor Neuron Lesions

Injuries of the sacral spinal cord or nerve roots or branches may result in detrusor areflexia with or without sphincter areflexia. Atony of the detrusor muscle results in overdistension, which, if prolonged, may cause separation of the tight junctions and increased bladder capacity with large amounts of residual urine. If the pudendal nerve is damaged, the external urethral sphincter is incompetent. As the bladder fills and intravesical pressure increases, the sphincter is no longer able to maintain continence, and urine leakage occurs.

Non-neurological Causes of Urinary Incontinence

Congenital Abnormalities

The most common congenital abnormality resulting in urinary incontinence is ectopic ureter. Although ectopic ureters may occur in both male and female dogs and cats, the abnormality is primarily associated with incontinence in female dogs.[58] If the ectopic ureters empty distal to the external urethral sphincter, involuntary dribbling of urine occurs. Surgery may correct the urinary incontinence, depending on the location of the ectopic ureters. Although dogs with vaginal ectopic ureters often become continent following surgery, there is a high incidence of persistent urinary incontinence in female dogs whose ureters terminated in the urethra prior to surgery. This suggests inherent urethral incompetence.

Other congenital abnormalities that may result in urinary incontinence include patent urachus, urethrorectal fistulae, and urethrovaginal fistulae. In patients with patent urachus, urine is voided through the umbilicus, and surgical correction is warranted. Urethrorectal and urethrovaginal fistulae also require surgery for correction of the incontinence.

Hormone-Responsive Urinary Incontinence

Estrogen-responsive incontinence in female dogs is an uncommon and poorly understood sequela to ovariohysterectomy. It develops in dogs after a variable period of time following surgery. The reported mean age of dogs in which this type of incontinence has been recognized is 8.3 years.[58] The pathogenesis of this syndrome is unclear; it appears that the proper maintenance and function of urethral mucosa and musculature are dependent upon estrogen, and the removal of an important source of this hormone results in incontinence in some female dogs.[59]

Hormone-responsive incontinence has also been reported in a castrated male dog.[9] The time of onset after castration and response to testosterone therapy supported an endocrine etiology. This syndrome is apparently similar to estrogen-responsive incontinence in neutered bitches.

Incontinence Due to Cystitis, Urethritis, or Prostatic Disease

The urinary bladder, urethra, and prostate gland are subject to non-neurogenic diseases that may result in incontinence of varying magnitude. An inflamed or irritated bladder may become hyperactive or unstable, resulting in a syndrome called urge incontinence, which is characterized by detrusor contractions that cannot be voluntarily inhibited. The loss of urine by uncontrolled detrusor contraction occurs immediately after a sensation of bladder fullness. Urge incontinence is often accompanied by increased frequency of urination and nocturia.[17, 58] Urge incontinence in man is commonly associated

Urinary System

with neurological or psychological abnormalities,[17] but in the dog it is recognized most frequently as a sequela to cystitis.[58] It is also known as small bladder syndrome because the bladder is abnormally small and incapable of storing a normal volume of urine.

Chronic cystitis, urethritis, or prostatic disease can also cause urethral incompetence resulting in urinary incontinence. In these cases, as the bladder fills with urine and intravesical pressure increases, the diseased or damaged urethra is unable to prevent the flow of urine through its lumen. Dogs with urethral incompetence secondary to chronic prostatic disease may have a history of urethral obstruction during the acute phase of the disease.

Paradoxical Incontinence Due to Mechanical Obstruction of the Urethra

Mechanical obstruction of the urethra by calculi, foreign bodies, neoplasms, or strictures can result in paradoxical urinary incontinence. Resistance to urine flow through the urethra is increased by the obstruction, and normal micturition is hampered or cannot occur. As the bladder distends with urine, intravesical pressure exceeds the increased urethral resistance, and urinary incontinence results. Treatment of these disorders generally requires invasive techniques such as surgery or hydropropulsion of calculi.

Idiopathic Urinary Incontinence

Occasionally, the specific cause of urinary incontinence cannot be determined. Frequently, the urinary incontinence is due to urethral incompetence, but a neurological, hormonal, or inflammatory basis for the urethral weakness cannot be proven. These cases can be considered idiopathic, and therapy should be attempted, since results are often positive.

Diagnosis

An accurate history, recorded chronologically, is important in the diagnosis of the cause of urinary incontinence. The owner should be asked to describe the present problem and how the animal's urination habits have changed. Whether the onset of the micturition disorder paralleled or followed another disease or procedure should also be established. Knowledge of recent ovariohysterectomy, abdominal or neurological surgery, prostatic or urinary tract disease, or trauma could be important to the diagnosis.

Observation of the animal's urination, attempted urination, or lack of urination can provide important clues to the dysfunction. Measuring residual urine may provide additional information. Normally, residual urine volume should be less than 10 ml.[57]

The presence of voluntary control of urination is important in the diagnosis of urinary incontinence. If the animal initiates and maintains urination until the bladder is emptied, it can be assumed that a detrusor reflex is present and that functional urethral obstruction does not exist. If the animal dribbles urine, has a distended bladder, and does not voluntarily initiate urination, a denervated bladder is likely, and neurological examination helps localize the lesion. Dribbling of urine in an animal that can voluntarily urinate suggests urethral incompetence; normal initiation of urination followed by sudden interruption of urine flow and continued staining implies functional urethral obstruction or detrusor urethral dyssynergia. Increased frequency of urination, inappropriate urination, and urge incontinence may occur with inflammatory diseases of the bladder and urethra, such as cystitis and urethritis, or with certain neurological diseases.

In addition to observation of urination, a complete physical and neurological examination is essential to the correct diagnosis of disorders of continence. Palpation and careful manual expression of the bladder provide information about bladder and urethral tone. Expression of the bladder in a male dog is more difficult than in a female dog, but in either sex if the bladder can be easily expressed with only slight pressure, the intrinsic tone of the urethra is probably decreased.

If the physical examination reveals dribbling of urine and an easily expressed bladder, the urethral sphincter mechanism is inefficient. A neurological examination to assess concurrent deficits and localize the lesion should be done. Diseases of the sacral spinal cord, sacral roots, or pudendal nerves can cause these clinical signs, and examination of the animal's perineal region for intact sensation and anal sphincter tone and reflexes should support such a diagnosis.

If neurological disease cannot be documented, other causes of urethral incompetence should be considered, including ectopic ureter syndrome, hormone-responsive urinary incontinence in neutered animals, and inefficiency of the urethra following prostatic or urethral disease.

Difficulty in expressing the bladder in a dog with signs of bladder-urethral incoordination is further evidence that dyssynergia exists. It is difficult on the basis of physical examination to determine whether the dyssynergia is somatic, with urethral striated muscle contraction, or sympathetic, with urethral smooth muscle contraction, and response to therapy may provide the diagnosis. Strictly somatic dyssynergia is uncommon in human patients, and in those dyssynergics with somatic and sympathetic components the major urethral resistance is due to sympathetic overdischarge.[4]

Increased urethral tone via sympathetic discharge can occur in animals with cauda equina lesions such as intervertebral disc protrusion, lumbosacral instability, or cauda equina tumors. Interruption of the reflex pathway from the pelvic and pudendal nerve centers in the sacral spinal cord to the sympathetic center in the thoracolumbar cord can result in over-discharge of sympathetic impulses when the animal attempts to urinate or when manual expression of the bladder is attempted.[1, 7] The sympathetic tone in the urethra can increase rapidly and can be strong enough to cause a functional obstruction to urination. This obstruction is largely due to smooth muscle contraction, but striated urethral muscle via its sympathetic innervation will contribute to the obstruction as well.

In all continence disorders, thorough examination for urinary tract infection or mechanical obstruction to urination must be performed. Urinalysis and urine culture may provide important information. Although urinary tract infection alone infrequently causes incontinence, it often exists concurrently, may exacerbate the signs, and should be treated definitively.

If functional obstruction is suspected but mechanical obstruction cannot be excluded on the basis of physical and neurological examination, further examination of the urethra and bladder should be initiated. Catheterization of the bladder with no obstruction to passage of the catheter implies absence of mechanical obstruction of the urethra. Infrequently, urethral polyps or mucosal flaps can cause intermittent mechanical obstruction to urine flow but not to catheter passage, and these possibilities should be excluded before a diagnosis of functional obstruction is made. Plain and contrast radiography can provide valuable information about the bladder and urethra and the patency of the urethral lumen.

Other diagnostic tests that are usually available through referral centers and that may be necessary in making a definitive diagnosis include the electromyogram (EMG), the cystometrogram (CMG), and the urethral pressure profile (UPP). Electromyography of the anal sphincter provides indirect information on the integrity of the urethral sphincter, since branches of the pudendal nerve innervate both structures. The EMG of limb and paraspinal muscles may also aid in localizing a neurological lesion.

The CMG measures intravesical pressure during a detrusor reflex, and, besides documenting the presence or absence of a detrusor reflex, provides information on threshold volume and pressure capacity, elasticity, and function of the bladder.[60]

The UPP measures intraluminal urethral pressure and allows the effective closure pressure of the urethra at rest to be determined.[65] It can be a valuable tool in the diagnosis and management of certain types of urinary incontinence in the dog and may help identify the site and extent of urethral incompetence or obstruction. Only the resting urethral pressure is measured by the UPP, and conditions that are not problems during rest, such as functional urethral obstruction, may not be diagnosed by the UPP alone. However, clinical signs and the exclusion of mechanical obstruction by radiology and the UPP allow a presumptive diagnosis of functional obstruction.

Treatment

Once the cause of urinary incontinence or obstruction has been identified, a therapeutic plan can be established. Micturition disorders that are responsive to specific drug therapy are listed in Table 134–4. These pharmacological agents have been tested in the dog either clinically or experimentally and have demonstrated effectiveness in alleviating the disorders for which they are advocated. However, pharmacological manipulation of the lower urinary tract is a palliative measure.

Clinical effectiveness of the drugs depends greatly on accurate assessment of the voiding disorder and the patient's response to the dose of drug used. It should be emphasized that the drug dosages and maintenance intervals used are empirical: they have been established on the basis of uncontrolled clinical observations or were extrapolated from recommended children's dosages. Dosages should begin at the low end of the range given and increased gradually until the desired response is seen or the maximum dosage is reached. The duration of the therapeutic trial at maximum dosage depends on the individual drug but in general should be one to two weeks. If no response to the chosen drug is seen within this time period, the drug can be considered ineffective and discontinued.

Each drug mentioned has certain side effects related to its mode of action, and although the majority of adverse effects are inconsequential, they must be understood before therapy is implemented (see Table 134–4). Consulting a pharmacology text prior to use of an unfamiliar drug is axiomatic.

Hormone-responsive Urinary Incontinence

See Table 134–4 for recommended drugs and dosages, mode of action, and potential side effects. The dose and route of administration of testosterone to control incontinence in castrated male dogs are not well established. Oral testosterone is less effective than parenteral because of hepatic degradation.[9] Testosterone esters, such as testosterone cypionate, that are absorbed more slowly than testosterone itself are recommended.

Urethral Incompetence

Phenylpropanolamine is an alpha stimulant that is effective in increasing urethral pressure and resistance to urine leakage when given orally.[7] It is preferable to use products that contain phenylpropanolamine alone rather than those that contain antihistamines or caffeine. Ephedrine is another alpha stimulant that can be used for incontinence due to urethral incompetence.[7]

Urge Incontinence

Propantheline, an anticholinergic drug, is commonly the drug of choice in cases of detrusor hyper-

TABLE 134-4. Disorders of Micturition and Drugs Used in Their Management

Disorder	Drug	Brand Name and Manufacturer*	Dosage†	Mode of Action	Potential Side Effects‡
Estrogen-responsive incontinence	Estrogens: diethylstilbestrol	Stilbestrol, North American Pharmacol	Initially 0.1 to 1.0 mg/day for 3 to 5 days Maintenance 1 mg/wk	Unknown, thought to enhance alpha receptor response to sympathomimetics[12]	Bone marrow toxicity
Testosterone-responsive incontinence	Testosterone cypionate	Depo-Testosterone Cypionate, The Upjohn Co.	200 mg/mo IM	Unknown	None noted in the dog
Urethral incompetence due to: postprostatic or posturethral disease, ectopic ureter syndrome (see text), neurogenic disorders	Phenylpropanolamine OR	Dexatrim Capsules, Thompson Medical Co., Inc.	12.5 to 50.0 mg t.i.d., titrate to effect	Sympathomimetic alpha receptor stimulation and increased urethral resistance	Minimal; restlessness may be noted
	Ephedrine	Ephedrine Sulfate, Eli Lilly & Co.	20 to 50 mg b.i.d.	Same as that of phenyl propanolamine	Same as those of phenylpropanol-amine; may cause urine retention
Urge incontinence	Propantheline	Pro-Banthine, Searle & Co.	7.5 to 30 mg t.i.d. to q.i.d.	Anticholinergic: decreased uninhibited bladder contractions	Urine retention

	Drug	Manufacturer*	Dosage†	Mode of action‡	Adverse reactions‡
Functional urethral obstruction	Oxybutynin	Ditropan, Marion Laboratories, Inc.	5 mg b.i.d. to t.i.d.	Direct antispasmodic effect on smooth muscle to allow increased bladder capacity	Urine retention
	Flavoxate	Urispas, Smith Kline & French Laboratories	100 mg t.i.d. to q.i.d.		
Sympathetic	Phenoxybenzamine	Dibenzyline, Smith Kline & French Laboratories	2.5 to 30 mg s.i.d. or in divided doses	Sympatholytic: alpha receptor blockage and decreased urethral resistance	Postural hypotension, tachycardia
Somatic	Diazepam	Valium, Roche Laboratories	2 to 10 mg t.i.d.	Skeletal muscle relaxation and decreased external sphincter resistance	Sedation
	Dantrolene	Dantrium, Norwich-Eaton Pharmaceuticals	3 to 15 mg/kg daily in divided doses		Generalized muscle weakness hepatotoxicity (long-term use)
Detrusor atony	Bethanechol	Urecholine, Merck Sharp & Dohme	5 to 15 mg t.i.d.	Cholinergic: stimulation of detrusor contractions	Abdominal discomfort due to increased intestinal peristalsis
Detrusor atony with urethral resistance	Bethanechol and phenoxybenzamine	See above	As listed above	Stimulation of detrusor contraction and decreased urethral resistance	As listed above

*Products may be available from other manufacturers or as generic drugs.
†Dosage is for the dog and administered orally unless otherwise indicated.
‡Consult a pharmacopeia for a complete description of each drug and its mode of action, contraindications, and adverse reactions prior to use.

activity. It is effective in the dog.[50] Unfortunately, the therapeutic and toxic doses are similar, and side effects may be seen at therapeutically effective doses. Because of this, direct-acting smooth muscle relaxants may be more rewarding.

Oxybutynin and flavoxate are antispasmodic drugs with little or no anticholinergic action and fewer potential side effects than propantheline. They may require several weeks of therapy before maximum response is achieved.[7] The prototypical anticholinergic drug, atropine, is relatively ineffective in alleviating uninhibited detrusor contractions.[7]

Functional Urethral Obstruction

Sympathetically induced urethral obstruction can be treated effectively with the alpha-adrenergic blocking agent phenoxybenzamine.[6, 49] It has also been useful in alleviating functional urethral obstruction in human patients with prostatic disease.[29] Phenoxybenzamine is long acting, but therapeutic blood levels are attained slowly; several days to two weeks may be required for noticeable effect.

Somatically induced urethral obstruction can be treated with diazepam or dantrolene.[7, 47] Diazepam is a centrally acting muscle relaxant and provides nonspecific action in the treatment of somatic dyssynergia. Dantrolene is a more specific skeletal muscle relaxant, but it can cause generalized muscle weakness. It is effective in decreasing intraurethral pressure in dogs.[47]

Detrusor Atony and Detrusor Atony With Functional Urethral Obstruction

Bethanechol is a cholinergic agent that has been used successfully to stimulate detrusor contraction in neurogenic and non-neurogenic hypotonic bladder dysfunction.[7, 48] It is indicated in atony of the bladder with urine retention. Bethanechol is a potent drug that stimulates contractions of the detrusor muscle as well as contractions of the smooth muscle of the gastrointestinal tract. High parenteral doses can cause increased gastric motility, diarrhea, and abdominal discomfort. Atropine is the antidote. Although oral therapy is less successful in low doses, up to 50 mg is clinically effective while avoiding undue systemic effects in man.[67]

Since bethanechol stimulates the parasympathetic receptors of smooth muscle, it may cause increased urethral resistance, and its efficacy in improving bladder emptying depends on its effect on the detrusor exceeding its effect on the urethra.[68, 78] In cases of suspected outlet resistance or dyssynergia, phenoxybenzamine should be used concurrently with bethanechol. Combined administration allows increased intravesical pressure with lowered urethral resistance.[48, 78]

Bethanechol should not be used in patients with a mechanical obstruction to urination or defecation or if the integrity of the patient's urinary bladder or gastrointestinal wall is in question.

URINE SPRAYING AND MARKING IN CATS

Even though male cats are castrated to prevent urine spraying and female cats spray urine infrequently, this behavior remains a clinical problem in feline practice. In this section of the chapter, therapeutic approaches to problem spraying behavior will be described. These approaches range from advice on behavioral control to administration of progestins and, as a last resort, employment of neurosurgical techniques. Urine spraying is a serious behavioral problem. If therapy is not successful, often the only other solution is euthanasia. The clinician, therefore, has the leeway to utilize more extreme measures than may be advisable for other behavioral problems. The severity of the problem is indicated by the range of measures that have been employed to try to correct it. A number of hormonal preparations, including estrogen, testosterone, and progestins, have been advocated. Attempts to physically alter the animal's ability to spray by performing a perineal urethostomy have not been successful because the animal eventually regains the ability to direct a jet of urine in a spray (unpublished observations). None of the therapeutic approaches currently employed are 100 per cent effective. Progestin therapy is much more effective in males than females, but satisfactory results are obtained with olfactory tractotomy in virtually all females and 50 per cent of males.

Before describing the therapeutic approaches to the problem of urine spraying, the natural context of this condition and its differential diagnosis will be reviewed. Also, the incidence of urine spraying in cats that are neutered prepubertally is examined and some of the factors that may predispose cats to problem spraying are considered. Therapeutic measures to be discussed include attempts to (1) alter the animal's reaction to environmental stimuli through remote punishment or behavioral "tricks"; (2) suppress activation of spraying by the use of progestins; and (3) permanently alter the olfactory field and make the cat less responsive to olfactory stimuli by olfactory tractotomy.

Normal Urine Spraying and Urine Marking Behavior

Territorial Marking

Urine spraying is usually initiated by the cat smelling a vertical target and then turning around and directing a stream of urine toward the investigated target. Males and females spray using basically the same posture. The squatting posture is used in urine marking, but the urination is in places that would not be normal toilet areas, such as specific places on a carpet, the shoes or clothes of a family member, or an owner's bed. Some cats may alternate between spraying and marking with the squatting posture, or they may start spraying after engaging in horizontal marking for several weeks. Because the behavioral context for both urine marking and urine spraying is the same, they are considered here as being influenced by the same factors, and the term *urine spraying* is used to refer to both behavioral patterns unless indicated otherwise.

Cats have a tendency to spray particular objects in their environment, and this seems to be associated with an attempt to make their environment familiar.[27, 32, 75] By creating a recognizable olfactory field in the home environment, it is believed that the cat may feel more self-assured and confident, especially in regard to agonistic encounters with other cats.[26] Agitation or anxiety stemming from interactions between cats is one factor that evokes spraying. Since such interactions commonly occur near territorial boundaries, territorial border objects, such as trees or walls, may be sprayed most often.[75] This is not to say that a cat goes through an intentional boundary marking routine from time to time. Rather, they mark boundary areas because this is where the anxiety-evoking encounters occur.

Sexually Dimorphic Aspects

Spraying is a behavior normally associated with tomcats, and the onset is related to sexual maturation. Like sexual activity, spraying occurs most frequently during the breeding season,[75] presumably as a function of an increase in seasonal secretion of testosterone and also because of increased agonistic interactions with other male cats. Urine marks are undoubtedly useful in attracting sexually receptive females to a male's territory.

Like fighting, roaming, and sexual behavior, urine spraying is sexually dimorphic behavior that occurs less frequently in females than males. Under natural conditions, one would expect females to spray at estrus when the deposition of urine on prominent vertical objects would "advertise" their sexual condition.[27, 75]

It is helpful to envision spraying as being mediated by a type of neural circuitry that is basically innate. The neural circuitry exists in both males and females, but in females it is held under some sort of neural inhibition so that it is less likely to be displayed. In males, testosterone, either directly or indirectly, activates the neural circuitry, making it much more likely to be activated by certain environmental stimuli. When a male is castrated, activation of the neural cavity is reduced; however, the neural circuitry in castrated males and females can still be activated by strong environmental stimuli.

Differential Diagnosis of Problem Spraying

To effectively treat urine spraying it is imperative to distinguish urine spraying from other types of urination problems, namely, inappropriate urination and urinary disorders. When urine is found 1 to 2 feet above the ground on vertical objects, it is a result of spraying. In both urine spraying and marking, certain objects are usually selected and repeatedly hit. Usually the cat is still using a litterbox or the outdoors for most urinations and all defecations.

Inappropriate Urination

If a cat has an aversion to the litterbox or the outdoors, it often ceases using a litterbox or going outdoors entirely. Defecation as well as urination will occur in inappropriate areas. The treatment of inappropriate elimination involves some conditioning principles to induce the cat to use the litterbox or the outdoors again.[31]

Urinary Disorders

The presence of a urinary disorder is usually evident from the medical history. Problem urination stemming from a urinary infection should be indiscriminate in terms of target areas, and the pattern of urination is consistent with the behavior of an animal unable to make it to the litterbox or the outdoors. There might also be straining at the time of urination and frequent urination. A urinalysis may be conducted to differentiate spraying from a disease of the urinary tract.

It is not uncommon for a cat that has started urine spraying after one or more bouts with urinary cystitis with possible blockage to be presented. Perhaps some discomfort in the urinary tract is one of the factors that predisposes the cat to spraying.

Androgenic Steroids

An occasional cause of spraying may be administration of androgenic steroids to stimulate metabolism, increase muscle tone, or treat certain skin conditions. The steroids may have sufficient androgenic activity to activate the neural circuitry for spraying, similar to the activation that occurs as male cats go through puberty.

Multicat Households: Identification of Urine Source

One of the problems in diagnosing urine spraying that occurs in multicat households is determining which cat is actually doing the spraying. Even if one cat is observed in the act of spraying, there is a chance that another resident cat may be contributing as well. The owner can confine one or more cats; however, this may alter the environment enough that the cat doing the spraying may temporarily stop. The administration of sodium fluorescein dye, of the type used to diagnose corneal ulcers and test the patency of the nasolacrimal duct, may be given to the cat suspected of urine spraying.[41] When given orally or injected subcutaneously, the dye is readily excreted in the urine. The fluorescence of urine-soiled spots is retained for at least 24 hours; over the next few days the fluoresence gradually deteriorates. If given orally or subcutaneously the dye appears in the urine within two hours. It is water soluble and, when diluted in urine, does not discolor fabrics upon which the urine may be deposited.

The following recommendations for using sodium fluorescein as a marker to identify a source of spraying are suggested. The cat considered the most likely source of spraying should be given a simultaneous injection of 0.3 ml of sodium fluorescein (10%, equivalent to 100 mg/ml) in the late afternoon. This dye labels the urine deposited that night and the next morning. Alternatively, the dye can be administered orally at home by the client by giving 0.5 ml of the solution or six strips of ophthalmic test paper inserted in gelatin capsules. Following either subcutaneous or oral administration, the client can be given an ultra-violent (Wood's) lamp on loan and instructed in how to scan the house for urine spots while the house is darkened. Cats that are considered possible culprits for urine staining can be treated at two-day intervals until the owner determines which cat is spraying.[41]

Incidence of Urine Spraying

Effects of Postpubertal Castration

In tomcats the frequency of spraying usually increases during the feline breeding season, presumably as a result of seasonal increases in testosterone secretion as well as the higher level of sexual awareness and increased social interactions with other male cats. Tomcats vary in the degree to which they engage in spraying, and this seems to be influenced by the number of cats in the neighborhood. Some spray indoors as well as outdoors, others reportedly spray only outdoors. There are constituents of tomcat urine not present in the urine of females or castrated males that contribute to the offensive odor, and most people can readily identify such urine.

Castration of tomcats after puberty, even after spraying has begun, is quite effective in eliminating or markedly reducing spraying. We found that about 80 per cent of adult males castrated because of problem spraying underwent a rapid decline in the behavior with an additional 10 per cent experiencing a more gradual decline.[39] One could expect from these data that approximately 10 per cent of male cats castrated because of problem spraying persist indefinitely in the behavior.

The persistence in spraying following castration is not due to residual amounts of testosterone, since within 8 to 16 hours after castration the concentration of testosterone in the blood is reduced to castrate levels and is behaviorally insignificant.[34] The treatment of persistent urine spraying or urine marking in male cats that have been castrated as adults is the same as that described for prepubertally castrated male cats discussed hereafter.

Effects of Prepubertal Castration

It is common for male cats to be castrated before puberty, and there is an assumption among veterinarians and cat owners that prepubertal castration is more effective in preventing objectionable urine spraying, fighting, and roaming than postpubertal castration is in eliminating these behaviors once they have begun. However, urine spraying is common enough in prepubertally castrated males and spayed females that the administration of progestins in an attempt to control this behavior has become routine in feline practice.[34, 36] It is not unusual to find male or female cats, neutered at six months of age, begin spraying as late as three or four years of age. Often the onset of spraying is related to the introduction of new cats into a household with other cats, changing households, or altering a major aspect of the cat's lifestyle, such as making an outdoor cat an indoor cat.

The question arises as to whether prepubertal castration is actually more effective in preventing urine spraying than postpubertal castration is in eliminating the behavior. Another concern is whether neutered males are more or less likely to engage in spraying than females and also whether the age of the cat at the time of prepubertal gonadectomy is related to the likehood of spraying. Another issue is whether a female that existed *in utero* adjacent to one or two males may have been partially androgenized and is thus more predisposed to engage in male behavior, such as urine spraying, than females from all female litters. This type of prenatal androgenization of behavior has been documented for sexual and aggressive behavior in female rats and mice.[21, 76]

Given the intolerable nature of urine spraying in the house, the answers to these questions about prepubertally neutered cats would be useful in advising clients about the selection of a male or female for a pet and in advising about the age at which to castrate or spay the cat. These questions were addressed in a recent survey.[40] The survey included 136 male and 124 female cats gonadectomized between six and ten months of age. The study found no relationship between age of male cats at the time of castration and the likelihood of spraying; there was also no relationship between age at ovariohysterectomy in female cats and the incidence of spraying. Furthermore, there was no greater spraying tendency in females coming from litters in which all the other littermates were male and in which androgenization was likely than in females coming from all female litters.

Problem spraying in both male and female cats was categorized as occasional, defined as once a month, or frequent, defined as at least once a week. Cat owners differ in their tolerance of urine spraying in the house, and some find the occasional sprayer unacceptable, whereas others readily tolerate this level of spraying. Frequent spraying would probably be highly objectionable to most cat owners.

In our survey the incidence of frequent urine spraying by prepubertally castrated male cats was very close to 10 per cent, and the incidence of frequent spraying by prepubertally spayed females was 5 per cent. As only 10 per cent of male cats castrated in adulthood for spraying continue to spray, this survey revealed that prepubertal castration is not likely to be more effective in preventing objectionable spraying than postpubertal castration is in eliminating the behavior once it has started. This information may be of value in counseling cat owners who wish to allow their males to grow the larger head, heavier jowls, and general morphology characteristic of tomcats.

Therapy for Problem Spraying

Predisposing and Causal Factors

When treating urine spraying and marking, it is a good idea to determine why the cat started spraying and continues to spray. Did it begin with the onset of the breeding season? Did the owners recently move? Has the cat been especially nervous or anxious recently? Are there new cats in the household? Some of the factors provoking spraying may be transient, such as the breeding season or a move to a new house, and therefore the problem may resolve itself. Other causal factors may be more permanent and may continue to maintain spraying activity. Therapy is more difficult for these problems.

Therapeutic approaches at three levels are discussed here: behavioral and management approaches, use of synthetic progestins, and neurosurgical procedures. Of course, a combination of approaches may be attempted. For example, a cat for which progestin treatment did not satisfactorily suppress the behavior may be subjected to an olfactory tractotomy. If the operation is not completely effective, the additional use of a progestin may control the behavior.

Behavioral Approaches and Management

Prior to seeking the services of a veterinarian, cat owners have often tried punishment such as yelling or throwing something at the cat when it is caught in the act of spraying. In some instances this has been effective for a time. Most cat owners understand the futility of bringing the cat to the urine-soiled spot and either pointing it out or rubbing the cat's nose in it. This usually just makes the cat wary of the owner.

A remote punishment, such as upside-down mouse traps near the soiled areas, may be effective. Ambushing a cat with a squirt gun or water sprayer when it is beginning to spray is another technique. It is important that remote punishment be delivered without the cat knowing that the owner is involved in the punishment process. In this way the animal makes the association between the target areas and the punishment rather than between the owner and the punishment. Remote punishment is only useful if a cat is spraying very few objects. Obviously one cannot have an entire house booby-trapped with upside-down mouse traps. A comprehensive discussion of the use of remote punishment is available.[33, 35]

Another technique for dealing with spraying in just one or two spots in the house is to feed the animal at these spots during its regular mealtime. Cats are unlikely to eliminate in the same spot in which they eat.

Progestin Therapy

Synthetic progestins are related to the hormone progesterone; the progestins suppress malelike behavior, such as spraying, even when the behavior occurs in females. The long-acting progestins effective in correcting spraying include the commercially available medroxyprogesterone (MPA; Depo-Provera, The Upjohn Co.) and megestrol acetate (MA; Ovaban, Schering Corp.). MPA is given as an injection and MA orally. One injection or an oral treatment series may permanently eliminate the behavior, especially if transient environmental factors evoked the behavior. If the cat is continuously anxious or nervous or if other factors are continuously stimulating the behavior, only repeated injections or continuous oral therapy may be effective. In these instances the potential side effects of the progestin therapy must be noted. Given the objectionable nature of urine spraying, there may be no option but to continue progestin therapy despite the potential for adverse side effects.

Our clinical survey of the overall effectiveness of progestin therapy in gonadectomized cats revealed that problem spraying or urine marking was resolved for a month or longer in about 30 per cent of cats.[36] However, the sex of the cat and number of cats in the household were important considerations. Of males, 50 per cent responded favorably, compared with less than 20 per cent of spayed females. About 50 per cent of cats (both sexes) from single-cat households responded favorably compared with only 18 per cent of cats from multicat households. Thus, the prognosis for progestin therapy is highly dependent upon the sex of the cat and its home environment. Females from multicat environments appear to warrant the poorest prognosis and males from single-cat homes the most favorable prognosis.

Both MPA and MA were about equally effective in the initial treatment of spraying. However, as many as one-half of the cats not responding to MPA treatment were found to respond favorably to subsequent MA treatment.

Common side effects included an increase in appetite and signs of behavioral depression. These side effects, which developed shortly after initial administration of the drug, were more common with MA than with MPA, occurring in up to 30 per cent of patients after MA treatment. Mammary gland hyperplasia[25, 43] and tumors[36] have been reported after both MA and MPA treatment. The hyperplasia regresses after treatment is terminated. Other side effects have been reported in the literature, including precipitation of diabetes mellitus in prediabetic patients, depression of corticosteroid output, and corticosteroidlike effects.[36] One would expect these more serious side effects to follow rather long-term therapy.

Since MPA and MA seem to be about equally effective in the initial treatment of spraying but MA results in more depression and appetite stimulation than MPA, it is recommended that injectable MPA be used in most cases for initial treatment. The use of an injectable drug also eliminates the need for a client to follow a complex dosage regimen. A dosage of 10 to 20 mg/kg of MPA is recommended. Because of occasional loss of hair or change in hair pigmentation immediately over the site of injection, a subcutaneous injection into the inguinal region is recommended. For treatment with MA alone or following unsuccessful MPA treatment, the recommended initial oral dosage is 5 mg/kg/day. If the treatment is effective, the dosage should be gradually reduced over intervals of two weeks to a dosage of 5 mg once a week. This treatment should then be terminated in about two to six months depending on the severity of the problem. If the initial MA treatment is not effective in one week, no additional MA should be given.

Olfactory Tractotomy

When progestin therapy is not effective, many cat owners wish to consider more extreme measures to resolve the spraying or marking problem. Olfactory tractotomy has been used successfully to eliminate spraying in cats that do not respond to progestin treatment.[37, 38] The operation is a simple neurosurgical procedure, carrying little surgical and recovery risk, and requires little in the way of specialized instruments and neuroanatomical background. The rationale for the operation is that spraying is usually initiated by the cat smelling the target area. The cat then usually turns around and directs a stream of urine toward the investigated target. The operation is a modification of that used by other investigators in their study of the sensory control of sexual behavior.[3] The olfactory tracts and caudal parts of the olfactory bulbs are approached dorsally through the frontal sinus. No adverse behavioral changes have been noted.

The complications that have been reported include transient anorexia and occasional and transient subcutaneous emphysema over the incision site. Subcutaneous emphysema, if it does occur, is due to passage of air from the frontal sinus to the wound site and usually disappears within a day or two.

Transient anorexia occurs in about half of the patients, but one can usually stimulate a cat to start eating by placing chicken or turkey baby food in its mouth or smearing the food on its lips. After it has eaten baby food, a cat will usually accept its regular semimoist or dry food, but it may be necessary to mix the normal food with baby food for a period of time. To verify complete anosmia, cat owners can be asked to conduct a "hidden food" test by placing food (tuna) under paper towels and determining if the cat can find the hidden food.

Individual responses to the operation vary. Spraying in some cats is markedly reduced or eliminated on a permanent basis. In others it is reduced to an occasional level that is tolerable to the owner. One might find that a cat sprays inside the house while under postoperative confinement, but after it is allowed access to the outdoors no further spraying is seen. A number of cats show an increase in affection toward the owner. In other cats there is an increase in appetite or at least a willingness to consume a greater variety of food than preoperatively. Occasionally cats become more finicky eaters.

Our clinical evaluation of the effectiveness of this operation is 50 per cent for male cats and 80 to 90 per cent for female cats.

Another neurosurgical operation, the creation of bilateral hypothalamic lesions,[42] was found to be 100 per cent effective in eliminating spraying in male cats but completely ineffective in female cats. This operation is lengthy and requires equipment for stereotaxic brain surgery and is not reviewed here.

Surgical Procedure

Perhaps the greatest concern in performing this surgery is that one can miss completely severing the olfactory tracts bilaterally, thus leaving the animal with a sense of smell. It is suggested that the surgeon practice on a cadaver with subsequent dissection of the surgical area. The technique might also be performed at least once on a practice cat.

An inhalant anesthetic for general anesthesia is appropriate. The hair over the incision site should be clipped and a depilatory cream can be used for additional hair removal, especially if the area is to be draped with an adhesive plastic drape such as one designed for eye surgery (Fig. 134–2).

An opening into the frontal sinus, 6 to 8 mm in diameter, is made after making a midline incision through the skin (Fig. 134–3). Removal of the bone is best accomplished with a pneumatic drill. Care is taken to avoid cutting into the ethmoturbinates, which project into the frontal sinus. The midsagittal septum is removed to completely expose the floor of the frontal sinus, which overlies the olfactory (ethmoidal) fossa enclosing the olfactory bulbs and tracts

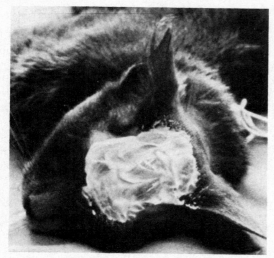

Figure 134–2. Depilatory cream used for hair removal, which is necessary for adhesion of a plastic drape. The cream, which is applied after the hair is clipped, should remain on the skin for five to ten minutes.

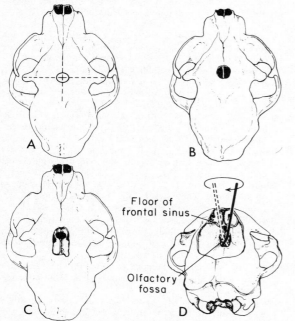

Floor of
frontal sinus

Olfactory
fossa

Figure 134–3. Surgical approach to olfactory tractotomy. *A,* A hole, 6 to 8 mm in diameter, is made in the roof of the frontal sinus at the intersection of the sagittal suture and a line passing through the tips of the zygomatic processes of the frontal bones. Dorsal view. *B,* The opening to the frontal sinus reveals a midsagittal septum, which must be removed. Dorsal view. *C,* A hole, 6 mm (transversely) by 3 mm (longitudinally), is made in the floor of the frontal sinus to expose the olfactory fossa and to allow lateral movement of the aspiration tube. In this illustration, the hole in the roof of the frontal sinus is enlarged to show the opening in the floor of the frontal sinus, which lies about 12 mm below the roof. Part of the septum of the sinus is evident. Dorsal view. *D,* In this caudal view, the relationship of the roof and floor of the frontal sinus to the olfactory fossa is shown. At the rostral end of the olfactory fossa is the cribriform plate, through which pass olfactory nerves to terminate in the olfactory bulb, which occupies the olfactory fossa. The range of movement of the aspiration tube (with the angled tip directed caudally) is illustrated. In this operation, the olfactory bulb cannot be completely removed, but the olfactory tracts passing along the floor of the olfactory fossa are completely severed. (Reprinted with permission from Hart, B. L.: Olfactory tractotomy for control of objectionable urine spraying and urine marking in cats. J. Am. Vet. Med. Assoc. *179*:231, 1981.)

(Fig. 134–4). A hole about 6 × 3 mm is made in the floor of the frontal sinus to allow access to the olfactory bulbs.

The caudal parts of the olfactory bulbs and the olfactory tracts can be removed by aspiration through a metal suction tube (No. 8 French). Although not necessary, it is best to modify the tube by bending the last 10 mm to about a 30° angle (see Fig. 134–4). The olfactory tracts are located on the ventral side of the olfactory fossa, and the tractotomy is accomplished by rubbing the aspiration tube across the floor and sides of the olfactory fossa. Visual inspection of the area is usually not possible because of seepage of blood into the fossa. To be sure that the tracts are completely severed, the bent part of the cannula should be directed caudally.

Minor hemorrhage can be controlled by packing the olfactory fossa with absorbable hemostatic material such as gelatin foam. Subcutaneous fascia and skin are closed separately. The surgery itself should take about 30 minutes. Minor bleeding from the nose may be seen in some cats. Since the frontal sinus communicates with the nasal cavity, it is recommended that one day before surgery cats be placed on a prophylactic (five-day) regimen of a broad spectrum antibiotic, such as ampicillin.

Graphic representation to highlight successive approaches to the treatment of urine spraying in gonadectomized female and male cats is shown (Fig. 134–5). Gonadectomy, which refers to prepubertal[40] and

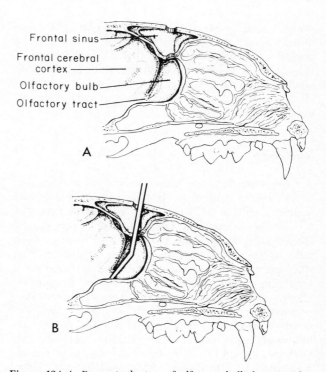

Frontal sinus
Frontal cerebral cortex
Olfactory bulb
Olfactory tract

Figure 134–4. Parasagittal view of olfactory bulb lying in the olfactory fossa. *A,* Anatomical relationships of cerebral cortex, olfactory bulb, and olfactory tract. *B,* View of insertion of aspiration tube to perform the olfactory tractotomy. Reprinted with permission from Hart, B. L.: Olfactory tractotomy for control of objectionable urine spraying and urine marking in cats. J. Am. Vet. Med. Assoc. *179*:231, 1981.)

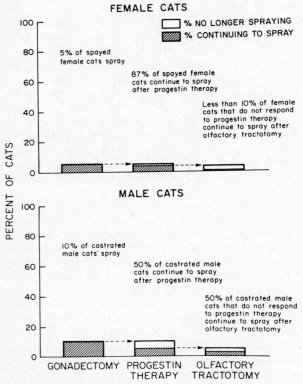

FEMALE CATS

□ % NO LONGER SPRAYING
▨ % CONTINUING TO SPRAY

5% of spayed
female cats spray

87% of spayed female
cats continue to spray
after progestin therapy

Less than 10% of female
cats that do not respond
to progestin therapy
continue to spray after
olfactory tractotomy

MALE CATS

10% of castrated
male cats spray

50% of castrated male
cats continue to spray
after progestin therapy

50% of castrated male
cats that do not respond
to progestin therapy
continue to spray after
olfactory tractotomy

PERCENT OF CATS

GONADECTOMY   PROGESTIN   OLFACTORY
                THERAPY   TRACTOTOMY

Figure 134–5. Clinical results of successive approaches to treatment of urine spraying in neutered female and male cats.

postpubertal[39] castration of male cats or spaying of female cats,[40] is tried first. For those that do not respond, progestin therapy with either MPA or MA[36] is used. Neurosurgery is tried last, not first. Data on olfactory tractotomy include previously published clinical trials[37, 38] substantiated by more recent unpublished clinical results.

SUMMARY

Urine spraying is an innate behavioral pattern that is difficult to control by training, punishment, and management procedures. Even when causative factors in the environment can be identified, clients are often unable or unwilling to alter their own or their pet's habits that lead to the problem urination. The simplest measures are management and punishment techniques, but these are often only temporarily effective, if at all. The second level of therapy, i.e., progestin treatment, is effective in some cats, depending on sex and number of cats in the home. The neurosurgical approach is the third level of treatment. Surgical placement of bilateral hypothalamic lesions reliably eliminates urine spraying in male cats. However, this operation is lengthy and requires specialized equipment for stereotaxic brain surgery. Olfactory tractotomy, a much more practical operation requiring little in the way of specialized equipment,

is rapid and carries minimal surgical risk. Viewed in the light of an alternative to euthanasia, elimination of a cat's sense of smell cannot be considered inhumane. It should be emphasized, however, that the neurosurgical approach described here represents the end of a continuum of therapeutic measures aimed at treating the problem behavior.

1. Albert, N. E., Sparks, F. C., and McGuire, E. J.: Effect of pelvic and retroperitoneal surgery on the urethral pressure profile and perineal floor electromyogram in dogs. Invest. Urol. *15*:140, 1977.
2. Appel, G. B., and New, H. C.: Gentamicin in 1978. Ann. Intern. Med. *89*:528, 1978.
3. Aronson, L. R., and Cooper, M. L.: Olfactory deprivation and mating behavior in sexually experienced male cats. Behav. Biol. *11*:459, 1974.
4. Awad, S. A., and Downie, J. W.: Sympathetic dyssynergia in the region of the external sphincter: A possible source of lower urinary tract obstruction. J. Urol. *118*:636, 1977.
5. Awad, S. A., Downie, J. W., and Kiruluta, H. G.: Alpha adrenergic agents in urinary disorders of the proximal urethra. Part I. Sphincteric incontinence. Br. J. Urol. *50*:332, 1978.
6. Awad, S. A., Downie, J. W., and Kiruluta, H. G.: Alpha adrenergic agents in urinary disorders of the proximal urethra. Part II. Urethral obstruction due to sympathetic dyssynergia. Br. J. Urol. *50*:336, 1978.
7. Awad, S. A., Downie, J. W., and Kiruluta, H. G.: Pharmacologic treatment of disorders of bladder and urethra: a review. Can. J. Surg. *22*:515, 1979.
8. Balint, P., Laszlo, K., Szocs, E., and Tayan, E.: Renal haemodynamics in dogs with dehydration azotemia. Acta Med. Acad. Sci. Hung. *32*:193, 1975.
9. Barsanti, J. A., Edwards, P. D., and Losonsky, J.: Testosterone responsive urinary incontinence in a castrated male dog. J. Am. Anim. Hosp. Assoc. *17*:117, 1981.
10. Baylis, C., Rennke, H. G., and Brenner, B. M.: Mechanisms of the defect in glomerular ultrafiltration associated with gentamicin administration. Kidney Int. *12*:344, 1977.
11. Bercovitch, D. D., Kasen, L., Blann, L., and Levitt, M. F.: The postobstructive kidney. Observations on nephron function after the relief of 24 hours of ureteral ligation in the dog. J. Clin. Invest. *50*:1154, 1971.
12. Bovee, K. C.: Functional responses to nephron loss. *In* Bovee, K. C. (ed.): *Canine Nephrology.* Harwal Publishing Co., Media, PA, 1983.
13. Bovee, K. C.: Metabolic disturbances of uremia. *In* Bovee, K. C. (ed.): *Canine Nephrology.* Harwal Publishing Co., Media, PA, 1983.
14. Bovee, K. C., Pass, M. A., Wardley, R., Biery, D., and Allen, H. L.: Trigonal-colonic anastomosis: A urinary diversion procedure in dogs. J. Am. Vet. Med. Assoc. *174*:184, 1979.
15. Burke, T. J., Cronin, R. E., Duchin, K. L., Peterson, L. N., and Schrier, R. W.: Ischemic and tubule obstruction during acute renal failure in dogs: Mannitol in protection. Am. J. Physiol. *238*:F305, 1980.
16. Burrows, C. F., and Bovee, K. C.: Characterization and treatment of acid-base and renal defects due to urethral obstruction in cats. J. Am. Vet. Med. Assoc. *172*:801, 1978.
17. Cardozo, L. D., and Stanton, S. L: An objective comparison of the effects of parenterally administered drugs in patients suffering from detrusor instability. J. Urol. *122*:58, 1979.
18. Chander, M., Stacey, W. K., Haden, H. T., and Falls, W. F.: The influence of extracellular fluid volume expansion on postobstructive diuresis in the dog. Invest. Urol. *11*:114, 1973.
19. Chew, D. J., and Capen, C. C.: Hypercalcemia nephropathy and associated disorders. *In* Kirk, R. W. (ed.): *Current Veterinary Therapy VII.* W. B. Saunders, Philadelphia, 1980.

20. Christie, B. A.: Vesicoureteral reflux in dogs. J. Am. Vet. Med. Assoc. *162*:772, 1973.
21. Clemens, L. G.: The neurohormonal control of masculine sexual behavior. *In* Montagna, W., and Sadler, W. A. (eds.): *Reproductive Behavior*. Plenum Press, New York, 1974, p. 23.
22. Cowgill, L.: Acute renal failure. *In* Bovee, K. C. (ed.): *Canine Nephrology*. Harwal Publishing Co., Media, PA, 1983.
23. Crane, S. W., and Waldron, D. R.: Ureteral function and healing following microsurgical transureteroureterostomy in the dog. Vet. Surg. *9*:108, 1980.
24. Cronin, R. E., de Torrente, A., Miller, P. D., Bulger, R. E., Burke, T. J., and Schrier, R. W.: Pathogenic mechanisms in early norepinephrine-induced acute renal failure: Functional and histological correlates of protection. Kidney Int. *14*:115, 1978.
25. Dorn, A. S., Legendre, A. M., and McGavin, M. D.: Mammary hyperplasia in a male cat receiving progesterone. J. Am. Vet. Med. Assoc. *182*:621, 1983.
26. Eisenberg, J. F., and Kleiman, D. G.: Olfactory communication in mammals. Ann. Rev. Ecol. Syst. *3*:1, 1972.
27. Ewer, R. F.: *The Carnivores*. Cornell University Press, Ithaca, 1973.
28. Fletcher, T. E., and Bradley, W. E.: Neuroanatomy of the bladder-urethra. J. Urol. *119*:153, 1978.
29. Gerstenberg, T., Blaaberg, J., Nielson, M. L., and Clausen, S.: Phenoxybenzamine reduces bladder outlet obstruction in benign prostatic hyperplasia. Invest. Urol. *18*:29, 1980.
30. Gillenwater, J. Y., Westervelt, F. B., Jr., Vaughan, E. D., Jr., and Howards, S. S.: Renal function one week after release of chronic unilateral hydronephrosis in man. Kidney Int. *7*:179, 1975.
31. Hart, B. L.: Inappropriate urination and defecation. Feline Pract. *6*:6, 1976.
32. Hart, B. L.: *Feline Behavior*. Veterinary Practice Publishing Co., Santa Barbara, 1978.
33. Hart, B. L.: Water sprayer therapy. Feline Pract. *8*:13, 1978.
34. Hart, B. L.: Problems with objectionable sociosexual behavior of dogs and cats: Therapeutic use of castration and progestins. Comp. Cont. Ed. *1*:461, 1979.
35. Hart, B. L.: Behavioral therapy with mousetraps. Feline Pract. *9*:10, 1979.
36. Hart, B. L.: Objectionable urine spraying and urine marking in cats: Evaluation of progestin treatment in gonadectomized males and females. J. Am. Vet. Med. Assoc. *177*:529, 1980.
37. Hart, B. L.: Olfactory tractotomy for control of objectionable urine spraying and urine marking in cats. J. Am. Vet. Med. Assoc. *179*:231, 1981.
38. Hart, B. L.: Neurosurgery for behavioral problems. A curiosity or the new wave? Vet. Clin. North Am. *12*:707, 1982.
39. Hart, B. L., and Barrett, R. E.: Effects of castration on fighting, roaming, and urine spraying in adult male cats. J. Am. Vet. Med. Assoc. *163*:290, 1973.
40. Hart, B. L., and Cooper, L.: Factors relating to urine spraying and fighting in prepuberally gonadectomized male and female cats. J. Am. Vet. Med. Assoc. *184*:1255, 1984.
41. Hart, B. L., and Leedy, M.: Identification of source of urine stains in multi-cat households. J. Am. Vet. Med. Assoc. *180*:77, 1982.
42. Hart, B. L., and Voith, V. L.: Changes in urine spraying, feeding and sleep behavior of cats following medial preoptic-anterior thalamic lesions. Brain Res. *145*:406, 1978.
43. Hinton, M., and Gaskell, C. J.: Non-neoplastic mammary hypertrophy in the cat associated with pregnancy or with oral progestational therapy. Vet. Rec. *100*:277, 1977.
44. Janknegt, R. A.: Abosrption of urine products in jejunum, ileum, and sigmoid loops. Urol. Int. *22*:435, 1967.
45. Kamizaki, H., and Cass, A. S.: Conduit and renal pelvic pressures after ileal and colonic urinary diversion in dogs. Invest. Urol. *16*:27, 1978.
46. Kaplan, M. A., Canterbury, J. M., Gavellas, G., Jaffe, D., Bourgoignie, J. J., Reiss, E., and Bricker, N. S.: Interrelations between phosphorus, calcium, parathyroid hormone, and renal phosphate excretion in response to an oral phosphorus load in normal and uremic dogs. Kidney Int. *14*:207, 1978.
47. Khalaf, I. M., Foley, G., and Elhilali, M. M.: The effect of Dantrium on the canine urethral pressure profile. Invest. Urol. *17*:188, 1979.
48. Khanna, O. P.: Disorders of micturition. Neuropharmacologic basis and results of drug therapy. Urology *8*:316, 1976.
49. Khanna, O. P., and Gonick, P.: Effects of phenoxybenzamine hydrochloride on canine lower urinary tract: Clinical implications. Urology *6*:323, 1975.
50. Khanna, O. P., Heker, D., and Gonick, P.: Cholinergic and adrenergic neuroreceptors in urinary tract of female dogs: Evaluation of function with pharmacodynamics. Urology *5*:616, 1975.
51. Larrain, C., and Langdell, R. D.: The hemostatic defect of uremia. II. Investigation of dogs with experimentally produced acute urinary retention. Blood *11*:1067, 1956.
52. Lindner, A., Cutler, R. E., Goodman, W. G., et al.: Synergism of dopamine plus furosemide in preventing acute renal failure in the dog. Kidney Int. *16*:158, 1979.
53. Madsen, P. O.: The etiology of hyperchloremic acidosis following intestinal anastomosis: An experimental study. J. Urol. *92*:448, 1964.
54. Maydl, I.: Neue beobachtungen von ureterenimplantation die flexura romana bei ectopia vesicae. Wien. Med. Wochenschr. *46*:1241, 1896.
55. Miller, J. B., Marion, D. M., and Gillenwater, J. Y.: Patterns of recovery of renal function after surgical relief of chronic bilateral partial ureteral obstruction. Invest. Urol. *17*:69, 1979.
56. Morris, C. R., Alexander, E. A., Burns, F. J., and Levinsky, N. G.: Restoration and maintenance of glomerular filtration by mannitol during hypoperfusion of the kidney. J. Clin. Invest. *51*:1555, 1972.
57. Oliver, J. E.: Diseases of micturition. *In* Hoerlein, B. F. (ed.): *Canine Neurology: Diagnosis and Treatment*. W. B. Saunders, Philadelphia, 1978, p. 461.
58. Osborne, C. A., Oliver, J. E., and Polzin, D. E.: Non-neurogenic urinary incontinence, *In* Kirk, R. W. (ed.): *Current Veterinary Therapy VII*. W. B. Saunders, Philadelphia, 1980, p. 1128.
59. Osborne, C. A., and Polzin, D. J.: Canine estrogen responsive incontinence: An enigma. DVM Newsmag. *10*:42, 1979.
60. Oliver, J. E., and Young, W. O.: Air cystometry in dogs under xylazine induced restraint. Am. J. Vet. Res. *34*:1433, 1973.
61. Parker, H. R.: Peritoneal dialysis and hemoperfusion. *In* Bovee, K. C. (ed.): *Canine Nephrology*. Harwal Publishing Co., Media, PA, 1983.
62. Pond, H. S., and Texter, J. H.: Trigonal-ileal anastomosis: Experimental studies. J. Urol. *103*:746, 1970.
63. Porter, G. A., and Bennett, W. M.: Toxic nephropathies. *In* Brenner, B. M., and Rector, F. C. (eds.): *The Kidney*, 2nd ed. W. B. Saunders, Philadelphia, 1981, p. 2045.
64. Richie, J. P., Skinner, D. G., and Waisman, J.: The effect of reflux on the development of pyelonephritis in urinary diversion: An experimental study. J. Surg. Res. *16*:256, 1974.
65. Rosin, A., Rosin, E., and Oliver, J.: The canine urethral pressure profile. Am. J. Vet. Res. *41*:1113, 1980.
66. Selkurt, E. E.: Changes in renal clearance following complete ischemia of the kidney. Am. J. Physiol. *144*:395, 1945.
67. Sonda, L. P., Gershon, C., Diokno, A. C., and Lapides, J.: Further observations on the cystometric and uroflowmetric effects of bethanechol chloride on the human bladder. J. Urol. *122*:775, 1980.
68. Spence, B., Esho, J., and Cass, A.: Bacteriuria in intestinal conduit urinary diversion in dogs. Invest. Urol. *10*:290, 1973.
69. Sporer, A., Leyson, J. F., and Martin, B. F.: Effects of bethanechol chloride on the external urethral sphincter in spinal cord injury patients. J. Urol. *120*:62, 1978.
70. Sprangler, W. I., Gribble, D. H., and Lee, T. C.: Vitamin D intoxication and the pathogenesis of Vitamin D nephropathy in the dog. Am. J. Vet. Res. *40*:73, 1979.

71. Starr, A., Rose, D. H., and Cooper, J. F.: Antireflux ureter-oileal anastomosis: Two experimental techniques. Invest. Urol. *12*:165, 1974.

72. Thornhill, J. A.: Hemodialysis. *In* Bovee, K. C. (ed.): *Canine Nephrology.* Harwal Publishing Co., Media, PA, 1983.

73. Van Stone, J. C., and Max, P.: Effect of erythropoietin on anemia of peritoneally dialyzed anephric rats. Kidney Int. *15*:370, 1979.

74. Vaughan, E. D., Jr., Sorenson, E. J., and Gillenwater, J. Y.: The renal hemodynamic response to chronic unilateral complete ureteral occlusion. Invest. Urol. *8*:78, 1970.

75. Verberne, G., and Leyhausen, P.: Marking behavior of some viverridae and felidae. Time-interval analysis of marking pattern. Behaviour *58*:192, 1976.

76. Vom Saal, F. S., and Bronson, F. H.: Sexual characteristics of adult female mice as correlated with their blood testosterone levels during female development. Science *208*:597, 1980.

77. Walls, J., Buerkert, J. E., Pukerson, M. L., and Klahr, S.: Nature of the acidifying defect after the relief of ureteral obstruction. Kidney Int. *7*:304, 1975.

78. Westmore, D. D.: Urinary incontinence: Which drugs to use. Drugs *17*:418, 1979.

79. Wilson, D. R.: Micropuncture study of chronic obstructive nephropathy before and after release of obstruction. Kidney Int. *2*:119, 1972.

80. Yarger, W. E., Aynedjian, H. S., and Bank, N.: A micropuncture study of postobstructive diuresis in the rat. J. Clin. Invest. *51*:625, 1972.

81. Yarger, W. E., and Griffith, L. D.: Intrarenal hemodynamics following chronic unilateral ureteral obstruction in the dog. Am. J. Physiol. *227*:816, 1974.

82. Zetterstrom, R., Ericsson, N. O., and Winberg, J.: Separate renal function studies in predominantly unilateral hydronephrosis. Acta Paediatr. Scand. *47*:540, 1958.

83. Zincke, H., and Seruga, J. W.: Ureterosigmoidostomy: Critical review of 173 cases. J. Urol. *113*:324, 1975.

Chapter 135   Principles of Urinary Tract Surgery

Bruce A. Christie

PATIENT EVALUATION

The aim of patient evaluation is to determine the location and extent of any observed problem in order to recommend a definitive treatment.

History taking generates a number of diagnostic possibilities. The species, breed, sex, and age of the patient should immediately eliminate some disease conditions and provide a high index of suspicion for others. A method of proceeding diagnostically is outlined (Fig. 135–1). Urinary tract problems usually present as hematuria, altered voiding habits, or changes in demeanor. The duration of signs indicates whether the condition is acute or chronic. The possible association of the problem with a recent significant event such as trauma, parturition, or previous drug treatment should be eliminated.

The *physical examination* narrows the diagnostic possibilities down to probabilities and, with the history, supplies most of the information needed to make a diagnosis. The vital signs may indicate whether the condition is local or systemic. A general inspection gives information on nervous system function, dehydration, trauma, and the presence of congenital abnormalities. Abdominal palpation is usually possible in cats but more difficult in dogs. However, even in fat dogs, kidney trauma associated with flank swelling or pain can nearly always be detected. A larger bladder, a large cystic calculus, or the presence of fluid in the abdomen should not be missed. A digital rectal examination in adult male dogs reveals an enlarged or painful prostate. If the abnormality is related to altered voiding habits, a voiding episode should be observed to help differentiate frequent urination (pollakiuria) from difficult urination (dysuria).

Clinical chemistry and pathology tests confirm or rule out urinary tract bleeding or urinary tract infection and indicate the degree of compromise of renal function. When dealing with any potential or actual urinary tract abnormality, the baseline hemogram and urea nitrogen levels should be known, as this information can be used to monitor improvement or deterioration during the course of the disease.

A *radiographic examination* can confirm or suggest a diagnosis or provide data with which to plan surgical therapy. If removal of a kidney is contemplated, an excretory urogram, intravenous pyelogram (IVP), will indicate whether the other kidney is present and functioning. The IVP may show the position of an ectopic ureteral opening when viewed against negative contrast (air) in the bladder and urethra. If a pneumocystogram is to be performed, it should be kept in mind that such an examination can result in fatal air embolism.[99] Dyspnea and cyanosis can occur within a few minutes.

Air can enter the vascular system through bleeding capillaries. If this happens, the animal should be placed in left lateral recumbency with its head lowered. As the pulmonary artery is then ventral, trapped air is released into the pulmonary circulation, where it can be absorbed by the lungs. It is sometimes less expensive and more expedient to inspect the lesion at operation and decide then whether or

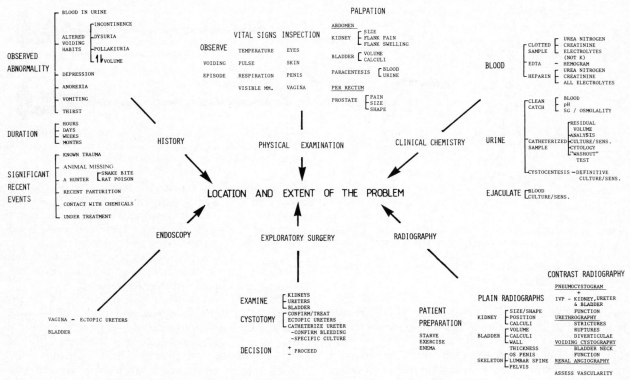

Figure 135–1. Method of diagnosing urinary tract abnormalities.

not to proceed. The location of ectopic ureters can be confirmed at operation, and ureteral catheterization can be done by direct vision through a cystotomy.

Endoscopes small enough to be inserted into the renal pelvis are available and can be used to evaluate unilateral hematuria.[40] Endoscopes can also be used to search for an ectopic ureteral orifice in the vagina. Most operations on the urinary tract are elective, but if the urinary tract is obstructed or ruptured or if there is severe bleeding, emergency surgery is justified.

SURGICAL PRINCIPLES

Surgical Instruments

A gentle touch with fine, good-quality equipment and minimal handling of the tissues minimize edema. Instruments used for basic surgery are those that permit cutting and grasping. A cut with a scalpel causes minimal trauma to the tissues. A scalpel can be used to make an incision in any part of the urinary tract. Crush is associated with an incision made with scissors; however, good-quality scissors can be very useful for making incisions in ureters or the urethra.

The electroscalpel is a very useful tool for incising the bladder and urethra and for achieving hemostasis by coagulation of small bleeders. When an electric current with radiofrequency (rf) is applied to tissues,

it produces heat proportional to the frequency of oscillation and inversely proportional to the contact area of the electrode used.[10] Needle electrodes are used, and tips should be kept clean of carbonized biological material. Parting of the tissues is due to the generation of steam bubbles, which rupture cells in the vicinity of the tip of the cutting electrode.[44] Healing of skin wounds is delayed a few days when compared with healing of sharp incisions made with a scapel.[49] This disadvantage is offset by the precision and ease with which the tissue can be cut and the capacity for rapid hemostasis.

Grasping instruments with strong jaws and large teeth are not required for operating on delicate urinary tissues. Smooth-tipped dissecting forceps can be used to manipulate tissue gently without crushing it. Such instruments are also valuable for controlling fine suture needles, which are too small to be easily manipulated by the fingers.

Mosquito forceps are sometimes needed to control hemorrhage but are also useful for grasping suture material for tissue retraction. Often the most gentle way to stabilize and retract the kidneys and the bladder is to use the fingers and thumb. The renal vascular pedicle can also be gently occluded by digital pressure. Hemostats should never be used for temporary vascular occlusion, as they crush vessels and promote clotting and stricture. Bulldog clamps (serrefines) or, preferably, vascular clamps (Fig. 135–2) can be used when adjustable closing pressure is needed. Needle holders must have fine jaws when

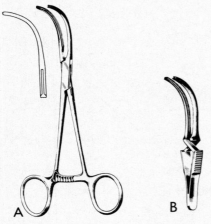

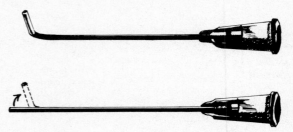

Figure 135–4. A disposable hypodermic needle modified to irrigate the diverticula of the renal pelvis. The sharp tip has been ground off and the distal 5 mm bent approximately 70°.

Figure 135–2. Peripheral vascular clamps. *A,* Adjustable pressure clamp. When the ratchet is engaged in the first notch, the jaws are still open. Enough pressure is applied to just occlude the blood vessel. *B,* Bulldog clamp. These clamps can be purchased with a specific pressure rating.

small needles are used to maximize effective needle length and minimize the straightening stress as the needle holder is applied (Fig. 135–3).

Nylon catheters with rounded, sealed ends and a side hole in a range of sizes from 3 to 8 French gauge (F) can be used for catheterizing the urethra or ureters of cats and dogs. Catheters can be used to test patency, to flush the urinary tract, and to act as a landmark to help locate the urethra when performing urethrotomy and as a splint or stent during urethral and ureteral surgery. For irrigating the renal pelvis during nephrotomy, a lacrimal needle or a modified disposable hypodermic needle can be used (Fig. 135–4). Some type of suction apparatus is very useful to aspirate urine and flushing solutions. For fine work on ureters, operating loupes with 2 to 4× magnification are helpful (Fig. 135–5).

Suture Materials

The choice of suture material depends on the normal strength of the tissues, the rate at which the wound recovers strength, the strength of the suture material, the rate at which the suture material loses strength in tissues, and the interactions that occur between sutures and tissues.[89] The bladder, along with the proximal colon, is one of the weakest organs in the body.[89] However, its regenerative capacity after injury is high, with the repair being virtually complete in 14 days.[75] Sutures should be at least as strong as the tissue through which they are placed. Nonabsorbable sutures cannot be used in the urinary tract because they provide a nidus for the formation of urinary calculi. The following remarks, therefore, concern absorbable suture materials only.

When 5/0 (1M-Metric) polyglycolic acid (PGA), 6/0 (0.7M) plain surgical gut, and 7/0 (0.5M) chromic gut were used to close an incised rat bladder, all three suture materials retained tensile strength long enough for the bladder to heal.[1] During burst strength tests, pressures of up to 550 mm Hg were reached. Some bladders burst, but this was due to sutures cutting through tissues and not to breaking.[1] Since a "desire to void" reflex is triggered at approximately 17 mm Hg and voiding pressures are usually on the order of 20 to 40 mm Hg in normal dogs,[18] there is little justification for using suture materials much outside the previously mentioned diameter range. Polyglycolic acid sutures have a greater tensile strength than surgical gut of the same diameter,[89] but when placed in tissues this material loses tensile strength more rapidly than surgical gut.[89] It is reasonable, therefore, to equate 5/0 PGA with 7/0 surgical gut.

Most suture materials in contact with urine for any length of time can act as a nidus for calculus formation,[47, 96] but when concretions occurred on PGA suture material used to close cystotomy incisions in rabbits, the suture material was suspected.[8] This

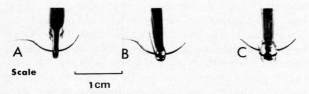

Figure 135–3. Three different size needle holders are applied to the same size needle. The effective working length of the needle from the needle tip to the needle holder decreases from *A* to *C.* As the largest needle holder (*C*) is applied, the curved needle is stressed as it straightens out.

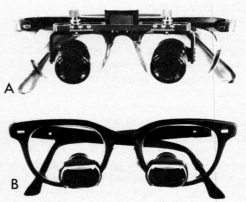

Figure 135–5. *A,* Keeler 2× operating loupe. *B,* Zeiss 2× operating telescope mounted on plain glass lenses.

conclusion prompted further work by other investigators in rabbits,[47] rats,[62] dogs,[14, 16, 47] and cats.[77] The results substantiated the previous findings in rabbits, but it was found that PGA was superior to surgical gut in the rat, dog, and cat.[14]

There are two common synthetic absorbable suture materials: polyglycolic acid (Dexon [Davis & Geck]) and polyglactin 910 (Vicryl [Ethicon]). Both are braided polyester sutures degraded by hydrolysis and absorbed by the body with minimal tissue reaction. Mechanical performance tests of these two suture materials showed that 4/0 polyglactin was significantly thicker than 4/0 PGA.[77] Since the strength of a suture thread is proportional to its cross-sectional area, it was not surprising that 4/0 polyglactin had a breaking strain of 2.1 kg, whereas 4/0 PGA had a breaking strain of only 1.4 kg. However, when the diameters were equalized, the breaking strain for PGA was 49.9 kg/mm^2 and for polyglactin 44.6 kg/mm^2. As with all suture materials, knotting decreases the breaking strain. The reduction in strength was 40 per cent for polyglactin and 32 per cent for PGA. These materials have a high coefficient of friction, and square knots are secure. From a practical point of view, a granny knot with a double first throw should be tied first to allow the knot to be set and advanced until snug; then a square knot can be tied on top to ensure knot security.

The breaking strength of skin wounds in guinea pigs closed with PGA and polyglactin showed that at seven days the polyglactin closure was stronger, but by 14 days the disruption strain was the same for both materials. These findings suggested that the absorption rate of the two materials was independent of suture size. In another experiment, 2/0 PGA or polyglactin was degraded at approximately the same rate as 4/0 material.[24]

Accelerated hydrolysis of PGA sutures has been reported in the presence of *Proteus* infection and high urine pH. This observation was confirmed in an experimental study that compared the effect of pH on hydrolysis of Dexon and Vicryl. It was found that in an acid environment there was very little difference between the two, but in a neutral or alkaline environment Vicryl sutures retained tensile strength longer than Dexon sutures. Therefore, with respect to pH of the environment, Vicryl sutures are more versatile than Dexon. A new monofilament, synthetic absorbable suture material, polydioxanone (Ethicon), has become available.[76] Early clinical experience with this material in general surgery suggests that it may be used whenever there is a need for an absorbable suture material. Its major advantage over the braided synthetic absorbable materials is its lack of suture drag.

Splinting (Stenting) in Urethral and Ureteral Surgery

Epithelium is damaged by indwelling urethral catheters.[31] Stomal stricture after perineal urethros-tomy in cats has been attributed to early use of catheters postoperatively.[83] As a general rule, if primary intention healing is being sought, splinting catheters should be avoided because (1) they might interfere with healing, and (2) there is the risk of ascending infection.[48, 52, 87] Urine leakage at the anastomosis can delay healing; if this is considered a possibility, urine can be diverted during healing by placing a Foley catheter in the bladder and exteriorizing it in the antepubic position.[78] An absolute indication for a splinting catheter is repair of a urethral injury in which there is loss of tissue. If the splinting catheter can be left in place for three weeks, the fibrous tissue reaction around the catheter becomes lined by regenerating urethral mucosa. It requires that, initially, there be some continuity of mucosa over the defect.[93]

It is much more difficult for mucosa to bridge a complete urethral defect. Ureteral epithelium also has the capacity to regenerate over a splint, as does urethral epithelium.[63] Although ureteral splints are not necessary in uncomplicated ureteroneocystostomy, most medical urologists routinely use ureteral splints and believe that they do little or no harm.[88] The duration of splinting can range from 4 to 5 days for ureteral re-implantation to 10 to 15 days for ureteral anastomosis and up to 45 days for ureteral regeneration. In animals, lack of patient cooperation makes management of indwelling catheters difficult. If sound microsurgical techniques are used for ureteral anastomosis in the dog, splinting catheters are not required.[26, 45]

Altered Renal Function Due to Anesthesia, Surgery, and Drugs

At the beginning of this century it was known that ether anesthesia caused urine flows to drop from 50 ml/hr to 1.2 ml/hr during the course of the operation and that the urine flow returned to normal postoperatively, usually within a few hours.[22, 74] After extensive surgery and prolonged anesthesia, direct and indirect secondary effects were seen.

Indirect Effects of Anesthesia

Circulation. Renal blood flow (RBF) is decreased owing to renal vasoconstriction and hypotension. Catecholamine release with renal vasoconstriction is pronounced with cyclopropane and ether.[73] Thiopentone and halothane do not provoke a catecholamine response but cause myocardial depression and peripheral vasodilation. The result is hypotension, which provokes some compensatory renal vasoconstriction.[28]

Sympathetic Nervous System. Renal blood vessels are innervated by celiac and renal plexes with sympathetic constrictor fibers. In response to moderate stress, efferent arteriolar constriction occurs. So although RBF has decreased, glomerular filtration rate

(GFR) remains constant. With further stress, afferent arteriolar constriction occurs and GFR drops (see Chapter 133). When the kidney is denervated, anesthetic stress does not affect renal function.[9]

Endocrine Effects. These are significant and are closely related to circulatory changes. Signals from baroreceptors in the right atrium mediate antidiuretic hormone (ADH) release and antidiuresis. Angiotensin II, a potent vasoconstrictor, is produced by the action of renin on renin substrate (angiotensinogen). Control of renin release is multifactorial, and these factors (sodium content of tubular fluid, catecholamine levels, sympathetic nervous system impulses, and pressure within the afferent arterioles[39]) are all influenced by anesthesia.

Direct Effects of Anesthesia

Immediate effects are masked by the indirect effects outlined previously. Delayed effects are related to direct nephrotoxicity and the use of methoxyflurane anesthesia.[25] Affected patients are unable to concentrate urine, resulting in high-output renal insufficiency. The effect is usually transient but sometimes can lead to renal failure. Methoxyflurane is a fluorinated hydrocarbon, and two of its metabolites are inorganic fluoride and oxalate. Inorganic fluoride has been suggested as the toxic agent,[61, 85] but oxalic acid might also be a factor in patients that develop permanent renal insufficiency.[38, 60] If the duration of methoxyflurane anesthesia is limited to less than two hours, nephrotoxicity is unlikely. If anesthesia must continue beyond two hours, the use of narcotics, nitrous oxide, and muscle relaxants is recommended.[22] Other fluorinated anesthetics causing direct renal toxicity can be arranged in decreasing order of toxicity: methoxyflurane, enflurane, isoflurane, and halothane. Halothane is metabolized to fluoride to a negligible extent.[57] Light anesthesia and an adequate intraoperative fluid regimen with a balanced electrolyte solution will ensure that patients have only minimal and transient depression of renal function.[22] Premedication with drugs with mild α blocking properties, such as the neuroleptics acetylpromazine and droperidol, will help to prevent catecholamine-induced vasoconstriction and, therefore, depressed renal function during anesthesia.[22]

Certain antimicrobial agents, analgesics, and contrast agents are potentially nephrotoxic.

Antimicrobial Agents

The kidney is a major excretory pathway for many antibiotics. Nephrons are exposed to high concentrations by glomerular filtration, tubular re-absorption, and secretion. The relative nephrotoxicity of various antimicrobials[3] is listed in Table 135–1. Of the *cephalosporins*, cephaloridine is much less protein bound than cephalothin or cephazolin. It achieves a higher serum concentration and therefore is more nephrotoxic than cephalothin or cephazolin. There is consid-

TABLE 135–1. Nephrotoxicity of Antibiotics*

Agent	Frequency of Nephrotoxicity†
Amikacin	S
Amoxicillin	N
Ampicillin	R
Carbenicillin	R
Cefazolin	N
Cephalexin	R
Cephaloridine	S
Cephalothin	R
Chloramphenicol	N
Chlortetracycline	R
Cloxacillin	N
Colistin	S
Erythromycin	N
Gentamicin	S
Kanamycin	S
Lincomycin	N
Methenamine mandelate	N
Methicillin	R
Nalidixic acid	N
Neomycin	S
Nitrofurantoin	N
Oxacillin	R
Oxytetracycline	R
Penicillin G	R
Polymyxin	S
Streptomycin	S
Sulfadiazine	R
Sulfamethoxazole	R
Sulfisoxazole	R
Tetracycline HCl	R
Ticarcillin	N
Trimethoprim	R
Tobramycin	S

*Modified from Appel, G. B., and Neu, H. C.: The nephrotoxicity of antimicrobial agents (first of three parts). N. Engl. J. Med. 296:663, 1977.

†N = none reported; R = rare; S = substantial.

erable species variation in renal handling of the cephalosporins, and they are not considered nephrotoxic in the cat and dog.[72]

Degradation products from outdated *tetracycline* may cause a reversible Fanconi syndrome, and demethylchlortetracycline produces a reversible nephrogenic diabetes insipidus.[3] These drugs also have an antianabolic effect and can lead to progressive azotemia. Anabolic steroids prevent these effects,[30] whereas concurrent use of diuretics exacerbates them.[86] Tetracyclines are reported to potentiate the nephrotoxicity of methoxyflurane in man,[15] but in an experiment in which this combination of drugs was administered to ten healthy dogs, nephrotoxicity was not observed.[64] Nephrotoxicity is a well-recognized side effect of treatment with polymyxins B and E.[90] These drugs should only be used if less toxic antibiotics are not available.

The *sulfonamides* had a reputation for crystallization within the renal parenchyma.[3, 29] When it was found that a mixture of sulfonamides could be dissolved to the limits of their individual solubilities and that the combination had antibacterial effectiveness, crystallization was no longer a real problem. Since the 1950s, the availability of short-acting, highly soluble sulfonamides such as sulfisoxazole and sulfamethizole has all but eliminated crystallization problems. In burn therapy, topical silver sulfadiazine produces the nephrotic syndrome in man by inducing immune-complex glomerulonephritis.[69] When combined with trimethoprim, which has no reported nephrotoxicity associated with its use, the renal handling of the sulfa drugs is the same. However, azotemia has been reported with this combination,[46] possibly owing to altered renal handling, which does not affect glomerular filtration rate.

Aminoglycoside antibiotics are not absorbed orally but, after parenteral administration, distribute within the extracellular space. The aminoglycosides are not metabolized and are excreted 99 per cent by the kidney and 1 per cent in the bile. They are filtered and have a predilection for uptake by the proximal tubules and retention within the renal cortex.[94] The proximal tubule is the specific site for nephrotoxicity. In addition to the kidney, the inner ear and neuromuscular junction are target sites for toxicity. Streptomycin is the least nephrotoxic of this class,[3, 34] and neomycin is the most nephrotoxic.[17] The toxicities of other aminoglycosides—kanamycin,[34] gentamicin,[92] tobramycin,[27] and amikacin[3]—are within these limits. If any of the more toxic antibiotics have to be used during treatment, monitoring of renal function is essential. If changes are detected, administration of the drug should be stopped.

Analgesic Nephropathy

In man, nephropathy after administration of non-steroidal anti-inflammatory drugs has been recognized since 1953. Phenacetin was incriminated, but this finding is still controversial, since phenacetin was always taken in conjunction with aspirin, codeine, or caffeine. Paracetamol, a metabolite of phenacetin, in massive doses can cause papillary necrosis. Toxicity has been reported in cats.[13] Aspirin in high doses produces papillary necrosis in rats.[66] It has a long half-life in cats (36 hours) and can cause cumulative toxicity.[13] Phenylbutazone and indomethacin can also produce toxic renal effects.[4] Aspirin, phenylbutazone, and indomethacin interfere with prostaglandin synthesis. It has been suggested that vasodilatory renal prostaglandins may function to offset ischemic vasoconstriction resulting from sympathetic stimuli associated with anesthesia, surgery, and other stresses.[6] This protective effect is lost with prolonged antiprostaglandin therapy.

Radiographic Contrast Agents

Acute renal failure has been reported in man following contrast studies of the kidney, heart, and brain.[91] The duration of acute failure was three to five days. If iodinated contrast agent is injected through a catheter wedged tightly enough into the artery to cut off blood flow, organ damage results.[12] The damage is indicated by prolonged and intense accumulation of contrast agent within the perfused organ. This is called contrast staining. Such a result might be unintentional or can be used for therapeutic "nephrectomy."[12] Renal atrophy occurs because of diffuse infarction of the renal arteries.

Urinary Tract Infection

Most urinary tract pathogens originate in the gut or on the skin. Organisms ascend from the urethral orifice.[64, 68] Most are mechanically cleared by normal voiding.[23] The long urethra of the male provides real protection against infection. If normal voiding is impaired for any reason, or, if after voiding, there is residual urine, the establishment of a urinary tract infection is possible. The bladder does, however, have an intrinsic defense mechanism. The bladder mucosa resists the binding of microorganisms, and if organisms do become established in the bladder wall they are engulfed by phagocytes and are acted upon by humoral defense mechanisms.[67] Although urine has been described as an excellent culture medium,[23] it is also true that in rabbits bacterial multiplication is inhibited on either side of the pH range of 5 to 8 and by osmolality in excess of 800 mOsm.[65, 80] A 4 per cent urea concentration is bacteriostatic for most urinary tract pathogens. This concentration is reached in the renal medulla during antidiuresis.[80] Cat urine appears to have enhanced bactericidal properties.[51]

By well-meaning diagnostic endeavors, a veterinary surgeon might be responsible for establishing a significant urinary tract infection where one was not previously present. Quantitative urine cultures indicate if an infection has become established. The number of organisms present depends on the method[15] and time[84] of urine collection, whether or not the patient is undergoing diuresis and, therefore, diluting the urine, and whether or not the patient is on antibacterial therapy.

The method of *urine collection* may be either clean catch of voided urine or expression by bladder compression into a sterile container. The container is moved into the urine stream once voiding has commenced. This is a midstream clean catch, and is quite adequate for a screening urine analysis. Manual compression of the bladder with sufficient force to initiate voiding induced vesicoureteral reflux in five of ten mature dogs and four of ten mature cats.[35] Therefore, manual compression of the urinary bladder for urine collection is not recommended for patients suspected of having cystitis for fear of producing pyelonephritis.[19] The other alternatives for urine collection are a catheterized sample and cystocentesis.

Urine contamination can occur from the urethra, prepuce, or vagina when a clean catch or catheterized specimen is obtained. Contamination can be minimized by first cleansing the external genitalia or flushing the preputial cavity or vagina with sterile water or saline. Cleansing the external genitalia with antiseptics such as 0.05% aqueous chlorhexidine is recommended prior to catheterization so long as a urine culture is not contemplated. Even very small traces of antiseptic can interfere with colony counts.[84] The risk of mechanically seeding the bladder with organisms from the preputial cavity or perineum is greater in females than in males.[11] If contamination occurs and the catheterization attempt was rough, the mucosal injury provides an opportunity for contaminating organisms to become established within the bladder wall and to produce an infection. For this reason, a bladder rinse with 0.2% neomycin prior to removing the catheter significantly decreases the incidence of postcatheterization bacteriuria.[21]

Open indwelling urethral catheters are frequently used for temporary urine diversion in animals and man. Their use has to be weighed against the known risk of infection. Organisms can ascend the lumen of the drainage tubes,[87] and most patients with previously sterile urine have bacteriuria within 24 hours of catheterization.[48, 52] Closed catheter drainage systems with nonreturn valves prevent catheter-associated urinary tract infection for short periods.[87] EDTA-tris-lysozyme lavage has been advocated to treat *Pseudomonas* sp. infections and coliform cystitis associated with indwelling catheters.[41, 96] If examination of uncentrifuged urine[58] or sediment shows bacteria, urine cultures should be done. Contamination of voided urine does not usually result in sufficient numbers of bacteria in the sediment. On the other hand, absence of bacteria by direct examination does not rule out urinary tract infection.[2]

For quantitative urine culture, the number of colony-forming units per ml of urine is recorded.[17] The greater the interval between voiding episodes, the greater the number of bacterial multiplications. This means that first morning specimens usually have a higher colony count than second and subsequent specimens during the day. Therefore, for the greatest chance of detecting significant urinary tract infection, specimens for culture should always be taken from first morning samples. In man, colony counts of 10^5 colony-forming units (cfu) per ml of urine have an 80 per cent likelihood of indicating significant infection in the midstream sample and a 95 per cent chance of indicating signficant infection in a catheterized sample.[2] In animals, greater than 10^4 cfu/ml in the catheterized sample may represent a significant urinary tract infection.[17] If there is doubt about the significance of the result or if it is important to have very accurate results, the sample should be collected by cystocentesis after surgical preparation of the skin. Using this technique, any growth of organisms is considered abnormal, since normal bladder urine is sterile.[68]

There should be no delay in processing urine once

TABLE 135–2. Organisms Commonly Isolated From Dogs and Cats With Urinary Tract Infection

Dogs	Cats
Escherichia coli	*Escherichia coli*
Proteus sp.	Enterococci
Staphylococcus aureus	*Proteus* sp.
Enterococci	*Pasteurella*
Klebsiella	β hemolytic streptococci
Enterobacter	
Pseudomonas sp.	

it has been collected because bacterial numbers can double at room temperature in 45 minutes.[5] If the specimen is refrigerated at 4°C, it can be stored for 24 hours and meaningful results can still be expected from the cultures.[17] The test to confirm renal infection is culture of ureteric urine. In animals, this is usually done by exposing the ureteric orifices by cystotomy. It is, however, possible to sample urine from the renal pelvis by percutaneous nephropyelocentesis.[53] An indirect method used in man is the bladder washout test.[33] Serial quantitative urine cultures are performed, first on a catheterized urine sample. The bladder is sterilized by infusing enzymes and antibiotics, which are then washed out with sterile saline. Urine is then sampled at regular intervals and cultured. If successive cultures remain sterile, the infection can be assumed to have arisen from the bladder. If colony counts rise with successive cultures, the infection is seated in the kidneys. This test is simple but time-consuming and costly and in animals might be unreliable.[36, 37] Organisms that commonly infect the urinary tract of dogs and cats are shown in Table 135–2. *Escherichia coli*, *Proteus* sp., and *Staphylococcus aureus* account for 80 per cent of isolates in dogs.[95] The prevalence of urinary tract infection in cats is less than that in dogs.[17] This might be related to better antibacterial qualities of cat urine.[51]

Antibiotic, Antibacterial, and Analgesic Therapy (Table 135–3)

Antibiotics

Penicillins. These drugs are bactericidal and, except for cloxacillin and oxacillin, are destroyed by bacterial penicillinase. As a group, the penicillins are generally active against gram positive organisms. Penicillin G and ampicillin, when given orally, reach urine concentrations 100 times greater than serum concentrations and can be effective against gram negative as well as gram positive organisms.[55] Food in the stomach interferes with penicillin absorption; therefore, food should be withheld for 20 minutes after dosing to aid absorption.

Voiding opportunities should be limited to 15 to 20 minutes before the next dose is due to maintain

TABLE 135–3. Antibiotic, Antibacterial, and Analgesic Therapy for Urinary Tract Infection

Therapy	Oral	Intramuscular	Dose Frequency/ day
Antibiotic			
Penicillin G	12*	12	6
Penicillin V	8		3
Ampicillin	10	7	3
Amoxicillin	10	7	3
Streptomycin		20	1
Gentamicin		2	3
Neomycin	0.2% solution for bladder infusion		
Cephalexin	10		2
Cephaloridine		11	2
Tetracycline	20		3
Oxytetracycline	27		2
		10	1
Chloramphenicol	40		3 (dog)
			2 (cat)
Antibacterial			
Sulfamethizole	50		4
Sulfisoxazole	50		4
Trimethoprim/	15		2 (dog)
Sulfadiazine (1:5)	30		1 (cat)
Nitrofurantoin	4		3
Methenamine	25		2
Methenamine mandelate or hippurate	25		2
Analgesic			
Phenazopyridine	5		2

*1,595 units penicillin G/mg.

high urine levels of the drug. Amoxacillin is an analogue of ampicillin and has the same antibacterial spectrum but is better absorbed in the presence of food.[13] Carbenicillin and ticarcillin are semisynthetic penicillins with activity against *Pseudomonas* sp. and are synergistic with gentamicin.[13]

Aminoglycosides. Streptomycin at the recommended concentrations is bactericidal against many gram negative organisms including *Proteus* sp. and *Pseudomonas* sp. Pencillin/streptomycin mixtures are, therefore, compatible and have a broad spectrum of activity. Streptomycin resistance can develop very quickly—within a week.[13] Neomycin is bactericidal and has a broad spectrum of activity. It is not recommended for parenteral use because of the risk of nephrotoxicity and ototoxicity. It is useful for local instillation into the bladder after catheterization. Gentamicin is bactericidal and has a broad spectrum of activity. It is particularly effective against *Pseudomonas* sp. Resistance occurs in proportion to usage, so, as a rule, this drug should not be used as a "first line" antibiotic. Ototoxicity, renal toxicity, and neuromuscular blockade with the risk of respiratory paralysis can occur with this drug. Cats are most at risk.[13] Tobramycin is like gentamicin and is active against *Pseudomonas* organisms.

Cephalosporins. These antibiotics are bactericidal with a spectrum of activity similar to that of ampicillin. Many cephalosporins have been synthesized, including cephalothin, cephaloridine, and cephazolin as intramuscular preparations and cephalexin and cephradine as oral preparations. These drugs can cause nephrotoxicity in man but are not nephrotoxic in dogs and cats.[72]

Tetracyclines. These antibiotics have a broad spectrum of activity and are bacteriostatic at the usual concentrations. They are absorbed in the gut and undergo enterohepatic circulation but are not metabolized and are mainly excreted in urine. Oxytetracycline is more freely excreted in the urine than chlortetracycline. Tetracycline, from which chlor- and oxytetracycline are derived, is absorbed well from the gastrointestinal tract. Blood levels are higher and are maintained longer than with the other tetracyclines. This drug is inexpensive and has a high cure rate against *Pseudomonas* sp. urinary tract infections in dogs.[54] Nephrotoxicity has been reported when degraded, out-of-date tetracycline was used in conjunction with methoxyflurane anesthesia in a stressed patient.[50]

Chloramphenicol. This antibiotic is bacteriostatic with a broad spectrum of activity. It is rapidly absorbed after oral dosing. Up to 45 per cent of the drug adsorbs to serum proteins.[13] It is effective in treating urinary tract infections in dogs, including *Proteus* sp. and *Pseudomonas* sp. infections. This drug affects bone marrow and interferes with hematopoiesis, particularly in cats. It also depresses liver mitochondrial activity, which means that animals being treated may show greatly delayed recovery after barbiturate anesthesia.[13]

Polymyxins. These antibiotics have a gram negative spectrum of activity and are synergistic with oxytetracycline. Therefore, the doses of each can be cut by one-half to one-sixteenth.[13] These drugs are known nephrotoxins and should only be used if other less toxic drugs are unavailable.[90]

Antibacterials

Sulfonamides. These drugs are bacteriostatic with a gram positive spectrum of activity. Sulfacrystalluria can occur in acid urine and at low urine flows but is not likely with the more soluble sulfonamides such as sulfisoxazole and sulfamethizole. There is a tendency for resistant strains to develop following the use of sulfa drugs.

Enhanced Sulfonamides. When sulfonamide is combined with another bacteriostatic drug trimethoprim, the combination is bactericidal and has a broad spectrum of activity.[13] Antibacterial effects are enhanced because each drug inhibits a different step in the synthesis of folic acid, which is needed by the microorganisms.[56]

Nitrofurans. These agents are bactericidal and have a broad spectrum of activity in acid urine. If there is oliguria or anuria, toxic levels can be reached.

Many urinary tract pathogens are resistant to this drug.[81]

Methenamine and its Salts. Methenamine is excreted in the urine, where, in the pH range of 5 to 6, it breaks down to form ammonia and formaldehyde. To provide the acid medium, methenamine has been coupled with the organic acids mandelamine and hippuric acid. Methenamine mandelate and hippurate are absorbed as individual components, and *in vitro* tests suggest that if the pH is maintained between 5 and 6, methenamine by itself is not inferior to the combination with acid salts.[42] Bacterial resistance to methenamine has not been demonstrated; therefore, it can be used with its acid salts for long-term therapy. If necessary, urine pH can be adjusted to between 5 and 6 with ammonium chloride or sodium acid phosphate.

Some urinary antiseptics contain methylene blue. These agents should not be used in cats, as severe hemolytic anemia can result.[79]

Urinary Tract Analgesia

Phenazopyridine is an azo dye that, when excreted in the urine, has a topical analgesic effect. It also turns urine a bright orange color. This drug is therapeutically hazardous in cats, as it can cause methemoglobinemia and Heinz body hemolytic anemia,[43] and should never be used in dogs, as it produces acute keratoconjunctivitis sicca owing to lacrimal gland damage. This drug is not recommended for use in animals with renal or hepatic insufficiency.

1. Adams, H., Barnes, R., Small, C., and Hadley, H.: Sutures and bladder wound healing in the experimental animal. Invest. Urol. *12*:267, 1975.
2. Andriole, V. T.: Urinary tract infections in pregnancy. Urol. Clin. North Am. *2*:486, 1975.
3. Appel, G. B., and Neu, H. C.: The nephrotoxicity of antimicrobial agents. Parts 1, 2, and 3. N. Engl. J. Med. *296*:663, 722, 784, 1977.
4. Arnold, L., Collins, C., and Starmer, G. A.: Further studies of the acute effects of phenylbutazone, oxyphenbutazone and indomethacin on the rat kidney. Pathology *8*:135, 1976.
5. Asscher, A. W., Sussman, M., Waters, W. E., Davis, R. H., and Chick, S.: Urine as a medium for bacterial growth. Lancet *2*:1037, 1966.
6. Attallah, A. A., and Lee, J. B.: Prostaglandins, renal function and blood pressure regulation. *In* Lee, J. B. (ed.): *Prostaglandins*. Elsevier New Holland Inc., New York, 1982.
7. Berglund, F., Killander, J., and Pompeius, R.: The effect of trimethoprim-sulfamethoxazole on the renal excretion of creatinine in man. J. Urol. *114*:802, 1975.
8. Bergman, F. O., Borgstrom, S. J. H., and Holmund, D. E. W.: Synthetic absorbable suture material (P.G.A.). Acta Chir. Scand. *137*:193, 1971.
9. Berne, R. M.: Hemodynamics and sodium excretion of denervated kidney in anesthetized and unanesthetized dog. Am. J. Physiol. *171*:148, 1952.
10. Bierman, W.: Electrosurgery. Am. J. Surg. *50*:768, 1951.
11. Biertuempfel, P. H., Ling, G. V., and Ling, G. A.: Urinary tract infection resulting from catheterization in healthy adult dogs. J. Am. Vet. Med. Assoc. *178*:989, 1981.
12. Brady, T. M., Singer, D., Weiss, C. A., Smolin, M. F., Brinker, R. E., and Cho, K. J.: Angiographic nephrectomy using iodinated contrast agent. Invest. Radiol. *17*:479, 1982.
13. Brander, G. C., Pugh, D. M., and Bywater, R. J.: *Veterinary Applied Pharmacology and Therapeutics*, 4th ed. Balliere Tindall, London, 1982, pp. 228, 383, 392.
14. Brannan, W., Ochsner, M. G., Pond, H. S. III, Fuselier, H. A., Jr., and Scharfenberg, J. C.: Laboratory and clinical experience with polyglycolic acid suture in urogenital surgery. J. Urol. *110*:571, 1973.
15. Carter, J. M., Klausner, J. S., Osborne, C. A., and Bates, F. Y.: Comparison of collection techniques for qualitative urine collection in dogs. J. Am. Vet. Med. Assoc. *173*:296, 1978.
16. Case, G. D., Glenn, J. F., and Postlethwait, R. W.: Comparison of absorbable sutures in urinary bladder. Urology *7*:165, 1976.
17. Chew, D. J., and Kowalski, J. P.: Urinary tract infection. *In* Bojrab, M. J. (ed.): *Pathophysiology in Small Animal Surgery*. Lea & Febiger, Philadelphia, 1981.
18. Christie, B. A.: Incidence and etiology of vesico-ureteral reflux in apparently normal dogs. Invest. Urol. *9*:184, 1971.
19. Christie, B. A.: The occurrence of vesicoureteral reflux and pyelonephritis in apparently normal dogs. Invest. Urol. *10*:359, 1973.
20. Chu, C. C.: A comparison of the effect of pH on the biodegradation of two synthetic absorbable sutures. Ann. Surg. *197*:55, 1982.
21. Clark, L. W.: Neomycin in the prevention of postcatheterization bacteriuria. Med. J. Aust. *1*:1034, 1973.
22. Cousins, M. J., and Mazze, R. I.: Anaesthesia surgery and renal function. Anaesth. Intensive Care *1*:355, 1973.
23. Cox, C. E., and Hinman, F., Jr.: Experiments with induced bacteriuria, vesical emptying and bacterial growth on the mechanism of bladder defence to infection. J. Urol. *86*:739, 1961.
24. Craig, P. H., Williams, J. A., Davis, K. W., Magoun, A. D., Levy, A. J., Bogdansky, S., and Jones, J. P., Jr.: A biological comparison of polyglactin 910 and polyglycolic acid synthetic absorbable sutures. Surg. Gynecol. Obstet. *141*:1, 1975.
25. Crandell, W. B., Pappas, S. G., and MacDonald, A.: Nephrotoxicity associated wtih methoxyflurane anaesthesia. Anesthesiology *27*:591, 1966.
26. Crane, S.: Transureteroureterostomy in the dog. Vet. Surg. *9*:108, 1980.
27. DeRosa, F., Buoncristiani, U., Capitanucci, P., and Frongillo, R. F.: Tobramycin: toxicological and pharmacological studies in animals and pharmacokinetic research in patients with varying degrees of renal impairment. J. Int. Med. Res. *2*:100, 1974.
28. Deutsch, S., Pierce, E. C., Jr., and Vandam, L. D.: Effects of anaesthesia with thiopental, nitrous oxide, and neuromuscular blockers on renal function in normal man. Anesthesiology *20*:184, 1968.
29. Dowling, H. F., and Lepper, M. H.: Toxic reactions following therapy with sulfapyridine, sulfathiozole, and sulfadiazine. JAMA *121*:1190, 1943.
30. Editorial: The danger of giving tetracyclines to patients with kidney disease. N.Z. Med. J. *77*:397, 1973.
31. Edwards, L., and Trot, P. A.: Catheter-induced urethral inflammation. J. Urol. *100*:678, 1973.
32. Einspruch, B. C., and Gonzalez, V. V.: Clinical and experimental nephropathy resulting from the use of neomycin sulphate. JAMA *173*:809, 1960.
33. Fairley, K. F., Bond, A. G., Brown, B. B., and Haffersberger, P.: Simple test to determine the site of urinary tract infection. Lancet *2*:427, 1967.
34. Falco, F. G., Smith, H. M., and Arcieri, G. M.: Nephrotoxicity of the aminoglycosides. J. Infect. Dis. *119*:406, 1969.
35. Feeney, D. A., Osborne, C. A., and Johnston, G. R.: Vesicoureteral reflux induced by manual compression of the urinary bladder of dogs and cats. J. Am. Vet. Med. Assoc. *182*:795, 1983.
36. Finco, D. R., and Kern, A.: Pyelonephritis. *In* Kirk, R. W. (ed.): *Current Veterinary Therapy VI*. W. B. Saunders, Philadelphia, 1977.
37. Finco, D. R., Shotts, E. B., and Crowell, W. A.: Evaluation of methods for localization of urinary tract infection in the female dog. Am. J. Vet. Res. *40*:707, 1979.
38. Franscino, J. A., Vanamee, P., and Rosen, P. P.: Renal

oxalosis and azotaemia after methoxyflurane anaesthesia. N. Engl. J. Med. *283*:676, 1970.

39. Ganong, W. F.: *Review of Medical Physiology,* 8th ed. Lange Medical Publications, Los Altos, CA, 1977, p. 346.

40. Gittes, R. F., and Varady, S.: Nephroscopy in chronic unilateral hematuria. J. Urol. *126*:297, 1981.

41. Goldschmidt, M. C., Kuhn, C. R., Perry, K., and Johnston, D. E.: EDTA and lysozyme lavage in the treatment of pseudomonas and coliform bladder infections. J. Urol. *107*:969, 1972.

42. Hamilton-Miller, J. M. T., and Brumfitt, W.: Methenamine and its salts as urinary tract antiseptics. Invest. Urol. *14*:287, 1977.

43. Harvey, J. W., and Kornick, H. P.: Phenazopyridine toxicosis in the cat. J. Am. Vet. Med. Assoc. *169*:327, 1976.

44. Honig, W. M.: The mechanisms of cutting in electrosurgery. IEEE Trans. Biomed. Eng. *22*:58, 1975.

45. Jonas, D., Kramer, W., and Weber, W.: Splintless microsurgical anastomosis of the ureter in the dog. Urol. Res. *9*:271, 1981.

46. Kalowsky, S., Nanra, R. S., Mathew, T. H., and Kincaid-Smith, P.: Deterioration of renal function in association with co-trimoxazole therapy. Lancet *1*:394, 1973.

47. Kaminski, J. M., Katz, A. R., and Woodward, S. C.: Urinary bladder calculus formation on sutures in rabbits, cats, and dogs. Surg. Gynecol. Obstet. *146*:353, 1978.

48. Kass, E. H., and Sossen, H. S.: Prevention of infection of urinary tract in the presence of indwelling catheters. JAMA *169*:1181, 1959.

49. Knecht, C. D., Clark, R. L., and Fletcher, O. J.: Healing of sharp incisions and electroincisions in dogs. J. Am. Vet. Med. Assoc. *159*:1447, 1971.

50. Kuzucu, E. Y.: Methoxyflurane, tetracycline and renal failure. JAMA *211*:1162, 1970.

51. Lees, G. E., and Osborne, C. A.: Antibacterial properties of urine: A comparative review. J. Am. Anim. Hosp. Assoc. *15*:125, 1979.

52. Lees, G. E., Osborne, C. A., Stevens, J. B., and Ward, G. E.: Adverse effects of indwelling urethral catheterization in clinically normal male cats. Am. J. Vet. Res. *42*:825, 1981.

53. Ling, G. V., Ackerman, M., Lowenstine, L. J., and Cowgill, L. D.: Percutaneous nephropyelocentesis and nephropyelostomy in the dog: A description of the technique. Am. J. Vet. Res. *40*:1605, 1979.

54. Ling, G. V., Creighton, S. R., and Ruby, A. L.: Tetracycline for oral treatment of canine urinary tract infections caused by *Pseudomonas aeruginosa.* J. Am. Vet. Med. Assoc. *179*:578, 1981.

55. Ling, G. V., and Gillmore, C. J.: Penicillin G or ampicillin for oral treatment of canine urinary tract infections. J. Am. Vet. Med. Assoc. *171*:358, 1977.

56. Ling, G. V., and Ruby, A. L.: Chloramphenicol for oral treatment of canine urinary tract infections. J. Am. Vet. Med. Assoc. *172*:914, 1978.

57. Loew, G., Motulsky, H., Trudell, J., Cohen, E., and Hjelmeland, L.: Quantum chemical studies of the metabolism of the inhalation anesthetics methoxyflurane, enflurane and isoflurane. Mol. Pharmacol. *10*:406, 1974.

58. Long, G. R., and Levin, S.: Diagnosis and treatment of urinary tract infection. Med. Clin. North Am. *55*:1439, 1971.

59. Malnati, G. A., and Stone, E. A.: Clinical experience with polydioxanone suture material. Vet. Surg. *12*:24, 1983.

60. Mazze, R. I., Cousins, M. J., and Kosek, J. C.: Strain differences in metabolism and susceptibility to the nephrotoxic effects of methoxyflurane in rats. J. Pharmacol. Exp. Ther. *184*:481, 1973.

61. Mazze, R. I., Trudell, J. R., and Cousins, M. J.: Methoxyflurane metabolism and renal dysfunction: Clinical correlation in man. Anesthesiology *35*:247, 1971.

62. Milroy, E.: An experimental study of the calcification and absorption of polyglycolic acid and catgut sutures within the urinary tract. Invest. Urol. *14*:141, 1976.

63. Mobley, D. F.: Studies in ureteral regeneration. Invest. Urol. *14*:269, 1976.

64. Mulholland, S. G.: Lower urinary tract antibacterial defense mechanisms. Invest. Urol. *17*:93, 1979.

65. Mulholland, S. G., Perez, J. R., and Gillenwater, J. Y.: The antibacterial effects of urine. Invest. Urol. *6*:569, 1969.

66. Nanra, R. S., and Kincaid-Smith, P.: Papillary necrosis in rats caused by aspirin and aspirin containing mixtures. Br. Med. J. *3*:559, 1970.

67. Orikase, S., and Hinman, F., Jr.: Reaction of the vesical wall to bacterial penetration. Invest. Urol. *15*:185, 1977.

68. Osborne, C. A., Lowe, D. G., and Finco, D. R.: *Canine and Feline Urology.* W. B. Saunders, Philadelphia, 1972.

69. Owens, J. C., Yarborough, D. R. III, and Brackett, N. C., Jr.: Nephrotic syndrome following topically applied sulfadiazine silver therapy. Arch. Intern. Med. *134*:332, 1974.

70. Pedersoli, W. M., and Jackson, J. A.: Tetracycline, methoxyflurane anesthesia, and severe renal failure in dogs. J. Am. Anim. Hosp. Assoc. *9*:57, 1973.

71. Perez, J. R., Grieco, E. R., and Gillenwater, J. Y.: Evidence for bladder bacteriocidal factor. Invest. Urol. *11*:489, 1974.

72. Perkins, R. L., Apicella, M. A., Lee, I. S., Cuppage, F. E., and Saslaw, S.: Cephaloridine and cephalothin: Comparative studies of potential nephrotoxicity. J. Lab. Clin. Med. *71*:75, 1968.

73. Price, H. L., Linde, H. W., Jones, R. E., Black, G. W., and Price, M. L.: Sympathoadrenal responses to general anesthesia in man and their relation to hemodynamics. Anesthesiology *20*:563, 1959.

74. Pringle, H., Maunsell, R. C. B., and Pringle, S.: Clinical effects of ether anesthesia on renal activity. Br. Med. J. *2*:542, 1905.

75. Rasmussen, F.: Biochemical analysis of wound healing in the urinary bladder. Surg. Gynecol. Obstet. *124*:553, 1967.

76. Ray, J. A., Doddi, N., Regula, D., Williams, J. A., and Melveger, A.: Polydioxanone (PDS): a novel monofilament synthetic absorbable suture. Surg. Gynecol. Obstet. *153*:497, 1981.

77. Rodeheaver, G. T., Thacker, J. G., and Edlich, R. F.: Mechanical performance of polyglycolic acid and polyglactin 910 synthetic absorbable sutures. Surg. Gynecol. Obstet. *153*:835, 1981.

78. Rosenberg, M.: Experience with extended use of Foley Catheter following repair of the bladder. Surg. Gynecol. Obstet. *141*:734, 1975.

79. Schechter, R. D., Schalm, O. W., and Kaneko, J. J.: Heinz body hemolytic anemia associated with the use of urinary antiseptics containing methylene blue in the cat. J. Am. Vet. Med. Assoc. *162*:37, 1973.

80. Schlegel, J. U., Cuellar, J., and O'Deu, R. M.: Bacteriocidal effect of urea. J. Urol. *86*:819, 1961.

81. Seneca, H., Peer, P., and Warren, B.: Efficacy of drugs in Gram negative urinary pathogens. J. Urol. *99*:337, 1968.

82. Siegel, C. W., Ling, G. V., Bushby, S. R. M., Woolley, J. L., DeAngelis, D., and Eure, S.: Pharmacokinetics of trimethoprim and sulfadiazine in the dog. Urine concentrations after oral administration. Am. J. Vet. Res. *42*:996, 1981.

83. Smith, C. W., and Schiller, A. G.: Perineal urethrostomy in the cat. A retrospective study of complications. J. Am. Anim. Hosp. Assoc. *14*:225, 1978.

84. Stamey, T. A., and Pfau, A.: Urinary infections. A selective review and some observations. Calif. Med. *113*:16, 1970.

85. Taves, D. R., Fry, B. W., Freeman, R. B., and Gillies, A. J.: Toxicity following methoxyflurane anesthesia. JAMA *214*:91, 1970.

86. Tetracycline and drug attributed rises in blood urea nitrogen. A report from the Boston Collaborative drug surveillance program. JAMA *220*:377, 1972.

87. Thornton, G. F., and Andride, V. T.: Bacteriuria during indwelling catheter drainage. JAMA *214*:339, 1970.

88. Turner, M. D., Witherington, R., and Carswell, J. J.: Ureteral splints: Results of a survey. J. Urol. *127*:654, 1982.

89. Van Winkle, W., and Hastings, J. C.: Considerations in the choice of suture material for various tissues. Surg. Gynecol. Obstet. *135*:113, 1972.

90. Vinnicombe, J., and Stamey, T. A.: The relative nephrotoxicity of polymyxin B sulfate, sodium sulfomethyl-polymyxin B, sodium sulfamethyl-colistin (Colymycin) and neomycin sulfate. Invest. Urol. 6:505, 1969.

91. Wagoner, R. D.: Acute renal failure associated with contrast agents. Arch. Intern. Med. 138:353, 1978.

92. Waitz, J. A., Moss, E. L., Jr., and Weinstein, M. J.: Aspects of chronic toxicity of gentamycin sulphate in cats. J. Infect. Dis. 124:Suppl. 125, 1971.

93. Weaver, R. G., and Schulte, J. W.: Experimental and clinical studies of urethral regeneration. Surg. Gynecol. Obstet. 115:729, 1962.

94. Whelton, A., and Solez, K.: Aminoglycoside nephrotoxicity. J. Lab. Clin. Med. 99:148, 1982.

95. Wooley, R. E., and Blue, J. L.: Quantitative bacteriological studies of urine specimens from canine and feline urinary tract infections. J. Clin. Microbiol. 4:326, 1976.

96. Wooley, R. E., Schall, W. D., Eagon, R. G., and Scott, T. A.: Efficacy of EDTA-tris-lysozyme lavage in the treatment of experimentally induced *Pseudomonas aeruginosa* cystitis in the dog. Am. J. Vet. Res. 35:27, 1974.

97. Yodofsky, S. C., and Scott, F. B.: Urolithiasis on suture materials. J. Urol. 102:745, 1969.

98. Zimmerman, L. M., and Veith, I.: *Great Ideas in the History of Surgery.* Williams & Wilkins, Baltimore, 1961.

99. Zontine, W. J., and Andrews, L. K.: Fatal air embolism as a complication of pneumocystography in two cats. Vet. Radiol. 29:8, 1978.

Chapter **136**

Kidneys

Bruce A. Christie

CONGENITAL ABNORMALITIES

The embryological basis for the occurrence of congenital abnormalities affecting the urinary tract is discussed in Chapter 132.

Number. If the metanephrogenic blastema fails to produce nephrons, renal aplasia or agenesis results. Bilateral agenesis is incompatible with life. Unilateral agenesis (Fig. 136–1) occurs infrequently in dogs and cats[25, 36, 63] and is often associated with ipsilateral abnormalities of the genitalia (Fig. 136–2). The remaining kidney is usually hypertrophied and is capable of maintaining normal function throughout life. If renal surgery, particularly nephrectomy, is contemplated, it is vital to know in advance that a second kidney is present and functioning. Removal of a solitary kidney is indefensible. Supernumerary kidneys can develop as a consequence of ureteric bud malformation. This abnormality is discussed in Chapter 137.

Volume. Hypoplasia or dysgenesis means arrested development or maldevelopment and results in a very small kidney. Histological examination is necessary to confirm the diagnosis, since a previously normal kidney that suffers repeated insults can become scarred and shrunken. The glomeruli and tubules in a hypoplastic kidney should have comparatively normal architecture with no interstitial scar tissue. Hypoplasia is more common than aplasia. In dogs, hypoplasia may be unilateral (Fig. 136–3), but it more often affects both kidneys.[36] The cocker spaniel is the most frequently affected breed, but this disease has also been reported in the German shepherd, Doberman pinscher, Norwegian elkhound, and malamute.[32, 37, 40] The prognosis is poor. Affected dogs usually die of renal failure before two years of age. The clinical signs are those of chronic renal failure. In cats, the condition is usually asymmetrical, affecting the left kidney, and is accompanied by compensatory hypertrophy of the right kidney. Hypertrophy of the kidney occurs in response to the loss or nonfunction of renal tissue. Increase in mass is due mainly to increase in cell size. No new nephrons are formed, but tubular cell multiplication (hyperplasia) does occur.[35] Renal hypertrophy can be induced in many ways, including partial or complete nephrectomy, ureteral ligation, high-protein diet, high-sodium diet, and exposure to cold and certain hormones.[28] Experiments in rats have shown that the stimuli that trigger hypertrophy are humoral.[75] These

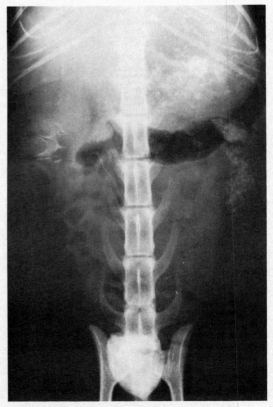

Figure 136–1. Unilateral renal agenesis in a dog. An intravenous pyelogram outlines the right kidney, but there is no evidence of a left kidney.

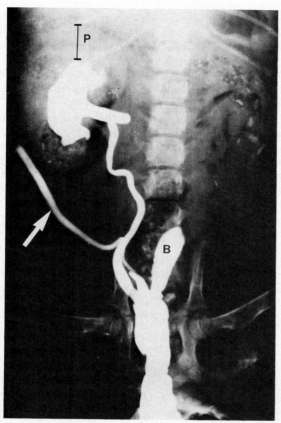

Figure 136–2. Unilateral renal agenesis and ipsilateral absence of the uterus in a dog demonstrated by vaginography. The right ureter has an ectopic opening into the uterus. The bladder (B) is infantile, and the ureter and renal pelvis of the right kidney are outlined by retrograde flow of contrast agent. The right uterine horn is visible (*arrow*). The kidney is enlarged. There is mild hydronephrosis, but the thickness of the renal parenchyma (P) indicates that hypertrophy of the kidney has occurred.

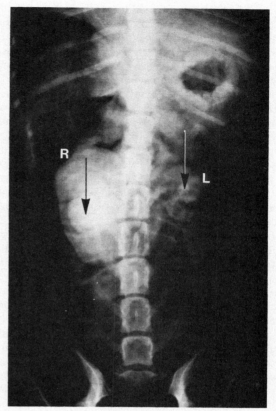

Figure 136–3. Unilateral renal hypoplasia in a dog. The left kidney (L) is much smaller than the right (R), and both kidneys contain calculi (*arrows*).

so-called renotrophins are produced by the kidneys and inactivated by the liver.[8]

Position. Renal ectopia has been described in the dog[78] and the cat.[34] The kidney is found in its embryonic position near the pelvis and fails to ascend (see Chapter 132). The diagnosis of ectopic kidney is usually made radiographically, during investigation of a caudal abdominal mass. Occasionally the condition is noted as an incidental finding during abdominal surgery. Kidney function is not usually compromised, but pressure exerted by the kidney could compress the colon or uterus, producing constipation or dystocia. The incidental finding of an ectopic kidney is probably no cause for concern unless the malposition is causing a clinical problem.

Fusion. During the early stages of development, the kidneys lie close to each other near the origin of the iliac arteries. Fusion anomalies can occur at this time and are seen in all species.[36] The commonest abnormality is horseshoe kidney with fusion at the caudal pole.[25] The fusion may involve only a portion of the capsule or parenchyma[57] or may be so extensive that a common pelvis if formed. When fusion is extensive, the renal mass cannot ascend normally and

remains in the pelvic cavity.[65] Fusion per se is unlikely to be clinically significant.

Cysts. Cysts can develop in any part of the nephron and collecting duct system. Some cystic lesions are heritable and arise during organogenesis. Others develop in normal renal tissue after the kidneys are fully formed. Cysts may be few and large or multiple and small. Solitary cysts are infrequently reported and are rarely of pathological consequence.[69] The boundaries of this type of cyst show up well against the contrast of the nephrogram phase of an intravenous pyelogram.[45] Polycystic disease affecting the kidney and liver has been reported in Cairn terriers[48] and long-haired cats.[20] In both instances the lesions were bilateral and appeared as abdominal distension in very young animals. In another form of this disease in cats, some affected animals with bilateral lesions lived up to three years before renal failure occurred.[53] Polycystic disease can also be unilateral. Removal of the affected kidney is advised as it is predisposed to infection and its presence is known to cause abdominal discomfort.[4]

ACQUIRED ABNORMALITIES

Trauma

The automobile inflicts most injuries to the urinary tracts of dogs and cats. The most common injury is rupture of the urinary bladder, followed by rupture of the kidney, urethra, and ureter. A kidney lesion that stops short of total rupture is perirenal hematoma.[62] A sharp blow may rupture abdominal wall muscles. If this occurs, the kidney may herniate into a subcutaneous position,[17, 79] and still continue to function normally. Sometimes the displacement through the abdominal wall (or even through the diaphragm) may be so great that the renal vascular pedicle is avulsed, leaving a nonfunctional organ. Reports of foreign body penetration of the kidney have included a rifle bullet lodged in the renal pelvis of a dog,[44] an airgun pellet in the renal parenchyma of a cat,[5] and a 5-cm long sewing needle that penetrated the duodenum of a dog and entered the right kidney.[22]

In blunt abdominal trauma, renal parenchymal damage can vary from minor subcapsular bleeding with hematuria to a shattered kidney from which death from exsanguination, hemorrhagic shock, or acute renal failure is possible. If the peritoneum remains intact, the expanding perirenal hematoma produces a flank swelling with local pain. If the peritoneum is traumatized as well, blood can accumulate in the abdominal cavity. If the patient survives and the renal parenchymal injury communicates with the collecting duct system, or if the ureter has been avulsed, then perirenal extravasation of blood and urine can occur. Such lesions have been called pararenal or perinephric pseudocysts.[31]

The diagnosis of renal trauma is based on history, clinical examination, laboratory findings, radiographic findings, and sometimes exploratory surgery (Chapter 135). The presence of renal injury is confirmed by excretory urography with the demonstration of extravasated contrast agent.[62] Rapid administration of an organic iodine contrast agent at the rate of 880 mg iodine/kg body weight is recommended.[62] If the kidney is not excreting the contrast agent within 20 minutes, the renal blood supply should be evaluated by renal arteriography.[18] Renal angiography is used frequently in human medicine to detect traumatic lesions such as aneurysms, infarcts, and arteriovenous fistulae.[41]

The therapeutic objectives in renal trauma are to control hemorrhage, excise devitalized tissue, and repair injured structures. Most renal lesions respond to rest and osmotic diuresis. If major renal damage is suspected, shock should be stabilized by fluid therapy and exploratory surgery undertaken. Parenchymal tears can be packed with a topical hemostatic agent such as gelatin sponge* or polymerized methyl cellulose.† If the damage is confined to one pole, partial nephrectomy may be considered. If the kidney is shattered, it should be removed, provided the other kidney is present and functioning.

---

*Gelfoam, Upjohn Company, Kalamazoo, MI.
†Oxycel, Parke-Davis, Morris Plains, NJ.

Nephrectomy

The kidneys are attached to the sublumbar region by peritoneum and renal fascia and are embedded in varying amounts of perirenal fat. The renal artery of dogs, particularly the left renal artery, is often paired, whereas multiple renal veins are frequently found in cats (Chapter 132).

The kidney can be exposed through a retroperitoneal flank or ventral midline approach. The abdominal approach is favored because both kidneys and the abdomen can be thoroughly examined. The incision starts in the cranial abdomen and extends as far caudally as necessary. The left kidney is exposed by packing abdominal viscera behind the mesentery of the descending colon (Fig. 136–4A). The right kidney is exposed by using the mesoduodenum in a similar fashion (Fig. 136–4B) and retracting the viscera to the left. The kidney is freed from its sublumbar attachment by a combination of sharp dissection with scissors and blunt dissection with a finger or gauze sponge (Fig. 136–5). Minor hemorrhage may be encountered from hypertrophied capsular vessels,[16]

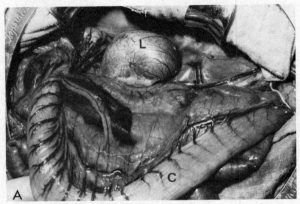

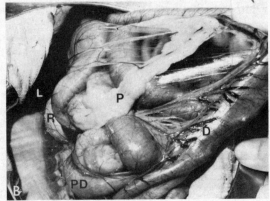

Figure 136–4. Transperitonal approach to the kidney. *A,* The left kidney (*L*) is exposed by retracting the colon (*C*) to the right and packing the abdominal viscera behind the mesocolon. *B,* The cranial part of the right kidney (*R*) is embedded in the caudate lobe of the liver (*L*). The duodenum (*D*) has been retracted to the left. The pancreas (*P*) is visible and viscera has been packed behind the mesoduodenum. The kidney is exposed completely by retracting the proximal duodenum (*PD*) to the left.

decreases the risk of spread from a renal tumor. Unless the patient is uremic or in shock, no special care is required following unilateral nephrectomy.

Partial Nephrectomy

The desire to salvage viable renal mass, if possible, was no doubt on the mind of Czerny when he performed the first human partial nephrectomy in 1887.[27] Wedge resection and transverse resection have been used since that time.[49] Partial nephrectomy was not popular, however, because postoperative hemorrhage, infection, and urine fistula were common complications. Nevertheless, the operation became a necessity as a treatment for renal tuberculosis. Newer techniques for partial nephrectomy have been developed that use either a single,[81] or triple thread[39] to cut through the renal parenchyma and simultaneously control the hemorrhage. The multiple suture method is preferred, as there is less chance of the ligatures slipping (Fig. 136–6).

The renal capsule is stripped back from the area to be resected, then two long, straight needles threaded with No. 1 chromic catgut are inserted into the kidney at the proposed site of resection. The needles and thread are passed through the kidney. The thread is cut to make three separate nooses, which are tied. Guillotine amputation is performed distal to these ligatures. Bleeding points or open diverticula are closed with suture ligatures of 3/0 synthetic absorbable suture material. The capsule is approximated over the amputated section, and some additional stitches are placed to anchor the capsule

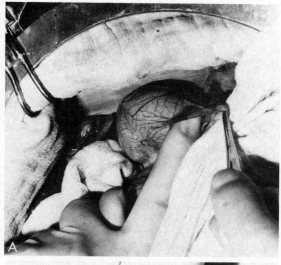

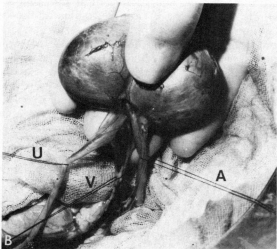

Figure 136–5. Mobilization of the left kidney of a dog. *A,* The peritoneum and caudal renal fascia have been elevated with forceps and cut with scissors. They are peeled from the kidney with a finger and gauze sponge. *B,* When mobilized, the kidney can be elevated from its sublumbar position to expose the renal artery (*A*), vein (*V*), and ureter (*U*).

but this soon stops or is easily controlled by cautery or ligation. The arterial supply is isolated close to the aorta proximal to any interlobar branches. In the dog, the left ovarian vein should be identified as it does not drain into the posterior vena cava but into the renal vein. The ureter is freed as far as the bladder. Mass ligation of the renal artery and vein is convenient but is not recommended because of the possibility of an arteriovenous fistula developing with its consequence of high output cardiac failure.[15] Cardiovascular silk (2/0 to 1 for cats and 0 to 1 for dogs) is an excellent material for ligation of blood vessels. Ligatures can be placed and tied directly around the blood vessels or tied around previously placed vascular clamps. The ureter is ligated and divided close to the bladder. This removes any possibility of a urine cul-de-sac that could promote infection and also

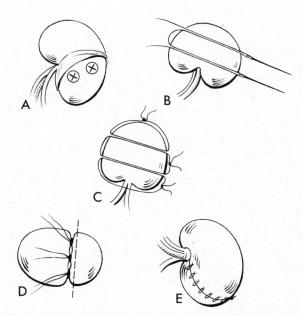

Figure 136–6. Partial nephrectomy. *A,* The kidney capsule is peeled back, and the points of insertion of the needles are indicated by crosses. *B,* The needles are drawn through the kidney parenchyma. *C,* The thread is cut to make three separate nooses. *D,* The nooses are tightened and tied and guillotine amputation (*dotted line*) performed. *E,* The capsule is reapproximated.

to the abdominal wall to prevent accidental rotation of the kidney.

Idiopathic Hematuria

Hematuria is expected with accidental or iatrogenic renal trauma or renal infection. It can also occur as a consequence of discrete renal hemangioma.[12, 43] Sometimes, however, no reason can be found for renal bleeding. In one case of human hematuria, the bleeding was traced to herniation of collecting ducts into renal veins caused by back pressure from urine obstruction.[32] Hemorrhage was intermittent. It appeared only during periods of raised venous pressure such as during exercise. In another case in a 16-year-old girl, severe renal bleeding was treated by selective embolization of the renal artery branch leading to the lesion with a saline suspension of gelatin sponge.[9] Gross bleeding continued but gradually decreased in intensity over three to four days. The fact that hemorrhage was not immediately controlled suggested that the bleeding was not arterial.

Selective embolization of an interlobar artery has been used to treat traumatic renal hemorrhage.[2] A suspension of gelatin sponge was not successful because it passed directly into the collecting duct system. In this case hemorrhage was controlled by placing a 5-mm wide steel coil* into the interlobar artery feeding the lesion.[77] In a case I saw of intermittent renal hemorrhage of unknown etiology in a dog, the diagnosis of renal hemorrhage was made by cystotomy and catheterization of the ureters. Blood-stained urine indicated the affected side, and the treatment was nephrectomy.

Nephrolithiasis

Results of surveys in dogs have indicated that calculi may form anywhere along the urinary tract, but the kidneys are involved in only 4 per cent of cases.[10] Urolithiasis in cats, with accumulation of mineral aggregates in the bladder, does occur and occasionally the kidneys are also involved.[66] For a detailed account of canine and feline urolithiasis, including medical management, see Chapters 140 and 141. Clinical signs of nephrolithiasis are often lacking, but if the calculi are associated with significant urinary tract infection, depression, anorexia, hematuria, and flank pain probably will be present. In bilateral nephrolithiasis, kidney function can be compromised to such a degree that signs of uremia may be seen. The diagnosis is confirmed by radiography. If the affected kidney or kidneys still have adequate function, medical dissolution may be attempted (Chapter 140). If renal function is already depressed, surgical removal of the calculi probably will be life-saving.

The dog whose kidney radiographs are shown in Figure 136–3 had a history of anorexia and vomiting and was azotemic. Calculi were present in both kidneys. The shrunken left kidney was removed, and a histological examination showed that the small size was due to primary renal hypoplasia. The right kidney was hypertrophied, but the azotemia indicated that the calculus was causing significant outflow obstruction. The calculus was removed, the dog improved rapidly, and it lived happily for a further four years.

Nephrotomy

Nephrotomy temporarily decreases renal function by 20 to 40 per cent.[26] If calculi are present in both kidneys and a decision is made to remove them, a choice of one operation or two operations a few weeks apart has to be made. Bilateral nephrotomy can be performed at one operation, but if the patient is severely azotemic or if surgical trauma at the first operation was judged to be excessive, the operations should be spaced. The safest route into the canine renal pelvis is by a longitudinal sagittal incision through the convex lateral surface of the kidney. If the calculus is spindle-shaped and the pelvis and proximal ureter have dilated, the calculus may be removed through a pyelotomy. Pyelotomy is not usually recommended in dogs and cats, however, because they have small renal pelves and there is an increased risk of hitting an interlobar vessel.

The best access to the kidney is via a long, ventral, transperitoneal abdominal incision. The renal artery and vein can be temporarily occluded with vascular clamps (Chapter 135). Both kidneys are sufficiently mobile to be held between thumb and fingers to expose their convex lateral surfaces. This is preferred to dissecting the kidney from its sublumbar attachments as it avoids rupturing functional collateral vessels, thus surgical trauma is kept to a minimum.

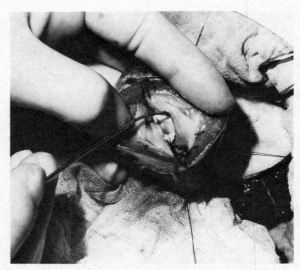

Figure 136–7. Sagittal nephrotomy exposing the renal pelvis of a dog. The renal crest has been elevated with a probe.

---

*Gianturco coil, Cook Bloomington, Markham, Ontario.

An incision is made with a scalpel into the renal pelvis through the cortex and medulla (Fig. 136–7). Passive blood flow is sponged away to expose the calculus, which is removed. Mineral aggregates can be flushed from each diverticulum with saline, using a modified hypodermic needle (Chapter 135). The ureteral orifice is catheterized with a 3.5 French catheter, and saline is gently flushed through the ureter to confirm its patency. The nephrotomy is closed by apposing the two renal parenchymal flaps. This can be done with gentle thumb and finger pressure while the clamps on the vascular pedicle are released. Hemorrhage from the nephrotomy site is minimal as this approach does not cut any major blood vessels. Within five minutes the clotted blood has virtually glued the two halves of the kidney together (Fig. 136–8). This method has been called the sutureless nephrotomy closure. It has been successfully used in humans[60] and experimental dogs.[26] I have used this technique successfully in clinical situations in dogs; although dispensing with the usual parenchymal mattress stitches, the capsular row has been retained (see Fig. 136–8).

Following nephrotomy, there may be minor hematuria for a few days. Intravenous fluids given during surgery and in the immediate postoperative period encourage diuresis and help flush blood clots from the urinary tract. If hematuria persists beyond

a few days, treatment with a hemostatic agent such as aminocaproic acid* could be tried.[67] This drug promotes clotting by inhibiting urokinase, which is an activator of plasminogen and plasmin (fibrinolysin). Tranexamic acid† has the same action and uses an aminocaproic acid, but it is ten times more potent and is less toxic. It is given at a dose rate of 25 mg/kg body weight initially, then 10 mg/kg every six hours.

Hydronephrosis

This condition results in the progressive dilation of the renal pelvis and progressive atrophy of the renal parenchyma.[56] Dogs are more often affected than cats.[30, 52] When urine outflow obstruction affects both kidneys, the animal will die before pressure atrophy can cause much reduction in renal mass. When the obstruction is unilateral, the degree of hydronephrosis can reach such proportions that the renal parenchyma is only a shell (Fig. 136–9). As a general rule, when the duct of a gland becomes obstructed, the gland immediately stops secreting and the organ atrophies. The kidney might also act in this manner,[68] but usually urine production continues after the lower urinary tract is obstructed. This is because the obstruction is not complete. Urine is reabsorbed through the renal vein and the renal hilar lymphatics.[50] If the obstruction is relieved within one week, the renal damage is totally reversible. Even after four weeks total obstruction, 25 per cent of normal renal function can be expected to return.[76]

Since the renal tubules are metabolically very active, they are the major sites of pathological change during the early course of hydronephrosis. Eventually, however, even the glomeruli are destroyed. Urine outflow obstruction can be congenital. Torsion,

*Amicar, Lederle Laboratories, Wayne, NJ.
†Vasolamin, Troy Laboratories, Smithfield, N.S.W. Australia.

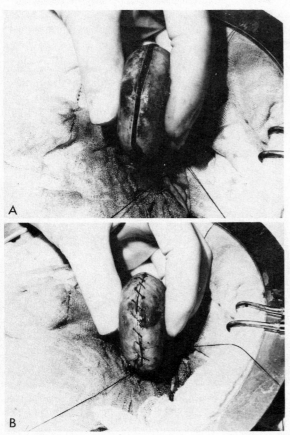

Figure 136–8. Sutureless nephrotomy closure. *A,* The renal parenchymal flaps are united by a fibrin bond. *B,* The capsule is apposed with a continuous suture.

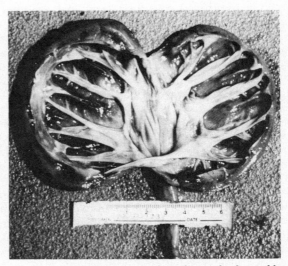

Figure 136–9. Hydronephrosis in a dog. The renel pelvis is dilated and the parenchyma remains as a thin shell. (Courtesy of R. Mitten.)

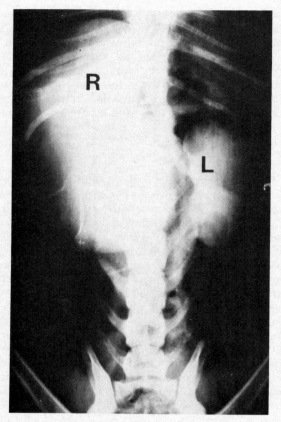

Figure 136–10. Unilateral hydronephrosis in a dog demonstrated radiographically against the contrast of a pneumoperitoneum. The dimensions of the left kidney (L) are normal, but the right kidney (R) is enlarged.

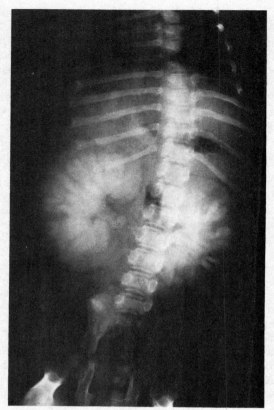

Figure 136–11. Bilateral hydronephrosis in a one-week-old pup with urethral obstruction. Excretory urography shows that both renal pelves are dilated.

kinking, stenosis, and atresia of the ureters or urethra or aberrant renal vessels that constrict the ureters have been reported.[56] Hydronephrosis may also be acquired as a result of compression of the ureters or urethra by neoplastic or other masses, such as hematoma, cysts, or abscesses. It will also follow obstruction by urinary calculi or accidental ligation of the ureter during ovariohysterectomy.[72]

The clinical signs and pathophysiology of urinary tract obstruction are discussed in Chapter 134. The usual clinical sign of uncomplicated unilateral hydronephrosis is an enlarged abdomen. Abdominal radiographs show an enlarged renal shadow (Fig. 136–10). The degree of dilation can be seen with excretory urography as long as sufficient functioning nephrons are present in the kidney (Fig. 136–11). If the kidney is not excreting contrast agent, renal angiography could indicate hydronephrosis by the appearance of an attenuated vascular pattern (Fig. 136–12). However, palpation of an enlarged kidney and lack of kidney function on an excretory urogram are sufficient justification to explore the abdomen to confirm the diagnosis and effect a treatment. In recent acute ureteral obstruction, the affected kidney is tense, and the renal hilar lymphatics are prominent.

A condition called capsular hydronephrosis has been described in cats, in which the kidney capsule is separated from the renal parenchyma by a large collection of fluid.[1, 14, 64, 73] Capsular hydronephrosis is possibly related to lymphatic obstruction and is effectively treated by excising the wall of the pseudocyst.[1, 14, 56] If the hydronephrosis is well advanced and the kidney is only a fluid-filled sac, the prognosis is hopeless and the remains of the kidney should be

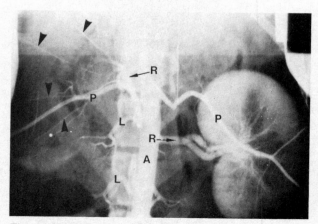

Figure 136–12. Unilateral hydronephrosis seen as an incidental finding during arteriography of the infrarenal aorta. Contrast agent has passed into both renal arteries. The left kidney shows a normal vascular pattern. The interlobar vessels of the right kidney (arrows) are regular but attenuated, and the right renal shadow is enlarged. Vessels opacified are the aorta (A), renal artery (R), phrenicoabdominal artery (P), and lumbar arteries (L).

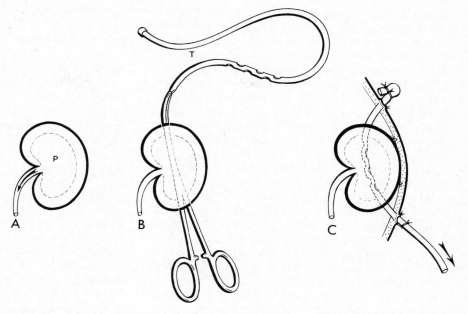

Figure 136–13. Nephrostomy. *A,* Increased resistance to urine outflow (arrow) results in dilatation of the renal pelvis (*P*). *B,* A fenestrated tube (*T*) is drawn into the renal pelvis with a narrow, long-jawed forceps passed through the renal parenchyma and pelvis in a sagittal plane. *C,* Each end of the tube is exteriorized through the abdominal wall. One end is sealed and the other end is connected to a closed urine drainage system. The kidney is anchored to the abdominal wall muscles with a few capsular stitches, and the nephrostomy tube is anchored to the skin.

removed. If some kidney function is evident on excretory urography, and if the cause of the urine obstruction can be identified and corrected, it is vital, particularly if the other kidney is also damaged, to try to save that kidney.

Nephrostomy drainage of urine will immediately relieve pressure. The kidney is mobilized, and a length of fenestrated latex or silicone rubber tubing 5 or 6 mm in diameter is positioned in the dilated renal pelvis (Fig. 136–13). The catheter is exteriorized through the abdominal wall and the urine diverted into the closed container. Drainage can be maintained until the cause of the obstruction has been corrected. The kidney is anchored to the abdominal wall with a few capsular sutures. This type of nephrostomy tube can be replaced.[80] When the tube is removed, a urine fistula will be created for a short while. If distal obstruction still exists, the fistula persists.

Purulent Nephritis

Experiments in cats have shown that if the ureter is obstructed and a systemic bacterial infection is established, the kidney associated with the obstructed ureter will become infected.[38] Clinical experience has shown that bacterial infection by the hematogenous route is a common complication of obstructive uropathy.[19, 24] Renal injury also predisposes the kidney to a bloodborne infection.[24] Purulent nephritis also can occur as an ascending infection from the lower urinary tract, particularly in the presence of an incompetent ureterovesical junction and vesicoureteral reflux.[24] The treatment of urinary tract infection is discussed in Chapter 135.

When both kidneys are infected, the relative contribution of each kidney to total renal function is important. In humans, this is determined by renal scans after the injection of radioactively labelled substances that are excreted by the kidneys. These techniques are now becoming available in some veterinary hospitals.[18] In bilateral renal infection, it is feasible to remove foreign bodies or excise focal abscesses. If an abscess is unilateral, partial or total nephrectomy is an effective treatment in conjunction with systemic antibiotic therapy.

Kidney Worm

Dioctophyma renale, the giant kidney worm, is found sporadically in dogs and wild fish-eating carnivores, particularly mink. Cats are resistant to this parasite.[58] Dogs become infected by eating fish or frogs that contain infective larvae. The larvae penetrate the gut wall of the host and mature into adults usually within the peritoneal cavity. Often, however, they penetrate the kidney and may completely destroy the renal parenchyma. The presence of the giant kidney worm is usually discovered incidentally after *D. renale* ova are found in the urine. Alternatively, adult worms are found in the peritoneal cavity during abdominal surgery. The treatment is nephrectomy or nephrotomy, depending on the degree of renal damage and whether one or both kidneys are harboring parasites. Prevention depends on blocking access to raw fish, particularly the North American catfish.

Acute Renal Failure

This is characterized by the rapid onset of oliguria or anuria, reduced renal blood flow, reduced glomerular filtration rate, and sudden azotemia. Acute renal failure is potentially reversible, but invariably some renal tubular damage will have occurred. Recovery depends on the quantity of renal mass injured and on whether the remaining nephrons can repair enough to increase their functional capacity. A consideration of the pathophysiology and management of acute renal failure can be found in Chapter 134.

The two major predisposing factors that might initiate acute renal failure are reduced renal hemodynamics and exposure of the kidneys to nephrotoxic agents, such as heavy metals, organic compounds, and antimicrobial drugs. Reduced renal hemodynamics can occur in many ways, including hemorrhage, trauma, prolonged anesthesia, extensive surgery, and reduced cardiovascular function. Any or all of these inciting factors are present in varying proportions in all surgery. In elective surgery on patients with no preoperative renal disorder, the infusion during surgery of a balanced salt solution such as lactated Ringer's at the rate of 15 ml/kg body weight minimizes the anesthetic and surgical depression of renal function.[29]

If surgery must be performed on animals with renal disease, the anesthetist has a very responsible job.[33] Attention must be paid to fluid balance, since dehydration usually accompanies acute renal failure. Electrolyte abnormalities will be present, e.g., hyperkalemia in acute renal failure and hyponatremia in chronic failure. Metabolic acidosis accompanies the impaired ability to excrete hydrogen ion. Acidosis causes myocardial irritability and also results in decreased barbiturate binding to plasma protein. This means that the barbiturate becomes more potent. If albuminuria has been present for any length of time, hypoproteinemia will be seen. Fluid replacement in hypoproteinemic animals should be given in the form of colloid (plasma) rather than crystalloid. Furthermore, as protein is lost from the plasma, more barbiturate and narcotic remain unbound, and so the concentration of these drugs rises. This is another cause of the increased potency of anesthetic agents.

Patients with chronic renal failure are anemic. If the blood oxygen saturation is less than 70 gm/L, adequate oxygenation under anesthesia will not be possible. The patient will require a blood transfusion with crossmatched blood, for even minor transfusion reactions cannot be tolerated by animals with renal disease.

Since it is possible for animals with compensated chronic renal failure to decompensate and experience a uremic crisis, it is important for therapeutic and prognostic reasons to first distinguish between acute and chronic renal failure (Chapter 134). One of the ways of doing this is by renal biopsy.[59] Even in kidneys with diffuse lesions, histological examination is not a reliable way to predict reversibility and functional compensation. In focal lesions, chance sampling errors obviously can lead to diagnostic and prognostic mistakes. A biopsy could mean total or partial removal or core sampling with a needle. Nephrectomy and partial nephrectomy are biopsy methods that have already been described.

Needle Biopsy

With this technique, it is possible to obtain a kidney tissue sample without having to open the abdomen. In most instances, however, there is more merit in exposing the two kidneys and sampling from one or both under direct vision than in blind percutaneous biopsy or even the "key hole" technique.[59] Before proceeding with a biopsy, the benefits must be weighed against the risks. Absolute contraindications to needle biopsy are hemorrhagic tendencies, inexperienced diagnosticians, and damaged equipment.[54]

Two types of needle are currently in use, the modified pediatric Franklin-Silverman biopsy needle* (Fig. 136–14) and the Vim Tru-cut.† The Franklin needle is reusable and can be resharpened. There is economic merit in having this needle in a hospital unit that performs many biopsies on a regular basis. However, if it is not cared for, much damage is done to the kidney and the sample is often unsatisfactory. The Tru-cut needle is disposable, very sharp, and easy to use, so it is ideal for the occasional biopsy. If required, this needle can be cleaned and resterilized with ethylene oxide gas.[54]

The components of the Vim Tru-cut needle are shown in the retracted and fully advanced positions (Fig. 136–15). To use this instrument, the obturator specimen rod is fully retracted within the outer cannula. The tip of the instrument is placed on the surface of the lesion and the specimen rod is thrust into the lesion by depressing the plastic handle. The outer sheath of the needle is now advanced. This action cuts the surrounding tissue, which is retained in the specimen notch. As the needle is withdrawn, hemorrhage is often profuse for a short while. It is

*Mueller Company, Chicago, IL.
†Travenol Laboratories, Deerfield, IL.

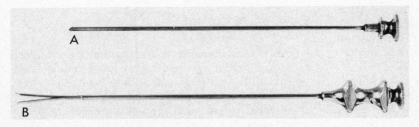

Figure 136–14. The Franklin-modified Vim Silverman biopsy needle. *A*, Obturator. *B*, The obturator has been removed from the sheath and replaced by cutting prongs, which are thrust into the tissue to be sampled. When the sheath is advanced over the cutting prongs, the specimen is retained and the needle can be withdrawn.

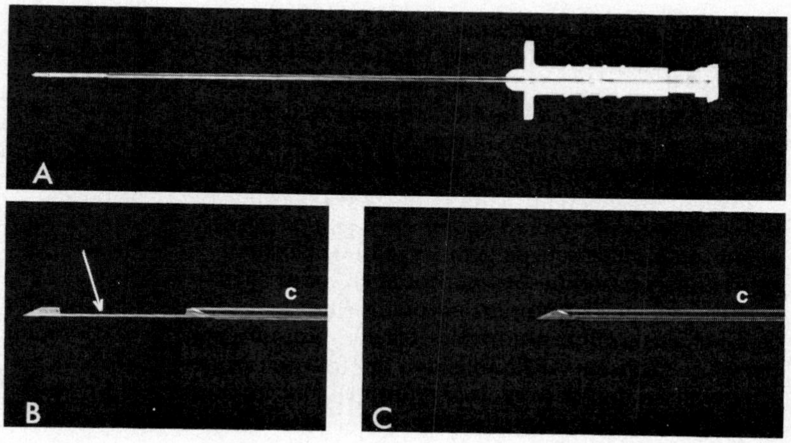

Figure 136–15. *A*, Vim Tru-cut biopsy needle. *B*, When the obturator specimen rod is advanced tissue fills the specimen notch (arrow). *C*, When the sheath (*C*), with its sharp cutting tip is advanced, a core of tissue is cut and retained in the specimen notch as the needle is withdrawn.

controlled by finger pressure and soon stops. If gross hematuria persists beyond 24 hours, the animal can be treated with a hemostatic agent such as tranexamic acid (refer to nephrotomy).

Arteriovenous fistulae have been reported as complications following renal biopsy in humans[23, 74] but have not been encountered in dogs and cats.[55]

Dialysis

Part of the management of acute renal failure includes dialysis. Dialysis makes it possible to rid the body of metabolic waste products that contribute to the signs of uremia.

Two techniques are available, hemodialysis and peritoneal dialysis. Alterations in the volume and composition of the extracellular fluid take place across a semipermeable membrane. This membrane is cellulose in hemodialysis and the peritoneum in peritoneal dialysis. Hemodialysis is more efficient, but it requires special equipment and trained staff as the blood has to be removed from the body, circulated through an artificial kidney, and returned to the body. For chronic hemodialysis, an arteriovenous fistula or vascular shunt must first be inserted in the patient. A disadvantage of hemodialysis is the need for anticoagulation therapy to be given for the life of the shunt. The patient also has to face the risks of hemorrhage resulting from the reduction of platelets during extracorporeal circulation, hypotension and hemolysis during each dialysis, and infection at the site of the vascular access.[71]

Peritoneal dialysis is quite feasible in dogs and cats.[61] It is performed with commercial dialysing fluid containing at least 1.5% glucose* to prevent rapid water absorption caused by the hyperosmotic state of the uremic plasma. Hyperosmotic dialysis solutions with 4.25 and 7% glucose are also available, and their use effectively reduces plasma volume in edematous patients. In an emergency, lactated Ringer's solution can be used by adding 30 ml of 50% dextrose per liter of fluid to make a 1.5% solution. A disadvantage

*Dianeal, Travenol Laboratories, Deerfield, IL.

of Ringer's solution is its low sodium content. It also contains potassium and phosphate, two of the electrolytes already present in excess in renal failure. Warming the dialysate to 40 to 42°C promotes vasodilation and enhances blood flow to the peritoneal membrane. Intraperitoneal vasodilators such as isoproterenol increase urea clearance by approximately 25 per cent.[51]

The major difficulty with peritoneal dialysis has been to remove the bulk of the fluid that is instilled. This problem has largely been overcome by the development of two efficient silicone rubber peritoneal dialysis cannulae, one by Parker[61] and the other by Thornhill.[70] These catheters are flexible and are designed to be attached to the abdominal wall. They can be maintained in place for a number of weeks during the period of chronic intermittent dialysis. The expected drainage rate by gravity alone with these catheters is about 100 ml/min, with a recovery rate of 90 to 100 per cent.[7]

The recommended volume of dialysis fluid to infuse is 40 ml/kg body weight. This should be allowed to dwell for 30 minutes. A cycle of infusion, dwell, and recovery should take about one hour. During the first exchange, up to 20 per cent of the dialysate may be lost to the interspaces of the intestines. The first few exchanges may be blood-tinged from hemorrhage that may have occurred during insertion of the cannula. Six to eight exchanges can be completed in 24 hours. After each session the cannula is flushed with heparinized saline and 100 to 500 mg of ampicillin is instilled into the peritoneal cavity. Records must be kept of fluid balance and plasma chemistry before the commencement of treatment and after every 12 to 24 hours of treatment.

Chronic Renal Failure

This is the result of progressive nephron loss, regardless of etiology, leading eventually to uremia when the process has reached its end stage (Chapter 134).

Dietary Therapy

Conservative management that helps delay progression of chronic renal disease includes attention to diet. Although the principles may apply to all species, the only available data relate to dogs. The following factors need to be considered.

Protein Restriction. This is introduced when the blood urea nitrogen levels are greater than 80 mg/dl. Protein intake should be restricted to 0.6 to 1.2 gm/kg body weight per day. As much of the protein as possible should be in the form of cooked eggs.[6] Within a few weeks the dog should experience less nausea and vomiting and be more active.

Caloric Requirement. Calories must be kept up in animals on a protein-restricted diet, or catabolism of body protein for energy will occur. The recommended level is 70 kcal/kg body weight per day. A diet can be constructed from the foods listed in Table 136–1 with the addition of a multivitamin supplement. The daily food intake should be divided into three or four feedings.

Electrolyte Balance. Sodium intake should be maintained at normal levels since dogs can maintain sodium balance throughout the course of chronic renal failure.

Metabolic acidosis is not a feature of chronic renal failure in dogs until the very late stages of the disease. This is because enhanced bicarbonate reabsorption occurs in uremic dogs independent of the state of extracellular fluid volume or the presence of parathyroid hormone.[3]

Hyperphosphatemia is usually a feature of dogs with chronic renal failure. Restricting phosphate intake abolishes hyperparathyroidism. Phosphate restriction occurs automatically with protein restriction when foods from the diet in Table 136–1 are used. However, the level of hyperphosphatemia varies with the degree of renal failure and the amount of dietary phosphate. It is necessary, therefore, to monitor plasma phosphate on a regular basis. If hyperphosphatemia persists, aluminum hydroxide gel, 5 to 10 ml orally three times daily before meals, can be given to bind phosphate in the lumen of the bowel and inhibit its absorption.

Calcium carbonate supplements at 100 mg/kg body weight help combat renal osteodystrophy. This should be coupled with oral vitamin D, which may be administered as 24,25 $(OH)_2$-cholecalciferol (1 μg daily).[13]

Protein restriction also means potassium restriction. Potassium retention is uncommon until the very late stages of chronic renal failure in dogs.

Dialysis

This technique, described under acute renal failure, is recommended for chronic renal disease only with acute decompensation that can be reversed. There is no justification for dialysis of an animal in terminal renal failure unless renal transplantation is being contemplated.

Renal Transplantation

Renal allografting is a therapeutic procedure that has not been applied to clinical situations in animals to the extent it has been in humans. Currently a vast amount of knowledge about antigens, graft rejection, and immunosuppression is available for dogs, but graft rejection is still a major obstacle. It is possible to perform major and minor crossmatching of red blood cell antigens in dogs and look at their serological and cell-mediated histocompatibility antigens. Even if a good match is found, immunosuppressive therapy is still required to suppress the immune response to other histocompatibility antigens present but not yet detected.[11] Cyclosporin A is an immunosuppressive agent that seems to have the best chance of abrogating graft rejection.[21]

In renal transplantation experiments in which the lymphocyte antigens (DLA) of sibling dogs were fully matched, 2 of 11 transplants were maintained in excess of 100 days without the need for immunosuppression. On the other hand, in another group of siblings in which DLA antigens were totally incompatible, 1 in 12 grafts was accepted, again without the need for immunosuppression. The cost of performing a clinical, living, related, full sibling canine renal transplant, including histocompatibility testing and preoperative and postoperative care, was $1,685.[21] If a compatible unrelated donor would have had to be found, it was estimated that the fee would have doubled.

The operative technique of renal transplantation is straightforward. The donor kidney is obtained and infused with heparinized saline at 4°C to wash out donor blood and cool the organ. Cooling the kidney prolongs ischemia time before excessive pathological

TABLE 136–1.   Foods Used in Renal Failure

	Protein (gm)	Energy (kcal)
Bread, toast, 1 slice	2.0	60
Butter, margarine, 1 tsp	—	40
Cake, cupcake	2.6	130
pound, 1 slice, $2 \times 3 \times 5$	2.1	130
sponge, 2" slice	3.2	120
Cream cheese, 1 oz	2.6	106
Cream, light, 1 oz	—	50
Doughnut, 1	2.1	130
Egg, cooked, 1	7.0	120
Gravy, 1 Tbsp	—	80
Ice cream, 1 oz	1.2	62
Jelly, 1 tsp	—	60
Milk, whole, 2 oz	2.0	40
Pancakes, wheat, 4" diameter	1.8	60
Sweet roll, 4×1", 50 gm	4.2	160
Rice, cooked, 1 cup	4.2	200
Soups: bouillon, consomme, 1 cup	2.0	9
chicken, 1 cup	3.5	75
Spaghetti, cooked, 1 cup	7.4	220
Sugar, honey, 1 tsp	—	20

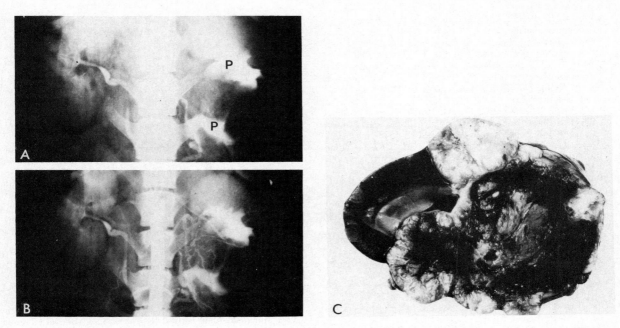

Figure 136–16. Renal carcinoma in a dog. *A,* An intravenous pyelogram shows contrast agent being excreted by both kidneys. The left kidney is enlarged, and its pelvis (*P*) is misshapen and contains a large filling defect. *B,* A renal angiogram shows increased vascularity of the caudal pole. *C,* The excised surgical specimen.

changes occur in the tubules. The kidney is implanted in the iliac fossa of the recipient with the renal artery anastomosed end-to-end with the external iliac artery and the renal vein anastomosed end-to-side to the common iliac vein. The ureter is implanted into the bladder using techniques outlined in Chapter 138.

Renal Autotransplantation

In this operation the kidney is removed from its orthotopic position and transferred to a heterotopic position, such as the iliac fossa. This procedure could be an alternative to nephrectomy if a damaged distal ureter were too short to be reimplanted into the bladder. The technique is as outlined for allotransplantation. As an adjunct to autotransplantation, extracorporeal or "work bench" surgery has become established as a technique to treat certain human renal vascular lesions.[42] The kidney is excised and cooled, the lesion dealt with on the bench top, then the kidney is reimplanted—usually in a heterotopic site. This technique has also been used in selected cases of renal tumor and stone disease.[42] An experimental study in dogs comparing bench surgery with *in situ* repair of induced renal trauma showed that both methods were equally good.[47] It was concluded that hilar injuries with segmental artery involvement would benefit most from bench microsurgery and bench angiography.

Renal Neoplasia

A wide range of tumors occur in the kidneys of dogs and cats. Their diagnosis, biological behavior, and details of treatment are covered in Section XIX. It is important not to be too pessimistic when a space-occupying lesion is detected in the kidney. It may be benign, in which case partial or total nephrectomy has an excellent prognosis. Even if a carcinoma were diagnosed (Fig. 136–16), nephrectomy should be tried as long as radiographs of the chest show clear lung fields and exploratory surgery does not reveal enlarged regional lymph nodes. Extended survival of up to four years has followed excision of a renal carcinoma in a dog.[46]

1. Abdinoor, D. J.: Perinephric pseudocysts in a cat. J. Am. Vet. Med. Assoc. *16:*763, 1980.
2. Ankenman, G. J., and Murray, J. B.: Control of post operative renal hemorrhage by embolization with a Gianturco coil. Can. J. Surg. *25:*269, 1982.
3. Arruda, J. A. L., Carrasquillo, T., Cubria, A., Rademacher, D. R., and Kurtzman, N. A.: Bicarbonate reabsorption in chronic renal failure. Kidney Internat. *9:*481, 1976.
4. Battershell, D., and Garcia, J. P.: Polycystic kidney in a cat. J. Am. Vet. Med. Assoc. *154:*665, 1969.
5. Borthwick, R.: Foreign body in a cat's kidney. J. Small Anim. Pract. *12:*623, 1971.
6. Bovee, K. C.: Dietary therapy in renal failure. *In* Nephrology, Urology and Diseases of the Urinary Tract. Univ. of Sydney Post Grad. C'ttee in Vet. Sci. Proceedings No. 61, 1982, p. 273.

7. Bovee, K. C.: Peritoneal dialysis, hemodialysis and prospects of renal transplantation. *In* Nephrology, Urology and Diseases of the Urinary Tract. Univ. of Sydney Post Grad. C'ttee in Vet. Sci. Proceedings No. 61, 1982, p. 299.

8. Bricker, N. S., and Fine, L. G.: The renal response to progressive nephron loss. *In* Brenner, B. M., and Rector, F. C. (eds.): *The Kidney.* Vol. 1, 2nd ed. W. B. Saunders, Philadelphia, 1981.

9. Brooker, W. J., Ahrens, C. F., and Hutchens, H. C.: Renal bleeding due to congenital vascular malformation: Control by arterial embolization. J. Urol. *119*:261, 1978.

10. Brown, N. O., Parks, J. L., and Green, R. W.: Canine urolithiasis: Retrospective analysis of 438 cases. J. Am. Vet. Med. Assoc. *170*:414, 1977.

11. Bull, R. W.: Antigens, graft rejections and transfusions. J. Am. Vet. Med. Assoc. *181*:1115, 1982.

12. Cadwallader, J. A., Goulden, B. E., Wyburn, R. S., and Jolly, R. D.: Renal haemangioma in a dog. N.Z. Vet. J. *21*:48, 1973.

13. Canterbury, J. M., Gavellas, G., Bourgoignie, J. J., and Reiss, E.: Metabolic consequences of oral administration of 24,25-dihydroxy-cholecalciferol to uremic dogs. J. Clin. Invest. *65*:571, 1980.

14. Chastain, C. B., and Grier, R. L.: Bilateral retroperitoneal perirenal cysts in a cat. Feline Pract. *5*:41, 1975.

15. Chew, Q. T., and Madayag, M. A.: Post nephrectomy arteriovenous fistula. J. Urol. *109*:546, 1973.

16. Christie, B. A.: Collateral arterial blood supply to the normal and ischemic canine kidney. Am. J. Vet. Res. *41*:1519, 1980.

17. Churchward, R. E.: Subcutaneous herniation of a kidney of a dog. Aust. Vet. J. *47*:178, 1971.

18. Cowgill, L. D.: Diseases of the kidney. *In* Ettinger, S. J. (ed.): *Textbook of Veterinary Internal Medicine.* Vol. 2, 2nd ed. W. B. Saunders, Philadelphia, 1983, p. 1812.

19. Crow, S. W., Lauerman, L. H., and Smith, K. W.: Pyonephrosis associated with Salmonella infection in a dog. J. Am. Vet. Med. Assoc. *169*:1324, 1976.

20. Crowell, W. A., Hubbell, J. J., and Riley, J. C.: Polycystic renal disease in related cats. J. Am. Vet. Med. Assoc. *175*:286, 1979.

21. Deeg, H. J., Storb, R., Gerhard-Muller, L., Shulman, H. M., Weiden, P. L., and Thomas, E. D.: Cyclosporin A, a powerful immunosuppressant in vivo and in vitro in dogs, fails to produce tolerance. Transplantation *29*:230, 1980.

22. Dorn, A. S., and Stoloff, D.: Renal foreign body in a dog. J. Am. Vet. Med. Assoc. *167*:755, 1975.

23. Ekelund, L., Gothlin, J., Lindholm, T., Lindsteal, E., and Mattsson, K.: Arteriovenous fistulae following renal biopsy with hypertension and hemodynamic changes. J. Urol. *108*:373, 1972.

24. Finco, D. R., and Barsanti, J. A.: Bacterial pyelonephritis. Vet. Clin. North Am. *9*:645, 1979.

25. Finco, D. R., Kneller, S. K., and Crowell, W. A.: Diseases of the urinary system. *In* Catcott, E. J. (ed.): *Feline Medicine and Surgery,* 2nd ed. American Veterinary Publications Inc., Santa Barbara, 1975, p. 263.

26. Gahring, D. R., Crowe, D. T., Powers, T. E., Powers, J. D., Krakowka, S., and Wilson, G. P., III: Comparative renal function studies of nephrotomy closure with and without sutures in dogs. J. Am. Vet. Med. Assoc. *171*:537, 1977.

27. Goldstein, A. E., and Abeshouse, B. S.: Partial resection of the kidney. J. Urol. *38*:15, 1937.

28. Goss, R. J., and Dittmer, J. E.: Compensatory renal hypertrophy: Problems and prospects. *In* Nowinski, W. W., and Goss, R. I. (eds.): *Compensatory Renal Hypertrophy.* Academic Press, New York, 1969, p. 305.

29. Gourley, I. M. G.: Prevention and treatment of acute renal failure in the canine surgical patient. J. Am. Vet. Med. Assoc. *157*:1722, 1970.

30. Hall, M. A., Osborne, C. A., and Stevens, J. B.: Hydronephrosis with heteroplastic bone formation in a cat. J. Am. Vet. Med. Assoc. *160*:857, 1972.

31. Hurwitz, S. P., and Weisenthal, C. L.: Pararenal pseudocysts. J. Urol. *97*:8, 1967.

32. Iliff, W. J., and Galdabini, J. J.: Massive intratubular hemorrhage with herniations into renal veins requiring nephrectomy. J. Urol. *108*:44, 1972.

33. Ilkiw, J.: Anaesthesia and renal failure. *In* Nephrology, Urology and Diseases of the Urinary Tract. Univ. of Sydney Post Grad. C'ttee in Vet. Sci. Proceedings No. 61, 1982, p. 145.

34. Johnson, C. A.: Renal ectopia in a cat. J. Am. Anim. Hosp. Assoc. *15*:599, 1979.

35. Johnson, H. A.: Cytoplasmic response to overwork. *In* Nowinski, W. W., and Goss, R. I. (eds.): *Compensatory Renal Hypertrophy.* Academic Press, New York, 1969, p. 14.

36. Jubb, K. V. F., and Kennedy, P. C.: *Pathology of Domestic Animals.* Vol. 1, 2nd ed. Academic Press, New York, 1970, p. 288.

37. Kaufman, C. F., Soirez, R. F., and Tasker, J. P.: Renal cortical hypoplasia with secondary hyperparathyroidism in the dog. J. Am. Vet. Med. Assoc. *155*:1679, 1969.

38. Kelly, D. F., Lucke, V. M., and McCullagh, K. G.: Experimental pyelonephritis in the cat. J. Comp. Pathol. *89*:125, 1979.

39. Kim, S. K.: New techniques of partial nephrectomy. J. Urol. *102*:165, 1969.

40. Klopfer, U., Nobel, T. A., and Kaminski, R.: A nephropathy similar to renal cortical hypoplasia in a Yorkshire Terrier. Vet. Med./Small Anim. Clin. *73*:327, 1978.

41. Lang, E. K., Trichel, B. E., Turner, R. W., Fontenot, R. E., Johnson, B., and Martin, E. C.St.: Renal arteriography in the assessment of renal trauma. Radiology *98*:103, 1971.

42. Lawson, R.: Extracorporeal renal surgery. J. Urol. *123*:301, 1980.

43. Lee, R., Weaver, H. D., and Robinson, P. B.: Persistent haematuria in a dog due to discrete renal haemangioma. J. Small Anim. Pract. *15*:621, 1974.

44. Lipson, M. P., Ellingwood, J., and Field, P. J.: Bullet lodged in the kidney of a dog. J. Am. Vet. Med. Assoc. *161*:293, 1972.

45. Lord, P. F., Scott, R. C., and Chan, K. F.: Intravenous urography for evaluation of renal disease in small animals. J. Am. Anim. Hosp. Assoc. *10*:139, 1974.

46. Lucke, V. M., and Kelly, D. F.: Renal carcinoma in the dog. Vet. Pathol. *13*:264, 1976.

47. McAninch, J. W., Rodkey, W. G., Stutzman, R. E., and Peterson, L. J.: Experimental penetrating renal trauma: A comparison of bench and in situ repair. Invest. Urol. *17*:33, 1979.

48. McKenna, S. C., and Carpenter, J. L.: Polycystic disease of the kidney and liver in the Cairn Terrier. Vet. Pathol. *17*:436, 1980.

49. Murphy, J. J., and Best, R.: The healing of renal wounds. 1. Partial nephrectomy. J. Urol. *78*:504, 1957.

50. Nabar, K. G., and Madson, P. O.: Renal function during acute total ureteral occlusion and the role of the lymphatics. An experimental study in dogs. J. Urol. *109*:330, 1973.

51. Nolph, K. D., Ghods, A. J., Van Stone, J., and Brown, P. A.: The effects of intraperitoneal vasodilator on peritoneal clearances. Trans. Am. Soc. Artif. Intern. Organs *22*:586, 1976.

52. North, D. C.: Hydronephrosis and hydroureter in a kitten. J. Small Anim. Pract. *19*:237, 1978.

53. Northington, J. W., and Juliana, M. M.: Polycystic kidney disease in a cat. J. Small Anim. Pract. *18*:663, 1977.

54. Osborne, C. A.: General principles of biopsy. Vet. Clin. North Am. *4*:213, 1974.

55. Osborne, C. A., Low, D. G., and Finco, D. R.: *Canine and Feline Urology.* W. B. Saunders, Philadelphia, 1972, p. 114.

56. Osborne, C. A., Low, D. G., and Finco, D. R.: *Canine and Feline Urology.* W. B. Saunders, Philadelphia, 1972, p. 198.

57. Osborne, C. A., Quast, J. F., Barnes, D. M., and Stockner,

P.: Congenital fusion of kidney in a dog. Vet. Med./Small Anim. Clin. 67:39, 1972.

58. Osborne, C. A., Stevens, J. B., Hanlon, G. F., and Rosin, E.: *Dioctophyma renale* in the dog. J. Am. Vet. Med. Assoc. 155:605, 1969.

59. Osborne, C. A., Stevens, J. B., and Perman, V.: Kidney biopsy. Vet. Clin. North Am. 4:351, 1974.

60. Paramo, P. G., D'Ocon, M. Y., and De La Pena, A.: Sutureless nephrotomy. J. Urol. 98:456, 1967.

61. Parker, H. R.: Current status of peritoneal dialysis. *In* Kirk, R. W. (ed.): *Current Veterinary Therapy VII*, W. B. Saunders, Philadelphia, 1980.

62. Pechman, R. D.: Urinary trauma in dogs and cats: A review. J. Am. Anim. Hosp. Assoc. 18:33, 1982.

63. Robbins, G. R.: Unilateral renal agenesis in the Beagle. Vet. Rec. 77:1345, 1965.

64. Robotham, G. R.: Unilateral hydronephrosis in a cat. Feline Pract. 8:23, 1978.

65. Ryan, C. P.: Fused pelvic kidney. Feline Pract. 9:32, 1979.

66. Ryan, C. P., and Smith, R. A.: Bilateral nephrolithiasis in a cat. J. Am. Vet. Med. Assoc. 158:1946, 1971.

67. Silverberg, D. S., Dosetor, J. B., Eid, T. C., Mant, M. J., and Miller, J. D. R.: Arteriovenous fistula and prolonged hematuria after renal biopsy: Treatment with epsilon amino caproic acid. Can. Med. Assoc. J. 110:671, 1974.

68. Smith, H. A., Jones, T. C., and Hunt, R. D.: *Veterinary Pathology*. Lea & Febiger, Philadelphia, 1972, p. 1283.

69. Stowater, J. L.: Congenital solitary renal cyst in a dog. J. Am. Anim. Hosp. Assoc. 11:199, 1975.

70. Thornhill, J. A.: Peritoneal dialysis in the dog and cat: An update. Comp. Cont. Ed. 3:20, 1981.

71. Thornhill, J. A.: Hemodialysis. *In* Bovee, K. C. (ed.): *Canine Nephrology*. Harwell Publishing Company, Media, 1983.

72. Thun, R., Smith, C. W., Goodale, R. H., McCracken, M. D., and Stowater, J. L.: Iatrogenic hydronephrosis in a bitch. J. Am. Vet. Med. Assoc. 167:388, 1975.

73. Ticer, J. W.: Capsulogenic renal cyst in a cat. J. Am. Vet. Med. Assoc. 143:613, 1963.

74. Tynes, W. V., Devine, C. J., Jr., Devine, P. C., and Poutasse, E. F.: Surgical treatment of renal arteriovenous fistulas. J. Urol. 103:692, 1970.

75. Van Vroonhoven, T. J., Soler-Montesinos, L., and Malt, R. A.: Humoral regulation of renal mass. Surgery 72:300, 1972.

76. Vaughan, E. D., Jr., Sweet, R. E., and Gillenwater, J. Y.: Unilateral ureteral occlusions: Pattern of nephron repair and compensatory response. J. Urol. 109:979, 1973.

77. Wallace, S., Gianturco, C., Anderson, J. H., Goldstein, H. M., Davis, L. J., and Bree, R. L.: Therapeutic vascular occlusion utilizing steel coil technique: Clinical applications. Am. J. Roentgenol. 127:381, 1976.

78. Webb, A. I.: Renal ectopia in a dog. Aust. Vet. J. 50:519, 1974.

79. Wells, M. J., Coyne, J. A., and Prince, J. L.: Ectopic kidney in a cat. Mod. Vet. Pract. 61:693, 1980.

80. Weyrauch, H. M., and Rous, S. N.: U-tube nephrostomy. J. Urol. 97:225, 1967.

81. Williams, D. F., Schapiro, A. E., Arconti, J. S., and Goodwin, W. E.: A new technique of partial nephrectomy. J. Urol. 97:955, 1967.

Chapter	**137**	# Ureters

Bruce A. Christie

CONGENITAL ABNORMALITIES

The anatomical basis for the occurrence of congenital abnormalities affecting the urinary tract is discussed in Chapter 132.

Absence or Duplication of Ureters

During embryonic development, penetration by the growing ureteric bud into the metanephrogenic tissue stimulates development of nephrons. If the ureteric bud fails to form, the consequence is renal agenesis. If two ureteric buds grow out of the same mesonephric duct, or if division of the ureteric bud is faulty, separate renal development is induced around each duct system. Each moiety fuses to form a duplex kidney. The ureter associated with the more cranial part of the duplicated kidney usually migrates with the mesonephric duct to the urethra[13]; that is, it is ectopic, and will usually be associated with urinary incontinence.

Although renal or ureteral duplication is the most common congenital abnormality of the urinary tract in humans,[17] the only veterinary case of this condition occurred in an English bulldog with a history of intermittent hematuria and urine incontinence since six months of age.[46] The diagnosis was made by excretory urography, and pyelonephritis due to gram-negative bacteria was present in both normal and duplex kidneys. Although the ureter that drained the cranial part of the duplex kidney was ectopic, the orifice was intravesicular. It is difficult to diagnose duplex kidneys at postmortem examination, since there is probably a common capsule, a common renal artery, and a common peritoneal fold around the two ureters.[46] Perhaps the prevalence of this abnormality is greater than suspected. In humans, most duplex kidneys remain healthy, but sometimes the caudal part—the part that is not usually ectopic—becomes associated with megaureter and pyelonephritis.[46]

Ureteral Ectopia

Faulty differentiation of the mesonephric and metanephric ducts results in ureteral ectopia (see Chapter 132). Although 70 per cent of ureteral ectopia in humans are associated with ureteral and renal duplication,[13, 20] ureteral ectopia occurs sporadically in dogs and cats, and most affected animals are presented for treatment of persistent urinary incontinence. Females are more likely to exhibit incontinence than males because the ectopic ureter terminates in the proximal urethra, uterus, or vagina, whereas in the male, the ureter usually terminates proximal to the external urethral sphincter.[47]

Ureteral ectopia has been reported in at least 24 different breeds of dogs, and 14 per cent of reported cases occurred in cross-bred dogs,[31, 32, 49, 60] suggesting that ureteral ectopia is not inherited. A familial tendency has been reported in Golden retrievers,[32] Labradors,[32] and Siberian huskies.[36]

Ureteral ectopia is not as common in cats as in dogs. The first case in a cat, reported in 1959, was discovered during a laboratory dissection session.[55] The first clinical case was described in 1977,[4] and since that time there have been three more reports.[7, 27, 59] Both sexes were represented, and all cats were presented with a history of urinary incontinence. The diagnosis and surgical treatment of ectopic ureter in the dog are discussed in Chapter 138. The same principles are applied to the management of ureteral ectopia in cats.

If the ureter is massively dilated, the usual methods of reimplantation are unsuitable. An alternative method developed in dogs[25] has been used successfully in human clinical urology.[26] The ureter is spatulated, and a V-shaped incision is made in the bladder epithelium to match the inverted V of the spatulated ureter. The two margins of the incised intravesical ureter are sutured into the two limbs of the V-shaped incision in the bladder floor.

Ureterocele

A ureterocele is a cystic dilation of the submucosal segment of the intravesical ureter (Fig. 137–1). This abnormality in humans is often associated with small pinpoint ureteral orifices, but it can occur in an apparently unobstructed ureter.[63] Ureteroceles have also been reported in dogs,[50, 58, 65] and may be associated with urinary incontinence when the affected ureter is also ectopic. Periodic straining to urinate occurs when the dilated segment achieves such proportions that the bladder neck is obstructed.[24] The result is hydronephrosis, which leads to renal parenchymal atrophy. The diagnosis can be made radiographically by intravenous urography. The rate of excretion of contrast agent by the affected kidney depends upon the severity of hydronephrosis. Assuming normal function in the opposite kidney, contrast agent accumulates in the bladder neck, and the ureterocele appears as a filling defect.[65] As contrast agent from the hydronephrotic kidney is gradually excreted, the ureterocele becomes more opaque and then invisible. Other complications of urinary stasis include increased predisposition to infection and calculus formation.[58] If the diagnosis is made when functional renal tissue still remains, it is feasible to excise the ureterocele and reimplant the ureter into the bladder.[7] If hydronephrosis is advanced, the ureterocele is excised and nephroureterectomy is performed.

Ureteral Valves

Ureteral valves are very rare in humans[13] and animals.[53] In the only report in a dog, the valves appeared as transverse filling defects in the ureter during excretory urography.[53] However, because ureteral kinking and constriction by periureteral fibrous bands or blood vessels could also have this radiographic appearance, surgical exploration is indicated. Urinary incontinence was the presenting sign in the dog, but ectopic ureter was ruled out because the vesicoureteral junction was proximal to a well-defined bladder neck and urethra.[53] It was not clear from the account given whether or not the bladder was opened. If the ureteral orifices were not observed, ureteral ectopia could not be ruled out simply by observing the ureterovesical junctions. Many ectopic ureters appear from without to be in a correct anatomical position, but their submucosal segment is long and the orifice is ectopic (see Chapter 138). In humans, ureteral valves are seldom the cause of a urological problem.[13] If the ureter becomes nonfunctional, the possibility of providing a replacement urine conduit could be considered.

Ureteral Replacement

When faced with ureteral replacement, urologists can lower the kidney (see Chapter 136),[54] elevate the ureterovesical junction with a bladder flap,[67] perform a two-stage bladder flap ureteroplasty,[35] or construct pedicle grafts of intestine[30] or bladder mucosa.[34]

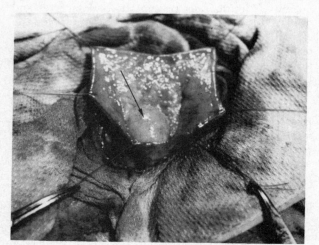

Figure 137–1. Ureterocele (arrow) in a dog, exposed by incising the ventral wall of the bladder. (Courtesy of Dr. D. E. Johnston.)

Intestinal grafts have the disadvantage of producing mucus. If the mucous membrane is removed, it regenerates. If the submucosa is also removed, the graft becomes lined with urothelium but consistently produces extensive osteoid.[59] Free autologous bladder mucosal grafts 5 to 20 cm in length have functioned satisfactorily as ureters in dogs. These grafts regenerate a smooth muscle coat, presumably from submucosal cellular elements in the graft.[34] Aggregates of lymph follicles and osteoid tissue, which are believed to develop from pleuripotential submucosal cellular elements in the graft, are also seen.

Other materials, including glass, metals, plastics, skin, fallopian tube, vermiform appendix, arteries, and veins, have been tried as prosthetic ureters, but none has proved satisfactory.[3, 33] Complications from their use have included luminal incrustations, calculus formation, urine leakage, infection, vesicoureteral reflux, graft dislodgment, and hydronephrosis. An autogenous fibroelastic tube reinforced with a polyester mesh endoskeleton (Sparks' mandril), developed for use as a vascular graft, was tried as a urine conduit but was not successful.[10] Excessive fibrosis and stricture developed at the anastomoses, and although urothelium grew into the conduit, the polyester mesh was extruded into the lumen. Expanded (microporous) polytetrafluoroethylene (PTFE) (Gore-Tex), a new form of Teflon developed as a vascular substitute, has been tried in the urinary tract of dogs.[19, 66] Segmental replacement of the ureter with 5-mm PTFE grafts anastomosed with a running suture of 6-0 polypropylene functioned well during a mean observation time of 7.5 months. However, partial replacement of the ureter including the ureterovesical junction was not successful. The anastomoses broke down, the graft migrated into the bladder, infection was a problem, and calcium salts accumulated in the wall of the conduit.

FUNCTIONAL ABNORMALITY

Vesicoureteral Reflux

Retrograde flow of urine from the bladder to the renal pelvis can occur if the normal flap valve associated with the ureterovesical junction is incompetent (Fig. 137–2). Vesicoureteral reflux is common in immature dogs but declines in prevalence with age.[15] The phenomenon is transient and apparently is related to growth and maturation of the ureterovesical junction. Urinary reflux can also occur in an otherwise normal urinary tract during episodes of cystitis, bladder neck obstruction, or neurogenic bladder disease. Vesicoureteral reflux has been observed in cats with urological disease, and although the prevalence in normal cats has not been studied, it is low.[38]

In the absence of infection, vesicoureteral reflux has little effect on renal function and renal maturation,[61] but with intermittent cystitis and reflux, repeated episodes of pyelonephritis may eventually destroy the kidney.[15] Manual compression of the

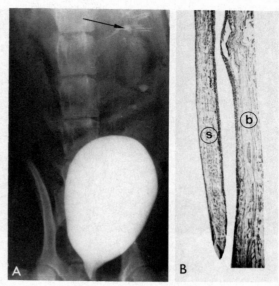

Figure 137–2. A, Unilateral vesicoureteral reflux in a dog demonstrated by voiding cystourethrography. Contrast agent, which had run back to the renal pelvis (arrow), is being cleared by ureteral peristaltic action. B, A normal ureterovesical junction showing the submucosal ureter (S), which is compressed against the bladder wall (B) as pressure in the bladder rises. (H&E ×10.)

urinary bladder to obtain a urine sample induces vesicoureteral reflux in 50 per cent of dogs and 40 per cent of cats.[21] This fact should be considered when collecting a urine sample from a dog or cat that may have a lower urinary tract infection (see Chapter 135).

ACQUIRED ABNORMALITIES

Ureteral Rupture

Trauma is the most common cause of ureteral rupture, but rupture can also occur as a sequel to impacted ureteral calculi.[12]

A study of the patterns of trauma in urban dogs and cats showed that motor vehicle accidents, animal fights, and injuries from unknown causes accounted for 75 per cent of all accessions.[40] Approximately one-third of the animals injured by motor vehicles suffered trauma to the abdomen or pelvis leading in many instances to involvement of the urinary system. The ureter is much less likely to be lacerated or ruptured than the bladder, but when it is injured the damage will probably occur in the proximal 4 cm of its length. Mid-ureteral and distal ureteral tears and ruptures have been recorded.[29, 39, 41]

Diagnosis of Ureteral Trauma

Excretory Urography. The most reliable noninvasive method of establishing the exact site, nature, and extent of traumatic injury to the urinary tract is

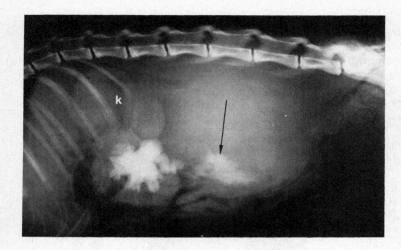

Figure 137–3. Ruptured ureter in a dog (arrow) demonstrated by excretory urography. There is a retroperitoneal accumulation of fluid in the sublumbar region. The right kidney (*k*) is nonfunctional.

by excretory urography.[44, 51] If the kidney is functioning, the contrast agent will escape at the site of rupture and collect in the adjacent tissue or tissue space (Fig. 137–3). Rapid intravenous administration of a solution of aqueous organic iodide at a dose rate of 880 mg of iodide per kg body weight is recommended.[22] A wide variety of contrast media can be used (Table 137–1). Sodium salts give better definition than methylglucamine (meglumine) at the same concentration but can stimulate vomiting in unanesthetized animals and humans. If the patient has sodium retention, meglumine is the alternative cation. Meglumine salts are more viscous than sodium salts, so to make their injection easier (and faster), larger catheters are used and the solution is warmed to body temperature.

The first exposure is made ten seconds after starting the injection and a second exposure is made as soon as possible after the first. The ten-second exposure usually shows the bolus of contrast agent as an intravenous aortogram, which should reveal any abnormality of the renal vascular pedicle. The renal outline is visible in the second radiograph during the nephrogram phase. If the kidney is functioning normally the ureters are best evaluated in the five-minute film. Opacification of the renal pelvis is optimum ten to 20 minutes after the contrast agent has been injected. If excretory urography does not demonstrate the urinary tract, renal angiography should be tried.

Renal Angiography. A specially designed catheter is maneuvered into the renal artery using fluoroscopic monitoring, and a small volume of contrast agent is injected to outline, in turn, the major renal artery branches, the veins, and the collecting duct system. A method for exposing serial radiographs rapidly is also required. The major disadvantage of this method is the cost of the equipment needed to perform the study. Non-selective renal angiography can be performed with less equipment.[16] A radiopaque intra-

TABLE 137–1. Radiographic Contrast Agents for Urography and Renal Angiography

Contrast Medium			Iodide Content (mg/ml)	Viscosity at 37°C (Centipoises)
Generic Name	*Trade Name*	**Manufacturer**		
Sodium iothalamate	Conray 420	May & Baker, Australia Pty. Ltd.	420	5.2
	Conray 400	Mallinckrodt, Inc., St. Louis, MO.	400	4.7
Methylglucamine iothalamate	Conray 280	May & Baker, Australia Pty. Ltd.	280	4.0
	Conray 60	Mallinckrodt, Inc., St. Louis, MO.	282	3.8
Methylglucamine (66%) and sodium (10%) diatrizoate combination	Renografin-76	E. R. Squibb & Sons, Inc., Princeton, NJ.	370	8.4
	Urografin-76	Schering Corp., Kenilworth, NJ.	370	9.0
	Hypaque-76	Winthrop Aust., Ermington, NSW.	370	9.0

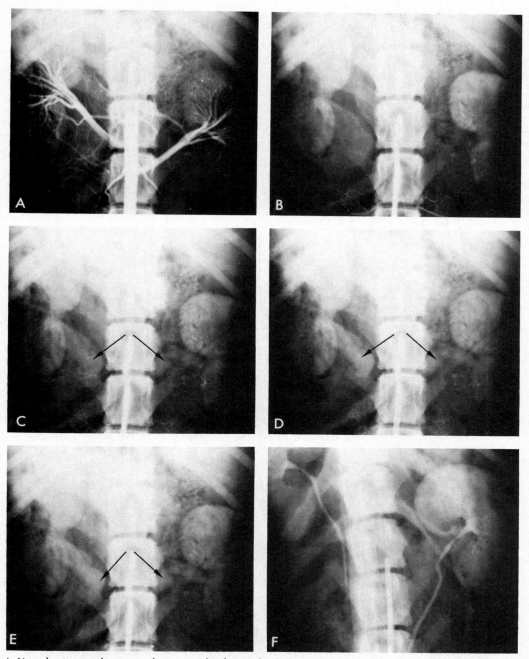

Figure 137–4. Nonselective renal angiography in a 15-kg dog. Individual 5-ml boluses of contrast agent were given and radiographs exposed 1.5 (A), (B), 6 (C), 8 (D), and 10 seconds (E) after commencing each injection. The five exposures were all taken within one minute. Features visible include renal artery and major branches (A), renal veins (arrows in C through E), and, after 3 minutes, the origin of the ureter (excretory urogram) (F).

venous catheter is passed retrograde along the aorta through a femoral artery venipuncture, and its tip is positioned in the mid-lumbar region. An abdominal survey radiograph is taken, and the tip of the catheter is adjusted to be level with the caudal edge of the fourth lumbar vertebra for cats and small dogs, midway along the third lumbar vertebra for medium-sized dogs, and at the caudal edge of the second lumbar vertebra for large dogs. A 5- to 10-ml bolus of contrast agent is injected as rapidly as possible. One radiograph is exposed one-half to one second after the start of the injection to outline the renal artery and its branches, and a second is exposed approximately five to ten seconds later, when the contrast agent is in the renal vein (Fig. 137–4).[6]

Antegrade Ureterography. The technique of percutaneous nephropyelocentesis has been perfected in dogs,[42] and is recommended for sampling renal pelvic urine and for performing antegrade ureterography.[1] A catheter is passed through the renal parenchyma into the pelvis or ureter, and contrast agent is injected. This method of examination of the ureters gives more anatomical detail than excretory urography and does little damage to the kidney.[42] To monitor the position of the catheter, facilities for fluoroscopy, ultrasonography, or computerized tomography are required.

Management of Ureteral Trauma

A common solution to ureteral trauma in veterinary medicine is to perform ureteronephrectomy. In humans, the surgical approach to trauma of the urinary tract has become more conservative.[45] Extravasation of sterile urine is relatively harmless for 24 to 36 hours. Extravasation of infected urine, however, results in rapidly spreading cellulitis. Therefore, in suspected ureteral or renal injury, a broad-spectrum antibiotic should be commenced immediately (see Chapter 135). Small ureteral tears will ultimately heal completely,[45] so extravasation of urine is not an absolute indication for immediate surgery. In humans, percutaneous nephrostomy drainage has become a valuable method of diverting urine in the

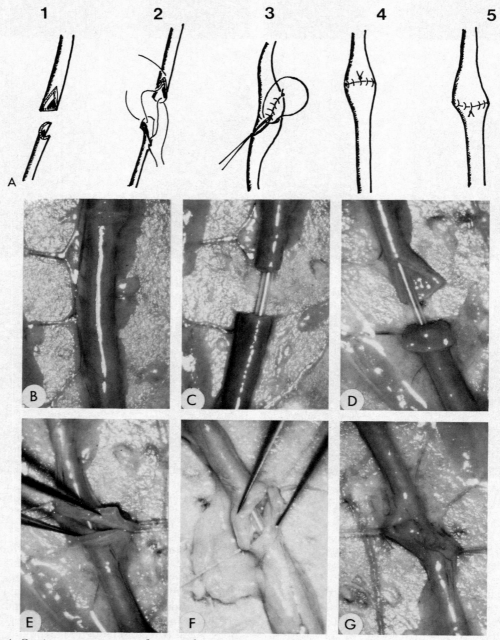

Figure 137–5. *A*, Continuous suture pattern for ureteral anastomosis. *1*, Spatulate ureter. *2*, Place stay sutures. *3*, Insert running stitch. *4* and *5*, Finished anastomosis viewed from opposite sides. *B*, Normal dog ureter viewed through an operating microscope using ×6 magnification. Longitudinally oriented blood vessels in the adventitia supply regular transversely oriented blood vessels to the wall of the ureter. *C*, Ureter cut and splinted with vinyl tubing. *D*, Ureters spatulated. *E*, Stay sutures placed. *F*, First row of stitches completed and ureter rolled through 180 degrees. *G*, Anastomosis completed.

management of ureteral injury.[52] In animals, for economic but also humane reasons, early exploratory surgery and definitive therapy if possible is preferred to protracted conservative management.

Ureteral Anastomosis. If a small segment of the ureter is damaged, one or two centimeters can be resected and the severed ends can be spatulated and anastomosed. Sutures are placed to connect the toe (apex) and heel (base) of the approximated ends. The sutures are tied and the anastomosis is completed with a running suture (Fig. 137–5) using 5-0 to 7-0 polyglycolic acid or polygalactin.[14] A more gentle and more accurate approximation is possible if the sutures are placed with the aid of a magnifying loupe or operating microscope. In traumatic avulsion of the ureter from the renal pelvis, anastomosis is achieved with a splinting catheter (Fig. 137–6). For a discussion of choice of suture material and the advantages and disadvantages of intraluminal stents or splints, see Chapter 135. After completion of the anastomosis, the suture line can be checked for leaks by compressing the distal ureter for a few minutes to build up intraluminal urine pressure or by injecting a small volume of sterile water through a fine needle directly into the ureteral lumen. A small leak is probably of little concern, but the suture line can be sealed with a thin film of the fluorinated tissue adhesive fluoralkyl cyanoacrilate.*[68] This tissue adhesive is less toxic than other cyanoacrilates, invokes only a mild inflammatory reaction, and does not interfere with normal ureteral healing.

Iatrogenic Ureteral Injury

Inadvertent cutting, crushing, or devascularizing injuries do occur in humans during abdominal surgery[45, 56] and certainly occur from time to time in animals. In veterinary medicine the options are

---

*Flucrylate, 3M Company, St. Paul, MN.

straightforward if the ureter is accidentally transected or a portion is inadvertently resected. Either an attempt is made to perform ureteroureteral anastomosis or the affected kidney and ureter are removed. The decision is not so easy to make if the ureter is crushed or has suffered a devascularizing injury. In experiments in dogs in which the ureters were crushed within the jaws of a Kelly forceps closed to maximum pressure for periods of one, five, ten, 30 and 60 minutes, it was found that the duration of crush injury did not influence the degree of injury.[9] During the first week, radiographic findings invariably showed localized narrowing at the crush site and increased tortuosity along the length of the ureter, but by the 12th post-traumatic week, 90 per cent of strictures had resolved and 41 per cent had formed aneurysmal dilations. It was recommended that crush injuries not be treated at the time of wounding but that they be evaluated from time to time by excretory urography and treated only if persistent or progressive changes were seen. Experimental devascularizing trauma in dogs was achieved by dissecting 2 or 3 cm of adventitia from the ureter. This injury was more serious than crush injury. Forty per cent of damaged ureters developed early strictures and 50 per cent of the strictures persisted, leading in many instances to hydronephrosis, calculus, and urine fistula formation.[9] For these reasons, prompt resection of the compromised segment and anastomosis are the recommended treatment.

Ureteral Obstruction

Apart from iatrogenic ureteral trauma already mentioned, ureters can be occluded by intramural obstruction and by mural or extramural compression. Intramural obstruction by calculi is only rarely reported in dogs,[11, 12] and cats,[71] probably owing to the abrupt, nontapered origin of the proximal ureter in these species (Fig. 137–4F). Experiments with arti-

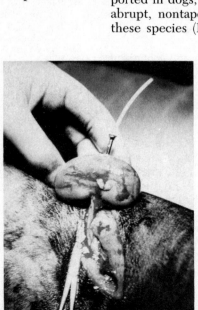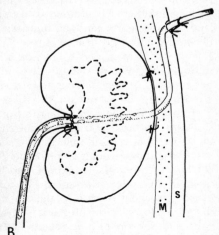

Figure 137–6. Splinting an avulsed ureter. A trocar and cannula are passed into the renal pelvis through the parenchyma (A). The trocar is withdrawn and a No. 5 French gauge fenestrated flexible catheter is inserted into the renal pelvis. The cannula is then withdrawn. The catheter is advanced into the distal ureter. The ureter is anchored to the kidney adjacent to the site of avulsion. The catheter is exteriorized through a subcutaneous tunnel and anchored to the skin (S). Nephropexy is performed with a few capsular sutures to anchor the kidney to the abdominal wall muscles (M).

ficial calculi in dogs have shown that solid spheres with diameters of 2.3 mm were freely passed, those of 2.8 mm became firmly impacted, and when the diameter was 3.9 mm or greater, the calculi could not even be introduced into the ureter.[37] Mural lesions causing obstruction are also rare, but benign[43] and malignant[5] tumors of the ureter have been described in dogs, and a malignant transitional cell tumor of the renal pelvis has been recorded in a cat.[48] Extramural causes of compression, apart from tumors, include intrapelvic cysts, which are developmental abnormalities,[70] and uterine stump granulomas, which occur as sequelae of ovariohysterectomy.[2]

One constant feature of ureteral obstruction is dilation of the proximal segment. It is due to dilation of the lumen and a moderate degree of hyperplasia and hypertrophy of smooth muscle in the ureteral wall.[18]

Alteration in renal function occurs during and after release of acute ureteral occlusion. The pathophysiology of these changes is discussed in Chapter 134.

Treatment

Experimental studies in dogs have shown that if ureteral obstruction is relieved within ten weeks of its occurrence, the dilated segment returns to its normal size and shape.[69] If this return does not occur, or if the dilation is not related to obstruction, ureteral plication can be tried.[62] The plication technique was perfected in dogs to reduce the caliber of dilated ureters without disrupting their blood supply and so to restore normal coaptation and propulsion of urine into the bladder. The plication is performed over a 10F- to 12F-gauge catheter by inserting interrupted Lembert stitches of 4-0 to 5-0 chromic catgut through the medial and lateral walls of the ureter. The sutures are placed about 1 cm apart and are reinforced with simple interrupted stitches placed between them. When the plication has been completed the catheter is removed.

Ureterotomy. Ureteroliths are seldom recognized in animals.[12] If a ureteric calculus is detected, its position should be noted radiographically and treatment should be commenced by administering a smooth muscle relaxant and increasing dietary intake of fluids. Ureteral transit time for solid artificial calculi varies from one to 24 hours.[37] If there is no radiographic evidence within this time that the stone has moved, ureterotomy is indicated. The ureter is incised over the calculus with either a longitudinal[28] or transverse[64] incision. Longitudinal incisions heal well, but sutures tend to tear out easily. Transverse incisions heal well if one-third to one-half of the ureteral circumference is left intact.[23] After removal of the calculus, the proximal and distal ureter is flushed with saline through a 3F- to 4F-gauge catheter or lacrimal needle to ensure its patency. The defect is closed with interrupted 4-0 to 5-0 polyglycolic acid (Dexon) or polygalactin (Vicryl) sutures (see Chapter 135). The needle is passed through all layers

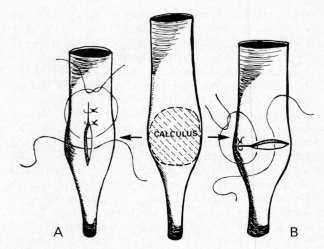

Figure 137–7. Longitudinal (A) or transverse (B) ureterotomy over a calculus. Closure may be by interrupted (illustrated) or continuous sutures to bring the edges of the ureteral wall into loose apposition.

of the ureteral wall, and sutures are tied so that the edges of the incision are brought into loose apposition (Fig. 137–7). If the calculus has been impacted for some time, the damaged segment of ureter should be resected. Alternatively, the ureter can be allowed to heal around a splinting catheter (see Chapter 135).

1. Acherman, N., Ling, G. V., and Ruby, A. L.: Percutaneous nephropyelocentesis and antegrade ureterography. A fluoroscopically assisted diagnostic technique in canine urology. Vet. Radiol. 21:117, 1980.
2. Bartells, J. E.: Radiology of the genital tract. In O'Brien, T. R. (ed.): Radiographic diagnosis of abdominal disorders in the dog and cat. W. B. Saunders Co., Philadelphia, 1978.
3. Baum, N., Mobley, D. F., and Carlton, C. E., Jr.: Ureteral replacements. Urology 5:165, 1975.
4. Bebko, R. L., Prier, J. E., and Biery, D. N.: Ectopic ureters in a male cat. J. Am. Vet. Med. Assoc. 171:738, 1977.
5. Berzon, J. L.: Primary leiomyosarcoma of the ureter in a dog. J. Am. Vet. Med. Assoc. 175:374, 1979.
6. Biery, D. N.: Upper urinary tract. In O'Brien, T. R. (ed.): Radiographic Diagnosis of Abdominal Disorders in the Dog and Cat. W. B. Saunders Co., Philadelphia, 1978.
7. Biewenga, W. J., Rothuizen, J., and Voorhout, G.: Ectopic ureters in a cat—a report of two cases. J. Small Anim. Pract. 19:531, 1978.
8. Boatwright, D. C.: Ureterocele: surgical treatment. J. Urol. 106:48, 1971.
9. Brodsky, S. L., Zimskind, P. D., Dure-Smith, P., and Lewis, P. L.: Effects of crush and devascularizing injuries to the proximal ureter. An experimental study. Invest. Urol. 14:361, 1977.
10. Brothers, L. R., III, Picket, J. D., Weber, C. H., Jr., et al.: Segmental replacement of the ureter using Sparks' mandrils. Invest. Urol. 14:460, 1977.
11. Brown, N. O., Parks, J. L., and Greene, R. W.: Canine urolithiasis: Retrospective analysis of 438 cases. J. Am. Vet. Med. Assoc. 170:414, 1977.
12. Campbell, K. L.: Ureteral rupture associated with struvite nephrolithiasis and ureterolithiasis. Canine Pract. 8:41, 1981.
13. Campbell, M. F.: Anomalies of the ureter. In Campbell, M. F., and Harrison, J. H. (eds.): Urology. 3rd ed. Vol. 2. W. B. Saunders Co., Philadelphia, 1970.
14. Cass, A. S., Schmaelzle, J. F., and Hinman, F., Jr.: Ureteral anastomosis in the dog comparing continuous sutures with interrupted sutures. Invest. Urol. 6:94, 1968.

15. Christie, B. A.: Vesicoureteral reflux in dogs. J. Am. Vet. Med. Assoc. *162*:772, 1973.

16. Christie, B. A., and Wood, A. K. W.: Renal angiography in dogs. *In*: Proceedings, 5th International Veterinary Radiology Congress, Munich, 1979.

17. Currarino, G., and Allen, T. D.: Congenital anomalies of the upper urinary tract. Prog. Pediatr. Radiol. 3:179, 1970.

18. Cussen, L. J.: The effect of incomplete chronic obstruction on the ureteric muscle of a dog. Invest. Urol. *10*:208, 1972.

19. Dreikhorn, K., Loblenz, J., Horsch, R., and Rohl, L.: Alloplastic replacement of the canine ureter by expanded polytetrafluoroethylene (Gore-Tex) grafts. Eur. Urol. *4*:379, 1978.

20. Emmett, J. L.: *Clinical Urography.* 2nd ed. W. B. Saunders Co., Philadelphia, 1964.

21. Feeney, D. A., Osborne, C. A., and Johnston, G. R.: Vesicoureteral reflux induced by manual compression of the urinary bladder in dogs and cats. J. Am. Vet. Med. Assoc. *182*:795, 1983.

22. Feeney, D. A., Thrall, D. E., Barber, D. L., et al.: Normal canine excretory urogram: Effects of dose, time, and individual dog variation. Am. J. Vet. Res. *40*:1596, 1979.

23. Gil-Vernat, J. M.: Transverse ureterotomy. J. Urol. *111*:755, 1974.

24. Gingell, J. C., Gordon, I. R., and Mitchell, J. P.: Acute obstructive uropathy due to prolapsed ectopic ureterocele: case report. Br. J. Urol. *43*:305, 1971.

25. Girgis, A. S., and Veenema, R. J.: Triangular flap ureterovesicoplasty: a new technique for the correction of ureteral reflux; a preliminary report. J. Urol. *94*:233, 1965.

26. Girgis, A. S., Veenema, R. J., and Lattimer, J. K.: Triangular flap ureterovesical anastomosis. A new technique for correction or prevention of ureteral reflux. J. Urol. 95:19, 1966.

27. Grauer, G. F., Freeman, L. F., and Nelson, A. W.: Urinary incontinence associated with an ectopic ureter in a female cat. J. Am. Vet. Med. Assoc. *182*:707, 1983.

28. Greene, R. W., and Greiner, T. P.: The Ureter. *In* Bojrab, M. J. (ed.): *Current Techniques in Small Animal Surgery.* Lea & Febiger, Philadelphia, 1975.

29. Gumbrell, R. C., and McLeavey, B. J.: Traumatic atresia of a ureteral orifice in a dog. N. Z. Vet. J. *20*:59, 1972.

30. Hatch, C. S.: Intestinal seromuscular pedicle graft to defects of the ureteropelvic junction. J. Urol. 95:764, 1966.

31. Hayes, H. M., Jr.: Ectopic ureter in dogs: epidemiological features. Teratology *10*:129, 1974.

32. Holt, P. E., Gibbs, C., and Pearson, H.: Canine ectopic ureter—a review of twenty-nine cases. J. Small Anim. Pract. 23:195, 1982.

33. Hovnanian, A. P.: Ureteral replacements. Surg. Gynecol. Obset. *135*:801, 1972.

34. Hovnanian, A. P., and Kingsley, I. A.: Reconstruction of the ureter by free autologous bladder mucosa graft. J. Urol. 96:167, 1966.

35. Ivancevic, L. D., Hohenfellner, R., and Wulff, H. D.: Total replacement of the ureter using a bladder flap and cinematographic studies on the newly constructed ureter. J. Urol. *107*:576, 1972.

36. Johnston, G. R., Osborne, C. A., Wilson, J. W., and Yano, B. L.: Familial ureteral ectopia in a dog. J. Am. Anim. Hosp. Assoc. *13*:168, 1977.

37. Kim, H. L., Labay, P. C., Boyarsky, S., and Glenn, J. F.: An experimental model of ureteric colic. J. Urol. *104*:390, 1970.

38. Kipnis, R. M.: Vesicoureteral reflux in a cat. J. Am. Vet. Med. Assoc. *167*:288, 1975.

39. Kleine, L. J., and Thornton, G. W.: Radiographic diagnosis of urinary tract trauma. J. Am. Anim. Hosp. Assoc. 7:318, 1971.

40. Kolata, R. J., Kraut, N. H., and Johnston, D. E.: Patterns of trauma in urban dogs and cats: a study of 1000 cases. J. Am. Vet. Med. Assoc. *164*:499, 1974.

41. Leeds, E. B.: The diagnosis and treatment of ruptured ureters in the dog. Arch. Am. Coll. Vet. Surg. 3:45, 1973.

42. Ling, G. V., Acherman, N., Lowenstein, L. J., and Cowgill, L. D.: Percutaneous nephropyelocentesis and nephropyelostomy in the dog: A description of the technique. Am. J. Vet. Res. *40*:1605, 1979.

43. Liska, W. D., and Patnaik, A. K.: Leiomyoma of the ureter of a dog. J. Am. Anim. Hosp. Assoc. *13*:83, 1977.

44. Lord, P. F., Scott, R. C., and Chan, K. F.: Intravenous urography for evaluation of renal diseases in small animals. J. Am. Anim. Hosp. Assoc. *10*:139, 1974.

45. Mitchell, J. P.: Trauma to the urinary tract. New Engl. J. Med. *288*:90, 1973.

46. O'Handley, P., Carrig, C. B., and Walshaw, R.: Renal and ureteral duplication in a dog. J. Am. Vet. Med. Assoc. *174*:484, 1979.

47. Osborne, C. A., and Perman, V.: Ectopic ureter in a male dog. J. Am. Vet. Med. Assoc. *154*:273, 1969.

48. Osborne, C. A., Quast, J. F., Barnes, D. M., and Fitz, C. R.: Renal pelvic carcinoma in a cat. J. Am. Vet. Med. Assoc. *159*:1238, 1971.

49. Owen, R. ap R.: Canine ureteral ectopia—a review. 1: Embryology and aetiology. J. Small Anim. Pract. *14*:407, 1973.

50. Pearson, H., and Gibbs, C.: Urinary tract abnormalities in the dog. J. Small Anim. Pract. *12*:67, 1971.

51. Pechman, R. D., Jr.: Urinary trauma in dogs and cats: a review. J. Am. Anim. Hosp. Assoc. *18*:33, 1982.

52. Persky, L., Hampel, N., and Kedia, K.: Percutaneous nephrostomy and ureteral injury. J. Urol. *125*:298, 1981.

53. Pollock, S., and Schoen, S. S.: Urinary incontinence associated with congenital ureteral valves in a bitch. J. Am. Vet. Med. Assoc. *159*:332, 1971.

54. Popesco, C.: Replacement of the pelvic ureter by lowering the kidney. Presse Med. 77:2061, 1969.

55. Reis, R. H.: Renal aplasia, ectopic ureter and vascular anomalies in a domestic cat. Anat. Rec. *135*:105, 1959.

56. Schapira, H. E., Li, R., Gribetz, M., et al.: Ureteral injuries during vascular surgery. J. Urol. *125*:293, 1981.

57. Shoemaker, W. C.: Reversed seromuscular grafts in urinary tract reconstruction. J. Urol. 74:453, 1955.

58. Scott, R. C., Greene, R. W., and Patnaik, A. K.: Unilateral ureterocele associated with hydronephrosis in a dog. J. Am. Anim. Hosp. Assoc. *10*:126, 1974.

59. Smith, C. W., Burke, T. J., Froehlich, P., and Wright, W. H.: Bilateral ureteral ectopia in a male cat with urinary incontinence. J. Am. Vet. Med. Assoc. *182*:172, 1983.

60. Smith, C. W., Stowater, J. L., and Kneller, S. K.: Ectopic ureter in the dog—a review of cases. J. Am. Anim. Hosp. Assoc. *17*:245, 1981.

61. Stamey, T. P.: Urinary infections. Williams & Wilkins Co., Baltimore, 1972.

62. Starr, A.: Ureteral plication. Invest. Urol. *17*:153, 1979.

63. Stephens, D.: Caecoureterocele and concepts on the embryology and aetiology of ureteroceles. Aust. N. Z. J. Surg. *40*:239, 1971.

64. Stone, E. A.: Surgical management of urolithiasis. Comp. Cont. Ed. 3:627, 1981.

65. Stowater, J. L., and Springer, A. L.: Ureterocele in a dog. Vet. Med. Small Anim. Clin. 74:1753, 1979.

66. Varady, S., Freidman, E., Yap, W. T., et al.: Ureteral replacement with a new synthetic material: Gore-Tex. J. Urol. *128*:171, 1982.

67. Vargas, A. D., and Silva, E. I.: Mobilization of the ureter by a posterior vesical flap in dogs: preliminary report of a new technique. J. Urol. *107*:742, 1972.

68. Vargas, A. D., Starr, A., and Cooper, J. F.: Experimental use of fluoroalkyl cyanoacrilate in ureteral anastomosis. Invest. Urol. 15:416, 1982.

69. Wan, S. P., Goodwin, B. S., Uechi, M. D. S., and Blight, E. M., Jr.: A second look at ureteral plication. J. Urol. *127*:803, 1982.

70. Weaver, A. D.: Intrapelvic cyst as a urinary obstruction in a bitch. J. Am. Vet. Med. Assoc. *169*:798, 1976.

71. Wolf, A. M., Leighton, R. L., and Watrous, B. J.: Uric acid ureteral calculus and pararenal cyst in a cat. J. Am. Anim. Hosp. Assoc. 15:767, 1979.

Chapter 138

Surgery of the Bladder

H. Philip Hobson and Philip Bushby

Anatomy

In the dog and the cat, the distended bladder lies in the posterior ventral abdomen. In the cat the empty bladder remains in the abdomen, whereas in the dog the empty bladder or the congenitally hypoplastic bladder may lie partially or entirely within the anterior pelvic cavity. The blood supply to the bladder is dual. The variably patent cranial vesicular arteries originate from the umbilical arteries and pass to the bladder in the lateral ligaments. The main blood supply to the bladder is provided by the caudal vesicular arteries, which originate from the vaginal or prostatic arteries. Motor innervation to the bladder is provided by fibers of the pelvic (parasympathetic) and hypogastric (sympathetic) nerves located in the lateral ligaments in close proximity to the caudal vesicular arteries. (For more information on anatomy of the urinary tract, see Chapter 132.)

Clinical Signs and Diagnostic Techniques

The clinical signs that indicate bladder disorders include hematuria, pyuria, stranguria, frequent attempts to urinate with or without the passage of urine, anuria, and signs of uremia: anorexia, lethargy, vomiting, dehydration, urinary incontinence, pain in the posterior abdomen, and abdominal distension. Physical examination may reveal that the patient is wet with urine, often with accompanying urine scald, and has a distended bladder, a thickened bladder wall (Fig. 138–1A), or perhaps no detectable bladder on abdominal or rectal palpation. Bladder stones (Fig. 138–1B) may be palpable through the abdominal wall of conscious or sedated patients.

Hematuria in a urine sample obtained by cystocentesis usually indicates bladder involvement, although the source of bleeding may be still higher up the urinary tract or even, by reflux, from the proximal urethra or prostate gland. A culture taken from urine obtained by cystocentesis is less likely to be inadvertently contaminated during collection than is a catheterized sample or a "clean catch," provided standard precautions are taken to prepare the skin. Thus, the culture results are much more meaningful when the urine is collected by cystocentesis.

Exfoliated cells quickly undergo morphological changes in the urine, so cytological preparations from urine sediment are difficult to evaluate. When neoplasia is suspected, the bladder should be catheterized and emptied of urine. Approximately 5 to 10 ml of sterile saline should be infused, the bladder massaged, and the fluid aspirated. Additional negative pressure should be applied to the syringe with the tip of the catheter located in the suspicious area of the bladder. The catheter should be withdrawn under light negative pressure, and the contents of the syringe and catheter used to make slide preparations for cytological examination.

The bladder is usually outlined well by plain radiographs. The bowel should be emptied prior to performing diagnostic radiographic procedures, especially when discrete lesions are suspected. Most cystic calculi are radiopaque and are easily seen (see Fig. 138–1B). The kidneys should also be checked when calculi are seen in the bladder. Radiolucent calculi may be demonstrated with a pneumocystogram (Fig. 138–2A). If the radiolucent stones are large enough, they may be recognized as filling defects in an intravenous urogram (Fig. 138–2C). Occasionally a double contrast urogram may outline the stones best (Fig. 138–2B).

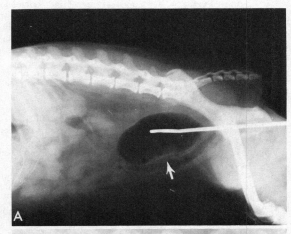
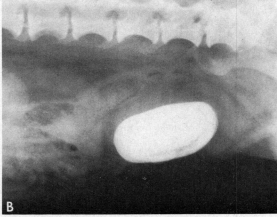

Figure 138–1. A, A thickened bladder wall (arrow) demonstrated radiographically by a pneumocystogram. B, A large layered cystic calculus. A stone of this size can be palpated through the abdominal wall.

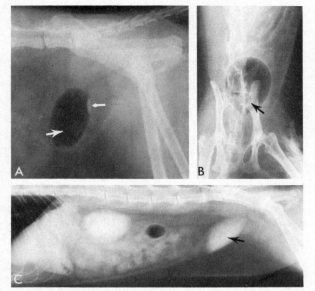

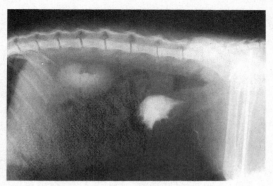

Figure 138–4. Blood clots in the bladder on an intravenous urogram as multiple filling defects in the bladder lumen.

Figure 138–2. *A,* Radiolucent stone *(large arrow)* and radiopaque stone *(small arrow)* demonstrated by a pneumocystogram. *B,* Radiolucent stone *(arrow)* demonstrated radiographically by a double contrast technique. *C,* Radiolucent stone *(arrow)* demonstrated with an intravenous urogram.

Space-occupying lesions, such as tumors (Fig. 138–3), blood clots (Fig. 138–4), or cysts, can be demonstrated by intravenous urography. This same technique also outlines impingement on the bladder by

masses in the adjacent area (Fig. 138–5) as well as demonstrates congenital or acquired anomalies. Vesicoureteral reflux can best be demonstrated by infusion of a radiopaque contrast agent directly into the bladder. If reflux is present, a cystogram will show contrast agent in the ureters.

Bladder rupture may be demonstrated by leakage of positive contrast media into the surrounding tissue or the abdominal cavity. A barium infusion should never by used for this procedure, nor should air (see Chapter 135). A twofold or greater increase in creatinine in fluid aspirated from the abdomen, compared with serum creatinine, is diagnostic of a ruptured bladder.

Cystoscopy is possible in large female dogs. The bladder is emptied of urine and refilled to a minimal degree with sterile water. An arthroscope, fiberoptiscope, or human urethroscope may be inserted into the bladder through the urethra and the bladder wall observed.

CONGENITAL ANOMALIES

Persistent Urachus

Embryologically, the bladder is connected to the allantois by a tubular structure termed the *urachus,*

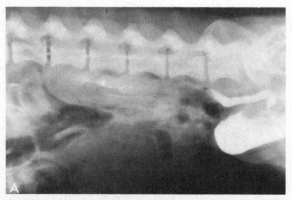

Figure 138–3. *A,* Neoplasia of the trigonal area of the bladder, seen as a space-occupying lesion with the aid of intravenous urography. A stricture of the ureteral orifice, caused by the neoplasm, is resulting in a hydroureter. *B,* Neoplasia of the neck of the bladder, demonstrated by pneumocystogram.

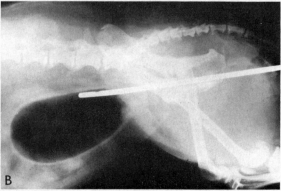

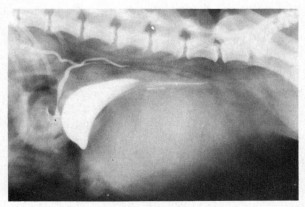

Figure 138–5. Massive distension of the prostate due to abscess formation. The severe anterior displacement of the bladder is demonstrated by an intravenous urogram.

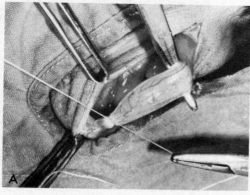
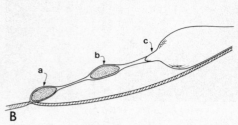

Figure 138–6. A, A persistent urachus in a two-week-old puppy. Urine dripped from the umbilicus prior to surgery. B, Failure of the urachus to close completely may result in *(a)* cyst formation at the umbilicus; *(b)* cyst formation between the umbilicus and the bladder; *(c)* diverticulum of the anterior pole of the bladder.

which normally closes at birth. If the entire tube remains patent (Fig. 138–6A), urine collecting in the bladder discharges at the umbilicus. Viewed grossly, the bladder may simply appear stretched anteriorly and attached at the umbilicus. Failure of the urachus to close completely at the bladder may result in a diverticulum of the apex of the bladder. This may result in incomplete emptying of the bladder, thus predisposing it to inflammation and infection. Cysts may also occur anywhere along the closed urachus, including the umbilical area (Fig. 138–6B). These later defects are usually clinically silent and are seen as incidental findings. They may become infected, however, and produce clinical signs associated with an abscess.

The surgical correction of urachal abnormalities involves excision of the cystic structures or excision of the entire urachus. A posterior ventral midline incision allows exposure of the bladder and its communication with the umbilicus. The patent urachus may be ligated at the umbilicus and the bladder and excised. To remove the possibility of cyst formation at either the umbilical or bladder ends of the urachus, total excision is advised, in which the umbilicus and part of the bladder wall are excised with the urachus. A diverticulum in the wall of the bladder can be excised and the bladder wall closed in the usual fashion, or the thin-walled area can be invaginated with a single or double layer of inverting sutures, using 3–0 chromic catgut to promote an inflammatory response.

Exstrophy of the Bladder

Developmental deformities involving the bladder are common in humans but uncommon in animals.[1, 17, 26, 41, 43, 52, 54] Exstrophy of the bladder has been reported only once in a cat[31] and once in a dog.[25] The latter abnormality was in a female bulldog (Fig. 138–7A), in which the dorsal bladder wall formed the ventral body wall. The ureters discharged from the bladder wall directly to the exterior. An intravenous urogram (Fig. 138–7B) demonstrated a

dilated renal pelvis in each kidney and bilateral megaureters with additional ectasia at their distal ends. No strictures were present. The urethra was short and dilated, and the ventral aspect of the vulva was cleft ventroanteriorly. The pubis was absent but locomotion was normal.

Repair of the bladder was accomplished by carefully dissecting the bladder wall free from the surrounding tissues and reconstructing the wall with a Cushing followed by a Lembert suture pattern. The newly formed viscus was quite small and irregularly shaped (Fig. 138–7C), and when saline was infused into the lumen it was retained poorly, suggesting poor spincter tone with the likelihood of innervation deficiencies. (See Chapter 134 on pathogenesis of urinary incontinence.)

The defect in the body wall was approximated with little difficulty. The puppy recovered but remained incontinent. Three months later, pyelonephritis was diagnosed. Response to therapy was temporary and the puppy was euthanized.

Ectopic Ureters

This condition is uncommon in dogs[47] and even more uncommon in cats.[46] The correction of ureteral ectopia is primarily a surgical exercise on the bladder.[15, 24, 42] A dog with an ectopic ureter is one that has dribbled urine continuously since birth. Most such dogs urinate normally, since bilateral ureteral ectopia occurs much less frequently and adequate sphincter tone is usually present. Occasionally the sphincter action is inadequate, and the dog may remain incontinent following surgery.

The anatomical explanation for this developmental abnormality is given in Chapter 132. Most clinical cases are seen in female dogs. The ectopic ureter approaches and enters the bladder wall normally but fails to open into the lumen of the bladder at the base of the trigone. Instead, it continues posteriorly to open into the distal urethra or the proximal vagina.

Examination of the vagina through a speculum or endoscope may reveal the orifice of the ectopic

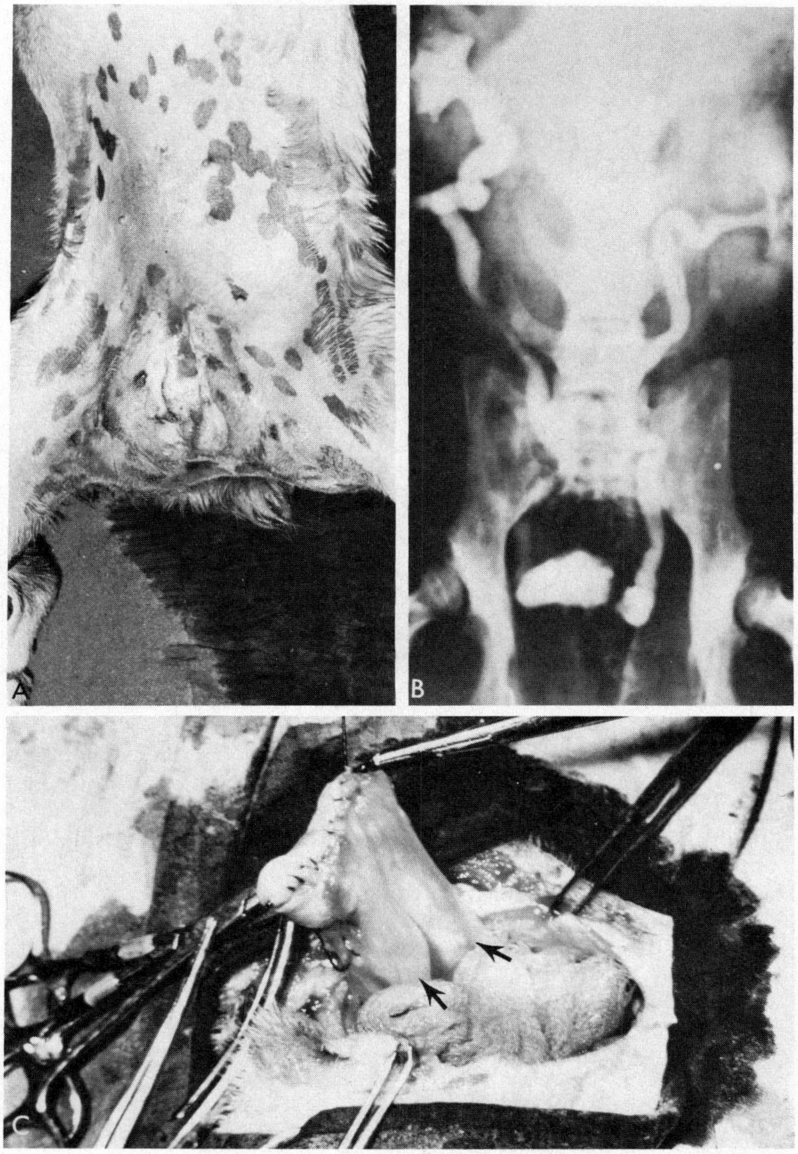

Figure 138–7. *A,* Exstrophy of the bladder in a female bulldog pup. This congenital malformation resulted in the dorsal bladder wall serving as the ventral body wall, with the ureters discharging directly to the outside. Extensive urine scalding is present on the ventral abdominal wall. *B,* An intravenous urogram demonstrating dilation of the renal pelves and bilateral tortuous megaureters that terminate with an even greater ectasia. Note also the absence of the pubis. *C,* Reconstruction of the bladder. The grossly dilated ureters (arrows) give the "bladder" the appearance of a pair of pants.

ureter. In most dogs, however, visual examination is difficult because of the small size of the pup and the presence of the hymen. Pooling of urine in the proximal vagina or thickening of the vaginal mucosa may be all that is seen. Intravenous urograms (Figs. 138–8 and 138–9) may be of diagnostic value. A common finding is megaureter, which is often tortuous and may show additional ectasia at its distal end and occasionally may show a well-defined entry posterior to the bladder neck. A definitive diagnosis, however, might not be made prior to exploratory surgery.

In some dogs in which both ureters are ectopic, the bladder never fills. It remains infantile (hypoplastic) and is positioned well posteriorly within the pelvic cavity (Fig. 138–9B). In such cases, the bladder must be dilated with saline before surgical relocation of the ureteral orifices can be performed. Distending the bladder with saline also checks the integrity of the bladder sphincter. If it is competent, one could predict frequent voiding episodes soon after surgery but expect more normal voiding intervals as bladder capacity expands.

Where the ectopic ureter approaches the bladder in the normal location, surgical correction is accomplished by making a ureterovesicular stoma at the place of the normal orifice (Fig. 138–10). The bladder wall is incised on the ventral midline from the midbody area, posteriorly through the neck of the bladder to the proximal urethra. The bladder walls are retracted laterally, exposing the trigone. The left index finger of the right-handed surgeon is placed over the ureter on the external side of the bladder, pushing it ventrally. The ectopic ureter is seen as a ridge in the bladder wall. A longitudinal incision with a #15 Bard-Parker blade is made through the bladder mucosa into the lumen of the ureter near the normal orifice. Only when the bladder wall is thickened as a

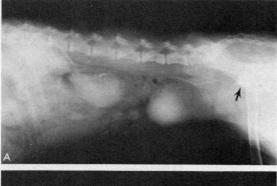

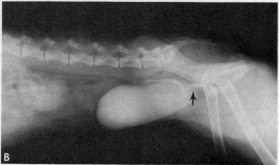

Figure 138–8. *A,* A three-minute urogram of a dog with an ectopic ureter. Note the ectasia at the terminal end of the ureter *(arrow).* *B,* This urogram was taken at ten minutes. Note the dilated segment of ureter *(arrow).*

result of a chronic cystitis is there likely to be any difficulty in locating the ureter. However, excessive handling of the bladder can result in swelling of the bladder wall and hemorrhage in the mucosa, making it more difficult to identify tissues accurately. A magnifying head loupe (2.5×) or operating telescope (see Chapter 135) may be helpful.

Once the ureteral lumen has been incised, patency

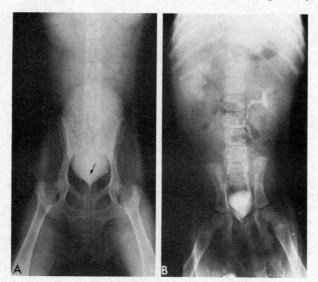

Figure 138–9. *A,* A ventrodorsal radiograph of the dog in Figure 138–8. The arrow indicates the ballooned end of the ectopic ureter. *B,* A urogram of a dog with bilateral ectopic ureters. Note the tortuous course of the ureters, especially the left, which also shows a greater degree of dilation. Note also the relatively small bladder.

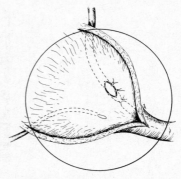

Figure 138–10. The creation of a new stoma into the bladder of the ectopic megaureter. An incision is made through the bladder mucosa into the lumen of the ectopic ureter. The bladder mucosa is sutured to the ureteral mucosa. The ectopic ureter is ligated distal to the new stoma.

of the new lumen is verified by passing a lubricated tomcat catheter proximally into the ureter. With the catheter still in place, the ureteral mucosa is sewn to the bladder mucosa with six interrupted sutures of 7–0 collagen or 7–0 coated vicryl (see Fig. 138–10). The tomcat catheter is withdrawn from the proximal ureter and redirected distally down the ectopic ureter from the new orifice. Just distal to the new orifice, a 3–0 double-armed chromic catgut suture is placed around the ectopic ureter by passing the needle through the bladder wall, from the mucosal side, on either side of the ureter. The ligature is tied on the outside of the bladder as the catheter is removed, to

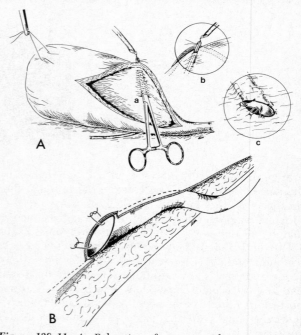

Figure 138–11. *A,* Relocation of a transected ureter into the bladder wall. The bladder mucosa is undermined from a small incision through the mucosa with forceps, which are driven through the musculature and serosa of the bladder wall *(a).* The stay suture in the end of the ureter is grasped with forceps *(b),* and it plus the ureter are delivered gently through the tunnel. The spatulated tip of the ureter is sutured to the bladder mucosa *(c).* *B,* Diagram of the ureter passing beneath the mucosa and out through the muscular wall of the bladder.

keep the knot away from the new orifice. If the length:diameter ratio of the submucosal ureter is less than 6:1, an inadequate valvelike closure of the ureteral orifice as the bladder fills is likely.[11, 16] It is possible to improve the passive flap valve effect by incising the bladder musculature adjacent to the extravesical ureter and closing the muscle over the ureter with sutures.[15]

The bladder wall, the neck of the bladder, and the proximal urethra are closed with a double row of simple, continuous, 4–0 chromic catgut sutures. The diameters of the neck of the bladder and proximal urethra are usually too small to justify an inverting pattern. However, if the diameter of this area is considered too large, then inversion of the wall is indicated to improve action and tone. Female pups of toy breeds may require this operation. A 10 French gauge, sterile, soft rubber catheter is threaded out of the urethra, and the wall is inverted over it. The catheter is sutured to the vulva and left in place for five to seven days to ensure patency during healing.

If the ectopic ureter empties into the reproductive tract, surgical relocation into the bladder is required. Various techniques, both intra- and extravesicular, have been described for this procedure.[2, 4, 30] One simple method follows. The distal end of the ureter is ligated. A fixation suture is passed through the ureter, and the ureter is incised just distal to the fixation suture and proximal to the ligation suture. The bladder wall is opened on the ventral midline (Fig. 138–11A). A 5-mm incision is made through the bladder mucosa at the reimplantation site. The location of the incision is determined largely by the length of the ureter to be translocated. A hemostat is used to bluntly dissect a tunnel beneath the bladder mucosa for a distance of at least 1 cm. The forceps is forced through the bladder wall. The distal end of the ureter is dissected free from the surrounding tissue, preserving as much of its blood supply as possible. The fixation suture through the end of the ureter is grasped with the hemostat, and by gentle traction, the thread and the ureter are both delivered through the bladder wall. The orifice of the transected ureter is trimmed in an oblique fashion and sutured to the bladder mucosa with six interrupted 7–0 collagen or 7–0 coated vicryl sutures (see Fig. 138–11).

Interrupted sutures are placed to close the bladder mucosa around the new stoma and to tack the ureter to the serosa and musculature of the outer bladder wall. Care must be taken not to occlude the lumen of the transplanted ureter. Urine should flow freely through the ureter. This can be assessed immediately if the intravesicular technique is used. If the viability of the transplanted ureter or a possible swelling in the bladder wall occluding the ureter is a concern, it may be desirable to leave a stent in place for five to seven days. This is accomplished by threading one end of a small, sterile, open-ended polyethylene tube a few centimeters up the ureter. The other end is passed down the urethra to the exterior. The tip of

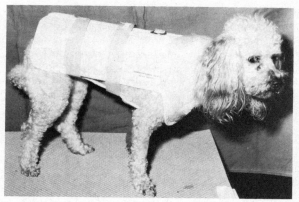

Figure 138–12. Side bar–type restraint device used to prevent the patient from licking or chewing at sutures.

this "catheter" is sutured to the lip of the vulva in the female or directly to the tip to the penis in the male to prevent dislodging. Side bar restraint devices (Fig. 138–12) should also be used to keep the patient from licking at the area. (For a further discussion of splinting catheters, see Chapter 135.)

Cystic Agenesis

Total absence of the bladder in which the ureters emptied directly into the vagina has been reported.[39] Transplantation of the distal ureters into the bowel[2, 5, 30] in a fashion similar to transplantation of the ureters into the bladder wall (Fig. 138–11B) is possible, but the risk of ascending infection is high. Also, metabolic changes are induced (Chapter 134). Indications are that infection is less if the ureters are anastomosed into an isolated section of bowel, which is then anastomosed into the main bowel.[2, 4, 30]

An isolated rectum can be used as a substitute bladder in conjunction with a colostomy.

Mechanical valves to achieve bladder control have not yet achieved long-term success.[49]

ACQUIRED LESIONS

Chronic Cystitis

Chronic inflammatory lesions of the bladder that do not respond to medical therapy can sometimes be treated successfully surgically.[28, 34] Mineralized plaques or small ulcerated areas can be excised. Pseudomembranous necrotic material can be removed from the lining of the bladder either by rubbing the lining with a gauze sponge or by scraping it off with a metal curette.

Cystic Calculi

The most common reason for performing a cystotomy in dogs is for removal of calculi from the lumen of the bladder (see Chapter 140). Calculi are found most commonly in the middle-aged dog but may be found at any age. The most common stones are the phosphates, usually magnesium ammonium phosphate, also referred to as struvite. In recent years these stones have been dissolved by dietary management.[35] Prescription diets for dissolution of struvite calculi are very low in protein and minerals and are high in salt. They therefore should be used with caution in growing animals and are not recommended for prevention of recurrence of calculi. When infections are present, the appropriate antibiotics are indicated (see Chapter 135).

Medical management of such nonstruvite calculi as urate, cystine, and oxalate has been less rewarding. Positive identification of the composition of the uroliths is always indicated, as medical therapy can be based on a definitive diagnosis. When no stones are available, conservative therapy is based primarily on deduction from the history and clinical findings. Serious consideration should be given to performing an initial cystotomy for immediate relief as well as to obtain uroliths for identification. Surgery is always indicated in patients with obstructed outflow that cannot be relieved by nonsurgical methods,[36] in patients with calculi located in kidneys without adequate function, and in patients with anatomical defects that predispose them to infection and obstruction.

Small stones may be passed readily from the bladder during normal urination and rarely produce an occlusion in the urethra in female animals. In male dogs, however, the urethra narrows as it enters the groove in the os penis. Small calculi can lodge and impact in this area and produce obstruction. Dislodging of these stones, either by flushing[39] or urethrotomy, is indicated before a cystotomy. Attempts to push the stones back into the bladder with a catheter may result in considerable damage to the urethra, with possible stricture formation. Urohydropulsion[39] should be tried. The urethra is first dilated by infusing a sterile lubricating solution while occluding the urethral orifice and the pelvic urethra with digital pressure. Sudden release of the pelvic urethral pressure may allow the stones to be carried back into the bladder, from which they can be removed by cystotomy.

When surgery is indicated, the bladder is approached through a posterior ventral midline incision. In male animals, the skin incision is made parallel and adjacent to the penis. On occasion, the incision may need to be carried farther anteriorly. In these cases, the incision is curved toward the midline anterior to the penis and continued anteriorly on the ventral midline as far as desired. Care should be taken to identify the preputial branches of the caudal superficial epigastric vessels in the subcutis and to ligate them. The incision into the abdomen is made through the body wall on the ventral midline, as the penis is retracted laterally, and should extend to the brim of the pelvis.

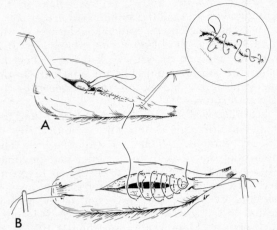

Figure 138–13. *A,* Closure of a cystotomy incision in a thin-walled bladder. A Cushing or Connell pattern is used for the first row of sutures, followed by a Lembert pattern *(inset)* as the second row. Note the use of stay sutures at either end of the cystotomy to manipulate the bladder during surgery. *B,* The first row in a double simple continuous suture pattern closure of a cystotomy incision of a thick-walled bladder. These sutures can be placed without entering the lumen of the bladder.

The bladder is elevated from the abdominal cavity, isolated from it, and "packed off" with moistened soft cotton abdominal packs to minimize contamination. Stay sutures (Fig. 138–13) are placed at either end of the anticipated incision to manipulate the bladder atraumatically. Classically, the incision has been made in the dorsum of the bladder because of concern that sediment might form calculi on exposed sutures if it were made on the ventral aspect. In our opinion, this is not a valid assumption when absorbable sutures are used;[27] location of the incision site should be determined by vascularity and optimal exposure of the suspected lesion. When uroliths are to be removed, the logical incision site is the anterior pole of the bladder, which is usually less vascular than other regions.

Once the bladder is incised, multiple small stones usually can be removed gently and easily with a sterile teaspoon. A human gallbladder scoop is excellent for removing small stones from the neck of the bladder and the proximal urethra. Repeated retrograde flushing and aspiration may be required to remove all stones. Free "urine" flow is checked by flushing from the bladder outward and observing the "urine" stream. This can be accomplished by gently wedging a syringe filled with sterile water into the neck of the bladder and then forcing the water out through the urethra.

The bladder is closed (see Fig. 138–13) with a double row of continuous absorbable suture material. If the bladder wall is thin (Fig. 138–13A), inverting patterns are advocated as this provides a more watertight closure. A Cushing or Connell suture pattern is used, followed by a Lembert suture pattern. If the bladder wall is thick (Fig. 138–13B), a double row of simple continuous sutures is used. When practical, it is still advisable to place the sutures outside the

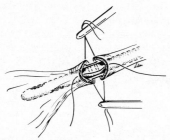

Figure 138–14. Anastomosing the urethra to the neck of the bladder with a catheter in place. Simple interrupted sutures are placed at the 12 (dorsal), 4, and 8 o'clock positions, and a simple continuous suture is placed between each two stay sutures.

lumen of the bladder. The suture line should be continuous to prevent leakage between sutures during bladder filling. If absorbable synthetic suture materials are used for bladder closure, additional attention must be paid to preventing the suture material from acting as a saw, as these materials do not pass through the tissue as easily as does chromic catgut.

Trauma to the Bladder

Small leaks in the bladder may go undetected during trauma and seal uneventfully. Partial tears may heal normally or may result in an abnormally contoured bladder. Diverticula created in this way may predispose the bladder to chronic infections through a residual urine problem. Even large tears in the bladder wall may go undetected for some time as the patient may still void small amounts of urine. Thus, the bladder should always be evaluated in any traumatic situation, especially those involving the abdomen or pelvis.

Tears in the bladder wall are debrided of avascular tissue and the wall closed as previously described. If the bladder neck is torn from the urethra, both ends are debrided and apposed with absorbable suture material over a stent. A triangulation technique (Fig. 138–14) is used in which interrupted sutures are placed at the 12, 4, and 8 o'clock positions. The ends of these sutures are left long and are grasped with hemostats. With the tissue under gentle tension, a simple continuous suture is placed between each of the stay sutures. The stent should be left in place for seven days.

Displacement of the Bladder

The bladder may be displaced laterally or ventrally through tears in the body wall or caudally as part of a perineal hernia (Fig. 138–15). If the urethra is kinked, obstruction to urine outflow occurs. Cystocentesis may be necessary before the bladder can be returned to its proper position. Surgical repair of the perineal diaphragm or defect in the abdominal wall maintains the bladder in its correct location.

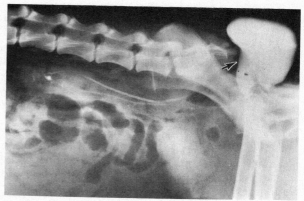

Figure 138–15. Displacement of the bladder (arrow) caudally into a perineal hernia demonstrated by intravenous urography.

Neoplasms of the Bladder

Benign neoplasms, such as papillomas, fibromas, or leiomyomas (Fig. 138–16A), may be removed by wide excision and the bladder closed as previously described. If the trigone or neck of the bladder is involved, reconstruction or urine diversion is needed. The bladder can adapt well to the loss of a considerable amount of wall.

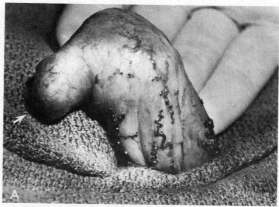

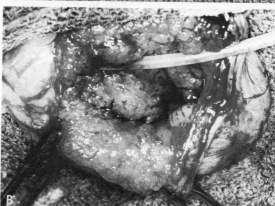

Figure 138–16. A, A leiomyoma involving the anterior pole of the bladder (arrow). B, A transitional cell carcinoma involving the wall of the entire bladder.

The most commonly reported malignant neoplasms are transitional cell carcinomas (Fig. 138–16B), squamous cell carcinomas, adenocarcinomas, fibrosarcomas, leiomyosarcomas, undifferentiated sarcomas, and rhabdomyosarcomas.[38] These tumors have most likely spread to regional lymph nodes and perhaps the lungs by the time they are detected. If the tumor is limited to an area of the bladder that can be sacrificed readily, resection should be tried. However, these tumors frequently involve the trigone, and transplantation of the ureters or bladder reconstruction is required.[30] A careful inspection of the hypogastric, middle iliac, and lumbar lymph nodes should be carried out before extensive reconstructive surgery is undertaken.

Impression smears and immediate evaluation of frozen sections may be valuable in determing treatment. Preoperative, operative, and postoperative radiotherapy in conjunction with chemotherapy may offer some hope for selected patients (personal communication from C. Barton) (see oncology section).

URINARY INCONTINENCE CAUSED BY BLADDER NECK MALFUNCTION

Urinary incontinence caused by bladder neck malfunction has neurogenic, non-neurogenic, or miscellaneous components (Table 138–1). Successful management of urinary incontinence depends on an accurate determination of the etiology and re-establishment of normal anatomical or physiological relationships that control urination.[37] If medical management of urinary incontinence (see Chapter 134) is unsuccessful, it may be combined with or replaced by surgical management. Only one report in the veterinary literature deals specifically with the surgical management of urinary incontinence caused by bladder neck and proximal urethral malfunction.[9]

However, the human medical literature provides much information relevant to this topic. The options for surgical management of urinary incontinence caused by bladder neck malfunction are (1) bladder neck sling, (2) sling urethroplasty, (3) bladder neck reconstruction, (4) perineal sling, and (5) artificial sphincter.

Bladder Neck Sling

The bladder neck sling provides a mechanical means of increasing proximal urethral resistance to urine flow. Bladder neck slings may be created using fascia,[3, 20, 32, 40, 48] polypropylene gauze,[8] and Teflon tape.[10] A fascial sling was first used with success in the management of human urinary incontinence in 1914.[20] Christie reported the fascial sling technique for control of urinary incontinence in dogs.[13]

Candidates for the bladder neck fascial sling should have a normal neurological ability to urinate. The incontinence must be due to decreased sphincter tone caused by a weakness of the muscles of the bladder neck or proximal urethra. Voiding cystourethrography[12] demonstrates a bladder of normal size and shape with the contrast agent escaping freely around a catheter.

A fascial strip 8 to 10 mm wide and 10 cm long is harvested from the external rectus abdominis sheath or from the fascia lata. A ventral midline approach to the bladder is made, with the incision in the skin extending from the umbilicus to the pubis. The bladder neck is mobilized and the sling passed dorsally over the junction of the bladder neck and the proximal urethra (Fig. 138–17). The posterior 4 cm of the incision in the linea alba is sutured to permit accurate anchoring of the sling. Bilateral stab incisions are made through the abdominal musculature 2 cm off the midline and 3 cm cranial to the brim of

TABLE 138–1. Classification of Urinary Incontinence

Classification	Definition	Characteristics	Examples
Neurogenic	Damage to or loss of nervous supply	Loss of voluntary micturition Overdistended bladder	Intervertebral disc protrusion, spinal fracture, tumor association with posterior paralysis
Nonneurogenic	Nerve supply to bladder is intact	Normal micturition is possible Bladder is not overdistended	Ectopic ureter Endocrine imbalance
Paradoxical	Increased intravesical pressure secondary to partial urinary obstruction	Dysuria Overdistended bladder	Urethral calculi Urethral stricture
Miscellaneous	Primary diseases of bladder or urethra or both	Small nondistensible bladder	Chronic cystitis with fibrosis Neoplastic infiltration Surgical trauma to bladder neck

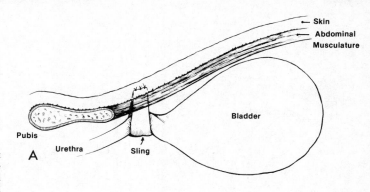

Figure 138–17. Bladder neck sling. *A*, Sagittal view, patient in dorsal recumbency. The fascial strip penetrates the abdominal musculature, passes dorsal to the urethra and bladder neck, and is sutured superficial to the abdominal musculature. *B*, Transverse view.

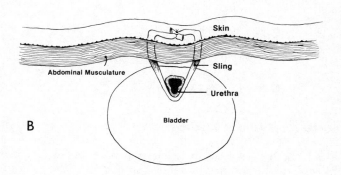

the pubis. The ends of the fascial strip are delivered through these stab incisions. When tension is applied to the fascial strip, the bladder neck is pulled cranially and ventrally, the urethra is elongated, and the junction of the bladder neck and urethra is compressed against the ventral abdominal wall.

The amount of tension applied to the fascial strip and, therefore, the degree of compression of the bladder neck and proximal urethra are critical to success of the procedure. Brown and Wickham have described the equipment and techniques required for precise measurement of urethral compression.[6] However, effective use of this measurement requires special equipment and trained personnel. Christie described a technique by which he estimated the amount of tension to apply.[13] While tension on the fascial strip is being adjusted, the bladder is catheterized. One hundred milliliters of sterile fluid are instilled and the catheter removed. The bladder is gently compressed until fluid begins to drip from the vulva. Tension is applied to the sling until the drip rate begins to decrease. The ends of the fascial sling are secured to each other, superficial to the linea alba, with nonabsorbable sutures. After the sling is secured, the tension is again checked by compressing the bladder. Compression should result in free flow of fluid, which should stop abruptly as the pressure is relaxed. The linea alba and the remainder of the abdominal closure are completed.

Sling Urethroplasty

The sling urethroplasty also provides a mechanical means of increasing proximal urethral resistance to

urinary flow.[9] In addition, contraction of musculature of the trigone supplements this resistance and decreases the lumen size of the proximal urethra. This procedure is indicated only in female patients that (1) have the ability to urinate, (2) show dilation of the proximal urethra confirmed by contrast radiography, and (3) are incontinent due to the urethral dilation or to weakened muscles of the bladder neck and proximal urethra.

The urinary bladder is approached through a ventral abdominal midline incision. The bladder and proximal urethra are reflected caudally, exposing the trigone of the bladder and the dorsal wall of the proximal urethra. Three parallel incisions 8 cm in length are made, approximately 1 cm apart, extending from the midtrigone area onto the dorsal wall of the urethra (Fig. 138–18). Care must be taken to avoid damaging the ureters. The incisions must not penetrate the mucosa. The distal ends of the longitudinal incisions are incised transversely. Blunt and sharp dissection superficial to the mucosa results in the harvesting of two seromuscular flaps that are attached to the midtrigone area. These flaps are reflected to either side, and the defect in the dorsal wall of the urethra is closed with fine absorbable suture material. Each flap is reflected laterally to meet on the ventral surface at the junction of the bladder neck and proximal urethra. The flaps are sutured to each other ventral to the vesicourethral junction, creating a constricting and compressive force. The tension on the sling is critical and may be adjusted by the placement of additional sutures. Measurement of the proper tension is performed by the technique described by Christie,[13] presented previously in this section under bladder neck slings.

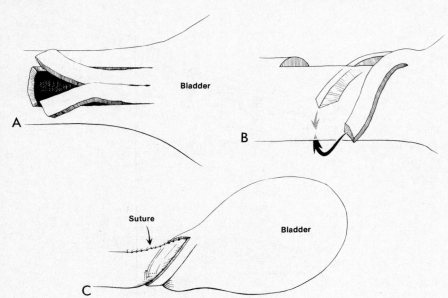

Figure 138–18. Sling urethroplasty. *A,* Three parallel incisions are made on the dorsal surface of the trigone and proximal urethra without penetrating the mucosa. *B,* The incisions are undermined and the seromuscular flaps reflected laterally. *C,* Suturing the flaps to each other ventral to the vesicourethral junction results in the creation of a supporting sling.

Bladder Neck Reconstruction

The bladder neck reconstruction procedures create a urethral tube from the ventral or dorsal walls of the bladder. Bladder neck reconstruction is indicated in those patients that are incontinent due to (1) congenital abnormalities of the bladder neck and proximal urethra, or (2) damage to the vesicourethral junction resulting from fracture of the pelvis, surgical prostatectomy, or other traumatic factors.

The use of the posterior (dorsal) bladder wall to create a urinary sphincter was first reported by Dees in 1949.[14] Others modified this technique by transplanting the ureters to the body of the bladder to allow construction of a longer urethra.[29, 33] Flocks and Culp introduced the anterior (ventral) bladder wall urethral tube in 1953 to lengthen the urethra following prostatectomy.[18] Tanagho and co-workers described the use of a similar technique for the treatment of urinary incontinence.[51] This and a modified technique[53] have specific applications to dogs and cats with urinary incontinence secondary to congenital abnormalities of the vesicourethral junction. The bladder neck reconstruction procedure may also be performed in conjunction with a total prostatectomy or following traumatic severance of the urethra owing to a fractured pelvis or other injuries. In these cases the only modification of the technique is that a complete anastomosis of the tube to the urethra is necessary.

The bladder is exposed through a caudal ventral midline approach. Stay sutures are placed in the apex of the bladder to allow cranial retraction of the bladder and proximal urethra. A full thickness incision is made 1 cm off the midline of the ventral surface of the bladder, extending from the midblad-

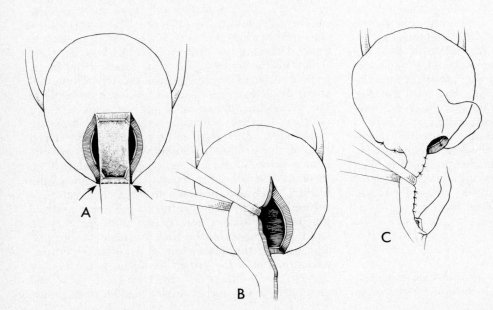

Figure 138–19. Bladder neck reconstruction. *A,* Two parallel longitudinal incisions are made in the ventral wall of the bladder. A transverse incision is made in the dorsal wall of the urethra at its junction with the neck of the bladder. *B,* The lateral edges of the ventral flap are sutured together, forming a tube. *C,* Anastomosis of the tube to the urethra (dorsally) and the bladder (dorsally) and repair of the bladder wall completes the bladder neck reconstruction.

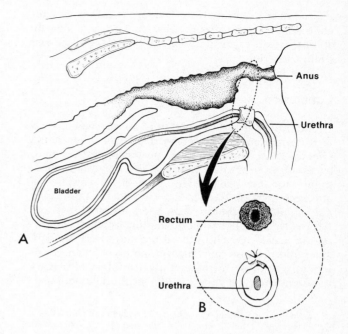

Figure 138–20. Perineal sling. *A*, Sagittal view. The sling is passed around the membranous urethra from incisions in each ischiorectal fossa. *B*, Transverse view.

der wall to the urethra (Fig. 138–19). A second incision of identical length is made 1 cm to the contralateral side of the midline. This creates a flap attached both cranially and caudally. A transverse incision is made on the dorsal wall of the urethra at the caudal aspect of the flap. The urethra is attached to the bladder only by the ventral flap. This 2-cm-wide flap is formed into a tube by suturing it dorsally around a urinary catheter. Distally, the dorsal wall of the urethra is sutured to the tube. Proximally, the defect in the bladder created by harvesting the flap is closed and the dorsal wall of the tube anastomosed to the bladder. The muscle fibers of the bladder wall act as a sphincter in the newly created urethral tube.

Perineal Sling

Christie described placement of a perineal fascial sling for correction of urinary incontinence in a male dog.[13] The indications for placement are the same as for the bladder neck sling. The effect of the procedure, as with the bladder neck sling, is to create increased mechanical resistance to the flow of urine.

The perineal sling is placed around the membranous urethra (Fig. 138–20). A fascial strip is harvested from the fascia lata or the rectus abdominis fascia. The membranous urethra is approached by an incision over each ischiorectal fossa. The fascial strip is passed ventral to the membranous urethra with the aid of forceps. Blunt dissection is used to create a subcutaneous tunnel ventral to the anus from one ischiorectal fossa to the other. The ends of the fascial strip are passed through the subcutaneous tunnel in opposite directions. Tension is placed on the sling until it just compresses the urethra. On palpation of slight compression of the urethra, the ends of the

sling are anchored to each other using nonabsorbable suture material.

Artificial Sphincter

The use of artificial bladder sphincters is well documented.[7, 19, 21, 22, 23, 44, 45] Although their clinical use in animals has not been reported, Swenson and Malinin reported the experimental use of implantable artificial sphincters* with a subcutaneous control unit in 17 female dogs.[50] This device may be indicated as a treatment for both neurogenic and nonneurogenic urinary incontinence. The artificial sphincter consists of a silastic-covered spring, a control device, and a connecting cable (Fig. 138–21). The artificial sphincter is controlled by a subcutaneous titanium control unit that must be activated by the owner. Dedicated owners could learn how to activate the artificial sphincter, allowing animals with nonneurogenic incontinence to urinate. Even more dedication would

*Codman and Shurtleff, Inc., Randolph, MA.

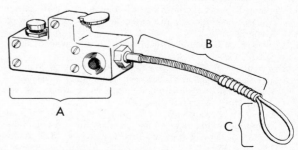

Figure 138–21. Artificial sphincter. Schematic representation of the artificial sphincter demonstrating (*a*) control device, (*b*) connecting cable, and (*c*) Silastic-coated spring.

be required in animals with neurogenic urinary incontinence, as owners would have to activate the sphincter and express the bladder or catheterize and drain the urine.

Conclusion

The procedures described here are not well known to veterinarians. No specific discussion concerning effectiveness, complications, or postoperative management is presented because the literature documents too few cases. The procedures can be an alternative to euthanasia and should be performed only if medical therapy has been unrewarding and only with full client understanding of their experimental nature. Each of these techniques shows considerable promise and may ultimately provide a satisfactory solution to the complex problem of urinary incontinence caused by bladder neck malfunction.

1. Adams, W. M., and DiBartola, S. P.: Radiographic and clinical features of pelvic bladder in the dog. J. Am. Vet. Med. Assoc. *182*:1212, 1983.
2. Ashken, M. H.: *Urinary Diversion.* Springer-Verlag, Berlin, 1982.
3. Beck, R. P., Grove, D., Arnusch, D., and Harvey, J.: Recurrent urinary stress incontinence treated by the fascia lata sling procedure. Am. J. Obstet. Gynecol. *120*:613, 1974.
4. Blandy, J. P.: *Urology.* Blackwell Scientific Publications, Oxford, 1976.
5. Bovée, K. C., Pass, M. A., Wardley, R., Biery, D., and Allen, H. L.: Trigonal-colonic anastomosis: A urinary diversion procedure in dogs. J. Am. Vet. Med. Assoc. *174*:184, 1979.
6. Brown, M., and Wickham, J. E. A.: The urethral pressure profile. Br. J. Urol. *41*:211, 1969.
7. Bruskewitz, R., Raz, S., and Kaufman, J.: Treatment of urinary incontinence with the artificial sphincter. J. Urol. *126*:469, 1981.
8. Bryans, F. E.: Marlex gauze hammock sling operation with Cooper's ligament attachment in the management of recurrent urinary stress incontinence. Am. J. Obstet. Gynecol. *133*:292, 1979.
9. Bushby, P., and Hankes, G.: Sling urethroplasty for the correction of urethral dilation and urinary incontinence. J. Am. Anim. Hosp. Assoc. *16*:115, 1980.
10. Cato, R. J., and Murray, A. G.: Teflon tape suspension for the control of stress incontinence. Br. J. Urol. *53*:364, 1981.
11. Christie, B. A.: Incidence and etiology of vesicoureteral reflux in apparently normal dogs. Invest. Urol. *9*:184, 1971.
12. Christie, B. A.: Vesicoureteral reflux in dogs. J. Am. Vet. Med. Assoc. *162*:772, 1973.
13. Christie, B. A.: A simple sling technique for the correction of urinary incontinence, presented at Am. Coll. Vet. Surg. Meeting, 1979.
14. Dees, J. E.: Congenital epispadias with incontinence. J. Urol. *62*:513, 1949.
15. Dingwall, J. S., Eger, C. E., and Owen, R. R.: Clinical experiences with the combined technique of ureterovesicular anastomosis for treatment of ectopic ureters. J. Am. Anim. Hosp. Assoc. *12*:406, 1976.
16. Feeney, D. A., Osborne, C. A., and Johnston, G. R.: Vesicoureteral reflux induced by manual compression of the urinary bladder of dogs and cats. J. Am. Vet. Med. Assoc. *182*:795, 1983.
17. Firth, L. K., and Owen, T. L.: Communiciation between bladder and vagina. J. Am. Vet. Med. Assoc. *166*:93, 1983.
18. Flocks, R. H., and Culp, D. A.: A modification of technique for anastomosing membranous urethra and bladder neck following total prostatectomy. J. Urol. 69:411, 1953.
19. Foley, F. E.: An artificial sphincter; A new device and operation for control of enuresis and urinary incontinence. J. Urol. 58:250, 1947.
20. Frangenheim, C.: Zür operativen behandlung der Inkontinenz der mannlichen Harnrohre. Verh. dt. Ges. Chir. 4310 Cong. 1914, 149.
21. Furlow, W. L.: The implantable artificial genitourinary sphincter in the management of total urinary incontinence. Mayo Clin. Proc. *51*:341, 1976.
22. Gonzales, R., and Dewolf, W. C.: The artificial bladder sphincter AS-721 for the treatment of incontinence in patients with neurogenic bladder. J. Urol. *121*:71, 1979.
23. Hald, T., Bystrom, J., and Alfthan, O.: Treatment of urinary incontinence by the Scott-Bradley-Timm artificial sphincter. Urol. Res. *3*:133, 1975.
24. Hobson, H. P.: Ectopic ureters. J. Texas Vet. Med. Assoc. *40*:14, 1978.
25. Hobson, H. P., and Ader, P. L.: Exstrophy of the bladder in a dog. J. Am. Anim. Hosp. Assoc. *15*:103, 1979.
26. Hoskins, J. D., Abdelbaki, Y. Z., and Root, C. R.: Urinary bladder duplication in a dog. J. Am. Vet. Med. Assoc. *181*:603, 1982.
27. Kaminski, J. M., Katz, A. R., and Woodward, S. C.: Urinary bladder calculus formation on sutures in rabbits, cats and dogs. Surg. Gynecol. Obstet. *146*:353, 1978.
28. Kunin, S., and Terry, M.: A complication following ovariohysterectomy in a dog. Vet. Med./Small Anim. Clin. 75:1000, 1980.
29. Leadbetter, G. W.: Surgical correction of total urinary incontinence. J. Urol. *91*:261, 1964.
30. Libertino, A., and Zinman, L.: *Reconstructive Urologic Surgery.* Williams & Wilkins, Baltimore, 1977.
31. Marshal, V. F., and Muecke, E. C.: Variations in exstrophy of the bladder. J. Urol. *88*:766, 1962.
32. McQuire, E. J., and Lytton, B.: Pubovaginal sling procedure for stress incontinence. J. Urol. *119*:82, 1978.
33. Michener, F. R., Thompson, I. M., and Ross, G.: Urethrovesical tubularization for urinary incontinence. J. Urol. 92:203, 1964.
34. Moldoff, D. L., and Gordon, R. P.: Pyogranuloma of a canine urinary bladder. J. Am. Anim. Hosp. Assoc. *12*:507, 1976.
35. Osborne, C. A.: Strategy for nonsurgical removal of canine struvite uroliths. Proc. 49th Ann. Mtg. Am. Anim. Hosp. Assoc., 1982, p. 211.
36. Osborne, C. A., Abdullahi, S., Klausner, J. S., Johnston, G. R., and Polzin, D. J.: Nonsurgical removal of uroliths from the urethra of female dogs. J. Am. Vet. Med. Assoc. *182*:47, 1983.
37. Osborne, C. A., Low, D. G., and Finco, D. R.: *Canine and Feline Urology.* W. B. Saunders, Philadelphia, 1972, p. 394.
38. Osborne, C. A., Low, D. G., and Perman, V.: Neoplasms of the canine and feline urinary bladder; Clinical findings, diagnosis, and treatment. J. Am. Vet. Med. Assoc. *152*:247, 1968.
39. Pearson, H., Gibbs, C., and Hillson, J. M.: Some abnormalities in the canine urinary tract. Vet. Rec. 77:775, 1965.
40. Petterson, S.: Free fascial sling to correct urinary incontinence after prostatic surgery. Scand. J. Urol. Neophrol. *9*:24, 1975.
41. Piermattei, D. L., and Osborne, C. A.: Nonsurgical removal of calculi from the urethra of male dogs. J. Am. Vet. Med. Assoc. *159*:1755, 1971.
42. Rigg, D. L., Zenoble, R. D., and Riedesel, E. A.: Neoureterostomy and phenylpropanolamine therapy for incontinence due to ectopic ureter in a dog. J. Am. Anim. Hosp. Assoc. *19*:237, 1983.
43. Schneck, C.: Duplication of the bladder. J. Am. Vet. Med. Assoc. *168*:523, 1976.
44. Scott, F. B., Bradley, W. E., and Timm, G. W.: Treatment of urinary incontinence by implantable prosthetic sphincter. Urology *1*:252, 1973.
45. Scott, F. B., Bradley, W. E., and Timm, G. W.: Treatment

of urinary incontinence by an implantable prosthetic urinary sphincter. J. Urol. *112*:75, 1974.

46. Smith, C. W., Burke, T. J., and Froehlich, P.: Bilateral ureteral ectopia in a male cat with urinary incontinence. J. Am. Vet. Med. Assoc. *182*:172, 1983.

47. Smith, C. W., Stowater, J. L., and Kneller, S. K.: Ectopic ureter in the dog—a review of cases. J. Am. Anim. Hosp. Assoc. *17*:245, 1981.

48. Studdiford, W. E.: Transplantation of abdominal fascia for the relief of urinary stress incontinence. Am. J. Obstet. Gynecol. *47*:764, 1944.

49. Swenson, O.: An experimental implantable urinary sphincter. Invest. Urol. *14*:100, 1976.

50. Swenson, O., and Malinin, T. L.: An improved mechanical device for control of urinary incontinence. Urology *15*:389, 1978.

51. Tanagho, E., Smith, D., Meyers, F. H., and Fisher, R.: Mechanism of urinary continence. II. Technique for surgical correction of incontinence. J. Urol. *101*:305, 1969.

52. Weaver, A. D.: Intrapelvic cyst as a urinary obstruction in a bitch. J. Am. Vet. Med. Assoc. *169*:798, 1976.

53. Williams, D., and Snyder, H.: Anterior detrusor tube for urinary incontinence in children. Br. J. Urol. *48*:671, 1976.

54. Zachary, J. F.: Cystitis cystica, cystitis glandularis, and Brunn's nests in a feline urinary bladder. Vet. Pathol. *18*:113, 1981.

Chapter **139**

Surgical Diseases of the Urethra

C. W. Smith

The urethra is the channel that carries urine from the bladder to the exterior. The male urethra is relatively long (10 to 35 cm in dogs) and consists of three portions: prostatic, pelvic (membranous), and cavernous (penile). The prostate gland encompasses the proximal portion of the male urethra at the neck of the bladder.[7] In the dog, the neck of the bladder is very short, whereas in the cat it is extremely elongated.[24] The prostatic portion of the urethra is U-shaped and passes through the prostate gland.[7] In dogs, diseases of the prostate gland (hyperplasia, cyst formation, prostatitis, abscess, and carcinoma) may affect this portion of the urethra. The pelvic urethra extends from the prostate gland to the bulb of the penis near the ischiatic arch.[7] Because of its relationship to the symphysis pubis, this portion of the urethra is vulnerable to injury from pelvic fractures. The cavernous portion of the urethra begins at the bulb of the corpus spongiosum and extends to the external opening of the penis. The corpus spongiosum and the penile urethra occupy the ventral groove of the os penis.[7] Distension of the urethra in this groove is very limited, so urethral obstruction with calculi generally occurs at this level. Fractures of the os penis can lead to urethral injury.

The female urethra corresponds to that portion of the male urethra that lies cranial to the prostatic utricle. In the dog, it is about 0.5 cm in diameter and 7 to 10 cm long. The urethra enters the genital tract approximately 0.5 cm caudal to the vaginovestibular junction. Its dorsal wall is in close apposition to the ventral wall of the vagina. The lumen can expand considerably when under pressure because of its folded mucous membrane.[7] As in the male dog, the close proximity of the urethra to the pubic symphysis makes it vulnerable to injury from pelvic fractures. Because of its relationship to the vagina,

disease processes in the genital system (vaginitis, vaginal neoplasia) may involve the urethra. Further discussion of the urethra may be found in Chapter 132 and Sections 13 and 14.

CONGENITAL OR HEREDITARY LESIONS AFFECTING THE URETHRA

Urethral anomalies in all species of animals are relatively uncommon.[25] Hypospadias, epispadias with exstrophy of the bladder, imperforate urethra, ectopic urethra, urethral aplasia (or agenesis), duplicated urethra, and urethrorectal fistula have been reported in dogs.[2, 10, 25] A few of these conditions, including hypospadias, epispadias with exstrophy of the bladder, and urethrorectal fistula, have been surgically corrected.[2, 9, 10, 25]

Hypospadias

This anomaly occurs when there is a fusion failure of the urogenital folds and incomplete formation of the penile urethra. Varying degrees of this abnormality can occur with fusion failure anywhere from the area of the penis to the perineal area. In humans, this condition is believed to result from inadequate production of androgens by the fetal testis.[22] Differences in the timing and degree of hormonal failure account for the variety of human types. In dogs, hypospadias is usually associated with fusion failure of the prepuce and underdevelopment or absence of the penis (Fig. 139–1).

Dogs with hypospadias are seen as puppies with irritated and urine-soaked skin and hair around the urethral opening. Remnants of the incomplete pre-

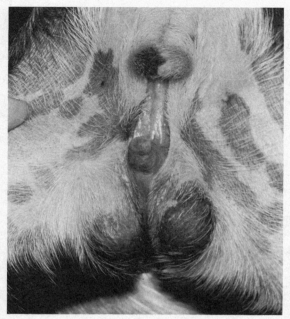

Figure 139–1. Canine hypospadias: fusion failure of the urethra, prepuce, and scrotum and the underdevelopment of the penis.

puce appear as unsightly defects. Corrective surgery, if performed, includes identification and preservation of the urethral opening, excision of the urethral groove and remnants of the prepuce and penis, and castration. Even after surgery, the perineum and ventral abdomen near the urethral opening may become excoriated by urine. Prognosis is generally good except that patients may be more prone to ascending infections because of the shorter urethra.

Epispadias

A rarer anomaly, which also represents fusion failure, occurs as an abnormally located urethral groove along the dorsal surface of the penis. In men, in whom it has been reported more commonly, it appears in combination with another anomaly known as exstrophy of the urinary bladder. In the latter malformation, the bladder lies wide open midventrally and the pubic arches fail to unite. The dorsal wall of the bladder thus becomes the ventral body wall with the ureters discharging urine directly to the exterior.[22] This combination of anomalies has been reported in a dog[10] (see Chapter 138).

Urethrorectal Fistula

This is a developmental anomaly of the fetal cloaca in which a communication between the urethra and rectum persists.[2, 9, 25] In humans, it is proposed that these fistulae develop as a result of failure of the urorectal septum to completely separate the cloaca into an anterior urethrovesical segment and a poste-

rior rectal segment.[5] They occur twice as frequently in boys as in girls and are associated with an imperforate anus and anomalies of other body systems.[16] In dogs, urethrorectal fistulae have been reported in both sexes. Clinical signs are associated with abnormal micturition, first observed shortly after weaning. Urine passes simultaneously through the urethra and anus. Generally, concurrent cystitis is present. Diagnosis is confirmed by physical examination, including rectal examination using a nasal speculum and positive contrast urethrogram demonstrating leakage of contrast media from the urethra into the rectum. Surgical correction is performed via ventral pubic symphysiotomy.[2] The pubic symphysis is split with an osteotome and distracted with retractors. The fistula is identified, double-ligated, and excised. The symphysis is stabilized using wire. Concurrent medical therapy for cystitis is necessary (see Chapter 135).

ACQUIRED NONTRAUMATIC LESIONS AFFECTING THE URETHRA

Acquired nontraumatic lesions of the urethra include urethritis, urethral prolapse; obstruction associated with urethral calculi and with stricture formation following inflammation, passage of calculi, and urethral surgery; and neoplasia.

Urethritis

Urethritis as an isolated clinical entity is uncommon. Generally, it is associated with other inflammatory diseases of the urogenital tract, such as cystitis, prostatitis, or vaginitis. Predisposing factors include trauma, catheterization, urolithiasis, and neoplasia.[31] Therapy for urethritis is directed at controlling infection and eliminating the identifiable factors. Although rare, urethritis can lead to urethral prolapse or stricture formation, necessitating surgical intervention.

Urethral Prolapse

Urethral prolapse has been reported in young male dogs of the brachycephalic breeds.[4, 11] Prolonged sexual excitement and urethral infection may be the cause, although the exact pathophysiology is unknown. Patients are observed to excessively lick the tip of the penis and preputial orifice. Diagnosis is based on observing the protruding mucosa (Fig. 139–2). With a urinary catheter in place, the prolapsed urethra is partially incised into the lumen just caudal to the prolapse and sutured circumferentially with 4-0 monofilament nylon by alternately incising and suturing. A splinting catheter is usually unnecessary following surgery. Sedation and an Elizabethan collar might be necessary for three to five days to prevent

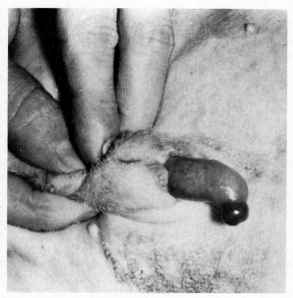

Figure 139–2. Prolapse of the penile urethra in a male dog. (Courtesy of Dr. A. G. Schiller.)

self-trauma. Systemic antibiotics are used to treat any urogenital infection present.

Urethral Obstruction

Obstruction of the urethra occurs with urethral calculi and stricture formation following inflammation, passage of calculi, and urethral surgery.

Urethral Calculi

Urethral calculi are the most common cause of urethral obstruction in male dogs.[4] Less-organized

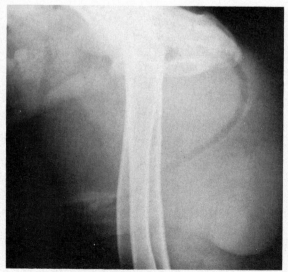

Figure 139–3. A lateral radiograph of a male dog with cystic and urethral calculi. Note several calculi in the urethra of the os penis. (Courtesy of Drs. S. Kneller and J. Stowater.)

debris causes obstruction in male cats.[26] A detailed discussion of canine urolithiasis and feline urolithiasis may be found in Chapters 140 and 141, respectively. This discussion is limited to understanding when surgical intervention is indicated and the surgical procedures used. Urethral obstruction may be complete or incomplete and most often occurs just behind the os penis (Fig. 139–3). Clinical signs vary with the degree and duration of obstruction and include dysuria and anuria, hematuria, and distended or turgid abdomen. Signs of uremia may be present if complete obstruction has been present for at least 48 hours.[26] Diagnosis is based on palpation of calculi, obstruction met in passage of a urethral catheter, and radiological demonstration of stones.

Once the diagnosis has been established, nonsurgical techniques to improve a patient's status and to overcome the blockage should be attempted before utilizing surgical techniques (Chapter 140). Urethral calculi that cannot be moved either by catheterization or urohydropulsion[30] to the exterior or into the bladder require urethral surgery. If the calculus cannot be dislodged and if the patient's condition permits anesthesia, the calculus can be removed via a urethrotomy performed at the obstruction. Cystocentesis and fluid therapy may be necessary to improve the patient's ability to tolerate anesthesia.

Urethrotomy/Cystotomy

With a urethral catheter in place to the point of obstruction, a 3- to 4-cm ventral midline skin incision is made over the obstruction. The subcutaneous tissue is incised down to the retractor penis muscle over the urethra in the midline. After its fascial attachment is freed, the muscle is retracted laterally to expose the ventral portion of the urethra. A longitudinal incision is made over the calculus (or catheter tip), and the stone is carefully removed. The catheter is advanced and the remaining calculi are flushed into the bladder with a stream of saline. These calculi and any other cystic calculi are removed via cystotomy. Radiographs may be necessary to determine whether the urethra is free of calculi and whether any cystic calculi remain.

If the urethra has not been severely traumatized by the calculus or the surgical incision, the urethrotomy can be closed with 4-0 polyglycolic acid sutures using an interrupted pattern. Sutures are anchored in the corpus spongiosum and, if possible, the urethral mucosa as well.[2] An indwelling catheter makes it easier to place these sutures carefully, since stricture of the lumen may result if too great a "bite" is taken. If trauma to the urethra is excessive, the urethrotomy incision is not sutured but is allowed to granulate. Urine leaks through the wound for several days, and hemorrhage from the corpus spongiosum may be a problem when the dog urinates or becomes excited.

The major complication associated with urethrotomy is urethral stricture formation. For this reason a concerted (but gentle) effort should be made to move the calculi by catheterization or urohydropulsion first before performing urethral surgery. A laparotomy with cystotomy is much less likely to result in complications.

Urethrostomy

The creation of a permanent opening into the urethra can be used for (1) calculi that cannot be removed by flushing; (2) chronic stone formers that cannot be kept free of calculi medically; (3) strictures of the urethra resulting from one or more episodes of prior urethral surgery or trauma; and (4) severe penile trauma when penile amputation is required.

Canine Urethrostomy. In dogs, four levels of urethrostomy can be performed: prescrotal, scrotal, perineal, and antepubic. The level selected is based on the site of obstruction and the surgeon's preference.

If a choice exists, and if the patient can be castrated, scrotal urethrostomy is recommended. The advantages of a scrotal urethrostomy are that the urethra is wide and more superficial at this level and surrounded by less cavernous tissue, therefore decreasing the possibility of hemorrhage. Higher obstructions require perineal or antepubic urethrostomy.

A scrotal urethrostomy is performed with the dog in dorsal recumbency (Fig. 139–4). If possible, a catheter is passed to facilitate identification and incision of the urethra. If the dog is intact, castration is performed and the scrotum excised. The retractor penis muscle is isolated and sutured in a lateral position to expose the ventral aspect of the urethra. This is incised for 3 to 4 cm, and the urethra is sutured to the skin with 3-0 or 4-0 monofilament nylon or prolene suture material in a simple interrupted pattern. Skin not sutured to the urethra is closed in the usual fashion. The catheter is removed.

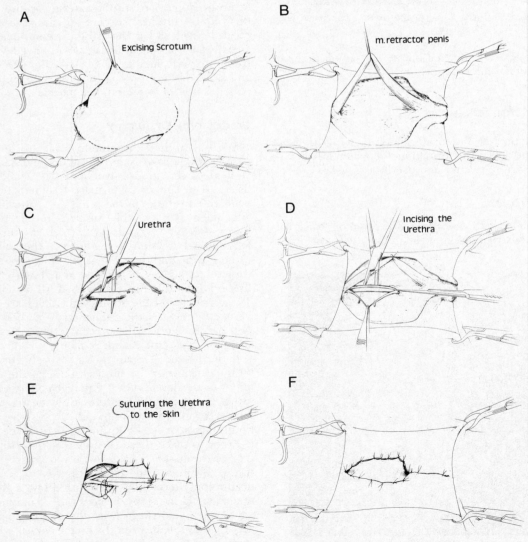

Figure 139–4. Scrotal urethrostomy. *A,* An elliptical skin incision is made around the scrotum, which is excised. The dog is castrated. *B,* The retractor penis muscle is isolated and retracted laterally. *C,* The retractor penis muscle is sutured laterally, and the urethra is located. *D,* The ventral aspect of the urethra is incised for 3 to 4 cm. *E,* The urethra is sutured to the skin. *F,* The remaining skin incision is sutured closed.

Complications include hemorrhage from the cavernous tissue for up to ten days and urethral strictures. An Elizabethan collar and sedation are helpful in preventing self-mutilation during the initial healing period. Sedation of the patient at discharge prevents excitement and reduces the risk of hemorrhage.

Feline Urethrostomy. Techniques of urethrostomy are many in male cats,[12, 35] but perineal urethrostomy using the Wilson and Harrison technique[43, 44] is my preferred method (Fig. 139–5). The patient may be positioned in dorsal or ventral recumbency. A purse-string suture is placed around the anus, an elliptical incision is made around the scrotum and prepuce, and the cat is castrated. The penis is isolated and the ischiocavernosus muscles exposed by blunt dissec-

tion. These muscles are transected at their attachment to the ischium. Incision through the muscle belly causes hemorrhage from the muscle and the underlying crura of the penis. The penis has a fibrous pubic attachment that must also be transected. Blunt dissection with a finger ventrally and laterally permobilization and posterior displacement of the penis and pelvic urethra. The loose tissue near the penis is carefully excised to expose the retractor penis muscle, bulbospongiosus muscle, and bulbourethral glands. The retractor penis muscle is transected near the external anal sphincter muscle, dissected from the urethra, and excised. Care should be exercised in this dissection to prevent damage to the rectum and pelvic nerves (Fig. 139–6). The penile urethra is

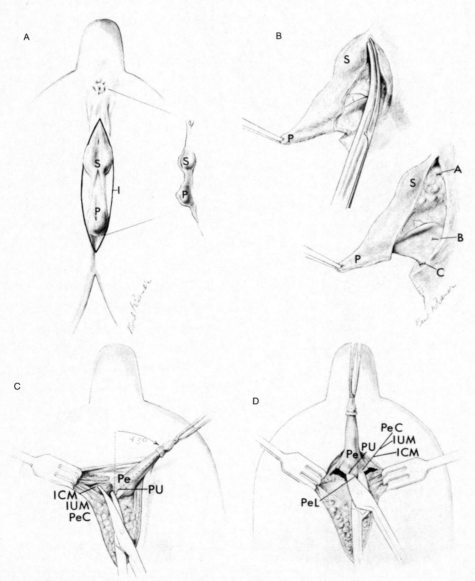

Figure 139–5. *A,* Elliptical incision incorporating the scrotum and prepuce. S, scrotum; P, prepuce; I, skin incision. *B,* Removal of prepuce and scrotum. A, caudal scrotal artery; B, cranial scrotal artery; C, dorsal artery and vein of penis, prostatic artery. *C,* Dissection of penis from surrounding tissue to its pelvic attachments on the ischium. ICM, ischiocavernosus muscle; IUM, ischiourethralis muscle; PeC, crus of penis; Pe, penis; PU, pelvic urethra. *D,* Incision of ligament of penis. PeL, ligament of penis.

Illustration continued on following page

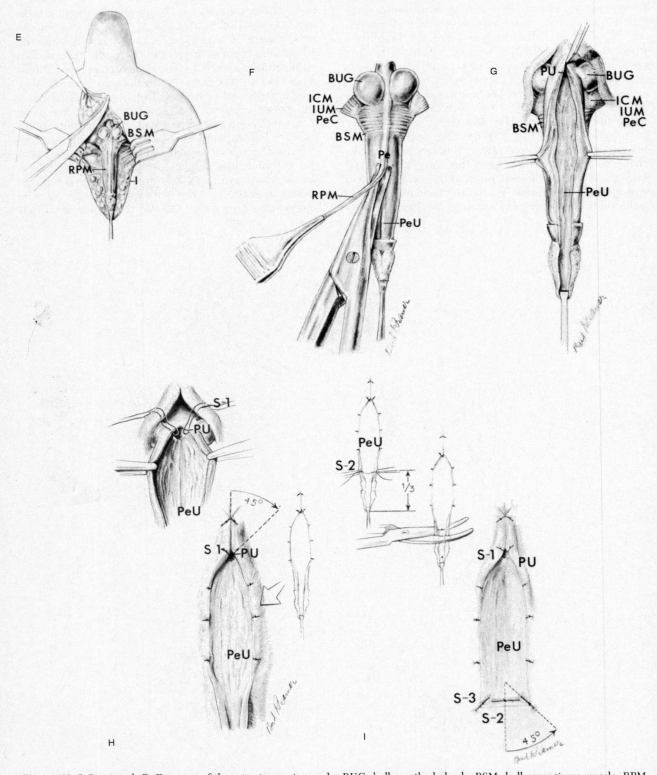

Figure 139–5 *Continued. E,* Exposure of the retractor penis muscle. BUG, bulbourethral glands; BSM, bulbospongiosus muscle; RPM, retractor muscle of penis. *F,* Insertion of probe into penile urethra. PeU, penile urethra. *G,* Incision of the penile urethra through the glans penis to the pelvic urethra. *H,* Suture of the pelvic and penile urethral mucosa to the perineal skin. S-1, initial sutures. *I,* Placement of through-and-through suture through body of penis; S-1, Initial sutures; S-2, through-and-through mattress suture; S-3, mucosa-to-skin sutures. (Reprinted with permission from Wilson, G. P., and Kusba, J. K.: Perineal urethrostomy in the cat. *In* Bojrab, M. J. (ed.): *Current Techniques in Small Animal Surgery.* Philadelphia, Lea & Febiger, 1983; modified from Wilson, G. P., and Harrison, J. W.: Perineal urethrostomy in cats. J. Am. Vet. Med. Assoc. *159:*1789, 1971.)

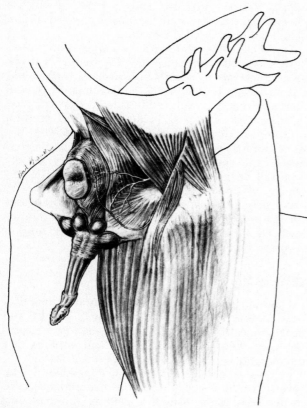

Figure 139–6. Pelvic nerves and rectum in relation to the penis and pelvic musculature. (Reprinted with permission from Wilson, G. P., and Kusba, J. K.: Perineal urethrostomy in the cat. *In* Bojrab, M. J. (ed.): *Current Techniques in Small Animal Surgery,* 2nd ed. Lea & Febiger, Philadelphia, 1983, pp. 325–333.)

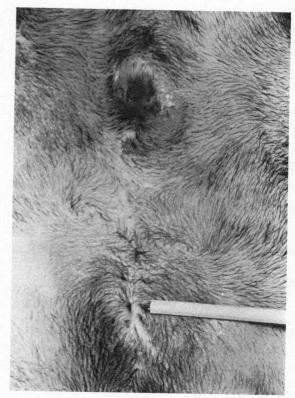

Figure 139–7. The perineal area of a cat with a urethral structure following perineal urethrostomy. Note pinpoint urethral opening.

incised on its ventral aspect to the level of the bulbourethral glands. In this location, the urethral opening is about 4 mm in diameter. The incised pelvic urethra and two-thirds of the penile urethra are sutured to the skin with 4-0 monofilament nylon or prolene with interrupted sutures or 5-0 synthetic absorbable sutures.[17] The remaining urethra and penis are amputated and discarded. A mattress suture may be placed through the body of the retained penile shaft to control the hemorrhage, and the remaining skin incision is closed. The purse-string suture around the anus is removed. An Elizabethan collar is used to prevent self-trauma. No indwelling catheter is used postoperatively. Shredded paper may be used instead of litter until healing occurs. Complications include hemorrhage from erectile tissue, which subsides in a few days, cystitis, and urethral strictures (Fig. 139–7).[38]

To treat postoperative strictures, the urethra is freed from surrounding scar tissue and mobilized additionally to permit suturing of healthy urethra to a fresh skin incision. Usually the urethra was not adequately mobilized or the pelvic urethra was not incised far enough in the beginning. When strictures occur more cranially, an antepubic urethrostomy[20] may be necessary. This technique uses the "urethra" between the bladder and the prostate gland to divert the urine through the ventral abdominal wall in front of the pubis.

Urethral Prostheses in Cats. Prosthetic conduits manufactured from steel and Teflon,[18] silicone rubber and Dacron velour,[36] and silicone rubber* alone[34] have been advocated as treatments for urethral stricture and urethral obsturction in cats (Fig. 139–8). The steel and Teflon prosthesis is inserted directly into the bladder to permit flushing and draining, but it promotes cystic calculi in 25 per cent of cases in which maintenance flushing of the prosthesis and bladder has been neglected. The silicone rubber and Dacron prosthesis is sutured to the bladder neck just cranial to the prostate gland and it replaces the pelvic and penile urethra. Problems with this implant have

---

*Richards all-silicone urethral shunt tube, Richards Manufacturing Co., Inc., Memphis, TN.

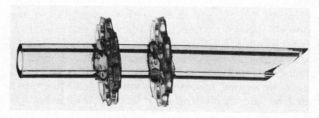

Figure 139–8. Richards all-silicone urethral shunt tube.

been perineal fistula, mineral encrustation of the lumen, and rejection as a foreign body. The silicone prosthesis is inserted into the pelvic urethra near the bulbourethral glands. However, urine leakage and mechanical irritation have not allowed even this prothesis to remain maintenance-free.

A well-done perineal urethrostomy remains the method of choice for treating cats with recurrent urethral obstruction.

Neoplasia

Neoplastic processes can involve the urethra, producing partial to complete obstruction. Tumors of the urinary tract are uncommon in cats.[3] In dogs, primary urethral tumors, although uncommon, are most likely to occur in females.[39, 41] Clinical signs vary in severity and include mild stranguria to anuria and hematuria. Radiographs, including pneumocystogram-cystogram with voiding urethrogram, are important in delineating the location and extent of lesions.[40] Survey radiographs of the abdomen and thorax are important in detecting metastatic lesions. In some cases urinary exfoliative cytology may be helpful in diagnosis, but more often excisional or incisional biopsy is necessary. Surgical excision is the treatment of choice when the lesion is discrete but may be impossible when the lesion is diffuse. Lesions that cannot be resected should be biopsied for diagnostic, prognostic, and chemotherapeutic planning purposes. For exploratory surgery, the caudal abdominal approach is recommended over the vaginal approach via episiotomy, because it permits better visualization of the urethra, periurethral tissues, bladder, and regional lymph nodes.[39] For further information regarding urethral neoplasms, see Chapter 183.

ACQUIRED TRAUMATIC LESIONS AFFECTING THE URETHRA

Acquired traumatic lesions of the urethra include contusion, laceration, rupture, and obstruction. Urethral contusions are associated with blunt trauma. Urethral lacerations and ruptures are associated with fractures of the pubis and os penis; penetrating wounds caused by knife, gunshot, or bite injuries; and iatrogenic injuries as a result of urethral examination, dilatation, catheterization, and surgery on and near the urethra. Traumatic urethral obstructions are usually associated with fractures of the pubis or os penis but can also occur with strangulation of the penis by foreign objects (rubber bands), phimosis/paraphimosis, herniation of the bladder into perineal and inguinal areas, and marked prostatic enlargement. An unusual cause of urethral obstruction has been described in a dog, in which an airgun pellet that had penetrated into the bladder lumen became

impacted in the urethra,[6] and in a cat, in which a plug of hair carried into the bladder by an airgun pellet had obstructed the urethra.[1]

The causes of traumatic urethral injuries are many, but the overall incidence is low. In one survey it was found that the most common urinary tract injury accompanying trauma to the abdomen and pelvis in dogs and cats was ruptured bladder.[28] Less common injuries were ruptured kidney, ruptured urethra, ruptured ureter, and perirenal hematoma. The ruptured urethras were most likely associated with pelvic fractures in male animals and the injury usually occurred near the urethrovesical junction. The frequency of urinary tract trauma that occurred with blunt pelvic trauma in another survey of 100 cases was 39 per cent.[37] Only 5 per cent of these injuries involved the urethra, and rupture of the urethra occurred exclusively in the male dog.

Clinical Signs

Clinical signs associated with urethral trauma may be masked by other problems or may be absent. The usual clinical signs include dysuria, anuria, hematuria, pain, fluid in the abdomen, and swelling and discoloration of the skin in the perineal area.[28, 33, 37] The range of clinical signs varies, depending on the severity of the lesion. Contusions may produce minimal clinical signs, whereas urethral ruptures may show all those listed. Although clinical signs may be helpful when present, their absence does not rule out the presence of urethral trauma. For example, a dog may void normally with a urethral tear. Selcer reported that clinical signs suggestive of urinary tract injury were absent in 59 per cent of the pelvic trauma cases with positively diagnosed urinary tract trauma.[37] One-third (13 of 39) of all urinary tract injuries in this series were clinically unsuspected. Sixty-nine per cent (9 of 13) of the clinically undetected urinary tract trauma was seen in female dogs. Hematuria was the most frequent clinical sign, but it occurred in only 36 per cent (14 of 39) of dogs with urinary tract trauma. The clinical signs that were consistently associated with urinary tract trauma were dysuria/anuria and external evidence of an abdominal or inguinal hernia.

If the urethra is ruptured, urine leakage produces a cellulitis that leads to fistula formation. Leukocytosis, with counts of 50,000 to 100,000 cells/mm^3, may occur when significant local infection is present.[33] If the patient is anorectic, signs of dehydration, hypoproteinemia, and hypoglycemia may occur. If the urethra is obstructed, signs of uremia are seen (see Chapter 134).

Diagnosis

Diagnosis is based on a high level of suspicion (abdominal or pelvic trauma), clinical signs, and positive contrast urethrography. Plain radiographs are rarely diagnostic.[28, 37] Positive contrast urethrography should be done prior to catheterization if urethral damage is suspected. Negative contrast studies with room air are contraindicated because of air emboli.[33] Obstruction and lacerations are demonstrated by obstruction or extravasation of contrast material. Furthermore, positive contrast urethrograms help distinguish incomplete from complete urethral ruptures, which need to be managed differently. An experimental study in dogs of partial versus complete division of the penile urethra just cranial to the scrotum revealed, in the partial tear group, extravasation of dye at the site of injury with some dye reaching the bladder; in the complete urethral tear group, extravasation of dye at the site of injury with no dye reaching the bladder was seen.[32] A positive contrast urethrogram usually delineates the distal boundary of the urethral obstruction or stricture well but may not identify its proximal border.

Treatment

Before specific treatment of urethral trauma can be instituted, the general condition of the patient must be assessed. Shock, anuria, dysuria, uremia, dehydration, electrolyte imbalances, and anorexia must be recognized and corrected prior to definitive repair of the urethra.

Treatment methods used for managing urethral trauma take advantage of the remarkable regenerative ability of the urethral mucosa. The entire length of the urethra regenerates from a longitudinal strip of mucosa if an intraurethral catheter is maintained for three weeks.[42] Following complete transection, however, the urethral muscle and mucosa retract. During healing the intervening space is usually filled by fibroblasts that produce fibrous connective tissue that contracts during maturation, producing stenosis.[19] Therefore, primary repair to prevent or delayed repair to excise the almost inevitable stenosis is essential in most complete urethral transections.

Contusions

Specific treatment is based on the type and severity of the injury. Minor urethral contusions and lacerations may heal spontaneously with conservative therapy, including systemic antibiotics and manual assistance in emptying the bladder to prevent urine retention. Healing can sometimes be improved by the placement of a soft, flexible, indwelling catheter,* which reduces delay in healing from urine leakage and acts as a urethral splint. Catheter size should not be so large that undue pressure is placed on the epithelium, as this may interfere with its regeneration.

---

*Brunswick Laboratories, St. Louis, MO.

Lacerations

Lacerations that permit extravasation of urine into the surrounding tissues should be explored and sutured with 3-0 or 4-0 synthetic absorbable suture material and the urine diverted with an intraurethral catheter for three to five days. Bite wounds of the extrapelvic urethra are treated similarly, with the addition of a soft Penrose drain to provide drainage for a few days. If gross infection is present, primary closure is delayed. The external wound is allowed to drain for three days while the urine is diverted through a urethral catheter. Culture and sensitivity testing and appropriate antibiotic administration are indicated.

Intrapelvic Urethral Partial Rupture

Incomplete rupture of the intrapelvic urethra without impingement by fracture fragments may be treated by diverting urine through the largest Foley catheter that can be comfortably passed and maintained in place for 7 to 21 days (depending on the size of the urethral tear). When passage of the catheter is impossible, a ventral midline approach for cystotomy and reflection of the fracture fragments may allow visual passage of the catheter across the tear. At this time suturing of the tear may be possible. If fracture fragments imping on the urethra, they are reduced and stabilized, using wire or other orthopedic techniques. The surgical site is flushed with sterile saline and the pelvic cavity drained to remove debris resulting from urine leakage, blood clots, and necrotic tissue. A urinary diversion catheter is passed and maintained in the urethra for three to five days (with tears that are sutured) or for up to three weeks (if the tears are left unsutured).

Complete Urethral Rupture

In complete rupture of the urethra, experience gained in humans[21, 23, 29] and experiments conducted in dogs[19] indicate that, where possible, primary suture repair is the best treatment. Through a midline symphysiotomy, the severed ends of the urethra are identified, debrided (1 to 2 mm), and sutured with about six interrupted synthetic absorbable sutures over a Foley catheter, which should remain indwelling for five to seven days. If there is severe trauma to the urethra and periurethral tissue, accumulations of blood, urine, and devitalized tissue may preclude primary suturing. In these cases, delayed urethral repair is indicated. A Foley catheter is passed up the urethra from the penis and directed into the bladder. If necessary, a cystotomy is performed and a smaller, more rigid catheter is passed from the bladder into the urethra to emerge at the traumatized area. The catheter tip is tied to the tip of the Foley catheter, which is pulled through the area of urethral damage into the bladder. The balloon of the Foley catheter is inflated and traction applied to the catheter, which is anchored to the penis at the urethral orifice. This approximates the severed ends and diverts the urine. Close approximation is extremely important because it may result in healing with a good urethral lumen or, if a stricture does develop, is more easily correctable.[29]

The cystotomy incision is closed, the surgical site is irrigated with sterile saline solution, and a Penrose drain is positioned. Wire fixation is used to stabilize the symphysiotomy defect, and monofilament nylon, prolene, or stainless steel wire is used to close the potentially infected laparotomy wound. The intraurethral Foley catheter can be left in place for three weeks or until delayed definitive repair is performed. An antepubic Foley catheter may also be used to divert the urine during healing.[33] Penrose drains are removed in three to five days or when drainage subsides. If healing is not satisfactory, a definitive repair involving debridement and anastomosis or excision of the stricture and anastomosis can be accomplished once the inflammatory process has subsided.

Urethral Obstructions

Urethral obstruction generally requires some temporary measures to decompress the bladder as well as fluid therapy to correct metabolic abnormalities before definitive diagnosis and treatment can be performed. Cystocentesis and urinary diversion through catheters, either urethral (with partial obstruction) or antepubic, are helpful life-saving techniques. If the obstruction is associated with a pubic fracture, exploration, reduction, and stabilization of the fracture are required. If the urethra is traumatized, it is treated as previously described.

Urethral impingement from fractures of the os penis (Fig. 139–9) can be treated by reducing the fracture by manipulation and splinting it with a urethral catheter.

Strangulation of the penis by foreign objects such as rubber bands, if discovered early, may require only removal of the constriction. If the penis becomes gangrenous, it will require amputation, castration, and urethrostomy. Phimosis can lead to paraphimosis with strangulation and necrosis of the penis and urethral obstruction. This also requires penile amputation, castration, and urethrostomy.

Urethral obstruction can occur when the bladder is herniated into the inguinal and perineal regions. Definitive treatment in these cases is prompt hernia repair. Some degree of urethral obstruction may occur with severe prostatic disease (see Section XII).

Urethral Strictures

Urethral obstruction may be due to stenosis or stricture following urethral trauma or urethral surgery. Extrapelvic urethral strictures are best managed using urethrostomy techniques, discussed earlier in this chapter. Intrapelvic urethral strictures of 1 cm or less are best managed by resection and anastomosis. Larger defects require heroic measures, such as extrapelvic cystourethral anastomosis;[15] antepubic urethrostomy;[20, 45] or urethral prostheses using silicone rubber,[8] silicone rubber and Dacron,[27] lyophilized human dural tubes,[13] or lyophilized vein homografts.[14] The prostheses serve as a guide for ingrowth of urethral mucosa. Lyophilized vein homograft appears to be the most promising grafting technique. The graft causes very little tissue reaction and consequently little fibrous tissue. The prosthesis be-

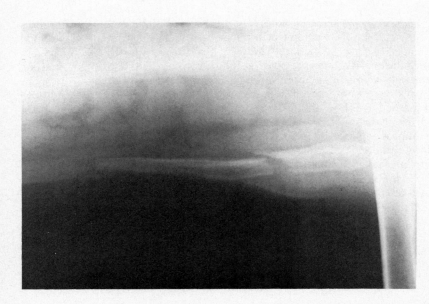

Figure 139–9. A lateral radiograph of a fracture of the os penis in a dog. (Courtesy of Drs. S. Kneller and J. Stowater.)

came lined with epithelium after four to eight weeks and eight of nine dogs showed no signs of obstruction during the six-month follow-up period.[14]

Urethral Trauma Aftercare

Urethral trauma cases often require extensive postoperative nursing care. To maintain urinary catheters in place without patient cooperation involves the use of Elizabethan collars or the incorporation of the urethral catheters in an abdominal bandage. The premature removal of the catheter by the patient and the subsequent blind replacement by the clinician can have disastrous consequences. Checking and maintaining the patency of the catheter is essential to assure proper decompression of the bladder. Frequent urinalysis helps determine the status of the bladder and kidneys. Because of the increased risk of ascending infections with indwelling urinary catheters, utilizing closed urinary drainage systems, taking periodic urine cultures, and using the appropriate antibiotic therapy are indicated. Drains should be protected with bandages, their exudate should be monitored, and they should be removed as soon as drainage subsides. Culturing of the drain detects persistent infection. Proper feeding and hydration encourages healing and speeds convalescence.

1. Andre, P. G., and Jackson, O. F.: An unusual cause of feline urethral obstruction. J. Small Anim. Pract. 11:563, 1970.
2. Archibald, J., and Owen, R. ApR.: Urinary system. In Archibald, J. (ed.): Canine Surgery, 2nd ed. Santa Barbara, American Veterinary Publications, Inc., 1974, pp. 693–701.
3. Barrett, R. E., and Nobel, T. A.: Transitional cell carcinoma of the urethra in a cat. Cornell Vet. 66:14, 1976.
4. Brown, S. G.: Surgery of the canine urethra. Vet. Clin. North Am. 5:457, 1975.
5. Campbell, M. F.: Anomalies of the genital tract. In Campbell, M. F., and Harrison, J. H. (eds.): Urology. Vol. 2, 3rd ed. W. B. Saunders, Philadelphia, 1970, pp. 1573–1625.
6. Denny, H. R.: An unusual cause of urethral obstruction in the dog. J. Small Anim. Pract. 13:339, 1972.
7. Evans, H. E., and Christensen, G. C.: Miller's Anatomy of the Dog, 2nd ed. W. B. Saunders, Philadelphia, 1979, pp. 578, 594.
8. Gilbaugh, J. H., Utz, D. C., and Wakim, K.: Partial replacement of the canine urethra with a silicone prosthesis. Invest. Urol. 7:41, 1969.
9. Goulden, B., Bergman, M., and Wyburn, R. S.: Canine urethrorectal fistulae. J. Small Anim. Pract. 14:143, 1973.
10. Hobson, H. P., and Ader, P. L.: Exstrophy of the bladder in a dog. J. Am. Anim. Hosp. Assoc. 15:103, 1979.
11. Hobson, H. P., and Heller, R. A.: Surgical correction of prolapse of the male urethra. Vet. Med/Small Anim. Clin. 66:1177, 1971.
12. Johnston, D. E.: Feline urethrostomy: A critique and new method. J. Small Anim. Pract. 15:421, 1976.
13. Kelami, A., Korb, G., Rolle, J., Schnell, J., and Lehnhardt, F. J.: Replacement of the total resected urethra with alloplastic materials: Experimental studies of dogs. J. Urol. 107:75, 1972.
14. Kjaer, T. B., Nilsson, T., and Madson, P. O.: Total replacement of part of the canine urethra with lyophilized vein homografts. Invest. Urol. 14:159, 1976.
15. Knecht, C. D., and Slusher, R.: Extrapelvic anastomosis of the bladder and penile urethra in the dog. J. Am. Anim. Hosp. Assoc. 6:247, 1970.
16. LeDuc, E.: Congenital rectourethral fistula: Report of a case without rectal anomaly. J. Urol. 93:272, 1965.
17. Leighton, R. L.: Surgical procedures. In Catcott, E. J. (ed.): Feline Medicine and Surgery. 2nd ed. Santa Barbara, American Veterinary Publications Inc., 1975, p. 570.
18. Manziano, C. F., and Manziano, J. R.: A bladder prosthesis to relieve urethral blockage in the male cat. J. Am. Vet. Med. Assoc. 151:218, 1967.
19. McRoberts, J. W., and Ragde, H.: The severed canine posterior urethra: A study of two distinct methods of repair. J. Urol. 104:724, 1970.
20. Mendham, J. H.: A description and evaluation of antepubic urethrostomy in the male cat. J. Small Anim. Pract. 11:709, 1970.
21. Meyers, R. P., and Deweerd, J. H.: Incidence of stricture following primary realignment of the disrupted proximal urethra. J. Urol. 107:265, 1972.
22. Moore, K. L.: The Developing Human. W. B. Saunders, Philadelphia, 1977, p. 231.
23. Morehouse, D. D., Belitsky, P., and MacKinnon, K.: Rupture of the posterior urethra. J. Urol. 107:255, 1972.
24. Nickel, R., Schummer, A., Seiferle, E., and Sack, W. D.: The Viscera of the Domestic Mammals. Verlag Paul Parey, Berlin, 1973, pp. 318–328.
25. Osborne, C. A., Engen, M. H., Yano, B. L., Brasmer, T. H., Jessen, C. R., and Blevins, W. E.: Congenital urethrorectal fistula in two dogs. J. Am. Vet. Med. Assoc. 166:999, 1975.
26. Osborne, C. A., Low, D. G., and Finco, D. R.: Canine and Feline Urology. W. B. Saunders, Philadelphia, 1972, p. 319.
27. Palleschi, J. R., and Tanagho, E. A.: Urethral tube graft in dogs. Invest. Urol. 15:408, 1978.
28. Peckman, R. D.: Urinary trauma in dogs and cats: A review. J. Am. Anim. Hosp. Assoc. 18:33, 1982.
29. Pierce, J. M.: Management of dismemberment of the prostatic-membranous urethra and ensuing stricture disease. J. Urol. 107:259, 1972.
30. Piermattei, D. L., and Osborne, C. A.: Nonsurgical removal of calculi from the urethra of male dogs. J. Am. Vet. Med. Assoc. 159:1755, 1971.
31. Polzin, D. J., and Jeraj, K.: Urethritis, cystitis, and ureteritis. Vet. Clin. North Am. 9:661, 1979.
32. Raney, A. M.: Radiographic findings immediately after urethral rupture: An experimental study and case report. J. Urol. 116:581, 1976.
33. Rawlings, C. A., and Wingfield, W. E.: Urethral reconstruction in dogs and cats. J. Am. Anim. Hosp. Assoc. 12:850, 1976.
34. Rickards, D. A.: The feline urethral shunt. Feline Pract. 6:48, 1976.
35. Rickards, D. A., and Hinko, P. J.: Feline urethrostomy: The Cleveland technique. Feline Pract. 4:41, 1974.
36. Robinette, J. D.: Silicone rubber prostheses for replacement of the urethra in male cats. J. Am. Vet. Med. Assoc. 163:285, 1973.
37. Selcer, B. A.: Urinary tract trauma associated with pelvic trauma. J. Am. Anim. Hosp. Assoc. 18:785, 1982.
38. Smith, C. W., and Schiller, A. G.: Perineal urethrostomy in the cat: A retrospective study of complications. J. Am. Anim. Hosp. Assoc. 14:225, 1978.
39. Tarvin, G., Patnaik, A., and Green, R.: Primary urethral tumors in dogs. J. Am. Vet. Med. Assoc. 172:931, 1978.
40. Ticer, J. W., Spencer, C. P., and Ackerman, N.: Positive contrast retrograde urethrography: A useful procedure for evaluating urethral disorders in the dog. Vet. Radiol. 21:2, 1980.
41. Ticer, J. W., Spencer, C. P., and Ackerman, N.: Transitional cell carcinoma of the urethra in four female dogs: Its urographic appearance. Vet. Radiol. 21:12, 1980.
42. Weaver, R. G., and Schulte, J. W.: Experimental and clinical

studies of urethral regeneration. Surg. Gynecol. Obstet. *115*:729, 1962.

43. Wilson, G. P., and Harrison, J. W.: Perineal urethrostomy in cats. J. Am. Vet. Med. Assoc. *159*:1789, 1971.

44. Wilson, G. P., and Kusba, J. K.: Perineal urethrostomy in the cat. *In* Bojrab, M. J. (ed.): *Current Techniques in Small Animal Surgery*, 2nd ed. Lea & Febiger, Philadelphia, 1983, pp. 325–333.

45. Yoshioka, M. M., and Carb, A.: Antepubic urethrostomy in the dog. J. Am. Anim. Hosp. Assoc. *18*:290, 1982.

Chapter **140**

Medical Dissolution and Prevention of Canine Uroliths

Carl A. Osborne, David J. Polzin, and Shehu Abdullahi

The urinary system disposes of waste products in soluble form. However, some waste products are sparingly soluble and occasionally precipitate to form crystals. Urolithiasis may be defined as the formation of calculi from less soluble crystalloids of urine as a result of multiple congenital or acquired physiological and pathological processes. If such crystalloids become trapped in the urinary system, they may grow to sufficient size to cause clinical signs.

Major deficits persist in our understanding of the causes of urolithiasis in animals. However, it appears that the pathophysiology of urolithiasis is similar in all species. Unfortunately, significant differences exist, resulting in an unpredictable risk associated with the formulation of generalities concerning one species on the basis of observations made in another. Pending further studies, application of the following principles to various animal species must be accompanied by appropriate caution.

CHEMICAL AND PHYSICAL CHARACTERISTICS

Summary

Uroliths are crystalline concretions that contain greater than 95 per cent organic or inorganic crystalloids and less than 5 per cent organic matrix (weight versus weight ratio). They may also contain a number of minor constituents. A variety of different types of uroliths may occur in dogs (Table 140–1). Uroliths typically are comprised of organized crystal aggregates with a complex internal structure. Cross sections of uroliths frequently reveal nuclei and laminations and, less frequently, radial striations. This probably reflects the fact that the composition of urine that bathes calculi varies in composition and degree of saturation with calculogenic crystalloids from day to day and perhaps from hour to hour.

Uroliths may be named according to mineral composition (Table 140–2), location (nephroliths, renoliths, ureteroliths, cystoliths, vesical calculi, urethroliths), or shape (smooth, faceted, pyramidal, laminated, mulberry, jackstone, staghorn, and so on).

Mineral Composition

The most common mineral types of calculi encountered in dogs are magnesium ammonium phosphate, ammonium acid urate, and calcium oxalate (monohydrate and dihydrate) (see Table 140–1). Less common types of calculi encountered in dogs include calcium phosphate, silica, sodium acid urate, cystine, carbonate, xanthine, tetracycline, and matrix uroliths. Trace elements including iron, copper, zinc, tin, lead, and aluminum have been identified in human uroliths[54] and may also occur in canine uroliths. Although a particular mineral usually predominates, the mineral composition of calculi is frequently mixed. On occasion the center of a urolith

TABLE 140–1. Quantitative Mineral Analysis of 410 Canine Uroliths*

Mineral	No.	Percentage
Magnesium ammonium phosphate	314	77
Calcium oxalate Monohydrate (19) Dihydrate (3)	22	5
Ammonium acid urate	16	4
Sodium acid urate	3	1
Calcium phosphate	12	3
Cystine	6	1
Silica	3	1
Matrix	2	1
Mixed	32	8

*Analysis performed by Urolithiasis Laboratory, P.O. Box 25375, Houston, TX 77005.

TABLE 140–2.   Crystalline Substances in Uroliths*

Chemical Name	Crystal Name	Formula
Oxalates		
Calcium oxalate monohydrate	Whewellite	$CaC_2O_4 \cdot H_2O$
Calcium oxalate dihydrate	Weddellite	$CaC_2O_4 \cdot 2H_2O$
Phosphates		
β-tricalcium phosphate (calcium orthophosphate)	Whitlockite	$\beta\text{-}Ca_3(PO_4)_2$
Carbonate-apatite	Carbonate-apatite	$Ca_{10}(PO_4 \cdot CO_3 \cdot OH)_6 \ (OH)_2$
Calcium hydrogen phosphate dihydrate	Brushite	$CaHPO_4 \cdot 2H_2O$
Calcium phosphate	Hydroxyapatite	$Ca_{10}(PO_4)_6 \ (OH)_2$
Magnesium ammonium phosphate hexahydrate	Struvite	$MgNH_4 \ PO_4 \cdot 6H_2O$
Magnesium hydrogen phosphate trihydrate†	Newberyite	$MgHPO_4 \cdot 3H_2O$
Uric Acid and Urates		
Anhydrous uric acid	Same	$C_5 \ H_4 \ N_4 \ O_3$
Uric acid dihydrate	Same	$C_5 \ H_4 \ N_4 \ O_3 \cdot 2H_2O$
Ammonium acid urate	Same	$C_5 \ H_3 \ N_4 \ O_3 \cdot NH_4$
Sodium acid urate monohydrate	Same	$C_5 \ H_3 \ N_4 \ O_3 \ Na \cdot H_2O$
Cystine	Same	$(SCH_2CHNH_2COOH)_2$
Silicone Dioxide	Same	$Si \ O_2$
Xanthine	Same	$C_5 \ H_4 \ N_4 \ O_2$

*Reprinted from Kirk, R. W.: *Current Veterinary Therapy, VIII*. W. B. Saunders, Philadelphia, 1983.
†Not a primary constituent; forms as a result of decomposition of struvite.

may be composed of one type of crystalloid (e.g., cystine), whereas outer layers are composed of a different crystalloid (especially struvite).

Matrix Composition

The nondialysable portion of calculi that remains after crystalline components have been dissolved with mild solvents is organic matrix. Calculi consistently contain small quantities of organic matrix substances in addition to crystalloids.[16, 49, 68] Organic matrix substances identified in human uroliths and uroliths experimentally produced in animals include matrix substance A, serum albumin, alpha and gamma globulins, and uromucoid.[49,84] Although calculi composed primarily of matrix have been reported in man and animals (primarily cats), they are uncommon.

In vitro studies using human urine revealed that Tamm-Horsfall protein (uromucoid) is related to the formation of calcium oxalate crystals.[74] On the other hand, heparin (a sulfated glycosaminoglycan) was found to prevent calcium oxalate adhesion to chemically injured rat bladder urothelium.[30]

In summary, organic matrix may affect urolith formation by one or more of several mechanisms providing: (1) a site for heterogeneous nucleation (refer to Etiology and Pathogenesis), (2) a template for organizing and modifying growth of crystals, (3) a binding agent that cements calculi particles together and promotes retention of crystals, and (4) protective colloids that prevent further growth of calculi.[76] Organic matrix could also be a passive substance with no effect on stone formation or growth.

ETIOLOGY AND PATHOGENESIS

Summary

Calculi formation is associated with two phases. The initial step is the formation of a crystal nidus (or crystal embryo). This phase, called *nucleation*, is dependent on supersaturation of urine with calculogenic crystalloids. Growth of the crystal nidus is dependent on (1) its ability to remain in the urinary system, (2) the degree and duration of supersaturation of urine with crystalloids identical or different from that of the nidus, and (3) physical characteristics of the crystal nidus.[13, 69]

Several theories have been proposed to explain the initiation of calculogenesis.

Precipitation-Crystallization Theory. According to this hypothesis, the production of urine excessively saturated with one or more urolith-forming crystalloids leads to spontaneous nucleation of the crystalloid. If nucleated crystalloids are trapped in the urinary system during continued supersaturation, urolith growth occurs. Protein matrix is thought to be nonspecifically incorporated into the urolith as calculus growth proceeds.

Supersaturation of urine with urolith-forming crystalloids may be associated with (1) increased renal excretion of crystalloids as a result of increased glomerular filtration, increased tubular secretion, or decreased tubular reabsorption (e.g., hypercalciuria, hyperuricosuria, hyperoxaluria, cystinuria, and xanthinuria), (2) negative body water balance associated with increased tubular reabsorption of water and subsequent urine concentration (e.g., excessive water loss via other routes, lack of water consumption, and living in a hot, dry climate), and (3) urine pH favoring crystallization (e.g., formation of alkaline urine by urease-producing bacteria, formation of alkaline urine as a result of renal tubular acidosis, and administration of alkalinizing or acidifying drugs).

Matrix-Nucleation Theory. This hypothesis is based on the assumption that preformed organic matrix forms an initial nucleus that subsequently permits urolith growth by precipitation of crystalloids. Opponents of the matrix nucleation theory cite data indicating that uroliths can acquire a large portion of organic matrix by physical absorption during urolith growth.

Crystallization-Inhibition Theory. This theory is based on the fact that urine is a metastable supersaturated solution. Several crystalloids, including calcium, are maintained in solution at concentrations significantly higher than is possible in water. The following substances have been reported to inhibit calcium salt crystallization: (1) organic acids (especially citrates) that form soluble chelates with calcium; (2) magnesium, which is thought to attach nonspecifically to crystal surfaces and thereby interfere with migration of the solute to crystal growth sites; (3) inorganic pyrophosphates (products of intermediary metabolism) that inhibit crystallization of calcium salts; however, the role that pyrophosphates play in the pathogenesis of urolithiasis has not been determined because similar quantities are excreted in normal and urolith-forming human patients; and (4) a variety of other substances, including urea, mucopolysaccharides, and some that are not yet identified.

Irrespective of the theory proposed for nucleation and nidus formation, an essential requirement is supersaturation of urine with a urolith-forming crystalloid. A crystal nidus cannot be formed if urine is undersaturated with the crystalloid in question.

Struvite Uroliths

Struvite uroliths are predominantly composed of magnesium ammonium phosphate (see Table 140–1). Struvite uroliths also have been called MAP (magnesium ammonium phosphate) calculi, phosphate calculi, "infection stones," "urease stones," and triple phosphate stones. Triple phosphate is a misnomer that originated because chemical analyses of uroliths revealed calcium, magnesium, ammonium, and phosphate (three cations and one anion). The name is incorrect, since struvite does not contain calcium. However, struvite uroliths frequently contain calcium phosphate (apatite) and may contain calcium carbonate. Several factors, which may be interrelated, appear to play a role in supersaturation of urine with struvite, including bacterial urinary tract infections, alkaline urine, and genetics. Of these factors, urinary tract infections appear to be most important in dogs.[65]

The solubility of struvite decreases in alkaline urine. Conversion of urea to ammonia as a result of bacterial urease appears to play an important role in causing urine to become supersaturated with magnesium ammonium phosphate as well as with calcium phosphate and carbonate-apatite crystals. Urease produced by bacteria catalyzes the formation of ammonia (NH_3) and carbon dioxide (CO_2) and subsequently carbonate (CO_3). Hydroxyl (OH^-) and ammonium (NF_4^+) ions are produced from the hydrolysis of ammonia. The results of these reactions are (1) alkalinization of urine, (2) increased availability of ammonium ions for formation of struvite crystals, and (3) an increase in the concentration of phosphate ion ($PO_4^=$) because of increased dissociation of phosphorus. Both urea and urease are required for alkalization, supersaturation, and subsequent precipitation of struvite (and apatite) crystals. Because of the importance of urease in the etiology of struvite uroliths, the name "urease stones" has been proposed.[32]

Staphylococci and *Proteus* spp. are both potent urease producers. For reasons that are unexplained, staphylococci are far more commonly associated with struvite uroliths in dogs than *Proteus* spp. (*Proteus* spp. are most commonly associated with struvite uroliths in man).[8, 10, 27, 42, 62, 78, 82] Evaluation of struvite uroliths removed from dogs revealed that staphylococci produce phosphatase in addition to urease[11] Bacterial phosphatase might increase the concentration of inorganic phosphorus by action on organic phosphates. Although other organisms such as *Klebsiella* and *Pseudomonas* spp. have the potential to produce varying quantities of urease, they are not commonly associated with initiation of struvite urolith formation. Likewise, *Escherichia coli* are not associated with initiation of struvite uroliths because they rarely produce urease.[32]

Infection of male or female dogs with ureaseproducing bacteria, primarily staphylococci, precedes the development of struvite uroliths. Struvite uroliths present in infected urine often grow rapidly. In one study, cystic calculi were detected by abdominal survey radiography two to eight weeks following infection of the urinary tract[43] Staphylococci have been cultured from inside canine struvite uroliths, suggesting their presence at the time the uroliths were formed. In contrast, bacteria have been uncommonly cultured from the inside of nonstruvite uroliths. After formation of struvite uroliths as a result of staphylococcal urinary tract infection, the bacterial flora of urine may change. This change may be associated with damage to local host defense mechanisms by uroliths, iatrogenic infection induced by urinary catheters, or administration of antimicrobial agents.

A substantial percentage of dogs with struvite urolithiasis have sterile urine. In some of these cases, however, bacteria have been isolated from the inside of calculi.[62] This observation indicates that bacterial infection of the urinary tract may undergo spontaneous remission after initiating urolith formation in some patients.

On occasion we have encountered dogs in which

urine and the inside of struvite uroliths have been sterile. The urine pH of these patients is frequently alkaline. The significance of these observations and their relationship to struvite uroliths initiated by bacterial infections is unknown. However, detection of a persistently high urine pH not explained by infection or medication is suggestive of renal tubular acidosis or consumption of a diet with reduced production of acid catabolites.

In contrast to struvite uroliths, bacterial infection of the urinary tract is not a consistent finding in dogs with nonstruvite uroliths. When infection does occur, it is a sequela rather than a predisposing cause of urolith formation.[8] If by chance staphylococci are the cause of the secondary urinary tract infection, however, layers of struvite may form around a nucleus composed of the nonstruvite (metabolic) calculus.

Urate Uroliths

Applied Biochemistry

Uric acid is the end product of purine metabolism in man.[20, 21, 29] In dogs, uric acid is further oxidized by the hepatic enzyme uricase to form allantoin. Uric acid is a weak acid that in undissociated freeform has limited solubility in urine (especially acid urine). In contrast, the salt of uric acid (sodium urate) and allantoin are much more soluble in urine.

Ammonium Acid Urate Uroliths In Dogs

Ammonium acid urate uroliths are far more common than uric acid stones in dogs.[71, 72] Although a high incidence of urate uroliths is seen in Dalmatians, they have also been detected in several other breeds and in cats. Urate uroliths have been more commonly reported in males than females.

Urate salts form lyophobic gels when they become supersaturated in urine. Ammonium ion, and to a lesser degree hydrogen ion, appears to be important in the flocculation of ammonium urate. In one study, acid urine was not commonly observed in stone-forming Dalmatians.[72] In contrast to uric acid, which becomes more soluble as urine pH becomes more alkaline, ammonium urate becomes less soluble in alkaline urine associated with increased ammonium concentration. This logically explains the common finding of phosphates in urate uroliths.

Ammonium ion appears to be more important in canine urate urolithiasis, whereas hydrogen ion appears to be more important in uric acid urolithiasis in man.

Ammonium Acid Urate Uroliths In Dalmatians

The definitive cause of urate urolith formation in Dalmatians is unknown. However, increased urate excretion is a predisposing factor rather than a primary cause. Whereas all Dalmatians excrete relatively high quantities of urate in their urine, only a small percentage form urate stones. In addition, stone-forming Dalmatians do not excrete greater quantities of urate in their urine than nonstone-forming Dalmatians. These observations indicate that other factors influence urate urolith formation.

The ability of Dalmatians to oxidize uric acid to allantoin is intermediate between that of humans and non-Dalmatian dogs. Humans have a serum uric acid concentration of approximately 3 to 7 mg/dl and excrete approximately 500 to 700 mg of uric acid in their urine per day. Non-Dalmatian dogs have a serum uric acid concentration of less than 0.5 mg/dl and excrete approximately 10 to 60 mg of uric acid in their urine per day. Dalmatians have a serum uric acid concentration two to four times that of non-Dalmatians and excrete approximately 400 to 600 mg of uric acid in their urine per day.

Studies of the fate of uric acid in Dalmatians have revealed that they have unique hepatic and renal pathways of uric acid metabolism. Of these two sites of unique purine metabolism, reciprocal allogenic renal and hepatic transplantations between Dalmatians and non-Dalmatians indicate that the hepatic mechanism is quantitatively the most significant.[2, 15, 45] Their liver does not completely oxidize available uric acid, even though it contains a sufficient concentration of urease to do so. Compared with non-Dalmatians, they convert uric acid to allantoin at a reduced rate. It has been hypothesized that hepatic cellular membranes are partially impermeable to uric acid.

The proximal renal tubules of Dalmatians re-absorb less uric acid than those of non-Dalmatians; a small amount is secreted by the distal tubules. In non-Dalmatian dogs, 98 to 100 per cent of the uric acid in glomerular filtrate is re-absorbed by the proximal tubules and returned to the liver for further metabolism. Uric acid present in the urine of non-Dalmatians is thought to be secreted by the distal tubules.

Portal Vascular Anomalies

A high prevalence of ammonium urate stones has also been observed in dogs with portal vascular anomalies.[50] The predisposition of dogs with portal vascular anomalies to develop ammonium urate uroliths probably is associated with concomitant elevations of ammonia and uric acid in blood and urine.

Cystinuria and Cystine Uroliths

Summary

Cystinuria is an inborn error of metabolism characterized by abnormal transport of cystine (a nonessential, sulfur-containing amino acid composed of two molecules of cysteine)[2] and other amino acids by the renal tubules. Cystine is normally present in low concentrations in plasma. Normally, circulating cystine is freely filtered at the glomerulus and most is actively re-absorbed in the proximal tubules. The solubility of cystine in urine is pH dependent. It is relatively insoluble in acid urine but becomes more soluble in alkaline urine. In dogs, the solubility of cystine at a urine pH of 7.8 has been reported to be approximately double that of a pH of 5.0.[81]

Canine Cystinuria

In dogs with cystinuria the exact pattern of amino aciduria reported by various investigators has varied.[11, 17, 18] Bovee and colleagues identified two populations of cystinuric dogs.[4, 5, 6] One group had cystinuria without loss of other amino acids, and the other had cystinuria and a lesser degree of lysinuria.

The exact mechanism of abnormal renal tubular transport of cystine in dogs is unknown. Plasma concentration of cystine in affected dogs is normal, indicating faulty tubular function rather than hyperexcretion.[4, 5] Plasma methionine has been found to be elevated in cystinuric dogs.[6]

Unless protein intake is severely restricted, cystinuric dogs have no detectable abnormalities of amino acid loss with the exception of formation of cystine uroliths. This is related to the fact that cystine is sparingly soluble at the usual urine pH range of 5.5 to 7.0. Cystinuria would probably be a medical curiosity if cystine were not the least soluble naturally occurring amino acid. The major causes of morbidity and mortality associated with this disorder are the sequelae of urolith formation.

The exact mechanism of cystine urolith formation is unknown. Since not all cystinuric dogs form uroliths, cystinuria is a predisposing factor rather than the primary cause of cystine urolith formation. In one study, 4 of 14 dogs with a history of cystine urolith formation had urine cystine concentrations that fell within the range of control dogs.[5] Many breeds have been reported to develop cystine uroliths, especially dachshunds.[62] With one exception, cystine uroliths have only been reported in male dogs[8] However, cystinuria has been observed in female dogs.[4] This observation suggests that lack of detection of cystine calculi in females may be related to the passage of small calculi through their relatively short, wide, and distensible urethra.

Calcium Oxalate Uroliths

Oxalate is a salt of oxalic acid. In man and animals, oxalate is a nonessential end product of metabolism and is excreted unchanged in urine. Oxalic acid is usually synthesized in small quantities from glyoxylic acid (which may be derived from glycine) and ascorbic acid. Oxalic acid is also commonly found in green leafy vegetables, including rhubarb, spinach, celery, and cabbage. Oxalic acid is poorly absorbed from the gastrointestinal tract, however, and under normal conditions does not contribute significantly to urinary oxalate. In man most of the oxalic acid excreted in urine is produced endogenously by the liver.[53]

Following excretion in urine, oxalic acid combines with calcium to form an insoluble salt of calcium oxalate. The specific conditions that govern crystallization of calcium oxalate (whewellite and weddellite) remain undetermined. Urine pH within physiological range (4.5 to 8.0) does not appear to affect the solubility of calcium oxalate significantly. Factors incriminated in the pathogenesis of calcium oxalate urolithiasis include hypercalciuria, hyperoxaluria, and hyperuricosuria.[63]

The reason for the high incidence of calcium oxalate uroliths in man and the comparatively low incidence of these uroliths in dogs and cats is unknown. However, differences may be related in part to veterinary use of insensitive qualitative urolith analysis kits to detect calcium.

Silica Uroliths

During recent years silica uroliths have been encountered with increased frequency in the urinary tract of dogs in the United States.[61] Perusal of the literature revealed a conspicuous absence of these calculi in dogs prior to 1976.[8, 62] Since that time we have had the opportunity to evaluate silica uroliths removed from the urinary bladder or urethra of 83 dogs. All geographic areas were represented. Twenty-five of 83 affected dogs were German shepherds; the remainder were of 26 different breeds.[61]

For undetermined reasons, 81 dogs in our series were males, whereas only two were females. Silica uroliths were detected in a high percentage (125 of 241) of native Kenyan dogs.[7] Both males and females were affected.

Most silica uroliths have a characteristic jackstone appearance.[61] Not all silica uroliths had a jackstone configuration, however, and not all jackstones are composed of silica.

Silica uroliths are not associated with characteristic crystals in urine sediment, presumably because they are composed of amorphous silica. There has been no obvious relationship between the occurrence of silica uroliths and urine pH.

The following observations prompt the hypothesis that development of silica uroliths may be related to diet: (1) Silica uroliths developed in male dogs fed experimental diets containing a high concentration of silicic acid for several months.[51] Elimination of silicic acid from the diet prevented further urolith development. (2) It was hypothesized that the high incidence of silica uroliths in native Kenyan dogs might be related to consumption of corn, a common ingredient in their diet.[7] (3) Silica is rapidly cleared by the kidneys from the plasma of dogs and other animals following absorption into the body.[3, 41] Silica uroliths are common in range cattle and sheep consuming forage grasses with a high concentration of silica.[83]

(4) Silica uroliths have been experimentally produced in rats fed diets containing a large quantity of tetra-ethylorthosilicate.[25] (5) Silica uroliths have been reported in humans consuming large quantities of magnesium trisilicate to alleviate signs of peptic ulcer.[39, 40] Whether or not change in the formulation of diets is associated with silica uroliths in dogs in the United States remains to be determined. The 83 affected dogs in the study mentioned previously were consuming a large variety of commercially manufactured moist and dry foods in addition to home-made diets.

Calcium Phosphate Uroliths

Calcium phosphate uroliths are commonly called apatite uroliths. The most common forms of calcium phosphate observed in uroliths are hydroxyapatite and carbonate-apatite (see Table 140–2). With the exception of brushite, calcium phosphates are least soluble in alkaline urine. In addition to hydrogen ion concentration, calcium phosphate solubility is influenced by calcium ion concentration and total inorganic phosphate concentration.[24]

Calcium phosphate is commonly found as a minor component of struvite and calcium oxalate uroliths. However, uroliths composed primarily of calcium phosphate are uncommon in dogs and man. When present, they usually occur in association with metabolic disorders such as primary hyperparathyroidism, renal tubular acidosis, and excessive dietary calcium and phosphorus.

DIAGNOSIS

Summary

Uroliths are usually suspected on the basis of typical findings obtained by history and physical examination. Urinalyses, urine culture, and radiography may be required to eliminate urinary tract infection, diverticula of the bladder, inflammatory polyps, and neoplasia as possible diagnoses.

A variety of methods have been used to determine the composition of uroliths including gross appearance, crystalluria, radiographic appearance, qualitative analysis, quantitative analysis, and urolith culture. Of these, quantitative analysis provides the most definitive diagnostic, prognostic, and therapeutic information.

Radiographic Characteristics

The primary objective of radiographic evaluation of patients suspected of having uroliths is to determine the site, number, density, and shape of calculi. Once urolithiasis has been confirmed, radiographic evaluation also is an important technique to detect predisposing abnormalities.

TABLE 140–3. Radiographic Characteristics of Common Canine and Feline Uroliths*

Mineral Type	Degree of Radiopacity	Shape
Cystine	+ to + +	Smooth; usually small; round to oval
Oxalate	+ + + +	Usually rough; round to oval
Phosphate (struvite)	+ + to + + + +	Smooth; round or faceted; sometimes assume shape of renal pelvis, ureter, bladder, or urethra; sometimes laminated
Phosphate (apatite)	+ + + +	Smooth; round or faceted
Urate	0 to + +	Smooth; round or oval; sometimes jackstone
Silica	+ + to + + + +	Typically jackstone

*Reprinted from Kirk, R. W.: *Current Veterinary Therapy VIII.* W. B. Saunders, Philadelphia, 1983.

The radiographic appearance of uroliths is dependent on their size and mineral composition. Very small calculi may not be visible. Most canine and feline uroliths have varying degrees of radiodensity and can be detected by survey abdominal radiography (Table 140–3). Oxalate, phosphate, and silica calculi are typically, but not invariably, more radiodense than cystine and urate calculi. This may be related to their calcium content. Urate uroliths may be radiolucent but usually are radiodense. Because of significant variation, the radiodensity of uroliths is not a reliable index of mineral composition.

Uroliths must be differentiated from (1) nephrocalcinosis associated with dystrophic or metastatic calcification of the renal parenchyma, (2) radiodense medications or ingesta in the gastrointestinal system, (3) calcified mesenteric lymph nodes, (4) osseous metaplasia of transitional epithelium or mineralization of a neoplasm, (5) radiodensities in the gallbladder (uncommon in dogs and cats), and (6) large thelia in female dogs. Calcifications of the renal parenchyma are typically near, but not within, the renal pelvis. Radiodense calculi within the excretory pathway may disappear or become radiolucent following excretion of radiopaque contrast agents. Radiodense objects outside the excretory pathway remain radiodense.

In our experience, radiolucent uroliths are very uncommon in dogs. Uric acid uroliths of man are typically radiolucent. However, in our experience, most (but not all) ammonium acid urate uroliths of dogs are radiodense. This may be related to the presence of a variable quantity of phosphates in urate uroliths of dogs. Matrix uroliths may be radiolucent. They have not been commonly recognized in dogs. Blood clots may be mistaken for radiolucent uroliths.

Calculi that appear radiodense by survey radiography may be radiolucent when evaluated by positive contrast radiography. This is related to that fact that many calculi are more radiodense than body tissue but less dense than the contrast material. A diagnosis of radiolucent stones should be based on their radiodensity compared with body tissues, not positive contrast material.

Following removal of uroliths, compare the number removed with the number detected by radiography. If the numbers of calculi determined by radiography are too numerous to count, postsurgical radiography is indicated to detect uroliths that have been inadvertently allowed to remain in the urinary tract (so-called pseudo recurrence). Immediate detection of calculi remaining in the urinary tract following surgery is important, since it has prognostic significance. If uroliths inadvertently missed during surgery performed to remove them are not detected for several weeks following surgery, it may be erroneously assumed that the patient is highly predisposed to recurrent urolithiasis.

Analysis of Calculi

Record the location of the uroliths removed from the urinary tract in addition to their size, shape, color, and consistency. Save all uroliths in a container (preferably a sterile one) for future analysis. Do not give them to owners. One or more uroliths may be placed into a container of 10 per cent buffered formalin if microscopic examination is desired.

Because many uroliths contain more than one mineral component, it is important to examine representative portions of them. The mineral composition of crystalline nuclei may be identical or different from that of the remainder of calculi. The nuclei of uroliths should be analyzed separately from outer zones when possible, since the underlying cause of its presence may be suggested by knowledge of the mineral composition of the nuclei.

Qualitative Analysis

We do not recommend analysis of uroliths by single qualitative chemical analysis. The major disadvantage of this procedure is that only some of the chemical radicals and ions can be detected. In addition, the proportion of the different chemical constitutents in the urolith cannot be quantified. One kit commonly used by veterinarians and veterinary laboratories is the Oxford Stone Analysis set.* In our hands, this chemical kit is unreliable in accurate detection of the composition of uroliths. It is not designed to detect infrequently occurring uroliths, including those composed of silica or xanthine. The kit is also unreliable in consistently detecting calcium in calculi and provides false positive results.

Quantitative Analysis

In contrast to chemical methods of analysis, physical methods have proved to be far superior in identification of crystalline substances. They also permit differentiation of various subgroups of minerals (i.e., calcium oxalate monohydrate and calcium oxalate dihydrate, or uric acid and ammonium acid urate) and allow semiquantitative determinations of various mineral components. Physical methods commonly used by laboratories in the United States that specialize in quantitative urolith analysis* include a combination of polarizing light microscopy, x-ray diffractometry, infrared spectroscopy, and thermogravimetry. Some laboratories are also equipped to perform elemental analysis with an energy dispersive–type x-ray microanalyzer (EDX). On occasion chemical methods of analysis and paper chromatography may be used to supplement information provided by the physical methods previously mentioned.

Caution must be used to avoid irrevocable loss of uroliths by unreliable qualitative chemical studies. If qualitative studies are performed, representative uroliths should be saved for subsequent quantitative analysis. Although the cost of routine quantitative urolith analysis is about double that of routine qualitative analysis (approximately $10 versus $20), it is minute compared with the costs of mismanagement based on erroneous results.

MEDICAL DISSOLUTION OF UROLITHS

Summary

Therapy of urolithiasis encompasses (1) surgical or nonsurgical relief of obstruction to urine outflow when necessary,[7, 70, 79] (2) elimination of existing calculi, (3) eradication or control of predisposing causes,[62] (4) eradication or control of urinary tract infections,[42] and (5) prevention of recurrence of uroliths.

As with selection of all forms of therapy, cautious and careful judgement is in order. The unpredictable and erratic rate at which canine uroliths form, grow, recur following removal, and undergo dissolution suggests that carefully designed and controlled experimental trials are mandatory before a particular regimen of therapy is judged to be of benefit. The following recommendations should not be used as a standardized approach to treatment, since no two patients have identical therapeutic needs. Within the guidelines outlined herein, individual therapy is essential.

---

*Oxford Laboratories, 107 North Bayshore Blvd., San Mateo, CA 94401.

*Urolithiasis Laboratory, P.O. Box 25375, Houston TX 77055. Veterinary Teaching Hospital, School of Veterinary Medicine, University of California, Davis, CA 95616.

Indications

Although surgery has been an effective and time-honored method of urolith removal, it is associated with several limitations, including (1) persistence of underlying causes and recurrence of uroliths despite surgery, (2) factors that enhance adverse consequences of general anesthesia or surgery, and (3) inability to remove all calculi or calculi fragments during surgery. In addition, situations occasionally arise in which owners will not consent to surgical therapy but will consider medical therapy. For these and other reasons, an effective noninvasive medical regimen that will induce urolith dissolution has been a desired but elusive goal. However, recent results of several experimental and clinical investigations support the feasibility of medical dissolution of uroliths, especially canine struvite uroliths.[44, 58, 60, 65] Results of human studies suggest the feasibility of medical dissolution of cystine uroliths.[75] Attempts to induce dissolution of human and canine calcium oxalate uroliths have been unrewarding.

Objectives

The objectives of medical management of uroliths are to arrest further urolith growth or promote urolith dissolution by correcting or controlling underlying abnormalities. For therapy to be effective it must induce undersaturation of urine with calculogenic crystalloids by (1) increasing the solubility of crystalloids in urine, (2) increasing the volume of urine in which crystalloids are dissolved or suspended, and (3) reducing the quantity of calculogenic crystalloids in urine. For example, attempts to increase the solubility of crystalloids in urine often include administration of medications to change urine pH in an effort to create a less favorable environment for crystallization. Likewise, induction of diuresis is a time-honored method of increasing the volume of urine in which crystalloids are dissolved or suspended. Examples of methods used to reduce the quantity of calculogenic crystalloids in urine include changes in diet, administration of allopurinol to decrease the formation of uric acid, and administration of cellulose phosphate to minimize intestinal absorption of calcium.

These objectives may be hampered because the underlying causes, and therefore the treatment, of different types of uroliths are dissimilar. They may also be hampered by uroliths that are not homogeneous in composition. This has not been a problem in dogs with uroliths composed primarily of magnesium ammonium phosphate with lesser degrees of calcium phosphate, because the solubility characteristics of the two minerals are similar. However, it is logical to expect difficulty in inducing dissolution of a urolith with a nucleus of cystine and a shell of struvite because the solubility characteristics of these two minerals are dissimilar. This phenomenon should be considered if medical therapy seems to become ineffective after initially reducing the size of a urolith.

Increasing Urine Volume

Diuresis induced by augmenting water consumption is a logical way to decrease the urine concentration of calculogenic substances. Depending on the size of the patient, the quantity of urine produced, the status of the cardiovascular system, and the composition of their diet, we recommend oral administration of 0.5 to 10 grams of sodium chloride per day to stimulate thirst. CAUTION: additional salt should not be given to patients being fed calculolytic diets that have already been supplemented with sodium chloride.

It is mandatory to the success of this procedure that drinking water be available at all times. Alternatively, water, gravy, or other liquids may be mashed into the food.

The effectiveness of diuresis in medical dissolution or prevention of uroliths appears to be directly proportional to the volume of urine formed and eliminated. A satisfactory compensatory increase in urine volume is indicated by formation of urine with a specific gravity of less than 1.020.

Definition of Urolith Composition

With the exception of diuresis, therapy to reduce the composition of specific calculogenic crystalloids in urine depends on knowledge of the composition of uroliths. For example, the administration of d-penicillamine would be of no benefit in patients with calcium oxalate uroliths. Likewise, administration of ascorbic acid, a commonly used acidifier, might potentiate calcium oxalate urolithiasis since it is a precursor of oxalic acid. In situations in which consideration is being given to medical therapy but uroliths that have been surgically removed are not available for analysis, one may be forced to make an educated guess about their composition (Table 140–4).

Struvite Urolithiasis

Summary

Experimental and clinical studies of canine struvite urolithiasis have confirmed the feasibility of inducing dissolution by medical therapy.[44, 58, 60, 65] Current recommendations include the following.

Eradication or Control of Urinary Tract Infections. Sterilization of urine appears to be an extremely important prerequisite in creating a state of struvite undersaturation that may prevent further growth of uroliths or promote their dissolution.

Appropriate antimicrobial agents selected on the basis of susceptibility or minimum inhibitory concen-

TABLE 140–4. Factors That May Aid in Estimation of Mineral Composition of Uroliths*

Radiographic density and physical characteristics of uroliths (see Table 140–3)

Urine pH
  Struvite and apatite uroliths: usually alkaline
  Ammonium urate uroliths: variable
  Cystine uroliths: acid
  Calcium oxalate uroliths: variable
  Silica uroliths: variable

Identification of crystals in urine sediment

Type of bacteria, if any, isolated from urine
  Urease-producing bacteria, especially staphylococci, are commonly associated with struvite uroliths
  Urinary tract infections often are absent in patients with calcium oxalate, cystine, ammonium urate, and silica uroliths
  Calcium oxalate, cystine, ammonium urate, and silica uroliths may predispose patients to urinary tract infections; if infections are caused by urease-producing bacteria, struvite may precipitate around them

Serum chemistry evaluation
  Hypercalcemia may be associated with calcium-containing uroliths
  Hyperuricemia may be associated with urate uroliths

Breed of dog and history of occurrence of uroliths in patient's ancestors or littermates

Analysis of uroliths fortuitously passed and collected during micturition

*Reprinted from Kirk, R. W.: *Current Veterinary Therapy VIII*. W. B. Saunders, Philadelphia, 1983.

---

tration tests should be used at therapeutic dosages. Higher dosage ranges should be considered, since forced diuresis may reduce the concentration of antimicrobial agents in urine.

Antimicrobial agents should be administered as long as the uroliths can be identified by survey radiography. This recommendation is based on the fact that bacterial pathogens harbored inside calculi may be protected from the effects of antimicrobial agents. Whereas the urine and surface of calculi may be sterilized following appropriate antimicrobial therapy, the original infecting organisms may remain viable below the surface of the urolith. Discontinuation of antimicrobial therapy may result in relapse of bacteriuria and infection.

Although the use of antimicrobial agents alone may result in dissolution of struvite uroliths in some patients, experimental studies in rats[46] and clinical studies in humans and dogs have revealed that this phenomenon represents the exception rather than the rule. In addition, the time required to induce urolith dissolutions is usually measured in months rather than weeks.

Calculolytic Diets. Experimental and clinical studies in man and dogs revealed that inhibition of bacterial urease with a urease inhibitor was effective in inhibiting struvite urolith growth and in some instances induced struvite urolith dissolution. This led to the hypothesis that reduction of the urine concentration of urea (the substrate of urease) would provide similar results.[58, 60] To test this hypothesis, a calculolytic diet* was formulated that contained a reduced quantity of high-quality protein (1.6 per cent) and reduced quantities of phosphorus (0.048 per cent) and magnesium (0.006 per cent). The diet was supplemented with salt to stimulate thirst and induce compensatory polyuria. Reduction in the hepatic production of urea from dietary protein was hypothesized to reduce medullary urea solute concentration and further contribute to diuresis. This calculolytic diet was found to be highly effective in inducing struvite urolith dissolution in five of six experimental dogs despite persistent infection with urease-producing bacteria. The uroliths underwent dissolution in about 3.5 months (range 8 to 20 weeks). The urolith in the remaining dog decreased to less than one-half its pretreatment size at the termination of the study, six months following initiation of dietary therapy. Urinary tract infections persisted in these dogs until the uroliths dissolved, at which time they underwent remission in three dogs. In the corresponding control group fed a popular maintenance diet (10 per cent protein, 0.19 per cent phosphorus, and 0.06 per cent magnesium), calculi increased in size by a mean of 5.5 times their pretreatment size (range 3 to 8 ×). A urolith developed in the renal pelvis of one of these dogs. Urinary tract infections persisted in control dogs throughout the six-month study.

In a related experimental study of sterile struvite uroliths, consumption of the calculolytic diet induced urolith dissolution in a mean of 3.3 weeks (range 2 to 4 weeks). In a corresponding control group fed a maintenance diet, four uroliths dissolved over a mean period of 14 weeks (range 2 to 5 months). In the remaining two control dogs, the uroliths were one-fifth of their initial size at the termination of the study.

When a combination of calculolytic diet and antimicrobial agents was given to dogs with naturally occurring urease-positive urinary tract infections and uroliths presumed to be composed of struvite, similar results were obtained.[60] Likewise, use of a calculolytic diet to induce dissolution of uroliths presumed to be struvite in nine dogs without urinary tract infection has also been extremely effective. A combination of calculolytic diet, antimicrobial agent, and acetohydroxamic acid given to dogs with experimentally induced staphylococcal urinary tract infection and struvite urolithiasis induced stone dissolution in six weeks.

Because calculolytic diets stimulate thirst and promote diuresis, owners should be informed that dogs with uroliths located in the urinary bladder may develop pollakiuria for a variable time following initiation of dietary therapy. The pollakiuria will usually subside as the infection is controlled and the uroliths decrease in size.

---

*S/D, Hills, Division, Riviana Foods, Inc., Topeka, KS.

Consumption of calculolytic diets by dogs with experimentally induced staphylococcal urinary tract infection and struvite uroliths was associated with a marked reduction in the serum concentration of urea nitrogen (baseline 21.8 mg/dl ± 2.9; posttreatment 3.5 mg/dl ± 2.4) and mild reductions in the serum concentrations of magnesium (baseline 2.2 mg/dl ± 0.2; posttreatment 1.8 mg/dl ± 0.2), phosphorus (baseline 4.6 mg/dl ± 0.6; posttreatment 3.8 mg/dl ± 0.8), and albumin (baseline 3.1 gm/dl; posttreatment 2.1 gm/dl ±0.3). A mild increase in the serum activity of hepatic alkaline phosphatase isoenzyme (baseline 31.8 mμ/ml ± 1.50; posttreatment 147.7 mμ/ml ± 48.1) was also observed. These alterations in serum chemistry values were of no detectable clinical consequence during six-month experimental studies or during clinical studies. They have been used during clinical studies as one index of client compliance with dietary recommendations.

Diuresis. As mentioned previously, diuresis induced by augmenting water consumption appears to be a logical way to decrease the urine concentration of struvite and other calculogenic substances. However, additional salt is not recommended for dogs fed the calculolytic diet previously described because it has been formulated to contain supplemental sodium chloride. The mean urine specific gravity value of dogs fed the calulolytic diet was 1.008 ± 0.003 compared with a baseline value of 1.028 ± 0.01. The mean 24-hour urine volume of dogs fed the calculolytic diet was 549 ml ± 223 ml compared with a baseline value of 352 ml ± 107 ml.

Acidification of Urine. Because acidification of urine dramatically increases the solubility of struvite, it is an important therapeutic goal in the medical management of struvite urolithiasis. Since dogs fed the calculolytic diet develop aciduria, however, supplemental urine acidifiers are not recommended. The mean urine pH of dogs with staphylococcal urinary tract infections fed the calculolytic diet was 6.2 ± 0.7 compared with a baseline value of 7.6 ± 0.5.

If urine acidifiers such as DL-menthionine or ammonium chloride are deemed appropriate, they must be selected and administered with appropriate caution.[64] The dosage of urine acidifiers should be adjusted for each patient on the basis of urine pH. The pH of urine obtained a few hours following eating is most likely to be altered by the postprandial alkaline tide. If postprandial urine is acidic, therapy is likely to be effective. The most reliable data, however, are obtained by periodically monitoring urine pH throughout the day. Ideally, urine acidifiers should be administered three to four times per day to maintain a consistent acidic environment in the urinary tract.

Urinary acidifiers may be ineffective in some patients with urinary tract infections caused by urease-producing bacteria (*Proteus* spp., staphylococci, and so on) because therapeutic dosages may be insufficient to overcome the continuous production of ammonia by bacterial urease. Combination therapy with appropriate antimicrobial agents is recommended.

Acidifiers should not be administered to uremic animals, since they will aggravate the severity of metabolic acidosis typically associated with renal failure.

Urease Inhibitors. Studies of a urease inhibitor, acetohydroxamic acid (AHA),* in dogs with infection-induced struvite urolithiasis indicate that the drug is of value in the medical management of this disorder. AHA is rapidly and completely absorbed from the gastrointestinal tract of dogs and is excreted and concentrated in urine. When given orally at pharmacological doses, AHA retards the alkalinization of urine caused by the growth of urease-producing bacteria. Its urease-inhibiting activity is effective at a urine pH of between five and nine but is most effective at pH 7. AHA appears to have a dose-related bacteriostatic effect against gram-positive and gram-negative bacteria and may potentiate the antimicrobial effect of antibiotics.[44]

Experimental studies performed at the University of Minnesota revealed that struvite uroliths experimentally induced in dogs were prevented from undergoing further growth, or underwent dissolution, following oral administration of AHA at a dosage of 100 mg/kg/day divided into two doses.[44] The dogs had normal renal function. Unfortunately, administration of the drug at a dosage (100 mg/kg/day) sufficient to induce dissolution of uroliths resulted in a mild hemolytic anemia (mean PCV = 37 per cent compared with pretreatment value of 47 per cent). The anemia rapidly underwent amelioration when the daily dosage of AHA was reduced from 100 to 25 mg/kg. Although urolith growth was retarded at this dosage, they did not dissolve. Similar results were obtained when AHA was administered at a daily dosage of 50 and 75 mg/kg. Studies to evaluate the efficacy of AHA in causing stone dissolution when combined with antimicrobial agents or calculolytic diets have revealed that these combinations substantially reduce the time required to cause litholysis.

Monitoring Response to Medical Therapy. The size of uroliths should be periodically monitored by survey radiography. We recommend radiography at monthly intervals. Survey radiography is preferable to retrograde contrast radiography to monitor urolith dissolution, because the use of catheters during retrograde radiographic studies may result in iatrogenic urinary tract infection. Alternatively, intravenous urography may be considered.

Periodic evaluation of urine sediment for crystalluria may also be considered. Struvite crystals should not form if therapy has been effective in promoting formation of urine that is undersaturated with magnesium ammonium phosphate.

Urine collected by cystocentesis should be quantitatively cultured during therapy and five to seven

---

*Urostat, Mission Pharmaceutical Company, San Antonio, TX

days following discontinuation of antimicrobial therapy. It is emphasized that the results of urine culture may not be the same as those obtained prior to therapy or from cultures of the inside of uroliths. Rapid recurrence of urinary tract infection caused by the same type of organism (relapse) or a different type of bacterial pathogen (re-infection) following withdrawal of antimicrobial therapy may indicate residual calculi within the urinary tract or other abnormalities in local host defense mechanisms that predisposed to urinary tract infection and subsequent urolithiasis.

In patients with urinary tract infections without concomitant uroliths, persistence of bacteriuria during antimicrobial therapy suggests infection with a resistant organism.[42] In our experience with treatment of naturally occurring and experimentally induced infection-related struvite uroliths of dogs, however, it has been difficult to eradicate bacteriuria with antimicrobial agents in some patients. In this situation, we hypothesize that concomitant induction of diuresis with calculolytic diets may have impaired the natural antimicrobial activity of urine[66] or reduced the concentration of antimicrobial agents in urine. Despite persistent bacteriuria during antimicrobial and dietary treatment of infected patients with struvite uroliths, however, we have had excellent success in inducing urolith dissolution. As previously discussed, concomitant use of calculolytic diets, antimicrobial agents, and AHA in this situation provided the most effective method of inducing urolith dissolution.

In our experience with naturally occurring struvite uroliths, use of the regimen described herein has induced urolith dissolution in as short a period as two weeks. In one miniature schnauzer with bladder uroliths estimated to be in excess of 100, complete dissolution induced with calculolytic diet and antimicrobial agents required seven months (Fig. 140–1).

Since small uroliths may escape detection by survey radiography, we recommend that the calculolytic diet and (if necessary) antimicrobial agents be continued for at least one month following radiographic documentation of urolith dissolution.

If uroliths increase in size during therapy or do not begin to decrease in size after approximately eight weeks of appropriate medical therapy, alternative methods of management should be considered. Small uroliths that become lodged in the urethra of male or female dogs during therapy may be readily returned to the urinary bladder lumen by urohydropropulsion.[50, 70] Complete obstruction of a ureter or renal pelvis, especially in the face of concomitant urinary tract infection, is an absolute indication for surgical intervention.

Difficulty in inducing complete dissolution of uroliths by creating urine that is undersaturated with the suspected calculogenic crystalloid should prompt consideration that (1) the wrong mineral component was identified, (2) the nucleus of the urolith is of

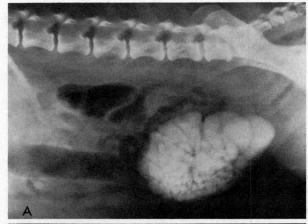

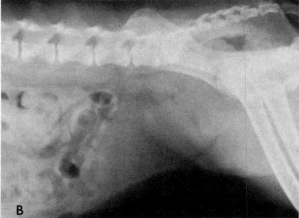

Figure 140–1. A, Lateral survey abdominal radiograph of the abdomen of a two-year-old female miniature schnauzer with urease-positive staphylococcal urinary tract infection and urolithiasis. B, Seven months following initiation of therapy with a calculolytic diet and orally administered ampicillin.

different mineral composition than outer portions of the urolith, and (3) the owner or the patient is not complying with therapeutic recommendations.

Medical Versus Surgical Management. Despite the development of effective medical regimens to induce dissolution of struvite uroliths in dogs, surgical intervention will continue to play a role in some patients. Surgical candidates include those with obstruction to urine outflow that cannot be corrected by nonsurgical techniques, those with renal calculi located in the kidneys without adequate function, and those with anatomical defects of the urogenital tract that predispose to urinary tract infection. Eradication or control of infections of the urinary tract with urease-producing bacteria is the most important factor in preventing recurrence of most struvite uroliths. Development of urinary tract infections is dependent on the balance between infectious agents (analogous to seeds) and host resistance (analogous to soil). In order for microbial "seeds" to grow, a suitable "soil" must be present. Although pathogenic bacteria must gain access to the urinary tract to induce infection, entrance of bacteria into the urinary tract is not synonymous with infection. Current evidence indicates that host defense mechanisms must be transiently or persistently abnormal for bacterial colonization of the urinary tract to occur. Although antimicrobial agents remain the cornerstone of therapy, the status of host defense mechanisms appears to be the most important factor in the pathogenesis of urinary tract infections. Permanent eradication of infection is often impossible unless the abnormality in host defense mechanisms is identified and eliminated. Examples of surgical disorders that predispose to urinary tract infections by altering local host defense mechanisms include diverticulae of the bladder, strictures that impede urine outflow, metabolic uroliths (silica, ammonium urate, calcium oxalate, and so on) that damage the mucosal lining of the urinary tract, and benign or malignant neoplasms that damage the mucosal lining or impede urine outflow.

Summary of Recommendations for Medical Dissolution of Struvite Uroliths

The following recommendations apply to adult dogs with urinary tract infections and suspected struvite uroliths.

1. Eradicate or control urinary tract infections with appropriate antimicrobial therapy. Maintain antimicrobial therapy during and for four weeks following urolith dissolution.

2. Initiate therapy with calculolytic diets. No other food or mineral supplements should be fed to the patient. Compliance with dietary recommendations is suggested by a reduction in the serum concentration of urea nitrogen (usually below 10 mg/dl. Maintain affected animals on the diet for one month following disappearance of uroliths as detected by survey radiography. Avoid retrograde radiographic studies requiring catheterization.

3. Induce diuresis only if polyuria does not occur while the patient is consuming the calculolytic diet.

4. Administer AHA (25 mg/kg per day divided into two doses) to patients with persistent urease-producing bacteriuria despite use of antimicrobial agents and calculolytic diets.

The following recommendations pertain to adult dogs with sterile uroliths presumed to be struvite.

1. Follow the same procedure recommended for dogs with concomitant urinary tract infections and uroliths but do not administer antimicrobial agents or AHA.

2. Periodically culture urine samples obtained by cystocentesis to detect secondary bacterial urinary tract infections. If they develop, eradicate them with appropriate antimicrobial agents.

For immature dogs with struvite uroliths use caution in consideration of the use of calculolytic diets since they have not been extensively evaluated in normal growing pups or in immature dogs with struvite urolithiasis. Although it is likely that they would induce struvite urolith dissolution, if consumed for prolonged periods these low-protein diets

would probably impair normal growth. We were able to induce dissolution of a sterile urolith presumed to be struvite in a 12-week-old dachshund after two weeks of therapy with the calculolytic diet. Pending further studies, however, we recommend that the use of low-protein calculolytic diets be avoided in immature dogs unless the alternative is no treatment or euthanasia. AHA has not been evaluated in growing pups.

Ammonium Urate Urolithiasis

Summary

Uric acid uroliths in man may be dissolved by reducing urine uric acid supersaturation.[28, 36, 56, 75] The regimen usually consists of (1) alkalinizing urine with sodium bicarbonate or Polycitra,* (2) enhancing the formation of dilute urine, and (3) the administration of allopurinol.

Uric acid nephroliths in human beings have also been dissolved by irrigation of the renal pelvis with litholytic agents introduced through percutaneous nephrostomy tubes or retrograde ureteral catheters.[23, 31,77] It is emphasized, however, that results of studies in man may not be applicable to dogs because (1) human beings typically form uric acid calculi rather than ammonium acid urate calculi, and (2) ammonium ions appear to be of greater significance in flocculation of urate crystals in dog urine than hydrogen ions.[71-73]

Diuresis. Increasing the volume of urine produced by increasing water consumption appears to be a logical recommendation.

Diets. Low-purine diets (i.e., those low in kidney, liver, and other glandular organs) appear to be a logical consideration but are uncommonly utilized by physicians or veterinarians. It has been the general consensus of opinion that they are cumbersome to formulate (vegetable proteins tend to be lower in purine than animal proteins) and that they are not very effective in preventing recurrence of urate uroliths or prompting their dissolution.

Ultra low-protein diets (2.5 per cent protein) have been recommended for the treatment of dogs with urate uroliths.[55] Numerous small uroliths presumed to be ammonium urate disappeared from the urinary bladder in a two-year-old male Dalmatian consuming the calculolytic diet previously described (S/D). The precise mechanism of their disappearance was not established but may have been related to (1) dissolution caused by diuresis and reduced formation of uric acid from dietary purines, or (2) diuresis that caused them to be flushed through the urethra. These mechanisms apparently counteracted any deleterious effect caused by production of aciduria during consumption of the calculolytic diet.

We have also observed dissolution of an ammonium

---

*Willen Drug Co., Baltimore, MD.

urate urolith in a two-year-old female miniature schnauzer with a portal vascular anomaly during consumption of a low-protein diet designed for treatment of renal failure (K/D). The mechanisms involved may have been decreased endogenous production of ammonium from urea, reduced formation of uric acid from dietary purines, and diuresis.

Urine pH. Because ammonium and hydrogen ions have been shown to flocculate ammonium urate crystals in dog urine, administration of alkalinizing agents, such as oral sodium bicarbonate, would appear to be of value in preventing acid urine from increasing renal tubular production of ammonia. Maintenance of urine pH between 6.5 and 7.0 is suggested.

Eradication or Control of Urinary Tract Infection. Reduction of the concentration of ammonium ions by eradicating infection with urease-producing bacteria appears to be a logical recommendation. The role, if any, however, that ammonium ions produced by reduction of urea via bacterial urease plays in the production of urate uroliths has not been established.

Allopurinol. Allopurinol is a synthetic isomer of hypoxanthine. It inhibits the action of xanthine oxidase in the liver and thereby decreases the production of uric acid by inhibiting the conversion of hypoxanthine to xanthine and xanthine to uric acid. Although allopurinol has a short half-life (90 minutes), its metabolic derivative oxypurinol is also a xanthine-oxidase inhibitor and is slowly excreted.[67, 80] Iatrogenic xanthine calculi are a potential problem in patients receiving allopurinol but are rare in man and have not been reported in dogs.

The dosage of allopurinol commonly recommended for prevention of ammonium urate uroliths in dogs is 30 mg/kg/day in two or three divided doses for one month and then 10 mg/kg/day.[26, 57] Prolonged maintenance doses of 0.8 mg/kg/day have been advocated for long-term control.[57] The dosage should be reduced if the patient has renal failure. Allopurinol is sold commercially in 100-mg tablets.* The therapeutic value, if any, of combining allopurinol with calculolytic diets is unknown.

Calcium Oxalate Urolithiasis

The literature pertaining to calcium oxalate urolithiasis is voluminous. Unfortunately, the vast majority of it pertains to humans and laboratory animals. Knowledge of the etiology, pathogenesis, and treatment of calcium oxalate uroliths in dogs is virtually nonexistent. Attempts to dissolve calcium oxalate stones in humans have been extremely disappointing.[1, 75] Surgery remains the most effective method of removing calcium oxalate uroliths.

---

*Zyloprim, Burroughs Wellcome Co., Research Triangle Park, NC.

Calcium Phosphate Urolithiasis

The solubility of calcium phosphate in urine is dependent on hydrogen ion concentration, calcium ion concentration, and total inorganic phosphate ion concentration. Although the use of effective acidifiers to reduce urine pH would be expected to be of value, this treatment alone has been ineffective in humans.[75] Likewise, the use of AHA in an in vitro study to promote urine acidification was not as effective in promoting calcium phosphate dissolution as it was in promoting magnesium ammonium phosphate dissolution.[33] It has been suggested that the administration of citric acid may increase the solubility of calcium phosphate by the formation of soluble calcium complexes.[24]

Although the use of calcium chelating agents has been reported to be of value in inducing dissolution of calcium phosphate uroliths in man,[75] there have been no controlled studies reported concerning the feasibility of medical dissolution of calcium phosphate uroliths in dogs. Since uroliths primarily composed of calcium phosphate are most likely to be encountered in dogs with diseases associated with hypercalcemia or renal tubular acidosis, it is tempting to speculate that correction of these metabolic abnormalities might be associated with the formation of urine undersaturated with calcium phosphate crystalloids. If this hypothesis is accurate, calcium phosphate uroliths would dissolve. However, we did not observe dissolution of calcium phosphate uroliths in an eight-year-old female Welsh corgi with hypercalcemic hyperparathyroidism nine months following surgical removal of a parathyroid adenoma.

Cystine and Silica Urolithiasis

There have been no published reports of studies evaluating the medical dissolution of cystine or silica uroliths in dogs. However, combinations of oral fluids, urine alkalinizing agents, and D-penicillamine are effective in inducing cystine urolith dissolution in man.[19]

Regimen to Dissolve Uroliths

1. Determine precise location, size, and number of uroliths.
2. If possible, determine mineral composition of uroliths or estimate their composition by evaluating appropriate clinical data (see Table 140–4).
3. Give appropriate therapy to eradicate urinary tract infection. Consider surgical correction if a predisposition to urinary tract infection is identified via radiography or other means.
4. Consider dietary alterations to reduce excretion of calculogenic substances in urine.

5. Promote formation of a large volume of dilute urine.
6. Adjust urine pH to enhance solubility of calculogenic crystalloids.
7. Administer specific agents that will:
   a. Reduce the quantity of crystalloids in urine.
   b. Increase the solubility of crystalloids in urine.
8. Follow periodically with:
   a. Serial urinalyses for urine pH, specific gravity, and microscopic examination of sediment for crystals. Crystals formed in stale urine at room or refrigeration temperatures may be artifacts.
   b. Serial radiography to evaluate stone location, number, size, density, and shape.
   c. Quantitative urine culture where indicated.
9. Be certain that owners are informed about dosages of medication, methods to monitor responses to therapy, and duration of therapy.

PREVENTION OF RECURRENT UROLITHIASIS

Summary

Calculi of all types have a tendency to recur following surgical removal or medical dissolution.[9] Unfortunately, recurrence is unpredictable and may be related to (1) persistence of the underlying causes of urolithiasis, (2) failure to remove all uroliths from the urinary tract, especially those that are small, (3) persistence of urinary tract infection with urease-producing bacteria, and (4) lack of owner or patient compliance with therapeutic or prophylactic recommendations.

Recurrent calculi are usually similar in mineral composition to those present during the initial episode, except when urinary tract infection with urease-producing bacteria (especially staphylococci) persists or develops. In this instance, stones originally composed of urate, cystine, oxalate, or silica may be followed by struvite uroliths.

Increasing Urine Volume

Induction of polyuria is generally recommended for all types of uroliths. Occurrence of recalcitrant urinary tract infection represents the only exception to this generality. Production of polyuria minimizes stagnation of urine by promoting increased urine volume and more frequent micturition and dilutes calculogenic crystalloids that cause uroliths. (Consult the section on increasing urine volume under Medical Dissolution of Struvite Uroliths for further details.)

Long-term administration of diuretics to induce polyuria in patients with recurrent urolithiasis has not been evaluated in dogs by experimental studies or controlled clinical trials, and their efficacy in inducing diuresis is unquestionable. However, iatrogenic fluid and electrolyte abnormalities and alterations in the pattern of urinary excretion of electrolytes should be considered. Pending results of such trials, methods to stimulate polydipsia and compensatory polyuria remain the safest alternative.

Long-term administration of hydrochlorothiazide to minimize the recurrence of calcium oxalate uroliths in man is commonly employed.[86] This diuretic is selected because it decreases urinary excretion of calcium.[12] However, it also increases the urinary excretion of magnesium. Although hydrochlorothiazide has been used with some success in the management of calcium oxalate uroliths in man,[85] its use in an attempt to prevent experimentally induced infection (struvite) uroliths in rats resulted in a higher incidence of calculi (67 per cent) than in controls (43 per cent).[46]

Prevention of Recurrent Struvite Uroliths

Eradication or control of infections of the urinary tract with urease-producing bacteria is the most important factor in preventing recurrence of most infection-induced struvite uroliths. If recurrent urinary tract infection persists, indefinite therapy with prophylactic dosages of antimicrobial agents eliminated in high concentrations in urine is indicated.[48] These include nitrofurantoin, ampicillin, and trimethoprim-sulfa (see Chapter 135).

In light of the effectiveness of diets in inducing struvite urolith dissolution, some form of dietary modification to prevent recurrence of uroliths would appear to be both logical and feasible. However, further studies must be performed to evaluate the long-term effects of low-protein calculolytic diets in dogs before reliable recommendations about their use can be established. Because they induce polyuria, varying degrees of hypoalbuminemia, and mild alterations in hepatic enzymes and morphology, diets designed for the management of renal failure that contain less salt and more protein (U/D, K/D) should be considered.[55] This recommendation has not been evaluated by controlled experimental and clinical trials.

Studies to evaluate the effectiveness of AHA in the prevention of struvite urolithiasis in dogs with persistent urinary tract infection by urease-producing bacteria have been encouraging. Administration of 25 mg AHA/kg/day to dogs with urinary bladder foreign bodies (zinc discs) and experimentally induced urease-positive staphylococcal infections has been effective in preventing urolith formation in most and minimizing the rate of urolith growth in others. AHA has also been reported to be effective in preventing struvite uroliths induced by urease-producing mycoplasma in rats.[46] (Consult the appropriate section under Medical Dissolution of Struvite Uroliths for specific details.)

Caution must be used in deciding whether or not to induce prophylactic diuresis in patients with struvite uroliths induced by recurrent urinary tract infections. Although formation of dilute urine minimizes supersaturation of urine with calculogenic crystalloids, it may counteract innate antimicrobial properties of urine.[66] Experimental studies performed in cats indicate that diuresis minimizes pyelonephritis but enhances lower urinary tract infections.[47]

If the urine pH of patients with previous struvite urolithiasis remains alkaline despite antimicrobial or dietary therapy, administration of urine acidifiers should be considered. (See Acidification of Urine under Medical Dissolution of Struvite Uroliths.)

Prevention of Recurrent Urate Uroliths

Consult Medical Dissolution of Uroliths for the rationale of the following recommendations: (1) using calculolytic diets; (2) maintaining urine pH between 6.5 and 7.0 to minimize urate flocculation by hydrogen and ammonium ions, (3) inducing polyuria, if necessary; (4) administering allopurinol (Zyloprim), 30 mg/kg/day in two or three divided doses for the first month, then reducing the dosage to 10 mg/kg/day; and (5) eradicating urinary tract infection if present. In humans, allopurinol is usually administered only if uric acid stones recur despite fluid and alkali therapy.[14]

Prevention of Recurrent Calcium Oxalate Uroliths

Methods to reduce the degree of supersaturation of urine with calcium oxalate include (1) inducing diuresis, (2) reducing urinary excretion of calcium, oxalate, and uric acid, and (3) increasing the solubility of calcium oxalate in urine.[63] In addition to these measures, control of secondary urinary tract infection (when present) is also important.

Prevention of Recurrent Calcium Phosphate Uroliths

Consult Medical Dissolution of Uroliths for the rationale of the following recommendations: (1) controlling or eliminating the underlying cause of hypercalcemia and hypercalciuria (if present); (2) using a calculolytic diet (S/D); (3) eradicating or controlling urinary tract infection (if present); (4) inducing polyuria, if necessary; and (5) acidifying urine, if necessary.

Prevention of Recurrent Silica Uroliths

Since the causes of silica urolithiasis are unknown, only nonspecific measures designed to reduce the degree of supersaturation of urine with calculogenic substances can be recommended for prophylaxis. Increasing the volume of urine produced by increasing water consumption will increase the volume of urine in which calculogenic substances are dissolved or suspended. Diuresis induced by oral administration of salt or consumption of additional water in the form of milk has been effective in preventing or minimizing the growth of silicaceous uroliths in calves.[60]

Since information regarding the solubility of calculogenic substances in silica uroliths at acid, neutral, and alkaline pH is unavailable, recommendations regarding the alteration of urine pH cannot be formulated. In one report of bovine silica urolithiasis, it was implied that silica is less soluble in acid urine.[52]

Although the role of diet in canine silica uroliths is speculative, it seems reasonable to recommend that the diet of affected patients be changed, especially if the problem is recurrent. Although empirical, this maneuver is unlikely to be harmful and may be helpful.[61]

Prevention of Recurrent Cystine Uroliths

Currently available methods have been extrapolated from those designed for humans with cystine urolithiasis.

Alkalinization of Urine

To significantly increase the solubility of cystine in urine, the urine pH should be maintained as alkaline as possible (7.5 or higher throughout the day). Alkalinization may be achieved by administration of sodium bicarbonate tablets or baking soda mixed with food. Although the most effective dosage must be determined on the basis of evaluation of urine pH, the initial dosage is approximately 7 to 10 mg/kg three times per day (20 to 30 mg/kg/day).

D-Penicillamine and Other Thiol Derivatives

Penicillamine is dimethyl-cysteine. D-Penicillamine is a nonmetabolizable compound that reduces the concentration of insoluble cystine in urine by forming a dimer of cysteine-D-Penicillamine disulfide instead of a dimer of cysteine-cysteine.[62] The latter compound has been reported to be approximately 50 times more soluble than cystine. D-Penicillamine is most effective at a neutral to alkaline pH, indicating the need to maintain an alkaline urine.[22]

D-Penicillamine is available in 250-mg tablets.* The most commonly recommended dosage for dogs is 30 mg/kg/day divided into two doses and mixed with food or given at meal time.[4, 34] Unfortunately, dogs are unable to tolerate as large a dose of D-Penicillamine as humans (1 to 3 gm/day) without vomiting and anorexia. If vomiting or anorexia occurs, reduce the dosage to 10 mg/kg/day and attempt to gradually increase it. Antiemetics may also be considered.

---

*Cuprimine, Merck Sharp & Dohme, West Point, PA.

Anorexia and vomiting are the major undesirable effects of D-penicillamine in dogs. Reversible side effects of D-penicillamine in man include proteinuria associated with immune-complex glomerulonephropathy, dermatitis (epidermolysis), pruritus, fever, neutropenia, arthropathy, and abnormalities of taste and smell.[34] Because of adverse reactions frequently associated with D-penicillamine therapy in man, it is used only if forced diuresis and urine alkalinization are unsuccessful in controlling recurrent cystine urolithiasis.[34]

Alpha-mercaptopropionylglycine (MPG) affects cystine disulfide bonds in a manner similar to D-penicillamine. It has been reported to be effective in preventing cystine urolithiasis in man without the adverse effects caused by D-penicillamine.[37] There have been no reports of the effectiveness of MPG in dogs with cystine urolithiasis. Likewise, direct injection of tiopronin (x-mercaptopropionylglycine) into the urinary tract has been effective in dissolving cystine uroliths in man [38] but has not been evaluated in dogs.

Other Recommendations

Increasing the volume of urine produced by increased oral water consumption is recommended. Likewise, concomitant urinary tract infections should be eradicated or controlled. Feeding diets low in precursors of cystine is difficult and of questionable value in the prophylaxis of cystine calculi. However, animal proteins usually have more sulfur-containing amino acids than vegetable proteins.

1. Anonymous: Supersaturated urine. Lancet *1*:1219, 1979.
2. Appleman, R. M., Hallenbeck, G. A., and Shorter, R. G.: Effect or reciprocal allogeneic renal transplantation between Dalmation and non-Dalmation dogs on urinary excretion of uric acid. Proc. Soc. Exp. Biol. Med. *121*:1094, 1966.
3. Benke, G. M., and Osborn, T. W.: Urinary silicon excretion by rats following oral administration of silicon compounds. Food Cosmet. Toxicol. *17*:123, 1979.
4. Bovee, K. C.: Cystine urolithiasis. *In* Kirk, R. W. (ed.); *Current Veterinary Therapy VI*. W. B. Saunders, Philadelphia, 1977.
5. Bovee, K. C., and Segal, S.: Canine cystinuria and cystine calculi. 21st Gaines Veterinary Symposium, 1971.
6. Bovee, K. C., Thier, S. O., and Segal, S.: Renal clearance of amino acids in canine cystinuria. Metabolism 23:51, 1974.
7. Brodey, R. S., Thomson, R., Sayer, P., and Eugster, B.: Silicate renal calculi in Kenyan dogs. J. Small Anim. Pract. *18*:523, 1977.
8. Brown, N. O., Parks, J. L., and Greene, R. W.: Canine urolithiasis: Retrospective analysis of 438 cases. J. Am. Vet. Med. Assoc. *170*:415, 1977.
9. Brown, N. O., Parks, J. L., and Greene, R. W.: Recurrence of canine urolithiasis. J. Am. Vet. Med. Assoc. *170*:419, 1977.
10. Clark, W. T.: Staphylococcal infection of the urinary tract and its relation to urolithiasis in dogs. Vet. Rec. 95:204, 1974.
11. Clark, W. T., and Cuddeford, D.: A study of amino acids in urine from dogs with cystine urolithiasis. Vet. Rec. 88:414, 1971.
12. Coe, F. L.: Treated and untreated recurrent calcium nephrolithiasis in patients with idiopathic hypercalciuria, hyperuricosuria, or no metabolic disorder. Ann. Intern. Med. 87:404, 1977.
13. Coe, F. L.: *Nephrolithiasis: Pathogenesis and Treatment*. Year Book Medical Publishers, Inc., Chicago, 1978.
14. Coe, F. L.: Nephrolithiasis. Causes, classification, and management. Hosp. Pract. *16*:33, 1981.
15. Cohn, R., Dibbel, D. G., Laub, D. R., and Kountz, S. L.: Renal allotransplantation and allantoin excretion of Dalmatian. Arch. Surg. *91*:911, 1965.
16. Cornelius, C. E., and Bishop, J. A.: Ruminant urolithiasis. III. Comparative studies on the structure of urinary concretions in several species. J. Urol. 85:842, 1961.
17. Cornelius, C. E., Bishop, J. A., and Schaffer, M. H.: A quantitative study of amino aciduria in Dachshunds with a history of cystine urolithiasis. Cornell Vet. 57:177, 1967.
18. Crane, C. W., and Turner, A. W.: Amino acid patterns of urine and blood plasma in a cystinuric Labrador dog. Nature 177:237, 1956.
19. Dahlberg, P. J., Van Den Berg, C. J., Kurtz, S. B., Wilson, D. M., and Smith, L. H.: Clinical features of cystinuria. Mayo Clin. Proc. 52:533, 1977.
20. Duncan, H., and Curtiss, A. S.: Observations on uric acid transport in man, the Dalmatian, and the non-Dalmatian dog. Henry Ford Hosp. Med. J. *19*:105, 1971.
21. Duncan, H., Wakim, K. G., and Ward, L. E.: The effects of intravenous administration of uric acid on its concentration in plasma and urine of Dalmatian and non-Dalmatian dogs. J. Lab. Clin. Med. 58:876, 1961.
22. Earll, J. M., and Kolb, F. O.: Treatment of cystinuria and cystine stone disease. *In* Kolb, F. O. (ed.): *Modern Treatment*. Harper & Row, New York, 1977.
23. Eason, A. A., Sharlip, I. D., and Spaulding, J. T.: Dissolution of bilateral uric acid calculi causing anuria. J. Am. Med. Assoc. *240*:670 1978.
24. Elliott, J. S.: Calcium phosphate solubility in urine. J. Urol. 77: 269, 1957.
25. Emerick, R. J., Kugel, E. E., and Wallace, V.: Urinary excretion of silica and the production of siliceous urinary calculi in rats. Am. J. Vet. Res. *24*:610, 1963.
26. Finco, D. R.: Urate urolithiasis. *In* Kirk, R. W. (ed.): *Current Veterinary Therapy VI*. W. B. Saunders, Philadelphia, 1977.
27. Finco, D. R., Rosin, E., and Johnson, K. H.: Canine urolithiasis: A review of 133 clinical and 23 necropsy cases. J. Am. Vet. Med. Assoc. *157*:1225, 1970.
28. Freiha, F. S., and Hemady, K.: Dissolution of uric acid stones. Alternative to surgery. Urology 8:334, 1976.
29. Friedman, M., and Byers, S. O.: Observations concerning the causes of excess excretion of uric acid in the Dalmatian dog. J. Biol. Chem. *175*:727, 1948.
30. Gill, W. B., Jones, K. W., and Ruggiero, K. F.: Protective effects of heparin and other sulfated glycosaminoglycans on crystal adhesion to injured urothelium. J. Urol. *127*:152, 1982.
31. Gordon, M. R., Carrion, H. M., and Politano, V. A.: Dissolution of uric acid calculi with Tham irrigation. Urology *12*:393, 1978.
32. Griffith, D. P.: Struvite stones. Kidney Int. *13*:372, 1978.
33. Griffith, D. P., Bragin, S., and Musher, D. M.: Dissolution of struvite urinary stones experimental studies in vitro. Invest. Urol. *13*:351, 1976.
34. Halperin, E. C., Thier, S. O., and Rosenberg, L. E.: The use of D-pennicillamine in cystinuria: Efficacy and untoward reactions. Yale J. Biol. Med. *54*:439, 1981.
35. Hande, K., Reed, E., and Chabner, B.: Allopurinol kinetics. Clin. Pharmacol. Ther. *23*:598, 1978.
36. Hardy, B., and Klein, L. A.: In situ dissolution of ureteral calculus. Urology 8:444, 1976.
37. Hautmann, R., Terhorst, B., Stuhlsatz, H. W., and Lutzezer, W.: Mercaptopropionylglycine: A progress in cystine stone therapy. J. Urol. *117*:628, 1977.
38. Hayase, Y., Fukatsu, H., and Segawa, A.: The dissolution of cystine stones by irrigated tiopronin solution. J. Urol. *124*:775, 1980.
39. Herman, J. R., and Goldberg, A. S.: New type of urinary calculus caused by antacid therapy. J. Am. Med. Assoc. *174*:1206, 1960.

40. Joekes, A. J., Rose, G. A., and Sutor, J.: Multiple renal silica stones. Br. Med. J. *1*:46, 1973.

41. King, E. J., Stantial, H., and Dolan, M.: The biochemistry of silicic acid. III. The excretion of administered silica. Biochem. J. *27*: 1007, 1973.

42. Klausner, J. S., and Osborne, C. A.: Bacterial infections of the urinary tract. *In* Kirk, R. W. (ed.): *Current Veterinary Therapy VI*. W. B. Saunders, Philadelphia, 1977.

43. Klausner, J. S., Osborne, C. A., O'Leary, T. P., Muscoplat, C. M., and Griffith, D. P.: Experimental induction of struvite uroliths in Miniature Schnauzer and Beagle dogs. Invest. Urol. *18*:127, 1980.

44. Krawiec, D. R., Osborne, C. A., Leininger, J. R., and Griffith, D. P.: Effect of acetohydroxamic acid on dissolution of canine struvite uroliths. Am. J. Vet. Res., in press.

45. Kuster, G., Shorter, R. G., Dawson, B., and Hallenbeck, G.: Uric acid metabolism in Dalmatians and other dogs. Arch. Intern. Med. *129*:492, 1972.

46. Lamm, D. L., Johnston, S. A., Friedlander, A. M., and Gottes, R. F.: Medical therapy of experimental infection stones. Urology *10*:418, 1977.

47. Lees, G. E., Osborne, C. A., Stevens, J. B., and Ward, G. E.: Adverse effects of open indwelling urethral catheterization in clinically normal male cats. Am. J. Vet. Res. *42*:825, 1981.

48. Ling, G. V.: Choice of antimicrobial agents in the treatment of urinary tract infections. *In* Kirk, R. W. (ed.): *Current Veterinary Therapy VII*. W. B. Saunders, Philadelphia, 1980.

49. Malek, R. S., and Boyce, W. H.: Observation on the ultrastructure and genesis of urinary calculi. J. Urol. *117*:336, 1977.

50. Maretta, S. M., Pask, A. J., Greene, R. W., and Liu, S. K.: Urinary calculi associated with portosystemic shunts in six dogs. J. Am. Vet. Med. Assoc. *178*:133, 1981.

51. McCullagh, K. G., and Ehrhart, L. A.: Silica urolithiasis in laboratory dogs fed semisynthetic diets. J. Am. Vet. Med. Assoc. *164*:712, 1974.

52. McIntosh, C. H.: Urolithiasis in animals. Aust. Vet. J. *54*:267, 1978.

53. Menon, M., and Mahle, C. J.: Oxalate metabolism and renal calculi. J. Urol. *127*:148, 1982.

54. Meyer, J. L., and Angino, E. E.: The role of trace metals in calcium urolithiasis. Invest. Urol. *14*:347, 1977.

55. Morris, M. L., and Doering, G. G.: Diet and canine urolithiasis. Canine Pract. *5*:53, 1978.

56. Neto, M., Pilloff, B., and Simon, J. A.: Dissolution of renal uric acid calculus with alopurinol and alkalinization of urine: A case report. J. Urol. *115*:740, 1976.

57. Osbaldiston, G. W., and Lowrey, J. L.: Allopurinol in the prevention of hyperuricemia in Dalmation dogs. Vet. Med. Small Anim. Clin. *66*:711, 1971.

58. Osborne, C. A.: Strategy for nonsurgical removal of canine struvite uroliths. Proc. Am. Anim. Hosp. Assoc., 1982.

59. Osborne, C. A., Abdullahi, S., Klausner, J. S., Johnston, G. R., and Polzin, D. J.: Nonsurgical removal of uroliths from the urethra of female dogs. J. Am. Vet. Med. Assoc. *182*:47, 1983.

60. Osborne, C. A., Abdullahi, S. U., Leininger, J. R., Polzin, D. J., Hauer, N. E., Klausner, J. S., Hardy, R. M., Kuzma, A. B., and Gidlund, C. J.: Medical dissolution of canine struvite uroliths. Minn. Vet. *22*:14, 1982.

61. Osborne, C. A., Hammer, R. F., and Klausner, J. S.: Canine silica urolithiasis. J. Am. Vet. Med. Assoc. *178*:809, 1981.

62. Osborne, C. A., and Klausner, J. S.: War on urolithiasis: Problems and solutions. Proc. Am. Anim. Hosp. Assoc., 1978.

63. Osborne, C. A., and Klausner, J. S.: Calcium oxalate urolithiasis. *In* Kirk, R. W. (ed.): *Current Veterinary Therapy VII*. W. B. Saunders, Philadelphia, 1980.

64. Osborne, C. A., Klausner, J. S., Hardy, R. M., and Lees, G. E.: Ancillary treatment of urinary tract infections. *In* Kirk, R. W. (ed.): *Current Veterinary Therapy VII*. W. B. Saunders, Philadelphia, 1980.

65. Osborne, C. A., Klausner, J. S., Krawiec, D. R., and Griffith, D. P.: Canine struvite urolithiasis: Problems and their solution. J. Am. Vet. Med. Assoc. *179*:239, 1981.

66. Osborne, C. A., Klausner, J. S., and Lees, G. E.: Urinary tract infections: Normal and abnormal host defense mechanisms. Vet. Clin. North Am. *9*:587, 1979.

67. O'Sullivan, W. J.: Metabolic side effects of allopurinol. *In* Edwards, K. D. G. (ed.): *Progress in Biochemical Pharmacology Drugs and the Kidney*, Vol. 9. S. Karger, New York, 1974, p. 174.

68. Pak, C. Y. C.: Disorders of stone formation. *In* Brenner, B. M., and Rector, F. C. (ed.): W. B. Saunders, Philadelphia, 1976.

69. Pak, C. Y. C.: *Calcium Urolithiasis: Pathogenesis, Diagnosis, and Management*. Plenum Publishing Corp., New York, 1978.

70. Piermattei, D. L., and Osborne, C. A.: Nonsurgical removal of calculi from the urethra of male dogs. J. Am. Vet. Med. Assoc. *159*:1755, 1972.

71. Porter, P.: Physico-chemical factors involved in urate calculus formation. II. Colloidal flocculation. Res. Vet. Sci. *4*:580, 1963.

72. Porter, P.: Urinary calculi in the dog. II. Urate stones and urate metabolism. J. Comp. Pathol. 73:119, 1963.

73. Porter, P.: Colloidal properties of urates in relation to calculus formation. Res. Vet. Sci. 7:128, 1966.

74. Rose, A. G., and Sulaiman, S.: Tamm-Horsfall mucoproteins promote calcium oxalate crystal formation in urine: Quantitative studies. J. Urol. *127*:177, 1982.

75. Sheldon, C. A., and Smith, A. D.: Chemolysis of calculi. Urol. Clin. North Am. 9:121, 1982.

76. Smith, L. H., Boyce, W. H., Finlayson, B., et al.: Urolithiasis. *In Research Needs in Nephrology and Urology*, Vol. 5. U. S. Dept HEW, NIH, Bethesda, MD., 1978.

77. Spataro, R. F., Linke, C. A., and Barbaric, Z. L.: The use of percutaneous nephrostomy and urinary alkalinization in the dissolution of obstructing uric acid stones. Radiology *129*:629, 1978.

78. Stamey, T. A.: *Urinary Infections*. Williams & Wilkins, Baltimore, 1972.

79. Stone, E. A.: Surgical management of urolithiasis. Comp. Cont. Ed. 3:627, 1981.

80. Thomas, W. C.: Medical aspects of renal calculous disease treatment and prophylaxis. Urol. Clin. North Am. *1*:261, 1974.

81. Treacher, R. J.: Urolithiasis in the dog. II. Biochemical aspects. J. Small Anim. Pract. 7:537, 1966.

82. Weaver, A. D.: Relationship of bacterial infection in urine and calculi to canine urolithiasis. Vet. Rec. 97:48, 1975.

83. White, E. G., and Porter, P.: Urinary calculi. *In* Medway, W., Prier, J. E., and Wilkinson, J. S. (eds.): *Textbook of Veterinary Clinical Pathology*. Williams & Wilkins, Baltimore, 1969.

84. Wickham, J. E. A.: The matrix of renal calculi. *In* Williams, D. I., and Chrisholm, G. D., (eds.): *Scientific Foundations of Urology*, Vol. 1. Year Book Medical Publishers, Inc., Chicago, 1976.

85. Yendt, E. R., Guay, G. F., and Garcia, D. A.: The use of thiazides in the prevention of renal calculi. Can. Med. Assoc. J. *102*:614, 1970.

86. Zerwekh, J. E., and Pak, C. Y. C.: Selective effects of thiazide therapy on serum 1 & 25-Dihydroxyvitamin D and intestinal calcium absorption in renal and absorptive hypercalciurias. Metabolism 29:13, 1980.

Chapter 141

Feline Urologic Syndrome

David J. Polzin and Carl A. Osborne

DEFINITIONS AND CONCEPTS

Popular Concepts

Feline urologic syndrome (FUS) has been defined as a condition associated with dysuria, hematuria, and urethral obstruction.[1, 48] Although considerable effort has been expended searching for "the cause" of FUS, there is currently no generally agreed upon etiology. Many veterinarians currently believe that FUS is the result of a combination of primary and predisposing factors.[34] However, the current controversy seems to be primarily focused on whether FUS is initiated by a virus or diet-related factors. Considerable clinical and experimental data have been presented to support both views.[10–12, 20, 27] The common theme seems to be that FUS has to be initiated by one mechanism or the other.

The current concept that FUS represents a unique disease entity may be incorrect. Clinical studies to determine the role of various factors in the pathogenesis of FUS have generally assumed that cats with dysuria, hematuria, or urethral obstruction have a disorder caused by single agents or multiple interacting agents. However, these studies have failed to identify a consistently reproducible group of factors that cause FUS. Dietary and viral experimental models of "FUS" have failed to simulate the wide clinical spectrum of spontaneous FUS, suggesting that although these factors may play a role in some naturally occurring cases, they are unlikely to explain all aspects of the natural disease.

New Hypothesis

We hypothesize that FUS may be caused by single agents, multiple interacting agents, or fundamentally different agents (Table 141–1). We believe that it is likely that FUS represents a response to a group of distinct disease entities that have in common clinical signs referable to the lower urinary tract, especially dysuria, hematuria, crystalluria, and urethral obstruction. Diseases of the feline lower urinary tract that may cause FUS include viral, bacterial, fungal, and mycoplasmal urinary tract infections; urolithiasis; neoplasia; neurogenic disorders; congenital anomalies; noninfectious inflammatory conditions; prostatic disease; trauma; idiopathic disorders; and iatrogenic conditions.

The lack of specificity inherent in current definitions of FUS has led to confusion about which disorders of the feline lower urinary tract should be considered as FUS. Lack of specificity and the as-

sumption that FUS represents a single disease entity have led to the tendency to believe that all cats with clinical evidence of lower urinary tract disease have the same disease (FUS). This has resulted in the formulation of stereotyped treatment. Such an approach fails to recognize that some cats have disease entities that may be readily amenable to specific therapy (e.g., bacterial urinary tract infections, urolithiasis) (see Tables 141–1 and 141–6).

We propose that FUS be defined as encompassing all cats with evidence of lower urinary tract disease, regardless of the specific underlying disease. We define FUS in this manner to emphasize that it may result from many diverse lower urinary tract diseases rather than from a unique disease entity.

ETIOLOGY OF FELINE UROLOGIC SYNDROME

Urinary Tract Infection

Viral Urinary Tract Infection

Three different viruses, a calicivirus ("Manx virus"), a syncytium-forming virus belonging to the class Paramyxoviridae, and a cell-associated herpesvirus, have been isolated from urine of cats with naturally occurring FUS.[10–12] Recent studies in specific pathogen-free cats have indicated that the feline herpesvirus may play a primary role in some cases of

TABLE 141–1. Etiological Agents Associated with Feline Urologic Syndrome

Infection	Anomalies
Bacterial	Persistent urachus
Mycotic	Urethral strictures
Mycoplasmal	Other
Viral	
Parasitic (*Capillaria* spp.)	**Inflammation (noninfectious)**
Urolithiasis	
Struvite	**Trauma**
Calcium phosphate	Bladder
Calcium oxalate	Urethra
Ammonium urate	Herniated bladder
Uric acid	
Matrix	**Neurogenic Disorders**
Other	Urethral spasm
	Reflex dyssynergia
	Atonic bladder
Neoplasia	Other
Bladder	
Urethra	**Idiopathic Disorders**
Prostate	
Extraurinary—impinging on urinary tract	**Iatrogenic Conditions**

FUS.[10-12] Intravesicular administration of feline herpesvirus alone or in combination with the feline calicivirus was associated with the development of dysuria, hematuria, and urethral obstruction.[10] It appeared that the feline calicivirus alone did not induce clinical siigns of FUS but enhanced the onset and severity of clinical signs and lesions in cats concurrently infected with feline herpesvirus. The syncytium-forming virus is not required for development of clinical signs of FUS and is currently believed not to play a substantial role in the pathogenesis of FUS.[11, 15]

Intracellular and extracellular lipid and a variety of crystals have been observed in cell cultures infected with feline cell–associated herpesvirus.[11, 12] In addition, supernatant fluids of some of these cell cultures contained structures that resembled the crystals found in urethral plugs in some male cats with FUS. However, the mineral composition of the tissue culture crystals was not determined. The relationship between these *in vitro* observations and the development of crystalluria, urolithiasis, and urethral plugs in cats with FUS remains speculative.

Viruses might be responsible, directly or indirectly, for production of a unique but unidentified mucoprotein that has been detected in the urine and urethral plugs of male cats with naturally occurring FUS.[34, 45] These observations have led to the unproved hypothesis that virus-induced matrix protein may have crystal binding properties and therefore may play a role in the initiation or growth of urethral plugs.

Although a viral etiology appears promising for some cases of FUS, other researchers have been unable to isolate feline herpesvirus in urine from cats with naturally occurring FUS.[1, 15] However, it has been claimed that feline herpesvirus is strongly cell-associated and, therefore, must be cultured from tissue specimens rather than urine.[11] Gaskell and associates were unable to isolate the virus from urethral tissue in 26 cats submitted for urethrostomy.[15] The likelihood of finding virus in urethral tissue compared with bladder tissue is unknown. Efforts to demonstrate transmissibility of the virus using intravesicular injection of urine obtained from FUS-affected cats have failed. However, failure may have been associated with the fact that herpesvirus must be present in adequate numbers in urine to cause clinical signs.[1, 15] It may also be because urine collected from cats with naturally occurring FUS did not have the viral form of the disease. Because isolation of feline herpesvirus is difficult and may require bladder tissue samples for isolation, the incidence and significance of viral urinary tract infections in naturally occurring FUS remain unresolved.

Bacterial Urinary Tract Infection

It has been concluded that bacterial urinary tract infection (UTI) is not the primary cause of FUS.[1, 6, 9, 15, 45, 46] However, these studies have revealed a subpopulation of cats ranging from 10 to 52 per cent of those with FUS that had bacteriuria. Whether bacteriuria is the primary etiology of lower urinary tract disease, secondary infection, or contaminations in these cats has not been fully resolved. Frequently, urine bacteria counts in these cats were less than 10^5 colony-forming units per milliliter of urine (cfu/ml). It was concluded that the bacteria probably represented contamination rather than infection, despite the fact that cultures were obtained by cystocentesis in some studies.[1, 44]

The conclusion that bacterial UTI is not the primary cause of FUS in these cats is based on two assumptions: (1) FUS results from a single pathological factor, therefore bacteriuria would have been expected to be present in all cats if it were the primary cause of FUS, and (2) urine bacteria counts of less than 10^5 cfu/ml represent contamination rather than infection in cats. We believe the conclusion that bacterial UTI is not a primary cause of FUS may be incorrect because the assumptions underlying this conclusion are erroneous. FUS is probably a group of separate diseases that have common clinical signs. The observation that some cats with FUS have bacteriuria is consistent with bacterial UTI as a primary cause of FUS.

The assumption that urine bacteria counts of less than 10^5 cfu/ml represent contamination rather than infection in feline urine is unproven and may be erroneous. Definitions of significant bacteriuria developed for humans have apparently been applied to cats without consideration that cat urine might be a less favorable medium for bacterial growth than human urine. To the extent that cat urine inhibits the rate of bacterial growth, cats with urinary tract infections might not excrete urine containing the same number of bacteria as that observed in humans with urinary tract infections.[21-23] When urine is collected by cystocentesis, detection of low numbers of bacteria should be viewed with suspicion. In a recent study of 51 normal cats, bacteriuria was not detected when samples were collected by cystocentesis.[24] Further studies are needed to delineate the role of bacterial UTI in FUS and to determine the clinical and pathological significance of low numbers of bacteria in feline urine.

Mycoplasmal and Fungal Urinary Tract Infection

Currently, there is no evidence to support a substantial role for mycoplasma or fungi in FUS. In a recent study, mycoplasma were not detected in any of 48 cats with naturally occurring FUS.[1] There are currently no reports of fungal UTI in cats with clinical evidence of FUS. *Candida albicans* was isolated in 1 of 326 feline urine specimens in one study, but no information concerning clinical signs was given.[50] Despite the lack of evidence for an association between these infections and FUS, the possibility that these organisms may play a role in at least an occasional case of FUS should not be excluded.

Parasitic Infection

Although rare in cats, *Capillaria* infections of the urinary bladder may be associated with hematuria, dysuria, and pollakiuria.

Urolithiasis

Urolithiasis should be viewed as a sequela of one or more underlying disease processes rather than as a single disease entity. When uroliths are detected, the underlying disease responsible should be sought.

Urethral Plugs

Although feline urethral plugs presumably composed of struvite occur frequently in male cats, the composition and architecture of most urethral plugs appear to be dissimilar from those of struvite uroliths in other species and struvite uroliths in cats (Fig. 141–1). Urethral plugs appear to lack a definite structure. Most are thought to contain varying quantities of proteinaceous material, cellular debris, and crystals. Although there have been few documented studies of quantitative evaluation of the mineral and matrix composition of plugs, the general consensus of opinion is that the crystals of most plugs are composed of struvite.[18, 43] Unlike most struvite uroliths in dogs, humans, and mink, infection with urease-producing bacteria is uncommonly associated with struvite urethral plugs in cats. Viruses and dietary imbalances of calcium, phosphorus, and magnesium have been incriminated as possible etiological agents.[10–12, 27]

Feline Uroliths

Uroliths are polycrystalline concretions that contain greater than 95 per cent organic or inorganic crystalloids and have less than 5 per cent organic matrix (by weight). They may also contain a number of minor constituents. Although a particular mineral usually predominates, the mineral composition may be mixed. Unlike urethral plugs, uroliths are not disorganized precipitates of crystalline material. They are composed of organized crystal aggregates with a complex internal structure. Cross sections of uroliths often reveal nuclei and laminations and occasionally radial striations.

Uroliths similar in appearance to those in dogs and humans have been observed in the urinary system of male and female cats. In contrast to urethral plugs, most are radiodense.[3] Struvite calculi are the most common mineral form of feline uroliths (Table 141–2); ammonium urate, uric acid, and calcium oxalate calculi are encountered much less frequently. Cystine

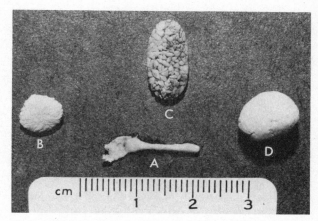

Figure 141–1. Photograph of a urethral plug (*a*), two waferlike sterile struvite uroliths (*b* and *c*), and an infected struvite urolith (*d*) removed from the urinary tract of male cats. One end of the urethral plug was crushed with an index finger to illustrate its friable nature.

and silica uroliths have not been observed in domestic cats.

Most calculi observed in cats occur in the bladder. On occasion, small calculi formed in the bladder may obstruct the urethra. Calculi located in the bladders of cats are frequently wafer- or disc-shaped; they are somewhat thicker at the center than at the periphery.

The etiology of most uroliths has not been determined. In some cats, especially those with wafer-shaped struvite calculi, urolith initiation and growth do not appear to be related to urinary tract infections. Affected patients typically have sterile urine. The gross appearance of these uroliths is similar to that of uroliths experimentally induced with high-magnesium diets.

Some cats may develop struvite uroliths as a sequela to urinary tract infections with urease-producing bacteria, especially staphylococci. The gross and microscopic appearance and the mineral composition of these "infection uroliths" are similar to those seen

TABLE 141–2. Quantitative Mineral Composition of Uroliths in 73 Male and Female Cats*

Mineral Composition	Number
100% Magnesium ammonium phosphate	68
> 70% Magnesium ammonium phosphate with calcium phosphate and/or ammonium urate	20
60% Magnesium ammonium phosphate; 40% ammonium urate	1
60% Calcium phosphate; 40% magnesium ammonium phosphate	1
100% Calcium phosphate	3
> 90% Calcium oxalate	3
100% Ammonium urate	2
100% Uric acid	2
Matrix	3
Cystine	0
Silica	0
Total	103

*Mineral composition determined by crystallography.

in dogs as sequelae to infection with urease-producing bacteria.

Like canine uroliths, feline uroliths have a tendency to recur. In a recent survey of uroliths in cats, there were 25 known recurrences in 131 patients.[3] Twenty-one cats had two episodes of recurrence, whereas three cats had three episodes and one cat had four episodes. Recurrence may be related to (1) persistence of the underlying cause, (2) failure to remove all uroliths from the urinary tract, especially those that are small in size, or (3) secondary urinary tract infection with urease-producing microbes, especially staphylococci.

We have observed three cases of *in vivo* dissolution of struvite uroliths in cats. Pilot studies of naturally occurring bladder uroliths have confirmed the feasilibility of therapeutic *in vivo* dissolution of natural struvite uroliths with low-magnesium diets and urinary tract acidifiers.

Influence of Diet

Dietary intake and urinary excretion of magnesium may be involved in the pathogenesis of urolithiasis and urethral obstruction. Results of several experimental studies have confirmed that feeding of high-magnesium diets (0.75 per cent on a dry weight basis) is associated with a substantial incidence (25 to 88 per cent) of urethral obstruction in male cats.[8, 20, 27] Postmortem examinations of these cats revealed cystic or urethral calculi, crystalline debris, and mucoid material. The composition of the calculi and crystalline debris produced in these studies has been reported as either magnesium phosphate or struvite. The clinical significance of these findings has been questioned because the mineral composition of the urethral plugs reported in earlier studies (magnesium phosphate) was not the same as that observed in the spontaneous disease (magnesium ammonium phosphate). However, the authors of these studies subsequently indicated that reports describing urolith composition as magnesium phosphate were in error and that uroliths and crystalline material produced in these studies were composed of magnesium ammonium phosphate.[26]

Although considerable experimental evidence linking high-magnesium diets to development of struvite uroliths and crystalluria exists, the association between these experimental observations and the natural disease remains controversial. Studies comparing the structure and composition of uroliths produced experimentally with those occurring in cats with natural diseases have not been published. However, it appears that uroliths experimentally induced with high-magnesium diets are similar to naturally occurring sterile struvite uroliths. We are doubtful that experimental uroliths are similar to urethral plugs.

The relationship between diet-induced increases in crystalluria and clinical signs of lower urinary tract disease in unobstructed male and female cats is unresolved. However, it has been reported that cats with naturally occurring "FUS" do not have larger numbers of struvite crystals in their urine than unaffected cats.[44]

Neoplasia

Neoplasms of the urinary bladder, urethra, and prostate are rare in cats.[7, 38] When present, neoplasms may result in clinical and laboratory signs of feline lower urinary tract disease, including intermittent or persistent hematuria, dysuria, and urinary obstruction. Tumors of the lower urinary tract may also predispose cats to bacterial urinary infection and infection-induced urolithiasis. Although uncommon, compression of the urinary outflow tract by tumors outside the urogenital system may also result in dysuria, hematuria, and urinary obstruction.

Urinary Tract Anomalies

A high incidence of anatomical anomalies of the urinary tract has been reported in cats with clinical signs of lower urinary tract disease.[17, 19] The most common anomaly is persistent urachal diverticula. Diverticula of the urinary bladder may be congenital or acquired; however, congenital forms are more common. Although urachal diverticula have been proposed as a significant predisposing factor in lower urinary tract disease,[17] the relationship between urachal diverticula and clinical signs of lower urinary tract disease in cats is not clear. One possible explanation is that urachal diverticula result in urinary stasis and retention and therefore predispose to urinary tract infection. The significance of urachal diverticula in cats with FUS characterized by bacteriologically sterile urine is unknown.

Congenital or acquired urethral strictures may be associated with dysuria and partial or complete urinary obstruction. Identification of the location and cause of the urethral stricture is important in developing a therapeutic plan. Urethral strictures that are cranial to the penile urethra will not be corrected by perineal or preputial urethrostomy.

Noninfectious Inflammatory Factors

Several types of noninfectious inflammatory cystitis have been recognized in humans, including interstitial cystitis,[28] eosinophilic cystitis,[47] lupus cystitis,[31] and cyclophosphamide-induced hemorrhagic cystitis.[39] Although these diseases may be associated with secondary bacterial infections, they are not initiated by any recognized infectious agent. Clinical signs of these diseases are typical of those of lower urinary tract disease and may include varying combinations of hematuria, dysuria, and pollakiuria. It is not known whether similar diseases occur in cats, partly because bladder biopsies are uncommonly obtained in cats with lower urinary tract disease.

Trauma

Traumatic injuries resulting in contusion, laceration, or rupture of the urinary bladder or urethra may result in hematuria, dysuria, or obstruction to urine outflow. Trauma may result from a number of causes, including automobile accidents, falls, fights, and deliberate abuse. Urethral and bladder trauma may also be induced by careless palpation or inappropriate urinary catheterization. Traumatic disorders of the lower urinary tract are often self-limiting and nonrecurrent.

Neurogenic Disorders

Neurogenic disorders of micturition, such as urethral spasm, reflex dyssynergia, and bladder atony may cause clinical signs of lower urinary tract disease, including dysuria, reduced size and force of the urine stream, urinary retention, and urinary obstruction. Hematuria may be present and may result from such factors as secondary bacterial infection or iatrogenic trauma associated with bladder compression or catheterization. Urinary retention and obstruction may predispose to bacterial urinary tract infection.

Clinical and laboratory findings that suggest neurogenic disorders as causes of lower urinary tract disease include (1) absence of blood, inflammatory cells, and bacteria in the urine sediment, (2) absence of urethral plugs or crystalline debris in male cats with urethral obstructions, and (3) moderate to large bladder capacity in cats that strain to urinate but from which urine can readily be expressed.

Iatrogenic Causes

Diagnostic and therapeutic instrumentation or manipulation of the urinary tract may result in trauma or secondary infection, leading to clinical signs of lower urinary tract disease. Routine procedures that may result in urinary trauma or infection include careless cystocentesis, urethral catheterization, surgery of the urinary bladder or urethra, excessively vigorous palpation of the lower urinary tract, and manual expression of urine from the urinary bladder.

Idiopathic Factors

Despite careful clinical evaluation, there are cats with lower urinary tract disease the etiology of which cannot readily be assigned to one of the previously designated categories. This may result from (1) inaccuracy or lack of sensitivity of diagnostic endeavors, (2) failure to perform diagnostic tests necessary for

TABLE 141–3. Factors That May Influence Predisposition to Feline Urologic Syndrome

Seasonal variation	Activity
Breed	Diet
Age	Feeding frequency
Nutritional status	Fluid intake
Neutering	Urination habits

identification of the underlying disease process (e.g., viral culture, mycoplasma culture, bladder biopsy, radiography of the urethra, and so on), or (3) the possibility that a unique lower urinary tract disease exists in cats for which the etiological factors have not yet been identified.

EPIDEMIOLOGY

Numerous epidemiological surveys have been performed to delineate the cause of "FUS."[9, 14, 41, 48, 49] These studies have implicated several predisposing factors that may be related to the development of FUS (Table 141–3). However, controversy still exists regarding the influence of these predisposing factors on FUS.[34, 48]

CLINICAL FINDINGS

Common clinical signs of feline lower urinary tract disease are summarized in Table 141–4. Clinical signs are often recurrent and intermittent in unobstructed male or female cats with lower urinary tract disease. In one study of naturally occurring FUS, clinical signs resolved within five days in 70 per cent of affected cats[2] regardless of therapy. In this same study, 39 per cent of affected cats experienced recurrence of clinical signs within 18 months. A smaller percentage of cats had persistent clinical signs of

TABLE 141–4. Common Clinical Signs of Feline Urologic Syndrome*

Nonobstructed and Obstructed Cats	Obstructed Cats
Dysuria	Depression
Pollakiuria	Dehydration
Inappropriate micturition	Anorexia
Hematuria	Enlarged urinary bladder
Reduced size and force of urine stream	(unless bladder has ruptured)
Licking of penis and prepuce	Vomiting
Crying when using litter pan	
Abdominal discomfort	
Spontaneous voiding of small uroliths or "sand"	

*Not all of these signs occur in every patient.

lower urinary tract disease. Because urolithiasis and congenital anomalies are more prevalent in cats with persistent clinical signs, they should be properly evaluated with appropriate diagnostic techniques.

Cats with nonobstructive lower urinary tract disorders have small, contracted urinary bladders; cats with evidence of lower urinary tract disease and enlarged urinary bladders should be suspected of having structural or functional obstruction to urine outflow. Clinical findings typical of urethral obstruction in cats include repeated attempts to micturate, dysuria, sitting or lying in the litter box, abdominal pain, licking of the penis and prepuce, and distressful crying. If urethral obstruction persists, signs of uremia—anorexia, depression, vomiting, dehydration, cardiac arrhythmias, hypothermia, and terminal coma—occur. Laboratory evaluation may reveal azotemia, hyperphosphatemia, metabolic acidosis, or hyperkalemia. Death usually results from fluid, electrolyte, and acid-base disturbances.

URINARY TRACT OBSTRUCTION

Urinary tract obstruction associated with "FUS" occurs predominantly, although not exclusively, in male cats, presumably as a result of the longer, narrower, less distensible urethra of male cats. The diameter of the penile urethra of male cats is much smaller than the diameter of the pelvic and preprostatic urethra. Clinical experience indicates that the penile urethra is the most common site of urethral obstruction. Although this opinion is logical, the site and degree of urethral obstruction have not been carefully documented in a large series of cats with naturally occurring disease (Fig. 141–2).[32] This neglect has left a conspicuous void in our knowledge, especially when consideration is given to the frequency with which surgical removal of the penile urethra is recommended to treat this disorder.

Although it is generally believed that urethral plugs are the most common cause of obstruction, urethral spasm, urinary calculi, urethral strictures, urethritis, and urethral trauma may cause or contribute to obstruction. The relative frequencies with which these various causes produce obstruction in cats with naturally occurring FUS is unknown.

DIAGNOSIS

Cats with clinical and laboratory evidence of lower urinary tract disease are considered to have FUS. Unfortunately, FUS is often considered as a diagnostic endpoint. However, in our view, FUS should be viewed as a starting point for diagnostic evaluation of affected patients.

A recommended diagnostic approach to cats with FUS is summarized in Table 141–5 and Figure 141–3. Typical urine sediment findings in cats with FUS include hematuria and crystalluria; pyuria and bacteriuria are less commonly observed. Evaluation of the history and results of complete urinalyses are often useful in differentiating inappropriate micturition due to behavioral abnormalities from other forms of FUS.[4] A urine sediment without blood, bacteria, or inflammatory cells should prompt consideration of behavioral abnormalities, structural anomalies of the urinary tract, or neuromuscular abnormalities of the urinary tract (e.g., urethral spasms, reflex dyssynergia, bladder atony). In contrast, hematuria, pyuria, or bacteriuria in the absence of clinical signs of lower urinary tract disease should prompt consideration of renal disease.

It is recommended that urine cultures be performed on all cats with FUS because (1) identification of bacterial urinary tract infection as the primary cause of FUS permits development of a specific therapeutic plan, and (2) identification and appropriate treatment of iatrogenic or secondary bacterial infections in cats with FUS may be beneficial in preventing complications that may result from such

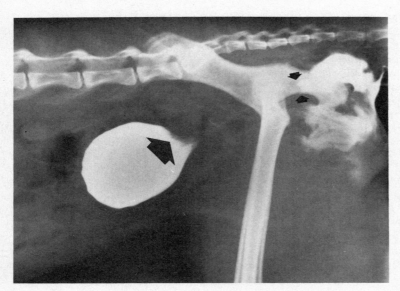

Figure 141–2. Positive contrast urethrocystogram of the lateral abdomen of a seven-year-old castrated male domestic long-haired cat with urethral obstruction. A perineal urethrostomy was performed three days previously. The lumen of the proximal urethra has been partially occluded by compression induced by a persistent uterus masculinus *(large arrow).* The lumen of the postprostatic urethra was completely obstructed by a stricture, presumably inflammatory in origin *(small arrows).*

TABLE 141–5.   Problem-Specific Data Base for Feline Urologic Syndrome

1. History checklist
   a. Changes in frequency and location of voiding?
   b. Apparent difficulty or pain upon voiding?
   c. Size and velocity of urine stream?
   d. Quantity of urine passed during each attempt at voiding?
   e. Changes in urine odor, color, or clarity?
   f. Presence of sand or calculi in urine?
   g. Changes in water consumption and overall urine production?
   h. Ability to void normally?
   i. Licking of vulva or prepuce?
   j. Duration of problem?
   k. Are problem(s) increasing in severity, decreasing in severity, or remaining the same?
   l. Other signs not directly related to the urinary system?
   m. Medications given? type? dose? response?

2. Physical examination checklist
   a. Kidneys
      (1) Position? Number?
      (2) Size? Shape? Consistency? Surface contour? Pain?
   b. Bladder
      (1) Position?
      (2) Size? Shape? Consistency?
      (3) Surface contour? Thickness of bladder wall?
      (4) Grating or nongrating masses within or adjacent to bladder lumen? If present, constant or variable in location?
      (5) Pain?
   c. Urethra
      (1) Position
      (2) Size? Shape? Consistency?
      (3) Uroliths or masses palpable?
      (4) Discharge or uroliths visible at urethral orifice?
      (5) Pain?
   d. Genital system
      (1) Prostate: position? size? shape? consistency? pain?
      (2) Penis and prepuce: size? shape? consistency? pain?
      (3) Vulva: size? shape? consistency? pain?

3. Laboratory and specialty examinations
   a. Complete blood count
   b. Urinalysis
   c. Quantitative urine culture
   d. Consider blood chemistry profile
   e. Consider quantitative urolith analysis
   f. Consider bladder biopsy
   g. Consider neurological examination
   h. Consider cystometrogram
   i. Consider special urine culture techniques (e.g., mycotic, mycoplasmal, or viral isolations)

4. Radiographic studies
   a. Survey abdominal radiographs
   b. Consider contrast urethrocystogram
   c. Consider double contrast cystogram

infections, e.g., pyelonephritis, systemic infections, and chronic urethrocystitis.

Radiographic studies are useful in detecting uroliths and structural lesions of the bladder that may be associated with FUS and in localizing the site of urethral lesions. Over 95 per cent of all uroliths in cats may be detected by survey radiography.[3] However, certain types of radiolucent uroliths or small uroliths may be detected only by contrast radiographic procedures.[19] In addition, structural or functional lesions of the urethra (urethral strictures, neoplasms, urethral spasms, and so on) or bladder (neoplasia, urachal diverticulae, and so on) may be detected only by contrast radiography. Survey abdominal radiographs should be performed on all cats with FUS to rule out urolithiasis. Retrograde or antegrade contrast urethrocystography and double contrast cystography should be considered in all cases in which the clinical signs of FUS are severe, protracted, or recurrent.

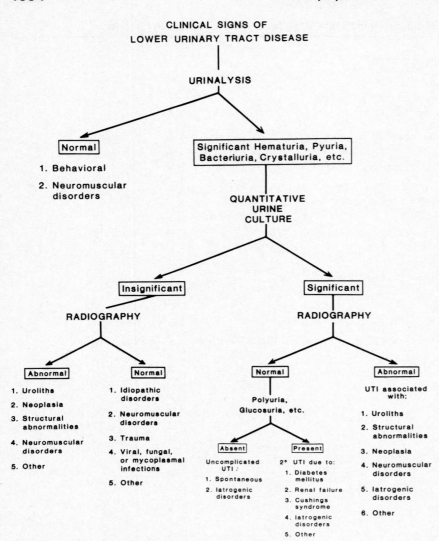

CLINICAL SIGNS OF
LOWER URINARY TRACT DISEASE

URINALYSIS

Normal
1. Behavioral
2. Neuromuscular disorders

Significant Hematuria, Pyuria, Bacteriuria, Crystalluria, etc.

QUANTITATIVE URINE CULTURE

Insignificant

RADIOGRAPHY

Abnormal
1. Uroliths
2. Neoplasia
3. Structural abnormalities
4. Neuromuscular disorders
5. Other

Normal
1. Idiopathic disorders
2. Neuromuscular disorders
3. Trauma
4. Viral, fungal, or mycoplasmal infections
5. Other

Significant

RADIOGRAPHY

Normal
Polyuria, Glucosuria, etc.

Absent
Uncomplicated UTI:
1. Spontaneous
2. Iatrogenic disorders

Present
2° UTI due to:
1. Diabetes mellitus
2. Renal failure
3. Cushings syndrome
4. Iatrogenic disorders
5. Other

Abnormal
UTI associated with:
1. Uroliths
2. Structural abnormalities
3. Neoplasia
4. Neuromuscular disorders
5. Iatrogenic disorders
6. Other

Figure 141–3. Urine cultures in cats should be obtained by cystocentesis. It is probable that data concerning significant bacteriuria in man and dogs represent overestimates for significant bacteriuria in cats, because cat urine normally inhibits the growth of commonly isolated aerobic bacterial pathogens. Recommended radiographic procedures include survey abdominal radiographs (which include the entire urinary tract from the penile urethra to the kidneys) and positive contrast urethrocystograms. Double contrast cystograms may be required to detect calculi less than 3 mm in diameter.

TREATMENT

Antibiotics, urinary acidifiers, low-magnesium diets, moist cat foods, increased dietary salt intake, free access to water, anti-inflammatory agents, urinary antiseptics, mineral chelators, hormones, and surgery, alone or in various combinations, have been recommended for the treatment of FUS.[13, 16, 18, 25, 35] These recommendations have generally been based on the premise that FUS represents a single disease entity. This error has been compounded by the fact that few controlled clinical studies have been performed to evaluate the effectiveness of these treatments. In those instances in which evaluation of therapeutic efficacy has been attempted, the etiological basis of the disorder being studied has generally not been sufficiently defined (see Table 141–5 and Fig. 141–3). Because the biological behavior and therapeutic responsiveness of various lower urinary tract diseases of cats are largely unknown, therapeutic recommendations for these disorders remain tentative (Table 141–6).

Consistently effective therapy of most feline lower urinary tract diseases must be based on an accurate diagnosis. It is beyond the scope of this chapter to discuss medical and surgical therapy of all feline lower urinary tract diseases. However, recommended therapies for various feline lower urinary tract diseases are summarized in Table 141–6. For additional information concerning treatment of these conditions, consult the references in the table and appropriate chapters in this text.

MEDICAL PROPHYLAXIS

Recurrence of urinary obstruction or clinical signs is a substantial problem in cats with lower urinary tract disease.[2, 5, 14] Numerous prophylactic measures have been recommended in attempt to minimize or prevent the incidence of recurrence, including dietary modifications (low-magnesium and high-moisture cat foods), administration or urine acidifiers, supplementation of dietary salt intake, administration

TABLE 141–6.   Usual Treatment of Lower Urinary Tract Diseases of Cats

Etiology	Recommended Treatment	References	Etiology	Recommended Treatment	References
Bacterial UTI	Appropriate antibiotics based on urine culture and antimicrobial susceptibility	40	Trauma	May require some combination of anti-inflammatory drugs, antibiotics, or surgery, depending on type and extent of trauma	
Mycotic UTI	Appropriate antimycotic agents (e.g., 5-fluorocytosine or ketoconazole)	40	Urethral spasm	Treat underlying cause of urethral spasm if identified; smooth muscle relaxants (e.g., phenoxybenza-mine) or skeletal muscle relaxants (e.g., diazepam) may be of benefit	29,30
Mycoplasmal UTI	Appropriate antibiotics				
Viral UTI	None available; prevent secondary bacterial UTI				
Struvite uroliths	Surgical removal or medical dissolution using low-magnesium diets and urinary acidifiers; urethral uroliths may be dislodged by flushing procedures		Reflex dyssynergia	Phenoxybenzamine; bethanecol chloride may also be necessary if detrusor function is decreased	29,30
Other uroliths	Surgical removal or medical dissolution		Bladder atony	Empty bladder by intermittent or indwelling urinary catheterization; bethanecol chloride may be indicated; phenoxybenzamine may be necessary if urethral pressure is not appropriately decreased during the voiding phase of micturition; antibiotic therapy is usually necessary because of urine stasis and urethral catheterization	29,30
Urethral plugs	Removal by appropriate techniques				
Neoplasia	Surgical resection, chemotherapy, immunotherapy, or radiation therapy, depending on type and behavior of neoplasm	7,38			
Anomalies	Surgical correction, if possible				
Capillaria plica infection	Albendazole		Idiopathic FUS	Symptomatic therapy to control discomfort or urge incontinence may be indicated	13,35

of crystallization inhibitors, and free access to water.[13, 24, 36, 37] These recommendations are directed primarily at altering urine struvite supersaturation and are based on the assumption that struvite crystalluria and urolithiasis play an importat role in the pathogenesis of recurrent FUS. Although this may be correct in some instances, it is improbable that this assumption is correct for all cats with lower urinary tract disease. As with selection of initial treatment, consistently effective prevention of recur-

rent "FUS" is dependent upon identification and elimination of the etiological factors that led to lower urinary tract disease. Patients should be carefully evaluated for abnormalities that may predispose to lower urinary tract disease. For example, cats with urinary tract infection should be examined for evidence of abnormal micturition, incomplete emptying of the excretory pathway, anatomical defects, alterations of the urothelium, impaired immunocompetence, and alterations in the volume, frequency, or

20. Kalkelz, F. A., and Bennett, J. D.: Urethral obstruction in random source and SPF male cats induced by high levels of dietary magnesium or magnesium and phosphorus. Feline Pract. 10:25, 1980.
21. Lees, G. E., and Osborne, C. A.: Antibacterial properties of urine: a comparative review. J. Am. Anim. Hosp. Assoc. 15:125, 1979.
22. Lees, G. E., Osborne, C. A., and Stevens, J. B.: Antibacterial properties of urine: studies of feline urine specific gravity, osmolality, and pH. J. Am. Anim. Hosp. Assoc. 15:135, 1979.
23. Lees, G. E., Osborne, C. A., and Stevens, J. B.: Urine: a medium for bacterial growth. Vet. Clin. North Am. 9:611, 1979.
24. Lees, G. E., Osborne, C. A., Stevens, J. B., and Ward, G. E.: Adverse effects of open indwelling urethral catheterization in clinically normal male cats. Am. J. Vet. Res. 42:825, 1981.
25. Lewis, L. D.: F.U.S., A Commentary on Nutritional Management of Small Animals. Mark Morris Associates, Topeka, KS, 1981.
26. Lewis, L. D.: Personal communication, 1983.
27. Lewis, L. D., Chow, F. H. C., Taton, G. F., and Hamar, D. W.: Effect of various dietary mineral concentrations on the occurrence of feline urolithiasis. J. Am. Vet. Med. Assoc. 172:559, 1978.
28. Messing, E. M., and Stamey, T. A.: Interstitial cystitis: early diagnosis, pathology, and treatment. Urology 12:381, 1978.
29. Moreau, R. M.: Neurogenic disorders of micturition in the dog and cat. Comp. Cont. Ed. 4:12, 1982.
30. Oliver, J. E., and Osborne, C. A.: Neurogenic urinary incontinence. In Kirk, R. W. (ed.): Current Veterinary Therapy VII. W. B. Saunders, Philadelphia, 1980, pp. 1122–1127.
31. Orth, R. W., Weisman, M. H., Cohen, A. H., Talner, L. B., Nachtsheim, D., and Zvaifler, N. J.: Lupus cystitis: primary bladder manifestations of systemic lupus erythematosus. Ann. Intern. Med. 98:323, 1983.
32. Osborne, C. A., Johnston, G. R., Polzin, D. J., et al.: Feline

Veterinary Therapy VII. W. B. Saunders, Philadelphia, 1980.
38. Osborne, C. A., Low, D. G., and Perman, V.: Neoplasms of the canine and feline urinary bladder: clinical findings, diagnosis, and treatment. J. Am. Vet. Med. Assoc. 153:247, 1968.
39. Plotz, P. H., Klippel, J. H., Decker, J. L., Grauman, D., Wolff, B., Brown, B. C., and Rutt, G.: Bladder complications in patients receiving cyclophosphamide for systemic lupus erythematosus or rheumatoid arthritis. Ann. Intern. Med. 91:221, 1979.
40. Polzin, D. J., and Jeraj, K.: Urethritis, cystitis, and ureteritis. Vet. Clin. North Am. 9:661, 1979.
41. Reif, J. S., Bovee, K. C., Gaskell, C. J., Batt, R. M., and Maguire, T. G.: Feline urethral obstruction: a case-controlled study. J. Am. Vet. Med. Assoc. 170:1320, 1977.
42. Rich, L. J., Dysart, I., Chow, F. H. C., and Hamar, D. W.: Urethral obstruction in male cats: experimental production by addition of magnesium and phosphate to diet. Feline Pract. 4:44, 1974.
43. Rich, L. J., and Kirk, R. W.: Feline urethral obstruction: mineral aspects. Am. J. Vet. Res. 29:2149, 1968.
44. Rich, L. J., and Kirk, R. W.: The relationship of struvite crystals to urethral obstruction in cats. J. Am. Vet. Med. Assoc. 154:153, 1969.
45. Rich, L. J., and Norcross, N. L.: Feline urethral obstruction: immunologic identification of a unique urinary protein. Am. J. Vet. Res. 30:1001, 1969.
46. Schecter, R. D.: The significance of bacteria in feline cystitis and urolithiasis. J. Am. Vet. Med. Assoc. 156:1567, 1970.
47. Sidh, S. M., Smith, S. P., Silber, S. B., and Young, J. D.: Eosinophilic cystitis: advanced disease requiring surgical intervention. Urology 15:23, 1980.
48. Willeberg, P.: Epidemiology of the feline urological syndrome. Adv. Vet. Sci. Comp. Med. 25:311, 1981.
49. Willeberg, P., and Priester, W. A.: Feline urologic syndrome: associations with some time, space, and individual patient factors. Am. J. Vet. Res. 37:975, 1978.
50. Wooley, R. E., and Blue, J. L.: Bacterial isolations from canine and feline urine. Mod. Vet. Pract. 57:535, 1976.

TABLE 141–7.   **Medical Prophylaxis of Feline Lower Urinary Tract Disease**

Etiology	Recommended Prophylaxis	References
Bacterial, mycotic, or mycoplasmal UTI	Appropriate specific therapy for the disease process; identification and elimination of predisposing factors, if possible	33,40
Viral UTI	?	
Struvite uroliths	Low-magnesium diets; urinary acidifiers; appropriate therapy for urinary tract infections, if present; identification of any predisposing factors, if possible	20,25,27
Other uroliths	? (insufficient numbers of cases have been examined to permit generalizations)	
Urethral plugs	If a large proportion of the plug is struvite, consider low-magnesium diets and acidifiers; there are no proven methods to specifically prevent formation of plug matrix, since its genesis and composition are unknown	
Capillaria plica infection	Prevent access to earthworms	
Neurogenic dysfunctions	Diagnosis and appropriate therapy of the neuromuscular disorder may prevent recurrences; in some cases, lifelong therapy may be necessary; preventing bladder atony is largely dependent upon preventing urinary retention due to urethral spasm, uroliths, etc.	
Idiopathic FUS	?	36,37

composition of urine.[33] Recommended prophylactic measures for various forms of feline lower urinary tract disease are summarized in Table 141–7.

Unfortunately, controlled studies to evaluate the efficacy of various prophylactic medial regimens in minimizing or eliminating clinical signs of lower urinary tract disease, including urethral obstruction, have not been performed in cats with idiopathic FUS. Until the results of such studies become available, recommendations concerning medical prophylaxis of this condition remain empirical. The therapeutic ef-

elimination behavior problems in cats. Vet. Clin. North Am. *12*:673, 1982.
5. Bovee, K. C., Reif, J. S., Maguire, T. J., Gaskell, C. J., and Batt, R. M.: Recurrence of feline urethral obstruction. J. Am. Vet. Med. Assoc. *174*:93, 1979.
6. Burrows, C. F., and Bovee, K. C.: Characterization and treatment of acid-base and renal defects due to urethral obstruction in cats. J. Am. Vet. Med. Assoc. *172*:801, 1978.
7. Caywood, D. D., Osborne, C. A., and Johnston, G. R.: Neoplasms of the canine and feline urinary tracts. *In* Kirk, R. W. (ed.): *Current Veterinary Therapy VII*. W. B. Saunders, Philadelphia, 1980, pp. 1203–1212.
8. Chow, F. C.: Dietary ...

Section XVI

Endocrine System

Anthony Schwartz
Section Editor

The History of Clinical Pituitary Diseases in Small Animals

Although descriptions of pituitary tumors in the dog appeared as early as 1935, it was not until 1939 that the first description of Cushing's disease in the dog appeared.[75] Clinical studies by Coffin and Munson (1953),[11] pathological studies by Capen and coworkers (1967)[6], and clinical, biochemical, and pathological studies by Rijnberk and associates (1968)[62] are milestones in the history of a now frequently recognized and treatable disease. Acromegalic features in a dog suffering from an eosinophilic adenoma were reported in 1923 by Luksch.[42] Acromegaly was again tentatively diagnosed by Groen and colleagues (1963) in a female dog having also a pituitary adenoma.[28] However, it was not until 1980 that Rijnberk and coworkers[63] conclusively diagnosed iatrogenic acromegaly in a dog and not until 1981 that Eigenmann and Venker-van Haagen[20] reported a large number of dogs suffering from either iatrogenic or spontaneous acromegaly.

Dwarfism in German shepherds was tentatively diagnosed to be of pituitary origin in 1953. It was not until recently that dwarfism in this breed was unequivocally determined to be of pituitary origin (growth hormone deficiency).[16, 69]

ANATOMY OF THE PITUITARY GLAND

Developmental Anatomy[24, 32, 45]

Contact between the oral and neural ectoderm occurs at an early stage of development. A small portion of oral ectoderm evaginates and contacts the ventral surface of the neural tube. This portion is ultimately freed entirely from the remaining ectoderm. With continued differentiation, a small evagination of the neural tube develops at the point of adhesion with the oral ectoderm. This structure becomes surrounded by the collapsing vesicle of oral ectoderm. Components of the surrounding mesenchyme develop into the stroma and blood vessels of the pituitary.

A portion of the neuroectoderm forms the neurohypophysis, consisting of the pars proximalis and pars distalis. The oral ectoderm surrounds the neurohypophysis. The surface of the oral ectoderm vesicle contacting the neurohypophysis develops into the pars intermedia. The remaining part of the vesicle, not being in direct contact with the neurohypophysis, evolves into the pars proximalis and the pars distalis of the adenohypophysis.

The size of the pituitary varies among breeds of dogs, and variation occurs even in the same breed. In 10-kg dogs, the weight of the pituitary ranges from less than 100 to about 300 mg. The larger the dog, the bigger the pituitary. This represents only an increase in absolute weight. The relative pituitary weight in a large dog is less than that in a small dog.[31, 73]

Macroscopic Anatomy[24, 32, 45]

The main part of the pituitary is embedded in a recess in the sphenoid bone. The recess is shallow in the dog but not in man. The cranial and caudal margins of the fossa are formed by the tuberculum sellae. Dorsally, the pituitary is confined by the dorsum sellae. Although the external or endosteal layer of the dura mater extends into the pituitary fossa and lines the fossa, the inner meningeal part does not enter and forms the diaphragma sellae (dorsum sellae). In the dog, in contrast to man, a large oval foramen is present in the center of the diaphragm, allowing dorsal expansion of tumor growth. Large cavernous sinuses can be found on both sides of the pituitary. In the dog, they are connected by a smaller caudal transverse sinus. Within each of the cavernous sinuses lie the rostral portion of the middle meningeal artery and the anastomotic ramus of the external ophthalmic artery. In addition, the internal carotid artery courses through each of the sinuses. In close proximity to the hypophysis pass the oculomotor, trochlear, and abducent nerves and the ophthalmic branch of the trigeminal nerve.

The Parts of the Pituitary

Proximal Part

This part consists of the infundibular portions of the neuro- and adenohypophysis. Together, they form a funnel-like structure enclosing the infundibular recess, the pituitary stalk. This structure consists of a neural and an epithelial component. The epithelial cells are of a cuboidal, undifferentiated nature. The infundibular part of the adenohypophysis contains the long portal vessels and some of the capillary network draining into the portal vessels. The neural tissue consists mainly of nonmyelinated nerve fibers from the hypothalamus, blood vessels, and pituicytes. The neural tissue is composed of distinct internal and external zones. The internal zone contains fibers extending from the supraoptic and paraventricular nuclei of the hypothalamus into the pituitary. The external zone is the site of termination of the tuberoinfundibular fiber system. The fiber system probably originates from the parvocellular nuclei located in the region called the hypophysiotrophic area.

Distal Part

This part consists of the pars distalis and pars intermedia of the adenohypophysis and the infundibular process of the neurohypophysis. The pars distalis adenohypophysis is composed of cuboidal epithelial cells and contains a network of sinusoids. The cells can be characterized according to content of granules, staining properties, and size as acidophils, basophils, and chromophobes. Sophisticated staining techniques have revealed that both basophils and acidophils consist of distinct classes of cell types. Among acidophils, growth hormone–(GH) secreting cells and prolactin-secreting cells are recognized. The latter can be differentiated from GH-producing cells by light microscopy. Basophils secrete thyroid-stimulating hormones (TSH), gonadotropins (luteinizing hormone, follicle-stimulating hormone), and adenocorticotropic hormone (ACTH). Of the anterior pituitary cells, depending on the staining techniques, 15 to 40 per cent are chromophobic by light microscopy. Depending on the stain, these cells resemble either basophils or acidophils and have been named amphophils. Although in the normal pituitary no hormonal secretory role for these cells has been identified, it is possible that they are either actively secreting or resting, degranulated cells. Moreover, in pituitary tumors these cells have been associated with hormone oversecretion. Cells of a given type tend to be clustered together in certain regions of the pars distalis.

Pars Intermedia

The pars intermedia varies considerably in extent and demarcation in various animal species. There is no distinct pars intermedia in the pituitary of the adult human. However, the pars intermedia does exist in the dog and consists of a broad band of epithelial cells. Although the cat also has a pars intermedia, the zone is not as prominent as that in the dog. The band is intimately attached to the infundibular process but is partly separated from the pars distalis by Rathke's cleft (the residual lumen of the Rathke's pouch).

There are two cell types in the pars intermedia, the A- and B-cells. These epithelial cells are either large and rounded or smaller and more angular. Together, these cells secrete melanotropin, ACTH, and B-lipotropin. Whereas the A-cells secrete all of these hormones, the B-cells secrete only ACTH and lipotropin.[29] There are few blood vessels and only occasional nerve fibers in the pars intermedia.

Infundibular Process

The infundibular process comprises the distal part of the neural component of the pituitary gland. The majority of nerve fibers of the supraoptic-paraventriculohypophyseal tract terminate here. Ramifications of these fibers extend into the posterior lobe. Stainable neurosecretory material containing vasopressin, oxytocin, and their carrier proteins is present, particularly around the blood vessels.

Vascularization of the Pituitary

The major arterial supply is provided by the internal carotid arteries and the caudal communicating arteries. Several branches that provide blood supply directly to the pituitary stem from the rostral and caudal intercarotid arteries and the caudal communicating arteries. Four to ten branches to the proximal part of the neurohypophysis stem from the rostral intercarotid artery. Another extensive group of vessels arises from the rostral communicating arteries. All of these vessels pass toward the proximal part of the neurohypophysis. Here, by anastomosing, they form the mantle plexus. On the cranial and lateral surfaces of the median eminence, major vessels arise from the mantle plexus or as direct branches of the intercarotid vessels, named the rostral hypophyseal arteries. Several of these provide capillaries to the median eminence and the proximal part of the neurohypophysis. The capillaries receive neurohumoral substances (releasing factors), subsequently carried from the hypothalamus, via the portal system, to the pituitary. The capillaries of the adenohypophysis form the secondary blood capillary network. The veins that connect the secondary with the primary (situated in the infundibulum) plexus are the portal vessels of the pituitary.

Hypothalamic-Hypophyseal Connections[14, 21, 37, 52, 72]

Both neural and neurovascular connections are found between the hypothalamus and the pituitary gland. Nonmyelinated axons arise from the supraoptic and paraventricular nuclei and pass through the infundibulum as the supraoptic-paraventriculo-hypophyseal tract. This tract conveys vasopressin, oxytocin, and their neurophysins (carrier proteins). This system is referred to as the magnocellular neurosecretory system.

The parvocellular system is represented by the tuberoinfundibular tract. This tract originates from the periventricular and infundibular nuclei and terminates on the portal vessels of the tuberal area of the infundibulum. This system is believed to transport corticotropin-releasing factor (CRF).

The portal system consists of a primary capillary plexus in the infundibulum that is continuous with both the vascular bed of the hypothalamus and the secondary capillary plexus situated within the pituitary. Connection is provided by the long portal vessels. A second, primary capillary plexus supplied by the inferior hypophyseal arteries is situated in the infundibular process. This plexus is connected with the adenohypophyseal plexus by short portal vessels.

Thus, all blood ultimately reaching the pituitary passes through one of the two primary plexuses.

PITUITARY HORMONES: CHEMISTRY AND PHYSIOLOGY

Growth Hormone (GH)

GH is a single-chain polypeptide with interchain disulfide linkages. Among different species, the molecular weight is fairly constant (approximately 22,000 daltons). Although subprimate GHs are biologically inactive in humans, human GH is biologically active in dogs. Moreover, there is immunological and biological cross-reactivity among most nonprimate, mammalian growth hormones.[77] In contrast to other pituitary hormones, GH's action is not confined to one single target tissue. The molecule displays two diametrically opposed biological activities, anabolic (growth-promoting) and catabolic (diabetogenic). It is widely assumed that the growth-promoting effect of GH is indirect. GH controls growth factors (somatomedins, insulinlike growth factors), which in turn stimulate growing tissues, thus mediating the effect of GH.[8, 74, 79] In addition, GH is a potent diabetogenic agent.[2, 78] In certain species, e.g., the dog and cat, the hormone evokes increased lipolysis and hyperglycemia characterized by insulin resistance and subsequent diabetes. It is possible that this dual nature of GH is due to different smaller fragments evolving from the large GH molecule. The regulation of GH secretion is mediated by both a releasing factor (GHRF) and an inhibiting factor (somatostatin, SRIF) of hypothalamic origin. GH secretion/suppression is governed by a multitude of stimuli. Stimulatory effects in man are sleep, exercise, stress, hypoglycemia, neurotransmitters (α-adrenergic substances, dopaminergic agonists), starvation, chronic renal failure, and TSH-releasing hormone in acromegaly. Suppression is induced by hyperglycemia, somatostatin, glucocorticoids, α-adrenergic antagonists, and severe hypothyroidism.[40, 58, 65] With some exceptions, similar factors are involved in the control of GH secretion in the dog.[18, 41]

Prolactin[39, 49, 51]

Prolactin is closely related to GH, and there are extensive interspecies similarities between GH and prolactin. The primary site of prolactin action is the breast, where, in conjunction with other hormones, mammary tissue development and lactation are stimulated. Prolactin is somehow involved in normal breast development in many species, although an essential role has yet to be demonstrated.

During pregnancy, the increase in prolactin in conjunction with sex steroid hormones and in the presence of insulin results in additional breast development, leading eventually to milk formation. Prolactin specifically stimulates the synthesis of milk proteins. Continued prolactin secretion is required to maintain lactation once it has begun. Metabolic actions of prolactin in hypophysectomized animals resemble those of GH, including stimulation of protein synthesis and chondroitin sulfate formation in cartilage. The stimulatory and inhibitory effects of prolactin are almost exactly the same as those for the regulation of GH. Additional stimuli include pregnancy, nursing, and nipple stimulation.

The neuroendocrine control of prolactin is predominantly inhibitory. The hypothalamic inhibitor (PIF) is under dopaminergic control. A hypothalamic factor that stimulates prolactin release has been described, although its specific identity and physiological role remain to be determined.

Thyroid-Stimulating Hormone (TSH)[12, 23, 56, 67, 72, 75]

TSH is a glycoprotein with a molecular weight of approximately 28,500 daltons. TSH is composed of subunits termed α and β, as are the other pituitary glycoprotein hormones (LH and FSH). Within a single species, including humans, the α subunits of LH, FSH, and TSH are identical. The β subunit varies, providing the biological specificity to each hormone.

The effects of TSH on the thyroid glands are largely the same as those of ACTH on the adrenal glands. TSH promotes thyroid hormone synthesis and, probably in conjunction with other serum factors, controls thyroid size. In the thyroid, TSH stimulates mRNA and protein synthesis. Chronic overstimulation by TSH leads to an increase in thyroid size (goiter).

TSH secretion is governed by two main factors, the feedback effect of thyroid hormones and central nervous system stimuli and TSH-releasing hormone. Both thyroxin (T_4) and triiodothyroxine (T_3) are potent feedback-regulating hormones at the level of the pituitary. Thus, in the presence of low T_3 but normal T_4 concentrations, e.g., in chronic illness, TSH levels remain within the normal range. T_4 appears to be efficiently and preferentially deiodinated to T_3 within the pituitary, providing evidence that T_3 is the major hormone exerting feedback inhibition for TSH secretion. The influence of TRH on TSH secretion is of a modulatory nature. TSH is further influenced by glucocorticoids, which suppress TSH secretion.

Follicle-stimulating (FSH) and Luteinizing Hormone (LH)

FSH stimulates ovarian follicular and testicular growth and spermatogenesis. LH acts to promote ovulation and luteinization of the ovarian follicle as well as to stimulate testicular interstitial (Leydig) cell function and enhance steroid production in both the ovaries and testes (progesterone and testosterone, respectively). The control of secretion is complex, involving the gonadal and hypothalamic system, and there are differences between species. For detailed information, the reader is referred to textbooks of reproductive endocrinology.[26, 64]

Adrenocorticotropic Hormone (ACTH)[29, 32, 36, 38, 47, 61, 66, 73]

ACTH is a single chain, 39 amino acid peptide. The N-terminal amino acids 1 to 24 are identical in all species thus far studied. For full biological activity, the first 18 amino acids are required. A number of related peptides share a portion of the ACTH molecule. Two of these are fragments of ACTH, α-melanocyte–stimulating hormone (α-MSH, identical to $ACTH_{1-13}$) and corticotropinlike intermediate lobe peptide (CLIP, identical to $ACTH_{18-39}$). Furthermore, β-lipotropin (β-LPH), a 91 amino acid peptide, contains a heptapeptide that is identical to $ACTH_{4-10}$. α-MSH and CLIP are primarily found in species with a more fully developed intermediate lobe (e.g., sheep and dog). β-LPH contains the structures of α-MSH and β-endorphin. It is now accepted that ACTH and other peptides are cleavage products from a common precursor glycoprotein molecule. This molecule has been variously named pro-ACTH/endorphin, pro-corticomelanotropin, pro-opiocortin, and pro-corticolipotropin.

The primary effects of ACTH are on the adrenal cortex, where the hormone stimulates the secretion of glucocorticoids, mineralocorticoids, and androgenic steroids. The effect of ACTH on mineralocorticoid synthesis is only transient. ACTH stimulates protein synthesis; if ACTH oversecretion persists, adrenal hypertrophy and hyperplasia result.

Three major control systems contribute to ACTH secretion: a feedback system responsive to cortisol, an inherent diurnal rhythm, and a neurally mediated stimulus commonly referred to as "stress." ACTH is secreted in a pulsatile manner, and, hence, diurnal rhythmicity is observed for both ACTH and cortisol secretion. Cortisol exhibits a negative feedback effect at the level of the central nervous system and the pituitary. Moreover, evidence exists that cortisol exerts a negative feedback effect on corticotropin-releasing factor (CRF) via both the hypothalamus and extrahypothalamic sites.

Measurement of Pituitary Hormones in the Dog

Plasma concentrations of most pituitary hormones can be reliably assessed by radioimmunoassay (RIA) techniques. Hormones that can be measured include GH, ACTH, FSH, LH, and prolactin.[5, 25, 41, 59] An RIA for canine TSH has recently been reported. However, data on spontaneous diseases affecting TSH levels are not available.[57]

PRIMARY PITUITARY DISEASES

Hypofunction[1]

Hypopituitarism is characterized by a failure of a single (monotropic failure), several (multitropic failure), or all pituitary hormones. The last-mentioned is also referred to as panhypopituitarism or, in adult man, Simmond's disease.[70] Pituitary failure leads to an impaired production of target gland hormones such as T_4, T_3, corticosteroids, and sex steroids. As a result, the same signs may appear as those observed in primary target gland deficiency. In adult humans, panhypopituitarism is associated with clinical signs and symptoms such as changes in menstruation, loss of libido, failure of lactation, loss of pubic hair growth, hypoglycemia, intolerance to cold, adynamia, oliguria, and somnolence. Diabetes insipidus may occur temporarily. Hypopituitarism is encountered in adulthood or childhood; in the latter instance, it causes dwarfism. In man, the incidence of panhypopituitarism in adulthood is very low (1 in 10,000).

Pituitary failure may be due to processes directly impairing the hypothalamic-pituitary system (e.g.,

TABLE 142–1. Etiology and Clinical Signs of Hypopituitarism

Etiology	
Hypothalamic/Pituitary Origin	Extrasellar Structural Disease
Congenital	Space-occupying lesions
Traumatic	
Degenerative	
Inflammatory	
Vascular	
Neoplastic	
Functional (systemic disease, thyroid/adrenal disorders, administration of thyroid hormones or glucocorticoids, neuropharmacological medication)	

	Clinical Signs	
Hormone	Puppyhood	Adulthood
Growth hormone	Short stature/hair loss	Hair loss
TSH	Signs of hypothyroidism	Signs of hypothyroidism
ACTH	Adrenal atrophy, signs of glucocorticoid withdrawal (e.g., weakness, hypotension)	
Gonadotropins	Failure of sexual maturation	Loss of libido, testicular atrophy, absence of estrus
Prolactin	None	Failure of lactation possible

congenital, traumatic, inflammatory, vascular, degenerative, neoplastic, functional impairment by drugs, excessive autonomous secretion of peripheral hormones, e.g., T_4/T_3 and corticosteroids) or structural diseases that are anatomically separate from the hypothalamic-pituitary region (e.g., space-occupying lesions, aneurysms, or meningiomas) (Table 142–1).

In the dog, hypopituitarism is most frequently encountered as a congenital defect resulting in dwarfism in German shepherds. Hypopituitarism in mature dogs, documented by endocrine function studies, has rarely been reported.

Hypopituitarism in German Shepherd Dwarfs[3, 17]

Dwarfism in German shepherds is characterized clinically by short stature and hyperpigmentation and fragility of the skin. Further possible skin changes include a variable degree of insufficient hair growth (absence of primary hair, alopecia) (Fig. 142–1). The disease is transmitted by autosomal, recessive inheritance. Most of the dogs studied at necropsy exhibit a pituitary cyst. Although most authors assume that the cyst, by exerting pressure on the surrounding tissue, leads to pituitary hypofunction, this hypothesis can be challenged. For example, it is possible that pituitary cells fail to differentiate and instead of secreting specific peptides (hormones) secrete proteinaceous material into the cleft. Such proteinaceous material, as shown in other species, may be osmotically active, thereby attracting water and enlarging the cyst. Although unlikely, it is possible that surgical

evacuation of the cyst might partially restore pituitary function. The consistent endocrine abnormality is GH-deficiency and, consequently, a lack of GH-dependent growth factors (somatomedin/insulin like growth factor). Some dogs suffer from secondary hypothyroidism (with subnormal T_4 levels), in which the thyroids remain responsive to TSH. Treatment involves growth hormone and thyroxine administration.

Hypopituitarism Associated with Pituitary Tumors

Hypopituitarism in adult dogs, caused by pituitary tumors and documented by hormonal studies, rarely has been reported. Most of the diagnoses have been based on clinical and pathological findings. Moreover, in some of the reported cases, the primary disease may not have been hypopituitarism *per se* but rather Cushing's syndrome or another disease.

Dystrophia adiposogenitalis (Fröhlich's syndrome) has been described in a number of dogs.[13, 44] The disorder is caused by a craniopharyngioma, which, in man, can appear at any age. Craniopharyngiomas alter pituitary function primarily by mechanical/functional impairment of the hypothalamus, which leads to a deficiency of hypophysiotropic hormone. Obesity associated with Fröhlich's syndrome is also a result of hypothalamic impairment. Diabetes insipidus commonly occurs as well. Common endocrine changes in man include failure of GH and gonadotropin secretion. ACTH and TSH failure appear to be less common. In dogs with craniopharyngioma, clinical and pathological findings similar to those of man are seen. Endocrine function studies, however, are lacking.

Nelson's syndrome, i.e., hypopituitarism caused by mechanical or functional impairment of remaining pituitary tissue by ACTH-producing tumors,[50] is also observed in dogs. Actually, such tumors may develop preferentially in individuals treated for Cushing's disease with o,p'-DDD or by adrenalectomy. Patients treated for Cushing's disease are deprived of endogenous glucocorticoids. Physiological levels of glucocorticoids decrease ACTH-releasing hormone and, in turn, may decrease tumor growth and ACTH secretion. Hence, treatment of Cushing's disease may increase the rate of formation of a pituitary tumor.

Endocrine studies of hypopituitary dogs are rare. Rijnberk described secondary hypothyroidism due to a pituitary tumor in two dogs.[60] Eigenmann and coworkers described panhypopituitarism (GH failure and secondary hypothyroidism/hypoadrenocorticism) associated with diabetes insipidus in an adult dog. This dog appeared to have a pure suprasellar tumor, possibly a craniopharyngioma.[19]

Clinical signs associated with hypopituitarism vary and include hypothyroidism, hypoadrenocorticism, hypogonadism, and GH failure (hair loss). Secondary

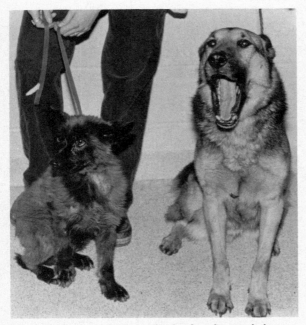

Figure 142–1. Dwarf German shepherd with growth hormone deficiency (left) and normal adult German shepherd. Note short stature and puppy haircoat in the dwarf.

hypoadrenocorticism in the dog does not lead to clinical signs, and hypoglycemia and electrolyte disturbances generally are not observed. If present, electrolyte disturbances, e.g., changes in serum sodium concentration, actually may be caused by hypothalamic derangement. Physiologically, the thirst center, located in the hypothalamus, is controlled by osmoreceptor cells situated in the anterior (cranial) hypothalamus. Changes in the structural or functional integrity of osmoreceptors may give rise to adipsia or exaggerated drinking behavior. This may be associated with impaired ADH secretion. At any rate, appreciable changes in hydration may induce hypernatremia as in ADH deficiency or adipsia or hyponatremia as in overdrinking.[68]

Isolated GH Deficiency in Mature Dogs

Recent investigations have shown that this disorder is not as uncommon as initially suspected. In the mature animal, signs of short stature are not observed. However, affected dogs are presented with severe alopecia and hyperpigmentation of the skin. The cause of GH failure remains unknown. Pathology reports from such dogs are not available. Treatment involves GH replacement.[54]

Pituitary Impairment Caused by Drugs[4, 7, 15, 22, 34, 53, 55]

Iatrogenic, drug-induced hypopituitarism may be a physiological or a pharmacological phenomenon. Administration of glucocorticoids or thyroid hormone, for example, invariably leads to suppression of ACTH and TSH secretion, respectively. However, aside from the latter physiological feedback mechanism, a few commonly used drugs suppress secretion of other pituitary hormones. In man, glucocorticoids are known to suppress GH and TSH levels. GH suppression in canine Cushing's disease has recently been documented. Thyroid hormone concentrations in dogs with iatrogenic or spontaneous Cushing's disease, not uncommonly, are low. It is possible that in the dog glucocorticoids, in addition to other effects, actually suppress TSH levels (TSH levels may be suppressed in humans suffering from glucocorticoid excess). Furthermore, megestrol acetate (Ovaban) commonly used in feline practice effectively suppresses pituitary-adrenal function, probably by virtue of intrinsic glucocorticoid activity.

DIAGNOSIS OF HYPOPITUITARISM

Accurate antemortem diagnosis of hypopituitarism should be based on the assay of pituitary hormones, e.g., GH. In normal individuals, however, resting plasma GH levels may be very low, even below the detection limit of the assay. Hence, a conclusive diagnosis has to be based on plasma GH measurements during a provocative test. Clonidine, an effective antihypertensive drug, with intrinsic α-adrenergic activity, is a reliable stimulus for this purpose in man and the dog.[18]

There are other means for direct assessment of pituitary integrity. However, no radioimmunoassay for the routine measurement of TSH in dog plasma is available. Measurements of dog plasma prolactin, FSH, or LH are performed in very few laboratories. Indirect assessment can be performed by stimulation of pituitary hormone secretion and subsequent estimation of the plasma concentration of target gland hormones such as T_4 and cortisol. Indirect tests, however, should be combined or preceded by assay of pituitary hormones, such as ACTH/TSH, to accurately assess the responsiveness of target glands.[19]

Secondary hypothyroidism is characterized by subnormal T_4 levels. However, in contrast to primary hypothyroidism, T_4 levels increase in response to TSH administration. Yet, multiple TSH administrations might be necessary. Administration of TSH-releasing hormone (TRH) in dogs lacking TSH is not followed by an appreciable increase in T_4 levels (normal increase: 0.5 to 2.0 μg/dl four hours after 0.2 mg TRH). Assessment of adrenal function is performed by ACTH testing. In secondary hypoadrenocorticism, basal cortisol levels are usually low, but, in contrast to primary hypoadrenocorticism, there is a distinct increase in cortisol levels in response to ACTH.[19] Indirect testing of pituitary ACTH secretory capacity can be performed by administering lysine-vasopressin (LPV), which possesses intrinsic ACTH-releasing activity. Cortisol is measured before and at multiple intervals after LVP injection.[45] Absent or subnormal response supports impaired ACTH secretion. Antidiuretic hormone secretory capacity is best evaluated in the modified water deprivation test.[48]

In man, because of expansion mainly within the sella, pituitary tumors may induce erosion of the bony sella. Such changes can be evaluated radiographically. In the dog, pituitary tumors do not lead to radiographically visible changes. Because of the incompletely developed diaphragma sellae, tumors in general expand dorsally into the third ventricle. However, more refined techniques such as computer-assisted tomographic (CAT) scanning are becoming more readily available.[35] CAT scanning should be an invaluable adjunct in the diagnosis of presumed pituitary tumors in small animals.

DISEASES INVOLVING HYPERFUNCTION OF THE PITUITARY GLAND

Recognized pituitary overproduction syndromes include acromegaly and Cushing's disease. Cushing's disease caused by either ACTH or primary cortisol oversecretion is discussed in Chapter 143.

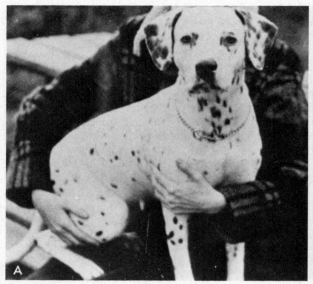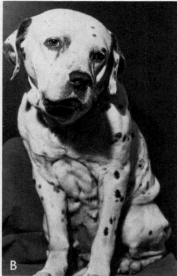

Figure 142–2. Acromegaly. *A,* Normal dog. *B,* After severe spontaneous acromegaly was diagnosed during a luteal phase. Note the general "heavy" appearance of the dog and the excessive skin folds.

Acromegaly[20]

Acromegaly in the dog is characterized mainly by an increase in soft tissue mass. This is readily visible as skin folds or abdominal enlargement and is radiographically evidenced by a diffuse increase in soft tissue mass in the orolingual/oropharyngeal/orolaryngeal region. As a result, acromegalic dogs almost invariably exhibit some degree of respiratory stridor (Fig. 142–2). Enlargement of interdental spaces also is encountered, although these changes are rather nonspecific. Other possible findings include poly-

TABLE 142–2.   Historical and Clinical Findings in 22 Acromegalic Dogs*

Age	4 to 11 years; mean 8.4 years
Progestogen treatment	15
Spontaneous occurrence during luteal phase	7
Breeds	Dachshund (4); Am. cocker spaniel (3); crossbreed (4); Dalmatian (3); German shepherd (2); Engl. cocker spaniel (2); springer spaniel (1); French bulldog (1); beagle, poodle (1)
Inspiratory stridor	19
Polyuria/polydipsia	10
Visible increase in soft tissue mass	19
Enlargement of interdental spaces	13

*Data from Eigenmann, J. E.: Diagnosis and treatment of pituitary dwarfism in dogs. *In* van Marthens, E. (ed.): Proc. Kal-Kan Symp. for the Treatment of Small Animal Diseases, 6:107, 1983.

uria/polydipsia, hyperglycemia, elevation of alkaline phosphatase, and lowered packed cell volume (Table 142–2). Elevation of GH levels is variable, ranging from 10 to 1500 ng/ml. Acromegaly thus far has been found to occur in intact female dogs during diestrus (progesterone phase) or in dogs treated with progestogens. Withdrawal of progestogens or ovariohysterectomy is invariably followed by reduction in GH levels and appreciable clinical improvement. GH elevation, therefore, is progesterone-controlled. It is unknown whether such dogs have pituitary tumors. If they were proven to have such a tumor, GH overproduction would still be progesterone/progestogen dependent. Hence, progesterone/progestogen withdrawal rather than hypophysectomy is the treatment of choice.

Acromegaly is accurately diagnosed by measurement of GH level. Single measurements of basal levels may be insufficient, since GH levels can be moderately elevated for a number of reasons. Hence, acromegaly is most reliably diagnosed by measuring GH before and during a suppression test, i.e., administration of an intravenous glucose load of 1 gm/kg. Using this test, GH levels should not become appreciably suppressed.

Hypophysectomy

Hypophysectomy is performed most often for the treatment of pituitary-dependent Cushing's disease (see Chapter 143).

Preoperative Preparation

No special preoperative preparation is required other than accepted clinical, biochemical, and he-

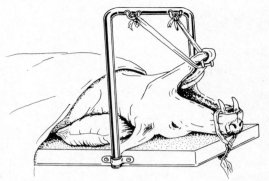

Figure 142–3. Positioning for hypophysectomy. The dog has been placed in dorsal recumbency with its mouth wide open.

matologic screening. Food is withheld for at least 12 hours before surgery, but water is provided.

Anesthesia and Monitoring during Surgery

One hour prior to surgery we prefer to premedicate dogs with methadone HCl SC (0.4 to 1.0 mg/kg), dehydrobenzperidol SC (0.5 to 1.2/mg/kg), and atropine SC (0.1/mg/kg). Anesthesia is induced with sodium thiopental and maintained with halothane/nitrous oxide. Artificial ventilation is necessary. Heart rate and respiratory function are continuously monitored.

Approach and Technique

Hypophysectomy has been performed experimentally in dogs and cats since 1881.[30] The most useful techniques are transoral, i.e., extracranial, in their approach. We have used the transoral technique of Markowitz and colleagues.[43] The patient is placed in dorsal recumbency at one end of the surgery table. The front legs are loosely fixed in a caudal direction. The upper jaw is fixed at the end of and parallel to the table. Horizontal positioning of the maxilla is very important. The mouth is almost maximally opened by fixing the mandible to a metal bar that

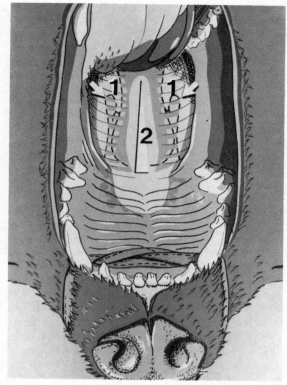

Figure 142–4. The dog's oral cavity. The dog is ready for hypophysectomy. Orientation is obtained by identifying the hamular processes (*l, arrow*). 2 = Incision line in the soft palate.

forms an arch over the dog (Fig. 142–3). The mouth and nasopharynx are disinfected with 70% alcohol. The surgical field is draped with four towels forming a square opening. A midline incision of 3 to 4 cm is made in the soft palate, starting just behind the hard palate (Fig. 142–4). Care must be taken not to extend the incision all the way to the hard palate because this can result in severe bleeding from the major palatine arteries. The incision is kept wide open with a small retractor. The mucoperiosteum covering the sphenoid bone is incised over a length of 3 cm on the midline between the hamular processes and is

Figure 142–5. Sagittal section through a dolichocephalic skull. Note the hamular process (*l, arrow*) and its position relative to the pituitary (*3, arrow*).

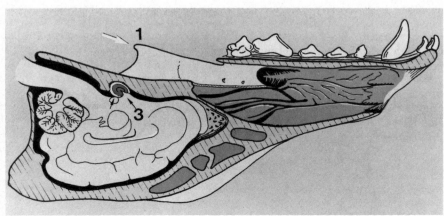

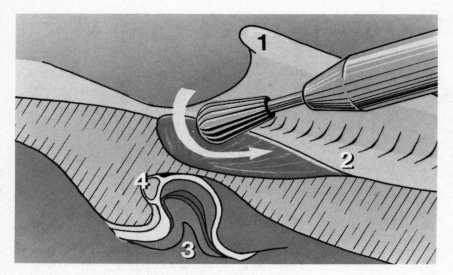

Figure 142–6. Sagittal section through part of a dolichocephalic skull and the relative position of the dental drill used in hypophysectomy. 1 = Hamular process; 2 = burr groove; 3 = pituitary; 4 = sinus venosus. Note that the dental drill is operating in a counterclockwise direction (arrow).

stripped aside. The pituitary, which is situated at the caudal base of the hamular processes (Fig. 142–5), is exposed using a slow-blurring dental drill with a 4-mm diameter burr, starting at the posterior end of the hamular processes. To control bleeding from the sphenoid bone, the burr grooves are filled with bone wax. The groove is carefully deepened and enlarged rostrally and caudally.

The shape of the groove is shown (Fig. 142–6). The caudal wall of the groove is made almost perpendicular to avoid damaging the venous sinus that forms a horseshoe-shaped arch around the pituitary gland. Rostrally, the groove is more flat. The position of the venous sinus makes it necessary to burr the groove exactly on the midline (in the center of the sphenoid). Damage to the venous sinus causes severe bleeding, and, although the bleeding can be controlled with gelatin foam* soaked with thrombin solution,† burring must cease and hence removal of the pituitary is not possible. When the groove is sufficiently enlarged, the pituitary is visible through the dorsal membrane as a yellowish-pink area that bulges slightly (the sphenoid bone is thinner where the pituitary is situated; see Figs. 142–5 and 142–6). The dural membrane is incised with a small dural knife, and the pituitary is removed by gentle suction. After incision of the dura, no further burring is possible. Therefore, it is important that the groove be made large enough to allow removal of the pituitary before the dura is incised. The pituitary is removed with fine forceps, usually in pieces. Removal of the gland generally does not cause severe bleeding. Sometimes, however, a few drops of cerebrospinal fluid are discharged. When the pituitary is completely removed, both the empty hypophyseal fossa and the pulsating artery of the circle of Willis can be seen. The burr hole is then closed with bone wax. After

cleaning the nasopharynx, the soft palate is closed with interrupted sutures in one or two layers with an absorbable suture material.*

An alternative technique to the one used by one of the authors (A.A.M.E.L.) has recently been employed in an experimental study.[30] This technique involves a transoral approach with concomitant mandibular symphysiotomy. These authors feel that their approach gives better exposure and ease of hypophysectomy. In addition, they employed a point 1 cm caudal to the intersphenoid suture as the site of the center of the drill hole and feel this gives an improved degree of accuracy over the use of the caudal extent of the hamular processes as described previously. With our technique, hypophysectomy has proved difficult in brachycephalic and dolichocephalic (long-headed) dogs. Hence, in these cases the transoral approach combined with mandibular symphysiotomy may be the only possible approach if hypophysectomy is warranted. We consider the transoral approach without mandibular symphysiotomy a generally adequate procedure for hypophysectomy for several reasons. (1) Most dogs affected by pituitary-dependent Cushing's disease in which this method has proved adequate are not brachycephalic or dolichocephalic dogs. Thus, symphysiotomy is only necessary in some cases. (2) Some dogs hypophysectomized experimentally by using the approach with symphysiotomy were either dolichocephalic or brachycephalic, and all were large.

Because of the very limited number of dogs studied with the symphysiotomy procedure[30] and because only large dogs, but not smaller dogs, were studied, it appears premature to us to generally recommend the procedure for the treatment of clinical patients even if they are dolichocephalic or brachycephalic.

During surgery lactated Ringer's solution is infused (100 ml/kg over three to four hours).

---

*Spongostan, Ferrosan, Denmark; Gelfoam, The Upjohn Co., Kalamazoo, MI.
†Thrombostat, Parke-Davis, Santurce, PR.

---

*Polyglycolic acid (Dexon), Davis and Geck, Pearl River, NY; Polyglactin 910 (Vicryl), Ethicon, Inc., Somerville, NJ.

Aftercare and Medication

During the first postoperative day, the following drugs are administered:

1. Prednisolone acetate, 0.4 mg/kg bodyweight SC every six hours.

2. A broad spectrum antibiotic SC (e.g., ampicillin).

3. 3 to 5 I.U. pitressin tannate in oil SC (to control postoperative diabetes insipidus).

As soon as the animal begins to eat (usually the first or second postoperative day), cortisone acetate or prednisolone is administered orally in a dose of 1 mg/kg (cortisone) or 0.2 mg/kg (prednisolone) every eight hours. If oral administration is not possible, the prednisolone acetate injections are continued. After four to five days the cortisone/prednisolone dose is decreased by half every eight hours during the first two weeks.

NOTE: Antibiotic administration is continued for ten days, and, as soon as oral administration is possible, thyroid hormone (L-thyroxin) substitution is started at a dosage rate of 200 μg/kg given once daily in the morning.

Maintenance therapy consists of 0.5 mg/kg cortisone or 0.1 mg/kg prednisolone given twice daily and 20 μg/kg L-thyroxin administered once daily in the morning.

Complications

The intra- and postoperative mortality rate is about 10 per cent, with most deaths occurring during the first 24 hours postoperatively. Although severe bleeding may be found at autopsy, in most cases no explanation for the death has been defined. Another complication is severe bleeding during surgery, making removal of the pituitary impossible. In addition, postoperative dyspnea may occur because of swelling of the soft palate and the mucosa of the nasopharynx. We have observed this, especially in toy poodles. Tracheotomy may be necessary in such cases. In a few cases, facial paralysis has occurred, without known cause, in combination with keratoconjunctivitis sicca, most commonly two to four weeks after surgery.

Severe polyuria may occur during the first few postoperative days (or weeks) owing to diabetes insipidus in combination with the high starting dose of cortisone. The administration of antidiuretic hormone may become necessary in such cases.

Prognosis

The therapeutic success of hypophysectomy is mainly dependent on the completeness of the removal of the pituitary gland. The pars distalis extends for a variable distance upward around the pituitary stalk, and if even minute remnants containing ACTH-producing cells remain *in situ*, signs of hyperadrenocorticism in dogs treated for Cushing's disease may recur, within a few weeks or few months of recovery

(see Chapter 143). The therapeutic failure rate is approximately 10 to 15 per cent. When surgery is successful, total recovery appears within two to three months.

The experience of one of the authors (A.A.M.E.L.) with hypophysectomies in approximately 260 cases over 13 years leads to the following conclusions. Hypophysectomy has proved to be very difficult or impossible in brachycephalic dogs because the thick, broad sphenoid bone in these breeds makes orientation difficult. The larger dolichocephalic breeds also present problems because the pituitary cannot be reached easily with this technique. In such cases, chemotherapy with o,p'-DDD is a possible treatment (see Chapter 143). However, perhaps mandibular symphysiotomy as previously discussed might be useful in both types of dogs, as has been suggested.[30]

Hypophysectomy has the advantage of preventing pituitary tumor growth. In addition, substitution therapy is simple and frequent clinical follow-up examinations are not necessary. The relative merits of hypophysectomy can be realized by a surgeon only after sufficient experience has been gained with the performance of the operation without complications.

We advise hypophysectomy in the following situations:

1. When a pituitary tumor is suspected,

2. In all dogs with pituitary-dependent Cushing's disease younger than ten years (brachycephalic and, perhaps, large dogs excluded unless mandibular symphysiotomy subsequently proves to aid the procedure).

3. If the owner prefers surgical therapy rather than lifelong treatment with o,p'-DDD (see Chapter 143).

1. Abboud, C. F., and Laws, E. R., Jr.: Clinical endocrinological approach to hypothalamic-pituitary disease. J. Neurosurg. *51:*271, 1979.

2. Altszuler, N.: Actions of growth hormone on carbohydrate metabolism. *In* Greep, R. O., and Astwood, E. B. (eds.): *Handbook of Physiology*, Section 7, Endocrinology, Vol. IV. Waverly Press, Inc., Baltimore, 1974, p. 233.

3. Andresen, E., and Willeberg, P.: Pituitary dwarfism in German Shepherds: Additional evidence of simple autosomal recessive inheritance. Nord. Vet. Med. 28:481, 1976.

4. Belshaw, B. E., and Rijnberk, A.: Hypothyroidism. *In* Kirk, R. W. (ed.): *Current Veterinary Therapy VII.* W. B. Saunders, Philadelphia, 1980, p. 994.

5. Boyns, A. R., Jones, G. E., Bell, E. T., Christie, D. W., and Parkes, M. F.: Development of a radioimmunoassay for canine luteinizing hormone. J. Endocrinol. 55:279, 1972.

6. Capen, C. C., Martin, S. L., and Koestner, A.: Neoplasms in the adenohypophysis of dogs. Pathol. Vet. 4:301, 1967.

7. Chastain, C. B., Graham, C. L., and Nichols, C. E.: Adrenocortical suppression in cats given megestrol acetate. Am. J. Vet. Res. 42:2029, 1981.

8. Check, D. B., and Hill, D. E.: Effect of growth hormone on cell and somatic growth. *In* Greep, R. O., and Astwood, E. B. (eds.): *Handbook of Physiology*, Section 7, Endocrinology, Vol. IV. Waverly Press, Inc., Baltimore, 1974, p. 159.

9. Chretien, M., Benjounet, S., Gossard, F., Gianoulakis, C., Crine, P., Lis, M., and Seidah, N. H.: From B-lipotropin to B-endorphin and pro-opio-melanocortin. Can. J. Biochem. 57:1111, 1979.

10. Christy, N. P.: Harvey Cushing as clinical investigator and laboratory worker. Am. J. Med. Sci. *281:*79, 1981.

11. Coffin, D. L., and Munson, T. D.: Endocrine diseases of the dog associated with hair loss. J. Am. Vet. Med. Assoc. *123*:402, 1953.

12. Connors, J. M., and Hedge, G. A.: Feedback regulation of thyrotropin by thryoxine under physiological conditions. Am. J. Physiol. *240*:E308, 1981.

13. Dämmrich, K.: Die morphologische und funktionelle Pathologie der Gewchwülste der Adenohypophyse bei Hunden. Zbl. Vet. Med. (A.) *14*:137, 1967.

14. Daniel, P. M., and Prichard, M. M. L.: Studies of the hypothalamus and the pituitary gland. Acta Endocrinol. [Suppl.] (Kbh) *80*:1, 1975.

15. Duick, D. S., and Wahner, H. W.: Thyroid axis in patients with Cushing's Syndrome. Arch. Intern. Med. *139*:767, 1979.

16. Eigenmann, J. E.: Diagnosis and treatment of dwarfism in a German Shepherd dog. J Am. Anim. Hosp. Assoc. *17*:798, 1981.

17. Eigenmann, J. E.: Diagnosis and treatment of pituitary dwarfism in dogs. *In* van Marthens, E. (ed.): Proc. Kal-Kan Symp. for the Treatment of Small Animal Diseases. *6*:107, 1983.

18. Eigenmann, J. E., and Eigenmann, R. Y.: Radioimmunoassay of canine growth hormone. Acta Endocrinol. (Kbh) *98*:514, 1981.

19. Eigenmann, J. E., Lubberink, A. A. M. E., and Koeman, J. P.: Panhypopituitarism caused by a suprasellar tumor in a dog. J. Am. Anim. Hosp. Assoc. *19*:377, 1983.

20. Eigenmann, J. E., and Venker-van Haagen, A. J.: Progestagen-induced and spontaneous canine acromegaly due to reversible growth hormone overproduction: Clinical picture and pathogenesis. J. Am. Anim. Hosp. Assoc. *17*:813, 1981.

21. El Etreby, M. F., Schilk, B., Soulioti, G., Tushaus, U., Wierman, H., and Gunzel, P.: Effect of 17-B-estradiol on cells of the pars distalis of the adenohypophysis in the beagle bitch: An immunocytochemical and morphometric study. Endokrinologie *69*:202, 1977.

22. Feldman, E. C.: Effect of functional adrenocortical tumors on plasma cortisol and corticotropin concentrations in dogs. J Am. Vet. Med. Assoc. *178*:823, 1981.

23. Florsheim, W. H.: Control of thyrotropin secretion. *In* Greep, R. O., and Astwood, E. B. (eds.): *Handbook of Physiology*, Section 7, Endocrinology, Vol IV. Waverly Press, Inc., Baltimore, 1974, p. 449.

24. Goldberg, R. D., and Chaikoff, I. L.: On the occurrence of six cell types in the dog anterior pituitary. Anat. Rec. *112*:265, 1952.

25. Graf, K.-J., Friedreich, E., Matthes, S., and Hasan, S. H.: Homologous radioimmunoassay for canine prolactin and its application in various physiological states. J. Endocrinol. *75*:93, 1977.

26. Greenwald, G. S.: Role of follicle-stimulating hormone and luteinizing hormone in follicular development and ovulation. *In* Greep, R. O., and Astwood, E. B. (eds.): *Handbook of Physiology*, Section 7, Endocrinology, Vol. IV. Waverly Press, Inc., Baltimore, 1974, p. 293.

27. Greep, R. O.: History of research on anterior hypophysial hormones. *In* Greep, R. O., and Astwood, E. B. (eds.): *Handbook of Physiology*, Section 7, Endocrinology, Vol. IV. Waverly Press, Inc., Baltimore, 1974, p. 1.

28. Groen, J. J., Frenkel, H. S., and Offerhaus, L.: Observations on a case of spontaneous diabetes mellitus in a dog. Diabetes *13*:492, 1969.

29. Halmi, N. S., Peterson, M. E., Colurso, G. J., Liotta, A. S., and Krieger, D. T.: Pituitary intermediate lobe in the dog: Two cell types and high bioactive adrenocorticotropin content. Science *211*:72, 1981.

30. Henry, R. W., Hulse, D. A., Archibald, L. F., and Barta, M.: Transoral hypophysectomy with mandibular symphysiotomy in the dog. Am. J. Vet. Res. *43*:1825, 1982.

31. Hewitt, W. F., Jr.: Age and sex differences in weight of pituitary gland in dogs. Proc. Soc. Exp. Biol. Med. *74*:781, 1950.

32. Hullinger, R. L.: The endocrine system. *In* Evans, H. I., and Christensen, G. C. (eds.): Miller's Anatomy of the Dog, 2nd ed. W. B. Saunders, Philadelphia, 1979, p. 602.

33. Johnston, S. D., and Mather, E. C.: Feline plasma cortisol (hydrocortisone) measured by radioimmunoassay. Am. J. Vet. Res. *40*:190, 1979.

34. Kemppainen, R. J., Lorenz, M. D., and Thompson, R. M.: Adrenocortical suppression in the dog after a single dose of methylprednisolone acetate. Am. J. Vet. Res. *42*:822, 1981.

35. Kricheff, I. I.: The radiologic diagnosis of pituitary adenoma. Radiology *131*:263, 1979.

36. Krieger, D. T.: Neuroendocrine physiology. *In* Felig, P., Baxter, J. D., Broadus, A. E., and Frohman, L. A. (eds.): *Endocrinology and Metabolism*. McGraw-Hill, New York, 1981, p. 125.

37. Krieger, D. T., and Liotta, A. S.: Pituitary hormones in brain: Where, how and why. Science *205*:366, 1979.

38. Krieger, D. T., Silverberg, A. I., and Rizzo, F.: Abolition of circadian periodicity of plasma 17-OHCS in the cat. Am. J. Physiol. *215*:959, 1968.

39. Li, C. H.: Chemistry of ovine prolactin. *In* Greep, R. O., and Astwood, E. B. (eds.): *Handbook of Physiology*, Section 7, Endocrinology, Vol. IV. Waverly Press, Inc., Baltimore, 1974, p. 103.

40. Locke, W.: Control of anterior pituitary function. Arch. Intern. Med. *138*:1541, 1978.

41. Lovinger, R., Boryczka, A. T., Shackelford, R., Kaplan, S. L., Ganong, W. F., and Grumbach, M.: Effect of synthetic somatotropin release inhibiting factor on the increase in plasma growth hormone elicited by L-DOPA in the dog. Endocrinology *95*:943, 1974.

42. Luksch, F.: Über Hypophysentumoren beim Hunde. Tierarztl. Arch. *3*:1, 1923.

43. Markowitz, J., Archibald, J., and Downie, H. G.: Hypophysectomy in dogs. *In* Experimental Surgery, Williams and Wilkins Co., Baltimore, 1964, p. 630.

44. McGrath, J. T.: *Neurologic Examination of the Dog with Clinicopathologic Observation*, 2nd ed. Lea & Febiger, Philadelphia, 1960.

45. Meijer, J. C., Lubberink, A. A. M. E., Rijnberk, A., and Croughs, R. J. M.: Adrenocortical function tests in dogs with hyperfunctioning adrenocortical tumors. J. Endocrinol. *80*:315, 1979.

46. Meyer, H.: The brain. *In* Evans, H. E., and Christensen, G. C. (eds.): *Miller's Anatomy of the Dog*. 2nd ed. W. B. Saunders Co., Philadelphia, 1979, p. 842.

47. Muller, J., and Baumann, K.: Multifactorial regulation of the final steps of aldosterone biosynthesis in the rat. J. Steroid Biochem. *5*:795, 1974.

48. Mulnix, J. A., Rijnberk, A., and Hendriks, H. J.: Evaluation of a modified water-deprivation test for diagnosis of polyuric disorders in dogs. J. Am. Vet. Med. Assoc. *169*:1327, 1976.

49. Neill, J. D.: Prolactin: Its secretion and control. *In* Greep, R. O., and Astwood, E. B. (eds.): *Handbook of Physiology*, Section 7, Endocrinology, Vol. IV. Waverly Press, Inc., Baltimore, 1974, p. 469.

50. Nelson, D. H., Meakin, J. W., and Thorn, G. W.: ACTH-producing pituitary tumors following adrenalectomy for Cushing's syndrome. Ann. Intern. Med. *52*:560, 1960.

51. Nicoll, C. S.: Physiological actions of prolactin. *In* Greep, R. O., and Astwood, E. B. (eds.): *Handbook of Physiology*, Section 7, Endocrinology, Vol. IV. Waverly Press, Inc., Baltimore, p. 253.

52. Palkovits, M.: Neural pathways involved in ACTH regulation. Ann. N.Y. Acad. Sci. *297*:455, 1977.

53. Pamenter, R. W., and Hedge, G. A.: Inhibition of thyrotropin secretion by physiological levels of corticosterone. Endocrinology *106*:162, 1980.

54. Parker, W. M., and Scott, D. W.: Growth hormone responsive alopecia in the mature dog: A discussion of 13 cases. J. Am. Anim. Hosp. Assoc. *16*:824, 1980.

55. Peterson, M. E., and Altszuler, N.: Suppression of growth hormone secretion in spontaneous canine hyperadrenocorticism and its reversal after treatment. Am. J. Vet. Res. *42*:1881, 1981.

56. Pierce, J. G.: Chemistry of thyroid-stimulating hormone. *In* Greep, R. O., and Astwood, E. B. (eds.): *Handbook of Physiology*, Section 7, Endocrinology, Vol. IV. Waverly Press, Inc., Baltimore, 1974, p. 79.

57. Quinlan, W. J., and Michaelson, S.: Homologous radioimmunoassay for canine thyrotropin: Response of normal and x-irradiated dogs to propylthiouracil. Endocrinology, *108*:937, 1981.

58. Reichlin, S.: Regulation of somatotrophic hormone secretion. *In* Greep, R. O., and Astwood, E. B. (eds.): *Handbook of Physiology*, Section 7, Endocrinology, Vol. IV. Waverly Press, Inc., Baltimore, 1974, p. 405.

59. Reimers, T. J., Phemister, R. D., and Niswender, G. D.: Radioimmunologic measurement of follicle stimulating hormone and prolactin in the dog. Biol. Reprod. *19*:673, 1978.

60. Rijnberk, A.: Iodine metabolism and thyroid disease in the dog. PhD thesis, University of Utrecht, 1971.

61. Rijnberk, A., DerKinderen, P. J., and Thijssen, J. H. H.: Investigations on the adrenocortical function of normal dogs. J. Endocrinol. *41*:387, 1968.

62. Rijnberk, A., Der Kinderen, P. J., and Thijssen, J. H. H.: Spontaneous hyperadrenocorticism in the dog. J. Endocrinol. *41*:397, 1968.

63. Rijnberk, A., Eigenmann, J. E., Belshaw, B. E., Hampshire, J., and Altszuler, N.: Acromegaly associated with transient overproduction of growth hormone in a dog. J. Am. Vet. Med. Assoc. *177*:534, 1980.

64. Sairam, M. R., and Papkoff, H.: Chemistry of pituitary gonadotrophins. *In* Greep, R. O., and Astwood, E. B. (eds.): *Handbook of Physiology*, Section 7, Endocrinology, Vol. IV. Waverly Press, Inc., Baltimore, 1974, p. 111.

65. Sandow, J., and Konig, W.: Chemistry of the hypothalamic hormones. *In* Jeffcoate, S. L., and Hutchinson, J. S. M. (eds.): *The Endocrine Hypothalamus*. Academic Press, London, 1978, p. 149.

66. Sayers, G., and Portanova, R.: Regulation of the secretory activity of the adrenal cortex: cortisol and corticosterone. *In* Greep, R. O., and Astwood, E. B. (eds.): *Handbook of Physiology*, Section 7, Endocrinology, Vol. IV. Waverly Press, Inc., Baltimore, 1975, p. 41.

67. Scanlon, M. F., Lewis, M., Weightman, D. R., Chan, V., and Hall, R.: The neuroregulation of human thyrotropin secretion. *In* Martini, L., and Ganong, W. F. (eds.): *Fron-tiers in Neuroendocrinology*, Vol. 6. Raven Press, New York, 1980, p. 333.

68. Schrier, R. W., and Berl, T.: Disorders of water metabolism. *In* Schrier, R. W. (ed.): *Renal and Electrolyte Disorders*. Little, Brown and Co., Boston, 1980, p. 1.

69. Scott, D. W., Kirk, R. W., Hampshire, J., and Altszuler, N.: Clinicopathological findings in a German shepherd with pituitary dwarfism. J. Am. Anim. Hosp. Assoc. *14*:183, 1978.

70. Simmonds, M.: Ueber Hypophyssisschwund mit todlichem Ausgang. Deutsche Med. Wschr. *40*:322, 1914.

71. Singer, M.: The brain of the dog in section. W. B. Saunders, Philadelphia, 1962.

72. Spaulding, S. W., and Utiger, R. D.: The thyroid: physiology, hyperthyroidism, hypothyroidism, and the painful thyroid. *In* Felig, P., Baxter, J. D., Broadus, A. E., and Frohman, L. A. (eds.): *Endocrinology and Metabolism*. McGraw-Hill, New York, 1981, p. 281.

73. Stockard, C. R.: Gross relative sizes of the pituitary glands in contrasted breed types and their hybrids.*In* Stockard, C. R. (ed.): *The Genetic and Endocrine Basis for Differences in Form and Behavior*. The Wistar Institute, Philadelphia, 1941.

74. Underwood, L. E., D'Ercole, A. J., and Van Wyk, J. J.: Somatomedin-C and the assessment of growth. Pediatr. Clin. North Am. *27*:771, 1980.

75. Verstraete, A., and Thoonen, J.: Twee Neiuwe gevallen van hypophysaire stoornissen big den hond. Vlaams Diergeneesk. Tijdschr. *8*:304, 1939.

76. Wartofsky, L., and Burman, K. D.: Alterations in thyroid function in patients with systemic illness: the "euthyroid sick syndrome." Endocrine Rev. *3*:164, 1982.

77. Wilhelmi, A. E.: Chemistry of growth hormone. *In* Greep, R. O., and Astwood, E. B. (eds.): *Handbook of Physiology*, Section 7, Endocrinology, Vol. IV. Waverly Press, Inc., Baltimore, 1974, pp. 5, 59.

78. Young, F. G.: Growth hormone and diabetes. Rec. Progr. Horm. Res. *8*:471, 1953.

79. Zapf, J., Rinderknecht, E., Humbel, R. E., and Froesch, E. R.: Nonsuppressible insulin-like activity (NSILA) from human serum: Recent accomplishments and their physiologic implication. Metabolism *27*:1803, 1978.

Chapter **143**

The Adrenals

J. E. Eigenmann and A. A. M. E. Lubberink

ANATOMY OF THE ADRENAL GLANDS[17]

The adrenal gland is unique in its structure and function. Each gland is composed of two functionally and morphologically different tissues, an outer cortex and inner medulla. The cortex consists of four zones: the outermost zona glomerulosa (arcuata), the zona intermedia, the zona fasciculata, and the innermost zona reticularis. The zona reticularis constitutes approximately 25 per cent, the zona intermedia less than 5 per cent, the zona fasciculata approximately 50 per cent, and the zona arcuata approximately 20 to 25 per cent of the adrenal cortex. The glands are craniomedial to the kidneys. In general, the adrenal cortex completely invests the adrenal medulla. On cut sections, the cortex appears white or slightly yellow in color, whereas the medulla is dark brown or black. In medium-sized, mature dogs, each gland weighs somewhat more than 1 gram, with the left being slightly larger than the right. Both glands are retroperitoneal in location and are surrounded by loose collagenous connective tissue and fat.

Macroscopic Anatomy

The left adrenal gland is ventral to the left psoas minor muscle and the lateral process of the second lumbar vertebra, near the craniomedial aspect of the left kidney. Medially, it is bounded by the descending aorta, just caudal to the origin of the cranial mesenteric artery. It is adjacent to the origin of the left phrenicoabdominal artery, which runs dorsal to the midpoint of the gland. The renal artery and vein form its caudal border. The phrenicoabdominal vein runs laterally over the ventral aspect of the middle of the gland.

The right adrenal gland is ventral to the right psoas minor muscle and the right crus of the diaphragm, beneath the lateral process of the last thoracic vertebra. It is closer to the renal hilus than is the left adrenal.

The caudal segment of the right adrenal gland is in close proximity to the right side of the caudal vena cava, the external tunic of the latter often being continuous with the capsule of the gland. The shorter cranial segment is close to the cranial pole of the right kidney. The right phrenicoabdominal artery crosses the dorsal surface and the phrenicoabdominal vein, the ventral surface of the gland. The right kidney covers a part of the lateral portion of the gland, and the cranial two-thirds of the gland are covered by the caudal portion of the right lobe of the liver.

Microscopic Anatomy

The stroma of the adrenal gland varies considerably, ranging from a thick fibrous capsule to fine reticular support fibers of the parenchymal cells in the medulla. The dog's adrenal capsule does not contain smooth muscle fibers. Septa and a few trabeculae arising from the capsule extend into the cortical parenchyma. The septa become confluent as thin sheets that envelop the parenchyma of the zona glomerulosa. From the zona intermedia, numerous fine reticular fibers project into the inner cortex. Most fibers end at the corticomedullary boundary. In contrast to the cortex, the adrenal medulla contains only a moderate number of fibers that support the parenchyma.

The zona glomerulosa is composed of vermiform palisades of columnar epitheloid cells resembling the arrangement of columnar cells of the villi of the small intestine. These cells produce mainly aldosterone, the essential hormone for electrolyte homeostasis. Small, polygonal cells of the zona intermedia appear between the parenchyma of the zona arcuata and zona fasciculata. The cells of this zone are not prominent in most other species. The cells of the zona fasciculata are polygonal in shape and are arranged in plates forming a murus complex. The zona reticularis is composed of cells similar to those of the zona fasciculata. The plates of this zone are direct continuations of the zona fasciculata but differ in that they are quite randomly arranged. Both the zona fasciculata and the zona reticularis produce glucocorticoids.

Cells of the medulla are larger than those of the cortex and are polygonal in shape. Occasionally, ganglionic cells are dispersed throughout the parenchyma. The major hormone synthesized in the adrenal medulla is epinephrine.

Developmental Anatomy

The adrenal cortex and adrenal medulla have different developmental origins. The cortex develops first from mesenchymal cells of the mesoderm. The medullary parenchyma arises from neural crest cells, which migrate from their point of origin into the developing mesodermal mass, finally assuming a central position characteristic of the adult medulla. By definition, the medulla is a sympathetic ganglion, and its development is similar to that of the ganglia of the sympathetic trunk. The adrenal capsule develops as a condensation of mesenchyme at the periphery of the cortex. Adrenal cortical tissue may occur randomly as accessory tissue, isolated or within another abdominal organ. Aggregates (isolates) associated with the gland may appear as nodules of increasing size with age.

Vascularization of the Adrenal Gland

Numerous arterial vessels supply the adrenal glands. Branches arise from the abdominal aorta, the arteriae adrenales mediae; from the phrenicoabdominalis artery, the rami adrenales craniales; and from the lumbar and renal arteries, the rami adrenales caudales. These provide 20 to 30 arterioles, approaching the gland from all surfaces. The arterioles enter the fibrous portion of the capsule and ultimately anastomose to form a network. From this network, numerous vessels penetrate the cortex. Some of these descend directly into the medulla. The sinusoids of the cortex are supplied via small arterioles. The sinusoids pass to and penetrate the corticomedullary junction, where they become confluent with sinusoids of the medulla. The resultant sinuses pass to the hilus of the adrenal gland to be ultimately drained via the adrenal vein. The adrenal veins of each gland terminate differently because of their position relative to the caudal vena cava. The right adrenal vein joins directly with the caudal vena cava, but the left enters the left renal vein.

Innervation of the Adrenal Gland

Multipolar nerve cells are present in all regions of the adrenal cortex. The parenchyma of the adrenal medulla is a sympathetic ganglion specialized for neurohumoral release. Some sympathetic preganglionic neurons innervate the adrenal medullae, which can be viewed as sympathetic postganglionic neurons with axons. The medullae release the catecholamine epinephrine along with smaller amounts of norepinephrine.

HORMONE SECRETION BY THE ADRENAL GLANDS

Adrenal Cortex[1]

Steroid hormones produced by the adrenal cortex are derived from cholesterol, much of which is not synthesized by the adrenal gland but is taken up by the gland from the periphery. Acute adrenocorticotrophic hormone (ACTH) stimulation causes a rapid release of newly synthesized steroids. These steroids are derived from a small pool of free glandular cholesterol, which in turn, comes from an increased hydrolysis of stored cholesterol esters. With prolonged stimulation, there is an accelerated uptake of cholesterol from plasma. Essential for adrenal cortex steroid synthesis are, in addition to cholesterol, acetyl coenzyme A and a number of enzymes. In contrast to the thyroid gland, adrenal glands are unable to store their hormones. Major hormones that are produced include pregnenolone, progesterone, corticosterone, cortisol, aldosterone, testosterone, and estrogens.

Whereas the synthesis of of aldosterone takes place primarily in the zona glomerulosa, the synthesis of cortisol occurs mainly in the zona fasciculata. The predominant glucocorticoid produced varies with the species. For example, in the rat, corticosterone is the major glucocorticoid, whereas in man or dog, cortisol is the major glucocorticoid hormone. ACTH is the most important control factor in adrenal function. Only if ACTH is present in sufficient amounts can the adrenals produce normal amounts of glucocorticoids and androgens.

In normal animals, an increase or decrease in the amount of glucocorticoids and androgens is invariably associated with parallel changes in ACTH concentration. ACTH is also somehow involved in aldosterone biosynthesis. However, this effect is only transient, so that in the hypophysectomized ACTH-lacking animal, aldosterone biosynthesis remains normal and no electrolyte imbalances are observed. In addition to the importance of ACTH in adrenal steroid biosynthesis, ACTH profoundly influences adrenal size. An ACTH deficit is associated with adrenal hypoplasia, whereas an ACTH excess is associated with adrenal hyperplasia.

It appears that ACTH stimulates adrenal steroid biosynthesis primarily by conversion of cholesterol to pregnenolone. Although ACTH action leads to an increase in cyclic AMP, exactly how ACTH influences steroid biosynthesis is not known. Additionally, it remains unknown how ACTH influences adrenal size. It appears that, in addition to ACTH, other humoral factors are important in the regulation of adrenal size.

Regulation of Adrenal Steroid Secretion[1, 23–27, 38, 52, 53, 62]

Cortisol

In humans as well as in many other species including the dog, plasma cortisol levels are subject to diurnal variation. In man, peak levels occur prior to awakening, whereas in nocturnal animals, peak levels occur in the evening. The circadian rise and fall of plasma ACTH and cortisol levels is not linear. These hormones are secreted in several bursts of 5 to 30 minutes duration. The periodicity of plasma cortisol levels reflects the periodicity of ACTH levels. The rhythms are endogenously provoked and appear not to be subject to environmental changes. However, they are entrained by environmental synchronizers such as light/dark transition or the offering of food/water at fixed times. In the dog, as in man, diurnal rhythm is characterized by maximal cortisol levels early in the morning (8 AM) and minimal cortisol levels at night (11 PM). The question of whether a diurnal rhythm also exists in the cat remains controversial. Some authors have been unable to demonstrate circadian variation of cortisol levels in cats, whereas others have found such variations. If a circadian rhythm exists in the cat, it appears that the highest cortisol levels occur sometime during the night rather than in the morning. Circadian rhythmicity also has been observed for hypothalamic corticotropin-releasing factor. It appears that the main neuroanatomical site responsible for cortisol periodicity and other diurnal rhythms is the suprachiasmatic nucleus.

Plasma cortisol does not circulate in free form but, depending on the concentration, is bound to carrier proteins. With higher cortisol concentrations, more cortisol appears in the free form, because carrier proteins become saturated. The proportion of the total free cortisol increases in a nonlinear fashion. In man, at a concentration of 10 μg/dl, approximately 10 per cent (i.e., 1 μg/dl) appears in the free form. Similar bound/free ratios are observed in the dog. However, in the dog, as in the case of thyroxine-binding globulin, the carrier protein that specifically binds cortisol (e.g., cortisol-binding globulin) has a much lower affinity for cortisol than does human cortisol-binding globulin. This may be associated with the lower plasma cortisol concentration in the dog than in man. Thus, in the dog, cortisol/corticosterone is bound to plasma proteins by a low-affinity, high-capacity binder. Depending on author and assay technique, basal plasma cortisol concentrations in normal dogs (8 AM) vary considerably. However, basal concentrations in general are below 10 μg/dl. The biological half-life of cortisol in the dog ranges from 28 to 88 minutes (mean 52 minutes).

Actions of Glucocorticoids[1, 30, 55]

Although glucocorticoids induce catabolic activity in most peripheral tissues (e.g., connective, lymphoid, adipose), they stimulate anabolic effects in the liver. The influence of glucocorticoids on carbohydrate metabolism is complex. In excess, glucocorticoids increase hepatic glycogen synthesis and gluconeogenesis and decrease peripheral glucose utilization by inducing insulin resistance. In adipose tissue, glucocorticoids increase lipolysis and enhance the actions of other lipolytic agents (e.g., catecholamines). In a number of tissues, glucocorticoids affect protein, RNA, and DNA synthesis more generally. The trend is to stimulate breakdown in many peripheral tissues such as skin, muscle, and adipose, lymphoid, and fibroblastic tissues. Glucocorticoid excess suppresses immunological and inflammatory responses. In the liver, glucocorticoids induce an alkaline phosphatase enzyme (steroid-induced AP). In addition, glucocorticoids affect the white blood cell component of the hemogram; lymphocytopenia, eosinopenia, and neutrophilia are classical changes associated with increased blood levels. Glucocorticoids also influence cardiac function, vasculature, water excretion, and electrolyte balance. In glucocorticoid deficiency, there is mineralocorticoid-independent hypotension and decreased cardiac output. Glucocorticoid effects on the heart may be direct. In some instances, glucocorticoids potentiate the effects of vasoconstrictor agents such as catecholamines. In addition, glucocorticoids appear to increase the glomerular filtration rate. They also may affect potassium balance by their mineralocorticoid activity.

Aldosterone[1]

Synthesis/secretion of aldosterone by the zona glomerulosa is governed by the renin-angiotensin system, potassium, sodium, ACTH, serotonin, and, possibly, other factors. A complex interrelationship exists between these factors. Aldosterone secretion is enhanced by sodium depletion, potassium overload, and hypovolemia (increase in angiotensin). ACTH affects aldosterone secretion only transiently. The release of aldosterone, like that of cortisol, follows a circadian rhythm and is episodic. In contrast to most other steroids or steroid like hormones, there is no protein in plasma known to specifically bind a substantial amount of aldosterone. Aldosterone promotes the reabsorption of sodium and the secretion of hydrogen and potassium in cortical collecting tubules. These effects require RNA and protein synthesis. The major effect of the hormone may be to increase enzyme activities in the kidney that generate ATP. This drives the sodium pump and increases the number of sodium channels for reabsorption.

Adrenal Medulla

The adrenal medullae release epinephrine along with smaller amounts of norepinephrine. The substrate for catecholamine synthesis is tyrosine. Synthesis occurs in the following sequence: tyrosine →

dihydroxyphenylalanine (dopa) → dopamine (DA) → norepinephrine (NE) → epinephrine (E). Catecholamines are degraded by two principal enzyme systems, catechol-o-methyl-transferase (COMT) and monoamine oxidase (MAO). A major degradation product of epinephrine and norepinephrine is vanillylmandelic acid (VMA).

To produce biological actions, hormones and neurotransmitters first interact with cellular receptors at the external surface of the target cell. There is now ample evidence for two catecholamine receptors, α and β. Although endogenous agonists such as epinephrine and norepinephrine are capable of interacting with both receptors, certain synthetic agonists are not, thus offering selective α- or β-adrenergic stimulation by drugs. Depending on the tissue, one or both classes of receptors may be present. Typical adrenergic, receptor-mediated responses include an increase in cardiac pacemaker rate or peripheral vasoconstriction and a generalized increase in oxygen consumption. Many endocrine glands, in addition to being controlled by substrate, pituitary hormone, or feedback mechanism, are subject to adrenergic control. The sympathetic nervous system is involved in a variety of homeostatic phenomena. In man, assumption of an upright posture causes an acute decrease in venous return to the heart. However, a compensatory mechanism exists. A baroreceptor-mediated neural reflex exists that evokes a sympathetic discharge, causing an increase in peripheral vascular resistance and limiting the fall in cardiac output.

The role of adrenergic mechanisms in physiological adaptation to metabolic stress is exemplified by the response to hypoglycemia. Adrenergic mechanisms, along with glucagon, appear to play a role in the return of plasma glucose concentration to normal following the production of absolute hypoglycemia. Postural stress, hypoglycemia, and vigorous physical exercise are examples of stimuli for an adrenergic response.

DISEASES INVOLVING THE PITUITARY OR THE ADRENAL GLAND

Cushing's Disease— Hyperadrenocorticism[31, 34]

Cushing's disease refers to the manifestations of glucocorticoid excess regardless of the specific underlying cause of the derangement. The disorder can occur spontaneously or may be the result of drug medication (iatrogenic Cushing's disease). Spontaneous Cushing's disease results from pituitary or adrenal hyperfunction, e.g., an adrenal tumor that produces glucocorticoids, or from ACTH overproduction, causing hyperplasia of the adrenal cortex and concomitant glucocorticoid oversecretion. ACTH overproduction may result from a pituitary tumor or, in man, from ectopic, tumorous tissue producing ACTH, e.g., a bronchogenic carcinoma. The latter condition has not been reported in the dog. Thus, spontaneous Cushing's disease in the dog only has been associated with pituitary or hypothalamic derangement or an adrenal tumor. Cushing's disease associated with pituitary-hypothalamic derangement, regardless of whether a pituitary tumor is found, is called pituitary-dependent (PD) Cushing's disease.

Although in normal dogs administration of either cortisol or dexamethasone is followed by suppression of endogenous glucocorticoid production over time, all forms of Cushing's disease share a relative nonsuppressibility in response to these steroids. Nonsuppressibility in the case of adrenal tumors can be ascribed to the fact that adrenal tumors secrete glucocorticoids in an ACTH-independent, autonomous fashion. In pituitary-dependent Cushing's disease, relative nonsuppressibility is the result of a decreased feedback action of cortisol on the pituitary-hypothalamic system. It is important to differentiate between pituitary-dependent Cushing's disease and Cushing's disease caused by an adrenal tumor. Pituitary dependent disease can be treated medically, whereas adrenal tumors should be removed surgically. The clinical signs of Cushing's disease can be ascribed mainly to excessive levels of glucocorticoid hormone.

Natural History

No sex predilection exists for canine Cushing's disease, although adrenocortical tumors occur predominantly in females.[58] Breeds relatively more at risk are terriers, dachshunds, poodles (toy/miniature), schnauzers, boxers, and mixed breeds. Lubberink found Cushing's disease in 19 different breeds and crossbreeds.[32] The age of presentation varied from 4 to 14 years (median 7 to 9 years). The time between the first clinical signs and presentation was eight weeks to three years. Common presenting complaints include polyuria/polydipsia (PU/PD), lethargy, and skin changes.[31, 32, 34, 36]

Routine Clinical and Laboratory Findings[2, 3, 7, 13, 18, 52]

Clinical findings in Cushing's disease are listed in Table 143–1. Frequent signs are abdominal enlargement, hepatomegaly, skin atrophy, and PU/PD. Frequently there is nonpruritic, bilaterally symmetrical alopecia. In some dogs, this may be the only sign of the disease. Skin changes include increased pigmentation, changes in hair color and texture, retarded hair growth, and gradual loss of hair on the flanks, rear legs, and ventral abdomen (Fig. 143–1). Hair loss may occur on the entire body except the head. Other manifestations of skin disease include thin, easily wrinkled skin and cutaneous striae. In the early stage of the disease, clinical changes may be mild and the diagnosis may be difficult. With increasing experience, the suspicion of Cushing's disease may arise early. In our experience, this is particularly true for large dogs having Cushing's disease. Large dogs

TABLE 143–1.   Clinical and Laboratory Findings in Canine Hyperadrenocorticism*

Clinical Findings
Abdominal enlargement
Hepatomegaly
Skin atrophy
Polydipsia/polyuria/polyphagia
Decreased exercise tolerance
Muscle atrophy
Increased panting
Lethargy
Obesity
Intolerance to hot environments
Exophthalmos
Anestrus
Testicular atrophy

Laboratory Changes
Elevated alkaline phosphatase, elevated alkaline
   phosphatase isoenzyme
Elevated SGPT
Hyperglycemia
Occasional hypokalemia
Lymphopenia
Eosinopenia
Neutrophilia
Nucleated red blood cells

*Modified from Meijer, J. C.: Canine hyperadrenocorticism. *In* Kirk, R. W. (ed.): *Current Veterinary Therapy VII.* W. B. Saunders, Philadelphia, 1980.

may have only mild or no classical signs such as PU/PD or extensive hair loss (Fig. 143–2). Such dogs, however, may be presented with primary complaints, such as decreased exercise tolerance, panting, and abdominal enlargement. Dogs with Cushing's disease frequently are presented because of fatigue and muscle weakness. These signs may result from the catabolic effects glucocorticoids exert on muscle. Moreover, glucocorticoids can cause muscle pathology directly by fiber splitting. Occasionally, dogs are

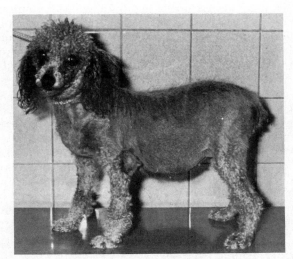

Figure 143–1. Pituitary-dependent hyperadrenocorticism in a poodle. Note the hair loss on the entire body except for the extremities and head, the enlarged abdomen, and the hyperpigmentation of the skin.

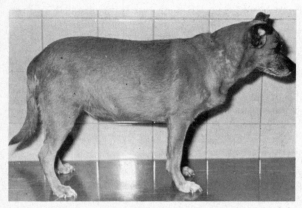

Figure 143–2. Hyperadrenocorticism in a large mixed breed dog. Note the "absence" of the classical signs seen in Figure 143–1. The enlarged abdomen is the most prominent sign.

presented with muscle stiffness, e.g., myotonia or continued contraction of muscles. Palpation of the abdomen may reveal an enlarged liver due to steroid-induced hepatopathy. Patients with Cushing's disease may have signs of hypertension, e.g., proteinuria or retinal hemorrhages.

Abnormal laboratory findings include elevation of alkaline phosphatase levels, eosinopenia, lymphopenia, neutrophilia, and presence of circulating nucleated red blood cells, elevation of SGPT, hyperglycemia, glucosuria (less frequent than hyperglycemia), and low thyroxine (T_4) concentrations. Hypokalemia (serum K^+ concentration less than 3.5 mmol/L) has also been seen in Cushing's disease but is invariably associated with an adrenal tumor. The frequency of laboratory changes is listed in Table 143–1. The urine specific gravity (SG) varies. In random samples, Meijer found the urine SG to be between 1.001 and 1.005 in 40 per cent of cases and between 1.007 and 1.012 in another 40 per cent.[36] As mentioned previously, glucosuria is present in approximately 10 per cent of cases. The urine SG may be normal or even high normal in this circumstance. Elevations of liver enzymes are likely to be the result of hepatotoxic effects of glucocorticoids or, in the case of alkaline phosphatase, the result of both hepatotoxicity and induction of an AP-isoenzyme by cortisol (steroid-induced AP) (see Table 143–1).

Low plasma T_4 concentrations result directly from glucocorticoid excess. It is unknown whether the same mechanisms as in man under cortisol exposure (lowered TSH, thyroxine-binding globulin, and lowered peripheral conversion) are responsible for the changes. The mechanism whereby cortisol excess induces PU/PD is only incompletely understood. In contrast to earlier beliefs, it now appears that, in the dog, cortisol does not inhibit ADH secretion but rather diminishes ADH action on the kidney.

Radiographic Findings

Commonly encountered radiographic changes include hepatomegaly, increased hepatic radiodensity, osteoporosis, and dystrophic calcification of soft tissues (e.g., the bronchial wall or the skin). Enlargement or calcification of the adrenals or a mass mimicking the adrenals may also be seen. Adrenal tumors cannot be accurately diagnosed by standard radiographic techniques, however, and other masses may occur in a location compatible with an adrenal tumor. In the dog, pituitary tumors cannot be seen by conventional radiography.[57]

Other newer imaging techniques may be useful. Two of these are gamma camera imaging and computerized axial tomographic (CAT) scanning. Gamma camera imaging is based on the administration and specific uptake of x-ray–emitting compounds by the adrenals. As a labelling substance, ^{131}I-29-iodocholesterol is used. Upon administration, ^{131}I-29-iodocholesterol is taken up by the adrenals. Several days after ingestion, the adrenal glands can be seen with a gamma camera. Since unilateral adrenal tumors (most adrenal tumors are unilateral) lead to suppression of the contralateral adrenal gland, gamma camera imaging may indicate both the presence or absence of an adrenal tumor and its location (left versus right). Gamma camera imaging is expensive because of the cost of the compounds and the procedure and because dogs have to be hospitalized for days or weeks (because of radiation safety regulations). If the equipment is accessible, CAT scanning may be a more feasible and less expensive means of diagnosing and localizing an adrenal or pituitary tumor.

Etiology

Adrenal tumors cause approximately 20 per cent of cases of spontaneous Cushing's disease.[36] The remaining 80 per cent are of pituitary origin (ACTH overproduction). Depending on the author, pituitary-dependent Cushing's disease is associated with a pituitary tumor in as few as 20 per cent[46] or as many as 84 per cent of cases.[44] This rather striking difference in the frequency of pituitary tumors in the two reports remains unexplained. It is unknown whether the two groups of dogs were studied at different stages of the disease, thus accounting for the discrepancy. It is possible that the high frequency observed in one of the studies was the result of more refined sectioning techniques and a more conscientious search for tumors.[44] Pituitary tumors in dogs suffering from Cushing's disease might arise from the pars distalis or, in contrast to other species, the pars intermedia.[4] Recently, it has been proposed that dogs, in contrast to other species, have an unusual number of pars intermedia cells capable of producing ACTH, thus explaining why canine Cushing's disease can be caused by tumors of the pars intermedia.[14]

The etiology of pituitary-dependent Cushing's disease remains largely unknown, and the tentative explanations are controversial. Recently, it has been suggested that hypothalamic norepinephrine depletion causing excessive corticotrophin-releasing factor (CRF) secretion and, hence, excessive ACTH release may be involved in the etiology of pituitary-dependent Cushing's disease. However, the importance of these findings remains questionable.

Actually, an important, insufficiently answered question is whether Cushing's disease is of primary pituitary or of primary central nervous system (CNS)/hypothalamic origin.[37, 40] Arguments in favor of a CNS/hypothalamic origin primarily stem from the fact that drugs known to primarily affect the CNS (e.g., cyproheptadine) are effective in the treatment of the disease in some cases.[11] Cyproheptadine is a serotonin-receptor blocker, and the drug has been shown to affect CNS control of ACTH secretion in animals. Recent results in humans subjected to transsphenoidal hypophysectomy have shown that, in most instances, a pituitary microadenoma is present and that removal of the microadenoma, in a majority of cases, is followed by improvement of Cushing's disease. More importantly, hypophysectomy is followed by reversal of many changes such as growth hormone (GH) and leutinizing hormone (LH) suppression or absent cortisol diurnal rhythmicity, previously thought to be the result of a primary hypothalamic derangement.[28, 29] Thus, it is likely that, in man, Cushing's disease is usually of primary pituitary origin. However, it cannot be discounted that both pituitary and CNS/hypothalamic Cushing's disease exist. The recent finding that as many as 84 per cent of dogs affected by pituitary-dependent Cushing's disease have pituitary adenomas[44] indicates that the situation in the dog may be similar to that in man.

Pathological Findings in Pituitaries or Adrenals[20, 37, 44, 60]

Depending on the etiology of the disorder, adrenal glands from dogs with Cushing's disease are either hyperplastic or neoplastic. Since approximately 80

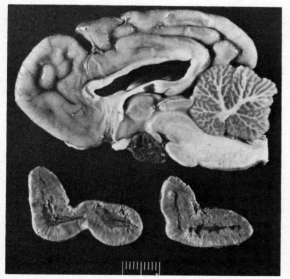

Figure 143–3. Pituitary chromophobe adenoma and hyperplasia of both adrenals in a dog with pituitary-dependent hyperadrenocorticism. Scale = 1 cm. (Courtesy Dr. C. C. Capen.)

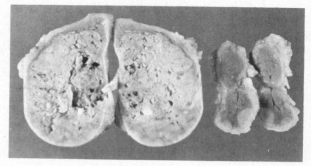

Figure 143–4. Unilateral adrenal carcinoma from a dog with hyperadrenocorticism.

per cent of all cases of Cushing's disease are caused by ACTH overproduction, adrenals are hyperplastic in approximately 80 per cent of cases (Fig. 143–3). Adrenal tumors are adenomas or carcinomas (Fig. 143–4). If they metastasize, adrenal tumors do so to regional lymph nodes or the liver. Pituitary changes include hyperplasia of ACTH-producing cells (basophils, chromophobes) and tumors. Pituitary tumors most frequently are adenomas. Malignant pituitary tumors (carcinomas) have been found occasionally, however. Some pituitary tumors are basophilic, but most are chromophobic. Adenomas arising from the pars intermedia may be found in as many as 29 per cent of the cases.

Diagnosis

A tentative diagnosis of Cushing's disease is based on one or several changes obtained from history, clinical and laboratory examination, and radiographic evaluation. As a rule, the diagnosis should never be rejected if at least one of the typical signs (PU/PD, hair loss, enlarged abdomen, decreased exercise tolerance) is present. Not infrequently, a tentative diagnosis can be made on the basis of history and clinical findings. However, when only a few signs are present, additional information from a urine examination or chemistry panel is needed. The number and kind of differential diagnoses are a function of the major presenting sign(s). For example, if PU/PD is the leading sign, the rule-out list should include those diseases associated with PU/PD (e.g., chronic renal failure, diabetes mellitus, hyperthyroidism, hypercalcemia, diabetes insipidus, liver disease, and so on). However, if decreased exercise tolerance exists, a rule-out list compatible with the latter sign has to be established. When the predominant or the only changes are in the skin, e.g., as in poodles, the rule-out list includes the causes of endocrine alopecia, e.g., hypothyroidism, sex hormone-related alopecia, and growth hormone deficiency-associated alopecia.

A disease that may be mistaken for Cushing's disease is acromegaly (see Chapter 142). Acromegalic dogs may present with PU/PD, decreased exercise tolerance, panting, and an enlarged abdomen. However, a thorough history and clinical examination are quite helpful in differentiating the two diseases. Acromegalic dogs, thus far seen, have been intact females recently in estrus or treated with progestogens. This is in contrast to intact female dogs with Cushing's disease, which frequently exhibit abnormal estrus cycling. Moreover, in acromegaly, there is thickening rather than thinning of the skin and general, rather than just "potbelly," abdominal enlargement. A tentative diagnosis has to be confirmed by specific function tests.

Function Tests in the Diagnosis of Cushing's Disease

ACTH Stimulation Test

The ACTH stimulation test is an evaluation of the cortisol secretory response to a defined ACTH stimulus. The magnitude of the response in general depends on the size of the adrenal. Since approximately 80 per cent of all cases of Cushing's disease are caused by ACTH oversecretion, approximately 80 per cent of all patients have enlarged adrenals and hence an exaggerated response to ACTH. In the remaining 20 per cent (adrenal tumors), response is highly variable. Theoretically (autonomous function), one would expect the adrenal tumors not to respond to ACTH at all. However, cortisol secretory response with an adrenal tumor in response to ACTH may be exaggerated, normal, subnormal, or absent.

An ACTH stimulation test is performed by inject-ing 0.25 mg synthetic α^{1-24} ACTH* IV or 2.2 IU of porcine$^{1-39}$ ACTH† /kg IM. Plasma cortisol is determined before ACTH administration and 60 or 90 minutes (Cortrosyn*) or two hours (Adrenocortgel-40†) after administration. The magnitude of increase is similar with both methods. There are, however, one theoretical and two factual reasons rendering ACTH testing less valuable than dexamethasone suppression for the diagnosis of Cushing's disease.

1. Cushing's disease is a condition characterized by hormone overproduction. Thus, it is more logical to prove abnormal function by attempting to suppress rather than stimulate plasma cortisol levels.

2. Cortisol increments in response to ACTH obtained in affected and normal dogs overlap appreciably. Thus, in some animals having Cushing's disease, the diagnosis would be missed.

3. Cortisol increment in response to ACTH in dogs with adrenal tumors is erratic. Some dogs do not respond, some respond normally, and some respond supranormally. Thus, there is overlap with normals, and a distinction between adrenal hyperplasia and adrenal tumor cannot be made.

In conclusion, we do not recommend the ACTH stimulation test for the diagnosis of Cushing's disease.

*Cortrosyn, Organon, West Orange, NJ.
†Adrenocortgel-40, Carlisle Labs, Inwood, NY.

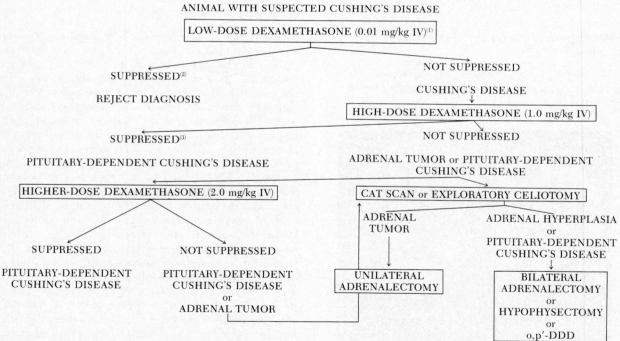

Figure 143–5. Functional diagnosis of spontaneous canine hyperadrenocorticism using dexamethasone suppression tests. Notes: 1. If, during the low-dose dexamethasone test (0.01 mg/kg), cortisol levels drop below 50 per cent of baseline but escape at eight hours above 2 µg/dl, the diagnosis is Cushing's disease caused by primary ACTH overproduction. In this case, Cushing's disease is not caused by an adrenal tumor; suppression is greater than 50 per cent baseline; thus, the high-dose dexamethasone test (1.0 mg/kg) is not necessary. 2. Suppressible (plasma cortisol level less than 1.5 µg/dl at eight hours after dexamethasone administration). 3. Suppressible (plasma cortisol level less than 50 baseline at either three or eight hours after dexamethasone administration). Adrenal tumors may fluctuate up to 30 per cent of baseline. Suppression of less than 50 per cent of baseline, therefore, is compatible with pituitary-dependent Cushing's disease but not with an adrenal tumor (errors are possible).

Dexamethasone Suppression Test (Figure 143–5)

Dexamethasone suppression tests are aimed at confirming the tentative diagnosis and establishing the etiology of Cushing's disease (pituitary-dependent versus adrenal tumor). Dexamethasone (DXM), rather than cortisol, is used to suppress ACTH secretion because it is more efficient than cortisol, does not crossreact in assay systems, and is readily available and inexpensive. In response to DXM administration, normal dogs suppress their cortisol concentrations over a certain period of time. Patients with Cushing's disease, because of decreased sensitivity at the level of the feedback system or because autonomous cortisol secretion is prevalent, either fail to suppress or, after initial suppression, exhibit a premature escape of cortisol levels.

Dexamethasone testing usually is performed in steps, using increasing doses of DXM. Plasma cortisol levels are measured before and three and eight hours after DXM administration. Whereas the first step is aimed at confirming the disease, subsequent steps are aimed at elucidating the etiology of the disorder. If Cushing's disease is confirmed, differentiation between pituitary-dependent Cushing's disease and Cushing's disease caused by an adrenal tumor becomes important, since treatment of the two conditions is fundamentally different.

Confirmation of presumed Cushing's disease is obtained by performing a low-dose DXM suppression test (0.01 mg DXM/kg IV). As a rule, adrenal tumors, because of the autonomous nature of cortisol secretion, do not suppress at any time. However, cortisol secretion may fluctuate, thereby mimicking pituitary-dependent Cushing's disease. In response to a low dose of DXM, cortisol levels in normal dogs decline below 1 μg/dl at three hours and remain suppressed for eight hours or more (<1.5 μg/dl). Dogs with cortisol levels greater than 1.5 μg/dl at eight hours have Cushing's disease. In pituitary-dependent Cushing's disease, there may be a distinct decrease at three hours (below 50 per cent of baseline) but by eight hours plasma cortisol levels may exceed 1.5 μg/dl. A lesser degree or absence of suppressibility does not exclude pituitary-dependent Cushing's disease.

High-Dose DXM Suppression Test[9, 10, 36, 42, 43, 47, 61]

High-dose testing is aimed at differentiating between pituitary-dependent Cushing's disease and Cushing's disease caused by an adrenal tumor. A DXM dose 100 times higher than the low dose, i.e., 1.0 mg/kg IV, is used. In most dogs affected by pituitary-dependent Cushing's disease, cortisol declines below 50 per cent of baseline at three and/or eight hours after DXM administration. However, even at this high dose some dogs with pituitary-dependent Cushing's disease may not have suppressed cortisol levels, mimicking laboratory features of an adrenal tumor. An even higher dose (2.0 mg/kg IV) may disclose suppression and, hence, pituitary-dependent Cushing's disease rather than Cushing's disease caused by an adrenal tumor. If no suppression is obtained at the 1.0 mg/kg dose, an alternative procedure is to stop testing and proceed to a laparotomy. Laparotomy will provide the diagnosis by inspection of the adrenal glands. Then, either bilateral adrenalectomy, in the case of adrenal hyperplasia, or unilateral adrenalectomy, in the case of an adrenal tumor, is performed.

Basal (Endogenous) Plasma ACTH Measurement

In some cases, plasma ACTH measurement is helpful in differentiating pituitary-dependent Cushing's disease from Cushing's disease caused by an adrenal tumor.[8, 42] There are a few drawbacks of the procedure, such as the difficulty of obtaining plasma ACTH measurements (only a small number of laboratories perform this test), the high technical sophistication involved in the procedure, and the high costs involved. Although some authors are more successful using this technique than others,[8] it appears that there is some overlap of plasma ACTH levels in dogs suffering from pituitary-dependent Cushing's disease and those in dogs suffering from an adrenal tumor.[40] Thus, as with any endocrine diagnosis based on hormone measurements, the measurement of basal levels alone is infrequently sufficient for a dependable diagnosis. Hence, in my opinion (J.E.E.), ACTH measurements before and after the attempt to suppress ACTH levels (e.g., intravenous Dexamethasone) potentially should be more helpful in the differential diagnosis of Cushing's disease. Yet such studies are not available. Furthermore, there is no study available comparing all the ancillary diagnostic techniques such as ACTH measurement, CAT scanning, and gamma camera imaging of the adrenals.

Other Diagnostic Methods

It is my belief (J.E.E.) that CAT scanning has the greatest potential. The procedure is relatively easily available, not too expensive, and, provided the tumor is detectable (size), will provide additional information concerning the location of the tumor. Selective blood sampling by catheterization of the adrenal vein and concomitant cortisol measurement such as that used in man to decide whether both adrenals secrete comparable amounts of cortisol (e.g., in the case of adrenal hyperplasia) or appreciably different amounts of cortisol (e.g., in the case of a unilateral tumor) is not possible in the dog; the dog has multiple adrenal veins, which does not allow catheterization.

Treatment [13, 15, 18, 32, 35, 36]

Treatment is aimed at lowering ACTH secretion in cases of primary ACTH oversecretion or lowering adrenal cortisol secretion by either drug medication or surgery. Since cortisol oversecretion, regardless of the etiology, is the hallmark of the disorder, adrenalectomy, either bilateral (hyperplasia) or unilateral (tumor), is potentially an effective means of treating all forms of Cushing's disease. Unilateral adrenalectomy is the treatment of choice in cases of adrenal tumors. Medical management of Cushing's disease with o,p'-DDD* (mitotane) is effective in cases of adrenal hyperplasia but not in cases of adrenal neoplasia. Hypophysectomy (Chapter 142) is effective in animals characterized by primary ACTH overproduction (adrenal hyperplasia). Each of the treatments has its drawbacks.

Medical Management[22, 32, 33, 42, 45, 50, 59]

For medical management, o,p'-DDD, which inhibits cortisol synthesis, is used. More importantly, however, o,p'-DDD causes adrenal atrophy, predominantly of the zona fasciculata and zona reticularis. After an initial daily treatment of 25 mg/kg b.i.d. for 10 to 14 days, o,p'-DDD treatment is continued once a week or, occasionally, once every two weeks at this dose. It is recommended that during daily treatment, prednisolone (0.1 to 0.2 mg/kg b.i.d. PO) or cortisone (0.5 to 1.0 mg/kg b.i.d. PO) be administered simultaneously. During the first few days of treatment, PU/PD usually disappears. Remission of other changes (e.g., skin changes) may not occur before a few months after initiation of treatment. Relapses are common. Several treatment schedules for relapsing cases have been described. In principle, they are the same as the initial treatment. A new initial course of treatment, lasting from 5 to 14 days, is instituted. Increasing the maintenance dose by approximately 50 per cent, i.e., 37.5 mg/kg b.i.d., may decrease the frequency of relapses.

The means of assessing the efficacy of treatment include clinical signs (PU/PD), laboratory parameters (serum AP levels or CBC), ACTH testing, or a combination of all three. Basal cortisol levels should be within the normal range, and cortisol increment in response to ACTH should be absent. The treatment, in many instances, provides sufficient control of the disease for a period of years. Side effects of o,p'-DDD include gastrointestinal signs such as vomiting and diarrhea and neurological signs such as staggering, collapses, and those that are due to the glucocorticoid withdrawal syndrome (weakness, lethargy, anorexia). If side effects occur, o,p'-DDD treatment should be stopped immediately and the steroid dose doubled. If insufficient improvement follows, fluid administration might become necessary. o,p'-DDD treatment occasionally may lead to an Addisonian crisis (see hereafter).

Comparison of Medical Management, Hypophysectomy, and Adrenalectomy in the Treatment of Pituitary-Dependent Cushing's Disease

Controlled studies comparing these three approaches to therapy have not been performed. Thus, recommendations are based on experience, logic, and assumptions. Some owners are reluctant to have their pet undergo long-term medical treatment or surgery owing to expense or other reasons. Additionally, many older animals may have geriatric problems, thus rendering them unsuitable candidates for surgery. The owner may reject surgery for subjective reasons. Lubberink has compared the results of medical management versus hypophysectomy.[32] From her study, it appears that hypophysectomy is superior to medical management in cases of pituitary-dependent Cushing's disease. This is in keeping with recommendations for the treatment of Cushing's disease in humans, in whom transsphenoidal hypophysectomy (for removal of an adenoma) is the treatment of choice. A major drawback is the initial high cost involved. However, medical management, including many follow-up visits and ACTH-testing procedures, ultimately may be more expensive than a surgical procedure. A major drawback of the hypophysectomy procedure is that it requires specific surgical skills. Although adrenalectomy also offers a predictable amelioration in contrast to hypophysectomy, it requires lifelong mineralocorticoid replacement. In addition, adrenalectomy does not prevent, and actually may speed up, the development of a pituitary tumor (see Chapter 142). More extensive, carefully controlled studies are necessary to determine the relative merit of these methods.

Cushing's Disease in the Cat [39, 56]

Although Cushing's disease is relatively common in dogs, the condition has only very rarely been reported in cats. One case of pituitary-dependent Cushing's disease has been reported. Meijer reported one case of feline Cushing's disease caused by an adrenal adenoma successfully treated by unilateral adrenalectomy.

Iatrogenic Cushing's Disease [51]

Iatrogenic Cushing's disease is the result of exposure to excessive amounts of exogenous glucocorticoids. The clinical signs are the same as those encountered in spontaneous Cushing's disease. The diagnosis is based on history, clinical findings, and no increase in the plasma cortisol level in response to exogenous ACTH. It must be emphasized that the diagnosis is based mainly on the finding of clinical signs of Cushing's disease. The negative ACTH Stimulation test is compatible with, but does not provide conclusive evidence for, the disorder. ACTH nonresponsiveness ensues as early as a few days after steroid administration when clinical signs of glucocorticoid excess are largely absent.

Addison's Disease [48, 58]

Addison's disease results from both glucocorticoid and mineralocorticoid deficiency. The signs of the

---

*Lysodren, Bristol Laboratories, Syracuse, NY.

disease are the circulatory and metabolic consequences of a deficiency of all steroid hormones derived from the adrenal cortex. Metabolic changes include low serum sodium and elevated serum potassium levels and acidosis. The sodium:potassium ratio is lowered ($\leq$ 25; normal 30). Blood glucose may be slightly lowered. A common finding is an increased level of serum calcium.

Many of the clinical signs can be related directly to hypotonic dehydration (low sodium in the face of dehydration). Hypotension is likely to result from dehydration, decreased cardiac output, and vasodilation caused by glucocorticoid deficiency.

Most frequently, young dogs are affected with Addison's disease. There appears to be a predilection for females. The history may reveal vomiting with or without diarrhea, anorexia, loss of thirst, and depression. The signs may be mild or intermittent or may be characteristic of episodic weakness. Clinical findings are variable and include signs of shock, dehydration, or normal skin turgor; variable body temperature; a weak pulse; cardiac arrhythmias; decreased peripheral perfusion; and, possibly, hyperventilation secondary to metabolic acidosis. Thoracic radiographs may reveal microcardia and esophageal dilatation. Laboratory findings include low serum Na^+, high serum K^+, possibly high serum Ca^{++}, increased BUN and creatinine levels, and elevated packed cell volume, serum total solids, and neutrophils. The urine specific gravity varies from low to normal. Electrocardiographic changes include tall T-waves, short or flat P-waves, increased P-R interval, and widening of the QRS complex in lead II.

Emergency treatment should be initiated. Fluid loss is restored within 12 hours by administering saline solution intravenously. A glucocorticoid (e.g., hydrocortisone, 50 to 100 mg, or dexamethasone, 2 to 5 mg) should be added to the first bottle of saline. Mineralocorticoids are replaced by injecting 1 to 5 mg of desoxycorticosterone acetate (DOCA) subcutaneously. Emergency treatment is continued by lowering the fluid administration rate and administering prednisolone acetate (5 to 10 mg) subcutaneously every six hours. Improvement usually occurs within a matter of hours. As soon as the dog is able to stand, drink, and eat, maintenance treatment can be instituted. This consists of 25 to 50 mg of desoxycorticosterone trimethyl acetate (pivilate*) every month subcutaneously and oral prednisolone at a maintenance dose (0.2 mg/kg or less b.i.d.). Oral maintenance medication also is possible, given as prednisolone (0.1 mg/kg or less b.i.d.), fluorohydrocortisone acetate (0.1 to 0.2 mg b.i.d.†), and twice daily NaC1 (1 to 6 mg b.i.d., depending on the dog's size). Na^+ and K^+ levels should be assessed routinely and, if needed, treatment adjusted. The diagnosis of Addison's disease is confirmed by an ACTH stimu-

lation test. An increase in the plasma level fails to occur after ACTH administration in Addison's disease.

DISEASES OF THE ADRENAL MEDULLA

Pheochromocytoma

Pheochromocytomas are tumors derived from chromaffin cells of the adrenal medulla. In most instances, the tumors become clinically recognizable because they release large quantities of catecholamines, including norepinephrine and epinephrine, into the circulation. This leads to a variety of manifestations of catecholamine excess, including hypertension, the most common sign in humans suffering from pheochromocytoma. Hypertension may be intermittent. However, even when it is sustained, paroxysmal increments in blood pressure may be clinically detectable. Headaches, excessive perspiration, and palpitations are commonly seen in humans with pheochromocytoma. Typically, such signs occur in paroxysms. Less common signs include pallor, anxiety, nausea, and weakness. Catecholamine-induced cardiomyopathy also may occur. In one study based on necropsy findings, the diagnosis of a pheochromocytoma was made in seven dogs. Three tumors were benign and four were malignant, as evidenced by metastases to liver, spleen, lungs, and nodes. Four of the seven dogs were boxers.

Clinical signs compatible with a pheochromocytoma included paroxysmal hypertension, locomotor disturbance, arteriolar sclerosis, and medial hyperplasia of the arterioles in the kidneys, lungs, and spleen.[16] Schaer reported a dog with signs similar to those seen in humans with pheochromocytoma.[49] Clinical signs included paroxysms of apparent anxiety, palpitations, whining, weakness, trembling, and dilated pupils. Prompt relief of the signs occurred when adrenalectomy (tumor removal) was performed.[49] In most cases, however, malignant pheochromocytomas are nonresectable. This is because early invasion of the venous system and distant metastasis via the caudal vena cava has often occurred by the time the diagnosis is made. Preoperatively, a beta-adrenergic blocker such as propanolol may have to be administered to correct the cardiotoxic effects produced by excessive amounts of catecholamines.

SURGICAL PROCEDURES

Adrenalectomy

Preoperative preparation

Food is withheld for 12 hours before surgery. Water should be available until two hours prior to anesthesia.

---

*Percorten M, Ciba Pharmaceutical Co., Summit, NJ.
†Florinef, E. R. Squibb & Sons Inc., Princeton, NJ.

One hour prior to surgery, premedication with methadone HC1* (0.4 to 1.0 mg/kg), dehydrobenzperidol† (0.5 to 1.2 mg/kg), and atropine sulfate (0.1 mg/kg) is given. Anesthesia is induced with thiopental sodium and maintained with halothane/nitrous oxide. Respiration and the electrocardiogram are monitored continuously, and central venous pressure recordings are suggested.

Surgical Approach

Adrenalectomy may be performed via either a ventral midline abdominal incision or a paracostal (retroperitoneal) approach. The ventral midline approach is satisfactory for exposing the left adrenal gland, but exposure of the right gland is more difficult. In addition, it is not as easy to assess the degree of invasiveness of the adrenal tumor if the midline approach is chosen. In Cushing's disease, the liver may be friable and manipulation during right adrenalectomy may cause damage resulting in bile leakage. Medial retraction of the vena cava, using umbilical tape or retraction, is necessary to allow sufficient exposure of the right adrenal gland. Therefore, although only a single midline abdominal incision is required to expose both glands, the paracostal approach, even if performed bilaterally, remains the technique of choice because of an appreciably better access to each adrenal associated with less manipulation and, hence, less chance of damage to the liver and other abdominal contents such as the pancreas, intestines, and so on.

The dog is placed in lateral recumbency with the surgeon working at the dorsal aspect of the patient and the assistant at the ventral aspect. An 8- to 12-cm incision is made, 1 cm caudal and parallel to the costal arch, just below the lumbar muscles. Dissection of the external and internal abdominal oblique and transverse abdominal muscles, followed by incision through the transverse fascia and peritoneum is performed in the same direction as the skin incision. Although dissection parallel to the muscle fibers causes less tissue damage and bleeding, the technique as described is preferred because of better exposure and access to the adrenals.

---

*Methadone, Eli Lilly and Co., Indianapolis, IN.
†Dehydrobenzpendol, Jansen Pharmaceuticals, Belgium.

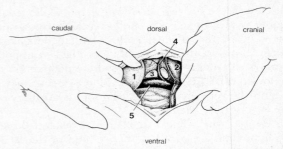

Figure 143–7. Approach to the right adrenal. The assistant gently pushes the liver cranial and the kidney and intestines caudally, exposing the adrenal. *1*, Kidney; *2*, liver; *3*, adrenal; *4*, phrenicoabdominal vein; *5*, postcava.

Right Adrenal Gland. When the abdomen is opened, the caudal pole of the kidney is visible. After division of the hepatorenal ligament (Fig. 143–6), the liver is gently retracted cranially by the assistant while the kidney and intestines are retracted caudally exposing the adrenal gland (Fig. 143–7). The phrenicoabdominal vein is occluded at the medial (and, if possible, the lateral) side by applying arterial clips.* The adrenal gland is carefully freed from the surrounding tissues. Special care is taken to avoid damage of the postcava. Peritoneum, fascia, and muscles are closed in one layer with interrupted sutures using 2–0 or 3–0 synthetic absorbable† material. The skin and subcutaneous tissues are closed routinely.

Left Adrenal Gland. The approach and surgical technique are almost identical to those for the right adrenal gland, except that the left adrenal gland can be exposed more easily. To do so, the stomach and the pancreas are moved cranially and the kidney caudally (Figs. 143–8 and 143–9).

Intraoperative Medication

During surgery, lactated Ringer's solution is infused at a rate of 100 ml/kg and 50 to 100 mg hydrocortisone is slowly infused intravenously over a period of about three to four hours (the cortisol is

---

*Ligaclip, Ethicon, Inc., Sommerville, NJ.
†Polyglycolic acid (Dexon), Davis & Geck, Inc., Pearl River, NY; polyglactin 910 (Vicryl), Ethicon, Inc., Sommerville, NJ.

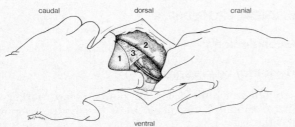

Figure 143–6. Approach to the right adrenal. *1*, Kidney; *2*, liver; *3*, hepatorenal ligament.

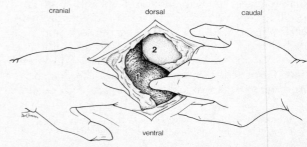

Figure 143–8. Approach to the left adrenal. *1*, Spleen; *2*, kidney.

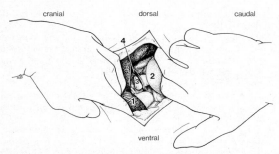

Figure 143–9. Approach to the left adrenal. The assistant pushes the stomach and pancreas cranially and the kidney caudally exposing the adrenal (3). 1, Spleen; 2, left kidney; 4, left phrenicoabdominal vein.

administered in a separate bottle of lactated Ringer's solution).

Care After Unilateral Adrenalectomy for a Cortical Tumor

During the first 24 hours postoperatively, the intravenous infusion of lactated Ringer's solution is continued via an indwelling catheter in the jugular vein. Hydrocortisone* is administered at a rate of 2 mg/kg SC every six hours starting at the end of the surgery. Assuming that dogs affected by Cushing's disease potentially have less resistance to infection and hence are at relatively high risk for postoperative complications, ampicillin therapy is initiated at the time of premedication and is repeated thereafter every eight hours. Monitoring of the patient is confined to the regular clinical observation.

As soon as the patient eats (most often the day after surgery), 2 mg/kg cortisone acetate or 0.4 mg/kg prednisolone is administered orally, divided into two daily doses. After one week, the dose is gradually decreased by one-half over the next two weeks. In the third and fourth weeks, half the initial dosage is given every other day and during the fifth week only twice. This regimen is used to allow the pituitary-adrenal system to recover from longstanding endogenous suppression by the hyperfunctioning adrenocortical tumor.

Prognosis—Adrenal Cortical Tumor

In malignant tumors, metastases in the adrenal gland, draining vessels, or liver may be observed. In these cases, euthanasia is recommended. Of 25 dogs thus adrenalectomized because of an adrenal tumor, 11 recovered completely. Eleven dogs, because of liver metastases, were euthanized intraoperatively. Two dogs died within 72 hours from surgery, and one dog, shortly after surgery, was euthanized on the owner's request.

If the tumor can be removed totally and no metastases are observed, the prognosis is good. Complete recovery from clinical signs usually occurs within two

to three months. However, in some patients, a period of malaise, which responds to corticosteroid administration, has been noted postoperatively.

Care After Bilateral Adrenalectomy (for Pituitary-Dependent Disease)

In addition to the previously mentioned administration of hydrocortisone, mineralocorticoid substitution is also necessary. After removal of both adrenals, a long-acting depot form of a mineralocorticoid, desoxycorticosterone trimethyl acetate, is given at a dose rate of 25 to 50 mg SC at monthly intervals or as indicated by the clinical status of the patient. Monitoring includes daily measurements of serum sodium and potassium and blood urea nitrogen levels until a stable clinical state exists. As soon as the animal eats, cortisone is administered orally at 2 mg/kg, divided into two daily doses. NaCl is given orally at 4 to 10 gm daily.

Maintenance Therapy

Lifelong corticosteroid substitution is necessary after bilateral adrenalectomy. We have given 1 mg/kg cortisone, divided in two daily doses, 4 to 10 gm NaCl daily, and 1/16 mg fluorhydrocortisone acetate twice daily for maintenance.

Prognosis—Bilateral Adrenalectomy

Hyperkalemia may occur, leading to muscle weakness and vomiting. These are the early signs of developing hypoadrenocorticism. Adjustment of the dose of NaCl and fluorhydrocortisone may be necessary to reverse this.

Surgical Procedure—Cat

The paracostal approach, technique, and aftercare in the cat, including medication, are identical to those in the dog. Anesthesia is induced with ketamine* (usually 15 mg/kg), xylazine (usually 0.5 mg/kg), and atropine (0.1 mg/kg body weight). Complete unilateral adrenalectomy was performed in one cat with an adrenal adenoma, and recovery was complete.

1. Baxter, J. D., and Tyrell, J. B.: The adrenal cortex. In Felig, P., Baxter, J. D., Broadus, A. E., and Frohman, L. A. (eds.): Endocrinology and Metabolism. McGraw-Hill Company, 1981, p. 385.
2. Braund, K. G., Dillon, A. R., and Mikeal, R. L.: Experimental investigation of glucocorticoid-induced myopathy in the dog. Exp. Neurol. 60:50, 1980.
3. Braund, K. G., Dillon, A. R., Mikeal, R. L., and August, J. R.: Subclinical myopathy associated with hyperadrenocorticism in the dog. Vet. Pathol. 17:134, 1980.
4. Capen, C. C., Martin, S. L., and Koestner, A.: Neoplasms in the adenohypophysis of dogs. Pathol. Vet. 4:301, 1967.

---

*Hydro-adreson, N. V. Organon Oss, The Netherlands.

*Ketaset, Bristol Laboratories, Veterinary Products, Syracuse, NY.

5. Cryer, P. E.: Physiology and pathophysiology of the human sympathoadrenal neuroendocrine system. N. Engl. J. Med. 313:436, 1980.

6. Cryer, P. E.: Diseases of the adrenal medullae and sympathetic nervous system. In Felig, P., Baxter, J. D., Broadus, A. E., and Frohman, L. A. (eds.): Endocrinology and Metabolism. McGraw-Hill Company, 1981, p. 511.

7. Duncan, I. D., and Griffiths, I. R.: Myotonia in canine Cushing's disease. Vet. Rec. 100:30, 1977.

8. Feldman, E. C.: Distinguishing dogs with functioning adrenocortical tumors from dogs with pituitary-dependent hyperadrenocorticism. J. Am. Vet. Med. Assoc. 183:195, 1983.

9. Feldman, E. C., and Stabenfeldt, G. H.: Comparison of ACTH response and dexamethasone suppression as screening tests in canine hyperadrenocorticism. Sci. Proc. Am. Coll. Vet. Intern. Med., 1982, p. 87.

10. Feldman, E. C., Stabenfeldt, G. H., Farver, T. B., and Addiego, L. A.: Comparison of aqueous porcine ACTH with synthetic ACTH in adrenal stimulation tests of the female dog. Am. J. Vet. Res. 43:522, 1982.

11. Fitzgerald, P. A., Aron, D. C., Findling, J. W., Brooks, R. M., Wilson, C. B., Forsham, P. H., and Tyrell, J. B.: Cushing's disease: Transient secondary adrenal insufficiency after selective removal of pituitary microadenomas; Evidence for a pituitary origin. J. Clin. Endocr. Metabl. 54:413, 1982.

12. Gaunt, R.: History of the adrenal cortex. In Greep, R. O., and Astwood, E. B. (eds.): Handbook of Physiology, Section 7, Endocrinology, Vol. IV. Waverly Press, Inc., Baltimore, 1974, p. 1.

13. Greene, C. E., Lorenz, M. D., Munnell, J. F., Prasse, K. W., White, N. A., and Bowen, J. H.: Myopathy associated with hyperadrenocorticism in the dog. J. Am. Vet. Med. Assoc. 174:1310, 1979.

14. Halmi, N. S., Peterson, M. E., Colurso, G. J., Liotta, A. S., and Krieger, D. T.: Pituitary intermediate lobe in dog: Two cell types and high bioactive adrenocorticotropin content. Science 211:72, 1981.

15. Henry, R. W., Hulse, D. A., Archibald, L. F., and Barta, M.: Transoral hypophysectomy with mandibular symphysiotomy in the dog. Am. J. Vet. Res. 43:1825, 1982.

16. Howard, E. B., and Nielsen, S. W.: Pheochromocytomas associated with hypertensive lesions in dogs. J. Am. Vet. Med. Assoc. 147:245, 1965.

17. Hullinger, R. L.: The endocrine system. In Evans, H. E., and Christensen, G. C. (eds.): Miller's Anatomy of the Dog, 2nd ed. W. B. Saunders, Philadelphia, 1979, p. 602.

18. Johnston, D. E.: Adrenalectomy via retroperitoneal approach in dogs. J. Am. Vet. Med. Assoc. 170:1092, 1977.

19. Joles, J. A., Rijnberk, A., Von den Brom, W. E., and Dogterom, J.: Studies on the mechanism of polyuria induced by cortisol excess in the dog. Vet. Q. 2:199, 1980.

20. Kelly, D. F., Siegel, E. T., and Berg, P.: Pathology of the adrenal in canine Cushing's Syndrome. Vet. Pathol. 8:385, 1971.

21. Kendrick, M. M., and Silverberg, G. D.: Transtemporal hypophysectomy in the dog. Surg. Neurol. 4:244, 1975.

22. Kirk, G. R., and Jensen, H. E.: Toxic effects of o,p'-DDD in the normal dog. J. Am. Anim. Hosp. Assoc. 11:765, 1975.

23. Krieger, D. T.: Regulation of circadian periodicity of ACTH and corticosteroids. Ann. N.Y. Acad. Sc. 297:561, 1971.

24. Krieger, D. T.: Rhythms of ACTH and corticosteroid secretion in health and disease, and their experimental modification. J. Ster. Bioch. 6:785, 1975.

25. Krieger, D. T.: Corticotropin releasing factor distribution in normal and Brattleboro rat brain, and effect of differentiation, hypophysectomy and steroid treatment in normal animals. Endocrinology 100:227, 1977.

26. Krieger, D. T.: Factors influencing the circadian periodicity of ACTH and corticosteroids. Med. Clin. North Am. 62:251, 1978.

27. Krieger, D. T., Liotta, A. S., Brownstein, M. J., and Zimmerman, E. A.: ACTH, B-lipotropin, and related peptides in brain, pituitary and blood. Rec. Progr. Horm. Res. 36:277, 1980.

28. Kuwayama, A., Kageyama, N., Nakane, T., and Watanabe, M.: Anterior pituitary function after transsphenoidal selective adrenomectomy in patients with Cushing's disease. J. Clin. Endocr. Metab. 53:165, 1981.

29. Lankford, H. B., Tucker, H. St. G., and Blackard, W. G.: A cyproheptadine-reversible defect in ACTH control persisting after removal of the pituitary tumor in Cushing's disease. N. Engl J. Med. 19:1244, 1981.

30. Lefer, A. M.: Corticosteroids and circulatory function. In Greep, R. O., and Astwood, E. B. (eds.): Handbook of Physiology, Section 7, Endocrinology, Vol. IV. Waverly Press, Inc., Baltimore, 1975, p. 191.

31. Ling, G. V., Stabenfeldt, G. H., Comer, K. M., Gribble, D. H., and Schechter, R. D.: Canine hyperadrenocorticism: Pretreatment clinical and laboratory evaluation of 117 cases. J. Am. Vet. Med. Assoc. 174:1211, 1979.

32. Lubberink, A. A. M. E.: Diagnosis and treatment of canine Cushing's Syndrome. Ph. D. thesis, University of Utrecht, 1977.

33. Lubberink, A. A. M. E.: Therapy for spontaneous hyperadrenocorticism. In Kirk, R. W. (ed.): Current Veterinary Therapy VII. W. B. Saunders, Philadelphia, 1980, p. 979.

34. Lubberink, A. A. M. E., Rijnberk, A., der Kinderen, P. J., and Thijssen, J. H. H.: Hyperfunction of the adrenal cortex: A review. Aust. Vet. J. 47:504, 1971.

35. Markowitz, J., Archibald, J. and Downie, H. G.: Hypophysectomy in dogs. In Experimental Surgery. Williams & Wilkins, Baltimore, 1964, p. 630.

36. Meijer, J. C.: Canine hyperadrenocorticism. In Kirk, R. W. (ed.): Current Veterinary Therapy VII. W. B. Saunders, Philadelphia, 1980, p. 975.

37. Meijer, J. C., Croughs, R. J. M., Rijnberk, A., Versteeg, D. H. G., and van Ree, J. M.: Hypothalamic catecholamine levels in dogs with spontaneous hyperadrenocorticism. Neuroendocrinology 32:197, 1981.

38. Meijer, J. C., DeBruijne, J. J., Rijnberk, A., and Croughs, R. J. M.: Biochemical characterization of pituitary-dependent hyperadrenocorticism in the dog. J. Endocrinol. 77:1048, 1978.

39. Meijer, J. C., Lubberink, A. A. M. E., and Gruys, E.: Cushing's syndrome due to adrenocortical adenoma in a cat. Tijdschr. Diergeneeskd. 103:1048, 1978.

40. Meijer, J. C., Mulder, G. H., Rijnberk, A., and Croughs, R. J. M.: Hypothalamic corticotropin releasing factor activity in dogs with pituitary-dependent hyperadrenocorticism. J. Endocrinol. 79:209, 1978.

41. Mulnix, J. A., Van den Brom, W. E., Lubberink, A. A. M. E., de Bruijne, J. J., and Rijnberk, A.: Gamma camera imaging of bilateral adrenocortical hyperplasia and adrenal tumors in the dog. Am. J. Vet. Res. 37:1467, 1976.

42. Peterson, M. E., and Drucker, W. D.: Advances in the diagnosis and management of canine Cushing's Syndrome. 31st Gaines Veterinary Symposium, 1981, p. 17.

43. Peterson, M. E., Gilbertson, S. R., and Drucker, W. D.: Plasma cortisol response to exogenous ACTH in 22 dogs with hyperadrenocorticism caused by adrenocortical neoplasia. J. Am. Vet. Med. Assoc. 180:542, 1982.

44. Peterson, M. E., Krieger, D. T., Drucker, W. D., and Halmi, N. S.: Immunocytochemical study of the hypophysis in 25 dogs with pituitary-dependent hyperadrenocorticism. Acta Endocrinol. (Kbh) 101:15, 1982.

45. Peterson, M. E., Nesbitt, G. H., and Schaer, M.: Diagnosis and management of concurrent diabetes mellitus and hyperadrenocorticism in thirty dogs. J. Am. Vet. Med. Assoc. 178:66, 1981.

46. Rijnberk, A., Der Kinderen, P. J., and Thijssen, J. H. H.: Spontaneous hyperadrenocorticism in the dog. J. Endocrinol. 41:397, 1968.

47. Saez, J. M., Tell, G. P., and Dazord, A.: Human adrenocortical tumors: Alterations in membrane-bound hormone receptors and cAMP protein kinases. In Sharma, R. K., and

Criss, W. E. (eds.): *Endocrine Control in Neoplasia.* Raven Press, New York, 1978, p. 53.

48. Schaer, M.: Hypoadrenocorticism. *In* Kirk, R. W. (ed.): *Current Veterinary Therapy VII.* W. B. Saunders, 1980.

49. Schaer, M.: Pheochromocytoma in a dog: A case report. J. Am. Anim. Hosp. Assoc. *16*:583, 1980.

50. Schechter, R. D., Stabenfeldt, G. H., Gribbe, D. H., and Ling, G. V.: Treatment of Cushing's syndrome in the dog with an adrenocorticolytic agent (o,p'-DDD). J. Am. Vet. Med. Assoc. *162*:629, 1973.

51. Scott, D. W.: Systemic glucocorticoid therapy. *In* Kirk, R. W. (ed.): *Current Veterinary Therapy VII.* W. B. Saunders, Philadelphia, 1980, p. 988.

52. Seal, U. S., and Doe, R. P.: Corticosteroid-binding globulin: species distribution and small scale purification. Endocrinology 73:371, 1963.

53. Seal, U. S., and Doe, R. P.: Vertebrate distribution of corticosteroid-binding globulin and some endocrine effects on concentration. Steroids 5:827, 1965.

54. Siegel, E. T., Kelly, D. F., and Berg, P.: Cushing's Syndrome in the dog. J. Am. Vet. Med. Assoc. *157*:2081, 1970.

55. Steele, R.: Influences of corticosteroids on protein and carbohydrate metabolism. *In* Greep, R. O., and Astwood, E.

B. (eds.): *Handbook of Physiology*, Section 7, Endocrinology, Vol. IV, Waverly Press, Inc., Baltimore, 1975, p. 135.

56. Swift, G. A., and Brown, R. H.: Surgical treatment of Cushing's syndrome in the cat. Vet. Rec. *99*:374, 1976.

57. Ticer, J. W.: Roentgen signs of endocrine disease. Vet. Clin. North Am. *7*:465, 1977.

58. Willard, M. D., Schall, W. D., McCaw, D. F., and Nachreiner, R. F.: Canine hypoadrenocorticism: Report of 37 cases and review of 39 previously reported cases. J. Am. Vet. Med. Assoc. *180*:59, 1982.

59. Willard, M. D., Schall, W. D., Nachreiner, R. F., and Shelton, D. G.: Hypoadrenocorticism following therapy with o,p'-DDD for hyperadrenocorticism in four dogs. J. Am. Vet. Med. Assoc. *180*:638, 1982.

60. Willeberg, P., and Priester, W. A.: Epidemiologic aspects of clinical hyperadrenocorticism in dogs (canine Cushing's syndrome). J. Am. Anim. Hosp. Assoc. *18*:717, 1982.

61. Wolfsen, A. R., and Odell, W. D.: The dose-response relationship of ACTH and cortisol in Cushing's disease. Clin. Endocrinol. *12*:557, 1980.

62. Yasuda, N., Greer, M. A., and Aizawa, T.: Corticotropin releasing factor. Endocrine Rev 3:123, 1982.

Chapter **144**

The Thyroid

Stephen W. Crane
and Michael Aronsohn

ANATOMY

Embryology

The histogenesis of thyroid cells and their organization into typical thyroid follicles occur during early embryonic life. Early endocrine function of the thyroid gland influences growth of cells, tissues, and organs as well as maturation and regulation of a wide variety of metabolic functions. Besides the discrete glands located near the larynx, accessory thyroid and parathyroid glandular remnants exist. Therefore, knowledge of the embryonic derivation of these structures has surgical relevance. The cell clusters that become the adult thyroid are derived from the endodermal epithelium that lines portions of both the third and fourth pharyngeal pouches. Neural crest cells that invade the endoderm give rise to the thyroid's parafollicular or C cells that later secrete calcitonin.[20] The parathyroid and thymus glands originate in close proximity to thyroid tissue, from other specific portions of both the third and fourth pharyngeal pouches. The external parathyroid glands arise from pharyngeal pouch III, and the internal parathyroid glands from pharyngeal pouch IV. Induction, differentiation, and fusion of specific embryogenic tissues, and migration of primordial cell populations in the third and fourth pharyngeal pouches have been mapped, and it is known that intermixture of the three differentiating tissue types commonly occurs.

Developmental migration of the embryonic thyroid gland starts from the base of the tongue and proceeds to the lower laryngeal area. During this process, the thyroid mass separates into two lobes, which move to lateral positions along the upper trachea. Thus, a large majority of dogs, and all cats, do not possess a grossly discernible isthmus between the two thyroid lobes. The thyroglossal duct, a stalk-like structure connecting the region of the embryonic pharyngeal pouches and the thyroid gland, normally degenerates into a fibrotic remnant. However, this structure rarely may persist postnatally as an abnormal opening at the base of the tongue.[20]

As the embryonic thymus gland migrates to the cranial mediastinum, the two pairs of parathyroid glands also move to their final anatomical positions within or upon the thyroid gland; further cell intermixture may also occur during this process.[20] Thyroid or parathyroid tissue may be included in the embryonic aortic sac. Thus, normal thymic and aortic sac migration, coupled with intermixing of cell types during organogenesis, explains the presence of accessory thyroid and parathyroid tissues in the neck and within the cranial or caudal mediastinum or the periaortic fat bodies in approximately 50 per cent of dogs.[19, 20] Accessory thyroid or parathyroid glandular fragments are clinically important because they may participate in physiological or pathological processes, such as primary or compensatory hormone secretion or carcinogenesis.

Gross Anatomy

In the medium-sized dog the thyroid glands are about 5.0 cm long, 1.5 cm wide, and 0.5 cm thick. They are paired, slightly lobulated structures lateral to the first five to eight tracheal rings. Moderate positional and size discrepancies between normal left and right glands are not uncommon, with the left lobe often being more caudal. The thyroid gland varies in size in different breeds. Brachycephalic dogs have relatively larger glands than mesocephalic breeds.[19] As a matter of mainly historical interest, iodine-deficient diets dramatically increase both gland size and blood supply.[2, 17] Thyroid size in the cat is consistent. Each thyroid lobe averages 2 cm long, 0.3 cm wide, and 0.3 cm thick. In both species, ramifications of a thin, fibrous, external capsule extend into the glandular parenchyma, resulting in septation of the parenchyma into lobules.

The parathyroid glands are closely associated with the thyroid glands. The external pair of glands (parathyroid glands III) are located on the lateral aspect of the thyroid capsule (Fig. 144–1). The internal parathyroid glands (parathyroids IV) usually are located within the parenchyma of the caudal pole of the thyroid gland, being invisible to inspection. They can be located only by sectioning of the thyroid gland. The internal parathyroids may also be located in an extraglandular, intracapsular position on the medial aspect of the gland.

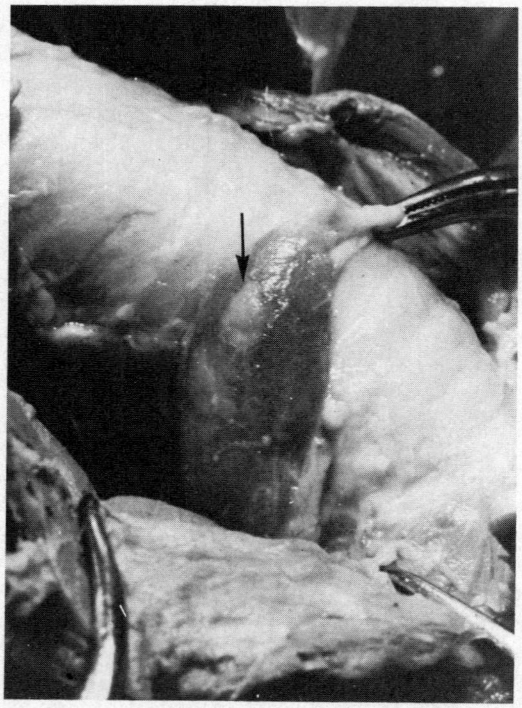

Figure 144–1. The right thyroid gland of a 6-year-old male mixed-breed dog (cadaver) has been mobilized and moved ventrally on the trachea to illustrate a normal external parathyroid gland (*arrow*) on the dorsolateral surface of the glandular capsule. The internal parathyroid glands are frequently imbedded in the parenchyma of the caudal pole of the gland (not shown). (Ventral approach, head to left.)

The blood supply of the thyroid glands is relatively large compared with other organs.[11] The major blood supply to both the thyroid and parathyroid glands of the dog and cat is from the cranial thyroid arteries, which consistently originate from the common carotid arteries, caudal to the larynx. They turn to run in a caudomedial direction, to the region of the proximal trachea, where they supply the thyroid glands (through thyroid branches) and the larynx (Fig. 144–2).[4, 19] One small branch of the cranial thyroid artery supplies the dorsal portion of the thyroid capsule and the external parathyroid gland.[19] The artery then continues dorsocaudally, lying medial and parallel to the gland and giving off branches that break through the medial aspect of the thyroid capsule. Once within the capsule, arterial branches follow the septae and ramify to become a distribution network characterized by highly muscular arterioles and extensive sinusoids.[5] With autonomically innervated arteriovenous shunts, these vascular channels indirectly aid in hormone release by regulating local blood flow.[17] The cranial thyroid artery continues past the thyroid gland, where it functions as an important source of blood for the esophagus and trachea (see Fig. 144–2).[4, 19]

In the dog and cat, the importance and distribution of the caudal thyroid artery, a branch of the brachiocephalic artery, is variable. The caudal thyroid artery is only occasionally a significant blood vessel in dogs and does not have the vascular or surgical importance of the inferior thyroid artery in humans.[4] Despite its name, the caudal thyroid artery participates only to a limited degree in perfusion of the thyroid gland in normal subjects, but it does anastomose with the termination of the cranial thyroid artery to supply the trachea and esophagus.[4]

Venous return from the thyroid glands is by the cranial and caudal thyroid veins (Fig. 144–3). The latter are not satellite structures of the caudal thyroid arteries. Rather, they usually drain into the internal jugular veins. In addition, a large unpaired vein is sometimes observed on the ventral aspect of the trachea. This vein drains the left thyroid lobe caudally into the brachiocephalic vein.[19]

Organized lymphatic drainage of the thyroid gland begins in intracapsular collection plexi. Lymph vessels emerge from the cranial portion of the capsule and proceed to the cranial and caudal deep cervical lymph nodes.[19] After exit from regional nodes, lymphatics on the right side drain toward the thoracic inlet, via the right lymphatic duct, and on the left side via the left tracheal duct. Additionally, some lymphatics enter directly into the internal jugular vein.

Nerve supply to the thyroids is from a combination of the external branch of the cranial laryngeal nerve (a branch of the vagus) and sympathetic fibers from the cranial cervical ganglion.[19] A major function of autonomic nervous supply is mediation of changes of vascular tone, to assist regulation of the blood supply to the glands.

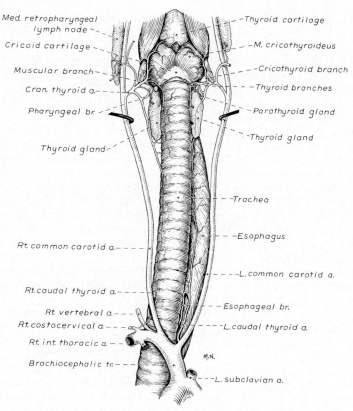

Med. retropharyngeal
lymph node

Cricoid cartilage

Muscular branch

Cran. thyroid a.

Pharyngeal br.

Thyroid gland

Rt. common carotid a.

Rt. caudal thyroid a.

Rt. vertebral a.

Rt. costocervical a.

Rt. int. thoracic a.

Brachiocephalic tr.

Thyroid cartilage

M. cricothyroideus

Cricothyroid branch

Thyroid branches

Parathyroid gland

Thyroid gland

Trachea

Esophagus

L. common carotid a.

Esophageal br.

L. caudal thyroid a.

M.N.

L. subclavian a.

Figure 144–2. Ventral view of the arterial blood supply to the laryngeal region, trachea, and esophagus of the dog, emphasizing the importance of the cranial thyroid artery and its distribution to the entire cervical region as well as the thyroid gland. The caudal thyroid artery is not an important source of arterial supply to the thyroid gland in companion animals. (Reprinted with permission from Evans, H. E., and Christensen, G.C.: *Miller's Anatomy of the Dog.* 2nd ed. W. B. Saunders, Philadelphia, 1979.)

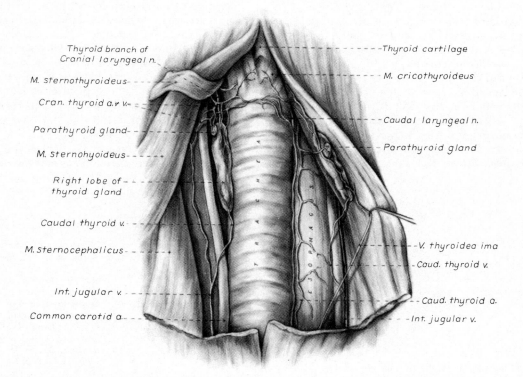

Thyroid branch of
Cranial laryngeal n.

M. sternothyroideus

Cran. thyroid a. r v.

Parathyroid gland

M. sternohyoideus

Right lobe of
thyroid gland

Caudal thyroid v.

M. sternocephalicus

Int. jugular v.

Common carotid a.

Thyroid cartilage

M. cricothyroideus

Caudal laryngeal n.

Parathyroid gland

V. thyroidea ima

Caud. thyroid v.

Caud. thyroid a.

Int. jugular v.

Figure 144–3. Surgical anatomy of the ventral cervical region of the dog is depicted following reflection of the ventral muscle bellies of the neck. Pertinent venous and nervous anatomy is included. (Reprinted with permission from Evans, H. E., and Christensen, G. C.: *Miller's Anatomy of the Dog.* 2nd ed. W. B. Saunders, Philadelphia, 1979.)

SURGICAL ANATOMY AND EXPLORATION OF THE NECK

Once a thyroid disorder is suspected, routine jugular sampling should be avoided to preclude hematoma formation near the intended surgical site. Prior to surgery, an intravenous catheter is aseptically placed into the cephalic vein for fluid therapy and postoperative blood specimen collection. Surgical exposure is made through a ventral midline incision extending from the larynx to the caudal third of the neck. This incision may be extended to the manubrium sterni or into the cranial sternabrae if exposure of the cranial mediastinum is necessary. Midline separation of the paired bellies of the sternohyoideus exposes all the major structures of the neck. The trachea, easily identified, serves as an anatomical landmark for locating the thyroid and parathyroid glands. The carotid sheaths (containing the common carotid arteries, the vagosympathetic trunk, and the internal jugular veins), both recurrent laryngeal nerves, the retropharyngeal lymph nodes, the lymphatic ducts and the esophagus are also found related to the trachea. Gentle traction and countertraction allow full exposure of the area.

The surgical area is lavaged at intervals with warm, sterile saline to remove blood clots and to keep tissues moist. All retraction is gentle, and the retractors are placed carefully over moistened cotton pads. Anatomical features that should be noted include the size, shape, color, texture, symmetry, and position of the thyroid and the external parathyroid glands. Internal parathyroid enlargement or asymmetry, if present, may be visible or palpable. The distribution of the cranial thyroid artery branches to the external parathyroid gland should be noted, because the appropriate vessel(s) must be preserved if partial or total thyroidectomy is anticipated.

Attention to the close proximity of the major portion of the laryngeal innervation is critically important during dissection of the thyroid region. The right recurrent laryngeal nerve is located on the right dorsolateral aspect of the trachea and is seen medial and deep to the right thyroid lobe when one is operating from the ventral aspect. The left recurrent laryngeal nerve is located between the left ventrolateral aspect of the trachea and the esophagus. The caudal laryngeal nerves leave the recurrent laryngeal nerves ventral or caudal to the thyroid and pass under the ventral edge of the cricopharyngeus to innervate all the muscles of the larynx except the cricothyroideus.[19, 27] Unilateral or bilateral laryngeal neuropraxia or neuroplegia can result from operative trauma, most likely during dissection of locally invasive neoplasms. Bilateral postoperative laryngeal dysfunction constitutes a disastrous surgical complication regardless of potential endocrinological improvement. A mental image of a transverse section of the neck at the level of the thyroid gland is useful for maintaining an appreciation of these relationships during difficult surgical dissections (Fig. 144–4).

PHYSIOLOGY: SYNTHESIS AND METABOLISM OF THYROID HORMONES

Secretion of thyroxin (T_4), triiodothyronine (T_3), and calcitonin occurs in the thyroid gland. Thyroglobulin is a glycoprotein molecule of 660,000 daltons MW secreted by thyroid cells into the follicular lumen. Hormone synthesis occurs within follicular thyroglobulin by enzymatically mediated iodination of the thyronine nucleus to yield monoiodotyrosine and diiodotyrosine. Two molecules of diiodotyrosine then combine to produce one molecule of T_4. In a similar manner, diiodotyrosine may couple with monoiodotyrosine to form T_3. Once synthesized, T_4 and T_3 remain bound to and stored with thyroglobulin.[17] Secretion of hormone occurs by the creation of surface membrane vesicles of colloid that extrude into the cytoplasm of thyroid cells. Enzymatic cleavage of the colloid into one of the iodothyronines and thyroglobulin occurs intracellularly. T_4 and T_3 are released through the external cell membrane into the extracellular spaces and capillaries.[17] The thyroglobulin protein and residual iodide anions resulting from the deiodination of T_4 into T_3 during secretion are retained for hormone resynthesis.[17]

There are major quantitative differences in T_4 and T_3 homeostasis between humans and the dog and cat.

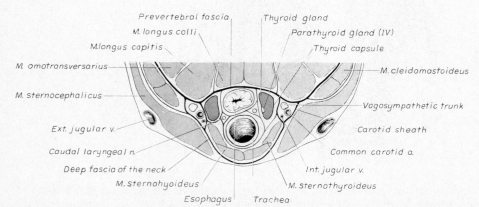

Prevertebral fascia
M. longus colli
M. longus capitis
M. omotransversarius
M. sternocephalicus
Ext. jugular v.
Caudal laryngeal n.
Deep fascia of the neck
M. sternohyoideus
Esophagus
Trachea
Thyroid gland
Parathyroid gland (IV)
Thyroid capsule
M. cleidomastoideus
Vagosympathetic trunk
Carotid sheath
Common carotid a.
Int. jugular v.
M. sternothyroideus

Figure 144–4. Transverse section of the neck of a dog, facing rostrally, illustrating the positions of vital structures in the neck. These relationships must be kept in mind during dissection for invasive neoplasms. (Reprinted with permission from Evans, H. E., and Christensen, G. C.: *Miller's Anatomy of the Dog.* 2nd ed. W. B. Saunders, Philadelphia, 1979.)

Normal circulating T_3 and T_4 levels of companion animals are considerably lower than those of humans, making it difficult to obtain an accurate determination of canine and feline thyroid function by using commercially available human laboratory tests or kit procedures.[2] For accuracy, the veterinarian should request that T_4 be quantitated by radioimmunoassay against diluted, known value standards, so that the less accurate extrapolation to a curve is avoided. A comprehensive discussion of the theory and practice of thyroid function testing in animals is presented by Belshaw.[2]

Although more T_4 than T_3 is synthesized, a considerable percentage of the production of T_3 occurs via deiodination of T_4 in the peripheral circulation.[17] T_4 has active hormone activity, but thyroxin may function as a circulating prohormone and the major endocrinological effect is derived from T_3.[1, 2] Although the mode of metabolic action of T_3 at the cellular level is not known, specific nuclear binding sites for T_3 have been identified. Because absence of thyroid hormones depresses basal metabolism by about 40 per cent, one hypothesis for the mechanism of action of T_3 is that it augments the efficiency of DNA and RNA transcription and translation and increases synthesis of enzymes and other proteins.[2, 17]

Control of hormone synthesis occurs mainly via negative feedback loops within a hypothalamic-pituitary-thyroid axis. The synthesis and release of thyroid-stimulating hormone (TSH) from the pituitary is caused by thyrotropin-releasing hormone (TRH), a neuropeptide secreted by the hypothalamus. TRH-induced release of TSH is inhibited by increasing levels of thyroid hormones and is also suppressed by endogenous or exogenous glucocorticoids. Inhibition of TSH release is also directly inhibited by circulating T_3. TSH is largely responsible for the anatomical and physiological status of the thyroid gland by augmenting iodine trapping, thyroglobulin and hormone synthesis, and T_3 and T_4 release into the circulation.[17]

Hypothyroidism is the most common thyroid disorder in dogs. On the basis of specific breed predisposition, it has a probable genetic basis.[1, 2, 9, 14, 15, 28, 31] Acquired idiopathic follicular atrophy accounts for nearly half of the cases of primary canine hypothyroidism. Autoimmune lymphocytic thyroiditis, associated with circulating thyroglobulin autoantibodies, also occurs in dogs.[14, 15] The clinical signs, diagnosis, and treatment of primary and secondary hypothyroidism are described elsewhere.[1, 2, 9]

SURGICAL DISEASES OF THE THYROID GLAND

Feline Hyperthyroidism

Hyperthyroidism in the cat, associated with adenomatous hyperplasia of the thyroid gland, has recently become a well-recognized clinical entity.[18, 35, 39] However, previous postmortem studies of feline thyroid glands suggested a possible correlation between thyroid lesions and clinical hyperthyroidism.[21] Case histories consistent with feline hyperthyroidism were published in 1964, and follicular nodules and "cystic adenomas" were found in 23 of 75 postmortem specimens.[25] Adenocarcinomas and solitary adenomas are infrequent causes of functional hyperthyroidism. Although the lesions of adenomatous hyperplasia may represent an emerging clinical entity, it is also possible that the currently more common diagnosis is due to increased professional awareness and testing of thyroid function.

Hyperthyroidism generally is seen in geriatric cats.[18, 39] In a study of 131 cats with thyrotoxicosis, the average age was 12.3 years with a range of six to 20 years.[35] There is no currently recognized sex predisposition. The disease occurs most commonly in mixed breed domestic short- or long-haired cats.[18, 35, 36, 39]

The most common presenting complaint is progressive weight loss to the point of emaciation in association with a ravenous appetite. Cats often cry constantly to be fed and may begin eating unusual foods or even stealing foods. In addition to polyphagia, polyuria and polydipsia are reported in about 50 per cent of cases.[18, 35] Restlessness, hyperactivity, heat intolerance, and panting are consistently mentioned by the client. Frequent defecation of soft, bulky, or watery stools may occur as well.

On physical examination, affected cats are observed to be thin or emaciated, often with a greasy, matted hair coat. They are usually restless and thus may be difficult to examine. The body temperature is often slightly elevated, and the mucous membranes may be hyperemic. The ears may be hyperemic and hot. In one study, careful palpation of the thyroid revealed enlargement of one or both lobes in nine of ten patients.[36] Lack of palpable enlargement does not rule out adenomatous hyperplasia, because a functional but nonpalpable lesion may exist. As mentioned previously, there also may be hyperfunctioning accessory thyroid tissue elsewhere in the cervical region or mediastinum.

In addition to body wasting, the most dramatic findings on physical examination are usually associated with cardiac function. Tachycardia is typical, with rates between 240 and 300 beats/min., owing to enhanced function of the beta receptor–catecholamine linkage associated with thyrotoxicosis.[35, 36] Ventricular hypertrophy, hypertension, arrhythmias, murmurs, and congestive heart failure have also been observed.[18, 35, 36, 39] ECG analysis of 45 cats with adenomatous hyperplasia frequently revealed sinus tachycardia and increased lead II R-wave amplitude.[36] Although the latter finding suggests left ventricular hypertrophy, the frontal plane mean electrical axis usually was normal.[18] One-half of the patients in a large series had cardiomegaly.[35] Conduction disturbances, including ectopic atrial and ventricular electrical activity, also occur with some frequency.[35, 36] Because cases of feline hyperthyroidism with thyrotoxicosis and the hypertrophic or

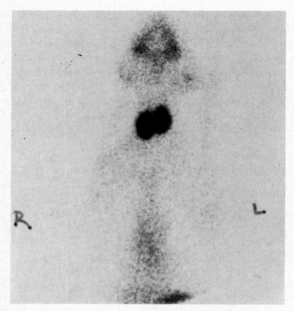

Figure 144–5. Ventrodorsal image produced by thryoid scintigraphy from a 13-year-old female domestic shorthaired cat, showing bilateral thyroid lobe hyperactivity. No evidence of ectopic thyroid gland hyperactivity is seen. Bilateral thyroid lobectomy was performed, and clinical signs of hyperthryoidism disappeared. The cat was maintained on sodium levothyroxine.

congestive forms of feline cardiomyopathy can be associated with similar cardiac problems, thoracic radiographs and an ECG should be performed in all cats with suspected hyperthyroidism. Cardiac ultrasonograms are useful if available.

Diagnostic aids, besides history and physical examination, include a complete blood count, urinalysis, and biochemical profile. Thyrotoxicosis may produce high levels of liver-specific enzymes.[35] Because diabetes mellitus should be considered in the differential diagnosis, a blood glucose determination and urinalysis should be done in every suspected case. Definitive diagnosis is based on elevated plasma levels of T_3 and T_4 by radioimmunoassay. Normal ranges for T_3 are 0.6 to 2 ng/ml, and for T_4, 15 to 50 ng/ml, but in hyperthyroid cats the T_3 level may be as high as 4 ng/ml, and T_4 level as high as 200 ng/ml.[39] Thyroid scans using sodium pertechnetate can be used to delineate adenomatous thyroid tissue and help locate functional ectopic thyroid tissue (Figs. 144–5 and 144–6).

Treatment of Feline Hyperthyroidism

Surgical removal of the affected thyroid tissues causes regression of clinical signs, including cardiac and behavioral manifestations, in days to weeks.[18, 39] In most cases, surgical intervention can be carried out promptly and without risk of "thyroid storm," which potentially complicates the surgical case of severely hyperthyroid human patients.[12, 13, 22, 39] In severe thyrotoxicosis with associated cardiac signs, presurgical stabilization with antithyroid drugs, beta-receptor blockade, or antiarrhythmogenic agents should be attempted.[12, 13, 18, 21, 22, 30, 39]

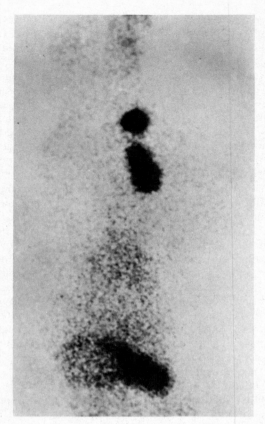

Figure 144–6. Ventrodorsal image produced by thyroid scintigraphy of a 10-year-old male domestic shorthaired cat that had undergone right thyroidectomy without remission of thyrotoxicosis. At surgery, the left thyroid lobe was found to be atrophied. Scintigraphy revealed a normal gastric mucosal image and two abnormal, functional masses of ectopic thyroid tissue at the thoracic inlet. Re-exploration was performed, and the accessory thyroid tissue was removed. The left thyroid lobe was still atrophied and was not removed. Clinical signs abated.

Iodides, given orally, have been used to block both the synthesis and the release of T_3 and T_4. Unfortunately, iodine therapy takes days to work, and any induced changes may be long-lasting.[17] In addition, iodides are unpalatable to cats. Propylthiouracil* blocks iodine incorporation into the thyronine precursor and decreases the quantity of new T_3 and T_4 synthesized. The oral dose in the cat is 50 mg given three times daily, but the drug should be used cautiously and only in the most serious cases. Propranalol (Inderal)† blocks the peripheral effects of thyroid hormone on cardiac beta receptors and effectively controls tachyarrhythmias at dosages of 2.5 mg, given orally, three times daily, for two to five days or until the heart rate is reduced to near-normal levels.[12, 18, 25, 29] If cardiac failure is present, concurrent treatment with iodides, furosemide,‡ total cage rest, and perhaps digoxin is indicated. Although propranalol may be safely used in congestive heart failure associated with thyrotoxicosis, it has a negative inotropic effect. Thyrotoxic cats usually are more

*Eli Lilly and Company, Indianapolis, IN.
†Ayerst Laboratories, New York, NY.
‡American Hoechst Corporation, Somerville, NJ.

stable following two to four weeks of medical treatment and are better anesthetic risks.

Routine anesthetic methods may be used, but premedication with atropine is contraindicated because it may potentiate sinus tachycardia and barbiturate-induced cardiac arrhythmias.[36] We use a regimen consisting of acetylpromazine or ketamine pretreatment, followed by induction with a short-acting barbiturate, and intubation and maintenance with gas anesthetics. Administration of inhalation anesthetic in a feline anesthesia chamber may also facilitate induction of anesthesia in a restless, hyperactive animal. Isoflurane, in particular, provides stable and controllable anesthesia with minimal depression of cardiac output and few arrhythmias. Continuous cardiac monitoring is mandatory during surgery, because cardiac dysrhythmias are the most common operative complication. Emergency cardiac drugs should be available.

Surgical Techniques

In neck exploration for hyperthyroidism in the cat, each thyroid lobe is individually and carefully evaluated. No thyroid tissue should be removed until both thyroid lobes and all visible parathyroid tissue are examined. Additionally, the recurrent laryngeal and caudal laryngeal nerves and carotid sheaths should be identified and protected. Throughout the procedure, hemostasis, using delicate instruments and fine ligatures, is recommended, because bleeding obscures the surgical field. Attempts to clamp and ligate bleeders with large instruments may damage normal tissues and vessels. Hemorrhage and tissue damage are minimized by the use of sterile cotton-tipped applicator sticks to develop tissue planes. Minor bleeding may be controlled by gentle pressure. To minimize tissue damage, electrocautery is contraindicated, although fine bipolar electrosurgical forceps may be used.

Feline adenomatous hyperplasia may be unilateral or bilateral; however, bilateral involvement is seen in 70 per cent of cases.[35] Unfortunately, a grossly normal lobe may reveal microscopic adenomatous hyperplasia or a premalignant lesion.[18, 21, 25] Cats undergoing unilateral thyroidectomy may develop subsequent hyperthyroidism owing to hyperplasia of the remaining lobe, requiring further surgery. Abnormal thyroid lobes are variably enlarged, mottled, cystic, or nodular.[18] The color is variable—dark brown, green, light brown, or yellow.

Because the etiology of this disease is not currently understood and no figures are available regarding recurrence of clinical signs after unilateral thyroidectomy, our preference, at this time, is to remove only those lobes that show an increased uptake of sodium pertechnetate on thyroid scan. If scanning is not available, only abnormal-appearing lobe(s) should be removed.

Following a midline incision as described previously, the thyroid lobes are located between the

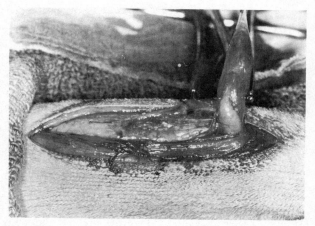

Figure 144–7. In a cat, the left thyroid gland is mobilized into the surgical incision following ligation of the caudal thyroid artery and division of loose connective tissue.

sternothyroideus muscles and the trachea. To remove one or both lobes, the branches of the caudal thyroid vessels that supply that lobe are ligated and divided, and the gland is mobilized into the incision (Fig. 144–7). The thyroid capsule is opened at the caudal pole. The parenchyma is gently dissected free by intracapsular teasing; this dissection is more difficult with very large lobes. The lobe is removed intact from within the capsule, leaving a cranial cuff of capsule with the external parathyroid gland and an intact local blood supply. After lavage and aspiration, total hemostasis is confirmed, and the muscle bellies are closed with 4-0 absorbable suture. Subcutaneous and skin closure is routine.

Following total thyroidectomy, lifetime supplementation with thyroid hormone is necessary. It should be started on the second to fourth day after operation. A dose of 0.2 mg of sodium levothyroxine (Synthroid)* is indicated on a daily basis. The T_3 and T_4 levels are monitored periodically thereafter, so that an appropriate maintenance dose may be determined.

Complications of Surgery

Postoperative hypocalcemia is the most serious potential complication of bilateral thyroidectomy. Inadvertent removal or destruction of all parathyroid glands results in hypocalcemia, which is characterized at first by restlessness and then by muscular tetany and convulsions. Hypocalcemia generally occurs within one to two days of operation, so it is necessary to monitor serum calcium. Operative trauma to the parathyroid glands or interference with their blood supply may also cause hypofunction and transient hypocalcemia (see Chapter 145). Other complications include hematoma and infection, which are treated by evacuation or drainage and hot compresses. Damage to the recurrent or caudal laryngeal nerves causes

---

*Flint Laboratories, Deerfield, IL.

temporary or permanent laryngeal and vocal cord paralysis on the affected side.

CANINE THYROID NEOPLASMS

Neoplasms are the most common indication for surgery of the canine thyroid gland. Epidemiological data based on five large studies indicate that the average age for thyroid neoplasia in dogs is nine to ten years, with a range of three to 18 years.[16] There is no sex predilection, but boxers, beagles, and golden retrievers are at greater risk than other breeds.[16] Approximtely one-third of all canine thyroid tumors are adenomas and two-thirds carcinomas.[21] However, because most adenomas are not detected antemortem, a very large majority of clinically apparent tumors are malignant.[37] Thyroid carcinomas are characterized by rapid growth, local invasion, and metastasis, and an advanced stage of tumor growth is frequently encountered at initial evaluation.

The most common presenting complaint is a palpable or visible neck mass.[7, 37] The mass may have been obvious for an extended period prior to examination. In one study of 13 dogs with thyroid carcinoma, the average period from when the mass was first noted by the owner until professional examination was sought was 6.8 months, with a range of one week to two years.[7]

Physical examination may reveal dyspnea due to compression of the trachea or from pulmonary metastases. Other physically detectable findings associated with malignant thyroid tumors include invasion into local soft tissues and spread to local and regional lymph nodes. Involvement of the skin and subcutaneous tissue, trachea, esophagus, muscle, neuromuscular structures, and parathyroid glands can occur (Fig. 144–8). If local invasion has occurred, the thyroid mass feels "fixed" in position and cannot be moved caudally down the trachea toward the thoracic inlet. This is not true of a thyroid adenoma, which remains freely mobile. In suspected thyroid tumor,

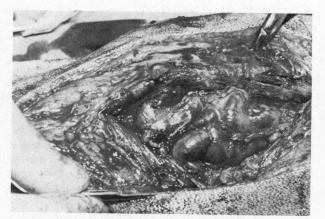

Figure 144–8. Surgical exploration of the region of the left thyroid gland in a dog, demonstrating thyroid adenocarcinoma.

a careful and complete neck palpation should be carried out from the angle of the mandible to the thoracic inlet.

Important clinical considerations for thyroid carcinomas include frequent occurrence of tumor emboli in the local draining veins and local lymph node involvement. Because of these features and the frequent occurrence of early pulmonary metastases, radiographic examination of the neck and thorax, in both lateral and ventrodorsal projections, should be performed. Other imaging techniques, available at referral centers, may include ultrasonography and thyroid scintigraphy. Ultrasonography is useful for determining the location and density of the tumor.[40] Morphological and functional studies useful for the diagnosis of both hypothyroid and hyperthyroid states can be obtained by thyroid scintigraphy, using sodium pertechnatate or ^{123}iodine.[6, 29]

Because dogs with thyroid carcinomas are variably hypothyroid, euthyroid, or hyperthyroid, every patient should be tested for T_3 and T_4 levels. Hyperthyroidism is present in about 20 per cent of cases and is often characterized by polydipsia, polyuria, and weight loss.[26, 37, 38] Definitive diagnosis is based on biopsy. Fine-needle biopsy may yield an adequate tissue specimen for cytological or histological diagnosis, but open exploration and biopsy is more definitive and safer because of better exposure.[32]

Parathyroid adenomas generally are not difficult to differentiate from thyroid carcinomas or adenomas, because they are smaller in size and noninvasive, and significant hypercalcemia is usually present.[20]

Pathology of Thyroid Tumors

Thyroid carcinomas are classified histologically as follicular, papillary, or compact.[21, 29, 33, 37, 38] Most carcinomas of the dog are mixed, having both follicular and compact elements.[21, 26, 33] Distinct papillary carcinomas are the most common human thyroid tumors but are rare in dogs. Medullary (C cell) and undifferentiated (anaplastic) carcinomas also have been reported, although less frequently.[24, 33] Local invasion is a postmortem finding in half, and metastatic disease in more than half, of dogs with thyroid carcinoma.[21] The lungs and local lymph nodes are the most common sites of metastasis; other sites include the adrenal glands, kidneys, liver, heart, and brain. The thyroid may also participate in the multiple endocrine neoplasia syndrome.[34] Metastasis of other primary neoplasms to the thyroid is uncommon despite the high blood supply of the gland.[11]

Therapeutic Techniques in Thyroid Neoplasia

Ideally, thyroid neoplasia is best treated by complete removal of all affected tissues. In thyroid adenoma, a total unilateral thyroparathyroidectomy is a curative and straightforward procedure. Following nerve identification and mobilization of the lobe by blunt manipulation, the local branches of the cranial thyroid artery are isolated and ligated for complete hemostasis. Surgical closure and recovery are routine. The results of surgery in animals with thyroid carcinoma have been variable. Tumor removal, if no local invasion or metastatic disease is evident, has been curative or has been associated with long-term remission of signs in some cases.[7, 37] Growth around or into the carotid sheath, the recurrent or caudal laryngeal nerves, or the epaxial musculature of the neck is difficult to manage and usually precludes further surgical manipulation. Similar findings may infrequently exist in association with other tumors, such as those of the carotid body.[10] In such instances, trial sectioning of the tumor mass or nodules down to a vital structure to expose the degree of invasion may help in deciding whether or not to abandon the operation. Radical unilateral *en bloc* excisions of the tumor and the carotid sheath may be successful in some instances if invasion is limited.[37]

If postoperative chemotherapy, such as with doxorubicin (Adriamycin),* or radiotherapy is anticipated, extensive tumor debulking consistent with the preservation of vital structures is an alternative method of treatment. Radiotherapy with [131]iodine and [60]cobalt has been used in the dog but is currently considered experimental.[27] Adjunctive therapy may include partial pharmacological suppression of autonomous tumor activity by administration of exogenous thyroid hormones. In functional hyperthyroidism associated with a malignant tumor, iodides or antithyroid drugs such as propylthiouracil may be considered to reduce signs of thyrotoxicosis.[29]

1. Belshaw, B. E., and Rijnberk, A.: Hypothyroidism. *In* Kirk, R. J. (ed.): *Current Veterinary Therapy VII: Small Animal Practice.* W. B. Saunders, Philadelphia, 1980.
2. Belshaw, B. E.: Thyroid diseases. *In* Ettinger, S. J. (ed.): *Textbook of Veterinary Internal Medicine.* 2nd ed. W. B. Saunders, Philadelphia, 1982.
3. Birchard, S. J.: Neoplasia of the thyroid gland in the dog: a retrospective study of 16 cases. J. Am. Anim. Hosp. Assoc. 17:369, 1981.
4. Booth, K. K., and Ghoshal, N. G.: Is there a caudal thyroid artery in the dog? Acta Anat. 99:183, 1977.
5. Booth, K. K., and Ghoshal, N. B.: Angioarchitecture of the canine thyroid gland. Anat. Anz. 145:32, 1979.
6. Branam, J. E., Leighton, R. L., and Hornof, W. J.: Radioisotope imaging for the evaluation of thyroid neoplasia and hypothyroidism in a dog. J. Am. Vet. Med. Assoc. 180:1077, 1982.
7. Brodey, R. S.: Thyroid neoplasms in the dog. Cancer 11:406, 1959.
8. Carillo, J. M., Burk, R. L., and Bode, C.: Primary hyperparathyroidism in a dog. J. Am. Vet. Med. Assoc. 174:67, 1979.
9. Chastain, C. B.: Canine hypothyroidism. J. Am. Vet. Med. Assoc. 181:349, 1982.
10. Cheville, N. F.: Ultrastructure of canine carotid body and aortic body tumors. Vet. Pathol. 9:166, 1972.
11. Czech, J. M., Lichtor, T. R., Carney, J. A., and Van Heerden, J. A.: Neoplasms metastatic to the thyroid gland. Surg. Gynecol. Obstet. 155:503, 1982.
12. Dial, P., and Hastings, P. R.: The use of selective beta-adrenergic receptor blockers for the preoperative preparation of thyrotoxic patients. Ann. Surg. 196:6:633, 1982.
13. Feely, J., Crooks, J., Forrest, A. L., et al.: Propranolol in the surgical treatment of hyperthyroidism, including severely thyrotoxic patients. Br. J. Surg. 68:12:865, 1981.
14. Gosselin, S. J., Capen, C. C., and Martin, S.: Histologic and ultrastructural evaluation of thyroid lesions associated with hypothyroidism in dogs. Vet. Pathol. 18:299, 1981.
15. Gosselin, S. J., Capen, C. C., Martin, S. L., and Krakowka, S: Autoimmune lymphocytic thyroiditis in dogs. Vet. Immunol. Immunopathol. 3:185, 1982.
16. Hayes, H. M., and Fraumeni, J. F.: Canine thyroid neoplasms: epidemiologic features. J.N.C.I. 55:931, 1975.
17. Haynes, R. C., and Murad, F.: Thyroid and antithyroid drugs. *In* Gilman, A. G., Goodman, L. S., and Gilman, A. (eds.): *Goodman and Gilman's The Pharmacological Basis of Therapeutics.* 6th ed. Macmillan, New York, 1980.
18. Holzworth, J., Theran, P., Carpenter, J. L., et al.: Hyperthyroidism in the cat: ten cases. J. Am. Vet. Med. Assoc. 176:345, 1980.
19. Hullinger, R. L.: The endocrine system. *In* Evans, H. E., and Christensen, G. C. (eds.): *Miller's Anatomy of the Dog.* W. B. Saunders, Philadelphia, 1979.
20. Langman, J.: *Medical Embryology.* Williams & Wilkins, Baltimore, 1975.
21. Leav, I., Schiller, A. I., Rijnberk, A., et al.: Adenomas and carcinomas of the canine and feline thyroid. Am. J. Pathol. 83:61, 1975.
22. Lee, T. C., Coffey, R. J., Currier, B. M., Ma, X., Canary, J. J.: Propranolol and thyroidectomy in the treatment of thyrotoxicosis. Ann. Surg. 195:6:766, 1982.
23. Legendre, A. M.: Primary hyperparathyroidism. *In* Kirk, R. J. (ed.): *Current Veterinary Therapy VII: Small Animal Practice.* W. B. Saunders, Philadelphia, 1980.
24. Long, G. C., Clemmons, R. M., and Heath, H.: Metastatic canine medullary thyroid carcinoma. Vet. Pathol. 17:323, 1980.
25. Lucke, V. M.: A histological study of thyroid abnormalities in the domestic cat. J. Small Anim. Pract. 5:351, 1964.
26. Madewell, B. R., and Mulnix, J. A.: Neoplasms of endocrine glands. Vet. Clin. North Am. 7:197, 1977.
27. McClure, R. C.: The cranial nerves. *In* Evans, H. E., and Christensen, G. C. (eds.): *Miller's Anatomy of the Dog.* W. B. Saunders, Philadelphia, 1979.
28. Milne, K. L., and Hayes, H. M.: Epidemiologic features of canine hypothyroidism. Cornell Vet. 71:3, 1981.
29. Mitchell, M., Hurov, L. I., and Troy, G. C.: Canine thyroid carcinomas: clinical occurrence and staging by means of scintiscans and therapy of 15 cases. Vet. Surg. 8:112, 1979.
30. Muir, W. J., and Bonagura, J.: Aprindine for the treatment of ventricular arrhythmias in the dog. Am. J. Vet. Res. 43:1815, 1982.
31. Nesbitt, G. H., Izzo, J., Peterson, L., and Wilkins, R. J.: Canine hypothyroidism: a retrospective study of 108 cases. J. Am. Vet. Med. Assoc. 177:1117, 1980.
32. Norton, L. W., Wagensteen, S. L., Davis, J. R., et al.: Utility of thyroid aspiration biopsy. Surgery 92:700, 1982.
33. Patnaik, A. K., Lieberman, P. H., Erlandson, R. A., et al.: Canine medullary carcinoma of the thyroid. Vet. Pathol. 15:590, 1978.
34. Peterson, M. E., Randolph, J. F., Zaki, F. A., and Heath, H.: Multiple endocrine neoplasia in a dog. J. Am. Vet. Med. Assoc. 180:1476, 1982.
35. Peterson, M. E., et al.: Feline hyperthyroidism: Pretreatment clinical and laboratory evaluation of 131 cases. J. Am. Vet. Med. Assoc. 183:103, 1983.
36. Peterson, M. E., Keene, B., Ferguson, D. C., and Pipers, F. S.: Electrocardiographic findings in 45 cats with hyperthyroidism. J. Am. Vet. Med. Assoc. 180:934, 1982.
37. Rijnberk, A., and Leav, I.: Thyroid tumors. *In* Kirk, R. J.

*Adria Laboratories, Wilmington, DE.

(ed.): *Current Veterinary Therapy VI: Small Animal Practice*. W. B. Saunders, Philadelphia, 1977.

38. Susaneck, S. J.: Thyroid tumors in the dog. Comp. Cont. Ed. 5:35, 1983.

39. Theran, P., and Holzworth, J.: Feline hyperthyroidism. *In*

Kirk, R. J. (ed.): *Current Veterinary Therapy VII: Small Animal Practice*. W. B. Saunders, Philadelphia, 1980.

40. Van Heerden, J. A., James, E. M., Karsell, P. R., et al.: Small part ultrasonography in primary hyperparathyroidism: initial experience. Ann. Surg. *195*:774, 1982.

Chapter **145**

The Parathyroid

Teresa Nesbitt, Stephen W. Crane, and Michael Aronsohn

ANATOMY

The anatomy of the parathyroid glands is described in Chapter 144.

PHYSIOLOGY OF CALCIUM-PHOSPHORUS HOMEOSTASIS

Parathyroid hormone (parathormone, PTH), calcitonin, and dihydroxycholecalciferol are the principal hormones involved in the homeostasis of calcium, phosphate, pyrophosphate, citrate and magnesium metabolism. These hormones also have a major regulatory role in bone homeostasis.

Calcium is the predominant cation in the body, with about 99 per cent captured in the hydroxyapatite crystals of the skeletal system.[49] The total serum calcium of mammals is approximately 10 mg/dl and is composed of protein-bound and diffusible fractions. Diffusible calcium consists of calcium bound to anions such as phosphate and citrate, plus the biologically active "free" (ionized) calcium. The amount of ionized calcium in the serum is accurately maintained despite an enormous reservoir of calcium in the skeleton and wide fluctuations in intake and excretion. Although the concentration of calcium in the body fluids is low, ionized calcium is critically maintained for neuromuscular excitability, membrane permeability, enzyme activity, blood clotting, and assistance in acid-base balance.

Elemental phosphorus is highly toxic and is present in the body only as organic or inorganic phosphates. Although 85 per cent of phosphate is in the skeleton, the phosphate radical is present in every cell and is important in many biochemical processes.[49]

Precise endocrine control mechanisms of calcium-phosphorus metabolism involve the balanced interactions of three primary hormones: parathyroid hormone, vitamin D, and calcitonin. The first two hormones are major control mechanisms, calcitonin being relatively less important. All three hormones are responsible for the regulation of calcium and phosphorus metabolism through their action on kidney, bone, and intestine, with the result that serum calcium is precisely maintained within narrow limits. Secondary hormones such as adrenal corticosteroids, reproductive steroids, thyroxine, somatotropin, and glucagon also contribute directly or indirectly to the maintenance of calcium homeostasis.

Parathyroid hormone is synthesized in the chief cells of the parathyroid gland from precursor and proparathyroid hormone intermediates.[21] Biologically active PTH is a straight-chain polypeptide consisting of 84 amino acid residues. Molecular fragments (carboxy- and amino-terminal) of PTH create immuno-heterogeneity, which causes significant problems in the development and application of highly specific radioimmunoassays for its measurement in serum. Studies with the native hormone and synthetic fragments have demonstrated that the amino-terminal region of the molecule contains the structural component required for biological activity.[48]

Control of Parathyroid Hormone Secretion

Small amounts of active PTH stored in the parathyroid glands allow a quick response to fluctuations in calcium concentration through rapid alteration in secretion rates.[38] Alteration of the rate of PTH synthesis is another mechanism of response to varying calcium concentration, but it occurs more slowly.[40] The concentration of ionized calcium in the extracellular fluid is the principal factor that controls the secretion of PTH from the parathyroid gland.[41] Experimentally, infusion of calcium results in reduction of the circulating level of immunoreactive parathyroid hormone (iPTH). Conversely, if the calcium level is lowered, there is substantial increase in the iPTH level.[7] There is no direct effect on the synthesis and secretion of PTH by serum phosphorus. Elevated serum phosphorus may indirectly stimulate PTH release, through the lowering of the serum calcium level, according to the law of mass-action, when the

HORMONAL RESPONSE TO LOW BLOOD CALCIUM

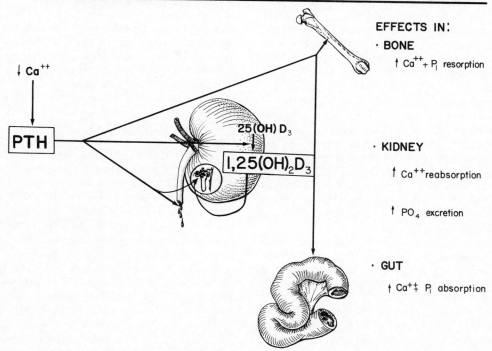

Figure 145–1. Homeostatic mechanisms that control blood calcium levels through the actions of parathyroid hormone.

serum is saturated with respect to these two ions.[29] Magnesium affects parathyroid hormone secretion as calcium does, but with lesser magnitude.[35]

Parathyroid hormone is the principal hormone involved in regulation of serum calcium, primarily through its actions on target cells in bone, kidney, and intestine (Fig. 145–1). In bone, calcium is mobilized from crystalline skeletal depots into extracellular fluids by the interaction of PTH with osteoclasts and osteocytes. This response of bone to PTH is biphasic.[37] First, there is increased activity of existing osteoclasts and osteocytes, which promotes movement of calcium from bone fluids to the extracellular fluid. Longer-term effects of PTH on bone are potentially greater and result from osteoclastic bone resorption and bone remodelling. Chronic elevation of PTH secretion may also result in increased numbers of osteoblasts, causing increased bone formation. There is a net negative skeletal balance because bone resorption is greater than bone formation. Parathyroid hormone inhibits phosphate transport in the proximal renal tubules[27] and produces phosphaturia. PTH also directly enhances renal reabsorption of calcium in the distal convoluted tubules.

The other major renal effect of PTH is on vitamin D metabolism. PTH regulates the rate of synthesis of 1,25-dihydroxycholecalciferol, the principal metabolically active form of vitamin D. This vitamin D metabolite sensitizes bone to the direct effects of PTH and greatly enhances gastrointestinal absorption of calcium. These two mechanisms amplify the effect of PTH on serum calcium.[39]

Calcitonin

Calcitonin (CT) is a major calcium-regulating factor because it lowers serum calcium and phosphate levels.[4] Thus, along with PTH and vitamin D, CT secretion forms a system of dual negative feedback loops for the precise control of calcium-phosphorus levels.[11] Calcitonin is secreted by the parafollicular (C) cells of the mammalian thyroid gland as a polypeptide hormone composed of 32 amino acid residues with one to seven disulfide linkages. The complete sequence of 32 amino acids and the disulfide bond are essential for full activity.[11] In experiments in which the thyroid and parathyroid glands were perfused with high-calcium blood, there was a prompt fall in systemic serum calcium that could not be explained on the basis of suppressed parathormone, because the effect was significantly different from that of total parathyroidectomy.[12] These and subsequent experiments led to the hypothesis that a hypocalcemic hormone was secreted by the parathyroid-thyroid complex in response to hypercalcemia.

The concentration of calcium ion in serum is the principal stimulus for the secretion of CT by C cells, and large amounts of preformed CT are stored in C cells and released in response to an elevation in serum calcium.[11] It is also released after a high-calcium meal, even before significant elevations in serum calcium levels can be detected. The cause of this increase in CT secretion may be due to a small undetectable rise in serum ionized calcium or to direct stimulation of certain gastrointestinal hormones.[10] Gastrin, pancreozymin, and glucagon all stimulate CT release.[8] Thus, the gastrointestinal hormones may be important in triggering the early release of CT to prevent hypercalcemia following ingestion of a high-calcium meal.[20] CT exerts both hypocalcemic and hypophosphatemic effects,[41] which are exerted primarily through the interactions of target cells in bone, kidney, and, to a lesser extent, intestine. The hypocalcemic effects of CT primarily are the result of a temporary inhibition of PTH-stimulated bone resorption.[1] The hypophosphatemia develops from a direct action of CT, increasing the rate of movement of phosphate out of plasma into soft tissue and bone, and from an inhibition of bone resorption.[44] In addition, CT decreases renal tubular reabsorption of phosphate, both in the ascending limb of the loop of Henle and in the distal convoluted tubule, leading to phosphaturia.[7]

PTH is the major factor in the regulation of serum calcium under normal conditions, since most mammalian diets are low in calcium and high in phosphorus. Calcitonin functions as an "emergency" hormone to prevent hypercalcemia during the postprandial absorption of calcium. Although calcitonin acts as an antihypercalcemic agent, hypercalcemia due to primary or secondary hyperparathyroidism, pseudohyperparathyroidism or other internal disorders is usually not prevented by calcitonin.[46]

Vitamin D

Cholecalciferol, or vitamin D, is an important factor in mineral and skeletal homeostasis. Cholecalciferol became an essential trace dietary constituent and therefore by definition a vitamin, only because of human predilection for clothing, industrial air pollution, and indoor activities which reduce exposure to ultraviolet (UV) radiation.[36] When adequate amounts of UV radiation are present, the epidermal cutaneous reservoir of the provitamin, 7-dehydrocholesterol, which is largely present in the Malpighii layer, is readily converted into vitamin D by an endogenous endocrine mechanism (Fig. 145–2).[36] This conversion obviates the necessity for a dietary source of vitamin D and explains the logic of studying its mode of action as a steroid. Vitamin D may be similar to the classic steroid hormones, e.g., aldosterone, testosterone, estrogen, hydrocortisone, and ecdysterone. The current concept of the mechanism of action of steroid hormones is that their cellular effects depend on interaction with the genome to induce biosynthesis of specific proteins.[2]

Initially, vitamin D must be metabolically activated, and it exerts its biological responses as a consequence of its further metabolism to more polar metabolites (see Fig. 145–2).[7, 13, 36] First, the parent molecule is transported by alpha globulins from the gut or skin to the liver, where it is hydroxylated to 25-hydroxycholecalciferol.[36] This first metabolite of cholecalciferol—25(OH)D—is transported to the kid-

ney where it undergoes transformation to the most biologically active form of vitamin D, 1,25 dihydroxycholecalciferol—$1,25(OH)_2D$.[22, 24] This reaction is catalyzed by 25-hydroxycholecalciferol-1-alpha-hydroxylase, which is present in the mitochondrial fraction of the renal cortex.[6, 33] The conversion of hydroxylated to dihydroxylated vitamin D is the rate-limiting step in the metabolic pathway and the primary reason for the delay between vitamin D administration and the expression of its effects.[19] The renal conversion to the 1,25-dihydroxylated vitamin D is complex and is regulated by several factors, including PTH, phosphate, and the quantity of $1,25(OH)_2D$ hormone. Parathyroid hormone determines $1,25(OH)_2D$ production in response to low dietary calcium availability. Conversely, low serum phosphate is a potent stimulus for active vitamin D production independent of PTH. Suppression of the renal enzyme conversion occurs with high levels of serum phosphate, calcium, vitamin D, and 1,25-$(OH)_2D$.[23] Apart from dietary factors such as calcium, phosphorus, and vitamin D deprivation, growth, pregnancy, and lactation enhance $1,25(OH)_2D$ production. Hormones that increase the production of active metabolites include prolactin, estradiol, placental lactogen, and, possibly, somatotropin.[32]

A second dihydroxylated metabolite, $24,25(OH)_2D$, may also play an important role in mediating biological responses of vitamin D. Twenty chemically characterized metabolites of vitamin D are known to be enzymatically hydroxylated in the kidney.[36]

Effects of Vitamin D

The major target tissue for $1,25(OH)_2D$ is the mucosa of the small intestine, where it increases both calcium and phosphorus absorption. After association of the active vitamin D hormone with its cytoplasmic receptor in target cells, the steroid-receptor complex becomes associated with the chromatin in the nucleus.[36] This association results in the synthesis of messenger RNA coding for the synthesis of calcium-binding proteins. Induction of these proteins alters cell function and enhances calcium and phosphate absorption from the intestinal lumen. The absorptive capacity of the intestine for calcium is a direct function of the amount of calcium-binding protein present.[50]

Other tissues in which the mechanism of $1,25(OH)_2D$ have been studied include bone, kidney, and parathyroid gland. In young animals, vitamin D is required for the orderly growth and mineralization of cartilage in the growth plate. Young animals fed diets deficient in vitamin D or without exposure to ultraviolet light may develop rickets, as a result of a failure of mineralization of osteoid on bone surfaces and at the growth plates.[7] Vitamin D is also necessary to permit osteolytic cells to respond to PTH (a "permissive effect") for osteoclastic resorption and calcium mobilization from bone. This latter effect is of obvious importance in calcium homeostasis. Much

VITAMIN D ENDOCRINE SYSTEM

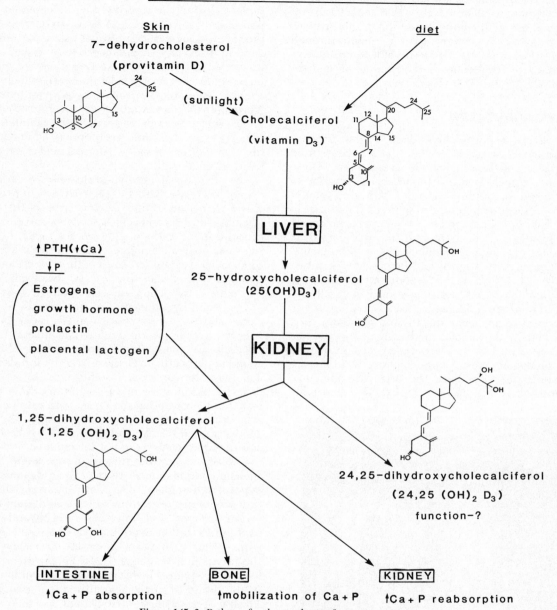

Figure 145–2. Pathway for the synthesis of active vitamin D.

less is known about the renal functions of vitamin D and its active metabolites. It stimulates the retention of calcium by increasing renal tubular absorption.[43] The role of $1,25(OH)_2D$ in the parathyroid gland is controversial, but cytoplasmic receptors for this hormone have been demonstrated. It may assist calcium in the feedback system for PTH secretion or synthesis.[23]

Calcium is absorbed largely from the upper part of the small intestine, and factors that hasten the passage of intestinal contents through this part of the tract reduce the amount of calcium that can be absorbed. The presence of alkali, excess fat, or a high

calcium to phosphate ratio in the diet makes calcium absorption difficult and may raise the requirement for $1,25(OH)_2D$. Because hydrochloric acid has a solubilizing effect on dietary calcium, the efficiency of calcium absorption may also be influenced by the reservoir function of the stomach and its frequency of emptying. Gastrectomy of puppies leads to skeletal deformities similar to those of rickets, which become apparent as the animal ages.[49] The achlorhydria after gastrectomy interferes with the absorption of calcium from the upper intestine. In the absence of a stomach, incompletely digested food passes so rapidly along the intestine that insufficient amounts of calcium and phosphorus are absorbed. On the other hand, an excess of dietary phosphate has no striking effect on the absorption of calcium; factors that reduce calcium absorption generally impede phosphate absorption. There is practically no movement of calcium through the intestinal mucosa of parathyroidectomized animals, because PTH controls the production and secretion of $1,25(OH)_2D$ by the kidney.

HYPERPARATHYROIDISM

In primary hyperparathyroidism, excess parathyroid hormone is produced because of parathyroid hyperplasia, adenoma, or adenocarcinoma. These conditions usually respond to surgical extirpation of the affected parathyroid glands. The surgical approach to the parathyroid glands is similar to that to the thyroid (see Chapter 144). When primary hyperparathyroidism is encountered in middle-aged to older dogs, it is more commonly the result of a chief cell adenoma of the parathyroid gland that is secreting excessive PTH.[8a, 17, 30a, 37b, 50a] Adenocarcinomas of the parathyroid gland are extremely rare in small animals.[37a] Parathyroid adenomas usually are located in the cervical region near the thyroid gland but may be present in the cranial mediastinum or near the heart base (Fig. 145–3). These tumors are uncommon in companion animals. A large majority of tumors are confined to one gland, and the larger the adenoma, the more likely it is to be ectopic.[47] Elevated para-

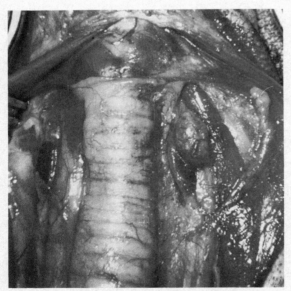

Figure 145–3. A parathyroid cleft adenoma in a 10-year-old spayed keeshond. Clinical signs included polydipsia and occasional vomiting associated with serum calcium level of 16.1 mg/dl and a serum creatinine level of 5.2 mg/dl. Radiographs of the skull and mandible showed generalized loss of bone density with destruction of the lamina dura. Following excision of the tumor, the dog developed postoperative hypocalcemia (6.2 mg/dl), which was treated successfully with intravenous calcium gluconate. At the time of writing, the dog had been maintained for six months on oral calcium lactate, her general clinical state was good, but the serum creatinine level was still elevated (3.7 mg/dl) and she continued to show polyuria and polydipsia.

thyroid hormone production causes increased bone resorption, decreased bone formation, fibrous tissue replacement of the resorbed bone, decreased serum phosphorus, increased 1,25-dihydroxycholecalciferol production, increased intestinal calcium absorption, and, in the early stages, decreased renal calcium excretion. The effect of these alterations is a dramatic increase in the serum calcium level, which is the clinical hallmark of primary hyperparathyroidism. Normally, the increased serum calcium would both inhibit PTH secretion and stimulate calcitonin secretion. Because hormone secretion is autonomous in this case, neither of the two normal negative feedback loops is functional.[3]

The clinical signs of hypercalcemia are varied and do not correlate with the degree of serum calcium elevation because other factors, such as the rate of calcium elevation and acid-base status and electrolyte concentrations, influence the clinical signs.[14] Clinical signs of hypercalcemia are related to decreased neuromuscular excitability. In smooth muscle, decreased excitability may lead to anorexia, dysphagia, vomiting, and constipation, and in skeletal muscle, to asthenia and hypotonicity. In cardiac muscle, bradycardia and, in severe cases, ventricular arrhythmias may occur.[5] Long-term nephrotoxic effects of hypercalcemia are potentially life-threatening. Hypercalcemic nephropathy is characterized by tubular injury and may lead to renal insufficiency. Injury to the distal nephron impairs the countercurrent mechanism for concentrating the urine, with resultant polyuria and polydypsia.[31] With prolonged hypercalcemia, azotemia may develop, and nephrolithiasis and nephrocalcinosis are not uncommon.

Unfortunately, the results of no single test or specific combination of tests are pathognomonic for hyperparathyroidism. The most important and practical laboratory test is the serial quantitation of total serum calcium. Calcium values consistently above 11.5 to 12 mg/dl in an adult dog are elevated. Animals with primary hyperparathyroidism usually have serum calcium levels of 12 to 20 mg/dl or more.[7] Serum phosphorus levels may be normal or low owing to inhibition of renal reabsorption of phosphorus. Alkaline phosphatase activity may be increased in animals with overt bone disease. Diagnostic alternatives include secondary hyperparathyroidism due to end-stage renal disease, pseudohyperparathyroidism, dietary imbalance of Ca to P (e.g., organ meat diets), hypervitaminosis D, and laboratory error.

Characteristic radiographic findings include generalized decrease in bone density, subperiosteal bone resorption, bone cysts, and loss of the dental lamina dura (Fig. 145–4). In advanced cases, pathological skeletal fractures, soft tissue mineralization, and nephrolithiasis may be present. Although primary hyperparathyroidism can be tentatively diagnosed on the basis of clinical signs and serum calcium levels, the definitive diagnosis depends upon histological confirmation. The serum PTH level, obtained by radioimmunoassay or perferably by bioassay, aids

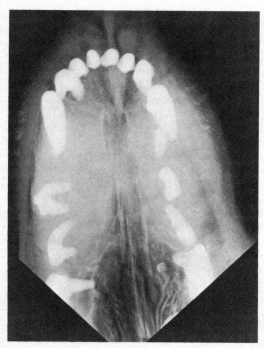

Figure 145–4. Chronic primary hyperparathyroidism in this 12-year-old Scottish terrier (serum Ca 16 mg/dl) resulted in nearly total resorption of the *lamina dura dentes* and hyperostotic replacement of the maxillofacial bones with fibrous connective tissue. A ventrodorsal open-mouthed view is presented. Rostral is up.

early diagnosis of hyperparathyroidism in humans. The measurement of renal cyclic AMP also is useful in the differential diagnosis of calcium disorders in humans.[15, 17] Renal cyclic AMP levels may better reflect functional PTH activity than radioimmunoassay of PTH, because of the carboxy- and amino-terminal fragments of PTH that circulate, resulting in immunochemical heterogeneity.[15]

PSEUDOHYPERPARATHYROIDISM

Pseudohyperparathyroidism occurs when a non-parathyroid tumor secretes a parathormone-like substance. Pseudohyperparathyroidism usually is associated with a malignant tumor unassociated with bony metastasis. This syndrome is frequently part of a paraneoplastic syndrome and is a more common cause of hypercalcemia in the dog than all other causes combined. Neoplasms that elaborate parathormone-like substances in dogs include lymphosarcoma, apocrine gland adenocarcinoma of the anal sac, and mammary adenocarcinoma.[5] In cats, the disorder has been reported secondary to thymic lymphoma and to a myeloproliferative disease associated with feline leukemia virus infection.[9] About 10 per cent of dogs with lymphosarcoma have concurrent hypercalcemia.[31] The nature of the hypercalcemic humoral factors that tumors secrete has been investigated. These chemical factors include prostaglandin E_2, osteoclast-activating factor (OAF), parathyroid hormone

of ectopic origin, parathyrotrophic factor, and other hypercalcemic agents such as osteolytic sterols and vitamin D metabolites.[43, 51] A parathormone-like polypeptide has been isolated in humans.[9] Elevations in serum calcium and alkaline phosphatase and decreases in serum phosphorus are in ranges similar to those in primary hyperparathyroidism. Accordingly, the preoperative work-up for a patient with a suspected tumor should include serum calcium. Conversely, hypercalcemia in the dog and cat together with nonspecific signs of polydypsia-polyuria, vomiting, and weakness requires an extensive evaluation of malignancy.[31] Differentiation between primary hyperparathyroidism and pseudohyperparathyroidism is difficult in the absence of gross neoplasia.

HYPOPARATHYROIDISM

Primary hypoparathyroidism results in a decreased concentration of circulating PTH and probably has an autoimmune basis.[7, 41, 43] Although attempts to detect circulating antibodies against parathyroid tissue in the dog have been unsuccessful, the morphological changes of canine hypoparathyroidism suggest an autoimmune pathogenesis. Furthermore, lymphocytic parathyroiditis has been produced experimentally in dogs by repeated injections of parathyroid tissue emulsions.[30] In puppies, agenesis of both pairs of parathyroid glands is a rare cause of congenital hypoparathyroidism.[7] Pseudohypoparathyroidism is another clinically recognized disorder in which a lack of end-organ responsiveness to parathyroid hormone exists in bone and kidney. Neither endogenous nor exogenous parathyroid hormone administration engenders a response in these situations.[15, 28]

Hypoparathyroid patients are unable to mobilize calcium from their bone fluid compartment to support plasma calcium levels, and because the production of 1,25-dihydroxycholecalciferol is PTH-dependent, there is a decreased capacity for intestinal calcium absorption.[13] In addition, a lack of PTH leads to hyperphosphatemia owing to increased renal tubular reabsorption of phosphorus. The clinical manifestations of hypoparathyroidism are due to a decreased serum calcium concentration, which increases the nerve membrane permeability to sodium, leading to hyperexcitability and spontaneous nerve action potentials. Total serum calcium levels decrease to 4 to 6 mg/dl, and hyperphosphatemia is present. Restlessness, muscle fasciculation, and tonic-clonic convulsions occur when the serum ionized calcium is less than 2.5 mg/dl.[28] Myocardial effects of hypocalcemia include decreased force of contraction and, in severe cases, bradycardia.

Management of Postoperative Hypoparathyroidism

Iatrogenic injury or intentional removal of parathyroid tissue during thyroid surgery (see Chapter 144) is the most common cause of hypoparathyroidism. When both lobes of the thyroid gland must be removed, every effort should be made to spare one or both of the external parathyroid glands together with their blood supply. Fortunately, functional ectopic parathyroid tissue is frequently present.[25, 26]

Following successful parathyroidectomy for primary hyperparathyroidism, the serum calcium level should return to normal within 18 to 36 hours,[16] but it may fall below normal in some patients. Profound hypocalcemia is more likely to occur in patients with severe skeletal demineralization,[18] owing to the strong affinity of the depleted skeleton for the available circulating calcium ("bone hunger syndrome").[16] Early postoperative management after thyroparathyroidectomy should include frequent determination of serum calcium levels. Hypocalcemia secondary to parathyroidectomy usually occurs within one to five days after surgery. The postoperative signs are determined both by the rate of fall and by the absolute level of ionized calcium in the serum. Acute hypoparathyroid tetany is a medical emergency, and management of chronic hypoparathyroidism requires frequent reevaluation and adjustment of therapy.[34] Parathyroidectomized animals should be observed continuously during the early and intermediate postoperative periods.

The principal aim of postoperative medical therapy in treating acute hypoparathyroidism is to restore and maintain normal serum concentrations of ionized calcium. Although treatment must be individualized, some generalizations can be made. An acute hypocalcemic crisis can be relieved by the intravenous administration of 10 per cent calcium gluconate,* 0.5 to 1.5 ml/kg body weight, not to exceed 10 ml.[28] It is added to 5 per cent dextrose and the mixture is administered by a slow drip over 15 to 30 minutes. Cardiac monitoring is performed by auscultation or electrocardiogram, and the calcium therapy is discontinued if abnormalities such as bradycardia or heart block develop.

Long-term maintenance of serum calcium in the absence of PTH secretion should be attempted by feeding diets high in calcium, low in phosphorus, and supplemented with calcium and vitamin D.[7, 33] Calcium lactate tablets† or a calcium elixir‡ can be used at dosages of 300 to 600 mg calcium/day.[28] A variety of forms of vitamin D are available for therapy. Because the renal production of 1,25-dihydroxycholecalciferol is PTH-dependent, pharmacological amounts of vitamin D must be given unless a biologically active metabolite is used. Vitamin D dosage is adjusted frequently by determining the serum calcium level, in order to preclude hypervitaminosis D with its sequelae of hypercalcemia and soft tissue mineralization. Unfortunately, the amount of vitamin D necessary to correct hypocalcemia is unpredict-

able, and fluctuations in serum calcium may occur even though treatment remains unchanged. Because the full effect of vitamin D is slow in onset, several weeks may elapse before the action of a particular dose is established or the effects of overdosage can be reversed.[42] Treatment with vitamin D_3§, 25,000 to 50,000 IU/day, has been recommended.[7] Alternatively, vitamin D_2, ‖ at dosages of 12,500 to 25,000 IU/day, may be used in dogs.[7, 28] Dihydrotachysterol** has the advantage that it is more rapidly converted to an active metabolite than either vitamin D_2 or vitamin D_3. After hydroxylation by the liver, dihydrotachysterol does not require further PTH-dependent renal hydroxylation. A dosage of 0.01 mg/kg/day has been recommended.[28] A synthetic form of the active metabolite, 1,25-dihydroxycholecalciferol,†† is the most potent form of vitamin D available. This compound has been used in humans and dogs, but a treatment regimen in dogs has not yet been established. It is important to recognize the potential difficulty in the maintenance therapy of chronic hypoparathyroidism, because the difference between the controlling and intoxicating doses of vitamin D may be small. Serum calcium levels should be determined frequently.

Replacement therapy with PTH is expensive and ineffective on a long-term basis because of the development of anti-PTH antibodies; however, the use of synthetic PTH is a prospect for the future.[42] In addition to vitamin D and calcium supplementation, the use of aluminum hydroxide may be indicated to bind phosphorus in the gut and to increase fecal phosphorus losses.

1. Aliapaulios, M. A., Goldhabner, P., and Munson, P. L.: Thyrocalcitonin inhibition of bone resorption induced by parathyroid hormone in tissue culture. Science 151:330, 1966.
2. Armbrecht, H. J., Zenser, T. V., and Davis, B. B.: Conversion of 25-hydroxyvitamin D_3 to 1,25-dihydroxyvitamin D_3 and 24,25-dihydroxyvitamin D_3 in renal slices from the rat. Endocrinology 109:218, 1981.
3. Arnaud, C. D.: Calcium homeostasis: regulatory elements and their integration. Fed. Proc. 37:2557, 1978.
4. Austin, L. A., and Heath, H.: Calcitonin: physiology and pathophysiology. N. Engl. J. Med. 304:269, 1982.
5. Blank, R. E.: Differential diagnosis of hypercalcemia in dogs. Comp. Cont. Ed. 1:220, 1979.
6. Brunette, M. G., Chan, M., Ferriere, C., and Roberts, K. D.: Site of 1,25(OH)$_2$ vitamin D3 synthesis in the kidney. Nature 276:287, 1978.
7. Capen, C. C., and Martin, S. L.: Calcium regulating hormones and diseases of the parathyroid glands. In Ettinger, S. J. (ed.): Textbook of Veterinary Internal Medicine. W. B. Saunders, Philadelphia, 1983.
8. Care, A. D., Bates, R. F., Phillippo, M., et al.: Stimulation

---

*Calcium gluconate, The Upjohn Co., Kalamazoo, MI 49001.
†Calcium lactate, Parke-Davis, Morris Plains, NJ 07950.
‡Neo Calglucon, Dorsey Laboratories, Lincoln, NB 68501.

§Vitamin D_3 solution, Grand Island Biological Co., Grand Island, NY 14072.
‖ Calciferol, Kremers-Urban Co., Milwaukee, WI 53201.
**Dihydrotachysterol, Philips Roxane Laboratories, Inc., Columbus, OH 43216.
††Rocaltrol, Hoffmann–La Roche Laboratories, Nutley, NJ 07110.

of calcitonin release from bovine thyroid by calcium and glucagon. J. Endocrinol. 48:667, 1970.

8a. Carillo, J. M., Burk, R. L., and Bode, C.: Prmary hyperparathyroidism in a dog.

9. Chew, D. J., Schaer, M., Liu, S., and Owens, J.: Pseudohyperparathyroidism in a cat. J.A.A.H.A. 11:46, 1975.

10. Cooper, C. W., Schwesinger, W. H., Ontjes, D. A., et al.: Stimulation of secretion of pig thyrocalcitonin by gastrin and related hormonal peptides. Endocrinology 91:1079, 1972.

11. Copp, D. H.: Endocrine regulation of calcium metabolism. Ann. Rev. Physiol. 32:61, 1970.

12. Copp, D. H., Cameron, E. C., Cheney, B. A., et al.: Evidence for calcitonin—a new hormone from the parathyroid that lowers blood calcium. Endocrinology 70:638, 1962.

13. DeLuca, H. F.: The kidney as an endocrine organ for the production of 1,25-dihydroxyvitamin D_3, a calcium mobilizing hormone. N. Engl. J. Med. 289:359, 1973.

14. Drazner, F. H.: Hypercalcemia in the dog and cat. J. Am. Vet. Med. Assoc. 178:1252, 1981.

15. Drezner, M. K., Neelon, F. A., Curtis, H. B., and Lebovitz, H. E.: Renal cyclic adenosine monophosphate: an accurate index of parathyroid function. Metabolism 25:1103, 1976.

16. Edis, A. J., Ayala, L. A., and Egdahl, R. H.: Manual of endocrine surgery. Springer-Verlag, New York, 1975.

17. Feldman, E. C., and Krutzik, S.: Case reports of parathyroid levels in spontaneous canine parathyroid disorders. J. Am. Anim. Hosp. Assoc. 17:393, 1981.

18. Friesen, S. R., and Bolinger, R. E.: Surgical Endocrinology: Clinical Syndromes. J. B. Lippincott, Philadephia, 1978.

19. Gray, R. W., Omdahl, J. L., Ghazarian, J. G., and DeLuca, H. F.: 25-Hydroxycholecalciferol-1-hydroxylase: subcellular location and properties. J. Biol. Chem. 247:7528, 1972.

20. Gray, T. K., and Ontjes, D. A.: Clinical aspects of thyrocalcitonin. Clin. Orthop. 111:238, 1975.

21. Habner, J. F., and Kronenberg, A. M.: Parathyroid hormone biosynthesis: structure and function of biosynthetic precursors. Fed. Proc. 37:2561, 1978.

22. Haussler, M. R., Boyce, D. W., Littledike, E. T., and Rasmussen, H.: A rapidly acting metabolite of vitamin D_3. Proc. Natl. Acad. Sci. 68:177, 1971.

23. Haussler, M. R., and McCain, T. A.: Basic and clinical concepts related to vitamin D metabolism and action. N. Engl. J. Med. 297:974, 1977.

24. Holick, M. F., and Clark, M. B.: The photobiogenesis and metabolism of vitamin D. Fed. Proc. 37:2567, 1978.

25. Holzworth, J., Theran, P., Carpenter, J. L., et al.: Hyperthyroidism in the cat: ten cases. J. Am. Vet. Med. Assoc. 176:345, 1980.

26. Hullinger, R. L.: The endocrine system. In Evans, H. E., and Christensen, G. C. (eds.): Miller's Anatomy of the Dog. W. B. Saunders, Philadelphia, 1979.

27. Kimura, S., Yamamoto, M., Itakura, M., et al.: Paradoxical response to parathyroid hormone or renal handling of phosphate in hyperthyroid rats. Endocrinology 111:1666, 1982.

28. Kornegay, J. N.: Hypocalcemia in dogs. Comp. Cont. Ed. 4:103, 1982.

29. Krook, L., and Lowe, J. E.: Nutritional secondary hyperparathyroidism in the horse with a description of the normal equine parathyroid gland. Pathol. Vet. 1(Suppl 1):1, 1964.

30. Lapelescu, A., Potorac, E., Pop, A., et al.: Experimental investigation on immunology of the parathyroid gland. Immunology 14:475, 1968.

30a. Legendre, A. M., Merkley, D. F., Carrig, C. B., and Krehbiel, J. D.: Primary hyperparathyroidism in a dog. J. Am. Vet. Med. Assoc. 168:694, 1976.

31. MacEwen, E. G. and Siegel, S. D.: Hypercalcemia: a paraneoplastic disease. Vet. Clin. North Am. 7:187, 1977.

32. MacIntyre, I., Colston, K. W., Szelke, M., and Spanos, E.: A survey of the hormonal factors that control calcium metabolism. Ann. N.Y. Acad. Sci. 307:345, 1973.

33. Midgett, R. J., Spielvogel, A. M., Coburn, J. W., and Norman, A. W.: Studies on calciferol metabolism. VI. The renal production of the biologically active form of vitamin D, 1,25-dihydroxycholecalciferol; species, tissue and subcellular distribution. J. Clin. Endocrinol. Metab. 36:1153, 1973.

34. Meyer, D. J.: Primary hypoparathyroidism. In Kirk, R. J. (ed.): Current Veterinary Therapy VII. W. B. Saunders, Philadelphia, 1980.

35. Morrissey, J. J., and Cohn, D. V.: The effects of calcium and magnesium on the secretion of parathormone and parathyroid secretory protein by isolated porcine parathyroid cells. Endocrinology 103:2081, 1978.

36. Norman, A. W., Roth, J., and Orci, L.: The vitamin D endocrine system: steroid metabolism hormone receptors, and biological response (calcium binding proteins). Endocr. Rev. 3:331, 1982.

37. Parsons, J. A., and Robinson, C. J.: Calcium shift into bone causing transient hypocalcemia after injection of parathyroid hormone. Nature 230:581, 1971.

37a. Patnaik, A. K., MacEwan, E. G., Erlandson, R. A., et al.: Mediastinal parathyroid adenocarcinoma in a dog. Vet. Pathol. 15:55, 1978.

37b. Pearson, P. T., Dellman, H-D., Berrier, H. H., et al.: Primary hyperparathyroidism in a beagle. J. Am. Vet. Med. Assoc. 147:1201, 1965.

38. Potts, J. T., Jr., Murray, T. M., Peacock, M., et al.: Parathyroid hormone: Sequence synthesis, immunoassay studies. Am. J. Med. 50:639, 1971.

39. Rasmussen, H., and Bordier, P.: The physiological and cellular basis of metabolic bone disease. Williams & Wilkins, Baltimore, 1974.

40. Roth, S. I.,and Raisz, L. G.: Effect of calcium concentration on the ultrastructure of rat parathyroid in organ culture. Lab. Invest. 13:331, 1964.

41. Rothstein, M., Morrissey, J., Slatopolsky, E., and Klahr, S.: The role of Na^+-Ca^{++} exchange in parathyroid hormone secretion. Endocrinology 111:225, 1982.

42. Sherding, R. G., Meuten, D. J., Chew, D. J., et al.: Primary hypoparathyroidism in the dog. J. Am. Vet. Med. Assoc. 176:439, 1980.

43. Singer, F. R., Sharp, C. F., and Rude, R. K.: Pathogenesis of hypercalcemia in malignancy. Mineral Electrolyte Metab. 2:161, 1979.

44. Stumpf, W. E., Sar, M., Reid, F. A., et al.: Target cells for 1,25 dihydroxyvitamin D_3 in intestinal tract, stomach, kidney, skin, pituitary and parathyroid. Science 206:1188, 1980.

45. Talmage, R. V., Anderson, J. J. B., and Cooper, C. W.: The influence of calcitonins on the disappearance of radiocalcium and radiophosphorus from plasma. Endocrinology 90:1185, 1972.

46. Talmage, R. V., Grubb, S. A., Norimatsu, H., and Vanderwiel, C. J.: Evidence for an important physiological role for calcitonin. Proc. Natl. Acad. Sci. USA 77:609, 1980.

47. Thompson, N. W., Eckhauser, F. E., and Harness, J. K.: The anatomy of primary hyperparathyroidism. Surgery 92:814, 1982.

48. Tregear, G. W., Van Rietschoten, J., Greene, E., et al.: Bovine parathyroid hormone: minimum chain length of synthetic peptide required for biological activity. Endocrinology 93:1349, 1973.

49. Turner, C. D., and Bagnara, J. T.: General Endocrinology. W. B. Saunders, Philadelphia, 1976.

50. Wasserman, R. H., and Taylor, A. N.: Metabolic roles of fat soluble vitamins D, E and K. Ann. Rev. Biochem. 41:179, 1972.

50a. Wilson, J. V., Harris, S. G., Moore, W. D., and Leipold, H. W.: Primary hyperparathyroidism in a dog. J. Am. Vet. Med. Assoc. 164:942, 1974.

51. Zenoble, R. D., and Rowland, G. N.: Hypercalcemia and proliferative myelosclerotic bone reaction associated with feline leukovirus infection in a cat. J. Am. Vet. Med. Assoc. 175:591, 1979.

146 Surgical Diseases of the Endocrine Pancreas

Richard Walshaw

Surgical diseases of the canine endocrine pancreas are limited to neoplastic lesions of islet cells. The islet cells of the pancreas, certain cells in the gastrointestinal tract, the ACTH-producing cells of the pituitary, the parafollicular cells of the thyroid and the adrenal medulla, and the chemoreceptor cells of the sympathetic nervous system are all thought to originate from the embryonic neural crest.[8] These cells secrete polypeptide hormones and possess certain common characteristics. The terms used to describe these functional characteristics are *amine, precursor, uptake*, and *decarboxylation*, the acronym for which is APUD. The term *APUDoma* is used in human beings to describe neoplasms derived from these cells, which usually become clinically detectable because of the pathophysiological effects of uncontrolled hormone production.[30] The islet cells of the pancreas give rise to a number of APUDomas, the two most significant of which in the dog are functional beta cell tumors (insulinomas) and functional non-beta cell tumors (gastrinomas).

FUNCTIONAL BETA CELL NEOPLASIA

Functional neoplasms of the beta cells of the canine pancreas are well recognized. Numerous reports have appeared in the veterinary literature in recent years describing the diagnosis and treatment of these tumors.[2, 3, 12, 14, 16–18, 20, 23, 27] These neoplasms also are referred to as insulinomas, islet cell adenocarcinomas, and beta cell carcinomas. Functional beta cell tumors are extremely rare in the cat; I have discovered only one reported case in the veterinary literature.[24] The incidence of functional beta cell neoplasia in dogs is unknown, but the tumor is regarded as rare. Middle-aged to older dogs are generally affected, with no noted sex predisposition. Although a wide variety of breeds have been reported to be affected with the disease, there are some indications that boxers and German shepherd dogs may have a greater predisposition than other breeds.[12, 14, 17, 18, 27]

Beta cell neoplasms produce excessive quantities of insulin, resulting in an increased entry of glucose into cells. This causes periods of hypoglycemia and resultant clinical signs.[14] A presumptive diagnosis of beta cell neoplasia can be made by demonstrating Whipple's triad; i.e., neurological disturbances associated with hypoglycemia, a fasting plasma glucose concentration below 50 mg/dl, and relief of neurological signs by feeding or the parenteral administration of glucose.[2, 14]

Nearly 100 per cent of beta cell tumors in the dog are malignant.[2, 3, 12–14, 16–18, 20, 23, 27] This is in sharp contrast to such neoplasms of human beings, approximately 80 per cent of which are benign.[8] In the dog, this malignant neoplasm behaves as a slowly progressive primary pancreatic lesion with early metastases to the regional lymph nodes and the liver. The primary lesion generally is small (2 to 4 cm), but extensive metastatic disease may already be present by the time of diagnosis. Even though gross evidence of metastasis is not present at the time of exploratory surgery, biopsy specimens of the regional lymph nodes and the liver should be evaluated histologically. There is almost a 100 per cent rate of recurrence of clinical signs following removal of the primary lesion, confirming that early metastasis occurs.[2, 27] Occasionally a primary neoplasm is not found at the time of exploratory surgery, in which case careful examination of the draining lymph nodes and liver is essential.[14]

History

Often the history of the present illness extends over a period of several months. Neurological abnormalities are often reported to be triggered by various stimuli such as fasting, exercise, and excitement, and to follow postprandial hyperglycemia that results in a further increase in insulin release. Generalized (grand mal) seizures, weakness, rear limb paresis, generalized muscle twitching, and disorientation with incoordination and apparent blindness may be noted. Other unusual local or generalized neurological abnormalities, ranging from barking and hysteria to localized twitching of facial muscles, may be reported.[2, 12, 14, 18, 27]

It has been noted that generalized seizures alone are not a consistent finding. Vague neurological abnormalities are often reported to have occurred early in the course of the disease, whereas generalized seizures tend to occur later. The frequency and severity of the clinical signs also appear to increase as the disease progresses. The occurrence of neurological signs correlates with the rate at which hypoglycemia develops rather than with the actual degree of hypoglycemia. Therefore, the severity of signs is not necessarily predictable from the measured blood glucose levels at any one time. Thus, a gradually produced steady state of hypoglycemia often can be well tolerated clinically by the patient.[14, 18]

Clinical Findings

If a hypoglycemic crisis exists at the time of presentation, neurological abnormalities such as those described previously will be noted. As stated previously, however, the patient may show few or no signs if a steady state of hypoglycemia or normoglycemia is present. Although malignant in its biological behavior, beta cell neoplasms usually are small; therefore, cachexia and mechanical bowel obstruction are not associated with this type of neoplasm.

Laboratory Evaluations

The results of abdominal and thoracic radiographs, a hemogram and most blood chemistry analyses generally are within normal limits.[14] Some controversy exists in the veterinary literature as to which laboratory tests give results that most consistently aid in the diagnosis of beta cell neoplasia.[18, 25] Therefore, each will be briefly outlined.

Fasting Blood Glucose

Twenty-four-hour fasting blood glucose levels generally are profoundly below normal, i.e., < 50 mg/dl. However, hypoglycemia does not always develop after a 24-hour fast, and, therefore, an extended fast or repeated testing may be required.[6, 14] The demonstration of hypoglycemia does not definitely confirm the diagnosis of beta cell neoplasia because there are other possible causes of hypoglycemia in the adult dog, such as hypoadrenocorticism, hepatic lipidosis, hepatic glycogen storage disease, hepatic cirrhosis, inanition, and cachexia.[14]

Plasma Insulin

Plasma insulin is measured by an immunoreactive technique (immunoreactive insulin—IRI). The normal mean fasting IRI level of dogs at one reference laboratory is 24 ± 9 µU/ml.[22] A high level of IRI in the plasma in association with marked hypoglycemia in a fasting dog is highly suggestive of a beta cell neoplasm. The causes of fasting hypoglycemia, other than beta cell neoplasia, generally result in normal or subnormal plasma IRI levels.[14] Some patients with beta cell neoplasia may have an apparently normal fasting plasma IRI level, possibly due to its precirculation removal by the liver. Therefore, a "normal" IRI level does not completely rule out the existence of a beta cell tumor (see hereafter). If the fast is continued and hypoglycemia progresses, the plasma IRI level should remain constant or rise in a patient with a beta cell neoplasm. This demonstrates the presence of autonomous insulin-producing tissue.[6]

Plasma IRI:Glucose Ratio and the Amended Plasma IRI:Glucose Ratio

Because some patients with beta cell neoplasia have plasma IRI levels within the normal range, yet are hypoglycemic, it has been suggested that comparing the fasting plasma IRI level with the glucose level will provide evidence of excessive insulin secretion. In such patients a significantly elevated ratio persists throughout an extended fast.[6, 14]

An "amended plasma IRI:glucose ratio" has been devised for use in human patients based on the assumption that, in normal individuals, plasma IRI levels approach O if the plasma glucose is 30 mg/dl or less.[17, 26] Proven cases of human insulinoma generally exhibit amended ratios of more than 200 µU/mg.[26] Whether the calculation of this amended radio aids in the diagnosis of beta cell neoplasia in the dog has been questioned.[23, 26] It must be emphasized that the actual "normal range" of the amended ratio depends on the laboratory test methods used. Therefore, normal and abnormal values must be established for each clinical laboratory.[6, 26]

Intravenous Glucagon Tolerance Test

Although it is rarely necessary to use a provocative test of insulin secretion to diagnose beta cell neoplasia,[6, 14] a glucagon tolerance test may be utilized if equivocal results are obtained from the previously mentioned tests. The insulinogenic effects of glucagon are exaggerated in the presence of a beta cell neoplasm, which results both in an excessive plasma insulin concentration and a subnormal blood glucose concentration. The diagnostic criteria for the glucagon tolerance test in dogs with beta cell neoplasia have been stated to be (1) a decrease in blood glucose concentration one to two minutes after injection (due to the rapid release of insulin from the tumor); (2) a peak blood glucose concentration of less than 135 mg/dl in the absence of liver disease; (3) hypoglycemia (<50 mg/dl) by 60 to 120 minutes; (4) a plasma IRI level of greater than 50 µU/ml or an increase of greater than 18 µU/ml from fasting levels after one minute; and (5) an IRI:glucose ratio of greater than 75 µU/mg at one minute after injection.[14]

Additional tests, such as insulin infusion with C-peptide suppression or insulin infusion with proinsulin suppression, or provocative tests, such as the tolbutamide test or glucose tolerance test, are occasionally used in human beings to confirm the presence of a beta cell neoplasm. Such tests appear to be unnecessary in the dog.[6]

Diagnosis

A presumptive diagnosis of beta cell neoplasia is made based on the presence of Whipple's triad (see previous discussion). The diagnosis is supported by the demonstration of an inappropriately elevated level of plasma IRI when hypoglycemia is present. Provocative tests frequently are unnecessary. Final confirmation depends on surgical exploration of the pancreas, adjacent lymph nodes, and liver, with removal and/or biopsy and histological evaluation of suspicious lesions.

Treatment

Surgery is an integral part of the therapy for beta cell neoplasia, providing both a confirmatory diagnostic tool and a therapeutic benefit. However, owing to the almost 100 per cent incidence of malignancy and early metastasis, surgery often is only palliative.[2, 14]

Because these patients generally are in critical condition at the time of presentation, careful preoperative stabilization is necessary prior to surgical exploration.

Preoperative Patient Stabilization

Irreversible hypoxic brain damage can result from prolonged, severe hypoglycemia as a result of a decreased metabolic rate. Whereas dogs with single seizures or other minor neurological signs have minimal neuronal damage, continued seizures or hypoglycemic coma may well predispose to cerebral edema and necrosis.[14] Therefore, to protect the patient, normoglycemia should be maintained during the preoperative period. This is accomplished by careful monitoring, frequent feeding of small amounts of food, and the continuous intravenous administration of 10 to 20% dextrose solutions. Intermittent bolus injections of 50% dextrose may also be required. To facilitate glucose administration, a central venous catheter should be placed and maintained aseptically to avoid sepsis and thrombophlebitis. Broad spectrum antibiotic therapy is also indicated. The blood glucose level should be followed carefully during this period, using reagent strips designed to detect glucose in whole blood. During the 12 hours prior to surgery when food is withheld, careful monitoring of the blood glucose level is required.[14, 18]

Fluid and electrolyte balance should be maintained using isotonic balanced electrolyte solutions. Hypokalemia has been reported to occur during this period of dextrose infusion owing to the transfer of potassium from the extracellular to the intracellular fluid. Therefore, careful potassium supplementation via intravenous fluids may be necessary.[14]

Continuous seizures and hypoglycemia-induced coma that do not respond to intravenous dextrose administration should be aggressively treated to minimize cerebral damage. Diazepam, phenobarbital, corticosteroids, and mannitol should be used if considered appropriate. Local hypothermia, by ice packing the head, also has been suggested.[14, 18] Preoperative administration of diazoxide may be helpful in the patient with hypoglycemia refractory to normal corrective therapy[18] (see Medical Therapy of Malignant Insulimona). Preoperative glucocorticoid therapy has also been suggested.[14]

Surgical Therapy

During surgery, blood glucose monitoring and dextrose infusions are continued. The abdomen is explored through an anterior ventral midline incision. A thorough examination is made of both limbs of the pancreas, the draining lymph nodes, the liver, the duodenum, the mesoduodenum, the root of the mesentery, and the omentum. The lymph nodes to be examined include the hepatic, splenic, gastric, duodenal, and cranial mesenteric nodes.

To locate the primary lesion, the entire pancreas should be examined and palpated carefully. Usually, a single, firm, circumscribed mass is visible and palpable in one of the limbs, although multiple masses may be discovered. Neither limb of the pancreas has a greater prevalence for tumor development. Rarely, ectopic tumor foci are found in the duodenal wall and mesoduodenum. In most cases, a primary lesion is located. Failure to do so may occur if the primary lesion is too small to see or palpate or if multiple microscopic tumors are present within the substance of the pancreas.[14]

Owing to the biological behavior of this tumor (i.e., early metastasis), radical pancreatic resection is not indicated. Surgery should be aimed at removing all obvious tumor tissue, including grossly involved lymph nodes and liver masses. In the few cases of benign disease in the dog, tumor excision will be curative. "Blind" pancreatic resection, when a tumor mass is not grossly detectable, no longer is a universally accepted approach to therapy.[8] The surgical techniques for pancreatectomy are described in Chapter 55 (Exocrine Pancreas). Care must be taken in handling the pancreas to avoid iatrogenic traumatic pancreatitis. Careful attention should be paid to the duct system to avoid occluding or disrupting the drainage of the remaining pancreas. During the resection of lesions of the right lobe, it is essential that the cranial and caudal pancreaticoduodenal vessels be preserved, thereby ensuring adequate blood supply to the duodenum and the remaining pancreas.

Extensive lesions of the right lobe of the pancreas, involving the duodenum, pylorus, bile duct, and adjacent tissue, are frequently unresectable. However, if resection is to be undertaken, it is likely that pancreaticoduodenectomy and partial gastrectomy will be necessary. Reconstruction involves a gastrojejunostomy and cholecystojejunostomy. Postoperative exocrine and endocrine pancreatic replacement therapy is required in these cases. If the primary lesions cannot be excised, representative biopsies should be taken for histological diagnosis.

Resection of all grossly involved draining lymph nodes and, if possible, affected liver lobes, should be undertaken. If the lymph nodes are not obviously involved, representative lymph node biopsies should be obtained for staging purposes, and suspicious liver lesions should be evaluated histologically.

Postoperative Care

The two aspects of immediate postoperative care that require careful attention are stabilization of the patient's blood glucose level and treatment of iatrogenic pancreatitis.[14]

Postoperatively, either hypo- or hyperglycemia may be present. If complete tumor excision was impossible, hypoglycemia may persist. In these cases, continued intravenous dextrose infusions and careful blood glucose monitoring are required until the patient has returned to normal oral feeding. Multiple small feedings of a diet high in carbohydrates and protein should be instituted. Diazoxide therapy also may be considered.[18]

Transient postoperative hyperglycemia may be present owing to residual suppresion of normal beta cell activity. This problem frequently resolves in three to five days and usually requires no specific therapy except the avoidance of dextrose-containing intravenous solutions.[1, 18] Insulin therapy should be instituted only if marked hyperglycemia and glycosuria persist.[7]

Owing to the possibility of iatrogenic pancreatitis, serum amylase and lipase levels should be monitored; if vomiting occurs, food and water should be withheld. Serum electrolytes should be monitored and fluid and electrolyte requirements met using an isotonic multiple electrolyte replacement fluid given intravenously. Fluid administration usually can be decreased gradually by the second or third postoperative day as oral feeding returns to normal.[14, 18]

Antibiotic therapy is not indicated postoperatively, except in the presence of sepsis.

Medical Therapy of Malignant Insulinoma

As has been stated previously, practically 100 per cent of beta cell neoplasms in dogs are malignant. Because they metastasize early in the course of the disease, clinical signs almost always recur following surgical removal, even in those cases in which resection appeared complete. Therefore, medical therapy probably is indicated in nearly all patients with malignant disease to allow them an extended period of symptom-free, good quality life. However, there are few reports of antineoplastic therapy of malignant beta cell tumors in the veterinary literature.[14, 19, 20, 23] Without medical therapy, there is a variable period before clinical signs recur, usually only a few months, but occasionally a year or more. This symptom-free period obviously depends on the amount of tumor remaining at the end of surgery.[2, 3, 12–14, 16–18, 20, 23, 27]

The medical management of malignant beta cell neoplasia consists of dietary control and both antihormonal and antineoplastic therapy. The following drugs have been shown to be effective.

Antihormonal Drugs

Diazoxide. A drug related to the thiazide diuretics, diazoxide possesses potent hyperglycemic properties. It increases blood glucose by directly inhibiting the release of insulin by the beta cells and by its extrapancreatic hyperglycemic effects, which include an increased hepatic release of glucose and peripheral inhibition of glucose utilization.[6, 7] Therefore, this drug can be used to temporarily correct hypoglycemia. The dose required to control hypoglycemia in dogs varies from 10 to 40 mg/kg/day, depending on the tumor size.[7, 14, 22] After a period of up to one year, diazoxide therapy generally is unable to suppress insulin release from the neoplasm, owing to either tumor cell tolerance or an overwhelming production of insulin by the tumor.[6, 7]

The benzothiadiazide diuretic trichlormethiazide has been shown to act synergistically with diazoxide to increase its hyperglycemic effects. Therefore, it can be used in refractory cases, although increased toxicity may result.[6, 7] At higher doses, diazoxide causes sodium retention and edema. The diuretic can also correct or prevent this side effect.[6] A number of descriptions of the beneficial effects of using diazoxide have appeared in the veterinary literature.[7, 14, 18, 23]

Propranolol. In human beings, use of propranolol has been associated with a reduction in plasma insulin levels and, therefore, a correction of hypoglycemia.[6] Whether this is also true in dogs is unknown.

Antineoplastic Drugs

5-Fluorouracil (5-FU). There are several reports describing occasional favorable responses to 5-FU in human patients with islet cell malignancies. The rate of response is similar to that seen with 5-FU in other gastrointestinal carcinomas.[6]

Adriamycin. Significant decreases in both the insulin level and measurable disease have been noted in human beings with malignant beta cell neoplasia following the use of Adriamycin.[6]

Streptozotocin. To date, this is the most effective single antineoplastic agent used for treating malignant beta cell neoplasia in human beings. Streptozotocin is a broad spectrum antibiotic and a naturally occurring nitrourea produced by *Streptomyces achromogenes.* Its mode of action is selective destruction of beta cells.[6] Unfortunately, this drug is nephrotoxic. By careful monitoring of the patient and correct timing of treatments, renal tubular toxicity in human beings has been minimized and is usually reversible.[6] In reports on the use of streptozotocin in two dogs, temporary remission of hypoglycemia was achieved, but renal tubular toxicity and hepatotoxicity were noted.[19, 20]

It has been demonstrated in human beings that a combination of 5-FU and streptozotocin is more effective than streptozotocin alone in controlling the malignant disease. Although notable gastrointestinal side effects are detected during the course of chemotherapy, the overall toxicity of the combination is not significantly greater than that of streptozotocin alone.[21]

In summary, the long-term medical management of malignant beta cell neoplasia should include dietary control and diazoxide therapy to allow the patient to remain symptom free for as long as possible. Unfortunately, there have been no clinical trials in dogs demonstrating which combination of antineoplastic agents is most successful in causing regression of beta cell neoplasia.

Both 5-FU and Adriamycin are well tolerated in the dog if therapy is closely monitored. These drugs can be used alone or in combination. More experience also needs to be gained with the use of streptozotocin in dogs to avoid or cope with the associated toxicity. Because of the small number of cases available for study, well-designed, multicenter clinical trials are required to determine whether aggressive chemotherapy can increase the symptom-free period of these patients.

Prognosis

The long-term prognosis in cases of malignant beta cell neoplasia in dogs is poor. Aside from the exceptional case, it is unrealistic to expect a surgical cure. However, it is possible to provide an extended period of symptom-free life with early diagnosis, surgical intervention, and appropriate adjunctive medical therapy. Postoperative survival periods of two years or more are possible in many cases.

FUNCTIONAL NON-BETA CELL NEOPLASIA (GASTRINOMA)

A clinical syndrome has been described in human beings that consists of gastric hypersecretion and multiple gastrointestinal ulcers. The syndrome was first described by Zollinger and Ellison and is associated with a non-beta cell neoplasm of the pancreas.[31] This islet cell tumor (gastrinoma) produces excessive quantities of gastrin, and it is this hormone that is responsible for the clinicopathological features of the syndrome.[9, 10] Zollinger-Ellison syndrome is considered to be a rare cause of peptic ulceration in human beings,[15] and only four reports have appeared in the veterinary literature describing a similar syndrome in a total of six dogs.[5, 11, 15, 28] In half of the dogs the diagnosis was made at necropsy.

In human beings, gastrinoma is a slowly progressive malignant neoplasm, with metastasis to the regional lymph nodes and liver occurring in more than 50 per cent of persons by the time of diagnosis.[31] The biological behavior appears to be similar in the dog in that all but one of the reported canine cases had metastatic lesions in the regional draining lymph nodes, and most had liver metastases as well.[5, 11, 15, 28]

About 25 per cent of human patients with Zollinger-Ellison syndrome also have tumors of other endocrine organs. This has been termed *multiple endocrine adenomatosis* type I. For example, the existence of a parathyroid adenoma, resulting in hypercalcemia, has been associated with the occurrence of non-beta cell neoplasia in man.[29] Although in one report two of three dogs with a gastrinoma also had nodular transformation of the zona fasciculata of the adrenal glands, and all three had C-cell hyperplasia of the thyroid glands, it is not clear that this represents endocrine adenomatosis.[11]

Primary peptic ulceration is rare in dogs and is usually associated with or secondary to other disease processes such as mast cell neoplasia or severe liver disease.[15] It is appropriate, therefore, to consider Zollinger-Ellison syndrome when evaluating a dog with unexplained peptic ulceration.

The pathophysiological effects of continued release of high levels of gastrin are[29] (1) thickening, hyperplasia and edema of the gastric mucosa; (2) greatly increased gastric secretion of hydrochloric acid; (3) duodenal and jejunal ulceration; in the dog, reflux esophagitis also has been described; (4) villous atrophy, mucosal infiltration, and edema of the small intestine; (5) severe diarrhea due to massive gastric ionic input into the small bowel, which increases intestinal motility; and (6) steatorrhea due to acid inactivation of pancreatic lipase.

History

Dogs with gastrinoma are presented with historical findings that include progressive anorexia, weight loss, intermittent diarrhea, depression, and vomiting. The vomitus may contain blood. The history usually extends over several months, and previous attempts at symptomatic therapy are usually reported to be unsuccessful or to provide only temporary relief from signs.[5, 11, 15, 28]

Clinical Findings

Clinical findings include dehydration, weight loss, depression, vomiting, and diarrhea. Melena and hematemesis may be present. Epigastric pain, which occurs in human patients, has not been detected in dogs with Zollinger-Ellison syndrome. Abdominal palpation is unlikely to reveal any significant findings.[5, 11, 15, 28] As the clinical findings are not specific for a gastrinoma, additional procedures and laboratory evaluations are required to confirm the diagnosis.

Diagnostic Procedures

Endoscopy

On esophagoscopy, distal reflex esophagitis with erosive and ulcerative lesions may be noted. At gastroscopy, large quantities of gastric fluid; irregular, thickened rugal folds, particularly in the antral region; and, possibly, mucosal hemorrhages may be observed. Histological evaluation of an antral mucosal biopsy may reveal hyperplastic changes. If the duodenum can be entered with the endoscope, peptic ulcers may be observed as well.[11, 28]

Radiography

An upper gastrointestinal barium series may show evidence of thickened gastric mucosa and large rugal folds. The small intestine will often show signs of thickening and hypermotility. The tumors thus far described have been too small to be detected radiographically.[29]

Laboratory Evaluation

A hemogram may demonstrate mild anemia and a slightly elevated white blood cell count. Serum alkaline phosphatase and glutamic pyruvic transaminase levels may be elevated owing to liver involvement. Hypoproteinemia, with a significantly low albumin level, is a consistent finding in reported cases, probably owing to protein-losing enteropathy and defective digestion. Hypokalemia and hypochloremia also may be present. Steatorrhea may be demonstrable on fecal examination.[11, 28]

Two specific diagnostic tests are required to help confirm the diagnosis of Zollinger-Ellison syndrome:

Basal Gastric Acid Secretion. In human patients, basal gastric acid secretion levels of greater than 15 mEq/hour are usually found.[29] In one report, nine normal dogs had no measurable basal gastric acid secretion (dogs do not constantly secrete hydrochloric acid).[11] These results are in contrast to those in two dogs with Zollinger-Ellison syndrome; one secreted 3 mEq/hour[11] and the other, 15 to 17 mEq/hour of hydrochloric acid.[28]

Serum Gastrin Levels. An immunoreceptive assay is available for the measurement of canine serum gastrin levels.[22] Normal levels in the dog at one reference laboratory have been 12 to 34 pg/ml.[22] A greatly increased level of gastrin, i.e., over 1000 pg/ml, is considered diagnostic of Zollinger-Ellison syndrome. If the basal serum level of gastrin is not diagnostic, provocative tests using oral protein administration (½ can of beef broth + ½ can of meat dog food) or the intravenous infusion of secretin (4 μg/kg) or calcium (2 mg/kg calcium gluconate) can be performed.[8, 28, 30] In normal dogs and human beings, secretin, given intravenously, causes a slight decrease in serum gastrin levels. However, in patients with gastrinomas, gastrin levels are paradoxically increased. Calcium, given intravenously, results in little, if any, increase in serum gastrin level in normal dogs and human beings but causes a significant rise in the presence of Zollinger-Ellison syndrome.[8, 28, 30]

Diagnosis

The diagnosis of Zollinger-Ellison syndrome is based on the demonstration of hypergastrinemia and an elevated rate of gastric acid secretion. Provocative tests to stimulate gastrin secretion may be required in equivocal cases. Mild elevations of serum gastrin in human beings can be found in certain other disorders, such as antral G-cell hyperplasia, atrophic gastritis, short bowel syndrome, hyperthyroidism, retained gastric antrum, and renal insufficiency. Circulating gastrin levels are not greatly increased by provocative testing in these diseases.[8, 30]

Treatment

The primary goal of the initial therapy of patients with severe clinical signs is to control excessive gastric acid secretion, the cause of the pathophysiological disturbances characteristic of this syndrome. This can be attempted by medical or surgical therapy. Control of the malignant neoplasm is attempted thereafter because patients suffering from fulminating disease are in very unstable condition owing to severe gastric hypersecretion and induced fluid and electrolyte losses. Administration of balanced multiple electrolyte replacement solutions and plasma is required to restore fluid and electrolyte balance and to correct the marked hypoproteinemia. This is particularly essential if surgery is being considered.[29]

In patients with mild to moderate signs, control of gastric acid secretion can be attempted with cimetidine, a histamine$_2$ receptor antagonist.[8, 29] At least one canine patient with the syndrome has transiently responded to cimetidine therapy, but for a period of less than two months.[5] The long-term success of cimetidine therapy is still unknown in human beings.[8, 29] It has been shown, however, to be useful in controlling gastric acid hypersecretion during the period of evaluation and stabilization prior to surgery.[8]

The treatment originally recommended by Zollinger and Ellison for human patients was total gastrectomy, that is, removal of the targets of gastrin, the parietal cells.[31] For human patients with more severe symptoms and those that have failed to respond to cimetidine therapy, this remains the treatment of choice. It is reported that these patients tolerate total gastrectomy extremely well, with a very low mortality rate.[8, 29]

It has been suggested that every human patient who is considered a good surgical risk should undergo abdominal exploration for possible tumor removal.[8, 29] Often, metastatic disease is present, but reducing the size of the tumor mass may help alleviate the symptoms of the disease. In the reported canine cases, an aggressive approach to therapy has not been tried. Treatment was attempted in only three dogs, with short-term palliation of symptoms.[5, 11, 28] An exploratory laparotomy should be performed in dogs with this syndrome and the pancreas, duodenum, and adjacent mesentery carefully examined for a tumor. Multiple primary lesions may be found. The draining regional lymph nodes and liver should be carefully examined for evidence of metastatic disease. If possible, all gross tumors should be resected. The surgical techniques for pancreatectomy are described in Chapter 55 (Exocrine Pancreas). If the disease is too widespread for resection to be feasible, biopsy specimens should be taken for histological evaluation and total gastrectomy should be considered as described previously.

Even though the symptoms of the disease in human beings can often be suppressed for considerable periods of time (approaching ten years), the progressing malignant disease eventually results in death. Therefore, adjunctive antineoplastic therapy is indicated. Streptozotocin has been advocated as the chemotherapeutic agent of choice.[8, 29] Some reports indicate that approximately 50 per cent of human patients with metastatic neoplasia benefit from such therapy.[8] However, other investigators report a very poor response to streptozotocin.[4]

Prognosis

The dogs with Zollinger-Ellison syndrome reported in the veterinary literature all were euthanized owing to extensive or progressive disease. Aggressive therapy was not undertaken. Therefore, the possible benefits of such an approach are unknown. Perhaps, as in man, long-term survival in the face of known metastatic disease can be achieved by target organ removal, i.e., total gastrectomy, and, therefore, allevation of the signs of disease.[29]

1. Caywood, D. D., and Wilson, J. W.: Functional pancreatic islet cell adenocarcinoma in the dog. In Kirk, R. W. (ed.): Current Veterinary Therapy VII, W. B. Saunders, Philadelphia, 1980, pp. 1020–1023.
2. Caywood, D. D., Wilson, J. W., Hardy, R. M., and Shull, R. M.: Pancreatic islet cell adenocarcinoma: Clinical and diagnostic features of six cases. J. Am. Vet. Med. Assoc. 174:714, 1979.
3. Chrisman, C. L.: Postoperative results and complications of insulinomas in dogs. J. Am. Anim. Hosp. Assoc. 16:677, 1980.
4. Dimitrov, N. V.: Department of Oncology, Michigan State University. Personal communication, 1982.
5. Drazner, F. H.: Canine gastrinoma: A condition analogous to Zollinger-Ellison syndrome in man. Cal. Vet. 35:6, 1981.
6. Fajans, S. S., and Floyd, J. C.: Diagnosis and medical management of insulinomas. Ann. Rev. Med. 30:313, 1979.
7. Feldman, E. C.: Diseases of the endocrine pancreas. In Ettinger, S. J. (ed.): Textbook of Veterinary Internal Medicine, Vol. II. W. B. Saunders, Philadelphia, 1983, Ch. 68, pp. 1615–1649.
8. Friesen, B. R.: Tumor of the endocrine pancreas. N. Engl. J. Med. 306:580, 1982.
9. Gregory, R. A., et al.: Extraction of a gastrin-like substance from a pancreatic tumor in a case of Zollinger-Ellison syndrome. Lancet 1:1045, 1960.
10. Gregory, R. A., et al.: Nature of the gastrin-like secretagogue in Zollinger-Ellison tumors. Lancet 2:543, 1967.
11. Happe, R. P., van der Gaag, I., Lamen, C. B., et al.: Zollinger-Ellison syndrome in three dogs. Vet. Pathol. 17:177, 1980.
12. Hill, F. W. G., Pearson, H., Kelly, D. F., et al.: Functional islet cell tumor in the dog. J. Small Anim. Pract. 15:119, 1974.
13. Huxtable, C. R., and Farrow, B. H.: Functional neoplasms of the canine pancreatic islet beta cells: A clinical pathological study of three cases. J. Small Anim. Pract. 20:737, 1979.
14. Johnson, R. K.: Insulinoma in the dog. Vet. Clin. North Am. 7:629, 1977.
15. Jones, B. R., Nicholls, M. R., and Badman, R.: Peptic ulceration in a dog associated with an islet cell carcinoma of the pancreas and an elevated plasma gastrin level. J. Small Anim. Pract. 17:593, 1976.
16. Kruth, S. E., Feldman, E. C., and Kennedy, P. C.: Insulin secreting islet cell tumor: Establishing a diagnosis and the clinical course for 25 dogs. J. Am. Vet. Med. Assoc. 181:54, 1982.
17. Mattheewws, D., Rottiers, R., DeRijcke, J., et al.: Hyperinsulinism in the dog due to pancreatic islet cell tumors: A report on three cases. J. Small Anim. Pract. 7:313, 1976.
18. Mehlhaff, C. J.: Surgical management of islet cell tumors. Resident paper, Animal Medical Center, 1981.
19. Meyer, D. J.: A pancreatic islet cell carcinoma in a dog treated with streptozotocin. Am. J. Vet. Res. 37:1221, 1976.
20. Meyer, D. J.: Temporary remission of hypoglycemia in the dog with an insulinoma after treatment with streptozotocin. Am. J. Vet. Res. 38:1201, 1977.
21. Moertel, C. G., Manley, J. A., and Johnson, L. A.: Streptozotocin alone compared with streptozotocin plus fluorouracil in the treatment of advanced islet cell carcinoma. N. Engl. J. Med. 303:1189, 1980.
22. Nachreiner, R.: Clinical Endocrinology Laboratory, Veterinary Clinical Center, Michigan State University. Personal communication, 1983.
23. Parker, A. H., O'Brien, D., and Musselman, E. E.: Diazoxide treatment of metastatic insulinoma in a dog. J. Am. Anim. Hosp. Assoc. 18:315, 1982.
24. Priester, W. A.: Pancreatic islet cell tumors in domestic animals. Data from II College of Veterinary Medicine in the United States and Canada. J. Nat. Can. Inst. 53:227, 1974.
25. Schall, W. D.: Personal communication, 1982.
26. Schall, W. D.: Personal communication, 1983.
27. Steinberg, H. S.: Insulin secreting pancreatic tumors in the dog. J. Am. Anim. Hosp. Assoc. 16:695, 1980.
28. Straus, E., Johnson, G. F., and Yalow, R. S.: Canine Zollinger-Ellison syndrome. Gastroenterology 72:380, 1977.
29. Thompson, J. C.: The stomach and duodenum. In Sabiston, D. C., Jr. (ed.): Davis-Christopher Textbook of Surgery, 12th ed. W. B. Saunders, Philadelphia, 1981, Ch. 31, pp. 896–940.
30. Willard, M. D., and Schall, W. D.: APUDomas. In Kirk, R. W. (ed.): Current Veterinary Therapy VIII. W. B. Saunders, Philadelphia, 1983.
31. Zollinger, R. M., and Ellison, E. M.: Primary peptic ulcerations of the jejunum associated with islet cell tumors of the pancreas. Ann. Surg. 142:709, 1955.

Section XVII

The Ear

Colin E. Harvey
Section Editor

ANATOMY AND PHYSIOLOGY

Concave and *convex* are used here to refer to the surfaces of the external ear. These correspond to the hairless, rostrolateral and haired, caudomedial surfaces of the auricle (pinna), respectively (Fig. 147–1).[6]

The auricular and scutiform cartilages form the external ear canal opening and ear pinna. The large, convoluted auricular cartilage is cone-shaped from its origin at the annular cartilage to where it flares to form the pinna distally.

Important surgical landmarks of the auricular cartilage are the helix, anthelix, tragus, antitragus, scapha, and cavum conchae (Fig. 147–1).

The helix is the free margin of cartilage around the pinna bordering the scapha on three sides. The scapha is bordered on the fourth side by a ridge and prominent tubercle termed the anthelix, which is on the medial concave aspect of the auricular cartilage at the entrance to the vertical canal. The tragus forms the lateral rim of the vertical canal meatus and is directly opposite the anthelix. The tragohelicine incisure separates the tragus and helix. The antitragus is caudal to the tragus and separated from it by the intertragic notch. The funnel-shaped cavum conchae forms the vertical canal, and along with the tragal, antitragal, and anthelicine borders it forms the external auditory meatus (Fig. 147–1).[7]

The boot-shaped scutiform lies medial to the auricular cartilage and muscles and assists in attachment of the auricular cartilage to the head. This cartilage is important in correcting ear carriage but not in reconstructive procedures.[17]

The great auricular arteries and veins arborize over the pinna. These vessels are branches of the external carotid artery and the internal maxillary vein. The lateral, intermediate, and medial vascular rami pass along the convex surface and wrap around the helicine margins as well as directly penetrate the scapha to supply the concave epithelium.[7]

The second cervical nerve is the principal caudodorsal sensory innervation on the convex surface, and the auriculotemporal branches of the trigeminal nerve are the principal sensory innervation on the concave surface. The external ear muscles are supplied by the auricular branch (auriculopalpebral trunk) of the facial nerve.[7]

The skin is closely adherent to the concave aspect of the perichondrium, and thus is difficult to undermine for suturing. The convex surface has subcuticular (areolar) tissue interposed between the skin and perichondrium; this skin is easy to undermine, and small defects are easily closed.

PHYSICAL INJURIES

Aural Hematoma

Aural or auricular hematoma is the most common physical injury to the dog's ear. It is self-inflicted and caused by scratching and head-shaking. This injury is seen most commonly in pendulous-eared dogs but is also seen in the erect-eared breeds and occasionally in cats. Underlying causes of the condition are acute or chronic inflammation, parasites such as ear mites or ticks, and foreign bodies in or near the ear canal.

Hematomas are normally confined to the concave surface of the ear (Fig. 147–2), although they may be on either or both sides of the auricular cartilage, depending upon the severity and duration of trauma. The hematoma does not, however, extend to the helix.

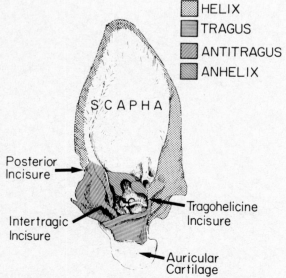

HELIX
TRAGUS
ANTITRAGUS
ANHELIX

SCAPHA

Posterior Incisure

Intertragic Incisure

Tragohelicine Incisure

Auricular Cartilage

Figure 147–1. Anatomy of the concave surface of the auricular cartilage, showing the important anatomical divisions. The intertragic notch and tragohelicine incisure are surgical landmarks.

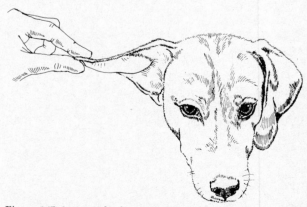

Figure 147–2. Auricular hematoma of the concave surface of the ear.

The great auricular artery is the source of hemorrhage, which accumulates within the cartilage plate as a result of shearing—the hematoma is lined by cartilage on both sides. When the arterial pressure equals the intrahematoma pressure, bleeding ceases. Additional pressure on the hematoma during head-shaking or scratching causes further separation of the tissues and allows hemorrhage to resume. Fibrin is deposited on the walls of the hematoma, leaving a central sanguineous seroma. With chronicity, the ear becomes thickened and deformed. Fibrous reorganization of the ear and secondary "cauliflower" contracture results.[14, 15]

Treatment

The therapeutic objectives for management of an auricular hematoma are: to identify the source of irritation, to maintain tissue apposition, to reduce fibrin deposition, and to prevent recurrence.

Conservative Management. Needle aspiration may be effective when the diagnosis is made soon after hematoma formation. The causative irritant must be eliminated and the tissues apposed. The contents of the hematoma must be removed aseptically. If the hematoma reforms, repeat aspiration is rarely successful. Cortisone instillation is dangerous, because it suppresses the inflammation that causes reattachment of the walls of the hematoma. Injection of any medication separates the tissues. A pressure bandage should be applied following aspiration.

Longer-standing hematomas in which minimum fibrin is present may be treated by placing a self-retaining, disposable teat cannula rather than relying upon multiple needle aspirations. The cannula is aseptically placed via a small stab incision in a dependent portion of the hematoma.[18] The application of continuous pressure for five to seven days decreases recurrence. Recurrence is fairly common following either conservative method.

Management by Incision. Large, severe or chronic (thick-walled) hematomas should be treated by surgical incision and suturing. The therapeutic objectives include elimination of the inciting irritant, removal of clot, and reapposition of tissues under aseptic conditions. Hematomas may be opened via straight, cruciate, or S-shaped incisions, depending upon the surgeon's preference or the size of the hematoma.

It has been suggested that the hematoma be allowed to organize for ten to 14 days prior to incision.[13] Delay may allow the hematoma to enlarge. It is acceptable and effective to incise the hematoma immediately after the diagnosis is made, but the sanguineous drainage is heavier in the early postoperative period than when incision is delayed.

When one is incising a hematoma, the incision should be bold, exposing the hematoma cavity from end to end. The clot is thoroughly curetted, and the hematoma is copiously irrigated. These measures

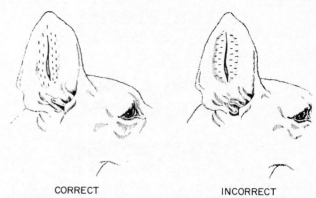

CORRECT   INCORRECT

Figure 147–3. Sutures to obliterate dead space in an auricular hematoma. Sutures are correctly placed when parallel to and not including the blood vessels. Incorrectly placed sutures may cause avascular necrosis.

promote better drainage and reduce the scarring and potential for infection. Dead space and pockets are obliterated, preventing the hematoma from reforming in small areas.[15] Although a pressure bandage with the ear pressed over the dorsum of the neck is effective alone in reducing hematoma reformation, drainage may not be adequate. Mattress sutures should be placed through the ear, parallel to the major vessels (Fig. 147–3). The three main great auricular branches are visible on the convex surface and should be avoided. The incisional edges are not apposed or sutured, because drainage must pass through this area. One should avoid leaving areas of hematoma cavity closed off from the incision by a line of sutures. If desired, a reinforcing stent such as radiographic film may be placed on the convex surface, but this is not usually necessary if the sutures are not greater than 0.5 cm in breadth and if they are not tied tightly.

A light, protective bandage may be applied, immobilizing the ear against the dorsum of the neck. The bandage is changed after three days, and sutures are removed in seven to ten days.

Alternatively, a sterile leather punch can be used to create 0.3- to 0.4-cm holes 0.75 cm apart; a tongue depressor is inserted through a small skin incision to protect the cartilage. A pressure bandage is placed for five days, and the ear is cleaned and bandaged for another five days. Healing of the epithelial defects is by contraction and epithelialization.[3]

Wounds of the Pinna

Therapeutic Objectives and General Management

The ear is commonly injured during fights because of its unprotected position. Regardless of the severity of the wound, the therapeutic objectives are: cleansing, debridement, apposition of tissues, protection, and prevention of secondary infection.

Following an initial rinse, the wound is packed

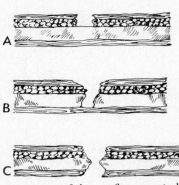

Figure 147–4. Lacerations of the ear flaps may include the skin only (*A*, convex surface), skin and cartilage (*B*), or cartilage and both skin surfaces (*C*).

with sterile water-soluble ointment or lubricant, and a razor blade or clippers are used to remove the hair from the area. Loose hair clippings are trapped in the lubricant rather than the wound and are more easily washed away.

While the lubricant is still protecting the wound, clean gauze, a balanced pH soap, and saline or tap water are used to wash the periphery of the wound and matted hair. The cleansing is continued to the wound margins, and finally to the depths of the wound. Gauze is changed and the wound is irrigated frequently.

The tissues may require sutures for apposition, or second-intention healing (contraction and epithelialization) may be adequate. Fresh wounds with minimal contamination may be apposed following cleansing, whereas more contaminated or infected wounds may be bandaged for 24 hours before closing. Small wounds, wounds in which the tissues remain in good apposition, and grossly infected wounds may be left unsutured.

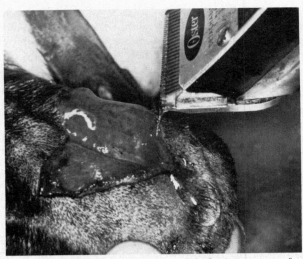

Figure 147–6. A traumatically raised pedicle flap on convex surface of an ear. This wound must be sutured to prevent contracture and a hairless scar. (Sterile lubricant is present to protect the wound during clipping.)

Ear Lacerations

Three types of lacerations of the ear may be distinguished on the basis of wound depth or structures involved. A laceration may involve the skin only (single surface skin wound), the skin and underlying cartilage, or the skin, contralateral skin, and interposed cartilage (perforating wound) (Fig. 147–4).

Single-Surface Skin Wound. Lacerations involving only the skin (Fig. 147–5) usually heal adequately by second intention because the rigid cartilaginous template underlies the wound, maintaining tissue apposition. Although not required, careful suturing may improve the cosmetic appearance.

Suturing is mandatory, however, when a two- or three-sided flap has been formed (Fig. 147–6). If not

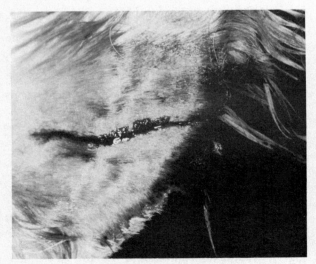

Figure 147–5. Lacerations of the concave ear skin superficial to the scapha and helix. The cartilage is intact, and the tissue apposition is excellent because of adherence of skin to the cartilage template.

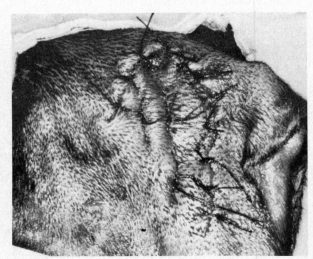

Figure 147–7. Sutured pedicle flap shown in Fig. 147–6. The dead space has been obliterated with three through-and-through mattress sutures as with aural hematoma obliteration.

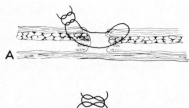

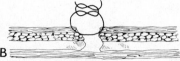

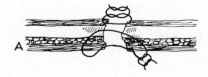

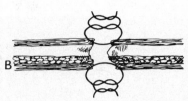

Figure 147–8. Suturing partial ear lacerations. *A*, Vertical mattress sutures may be used to align and stabilize the cartilage and skin. *B*, If the cartilage is stable, the wound may be closed with sutures in the skin surface only.

Figure 147–10. Suturing full-thickness ear lacerations. A vertical mattress suture may be used to align and stabilize the cartilage and the skin on one side of the ear. *A*, Simple interrupted sutures are placed in the skin on the remaining side of the ear. *B*, The wound may also be closed by simple interrupted sutures placed only through the skin on both ear surfaces.

sutured, the flap contracts during healing, creating an area that either cannot epithelialize or does so without haired covering. These wounds must be sutured at the margin as well as through the center of the flap as with aural hematomas, to obliterate dead space (Fig. 147–7).

Single-Surface Skin and Cartilage Wound. Wounds of this type respond similarly to single-surface wounds of skin only, except that in longer wounds, cartilaginous support is lost, and healing is delayed until fibrous union occurs. This delay results in malalignment of the cartilage margins and disfigurement of the ear. For best results, the skin is sutured, a vertical mattress suture being placed with the deeper bite aligning cartilage and the superficial bite aligning skin (Fig. 147–8).

Perforating Wound. Punctures or tears that extend through the pinna, but not through the helical border, heal adequately with conservative protection (Fig. 147–9). An improved cosmetic appearance is obtained by suturing, particularly with long tears (Fig. 147–10A).

The most serious lacerations are those in which the full thickness of the ear is lacerated through a helical border (Fig. 147–11). When left untreated, the margins of these wounds epithelialize, forming a permanent defect. Contraction during healing separates the wound edges. Such lacerations should be sutured soon after injury. A line of simple interrupted sutures is placed on each surface, beginning at the helical margin, or one row of simple interrupted sutures is placed on one side and a vertical mattress suture aligns both skin and cartilage from the other side (see Fig. 147–10B).

Avulsions of a Portion of the Pinna

The margins of untreated avulsion wounds of the pinna heal in the same manner as through-and-through lacerations, by contracture and epithelialization. These defects widen as a result of chronic wound contraction. Rarely is the avulsed portion narrow enough to suture without causing obvious cupping or folding.

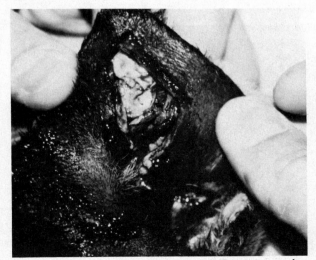

Figure 147–9. Contaminated wound through the entire ear, but not through the helical border. This wound may be adequately managed with chemical debridement and second intention healing. Pendulous-eared dogs may have more tendency toward contractural deformity.

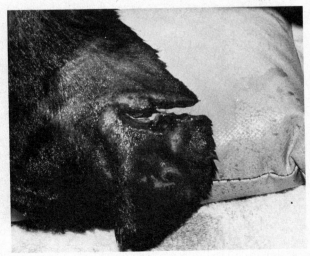

Figure 147–11. Auricular full-thickness lacerations through the helical border must be sutured.

The primary therapeutic objectives for treating a partially avulsed pinna are: to control hemorrhage, to prevent infection, and to allow wound epithelialization. These objectives are simply achieved, but the result of this treatment is an ear with a cosmetic defect. Several methods can be used to correct the defect.

Partial Amputation. Ears with shallow auricular avulsions may be improved by partial amputation of the auricle. The amputation need not include the

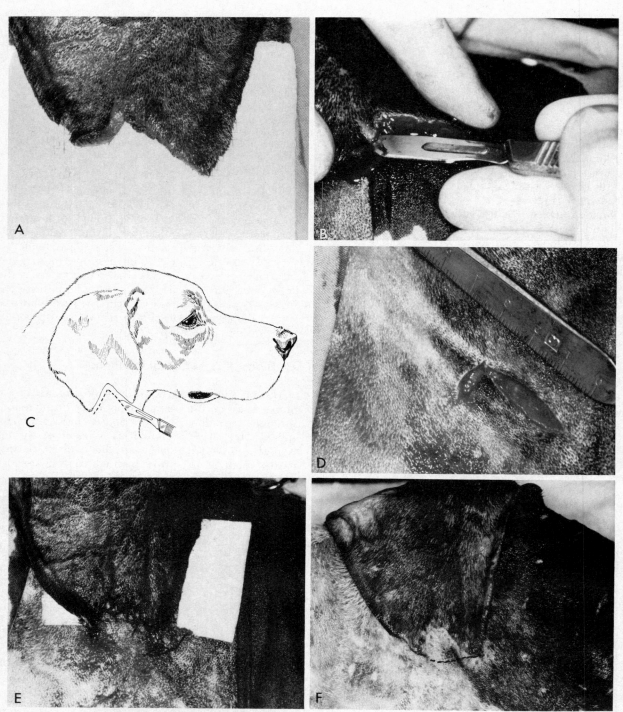

Figure 147–12. A, Marginal auricular defect to be corrected with a pedicle flap. *B*, Spliting the margin of the defect and debriding the edges. *C*, Ear in position over cervicobuccal area with defect being outlined on the skin. *D*, Pedicle flap formation. The pedicle flap shape is inscribed on the donor site by direct super-imposition of the recipient site defect. The incisional lengths are 0.5 cm longer than those of the recipient's margin. *E*, The pedicle is sutured into the defect with simple interrupted sutures. *F*, Two weeks after pedicle transposition. The healed flap is ready for transfer. Proposed line of excision *(dotted line).*

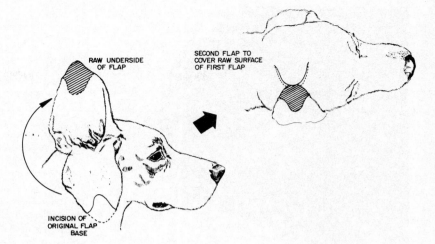

Figure 147–13. A technique for completing an auricular defect correction with a second flap.

apex of the avulsion, and the absolute minimum of tissue should be excised (see "Ear Fissures and Ear Tip Dermatitis").

Pedicle Flaps. An auricular margin defect may be restored by transposing a pedicle flap from the lateral cervicobuccal region. Both the concave and convex epithelial surfaces are replaced.

After the area around the auricular defect is clipped and cleaned, sharp scissors are used to debride and straighten the margins of the defect, removing as little tissue as possible. An antibacterial ointment is applied, and the ear is bandaged. The bandage is changed after three days. At seven days after site preparation, the ear epithelium is more vascular and thicker, facilitating acceptance of the graft. The skin of the cervicobuccal region is loose, vascular, and easily transferred. The direction of hair growth in this area is generally similar to that on the convex surface of the ear, except near the ventral midline where the hair pattern is lateral and caudal. However, the direction of hair growth in this area varies among dogs.

The donor (cervicobuccal) area and the recipient (ear) area are clipped and scrubbed 24 hours in advance of surgery. The auricular defect is evaluated and measured (Fig. 147–12A). The defect skin margins are split and are sharply but sparingly debrided (Fig. 147–12B). The ear is placed over the cervicobuccal area in a comfortable position, and a skin marker or light incision is used to outline the shape of the auricular defect on the cervicobuccal skin (Fig. 147–12C). Full-thickness incisions are made along these lines, extending five millimeters further (Fig. 147–12D). The flap is sutured beginning at the center of the wound, using simple interrupted sutures of 4-0 polypropylene placed three to five millimeters apart (Fig. 147–12E).

Postoperatively, the ear is protected under bandages for two weeks (Fig. 147–12F). A bactericidal ointment is applied topically prior to the initial bandaging. Ideally, this bandage should suffice for the first week. Changing the bandage sooner may disrupt the epithelial anastomosis and endanger the blood supply.

Transfer of the pedicle flap may be completed by several methods. First, the flap is severed from the donor site at its base, and a pedicle flap from another site is used to cover the concave auricular surface (Fig. 147–13). Second, after being severed, the concave surface may be left to heal by second intention if the area is not too large. Third, the pedicle origin may be incised in the shape of the contralateral

Figure 147–14. A second technique for completing an auricular defect correction with a folded pedicle. Vascular kinking and necrosis is more likely with this technique.

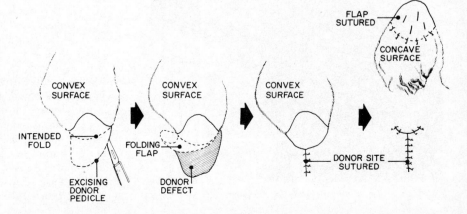

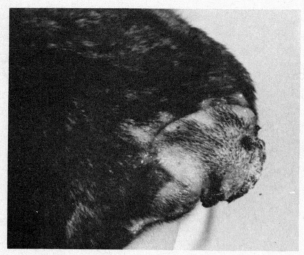

Figure 147–15. Completed pedicle flap after two weeks (convex surface).

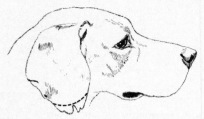

Figure 147–17. Partial amputation of auricle. As little tissue as possible is removed during amputation of a portion of the auricle, except when a neoplasm is present.

defect, folded upon itself, and sutured (Fig. 147–14); however, vascular necrosis may result from crimping vessels supplying the folded flap.

Sutures are removed in ten days, and unhealed surfaces are allowed to heal by second intention (Fig. 147–15).

Ear Fissures and Ear Tip Dermatitis

Fissure wounds of the ear begin along the distal helical border and extend for differing lengths toward or into the scapha portion of the auricle (Fig. 147–16). They are seen most commonly in pendulous-eared dogs, are caused by continuous abrasion, and are often associated with the ear margin seborrhea seen in dachshunds.[12] Because they are chronic, different areas of a lesion may show different stages of healing.[12] Although dissimilar in cause, the ear tip der-

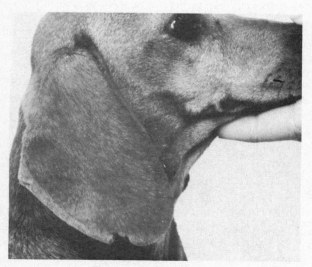

Figure 147–16. Ear fissure.

matitis of erect ears caused by biting flies may be similar to ear fissures in effect.

The primary therapeutic objective is to treat the cause of head-shaking. Insect barriers or repellents usually resolve ear tip dermatitis. Resolution of chronic skin disease causing ear fissure is less successful. Small fissures may be debrided, trimmed, and sutured, as may recently occurring long fissures that have little tissue loss. Chronic long fissures usually are contracted, making suture apposition of the wound edges impossible; they are removed by partial amputation.

Partial Amputation of the Pinna

The ear is amputated through normal tissue as distally as possible with scissors, curving the wound to approximate normal ear shape (Fig. 147–17). Bleeding vessels are crushed and twisted rather than ligated when possible. The skin edges are apposed with a simple continuous 3-0 or smaller suture. The shortened ear may be cosmetically acceptable to the owner, or the owner may wish the other ear to be shortened to match. Single deep fissures can also be treated by pedicle flaps from the neck and head, as with avulsion wounds of the auricle. Regardless of the therapy, the ears must be protected from trauma until completely healed. Recurrence is common.

SOLAR, THERMAL, AND PRESSURE TRAUMA

Solar Dermatitis of White Feline Ears

The white ears of cats are predisposed to auricular solar dermatitis.[12] The skin of the ear tip is exposed to more direct sunlight owing to lack of hair coverage.

The initial lesion appears as a mild sunburn and results in alopecia. A reduction in hairs protecting the lesion allows increased exposure. Over a period of years, the cartilage and overlying skin begin to deform. Ulceration of the skin overlying the helix is not uncommon. Solar dermatitis may lead to squamous cell carcinoma (Figs. 147–18 and 147–19).

The therapeutic objectives are: to decrease the exposure of the ear to direct sunlight by keeping the animal indoors during daylight or by applying sunscreening ointment to protect the ear margins, and

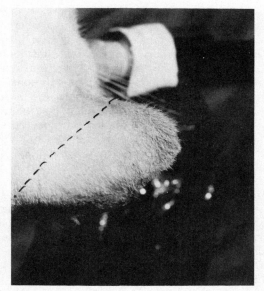

Figure 147–18. Feline solar dermatitis. Solar changes (distal to dotted line), most common on the white ears of cats, are caused by chronic sunburn.

to amputate progressive ulcerative lesions (see "Ear Fissures and Ear Tip Dermatitis"). Small early lesions may be treated by careful cryotherapy. Measures to reduce exposure to sunlight are continued following surgery. The protective effect of tattooing the affected area has not been evaluated, but this procedure may be useful.

Cold Injuries of the Auricle

The auricle is subjected to greater variation in temperature than other parts of the body because of its thinness and dependent position.

Cold injury may occur when the environmental

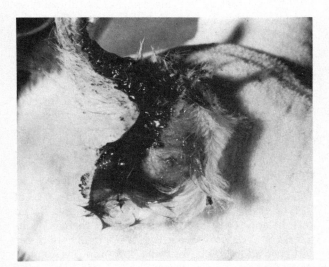

Figure 147–19. Squamous cell carcinoma. The contralateral ear of the cat in Fig. 147–18 is shown with a squamous cell carcinoma. The lesion is crateriform, appears as a chronic wound, and resulted from chronic solar exposure.

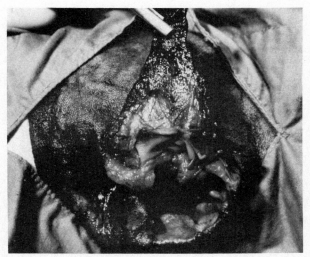

Figure 147–20. Avascular necrosis of the auricle resulting from a bandage that was applied too tightly following cosmetic auriculoplasty.

temperature is well above freezing, because of the wind chill or exposure to water, although the haired dog ear is well-insulated. This condition is fairly common in the northern regions of the United States and in Canada.* In acute cold injury, the auricle may feel hard, and there may be no response to painful stimuli. The most severe cases have clinical signs of avascular necrosis.[15] Systemic signs are rare. The frozen portion forms a dry eschar and desquamates. White hair regrows on the margin, and the cosmetic appearance is generally acceptable.

If gangrene is already apparent, amputation of the line of demarcation is contraindicated because less tissue than expected may slough. The gangrenous area should be protected with sterile dressings. Healed tissues are more susceptible to subsequent exposure to cold[15] and may be predisposed to neoplasia.[11]

Pressure Necrosis

Bandages that are applied to ears too tightly can impair auricular circulation, causing avascular necrosis (Fig. 147–20).

NEOPLASIA OF THE EXTERNAL EAR

Neoplasms arising from the external ear originate from skin, adnexa, connective tissue, or cartilage. The neoplasms commonly found in the external ear are: ceruminous gland or sebaceous adenoma or adenocarcinoma, papilloma, squamous cell carcinoma, histiocytoma, mastocytoma and mast cell sarcoma, basal cell carcinoma, and melanoma or melanosarcoma.

---

*Winthrow, S. J.: Personal communication, 1983.

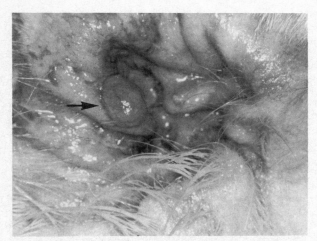

Figure 147–21. Ceruminous gland adenoma (arrow). Small tumors such as this one as well as hyperkeratotic epithelium may be surgically removed with very little hemorrhage.

Ceruminous Gland Adenomas and Carcinomas. The ceruminous gland tumors arise from the apocrine glands of the ear canal at any point within the ear. They are small, rounded, nodular or pedunculated lesions with a smooth surface and pinkish coloration (Fig. 147–21). They remain small but recur readily after incomplete excision. Carcinomas may metastasize to the regional lymph nodes and lungs.[1, 11]

Sebaceous Adenomas and Carcinomas. Sebaceous adenomas are common in the external ears of older dogs. They are usually small, firm, smooth, and pedunculated. Their usual color is grayish white. Carcinoma is rare, and metastasis is unlikely. Surgical resection usually results in a cure.

Papilloma. Papillomas may arise from any skin surface and appear as small (2–20 mm), horny projections that are pedunculated or sessile. The surface is irregular and cauliflower-like in appearance. Papillomas are usually single on the ear. They do not metastasize and are not locally invasive.[1] Surgical excision is indicated.

Squamous Cell Carcinoma. This tumor is most often seen on the white pinna of cats but may arise from any epidermal tissue on the ear. It appears as a chronic granulating, infected wound with an ulcerating center and proliferative margins (see Fig. 147–19). This tumor is slow to metastasize but is locally invasive.[1, 9] It is sensitive to radiation therapy.

Histiocytomas and Mastocytomas. These two tumors are impossible to differentiate on gross examination. When arising from the ear, they are usually located on the convex surface of the pinna, where they arise in the thin hypodermal or dermal tissues. They are reddish, raised, round, and dome-shaped as they displace the epidermis and become noticeable. Histiocytomas may regress spontaneously, whereas mastocytomas may become invasive and metastasize to regional lymph nodes. Surgical excision of single nodules is usually curative. Mastocytomas are radiosensitive and may temporarily regress with prednisone therapy.[1]

Basal Cell Tumors. Basal cell tumors arise from the stratum basale of the epidermis and are common on the head. They usually are raised hard plaques but may ulcerate and become infected. These tumors may recur after incomplete surgical excision but do not metastasize.[1] Carcinomas are often radiosensitive.

Round, raised, dome-shaped neoplasms, melanomas are common on the head. Depending upon the degree of malignancy, the growth rate may be slow or rapid and invasive. The color may vary from black to pink, the more anaplastic tumors being less pigmented. Heavily pigmented basal cell tumors may be confused clinically with melanomas.

Non-neoplastic Mass Lesions. Non-neoplastic inflammatory polyps and papillary verrucose hyperkeratosis[6] are commonly confused with neoplasms. Verrucose lesions are epithelial exuberances caused by chronic infection or local metabolic changes. Ultimately, such a lesion obstructs the vertical canal.

Inflammatory polyps are more common in cats than dogs and are restricted to the horizontal canal or middle ear cavity.

Treatment by Excision

Excision of part or all of the pinna is often avoided because of the fear of disfigurement.

Neoplasms that arise in the central portion of the pinna are more common on the convex surface. Small tumors on this surface are easily excised, because the skin is mobile and the skin defect can be closed after undermining. When one is undermining for closure, the dissection should remain close to the cartilage in order to avoid vessels. Usually, only the skin needs to be sutured. If a tumor has been removed from the concave ear surface and there is adequate tissue for closure, second-intention healing under a light bandage is usually cosmetically acceptable.

Neoplasia of the ear margin is managed like ear fissures, by partial amputation (see "Ear Fissures and Ear Tip Dermatitis"). Wide excision is indicated, as no pinna is preferable to a partial pinna with neoplasia.

MANAGEMENT OF DEVELOPMENTAL DEFORMITIES

Developmental deformities of the pinna are uncommon. Excessively small (microtia) or excessively large (macrotia) pinnae may be part of a more widespread deformity. Surgery is rarely indicated.

COSMETIC OTOPLASTY*

Cosmetic otoplasty is performed on the ears of certain breeds to meet breed specifications. The desired appearance for all breeds has changed considerably over the years, from a relatively short ear with considerable bell at the bottom to a longer, narrower ear.

*Editor's Note: This technique is not considered ethical or legal in some areas. Local details should be sought.

TABLE 147–1. Practical Schedule for Ear Trimming in Dogs

Breed	Age	Ear Length
Schnauzer	10 wks	⅔ of ear left
Boxer	9–10 wks	⅔–¾ of ear left
Doberman	8–9 wks	¾ of ear left
Great Dane	9 wks or 8–10 kg	¾ of ear left
Boston terrier	4–6 mos	Full trim

with considerable bell at the bottom to a longer, narrower ear.

Standards of Ear Trimming

Regardless of the trimming standard, all ears cannot be trimmed alike. Variations are justified in any breed, shape and length of the ear varying with the sex and conformation of the breed. Females generally are trimmed to have a finer ear than males. The ear is cut straight, narrower, and three to six millimeters shorter, little bell is left, and the tragus and the antitragus cartilages are trimmed sufficiently so that the ear blends into the head. Females of breeds that normally have a broad head, such as the boxer or schnauzer, can carry a little larger and wider ear than the Doberman or the Great Dane. No attempt should be made to trim the ear too short in the belief that it may fail to stand if trimmed to the preferred length. Short blocky ears detract from the appearance of the dog, with the exception of the bull terrier. One should also consider the dog's sire and dam. In females likely to be large and masculine in appearance or thin-boned with fine features, and males likely to be larger and more heavily muscled, the ear trim should be adjusted accordingly.

General Considerations

Ear trimming of a puppy that is malnourished, heavily parasitized, and in poor condition should be

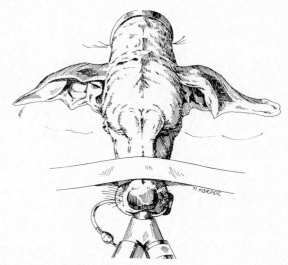

Figure 147–23. Proper position of the head so as to avoid undue pressure on the cervical area. The sandbag should not be placed too far caudally, so it does not put undue pressure on the auricular area.

delayed until the general health of the puppy is improved. The stress of anesthesia and surgery may suppress immune system responses and increase susceptibility to infection. Puppies should be vaccinated before having their ears trimmed.

Age. Ear trims have been performed on dogs as old as nine to 12 months, but this is not advisable, as the chance of success decreases with age. A practical schedule is presented in Table 147–1.

Young puppies, especially those in less than ideal physical condition, should not be anesthetized with barbiturates alone. Induction with a short-acting barbiturate such as thiopentyl or thiamylal sodium is followed by intubation and maintenance of anesthesia with halothane and nitrous oxide or methoxyflurane. Atropine sulfate is given. Local injection of epinephrine, recommended by some to control bleeding along the incision site, should be discouraged owing to its systemic effect.

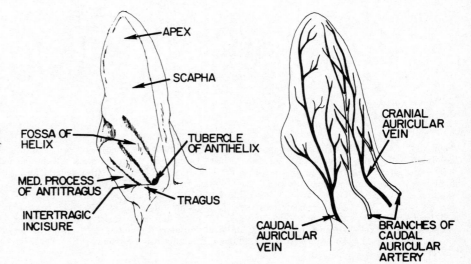

Figure 147–22. Anatomy and vasculature of the ear showing the tragus and antitragus cartilages and branches of the caudal auricular vein.

APEX

SCAPHA

FOSSA OF HELIX

TUBERCLE OF ANTIHELIX

MED. PROCESS OF ANTITRAGUS

TRAGUS

INTERTRAGIC INCISURE

CRANIAL AURICULAR VEIN

CAUDAL AURICULAR VEIN

BRANCHES OF CAUDAL AURICULAR ARTERY

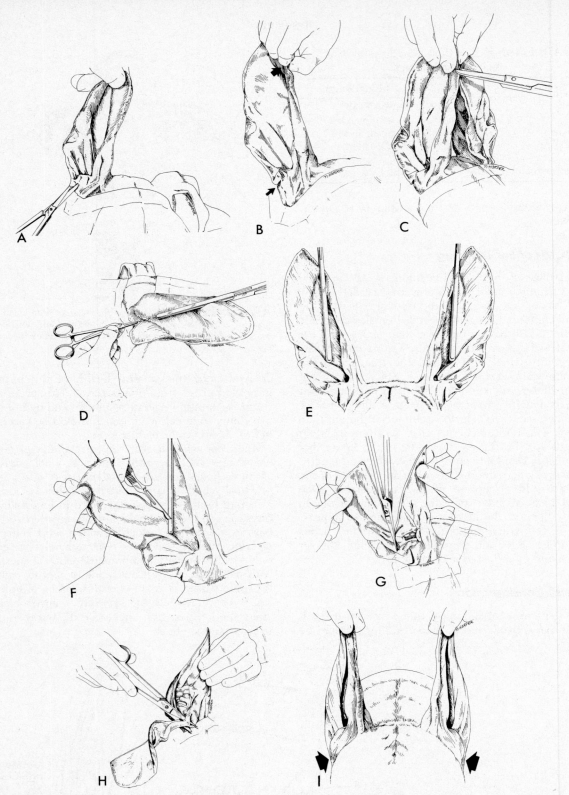

Figure 147–24. *A*, Initial skin incision beneath the tragus and antitragus cartilages serves as a future landmark. *B*, Position of the ear for determining the proper length. A small "pinch" mark is made on the rostal border of the ear with the index finger. *C*, Ears extended fully with the tips together. A small knick is made in both ears to insure identical length. *D*, Position of the ear for placing the intestinal forceps in an identical manner. The dotted line indicates the natural fold in the ear. *E*, Position of the forceps when viewed from a cranial position. The ears should be closely observed to insure that both forceps are placed in an identical position. *F*, Initial cut outside the forceps, stopping short of the end of the forceps. *G*, Continuation of the incision after removal of the forceps. No attempt is made to put a distinct "bell" in the distal one-third of the ear. *H*, Completion of the incision blending the ear to the side of the head. Portions of the tragus and antitragus cartilages are removed. The final portion of the incision joins the initial incision (see Fig. 147–29). *I*, Observation of the ears to insure that both are identical. Additional trimming may be necessary. Notice how the ears blend into the sides of the head *(arrows)*

Surgical Technique

Instruments such as ear trimming forms are often not satisfactory because placement is difficult and they usually fail to provide the type of trim desired. Finely serrated cartilage scissors are essential for performing the final trimming of the cartilage. With the dog in sternal recumbency and the head raised with a towel placed beneath it, the pinna and top of the head are prepared and draped for aseptic surgery (Figs. 147–22 and 147–23). Tape is placed across the muzzle to hold the head. Small pieces of cotton are placed in the external ear canal.

A triangular skin incision is made just beneath the tragus and antitragus cartilages where the ear joins the head; this landmark identifies the point where the ear blends to the dog's head (Fig. 147–24A). With one ear extended a ruler is used to measure along the rostral border of the ear, and a small nick is made at the desired length (Fig. 147–24B). Both ears are extended fully with the tips together, and a second nick is made in the other ear to insure identical length (Fig. 147–24C).

With one ear pulled forward and held in a stretched position to avoid wrinkling of the incision edge (Fig. 147–24D), Doyen intestinal forceps are placed on the ear, extending approximately two-thirds of the way from the "desired length" notch to the tragus cartilage. The forceps are placed so that the outside edge of the forceps is even with the knick at the top of the ear and the natural fold of the ear distally (Fig. 147–24D). Following placement of forceps on both ears, the ears are compared to insure identical positioning (Fig. 147–24E) and a straight cut from the proximal aspect to the junction of the middle and distal one-third. With the blade directed toward the edge of the intestinal forceps, the ear is incised with a scalpel. The incision stops just short of the rounded edges of the intestinal forceps, at the junction of the middle and distal thirds of the ear (Fig. 147–24F). The forceps are removed, and bleeding vessels are clamped with mosquito forceps, twisted, and pulled; they are not ligated. A branch of the caudal auricular artery is usually transected one-half of the distance from the ear tip to the tragus cartilage (see Fig. 147–23).

The distal third of the incision is made with finely serrated cartilage scissors. With the part of the ear to remain held in a normal standing position (Fig. 147–24G), the incision is continued to blend the distal one-third of the ear into the dog's head using a smooth, even cut (Fig. 147–24H), until the initial skin incision at the level of the tragus cartilage is reached. Rough edges are trimmed, and parts of the tragus and antitragus cartilages are removed to insure a smooth appearance. The opposite ear is trimmed in the same manner, the ears are compared (Fig. 147–24I), and adjustments are made as necessary, usually in the distal third of the cut.

Interrupted sutures are used to close the skin over the cut portion of the tragus cartilage and the skin defect distal to these cartilages (Figs. 147–25A and B). The main incision is closed with a simple continuous nonabsorbable suture, beginning at the ventral aspect of the incision. This suture passes through the skin edges only. Placement is from the inside out, so that the loose skin on the outside of the cartilage is rolled over the edge of the cartilage, allowing faster healing and less scar formation. The incision is closed to within six to 12 mm of the tip of the ear. The sutures are placed loosely and are left untied at the tips of the ear (Fig. 147–25C) to allow for postoperative swelling.

Postoperative Care

Many ears fail to stand because of improper aftercare. Scarring of the cut edge can produce undesirable effects such as contraction of the ear margin or unsightly blemishes. Some clients prefer the smooth, scarred hairless margin. The ears must be pulled above the head and stretched when taped or braced to obtain proper ear carriage, and examined closely for exudates, odors, and malpositioning.

Owners can be taught to tape their puppies' ears, although periodic examination by the veterinarian is essential. Tongue depressors, cotton-tipped applicators, foam inserts, wire racks,* wire ear implants,† and various other materials have been used for supporting the ear during the postoperative phase. Successful methods are as follows.

Rolled Gauze Sponge and Tape. After operation, the ears are cleaned of blood. Gauze sponges are formed into a cone and placed inside the ear, filling the base of the ear. A strip of gauze is placed along the suture line to prevent tape from contacting the incision. With the gauze cone in place and the ear held erect, tape is applied to the ear in a dovetail fashion. A brace formed of adhesive tape in a figure-of-eight around the base of the two ears keeps them parallel to each other (Fig. 147–26). This type of support for the ear is used for about two weeks—on for three days, off for one, on for three days, and so on. Sutures are removed at seven to ten days.

If the ears are not standing at two weeks, they are rolled in the direction opposite to that in which they are falling, and the tape is left in place for as long as five days at a time.

Cardboard Tube. After the sutures are removed at seven to ten days, the ears are held erect by using the cardboard tube of a regular tampon‡ with the cotton tampon left in place and the cotton end of the cardboard tube placed in the base of the ear. The ear is pulled or stretched above the head, and two strips of adhesive tape are used to secure the ear to the tube; one strip is placed around the base of the ear and the other is placed close to the tip. After two

---

*Shannon Ear Rack, Bayvet Corp., Shawnee Mission, KA.
†Behaney Ear Implant, Jorgenson Lab, Inc., Loveland, CO.
‡Tampax, Tampax, Inc., Palmer, MA.

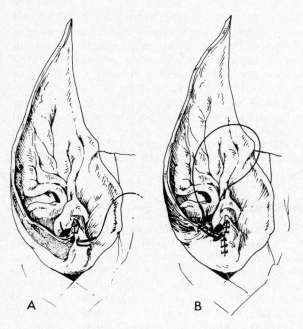
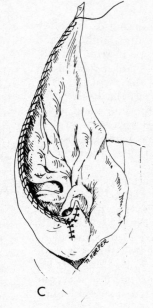

Figure 147–25. A and B, Initial closure with sutures placed through the skin edges only. C, Completion of the closure with interrupted sutures placed at the base of the ear and a continuous suture along the edge of the ear, stopping one-half inch from the tip. No attempt is made to tie the suture.

weeks, the cardboard tubes are discarded. Air foam with a piece of tape applied inside out is used to fill the bell at the base of the ear. The inside-out tape and a single strip of tape around the base of the ear are used to hold the foam in place. Another strip of tape close to the ear tip holds the ear in a rolled erect position. The foam is used repeatedly as needed until the ears stand permanently; it is changed when the ears become dirty or inflamed and as needed to check progress. The ears are cleaned each time the tapes are changed.

Styrofoam Cups. Immediately following surgery, while the dog is still anesthetized, a stand consisting of three styrofoam cups, one inside the other, is placed on the dog's head. A notch is cut into the cups at the base of the ears to accommodate the scutiform cartilage. A strip of tape is placed inside-out down the side of the cup, over the base, and down the other side. Strips of tape secure the inside-out tape in place. Elasticon* is applied to the front and rear edges of the cups to prevent slipping and rubbing of the cups on the head. Skin Bond† is applied to the medial and lateral surfaces of the ears, which are pulled high on the head and adhered to the cup stand. A final piece of tape is applied vertically on each ear and over the top of the cup to secure the ear in place.

The ears are left in the cup stand until they have healed completely. During this time, antibiotic ointment is applied to the healing edges of the ears to facilitate removal of scabs.

After the cup stand is removed, the cardboard tubes from coathangers are used for support. The tubes are cut long enough to extend from the tubercle of the anthelix to just past the end of the ear. The tube is padded at one end with Elasticon and placed in the ear, resting on the shelf formed by the tubercle of the anthelix. Tape is applied around the ear and tube both at the base and distally, and as a bridge between the ears.

The ear can remain taped in this way for as long as two weeks before retaping.

Complications

During recovery, bleeding should be controlled to prevent postoperative hematomas. Sutures should be snug but not tight.

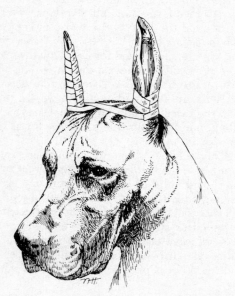

Figure 147–26. A 4 × 4 gauze sponge folded tightly in the shape of a cone is placed in the external ear canal. Short strips of one-inch adhesive tape are placed around the ear. A piece of tape is placed around the top of the head in a figure-of-eight fashion to hold the ears erect.

---

*Elasticon, Johnson & Johnson, New Brunswick, NJ.
†Skin Bond Cement, Skin Bond, Largo, FL.

The most severe problem, at least in the owner's eyes, is failure of the ears to stand. External support may be required for as long as 20 weeks. Despite prolonged efforts, ears may fail to stand. The most common problems are medial and lateral deviation of the tip of the ear (see later). Ear supports based inside the ear are particularly prone to cause otitis externa, which must be treated.

Corrective Ear Surgery

Ears that have been trimmed surgically may deviate laterally or medially. If discovered early, faulty ear carriage may be corrected by proper taping procedures, particularly in dogs less than six months of age.

Numerous techniques have been used to correct faulty ear carriage, most of which result in only slight improvement. Prosthetic devices such as stainless steel wire, Parham Martin bone bands, and collar stays have been inserted between the skin and cartilage to hold the ear erect. Scarification of the cartilage in the area of the break has also been used commonly, often resulting in a thickened cartilage and a worse ear carriage. Heterologous cartilage grafts have been used with varying degrees of success; infection is a problem and many cartilage grafts have had to be removed.

If the owner and veterinarian are patient and willing to put the animal through one or more surgical procedures, faulty ear carriage can usually be corrected. The direction of the break in the cartilage, the location of the break, and the position of the scutiform cartilage determine the surgical technique to be used and whether two or more procedures may be necessary.

Conservative Treatment

Conservative treatment must be started as soon as possible. The ear is rolled opposite to the way it is breaking. When the ear is deviated over the top of the head, or stands so that it is carried too far medially, it must be rolled away from the dog's head. The ear is grasped and pulled upward as tightly as possible. The index finger is placed in the external ear canal, and the ear is rolled away from the head around the finger. Starting close to the base of the ear, one-inch adhesive tape or masking tape in three- to five-inch strips is applied to the ear in the same direction as the roll. The tape is carried approximately two-thirds of the way from the base to the tip of the ear. The ear must be stretched tightly, pulling the scutiform cartilage toward the center of the head. Tape is left on the ear for five days, and the ear is observed for one day to see if improvement has occurred. Often, it is necessary to replace the tape for another week before faulty ear carriage is corrected. If there is little improvement after two weeks, corrective surgery is necessary.

With a lateral deviation of the ear, the index finger is inserted into the external canal, and the ear is pulled as tightly as possible and rolled toward the center of the head. Again, the tape is applied in the same direction as the roll. The ears look extremely awkward when taped in this position, but the end result is often good.

Surgical Correction

The ears are prepared and the animal is positioned as for ear trimming (Fig. 147–27).

Medial Deviation. In most instances, only one procedure is necessary. Usually, when the ear breaks toward the head, the scutiform cartilage has dropped ventrally, and there is a distinct fold in the cartilage on the medial aspect of the ear (Fig. 147–28A).

A longitudinal incision is made through the skin at the junction of the ear and the base of the skull, extending from approximately six millimeters caudal to the rostral edge of the ear to 12 to 16 mm cranial to the border of the ear (Fig. 147–28B). The incision is carried through the subcutaneous tissues, and the scutiform cartilage is exposed by blunt dissection (Fig. 147–28C). The cartilage is dissected free of its muscular attachments, pulled medially and slightly rostrally, and sutured to the temporal fascia using nonabsorbable sutures in a horizontal mattress pattern (Fig. 147–29). If this maneuver does not correct the deformity, it is necessary to remove an elliptical piece of skin at the break in the cartilage on the medial aspect of the ear. This latter procedure should be reserved for a later time, as often it is unnecessary. The subcutaneous tissues and skin are closed in routine fashion. A gauze sponge rolled into a cone is inserted into the ear. If necessary, a small strip of gauze sponge is placed over the incision site, and the ear is taped from the base to the tip while rolled away from the head.

Lateral Deviation. When the ear sits high on the head and the dog has good control of its base, the

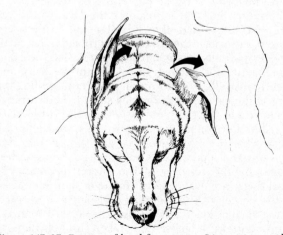

Figure 147–27. Position of head for surgery. Support is provided by placing a sandbag underneath the head. Note the lateral deviation of the left ear and medial deviation of the right ear (*arrows*).

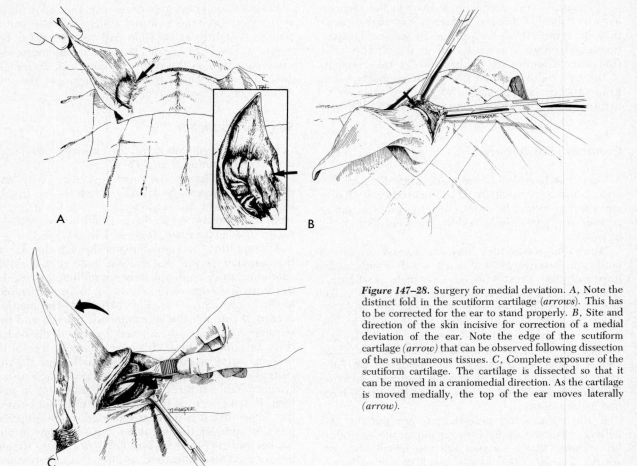

Figure 147–28. Surgery for medial deviation. *A*, Note the distinct fold in the scutiform cartilage *(arrows)*. This has to be corrected for the ear to stand properly. *B*, Site and direction of the skin incisive for correction of a medial deviation of the ear. Note the edge of the scutiform cartilage *(arrow)* that can be observed following dissection of the subcutaneous tissues. *C*, Complete exposure of the scutiform cartilage. The cartilage is dissected so that it can be moved in a craniomedial direction. As the cartilage is moved medially, the top of the ear moves laterally *(arrow)*.

only procedure necessary is removal of an elliptical piece of skin on the external surface at the level of the break (Fig. 147–30). The amount of skin to be removed is critical, since it is possible to create a medial deviation if too much is removed.

When the ear breaks at the base of the skull, a more involved surgical procedure is necessary. A longitudinal incision is made at the base of the ear (Fig. 147–30A) and the subcutaneous tissues are incised to expose the scutiform cartilage. The cartilage is partially dissected free from its muscular attachments and moved 12 to 16 mm medially and slightly rostrally from its original position, pulling the base of the ear closer to the dog's head. The cartilage is sutured to the temporal muscle fascia with nonabsorbable horizontal mattress sutures. An elliptical piece of skin is removed at the site of the skin incision, the amount of skin removed being determined by the severity of the lateral deviation. In most dogs, removal of 12 to 16 mm of skin, measured at the center of the elliptical incision, is necessary. The skin incision is closed using a vertical mattress suture pattern: a deep bite is taken through the skin on the skull, and the suture material is carried through the subcutaneous tissue, between the skin and scutiform cartilage, partially through the cartilage

itself, through the subcutaneous tissue between the skull and the ear, and then through the skin on the ear (Fig. 147–30B). The suture is continued by taking shallow bites through the skin edges. Tension is placed on the suture and the ear is pulled upward. One can determine the amount of tension to be placed on the suture material and the depth of the deep bites of the vertical mattress suture pattern by the position of the ear, which should stand with approximately a ten-degree lateral deviation (Fig. 147–30C). Usually three such sutures are needed to insure correct ear carriage. Either a vertical mattress or a simple interrupted suture pattern is used to complete the closure of the skin incision. A gauze sponge rolled into a cone is placed over the incision site and the ear is bandaged from the base to the tip (Fig. 147–30C).

The ear is left taped for three to five days and then rebandaged for five more days. If the operation has been successful, the ear should be standing in a relatively normal position at eight to ten days. If the ear fails to stand properly it may be necessary to remove another elliptical piece of skin. This incision should be made directly over the old scar. The skin edges are approximated with either vertical mattress or simple interrupted sutures. The second procedure

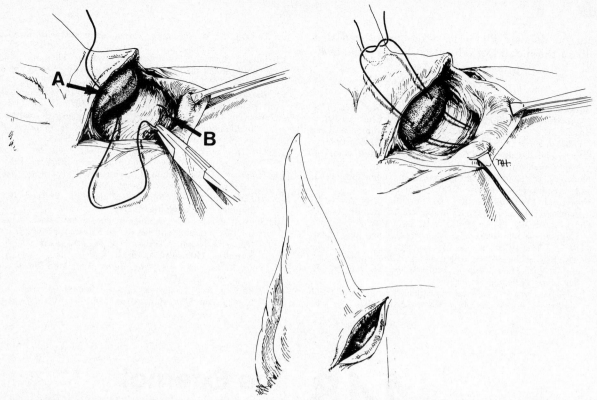

Figure 147–29. Proper placement of the mattress suture. The suture is placed through the cartilage and into the temporal fascia using a horizontal mattress suture pattern (*A* and *B*). When the suture is tied, the ear assumes the correct position. Closure is routine.

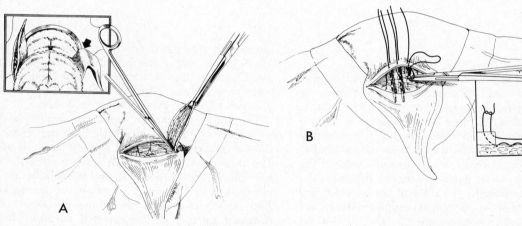

A

B

Figure 147–30. *A,* Location and direction of the skin incision for correction of a lateral deviation of the ear. Note that the incision is made directly over the "break" in the ear *(inset, arrow).* The amount of skin to be removed is determined by the severity of the deviation; it is better to remove too little than too much. *B,* Proper placement of three vertical mattress sutures. Note that the deep bite is carried through the subcutaneous tissues *(inset).* This is perhaps the most important step in the closure and ensures, in most instances, the correction of a lateral deviation. Proper tension on the sutures can be judged by the position of the ear when the sutures are tightened. *C,* Complete closure of the skin defect. Note that the ear stands with approximately a 10-degree lateral deviation. This is important because scar tissue will usually pull the ear medially. *Lower inset,* The ear is bandaged by placing a gauze sponge rolled in the shape of a cone in the external ear canal. The ear is folded around the sponge from both a cranial and caudal direction. Tape is applied in a "dovetail" fashion. The bandage is applied for three days. In most instances further bandaging is unnecessary.

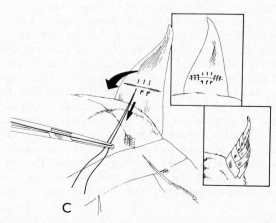

C

should be delayed for at least one month so that results of the initial procedure can be properly evaluated.

1. Bostock, D. E., and Owens, L. N.: *Neoplasia in the Cat, Dog and Horse*. Year Book Medical Publishers, Chicago, 1975.
2. Brodey, R. S., and Harvey, C. E.: Atresia of the vertical ear canal in a dog. J. Am. Vet. Med. Assoc. *155*:1457, 1969.
3. Cowley, F.: Treatment of hematoma of the canine ear. Vet. Med./Small Anim. Clin. *71*:283, 1976.
4. Dorn, C. R.: Epidemiology of canine and feline tumors. J. Am. Anim. Hosp. Assoc. *12*:307, 1976.
5. Fraser, G., Withers, A. R., and Spreull, J. S. A.: Otitis externa in the dog. J. Small Anim. Pract. *2*:32, 1961.
6. Getty, R., Foust, H. L., Presley, E. T., and Miller, M. E.: The macroscopic anatomy of the ear of the dog. Am. J. Vet. Res. *17*:364, 1956.
7. Getty, R. G.: The ear. *In* Miller, M. E., Christensen, G. C., and Evans, H. E. (eds.): *Anatomy of the Dog*. W. B. Saunders, Philadelphia, 1964.
8. Hardy, W. D., Jr.: General concepts of canine and feline tumors. J. Am. Anim. Hosp. Assoc. *12*:295, 1976.
9. Hayden, D. W.: Squamous carcinoma in a cat with intraocular and orbital metastases. Vet. Pathol. *13*:332, 1976.
10. Jabara, A. G.: A mixed tumor and an adenoma both of ceruminous gland origin in a dog. Aust. Vet. J. *52*:590, 1976.
11. Katsas, A., Agnantis, J., Smyrnis, S., et al.: Carcinomas on old frostbites. Am. J. Surg. *133*:377, 1976.
12. Mueller, G. H., and Kirk, R. W.: Feline solar dermatitis. *In*: *Small Animal Dermatology*. 2nd ed. W. B. Saunders, Philadelphia, 1976.
13. Ott, R. L.: Ears. *In* Archibald, J. (ed.): *Canine Surgery*. American Veterinary Publications, Santa Barbara, 1965.
14. Pandy, N. J.: Experimental production of "cauliflower ear" in rabbits. Plast. Reconstr. Surg. *53*:534, 1973.
15. Shambaugh, G. E.: *Surgery of the Ear*. 2nd ed. W. B. Saunders, Philadelphia, 1967.
16. Snow, J. B., Jr.: Surgical disorders of the ears, nose, paranasal sinuses, pharynx, and larynx. *In* Sabiston, D. C., Jr. (ed.): *Davis-Christopher Textbook of Surgery*. 12th ed. W. B. Saunders, Philadelphia, 1981.
17. Vine, L. L.: Corrective ear surgery. Vet. Med./Small Anim. Clin. *69*:1015, 1974.
18. Wilson, J. W.: Treatment of aural hematoma, using a teat tube. J. Am. Vet. Med. Assoc. *182*:1081, 1983.

Chapter **148**

The External Ear Canal
L. R. Grono

ANATOMY

The external ear canal is a cartilaginous tube lined by epithelium and extending from the auricle or pinna to the tympanic membrane (Fig. 148–1). At its proximal opening, the cartilaginous pinna is funnel-shaped. Proximally and medially, the aditus of the external auditory meatus, which faces dorsolaterally, is marked by the anthelix, a cartilaginous ridge of the conchal cartilage that has a prominent tubercle, the tubercle of the anthelix. The lateral border is formed by the tragus, and the antitragus completes the caudal border. The intertragic incisure marks the junction of the tragus and antitragus.

The external ear canal in the dog is long, about five to ten centimeters, and narrow, about four to seven millimeters in diameter.[33, 38] From the external aditus, the vertical canal runs ventrally and slightly rostrally before bending to become a horizontal canal that runs medially to the osseous external ear canal (Fig. 148–2). The vertical section is longer than the horizontal section. The horizontal canal is attached to the circular annular cartilage by ligamentous tissue, and the annular cartilage in turn is loosely connected to a short osseous external ear canal, a projection from the petrous temporal bone. The short osseous external ear canal, like the cartilaginous canal, is lined with epithelium and conducts sound waves and vibrations to the tympanic membrane, which forms part of the lateral border of the middle ear. The canal is not a smooth-sided tube; cartilaginous prominences partially occlude the lumen and may rub together when the ear is shaken.

The lining of the ear canal consists of stratified squamous epithelial cells with both sebaceous and tubular apocrine glands and varying amounts of hair. The sebaceous glands, which may be associated with hair follicles, are superficial, and the tubular apocrine glands are in the deeper connective tissue layer.[3] Both types of glands are more prevalent in the proximal portion of the external ear canal but do occur in the lining of the osseous canal. Ear wax is a mixed brown secretion from both of these glands that protects the canal and keeps the tympanic membrane moist and pliable.[1]

A greater number of sebaceous apocrine glands have been reported in long-eared dogs, such as cocker spaniels, than in short-eared dogs.[15]

The blood supply to the ear is via the great auricular artery, which arises from the external carotid artery medial to the dorsal apex of the parotid salivary gland. The great auricular artery gives rise to the intermediate, deep, lateral, and medial auricular vessels, which run on the convex side of the ear and anastomose at the tip of the pinna. The rostral/cutaneous base of the ear is supplied by the

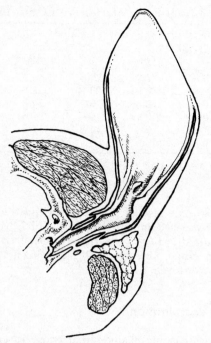

Figure 148–1. Anatomy of the external ear canal.

cranial auricular artery, which is a branch of the superficial temporal artery.

The great auricular nerve, a branch of the second cervical nerve, supplies the base of the concha and skin overlying the back of the neck. The retro-auricular nerve and auriculotemporal nerves are branches of the facial nerve, which lies under the proximal portion of the parotid gland in close proximity to the annular cartilage and its attachment to the osseous external ear canal. The sensory nerve supply to the external ear canal is via the auricular branch of the vagus nerve.

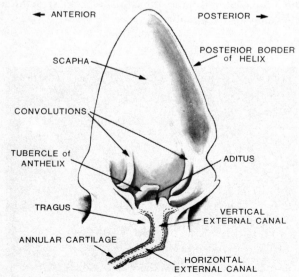

Figure 148–2. Sagittal section through external ear canal, showing auricular cartilage and the angular formation of the ear canal.

OTITIS EXTERNA

Otitis externa has been defined as an inflammation of the epithelium of the external auditory canal. The inflammation commonly involves the convolutions of the anthelix and the tubercle of the anthelix and may extend to involve the pinna. Otitis externa may also extend through the tympanic membrane to involve the middle ear.[36]

Incidence

Otitis externa is a common condition in the dog and cat. An incidence of three to 16 per cent has been recorded.[18, 30, 34] The condition has a worldwide occurrence, being prevalent in both temperate and tropical climates. In humans, a high incidence has been recorded in tropical environments[39] and in the warmer months of the year. No significant seasonal incidence has been recorded in the dog, although in two surveys the greatest number of cases was presented for treatment in the warmer months of the year.[18, 29]

Breeds with dependent ears or with hairy external auditory meatus, such as the cocker spaniel, Labrador retriever, and miniature poodle, develop otitis externa more commonly than other breeds.[15, 24, 29]

There does not appear to be any sex predisposition to the disease,[18] but the highest incidence appears to be in dogs between three and seven years of age.[15, 18, 29]

Pathophysiology

The microbiological populations of normal external ear canals and of ears with canine otitis externa have been widely reported in the literature.[4, 16, 31, 32, 37] Some of these findings are summarized in Table 148–1.

The gram-negative organisms *Pseudomonas* spp. and *Proteus* spp. are not commonly cultured from the normal external auditory meatus but are common in a large number of chronic cases of otitis externa, particularly in the Labrador retriever and cocker spaniel. Their exact role in the etiology is not clear, because attempts to produce the condition with these organisms have not been significantly successful.[19] These organisms are resistant to treatment (Table 148–2). They cause extensive pathological changes and render treatment more difficult. Ear mites, fungi, and foreign bodies have also been reported to cause otitis externa.[20, 38]

The microclimate of the external ear canal is favorable for the existence and proliferation of bacteria and fungi. The external ear canal in humans, which is much shorter (approximately 35 mm)[38] and less tortuous than that in the dog, has been described as a skin-lined test tube with an adequate blood supply.[11]

The microclimate in the canine ear canal has been investigated.[21–23] The mean temperature in the clinically normal external ear canal of 148 dogs was found

TABLE 148–1. Organisms Isolated from Normal Ear Canals and from Ears Affected with Otitis Externa

	Percentage of Ear Canals from Which Organisms Isolated*								
	Ref. 37		Ref. 31		Ref. 16		Ref. 32		Ref. 4
Organism	N	OE	N	OE	N	OE	N	OE	OE
Staphylococcus aureus	15.0	30.4	1.7	38.0	9.9	17.7	28.6	40.5	30.4
Pityrosporum spp.	6.0	23.0	28.3	86.2	16.8	56.9	20.6	34.8	44.3
Pseudomonas spp.	4.0	5.0	0	16.4	0	12.6	0	20.2	16.5
Proteus spp.	0	5.0	0	3.4	0	0.6	0	24.6	9.9
Streptococcus spp.	2.0	6.0	0	8.6	1.9	6.8	14.3	14.2	4.3
Aspergillus	—	—	—	—	0	0.6	—	—	1.1

*N = clinical normal ear canals; OE = ears affected by otitis externa.

to be 38.2°C, and the mean rectal temperature 0.6°C lower. Changes in environmental temperature had little effect on temperature of the external ear canal. No significant temperature difference was found between dogs with dependent ears and those with erect ears, but resection of the lateral wall of the vertical ear canal produced a drop in aural temperature of 0.6 to 1.0°C.

The pH of the clinically normal meatal surface in the dog has been recorded. The mean was 6.1, but that found in chronic purulent otitis externa was 6.8 to 7.4. The use of acid solutions to alter this pH resulted in a change of short duration. A 1.0 per cent solution of acetic acid in propylene glycol (pH 4.0) instilled into the meatus changed the pH for less than 60 minutes.

The relative humidity in the normal ear canal was 80 per cent. A rise of 24 per cent in atmospheric humidity was accompanied by a rise of 2.3 per cent in the humidity in the external ear canal. Humidity was, on average, nine per cent higher in ears affected with otitis externa.

Clinical Examination

The macroscopic changes that occur in ears with otitis externa are the result of inflammation. In some cases, the changes are hyperplastic, and the lumen of the ear canal is partially or completely blocked (Fig. 148–3). In other cases, the meatal epithelium is devitalized and ulcerated (Fig. 148–4).

Copious secretions from the sebaceous and apocrine glands, devitalized and necrotic epithelial cells, and debris accumulate in the meatus of affected ear canals. This secretion and debris plus the length and tortuous nature of the external meatus make thorough examination of the meatus difficult. Sedation or general anaesthesia is necessary to avoid further injury to the devitalized or ulcerated epithelium. A 6.0-cm speculum with a good light source that focuses at the end of the speculum is necessary to examine the horizontal external ear canal. Gentle traction to pull the pinna laterally and dorsally helps to straighten the canal for examination.

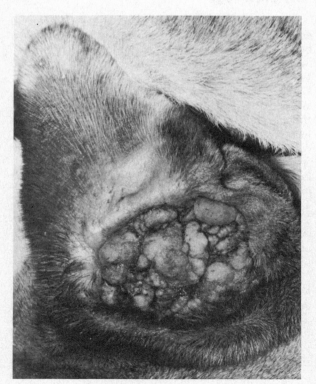

Figure 148–3. Severe hyperplastic otitis externa obstructing the external ear canal opening of a dog.

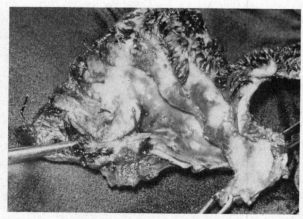

Figure 148–4. Widespread ulceration of the ear canal epithelium in a dog with otitis externa.

TABLE 148–2. Results of Sensitivity Tests of 467 Swabs from Canine Ears Affected with Otitis Externa

Drug	Sensitivity*	Percentage of Organisms						
		Pseudomonas	Proteus	S. aureus	Coliforms	Streptococci	Diphtheroids	Micrococci
Penicillin	S	0.0	11.8	60.9	0.0	100.0	75.0	50.0
	R	100.0	88.2	39.1	100.0	0.0	25.0	50.0
Streptomycin	S	46.2	52.9	95.4	66.7	60.0	50.0	100.0
	R	53.8	47.1	4.6	33.3	40.0	50.0	0.0
Chloramphenicol	S	3.8	58.8	97.7	55.6	100.0	100.0	100.0
	R	96.2	41.2	2.3	44.4	0.0	0.0	0.0
Tetracyclin	S	25.0	17.6	92.0	44.4	100.0	100.0	100.0
	R	75.0	82.4	8.0	55.6	0.0	0.0	0.0
Ampicillin	S	0.0	11.8	69.0	0.0	100.0	75.0	100.0
	R	100.0	88.2	31.0	100.0	0.0	25.0	0.0
Trimethoprim/sulfadiazine	S	3.8	29.4	66.7	33.3	20.0	50.0	100.0
	R	96.2	70.6	33.3	66.7	80.0	50.0	0.0
Neomycin	S	86.5	76.5	97.7	77.8	80.0	50.0	100.0
	R	13.5	23.5	2.3	22.2	20.0	50.0	0.0
Polymyxin B	S	86.5	0.0	97.7	77.8	80.0	75.0	100.0
	R	13.5	100.0	2.3	22.2	20.0	25.0	0.0
Gentamycin	S	100.0	88.2		100.0			
	R	0.0	11.8		0.0			
Carbenicillin	S	64.7	82.4		100.0			
	R	35.3	17.6		0.0			

*S = sensitive; R = resistant. (Reprinted with permission from Grono, L. R.: Otitis externa. In Kirk, R. W. (ed.): *Current Veterinary Therapy VII.* W. B. Saunders, Philadelphia, 1980.)

1. History—with special reference to:
   a. Other skin conditions.
   b. Previous treatment.
   c. Response to treatment and relapse.
2. General clinical examination, looking especially for:
   a. Head tilt.
   b. Local pain.
   c. Fluid in meatus
3. Sedation or anaesthesia.
4. Swab for culture and sensitivity testing.
5. Examination with otoscope for:
   a. Mites.
   b. Foreign bodies.
6. Irrigation and drying of meatus.
7. Reexamination with otoscope of:
   a. Vertical canal.
   b. Horizontal canal.
   c. Tympanic membrane.
8. Decision as to medical or surgical treatment.
   a. Surgical treatment—see text.
   b. Medical treatment:
      (1) Treatment according to etiology obtained or clinical picture.
      (2) Reassessment in seven to ten days.
      (3) Treatment according to results of culture and sensitivity testing.
      (4) If no response or response and then relapse, surgical treatment should be used.

Figure 148–5. Plan for examination and treatment of otitis externa.

Examination of the external ear canal and the medical treatment of otitis externa have been reviewed recently.[24, 26] The plan outlined in Figure 148–5 may be used to aid the diagnosis and treatment of otitis externa. Procedures 1 to 7 are used on all cases presented; the clinical findings then determine whether medical or surgical treatment is adopted.

Surgical Treatment

The need for surgical treatment of otitis externa has been recognized for some time. The surgical treatment of both ulcerative and proliferative otitis externa in 14 dogs was reported by Berge[2] in 1922, and removal of a V-shaped piece of tragus was recorded in 1931 by Formston and McCunn.[14] Hinz[28] in 1936 described techniques used in 1853 and 1892. The history of the surgical treatment of otitis externa has been reviewed recently.[27]

Surgical treatment of otitis externa is indicated in those cases in which:

(1) The disease has failed to respond to medical treatment; (2) the disease has responded to treatment but a relapse has occurred; (3) extensive pathological changes, such as hyperplasia or severe ulceration of the meatal epithelium or ossification of the meatal cartilage,[5, 8] have developed; (4) there are well-developed predisposing factors for the condition, such as a very hirsute meatus or narrow lumen; and (5) neoplasia[42] or congenital malformation[6] is present.

Three basic surgical procedures are used: resection of the lateral cartilaginous wall of the vertical canal with formation of a ventral cartilaginous flap (Zepp's

operation), total resection of the vertical external ear canal, and total ablation of the cartilaginous ear canal with or without drainage of the middle ear.[8]

Preparation for Surgery

The pinna and an extensive area of the lateral and ventral surface of the ear and face should be clipped. The pinna and aditus of the external ear canal are cleaned with chlorhexidine, cetrimide, or povidone-iodine solution. The external ear canal is thoroughly irrigated with one of these solutions using a five-milliliter syringe and polythene tubing. Povidone-iodine, one per cent (1 in 4) solution, has been reported to be ototoxic, but a 1 in 10 solution is not.[35] Excess solution is aspirated from the meatus prior to surgical intervention. With the dog in lateral recumbency, the pinna and skin over the lateral surface of the external ear canal should receive a final preparation for surgery.

Operative Procedures

The indications for each operation are summarized in Table 148–3.

Resection of the Lateral Cartilaginous Wall of the External Ear Canal with the Formation of a Ventral Cartilaginous Flap (Zepp's Procedure). This is the most common surgical procedure performed.

A probe is introduced into the canal to mark the direction and extent of its vertical section (Fig. 148–6). Allis tissue forceps are placed on the tragus at the aditus to apply gentle dorsal traction. Two parallel skin incisions are made over the ventral and caudal borders of the external surface of the vertical canal and extended below the junction of the vertical and horizontal canals. These incisions should extend approximately half the length of the vertical canal below the junction of vertical and horizontal skin incisions. The skin flap is dissected free dorsally to the aditus and excised at the proximal edge of the

TABLE 148–3. Indications for Surgical Procedures in Otitis Externa

Procedure	Indications
Zepp's operation	Congenital atresia or occlusion of the meatus
	Excessively hairy or narrow meatus
	Severe ulceration
	Proliferative or verrucous meatus with occluded lumen
	Inflammatory polyp
Ablation of vertical canal	Neoplasia
	Proliferation of vertical canal
	Partial failure to canalize
Total ablation of external ear canal	Failure of response to Zepp's operation
	Neoplasia

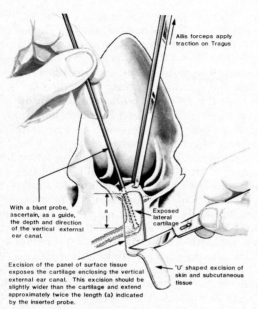

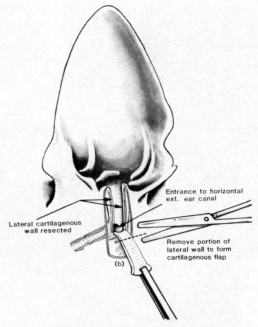

Figure 148–6. Zepp's procedure: extent of vertical section of external ear canal.

Figure 148–8. Zepp's procedure (continued).

tragus. Care should be taken to avoid the cranial auricular artery. Traction is reapplied on the tragus and, keeping close to the cartilaginous canal, blunt dissection is used to free overlying cutaneous tissue, part of the depressor auricularis muscle, and the dorsal apex of the parotid gland to expose the annular cartilage. Straight scissors are used to incise the lateral cartilage at its rostral and caudal borders (Fig. 148–7). The full lateral width of the cartilage can be incised once the canal has been exposed. The parallel incisions terminate just beyond the junction of vertical and horizontal sections of the canal. This flap is reflected ventrally, the dorsal half of the portion reflected is excised (Fig. 148–8), and the remaining portion is pulled ventrally so that the surgeon looks

straight into the horizontal section of the external ear canal. The ventral flap is sutured into position using a nonabsorbable, nonirritant suture material, such as 3-0 or 4-0 monofilament polypropylene or nylon. Simple interrupted sutures unite the edges of the skin incision and edges of the cartilage. The cartilaginous flap should be sutured so that it does not occlude the newly formed aditus (Figs. 148–9 and 148–10). All sutures should take a firm bite of cartilage and skin and should not be tied tightly, because some postoperative inflammation will occur. The following results of Zepp's operation have been re-

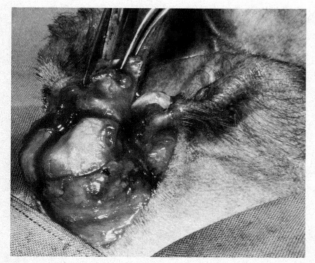

Figure 148–7. Straight Mayo scissors are used to incise the ear canal cartilage.

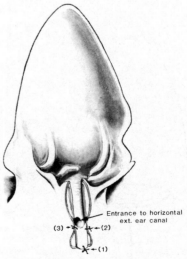

Figure 148–9. Suturing is commenced with a main "holding suture" (1), which maintains moderate tension on the flap of cartilage, ensuring that the entrance to the horizontal canal is permanently exposed. Sutures (2) and (3) further ensure that the lower end of the vertical canal remains open.

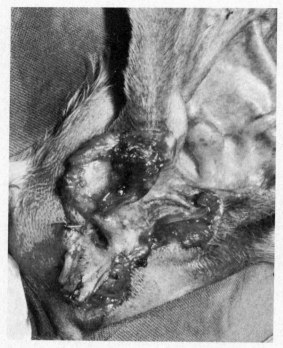

Figure 148–10. Unobstructed new aditus into the horizontal external ear canal.

ported: between 41 and 66 per cent cured, between 12 and 33 per cent with some improvement, and between 14 and 35 per cent with no improvement.[15, 17, 18, 26, 44]

Total Resection of the Vertical External Ear Canal. This procedure is indicated when hyperplasia of the meatal epithelium of the vertical canal has occurred but the horizontal canal is not involved or when neoplasia involves the vertical canal.

Preparation and placement for surgery are as for lateral resection.

A T-shaped incision is made, extending beyond the length of the vertical canal. The dorsal arm of the T is made parallel to the proximal edge of the tragus (Fig. 148–11). Two skin flaps are formed and reflected. The cartilaginous canal is exposed down to the annular cartilage. A hand retractor may be used to retract the proximal portion of the parotid gland. The vertical canal is freed by dissecting around its medial aspect, keeping close to the cartilage. A transverse incision is made across the canal above the level of the annular cartilage. Allis tissue forceps are used to grip the lateral distal edge of the vertical canal, and gentle upward traction is applied while the vertical canal is freed medially. The proximal arm of the initial T-shaped incision is extended to pass around the concave surface of the conchal cartilage above the anthelix and tubercle of the anthelix. This incision should pass just through cartilage, because the blood vessels previously described run along the convex surface of this cartilage. The funnel-shaped cartilage is excised. The horizontal canal is sutured to the ventral portion of the skin incision using simple interrupted sutures. The remainder of the T-shaped incision is closed with similar sutures.

This procedure can be modified to form a ventral flap to avoid stricture and hair regrowth at the new aditus to the horizontal canal. One author reported that total resection of the vertical canal for the treatment of chronic otitis externa in 75 dogs resulted in 72 being asymptomatic within 12 weeks postoperatively.[41]

Total Ablation of the Cartilaginous External Ear Canal. This procedure has been reported in the literature but it should be used as a last resort. It is indicated when marked hyperplasia or ulcerative changes are present in the horizontal ear canal. When coexisting otitis media is present, a bulla-osteotomy should be performed.

The procedure is the same as that for removal of

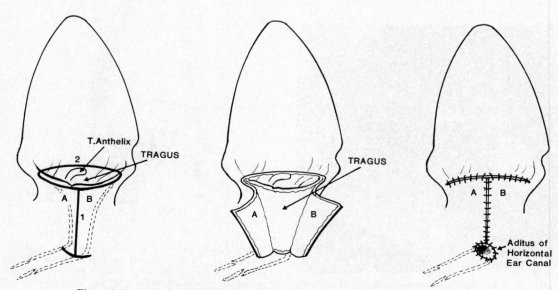

Figure 148–11. Total resection of the vertical external ear canal. See text for explanation.

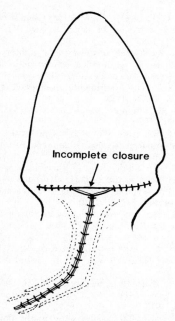

Figure 148–12. Total ablation of cartilaginous external ear canal. See text for explanation.

the vertical canal, except that the horizontal canal together with the annular cartilage is removed from its ligamentous attachment to the short osseous external ear canal. A small curette is used to remove the epithelial lining of the osseous canal.

The vertical arm of the T-shaped incision is closed with simple interrupted sutures, and both rostral and caudal edges of the dorsal horizontal arm are sutured, but the center of the incision is not closed (Fig. 148–12). This permits broad-spectrum antibiotic preparations (neomycin, polymyxin B, and bacitracin or gentamicin) to be instilled daily for four to five days postoperatively. The area is then allowed to fill with granulation tissue (Fig. 148–13). Complete clo-

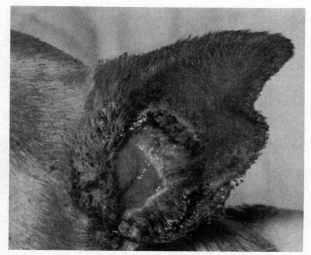

Figure 148–13. External ear canal ablation. The incision is left open dorsally to heal by granulation.

sure of the skin incision may lead to sinus formation in some cases.

Care should be taken not to injure the facial nerve and great auricular artery, which are medial to the parotid gland and close to the osseous external canal.

The results of total ablation reported in the literature vary from consistently good to postoperative sinus formation. Total ablation of the external ear canal in eight dogs resulted in seven being cured and sinus formation developing nine weeks postoperatively in one.[18, 40, 43] Total ablation of 26 ear canals with severe hyperplastic otitis externa combined with a lateral bulla-osteotomy was performed on 13 dogs: no sinus formation had developed in these dogs six months postoperatively.[8]

Postoperative Care

The indications for surgical treatment have been considered, and most surgical cases are those that have failed to respond to medical treatment. The results of a bacterial culture and sensitivity tests should be available prior to surgery so that the appropriate antibiotic can be used. When possible, the antibiotic should be administered immediately prior to surgery, given in high dosage and for a short duration. The aminoglycoside antibiotics (gentamicin, streptomycin) have disadvantages, in that the potentially toxic blood levels are only slightly higher than the levels required to inhibit the organisms for which they are prescribed. The use of antibiotics is not a substitute for good surgical technique.[7] The area is infected and tissues are devitalized and necrotic, so that removal of foreign material, debridement, the establishment of good drainage, and the control of hemorrhage are particularly important.

Postoperative care following both Zepp's operation and total resection of the vertical canal have been reviewed.[9, 10] Sedation, bandaging, and the use of Elizabethan collar and plastic buckets to protect the site from patient-inflicted trauma have been recommended. The minimum of postoperative restraint is desirable and varies with the temperament of the individual patients. Sutures should be removed ten to 14 days postoperatively.

Complications

Untoward sequelae that may occur following lateral resection are:

1. Poor exposure of the horizontal canal due to puckering of the ventral flap and occlusion of the new aditus, or stricture at the new aditus. Partial occlusion may be corrected by freeing the drainage flap from surrounding tissue, removing more skin ventrally, and resuturing the flap. The surgeon should now be able to look straight into the horizontal canal. Repositioning the flap may correct partial stricture; rarely, ablation of the meatus is required.

2. Wound dehiscence and poor subsequent ventilation. Poor healing and suture breakdown may occur as meatal epithelium is commonly devitalized and infection may be difficult to control. Sutures should be removed and the area allowed to granulate.

Following total resection of the vertical canal, stricture at the aditus to the horizontal canal or partial occlusion of the new aditus due to hair growth may occur. A ventral cartilaginous flap, as in Zepp's procedure, may be used to overcome these sequelae.

Total ablation of the cartilaginous external ear canal may cause sinus formation or facial nerve damage. Sinus formation is due to a focus of infection remaining in the osseous canal, or otitis media. Ventral drainage via bulla-osteotomy and irrigation of the sinus and middle ear is required. Facial nerve damage is not common and may be due to postoperative swelling. Mild facial nerve damage normally is of temporary duration.

Otitis Externa in the Cat

Otitis externa occurs less commonly in the cat than the dog, possibly because the cat's erect pinna gives better ventilation and drainage.[13] Etiology and clinical types are similar to those in the dog. Both inflammatory polyps and neoplasms have been recorded.[25] Surgical treatment and management are the same as in the dog.

1. Banks, W. J.: *Applied Veterinary Histology.* Williams & Wilkins, Baltimore, 1981.
2. Berge, E.: Ueber die otitis externa des hundes. Berl. Tierarztl. Wschr. *38*:38, 1922.
3. Bojrab, M. J., and Renergar, W. R.: The ear. *In* Bojrab, M. J. (ed.): *Pathophysiology in Small Animal Surgery.* Lea & Febiger, Philadelphia, 1981.
4. Deleted during publication.
5. Brizard, A., and Pomies J. L.: Ossification of the ear cartilages. Rev. Med. Vet. *114*:269, 1963.
6. Brodey, R. S., and Harvey, C. E.: Atresia of the vertical ear canal in a dog. J. Am. Vet. Med. Assoc. *155*:1457, 1969.
7. Burnett, W.: *Clinical Science for Surgeons.* Butterworths Pty Ltd., Sydney, 1981.
8. Cechner, P.: Total ablation of the ear canal and middle ear drainage. Ann. Mtg. Am. Coll. Vet. Surg., 1982.
9. Coffey, D. J.: Observations on the surgical treatment of otitis externa in the dog. J. Small Anim. Pract. *11*:265, 1970.
10. Coffey, D. J.: Lateral ear drainage for otitis externa. *In* Bojrab, M. J. (ed.): *Current Techniques in Small Animal Surgery.* Lea & Febiger, Philadelphia, 1975.
11. Collins, E. G.: Certain observations of the anatomy, histopathology and physiology of the external auditory meatus. J. Laryngol. Otol. *65*:112, 1951.
12. Elkins, A. D., Hedlund, C. S., and Hobson, H. P.: Surgical management of ossified ear canals in the canine. Vet. Surg. *10*:163, 1981.
13. Ellett, E. W., and Bowen, J. A.: *Feline Medicine and Surgery.* American Veterinary Publications, Santa Barbara, 1964.
14. Formston, C., and McCunn, J.: A surgical treatment for chronic otorrhoea in the dog. Vet. J. 87:112, 1931.
15. Fraser, G., Gregor, W. W., Mackenzie, C. P., et al.: Canine ear disease. J. Small Anim. Pract. *10*:725, 1970.
16. Gedek, B., Brutzel, K., Gerlach, R., et al.: The role of *Pityrosporum pachydermatis* in otitis externa in the dog. Vet. Rec. *104*:138, 1979.
17. Gregory, C. R., and Vasseur, P. B.: Clinical results of lateral ear canal resection in dogs. J. Am. Vet. Med. Assoc. *182*:1087, 1983.
18. Grono, L. R.: A study of the external auditory meatus in the dog with reference to inflammatory conditions. Ph.D. thesis, University of Queensland, 1967.
19. Grono, L. R.: The experimental production of otitis externa. Vet. Rec. *94*:34, 1969.
20. Grono, L. R.: Studies of the ear mite, *Otodectes cynotis.* Vet. Rec. *95*:6, 1970.
21. Grono, L. R.: Studies of the microclimate of the external auditory canal in the dog. I: Aural temperature. Res. Vet. Sci. *11*:307, 1970.
22. Grono, L. R.: Studies of the microclimate of the external auditory canal in the dog. II: Hydrogen ion concentration of the epithelial surface of the external auditory meatus. Res. Vet. Sci. *11*:312, 1970.
23. Grono, L. R.: Studies of the microclimate of the external auditory canal in the dog. III: Relative humidity within the external auditory meatus. Res. Vet. Sci. *11*:316, 1970.
24. Grono, L. R.: Otitis externa. *In* Kirk, R. W. (ed.): *Current Veterinary Therapy VII.* W. B. Saunders, Philadelphia, 1980.
25. Harvey, C. E., and Goldschmidt, M. H.: Inflammatory polypoid growths in the ear of cats. J. Small Anim. Pract. *10*:669, 1978.
26. Harvey, C. E.: Ear canal disease in the dog. J. Am. Vet. Med. Assoc. *177*:136, 1980.
27. Harvey, C. E.: A history of surgical management of otitis externa. Vet. Surg. 9:150, 1980.
28. Hinz, W.: Contribution to the operative treatment of otitis verrucosa in the dog. Vet. J. 92:6, 1936.
29. Karatzias, C., and Sarris, K.: Otitis externa in the dog. Hellenic Vet. Med. 23:175, 1980.
30. Kral, F., and Schwartzman, R. M.: *Veterinary and Comparative Dermatology.* J. B. Lippincott, Philadelphia, 1964.
31. Marshall, M. J., Harris, A. M., and Horne, J. M.: The bacteriological and clinical assessment of a new preparation for the treatment of otitis externa in dogs and cats. J. Small Anim. Pract. *15*:401, 1974.
32. McCarthy, G., and Kelly, W. R.: Microbial species associated with the canine ear and their antibacterial sensitivity patterns. Irish Vet. J. *36*:53, 1982.
33. Moltzen, H.: Otitis media in the dog and cat. *In* Catcott, E. J. (ed.): *Advances in Small Animal Practice III.* Pergamon Press, Oxford, 1962.
34. Moltzen, H.: Canine ear disease. J. Small Anim. Pract. *10*:589, 1969.
35. Morizono, T., and Sikoro, M. A.: The ototoxicity of topically applied povidone-iodine preparations. Arch. Otolaryngol. *108*:210, 1982.
36. Neer, M. T., and Howard, P. E.: Otitis media. Comp. Contin. Ed. *4*:410, 1982.
37. Sampson, G. R., Bowen, R. E., Murphy, C. N., and Schneider, J.: Clinical evaluation of a topical ointment. Vet. Med. Small Anim. Clin. 68:978, 1973.
38. Scott, D. W.: The ear. *In* Catcott, E. J. (ed.): *Canine Medicine IV.* American Veterinary Publications, Santa Barbara, 1979.
39. Senturia, B. H.: *Diseases of the External Ear.* Charles C Thomas, Springfield, 1957.
40. Seward, C. O., Blackmore, W. M., and Ott, R. L.: Treatment of chronic otitis externa by ablation of the ear canal. J. Am. Vet. Med. Assoc. *133*:417, 1958.
41. Siemering, G. H.: Resection of the vertical ear canal for treatment of chronic otitis externa. J. Amer. Hosp. Assoc. *16*:753, 1980.
42. Swaim, S. F.: *Surgery of Traumatized Skin.* W. B. Saunders, Philadelphia, 1980.
43. Spreull, J. S. A.: Ablation of the ear canal. *In* Bojrab, M. J. (ed.): *Current Techniques in Small Animal Surgery.* Lea & Febiger, Philadelphia, 1975.
44. Tufvesson, G.: Operation for otitis externa in dogs according to Zepps' method. Am. J. Vet. Res. *16*:565, 1955.

ANATOMY

The middle ear is a cavity lined by ciliated columnar epithelium, surrounded by bone, and situated on the caudoventrolateral aspect of the skull. The major, ventral part of the cavity is formed by the tympanic bulla, a rounded prominence consisting of thin bone. This part of the cavity is normally empty. A smaller, dorsal extension of the cavity is formed by the petrous part of the temporal bone and contains the ear ossicles. There are several openings. The largest is the lateral opening, which is covered by the tympanic membrane, which separates the middle ear cavity from the horizontal canal. One of the ear ossicles, the malleus, is partly embedded in the medial surface of the tympanic membrane.

On the medial surface of the middle ear cavity is the opening of the auditory tube (eustachian tube), which takes a short, angled pathway to the nasopharynx; there is no membranous covering to the opening of the auditory tube. Smaller openings are concerned with the neurological function of the ear. The cochlear (round) window is covered with a membrane similar to the tympanic membrane, and the vestibular (oval) window is occupied by the base of the stapes, thus forming an articulated bony chain from the tympanic membrane to the inner ear. The middle ear also contains muscles to tense the tympanic membrane and is traversed by a nerve, the chorda tympani, that goes from the facial to the lingual (trigeminal) nerve, carrying parasympathetic efferent fibers controlling the glands of the head. Several important structures run in bony channels or in soft tissue adjacent to the middle ear; these include the facial, auditory, and vagus nerves and the carotid (maxillary) and lingual arteries.

The two major functions of the ear are reception of auditory signals and maintenance of balance. These functions are carried out in the inner ear, a series of fluid-filled spaces where vibrations are converted into neural impulses. The three ear ossicles in the middle ear amplify sound waves received by the tympanic membrane and transmit them to the vestibular window.

METHODS OF EXAMINATION

Examination of the middle ear is difficult. Abnormalities are palpable only if there is gross swelling; most middle ear disease is confined to within the bullae and thus is not palpable. Generally, the bullae are palpable only through the pharynx by sliding a finger caudally from the hard palate. The first struc-

tures met are the hamular processes of the pterygoid bones, which form the lateral support of the caudal end of the nasal cavity. The bullae lie just caudal and lateral to the hamulae. The bullae normally feel rounded and smooth and are about the size of the tip of a finger. They are palpated for asymmetry and surface roughness.

The tympanic membrane can be examined with an otoscope through the ear canal, although this is often less than satisfactory.[21] A rigid fiberoptic telescope may give a better view of the tympanum.[20] It is almost impossible to examine the tympanic membrane thoroughly without anesthesia, even in a cooperative animal, as there is often some discharge in the horizontal canal that requires suction for effective removal. The normal tympanic membrane consists of two parts. The larger pars tensa is a thinly stretched membrane that appears translucent everywhere except dorsocranially, where the base of the malleus is visible through it. The crescent-shaped, dense, white malleus is surrounded by a visible blood vessel that gives off radiating branches. The smaller pars flaccida is an opaque, pink membrane located dorsocranial to the pars tensa that billows laterally.

Ear canal disease is very common in dogs in which tympanic membrane examination is indicated, and hyperplasia or stricture may obscure the tympanic membrane. When the tympanic membrane can be seen, it prevents examination of the cavity of the middle ear; unfortunately, an intact tympanic membrane does not eliminate the possible presence of middle ear disease. Examination of the tympanic membrane with an otoscope does allow collection of specimens for bacterial and fungal culture and, occasionally, biopsy.

The other opening in the middle ear cavity, the auditory tube, is of no help clinically; it is hidden above the soft palate, requiring anesthesia even for access. It can be cannulated with thin plastic tubing to obtain samples by aspiration or for irrigating the middle ear cavity,[10] although for both of these purposes the tympanic membrane route is simpler and more direct.

Radiographs are often used to examine the middle ear,[7] although here also there are many limitations. Gross bony changes on the surface of the bullae are often visible on oblique or lateral views of the skull (Fig. 149–1A). An open mouth projection made with the animal under anesthesia is necessary to show details of the cavity of the bullae (Fig. 149–1B). A ventrodorsal view may show bony changes of the more deeply situated petrous temporal area (Fig. 149–1C). Contrast radiography (injection of an aqueous contrast medium into the external ear canal)

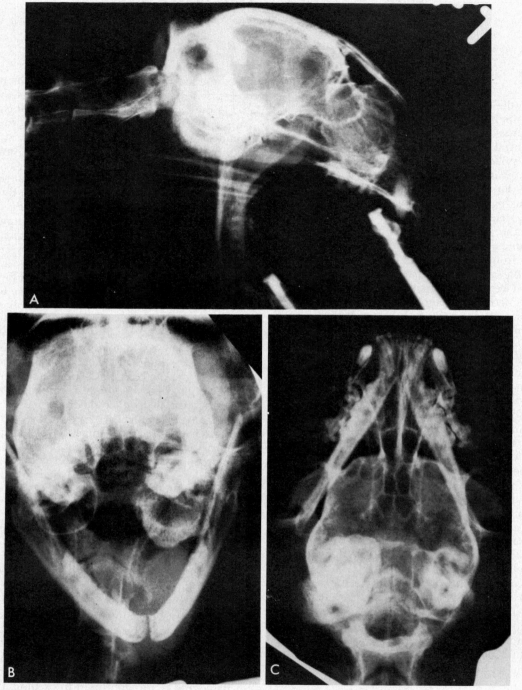

Figure 149–1. Unilateral middle ear disease in a cat. *A,* Lateral projection. *B,* Open mouth projection. *C,* Ventrodorsal projection.

is useful in occasional cases to show the position and size of the ear canal and may indicate rupture of the tympanic membrane in an animal in which the tympanic membrane cannot be adequately examined with an otoscope. Injection of contrast medium into a fistula on the side of the face may demonstrate that the middle ear is the site of chronic infection causing the fistula. There remain many dogs with middle ear

disease in which the diagnosis is not greatly assisted by radiographic examination.

Animals with obvious neurological deficits, such as circling, nystagmus, or inability to maintain an upright posture (all generally referred to as vestibular abnormalities) are easy to diagnose. However, there are many, indeed probably the majority of dogs, with middle ear disease that do not show neurological

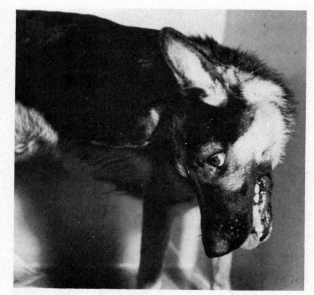

Figure 149–2. Severe head tilt in a dog with acute middle ear disease.

deficits. Head tilt (Fig. 149–2) is not included in the previous list of vestibular abnormalities, as it is not always clear whether the head tilt is due to interference with the sense of balance or, as in many dogs, the result of pain caused by external ear canal disease.

Objective, electronic means of evaluating middle ear anatomy and function include tympanometry and measurement of auditory-evoked brain stem potentials.[19] The clinical relevance of these tests in dogs is under investigation.

MIDDLE EAR DISEASES

Congenital Abnormalities

Congenital abnormalities affecting the middle ear are rarely diagnosed. Congenital deafness of dogs and cats caused by inner ear abnormalities is not treatable by surgery.

Trauma

The most common cause of injury affecting the middle ear cavity is rupture of the tympanic membrane by otitis externa or its treatment. Disease resulting from rupture of the tympanic membrane is considered hereafter under Infection. External trauma occasionally causes fracture or crushing injury of the bones of the middle ear. Initial treatment is conservative. Long-term effects usually present as chronic external ear canal disease or head tilt. Bony disruption is obvious on radiographs but may not appear as an obvious fracture, as periosteal response to the injury or chronic infection may cause blurring

of the edges. The only treatment presently available is decompression of the middle ear cavity by bulla osteotomy. This is described hereafter.

Infection

Infection is the major category of disease of the middle ear, although it is unclear in most cases whether the infection is primary or secondary to trauma. The most common cause of middle ear disease in the dog is extension of external ear canal disease through a damaged tympanic membrane; most of these animals do not show clinical signs referrable to the middle ear. Many dogs with chronic external ear canal disease develop recurrent disease because of an unrecognized focus of infection in the middle ear that periodically spills over into the external ear.[21] This avenue for discharge prevents the build-up of sufficient pressure in the middle ear cavity to cause the neurological deficits classically associated with middle ear disease. Occasionally, infection escapes from the bulla and spreads ventral to the skull (Fig. 149–3), appearing as a fistula on the side of the face.

Clinical Signs

The clinical signs of infection of the middle ear are chronic or recurrent discharge from the external ear canal, with or without pain on manipulating the ears, and head tilt. There is often some response to medication instilled into the affected ear, although there is also gradual development of resistant infections as different antibiotics are used. The end result is often a severe, nonresponsive *Proteus* or *Pseudomonas* infection. The severity of clinical signs and rapidity

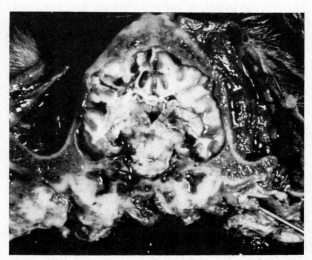

Figure 149–3. Skull of a dog with spreading middle ear infection causing osteomyelitis of the base of the skull (white areas at bottom). A probe is in the ear canal on one side.

of recurrence are often a function of the severity of pathological change in the horizontal ear canal. Head tilt does not automatically indicate active disease of the inner ear but may result from external ear canal pain; inflammation, granulation, or scarring of the middle ear epithelium covering; or reactive periosteal new bone formation around the cochlear window. When there are no neurological abnormalities, treatment is based on clinical intuition. Middle ear disease should always be suspected in dogs with chronic or frequently recurrent external ear canal disease, particularly when attempts at cleaning the ears have included instrumentation of the ear canal. Careful examination under anesthesia is essential; suction is necessary to clear the horizontal ear canal.

TREATMENT OF MIDDLE EAR DISEASES

Options for treatment include the following:
1. Administration of systemic and local antibiotics only.
2. Flushing of the middle ear cavity (via myringotomy if the tympanic membrane is intact at the time of treatment), followed by systemic and local antibiotics.
3. Curettage of the middle ear cavity.
4. Surgical drainage of the middle ear cavity (bulla osteotomy).

The value of external ear canal resection (see page 1912) as an adjunct to conservative management of otitis media has been shown.[18, 21]

In most cases, there is no reason not to proceed with the most conservative approach first, particularly if the condition of the horizontal ear canal would suggest the need for ablation of the ear canal as part of the procedure, since ablation and lateral bulla osteotomy result in almost complete hearing loss.

For conservative medical treatment, the choice of antibiotic is based on bacterial culture and sensitivity testing and fungal culture of ear discharges. The antibiotic is given systemically as well as locally, so that it is more likely to penetrate into the middle ear cavity. Chloramphenicol and gentamicin are likely choices for *Proteus* or *Pseudomonas* infections. Local medications are also given, or dilute antiseptics are used to help flush out the ear canal so that it can be cleaned. This regimen should be continued for at least seven to ten days. If there is no improvement in the clinical signs, middle ear flushing is indicated. Evidence of clinical improvement includes lessening of discharge and decreased severity of neurological signs. Head tilt is often the last sign to disappear and may remain for many weeks, although the dog is normal in all other respects. When head tilt persists after other signs of disease have resolved, oral prednisolone may speed its resolution. Prednisolone is also indicated to hasten resolution of severe acute vestibular signs that are interfering with the animal's ability to balance or eat.

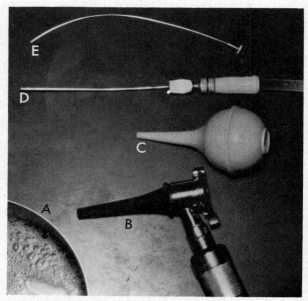

Figure 149–4. Equipment needed for middle ear flushing. *A*, Bowl of dilute antiseptic solution; *B*, otoscope; *C*, rubber ear irrigation syringe; *D*, suction cannula with metal tip; *E*, stylet to clear cannula of obstructing debris.

Myringotomy and Middle Ear Cavity Irrigation

Middle ear irrigation is performed under anesthesia. A specimen is obtained for bacterial culture prior to flushing. The external ear canal is cleaned first, flushing with saline or dilute povidone-iodine and suctioning as necessary, and the tympanic membrane is examined. If the tympanic membrane is ruptured or not observed before the suction tip meets the medial wall of the bulla, which is recognizable by its unyielding feel, the suction tip is left deep in the middle ear while the external ear canal is flushed copiously with a dilute antiseptic solution (Fig. 149–4). If the tympanic membrane is intact, a myringotomy must be performed first. This is most simply performed with the suction tip, advancing it into the middle ear cavity through the tympanic membrane in an area caudal to the malleus. Space is formed around the suction tube by moving the tube so that it lacerates the membrane. This allows the flushing fluid to enter the middle ear cavity. The middle ear cavity is then flushed as previously described.

Auditory Tube Insufflation

This can be done by pressing an air-filled rubber syringe into the external ear canal or by inserting a tube into the auditory tube through an otoscope placed across the tympanic membrane into the middle ear cavity.[15, 16] For the latter technique, discharge in the middle ear cavity is removed and the opening of the auditory tube is identified. The tip of a soft rubber tube is inserted into the opening, and the tube is cleared of debris by insufflation or irrigation. The auditory tube exits from the middle ear cavity about midway from dorsal to ventral; thus, under normal standing or sternal recumbency conditions, gravity drainage from the auditory tube is very inefficient.

Middle Ear Cavity Curettage

Lateral ear canal resection is performed first, the horizontal ear canal is flushed, and a curette is inserted through the tympanic membrane. The middle ear cavity is curetted extensively, and debris is flushed from the cavity. Systemic antibiotics and anti-inflammatory steroids are given for several weeks following surgery.[18]

Bulla Osteotomy

Drainage of infection or debris from the middle ear cavity can be achieved by several routes, although most are of limited usefulness. Myringotomy combined with local and systemic antibiotics resolves most cases treated. Unfortunately, it provides drainage only until the tympanic membrane is healed (usually four to ten days), and it does not drain the most dependent part of the bulla when the animal is standing or lying sternally.

Because of the limitations of these two conservative approaches, more radical means of surgical drainage were developed. Two early techniques that are rarely used now required chiselling of the ventral part of the bulla through the pharynx[6] and penetration of the tympanic membrane and ventromedial wall of

the bulla with a Steinmann pin.[13] With this latter technique, a hole was made in the tip of the pin so that a length of wire could be inserted from the external ear canal to the pharynx. The wire was then used to pull a rubber drainage tube through the middle ear cavity. With both of these techniques, the size of the opening in the wall of the bulla could not be controlled, and the cavity could not be inspected and cleaned directly. There was also a risk of damaging adjacent soft tissue structures that could not be seen during the procedure.

Ideally, the surgery should allow controlled resection of as much or as little of the bulla as seems necessary and inspection and cleansing of the bulla cavity under direct vision. The first approach that permitted these options was ventral bulla osteotomy, described in 1930.[14] A lateral approach to the bulla was described subsequently.[1]

Ventral Bulla Osteotomy

A paramedian skin incision is made just medial to the mandibular salivary gland (Fig. 149–5A). The platysma muscle is incised and reflected, a branch of the lingual-facial vein exiting medially from the salivary gland is ligated and transected, and the plane between the salivary gland and the digastricus muscle is dissected bluntly (Fig. 149–5B). As the digastricus muscle and mandibular gland are separated, the large superficial hypoglossal nerve becomes visible. This nerve must be identified and protected from damage, including that resulting from excessive pressure from retractors. The dissection proceeds deeper until the external carotid artery and its lingual artery branch (which runs with the hypoglossal nerve to the tongue) are seen (Fig. 149–5C). The bulla is found in the triangle formed by these structures. It can be iden-

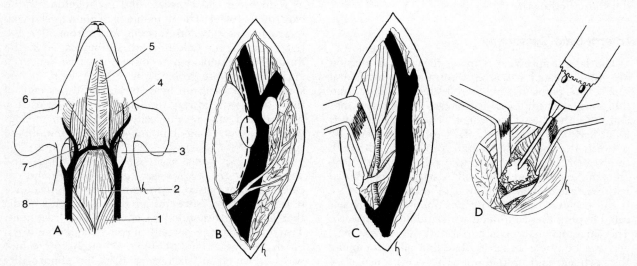

Figure 149–5. Ventral bulla osteotomy. *A,* Superficial structures of the ventral neck area. 1, Sternocephalic muscle; 2, sternohyoid muscle; 3, mandibular salivary gland; 4, digastric muscle; 5, mylohyoid muscle; 6, hyoid venous arch; 7, mandibular lymph nodes lying on either side of the facial vein; 8, jugular vein. *B,* Plane of dissection (dashed line) between the mandibular salivary gland and the linguofacial vein. A superficial branch of the second cervical nerve crosses the vein caudally. *C,* The digastric muscle and mandibular gland are retracted laterally to reveal the hypoglossal nerve and carotid and lingual arteries. *D,* The bulla, located in the triangle between the carotid artery laterally and the hypoglossal nerve and lingual artery medially, is penetrated with a Steinmann pin.

tified by following the stylohyoid bone (palpable as a thin, sticklike structure) dorsally, as this bone attaches to the skull on the lateral aspect of the bulla. If the bulla cannot be identified by these means, a nonscrubbed assistant can insert a finger into the mouth, palpate the hamular processes, and slide the finger caudally and laterally onto the bulla; the finger is then palpated by the surgeon, who displaces the finger with his own to locate the bulla. The thin covering of muscle is penetrated by scissors, and the periosteum is scraped off with a periosteal elevator for about 1 cm diameter. The bulla is penetrated with a Steinmann pin in a Jacob's chuck or a hand-driven orthopedic drill bit (Fig. 149–5D), proceeding gently so that when the pin or bit finally penetrates the normally thin-walled bulla, it does not lurch dorsally and cause damage. The area resected is enlarged with further holes and a rongeur. The extent of resection can be assessed by placing a curved mosquito hemostat into the bulla cavity to determine the extent of overhang available. When the cavity is fully exposed, abnormal contents are resected by gentle use of forceps or by irrigation and suction. When the bulla cavity is clean, a drain is placed, either by inserting a Penrose drain into the hole in the bulla and exiting it ventrally, with the risk that it will rapidly become displaced, or by inserting it through the external ear canal and tympanic membrane and out the incision so that it forms a loop. This latter method ensures that the periosteum will not rapidly seal over the opening in the floor of the bulla. To place a drain through the ear canal, a mosquito hemostat or alligator forceps is placed through the external ear canal opening and tympanic membrane into the bulla cavity, the jaws are opened, and the drain is fed into the jaws through the incision. The drain can be left in for 10 to 14 days to ensure soft tissue ingrowth.

Lateral Bulla Osteotomy

The lateral approach is made through an incision over the ear canal, extending ventral to the horizontal canal. The parotid gland is reflected ventrally, and the horizontal ear canal cartilages are followed medially to the bony ear canal. The facial nerve is identified and protected. This procedure can be performed either as a separate procedure (although the ventral approach is preferred as being more efficient in exposing the bulla cavity) or combined with ear canal ablation. The combination procedure is the preferred method for treatment of severe ear canal hyperplasia combined with middle ear disease. The ear canal ablation is performed (see Chap. 148), and the bony ear canal is identified after removing the cartilage and epithelium. The ventral aspect of the bony canal is resected with a rongeur, extending the excision gradually medially until the lateral and ventral walls of the bulla have been removed. If the external ear canal is to be left intact, the bulla is

penetrated with a Steinmann pin as for the ventral approach. Following exposure of the cavity and cleansing of its contents, a drain is placed, and the soft tissues are closed around the drain.

RESULTS AND COMPLICATIONS

In a review of the results of insufflation of the middle ear cavity to clear the tympanic tube in 104 dogs with otitis media, all 31 acute cases were cured and nearly all (89 per cent of 73) of the chronic cases were improved, although 25 per cent subsequently had recurrences.[16] Nystagmus, head tilt, and reduced ability to hear were observed in four of the chronic cases for one to two weeks following treatment. The definition of otitis media and duration of follow-up were not stated. In another report of 150 dogs, 114 were reported as excellent, 28 as good, and 8 as poor six months following treatment.[15] It is surprising, considering these results, that this technique is not used more generally. In another report, there was no improvement when the auditory tube was insufflated in addition to simple drainage and irrigation of the middle ear cavity.[21] Perhaps the good results reported are merely a reflection of the cleaning of the middle ear cavity that is part of the process. From my own observations, it is often very difficult to view the middle ear cavity at all, let alone the opening of the auditory tube, and I have been reluctant, as have others,[11, 17] to use high irrigation pressures in the middle ear cavity because of the danger of severe or permanent damage to the inner ear structures.

Flushing of the middle ear cavity is the initial treatment of choice in most reports, combined with a lateral ear canal resection procedure to eliminate or reduce ear canal disease and myringotomy if the eardrum is intact. The percentage of animals showing improvement in reported series varies from 50 to 100 per cent[9, 21]; the addition of antibiotics after the flushing and drainage procedures increased the cured or improved rate from 50 to 80 per cent in one series.[21] The eardrum heals in about 50 per cent of these animals following drainage. Hearing is usually present and may be clinically normal even in dogs with bilateral, long-standing tympanic membrane rupture.

Lateral ear canal resection, myringotomy, and curettage of the middle ear cavity through the ear canal opening caused improvement or disappearance of the head tilt in seven of ten dogs with otitis media that had not responded to conservative treatment. Two other dogs temporarily improved and then worsened, and one did not improve. When this procedure was performed on six normal dogs, no abnormality was found in five, and one developed a head tilt; hearing was not evaluated because the surgery was performed unilaterally.[18] This particular treatment regimen appears to have little advantage over the more conservative middle ear irrigation. If conservative treatment does not resolve the condition, I recommend proceeding to bulla osteotomy.

Ventral bulla osteotomy provided excellent long-term results in 20 of 22 dogs in two reports.[5, 13] Possible complications include hypoglossal nerve damage (causing tongue paralysis) and chorda tympani or petrosal nerve damage (causing potential loss of parasympathetic supply to the glands of that side of the head and keratoconjunctivitis sicca, or dry nose and nasal discharge). Continued or recurrent disease may result in abscessation through the side of the face in an occasional dog. Placement of a drain through the external ear canal and across the tympanic membrane does not seriously interfere with hearing following surgery.

Lateral bulla osteotomy combined with ear canal ablation resulted in elimination of severe hyperplastic otitis externa in 23 ears treated in 13 dogs; fistulae did not develop on the side of the face in any of the dogs; however, all 13 were deaf following surgery.[4] Results of using the lateral approach without ear canal ablation have not been reported.

Radical surgical treatment may be necessary to manage the effects of bone proliferation of the external surface of the bulla, preventing normal range of motion of the temporomandibular joint. This proliferative bone can be sufficiently removed during ventral bulla osteotomy with rongeurs to allow normal mouth opening. Adjacent neurovascular structures must be identified and protected.

MIDDLE EAR TUMORS

Neoplastic disease of the structures surrounding the middle ear cavity is uncommon.[3, 5] Several tumor types have been found sporadically. The clinical signs are initially those of inflammatory ear disease, or more diffuse neurological signs may be present if a brain tumor is invading the inner or middle ear (Fig. 149–6).

Diagnosis is by biopsy. Because of the anatomy involved, radical resection is not practical. Occasionally, combination therapy (surgical biopsy or debulking, with radiation therapy or chemotherapy) may be useful in extending comfortable life.

MIDDLE EAR DISEASES IN CATS

Chronic severe otitis externa is less common in cats than in dogs; middle ear disease secondary to otitis externa is also less common. Middle ear disease without external ear canal disease occurs occasionally in cats, more so than in dogs.[16] Possible reasons for this disparity are the incidence of inflammatory ear polyps in cats (see hereafter) and possible anatomical differences in the auditory tube that predispose cats to secretory middle ear disease (Fig. 149–7), as seen in children. If detailed examination of the ear canal and pharynx fails to show a polyp, initial treatment should be conservative, including systemic antibiotics and corticosteroids for two weeks. Serous effusions in the middle ear cavity can be aspirated through the tympanic membrane. Bulla osteotomy can be performed on cats using techniques similar to those described for dogs. Structures are easier to identify, and the route to the bulla is more shallow, making the approach easier than in most dogs.

Inflammatory Polyps of the Middle Ear Cavity of Cats

Inflammatory masses occasionally arise from the middle ear cavity or auditory tube of cats.[8] Affected cats vary in age and breed. The mass may extend through the tympanic membrane into the horizontal ear canal[8] or from or through the auditory tube into the nasopharynx.[2, 12] Clinical signs are chronic discharge from the external ear canal and noisy respiration and snoring, with occasionally dysphagia if the mass extends into the pharynx. Neurological abnormalities are rare. Diagnosis is by otoscopic or pharyngoscopic examination; a rounded, red-surfaced

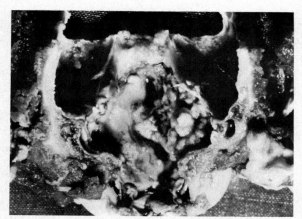

Figure 149–6. Skull of a dog with a carcinoma invading the brain from the middle ear.

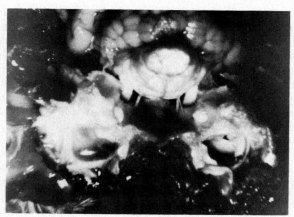

Figure 149–7. Unilateral (left side) serous otitis media in a cat. Both bullae have been opened to show their contents.

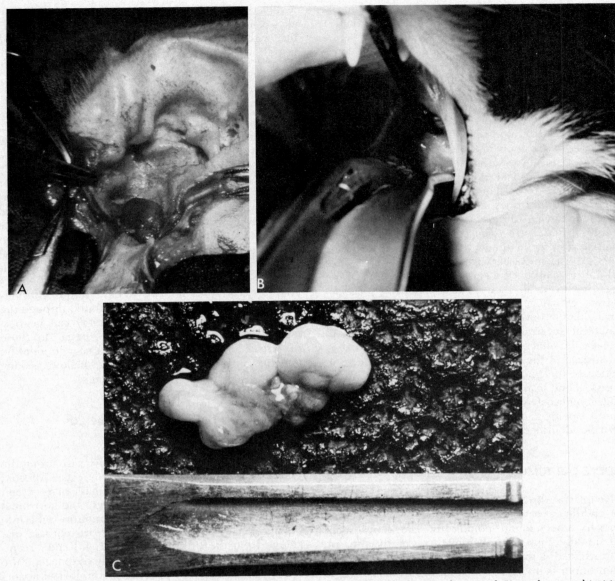

Figure 149–8. Inflammatory polyps arising from the middle ear in cats. *A*, Polyp in the horizontal ear canal. Vertical ear canal incisions have been made but not sutured. *B*, Polyp in the nasopharynx revealed by retracting the soft palate rostrally. *C*, Polyp removed from the horizontal ear canal. Scalpel handle indicates size.

mass, distinctly different from the surrounding epithelium, is seen in the ear canal or is palpated above the palate. On microscopic examination, the tissue is seen as chronic inflammation, sometimes with a covering of stratified squamous or ciliated columnar epithelium. Affected cats generally show a negative response to the fluorescent antibody test for feline leukemia virus, and no explanation for the localized nature of the disease has been suggested.

Treatment is by resection, either by lateral ear canal resection for access to the horizontal ear canal (Fig. 149–8A) or by reflecting the soft palate ventrorostrally for lesions in the pharynx (Fig. 149–8B). The polyp is grasped with a hemostat and pulled out (Fig. 149–8C). Following conservative resection, about 50 per cent of polyps recur.[8] Bulla osteotomy

may allow more accurate resection of the origin of the mass; long-term results in a series of cats following bulla osteotomy have not been reported.

1. Barrett, R. E., and Rathfon, B. L.: Lateral approach to a bulla osteotomy. J. Am. Anim. Hosp. Assoc. *11*:203, 1975.
2. Bedford, P. G. C.: Origin of the nasopharyngeal polyp in the cat. Vet. Rec. *110*:541, 1982.
3. Berzon, J. L., and Bunch, S. E.: Recurrent otitis externamedia secondary to a fibroma in the middle ear. J. Am. Anim. Hosp. Assoc. *16*:73, 1980.
4. Cechner, P.: Combined ear canal ablation and lateral bulla osteotomy in the dog. Abstract. Ann. Mtg. Am. Coll. Vet. Surg., 1982.
5. Denny, H. R.: The results of surgical treatment of otitis media and interna in the dog. J. Small Anim. Pract. *14*:585, 1973.
6. Ehmer, E. H.: Modified bulla ossea operation. North Am. Vet. *15*:44, 1934.

7. Gibbs, C.: Radiological refresher—ear disease. J. Small Anim. Pract. *19*:539, 1978.
8. Harvey, C. E., and Goldschmidt, M. H.: Inflammatory polyps of the horizontal ear canal of the cat. J. Small Anim. Pract. *19*:669, 1978.
9. Helfand, J., and Knecht, C. D.: Surgical treatment of otitis media in the dog. Illinois Vet. *9*:7, 1966.
10. Hopwood, P. R., and Bellenger, C. R.: Cannulation of the canine auditory tube. Res. Vet. Sci. *28*:382, 1980.
11. Knecht, C. D.: Diseases of the middle and inner ear in the dog and cat. Vet. Med. Update Ser 5:1, 1977.
12. Lane, J. G., Orr, C. M., Lucke, V. M., and Gruffydd-Jones, T.: Nasopharyngeal polyps arising in the middle ear of the cat. J. Small Anim. Pract. *22*:511, 1981.
13. McBride, N. L.: Persistent otorrhea in the dog. Proc. Ann. Mtg. Am. Vet. Med. Assoc. *123*:247, 1954.
14. McNutt, G. W., and McCoy, J. E.: Bulla osteotomy in the dog. J. Am. Vet. Med. Assoc. 77:617, 1930.
15. Meynard, J. A.: Traitement de l'otite moyenne du chien— insufflation de la trompe d'Eustache. Rev. Vet. Med. *111*:119, 1960.
16. Moltzen, H.: Otitis media in the dog and cat. Adv. Small Anim. Pract. 3:56, 1961.
17. Ott, R. L.: Diagnosis and correction of otitis media. Mod. Vet. Pract. *45*:39, 1964.
18. Parker, A. J., Schiller, A. G., and Cusick, P. K.: Bulla curettage for chronic otitis media and interna in dogs. J. Am. Vet. Med. Assoc. *168*:931, 1976.
19. Penrod, J. P., and Coulter, D. B.: Diagnostic uses of impedance audimetry in the dog. J. Am. Anim. Hosp. Assoc. *16*:941, 1980.
20. Sato, T.: Canine membrana tympani normal and diseased as observed by arthroscopy. J. Jap. Vet. Med. Assoc. *32*:694, 1979.
21. Spreull, J. S. A.: Treatment of otitis media in the dog. J. Small Anim. Pract. 5:107, 1964.

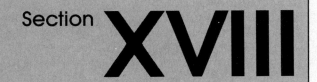

Section XVIII

Musculoskeletal System

Steven P. Arnoczky
Section Editor

Chapter 150

Connective Tissues of the Musculoskeletal System

Adele L. Boskey

Connective tissues serve many functions in the body: they hold it together, organize its compartments, and provide cohesion and internal support. Differing in form and function, the connective tissues—skin, tendon, ligaments, cartilages, bone, teeth, spleen, capsules and sheaths of muscles, blood vessels, lungs, and so forth—have several common features. All consist of cells, fibers, and nonstructured, amorphous ground substances; all are derived from mesenchyme; and all show the characteristic presence of banded fibers (collagen) under the light microscope (Fig. 150–1). The presence of a variety of extracellular fibers is the most characteristic feature of the connective tissues. The density and arrange-

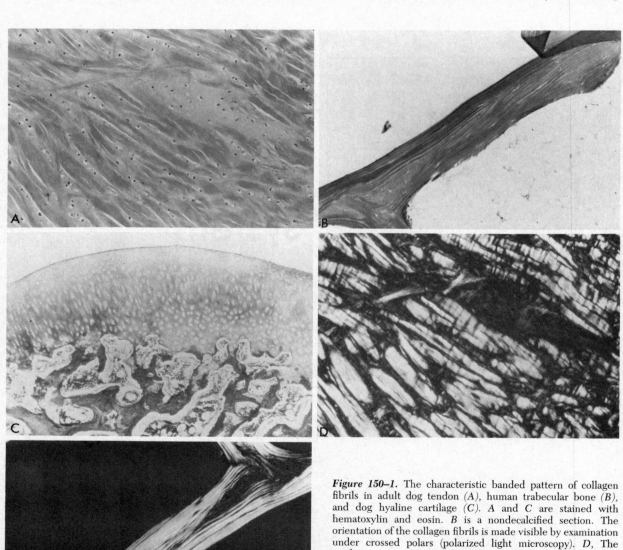

Figure 150–1. The characteristic banded pattern of collagen fibrils in adult dog tendon (*A*), human trabecular bone (*B*), and dog hyaline cartilage (*C*). *A* and *C* are stained with hematoxylin and eosin. *B* is a nondecalcified section. The orientation of the collagen fibrils is made visible by examination under crossed polars (polarized light microscopy). *D,* The tendon specimen in *A* under polarized light. Note the parallel arrangement of the fibers. *E,* A view of human trabecular (cortical lamellar) bone. Note the way the collagen fibers swirl around the osteone's vascular canal. (*A, C,* and *D* courtesy of Dr. Steven Arnoczky. *B* and *E* courtesy of Dr. Peter Bullough.)

ment of these fibers relative to the cells that produce them determine the function of the tissue.

In this chapter, the structure and composition of the connective tissues of the musculoskeletal system and their component macromolecules are considered to illustrate (1) how the tissues perform their functions and (2) the molecular basis of connective tissue disease. Muscles, not generally considered to be connective tissues, contain fibrous components, but in contrast to the extracellular fibrils and fibers of the connective tissues, the fibrous components are found within the muscle cell. Because muscle cells do secrete an extracellular matrix containing connective tissue elements, and because muscles are essential for the functioning of the skeletal system, they are also considered in this chapter.

STRUCTURE AND FUNCTION

Connective tissues are usually categorized according to the arrangement of their fibrous elements. Since the arrangement of the fibers is related to tissue function, this classification also provides functional categories of connective tissues. The connective tissues of the musculoskeletal system generally fall into the category "dense connective tissues." These tissues, owing to their organization, are able to perform structural and mechanical functions. In contrast to the loosely woven fibers and abundant cells found in the "loose connective tissues," which serve as packing materials and lubricants, ordered, closely packed fibers, few cells, and little non-fibrous material are found in dense connective tissues. These dense connective tissues can be further categorized according to the geometric packing of fibers.

Tissues that provide tensile strength and have the ability to withstand stress contain long, parallel bundles of fibers. The regular parallel arrangement of fibers in tendons and ligaments makes these tissues both flexible and resistant to pulling forces (Fig. 150–2). The tendon, which is inserted into bone at both ends, has a more spiral arrangement of fibers than the ligament, which inserts into bone at one end and into muscle at the other. The ability of ligaments and tendons to stretch depends on the presence of an additional protein—rubbery, expansible elastin.

Two- and three-dimensional networks of fibers exist in tissues that serve protective functions. The periosteum, which covers the surface of bone, the perichondrium, which coats the cartilage surface, and the membrane fibrosa of the joint capsule are all both elastic and resistant to tensile forces. These tissues contain considerably more nonfibrous, nonstructural material (ground substance) than other connective tissues.

Even more complicated patterns of fibers are found in tissues such as the arterial wall and the healing incised wound, which are exposed to pulsing fluids and lesser stresses and thus require greater flexibility. In these tissues, relatively short fibers appear in a circular arrangement, in close contact with elastin fibers and smooth muscle. In cartilage, the collagen fibrils are spaced farther apart, with a more random orientation, to provide mechanical strength and resilience while giving the tissue flexibility.

Cartilage is a special type of dense connective tissue, and there are three major types of cartilage: hyaline, elastic, and fibrous. All cartilages, with the exception of sections of the joint capsule, are covered by the perichondrium (another dense connective tissue). Hyaline is a semi-transparent cartilage found at the bone-joint surface, on the ventral ends of ribs, and in the respiratory system (Fig. 150–3A). It is extremely flexible owing to the presence of high-molecular-weight macromolecules known as proteoglycans. Hyaline cartilage contains a high proportion of water (more than 70 per cent of the tissue's wet weight). The other principal molecular components of hyaline cartilage are collagen (15–20 per cent of wet weight) and proteoglycans (2–10 per cent of wet

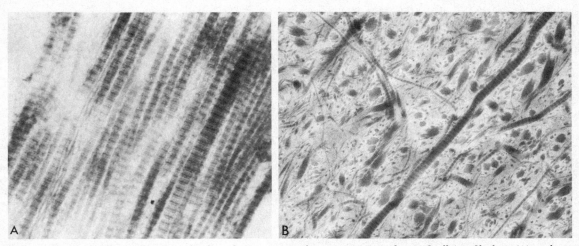

Figure 150–2. Transmission electron micrographs show the variation in the arrangement and size of collagen fibrils in (*A*) tendon and (*B*) cartilage. (*A* courtesy of Dr. Steven Arnoczky. *B* courtesy of Dr. Peter Bullough.)

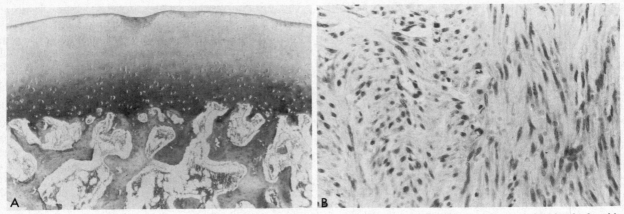

Figure 150–3. *A,* Light micrograph showing the hyaline (articular) cartilage of a dog's femur. The section was stained with toluidine blue to reveal territorial staining for proteoglycans. *B,* Light micrograph showing fibrocartilage of the medial meniscus from an adult dog. (Courtesy of Dr. Steven Arnoczky.)

weight). Elastic cartilage in the external ear has even greater elasticity and opacity than hyaline cartilage. The major fibrous element in elastic cartilage is elastin, not collagen. Fibrocartilage found in the intervertebral disc and in close association with joints contains dense collagen fibers (Fig. 150–3*B*). Fibrocartilage contains a lower proportion of proteoglycans and water than hyaline cartilage. However, proteoglycans in fibrocartilage are similar but not identical to those in hyaline cartilage. The functional differences between these cartilages are due to the differ-

ent interactions among proteoglycans, collagen, and other matrix components.

Bones and teeth are mineralized connective tissues that differ from the other connective tissues through the presence of calcium phosphate mineral crystals, which are deposited in an oriented fashion on the collagen fibers. These crystals make the tissue strong and rigid, providing the capacity for locomotion and protection. They also serve as storage sites for mineral deposition and are important in controlling calcium and phosphate homeostasis.

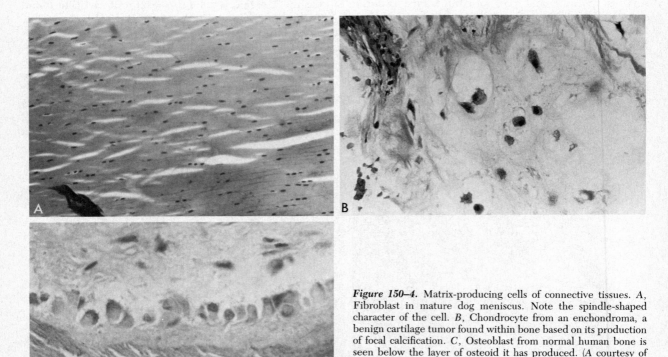

Figure 150–4. Matrix-producing cells of connective tissues. *A,* Fibroblast in mature dog meniscus. Note the spindle-shaped character of the cell. *B,* Chondrocyte from an enchondroma, a benign cartilage tumor found within bone based on its production of focal calcification. *C,* Osteoblast from normal human bone is seen below the layer of osteoid it has produced. (*A* courtesy of Dr. Steven Arnoczky. *B* and *C* courtesy of Dr. Vincent Vigoritta.)

COMPOSITION

All connective tissues are composed of cells, extracellular fibers, and "ground substance" (the nonstructured components of the matrix). The principal cells producing connective tissue matrices are fibroblasts. These long, spindle-shaped cells stretch across bundles of collagen fibers (Fig. 150–4A). Fibroblasts, which synthesize the matrix of loose connective tissues, are closely related to the chondrocyte (Fig. 150–4B), which produces cartilaginous matrices, the osteoblast (Fig. 150–4C), which produces bone matrix, and the odontoblast, which produces dentin matrices. Numerous other cells—macrophages, adipose cells, mast cells, monocytes, lymphocytes, plasma cells, and muscle cells—also produce connective tissue elements.

Collagen

The major fibrous component synthesized by connective tissue cells is collagen.[13, 30] Collagen is the most abundant mammalian protein, accounting for 20 to 50 per cent of the dry weight of adult long bones, for 67 to 71 per cent of the dry weight of skin, and for 87 to 92 per cent of the dry weight of tendons. Because collagen is a blood vessel constituent, it is found in low levels in all tissues.

Because of its unique fibrous structure collagen provides strength and integrity. Several different types of collagen are found in connnective tissues. All collagens are composed of three tightly folded polypeptide chains, consisting of about 1,000 amino acids and each known as alpha chains. The alpha chains are twisted about one another in a triple helical configuration. It is this long (300 nm), narrow (1.5 nm) structure that gives individual collagen molecules

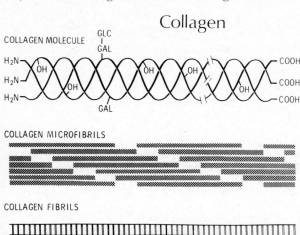

Figure 150–5. The triple helical *collagen molecule*, glycosylated by the addition of galactose or glucose-galactose to hydroxylysine residues; the *collagen fibril*, formed by the alignment of individual collagen molecules in a quarter-staggered array; and the type I or III *collagen fiber*, which gives the typical cross-striated banding pattern seen in the electron microscope. Type II, IV, and V collagens lacking thick fibrils do not give this pattern of cross striations.

their stability. The stability of individual fibrils (sets of collagen molecules aligned in a quarter-staggered array) and fibers (groups of collagen fibrils) is further increased by the presence of intramolecular and intrafibrillar cross-links. Structure of the collagen molecule, fibril, and fiber is shown in Figure 150–5.

The individual alpha chains of the collagen molecules, for the most part, consist of the repeating tripeptide $(GLY-X-Y)n$. Glycine accounts for one-third of all the constituent amino acids, because it is the only amino acid small enough to fit in the center of the collagen triple helix. Proline, alanine, hydroxyproline, and 5-hydroxylysine occur frequently in the X and Y positions, although 4-hydroxyproline and 5-hydroxylysine are confined to the Y position.

Hydroxylysine is frequently glycosylated with galactose or glucose and galactose. Proline, which owing to its rigid structure has a destabilizing effect in globular proteins, has a stabilizing effect on the fibrous collagens for exactly the same reason, i.e., it keeps the fibrous structure rigid. Hydroxyproline, an unusual amino acid that is not coded for by the genetic code and must be formed by post-translational modifications (see later discussion), is an essential component of collagen, because it participates in interchain hydrogen bonding required for stabilization of the collagen triple helix.

The most abundant collagen type, type I, is found in skin, bone, tendon, and ligament. Type I collagen consists of two identical alpha chains and one alpha chain of different amino acid composition— $[\alpha 1 \ (I)]_2 \alpha 2$. Type I collagen has a relatively low content of hydroxylysine and glycosylated residues compared with the three identical alpha chains found in type II $[\alpha 1(II)_3]$ collagen, characteristic of cartilage, the nucleus pulposus, and vitreous. Type III collagen $[\alpha 1 \ (III)_3]$ is found in blood vessels and in embryonic bone and skin. It differs from type I collagen, containing more than one-third glycine per alpha chain and its helical region terminating with a reducible disulfide bridge. Types IV and V collagens are basement membrane components, which unlike the other collagens do not form large cross-linked fibrils.

Although the triple helical structure of collagen molecules is quite simple, the manner in which these proteins are processed within the animal are quite complex. The type I collagen genes are the most complex genes that have been sequenced to date, containing more than 30 introns (noncoding regions) and more than 40 kilo bases.[28] The genes for types II and III appear to be equally complex. Transcription of DNA into messenger RNA (mRNA) therefore is a multistep process involving the cleavage and splicing of numerous fragments. Translation of mRNA produces individual polypeptide chains (pre-pro-alpha chains), which are much larger and structurally different from the individual alpha chains in the collagen molecule. At least nine enzymatically catalyzed post-translational modifications and several reactions that probably occur spontaneously are needed to hydroxylate, glycosylate, and process the triple helical molecules into insoluble, extracellular fibrils. A defect in

TABLE 150–1. Collagen Biosynthesis

Event	Enzymes and Cofactors	Product(s) and Function	Associated Conditions	Notes
Intracellular Events				
Translation of collagen mRNAs	All enzymes needed for eukaryotic transcription, translation, and protein synthesis	Soluble, extended collagen pre-pro-alpha chains	Osteogenesis imperfecta (OI) Ehlers-Danlos syndrome (IV)	Simultaneous for $\alpha 1$ and $\alpha 2$ of type I
Hydroxylation of proline	4-prolyl hydroxylase: O_2, Fe, ascorbic acid, alpha-keto-glutarate	Gly-Pro-4-OHPro. Forms H-bonds that stabilize triple helix	Scurvy (Vitamin C deficiency)	Essential for the formation of stable collagen Amount of OH-Pro varies with tissue
	3-prolyl hydroxylase: O_2, Fe, alpha-keto-glutarate and any reducing agent	Gly-3-OHPro-Pro ?	?	
Hydroxylation of lysine	Lysyl hydroxylase: O_2, Fe, alpha-keto-glutarate, and any reducing agent	Gly-X-5-OH-Lys Glycosylated	Hydroxylysine deficiency disease (OI)	
Glycosylations	Collagen UDP-galactosyl transferase Mn^{+2}	Gly-X-OH-Lys	Diabetes	
	Collagen UDP-glucosyl-transferase Mn^{+2}	Gal		
		[Glc-]		
	Mannose transferase	Mannose in nonhelical region	OI	
Self-assembly		Soluble triple helix-procollagen		
Extracellular events				
Cleavage of pro-peptides	N-pro-collagen peptidase C-pro-collagen peptidase	Collagen molecule	Ehlers-Danlos syndrome (VII) Dermatosparaxis	Sites differ in different collagen types
Packing of collagen	Spontaneous	Fibrils	Ehlers-Danlos syndrome (I) Dominant EDS (cats, mink, dogs)	
Cross-link formation aldehyde formation	Lysyloxidase: O_2, Cu^{+2}	Allysine Hydroxyallysine	Lathyrism treatment (βAPN) Penicillamine treatment X-linked cutis laxa Aneurysm (mice) Menke's kinky-hair syndrome Alcaptonuria	Formation of active aldehydes
Aldol condensation: aldimine formation, rearrangement	Spontaneous	Interchain and intrachain Schiff bases and aldol condensation products		Number of cross-links increases with age

any of these steps, whether it is inherited or caused by specific inhibition of a step, could cause serious, widespread changes in the properties of the final collagen fibrils. Study of the defects present in animals with the so-called collagen diseases has provided much of our current knowledge of functions of components of the collagen molecule.

Collagen biosynthesis begins with the processing of the collagen gene (Table 150–1). There are at least nine collagen genes; two type I, one each type II and type III, two type IV, and a minimum of three type V. Errors in formation of mRNAs from collagen genes, defects in the genes themselves, and abnormalities in gene frequency have all been associated with various forms of osteogenesis imperfecta (a heterogeneous group of connective tissue diseases characterized by bone fragility) in both humans and animals.

The initial pre-pro-collagen alpha chains that are synthesized in the cell are appreciably larger than the alpha chains of the final collagen molecules found in connective tissues. Amino and carboxyl pro-alpha terminal extensions, 15,000 to 40,000 daltons in molecular weight, do not form triple helixes but are essential for keeping the individual chains soluble, directing assembly of the collagen molecules, and facilitating transport from the site of synthesis into the cell.

While alpha chains are being synthesized, prior to triple helix formation, specific proline and lysine residues are hydroxylated in a series of reactions requiring molecular oxygen, iron, alpha-keto-glutaric acid, and vitamin C (ascorbic acid). This is the explanation for the connective tissue abnormalities seen in scorbutic (vitamin C–deficient) animals. The formation of hydroxyproline is essential for synthesis of a stable collagen molecule. The absence of the enzyme 4-prolyl-hydroxylase is not compatible with life.

Lysine hydroxylation does not require vitamin C, but similar to the enzymes that hydroxylate proline, lysyl hydroxylase has an absolute requirement for ferrous iron and molecular oxygen. The fact that wounds heal at a rate directly related to the oxygen tension in their environment can be interpreted in terms of the oxygen requirements of collagen synthesis. After lysine hydroxylation occurs, galactose or galactose and then glucose are added to some of the hydroxylated residues. The precise function of the hydroxylation and glycosylation of lysine is not known, although there is some data from individuals with hydroxylysine deficiency and from diabetic animals suggesting that these steps regulate fibril size. In another set of glycosylation reactions, mannose is added to specific sites in the C-terminal, non-helical end of the molecule.

All of the preceding modifications occur within the cell on individual alpha chains prior to triple helix formation. The final step in the intracellular processing of collagen is self-assembly, via the formation of disulfide bridges and other noncovalent interactions, of the three alpha chains into a triple helical molecule. The nonhelical terminal extensions are essential for this process, permitting recognition of the proper alpha chains (in type I collagen there are always two $\alpha 1$ chains, and one $\alpha 2$ chain), directing the formation of disulfide bridges, and keeping the helical molecule in soluble form.

Secretion of the collagen molecule, which occurs only after triple helix formation, is followed by the cleavage of the N- and C-terminal nonhelical domains by two peptidases. In types III and IV, the sites of such cleavage, if they exist, are quite different, because these types of collagen retain disulfide links in their C-terminals. In the absence of pro-collagen peptidase, the type I collagen fibrils formed are so soluble that skin and joints are extremely flexible and hyperextensible. A manifestation of this property is seen in dermatosporaxis in sheep and cattle and in Ehlers-Danlos (VII) syndrome in humans. (The Ehlers-Danlos syndromes are a heterogeneous group of diseases characterized by skin fragility, hyperextensibility, joint hypermobility, easy scarring, and various orthopedic problems.)[24] In both these diseases, electron-microscopic examination reveals the presence of abnormally thin, ribbon-like collagen fibrils outside the cell. These fibrils do not thicken, since in the absence of cleavage of the terminal extensions, the following extracellular modifications leading to stable fibril formation do not occur properly.

The final steps in collagen biosynthesis and maturation result in the formation of stable fibers and fibrils. Individual collagen molecules line up in a quarter-staggered array, forming thick threads. These fibrils are stabilized by intermolecular and intramolecular cross-links. Aldehydes, formed by the oxidative deamination of lysine and hydroxylysine residues, spontaneously react with other aldehydes (aldol condensation) or free-NH_2 groups (aldimine formation), gradually forming three-dimensional cross-links. Blockage of aldehyde formation (either inherited or induced by the chelation of copper ions—one of the cofactors of the enzyme lysyl oxidase) may produce bone deformities (lathyrism), joint dislocations, and aortic aneurysms, as a direct result of the inability of the collagen and elastin to cross-link. Compounds such as penicillamine, which interact with reactive aldehydes in collagen, cause similar abnormalities.

Elastin

The other fibrous component of the connective tissue matrix is elastin. The rubber-like component of elastic ligaments, blood vessels, skin, and lungs, elastin accounts for only a small amount of the matrix in nonextensible tissues (2.6 per cent elastin *versus* 32 per cent collagen in tendon) and a major proportion of the matrix of deformable tissues (32 per cent elastin *versus* 7 per cent collagen in ligaments).[32] In contrast to the highly oriented, regularly arranged

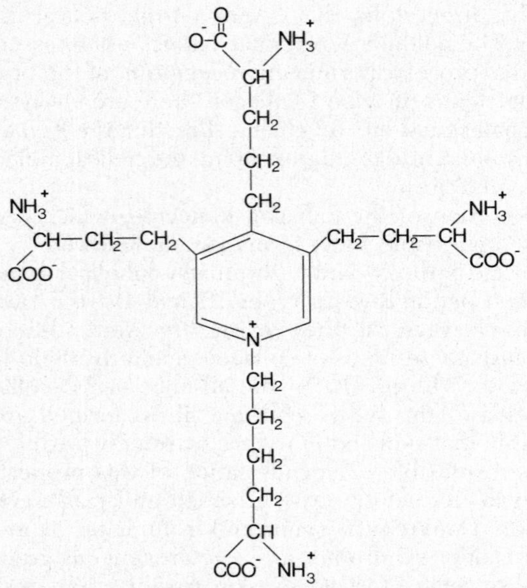

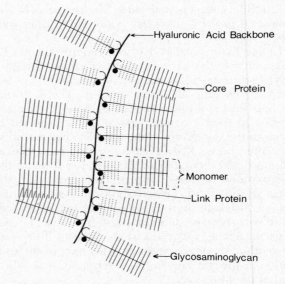

Figure 150–6. Desmosine, one of the unique amino acids that form the stabilizing cross links in elastin. Two lysines on two neighboring elastin molecules form aldehyde moieties and then react to provide this cross-linked structure.

collagen fibrils, elastin generally occurs in a compacted nonstructured (amorphous) form that is rubbery and soft and can be extended to double its length. Although the detailed molecular structure of elastin is still under investigation, the structural features that distinguish this rubber-like protein from collagen reflect the differences in functions of the two macromolecules.

Like collagen, elastin contains a high percentage of glycine (27 per cent) and a fair amount (10 per cent) of proline, but elastin is much more hydrophobic than collagen and hence is more insoluble. The repeating unit in elastin is a pentapeptide, distinct from the Gly-X-Y tripeptide of collagen. Elastin contains no hydroxylysine and little hydroxyproline.

Elastin is also similar to collagen in that it is synthesized in a high-molecular-weight, soluble form. After conversion to tropoelastin, lysyl oxidase, the same copper-dependent enzyme required for collagen cross-linking, causes the majority of the lysines of elastin to be oxidatively deaminated. Spontaneous reaction of specific active lysyl aldehydes results in the formation of two unique cross-linked amino acids, desmosine and isodemosine throughout the molecule (Fig. 150–6). These cross-links are important factors stabilizing the compact (or random) structure of elastin, making the compact structure the energetically more favorable one to which the molecule always returns after expansion.

Proteoglycans[9, 15]

One of the principal components of the "ground substance," the nonstructured component of the connective tissues, the high-molecular-weight proteogly-

cans with their component acidic glycosaminoglycans provide flexibility and resilience to the connective tissue matrix (Fig. 150–7). Although proteoglycan structure differs among the connective tissues, all proteoglycans consist of a central protein core to which acidic glycosaminoglycan chains are covalently attached. The individual glycosaminoglycans, formerly called mucopolysaccharides, are large anionic molecules consisting of repeating disaccharides—one acidic sugar (glucuronic or iduronic acid) and one basic monosaccharide (2-amino 2-deoxy glucose or galactose), which is made anionic by N-acetylation or N- or O-sulfation. Proteoglycans are synthesized by connective tissue cells and secreted into the matrix, where they interact with other matrix components, affecting the mechanical and physical properties of the tissues. In many, but not all tissues, proteoglycans monomers form giant (very-high-molecular-weight) aggregates, by association of specific hyaluronic acid binding regions on the core protein with hyaluronic acid. These aggregates, owing to their high charge density and branched configuration, are responsible for the viscoelastic, semipermeable nature of cartilage, synovium, and intervertebral disc. The interaction of proteoglycans with collagen is poorly understood, but there are data suggesting that proteoglycans, locked into place by the presence of collagen fibrils, enable the tissues to hold water, control the transport of molecules and ions, and resist deformation.

All the connective tissues contain highly anionic, viscous proteoglycans. However, the nature and size of these proteoglycans differ with the function of the tissue. For example, hyaline cartilage, fibrocartilage, and blood vessels, which must be resilient, contain

Figure 150–7. A typical cartilage proteoglycan aggregate. The hooked end of the core protein contains a hyaluronate binding region, which facilitates interaction of proteoglycan monomers with the hyaluronic acid backbone. The link proteins stabilize this interaction. Individual, repeating disaccharides—the glycosaminoglycans, keratin sulfate, and (predominantly) chondroitin sulfate—are covalently linked to serine groups on the core protein.

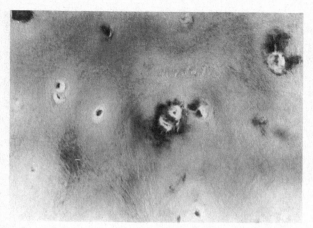

Figure 150–8. In degenerative joint disease, destruction of carti-lage proteoglycans is accompanied by mineral deposition. Elec-tron-dense calcium phosphate deposits can be seen on the periph-ery of the chondrocytes. (Courtesy of Dr. Vincent Vigoritta.)

higher proportions of large, high-molecular-weight proteoglycans than do lungs, calcified cartilage, and bone.

Modification of proteoglycan structure has marked effects on tissue properties. For example, in severe osteoarthritis, loss of proteoglycan from articular car-tilage, results in fibrillation of the tissue, and occa-sional ectopic mineralization (Fig. 150–8).[1, 3] Simi-larly, injection of papain, an enzyme that digests the protein core of proteoglycans and causes release of individual glycosaminoglycans into the matrix, causes rapid calcification of normally uncalcified tissues.[12] In the brachymorphic mouse, deficiency of sulfate groups on the proteoglycans causes severe dwarfing.[29] Similar shortening of stature is seen in the cartilage matrix deficiency mouse, in which core protein ab-normalities results in abnormal collagen-proteoglycan interactions.[21] Proteoglycan modification also occurs during endochondral ossification (see later).

Glycoproteins[14]

Included within the ground substance of the con-nective tissue matrix are several glycoproteins whose presence is also essential for tissue function. Glyco-proteins, as distinct from proteoglycans, are protein compounds that contain no large repeating sugar units and that tend to have a high protein-to-sugar ratio. Collagen itself is a glycoprotein. Among the less abundant but equally important connective and related tissue glycoproteins are: fibronectin, laminin (basement membranes only), osteonectin (bone only), and chondronectin (cartilage only). Each of these proteins functions to regulate cell adhesion, motility, and alignment.

Fibronectin, synthesized by fibroblasts and other connective tissue cells in culture, is found throughout the body in plasma, and some basement membranes (the continuous sheets of extracellular matrix mate-rials that separate cells other than connective tissue cells from matrix), as well as in all connective tissue matrices characterized to date.[19] Fibronectin, which has a high affinity for the clotting proteins fibrin and fibrinogen and for collagen, actin, and other fibrous proteins, is believed to control cell adhesion, mor-phology, motility, and growth via interaction with the cytoskeleton (fibrous, insoluble proteins in the cytoplasm). Fibronectin is being extensively studied, because transformed, oncogenic cells do not produce this protein. In tissue culture, chondrocytes bind to type I collagen when the interaction is mediated by fibronectin, but binding to type II collagen requires the presence of a different glycoprotein, chondronec-tin. Chondronectin is the cartilage analog of these cell and collagen binding proteins, having a specific affinity for type II (cartilage) collagen.[18]

Osteonectin, a glycoprotein found in bone and absent from cartilage and other connective tissues, binds strongly to both type I collagen and bone mineral and inhibits bone mineral crystal growth *in vitro*.[34] It, therefore, is thought to play a role in bone calcification. Recently, the absence of this protein has been associated with a form of osteogenesis imperfecta in cattle.

Numerous other glycoproteins present in the ex-tracellular matrix, in cell membranes, and in the cells themselves serve as enzymes and regulators of matrix protein function. They also serve protective, perm-selective, and messenger functions: controlling the flow of water, ions, and low molecular weight sub-stances into and out of the cell.

Other Components

Like other body tissues, the connective tissues contain nucleic acids, carbohydrates, regulatory pro-teins, enzymes, hormones, peptides, and membrane and depot lipids. These components serve functions similar to those in the other nonconnective tissues and are not discussed here.

ANATOMY AND PHYSIOLOGY OF SPECIALIZED CONNECTIVE TISSUES

Bone

Bones form an essential part of the locomotor system, acting as lever arms during motion and resisting the force of gravity. Bones also protect and support adjacent tissues and organs. In addition to these mechanical functions, bones serve an important chemical function, providing a reservoir for mineral homeostasis.

Bone consists of several functionally distinct re-gions (Fig. 150–9). At the articulating surfaces is articular cartilage. Surrounding the entire bone is a membranous structure, the periosteum. Below the articular cartilage, in the epiphysis, lies the secondary center of ossification, and below that, in growing

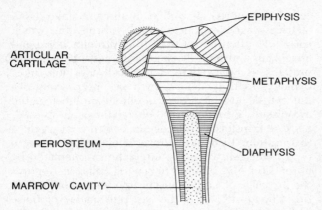

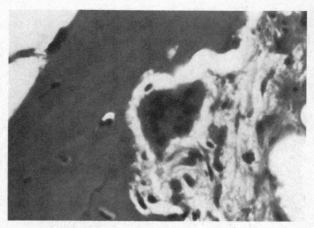

Figure 150–9. A long bone showing the joint surface, the articular cartilage, the secondary ossification center, the growth plate, and metaphyseal (cancellous) and diaphyseal (cortical) bone surrounding the marrow cavity.

Figure 150–11. Osteoclasts are easily recognized by three features: large size, many nuclei, and the presence of a ruffled border adjacent to a mineralized surface.

animals, the physis, or growth plate. Woven, lamellar, cancellous bone lies below the physis in the metaphysis, and the compact, cortical bone surrounds a marrow cavity in the diaphyseal region.

There are three principal cell types in all bones: osteoblasts, osteoclasts, and osteocytes.[26, 33] The osteoblasts, round, plump cells with abundant endoplasmic reticulum, are the bone cells responsible for laying down the matrix (see Fig. 150–9C). They are found on the surface of bone-forming regions, known as Haversian systems, which surround blood vessels within the matrix of woven bone. Once encased in mineral, these cells do not die but rather communicate via long processes with other mineral-encased cells and with unencased osteoblasts on the surface of the osteoid. These mineral-encased cells with long communicating processes are the osteocytes (Fig. 150–10). The large multinucleated cells with ruffled borders that lie on the surface of the mineralized matrix are osteoclasts (Fig. 150–11). These giant cells (20–100 μm in diameter), are directly responsible for removing mineral and matrix (bone resorption).

Examination of the shape and organization of bone

in radiographs or in slab sections reveals a pattern designed to withstand stress (Fig. 150–12). In a weight-bearing bone, they would correspond to the radiographic pattern of bone organization. The arrangement of this pattern corresponds to the nature and type of stresses applied to the bone. The ability of bone to adapt its architecture and external form in response to such stresses (Wolff's law) is one of the unique properties of bony tissues.[16]

All bones—long bones, flat bones, intramembranous bones, woven and compact bones—are specialized forms of connective tissue, and their form and function, like those of other connective tissues, depend upon the arrangement and interactions of the

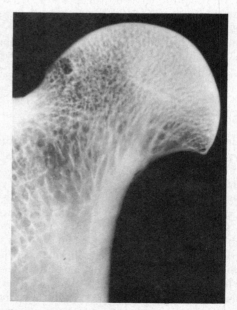

Figure 150–12. Radiograph of a canine femur illustrates the relationship between form and function (Wolff's law). The ball-and-socket arrangement of the joint provides a wide range of motion. The shape of the bone is such that there is sufficient mechanical strength to support the weight of the animal. The arrangement of the trabeculae matches the theoretical planes of force. (Courtesy of Dr. Steven Arnoczky.)

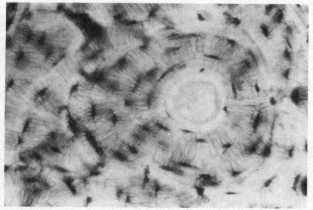

Figure 150–10. Osteocytes buried in calcified bone matrix communicate with other osteocytes and osteoblasts by long processes known as canaliculae. The precise function of the osteocyte is unknown. (Courtesy of Dr. Vincent Vigoritta.)

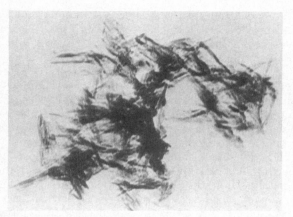

Figure 150–13. Electron micrographs of mineral crystals from immature rabbit bone, released from the collagen matrix by low temperature hydrazine deproteination. Individual crystals range in length from 15 to 40 nm.

elements of the extracellular matrix. The component of the extracellular bone matrix that distinguishes bones from other connective tissue matrices and enables it to perform its unique functions is the mineral.

The mineral found in bone is an analog of the naturally occurring mineral hydroxyapatite, $Ca_{10}(PO_4)_6(OH)_2$.[7] Bone mineral crystals, in contrast to the large geological apatite crystals, are extremely small (20–40 nm in largest dimension) (Fig. 150–13). The microscopic crystals found in bone mineral, as a consequence of their small size, are more soluble than geological apatites and contain more impurities than pure hydroxyapatite crystals. Bone mineral contains variable amounts of carbonate, magnesium, fluoride, and citrate, in addition to calcium and phorphorus. Bone mineral, as well as the entire bone matrix, is constantly being removed (by osteoclasts) and reformed (by osteoblasts) in response to normal mechanical, biochemical, and physiological stress. This remodelling of bone strengthens those areas subject to the most stress. Like other tissues, bone is in equilibrium with body fluids, and demineralization of bone occurs when the intake of minerals (calcium, magnesium, phosphorus) necessary for bone formation is inadequate, as in rickets, or when there is excessive loss of calcium and magnesium ions, as in hyperparathyroidism.

Mineral turnover (homeostasis) is principally controlled by three hormones:[11, 31] parathyroid hormone, calcitonin, and vitamin D.[11, 31] Parathyroid hormone is a peptide produced by the parathyroid gland, which maintains (increases) circulating calcium ion levels. It acts on three target organs: the kidney, where it increases calcium ion absorption and decreases phosphate absorption in the tubules; the intestinal tract, where it increases calcium absorption; and bone, where it causes demineralization. In each of these tissues, parathyroid hormone interacts with vitamin D metabolites to produce these effects. Calcitonin, a thyroid peptide hormone, is a parathyroid hormone antagonist, in that it directly affects osteoclasts, preventing the release of calcium ions from

bone. Vitamin D is now known to be a hormone, since it can be produced in one tissue (the skin) and is transported to other tissues (bone, intestine, kidney), where it binds to specific receptors and causes protein synthesis.[22] Several different vitamin D metabolites exist in normal sera, but the active metabolite which has been most thoroughly characterized is 1,25-dihydroxy-cholecalciferol $(1,25D_3)$. The 25-hydroxylation of this metabolite occurs in the liver, whereas 1-hydroxylation, under the influence of parathyroid hormone, occurs in the kidney. Animals with kidney disease, or anephric animals, lack this active metabolite and show severe bone problems characterized by decreased mineralization of osteoid (osteomalacia) and defective cartilage calcification. The bones of these animals are weakened, deformed, and unable to bear weight. Treatment with $1,25D_3$ or a mixture of $1,25D_3$ and a newly characterized metabolite, $24,25D_3$, rapidly reverses the process. The 24,25-dihydroxy metabolite, whose functions are still being investigated, may influence the formation of a calcifiable matrix.

Endochondral Ossification[2, 8]

Bone forms, for the most part, by transformation of cartilage into an ossified structure. In the embryo,

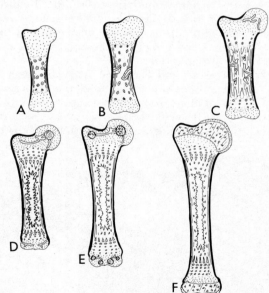

Figure 150–14. The embryonic (A–C) and neonatal (D–F) development of long bones. A, Initially the long bone is predominantly cartilaginous. Calcifying hypertrophic chondrocytes in the center of the bone are surrounded by a thin collar of cancellous periosteal membranous bone (primary ossification center). B, As development proceeds, canals enable vascular invasion of the calcified cartilage. Hyaline cartilage persists at the proximal and distal ends of the bone. C, Vascular invasion is followed by the deposition of endochondral bone on the calcified cartilage matrix. Epiphyseal capillaries begin to invade the hyaline cartilage. D, At birth, a secondary ossification center within the hyaline cartilage and a central marrow cavity appear, surrounded by newly formed compact bone. E, With further development the cartilaginous matrix narrows and more compact bone is laid down. F, A well-defined growth plate appears below the bone of the proximal and distal epiphysis. Growth in width occurs by periosteal bone formation, whereas longitudinal growth occurs by endochondral ossification.

mesenchymal cells condense to form a cartilage model, which later transforms into bone (Fig. 150–14). The cells in this cartilage model differentiate into chondroblasts. These chondroblasts secrete a cartilaginous matrix. Division of chondrocytes, developed as the chondroblasts were trapped within the matrix they themselves secreted, and apposition of new chondrocytes from the periosteum allow growth of this primitive bone form. The formation of a calcified osseous collar (periosteum) is followed by vascular invasion, resulting in the formation of the primary ossification center, which becomes the diaphysis and metaphysis of bone. Bone continues to grow by vascular-mediated ossification of the epiphysis, resulting in the formation of a secondary ossification center. Longitudinal growth proceeds via endochondral ossification, the conversion of rapidly growing cartilage in the physis (the area between primary and secondary ossification centers) into calcified cartilage and bone. The cartilage of the original model persists at the articular surface and as discs of cartilage (physis) separating the two calcifying regions.

Some bones (the perichondrium-derived, intramembranous bones of the bony collar and cranial and facial skeleton) form directly, without going through the process of endochondral ossification. In direct formation, osteoblasts, as they differentiate, form a quickly spreading fibrous intercellular matrix, which rapidly ossifies and provides sites upon which additional bone is deposited.

The process of endochondral ossification can be understood most easily in terms of the changes in the epiphyseal plate. The epiphyseal plate, or growth plate, extends from the resting or reverse cell zone to the calcified cartilage zone (Fig. 150–15). In the

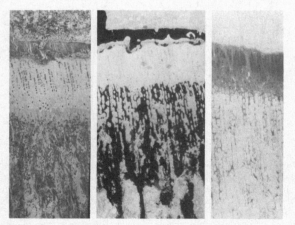

Figure 150–15. Growth plate of a 21-day-old rat, nondecalcified section, stained with H & E (left), von Kossa's stain (center), and safranin O (right). The cells of the growth plate extend from the bony spicules in the proximal area to the newly forming mineral spicules in the distal metaphyseal region. The widely spaced small cells at the top of the growth plate are the resting, or reserve, cells. These cells then line up in columns (columnar or proliferating cells) and begin to swell (hypertrophic cells). Calcification, shown in the von Kossa–stained section, occurs around the lowest hypertrophic cells. It is in this region that safranin O staining for proteoglycans is diminished. Staining for proteoglycans persists well into the calcified regions.

resting cell zone, the cells show less frequent mitosis and provide the stem cells for the process. Each of these cells divides to form another stem cell and a proliferating cell. Proliferating cells divide rapidly, lining up in long columns. The columns of cells are separated by wide longitudinal partitions of cartilage, and individual cells are separated by thin transverse septa. As the columns approach the metaphyseal area, the columnar cells enlarge, forming hypertrophic cells. In the lower half of the hypertrophic cell zone, mineral deposition begins. The most hypertrophic lowest cell is the only cell that dies in the process. After cartilage calcification, there is an invasion of blood vessels into the calcified cartilage, resulting in removal of the initial calcified deposits and concomitant deposition of woven bone (primary spongiosa) by osteoblasts on a type I collagen matrix. The importance of vascular invasion for triggering this osteogenesis has long been known.[35] The earliest-formed woven bone is subsequently remodelled to yield cortical bone with a well-developed marrow cavity.

Certain additional morphological changes can be seen in the cartilage matrix during endochondral ossification. In the proliferating zone, the cells are rich in rough endoplasmic reticulum, indicating their high metabolic activity. The mitochondria of the chondrocytes in the proliferating zone contain numerous electron-dense calcium-phosphate granules,[8] whereas the cells in the more distal zone of provisional calcification contain few such granules. The disappearance of calcium phosphate from the mitochondria when mineral crystals first appear in the extracellular matrix suggests a causal relationship between these intracellular and extracellular deposits.

Much of the first mineral to appear outside the chondrocytes is associated with membrane-bound bodies called extracellular matrix vesicles.[2, 6] These vesicles provide a preferential site for mineral deposition within the growth plate as well as in other mineralizing tissues.

Noncollagenous proteins, closely associated with cartilage or bone collagens, promote the initial deposition of apatite and regulate the size, orientation, and rate of growth of bone mineral crystals.

During endochondral ossification, cartilage proteoglycans are markedly altered.[9, 15] Although histochemical studies suggested proteoglycan loss during calcification, it is now clear that the size of the proteoglycan aggregates and the ability of proteoglycan monomers to form aggregates decrease from the resting zone to the hypertrophic zone. In addition, the spacing between individual monomers on the hyaluronic acid "backbone" increases as the calcification front is approached. Whether these changes are due to specific proteoglycan degradation or to synthesis of a different type of proteoglycans is not known. Bone cells do synthesize a proteoglycan quite different in composition from and smaller than growth plate proteoglycans.

In vitro studies show that at concentrations in

noncalcifying cartilage, the proteoglycan aggregate, and the subunit extracted from bovine nasal cartilage retards hydroxyapatite precipitation from a supersaturated calcium phosphate solution.[4] At these same concentrations, growth of hydroxyapatite crystals is inhibited.[7] These data support the thesis that proteoglycans are modified prior to calcification. The way these modifications take place and the mechanisms by which unmodified proteoglycans regulate mineral deposition remain to be determined.

Cartilage calcification also depends on an increase in the local calcium and phosphate concentration due to the action of enzymes and calcium-binding macromolecules. The formation of extracellular matrix vesicles and specific macromolecules such as phosphoproteins and Ca-phospholipid-phosphate complexes, which may serve as initiators of mineral deposition, are key steps in the mineralization process.[2, 5, 6, 26] Once the first mineral crystals form, the remaining mineral develops by growth on the initial crystals. The rate and extent of mineral growth depend on the interaction of mineral crystals with connective tissue elements, such as osteonectin, osteocalcin (a gamma-carboxyglutamic acid containing protein specific to bone), and, of course, collagen.

Muscle: The Contractile and Cytoskeletal Proteins[10, 20, 27]

Fibrous proteins occur intracellularly as well as in the extracellular matrix. Motion of single cells and whole tissues as well as of organelles within the cells depends on these intracellular proteins, called the cytoskeletal proteins because of their location (cytoplasmic) and structure (insoluble and fibrous). The cytoskeletal proteins are those fibrous elements that hold the cell intact, maintain its shape, and provide it with contractile, locomotive, and adhesive properties.[23] First characterized in muscle cells but known to exist in some form in all cells, the cytoskeleton consists, in order of decreasing size, of thick filaments

(40–45 nm in diameter), microtubules (24–25 nm in diameter), intermediate filaments (10–20 nm in diameter), and thin filaments (5–8 nm in diameter). The microtubules, which traverse the cytoplasm of all cells as continuous structures, are involved in mitosis. Consisting of a fibrous tubulin polymer with associated regulatory proteins, the microtubules can be disrupted by antimitotic drugs such as vinblastine and colchicine. Colchicine therapy is an effective treatment for "gouty" arthritis. The intermediate filaments, which differ in structure and composition in different tissues, are responsible for the maintenance of cell structure, and the anchorage of the nucleus during mitosis. Microfilaments, of which actin is a prime example, are essential for cell motility and, through postulated interactions with fibronectin, for cell-matrix interactions. The thick filaments contain myosin, a protein first isolated from muscle.

In the muscle cell, bundles of thick filaments (myosin), held in place by the intermediate filament protein (desmin), interact with the thin filaments (actin), contracting and producing mechanical work. These contractile proteins in the muscle cells produce work in the form of motion, sustenance of weight, balance, propulsion of blood, regulation of temperature, secretion, and excretion.

There are three types of muscle in vertebrates: skeletal, cardiac, and smooth. Skeletal muscle, also called striated muscle owing to its light-microscopic appearance, is attached to the bones by tendons and controls the voluntary movement of these bones (Fig. 150–16). Cardiac muscle is similar in appearance to striated muscle but is not under voluntary control. Smooth muscle, which for the most part is not under voluntary control, lacks the striations of the other muscle types. Examples of smooth muscles are the muscles of the intestinal wall, bile ducts, and blood vessels.

Cells of striated muscles are the best-characterized of the muscle cells (sarcomeres). Microscopic examination of these cells demonstrates many characteristic features. Each cell (two to three centimeters in

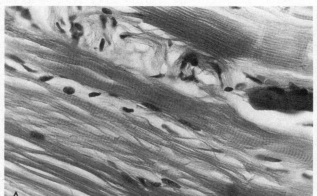
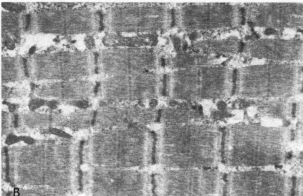

Figure 150–16. A, Light micrograph of striated muscle cells from a human rhabdomyosarcoma. The banded appearance is due to the overlap of thick and thin filaments as seen in *B*, an electron micrograph (× 72,000) from normal human skeletal muscle. (*A* courtesy of Dr. Vincent Vigoritta. *B* courtesy of Dr. P. Bullough.)

length), as seen in Figure 150–16*B*), is surrounded by a membrane, the sarcolemma or plasmalemma. There are discrete connections between this membrane and the fibrous elements of the cell, and tendons are attached to the outer surface of this membrane. The integrity of the membrane is essential for the maintenance of the electrical potential which controls the contractile process.

Within the boundaries of the cell membrane are the sarcoplasm (muscle cell cytoplasm), numerous cell nuclei, and mitochondria. The mitochondria, by the process of oxidative phosphorylation, produce the energy source of the cell, adenosine triphosphate (ATP). ATP is hydrolyzed during contaction to give adenosine diphosphate (ADP), inorganic phosphate, and energy. In the resting muscle, ADP can be converted to ATP by reaction with creatine phosphate. Skeletal muscle is often classified as fast (white) or slow (red), on the basis of the pattern of activity of the muscles and their energy requirements. Muscles that work continuously but slowly need a constant source of energy. This energy is produced by the coupling of the oxidation of glucose and oxidative phosphorylation. The red color of "slow muscle" is due to high concentrations of the heme-containing oxygen transport protein myoglobin. Muscles that work in bursts require rapid supplies of energy, generated by anaerobic glycolysis. These fast muscles, which do not depend on oxygen for energy production, contain less myoglobin and appear white.

The Contractile Process

The contractile process depends on interaction of four proteins: myosin, actin, troponin, and tropomyosin, with ionic calcium. In smooth muscle this interaction is mediated by a ubiquitous calcium-binding protein, calmodulin, which is structurally analogous to troponin.

Myosin is unique among the connective tissue fibrous proteins in that it is the only fibrous protein with enzymatic activity. The ATPase activity of myosin resides in a globular head at the end of the molecule. Each myosin molecule consists of two long alpha-helical rods coiled about each other, each ending in a globular region. A variety of proteins that regulate enzymic activity are associated with the globular regions.

Within the thick filaments, the myosin molecules are arranged tail-to-tail in a 1.5-μ long, cigar-shaped structure decorated with projections (globular heads) along its entire length. These thick filaments interdigitate with the actin-containing thin filaments to form the muscle fibers. It is this combination of fibers that gives striated muscle its characteristic appearance. The swivelling or rowing-like movements of the myosin cross-bridges towards the actin filaments result in a shortening of the fibers (contraction).

Actin is a globular protein found in numerous cells. Globular actin polymerizes to form a structure that resembles twisted two-stranded beads. Filamentous actin has the unique ability to activate the release of ADP from its binding site on the globular myosin heads. Thus, interaction of myosin head groups with actin thin filaments results in the activation of the multistep reaction:

$$\text{Myosin} + \text{ATP} \longrightarrow \text{Myosin}^* - \text{ATP} \rightarrow\rightarrow\rightarrow$$
$$\text{Myosin}^*\text{-ADP} - \text{P}_i \rightarrow \text{Myosin} + \text{ADP} + \text{P}_i + \text{energy}$$
$$\overset{\curvearrowright}{\underset{\text{actin}}{}}$$

in which the asterisk indicates an activated state of the enzyme. The trigger for the start of this set of reactions is calcium. Following transmission of an electrical signal, calcium ions flow into the cell, where they interact with troponin, a globular protein that has specific binding sites for this ion and for another protein, tropomyosin. Tropomyosin sits in the groove formed by the twisting chains of actin. Binding of calcium ions to troponin causes a series of conformational changes that result in the sliding of tropomyosin into the groove, permitting the myosin heads to interact with two actin subunits. After release of ADP and inorganic phosphate from myosin, the myosin heads return to their original positions. Following binding of a new ATP molecule, the muscle cell is ready for another calcium ion–triggered contraction.

Regulation of the contractile process and cell motility differs in smooth, skeletal, and cardiac muscle. For all these muscles, the process of contraction starts with a nerve signal that in turn levels to the release of calcium into the cytoplasm. In skeletal muscle, the increase in calcium ions results in the binding of calcium ions to troponin's calcium-binding subunit, which in turn causes a conformational change in the whole troponin molecule, which sat in the actin groove. This change results in the movement of a second regulatory fibrous protein, tropomyosin, into the actin groove, allowing the myosin-actin interaction to occur. Recently, tropomyosin has been shown to be a noncompetitive inhibitor of myosin. Because tropomyosin and myosin do not bind to the same sites on actin, this suggests that the control of the entire process resides in myosin. (The precise nature of this control is unclear.) The fact that myosin itself controls contraction is seen in all muscle systems. In the scallop adductor muscle, the direct binding of calcium activates myosin-ATPase. In cardiac muscle, calcium ion–triggered phosphorylation of a protein associated with the globular head causes the activation of myosin. Similar regulation via other calcium-binding proteins may occur in all cells.

1. Ali, S. Y., and Wisby, A.: Ultrastructural aspects of normal osteoarthritic cartilage. Ann. Rheum. Dis. *34*(Suppl. 2):21, 1975.
2. Anderson, H. C.: Vesicles associated with calcification in the matrix of epiphyseal cartilage. J. Cell Biol. *41*:58, 1969.
3. Axelsson, I., and Bjelle, A.: Proteoglycan structure of bovine articular cartilage. Variation with age and in osteoarthrosis. Scand. J. Rheumat. 8:217, 1979.
4. Blumenthal, N. C., Posner, A. S., Silverman, L. D., and

Rosenberg, L. C.: The effect of proteoglycans on in vitro hydroxyapatite formation. Calcif. Tissue Res. 27:75, 1979.

5. Boskey, A. L.: The role of Ca-PL-PO$_4$ complexes in tissue mineralization. Metab. Bone Dis. Rel. Res. 1:137, 1978.

6. Boskey, A. L.: Models of matrix vesicle calcification. Inorg. Persp. Biol. Med. 2:51, 1979.

7. Boskey, A. L.: Current concepts of the physiology and biochemistry of calcification. Clin. Orthop. 167:225, 1981.

8. Brighton, C. T., and Hunt, R. M.: The role of mitochondria in growth plate calcification as demonstrated in a rachitic model. J. Bone Jt. Surg. 60A:630, 1978.

9. Buckwalter, J. A.: Proteoglycan structure in calcifying cartilage. Clin. Orthop. 172:207, 1983.

10. Burke, J. M., and Ross, R.: Synthesis of connective tissue macromolecules by smooth muscle. Int. Rev. Connect. Tissue Res. 8:119, 1979.

11. Canalis, E.: The hormonal and local regulation of bone formation. Endocrine Rev. 4:62, 1983.

12. Engfeldt, B., Hielth, A., and Westerborn, O.: Effect of papain on bone. I. Histologic, autoradiographic, and microradiographic study on young dogs. Arch. Pathol. 68:600, 1959.

13. Eyre, D.: Molecular diversity in the body's protein scaffold. Science 207:1315, 1980.

14. Fisher, L. W., Whitson, S. W., Avioli, L. V., and Termine, J. D.: Matrix sialoprotein of developing bone. J. Biol. Chem. 258:12723, 1983.

15. Franzen, A., Heinegard, D., and Olsson, S. E.: Proteoglycans and calcification of cartilage in the femoral head epiphysis of the immature rat. J. Bone Jt. Surg. 64A:558, 1982.

16. Glimcher, M. J.: On the form and function of bone: from molecules to organs. In Veis, A. (ed.): The Chemistry and Biology of Mineralized Connective Tissues. Elsevier/North Holland, New York, 1982.

17. Handley, C. J., Brooks, P. R., and Lowther, D. A.: Extracellular matrix metabolism by chondrocytes. VI. Concomitant depression by exogeneous levels of proteoglycan of collagen and proteoglycan synthesis by chondrocytes. Biochim. Biophys. Acta 544:441, 1978.

18. Hewitt, A. T., Varner, H. H., Silver, M. S., et al.: Isolation and partial characterization of chondronectin, an attachment factor for chondrocytes. J. Biol. Chem. 257:2330, 1982.

19. Hynes, R. O.: Fibronectin and its relation to cellular structure and behavior. In Hay, E. D. (ed.): Cell Biology of the Extracellular Matrix. Plenum Press, New York, 1981.

20. Karpati, G.: Muscle: structure, organization, and healing. In Cruess, R. L. (ed.): The Musculoskeletal System. Embryology, Biochemistry, and Physiology. Churchill Livingstone, New York, 1982.

21. Kimato, K., Barrasch, H. J., Brown, K. S., and Pennypacker, J. P.: Absence of proteoglycan core protein in cartilage from the cmd/cmd (cartilage matrix deficiency) mouse. J. Biol. Chem. 256:6961, 1981.

22. Koshy, K. T.: Vitamin D: an update. J. Pharm. Sci. 71:137, 1982.

23. Lazarides, E.: Intermediate filaments, a chemically heterogenous, developmentally regulated class of proteins. Ann. Rev. Biochem. 51:219, 1982.

24. Leader, R. W., Hegreberg, G. A., Padgett, G. A., and Wagner, B. M.: Comparative pathology of connective tissue disease. In Wagner, B. M., Fleischmayer, R., and Kaufman, N. (eds.): Connective Tissue Diseases. Williams & Wilkins, Baltimore, 1983.

25. Linde, A., Jontell, M., Lundgren, T., et al.: Noncollagenous proteins of rat compact bone. J. Biol. Chem. 258:1698, 1983.

26. Marks, S. C., Jr.: The origin of osteoclasts: evidence, clinical implications and investigative challenges of an extra-skeletal source. J. Oral Pathol. 12:226, 1983.

27. Morent, D., Bertrane, R., Pantel, P., et al.: Structure of the actin-myosin interface. Nature 292:301, 1981.

28. Ohkubo, H., Vogeli, G., Mudry, M., et al.: Isolation and characterization of overlapping genomic clones covering the chicken α 2 (type I) collagen gene. PNAS US 77:7059, 1980.

29. Orkin, R. W., Williams, B. R., Cranley, R. E., et al.: Defects in the cartilagenous growth plates of brachymorphic mice. J. Cell Biol. 73:287, 1977.

30. Prockop, D. J., Kivirrkko, K. I., Tuderman, L., and Guzman, N. A.: The biosynthesis of collagen and its disorders. N. Engl. J. Med. 301:13, 1979.

31. Raisdz, L. G., and Kream, B. E.: Regulation of bone formation. N. Engl. J. Med. 309:29, 1983.

32. Sanberg, L. B., Soskel, N. T., and Leslie, J. G.: Elastin structure biosynthesis, and relation to disease states. N. Engl. J. Med. 304:566, 1981.

33. Simmons, D. J., Kent, G. N., Jilka, R. L., et al.: Formation of bone by isolated, cultured osteoblasts in millipore diffusion chambers. Calcif. Tissue Int. 34:291, 1982.

34. Termine, J. D., Belcourt, A. B., Conn, K. M., and Kleinman, H.: Mineral and collagen binding proteins of fetal calf bone. J. Biol. Chem. 256:10404, 1981.

Chapter **151**

Fractures and Fracture Biology

Steven P. Arnoczky, James W. Wilson, and Peter Schwarz

MECHANICAL PROPERTIES OF BONE

The mechanical characteristics of bone can be described in reference to its structural behavior or its material properties. Bone may be compressed (axial compression), stretched (axial tension), bent (bending), or twisted (torsion). The characteristics of bone can be expressed by qualitatively assessing the bone's response, or deformation, to the applied force or loads. To relate this principle to practical orthopedics, it is necessary to understand some of the basic concepts of structural analysis.

When sufficient forces are applied to any object, the object deforms from its original state. If the deformation is measured, a force-deformation curve can be constructed (Fig. 151–1). During the initial linear portion of the curve, the force is such that the object returns to its original dimensions when the force is removed; the object exhibits *elastic deformation*. If sufficient force is applied, a point is

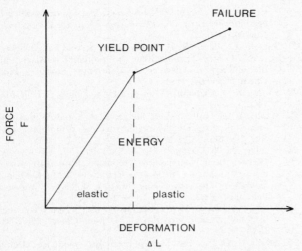

Figure 151–1. A force-deformation curve.

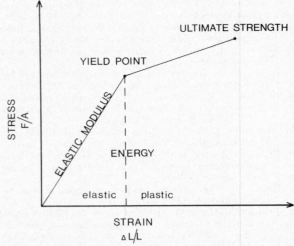

Figure 151–2. A stress-strain curve.

reached at which the tested object no longer returns to its original dimensions when the force is removed; this is the *yield point*. As more force is applied, the object undergoes progressive permanent deformation. The object is now undergoing *plastic deformation*. Further loading beyond the yield point results in more and more marked deformation, until the object breaks; this is the *failure point*. The area under the curve at any particular point is the energy absorbed by the test object when the indicated force is applied.

During loading, deformation occurs within the substance of the material, and internal forces are generated. The deformation created within the object is referred to as *strain*, and the resultant internal force intensities as *stress*. The strains at any point are mathematically related to the stresses at that point. There are two general types of stress and strain, normal and shear. *Normal stress* acts perpendicular to an object's surface and can be either compressive or tensile. *Normal strain* is the compressed or stretched change in an object. *Shear stress* acts parallel to an object's surface and tends to deform by deviation. *Shear strain* is the angular deformation expressed in radians. Measurement of stresses and strains during application of force to an object allows construction of a stress-strain curve (Fig. 151–2) with associated regions of elastic and plastic behavior, a yield point, an energy absorption, and a point of failure or *ultimate strength*. The slope of the elastic region of the curve is the *elastic modulus*, or *Young's modulus of elasticity*, and is a measurement of stiffness.

The relationships between stresses and strains are governed by the material properties of the object tested; thus, the stress-strain curve is a mechanical representation of the material properties. The force-deformation curve is related to the dimensional characteristics of the object being tested and is a mechanical representation of the structural properties. Application of these testing modes and terms to bone

allows the mechanical description of their structural and material properties.

The structural and material properties of bone are not static.[6] The bones of puppies and infants bend considerably before they break.[15,16] Immature bone resists overload failure not by its physical size and strength but by its ability to absorb energy through deformation. As bone matures there is an increase in the measured elastic modulus and yield stress at a rate parallel to growth.[6] Bone becomes stronger by becoming stiffer. As the material bone is made of becomes stiffer, the bones themselves adapt to the biological and physiological factors affecting them by optimizing their shape to resist the forces they are

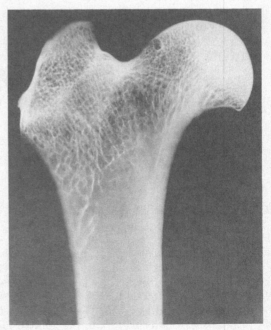

Figure 151–3. The proximal femur of a dog showing the orientation of the trabecular bone to reflect the stresses placed on this area.

subjected to. The principle of bone's adaptability to mechanical function is known as Wolff's law, which oversimplified states that bone is deposited where it is needed in response to mechanical stresses. This principle is best seen in the trabecular pattern of the proximal femur, and indeed, many of Wolff's original theories result from observations of this area (Fig. 151–3).[10, 19] Recent research suggests that this need for bone is transmitted by strain-related electrical potentials, a term preferable to piezoelectricity. As the skeleton matures, it adapts by increasing both the material and structural strength of its members. Once maturity is reached, bone appears to slowly and progressively deteriorate.

The position of cancellous bone at the ends of long bones suggests a specific function, possibly to support compressive loads (Fig. 151–4). Evaluation of a compression stress-strain curve for cancellous bone reveals initial elastic behavior; however, once the yield point is reached, a long plateau occurs owing to progressive fracture and collapse of trabeculae.[6] With increased load, the fractured trabeculae begin to compact and the specimen gains stiffness. In tension, cancellous bone fails at fairly low loads because of rapid trabecular fracture.[6] Thus, cancellous bone is mechanically strongest under compression.

The mechanical properties of cortical bone depend on the rate at which the bone is loaded during testing. A specimen loaded rapidly has a greater elastic modulus and ultimate strength and absorbs more energy than one loaded slowly.[6] Materials that are load

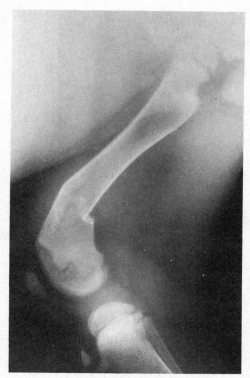

Figure 151–5. A pathological "folding" fracture of an immature dog with secondary nutritional hyperparathyroidism.

rate–dependent are *viscoelastic*. The mechanical properties also depend on the direction in which testing loads are applied.[6] Bone loaded perpendicular to the direction of the osteons fails in a brittle manner with less nonelastic deformation than bone loaded parallel.[6] Cortical bone is stronger, stiffer, and better able to resist stress along the axis of the bone than across the axis.[6] Materials whose properties depend on the direction of load are *anisotropic*. Cortical bone is thus a complex viscoelastic, anisotropic material. The rate of loading, the rapidity of deformation, or *strain rate*, and the direction of loading must be specified when one is describing material behavior.

Another important consideration in the material properties of bone is its biological composition. Alterations in this composition from secondary nutritional hyperparathyroidism, osteoporosis, and osteomalacia markedly alter the mechanical properties of bone (Fig. 151–5).

FRACTURE MECHANICS

Bone exhibits specific failure or fracture patterns associated with the different modes of loading (Fig. 151–6). When loaded in tension, a bone fails with a fracture plane oriented approximately perpendicular to the applied force (along the planes of high tensile stresses) (Fig. 151–7). If a bone is loaded in compression, the fracture plane is generally at an oblique angle to the applied force (along the planes of high

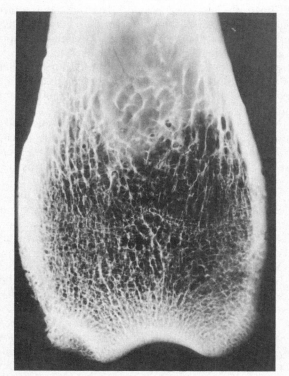

Figure 151–4. The distal femur of a dog showing the predominance of cancellous bone in this area.

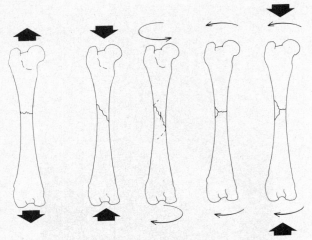

Figure 151–6. The fracture patterns created in cortical bone by tensile, compressive, torsional, bending, and combined bending and compressive forces. (After Carter, D. R., and Spengler, D. M.: Biomechanics of fracture. *In* Sumner-Smith, G. (ed.): *Bone in Clinical Orthopedics*. W. B. Saunders, Philadelphia, 1982.)

compressive stresses). When a bone is subjected to torsional loading the failure pattern is more complex. A fracture begins as a small crack on a plane of high shear stress parallel to the bone's axis, then runs in a spiral manner through the bone, following planes of high tensile stresses.[6] The final torsional fracture plane is a characteristic spiral (Fig. 151–8). Bending forces subject the bone to high tensile stresses on one side of the specimen and high compressive stresses on the other. Because bone is weaker in tension than in compression, the fracture plane usu-

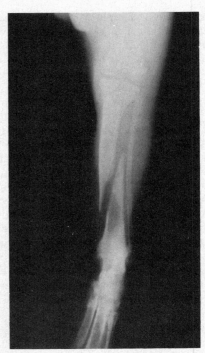

Figure 151–8. Classic spiral oblique fracture resulting from torsional forces.

ally originates transversely on the tension side of the specimen. In addition, an oblique fracture plane may be created on the compression side. If more than one oblique fracture plane is created on the compression side of the bone, a free, wedge-shaped fragment or "butterfly" may be created.[6] The oblique fracture planes may be accentuated in combined compressive and bending loading. Since bone is viscoelastic, rapid loading with higher strain rates causes the bone to absorb greater kinetic energy before failure.[6] When failure does occur, numerous fracture planes are propagated, resulting in the production of several butterfly fragments, or *comminution*.

Fracture lines always follow the path of least resistance. If changes in the bone structure occur, as with drill holes or osteolytic processes (neoplasia), these areas act as stress risers and the fracture line usually begins in or passes through them.

Bones in the body are seldom subjected to the idealized loading forces discussed in the previous paragraphs. Fractures seen clinically are usually a result of complex loading, and fracture patterns are likewise complex and numerous (Fig. 151–9). However, since clinical fractures result from overloading a bone to failure, evaluation of the patient's radiographs may provide insight into the type of loading that caused the fracture and a reasonable estimation of the magnitude and loading rate of the force. Fractures that resemble testing patterns are most likely due to applied forces similar to those in pure loading situations. Highly comminuted fractures indicate greater energy dissipation at failure most probably from a complex, rapidly applied force.

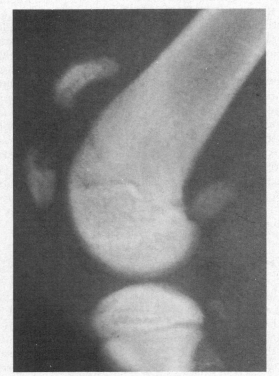

Figure 151–7. Fractured patella showing the fracture pattern resulting from tensile forces.

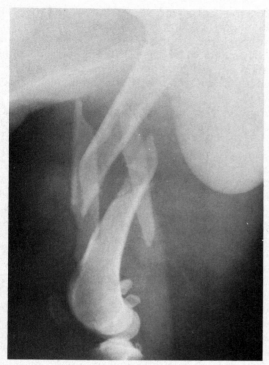

Figure 151–9. Comminuted fracture resulting from complex loading forces.

During trauma a tremendous amount of energy is transmitted to the body.[6] Most of this energy is absorbed by the soft tissue surrounding bones, principally muscle. Thus, when severe comminution is seen, a great deal of soft tissue injury usually accompanies the fracture. Appropriate measures need to be instituted to insure healing not only of the fracture but of the associated soft tissues as well. It is from these soft tissues that the normal blood supply to bone and the extraosseous blood supply of healing bone originate.

FRACTURE HEALING

"The healing of a fracture is one of the most remarkable of all the repair processes in the body since it results, not in a scar, but in the actual reconstruction of the injured tissue in something very much like its original form."[8]

Primary Bone Healing

Primary bone healing occurs with rigid internal fixation and results in bony union through direct growth of haversian systems across the fracture.[7, 8, 9, 13, 14] There is minimal to no external callus. Injury to the blood supply to osteons close to the fracture site stimulates intense activity in haversian systems in the area. Osteoclasts form "spearheads" at the ends of haversian canals close to the fracture site and become enlarged in preparation for the formation of a new system.[9, 14] The osteoclast "spear-

heads" (cutting cones) then advance at a rate of 50 to 80 μ per day, producing enlarged haversian canals that cross from one fragment to the opposite fragment.[9] Repair occurs when new osteons develop and cross the fracture site to replace old osteons that were deprived of their local blood supply. If a gap exists between the fracture fragments, or if there is not rigid immobilization, this type of healing does not occur. It is replaced by healing that is similar to that seen in the nonoperative management of fractures. In all probability, primary bone healing does not represent a qualitatively different form of healing but rather one that is quantitatively different owing to the mechanical environment.[3]

Secondary Bone Healing

When rigid internal fixation and excellent anatomic position do not exist, bone heals through a series of progressions known as secondary bone healing.

The classic stages of fracture repair encompass the progression of physiological events from fracture impact through fracture remodeling.[7] Although these can conveniently be considered as a series of phases occurring in sequence, they do overlap.

Stage of Fracture Impact. Bone absorbs energy until a failure occurs. The greater the rate of application of force, the greater the energy bone may absorb. The amount of energy absorbed is directly proportional to the volume of the bone. When fracture or failure occurs, this energy is "released" into the surrounding tissues. In severe comminution, a great deal of soft tissue injury may accompany the fracture.

Stage of Induction. This stage of fracture healing is perhaps the least differentiated because it occurs between fracture impact and the end of inflammation.[7] Following impact, cells in the area of the fracture are induced to form bone. The stimulus for this induction is probably multifactorial, involving enzymes, pH, and oxygen tension.[2] A bone morphogenic–stimulating substance (BMP) has also been described.[17]

Stage of Inflammation. In bone as in other tissues, the immediate responses to injury are inflammation and edema. The stage of inflammation begins immediately after the fracture occurs and persists until initiation of cartilage or bone formation. There is a disruption of blood supply within the bone and surrounding tissues with hemorrhage and hematoma formation. The exact role of the hematoma at the fracture site has been a subject of debate. Lexer believed that the fracture hematoma represented an inactive "stuffing" material between the ends of the fracture, without value for union, whereas Phemister believed that fibrin in the hematoma may stimulate cell regeneration and aid in immobilizing the fracture ends.[7, 10] Granulation tissue could advance into the hematoma and perform the same function as in soft tissue repair.[7] Most investigators agree that the active role of the hematoma is unimportant in the fracture healing process.[7] Studies have demonstrated that the hematoma between the fracture ends is virtually eliminated in rigid anatomical internal fixation, the condition in which primary bone healing occurs.[7]

Following fracture, there is gross disruption of the osteons and lacunae with release of lysosomal enzymes. The bone at the edge of the fracture site on both the periosteal and endosteal surfaces becomes necrotic, and a state of hypoxia exists with an acidic environment.[3, 5, 7, 13] The soft tissue in the region shows the usual changes of inflammation with vasodilatation and the exudation of plasma and leukocytes. Polymorphs, histiocytes, and mast cells soon make their appearance, and the process of clearing up the debris begins. Osteoclasts begin to mobilize, and osteolytic activity may be seen along the ruffled border of the cell.

Stage of Soft Callus. Within a few days following injury, fibroblasts proliferate, as in the fibroplastic phase of soft tissue healing. Simultaneously, osteogenic cells from the cambium layer of the periosteum and from the endosteum migrate and proliferate at the fracture site. This is a very active phase in which both an external callus and an internal soft callus are formed.[7] The external callus plays an important role by helping to immobilize the fracture and to load the bone long before union is complete.[18]

As the tissues of the callus form, each deposits its characteristic extracellular matrices. The production of collagen by the fibroblasts begins within days and reaches its peak at approximately one week.[3] Mucopolysaccharide production, characteristic of cartilage activity, also peaks at about one week and slowly decreases over many more weeks.[3] Calcium uptake similarly increases more slowly, within days after fracture, and does not reach a peak for at least several weeks. It may remain elevated for months or years.[3] The surface of the soft callus is electronegative and remains so throughout this stage, which usually lasts three to four weeks or until the bony fragments are united by fibrous and/or collagenous tissue.[7] The end of this stage is clinically evident when the osseous fragments are no longer grossly mobile and are at least in a "sticky" phase.[7]

Stage of Hard Callus. In this stage the callus is gradually converted into woven bone. In areas where cartilage is present, the conversion occurs through enchondral ossification.[3, 4, 5, 7, 8, 11] As enchondral ossification and mineralization of new osteoid progress, the healing becomes visible radiographically.[3] At one to three weeks, foci of mineralization are seen as flecks of radiodense material throughout the callus. The callus appears "fluffy" as these flecks coalesce, and as the callus matures and stiffens, the radiodensity begins to appear more uniform.[3] Eventually a trabecular pattern develops, and individual trabeculae may be seen crossing the fracture line.[3] This process may take a matter of weeks or sometimes months, even in normally healing fractures.[3] An increase in vascularity accompanies this stage along with a restoration of the endosteal and periosteal blood supply.[12]

Although the arbitrary end of this reparative stage is that point at which the fracture is "healed" enough to allow normal function, the fracture continues to strengthen and remodel during the final phase of healing.

Stage of Remodeling. The final stage of fracture repair is the longest and is characterized by a slow change in the shape of the bone to allow function and restore normal or near-normal strength. This process, which is an accelerated version of the normal deposition-resorption phenomenon, has been reported to occur as long as six to nine years after fracture.[3] The capability for remodeling is markedly greater in the immature animal than in the adult.[7] This effect is believed to be mediated through the epiphyseal plate, but the exact mechanism of its action has not been completely evaluated. It is not uncommon in the immature animal for a bone to heal in an angled position only to be actively remodelled and have the gross anatomical alignment of the bone restored some months later. Adult bone lacks this increased ability to actively remodel angular deformities at the fracture site, and thus fractures in the mature animal must be properly and accurately reduced if proper anatomical alignment is to be maintained.

1. Arnoczky, S. P., and Wilson, J. W.: The connective tissues. In Whittick, W. G. (ed.): Canine Orthopaedics. 2nd ed. Lea & Febiger, Philadelphia, 1985.
2. Bassett, C. A. L., and Herrman, I.: Influence of oxygen concentration and mechanical factors on differentiation of connective tissues in vitro. Nature 190:460, 1961.
3. Brand, R. A.: Fracture healing. In Albright, J. A., and Brand, R. A. (eds.): Scientific Basis of Orthopaedics. Appleton-Century-Crofts, New York, 1979.
4. Brown, S. G.: Secondary bone union. In Bojrab, M. J. (ed.): Pathophysiology in Small Animal Surgery. Lea & Febiger, Philadelphia, 1981.
5. Bryandt, W. M.: Wound Healing. Ciba Clinical Symposia, Vol. 29 no. 3, 1977.
6. Carter, D. R., and Spengler, D. M.: Biomechanics of fracture. In Sumner-Smith, G. (ed.): Bone in Clinical Orthopaedics. W. B. Saunders, Philadelphia, 1982.
7. Heppenstall, R. B.: Fracture healing. In: Fracture Treatment and Healing. W. B. Saunders, Philadelphia, 1980.
8. McKibbin, B.: The biology of fracture healing in long bones. J. Bone Jt. Surg. 60B:150, 1978.
9. Perren, S.: Primary bone healing. In Bojrab, M. J. (ed.): Pathophysiology in Small Animal Surgery. Lea & Febiger, 1981.
10. Perren, S. M., and Rahn, B. A.: Biomechanics of fracture healing. I: Historical review and mechanical aspects of internal fixation. Orthop. Surv. 2:108, 1978.
11. Rahn, B. A.: Bone healing: Histologic and physiologic concepts. In Sumner-Smith, G. (ed.): Bone in Clinical Orthopaedics. W. B. Saunders, Philadelphia, 1982.
12. Rhinelander, F. W.: The normal circulation of diaphyseal cortex and its response to fracture. J. Bone Jt. Surg. 50A:784, 1968.
13. Schatzker, J.: Concepts of fracture stabilization. In Sumner-Smith, G. (ed.): Bone in Clinical Orthopaedics. W. B. Saunders, Philadelphia, 1982.
14. Sevitt, S.: Healing of fractures. In Owen, R., Goodfellow, J., and Bullough, P. (eds.): Scientific Foundations of Ortho-

paedics and Traumatology. W. B. Saunders, Philadelphia, 1980.

15. Trozilli, P. A., Takebe, K., Burstein, A. H., and Heiple, K. G.: Structural properties of immature canine bone. J. Biomech. Eng. *103*:232, 1981.
16. Trozilli, P. A., Takebe, K., Burstein, A. H., et al.: The material properties of immature bone. J. Biomech. Eng. *104*:12, 1982.
17. Urist, M. R., Iwata, H., and Strates, B. S.: Bone morphogenic

protein and proteinase in the guinea pig. Clin. Orthop. *85*:275, 1972.
18. Urist, M. R., and Johnson, R. W.: Calcification and ossification; the healing of fractures in man under clinical conditions. J. Bone Jt. Surg. *25*:375, 1943.
19. Wolff, J.: Das Gesetz der Transformation der inneren Architectur der Knochen bei pathologischen Veranderungen der ausseren Knochenform. Dissertation, Stizungs Beericht Preuss, Akademie der Wissenschaften, 1884.

Chapter **152**

Fracture First Aid: The Open (Compound) Fracture

Daniel C. Richardson

The current terms *closed* and *open* fractures have replaced the terms "simple" and "compound" fractures. A fracture is *open* when it is exposed to the air through either a surgical incision or trauma. *Contaminated* is synonymous with *open*. Proper management is required to avoid progression from contamination to infection.

The most common cause for an open fracture is surgical open reduction of a closed fracture, which is generally undertaken with the attempt at "sterile" technique. Once a fracture is opened, the risks of contamination and subsequent infection increase. However, the benefits of open reduction and internal fixation usually surpass the risks of surgery.

The next most common cause for an open fracture is the fracture itself, as a result of "compounding" from within or of external forces. Further subdividing such fractures into first-, second-, and third-degree[11] or grades I, II, and III[9] allows a more concise description of severity and aids in a more accurate prognosis.

Grade I open fractures are those in which a bone fragment penetrates the muscle and skin from within outward. They may leave the bone exposed. Often, the bone penetrates and then returns to rest under the skin, leaving a skin wound of variable size. Clipping of the hair and careful inspection may be necessary to see the wound.

Grade II open fracture results when an external force penetrates the skin, exposing the bone to air. Degrees of skin wounds may be similar to those in grade I open fractures.

Open fractures classified as *grade III* are the result of external forces and have extensive loss of soft tissue, often because of gunshot wounds or degloving injuries from car-dog-pavement contact.

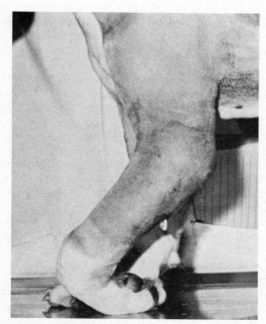

Figure 152–1. Grade I open fracture. The bone has penetrated the skin from within outward.

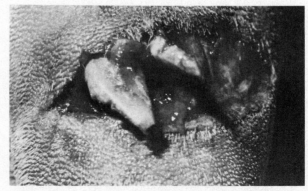

Figure 152–2. Grade II open fracture. An external force resulted in a skin laceration, soft tissue damage, and fracture of the underlying bone.

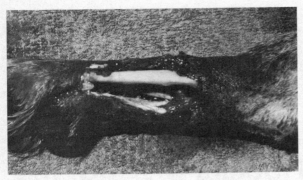

Figure 152–3. Grade III open fracture. Extensive soft tissue loss with underlying fractures of the metatarsals.

PATHOPHYSIOLOGY OF OPEN FRACTURES

Open fractures require accurate assessment and management of two factors, the fracture and the wound. The two factors are intimately related. Proper wound management generally allows uncomplicated bone healing. However, concentration on fracture reduction and stabilization without regard for the wound can result in failure of or, at best, delay in normal bone healing. The ultimate goal of fracture treatment is bony union and recovery of function.

Adequate circulation is of prime importance in fracture healing and infection control, both of which are involved in open fracture management. The first step in the fracture repair process is ingrowth of new capillaries and fibroblasts into the fracture hematoma.

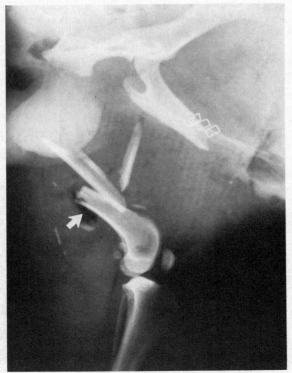

Figure 152–4. Radiographic evidence of air *(arrow)* in the soft tissues indicates an open fracture.

These vessels are fragile and rupture with the slightest motion. Rigid stability usually results in bone formation directly from mesenchymal (osteogenic) cells at the fracture site. With slight instability, fibrous tissue forms at the fracture, mineralizes, and undergoes necrosis. Through new vessels penetrating this tissue, macrophages enter to resorb necrotic debris, and mesenchymal cells (osteoblasts) lay down a bony callus. When even greater instability (with a resultant decrease in vascularity) exists, union occurs through an even slower process of endochondral ossification. All three processes can result eventually in bony union.

Infection results from the impairment of body defenses to combat a contaminated wound. Rapid quantitative techniques for bacterial count have been developed to aid in predicting when a contaminated wound can be closed. Less than 10^5 bacteria per gram of tissue is thought to be the "magic number" allowing tissue closure. However, more important than the number of bacteria is the culture medium (environment of the wound) in each case.

The presence of bacteria in or near a bone is insufficient to cause osteomyelitis,[10, 12, 13] an inflammation of the bone caused by a pyogenic organism.[4] For an open fracture to progress from contaminated to infected, pathogenic bacteria must be localized and have a suitable culture medium for growth.[8] Localization is readily accomplished by the mere definition of an open fracture. The bone has been exposed to the external environment and must be presumed to be contaminated. Because disruption of the vascular supply reduces the body's defenses, the contaminants are allowed time to multiply. The proper environment for bacterial growth is present owing to vascular stasis, plasma transudation, blood clot formation, and tissue necrosis. Thus, contamination proceeds to infection because of excessive bacteria, local ischemia (vascular stasis), tissue necrosis, and absence of drainage.[5] All of these detrimental factors can be corrected with early, aggressive therapy.

The average healing time of open fractures is significantly greater than that of closed fractures[11] because of impaired circulation and surrounding tissue infection.

Impairment of circulation in open fractures is generally more serious than in closed fractures, because of more energy dissipation in the bone and surrounding soft tissues. Another consequence of an open fracture is the penetration to the external environment that allows loss of fluids (e.g., the primary fracture hematoma) that would normally remain at the fracture site and aid in healing. The time required for subsequent reformation of the hematoma after the fracture site has been walled off may cause a diminution of osteogenic potential.[1]

An open fracture is contaminated. Contamination can readily lead to infection of the tissues. Just as loss of fluids can result in decreased osteogenic potential, entry of contaminants (bacteria) can result in tissue inflammation and necrosis, further delaying the healing process.

The overall goal in treatment of an open fracture is to combat the "negative factors" in order to allow normal healing. Cellular and bacterial debris must be encouraged to drain. Simultaneously, the fracture must be stabilized to encourage and preserve fibroblast infiltration, granulation tissue formation, and a new circulatory bed to promote progressive healing.[1, 6]

MANAGEMENT OF OPEN FRACTURES

Initial open fracture management is often performed at the accident by the owner or other concerned individual. The primary goals should be to avoid personal injury while handling an animal in pain, to stop active hemorrhage, and to prevent further wound contamination. Covering the wound with a clean cloth or first aid dressing and applying compression reduce contamination and hemorrhage. Upon presentation of the animal to the clinician, this dressing may be removed under clean conditions and replaced with a sterile bandage. This allows a rapid assessment of the wound primarily to stop active large-vessel hemorrhage requiring ligation. The compulsive urge to probe and explore the wound is avoided. Such maneuvers are of minimal to no value, no matter how well-intentioned. At best, they determine that there is communication from air to deeper tissues; at worst they introduce further contamination and damage tissues. The only good reason to introduce something into a wound is to promote drainage.[1]

Evaluation of the animal as a whole, system by system, is necessary. Often, the fracture is obvious but the associated and potentially life-threatening injuries are more subtle. A musculoskeletal and neurological examination is critical prior to repairing the fracture. Failure to detect concomitant ligamentous or nervous injuries may result in a healed bone but a nonfunctional limb.

Many open fractures have obvious skin lacerations. However, skin wounds indicating possible open fracture can be overlooked. Careful observation and clipping of the hair may be necessary to rule out an open fracture. Small puncture wounds from a grade I open fracture, left unattended, can result in purulent soft tissue infection within days.[11]

Manipulation of the fracture site is rarely indicated. If sufficient, temporary splinting materials are left in place. Inadequate immobilization should be replaced aseptically with a more functional bandage. Radiographs in two planes are generally adequate for initial planning of fracture management.

It is important to prevent rather than treat osteomyelitis. Culture and sensitivity testing in open fractures is of more diagnostic and therapeutic value in the obviously infected wound than in the "fresh" contaminated fracture. However, early cultures of contaminating organisms in wounds resulting in in-

fection included the infection-causing organism in 70 per cent of the cases in one large study in humans.[13] Consequently, early cultures of open fracture wounds showing increased potential for infection (e.g., grades II and III) may aid selection of future antibiotic therapy.

The use of systemic antibiotics is indicated in open fractures. Antibiotics are not a substitute for proper wound management. They are only an aid to the body's defense mechanisms. More importantly, resistance to infection and subsequent tissue healing depend on good blood supply. Owing to availability, relatively low cost, and common usage, ampicillin and penicillin have become less effective in treating bone infection, with more resistant strains of microorganisms emerging.[7] Consequently, other drugs or combination therapies are better suited for early treatment. Also, the incrimination of anaerobic bacteria in bone infections requires drugs that are effective in an anaerobic environment.[15, 16] The philosophy of using the cheaper, less effective antibiotics early and waiting for problems (resistant organisms and continued infection) to arise before using effective drugs is inappropriate in open fracture management. Culture specimens are best taken prior to antibiotic administration and should be taken at the fracture site to avoid skin contaminants. The next best alternative is surgical preparation of the wound and introduction of a sterile swab into the deep tissues. Chronic infections should be sampled for culture three to five days after antibiotic therapy has been discontinued.

Often, initial evaluation and management can be done without analgesics or anesthetics because of local wound analgesia from sensory nerve damage in the area. However, complete management requires cleansing and debridement, necessitating analgesia beyond that temporarily produced by trauma. Balanced anesthetic techniques as well as regional nerve blocks can be effective and avoid the depths of anesthesia that may be life-threatening in some cases. Hospital flora constitute the major contributor of contaminating organisms that produce infection.[11] Thus, aseptic technique should be adhered to as much as possible when evaluating, cleaning, debriding, and preparing the wound. This includes caps, masks, gloves, drapes, and sterile instruments. Gross contamination is removed, and the wound is covered with a moist sterile gauze or sterile, water-soluble ointment to avoid further contamination.[14] Hair is clipped from surrounding areas and the wound is thoroughly cleaned and debrided.

Debridement is "removal of foreign material and devitalized or contaminated tissue from or adjacent to a traumatic or infected lesion until surrounding healthy tissue is exposed."[7] Initial debridement involves the soft tissues. Obviously contaminated, devitalized tissues are removed. Subcutaneous fat, fascia, and muscle are removed, leaving a "saucerized" wound, the opening of which is wider than its base.

Copious lavage with sterile saline and gentle scrubbing using a sterile gloved hand aid in flushing out debris. Pulsating water jets and other "pressurized or pulsating irrigation" systems have been advocated.

Sharp dissection, combined with good anatomical knowledge, is the best means of removing devitalized tissues. Generally a scalpel is used, but on occasion scissors are useful. Excessive undermining and probing of tissues are avoided. Fresh, bleeding surfaces are probably the best indication of sufficient debridement. Sufficient debridement is often a difficult undertaking. The natural reaction is to leave as much tissue as possible. In gunshot wounds, for example, the entrance wound is generally small but the damage to the underlying tissues can be extensive. Often, if the wound is left unopened, underlying tissue necrosis eventually interferes with the best of orthopedic fixation techniques. It is better to be aggressive at debridement and leave the wound open (secondary closure or healing by second intention) than to close the wound early. If vascularity is impeded and the source of obstruction is not removed (dead space, fluid collection, foreign bodies, necrotic tissue), many surgical repairs fail. Drains may be used when early closure is instituted. This often allows remaining devitalized tissue to extrude.

In general, grades I and II fractures are treated with similar fixation methods and with the same degree of success as closed fractures. Grade III fractures rarely heal successfully without extensive preoperative and postoperative management efforts. The theory that a "golden period" of six to eight hours helps distinguish the contaminated wound from the infected wound may aid in the decision to close the wound or leave it open. Infected wounds should not be closed primarily. Contaminated wounds must be judged individually. Clean, sharply incised wounds may have a "golden period" longer than six hours. In severely contaminated, devitalized wounds such as seen with many open fractures, this period may be sharply reduced. If attempts at closure (primary closure) are initiated prematurely, complications associated with infection are likely to interfere with overall healing. All wounds, except fistulas, generally heal if the circulation is adequate and metabolism is normal. Healing cannot be imposed; it must be cultivated.[2]

Following adequate soft tissue debridement, the bone itself must be debrided. The maximum amount of bone that potentiates bone healing is maintained. Devascularized, contaminated fragments promote osteomyelitis.

Bone debridement may be done with initial soft tissue debridement or as a delayed procedure when skeletal fixation is instituted. Generally, grades I and II fractures require limited soft tissue debridement. Bone debridement can usually be carried out with skeletal fixation. Grade III fractures, requiring more extensive debridement of the soft tissues, often require removal of devitalized bone concurrent with initial soft tissue management.

Soft tissue attachments to bone fragments are preserved if possible, to help preserve blood supply and subsequent bone viability, allowing the fragment to take an active part in the healing process rather than being a scaffold at best and a sequestrum at worst. Small cortical fragments dislodged during debridement and lavage may be retained if their benefit to fracture repair and stabilization outweighs their potential function as a nidus of infection. If free fragments are retained, they should be carefully cleaned and lavaged to remove gross contamination.

The major fracture ends, proximal and distal, are cleaned in order to evaluate and remove gross contaminants that may have been lodged in the medullary canal. Excessive removal of healthy cancellous bone from the fracture ends is avoided. Bone ends are not "squared off" unless it is necessary for rigid fixation at the fracture site. It is better to maintain the maximum length possible in order to increase the chances of returning the bone to normal function by maintaining its biomechanical function in relation to the remainder of the skeleton.

Exposed cortical bone that has lost its soft tissue attachment (periosteum) dies if allowed to dry. If infection does not occur, this necrosis is usually relatively superficial, and healing continues. Exposed bone should not be allowed to dry. Management of many open wounds requires the bone to be exposed without soft tissue covering. In this case, the bone is kept moist with saline-soaked gauze, drainage of necrotic debris away from the bone is maintained, and tight bandages and topical medications that discourage revascularization are avoided. If kept moist, granulation tissue covers the exposed bone, beginning at the periphery and moving to the center.

Attempts at early covering of bone with relaxing incisions, local flaps, cross-leg pedicle flaps, and myocutaneous flaps are often advocated.[2] The cost can be great if bone and, more specifically, soft tissue are not ready to be closed. Healing of an open fracture is secondary to soft tissue wound healing and depends on removal of all tissues that will support bacterial growth.[1, 2]

Stability, whether attained with internal fixation, external coaptation, or percutaneous pin splints, is necessary for soft tissue and bone healing. Early (initial) stabilization is best achieved with large, padded bandages (e.g., Robert-Jones dressing). Following evaluation and initial treatment of the wound, support is necessary to allow repeated observation and treatment of the wound. This is usually best achieved in animals with percutaneous pin splints (Kirschner-Ehmer devices). The wound can be bandaged, ambulation is usually maintained, and minimal soft tissue disruption is necessary to apply the device. Casts, splints, and external coaptation bandages require repeated changes with risk of movement and disruption of the fragile capillary network that is forming. If adequate stability cannot be achieved with external devices, rigid internal fixation (intramedullary pins or plates) is required.

SUMMARY

Management and healing of open fractures, according to the precepts of Paré, Larrey, Orr, Trueta, Böhler, and Dehne, may be summarized as follows:

1. All healing depends upon good blood supply.

2. Resistance to and control of infection also depend on good blood supply and defense mechanisms. Antibiotics are no substitute.

3. Anything impeding vascularity (dead space, fluid collections, foreign bodies, devitalized tissue) must be removed or allowed to extrude.

4. Circulation of the wounded part as well as the wound site is enhanced by early return to function. This muscle activity reduces venous stasis and edema.

5. All wounds, fistulas excepted, heal if there is adequate circulation and normal metabolism. A wound cannot be surgically stimulated to heal; it must be cultivated to achieve healing.[2]

1. Brown, P. W.: The open fracture: cause, effect, and management. Clin. Orthop. Rel. Res. 96:254, 1973.
2. Brown, P. W.: The fate of exposed bone. Am. J. Surg. 137:464, 1979.
3. Crusfilo, R. B., and Anderson, J. T.: Prevention of infection in the treatment of 1025 open fractures of long bones. J. Bone Jt. Surg. 58A:453, 1976.
4. Dorland's Illustrated Medical Dictionary. 26th ed. W. B. Saunders, Philadelphia, 1981.
5. Dueland, R.: Emergency treatment of limb fractures. Vet. Clin. North Am. 5:305, 1975.
6. Heppenstall, R. B.: Delayed union, nonunion, and pseudoarthrosis. In Heppenstall, R. B. (ed.): Fracture Treatment and Healing. W. B. Saunders, Philadelphia, 1980.
7. Hirsch, D. C., and Smith, T. M.: Osteomyelitis in the dog: microorganisms isolated and susceptibility to antimicrobial agents. J. Small Anim. Pract. 19:679, 1978.
8. Kahn, D. S., and Pritzker, K. P. H.: The pathophysiology of bone infection. Clin. Orthop. Rel. Res. 96:12, 1973.
9. Müller, M. E., Allgöwer, M., and Willenegger, H.: Manual of Internal Fixation. Springer-Verlag, New York, 1970.
10. Norden, C. W.: Experimental osteomyelitis. I: A description of the model. J. Infect. Dis. 122:410, 1970.
11. Nunamaker, D. M.: Treatment of open fractures in small animals. Comp. Cont. Ed. 1:66, 1979.
12. Richardson, D. C., Walker, R., and Kincaid, S.: Production of a model for osteomyelitis. Unpublished data, University of Tennessee and Purdue University, 1981–83.
13. Robertson, D. E.: Acute hematogenous osteomyelitis. J. Bone Jt. Surg. 9:8, 1927.
14. Swaim, S. F.: Management of contaminated and infected wounds. In: Surgery of Traumatized Skin. W. B. Saunders, Philadelphia, 1980.
15. Walker, R. D., and Richardson, D. C.: Anaerobic bacterial infections: characteristics, diagnosis, treatment. Mod. Vet. Pract. April 1981, p. 289.
16. Walker, R. D., Richardson, D. C., Bryant, M. J., and Draper, C. S.: Anaerobic bacteria associated with osteomyelitis in domestic animals. J. Am. Vet. Med. Assoc. 182:814, 1983.
17. Withrow, S. J., and Moore, R. W.: Orthopedic emergencies in small animals. Vet. Clin. North Am.: Small Anim. Pract. 11:171, 1981.

Chapter **153** # Methods of Fracture Fixation

Methods of Internal Fracture Fixation

David J. DeYoung and Curtis W. Probst

Fracture repair in small animals is divided into three categories: closed reduction with external support, internal fixation alone, and internal fixation with secondary external support. The last category is further divided into internal fixation with minimal reliance on external support and internal fixation with heavy reliance on external support (Fig. 153–1). In this section, internal fixation as the sole means of fracture repair is discussed. However, the level of stability achieved with internal fixation may be inadequate, and secondary external support is often necessary. It should be stressed that whenever possible, the surgeon should strive to maintain fracture alignment and stability with internal implants and rely on minimal external support only when necessary. When fracture stability depends too heavily on external support, the incidence of complications dramatically increases. This situation most often arises from the improper choice of primary fixation.

Too often, the only immediate goal of fracture repair is to maintain anatomical reduction and fixation until the body's healing mechanisms restore the structural continuity of the bone. If one only considers bone union in fracture repair, long-term or permanent disabilities may develop owing to soft tissue complications (Fig. 153–2). Adhesions restrict or prevent the normal gliding motion in adjacent muscles and tendons. Joints of the affected limb may also stiffen because of capsular fibrosis and contracture, and disuse atrophy of articular cartilage may occur.[13] These disabling soft tissue complications, collectively referred to as "fracture disease," must be avoided during fracture repair and healing. Because the objective in fracture repair is an early return of the injured limb to full function, soft tissue as well as bone must be considered. An early return to function is achieved by anatomical reconstruction of the bone with stable internal fixation and strict adherence to

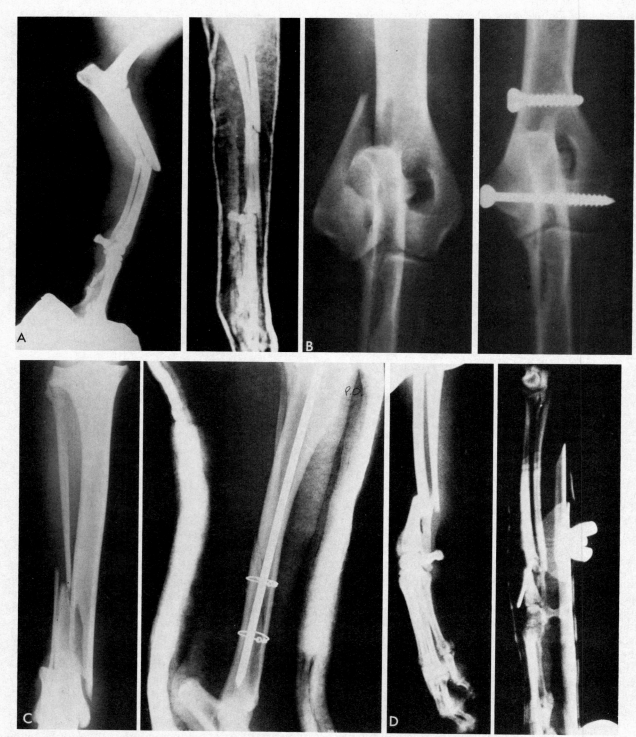

Figure 153–1. Three categories of fracture repair. *A,* Closed reduction with external support. *B,* Internal fixation alone. Internal fixation with secondary external support: *C,* minimal reliance on external support and *D,* heavy reliance on external support. In each part, the preoperative *(left)* and postoperative *(right)* views are shown.

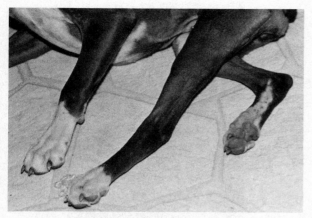

Figure 153–2. Fracture disease. Adhesions, capsular fibrosis, and contracture secondary to fracture repair resulting in hyperextension and permanent disability of the limb.

the basic principles of surgery, especially atraumatic soft tissue handling and preservation of blood supply to the bone. Satisfaction of these criteria precludes the use of restrictive coaptation devices and promotes early use of the muscles and joints of the affected limb. Stable internal fixation of fractures is achieved through two basic principles: the insertion of intramedullary pins and the application of bone plates.

CHOICE OF FIXATION

The method of fracture repair is based on the type and location of the fracture, the size and age of the animal, how many bones or limbs are involved, and concurrent soft tissue disease. Other factors to consider include the animal's behavior and environment, owner cooperation during the convalescent period, and the animal's expected level of performance after bone union. In addition, the veterinary surgeon must consider cost, surgical expertise, and the availability of equipment and technical assistance. The initial plan of fracture management should be based on sound medical judgment. Deviation from this plan because of economics or lack of expertise, equipment, or technical assistance may compromise the outcome. It is better to provide the optimum in fixation or to offer referral to a specialist than to compromise the principles of fracture repair. What begins as an apparently simple case may become a long, unpleasant ordeal.

Size, age, and temperament of the animal are obvious factors in the selection of the correct implant. Fractures in small or medium-sized animals may be adequately stabilized with intramedullary pins. However, if one considers other factors, this type of fixation may not be adequate. A small animal that is 12 years of age and housed outdoors without restriction of activity may require the more stable fracture fixation provided by a bone plate. A properly applied bone plate will withstand such an animal's additional activity and provide stability during the longer healing time required in the geriatric animal. In addition,

a plate may be indicated when a disease process is present in another limb, such as a fracture, dislocation, or even arthritis. The resulting early return to full function of the fractured limb enables the animal to walk sooner and allows the application of an Ehmer sling or similar device to another limb.

The type and location of a fracture may dictate using one implant over another. For example, it is technically easier to apply a bone plate to a pelvic fracture than to attempt fixation with alternative methods. Not only is the resulting stability much greater, but the return to function is almost immediate. Conversely, some fractures do not readily lend themselves to bone plate application. Certain metaphyseal and epiphyseal fractures may not leave enough bone length to allow plate fixation.

The degree of soft tissue damage may be a deciding factor in implant selection. A fracture associated with extensive soft tissue damage may require temporary stabilization with an external fixator such as a Kirschner apparatus.[1] Surgical invasion of such a fracture may cause further devitalization of tissues, resulting in delayed healing or wound infection. Application of an external fixation device stabilizes the bone until the soft tissues heal, at which time definitive fixation may be undertaken.

FRACTURE FORCES

In addition to the preceding criteria, it is necessary to consider the forces acting on the fracture site when selecting an implant. When force is applied to a limb during weight-bearing, the load is transmitted along the bone, resulting in stresses that tend to malalign or disrupt the fracture site. These stresses are also present in the absence of weight-bearing because of muscle tension.

For most purposes in clinical orthopedics, it is sufficient to consider four basic forces. These are rotational, bending, and shearing forces, and fragment apposition (Fig. 153–3). The last is not a true

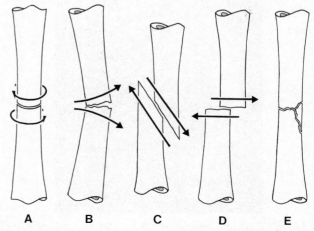

A   B   C   D   E

Figure 153–3. Basic fracture forces. *A,* Rotation. *B,* Bending. *C,* Angular shear. *D,* Horizontal shear. *E,* Fragment apposition.

fracture force, but it is necessary to consider fragment apposition for the purpose of implant selection. The fixation device, whether it involves external or internal stabilization, has to neutralize inherent forces acting on that particular fracture to prevent motion at the fracture site. It is not necessary for these forces to cause gross displacement of the fracture segments in order to adversely affect healing. Slight undetectable movement can impede the growth of small capillary buds across the fracture site. This vascular ingrowth is enhanced by stable fixation.[3] Lack of revascularization accounts for the nonunion in fractures with anatomical reduction and seemingly adequate fixation. If fracture forces are neutralized, soft tissue structures are preserved, vascular integrity is maintained, and infection is prevented, optimal conditions have been established for fracture healing.

Prior to surgical reconstruction of a fractured bone, the radiographic appearance of the fracture fragments is analyzed. The nature of the fracture fragments allows prediction of the forces acting at the fracture site and selection of an implant that will neutralize them.

Rotational force is present in most fractures. Rotation is most often a problem in transverse or slightly oblique long bone fractures that do not interdigitate. Fracture sites with interlocking ends that are anatomically reduced may withstand rotational forces. Fracture movement due to rotation, in addition to causing delayed union or nonunion, can result in rotational deformities of the distal limb (Fig. 153–4).

Bending forces are present in most fractures regardless of fracture type. Bending becomes a problem because of eccentric axial loading or the presence of

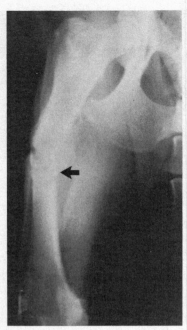

Figure 153–5. Enhancement of bending force due to a Schroeder-Thomas splint. In this fracture, the bar of the splint was acting as a fulcrum at the fracture site.

a cortical defect on the compression side, or with the application of an external unidirectional force. The common tendency is to use inadequate fixation where bending forces predominate. If the implants are unable to withstand the bending forces, implant failure (i.e., plate bending, pin breakage) and loss of reduction may occur. The angulation resulting from the implant failure further potentiates the bending force because of increased eccentric loading. A common error in fracture fixation is the application of an external coaptation device as secondary support for a femoral or humeral fracture. These devices seldom provide additional support for the implants and in fact may be detrimental because the top of a cast or the bar of a Schroeder-Thomas splint can act as a fulcrum to enhance the bending forces (Fig. 153–5).

Shearing forces are most commonly associated with oblique fractures. A shearing force causes the two bone ends to slide relative to each other in a direction parallel to their plan of contact, causing oblique fractures to override. However, shear force exists even in a simple transverse fracture, resulting in a tendency for the fracture ends to slide by each other in a horizontal plane. This horizontal shearing force is most frequently a problem when a single intramedullary pin is used for fixation. Shearing forces can have devastating effects on a fracture; therefore, every effort should be made to neutralize the impact of shear on the fracture site.

Fragment apposition is not a true fracture force. It is important to maintain fragment apposition in comminuted fractures, because accurate cortical contact helps the implants to withstand the rotational, shearing, and bending forces acting at the fracture site. During the healing period, tremendous forces are

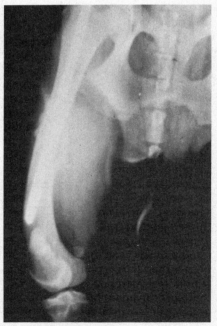

Figure 153–4. Rotational deformity. As a result of rotation at the fracture site, the distal fracture segment is rotated 90 degrees in relation to the proximal fracture segment.

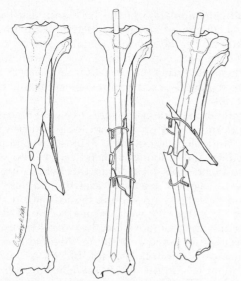

Figure 153–6. Fragment apposition. Failure of the primary fixation device as a result of loss of fragment apposition.

acting on reduced fracture fragments, which may be the major contributors to fracture stability. Therefore, fixation of fragments should be as secure as possible, since failure to maintain fragment apposition may result in failure of the primary fixation. Such fixation is most critical when a less stable type of primary fixation is used (Fig. 153–6).

It is difficult to classify each implant's ability to neutralize fracture forces because of the variety of fracture types. However, some generalizations can be made (Table 153–1). A particular implant may be effective in neutralizing a force, but such effectiveness does not assure a successful repair with that implant alone—especially with auxiliary fixation such as cerclage wire, lag screws, and Kirschner devices.

The ability of a single intramedullary pin to counteract horizontal shearing force in a transverse fracture or angular shearing force in an oblique fracture depends on the size of the pin in relation to the medullary cavity. If the pin is smaller than the medullary cavity, shearing may occur, resulting in

horizontal movement or overriding of the fracture segments. If the pin diameter equals that of the medullary cavity, shearing forces are effectively counteracted. However, since most bones are not perfect cylinders, the pin rarely fills the medullary cavity of both fracture segments. Therefore, either supplemental fixation or an alternative means of repair is required to neutralize the shearing forces.

The ability of an intramedullary pin to resist bending force is directly proportional to its diameter as well as to the ratio of the pin diameter to the medullary diameter. As the medullary diameter becomes excessively large, it is difficult to counteract the bending force solely with an intramedullary pin. It may be necessary in this case to add supplemental fixation such as a Kirschner apparatus to aid in resisting the bending force. In this situation, an alternative means of fixation such as a bone plate would be a better choice than "pushing" the pin and Kirschner device beyond their potential. This is obviously a subjective decision based on experience, but it may mean the difference between success and failure.

Rotation is not effectively counteracted by a single intramedullary pin regardless of its size. The cortical purchase at the end of the bone is insufficient to prevent rotation of the bone segments around the pin. Rotational forces may be counteracted by interlocking of fragments and by compression due to internal and external loading forces.[12] With the exception of a two-piece fracture, intramedullary pins do not maintain fragment apposition.

In summary, when using intramedullary pins, special care must be taken to counteract rotation, shear, and bending forces. If these criteria cannot be met, supplemental fixation must be used or an alternative implant chosen.

The use of two intramedullary pins aids in counteracting rotational forces. Two pins provide two-point fixation in the distal cancellous bone and emerge from two separate points in the proximal end of the bone.[15] In addition to the two-point fixation, the net effect of multiple pins is increased diameter of the implant in relation to the medullary canal, which aids in resisting bending and horizontal shearing forces. The use of multiple intramedullary pins is commonly referred to as "stack pinning."[5]

Properly applied, bone plates provide the most stable form of fracture fixation. They are effective in neutralizing rotational, shearing, and bending forces in addition to maintaining fragment apposition. Plates also increase the stability of fracture repair through active axial loading or compression of the bone fragments. As with other devices, success depends on selection and proper application of the appropriate-sized implant.

Lag screws and cerclage wire are not effective in neutralizing the major fracture forces. Their primary function is to maintain fragment apposition in order to facilitate application of the primary implant. These forms of auxiliary fixation are most often applied to

TABLE 153–1. Ability of Various Implants to Neutralize Fracture Forces*

Implant	Rotational Force	Bending Force	Shearing Force	Fragment Apposition
Single intramedullary pin	–	+	–	–
Multiple intramedullary pins	+	+	–	–
Bone plate	+	+	+	+
Kirschner splint	+	+	+	–
Cerclage wire	(+)	(+)	(+)	+
Lag screw	–	–	–	+

*A + indicates that neutralization is achieved; a – indicates that it is not.

oblique fractures or to maintain reduction of fragments. In these instances, shearing forces predominate and frequently result in failure of auxiliary fixation. These devices should be protected against shearing forces by the primary implant or by adding a secondary fixation device such as a Kirschner apparatus. If this is not possible, multiple cerclage wires of sufficient size and strength should be used to minimize the chance of breakage. Lag screws in cortical bone are especially prone to failure from shearing forces and should always be protected. Failure to realize the inherent weakness of these auxiliary devices, or improper application of them, is a common cause of fracture failure.

Wire is effective in neutralizing another fracture force that has not been discussed. This is the *tension* or *distracting force* that occurs at an apophysis such as the tibial tubercle, olecranon process, or trochanter major. A tension band device consisting of two parallel Kirschner pins and a figure-of-eight wire is used to repair fractures or osteotomies of these apophyses.

Various modifications of the Kirschner splint can be used for primary fracture fixation or as secondary fixation. In either case, this device is very effective in neutralizing the basic fracture forces.[1] Applied to the tension side of a bone, a Kirschner splint aids in counteracting bending forces and is an effective antirotational device.[1] In addition, when applied to an oblique or comminuted fracture as secondary fixation, the splint protects lag screws or cerclage wires from shearing forces, although not to the same extent as a bone plate.[1]

The orthopedic surgeon must be aware of the inherent forces acting at the fracture site and the potential of each implant to neutralize these forces. In selecting an implant to counteract fracture forces, the size, age, and temperament of the animal must also be considered. The size and behavior determine the magnitude of the force acting at the fracture site, and the age determines the length of time that fracture stability depends on the implants. The method of fixation of fractures varies considerably, but the basic principles of fracture repair are the same in every case.

SURGICAL CONSIDERATIONS

During open reduction for internal fixation of a fracture, strict aseptic conditions must be maintained. The surgical team must be properly attired and correct procedures for scrubbing, gowning, and gloving should be followed. The hair must be carefully removed from a liberal area surrounding the surgical site, and the skin prepared with an effective surgical germicide. Prior to draping, the surgical site should receive a final application of germicidal solution. It is advantageous in long bone fracture repair to prepare and drape the patient so the entire limb is accessible during the surgery. This arrangement facilitates manipulation of the limb and visual inspection of alignment during reduction. Skin towels or stockinette can be used to minimize wound contamination from the surrounding skin. If wound lavage is to be used during the procedure, a moisture barrier drape should be used to prevent contamination by wet drapes.

Atraumatic tissue handling is essential to minimize complications and promote an early return to function. Meticulous attention to hemostasis is important to reduce the amount of blood left in the wound. These blood clots provide an excellent culture medium to support bacterial growth and may delay wound healing by preventing tissue apposition. Frequent wound lavage with warmed saline or Ringer's solution helps promote a healthy wound environment by preventing tissue desiccation.[9] Wound lavage also mechanically removes bacteria, blood, and other debris from the surgical site. Every effort must be made to preserve the blood supply to fracture fragments, since bone healing and resistance to infection depend on a good vascular supply.[9]

THEORY AND TECHNIQUE OF INTRAMEDULLARY PINNING

Equipment

Round Steinmann pins are available in a variety of sizes. However, the most commonly used pins are nine and 12 inches in length and 1/16 to 1/4 inch in diameter. Smaller pins, called Kirschner wires, are available in .035, .045 and .062 inch diameters. These smaller pins are useful in auxiliary fixation devices such as the tension band and as intramedullary pins in very small bones. Both types of pins are available with several different points on either one or both ends. The double-pointed pins are the most versatile and economical to use because they can be inserted retrograde or can be cut in half and both ends used. Intramedullary pins are available with chisel, trocar, and threaded trocar points (Fig. 153–7). The nonthreaded trocar point is the most commonly used for intramedullary pinning because of its inherent ability to penetrate bone. The threaded trocar point is more difficult to insert and offers no advantage over the

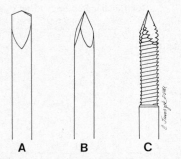

A   **B**   **C**

Figure 153–7. Steinmann intramedullary pin points: *A*, chisel; *B*, trocar; *C*, threaded trocar.

nonthreaded point.[12] Threaded pins are weaker at the thread shaft junction and are prone to breakage at this point. The chisel-pointed pin has a broad flat point that makes poor cortical penetration, which can be advantageous when pins are driven from the metaphyseal portion of soft bone into the diaphysis. The chisel point is less apt to engage the opposite cortex and leave the medullary canal prematurely.

A pin chuck is required to insert the pins into the bone, and a pin cutter is necessary to cut them to the proper length. Because intramedullary pinning does not always result in adequate fracture stability, auxiliary fixation devices such as cerclage wire and Kirschner splints should be available. As with any type of fracture repair, alignment and fixation of the fragments is greatly facilitated by bone forceps.

Principles of Intramedullary Pinning

One or more pins are inserted into the medullary canal to maintain fracture alignment and stability until union occurs. The pins can be placed by the closed or open technique. The closed method avoids surgical exposure and is applicable to stable fractures of palpable long bones. An open approach may expedite fracture repair and results in less soft tissue damage. The open method offers the advantages of direct exposure and manipulation of the bone fragments and allows application of auxiliary fixation such as cerclage wire. It also provides the opportunity to test and visually assess the degree of stability achieved with the implants.

Angular stability, or resistance to bending, is achieved by stable anchorage of the pin in the proximal and distal cortical or cancellous bone.[12] Theoretically, bending and horizontal shearing are prevented by firm contact of the pin with the endosteal surface of the cortex. To meet this ideal assumption, the pin diameter would have to equal the medullary diameter at the fracture site. Owing to the natural curvature of most long bones and variations in cross-sectional diameter, the pin rarely fills the medullary canal.[12] Therefore, bending and horizontal shearing forces cause instability. Filling the medullary canal at the fracture site may be undesirable, since the pin will interfere with the medullary blood supply. It also makes the application of a secondary fixation device, such as a Kirschner splint, difficult. A good compromise is to select a pin diameter that occupies approximately 60 to 70 per cent of the medullary cavity. Rotational stability depends on muscular compression and stability of the irregular cortex at the fracture site. Therefore, anatomical reduction of the fragments is important for healing as well as prevention of rotation. These concepts re-emphasize the importance of stable fixation of comminuted fragments with cerclage wire of sufficient strength to withstand the forces acting on the fracture. Cerclage wire should seldom be smaller than 20-gauge even for the smallest animals.

When the limitations of a single pin have been exceeded, it is necessary to use a multiple-pin technique or to add secondary fixation, such as with a Kirschner device. It is not advisable to combine external coaptation splints with internal skeletal fixation because of the fulcrum effect and restriction of limb use. Intramedullary pinning techniques should be restricted to small and medium-sized animals. The large and giant breeds have such a large medullary cavity that standard round pins are unable to maintain adequate alignment and stability. The size and weight of these large animals generate forces beyond the limitations of Steinmann pins. A bone plate is a better choice of fixation in these animals.

Technique of Application

Only the open method of fracture repair is described because it is more commonly used. The extent to which an approach is developed depends on the severity of the fracture. A simple transverse fracture requires only enough exposure to allow placement of reduction forceps on each fracture fragment. A long oblique or comminuted fracture requires a more extensive approach. The greater exposure facilitates fragment alignment and the application of cerclage wires. In spite of the additional time required for the approach and closure, a liberal exposure can result in decreased surgical time and better reduction and stability. Inadequate surgical exposure necessitates excessive retraction of the soft tissues, causing unnecessary trauma.

Following exposure, the pin may be inserted into the bone via either a normograde or a retrograde technique. With the normograde technique, the pin is started into the bone from an external landmark and advanced to the fracture site. With the retrograde method, the pin is started from the fracture site and advanced up the marrow cavity through the cortex and out of the skin. The pin chuck must then be removed and placed on the proximal end of the pin, and the pin retracted until the distal point is level with the fracture site. Regardless of the method used, the proximal bone fragment should be firmly held with bone forceps to prevent rotation as the pin is advanced. The pin is inserted into the medullary canal with steady pressure and back-and-forth quarter turns of the pin chuck. It is necessary to place the pin chuck in the palm of the hand while rotating the pin, in order to put the pin in line with the center of axial rotation of the wrist and prevent wobbling as the pin is rotated.

Once the pin has been placed in the proximal fragment, the bone is anatomically reduced with the aid of bone forceps and held in reduction while an assistant seats the pin into the distal fracture segment. It is helpful for the person seating the pin to place the free hand around the distal portion of the bone to provide counter-pressure. If the fracture is oblique, the fragments are reduced and alignment is

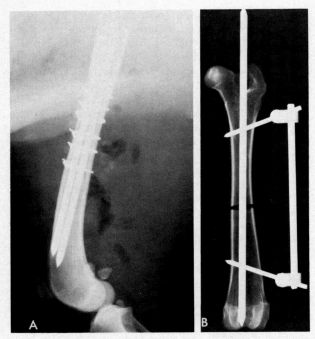

Figure 153–8. When instability exists following single intramedullary pin insertion, additional stability may be achieved with multiple intramedullary pins *(A)* or the addition of a half Kirschner splint *(B).*

handle a comminuted fracture is to convert it first to a two-piece fracture.

The pin is inserted into the distal segment until resistance is felt on the pin chuck. At this time, the chuck is removed, and a pin of equal length is placed beside the intramedullary pin to measure the distance of penetration into the distal fragment. Extreme caution must be taken to avoid penetration of the adjacent joint with the pin. It is often helpful to confirm the final pin placement with radiographs following operation.

Once the pin is seated in the distal fracture segment, the reconstructed bone is stressed to evaluate stability. Adjacent joints are also flexed and extended to determine whether the pin is interfering with normal joint motion. It is important at this time to visually examine the entire limb for rotational and angular alignment. Gross examination of the limb is facilitated if the entire leg has been aseptically prepared and pulled through the drape prior to surgery. If any malalignment or instability is present, the fragments must be correctly aligned, and additional fixation applied. Two common techniques are to add additional intramedullary pins or a two- or four-pin Kirschner splint (Fig. 153–8). The additional intramedullary pin may be added using the normograde method of pin insertion, or if its use was anticipated, it may be passed retrograde prior to fracture reduction.

Application of a two-pin Kirschner splint is a simple and effective means of providing additional fixation. This device can be applied after closure. However, application prior to closure allows visual evaluation of its effectiveness. The Kirschner clamps are available in three sizes, the small and medium sizes being used in small animals. The pins are inserted through the skin and soft tissues and into the bone with the

maintained with cerclage wires or a reduction clamp prior to seating of the pin. If the pin is seated without anatomical reduction, adjustments in alignment may be difficult, since the pin may have different axial alignment in each of the two fracture segments. If the fracture is comminuted, the fragments should be anatomically reduced, and reduction should be maintained with cerclage wire or reduction clamps while the pin is seated in the distal fragment. The way to

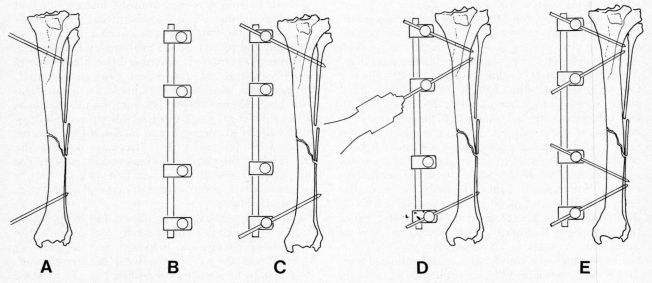

A   **B**   **C**   **D**   **E**

Figure 153–9. Full Kirschner splint with a single connecting bar configuration. *A,* The proximal and distal pins are inserted first. The connecting bar and single clamps are assembled *(B)* and connected to the pins *(C). D,* The third and fourth pins are inserted into the bone, through the clamp holes in the same plane as the first two. *E,* Final adjustments are made in fracture alignment and the clamps are tightened.

aid of a pin chuck. The pins are advanced through both cortices until the entire point protrudes through the far cortex. If the Kirschner pin strikes the intramedullary pin, the Kirschner pin often can be driven past the intramedullary pin by slight cranial or caudal angling. The pins should be placed at the proximal and distal extremities of the bone to be effective and to avoid placement in the incision.[1] Following insertion, the pins should be at a 35- to 45-degree angle to each other.[1] The angulation of the pins prevents the splint from being pulled out. It is important to insert the pins in the same axial plane, whenever possible, to prevent distraction of the fracture segments during loading. Following placement, the pins are connected by a single bar and held securely with two Kirschner clamps. Prior to tightening the clamps, final adjustments are made in the fracture alignment, and manual compression is applied to the bone. At this time, fracture stability should be further evaluated. If instability still exists or a cortical defect is present, more rigid fixation can be achieved by the addition of one or more pins to the splint. Regardless of the number of pins, they can usually be connected by a single connecting bar. This can be accomplished by placing the additional clamps on the bar and inserting the additional pins through the clamps and on into the bone. This ensures that all four pins are in the same plane (Fig. 153–9). A two-pin splint is commonly referred to as a half Kirschner, a three-pin splint as a three-quarter Kirschner, and a four-pin splint as a full Kirschner. The half Kirschner splint generally provides adequate secondary support to the intramedullary pin. The role of the Kirschner splint for secondary fixation is frequently underestimated.

Surgical Anatomy and Landmarks for Pin Placement

Femur

The femoral shaft is exposed from a lateral approach centered over the fracture site.[10] One obvious characteristic of the femur is the firm attachment of the adductor muscle to the caudal cortex. The fibers of this muscle blend with the periosteum and provide an important source of extraosseous blood supply to the healing fracture. Care should be taken to avoid stripping this important vascular supply away from the bone. Adductor muscle attachment to any major fragments should be left intact to promote rapid incorporation of these fragments during healing. The correct use of a wire passer minimizes the amount of muscle separation required to place cerclage wire around the bone.

Pin insertion in the femur is from the proximal end. The pin is inserted through the skin and underlying soft tissues, sliding along the medial surface of the trochanter major into the trochanteric fossa. At this point, the pin is inserted into the medullary cavity and down to the fracture site (Fig. 153–10). The pin chuck is held in axial alignment with the bone. During retrograde pin insertion, the hip is held in a normal position and the leg is adducted, in order to minimize soft tissue penetration and avoid the sciatic nerve as the pin emerges from the bone proximally. Normograde pin insertion requires more skill but has the advantages of trapping less soft tissue

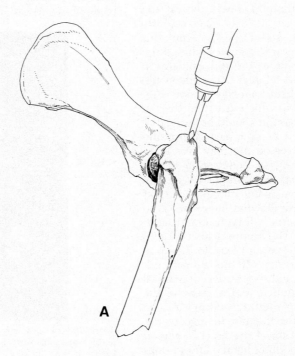
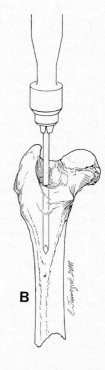

Figure 153–10. Normograde pin placement in the femur. *A*, The pin is inserted through the skin and soft tissues to the trochanter major. The pin is then "walked" medially until it slides into the trochanteric fossa. *B*, The pin is inserted into the medullary cavity with the pin aimed down the femoral shaft.

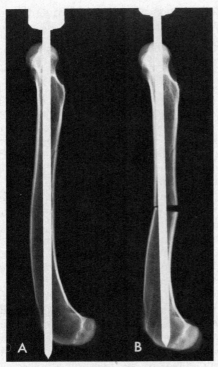

Figure 153–11. Pin placement in the distal femoral shaft. *A,* A pin seated in the intact or anatomically reduced femur engages the cranial cortex. *B,* A pin seated in the distal femur following cranial angulation of the distal fracture segment is directed caudally into the cancellous bone.

while avoiding the sciatic nerve and facilitates cutting the pin shorter. A shorter pin minimizes seroma formation and decreases patient discomfort.

Because of the cranial bowing of the canine femur, the intramedullary pin engages the cranial cortex near the patella. If an attempt is made to seat the pin the remaining distance, it may inadvertently enter the stifle joint (Fig. 153–11A). To avoid this possibility, the distal fracture segment should be angled slightly cranial to direct the pin caudally in the distal segment. The caudal angulation allows the pin to be seated into the distal cancellous bone (Fig. 153–11B). If it is not clear in which direction the pin is travelling, a lateral radiograph should be evaluated prior to final pin seating. Use of a second intramedullary pin alongside the seated pin may give erroneous information, resulting in penetration of the stifle joint. Once the pin has been properly seated in the distal fragment, the pin is cut off proximally as short as possible while still allowing for retrieval. If the pin is left too long, tissues will be traumatized as it moves back and forth. The trauma can result in seroma formation over the pin and lead to disuse of the limb during convalescence. If the animal suddenly stops using the limb and shows signs of unusual pain or a proprioceptive deficit, entrapment of the sciatic nerve should be suspected. If the hip is placed in flexion, it is possible for the pin to engage the sciatic nerve. Extreme flexion of the hip is common in cats because of their grooming habits, and in dogs as they scratch their ears. This complication may

necessitate careful surgical exploration of the area to remove the pin, if possible, or replacement of the nerve to its normal position and shortening of the pin. Entrapment of the sciatic nerve has led to amputation of the limb because of nerve paralysis and self-mutilation.

Tibia

The entire shaft of the tibia can be exposed from a medial approach.[10] The incision is centered over the fracture site and extended proximally and distally according to the extent of the fracture. An important point to remember about the tibia is that the pin must never be passed retrograde from the fracture site because it will emerge in the stifle joint, resulting in extensive destruction of articular cartilage, cruciate ligaments, and menisci and in permanent disability (Fig. 153–12). The proper point of pin insertion is on the medial side of the tibial tubercle, halfway between the attachment of the patellar tendon and the cranial edge of the medial femoral condyle (Fig. 153–13). The pin is started with the stifle joint in the flexed position and advanced toward the shaft of the tibia. If the pin is inserted at too acute an angle, it may emerge from the lateral or caudal cortex. Owing to the S shape of the tibia, it is necessary for the pin to curve slightly as it passes down the medullary canal. Also, if too large a pin is used, it may engage the cortex and leave the bone rather than bending and following the medullary cavity. If a large pin is required, it is helpful to insert a smaller pin first, then remove it and pass the larger pin through the established guide-hole.

The medial malleolus is the landmark for distal pin placement in the tibia. Because the malleolus protrudes beyond the articular surface of the tibia, it is

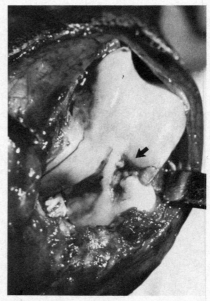

Figure 153–12. Damage to the articular cartilage of the femur *(arrow)* resulting from a retrograded pin in the tibia. Similar damage can result from not cutting the intramedullary pin short enough.

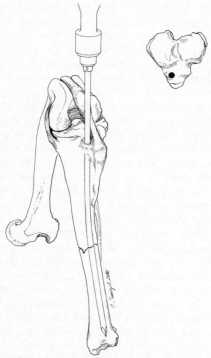

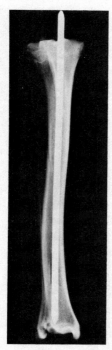

Figure 153–13. Normograde pin placement in the tibia. The point of pin insertion in the tibia is on the medial side of the tibial tubercle, halfway between the attachment of the patellar tendon and the cranial edge of the medial femoral condyle.

necessary to measure this distance from the antero-posterior radiograph and use that point as a reference for seating the pin (Figs. 153–14 and 153–15). Once the pin is properly seated, the proximal end must be cut off short enough so that the rest of the pin does not damage the articular cartilage of the femoral condyles during extension of the joint (see Figs. 153–12 and 153–15). One successful method is to seat the pin to the desired point, then retract it five to seven millimeters and cut it off close to the tibia. At this time, the distal limb is held firmly to provide support while the pin is driven the remaining five to seven millimeters with a mallet and countersinking device (Fig. 153–16).

Kirschner pin splints for secondary fixation are applied to the medial aspect of the bone.[1] The device is well tolerated in this position; however, it should be wrapped to prevent unnecessary trauma to the opposite limb.

Humerus

The humerus is a more difficult bone to approach because of the location and direction of the musculature and the close proximity of major nerves to the surgical site. Careful consideration must be given to selection of the appropriate surgical approach for a fracture of the humerus. The proximal shaft must be

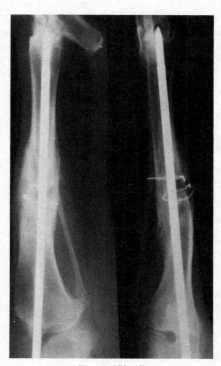

Figure 153–14   *Figure 153–15*

Figure 153–14. When the tip of the medial malleolus is used as a guide in final pin placement in the tibia, the distance from the tip of the malleolus to the joint surface must be considered.

Figure 153–15. Intramedullary pin cut too long, resulting in contact of the pin with the femoral condyle (refer to Fig. 153–12). Notice also that the distal point of the pin was incorrectly placed; it extends through the joint to the tip of the medial malleolus.

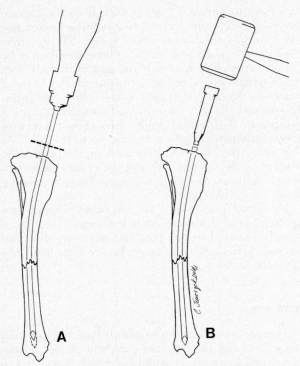

Figure 153–16. *A*, The pin is seated to the desired level, retracted, and cut. *B*, The pin is then driven to its previous position.

approached through a lateral skin incision.[10] The distal shaft, however, can be approached with either a medial or a lateral approach.[10] If it is necessary to do extensive reconstruction of the condylar region of the humerus, an osteotomy of the olecranon process is performed to expose the intercondylar region of the joint and the caudal surface of the distal humerus.[10]

Pins can be inserted into the humerus by either the normograde or the retrograde method. The landmark for normograde insertion is the anterior crest of the proximal greater tubercle (Fig. 153–17). If the retrograde method is chosen, care must be taken to avoid entering the shoulder joint. The pin is started at the medial cortex of the proximal fracture segment and aimed laterally as it passes up the medullary cavity. This angle directs the pin toward the greater tubercle and also positions it near the medial cortex at the fracture site. The medial location is advantageous, because the pin must be directed down into the medial condyle to avoid the elbow joint and gain the best anchorage. The pin is placed into the medial condyle because it is the larger condyle and is in direct axial alignment with the shaft (Fig. 153–18). The size of the medullary cavity in the medial condyle is the limiting factor in selection of pin size. When seating the pin, one must ascertain that the pin is entering the medial condyle, or it will enter the joint instead. It is sometimes helpful to bend the end of the pin slightly medially prior to inserting it in the distal fragment to aid entry into the medial condyle (see Fig. 153–18). With the tip of the pin bent, the pin should be inserted with shorter rotations of the chuck to ensure that the pin point stays directed medially. The distal fragment may also be angulated slightly laterally as the pin is advanced, to facilitate placement in the medial condyle. The pin can be advanced until it just penetrates the distal cortex of the medial condyle. Radiographic confirmation of pin

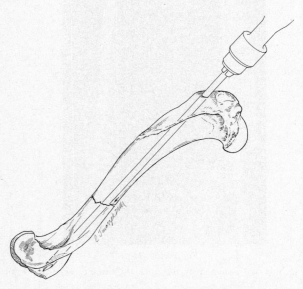

Figure 153–17. The landmark for normograde insertion of an intramedullary pin in the humerus is the anterior crest of the proximal greater tubercle.

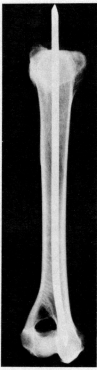

Figure 153–18. The distal pin point is seated into the medial condyle of the humerus. In this example, the end of the pin was curved slightly medially to facilitate placement in the medial condyle.

placement requires anteroposterior and lateral views to determine whether it is in the joint or the medial condyle.

The Kirschner device can be applied to the lateral aspect of the humerus for secondary fixation. If the fracture is distal, the distal Kirschner pin can be placed through the condyles. In distal fractures of the humerus, it is often desirable to insert a cross-pin from the lateral condyle up into the medial cortex of the shaft for additional fixation.

Radius and Ulna

Owing to the anatomical configuration of the radius, it is impossible to pass an intramedullary pin retrograde without its entering the proximal or distal joint. A pin can be inserted into the radius with a normograde technique. This specialized pinning method is discussed along with Rush pinning. Occasionally, it is necessary to pin the ulna to provide additional support for implants in the radius (Fig. 153–19) or for primary fixation of a fracture involving the articular surface of the proximal ulnar joint. The proximal ulna is exposed through a caudal approach, and the distal ulna through a caudal lateral approach.[10] The pin can be inserted by either a retrograde or a normograde technique. In a normograde technique, the pin is started in the top of the olecranon process, centered over the medullary cavity. As the pin is advanced, the lateral curvature of the proximal ulnar shaft must be palpated and the pin aligned accordingly. If this curvature is not accounted

for, the pin will leave the bone medially and just distal to the elbow joint. Prior to pin insertion, it is necessary to examine a radiograph to determine whether a medullary cavity exists at the fracture site, and which size pin will fit. Frequently, only small pins are used in the ulna, even in large dogs.

Advantages and Disadvantages of Intramedullary Pinning

Pins are less costly to purchase, are less time-consuming to use, require less exposure, and are easier to implant and remove than bone plates. These advantages must be considered along with the disadvantages of less stable fixation, slower return to function, secondary bone union, and more involved aftercare. These are generalizations that do not apply to all individuals or situations. For example, to an experienced surgeon, bone plate application may be just as fast as pinning, even in a transverse fracture. With a bone plate, return to full function is almost immediate, very few recheck examinations are required, and the chance of a successful outcome is greater—so the additional cost of the implant may be worthwhile.

Postoperative Management

Following surgery, fracture alignment and implant placement are evaluated by two radiographic views. Examination of postoperative radiographs not only allows assessment of the surgery but also provides documentation of implant positioning and fracture alignment for comparison with follow-up radiographs during the healing phase. Analysis of the radiographs provides an excellent opportunity for the surgeon to

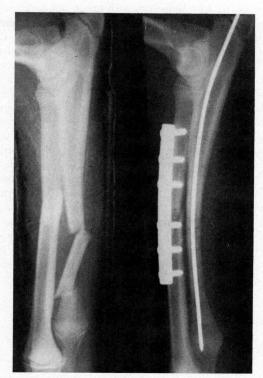

Figure 153–19. An intramedullary pin inserted in the ulna to maintain reduction of a segmental ulnar fracture and to provide additional support for the plated radial fracture.

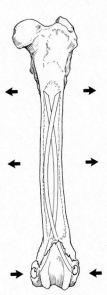

Figure 153–20. When properly inserted, Rush pins provide three-point fixation under spring-loaded tension. *Arrows* show the direction of the tension at the three points of fixation.

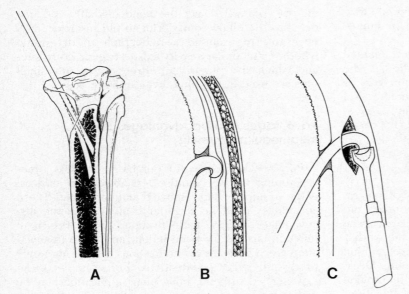

A   B   C

Figure 153–21. A, The point of the Rush pin is bevelled to allow it to slide along the inner cortex with less chance of penetration. B, The opposite end of the pin is hooked to engage the cortex (B) and facilitate removal (C).

improve surgical skills by critical evaluation of the reconstructed bone.

In many cases, a compression type bandage may be beneficial to reduce or prevent swelling immediately after surgery. It is usually removed prior to discharge. Most animals with uncomplicated fractures can be discharged on the second day after surgery. At discharge, it is beneficial to provide the client with written discharge instructions outlining the convalescent period. These notes should include instructions for medications, diet, and bandage care, exercise restrictions, and dates for follow-up examinations. The client should be told to restrict the animal's activity to leash exercise only until further instructed. It is advisable to prevent small breeds from jumping from furniture. This may re-

quire the client to purchase a cage or to confine the animal to an appropriate room when it is alone or at night. Regardless of size, it is best to avoid stairs unless the animal is restrained with a leash.

Following intramedullary pinning and half Kirschner application, the animal should be rechecked in ten to 14 days for suture removal. At this time, the limb should be evaluated for percentage of function, and joints adjacent to the fractured bone assessed for range of motion. The point where the pin emerges from the bone should be examined for swelling or evidence of pin migration. If gross appearance or physical examination fails to reveal any problems, radiographic evaluation is not necessary. The Kirschner splint should be examined for broken or bent pins and for skin irritation resulting from improper positioning of the clamps.

Implants are removed anytime from three to four weeks postoperatively in a puppy to six to 16 weeks in an adult. Implant removal is based on function, palpation of the fracture site, and radiographic confirmation of bone union. The half Kirschner splint can be removed in two to four weeks, depending on the age of animal and the type of fracture. Removal can be accomplished without anesthesia or tranquilization if the connecting bar is removed and each pin is pulled out in the same plane it was inserted in. In most cases, removal of the buried intramedullary pin is facilitated by having the animal anesthetized. This also allows careful palpation of the fracture site before and after pin removal.

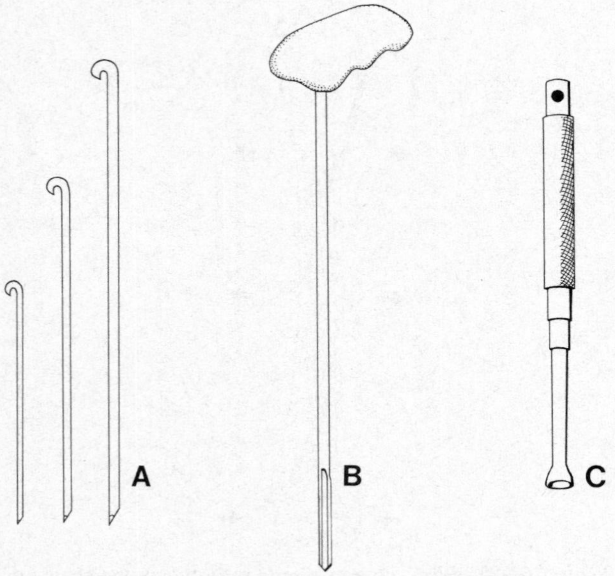

THEORY AND TECHNIQUE OF RUSH PINNING

Equipment

The Rush pin is a resilient stainless steel pin designed to be driven into bone to provide three-point fixation under spring-loaded tension (Fig.

Figure 153–22. A, Three sizes of Rush pins. B, The large awl used to start a guide-hole. C, The driver-extractor tool.

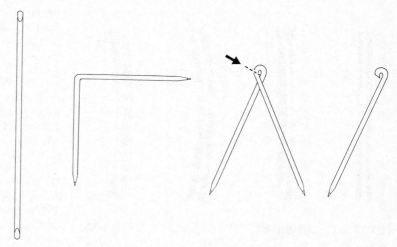

Figure 153–23. A Rush pin can be made from a chisel-pointed Steinmann pin by forming a tight loop at the desired length. One arm of the pin is then cut off close to the loop so a hook is formed.

153–20).[12, 17] The point of the Rush pin has a single bevel, which allows it to be deflected off the far cortex and slide along the inner cortical surface (Fig. 153–21A). The opposite end of the pin is hooked to grasp the outer cortex, preventing migration into the bone and facilitating removal (Fig. 153–21B and C). The pins are available in four different diameters: 3/32-inch, 1/8-inch, 3/16-inch, and 1/4-inch. Each pin diameter is supplied in several different lengths. Equipment required for insertion includes an awl to start a guide-hole, a driver-extractor, and a mallet (Fig. 153–22). Smaller pins can be made from Steinmann pins or Kirschner wires with chisel points. The Steinmann pin is bent until a tight loop is formed at

the required length, and one arm of the pin is then cut off close to the loop so a hook is formed (Fig. 153–23).[4]

Principles and Technique of Application

Rush pinning technique is restricted to fractures in the metaphyseal regions of bones. The pins are inserted into the metaphyseal region at an acute angle, passing obliquely through the cancellous bone and into the medullary cavity to the fracture site. Since the flat point of the Rush pin does not cut well through cortical bone, a guide-hole is made with the

Figure 153–24. *A,* The appropriate-size awl is used to start the guide-hole at a 30-degree angle to the long axis of the bone. *B,* Once both pins have been started, they are alternately driven into the opposite fracture segments with the aid of the driver-extractor tool and a mallet.

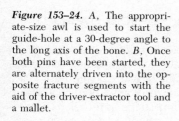
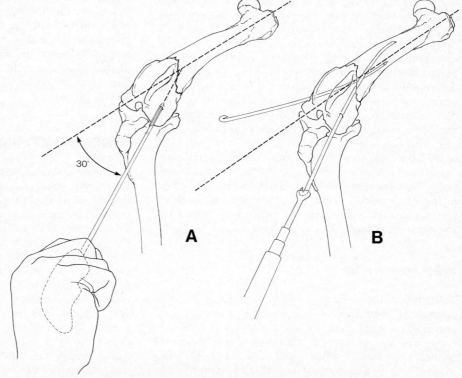

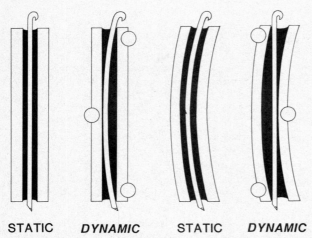

STATIC   *DYNAMIC*   STATIC   *DYNAMIC*

Figure 153–25. The shape of the bone in relation to the pin determines whether the pin merely acts as a static intramedullary pin or as a dynamic Rush pin.

awl reamer or a Steinmann pin of the same diameter. The angle of insertion of the pin is critical to avoid penetration of the opposite cortex and to provide adequate spring-loaded tension. Rush pins are inserted at a 30-degree angle to the axial plane of the bone for optimum results (Fig. 153–24A). The angle should not be greater than 40 degrees, because penetration of the opposite cortex may occur. If the angle is less than 20 degrees, spring-loaded tension is inadequate.

In most cases, two pins are used, one started on each side of the smaller fragment. After both pins are started, the fracture is held in reduction while the pins are alternately driven into the large fracture segment (Fig. 153–24B). Once the pins are driven across the fracture site, they glance off the opposite cortex and cross back toward the near cortex. It is helpful to bend the pins into a slight curve prior to insertion; this is called prestressing and helps prevent penetration of the opposite cortex. The end result is three-point fixation of the bone under spring-loaded tension without complete filling of the medullary cavity. To ensure spring-loaded tension, the shape of the bone must be considered when prebending the pin. The shape of the bone in relationship to the pin determines whether the pin acts merely as an intramedullary pin or as a dynamic Rush pin with three-point fixation (Fig. 153–25). This technique, when properly applied, is effective in resisting major fracture forces. Rush pins will not sufficiently counteract these forces if applied to a diaphyseal fracture.

Indications for Use

Rush pinning is limited in its application in small animals to fractures of the metaphyseal region of bones. Fractures most commonly repaired with this technique are transverse fractures of the proximal humeral, proximal tibial, and distal femoral metaphyses. Modifications of the Rush technique are frequently employed to repair fractures in the metaphysis and diaphysis of metacarpal and metatarsal bones as well as the radius. Often, in these instances, the only similarity to the Rush technique is the method of pin insertion. Since these bones have articular cartilage surfaces on both ends and no convenient prominences for pin insertion, the Rush method of pinning is the only acceptable means of gaining access to the medullary canal. Use in these cases may require external coaptation to help neutralize the forces acting at the fracture site.

When Rush pins are used to repair epiphyseal fractures in growing animals, premature closure of the growth plate may occur. Experimental use of Rush pins across the distal femoral epiphysis in normal puppies with no fracture resulted in premature closure and significant shortening of the limb if the pins were not removed. It was also noted that if the pins were removed after one month, no retardation of growth occurred.[14] Pin removal after one month is not a problem, because these fractures heal rapidly.

Postoperative Management

Management following Rush pinning is the same as that following routine intramedullary pinning. Because of the close proximity of metaphyseal fractures to the joint, it is advantageous to encourage early use of the limb to minimize joint stiffness. Pressure bandages should not be used for longer than one or two days, especially with epiphyseal fractures in young growing animals. The tremendous healing response in these animals often results in fibrous adhesions of the adjacent soft tissues, leading to a stiff joint, which can be a serious and debilitating complication. If the stifle joint of a growing animal becomes locked in hyperextension, the animal is unable to advance the limb and bear weight; therefore, self-rehabilitation does not occur (see Fig. 153–2).

THEORY AND TECHNIQUE OF BONE PLATING

The primary objective in fracture treatment is to return the injured limb to full function. Fracture disease is avoided through early active limb use made possible by stable internal fixation without coaptation. One method of obtaining stable internal fixation is through compression with bone plating techniques. A complete understanding of fracture forces is necessary to counteract these forces properly with bone plates and screws. A properly applied bone plate counteracts bending, rotational, and shearing forces and apposes fragments. The surgeon must also have a good knowledge of regional anatomy in order to select the best approach to a bone and disturb the blood supply and soft tissue the least.

Specialized training and equipment are required

to properly apply bone plates. A complete set of instruments, a full range of implants, and knowledge of their use are necessary before fracture repair is attempted. A less than thorough understanding of bone plating principles and techniques or a lack of equipment usually results in an unfavorable outcome of fracture repair. A plate may be used on any fracture where there is enough bone length on each side of the fracture site to adequately attach the plate. It may also be used on comminuted fractures provided that the fragments can be anatomically reconstructed with lag screw fixation or cerclage wire. The ASIF* System will be used to illustrate the principles; however, the same principles can be applied to any plating system. This material is not meant to provide all the information required for a thorough understanding of the principles and application of bone plating techniques. The authors encourage anyone interested in developing or improving their bone plating skills to refer to the appropriate references listed or attend a continuing education course in bone plating.

Interfragmentary Compression

Compression was initially thought to provide stimulus to bone healing, since compressed fractures healed without any visible callus.[11] It is now known that compression has no osteogenic properties. Compression of fractures increases fracture stability through frictional impact loading and narrowing the gap between fragments, thus providing optimum conditions for direct bone union.[8, 16] One of the features of bone healing under compression is that the removal of necrotic bone and the laying down of new bone can take place simultaneously and within

*Association for the Study of Internal Fixation, Synthes Ltd. (USA), Wayne, PA.

a few cells' distance of each other.[16] Therefore, there is no net resorption of bone in this type of bone healing.[13]

Fracture compression can be achieved through interfragmentary compression with lag screws or axial compression with a plate. Interfragmentary compression can be accomplished with either cortical or cancellous bone screws, although a screw has a lag effect only when it gains purchase in the far cortex and not in the cortex adjacent to the screw head. Since the cortical screw is fully threaded, the hole near the screw head must be overdrilled so the threads will not engage the near cortex. The overdrilled hole is called the glide hole, and the hole in the far cortex is called the thread hole. If a cortical screw is used as a lag screw and a gliding hole is not created in the near cortex, the screw threads maintain the fracture gap and compression is not obtained (Fig. 153–26). The cortical screw can be easily removed from cortical bone after fracture healing because it is fully threaded.[8, 11]

Cancellous screws have a nonthreaded portion near the head and threads near the tip. They have relatively thin core diameters and wide threads with two different thread lengths (Fig. 153–27). The cancellous screw is used in soft cancellous bone of the metaphysis and epiphysis. The bone in these areas has a thin cortical shell unlike the thicker cortex of diaphyseal bone. If cancellous screws are used in diaphyseal bone, they usually cannot be removed because cortical bone grows right up to the threadless shaft of the screw. If removal is attempted, the threads cannot cut a path through the threadless cortex, and the excessive torque generated may result in breakage of the screw. To achieve interfragmentary compression with a cancellous screw, it is important that only the smooth shank is within the near fragment and that the entire threaded portion is within the far fragment (Fig. 153–28). If threads are present

Figure 153–26. A, Compression of two fragments with a screw can occur only when the hole in the cortex adjacent to the screw head is at least as large as the outer diameter of the thread. This hole is called the gliding hole. The thread glides through this hole and only engages the opposite cortex in the thread hole. When the screw head contacts the cortex, interfragmentary compression is achieved. *B*, The screw cannot compress if both cortices are drilled and tapped, because the screw threads maintain the fracture gap. Either the bone or screw will break before there is the slightest approximation of the fragments.

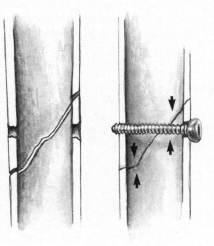

CORRECT

A

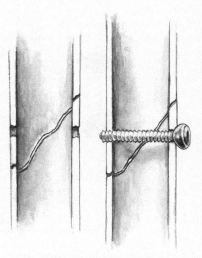

INCORRECT

B

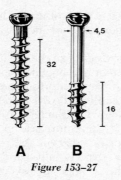

Figure 153–27

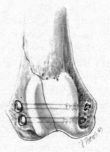

Figure 153–28

Figure 153–27. Two 6.5-mm ASIF cancellous screws with a 4.5-mm shaft. *A*, 32-mm thread. *B*, 16-mm thread.

Figure 153–28. Interfragmentary compression has been achieved with two cancellous screws. Note that the threads are present in the far fragment only. Compression will not occur if the threads are present on both sides of the fracture line. Washers may be necessary in young animals to prevent the screw head from sinking into the soft cancellous bone.

on both sides of the fracture, the threads maintain the fracture gap and compression cannot occur.[8, 13] Unlike cortical screws, cancellous screws in cancellous bone do not require tapping for the entire length of the hole. Only the first few millimeters of the hole are tapped to facilitate starting the screw. As the screw is advanced into the cancellous bone, the trabeculae are tightly compressed, resulting in greater holding power.[7, 8]

To achieve evenly distributed interfragmentary compression, it is necessary to center the screw in the middle of both fragments (Fig. 153–29). If the screws are placed eccentrically, they will produce shear instead of pure compression, often resulting in loss of reduction (Fig. 153–30). When one is lag-screwing a butterfly fragment, the screw should be inserted to bisect the angle subtended between a line perpendicular to the long axis of the bone and one perpendicular to the fracture plane (Fig. 153–31).[7, 8] Since lag screws are not effective in neutralizing fracture forces, they are rarely used as the sole means of fixation in diaphyseal fractures. The primary function of a lag screw is to provide fragment apposition through interfragmentary compression. The resulting fracture alignment and stability must be protected against the forces acting on the fracture with a bone plate. A plate that is applied for this purpose is called a neutralization plate.

Screws are available with either self-tapping threads or non–self-tapping threads. It was once thought that self-tapping screws provided poor holding power because their insertion caused bone necrosis, resulting in the screw's being embedded in fibrous tissue rather than bone. This has since been shown to be incorrect. The advantage of the non–self-tapping screw does not lie in its greater holding power, but in the ease and precision with which it can be inserted into bone.[13]

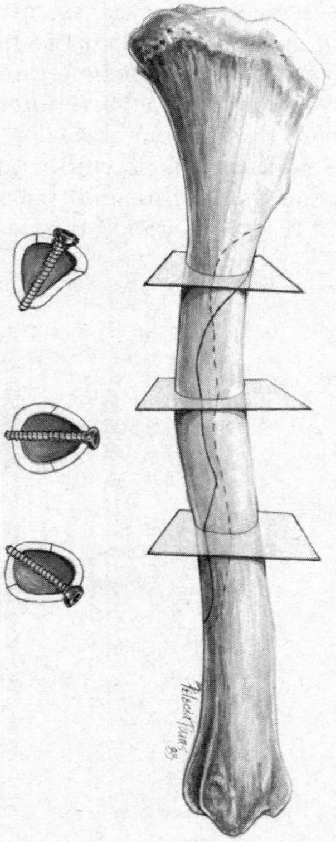

Figure 153–29. The orientation of lag screws used to compress an oblique fracture is shown. *Cross-sections,* The screws are ideally placed through the middle of both fragments to achieve maximal compression.

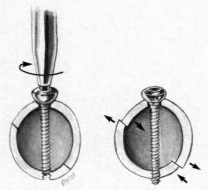

Figure 153–30. The effect of an eccentrically placed screw is shown. As the screw is tightened, it produces shear instead of pure compression, resulting in loss of reduction.

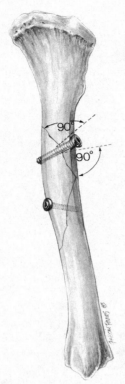

Figure 153–31. Lag fixation of a single butterfly fragment is shown. The screws have been inserted in such a way that they bisect the angle subtended by the perpendiculars dropped to the fracture plane and to the long axis of the bone.

Principles of Bone Plate Application

Bone plates are available in a variety of sizes and shapes. The surgeon must select the correct plate for any given fracture. Selection is based on many factors, including the size of animal, the bone involved, degree of comminution, presence of fissures, and location of the fracture within the bone. Plates should be large enough to neutralize the forces acting at the fracture·site, but not too thick or heavy for the bone they cover. If the plate is too heavy, complications may occur: A new fracture may occur at the end of the plate and the more elastic bone, or the bone may atrophy because the plate prevents the normal physiological stress necessary for maintaining normal bone composition. Lack of stress results in a loss of the axial haversian system, thus thinning and weakening the cortex.[8, 11] This cortical thinning due to overplating is called "stress protection." General guidelines have been suggested for selecting the proper size bone plate on the basis of the animal's weight.[2]

There are three types of plates: straight, special, and angled. The straight plates are used for the diaphysis, special plates for the epiphysis and metaphysis, and angled plates for the proximal and distal femur.[7, 8] Straight plates are the most commonly used plates in veterinary surgery because they can be contoured easily and used in most areas. In the AO system, plates are available in 2.0-mm, 2.7-mm, 3.5-mm, and 4.5-mm sizes. The millimeters denote the

size screw used with each plate. The 4.5-mm plates are available in two widths, narrow or broad. Most straight plates are available with either round or oval holes. Tubular plates are a specialized type of straight plate available in 2.7-mm, 3.5-mm, and 4.5-mm sizes and come with oval holes only.

The straight round-hole plate requires the use of a tension device that can be attached to the end of the plate to compress fractures. The plate is applied under tension, but the bone is in compression. Use of the tension device requires a greater surgical exposure than is necessary to apply the plate without tension. The round screw holes have recently been modified to allow cortical screws to be slightly angled and to allow cancellous screws to be inserted through all the holes.[7, 8]

The dynamic compression plate (DCP) is an improvement over the traditional round-hole plate. The special geometry of its oval screw holes has increased the potential uses of the plate. The DCP does not require a tension device for axial compression and can be used to compress fractures without additional surgical exposure. Compression is achieved through eccentric placement of the screws in the oval holes of the plate. Because of the sloping design of the screw holes, the plate moves as the screw head is seated. Movement of the plate results in axial compression. Drilling of the eccentric holes is done with the aid of a special drill guide, called a load guide. When compression is not desired, a neutral load guide is used. It is also possible to angle screws in any direction through the oval holes.[7, 8] These two features of the DCP make it a more versatile and popular implant among veterinary surgeons than the round-hole plate.

Semitubular plates can be used as self-compressing plates, but they are only 1 mm thick and easily deformable. Because they are so easily deformable, they should be used as tension band plates where the only deforming forces are those of tension. The advantage of tubular plates is their ability to provide rotational stability by their close adaptation to bone and by the digging of their edges into the bone. Their disadvantage is that the screw heads protrude deeply through the screw holes and may shatter the underlying cortex. The stability of tubular plates is considerably greater than that of other straight plates of equal thickness. The eccentric placement of screws in the oval holes accounts for the self-compressing properties of the plate.[8] The major indication for tubular plates is for fractures of the radius and ulna. However, regular straight plates function equally well.

The ability of a plate to provide rigid fixation is directly proportional to its distance from the fulcrum of the bending moment.[8] At least six cortices should be firmly engaged by screws on either side of the fracture.[8, 13] Deviation from this rule may be necessary, depending on the location of the fracture, because there may not be enough bone length beyond the fracture to engage six cortices. More screws may be placed on each side of the fracture if the animal is normally active and the ability of the owner to confine the animal postoperatively is uncertain.

Screws in a fracture or fissure line may result in distraction of fragments, worsening of the fissure, or stripping of the screw threads, necessitating screw removal. Placing a short screw through only one cortex or leaving a screw hole empty may be necessary to avoid this problem (Figs. 153–32 and 153–38).

Plates should be contoured to the original shape and curvature of the particular bone. They must be bent and twisted to fit the bone properly, requiring a bending press or bending irons. A radiograph of the normal opposite limb is useful as a template for contouring the plate. Malleable templates that can be easily bent and twisted with the fingers are available to facilitate contouring of the plate (Fig. 153–33).[8, 11] An improperly contoured plate will cause loss of fracture alignment when it is applied to the bone.

A plate can serve various functions, depending on the manner in which it is used. It may act as a "tension band plate" if it is placed on the tension side of a weight-bearing bone such as the lateral femur. It may act as a "neutralization plate" if it is used to protect a comminuted area that has been reconstructed with lag screws. It may also function as a "buttress plate" if it is used to bridge a diaphyseal defect.[8, 11] With a tension band, tensile forces are

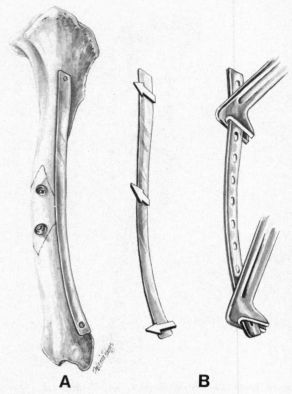

Figure 153–33. *A,* After reduction and lag screw fixation of the fracture, a malleable template is contoured to the shape of the bone. *B,* The contoured malleable plate serves as a template for the contouring of the bone plate.

counteracted and converted into compressive forces. Every eccentrically loaded bone is subjected to bending stresses, resulting in a distribution of stresses with tension on the convex and compression on the concave side of the bone (Fig. 153–34). To restore the load-bearing capacity of an eccentrically loaded bone, the tensile forces must be absorbed by the tension band (plate) and the bone itself must be able to withstand axial compression. Plates used as tension bands are intended to convert tensile forces of eccentrically loaded bones, such as the femur, into compressive forces (Fig. 153–35A). If a plate is placed on a side of the bone where compressive forces predominate, it cannot act as a tension band to stabilize the fracture. Because the plate may be unable to withstand or counteract the bending forces on the compression side of the bone, it fatigues under cyclic loading and soon breaks (Fig. 153–35B). If a plate is applied to the lateral side of the femur and a portion of the medial cortex is absent, the requirements of the tension band plate have not been met because the bone cannot absorb compression.[7, 8]

In vivo strain analysis indicates that the tension band side of the femur or tibia is anterolateral and that of the humerus is anteromedial; however, plates are not always applied to these areas.[6] The tension band side of weight-bearing bones may change, depending on the phase of stride. The tension band side of a fractured bone (e.g., humerus) may vary,

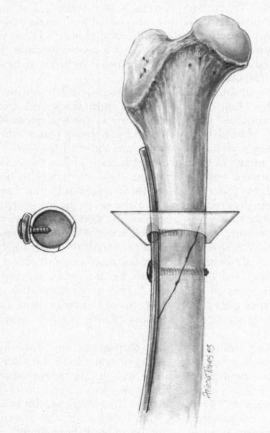

Figure 153–32. A short screw through the plate is used to prevent the screw from entering the fracture line.

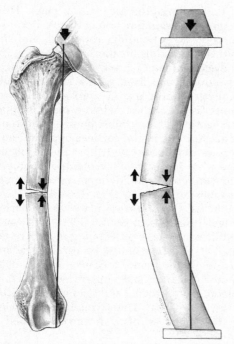

Figure 153–34. Long bones are subjected to eccentric loading. The femur, for example, can be compared to a bent column. As the load is applied, tension on the convex side and compression on the concave side of the column results.

depending on the location of the fracture within the bone. These factors, as well as the difficulty of the surgical approach, should be considered when deciding where the plate is to be applied to the bone.

Plates are usually applied to the medial aspect of the tibia, since the lateral approach is more difficult. The femur is usually plated on the lateral side rather than on the anterolateral aspect, so the plate will not interfere with gliding of the quadriceps muscle. The humerus may be plated caudally, medially, cranially, or laterally, depending on the fracture location and the surgeon's preference. The radius is usually plated cranially, and the proximal ulna may be plated caudally, laterally, or medially. When the true tension side of a bone is not plated, stability relies heavily on the inherent strength of the plate to overcome the forces due to axial loading.

Tension band plates are usually used to repair transverse or short oblique two-piece fractures and nonunited fractures. Theoretically, a plate applied to a bone on its tension side acts as a tension band when tension is applied during weight-bearing. The tension in the plate results in axial compression of the bone. However, to have axial compression present during periods of rest as well as activity, the plate must be pre-bent so that after it is applied, it is under tension.[8] If a straight plate is applied to a straight bone, a gap occurs in the opposite cortex as tension is applied to the plate. To overcome this, the plate must be pre-bent or contoured to a slight convexity at the fracture site. When a contoured plate is applied, the opposite cortices come in contact and a slight gap occurs in the cortices under the plate. As axial compression is generated by applying tension to the plate, the cortices under the plate come in contact and compressive force is evenly distributed across the entire fracture surface (Fig. 153–36). A similar effect is

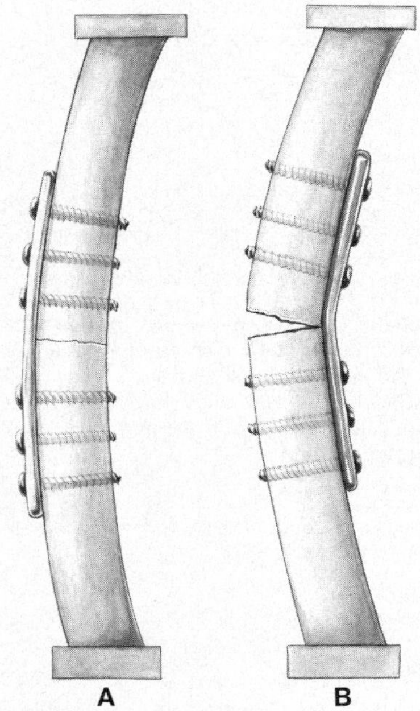

Figure 153–35. *A*, The result of a plate applied to the convex side of the column. The plate converts the tensile forces into compressive forces. *B*, The result of a plate applied to the concave side of the column. The plate cannot convert the tensile forces but is subject to bending forces and would soon fatigue and break.

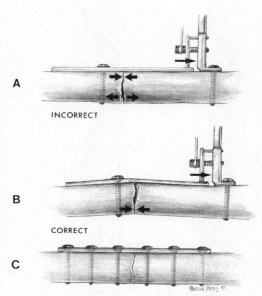

Figure 153–36. *A*, The result of applying a straight plate to a straight bone. As tension is applied to the plate, a gap occurs in the cortices opposite the plate. *B*, As the pre-bent plate is applied to the bone, the opposite cortices come in contact, and a slight gap occurs in the cortices under the plate. *C*, As the remaining screws are inserted and tension is applied to the plate, the cortices under the plate come in contact, and the compressive force is evenly distributed across the entire fracture surface.

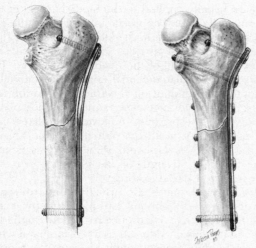

Figure 153–37. The effect of applying a straight plate to a concave bone. Although the plate has been contoured, it is straighter than the underlying cortex, such that there is a 1- to 2-mm gap between the plate and the bone at the fracture. Application of the plate results in compression of the opposite cortex.

obtained when a plate is applied to a concave bone such as the femur (Fig. 153–37).[8, 16]

Neutralization plates are used to stabilize comminuted fractures in which the butterfly fragments have been reconstructed with lag screws. Screw fixation alone provides poor resistance to shearing forces from axial loading or weight-bearing, necessitating protec-

tion of the comminuted area with a plate. This is by far the most common function of plates. Because such a plate neutralizes bending, rotational, and shearing forces that are acting on the fracture, it is called a "neutralization plate." First, the comminuted fracture is reduced and fixed with lag screws, and then a carefully contoured plate is applied to the two main fragments (Fig. 153–38). When a plate is applied as a neutralization plate, it must be pre-bent to prevent gaps from forming in the cortices opposite the plate. Lag screws can be inserted through the plate when necessary.[8, 13] Even in short oblique fractures, one oblique lag screw should be inserted through the plate to increase stability (Fig. 153–39).[8]

In animals, the "buttress plate" is primarily used to bridge a diaphyseal defect filled with cancellous bone graft while the graft is being incorporated (Fig. 153–40).[8, 11] The plate must be carefully adapted to the shape of the bone, because it is functionally designed to distract and support, not to compress. Its function is to prevent the fracture from collapsing until the diaphyseal defect can be filled with new bone. The buttress plate is never applied under tension.[8]

Postoperative Management

Achieving stable internal fixation is only one aspect of fracture management. The postoperative and con-

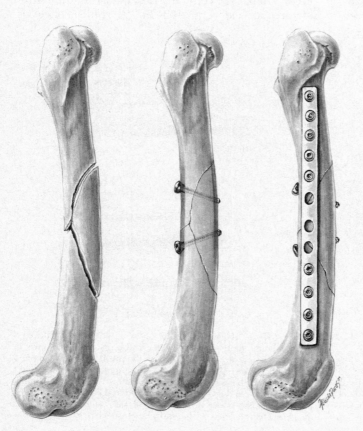

Figure 153–38. The use of a neutralization plate to protect the lag screw fixation of a comminuted area. The fracture is first reduced and stabilized with lag screws, and the plate is then applied to the two main fragments. Note that three screw holes have been left empty to keep screws from entering fracture lines.

tone and gliding function of muscles and tendons and to prevent fibrous adhesions from forming, thus preventing fracture disease. The early postoperative period must be closely supervised to prevent excessive activity that may result in implant failure.

Client education is another important aspect of fracture management. The client must be advised how to care for the convalescing pet properly. The animal's activity must be restricted until the fracture has healed. The owner must be made aware that the animal should begin using the affected limb normally long before the fracture has completely healed. Unsupervised activity during this period may result in implant failure. The animal should be periodically returned to the hospital for follow-up radiographs to assess fracture healing.

Stress Protection and Implant Removal

Plate removal is advised after bone union, not only because of possible corrosion, but also because bone under a plate never becomes biomechanically normal. The rigid plate prevents the bone from responding to normal physiologic stimuli because of the difference in the modulus of elasticity between the bone and the implant.[8] If a plate is too rigid, thinning of the underlying cortices may result. Because this response, known as "stress protection," is partially the result of improper implant selection, it is important not to "overplate" a fracture.

Usually, implants should not be removed before the architecture of the bone has become radiographically normal. The pre-stress of the implant slowly dissipates as bone healing and remodelling take place, and some loosening of implant may occur. This is an advantage because it results in physiological loading of the bone, and with it, a return to normal architecture. This process, however, requires time. The time required between implant application and removal varies, but it generally takes 12 to 18 months for complete bone remodelling to occur.[8]

There are some exceptions to the rule of implant removal.[8] Plates are usually not removed from healed pelvic fractures, because stress protection of this bone seldom occurs. Plates are not removed from many humeral fractures, if there is no evidence of stress protection, because the approach is difficult and the likelihood of damaging major nerves is increased because they are more difficult to identify in the scar tissue that forms after fracture repair. Single screws in the metaphysis or epiphysis need not be removed.[8] Plates are often not removed from old animals.

A diaphysis loses 50 per cent of its torsional resistance from the mere insertion or removal of a single screw. Animal experiments have shown that this reduction in strength lasts one to two months.[8] Long bones must be protected from excessive stress following implant removal. The animal's activity must be restricted for eight to 12 weeks after plate removal to prevent refracture of the bone.

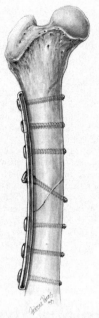

Figure 153–39. The insertion of a lag screw obliquely across a short oblique fracture. This procedure increases stability by creating interfragmentary compression.

valescent care is important to allow healing of the fracture before failure of the implant and to promote early function of the injured limb. After stable fracture fixation with a bone plate, the affected limb can be placed in a light support wrap, which helps prevent postoperative swelling and reduce any swelling present prior to the fracture repair. Prevention of postoperative swelling is beneficial in promoting early use of the limb. The animal is encouraged to use the limb as soon as possible to maintain muscle

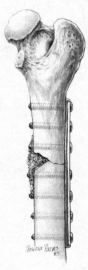

Figure 153–40. The use of a buttress plate to bridge a diaphyseal defect filled with cancellous bone graft. The function of the buttress plate is to support the cortex until the graft can be incorporated into the fracture.

1. Brinker, W. O., and Flo, G. L.: Principles of application of external skeletal fixation. Vet. Clin. North Am. 5:197, 1975.
2. Brinker, W. O., Flo, G. L., Lammerding, J. J., and Bloomberg, M. S.: Guidelines for selecting proper implant size for treatment of fractures in the dog and cat. J. Am. Anim. Hosp. Assoc. 13:476, 1977.
3. Butler, H. C.: Resumé of fracture healing. Vet. Clin. North Am. 5:147, 1975.
4. Campbell, J. R.: The technique of fixation of fractures of the distal femur using Rush pins. J. Small Anim. Pract. 17:323, 1976.
5. Chaffee, V. W.: Multiple (stacked) intramedullary pin fixation of humeral and femoral fractures. Am. Anim. Hosp. Assoc. 13:599, 1977.
6. Daly, R. W., Mills, E. J., and Hohn, R. B.: In vivo strain analysis of canine long bones and its application to internal fixation. Arch. Am. Coll. Vet. Surg. VI:11, 1977.
7. Muller, M. E., Allgower, M., and Willenegger, H. (eds.): Manual of Internal Fixation. Springer-Verlag, Berlin, 1970.
8. Muller, M. E., Allgower, M., Schneider, R., and Willenegger, H. (eds.): Manual of Internal Fixation. 2nd ed. Springer-Verlag, Berlin, 1979.
9. Nunamaker, D. M.: Management of infected fractures. Vet. Clin. North Am. 5:259, 1975.
10. Piermattei, D. L., and Greeley, R. G.: An Atlas of Surgical Approaches to the Bones of the Dog and Cat. 2nd ed. W. B. Saunders, Philadelphia, 1979.
11. Rosen, H.: Principles and application of bone plates. Vet. Clin. North Am. 5:229, 1975.
12. Rudy, R. L.: Principles of intramedullary pinning. Vet. Clin. North Am. 5:209, 1975.
13. Schatzker, J.: Concepts of fracture stabilization. In Sumner-Smith, A. G. (ed.): Bone in Clinical Orthopaedics. W. B. Saunders, Philadelphia, 1982.
14. Stone, E. A., Betts, C. W., and Rowland, G. N.: Effect of Rush pins on the distal femoral growth plate of young dogs. Am. J. Vet. Res. 42:261, 1981.
15. Whittick, W. G.: Fractures and dislocations of the pelvic limb. In: Canine Orthopedics. Lea & Febiger, Philadelphia, 1974.
16. Winstanley, E. W.: Aspects of compression treatment of fractures. Vet. Res. 95:430, 1974.
17. Wolf, E. F.: Rush pins in veterinary orthopedics—a review. Am. Anim. Hosp. Assoc. 11:756, 1975.

External Skeletal Fixation

Erick L. Egger and
Kenneth M. Greenwood

External skeletal fixation provides stable fixation of bone fragments without the need for implants in the fracture site or for immobilization of associated joints. Therefore, it is particularly useful in comminuted, open, or infected fractures and avoids the consequences of joint stiffness and muscle atrophy seen with coaptation splintage and the vascular damage associated with internal fixation. The relatively low initial cost, variety of uses, and ease of application make external skeletal fixation an attractive and valuable means of managing many orthopedic conditions.

DEFINITION

External skeletal fixation is a means of stabilizing fractures, osteotomies, or joints using percutaneous pins that penetrate the bone cortices internally and are connected together externally to form a rigid frame (Fig. 153–41).

HISTORY AND DEVELOPMENT

Parkhill[17] first reported on the use of external skeletal fixation in humans in 1897. Lambotte[13] used a design similar to current designs in 1907 (Fig. 153–42). In the 1930s Anderson, Hoffman, and Stader (a veterinarian) developed the basic designs still in use.[15] Ehmer[8] modified a human design specifically for veterinary use in the late 1940s. This is the design

currently manufactured by the Kirschner Company.* During World War II, many external skeletal fixation splints were applied incorrectly under battle conditions, with a high incidence of pin tract infection and

*Kirschner Company, Timonium, MD.

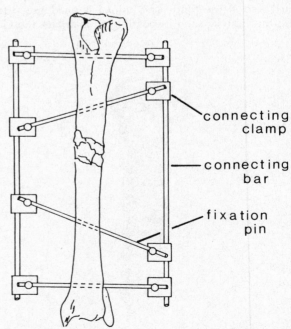

Figure 153–41. Components of external skeletal fixation in a full-pin type II configuration. (Reprinted with permission from Egger, E. L.: Static strength evaluation of six external skeletal fixation configurations. Vet. Surg. 12:130, 1983.)

connecting clamp

connecting bar

fixation pin

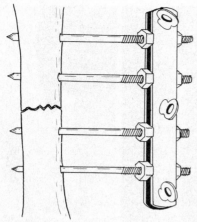

Figure 153–42. Lambotte's external fixator—1907.

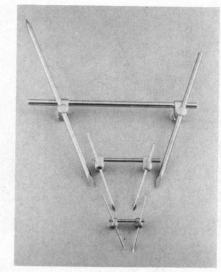

Figure 153–43. Large, medium, and small Kirschner apparatus.

nonunion.[19] Consequently, external skeletal fixation was discouraged as a form of fracture management until a rebirth of interest occurred in the 1970s. Currently, much effort is being devoted to improving both equipment and techniques of application.[9, 15, 16]

FRACTURE HEALING WITH EXTERNAL SKELETAL FIXATION

Spontaneous healing of a fracture depends on proliferation of connective tissue elements from multipotential mesenchymal cells. The type of connective tissue that proliferates depends on the oxygen tension of the area, which depends upon the vascularity. As the fracture area becomes progressively more stable, capillaries are better able to invade the fracture site, the oxygen tension rises, and the original tissues are replaced with stiffer and stronger tissues. Ultimately, bone is produced. This form of healing is referred to as callous healing. The rate and success of callous fracture healing and the amount of periosteal connective tissue callus produced are largely affected by instability that the callus must overcome and by the vascularity of the fracture fragments.[14] Also, stress across the fracture in the form of weight-bearing both speeds the production and improves the quality of callus formation.[16] The goals of fracture healing with external skeletal fixation are to stabilize the bone ends adequately with minimal damage to vascularity and to allow some stress on the fracture site to induce minimal callous healing.

CURRENT EXTERNAL SKELETAL FIXATION DEVICES

Kirschner Company makes the most popular veterinary external skeletal fixation device in three sizes (Fig. 153–43). The small apparatus utilizes 3/32-inch diameter or smaller fixation pins and 1/8-inch diameter connecting bars. It is suitable for use in cats, very small dogs, and some exotic animals such as

raptors. The medium-sized apparatus has 1/8-inch or smaller fixation pins and 3/16-inch connecting bars and is suitable for use in all but the smallest dogs. The large apparatus has 1/4-inch diameter fixation pins and 3/8-inch diameter connecting rods; it has been used on very large dogs, but its primary use is in horses and food animals. All three of the Kirschner external skeletal fixation sizes can use standard Steinmann pins for both fixation pins and connecting bars. Consequently, the addition of just a few clamps and wrenches can greatly expand the potential of most existing orthopedic instruments sets. Because the clamps are reusable, the implant costs are minimal.

Synthes* markets an external skeletal fixation system developed by the AO/ASIF† group for small animals. It has only one size clamp and connecting bar but can use 2.5-mm Kirschner wires as fixation pins in cats and small dogs or 4.0-mm Steinmann

---

*Synthes Ltd. (USA), Wayne, PA.
†Arbeitsgemeinschaft fur Osteosynthesefragen (Swiss)/Association for the Study of Internal Fixation.

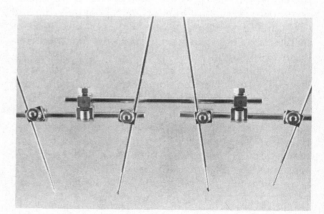

Figure 153–44. Small external fixator from Synthes in the double-clamp type I configuration.

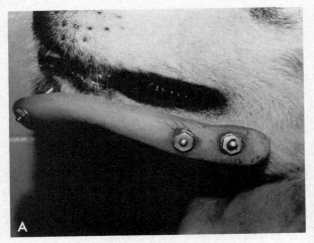

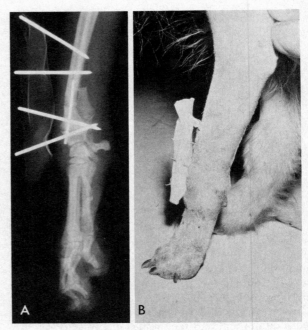

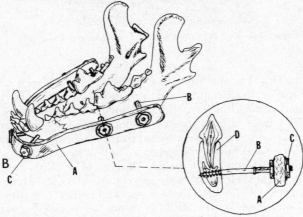

Figure 153–46. A, A distal radius and ulna fracture in a Pomeranian fixed with a small intramedullary Kirschner wire and a four-pin type I acrylic splint. *B,* A photograph of the splint, which was formed by injecting dental acrylic (polymethylmethacrylate) into a Penrose drain that was transfixed by the fixation pins.

Figure 153–45. A, Biphase splint in place on the mandible of a large dog. *B,* The screw-tipped bolts *(B)* are anchored directly into the mandibular body *(D).* The acrylic bar *(A)* connects the bolts together to form a rigid frame. A retaining nut *(C)* secures the acrylic bar to the bolt.

acrylic), either molded by hand or molded in a tube, for the connecting beam (Fig. 153–46).[1, 20]

NOMENCLATURE

The traditional nomenclature of external skeletal fixation is based on a combination of manufacturers' and surgeons' descriptive terms. Consequently, there is great variety and confusion in the nomenclature. In this discussion, we will categorize external skeletal fixation according to G. Hierholzer.[11]

Type I: half-pin splintage. Fixation pins pass through only one skin surface and through both bone

pins as fixation pins in larger animals (Fig. 153–44). The application and uses of this fixation system are similar to those for the Kirschner system.

Human external skeletal fixation devices such as Richard's Kronner* system or the mini Hoffman† system are marvels of biomechanical engineering and very effective but expensive. Occasionally, used or surplus devices are available from neighborhood clinics or hospitals.

The Biphase‡ splint, which uses acrylic cement as the connecting bar and screw-tipped bolts for bone fixation, is designed for fixing mandibular fractures. The device was developed for human patients but can be used on medium and large dogs (Fig. 153–45).[10] The fixation bolts are too large for cats and small dogs. Homemade versions of the splint are constructed of Steinmann pins or Kirschner wires for bone fixation and polymethylmethacrylate (dental

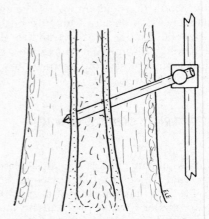

Figure 153–47. Type I half-pin splintage, in which pins penetrate only one skin surface and both bone cortices.

*Richards Manufacturing Company, Inc., Memphis, TN.
†Ets Jaquet Freres, Geneva, Switzerland.
‡Walter Lorenz Surgical Instruments, Inc., Jacksonville, FL.

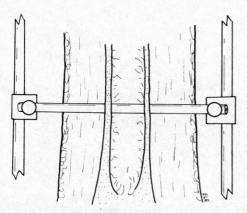

Figure 153–48. Type II full-pin splintage, in which the pins penetrate both skin surfaces and cortices.

cortices. The connecting clamps and bars are placed on one side of the leg only (Fig. 153–47).

Type II: full-pin splintage. Fixation pins pass through both skin surfaces and both bone cortices. The connecting clamps and bars are used on both sides of the leg (Fig. 153–48).

Type III: combination of half-pin and full-pin splintage. Type I and type II splints are placed at 90 degrees axial rotation to each other and are interconnected at both ends, creating a three-dimensional frame (Fig. 153–49).

External skeletal fixation can further be described

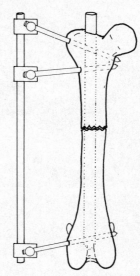

Figure 153–50. The two- or three-pin, single-bar type I configuration used to control rotation with an intramedullary pin.

by the type of connecting clamps used, the number of connecting bars that bridge the fracture site, and the number of fixation pins that hold the bone. A single connecting clamp (single clamp) connects a fixation pin to a connecting bar. A double connecting clamp (double clamp) connects two connecting bars. If needed, the fixation pins can also be described as either half-pin (penetrates only one skin surface) or full-pin (penetrates both skin surfaces).

CURRENT CONFIGURATIONS OF EXTERNAL SKELETAL FIXATION

Type I: Half-Pin Splintage

Two- or Three-Pin Single-Bar Type I. One or occasionally two pins are placed in each fragment and

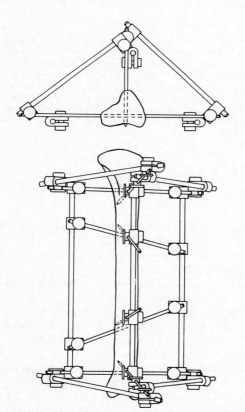

Figure 153–49. Type III three-dimensional configuration is a combination of half-pin and full-pin splintage. (Reprinted with permission from Egger, E. L.: Static strength evaluation of six external skeletal fixation configurations. Vet. Surg. *12:*130, 1983.)

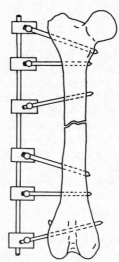

Figure 153–51. A six-pin, single-bar type I configuration is relatively simple and economical.

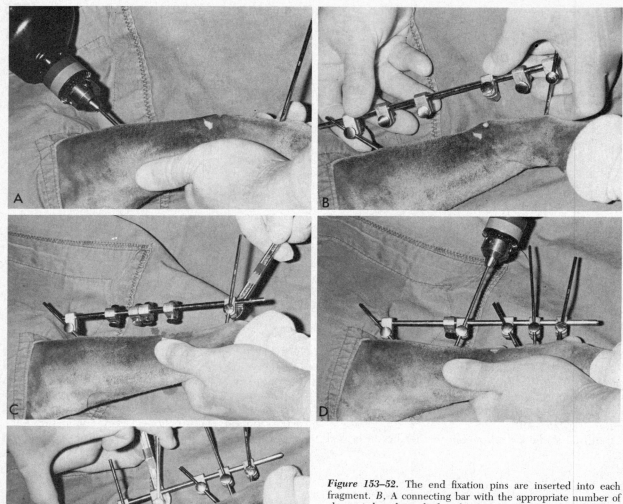

Figure 153–52. The end fixation pins are inserted into each fragment. *B,* A connecting bar with the appropriate number of clamps is loosely applied to the pins. *C,* The fracture is reduced and the end clamps are tightened. *D,* Fixation pins are driven through the open clamps and small skin incisions, and into the bone. *E,* The fixation pins can be squeezed together to obtain fracture compression or a spring-like grip on the bone, and the clamps are tightened.

connecting bar (Fig. 153–50). This form is useful as an adjunct to intramedullary pinning to control rotation and as some protection against fracture collapse. It is inadequate for fracture stabilization by itself.

Four (or More)-Pin Single-Bar Type I. At least two half pins per fragment are all attached to the same connecting bar (Fig. 153–51). It is an economical and the least complex configuration. It can be used above the elbow and stifle and does not interfere with the body wall. This configuration cannot be adjusted significantly after application. Consequently, the following procedure for application is usually followed:

1. The most proximal and distal fixation pins are placed in the two fragments at appropriate angles (Fig. 153–52A).

2. A single connecting bar is loosely attached to the pins with the anticipated number of "open" clamps in the middle (Fig. 153–52B).

3. The fracture is reduced and the two end clamps are tightened (Fig. 153–52C).

4. The remaining fixation pins are driven through the open clamps (Fig. 153–52D).

5. All the fixation pins are slightly squeezed together and all clamps are tightened (Fig. 153–52E).

6. Excess fixation pin and connecting bar length is removed with a pin cutter.

Double-Bar Type I. Two connecting bars are attached to the fixation pins on one side of the leg (Fig. 153–53). This provides significantly more resistance to compression in fractures with major defects or severe comminution in which the fragment ends provide no support.[7]

Quadrilateral Frame Type I. Two single-bar

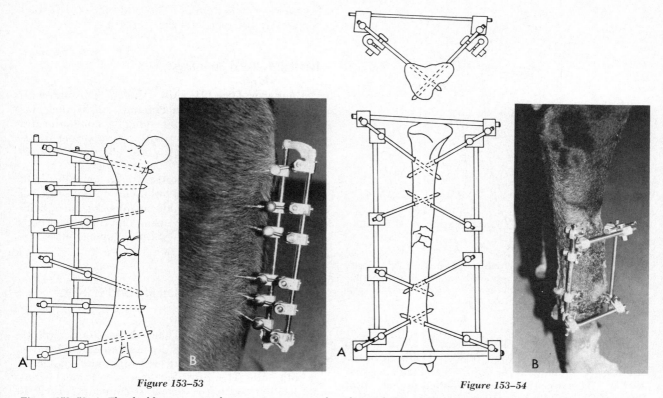

Figure 153–53   *Figure 153–54*

Figure 153–53. A, The double–connecting bar type I is stronger than the single-bar configuration but still useful proximal to the elbow and stifle. B, The double–connecting bar configuration applied to a fractured femur. (A reprinted with permission from Egger, E. L.: Static strength evaluation of six external skeletal fixation configurations. Vet. Surg. *12*:130, 1983.)

Figure 153–54. Drawing (A) and photograph (B) of the quadrilateral type I configuration. (Reprinted with permission from Egger, E. L.: Static strength evaluation of six external skeletal fixation configurations. Vet. Surg. *12*:130, 1983.)

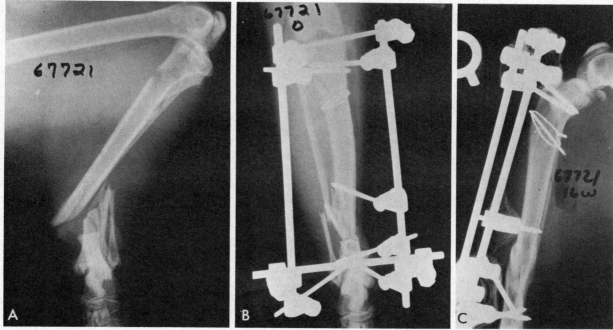

Figure 153–55. A, A segmental tibial fracture. B, Fixation of the same fracture with a quadrilateral frame. C, Radiographs of the healed fracture ten weeks after surgery.

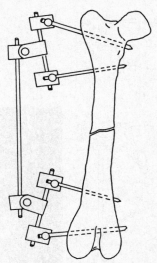

Figure 153–56. The double-clamp type I configuration is highly adjustable after placement. (Reprinted with permission from Egger, E. L.: Static strength evaluation of six external skeletal fixation configurations. Vet. Surg. *12*:130, 1983.)

splints are applied parallel and at 90-degree axial rotation to each other (Fig. 153–54). The ends of the splints are connected to form a triangular cross-section.[6] This apparatus can be applied to very short fragments (Fig. 153–55). Although it is not as resistant to compressive forces as full-pin splintage, it is more resistant to shear and bending forces.[7]

Double-Clamp Type I. Double clamps and a connecting bar are used to connect the two pin splints that are placed in each fragment (Fig. 153–56). This configuration is adjustable after the apparatus is applied, and the fixation pins can be placed in any order. In the Kirschner external skeletal fixation system, the double clamp is relatively weak.[7] This weakness limits its use to stable or rapidly healing

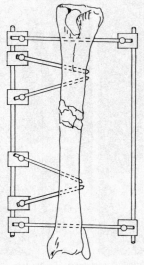

Figure 153–57. A modified type II configuration, in which only two fixation pins are applied as full pins, making application and adjustment of the apparatus easier.

fractures or osteotomies. The addition of a second connecting bar increases the strength.

Type II: Full-Pin Splintage

Standard Type II (Also Called Through-and-Through or Transfixation Pinning). All fixation pins are full and attached to connecting bars on both sides of the limb. This configuration is very strong but is limited to application below the elbow or stifle in small animals.[7]

Modified Type II. Because it can be difficult to get all of the fixation pins to line up on both sides of the limb without a pin guide, many surgeons modify the type II splint by only using one full pin in each fragment with additional half-pins for adequate stability (Fig. 153–57).[3]

Type III: Combination Half-Pin and Full-Pin Splintage

Standard Type III (Three-Dimensional Splint). Type I and type II splints are applied parallel and at 90 degrees axial rotation to each other and connected at both ends. This provides three-dimensional external fixation and is the strongest configuration.[7, 11] It is a potential means of effecting arthrodesis of joints and fixing fractures in larger animals.

PRINCIPLES OF APPLICATION

The first decision in the process of fracture treatment with external skeletal fixation is the choice of closed *versus* open reduction. Closed reduction causes less damage to soft tissue and osseous vascularity but it may not result in adequate fracture reduction, particularly of fractures proximal to the elbow or stifle. Open reduction achieves better fracture reduction but should be limited so as to avoid retarding the healing process. If fracture defects persist after open reduction, autogenous cancellous bone grafting is indicated. The graft can be obtained from the greater tubercle of the forelimb or from the dorsal ilial wing or proximal tibial crest of the hind limb.

The manner of fixation pin insertion is important. The pins are driven through small holes in intact skin, not through the incision site or open wounds. This practice eliminates problems with incision or wound management and decreases the incidence of pin tract infections. It also makes incision closure much easier. If possible, the fixation pin placement should avoid penetration of large muscle masses, which is often the cause of poor postoperative leg use.

Care must be taken when placing the pins in the cortical bone. If the pins are inserted with a hand chuck, wobbling can make the pin hole too large and result in premature pin loosening and fixation failure.

Also, hand placement of fixation pins into dense cortical bone can be mechanically difficult. For these reasons, many surgeons use power drills for pin insertion. Excessive pressure and high speeds should be avoided when inserting the pins, since thermal necrosis of the bone can occur and cause premature loosening.[18] Both half and full pins must be placed completely through both cortices of the bone to achieve secure fixation.

The angle of each pin should be carefully planned to contribute the most strength to the fixation yet obtain adequate purchase of the bone. Traditionally, an angle of 35 to 55 degrees between the outermost pins placed in each fragment has been used with type I (half-pin) splints.[5] Type II (full-pin) splints are mechanically strongest if the fixation pins are all placed parallel to one another and perpendicular to the long axis of the bone.[4] However, because the apparatus may loosen and slide back and forth on the leg, most surgeons place at least one of the pins in each fragment obliquely.[3]

The appropriate number of pins to be placed in each fragment has not been objectively determined. Traditionally, two pins have been placed in each fragment in veterinary applications.[5] Experimental work has shown that the bone-pin interface is the weakest length of most splints, and that increasing the number of fixation pins used significantly increases the devices' initial strength.[4] Premature loosening of the bone-pin interface is the most common limiting factor in the use of external skeletal fixation but this is much less a problem if more fixation pins are used. Perhaps using more pins reduces the stress placed on each bone-pin interface. We now use six to eight bone-pin interfaces (three or four pins) per fragment if at all possible.

Some clinicians have suggested the use of threaded pins when applying type I (half-pin) splints. However, the experience with threaded pins has been disappointing because of their tendency to break off or bend at the junction of the threaded and unthreaded shaft (stress riser effect) (Fig. 153–58).

Pin placement in the fragments relative to the fracture site and the bone ends also needs to be considered. It has been observed that the best mechanical advantage for neutralizing the forces exerted on a fracture is obtained by placing the fixation pins near the proximal and distal bone ends.[5] However, increasing the distance between the pins adjacent to a gap fracture significantly decreases the strength of type I (half-pin) configurations.[4] Consequently, pin placement is spread out over the entire fragment.

The distance from the connecting bar to the bone also greatly affects the overall strength of splintage. In experiments, doubling the distance reduced the resistance to compressive load by about 25 per cent.[4] However, the connecting bar and clamps must be placed far enough from the leg to allow for postoperative soft tissue swelling and callous formation. Therefore, the optimum bar-to-bone distance varies, depending upon the thickness of the involved soft tissues and the degree to which they have been traumatized.

SPECIFIC INDICATIONS FOR USE OF EXTERNAL SKELETAL FIXATION

Adjuncts to Other Internal Fixation

External skeletal fixation may be used in conjunction with certain forms of internal fixation. It can be effective in controlling axial rotation and collapse of the fracture site when used with intramedullary pins. It may also be used with cerclage wire, hemicerclage wire, or interfragmentary screws; these situations usually call for a two- or three-pin type I (half-pin) splint. This supplementary fixation can usually be removed in three to five weeks, when the callus becomes sufficiently organized to prevent rotation.

Nonunions

Nonunions are hypertrophic or atrophic. In hypertrophic nonunions, bone heals when the proper environment exists. Stabilization is all that is usually necessary and can be provided in many cases with closed reduction and application of external skeletal fixation. An atrophic nonunion has lost the capacity to heal. It is most commonly seen in fractures of avascular areas in miniature breeds that have poor leg use when treated with external coaptation (Fig. 153–59). Treatment requires open reduction, decortication of avascular bone, opening of the medullary canal, and packing with cancellous bone graft to stimulate vascular proliferation and callus production. External skeletal fixation can provide stabilization while allowing the stimulating stress of weight-bearing.

Comminuted Fractures

Severely comminuted fractures may be treated with external skeletal fixation when more exacting reconstruction is not possible (Fig. 153–60). External skeletal fixation requires minimal bone for fixation and can span large defects.[6] Care must be taken to avoid damage to osseous vascularity, since healing

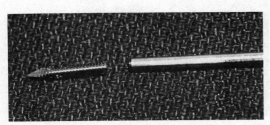

Figure 153–58. A threaded fixation pin that had broken off at the junction of the threaded and smooth shaft owing to the stress riser effect.

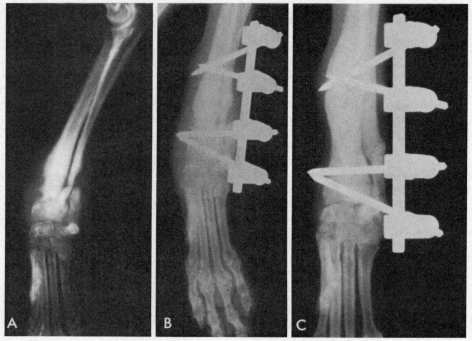

Figure 153–59. *A,* Radiograph of a distal radius and ulna fracture that had been treated with a cast for eight weeks. It has become an avascular, atrophic nonunion, as indicated by the sclerosis, loss of bone, and lack of periosteal response at the fracture site. *B,* Postoperative radiograph of the nonunion. The sclerotic bone has been resected, the medullary canal opened, and the area packed with cancellous bone graft from the proximal humerus. A four-pin single bar was used for fixation. *C,* An anteroposterior radiograph revealing solid healing 12 weeks after fixation.

relies on early callus formation. Consequently, a closed reduction or limited open reduction with massive cancellous bone graft is used. Overall alignment, but not necessarily perfect fracture reduction, is sought.

Open, Gunshot, and Infected Fractures

External skeletal fixation has the advantage of not invading the fracture site and spreading contamination or infection. The fixation pins can usually be

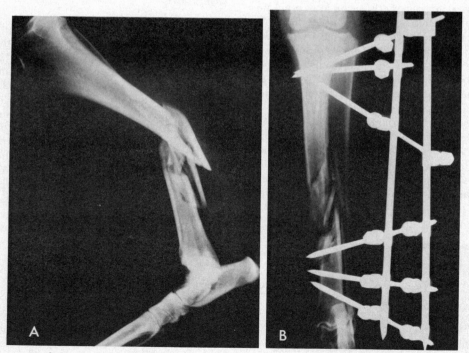

Figure 153–60. *A,* A severely comminuted tibial fracture in a large dog. *B,* The same fracture managed with a limited open reduction, cancellous bone graft, and a double–connecting bar type I splint.

Illustration continued on the opposite page

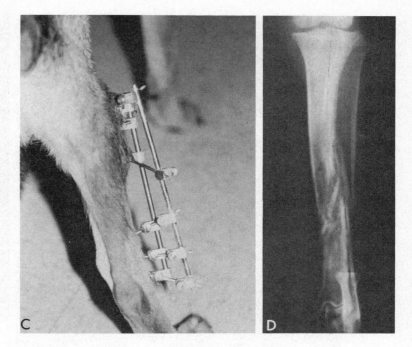

Figure 153–60 Continued. C, The limb and splint six weeks after placement. The dog was using the leg well. D, Final radiographic appearance of the limb 20 weeks after the fracture and six weeks after fixation removal.

applied away from the affected area, lessening the chance of premature bone lysis and early implant failure, which could result in nonunion (Fig. 153–61). External skeletal fixation is particularly useful for stabilizing severe open fractures because it supports the fracture and immobilizes soft tissue while leaving the traumatized area open for daily treatment (Fig. 153–62). External skeletal fixation is often applied as the definitive means of open fracture fixation. Occasionally, this method may be used as temporary stabilization while the infection is controlled. More rigid forms of internal fixation and bone grafting can be applied if needed.

Mandibular Fractures

External skeletal fixation avoids the placement of implants in open wounds and infected alveolar sockets. Mandibular fractures are often comminuted, and

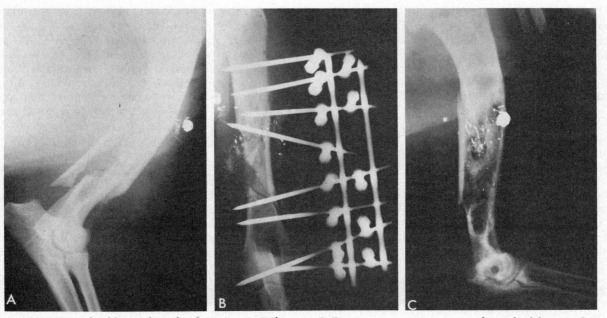

Figure 153–61. A, A distal humeral gunshot fracture in an Irish setter. B, Postoperative anteroposterior radiograph of the same fracture after stabilization with a double–connecting bar configuration. C, Final appearance of the limb 24 weeks after the fracture and eight weeks after fixation removal.

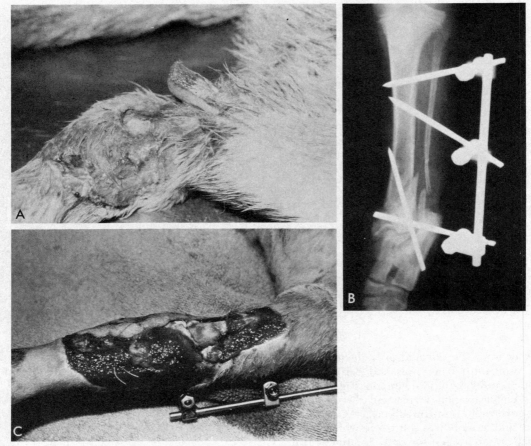

Figure 153–62. *A,* Massive soft tissue wound and contaminated open fracture from a shearing injury. *B,* Anteroposterior radiograph showing a distal tibial fracture stabilized with a cross-pin and external skeletal fixation. *C,* The same case three weeks after surgery, demonstrating external skeletal fixation's ability to immobilize a fracture while leaving the wound accessible for daily treatment.

external skeletal fixation allows preservation of remaining vascular supply to the multiple small fragments. The single–connecting-bar configuration is most often used.

Transarticular Stabilization

External skeletal fixation is occasionally used for transarticular stabilization.[2] It is ideal for ligamentous rupture associated with adjacent soft tissue injury. The ligament may be repaired and protected by external skeletal fixation while the open wound is being treated. External skeletal fixation may also be used for arthrodesis of certain joints (Fig. 153–63). It is especially useful with associated soft tissue damage or infection, in which the use of internal fixation would be less desirable.

Growth Deformities

External skeletal fixation can be useful for treating growth deformities. The adjustability of the double-clamp type I configuration after application is useful for correcting deformities in mature dogs.[5] An oblique osteotomy is performed on the deformed bone, and the tip of the distal segment is driven into the medullary cavity of the proximal segment. The external skeletal fixation is applied and adjusted until adequate correction is obtained (Fig. 153–64). A type II (full-pin) splint can be used as a spreading apparatus in the dynamic treatment of a progressive growth deformity.[12] The prematurely fused bone is cut and straightened. External skeletal fixation is applied and is stretched three times a week to maintain appropriate leg length and angulation. Care must be taken not to spread the osteotomy too fast, because fixation pins easily pull through the soft bone of young dogs. Six to eight weeks of spreading can be obtained before the osteotomy heals or the pins pull out. After termination of growth, definitive correction of any remaining deformity can be performed.

POSTOPERATIVE MANAGEMENT

Many clinical cases treated with external skeletal fixation require minimal postoperative care. In open wounds or where significant postoperative swelling

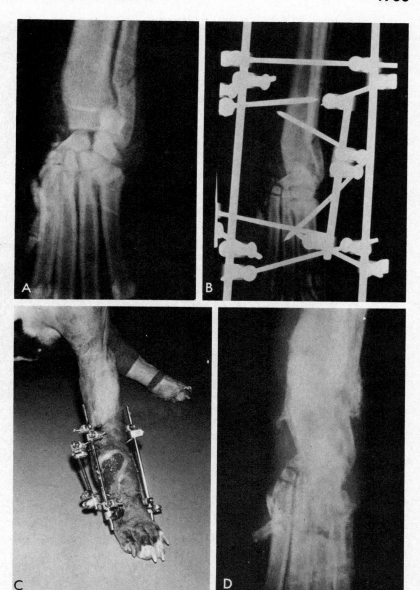

Figure 153-63. A, A severe shearing injury of the antebrachial carpal region. B, Postoperative radiograph of the same case. The articular cartilage was removed, cancellous bone graft was packed into the area, and a transarticular modified type II configuration was applied to induce arthrodesis. C, The same case two weeks after surgery, illustrating access for wound management. D, Final appearance of arthrodesis 20 weeks after surgery. (Courtesy of Dr. C. E. Blass.)

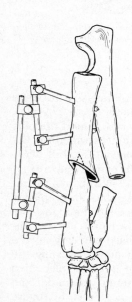

Figure 153-64. A double-clamp type I configuration applied to a radius and ulna after an oblique osteotomy for correction of a growth deformity.

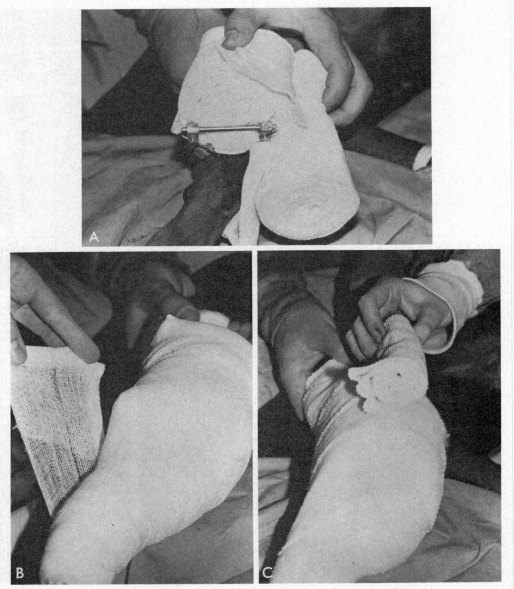

Figure 153–65. A postoperative compressive bandage may be indicated for management of open wounds or to control anticipated swelling. *A,* Padding is packed around the pins. *B,* Additional padding is applied around the whole leg from the toes to above the apparatus. *C,* Compressive gauze is used to compress the padding.

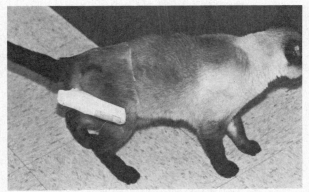

Figure 153–66. A gauze and tape cover placed over the connecting bar, clamps, and ends of fixation pins to protect the apparatus.

is anticipated, a postoperative compressive bandage may be used. The wounds or incisions are covered, and cotton or cast padding is packed around the pins (Fig. 153–65A). Additional padding is rolled on the leg from the toes to above the injury (Fig. 153–65B). The padding is compressed with elastic gauze (Fig. 153–65C) and fixed with tape. This bandage can usually be removed in four to five days and replaced with a gauze and tape cover that envelops only the apparatus (Fig. 153–66). The cover protects the animal and the owner from the sharp cut ends of the fixation pins and reduces the chance of catching the apparatus on fixed objects. The cover is placed so that it allows air circulation around and under the connecting clamps to keep the area dry. In severe tissue injury, external skeletal fixation maintains osseous stability while allowing easy access for wound management. Frequent bandage changes and debridement can be accomplished without traumatizing early vascular proliferation and callus formation. Once adequate granulation has occurred, the wound can be covered with skin grafts or allowed to heal by second intention.

Antibiotic treatment is not routinely used unless the fracture was open or infected, or soft tissue damage was so severe that its viability was in question. Most animals will not bother external skeletal fixation; however, some will lick or chew at incisions or wounds. In these animals, a collar or head bucket may be needed until the soft tissues heal.

CLIENT EDUCATION

Most patients treated with external skeletal fixation can be released to their owners within two to four days of surgery. The animal is released with instructions to restrict activity to leash-walking and to take particular care to avoid fencing or similar open structures that may catch the apparatus. Protection of the apparatus with a tape cover should be maintained until the apparatus is removed. Owners are advised to expect a small amount of crusty discharge to develop at the skin-to-pin interface (Fig. 153–67). A great diversity of opinion exists as to proper pin care,[9] but we advise not removing this material or cleaning the pin sites. Owners are instructed to inspect the apparatus daily and to return after ten to 14 days for evaluation for loose or broken clamps. Further re-

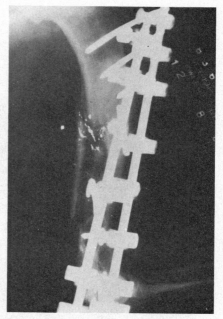

Figure 153–68. A fractured humerus five weeks after fixation with a double–connecting bar. The loss of fracture detail is characteristic of early bone healing.

checks are performed at three- to four-week intervals, depending on the anticipated rate of healing. A simple fracture in a young dog commonly heals in six weeks, whereas a comminuted fracture in a mature dog may require much longer. Loss in sharpness of detail of the fracture edges on radiographs is the earliest sign of fracture healing (Fig. 153–68).[14] External callus production is often minimal with external skeletal fixation.[9] However, young animals may produce a large callus because they have very active periosteum.[14] Complete healing is signified by the loss of discernible fracture lines and bony continuity on radiographs. In the severely comminuted fracture that is treated with a relatively rigid form of external skeletal fixation, staged removal of the fixation is often indicated. This allows increasing amounts of weight-bearing stress to stimulate bony proliferation and strengthening while providing some protection from excessive stress.[16] Staging can be by removing one side of a type II or type III splint or by removing alternating fixation pins of a type I splint (Fig. 153–69).

When fracture healing is complete, external skeletal fixation can usually be removed with minimal or no sedation. The connecting clamps or bars are removed and the fixation pins are pulled using a hand chuck or pin puller in a twisting motion. If threaded pins were used, they must be "unscrewed." A small amount of serosanguineous fluid often drains from the pin site, and a soft padded bandage may be used for a day. The owner is instructed to continue restricting activity for six to eight weeks while the fracture remodels and the bone hypertrophies.

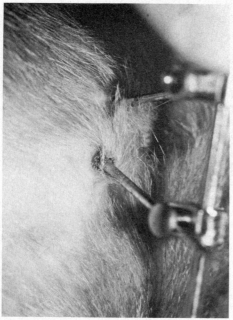

Figure 153–67. The typical crusty discharge at the skin-to-pin interface.

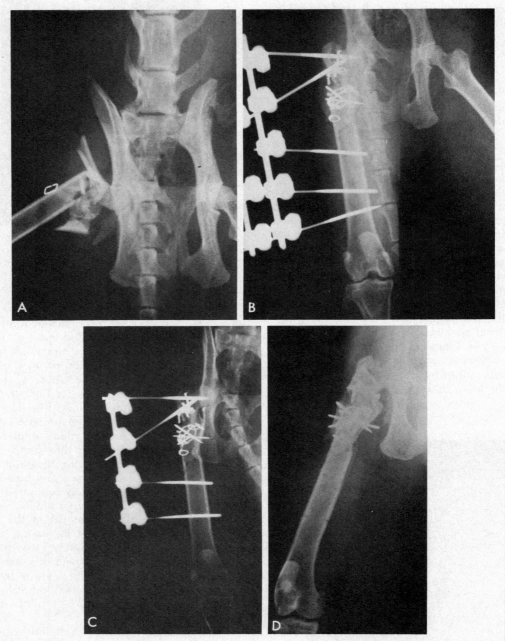

Figure 153–69. A, An extremely comminuted proximal femur fracture. B, Fixation of the same fracture with interfragmentary wires and double connecting bars. C, Staged removal of a connecting bar and fixation pin to allow more weight-bearing stress stimulation across the fracture. D, Final appearance of the healed fracture at the time of external skeletal fixation removal 16 weeks after surgery. Limited exercise was recommended for eight weeks more.

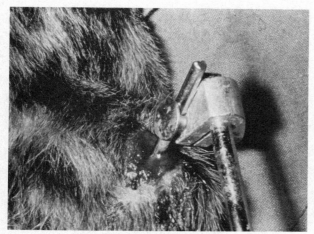

Figure 153–70. The most common problem associated with external skeletal fixation is drainage from the pin tract.

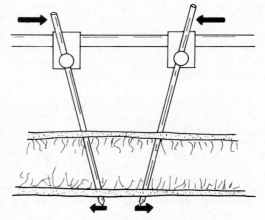

Figure 153–72. Squeezing loose fixation pins together will obtain a spring-like grip on the bone for a short period of continued fixation.

COMPLICATIONS

Probably the most common complication of fracture repair with external skeletal fixation is drainage around the pins (Fig. 153–70).[9] It may be caused by excessive skin and soft tissue movement or tension against the pins. Careful placement of the pins through nondisplaced tissue and avoidance of large muscle groups prevents this problem in most cases. If skin tension persists after pin placement, small relief incisions can be made. Drainage and pin tract infection may reflect loosening of the apparatus at the bone-pin interface (Fig. 153–71). Generalized osteomyelitis due to percutaneous pin fixation is rarely seen in animals, and pin tract infections usually

clear up rapidly after the loose pin is removed. The use of three or more pins per fragment reduces the incidence of premature loosening and drainage.

Loosening of pins may reduce leg use. In many cases, this lameness occurs at the same time as clinical fracture healing and resolves once the apparatus is removed. When continued support is required for a short time (one or two weeks), the fixation pins in each fragment can be squeezed together to obtain a spring grip on the bone (Fig. 153–72). Occasionally, pins must be replaced to maintain adequate stability. Although this usually requires general anesthesia, it can be done by closed insertion of a new pin at a new site.

An uncommon problem is iatrogenic fracture

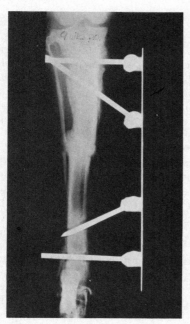

Figure 153–71. Drainage from the pin tract often reflects loosening of the pin as shown by lysis of the bone around the pin. (Courtesy of Dr. C. E. Blass.)

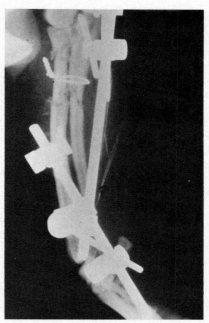

Figure 153–73. An iatrogenic fracture of the proximal radius managed by replacement of the fixation pins into the proximal ulnar fragment. (Courtesy of Dr. C. E. Blass.)

through the pin holes. This usually occurs when oversized pins are used or when pins are placed too close together or in fissure fractures. Unrestricted postoperative activity can also result in fracture through pin holes. Such problems are managed by replacement of pins in intact bone (Fig. 153–73).

1. Aron, J. D.: Using methyl methacrylate to make external fixation splints. J. Bone Jt. Surg. *58A*:151, 1976.
2. Bjorling, D. E., and Toombs, J. P.: Transarticular application of the Kirschner-Ehmer splint. Vet. Surg. *11*:34, 1982.
3. Bradley, R. L., and Rouse, G. P.: External skeletal fixation using the through-and-through Kirschner Ehmer splint. J. Am. Anim. Hosp. Assoc. *16*:523, 1980.
4. Briggs, B. T., and Chao, E. Y.: The mechanical performance of the standard Hoffmann-Vidal external fixation apparatus. J. Bone Jt. Surg. *64A*:566, 1982.
5. Brinker, W. O., and Flo, G. L.: Principles and application of external skeletal fixation. Vet. Clin. North Am. *2*:197, 1975.
6. Cooney, W. P.: Current management of fractures of the distal radius and forearm: experience with external pin fixation. *In* Booker, A. F., Jr., and Edward, C. C. (eds.): *External Fixation—The Current State of the Art*. Williams & Wilkins, Baltimore, 1979.
7. Egger, E. L.: Static strength evaluation of six external skeletal fixation configurations. Vet. Surg. *12*:130, 1983.
8. Ehmer, E. A.: Bone pinning in fractures of small animals. J. Am. Vet. Med. Assoc. *110*:14, 1947.
9. Green, S. T.: *Complications of External Skeletal Fixation: Causes, Prevention, and Treatment*. Charles C Thomas, Springfield, 1981.
10. Greenwood, K. M., and Creagh, G. B.: Biphase external skeletal splint fixation of the mandibular fractures in dogs. Vet. Surg. *9*:128, 1980.
11. Hierholzer, G., Kleining, R., Horster, G., and Zemenides, P.: External fixation—classification and indications. Arch. Orthop. Traumat. Surg. *92*:175, 1978.
12. Knecht, C. D., and Bloomberg, M. S.: Distraction with an external fixation clamp (Charnley apparatus) to maintain length in premature physeal closure. J. Am. Anim. Hosp. Assoc. *16*:873, 1980.
13. Lambotte, A.: *L'intervention operatoire dans les fracteurs*. Lamartins, Brussels, 1907.
14. McKibbin, B.: The biology of fracture healing in long bones. J. Bone Jt. Surg. *60B*:150, 1978.
15. Mears, D. C.: History of fixation. *In* Booker, A. F., Jr., and Edwards, C. C. (eds.): *External Fixation—The Current State of the Art*. Williams & Wilkins, Baltimore, 1979.
16. Mooney, V., and Claudi, B.: How stable should external fixation be? *In* Uhthoff, H. K. (ed.): *Current Concepts of External Fixation of Fractures*. Springer-Verlag, Berlin, 1982.
17. Parkhill, C.: A new apparatus for the fixation of bones after resection and in fractures with a tendency to displacement. Trans. Am. Surg. Assn. *15*:251, 1897.
18. Renegar, W. R., Leeds, E. B., and Olds, R. B.: The use of the Kirschner-Ehmer splint in clinical orthopedics. Part I. Long bone and mandibular fractures. Comp. Cont. Educ. *4*:381, 1982.
19. Siris, I.: External pin transfixation of fractures; an analysis of eighty cases. Ann. Surg. *120*:911, 1944.
20. Stambaugh, J. E., and Nunamaker, D. M.: External skeletal fixation of comminuted maxillary fractures in dogs. Vet. Surg. *11*:72, 1982.

External Coaptation and Bandaging

Steven P. Arnoczky, Charles E. Blass, and Louis McCoy

The proper use of casts, splints, slings, and padded bandages is an important part of small animal orthopedic surgery. They may be used as a primary method of immobilization of selected fractures, first aid or interim coaptation of severely traumatized limbs, postoperative support, or protection of repaired tissues.

BANDAGES AND SLINGS

Soft Padded Bandage

The soft padded bandage is probably the most versatile and most used dressing. It is used for support and protection of soft tissues. Although a well-padded bandage limits the motion of a joint or limb, it is not adequate for immobilization.

To apply the bandage, 2.54-cm (1-in.) adhesive tape stirrups are applied to the lateral and medial (or anterior and posterior) aspects of the distal limb and extended 15 to 20 cm (6 to 8 in.) beyond the limb (Fig. 153–74A). These stirrups help anchor the bandage to the limb. Cast padding (or cotton wadding) is applied to the limb. The padding is begun at the distal aspect of the limb, leaving the toes of the third and fourth digits exposed. The cast padding is wrapped up the limb proximally, overlapping the width by one-half. It is wrapped snugly to the limb and is taken as high above the elbow or stifle as possible (at least to the midshaft of the humerus or femur). Four to six layers of cast padding are used. More layers can be added if the animal is large or more support is desired. Although it is important to pad the pressure points of the limb (olecranon, tuber calcis, condyles, etc.), it is equally important to fill depressions between them to give a slightly tapered cylindrical shape (Fig. 153–74B). It is also important, especially in the rear limb, that the cast padding be placed with the limb in its functional position. Repositioning the limb to accommodate normal stifle or hock angles after the application of the cast padding may cause the padding to bunch up in the flexure crease of these joints, resulting in compression and vascular obstruction in these areas. Elastic or conforming gauze is then started at the distal end of the

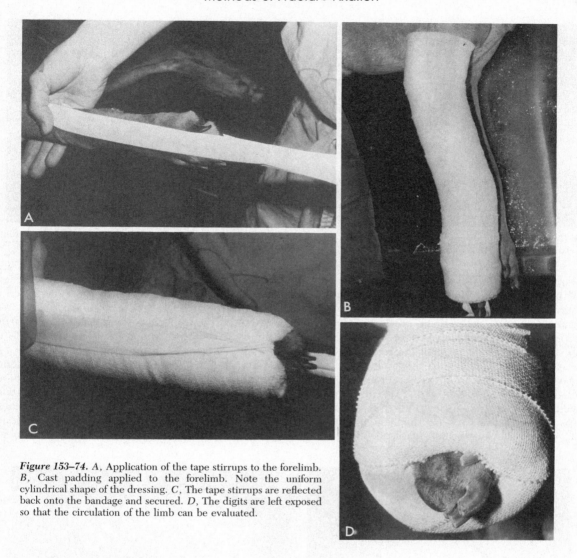

Figure 153–74. A, Application of the tape stirrups to the forelimb. *B,* Cast padding applied to the forelimb. Note the uniform cylindrical shape of the dressing. *C,* The tape stirrups are reflected back onto the bandage and secured. *D,* The digits are left exposed so that the circulation of the limb can be evaluated.

limb and wrapped up the limb, again overlapping by one-half. Care should be taken to apply the conforming gauze evenly and with equal tension to avoid areas of constriction. A firm fit that gently molds the cast padding to the limb is desirable. The tape stirrups are now reflected back on the bandage and secured to the dressing (Fig. 153–74C). These tapes help anchor the bandage to the limb and prevent the bandage from slipping distally. The dressing is then covered with an elastic tape, outer wrap, or adhesive tape. The digits are left exposed, because they are used to evaluate the circulation of the bandaged limb (Fig. 153–74D). Swollen or cold toes indicate vascular obstruction and dictate the removal of the dressing.

Robert-Jones Bandage

The Robert-Jones bandage is a heavily padded support bandage that provides excellent temporary stabilization of fractures or dislocations at or below the elbow or stifle.[1, 2] The bulky, compressive dressing prevents or minimizes soft tissue swelling and is an excellent dressing in the first aid treatment of fractures. The dressing decreases swelling, lessens pain, and minimizes additional trauma (e.g., laceration of vessels or nerves by fracture ends, conversion of a closed fracture to an open fracture, additional muscle trauma). The Robert-Jones bandage may also be used postoperatively to prevent or minimize soft tissue edema.

Prior to application of the bandage, soft tissue wounds are appropriately treated and covered with a nonadherent dressing. As with the soft padded bandage, tape stirrups are placed to help anchor the bandage to the limb. Cotton roll is then applied to the limb. Cotton roll supplies the bulk for the bandage, but because 12-inch rolls are often unwieldy, the rolls are usually cut into six-inch widths for application. The cotton is then wrapped circumferentially about the limb, beginning distally and continuing as proximally as possible (to midshaft of femur or humerus) (Fig. 153–75A). The cotton is wrapped up the limb as evenly and tightly as possible. Me-

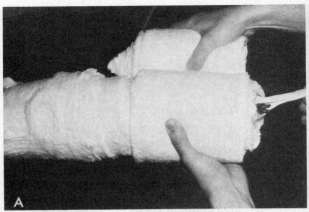
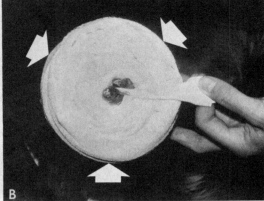

Figure 153–75. *A*, Cotton being wrapped up the limb on a Robert-Jones bandage. *B*, Cross-section of a Robert-Jones dressing. The compression applied by the tightly wrapped conforming gauze may be equally distributed through the bulk of the bandage.

dium-sized dogs usually require at least two one-pound rolls of cotton. Elastic (conforming) gauze is then wrapped around the cotton *as tightly as possible*. The gauze is begun at the distal portion of the limb and wrapped proximally. Because of the bulk of the cotton, the pressure exerted by the tightly wrapped gauze is distributed evenly to the limb surface and thus provides uniform compression and immobilization of the soft tissue, discouraging the development of swelling and edema (Fig. 153–75*B*). The tape stirrups are reflected back on the bandage and secured. As with the soft padded bandage, the toes are

left exposed for evaluation of circulation. The entire bandage (except the exposed toes) is wrapped with an elastic tape outer wrap or adhesive tape. When "thumped," a properly applied Robert-Jones bandage sounds like a ripe watermelon, owing to the compressive nature of the dressing.

The modified Robert-Jones bandage is essentially the same, except that cast padding is substituted for the cotton. This type of dressing is essentially a heavily padded soft padded bandage, and although it is effective in preventing and minimizing edema, it provides little or no immobilization for fractures.

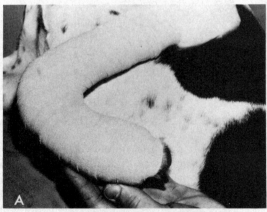
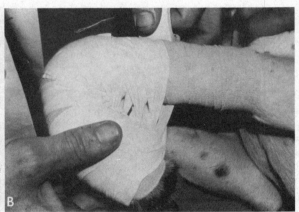
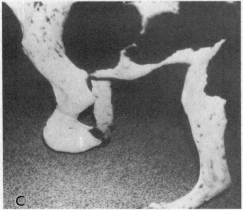

Figure 153–76. *A*, The carpus is maintained in flexion while the cast padding, conforming gauze, and outer wrap are applied. *B*, The figure-of-eight pattern of one-inch adhesive tape holds the carpus in flexion. *C*, The carpal flexion bandage prevents weight-bearing while allowing a full range of motion in the elbow and shoulder.

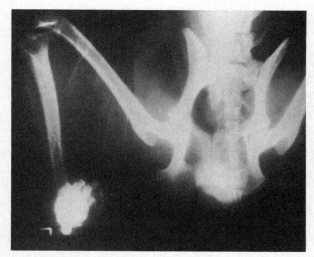

Figure 153–77. Radiograph showing how the Ehmer sling positions the femoral head in an abducted position, thus maximizing the coverage by the acetabulum.

Carpal Flexion Bandage

This bandage flexes the carpus (and relaxes the flexor tendons) and prevents weightbearing on the forelimb while permitting complete motion of the shoulder and elbow. The carpal flexion bandage is of value following repair of flexor tendon lacerations, in which relaxation of the tendon unit is desired and weightbearing is not allowed. This bandage can also be used following reconstructive surgery of the elbow, when joint motion without weightbearing may be desirable.

The carpus is flexed to the desired position and wrapped with two or three layers of cast padding. This padding should extend from the toes (which are left exposed) to the midshaft of the radius and ulna. A layer of conforming gauze is applied over the cast padding. It is important to remember to apply the cast padding and gauze to the limb with the carpus in the flexed position. To apply the dressing with the limb in a normal position and then flex the carpus results in bunching up of the material in the flexure crease of the carpus, with resulting compression and obstruction of the vasculature in that area. An outer wrap of elastic tape or adhesive tape is applied (Fig. 153–76A). One-inch adhesive tape is then applied in a figure-of-eight fashion from the metacarpus to the radius and ulna, spanning the flexed limb (Fig. 153–76B). This results in a series of cross-ties that hold the carpus in flexion. In this dressing, weightbearing on the forelimb is prevented but the shoulder and elbow are permitted free motion (Fig. 153–76C).

Ehmer Sling

The Ehmer sling prevents weightbearing by the pelvic limb. Because it also holds the hip in abduction

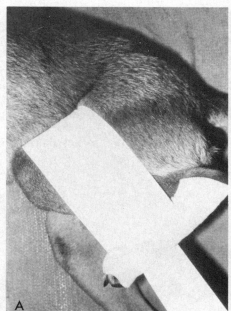

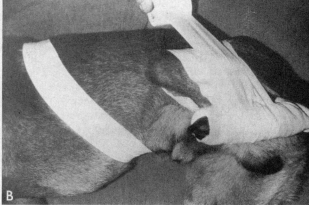

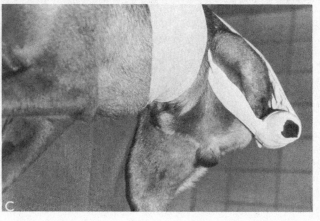

Figure 153–78. *A*, With the stifle and hock held in flexion, tape is passed around the flexed limb. *B*, To hold the limb in abduction, the tape is passed from the plantar surface of the metatarsus, over the lateral surface of the limb, and up over the dorsal midline. It is then passed around the cranial abdomen. Note that the tape is passed cranial to the prepuce in male dogs. *C*, The completed Ehmer sling holds the hip in abduction.

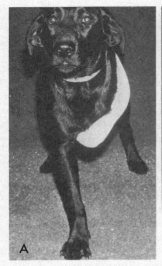
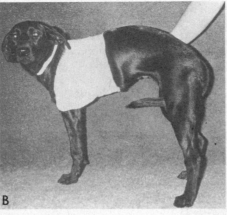

Figure 153–79. Cranial *(A)* and lateral *(B)* views of a dog with its forelimb in a Velpeau sling.

and internal rotation (a position that maximizes acetabular coverage of the femoral head), the sling is most commonly used after reduction of coxofemoral luxations (Fig. 153–77). The Ehmer sling may also be used to prevent weightbearing following open reduction of femoral head or neck fractures and acetabular fractures.

The metatarsal area is padded using cotton cast padding to prevent circulatory obstruction. With the stifle and hock hyperflexed, two- or three-inch adhesive tape is wrapped around the flexed limb (Fig. 153–78A). This wrap extends from the foot pad to the calcaneus. To place the limb in abduction, the tape is continued from the calcaneus across the lateral aspect of the limb and over the top of the lumbar spine, where it is held in place by a bellyband of circumferentially applied adhesive tape (Fig. 153–78B). (In male dogs it is important to avoid the prepuce when applying the bellyband.) When completed, the Ehmer sling holds the hip in an abducted position (Fig. 153–78C).

Velpeau Sling

The Velpeau sling prevents weightbearing on the thoracic limb. It is used for immobilization of the shoulder joint following surgery to correct shoulder luxation and of minimally displaced scapular fractures.

The limb is positioned so that the elbow is fully flexed and the carpus is touching the opposite shoulder. The limb is held in this position and wrapped to the trunk using elastic (conforming) gauze. The wrap may cross proximal to the carpus, allowing the paw to remain exposed, or may completely enclose the limb and paw with the carpus in full flexion and slight pronation. The gauze encircles the thorax, passing alternately in front of and behind the opposite thoracic limb (Fig. 153–79). The sling is completed by applying elastic tape in a similar manner.

Pelvic Limb Sling

The Ehmer sling is used to prevent weightbearing on the pelvic limb, but it also prohibits flexion and extension of the hip, stifle, and hock. The pelvic limb sling prohibits weightbearing but allows flexion and extension of these joints.[6] This is especially advantageous following a surgical procedure after which weightbearing is not desired but joint motion is permitted (Fig. 153–80).

A circular bellyband of two-inch adhesive tape is applied to the abdomen (caudal thorax in a male). The bellyband is approximately four inches wide and anchors the sling to the trunk. Next, a ten-foot strip of three-inch adhesive tape is doubled on itself, adhesive surfaces together. This results in a five-foot long, double-thickness piece of three-inch tape with no adhesive surface. The animal is placed in lateral recumbency and the tape is passed around the plantar surface of the metatarsus. With the limb in slight flexion (approximately 4 to 6 inches shorter than the

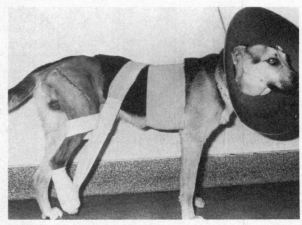

Figure 153–80. The pelvic limb sling prevents weight-bearing while allowing flexion and extension of the hip, stifle, and hock.

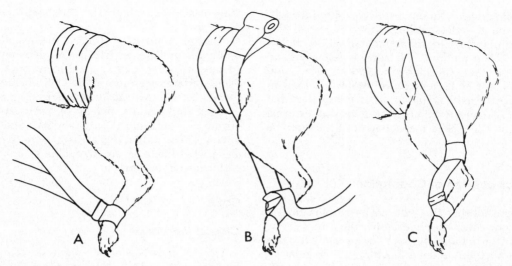

Figure 153–81. Application of the pelvic limb sling: *A*, With the bellyband in place, the double-thickness length of tape is placed around the plantar surface of the metatarsus. The tape is joined together on the dorsal surface of the metatarsus by a loop of tape. *B*, One end of the tape is passed medially to the limb and the other lateral to the limb. The limb is then flexed to make it six to eight inches shorter than the opposite limb, and the tape ends are incorporated into the bellyband by additional wraps of tape. *C*, The bandage is completed by taping the two arms of the sling together in back of the tibia, to prevent the limb from slipping out of the sling.

opposite limb), the two ends of the tape are passed, one each on the medial and lateral sides of the limb. The free ends of the tape are then passed over the dorsal aspect of the bellyband and secured with several wraps of adhesive tape. The free ends of the tape should be in a position to maintain the desired degree of limb flexion (Fig. 153–81). The two arms of the tape sling are taped together just above the dorsal surface of the metatarsus and just behind the midshaft area of the tibia, to prevent the tapes from slipping and to hold the sling in position.

EXTERNAL COAPTATION

Simple, closed, minimally displaced fractures of the long bones below the elbow and stifle are best suited for closed reduction and immobilization by external coaptation. Often, a highly comminuted, minimally displaced fracture of the radius/ulna or tibia that defies simple repair with internal fixation lends itself to immobilization with external coaptation (Fig. 153–82). External coaptation necessitates an understanding of the limitations and indications for

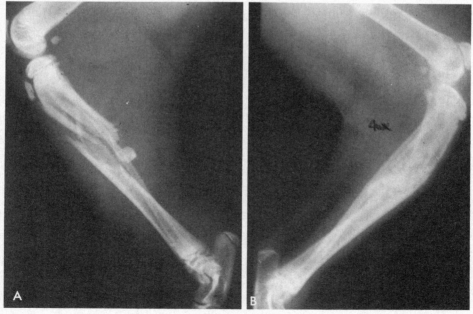

Figure 153–82. *A*, Preoperative radiograph of a severely comminuted tibial fracture in a cat. Note that the periosteal sleeve maintains the overall alignment of the fracture. Radiograph of same tibia four weeks after treatment by external coaptation (casting).

each specific device. No one rule can apply throughout, but a sound understanding of the basic principles allows one to adjust to almost any situation. It has been said, "The method of fixation is not nearly as important as the philosophy behind its use," and nowhere is this statement more applicable than in the use of external coaptation. It is paramount that some special considerations in the use of external coaptation in the closed management of fractures be examined.

Mechanics of External Coaptation

When considering the external immobilization of fractures, one must closely examine the forces acting upon a fracture. Basically, four forces can act alone or in combination upon a fracture: (1) angular or bending forces, (2) torsional or rotational forces, (3) compressive forces, and (4) tension or distractive forces (Fig. 153–83).

The effect of external coaptation on these forces must be considered before immobilization is attempted.

Angular or bending forces are readily neutralized by proper application of most rigid splints and casts by supporting the proximal and distal fracture segments and maintaining their proper alignment.

Torsional or *rotational forces* are never completely neutralized by external coaptation but are sufficiently overcome by immobilization of the joint above and below the fracture site. (Note: This is extremely difficult to achieve in fractures of the femur and humerus; see "Modified Spica Splint.")

Compressive forces are difficult to neutralize with external coaptation because they act in the longitudinal axis of the bone. The effect of these forces on the fracture site depends on the nature of the fracture (i.e., compressive forces on a transverse fracture are

more easily controlled than those on a long oblique fracture).

Tension or *distractive forces* are usually resultant to muscle pull (e.g., triceps on olecranon, gastrocnemius on tuber calcis, quadriceps on tibial tuberosity) and are therefore difficult if not impossible to overcome with external coaptation.

Casts and splints, when properly applied, can effectively neutralize only angular and rotational forces. These limitations are important when considering what fractures are amenable to immobilization with external coaptation.

Casts

Closed Reduction

The use of casts is usually limited to easily reduced fractures of the radius/ulna and tibia. The limited soft tissue covering of these bones makes reduction by closed manipulation possible. Closed reduction should always be carried out under general anesthesia, to allow relaxation of muscle forces and permit reduction to be carried out with as little trauma to the surrounding tissues and as little discomfort to the patient as possible. By observing two radiographs taken at right angles, one can determine the three-dimensional position of the fracture segments and reduce the fracture by using simple mechanics rather than applying brute force. Once it has been determined that the fracture can be reduced and held immobilized by external coaptation, a cast can be applied.

Cast Materials

Several materials are available for cast and splint construction. These range from the more traditional plaster of Paris to the newer thermo-moldable plastics

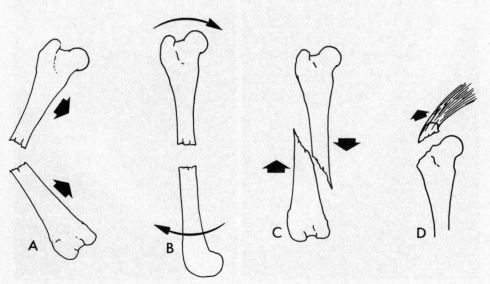

Figure 153–83. Schematic drawing of the forces that may act on a fracture: *A*, angular or bending; *B*, torsional or rotational; *C*, compressive; *D*, tension or distraction.

and polyurethane resins. These latter materials have the advantage of being light yet strong.

Plaster of Paris is a solid crystalline mineral, gypsum (calcium sulfate dihydrate), that is pulverized and heated to remove the water of crystallization. When water is added to the material, the process is reversed and the material hardens in an exothermic reaction. The time from when water is added to the material until the material becomes hard is known as the setting time. This time is affected by several factors: (1) the type of plaster used—fast-setting plaster usually requires five to eight minutes to set, whereas the extra-fast-setting plaster usually sets in about two to four minutes; (2) the temperature of the water—the warmer the water, the shorter the setting time; and (3) the amount of water left in the roll—obviously, the more water left in the roll, the longer the evaporation (and setting) time.

Thermo-moldable plastics usually require heating in a water bath to 160 to 170° F. The material then becomes pliable and is used like plaster of Paris.[5]

The polyurethane resins use cold water to initiate an exothermic chemical reaction that solidifies the material. This material is very light and strong.

Application of a Long-Leg Cast[1, 2, 3]

With the animal under general anesthesia and in lateral recumbency, strips of adhesive tape are applied to the medial and lateral (or anterior and posterior) aspects of the limb (Fig. 153–84A). These anchor the cast to the limb and discourage distal slippage of the cast. A stockinette is rolled up over the limb and held by an assistant at either end (Fig. 153–84B). Maintaining traction on each end of the stockinette allows the fracture to be supported and reduction maintained while the cast is being applied. Cast padding is applied to the limb, starting at the toes and progressing proximally, overlapping half the width of material with each turn (Fig. 153–84C). Although it is important to pad the pressure points such as the condyles and the olecranon or tuber calcis, excess cast padding is avoided. Excessive padding permits motion within the cast and may actually result in ulceration from movement of a loose cast on a pressure point. Also, secure conformation of the plaster to the limb may be prevented with an overly padded cast. In general, one layer of 50 per cent overlapped cast padding is sufficient. (Note: In obese animals this layer may be omitted and the cast applied directly over the stockinette.) Once the cast padding is in place, the plaster of Paris is applied to the limb. Beginning at the end of the second and fifth digits, leaving the end of the second and all of the third phalanges of the third and fourth digits exposed, the plaster of Paris is rolled up the limb, overlapping half the width on each turn. The plaster is applied firmly to the limb and at tapering parts of the limb. The turns are made to lie evenly by taking

small tucks and smoothing them into position. Above the elbow and the stifle, the plaster roll is pulled tightly to prevent a loose cast in this conical area of the limb (Fig. 153–84D). The heavy musculature on this area prevents compression of the underlying vasculature, and every effort should be made to maintain a compact cylindrical form in this area. The cast should be applied as high as possible on the femur or humerus (at least midshaft), and care should be taken to avoid undue discomfort due to pressure of the cast on the axillary or groin area.

The amount of cast material used varies with the size of the animal. One should apply only enough plaster to keep the fracture reduced while maintaining a strong and comfortable cast. This objective is easily accomplished in smaller animals, but large dogs require a cast that is strong enough to stand up to daily activities but not so bulky as to hinder mobility. This can be accomplished by adding plaster splints to the cast (Fig. 153–84E). After the first roll of plaster is applied, plaster splints are applied to the anterior and posterior aspects of the cast. Several of these splints may be folded in two to provide extra strength without added bulk.

Another roll of plaster is then applied, again starting at the toes, very firmly around the limb, molding each turn securely and blending it with the layers beneath (Fig. 153–84F). Constant smoothing and pressing movements are essential to blend all layers. In large dogs, a third layer of plaster may be rolled on for additional strength, although one should keep in mind that sufficient strength in the absence of additional weight is the ultimate goal.

During the application of the cast, it is important that every effort be made to apply the material evenly to avoid areas of constriction, which may structurally weaken the cast or cause vascular compression. The cast, when wet, should be supported only with the flat of the hand.

While the cast is setting, additional molding with wet hands may be done to adjust and align the cast (Fig. 153–84G). These corrections can only be minor, because excessive manipulations may disrupt the fracture site or compromise the soft tissues. The limb should be held in the desired position until the cast has sufficiently set.

After the plaster has become firm, the stockinette on each end of the cast is folded back over the cast for a distance of approximately two inches and cut. The tape stirrups are folded back over the cuffed stockinette and secured to the cast with a layer of plaster (Fig. 153–84H). The stockinette cuff on the proximal aspect of the cast is likewise secured.

The animal is observed for the 24 hours that the plaster takes to set completely (Fig. 153–84I). Also, discomfort from a cast that is too tight, irritates the axilla or groin, or is too loose can readily be detected the next day, and appropriate steps can be taken before the animal is sent home.

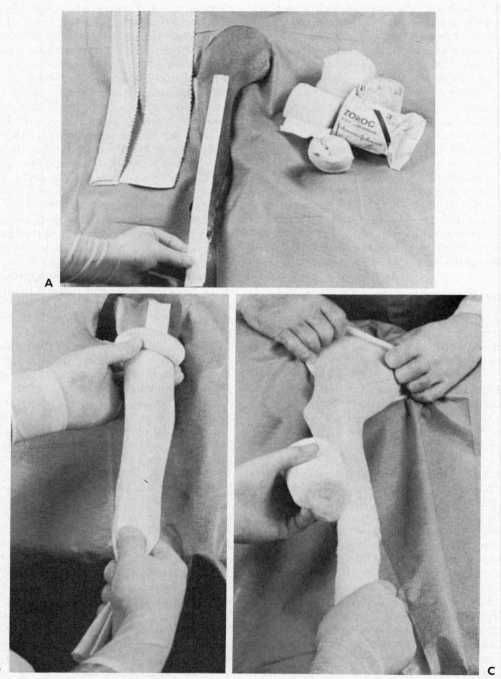

Figure 153–84. *A*, The forelimb of a dog with the tape stirrups in place. Note the plaster splints on the left and the stockinette, cast padding, and rolled plaster ready on the right. *B*, The stockinette is rolled up over the limb. *C*, The stretched stockinette holds the limb in normal position while the cast padding is applied.

Illustration continued on the opposite page

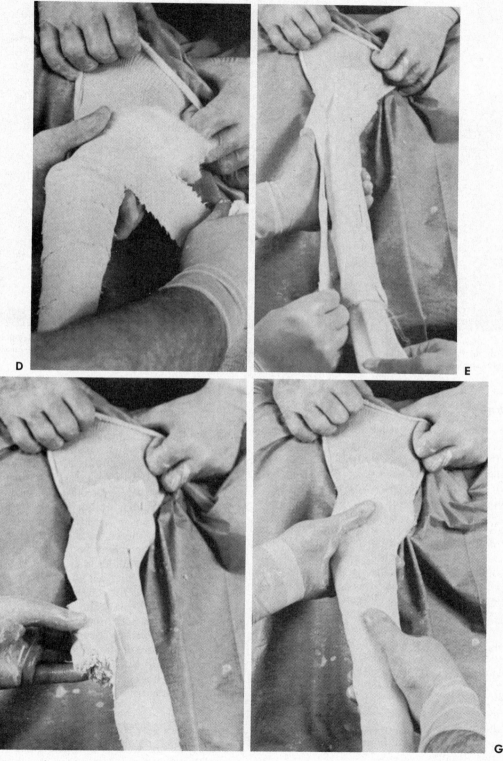

Figure 153–84 Continued. D, The plaster roll is applied firmly, especially above the elbow or stifle. *E*, Application of the plaster splints is effected anteriorly and posteriorly to provide extra strength along the stress lines but with less bulk. *F*, The second roll of plaster is applied to bind the splints firmly to the first layer of plaster. *G*, The cast is molded to the limb with wet hands while holding the limb in the desired position of reduction and function.

Illustration continued on the following page

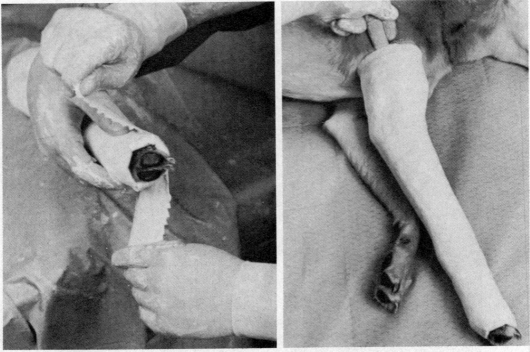

Figure 153–84 Continued. H, A plaster strip incorporates the tape and stockinette to the cast distally. *I,* Note the smooth surface of the finished cast, the high, tight fit of the cast proximally, and the amount of toe protruding distally. (Reprinted with permission from Hohn, R. B.: Principles and application of plaster casts. Vet. Clin. North Am. 5:291, 1975.)

Cast Management

The cast on an outpatient should be checked every two to three weeks (sooner in a young animal, which may outgrow the cast in that period). Palpation of the exposed toes gives some idea of the circulation of the limb. Swollen, cold toes signify vascular interference and should alert the clinician or owner to problems with the cast.

If a cast becomes too loose from muscle atrophy or reduction of edema, it should be replaced, as should a broken cast. Animals that chew excessively at one or more points on a cast usually do so because it is uncomfortable or perhaps has loosened enough to cause motion and subsequent ulceration. Such a cast should be removed and a new cast applied.

Periodic radiographic examination, first at two weeks postoperatively and then every three to four weeks, should be done to ensure that normal healing is progressing. A properly applied plaster cast should have an even thickness of the cast from end to end and should conform closely to the limb.

Except for circulatory or other soft tissue problems or external mutilation or breakage, the cast should not be removed until the fracture is shown to be healed by radiographs.

Walking Casts

Although long-leg casts are excellent for the immobilization of certain fractures of the radius/ulna and tibia, their design prohibits joint motion of the elbow or stifle, thus limiting or hampering walking. The walking cast allows motion of the elbow or stifle while providing some coaptation. The disadvantage of this cast is the inability to limit rotational forces on the radius or tibia because it doesn't immobilize the elbow or stifle. Thus, immobilization of greenstick fractures of the distal radius/ulna or tibia and fractures of the metacarpus or metatarsus, as well as temporary stabilization of the carpus and tarsus, can be accomplished with a walking cast.

The cast is applied in a manner similar to that described for a long-leg cast. However, the cast is not taken above the elbow or stifle, but rather is stopped at the level of the proximal radius or tibia to permit unrestricted motion of the joint. With close conformation of the cast to the limb, proper support and stability are maintained in the axial direction of the radius and tibia but rotational forces are free to act on the bone. For this reason, the cast is best suited for fractures of the metacarpus or metatarsus.

Special Considerations

Soft Tissue Injury. A cast should not be placed over an area of soft tissue damage, because the cast would hide the area from view. Making a window in the cast may alleviate this problem but structurally weakens the cast and is therefore less desirable. Also, a windowed cast may allow herniation of edematous tissue. Limbs with severe edema and open or infected wounds are best treated with a Robert-Jones dressing or Schroeder-Thomas splint. A cast may be applied when the infection or edema is under control.

Age. Casts in young growing animals may have to be changed to accommodate growth. Casts in younger animals should be checked weekly.

Client Communications. Daily checking of toes for swelling and general cast care is one of the most important considerations in the use of external coaptation. The owner should be instructed to keep the cast clean and dry at all times and to observe for signs of cast slippage, odor, or discomfort. Nothing is more frustrating than the return of the client with his or her pet's cast in hand or with an animal whose toes have been swollen in the cast for the past week because the owner "wasn't instructed" in cast care.

Splints

Lateral Splints

Lateral splints provide support and protection from angular or bending forces. Indications for a lateral splint include the immobilization of greenstick or nondisplaced fractures of the radius/ulna or tibia in very young animals; as an adjunct to internal fixation of the radius/ulna or tibia (the combined use of internal and external fixation is not advocated, but some instances arise in which internal fixation alone is not sufficient for adequate immobilization); and the immobilization of joints following reconstructive surgery (e.g., following ligament or tendon repair).

The animal is placed in lateral recumbency, and a

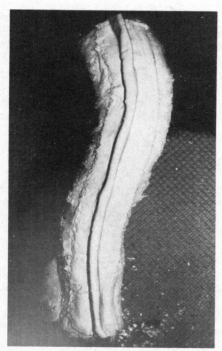

Figure 153–85. Lateral splint on a rear limb. A plaster "spine" has been added to strengthen the splint without adding additional bulk.

soft padded bandage is placed on the limb (see earlier description). Following the application of the elastic (conforming) gauze, splint material (plaster of Paris or one of the other cast materials) is placed on the lateral aspect of the limb. The plaster should extend from just below the top of the cast padding to the exposed phalanges of the digits. The thickness of the plaster depends on the size of the animal. The splint can be made structurally stronger by adding a "spine" of folded plaster splint and covering it with an additional layer of plaster (Fig. 153–85). In large dogs, an aluminum rod may be incorporated into the splint to add strength. The plaster is then molded to the contours of the limb. Again, it is important to place the limb in a functional position when this is done. The plaster of Paris is left to dry, and another layer of elastic gauze is used to firmly attach the splint to the padded bandage. The tape stirrups are reflected back on the dressing, and the entire splint is wrapped in an elastic tape outer wrap. It is important to be sure the plaster is dry before this is done; otherwise the excess water will not evaporate and the splint will never completely harden. As in cast application, the animal should be observed for 24 hours to check for swollen toes, slippage, or discomfort.

Modified Spica Splint[1]

The modified spica splint is a modification of a lateral splint that extends from the toes up over the shoulder or hip and applies immobilization to the shoulder, elbow, and carpus of the forelimb or the hip, stifle, and tarsus of the hindlimb. It therefore neutralizes bending and, to a degree, rotational forces in the femur or humerus as well as the other long bones of the extremity. Because the heavy musculature of the upper forelimb and thigh prevents as "rigid" a coaptation as is possible in the distal limb, the spica splint is indicated only as an interim fixation device in treatment of fractures of the femur and humerus. It can also be used as an adjunct to internal fixation of the femur or humerus and, in very young animals, as primary fixation of nondisplaced or greenstick fractures of the femur or humerus.

Tape stirrups and cast padding are applied in a manner similar to that described for the lateral splint. At the midshaft of the humerus or femur, the padding is continued up over the shoulder or hip joint and around the trunk of the animal in a continuous figure-of-eight pattern (Fig. 153–86A). As the cast padding passes over the shoulder or hip joint it forms a V pattern. This crossing V pattern resembles that in an ear of wheat, from the name of which the Latin word "spica" is derived. Several layers of cast padding are used to provide both support and protection from pressure sores over this area. An excessive amount of padding is contraindicated, and six to eight layers are usually enough. Lengths of plaster (or other material) are measured from the level of the toes to just beyond the dorsal midline and applied to the dressing. Again, the amount of plaster used depends

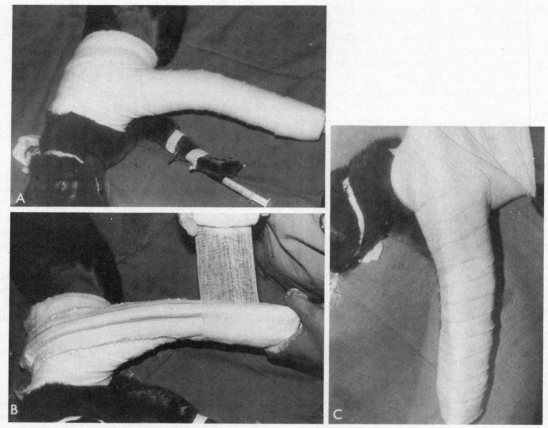

Figure 153–86. *A,* Cast padding applied to the limb and trunk. Note the "V" pattern of the padding over the shoulder. *B,* The plaster splint is wrapped to the limb and trunk using conforming gauze. Note the "spine" in the plaster to add strength. *C,* The completed splint immobilizes the shoulder, elbow, and carpus.

on the size of the animal and a plaster "spine" or aluminum rod can be incorporated into the splint to strengthen the structure. The plaster is permitted to dry, and the splint is firmly attached to the body with elastic (conforming) gauze (Fig. 153–86*B*). The gauze is wrapped around the trunk of the animal to attach the upper portion of the splint to the body. In over-the-hip spica in male dogs, care must be taken to avoid incorporation of the prepuce in the bandage. In these patients the gauze and cast padding are directed more cranially to encircle the cranial abdomen or caudal thorax. The tape stirrups are reflected back on the dressing, and elastic or adhesive tape is used to cover the splint (Fig. 153–86*C*). If it is properly applied, elevation of the splint in a laterally recumbent animal should rotate the entire fore or hind quarter and trunk of the animal as a unit.

Metal Rod Splints

Metal rod splints are similar in use and concept to the lateral splints previously described. They have the advantage of being light and are particularly useful in small animals or animals with multiple limb injury.

The affected limb is placed in a soft padded bandage, as described previously. Prior to covering the

bandage with an outer wrap, aluminum rods are placed on the anterior, posterior, and lateral aspects of the limb (Fig. 153–87*A*). These aluminum rods extend the length of the dressing and are bent to conform to the normal angulation of the limb (Fig. 153–87*B*). They are attached to the soft padded bandage by strips of tape, and the entire dressing is covered with an elastic tape outer wrap or adhesive tape.

Spoon Splints

Spoon splints are commonly used for fractures of the metacarpus, metatarsus, digits, and carpus and for nondisplaced or greenstick fractures of the distal radius and ulna in young dogs.

Aluminum or foam-padded plastic spoon splints are commercially available, or splints may be constructed from cast material (Fig. 153–88). A soft padded bandage is first applied to the limb. Enough cast padding should be applied to allow a firm fit of the spoon splint to the padded bandage. In the forelimb, the spoon splint should extend from the foot pad to the elbow, to provide uniform support to the distal limb. The splint is attached to the soft padded bandage by a layer of conforming gauze, and the tape stirrups of the soft padded bandage are reflected back and

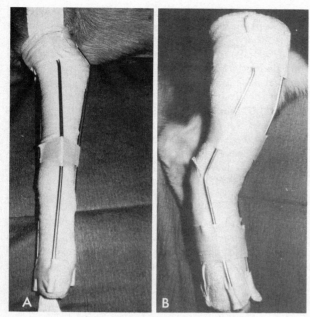

Figure 153–87. *A,* Aluminum rods placed on the anterior, posterior, and lateral aspect of the soft padded bandage. *B,* The aluminum rods are easily bent to conform to the normal angulation of the limb.

secured to the dressing. An outer wrap of elastic tape or adhesive tape is used to cover the dressing.

In the rear limb the padded bandage and splint should extend to the tuber calcis. Thus, in the rear limb, the spoon splint is applicable only to the closed treatment of metatarsal or digital fractures. As in all dressings, the toes are left exposed.

Schroeder-Thomas (Traction) Splints

The Schroeder-Thomas splint is a traction splint modified for use in animals by the adjustment of the configuration to conform to the shape of the animal's limb, on the basis of the location of the fracture.[4] A degree of reduction is possible using the Schroeder-Thomas splint because considerable traction is applied on the joints. Accurate and continued fixation of bone fragments results when the splint is applied properly.

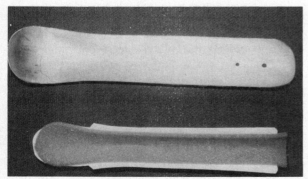

Figure 153–88. Spoon splints are fashioned from aluminum or plastic.

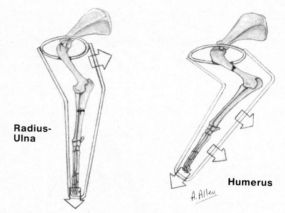

Figure 153–89. Configurations for fractures of the forelimb. (Reprinted with permission from Knecht, C. D.: Principles and application of traction and coaptation splints. Vet. Clin. North Am. 5:177, 1975.)

The materials needed for the construction of the splint include aluminum splint rods, combine roll (a laminated gauze-cotton-gauze roll), and adhesive tape. The aluminum splint rod is available in six-foot lengths with diameters of 1/8, 3/16, and 3/8 inch. A set of wooden ring blocks and a vice are useful in shaping the splints. Aluminum rods may be cut to length with bolt cutters or sawed with a hacksaw.

Although the Schroeder-Thomas splint consists of a padded elliptical ring and angled rods that join distally, the exact shape depends on the bone fractured. Tensions are applied to separate the joints at each end of the bone. The splint, as constructed for fractures of the radius and ulna, should be nearly straight, whereas a 90-degree angle is recommended for repair of the humerus (Fig. 153–89). Tension in the correct direction allows the fractured fragments to be separated and aligned. In the rear limb, the caudal aluminum rod is straight except in luxations and fractures of the hock. The angle at the stifle in

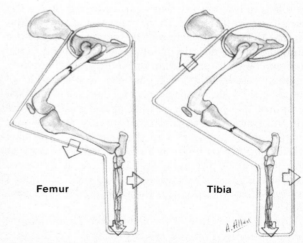

Figure 153–90. Configuration for rear limb fractures. (Reprinted with permission from Knecht, C. D.: Principles and application of traction and coaptation splints. Vet. Clin. North Am. 5:177, 1975.)

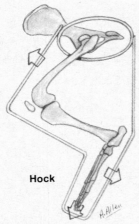

Hock

Figure 153–91. Modification for fracture-dislocation of the hock. (Reprinted with permission from Knecht, C. D.: Principles and application of traction and coaptation splints. Vet. Clin. North Am. 5:177, 1975.)

femoral fractures is placed ventral to the stifle, so that tension may be applied on the tibia, lessening overriding in the fractured femoral fragments (Fig. 153–90). For tibial fractures, the angle at the stifle is more proximal, permitting tension to be applied on the femur to distract the overriding fragments of the tibia. In fracture-luxation of the hock, the distal ends of both the cranial and caudal rods are bent forward in approximately the normal angle of walking (Fig. 153–91). This arrangement is necessary to prevent excessive extension of the hock should ankylosis occur. Splints structured in the latter conformation are not as strong as those built in the standard configuration and must be additionally supported.

The elliptical ring at the top of the splint closely approximates the size of the limb at the body. An excessively large ring permits slippage and accumulation of debris in the splint; too small a ring causes edema. Rubber rings made to fit the ring block are useful in determining proper size (Fig. 153–92A). Once structured, the ring is elongated from front to back and narrowed from top to bottom. It is bent medially on its ventral aspect to protrude under the standing animal. In addition, the entire ring is tilted so that the ventral portion of the ring rests under the animal and the dorsal portion is slightly lateral to the animal. This tilting, in addition to the ventral bending medially, helps the ring conform to the angle of departure of the limb from the body. The animal supports its weight by resting the sternum on the ventral ring in the forelimb and slightly ventrolateral to the pelvic symphysis in the rear limb. The ring itself is lightly padded because of excess pressure at the junction of the limb and the body if excessive padding is used. The padding is covered with neatly wound adhesive tape, as is the exposed dorsal unpadded ring.

Proper application of the Schroeder-Thomas splint requires tension on the joints proximal and distal to the fracture. Combine roll is excellent for this purpose because it is soft and has sufficient strength to allow tension without necrosis. Gauze or tape cannot be applied under similar tension without binding.

For either limb, the aluminum rod is structured and padded before the vertical rods are bent. The vertical rods are bent so that moderate to full extension of the limb is achieved when the foot is touched to the bottom of the splint rod. Adhesive tape is applied to the cranial and caudal surfaces of the foot and fixed with a spiral tape. The tape is joined distal to the foot and cut longitudinally. The lateral tape is placed medial to the distal splint rod and fixed with tape, and the medial half of the tape is rolled lateral to the rod and fixed with tape. The foot is rotated inward rather than outward.

Combine roll is placed on the limb and tightened in the nonfractured segments (Fig. 153–92B). In general, a single piece is placed at the distal end of either the front or rear limb first. In the forelimb, it may be cut, preplaced, and tightened as appropriate. A fracture of the humerus would be prepared by preplacing combine roll and then tightening the roll that encircles the radius and ulna from the foot to the elbow. Similarly, fractures of the radius and ulna would be repaired by fixation of the foot, preplacement of combine roll, tightening the roll that rests around the humerus, and finally, tightening the roll around the radius and ulna. In fracture of the tibia, the combine roll that encircles the femur is tightened following attachment of the foot; the reverse is true with fractures of the femur. The combine roll that covers the fractured bone is fixed under minimal tension, with the primary purposes of reducing lateral motion and maintaining even pressure on the limb.

A proper Schroeder-Thomas splint consists of more than a few pieces of tape and an aluminum rod. The finished splint is covered with adhesive tape, carefully and smoothly. Where angles are turned, a small flap of tape may be left and cut and the ends overlapped. A neat, completely covered, and smooth splint improves the attitude of the owner toward splint care (Fig. 153–92C). An aluminum stirrup distal to the end of the splint is essential to prevent wear and possible tearing of the distal tape.

Good aftercare is essential for the Schroeder-Thomas splint. The splint must be kept dry and clean. The underside of the ring must be checked daily and powdered with talc. When the animal is discharged, the owner should be instructed in splint care and made aware of potential complications.

Schroeder-Thomas splints adequately immobilize fractures of the radius and ulna and the middle and distal thirds of the humerus (provided that the fractures are minimally displaced and easily held in accurate reduction). In the rear limb, fractures of the tibia, except those involving the most proximal or distal aspects, are most often treatable with Schroeder-Thomas splints. The splint is also useful in the interim fixation of compound fractures to maintain alignment while the soft tissues are being treated.

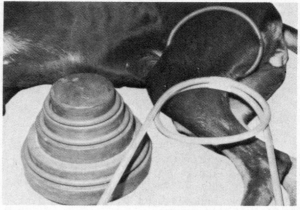

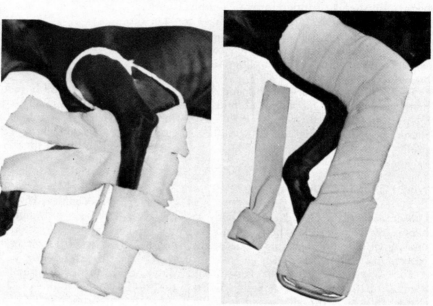

Figure 153–92. A, An elliptical ring is made to fit the limb. *B*, The nonfractured bones are placed under tension. *C*, Finished splint with aluminum stirrup. (Reprinted with permission from Knecht, C. D.: Principles and application of traction and coaptation splints. Vet. Clin. North Am. 5:177, 1975.)

1. Arnoczky, S. P., and Stoll, S. G.: External coaptation. *In: Proceedings, 46th Annual Meeting, American Animal Hospital Association,* 1979.
2. Hohn, R. B., Rosen, H., Bianco, A. J., and Jenny, J.: The principles and methods of application of plaster of Paris, modified Robert Jones dressing, and plastic coaptation splints. *In: Scientific Presentations and Seminar Synopses, 36th Annual Meeting, American Animal Hospital Association,* 1969.
3. Hohn, R. B.: Principles and application of plaster casts. Vet. Clin. North Am. 5:291, 1975.
4. Knecht, C. D.: Principles and application of traction and coaptation splints. Vet. Clin. North Am. 5:177, 1975.
5. Piermattei, D. L.: Hexcelite—a new cast material. *In: Scientific Proceedings, 45th Annual Meeting, American Animal Hospital Association,* 1978.
6. Robinson, G. W., and McCoy, L.: A pelvic sling for dogs. *In* Bojrab, M. J. (ed.): *Current Techniques in Small Animal Surgery.* Lea & Febiger, Philadelphia, 1975.

Wires in Long Bone Fracture Repair

William D. Liska

HISTORICAL ASPECT

The use of wire in fracture repair dates back to the advent of open reduction and internal fixation. Understanding and effective use of wires generally lagged behind the progress of orthopedic surgery until the last 10 to 15 years. Warnings that cerclage wires lead to delayed union and nonunion were published.[16]

Rhinelander, a human orthopedic surgeon and

researcher, kindled new interest in the use of wires in the 1960s. Using dogs, he examined the physiological response of bone to fractures. Using microradioangiography, he described bone healing with wires and other implants and showed that wires should be an effective fixation device.[17, 18, 19] The Association for the Study of Internal Fixation (ASIF) concurrently described bone healing and primary bone union following open reduction and rigid internal fixation. This group used plates and screws as their primary implants, but intramedullary devices and tension band wires were also used.[15]

Reports of successful clinical use of full cerclage wires began in 1975.[9] The proper use of tension band wires has also been described.[3, 8] Objective data have been published to support previous clinical impressions about such factors as variation of tension on wire applied by different instruments and surgeons,[20, 21] the effect of wire on the strength of cortical bone,[6] and the effect of twisting, bending, and cutting on wires.[20, 21]

The number of failures that occur should be minimal, and potential for failure should be recognized on postoperative radiographs. If failure occurs, the reason is usually violations of specific principles of use.

WIRE FOR IMPLANTATION

Metal implants placed in the body are put to a harsh test. They must be corrosion-resistant and biocompatible and must have adequate strength to withstand functional stress.

The American Society for Testing and Materials Standard F138, commonly called 316L Stainless Steel (Table 153–2), is the alloy used in orthopedic wire. Corrosion of the metal implants occurs because of the electrochemical activity of ions in body fluid. High-carbon steel corrodes rapidly. Lowering carbon content reduces the amount of corrosion. The low carbon content plus formation of an alloy of the iron with other metals such as chromium, nickel, and

TABLE 153–3. Conversion of Surgical Wire Sizes

Suture Material Size	Gauge	Size in Inches	Size in Millimeters
6-0	40	.0031	.079
6-0	38	.0040	.102
5-0	35	.0056	.142
4-0	34	.0063	.160
4-0	32	.0080	.203
3-0	30	.0100	.254
2-0	28	.0126	.320
0	26	.0159	.404
1	25	.0174	.455
2	24	.0201	.511
3	23	.0226	.574
4	22	.0254	.643
5	20	.0320	.813
7	18	.0403	1.016
—	16	.0492	1.25

molybdenum results in a highly corrosion-resistant substance. To further decrease corrosion, the surfaces are thoroughly cleaned and treated with a corrosion-resistant film. Scratching, marring, and excessive bending of the wire during implantation will increase the susceptibility to corrosion.[14]

The combination of chromium, nickel, and molybdenum (as in 316L Stainless Steel) provides superior mechanical strength and corrosion resistance. Chromium and molybdenum are hard metals that are highly corrosion-resistant and have good strength. Nickel decreases tensile strength but also decreases the tendency of the alloy to harden and become brittle with bending. Proportionately higher percentages of nickel also allow for the addition of more chromium and molybdenum with their desirable properties. The alloy cannot be magnetized.[2, 14]

Wire is available in a wide variety of diameters and lengths (Table 153–3). Wire most commonly used in veterinary orthopedics is 0.8 mm to 1.25 mm in diameter. Smaller diameter wire does not consistently withstand stress at the fracture site. Larger diameter wire is difficult to work with, especially in placing knots.

INSTRUMENTS OF APPLICATION

Only a few special instruments are necessary for using wire in fracture repair (Table 153–4). Wires are rarely used as the sole implant for internal fixation. Because intramedullary pins or Kirschner wires are commonly used, a Jacob's handchuck with extension and key plus an assortment of Steinmann pins and Kirschner wires are required.

Wires must be tight to maintain reduction with rigid internal fixation. The final amount of tension on the wire is greatly influenced by the instrument used to apply the tension and the type of knot (Fig. 153–93). Assuming that the same type of wire is applied with the same instrument, there is little

TABLE 153–2. Chemical Composition of Stainless Steel Bar and Wire for Surgical Implants (American Society for Testing and Materials)

Element	Composition (%)
Carbon	0.030 maximum
Manganese	2.00 maximum
Phosphorus	0.025 maximum
Sulfur	0.010 maximum
Silicon	0.75 maximum
Chromium	17.00 to 19.00
Nickel	12.00 to 14.00
Molybdenum	2.00 to 3.00
Nitrogen	0.10 maximum
Copper	0.50 maximum
Iron	Balance

TABLE 153–4. Instruments and Devices Available for Handling Wires in Fracture Repair

Trade Name	Manufacturer	Knot Type
Swiss Osteo	Richards Manufacturing Co., Inc., Memphis, TN	Loop
ASIF	Richards Manufacturing Co., Inc., Memphis, TN	Loop
Rhinelander	Richards Manufacturing Co., Inc., Memphis, TN	Twist
Richards	Richards Manufacturing Co., Inc., Memphis, TN	Twist
Bowen	Bowen and Co., Inc., Rockville, MD	Twist
Vise Grip	Peterson Manufacturing, Dewitt, NB	Twist
Pliers	Numerous manufacturers	Twist

difference in the tension created by different surgeons.

Data are available that compare the final tension produced on wire by various instruments.[20, 21] The loop-type knot instruments are superior. The initial mean tension the twist-type instruments create is about 60 per cent or less of that created by loop instruments, which provide a mechanical advantage with their two-step maneuver in applying the wire, i.e., the instrument pulls the wire tight first and then maintains the tension while the wire is bent 180 degrees back on itself. In contrast, with the twist-type instruments, except for the Rhinelander, the two maneuvers of creating tension and twisting are done simultaneously, giving less mechanical advantage. It is also technically more difficult to tighten and twist, and to avoid wobbling the knot in different planes. Wobbling should be avoided because it may lead to a weakening of the wire at the base of the twist.

Twisted knots must still be cut and bent over to minimize soft tissue irritation. Both cutting and bending result in significant loss of tension (32 to 70 per cent). With loop knots, cutting off excess wire does not result in tension loss. No bending is necessary because the wire is close to the bone. The final result is that twist-type instruments apply wires with about 40 per cent of the tension of wires applied with loop instruments.[20, 21] Less tension on twist knots is lost if the knot is bent over while the final twist is applied, but bending potentially weakens the wire.

If maximum tension is desired, e.g., full cerclages compressing fractures, a loop knot should be used. In most clinical situations when tension band wires, antirotation figure-of-eight wires, and hemicerclages are used, either loop knots or twist knots can be used.

BONE HEALING IN THE PRESENCE OF WIRE IMPLANTS

Adequate blood supply and fracture stabilization are essential for bone healing. Each may be compromised, but both must be present for consistently successful fracture repair. Delayed union results if reestablishment of blood supply is slower than normal or if fracture stabilization is not rigid. Nonunion occurs if the blood supply to a healing fracture does not reestablish itself or if fracture stabilization is inadequate. The reasons for delayed union and nonunion are discussed later.

Blood is supplied to normal long bones from three major sources, the afferent vascular system, the efferent vascular system, and the intermediate vascular system to cortical bone.[4, 10, 17, 18, 19] The *afferent vascular system* has three sources, as seen in Figure 153–94.

1. The nutrient artery enters the nutrient foramen of the diaphysis.

2. The metaphyseal arteries enter through ligamentous attachments in the ends of the bone. These arteries eventually anastomose with the nutrient artery proximally and distally via the medullary arteriole supply. The medullary arteriole system is the major blood supply to the diaphyseal cortex.

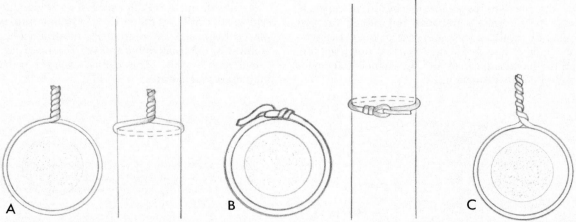

Figure 153–93. Twist (A) and loop (B) wire knots. In twist knots, the wires twist on each other. An incorrect twist knot (C) slips more easily because one wire twists around the other.

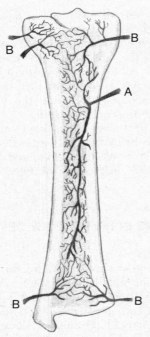

Figure 153–94. The afferent vascular system to bone has 3 sources. The nutrient artery *(A)* and the metaphyseal arteries *(B)* anastomose. Periosteal arterioles (not shown) enter via fascial attachments to supply the periosteum.

3. The periosteal arterioles enter through fascial attachments to supply the external third of the cortex. The periosteal vasculature is important during growth because it supplies the periosteal osteogenic layer for appositional growth. At maturity, the periosteal osteogenic layer atrophies as do the blood vessels. This system is reactivated when a bone is injured.

The *efferent vascular system* is a centrifugal one in a normal mature bone, i.e., blood flows from medullary canal to periosteum. The medullary contents are drained by large emissary veins that traverse the cortex and by vena comitans when a nutrient foramen is present. The metaphysis is drained by metaphyseal veins. The cortex is drained by cortical venous channels from its inner layers and by periosteal capillaries superficially.

The *intermediate vascular system* of cortical bone is not a true capillary network but rather vascular channels of capillary size coursing through the haversian canals. The links that convey nutrients between the haversian canals and the lacunar osteocytes are called cortical canaliculi.

The medullary arteriole system has an endosteal capillary pressure of 60 mm Hg. The periosteal capillary pressure is 15 mm Hg. Therefore, blood flow in the cortex is centrifugal. Rhinelander and Brookes have separately demonstrated microangioradiographically this unidirectional centrifugal flow from medullary canal through cortex.[4, 17, 18, 19] Blood does not flow longitudinally in the cortex for more than one or two millimeters in the haversian canals. When blood flow from the cortex is disrupted at the periosteum, as by periosteal stripping or a metal implant, normal blood flow through the cortex from the medullary vessels is also disrupted.

When a fracture is present, the blood supply to healing bone hypertrophies. There is active proliferation of both the medullary and the extraosseus vasculature. If the fracture is not displaced, the medullary arteries dominate, with active proliferation during the first week. If the fracture is displaced and is not rigidly repaired, the periosteal vasculature is important in early healing. Blood flow reverses and is centripetal to the outer third of the cortex. However, within three weeks, the medullary vasculature is reestablished and again becomes the major blood supply. If the displaced fracture is rigidly repaired, the medullary supply rapidly bridges the fracture and remains the primary cortical blood supply. Vessels course through the cortex to the periosteal osseus callus, where they are arranged perpendicular to the cortex.[17, 19, 25] Figure 153–95 illustrates the angiographic appearance of healing bone.

Following rigid fixation, a normal course of predictable events occurs. The periosteal vessels supply the external callus during the first three weeks. During this time, the central hematoma is organized and resolved while capillaries bud across the fracture gap. Increased cortical porosity allowing for increased cortical blood supply from the medullary vessels is also evident within three weeks. After this time, the medullary vasculature is the primary blood supply to both the internal and the external callus. It completely overshadows the periosteal vasculature. After about 20 weeks, the fracture should be healed and the blood supply returns to normal.[17, 19]

If callus forms it is either periosteal bridging callus, endosteal bridging callus (the first to unite in displaced fractures), or intercortical uniting callus. The amount of external callus reflects the need for additional stabilization. The callus enlarges only with increased vasculature.

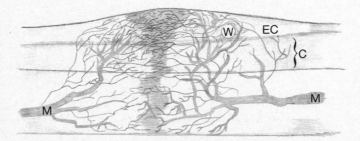

Figure 153–95. Medullary vessels *(M)* penetrate the cortex *(C)* and supply blood to the external callus *(EC)*. The vasculature will be unimpeded by the presence of a wire *(W)* tight on the cortex.

Wires have minimum contact with bone. They do not significantly interfere with the afferent, efferent, or intermediate vascular systems or with callus formation. They do not strangle bone or blood supply for several reasons:

1. External callus vessels originating from medullary vessels are directed perpendicular to the cortex and are unaffected by wires.

2. There are no consistent longitudinal periosteal arterioles that either may be strangled or are important for fracture healing. Capillaries in the periosteum rapidly grow around, and are unaffected by, the wires.

3. Extraosseous arterioles from fascial and muscle attachments enter bone perpendicularly to the cortex. Wires do not affect these arterioles.

4. The haversian system, which does run longitudinally, is in cortical bone and is not compressed by the wires. The longitudinal blood flow in the haversian system is not more than one or two millimeters.

Parham-Martin bone bands, with their wide surfaces, are different from wire loops.[1] They obstruct blood flow out of the cortex they contact. The 360-degree zone of cortical bone necrosis under the bands may lead to long-term complications, and their use is not recommended.

Other accompanying implants, such as intramedullary pins, are often used with wires in fracture repair. The effect these other implants have on blood supply to healing bone must also be considered. Intramedullary pins do not entirely fill the medullary canal. When the pin is placed, the medullary vasculature is temporarily disrupted but quickly reestablishes itself. The cortical vasculature is not affected. On the contrary, if intramedullary reaming is performed or an oversized intramedullary pin is used, blood flow from the medullary vessels into the cortex is adversely affected. Only the outer third of the cortex receives blood from periosteal vessels.

GENERAL INDICATIONS

Wire is used in fracture repair to neutralize forces along a fracture line so that healing can consistently progress to union. Figure 153–96 illustrates the forces involved: shearing, rotational, bending, and distraction. These forces are neutralized with varying efficiency, depending on the wire configuration used. The fracture must be carefully evaluated and the proper configuration chosen for that particular fracture. Because wires are usually used with another implant, such as an intramedullary pin, the pins and wires should be used to greatest mechanical advantage for additive effect. For example, a long oblique midshaft tibia fracture in a 20-kg dog is repaired with an intramedullary pin and four full-cerclage wires. The pin primarily neutralizes bending forces but has a minor effect on rotation and shear. The full-cerclage wires by themselves should not be relied on to neutralize bending forces. However, they have a

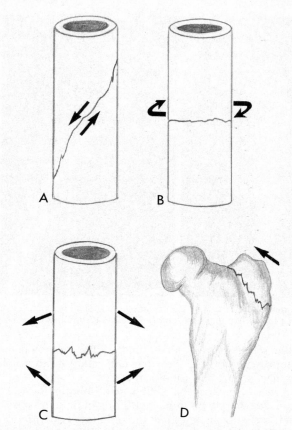

Figure 153–96. The arrows indicate the direction of the forces to be neutralized along fracture lines. The forces are those of shear (*A*), rotation (*B*), bending (*C*), and distraction (*D*).

major antirotation and antishear effect. Together, the pin and wires provide rigid internal fixation.

Wires can complement pins not only by helping neutralize forces but also by adding compressive forces. To accomplish this, a compressive load is applied to the fracture by wires placed under tension. In the preceding example the full-cerclage wires must be tight to compress all surfaces of the fracture. The tension-band wire is used to convert distracting forces (at an apophysis in this case) into compressive forces.

FULL-CERCLAGE WIRES

Indications

Full-cerclage wires are wire loops that pass 360 degrees around diaphyseal bone. The indications are limited. They are used in conjunction with other implants, primarily intramedullary pins, and are used most successfully on long cylindrical bones such as the femur (Fig. 153–97), tibia, and humerus. Their use in other bones is exceptional. The metaphyseal ends of the bone generally have irregular cross-sections or conical diameters that are not conducive to full-cerclage wiring. Full cerclages are not indicated in or near joints.[5, 7, 9, 12, 13, 23, 24] Properly applied

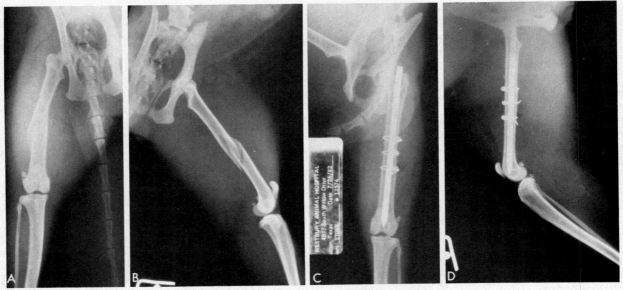

Figure 153–97. A and *B,* Two views of a long oblique femur fracture in a cat. The fracture was repaired using an intramedullary pin and three full cerclage wires. *C* and *D,* Postoperative radiographs show an anatomical reduction with rigid internal fixation.

full-cerclage wires serve four major functions—compression of the fracture and neutralization of angular, shear, and rotational forces.

A fracture must be sufficiently oblique for full-cerclage wires to be indicated. Long oblique or spiral fractures with the length of the obliquity two or more times the diameter of the diaphyseal shaft of the bone are candidates for cerclage fixation (Fig. 153–98). Full-cerclage wires are used to repair comminuted fractures only if every fracture and comminuted piece is anatomically reduced.

There are two other less commonly used circumstances in which full-cerclage wires are indicated. They can be used to hold fissures in the major proximal or distal segment (Fig. 153–99). They can also be used to hold a solitary comminuted piece of less than 90 degrees of the circumferences of the bone in a transverse irregular fracture (Fig. 153–100).

When a full-cerclage wire is used for fissures, the circumference of the bone is held intact in a barrel-stay fashion. In the second circumstance, the comminuted piece cannot move as long as the intramedullary device and wire remain in place.

Technique

Two methods exist for applying full-cerclage wires. The wires are generally passed around the bone after the reduction is complete. The knots are usually tied before the intramedullary pin is driven past the fracture and seated in the metaphysis.

One method involves the twist knot applied with wire twisters. The wire loop is tightened and the knot twisted simultaneously. The knot is bent over to the bone, and excess wire is cut off.

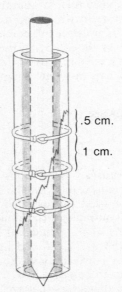

.5 cm.

1 cm.

Figure 153–98. This long oblique fracture is repaired with three full-cerclage wires.

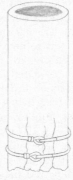

Figure 153–99. Full-cerclage wires are used to hold fissures in a barrel-stay fashion.

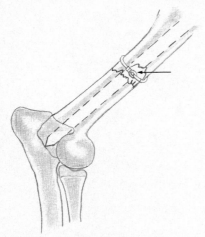

Figure 153–100. Occasionally, a narrow comminuted piece *(arrow)* will be present. It can be held in place with full-cerclage wires.

The second and preferred method of full-cerclage wire application uses a loop-knot applicator (Fig. 153–101). A wire with a preformed eye on one end is passed around the bone. The free end is passed through the eye, up the conical section of the wire applicator, and through the hole in the wire applicator crank. The wire loop is tightened with the crank. When the wire is tight, it is bent back 180 degrees on itself. The initial bending maneuver of 90 degrees or more is started with the loop under full tension. The crank is then loosened slightly to allow about one centimeter of wire to protrude from the tip of the conical portion of the applicator. The bend is completed by laying the wire 180 degrees back on

itself. Excess wire one centimeter beyond the bend is removed.

Basic Principles

Wire passers should be used to place the wire around the bone. They help prevent periosteal and fascial stripping and thus maintain blood supply. If the periosteum has not been stripped by the injury, the wire should lie directly on the periosteum. Fascia, muscle, vessels, and nerves must not be trapped between wires and bone.

Adequately strong wire that will not break because of stresses at the fracture should be used to ensure prolonged rigid fixation. The 0.8- to 1.2-mm wires are adequate for most canine and feline fractures. If orthopedic wire is used, 16- to 20-gauge wire should be used. Smaller diameter wire is too weak, often breaks, and can lead to undesirable results. Because suture material does not remain taut around the bone and does not have sufficient strength to resist the forces at a fracture, fine stainless steel suture wires are not adequate for full cerclage.

Each full-cerclage wire should go around the circumference of the bone at each cerclage site only once. If the wire goes around the bone at each site more than once, periosteal vessels and fascial attachments may be injured. In addition, the doubled or multiple loops cannot be tightened properly because of crossing, and looseness then results in instability.

Full-cerclage wires should take the shortest possible course around the circumference of the bone, directly perpendicular to the long axis (see Fig. 153–98). When cerclages are not perpendicular to a

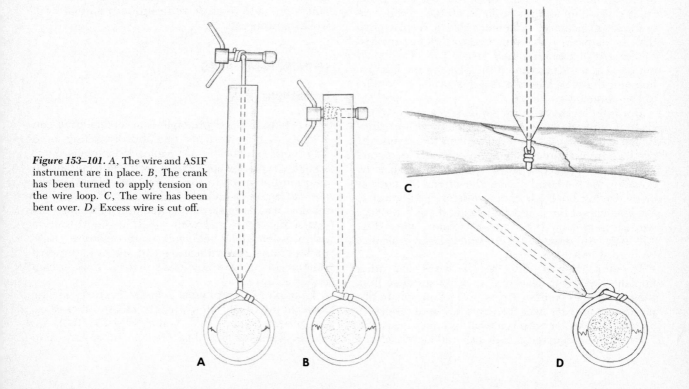

Figure 153–101. *A*, The wire and ASIF instrument are in place. *B*, The crank has been turned to apply tension on the wire loop. *C*, The wire has been bent over. *D*, Excess wire is cut off.

A   B   C   D

tubular piece of bone, a slight amount of slippage due to motion at the fracture site can result in decreased tension on the wire. Loop-knot full-cerclage wires are easier to apply perpendicular to the long axis of the bone. The twisting during tightening that occurs with twist-knot full-cerclage wires makes their perpendicular placement more difficult.

First the wire loop should be tightened and then the knot secured as a second maneuver. Only the loop-knot instruments and the Rhinelander wire twister perform this procedure properly so that maximum tension is left on the wires. As previously discussed, the cerclage loses tension when excess wire is cut from twist knots. Bending the free ends of the twist knot to avoid soft tissue irritation results in additional loss of tension. For these reasons, it is difficult to apply an optimum cerclage on long bone fractures with wire twisters.

A sufficient number of full-cerclage wires should be used. One of the greatest errors in full-cerclage fixation is using an inadequate number of loops. Cerclages are placed five millimeters from the proximal and distal tip of the obliquity (see Fig. 153–98). If the cerclage is too far from the tip of the fragment, it may act as a fulcrum for movement and may not neutralize shearing forces along the fracture.

The wires should be placed about one centimeter apart regardless of how many wires are required (see Fig. 153–98), to ensure adequate fixation. At least two full cerclages should always be used on long oblique or spiral fractures. The tension should be the same on all wire loops in a multiple-cerclage system, to distribute forces equally without overburdening one or two wires.

No portion of the wire loop should lie within a fracture line, i.e., no wire should lie within a plane created by the outermost limit of the cortex. An example of incorrect placement is a wire placed so that its course is traversing a cortical defect created by the loss of a comminuted piece. The wire should not lie near a fracture line if the plane of the fracture line and the wire loop are parallel or nearly parallel to each other.

If a full-cerclage wire is applied to a bone whose shaft is conical (e.g., proximal femur or proximal humerus), precautions must be taken to prevent the cerclage from slipping down the conical section and loosening. Slippage can be prevented either by notching the bone and placing the wire in the notches or by driving small Kirschner wires perpendicular to the long axis of the bone and placing the full-cerclage wire just proximal to the Kirschner wire (Fig. 153–102). An autogenous cancellous bone graft may be used if indicated.

In adult animals, full-cerclage wires and other implants are left in place unless problems arise from their presence. Neither stress protection nor predisposition to fracture near the wires has been observed. Special devices for wire removal[11] are not necessary.

Removing full-cerclage wires should be considered

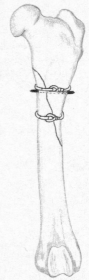

Figure 153–102. A Kirschner wire has been placed through a conical section of bone. The full-cerclage wire has been placed adjacent and just proximal to the Kirschner wire.

two to six weeks postoperatively in young animals with remaining radial appositional bone growth. If cerclages are not removed, they become encased in cortical bone and are retrievable with great difficulty. The disadvantages of a second operation for wire removal prior to total union of the fracture usually outweigh the advantages of removing the wires. Research indicates that cerclage wires on normal immature canine diaphyseal bone cause cortical bone thickening and increased weight. The bones initially become stiffer and fracture with less torsional, shear, and angular deformity than normal bones. The wired bone's strength tends to return toward normal by 12 weeks postoperatively.[6]

TENSION BAND WIRES

Indications

The tension band principle is an engineering concept used to convert bending and distracting forces into compression. This mechanical principle is ideally suited to repairing apophyseal, or traction epiphyseal, avulsion fractures. In such a fracture, pieces of bone are distracted by muscles, tendons, or ligaments. A tension band repair of the fracture neutralizes the distracting forces and with weightbearing results in compression along segments of the fracture. Early postoperative weightbearing and fracture compression are highly desirable goals that the tension band repair achieves.[3, 15]

Examples of apophyseal avulsion fractures include those of the tibial tuberosity, olecranon, tuber calcis, greater trochanter of the femur (Fig. 153–103), medial malleolus of the tibia, scapular tuberosity, acro-

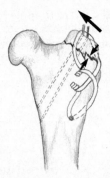

Figure 153–103. A tension band wire used to repair a fractured greater trochanter of the femur. Distracting forces in the direction of the gluteal muscle pull *(large arrow)* are neutralized. Compression is created by the wire along the fracture line *(small arrows).*

mion, greater tubercle of the humerus, and tuber ischii. Osteotomies of these structures, e.g., transolecranon approach to the elbow joint, are also indications for this repair method. The tension band principle may also be applied to transverse patellar fractures.

Technique

Even though tension band wires are applied in various locations, only minor technical variations exist from one fracture to another. After routine exposure of the fracture, the following procedure is used.

1. A hole is drilled transversely in the cortex on the diaphyseal side of the fracture. The hole is located as far from the fracture, or up to twice as far from the fracture, as the fracture is from the tip of the apophysis.

2. A wire that has been previously twisted to form a loop in its middle is passed through the hole.

3. The fracture is reduced anatomically.

4. One or two pins are placed across the fracture, starting at the tip of the apophysis and ending with the tips anchored in the diaphyseal side of the fracture. The pins are parallel to each other and approximately perpendicular to the fracture.

5. The wire is passed around the exposed ends of the pins adjacent to bone. The tension band wire should be touching bone and pins to avoid soft tissue entrapment. The wire is bent in a figure-of-eight with the preformed loop on one side and free ends of wire for twisting on the other side.

6. The wire is put under tension by interchangeably tightening the knots on both sides of the figure-of-eight wire.

7. The wire twists are cut and bent so as to avoid irritation of the soft tissues and skin.

8. The pins are bent slightly in the direction of the distracting force and cut short just beyond this bend.

Loop knots can be used in place of twist knots. If loop knots are used, two separate wires with preformed eyes form the figure-of-eight. One wire initially lies adjacent to bone and pin(s). The other is passed through the hole drilled in the diaphyseal cortex. The wires are bent to form the figure-of-eight, and a loop knot is tightened on both sides of the figure-of-eight. It is advisable to have two loop-knot wire tighteners so the knots can be placed under tension equally and simultaneously.

The advantages of loop over twist knots in tension band wires are ease of application and greater tension on the wires. The disadvantages include the need for two wire tighteners and a lower tensile force required for knot failure. The latter problem can be avoided by using large diameter wire to overpower the distracting forces at the fracture site.

Tension band repair for patellar fractures differs from that placed on apophyses. A small hole is drilled in the proximal and distal patella. A wire is passed through the holes and the free ends are twisted. The exposed wire lies on the anterior surface of the patella. Flexion of the patella results in compression of the fracture.

Basic Principles

Heavy (16- to 20-gauge) wire is most commonly used. If small fragments are involved, 22-gauge wire is satisfactory. A 0.062-inch Kirschner wire is a pin size commonly used.

Two pins provide optimum rotational stability at the fracture. If the fracture fragment is small, e.g., a medial malleolus fracture, one pin is adequate.

The knots on a tension band wire should be placed under equal tension. The temptation to tie only the free ends of the wire on one side of the figure-of-eight is to be avoided. If the wire is not tightened on both sides of the figure-of-eight, equal tension is not achieved and compression will not be equally distributed along the fracture line.

The tension band wire must be touching bone and pin on the apophyseal side of the figure-of-eight. If the wire is not touching both bone and pin, soft tissue is interposed between either the wire and the pin or bone and the pin. In either case, the wire can loosen as it passes through tendon, muscle, or ligament.

The tips of the pins must be anchored in cortical bone. If they are left in the medullary canal or in cancellous bone, migration may occur.

External support of the limb is necessary only to protect the soft tissues and the incision. Application of a soft padded bandage until suture removal is adequate. Early limited use of the leg is allowed.

Removal of the tension band in adult dogs is not necessary unless problems such as metal migration arise. In immature animals, the device compresses the physeal plate through which this type of fracture frequently occurs. Premature closure can occur, so early removal of the tension band wire should be considered. If reavulsion is a possibility, the pins can be left in longer.

FIGURE-OF-EIGHT ANTIROTATION WIRES

Indications

A figure-of-eight antirotation wire is applied with an intramedullary device to neutralize rotational forces along transverse diaphyseal fractures (Fig. 153–104). The fracture is usually in the middle two-thirds of the femur, tibia, or humerus. This antirotation device appears similar to a figure-of-eight tension band wire.

The figure-of-eight wire stops rotation in both directions. This is an advantage over a single wire such as a hemi-cerclage. A figure-of-eight wire applied on the tension band surface also helps provide axial compression with weightbearing.

Technique

Several steps are involved in applying the figure-of-eight antirotation wire.

1. After the fracture is reduced, two holes are drilled through the bone, one above and one below the fracture. The holes are perpendicular to the long axis of the bone and preferably perpendicular to the tension band surface of the bone. The holes are one to three centimeters from the fracture, depending on the size of the bone, and are located midway between the tension band surface and the thickest diameter of the cortex.

2. A wire of appropriate size is passed through each hole. If loop knots are used, the preformed eyes are on the same side of the bone.

3. The intramedullary pin is driven past the fracture and seated in the metaphysis with the fracture reduced.

4. The wires are crossed to form the figure-of-eight. The wires are tightened and a knot is completed. Loop or twist knots can be used.

Basic Principles

Adequate strength wire (16- to 20-gauge) must be used. The wires should be tight and the knots secure.

The wires should cross each other at about a 90-degree angle (see Fig. 153–104). The angle is chosen as a compromise between two angles. The antirotation plane is parallel to, and the tension band plane approximately perpendicular to, a transverse fracture. The 45-degree angles that split these angles are the planes in which the wires lie.

It is better to use two wires and cross opposite free ends than to use one long wire. Manipulation of a single wire and placement of the knots in the desired final location is difficult because both ends of the wire are passed through bone. Also, when one wire is used, several bends are made in it, rendering it more fragile.

Figure-of-eight antirotation wires are indicated for transverse fractures only. If applied to oblique fractures, they may actually exaggerate shear forces and have little effect on stopping rotation. When a figure-of-eight wire is applied properly, early limited weightbearing is allowed.

HEMI-CERCLAGE

Indications

A hemi-cerclage wire is used to help neutralize rotational and shear forces along a transverse or short oblique fracture. A hemi-cerclage wire stops rotation effectively in only one direction. As its name implies, the wire courses through and partially encircles the bone (Fig. 153–105). Hemi-cerclage wires can be used very effectively on flat bones.[22]

Technique

Hemi-cerclage is used primarily in conjunction with an intramedullary pin. The following steps are used to place the wire:

1. Holes are drilled in the bone above and below the fracture.

2. A wire is passed through the holes.

3. The fracture is reduced and the pin is driven and seated. It makes no difference whether the wire does or does not encircle the intramedullary pin.

4. The wire is tightened and the knot secured. Loop or twist knots may be used.

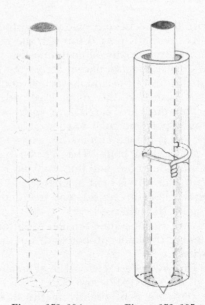

Figure 153–104   *Figure 153–105*

Figure 153–104. A figure-of-eight antirotation wire applied to a transverse irregular fracture.

Figure 153–105. A hemi-cerclage wire can be applied to a transverse irregular or short oblique fracture.

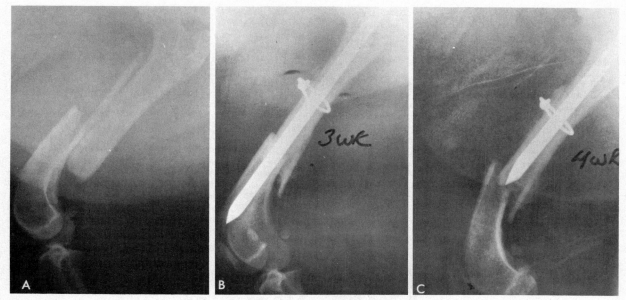

Figure 153–106. Violations of the principles of proper use of wire in fracture repair can lead to delayed unions and nonunions. A classical case of how complications arise is illustrated in preoperative *(A)* and three-week *(B)* and four-week *(C)* postoperative radiographs. An inadequate number *(1)* of cerclages was used to hold fissures and a long slender comminuted piece, the reduction was poor, and the fracture was a transverse irregular orientation with no antirotation device. The cerclage wire is not perpendicular to the long axis of the bone and can be expected to loosen or slip. The pin was originally driven too far (not shown) and was backed up. The pin was originally left protruding through the skin over the greater trochanter, the fracture became infected, and the patient was excessively active. The pin migrated out. All these factors led to failure. The full-cerclage wire was not the cause.

Basic Principles

As with other wires, large enough wire must be used and the wire must be tight. The other implant must be placed properly. When hemi-cerclage is used on transverse fractures, good interdigitation of the fracture ends with anatomical reduction is important. A figure-of-eight antirotation wire is a better device than a hemi-cerclage wire in most transverse fractures.

On short oblique fractures, a hemi-cerclage wire should be placed perpendicular to the fracture line. Shear and rotation forces are neutralized most effectively by a wire in this plane. Overtightening can result in opening of the fracture gap in the cortex on the side opposite the wire. If this occurs, it is best controlled by using two hemi-cerclage wires with knots on opposite sides of the bone.

COMPLICATIONS

Principal complications most commonly observed in one retrospective study of full-cerclage wiring in 60 cases were: insufficient number of cerclages (38 cases), faulty technique in applying the intramedullary pin (11 cases), full cerclages applied to transverse or short oblique fractures (seven cases), and loosely applied full cerclages (seven cases).[13] Of the nine delayed unions or nonunions that occurred, all had multiple principle violations. Of the four nonunions, all were vascular and involved fractures with four or more comminuted pieces. Repair of highly commi-

nuted fractures with pins and wires should be performed with utmost caution. Figure 153–106 illustrates a failed fracture repair using a wire, which did not cause the failure.

1. Annis, J. R.: The use of Parham-Martin bands in unstable fractures. Vet. Scope *17*:12, 1973.
2. Bechtol, C. O., Ferguson, A. B., and Laing, P. G.: *Metals and Engineering in Bone and Joint Surgery.* Williams & Wilkins Co., Baltimore, 1959.
3. Birchard, S. J., and Bright, R. M.: The tension band wire for fracture repair in the dog. Comp. Cont. Ed., *3*:37, 1981.
4. Brookes, M.: *The Blood Supply of Bone.* Butterworths, London, 1971.
5. Buhler, J.: Percutaneous cerclage of tibial fractures. Clin. Orthop. *105*:276, 1974.
6. Ellison, G. W., Piermattei, D. L., and Wells, M. K.: The effects of cerclage wiring on the immature canine diaphysis: a biomechanical analysis. Vet. Surg. *11*:44, 1982.
7. Gambardella, P. C.: Full cerclage wires for fixation of long bone fractures. Comp. Cont. Ed. 8:665, 1980.
8. Hauptman, J., and Butler, H. C.: Effect of osteotomy of the greater trochanter with tension band fixation on femoral conformation in beagle dogs. Vet. Surg. 8:13, 1979.
9. Hinko, P. J., and Rhinelander, F. W.: Effective use of cerclage in the treatment of long bone fractures in dogs. J. Am. Vet. Med. Assoc. 166:520, 1975.
10. Holden, C. E. A.: The role of blood supply to soft tissue in the healing of diaphyseal fractures. J. Bone Jt. Surg. 54A:993, 1972.
11. Johnson, R. A.: Fracture fixation by cerclage wiring utilizing cortical bone tacks and a pull-out tension device. J. Am. Anim. Hosp. Assoc. 13:105, 1977.
12. Liska, W. D.: The use of full cerclage wires in treating long bone fractures in dogs and cats (a retrospective study). Part I: Correct application of full cerclages and osteosynthesis with their use. Resident Paper, The Animal Medical Center, New York, 1976.

13. Liska, W. D.: The use of full cerclage wires in treating long bone fractures in dogs and cats (a retrospective study). Part II: Evaluation of clinical cases and discussion. Resident Paper, The Animal Medical Center, New York, 1976.
14. Medical metals. (Richards Publication No. 3922.) Richards Manufacturing Co., Inc., Memphis, 1980.
15. Muller, M. E., Allgower, M., and Willenegger, H.: *Manual of Internal Fixation.* Springer-Verlag, New York, 1970.
16. Newton, D. D., and Hohn, R. B.: Fracture nonunion resulting from cerclage appliances. J. Am. Vet. Med. Assoc. *165*:503, 1974.
17. Rhinelander, F. W.: The normal microcirculation of diaphyseal cortex and its response to fracture. J. Bone Jt. Surg. *50A*:784, 1968.
18. Rhinelander, F. W.: Circulation in bone. *In* Bourne, G. (ed.): *Biochemistry and Physiology of Bone.* Academic Press, New York, 1972.
19. Rhinelander, F. W.: Tibial blood supply in relation to fracture healing. Clin. Orthop. *105*:34, 1974.
20. Rooks, R. L., Tarrin, G. B., et al.: In vitro cerclage wiring analysis. Vet. Surg. *11*:39, 1982.
21. Rooks, R. L.: In vitro cerclage wiring analysis. Masters Thesis, University of Illinois, 1981.
22. Rudy, R. L.: Fractures of the maxilla and mandible. *In* Bojrab, M. J. (ed.): *Current Techniques in Small Animal Surgery.* Lea & Febiger, Philadelphia, 1975.
23. Withrow, S. J.: Use and misuse of full cerclage wires in fracture repair. Vet. Clin. North Am. 8:201, 1978.
24. Withrow, S. J., and Holmberg, D. L.: Use of full cerclage wires in the fixation of 18 consecutive long-bone fractures in small animals. J. Am. Anim. Hosp. Assoc. *6*:735, 1977.
25. Withrow, S. J.: Vascular and bone response to full cerclage wires. *In* Bojrab, M. J. (ed.): *Pathophysiology in Small Animal Surgery.* Lea & Febiger, Philadelphia, 1981.

Chapter **154**

Delayed Union and Nonunion

A. G. Binnington

The healing of a fracture has three end points: union, malunion, or nonunion. Delayed union, an intermediate stage, can proceed to union or nonunion depending on the skill and knowledge of the surgeon.

In delayed union healing is not completed in the normal time for a fracture of its type and location. The healing process has not stopped, as indicated by progressive callus formation and resorption of dead bone.

A nonunion is a fracture in which the apposed ends have failed to unite and all signs of repair have ceased. The healing that has occurred is variable, and it is highly unlikely that healing will take place without surgical intervention. However, a few slow-healing fractures may be judged as nonunion when in fact they are really delayed unions and will proceed slowly to fusion with sufficient time.

CLASSIFICATION

Weber and Čech classified nonunion fractures according to their biological reactions or osteogenic potentials.[20] They separated nonunions into two major categories: those capable of biological reaction, or viable, and those incapable of biological reaction, or nonviable.

The desired method of treatment of a nonunion is determined by the category into which it falls (Figs. 154–1 and 154–2).

Viable

1. The *hypertrophic* (or "elephant's foot") form of nonunion has an abundance of callus with a profusion of blood vessels (Fig. 154–3). The fracture gap remains owing to fibrocartilage in the space between the fragments. The usual cause is insufficient stabilization or premature weight-bearing.

2. The *slightly hypertrophic* ("horse hoof") is a milder form of hypertrophic nonunion with poor callus formation and a slight increase in density of

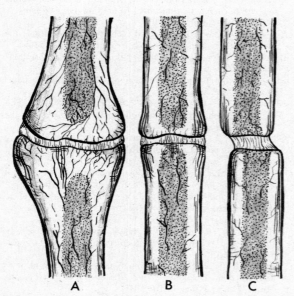

Figure 154–1. Weber and Čech classification of viable nonunion. *A,* Elephant's foot. *B,* Horse-hoof. *C,* Oligotrophic. (Reprinted with permission from Sumner-Smith, G.: *Bone in Clinical Orthopaedics.* W. B. Saunders, Philadelphia, 1982. Courtesy of Weber and Čech.)

A   B   C

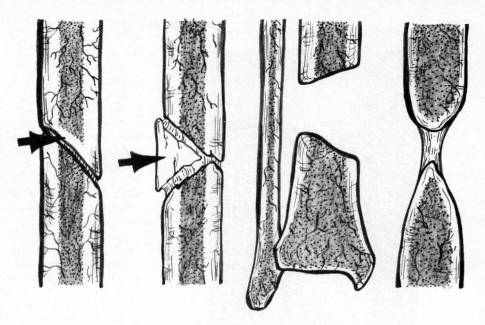

Figure 154–2. Weber and Čech classification of nonviable nonunion. *A*, Dystrophic. *B*, Necrotic. *C*, Defect. *D*, Atrophic. (Reprinted with permission from Sumner-Smith, G.: *Bone in Clinical Orthopaedics*. W. B. Saunders, Philadelphia, 1982. Courtesy of Weber and Čech.)

the fragment ends (Fig. 154–4). This form of nonunion is often the result of resorption beneath an orthopedic plate on an insufficiently stabilized fracture. With time and cycling the plate will fail unless sufficient callus forms to increase stability and allow eventual union.

3. *Oligotrophic* nonunion shows no evidence of callus; however, it is not atrophic as it is biologically still able to heal because the fragments are hypervascularized (Fig. 154–5). With time the ends round off, shorten, and decalcify through resorption. They may be joined by fibrous tissue. These fractures are usually the result of major displacement of the fracture

ends with too much extension or poor apposition or reduction of the fragments.

Nonviable

1. A *dystrophic* nonunion has an intermediate fragment with a comprised blood supply. The intermediate fragment has healed with one of the main fragments but not the other owing to interference

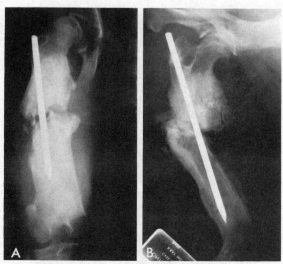

Figure 154–3. Lateral *(A)* and AP *(B)* radiographs of hypertrophic nonunion of two months duration due to inadequate alignment and stabilization of the fracture site. Note the subluxation of the coxofemoral joint in the AP view. At corrective surgery the pin was removed, sufficient tissue was excised to allow the fracture to mobilize and realign, and the site was placed under compression using a dynamic compression plate. Healing followed rapidly.

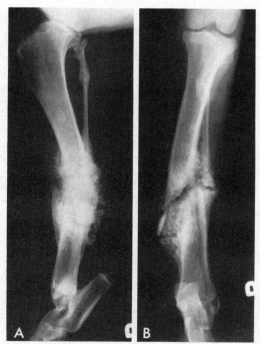

Figure 154–4. AP *(A)* and lateral *(B)* radiographs of slightly hypertrophic nonunion of the tibia and fibula due to inadequate stabilization and the presence of osteomyelitis. Note the presence of a sequestrum.

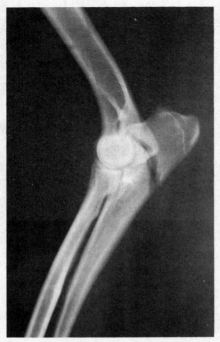

Figure 154–5. Oligotrophic nonunion of the olecranon, the fracture due to a direct blow to the area with a stick. The limb has been in a cast for 14 weeks. Healing followed the compression of the fracture site with a figure-of-eight tension band wire.

with its blood supply. The poorly vascularized fragment is incapable of sufficient osteogenesis in the face of instability to bridge the gap with the second major fragment. The major fragment may show callus formation, but the intermediate fragment does not.

2. A *necrotic* nonunion has numerous intermediate fragments, with some having insufficient blood supply to allow participation in callus formation. These fragments are often furthest from the main fragments and are more radiopaque than the surrounding fragments.

3. Nonunion of the *defect* occurs when a segment of bone is lost due to trauma, infection with subsequent sequestration, or the resection of neoplasms. The resultant gap between the bone ends is too great for bone bridging. Healing does not occur without surgical intervention.

4. *Atrophic* nonunion is the end result of one of the previously mentioned categories of nonviable nonunion (Fig. 154–6). Osteoporosis and muscular atrophy occur owing to inactivity of the limb. Finally, there is a loss of vascular supply to the fracture site with a subsequent loss of all osteogenic potential.

PATHOPHYSIOLOGY

Primary union of a fracture occurs when there is healing from fragment to fragment without a visible callus by both contact and gap healing. For this to occur, viable fracture fragments and stability are required. If insufficient stability is present, callus

forms in response to movement and provides increased stability, allowing the fracture to proceed to union. However, if the instability is greater than the ability of the callus to provide stability, a delayed union or nonunion may develop.[8]

If an adequate blood supply is available to the fracture site, fibrous tissue is laid down, and, with sufficient stability, this collagen acts as a scaffolding for osseous tissue development. With an inadequate blood supply cartilage is deposited at the fracture ends. With stability, a blood supply develops; capillaries invade the cartilage and chondroclasts remove the cartilage and allow osteons to form.[3]

The presence of callus is indicative of adequate blood supply to the fracture site.[8]

Any situation that leads to inadequate stability of the fracture ends and subsequent motion causes destruction of the delicate granulation tissue forming along with the invading capillary buds and developing osteocytes. If this continues delayed union occurs, and if instability persists a nonunion is the final outcome.

Delayed union is associated with slow osteogenic activity and, subsequently, prolonged healing time.[21] This may be due to instability as already noted or an inadequate blood supply failing to provide adequate mesenchymal cells and nutrients to the fracture site. The fracture site receives diaphyseal blood vessels from the nutrient artery via the medullary vessels as well as periosteal vessels. These may be damaged at the time of trauma and further compromised by various methods of fracture repair.

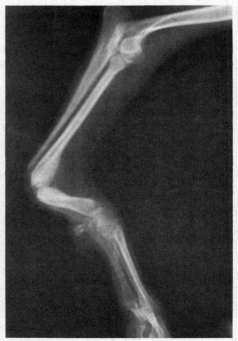

Figure 154–6. Atrophic nonunion of the radius and ulna of a three-year-old miniature poodle, five months post trauma. Note the disuse osteoporosis of the carpal bones, metacarpals, and phalanges. Union was not achieved despite bone grafting and plating attempts over a two-year period.

With delayed union there is an absence of sclerosis at the fracture ends. The fracture gap is filled with active granulation tissue and not scar tissue, and thus resorption of the bone ends occurs, leading to a widening of the fracture line with an ill-defined outline.[21]

ETIOLOGY

Normally fractured bones heal rapidly and become strong enough to permit functional use of the injured part shortly following the fracture. Therefore, those factors that are influential in producing a nonunion must become operational soon after injury. In many cases it is a combination of factors and not a single adverse condition that leads to nonunion.

A fundamental disturbance in the mesenchymal stem cell of certain individuals may lead to a failure to produce osteoblasts or chondroblasts in sufficient quantity for healing, and thus, a nonunion;[6] however, in the majority of cases it is a failure of the surgical repair and not of osteogenesis.[5]

Multiple forces act upon a fracture site; however, it is the rotational or torsional forces that are the primary cause of delayed union or nonunion, as they lead to tearing of the uniting fibroblastic network and developing capillary buds.[1, 5, 17] These forces come into play when there has been inadequate immobilization of the fracture fragments with a resultant instability at the fracture site.

Numerous authors[2, 3, 4, 6, 7, 9] have discussed factors that may contribute to nonunion or delayed union:[1, 8, 11, 17, 18, 21] inadequate reduction, interposition of soft tissue between fragment ends, comminution, distraction, bone loss, infection (primary or iatrogenic), inadequate immobilization time (too early weight-bearing and ambulation), ill-advised open surgery, loss of initial fracture hematoma due to surgical interference, stripping of the periosteum, reaction to metallic implants, improper use of cerclage wire, too much implanted material, osteoporosis, neoplasia, starvation, radiation, steroids, antimetabolic drugs, metabolic or nutritional disturbances, senile changes, anticoagulant drugs, hyperemia, ischemia, loss of soft tissue attachment to fragments, disuse of limb, and compression of fracture hematoma by unpadded cast. This last condition is more common where the bones are small and the soft tissue covering sparse, such as at the distal radius, ulna, tibia, fibular area of toy and small breeds of dogs.[5]

Delayed union and nonunion have been reported in a small number of human patients suffering from hyperparathyroidism. Healing rapidly followed excision of a parathyroid adenoma.[9]

DIAGNOSIS

The most common location for delayed and nonunion fractures (60 per cent) is the distal radius and ulna of small dogs.[5, 16] This is probably due to the difficulty in overcoming rotational and angular instabilities at this site. The next most common sites are the tibia and the femoral shaft (25 and 15 per cent, respectively).[16] Nonunions do occur; however, they are rare in the cat.

An animal suffering from a delayed union may exhibit pain and instability at the fracture site and may be reluctant to bear weight on the limb.[5, 8, 11] There may be evidence of muscular atrophy due to disuse.

The history provides the necessary time to allow an assessment of the rate of healing. Young animals may completely heal in four weeks, but animals over one year of age require at least eight weeks for healing to occur. Epiphyseal and metaphyseal areas heal more rapidly because of their high percentage of cancellous bone. Smaller bones usually heal faster than larger bones, with the exception of the metacarpal and metatarsal bones. In cats little callus formation may be seen with fractures of these bones for up to 16 weeks.[1]

Delayed union is usually diagnosed radiographically as there is no definite way of determining this clinically. Radiographically the fracture line is present, although it has usually widened and appears as a cavity with ragged or irregular edges.[11] There may be evidence of a nonbridging callus; however, the marrow cavities are still open. Adjacent bone shows no significant sclerosis.

The clinical signs of nonunion are similar to those of delayed union. In a longstanding nonunion, gross instability and possibly a deformity with progressive bowing or deviation may be present. Some weight-bearing may occur on a partially functioning limb owing to development of a pseudoarthrosis. At this point there is usually no pain at the fracture site.[5, 8, 11, 17]

A diagnosis of nonunion should not be made until at least two months after trauma and should be based on serial radiographs that show a cessation of healing. Radiographically the fracture gap remains and the medullary cavity is sealed off adjacent to the fracture site. The fracture ends may appear sclerotic due to an overproduction of well-vascularized bone rather than dead bone.[15] A well-developed but nonbridging callus may be present, and osteomalacia may be evident above and below the fracture area. If the nonunion is nonviable, little or no evidence of callus is present.[5, 8, 11, 17]

Osteomedullography is the intraosseous injection of contrast media to examine blood circulation within bone. This technique can be used in the diagnosis of delayed union and nonunion. Circulation across the fracture gap is evidence of healing, and noncrossing is evidence of delayed union or nonunion. Contrast media (3 to 5 ml of 45% meglumine amidotizoate) is injected into the distal fragment using a sternal puncture needle with the animal under general anesthesia. The soft tissue surrounding the fracture site is compressed and radiographs are taken at one-second intervals for five seconds following injection of the dye.

The dog should show a positive osteomedullograph (flow of contrast across the fracture gap) by three weeks post fracture. If there is no evidence of healing by four weeks, either clinically or on plain radiographs, osteomedullography is warranted. If the results are positive, continuation of the current therapy is appropriate. However, if the results are negative surgical intervention should be considered.[12]

TREATMENT

The treatment of delayed union implies that this condition was diagnosed before it had proceeded to nonunion. In most instances the treatment is directed toward continued or increased stabilization for a longer period. The animal's movements should be restricted until healing occurs.[1, 5, 21] Increased stabilization might take the form of bone grafting, removal and replacement of a loose implant, or the addition of supplemented support such as hemicerclage wiring or the use of half-pin splintage to stop rotational instability in conjunction with intramedullary pinning. If internal fixation has been used, the addition of external support, or vice versa, should be considered.

The animal should be carefully examined to differentiate between delayed union and nonunion, but once a diagnosis of nonunion is made, there is no advantage to any further delay. An aggressive approach to correcting the nonunion should be taken, as failure rate increases with successive operations. Each case should be considered and its own treatment regimen determined, taking into consideration present clinical and radiographic signs, past history (including postoperative management), and previous attempts at correction.

Consideration should be given to leaving a painless pseudoarthrosis if it is functionally acceptable. If monetary restraints preclude proper treatment, an amputation to salvage the animal or euthanasia, in certain circumstances, may be the action of choice.

With nonunion the bone fragments will not unite until some surgical interference occurs, as each bone fragment is already healed, although not to its neighbors. Early treatment is best, as soft tissue complications such as muscular atrophy and tendon contraction increase with time.[11]

A very conservative approach is the drilling of multiple small holes in the sclerosed fracture ends of an ununited fracture in good alignment. A new hematoma is formed with the bone decalcified by the traumatic hyperemia. With luck a bridging callus will be stimulated to form.[11]

In most cases, a more aggressive approach gives more consistent results. The use of bone plates, with or without bone grafting, affords rigid fixation and allows early but controlled ambulation during the healing period. This helps stimulate bone healing and maintains joint function and the surrounding soft tissues more satisfactorily.

In certain instances external fixation, such as with a Kirschner apparatus, may be the method of choice. It is invaluable in the presence of infection, especially if gross infection has developed after attempted stabilization by internal fixation. When poor skin and soft tissue viability are present from an old compound fracture, external fixation may be indicated. It may also be indicated when there is danger of disturbing the blood supply to the fracture area if internal fixation is used.

In determining treatment to be instituted, each nonunion should be assessed and categorized as viable or nonviable, infected or noninfected, and aligned or nonaligned.

With a viable, noninfected, aligned nonunion there is no need to resect fibrous tissue, nor is bone grafting necessary. Rigid fixation appropriate for the type and location of the fracture with the application of compression is usually all that is required to initiate healing.[1, 2, 10, 13, 17, 19] These nonunions are capable of reaction healing when stabilized, and following stabilization the intrafragmentary fibrocartilage mineralizes. As healing progresses there is substitution of the mineralized fibrocartilage by woven bone and then by lamellar bone and reconstruction of a compact cortex.[8]

Compression has a number of advantages in the treatment of nonunions. It assures rigid fixation and helps decrease the fracture gap. Early ambulation helps reduce fracture disease and speeds healing. Under compression, nonunion tissues can be stimulated to initiate primary bone healing.[1] However, compression is not the main ingredient of success, but rigid and stable fixation is of the utmost importance.

Alignment of the two fracture ends must be considered clinically, functionally, and radiographically. If alignment is good, no further work is necessary prior to plating, grafting, or any repair method, but if alignment is poor, the fracture ends must be realigned before further steps are undertaken. Only the callus required to achieve reduction is removed. The medullary canal proximal and distal to the fracture site is opened by reaming with a large drill or Steinmann pin. The fracture ends may be trimmed to achieve better alignment and stability, but care should be taken not to lose excessive bone length. If the fracture is atrophic an autogenous cancellous bone graft is used.[11, 17]

In nonviable nonunions both ends of the fracture are debrided to expose viable bone and the medullary canals re-established by reaming. The fracture should be compression plated and the surrounding cortical bone decorticated or shingled to expose additional osteocytes and stimulate osteogenesis. The final step is the packing of an autogenous cancellous bone graft into the fracture area, taking care to close the soft tissue layer by layer to maintain the new hematoma at the fracture site and to prevent loss of the cancellous graft into the surrounding tissue planes.[1, 8, 11, 13, 19]

The infected nonunion poses special problems. Not only has the bone failed to heal, but a chronic osteomyelitis plus or minus a surrounding deep-seated soft tissue infection is present. Bone will heal in the face of infection if it is properly immobilized by rigid fixation, either by internal or external means.[13]

The infected nonunion site is exposed surgically and all sequestra excised, fibrous tissue and dead bone removed by curettage, and samples taken for culture and sensitivity tests. The fracture is rigidly immobilized, with compression plating often proving the most satisfactory method. Any fistulous drainage tracts are excised. If the bone is large enough, decortication can be performed, but in almost all cases an autogenous cancellous graft should be packed into the area.[1, 10, 11, 17, 19] A cancellous graft will not form a sequestrum in the face of infection.[11] Drainage should be established by either suction or gravity, using Penrose or plastic tube drains.[11, 17, 19] In certain cases the installation of both infusion and suction tubing and the flushing of the site with copious quantities of saline with or without antibiotics or antibacterials may prove beneficial. In all cases the use of systemic antibiotics is warranted, starting with a broad spectrum antibiotic until sensitivity is known. The surgical site is closed routinely and rarely left open to drain.

In many cases healing occurs despite the ongoing infection. Once this point is reached, further saucerization and debridement of soft tissue can take place, implanted materials can be removed and autogenous cancellous bone grafts can again be used in areas where extensive necrotic bone has been removed. Either suction or gravity drainage should be established and systemic antibiotics chosen, depending on culture and sensitivity test results. This is usually sufficient to clear up the infection.[13]

During treatment of a nonunion, whether viable or nonviable, infected or noninfected, the amount of bone loss must be considered. An animal can stand a slight shortening of a limb with little gait abnormality, but a graft should always be considered when large amounts of bone are missing due to either the original trauma or subsequent infection. Autogenous cancellous bone grafts to bridge defects,[10] a rib graft,[11] or a full thickness graft from the iliac crest[14] can be used to re-establish proper limb length as well as promote osteogenesis.

In recent years, the use of electromagnetic and electrical stimulation of nonunions to initiate healing has been studied in human orthopedics. However, these methods are not currently practical for animals. Long-term treatment is required (three to six months or longer) with the patient undergoing as much as 12 hours treatment daily in the case of magnetic stimulation. With either method of treatment the affected limb has to remain non–weight-bearing for a minimum of three months.[3, 4, 7]

POSTSURGICAL REGIMEN

In most cases it is advisable to hospitalize the animal for seven to ten days unless the owner is extremely conscientious and trustworthy. If infection is involved, hospitalization is advisable until drainage has ceased and the drainage apparatus has been removed. Following release from the hospital, exercise is limited to short periods on the leash for elimination purposes only for a six-week period.

At six to seven weeks after surgery radiography is indicated to assess healing. If the evidence is favorable and the animal is using the limb well, more vigorous but controlled exercise can be instituted. The rate at which full exercise is allowed depends on assessment of healing noted on serial radiographs taken at four- to six-week intervals.

PREVENTION

The best method of handling a nonunion is to prevent its occurrence in the first place. Strict adherence to aseptic techniques and the correct usage of orthopedic apparatus are required. Rigid fixation with proper alignment, maintained for a sufficient period to allow healing as noted on serial radiographs, will prevent many cases of nonunion. A cancellous bone graft in the original repair can only improve the chances of success.

Wiber and Evans found that by delaying surgical correction of femoral shaft fracture in man until five days after trauma, there was a drastic reduction in the percentage of delayed unions and nonunions and postoperative infection rate was also significantly reduced.[22]

A nonunion is not just an ununited broken bone but an injured limb that may have additional problems such as shorting, angulation, joint stiffness, muscular atrophy, neural and vascular disorders, drainage, and infection present.[19] The whole animal must be evaluated and treated, not just the broken bone.

1. Aron, D. N.: Management of delayed union fractures in small animals. Comp. Cont. Ed. *1*:697, 1979.
2. Butler, H. C., and Henry, J. D., Jr.: The use of an ASIF compression plate for fixation of a nonunion fracture of nine years' duration. J. Am. Anim. Hosp. Assoc. 7:103, 1971.
3. Connolly, J. F.: Selection, evaluation and indications for electrical stimulation of ununited fractures. Clin. Orthop. *161*:39, 1981.
4. Day, L.: Electrical stimulation in the treatment of ununited fractures. Clin. Orthop. *161*:52, 1981.
5. DeAngelis, M. P.: Causes of delayed union and nonunion of fractures. Vet. Clin. North Am. 5:251, 1975.
6. Frost, H. M.: *Bone Remodelling and Its Relationship to Metabolic Bone Diseases.* Charles C Thomas, Springfield, 1973.
7. Heckman, J. D., Ingram, A. J., Loyd, R. D., Luck, J. V., and Mayer, P. W.: Nonunion treatment with pulsed electromagnetic fields. Clin. Orthop. *161*:35, 1981.
8. Hoefle, W. D.: Delayed union and nonunion of fractures. *In* Bojrab, M. J. (ed.): *Pathophysiology in Small Animal Surgery.* Lea & Febiger, Philadelphia, 1981.

9. Lancourt, J. E., and Hochberg, F.: Delayed fracture healing in primary hyperparathyroidism. Clin. Orthop. *124*:214, 1977.

10. Muller, M. E., and Thomas, R. J.: Treatment of nonunion in fractures of long bones. Clin. Orthop. *138*:141, 1979.

11. Piermattei, D. L.: *Canine Orthopedics: Fractures.* Lecture Notes, Colorado State University, Fort Collins, 1975.

12. Punto, L., Puronen, J., and Mokka, R. E. M.: Osteomedullography in the tibial shaft of the dog and pig. J. Am. Vet. Radiol. Soc. *19*:100, 1977.

13. Rosen, H.: Compression treatment of long bone pseudoarthrosis. Clin. Orthop. *138*:154, 1979.

14. Shelton, W. R., and Sage, F. P.: Modified Nicoll graft treatment of gap nonunions in the upper extremity. J. Bone Joint Surg. *63A*:226, 1981.

15. Solheim, K., and Vaogi, S.: Delayed union and nonunion of

16. Sumner-Smith, G.: Study of nonunion fractures in the dog. Master's Thesis, University of Guelph, 1969.

17. Sumner-Smith, G.: *Bone in Clinical Orthopaedics.* W. B. Saunders, Philadelphia, 1982.

18. Watson-Jones, R.: *Fractures and Joint Injuries,* 4th ed. E. and S. Livingston, Edinburgh, 1957.

19. Weber, B. G., and Brunner, C.: The Treatment of nonunions without electrical stimulation. Clin. Orthop. *161*:24, 1981.

20. Weber, H., and Čech, O.: Pseudoarthrosis. H. Huber Verlag, Bern, 1976.

21. Whittick, W. G.: *Canine Orthopedics.* Philadelphia, Lea & Febiger, 1974.

22. Wiber, M. C., and Evans, E. G.: Fracture of the femoral shaft treated surgically. J. Bone Joint Surg. *60A*:489, 1978.

fractures: Clinical experiences with the ASIF method. Trauma *12*:121, 1973.

Chapter **155**

Orthopedic Infections

William R. Daly

Infections in bones and joints represent a diagnostic and therapeutic challenge to the veterinary surgeon. Their manifestations vary depending on the intiating event, site of involvement, organism involved, treatment, and nature of the problem (i.e., acute or chronic). Early diagnosis and treatment are imperative to prevent many of the serious complications of infection.

An accurate description of bone and joint infections must first consider the mechanisms by which organisms can reach the osseous or articular tissues before considering the pathogenesis of the infective process itself. A discussion of the diagnosis of infection based on clinical features, radiographic signs, and laboratory findings is followed by consideration of methods of prevention and management of infection.

INFECTIONS INVOLVING BONE

The term *osteomyelitis* was introduced by Nelaton in 1844 to describe an inflammation of the bony cortex and marrow.[45] Most commonly this implies a bacterial infection; however, fungi, parasites, and viruses can infect bone and marrow. Osteitis, inflammation of the bony cortex, is generally recognized as a component of bacterial osteomyelitis. Panosteitis, a common affliction of young dogs, is an inflammation of uncertain origin, primarily of the bony cortex.

Periostitis is an inflammation of the periosteum that surrounds the bone. This may be an infectious (suppurative) periostitis, in which the accumulation of organisms under the periosteum frequently leads to osteitis and osteomyelitis, or it can be seen in the absence of infection with neoplastic, metabolic, or traumatic disorders. Soft tissue infections can lead to

inflammation of adjacent periosteal tissue without necessarily implying that the periosteum is contaminated.

Routes Of Contamination Of Bone

There are several mechanisms by which infective organisms can contaminate bone. There are two principal routes by which osseous (and articular) structures may be contaminated: (1) hematogenous spread, and (2) contamination from exogenous sources, including postoperative infections, infections in which bacteria reach the bone or joint through direct puncture wounds, and infections resulting from an extension of an adjoining soft tissue infection.

Hematogenous Spread Of Infection

The hematogenous spread of infection to bone is a reasonably common occurrence in man, comprising 19 per cent of all osteomyelitis cases.[52] In contrast, the hematogenous spread of infection in small animals is a rare occurrence seen only occasionally as an osteomyelitis in the metaphyseal or epiphyseal region of the bone or as a septic arthritis.[1,2,5,10,11,37,49]

Of particular importance in the hematogenous spread of infection to bones and joints is an understanding of the circulation to the bone and its varying patterns from birth to skeletal maturity.[45] The normal circulation to a growing tubular long bone consists of one or two nutrient arteries that pierce the diaphyseal cortex and divide into ascending and descending branches (Fig. 155–1). These branches continue to divide, becoming fine channels as they approach the ends of the bone. They are joined by metaphyseal

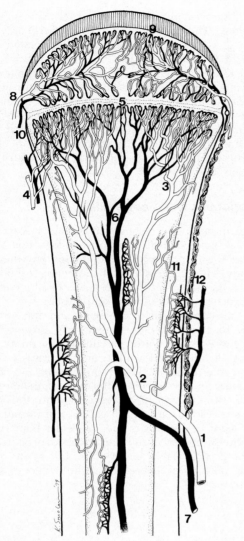

Figure 155–1. Normal osseous circulation to a growing tubular bone. Nutrient arteries (1) pierce the diaphyseal cortex and divide into descending and ascending (2) branches. These latter vessels continue to divide, becoming fine channels (3) as they appoach the end of the bone. They are joined by metaphyseal vessels (4) and, in the subepiphyseal (growth) plate region, form a series of end-arterial loops (5). The venous sinuses extend from the metaphyseal region toward the diaphysis, uniting with other venous structures (6) and eventually piercing the cortex as a large venous channel (7). At the ends of the bone, nutrient arteries of the epiphysis (8) branch into finer structures, passing into the subchondral region. At this site arterial loops (9) are again evident, some of which pierce the subchondral bone plate before turning to enter the venous sinusoid and venous channels of the epiphysis (10). At the bony surface, cortical capillaries (11) form connections with overlapping periosteal plexuses (12). In the growing animal, distinct epiphyseal and metaphyseal arteries can be distinguished on either side of the cartilaginous growth plate. Anastomoses between these vessels either do not occur or are infrequent. (Reprinted with permission from Resnick, D., and Niwayama, G.: *Diagnosis of Bone and Joint Disorders.* W. B. Saunders, Philadelphia, 1981.)

vessels, which originate from neighboring systemic vessels, and just below the epiphyseal plate form a series of end arterial loops. As the vessels turn back toward the diaphysis, they enter a system of large

sinusoidal veins with sluggish blood flow. The venous sinuses extend from the metaphyseal region toward the diaphysis, uniting with other venous structures and eventually piercing the diaphyseal cortex as a large venous channel.

At the ends of the bone, nutrient arteries to the epiphysis, which originate from periarticular vascular arcades, branch into finer structures that pass into the subchondral region. At this site, arterial loops are again present, some of which pierce the subchondral bone plate before turning to enter the venous sinusoids and venous channels of the epiphysis.

At the endosteal surface of the cortical bone capillaries penetrate the cortex to supply nutrients to the osteons via Haversian and Volkmann's canals. Vessels also enter the cortex from the periosteal surface and eventually anastomose with vessels from the endosteal surface. Thus, the cortices of tubular bones receive nutrition from both the periosteal and medullary circulations. The periosteal vessels nourish the outer third of the cortex, whereas the medullary vessels supply the inner two-thirds. The contribution of each may be age-dependent, and in the immature animal the contribution of the periosteal supply is greater.[45]

In growing bone separate epiphyseal and metaphyseal blood supplies exist (Fig. 155–2). Except in very young animals where an occasional vessel pierces the physeal plate, no metaphyseal vessel passes through the cartilage of the growth plate. As the bone matures and the growth plate fully ossifies, the metaphyseal vessels pass through the physeal area to anastomose with the epiphyseal vessels.

The changing blood supply is directly responsible for the various patterns of hematogenous osteomyelitis. In immature animals, hematogenous bacterial infections localize almost exclusively in the metaphyseal region. There have been several explanations proposed for this phenomenon.[50,53] The sudden change in diameter of the ascending metaphyseal capillary to a large sinusoidal vein results in considerably slower blood flow with increased turbulence. Bacteria in the blood tend to settle in this region,

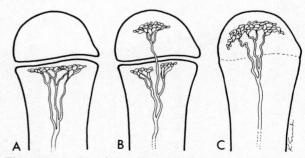

Figure 155–2. Normal vascular patterns of a tubular bone. *A,* In the juvenile animal the capillaries of the metaphysis turn sharply, without penetrating the open growth plate. *B,* In the newborn, some metaphyseal vessels may penetrate the open growth plate, ramifying in the epiphysis. *C,* In the adult, with closure of the growth plate, a vascular connection between metaphysis and epiphysis can be recognized. (Reprinted with permission from Resnick, D., and Niwayama, G.: *Diagnosis of Bone and Joint Disorders.* W. B. Saunders, Philadelphia, 1981.)

creating an initial imflammatory response and subsequent microthrombus formation. Because these vessels are end arterial branches of the nutrient artery, any obstruction that forms, whether by bacterial growth or thrombus, is likely to produce a small area of avascular necrosis. These factors combine to create an ideal medium for the growth and multiplication of organisms. In the newborn animal and in human infants less than one year of age, it is not uncommon for hematogenous osteomyelitis to involve the epiphysis directly, and frequently a septic arthritis develops as well.[13,27,45,50] An anatomical explanation for this is the fact that at this age some capillaries still perforate the epiphyseal growth plate.[53] A similar situation exists in the adult. Once the cartilaginous growth plate has been absorbed, extensive anastomoses exist between the metaphyseal and epiphyseal vessels, allowing infection to localize in the subchondral regions of the bone. Hematogenous osteomyelitis in the adult animal is exceptionally rare in long bones. There is considerable evidence that spondylitis and discospondylitis in adult dogs represent this type of infection.[20, 25]

Infections From Exogenous Sources

In veterinary practice, most osteomyelitis in small animals is due to contamination of bone from exogenous sources. There are several mechanisms by which this contamination can occur, including (1) open fractures, (2) closed fractures repaired by open reduction and internal fixation, (3) puncture wounds, e.g., animal bites or plant thorns, (4) gunshot wounds, (5) spread from contiguous sources of infection such as superficial surgical wound abscesses,

tooth abscesses, interdigital pyodermas, or nasal sinus infections. The most common cause of osteomyelitis in small animals is contamination associated with fractures or fracture repair.[11,49] In one study of 46 cases, 43 infections were found to follow either open fracture or open repair of a closed fracture and 3 were found to follow tooth abscessation.[49] In another review of 67 cases of osteomyelitis in the dog, bony infection in 91 per cent of the dogs resulted from open fractures (10 per cent), open reduction of closed fractures (55 per cent), or extension from a soft tissue infection (26 per cent).[11]

Pathogenesis Of Osteomyelitis

Regardless of the mechanism of contamination, a predictable physiological response follows that is the same as the response to contamination anywhere in the body. The progression of the infection is modified because the infection occupies a small volume of soft tissue surrounded by a rigid wall of bone.[27]

The initial reaction of the bone and surrounding tissues to bacterial contamination is inflammation with hyperemia, increased vascular permeability, diapedesis of phagocytic cells, and extravasation of serum proteins, antibodies, complement, and fibrin. In hematogenous osteomyelitis in the metaphyseal region, the inflammatory response and the small abscess that forms as a result cause local thrombosis, which leads to necrosis of the trabecular bone in the area. The periphery of such an abscess may be heavily infiltrated with viable neutrophils, but in the more central portion of the abscess the leukocytes are necrotic.

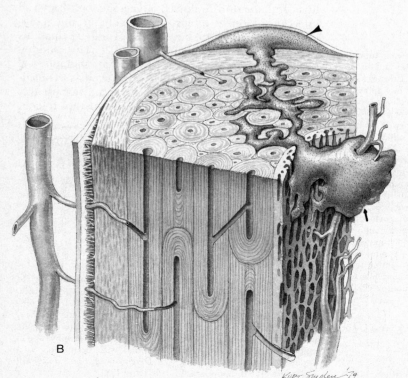

Figure 155–3. Diagram of the manner in which infection in the medullary canal (arrow) permeates the cortex and collects beneath the periosteal membrane (arrowhead). (Reprinted with permission from Resnick, D., and Niwayama, G.: *Diagnosis of Bone and Joint Disorders.* W. B. Saunders, Philadelphia, 1981.)

As in other tissues, the mere presence of bacteria in the bone does not always cause infection. Infection is a result of an imbalance between the bacteria and the normal host defense mechanisms. When the body is successful in overcoming the infection at an early stage, a chronic bone abscess (Brodie's abscess) may form. The abscess is generally small (1 to 3 cm), and its walls are lined with inflammatory granulation tissue. Toward the outer surface of the abscess the granulation tissue merges with a layer of connective tissue of varying thickness and density. This connective tissue represents the capsule of the abscess cavity, delimiting it from the neighboring bone. The cancellous bone bordering the abscess is compacted, although the sclerosis is more conspicuous in some areas than in others. The fluid content of the abscess varies. It may be purulent, oily, mucoid, or slimy. The infectious agent may be revealed by bacteriological examination of the fluid. If the abscess is not sterile, *Staphylococcus* or *Streptococcus* spp. or both are generally found.

If the body is unsuccessful in eradicating the infection, the abscess continues to expand, with further production of purulent exudate. Because of the limited volume of soft tissue space and the relatively rigid cortical walls, pressure in the area of the abscess increases dramatically, forcing the exudate deeper into the medullary cavity and the cortical bone. The exudate enters the cortical bone and spreads across it via Haversian and Volkmann's canals (Fig. 155–3). Inflammation near the abscess produces increased cortical porosity, at least in part by osteoclastic resorption, which encourages movement of the exudate through the cortex. In the metaphyseal area where the cortex is thin, particularly in the young animal, the inflammatory process rapidly reaches the outer surface of the cortex.

What happens when the developing abscess reaches the outer cortex of the bone depends on the age of the patient and the anatomical site. In the young animal the periosteum has a very loose attachment that allows the abscess to develop in the subperiosteal space. Elevation of the periosteum from the cortical bone further compromises the cortical blood supply, and necrosis of fragments of bone is likely.[27] This is one mechanism of the development of a *sequestrum*, as the dead fragment is called. These sequestra are eventually separated from the living bone and are surrounded by pus. As the body attempts to wall off the infection, fibrous tissue and new bone are produced on the medullary side of the sequestrum and a shell of new subperiosteal bone is produced by the cambium layer of the periosteum. This new bone is referred to as an *involucrum*. Although the involucrum walls off the infection, it also renders bacteria persisting around the sequestrum inaccessible to antibodies and antibiotics, as neither can penetrate a significant distance in the direction of the sequestrum. The sequestrum thus forms a constant source of re-infection and chronic low-grade osteomyelitis.

In adults, the periosteum is more tightly adherent to a thicker cortical wall. Infection that begins subchondrally tends to remain intramedullary. It can spread to large portions of the medullary canal before it is able to break through the cortex. As the exudate forces its way through Volkmann's canals, small subperiosteal abscesses form that rupture through the periosteum rather than lift it off the cortex. Soft tissue abscesses are more likely to form and sinus tracts develop that drain the infection through the skin. Such sinus tracts are referred to as *cloacae*. Since the periosteal blood supply generally remains largely intact, the formation of sequestra does not generally occur. Bone destruction (without sequestra), osteoporosity, and periosteal new bone formation are the features of adult hematogenous osteomyelitis.

In some joints, most notably the coxofemoral joint, a portion of the metaphysis is intra-articular. If the abscess erodes through the metaphysis in this region, a septic arthritis as well as the osteomyelitis develops.

When bone is contaminated from an exogenous source, the pathogenesis of bone infection is the same as that in endogenous infection. Particularly in animals that have suffered open fractures or open repair of fractures, the balance between bacteria, local environment, and host defense mechanisms (see Chapter 4) is very likely altered in favor of the bacteria.

Fracture patients obviously have suffered severe trauma and blood loss. In addition, many are in hypovolemic shock, and many receive large doses of corticosteroids. All of these factors tend to cause immunosuppression and reduce the animal's ability to resist bacterial challenge. Near the fracture there is tissue trauma, frequently with areas of avascular muscle, bone, and fascia. Hematoma formation is common. At surgery there is frequently further tissue trauma and blood loss with more avascular tissue produced. If the fracture was closed, open reduction and internal fixation introduce bacteria with a large foreign body (plates, pins, screws). The use of intramedullary pins can obliterate all medullary circulation, and bone plates have been shown to destroy all periosteal circulation under the area of the plate. Considered in this light, one cannot help but wonder why most fractures that are open or opened do not become infected. The credit must be given to the effectiveness of the host defense mechanisms. The surgeon is only able to help it function as effectively as possible.

The development of infection around a bone due to contamination from an exogenous source is physiologically no different from that of any wound infection. There is no evidence that the cellular and immune mechanisms differ between bone and other tissues.[27] The course and extent of the osteomyelitis depend in this circumstance on the degree of trauma to the skin, soft tissue, and bone (local environment); the resistance of the patient (host defense mechanisms); the virulence of the organisms (bacteria); but most of all the vascularization of the bone. In every fracture the blood supply to individual fragments is disturbed or even destroyed. Shattered bones with completely isolated fragments, necrotic tissue, and unavoidable hematomas offer organisms an ideal medium. Infection spreads over the entire area of the hematoma and encompasses necrotic soft tissue and avascular bone fragments. Periosteum, cortical bone, and the medullary space are all injured and bacteremia and sepsis become possible. In most cases the process is limited to the extent of the injury, especially if pus drains either spontaneously or through surgical intervention. Isolated dead bone fragments may be expelled spontaneously as sequestra or, if well-stabilized, may be revascularized and re-incorporated.[6]

When no drainage is allowed, pus retention may cause devastating consequences. Rapidly proliferating bacteria stimulate the production of a large volume of exudate, which damages more tissue by pressure and enhances the spread of infection. Bacterial by-products, enzymes liberated by destroyed leukocytes, and altered pH cause further damage to live tissue and disintegration of the bone matrix. Infection spreads from the surface through the bony cortex via Volkmann's and Haversian canals to strangle other vascular areas and destroy more osteocytes in their lacunae. This process corresponds closely to the progression of untreated hematogenous osteomyelitis.[6] Following complete drainage of pus, a defensive barrier of granulation tissue forms within a short time at the edge of the live tissue. The granulation tissue resists further extension of the infection and often overgrows and replaces dead tissue.

Persistence Of Infection

Although the mortality of acute osteomyelitis is quite low when treated effectively, 15 to 30 per cent of patients still develop chronic disease.[27,35,36,52,53,60] Chronic infection may occur in several ways. In those cases in which an acute suppurative osteomyelitis drained (or was surgically drained), the infection tends to resolve and newly formed bone and dense, avascular fibrous tissue isolate the area of infection. If any necrotic material (bone) persists, the process usually recurs at a later time. The body's limited resorptive capacity for the necrotic but still mineralized bone is responsible for recurrence.[27] As there is no biological enzyme that can digest mineralized bone in one stage, a phase of demineralization must precede matrix resorption. For this to occur, necrotic bone must be revascularized or in contact at its surface with viable cells or granulation tissue. For trabecular bone this does not present a significant problem because of the large peripheral surface area compared with its mass (9 cm²/gm). On the other hand, cortical bone has a surface area:mass ratio estimated to be 0.2 cm²/gm, or about 50 times smaller than that of cancellous bone.[27] For this reason the

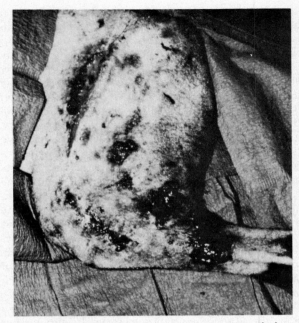

Figure 155–4. Multiple draining sinuses in association with chronic osteomyelitis. This patient had an open fracture of the femur that became chronically infected following plate fixation. Many draining sinuses were present, and the original surgical wound had opened spontaneously 16 months following the fracture repair. Removal of the plate and adequate debridement eliminated the problem.

resorption of detached necrotic cortical bone fragments (sequestra) is very slow. As mentioned previously, the presence of necrotic bone allows organisms to survive and proliferate free from challenge by the body's immune system or by systemically administered antibiotics. In time these organisms generally cause an acute exacerbation of the infection with inflammation, vascular thrombosis, and further necrotic bone production (including necrosis of the new bone produced previously as a result of prior acute infections). Eventually this process leads to draining sinuses, occasionally with severe mutilation (Fig. 155–4).

Diagnosis Of Osteomyelitis

Clinical Features

The clinical features of osteomyelitis vary depending on the stage of the disease and the method of contamination. In acute hematogenous osteomyelitis (rare), the patient is generally less than six months of age and is presented with a sudden onset of lameness with or without a history of trauma. Fever, anorexia, and local tenderness are present with a mild leukocytosis.

The acute onset of osteomyelitis from exogenous contamination is typical of that of any wound infection; it occurs within three weeks of the precipitating event (usually fracture repair) and commonly shows signs within the first five days. Acute suppurative osteomyelitis is characterized by pain, local heat, redness, swelling, fever, depression, anorexia, lameness, and the production of a purulent exudate, which either causes a wound dehiscence as it drains or remains localized as an abscess. Leukocytosis, occasionally with a degenerative shift, is common but not always present.

The diagnosis of chronic osteomyelitis is generally made following an unresolved infection that occurred as an acute suppurative osteomyelitis. It is possible in the case of relatively avirulent bacteria or with large metallic implants that the acute phase of the disease does not occur. The most consistent clinical signs of chronic osteomyelitis are pain, lameness, draining sinuses.[2,10,13,14,27,33,58]

Radiographic Features

The radiographic changes of bone infection are often nonspecific and limited primarily to local bone

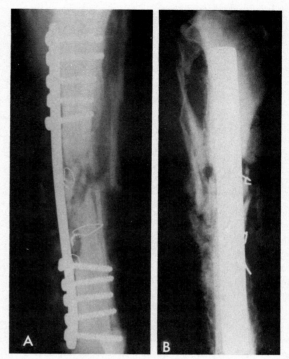

Figures 155–6. *A,* Anteroposterior and *(B)* lateral radiographs showing the usual signs of osteomyelitis. Bone lysis, periosteal elevations with exuberant periosteal new bone formation, and avascular bone without involucrum formation are present 50 days following repair of a highly comminuted open tibial fracture.

destruction and new bone formation.[7,10,11,40,49,54,58] Soft tissue changes such as swelling and loss of demarcation between fascial and muscle planes may be noticed early in the course of infection; however, bony changes do not appear for 10 to 14 days.

Classical radiographic changes revealing sequestra with involucrum formation are rarely encountered in the dog and cat (Fig. 155–5). Bone lysis, periosteal elevation with periosteal new bone formation, and avascular fragments of bone (sequestra without evidence of involucrum formation) are typical (Fig. 155–6).

The greatest difficulties in radiographically evaluating potentially infected fractures are the differentiation between normal bony and periosteal reactions following trauma, the reaction to instability at the fracture site, and infection. Instability following fracture stabilization can produce a radiographic appearance similar to that seen with posttraumatic osteomyelitis.[6] Zones of resorption occur around loose implants and periosteal deposits as a result of periosteal irritation caused by motion. One possible key to differentiation between infection and motion is the fact that resorption due to instability is usually sharply outlined and limited to the extent of the zone of movement of the loose foreign body (Fig. 155–7).

As a noninfectious stimulus, a reaction to the metal or reactions between dissimilar metals can be the cause of inflammatory alterations of the bone. Corrosion of metal can lead to osteolytic erosion and destruction of bones and subperiosteal and endosteal

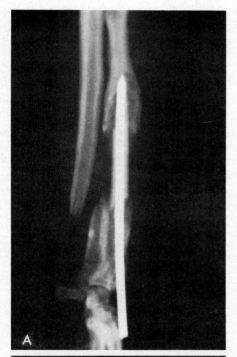
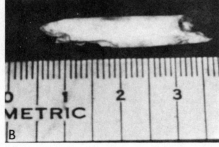

Figure 155–5. *A,* Classical radiographic changes revealing a large sequestrum of the radius and partial involucrum formation at the proximal and distal ends. This cat had suffered an open fracture of the radius and ulna with considerable soft tissue loss. The Steinmann pin provided insufficient stability and obliterated the intramedullary blood supply to the segment of bone, which later became a sequestrum. *B,* Photograph of the sequestrum.

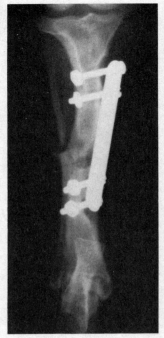

Figure 155–7. Nonunited fracture of the midshaft tibia with radiographic evidence of loose orthopedic implants. Bone lysis is visible under the plate, particularly at the ends. Note the lysis around the shafts of the proximal two screws.

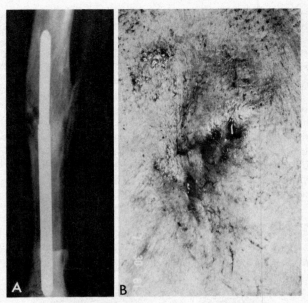

Figure 155–8. A, As a noninfectious stimulus for bony inflammation, corrosion of metal can lead to osteolytic erosion and destruction of bones and to subperiosteal and endosteal new bone formation with the presence of cavities and fistulae. This Jonas pin caused the late development of a draining fistula long after the fracture had healed. B, Draining fistula associated with the Jonas pin.

new bone formation with the presence of cavities and fistulae (Fig. 155–8).

Bacteriological Features

Several studies have been made of the organisms most commonly cultured from osteomyelitic lesions in the dog and cat (Table 155–1).[11,22,49] The organism most commonly found in all studies was *Staphylococcus aureus* (46 to 74 per cent of all cases studied). *Streptococcus, E. coli, Proteus, Pasteurella,* and *Pseudomonas* ssp. were the likely organisms in nonstaphylococcal osteomyelitis. Multiple species of organisms were recovered in 35 to 47 per cent of

TABLE 155–1. Bacterial Isolates from Osteomyelitis

Organism	Hirsch and Smith (15 dogs)		Smith et al. (39 dogs)		Caywood et al. (67 dogs)	
	No.	*(%)*	*No.*	*(%)*	*No.*	*(%)*
Staphylococcus spp.	10	(66)	18	(46)	50	(74)
Streptococcus spp.	2	(13)	3	(8)	20	(29)
E. coli					14	(21)
Proteus spp.			7	(18)	10	(15)
Pasteurella spp.	4	(26)			5	(7)
Pseudomonas spp.	2	(13)	3	(8)		
Micrococcus spp.			3	(8)	4	(6)
Klebsiella spp.	1	(7)				
Nocardia spp.					2	(3)
Corynebacteria spp.					2	(3)
Aerobacter spp.			1	(2.5)	2	(3)
Serratia spp.			2	(5)		
Clostridium spp.			1	(2.5)		
Enterococcus spp.			1	(2.5)		
Enterobacter spp.	1	(7)	1	(2.5)		
Bacteroides spp.	1	(7)				
Actinomyces spp.	1	(7)				
Eugonic Fermentor-4	1	(7)				
Moraxella spp.	1	(7)				

Notes: No. = number of isolates.
        % = percentage of total dogs.

cases. One study specifically cultured for anaerobic species and found 2 of the 17 cultures to be positive.[22] These results closely resemble the data collected from human osteomyelitis.[6,13,19,42,46,52,53]

Cultures of suspected osteomyelitis should be made from either fine needle aspiration or a debridement sample. Collecting samples for bacterial culture from draining sinus tracts is discouraged owing to the high number of contaminants found. A study in human patients compared cultures of operative specimens with sinus tract cultures in 40 cases of chronis osteomyelitis.[33] Thirty-five patients (87.5 per cent) had a single pathogen isolated from their operative specimens. Only 44 per cent of the sinus tract cultures contained the operative pathogen. This study concluded that the predictive value of common pathogens isolated from sinus tracts is low unless the pathogen is *S. aureus*. Less than one-half of the sinus tract cultures from patients with *S. aureus* osteomyelitis contained this organism.

Blood cultures should be taken in septic patients suspected of having hematogenous osteomyelitis. Blood cultures are positive in about 50 per cent of humans with hematogenous osteomyelitis, and if an organism is isolated from the blood it may be assumed to be responsible for the problem.

After a bacterium is isolated, standard antimicrobial disc sensitivity tests are performed. Without this vital information, the selection of a proper antimicrobial agent is difficult or impossible. It has been suggested that once disc sensitivity tests have been performed, the organism isolated should be tested by tube dilution methods to determine the minimum inhibitory and minimum bactericidal concentrations for the several antibiotics most likely to be used.[22,46] This can be important for several reasons: (1) there can be a great difference between the relative susceptibilities of an organism to several drugs that are equally effective on the basis of disc sensitivity results: (2) since bone does not have a rich supply of phagocytic and antibody-producing lymphocytic cells, a drug that is bactericidal in concentrations present is preferable to one that is bacteriostatic; this information can only be gained by tube dilution studies; and (3) some strains of *Staphylococcus aureus* are inhibited but not killed by semisynthetic penicillinase-resistant penicillins. These are only detected by tube dilution methods.

Treatment Of Osteomyelitis

Despite considerable progress in the understanding and treatment of osteomyelitis, this disease remains one of the most difficult and frustrating orthopedic problems for the veterinary surgeon. The treatment of osteomyelitis has undergone considerable change in recent years. Open treatments have included the application of sea sponges, carbolic acid, bichloride of mercury, Vaseline gauze, saline, topical antibiotics, and maggots.[31] The advent of antibiotics brought with it many attempts at closed treatment using systemic antibiotics.

The rational treatment of osteomyelitis requires an understanding of the pathological processes involved. Of fundamental importance is the understanding that the disease is not primarily one of bacterial infection, although this initiates the problem, but one of necrotic bone buried in poorly vascularized dense fibrous tissue. Consequently, successful treatment generally requires a combination of surgical and antibiotic treatment. Antibiotics alone may control the disease process; however, in most cases surgery is required to eradicate it.

Acute Osteomyelitis

If clinical signs and history suggest the presence of acute hematogenous osteomyelitis, appropriate antibiotics in adequate doses are the primary treatment. Blood cultures should be performed and antibiotics started while awaiting laboratory results. Since most osteomyelitis is a result of penicillinase-producing *S. aureus*, the antibiotic should be a synthetic penicillinase-resistant penicillin. Medullary bone is a highly vascular tissue, and until the infection progresses to produce vascular thrombosis and pus with increased marrow pressure, antibiotic treatment alone is effective. If after two to three days of appropriate parenteral antibiotic treatment significant clinical improvement has not occurred, surgical treatment is suggested.[46] An incision is made over the point of maximum tenderness, and the periosteum is exposed but not removed. Holes are drilled in several directions into the metaphysis from close to the growth plate to ensure decompression of the medullary canal. Cultures should be taken. If pus is encountered a small segment of cortex is removed to provide for adequate drainage.

If clinical signs and history suggest acute osteomyelitis of exogenous origin, treatment is the same as that for an infected wound. Treatment principles of wound infection have been discussed in Chapter 4. When a diagnosis of wound infection is made in any orthopedic wound, there are only four basic components of the treatment: (1) immobilization, (2) complete and careful debridement of the wound, (3) stability of the fracture, and (4) adequate drainage.

Unfortunately, most veterinary patients are unwilling to accept the restrictions of skeletal traction or elevation of the affected limb to reduce swelling. Application of a bulky but snug Robert-Jones bandage generally provides immobilization in the dog and cat. One goal of internal fixation of fractures is to allow early mobilization of the injured part and thus prevent or minimize "fracture disease." If an infection occurs in the postoperative course, immobilization must take precedence to prevent extension of the infection.[6]

Debridement of the infected wound is carried out in the operating room with the animal under anesthesia. This requires removal of the sutures and careful, systematic, gentle examination of the infected tissues. All fragments of necrotic tissue, hematomas, excess suture material, and heavy fascia are removed. Fragments of necrotic bone must either be removed or made stable, preferably by some means of interfragmentary compression (lag screws, cerclage wires). At the time of debridement the fracture fixation is evaluated. Any movement must be stabilized. This may mean complete revision of the original surgical repair, but, if necessary, this must be done without delay. Fracture instability leads to progression of the infection because the loose and poorly adapted fragments favor development of irreparable necrosis.[6] As with other infected wounds, closure of the incision is delayed unless the wound will heal without further complications. The surgeon who justifies closure of such wounds by pointing out that in the majority of cases he "got by with it" must be held fully accountable for the minority of wounds in which he did not "get by."[4] For the patient, the results are usually tragic.

The best method of providing drainage to an infected wound following adequate debridement is nonclosure. Drains, with or without suction or irrigation, can be used in some cases. This technique is discussed under Treatment of Chronic Osteomyelitis. Two common problems following fractures of the extremities are the development of hematomas and the presence of severely traumatized skin. If, despite correct surgical technique and hemostasis, a hematoma develops, an aggressive approach is required. A retrospective study of hematomas in the area of fracture fixation revealed that 20 per cent of the hematomas were contaminated by coagulase-positive *S. aureus*.[6] This suggests the possibility of infection developing at the fracture site due to a contaminated hematoma. Also, spontaneous perforation between the sutures often occurs over a hematoma, creating a new path for infection. Hematomas that develop over a subcutaneous orthopedic implant, such as on

the medial side of the tibia or the distal radius, are particularly dangerous.

Small hematomas should be evacuated by needle aspiration after thorough disinfection of the skin. The puncture wound should not be through the incision but through a point of entry away from it. The hematoma should be completely drained to permit the skin to adhere to soft tissue, bone, or the implant. A light bandage is applied to prevent re-accumulation.

Large hematomas require surgical removal of the clot. This entails complete surgical preparation, gentle evacuation of the wound, perfect hemostasis, and accurate re-apposition of the tissues. Generally several suction drains are used. Immobilization of the limb is essential until the soft tissue firmly adheres to the underlying bone.

Loss of skin in the fracture area due to trauma at the time of injury is usually of little consequence if the bone remains covered with healthy muscle. Problems arise, especially in areas where implants are placed subcutaneously, such as on the medial tibia, when at least part of the plate and bone is covered with necrotic skin only. It is important to preserve the dry necrotic skin as an impermeable biological dressing for as long as possible. With full thickness loss of skin and subcutaneous tissues, the metallic implant may be exposed. Even in this situation, infection can usually be prevented with appropriate wound treatment. The wound is treated until complete granulation or sufficient ossification of the fracture has occurred to permit removal of the implant (Fig. 155–9). Following implant removal the wound generally closes rapidly by granulation.

Chronic Osteomyelitis

Chronic osteomyelitis is a disease of ischemia more than infection. Organisms thrive in avascular bone and scar tissue, and frequently the surrounding scar

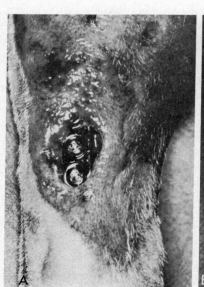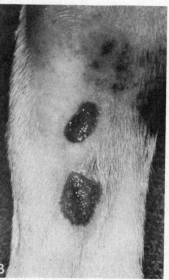

Figure 155–9. A, Full thickness loss of skin on the medial tibia following plate fixation. Even in this situation, infection can usually be prevented with appropriate treatment. The wound is treated until complete granulation or sufficient ossification of the fracture has occurred. *B,* Granulation tissue with partial epithelialization has formed over the exposed plate after three weeks of wound treatment.

and involucrum are impenetrable to antibiotics. Dead bone and scar tissue must be excised, effective antibiotic therapy provided, and dead space eliminated.[13]

The initial step in the treatment of chronic osteomyelitis is evaluation of the patient's general condition with a complete blood count. Osteomyelitis does not generally cause significant alterations in serum chemistries. Conditions such as anemia and hypoproteinemia should be corrected prior to surgical treatment.

A culture should be taken from the bone, not a draining sinus. Generally adequate culture material can be obtained with a needle aspiration of the infected site. Following isolation of an organism and determination of its antibiotic sensitivity, high levels of an appropriate parenteral antibiotic are given.

Radiographs should be taken before surgery to enable the surgeon to assess the infection and the stability of the fracture and any implants present. A sinogram (fistulogram) can be done with a radiopaque contrast material such as Renografin-76.* The sinogram can be of significant value in determining the extent of the pathological condition and allowing a surgical approach to be planned. The extent of the condition always exceeds that which is shown on the sinogram.[14]

All sinus tracts should be injected with a 1 per cent solution of methylene blue 12 to 24 hours prior to surgery. This dye stains the sinus walls and provides a guide for removal of diseased tissue. Methylene blue generally penetrates the entire fistulous tract. All tissues with poor vascularity are stained a deep blue, and after 12 hours tissues with significant blood supply are free of the dye and appear normal. The dye is excreted by the kidneys and liver.

The surgical procedure consists of careful and thorough debridement. If possible, this should be

carried out under a tourniquet to allow less blood loss and better exposure. The sinus tracts, abscess wall, and dead bone are excised, so that only normal, healthy skin, fat, muscle, and bleeding bone remain. The removal of all scar tissue is essential. At times it is necessary to approach the lesion from several directions. During and following debridement, the wound is flushed with copious volumes of isotonic fluids. The use of a pulsating jet lavage such as the SurgiLav* or a sterile dental Water-Pik† helps remove small fragments of debris from the wound.

Once the wound is cleaned and infected tissue removed, fracture stability should be evaluated. If the fracture has healed and implants are present, they are removed. If implants are present and are holding the fragments rigidly, they should be left in place until the fracture is healed. If the fragments are loose, metal implants should be removed and the fracture stabilized by another suitable means. In infected nonunions with no implant, metal plates and screws may be used to create stability and speed fracture union. Infection is not a contra indication to the use of metal implants, but plates and screws are preferred over intramedullary devices when dealing with infected nonunions for several reasons: (1) plates and screws provide better stability, which encourages more rapid fracture union, (2) the intramedullary device may spread a localized infection through the medullary canal, and (3) the chronically infected nonunion usually does not have an intact medullary canal, the ends of the nonunion closing the canal. Reestablishing the medullary canal may further reduce the vascularity of the fracture site.[37] Once the fracture is healed, the implants generally require removal to completely clear the infection.

The next step in the surgical procedure requires a

---

*E. R. Squibb & Sons, Princeton, NJ.

*Stryker Corporation, Kalamazoo, MI.
†Teledyne Aquatec, Ft. Collins, CO.

Figure 155–10. A, Following adequate debridement of chronic osteomyelitis, the wound may be left entirely open to promote the best drainage. The skin edges are sutured to the soft tissues near the bone, leaving a sizable defect in the cortex and the medullary canal exposed. *B,* Saucerized wounds are generally bandaged with either a bulky bandage, such as the Robert-Jones bandage, or gauze sponges secured to the wound margins.

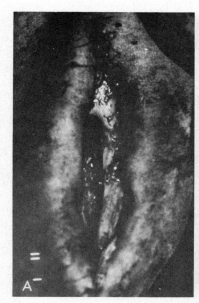
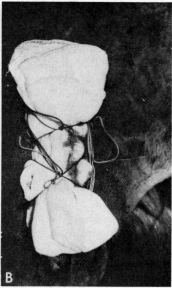

decision regarding closure or nonclosure of the wound. At this point the wound should contain only healthy tissue. If the procedure has been done under a tourniquet, the tourniquet is released to be sure all tissues have sufficient blood supply. Additional debridement is performed if necessary. Generally there is a sizable defect in the cortex of the bone with a large portion of the medullary canal exposed. Some advocate leaving the wound entirely open to promote the best drainage.[24,39,41,47,57,59] In this technique, known as "saucerization," the wound is left open but covered with a bandage (Fig. 155–10). The wound is examined daily and topical minor debridement performed as necessary. After the entire defect has filled with granulation tissue, generally 7 to 14 days, the wound is either closed or a secondary procedure is performed to fill the defect in the bone with a generous cancellous bone graft. In the case of a nonunion, the fracture is stabilized at the time of bone grafting and after the granulation tissue bed has formed.

A second popular technique involves primary wound closure over two or more drains to allow suction and irrigation of the dead space.[10,12,28,29,31,37,57,58] In this technique a system of drains is placed into the wound bed to leave the skin at a distant site. These tubes are used to flush the wound bed either continuously or intermittently with fluids containing antibiotics based on culture and sensitivity results or dilute antiseptics such as Betadine solution* (100 ml Betadine solution diluted into 900 ml saline). Some have advocated the addition of detergents such as tyloxapol† (30 ml/L) and enzymes such as streptokinase-streptodornase‡ (100,000 units streptokinase and 25,000 units streptodornase per liter).

Continuous fluid infusion is recommended to prevent occlusion of the tube perforations. Large volumes of fluids (3 to 10 liters per day) are used. This technique has the disadvantage of requiring suction and continuous monitoring in the usually uncooperative veterinary patient. Intermittent fluid infusion once or twice a day is more practical for animal patients.[2,37] The fluids are infused several times a day, allowed to remain in the wound for 15 minutes to 1 hour, and then removed. This process is repeated until the drains clot and cease to draw fluid. Radiographs can be taken to assess the size of the remaining dead space by administering contrast material into the wound via the entry tube.

Several precautions should be observed with suction-irrigation systems. If antibiotics are used in the irrigating fluid, care should be taken not to exceed the normal total parenteral daily dose for the patient. The antibiotics can be rapidly absorbed from the wound site and, particularly in the case of aminoglycosides, may have significant toxic effects. The system

should be kept sterile. It is not uncommon for secondary gram-negative bacteria to enter the wound via drains. The drains are best kept under a sterile bandage. Lastly, it is not uncommon for the drains to be removed prematurely by the patient. Whatever restraint is necessary should be used. Generally an Elizabethan collar and a heavy bandage work well.

Regardless of the technique used (saucerization-open drainage-delayed closure or suction-irrigation), some treatment is often required to restore the bone lost to infection. Once the infection is cleared, cancellous grafts placed into the defect provide the safest and most rapid method of encouraging filling of defects and return of weakened bone to a structurally sound state.[23,38,51] Bone grafting is discussed in Chapter 156.

SEPTIC ARTHRITIS

Septic arthritis is a relatively uncommon entity in small animals. However, when it does arise, it is frequently associated with devastating effects. As with osteomyelitis, an understanding of the problems associated with septic arthritis requires consideration of routes of contamination; physiological response to joint contamination; clinical, radiological, and laboratory features; and treatment alternatives.

Routes of Contamination

As in osteomyelitis, it is convenient to divide the potential routes of contamination of joints into two categories; hematogenous and exogenous. Hematogenous spread of infection to a joint indicates that the organism has been carried by the blood to lodge directly in the vasculature of the synovium. When bacteria are injected intravenously, they localize rapidly at two major sites; in the cells of the reticuloendothelial system all over the body, and in small deposits in the synovial membrane.[16] Bacteria also more readily gain access to the synovial fluid than to spinal fluid, aqueous humor, or urine.[16] Bacteremias that produce septic arthritis are commonly associated with pneumonia, diarrhea, umbilical infections, and endocarditis.[30] It is also possible for synovial membrane to be infected as a result of contamination through direct vascular anastomoses between an infected epiphysis and the synovial membrane (Fig. 155–11).

Hematogenous septic arthritis is most commonly seen in very young animals, particularly foals.[30,32] More commonly, septic arthritis is a result of direct contamination of the joint from exogenous sources. This can occur by several different methods (See Fig. 155–11). Penetrating wounds of the joint (bites, automobile accidents, surgery with poor aseptic technique, gunshot wounds, intra-articular injections) can lead to direct contamination. Corticosteroid injection into a joint is the most common predisposing cause

---

*Purdue Frederick Co., Norwalk, CT.

†Alevaire, Breon Laboratories Inc., New York NY

‡Varidase, Lederle Laboratories, Wayne, NJ. This product is no longer commercially available.

Figure 155–11. Septic arthritis: potential routes of contamination. *A*, Hematogenous spread of infection to a joint can result from direct lodgement of organisms in the synovial membrane *(1)* or, as illustrated in *B*, direct vascular continuity between an infected epiphysis and the synovial membrane. Spread into the joint from a contiguous source can occur from a metaphyseal focus that extends into the epiphysis and from there into the joint *(2)*; from the metaphyseal focus with extension into the joint when the growth plate is intra-articular *(3)*; or from a contiguous soft tissue infection *(4)*. Direct implantation following a penetrating wound *(5)* can also lead to septic arthritis. *B* and *C*, Hematogenous spread of infection to a joint can occur owing to vascular continuity between the epiphysis and the synovial membrane. In *B* the vessels shown include arterioles *(1)*, venules *(2)*, and capillaries *(3)*, of the capsule; periosteal vessels *(4)*; the nutrient artery *(5)*; and metaphyseal-epiphyseal anastomoses *(6)*. The synovial membrane may become infected from an osseous focus before the joint fluid is contaminated. This sequence of events is diagrammed in *C*. *D*, Spread from a contiguous osseous surface can result from penetration of the artilage *(1)* or pathological fracture with articular contamination *(2)*. In this situation, synovial fluid may become infected before the synovial membrane. (Reprinted with permission from Resnick, D., and Niwayama, G.: *Diagnosis of Bone and Joint Disorders.* W. B. Saunders, Philadelphia, 1981.)

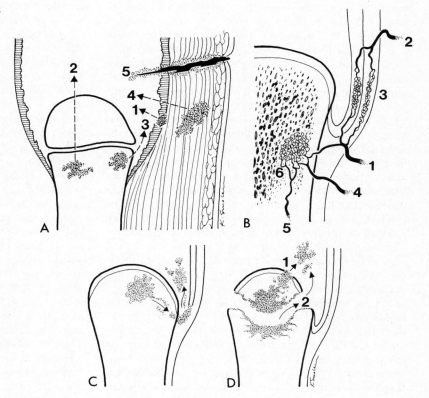

of joint infection in the horse.[30] Extension from a contiguous source of infection may also cause septic arthritis. This may occur from (1) a metaphyseal focus of osteomyelitis that extends into the epiphysis and into the joint, (2) a metaphyseal focus of infection that extends directly into the joint when the growth plate is intra-articular, such as the coxofemoral joint, and (3) a contiguous soft tissue infection.

Pathophysiology of Joint Infection

Regardless of the mechanism of contamination of the joint or synovial membrane, the infection and inflammatory response create considerable alterations in the normal physiology of the joint and are responsible for the pathological changes that occur.

The normal joint capsule consists of a tough fibrous outer layer and an inner layer, the synovial membrane or intima. The inner surface of the synovial membrane is thrown into processes or villi, the number and extent of which increase with increasing age and in inflammatory processes. Synovial tissue consists of an arrangement of intimal surface cells, subintimal cells, connective tissue fibers, ground substance, nerves, and lymphatics. Intimal cells lining the joint are generally divided into two subgroups, type A cells, which are thought to produce hyaluronate or mucin and have some phagocytic activity, and type B cells, which are more fibroblast like and have a protein-secreting function.

Synovial fluid is a protein-containing dialysate of plasma into which hyaluronate, secreted by the synovial cells, is added as plasma water diffuses through the synovial tissue spaces into the joint space. Hyaluronate is a sulfate-free mucopolysaccharide containing equimolar proportions of glucuronic acid and N-acetyl glucosamine, forming a long-chain compound of high molecular weight. Hyaluronic acid of synovial fluid is a highly polymerized coiled molecule with a molecular weight of 1 to 10 million. At physiological pH, the glucuronic acid units lose a H^+ ion so that the resulting molecule bears a strong negative charge. The coiled network of negatively charged hyaluronic acid is thought to act as a filter, repelling anionic proteins and thus decreasing the apparent permeability of the synovial membrane. Hyaluronate also lends special viscous properties to the synovial fluid. Normal synovial fluid also contains peptides, albumin, globulins, and other proteins of molecular weights of less than 160,000. None of the recognized factors of the blood clotting system, including fibrinogen and prothrombin, are found in normal synovial fluid. Perhaps the most obvious function of synovial fluid is to lubricate the cartilage surfaces. The coefficient of friction between cartilage surfaces coated with synovial fluid is 0.001 compared with 0.05 for steel sliding on ice and 0.005 for wet ice against ice.

When injury occurs in the synovial membrane, particularly bacterial infection, the inflammatory response that ensues is responsible for many changes that occur in the normal character of the joint fluid. When infected, the synovium becomes hyperemic, and there is an increased production of fluid, which has the characteristics of a transudate or exudate.

Synovial A cells increase the production of hyaluronate, but the hyaluronate is of a lower molecular weight owing to decreased polymerization. Increased permeability of the synovial capillaries allows fibrin, complement, blood clotting factors, and leukocytes to enter the joint. Neutrophils drawn into the joint may release their lysosomal contents, resulting in the production of highly reactive superoxide radicals, which can depolymerize hyaluronate as well as take part in other reactions. Fibrin deposits adhere to articular cartilage and can interfere with proper cartilaginous nutrition from the adjacent synovial fluid and impede the release of metabolic by-products from the cartilage.[45] Fibrin may attract more leukocytes to the joint chemotactically; these cells phagocytize fibrin, and degranulation of the leukocytes may accentuate further synovial inflammation. Of particular importance in septic arthritis is the fact that fibrin clots isolate bacteria from antibiotics, antibodies, and phagocytic cells.

Cartilage destruction occurs in septic arthritis as a result of several factors. It has been shown that leukocytic release of lysozymes can promote connective tissue breakdown.[21] Leukocytic collagenases, proteases that attack protein polysaccharides, elastases, cathepsins D and E, and acid peptidases have been isolated.[55] Cartilage destruction probably is a result of two mechanisms. First, collagen fibrils are directly attacked by collagenases of leukocytic and synovial origin. Synovial fluids from patients with septic arthritis occurring acutely in a joint not previously affected with arthritis have demonstrated active collagenase activity that disappeared when leukocytic counts dropped to low levels as the infection was cured.[21] Secondly, and possibly more importantly, enzymatic attack occurs on the cartilage matrix. Lysosomal enzymes of synovial and leukocytic origin break down the cartilage matrix (proteoglycans), leaving the collagen fibrils without support. These, theoretically, are broken off and fragmented by the pressure and grinding of the affected joint.[15]

Diagnosis of Septic Arthritis

The clinical signs of septic arthritis are heat, pain, redness, and swelling of the joint with loss of function. Generally the presenting complaint is lameness, and the patient may be depressed, anorexic, and febrile. Occasionally patients have normal temperatures and leukocyte counts. The most consistent clinical signs of septic arthritis are lameness and palpable evidence of joint effusion. Palpation of the shoulder, elbow, carpus, stifle, and hock usually reveal swelling. Palpation of the hip joint is nearly futile except in very thin or young patients and in cats.

Radiographs are of little help in the diagnosis of septic arthritis. Early radiographic signs are nonspecific and are limited to thickening of the synovial membrane and joint capsule, widening of the joint spaces because of exudate accumulation, and irregular swelling of adjacent soft tissues. Later changes with progression of the disease include joint destruction, periarticular rarefaction, irregular joint surfaces, and, in some cases, fibrous and bony ankylosis.[8,40] In most cases by the time radiographic changes are seen, irreversible joint changes have occurred and treatment is limited to salvage of a useful limb through arthrodesis. In spite of finding no radiographic changes, radiographs should not be omitted from the patient's initial examination because of their value in determining the extent of the disease or the chances of finding pre-existing degenerative joint diseases or articular fractures.

Fine needle aspiration of the affected joint is the most reliable method of determining if infection is present. No anesthesia or heavy sedation is required for most taps, and elaborate draping and even surgical gloves are not required.[43] For most joints a 1-inch, 22-gauge needle and a 3-ml syringe is sufficient. Taps of the hip joint require a longer needle.

Synovial fluid volumes, even in inflamed joints, are often quite small. A great deal of information can be gained from a very small sample. In the case of a small fluid sample in the suspected septic joint, the following priorities are given to the fluid tested:

1. Culture: a single drop of synovial fluid is streaked directly on blood agar and incubated.

2. Smears: smears are made for Gram and differential staining.

3. EDTA: a small sample of the fluid is placed in an EDTA tube (or a heparin tube) for total nucleated cell counts.

4. The remaining fluid is used for total protein, glucose, and mucin clot tests.

Color, clarity, and viscosity of the fluid can be

TABLE 155–2. Synovial Fluid Changes in Various Types of Canine Arthritis*

Condition	Nucleated Cells/mm³	Differential (%)	
		Mononuclear	*Neutrophils*
Normal	250–3000	94–100	0–6
Degenerative Joint Disease	1000–5000	88–100	0–12
Erosive Arthritis (Rheumatoidlike)	8000–38,000	20–80	20–80
Non Erosive Arthritis (All Types)	4,400–371,000	5–85	15–95
Septic Arthritis	40,000–267,000	1–10	90–99

*Reprinted with permission from Pedersen, N. C., and Pool, R.: Canine joint disease. Vet. Clin. North Am., 8:465, 1978.

determined from the initial drop of fluid as it is placed on the blood agar.

Culture and sensitivity is the single most important test run on synovial fluid samples from suspected septic arthritis patients. A negative culture should not be taken as proof of the absence of joint sepsis. Studies in man and horses have shown that only 50 per cent of synovial fluid cultures from proven septic joints were positive.[5,30] In horses, 80 per cent of the horses from which no organism was recovered had been on systemic or local antibiotics prior to joint culture. It is imperative to culture joints when they are first examined, not after response to "shotgun" antibiotic therapy has failed.[30] If available, anaerobic cultures should also be taken.

Smears made for Gram staining and differential nucleated cell counts can be useful in determining the approximate total count if fluid volumes are insufficient. At the very least an impression can be gained of the approximate cell count, i.e., normal, mildly elevated, or greatly elevated.[43] A differential exam of synovial fluid cells should reveal increased cellularity with a large predominance of polymorphonuclear leukocytes in an infected joint (Table 155–2).

In the infected joint, high levels of fibrinogen and clotting factor often cause rapid clotting of the fluid after aspiration (Fig. 155–12). EDTA or heparin prevents clotting, permitting a total nucleated cell count. The normal fluid for nucleated cell counting contains 2 per cent acetic acid to lyse red blood cells. This cannot be used for cell counting in synovial fluid, as the acetic acid causes immediate clumping of the hyaluronate in the fluid. This, in fact, is the mucin clot test, which is designed to determine the quantity of hyaluronate in the fluid. Synovial fluid cell counts are generally done by hand with saline as the diluting fluid.

Synovial fluid proteins may be measured. Protein levels generally increase with any synovitis. This is not a change specific for septic arthritis. Total protein in normal synovia is generally less than 1.0 gm/dl; 2 to 3 gm/dl suggests inflammation, whereas 4 to 5 gm/dl suggests infection.[9] Glucose levels can be measured in synovial fluid and serum simultaneously.

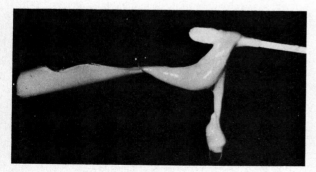

Figure 155–12. Joint aspirates from suspected septic joints must be placed into anticoagulants to prevent clotting. In the infected joint, a high fibrinogen and clotting factor content will often cause rapid clotting of the fluid.

Septic arthritis patients often have synovial glucose concentrations that are 50 per cent of the serum level.[56]

Treatment of Septic Arthritis

There are two equally important goals in the treatment of septic arthritis. The treatment must effectively sterilize the joint and remove the enzymes and fibrin debris that can potentially injure the articular cartilage. Both must be accomplished for satisfactory resolution of joint sepsis. One must act as soon as the diagnosis of septic arthritis is made, as early treatment is crucial to obtaining satisfactory results. All animals suspected of having septic arthritis are started on antibiotics immediately following arthrocentesis. Since over 50 per cent of all cases of septic arthritis are caused by S. aureus, a penicillinase-resistant synthetic penicillin or a cephalosporin is the usual choice while awaiting culture results.

In very early cases of septic arthritis a possible effective treatment is repeated needle aspirations or needle aspirations in conjunction with occasional distension-irrigation treatment. In this procedure the joint is injected with sterile saline until it is fully distended. If possible, distension is maintained for 10 to 15 minutes, then all fluids are aspirated from the joint. Some advocate the use of antiseptics, enzymes, detergents, and antibiotics in the lavage fluid; however, this remains controversial.[1,26,30,32,42,48] This type of lavage is rarely successful in well-developed cases because the fibrin clots quickly become too big and viscous to be removed by aspiration. In experimental staphylococcal gonitis in rabbits, the organization of the exudate by seven days was so advanced that surgical debridement was the only means of removal.[17]

Surgical debridement of the infected joint has many advantages: (1) it provides the best view of the extent of the joint injury, (2) it allows complete removal of the fibrin and pus from the joint, (3) it allows collection of a synovial membrane sample for culture, (4) it allows complete removal of any necrotic tissue, (5) it allows reconstruction of intra-articular fractures, (6) it allows accurate placement of irrigation tubes, and (7) it provides the best drainage of the joint.

Once good hemostasis has been achieved, all necrotic debris removed, and the joint lavaged, a decision must be made regarding closure of the joint. The goal following debridement is primary closure of the joint; however, this should only be done when debridement and lavage have eliminated all chances of recurring infection. In only a small minority of cases can the joint be primarily closed following debridement and lavage. Two options generally remain: (1) closure over drains and treatment with a distension-irrigation technique, and (2) nonclosure. There are advantages and disadvantages to both.

With the distension-irrigation treatment, at least two tubes are placed in the joint with exits through the skin at distant locations. The joint capsule is closed routinely with a nonabsorbable suture such as polypropylene. The joint is lavaged several times daily by gravity flow with a physiological fluid. The fluid of choice is a buffered isotonic, isosmotic fluid with a pH of 7.4. Normal saline (0.9%) has a pH of about 5.7, and lactated Ringer's solution has a pH of about 6.7. At each lavage the drainage tube is closed to allow fluid distension of the joint. After 10 to 15 minutes the fluid is thoroughly evacuated from the joint. There are several advantages to the distension-irrigation treatment: (1) repeated distension of the closed joint cavity tends to prevent and disrupt synovial adhesions that could later restrict joint motion, (2) without distension it has been shown that the fluid tends to take the most direct path to the drainage tube and does not adequately lavage the entire joint, (3) distension prevents the localization of pus and permits antibiotics to reach the farthest recesses of the joint cavity, and (4) distension can increase the amount of vascular synovium available for antibiotic absorption into the joint.[26]

Disadvantages of techniques that use suction-irrigation tubes are as follows: (1) they require more meticulous nursing care, (2) there is a substantial risk of introducing pathogenic organisms into a joint and the iatrogenic infection often involves highly resistant strains of gram-negative organisms such as *Pseudomonas* sp., and (3) tubes are often prematurely removed by uncooperative animal patients.

The techniques for nonclosure of the infected joint have several advantages. One common problem for which nonclosure is frequently indicated is shearing wounds of the carpus or tarsus. These wounds should never be closed for several reasons: (1) complete debridement is usually impossible with dirt ground into the bony tissues, (2) closure of the skin over these wounds usually results in excess tension in the skin, which is invariably followed by infection and wound dehiscence, and, possibly most importantly, (3) the ligamentous and capsular structures that have been ground away need the large granulation tissue bed that forms postoperatively. This tissue becomes dense fibrous tissue as it matures and provides excellent stability for the joints in place of the lost collateral ligaments (see Fig. 4–2 through 4–13).

When the joint is left open following thorough debridement and lavage, a fine mesh gauze is placed over the arthrotomy incisions. This is covered with a bulky absorptive dressing, which is covered with a cotton dressing. Daily bandage changes are required, and during this time the joint is moved passively through a complete range of motion to stimulate drainage of exudate and fibrin through the open incision. The wound is allowed to close by granulation and contraction.[5]

Following either distension-irrigation or nonclosure, the patient must be kept on antibiotics for at least two weeks after the cessation of all signs of joint disease. Caution should be taken in the consideration of local instillation of antibiotics into the affected joint. Numerous studies have shown that most antibiotics enter the joint fluid, particularly with synovitis, in levels equal to or greater than that of serum.[32] Intra-articular administration of antibiotics causes chemical synovitis, which may damage the cartilage.

Following resolution of a septic arthritis, prolonged rest is recommended. Passive motion only is given for the first seven to ten days, followed by a slow rehabilitation program. Three months should be allowed to pass before any vigorous exercise is allowed.

1. Alexander, J. W.: Septic arthritis: Diagnosis and treatment. J. Am. Anim. Hosp. Assoc. *14*:499, 1978.
2. Aron, D. N.: Pathogenesis, diagnosis, and management of osteomyelitis in small animals. Comp. Cont. Ed. *1*:824, 1979.
3. Ballard, A., Burkhalter, W. E., Mayfield, G. W., et al.: The functional treatment of pyogenic arthritis of the adult knee. J. Bone Joint Surg. *57A*:1119, 1975.
4. Brown, P. W.: The open fracture—cause, effect, and management. Clin. Orthop. Rel. Res. *96*:254, 1973.
5. Brown, S. G.: Infectious arthritis and wounds of joints. Vet. Clin. North Am. *8*:501, 1978.
6. Burri, C.: *Posttraumatic Osteomyelitis*. Hans Huber Publishers, Bern, 1975.
7. Butt, W. P.: The radiology of infection. Clin. Orthop. Rel. Res. *96*:20, 1973.
8. Butt, W. P.: Radiology of the infected joint. Clin. Orthop. Rel. Res. *96*:136, 1973.
9. Carb, A.: Suppurative arthritis. *In* Bojrab, M. J.: *Pathophysiology in Small Animal Surgery*. Lea & Febiger, Philadelphia, 1981.
10. Caywood, D. D.: Osteomyelitis in the dog. Small Anim. Vet. Med. Update Ser. *11*(2):1, 1979.
11. Caywood, D. D., Wallace, L. J., and Braden, T. D.: Osteomyelitis in the dog: A review of 67 cases. J. Am. Vet. Med. Assoc. *172*:943, 1978.
12. Clawson, D. K., Davis, F. J., and Hansen, S. T.: Treatment of chronic osteomyelitis with emphasis on closed suction-irrigation technique. Clin. Orthop. Rel. Res. *96*:88, 1973.
13. Clawson, D. K., and Dunn, A. W.: Management of common bacterial infections of bones and joints. J. Bone Joint Surg. *49A*:164, 1967.
14. Clawson, D. K., and Stevenson, J. K.: Treatment of chronic osteomyelitis. Surg. Obstet. Gynecol. *120*:59, 1965.
15. Curtiss, P. H., Jr.: Some uncommon forms of osteomyelitis. Clin. Orthop. Rel. Res. *96*:84, 1973.
16. Curtiss, P. H.: The pathophysiology of joint infections. Clin. Orthop. Rel. Res. *96*:129, 1973.
17. Daniel, D., and Akeson, W.: Lavage of septic joints in rabbits, effects of chondrolysis. J. Bone Joint Surg. *58A*:393, 1976.
18. Edlich, R. F., Rogers, W., and Kasper, G.: Studies in the management of contaminated wounds. Am. J. Surg. *117*:323, 1969.
19. Fitzgerald, R. H.: Laboratory diagnosis of postoperative sepsis of the musculoskeletal system. Orthop. Clin. North Am. *10*:361, 1979.
20. Gage, E. D.: Treatment of discospondylitis in the dog. J. Am. Vet. Med. Assoc. *166*:1164, 1975.
21. Harris, E. D., and Krane, S. M.: Collagenases. N. Engl. J. Med. *291*:557, 605, 652, 1974.
22. Hirsh, D. C., and Smith, T. M.: Osteomyelitis in the dog: Microorganisms isolated and susceptibility to antimicrobial agents. J. Small Anim. Pract. *19*:679, 1978.
23. Hogemann, K. E.: Treatment of infected bone defects with cancellous bone-chip grafts. Acta Chir. Scand. *98*:576, 1949.
24. Horwitz, T.: Surgical treatment of chronic osteomyelitis complicating fractures. Clin. Orthop. Rel. Res. *96*:118, 1973.

25. Hurov, L., Troy, G., and Turnwald, G.: Diskospondylitis in the dog: 27 cases. J. Am. Vet. Med. Assoc. 173:275, 1978.

26. Jackson, R. W., and Parsons, C. J.: Distension-irrigation treatment of major joint sepsis. Clin. Orthop. Rel. Res. 96:160, 1973.

27. Kahn, D. S., and Pritzker, K. P. H.: The pathophysiology of bone infection. Clin. Orthop. Rel. Res. 96:12, 1973.

28. Kawashima, M., Torisu, T., et al.: The treatment of pyogenic bone and joint infections by closed irrigation-suction. Clin. Orthop. Rel. Res. 148:240, 1980.

29. Kelly, P. J., Martin, W. J., and Coventry, M. B.: Chronic osteomyelitis II. Treatment with closed irrigation and suction. J. Am. Med. Assoc. 213:1843, 1970.

30. Koch, D. B.: Management of infectious arthritis in the horse. Comp. Cont. Ed. 1:s45, 1979.

31. Lawyer, R. B., and Eyring, E. J.: Intermittent closed suction-irrigation treatment of osteomyelitis. Clin. Orthop. Rel. Res. 88:80, 1972.

32. Leitch, M.: Diagnosis and treatment of septic arthritis in the horse. J. Am. Vet. Med. Assoc. 175:701, 1979.

33. Mackowiak, P. A., Jones, S. R., and Smith, J. W.: Diagnostic value of sinus-tract cultures in chronic osteomyelitis. J. Am. Med. Assoc. 239:2772, 1978.

34. Miller, J. B., Perman, V., Osborne, C. A., Hammer, R. F., and Gambardella, P. C.: Synovial fluid analysis in canine arthritis. J. Am. Anim. Hosp. Assoc. 10:392, 1974.

35. Norden, C. W.: Experimental osteomyelitis. I. A description of the model. J. Infect. Dis. 122:410, 1970.

36. Norden, C. W.: Experimental osteomyelitis. II. Therapeutic trials and measurement of antibiotic levels in bone. J. Infect. Dis. 124:565, 1971.

37. Nunamaker, D. M.: Management of infected fractures—osteomyelitis. Vet. Clin. North Am. 5:259, 1975.

38. deOliveira, J. C.: Bone grafts and chronic osteomyelitis. J. Bone Joint Surg. 53B:672, 1971.

39. Overton, L. M., and Tully, W. P.: Surgical treatment of chronic osteomyelitis in long bones. Am. J. Surg. 126:736, 1975.

40. Owens, J. M., and Ackerman, N.: Roentgenology of arthritis. Vet. Clin. North Am. 8:453, 1978.

41. Papineau, L. J., Alfageme, A., Dalcourt, J. P., and Pilon, L.: Ostéomyélite Chronique: Excision et Greffe de Spongieux à l'air Libre après Mises a Plat Extensives. Int. Orthop. 3:165, 1979.

42. Patzakis, M. J., Dorr, L. D., et al.: The early management of open joint injuries. J. Bone Joint Surg. 57A:1065, 1975.

43. Pedersen, N. C.: Synovial fluid collection and analysis. Vet. Clin. North Am. 8:495, 1978.

44. Pedersen, N. C., and Pool, R.: Canine joint disease. Vet. Clin. North Am. 8:465, 1978.

45. Resnick, D., and Niwayama, G.: *Diagnosis of Bone and Joint Disorders.* W. B. Saunders, Philadelphia, 1981.

46. Septimus, E. J., and Musher, D. M.: Osteomyelitis: Recent clinical and laboratory aspects. Orthop. Clin. North Am. 10:347, 1979.

47. Shannon, J. G., Woolhouse, F. M., and Eisinger, P. J.: The treatment of chronic osteomyelitis by saucerization and immediate skin grafting. Clin. Orthop. Rel. Res. 96:98, 1973.

48. Siemering, B.: Painful joints—A review of rheumatoid arthritis, systemic lupus erythematous (sic), infectious arthritis, and degenerative joint disease. Comp. Cont. Ed. 1:213, 1979.

49. Smith, C. W., Schiller, A. G., et al.: Osteomyelitis in the dog: a retrospective study. J. Am. Anim. Hosp. Assoc. 14:589, 1978.

50. Trueta, J.: The 3 types of acute hematogenous osteomyelitis. J. Bone Joint Surg. 41B:671, 1959.

51. Tuli, S. M.: Bridging of bone defects by massive bone grafts in tumorous conditions and in osteomyelitis. Clin. Orthop. Rel. Res. 87:60, 1972.

52. Waldvogel, F. A., Medoff, G., and Swartz, M. N.: Osteomyelitis: A review of clinical features, therapeutic considerations and unusual aspects. N. Engl. J. Med. 282:198, 260, 316, 1970.

53. Waldvogel, F. A., and Vasey, H.: Osteomyelitis: The past decade. N. Engl. J. Med. 303:360, 1980.

54. Walker, M. A., Lewis, R. E., et al.: Radiographic signs of bone infection in small animals. J. Am. Vet. Med. Assoc. 166:908, 1975.

55. Weissmann, G.: Lysosomal mechanisms of tissue injury in arthritis. N. Engl. J. Med. 286:141, 1972.

56. Werner, L. L.: Arthrocentesis and joint fluid analysis: Diagnostic applications in joint diseases of small animals. Comp. Cont. Ed. 1:855, 1979.

57. West, W. F., Kelly, P. J., and Martin, W. J.: Chronic osteomyelitis. I. Factors affecting the results of treatment in 186 patients. J. Am. Med. Assoc. 213:1837, 1970.

58. Wingfield, W. E.: Surgical treatment of chronic osteomyelitis in dogs. J. Am. Anim. Hosp. Assoc. 11:568, 1975.

59. Winter, F. E.: The surgical treatment of pyogenic osteomyelitis. Clin. Orthop. Rel. Res. 51:139, 1962.

60. Winters, J. L., and Cahen, I.: Acute hematogenous osteomyelitis: A review of sixty-six cases. J. Bone Joint Surg. 42A:691, 1960.

Chapter **156**

Bone Grafting

Sharon Stevenson

A properly applied bone graft is often the critical factor differentiating a successful fracture repair from a nonunion or the possibility of a limb salvage procedure from the necessity of an amputation. Considerable data have been accumulated since bone grafts were introduced into general surgical practice in 1915,[2] and the principles of bone grafting have been well established. Early grafts provided mechanical stability, but, since the development of metal implants, the bone graft has been valued more as a source of osteocytes and as a scaffold for the ingrowth of new host bone.[18] Many types of grafts are available, each with its own advantages and disadvantages. The most commonly used bone graft in veterinary surgery is the fresh cancellous autograft, which has the advantages of histocompatibility, live cells, and excellent osteogenic potential. If the graft must provide mechanical stability or fill large defects, cortical bone is preferable. Cortical bone grafts are often collected and preserved not only for convenience but also to reduce the immunogenicity of foreign donor cells implanted into the host. The various methods of preservation affect the properties of the bone graft and its rate of incorporation by the host differently.

This chapter discusses the various histological types of grafts and their normal incorporation. The methods of preservation of bone grafts and their effects on incorporation and antigenicity are presented. The specific indications for bone grafts in veterinary surgery are detailed, and the preferred techniques for harvesting and handling bone grafts are defined.

BONE GRAFT TERMINOLOGY

The terminology employed in clinical transplantation is quite exact, and, in the case of bone, is complicated by the various histological types of bone grafts.[82] The basic differentiation made is between *implants* and *grafts*. The term *graft* implies the transfer of living tissue, whereas *implant* refers to nonviable material placed in the body. Implant is also commonly used to describe nonbiological materials, such as metal or ceramic prostheses, in addition to dead bone, e.g., frozen or freeze-dried cortical bone. The next level of description refers to the origin of the graft. A graft moved from one site to another within the same individual is an autograft; the adjective is autologous, autogenous, or autochthonous. An allograft (adjective: allogeneic) is tissue transferred between two genetically different individuals of the same species. A xenograft is tissue of one species implanted into a member of a different species (adjective: xenogeneic).

Two special situations of grafting exist. When tissue from one twin is implanted into an identical, monozygotic twin, an isograft (adjective: isogeneic) occurs. Artificially inbred strains of mice are the second special situation. These animals are virtually identical genetically, and tissues transferred between them are also termed isografts (adjective: syngeneic).

The site of graft placement is either orthotopic (anatomically appropriate) or heterotopic (anatomically inappropriate). Additionally, bone grafts can constitute wholly cancellous bone, wholly cortical bone, corticocancellous bone, or bone and articular cartilage (osteochondral). The addition of fresh cancellous bone or bone marrow to a preserved alloimplant is known as a composite graft. Thus, fresh cancellous bone harvested from the proximal humerus and packed around a comminuted radial fracture in the dog is an orthotopic cancellous autograft. An example of an orthotopic cortical alloimplant is a frozen, banked, femoral diaphyseal graft replacing bone loss due to fracture comminution.

Bone grafts can be further described as fresh or preserved. Fresh grafts are transferred directly from the donor to the recipient site and are almost always autografts. Fresh grafts may be vascularized grafts, transferred with their blood vessels, which are then anastomosed to vessels at the recipient site. The more common fresh bone graft is the free graft. It is not vascularized and, therefore, depends on the ingrowth of host vessels for cellular nutrition.

Bone grafts may be preserved by freezing, freeze-drying, irradiation, autoclaving, or chemical preservation. Cell death results from all these techniques, and the graft functions mainly as a space filler and a scaffold for the ingrowth of new host bone. Maintenance of sterility is of primary concern with any of the preservation methods.

FUNCTIONS OF BONE GRAFTS

Osteogenesis

Bone grafts serve one or both of two main functions: as a source of osteogenesis and as a mechanical support. Osteogenesis refers to bone formation with no indication of cellular origin. When new bone is formed on or about a graft it may be either of graft origin, i.e., from cells that survived the transfer and are capable of forming bone, or from cells of host origin. Surface cells on cortical and cancellous grafts that are properly handled can survive and produce new bone.[5, 7, 39] (See Harvesting and Handling of Grafts/Implants.) This early bone formed by viable graft cells is often critical in callus formation[5] during the first four to eight weeks after surgery. Cancellous bone, with its very large surface area covered by quiescent lining cells or active osteoblasts, obviously has the potential for more graft-origin new bone formation than does cortical bone. However, heterotopically placed fresh isografts of rat femoral cortex did produce new bone as measured by radioactive strontium incorporation.[39] More than 50 per cent of the new bone was produced by endosteal lining cells and marrow stroma, 30 per cent was contributed by periosteal cells, and osteocytes accounted for only about 10 per cent of new bone formed. The absolute quantity of new bone formed by fresh cortical autografts is probably quite small compared with that formed by fresh cancellous autografts, but it may be helpful in graft incorporation.

The second way in which a bone graft may function as a source of osteogenesis is by being osteoinductive. Osteoinduction is the recruitment of mesenchymal-type cells, which then differentiate into cartilage- and bone-forming cells. Differentiation is probably modulated by bone morphogenic protein (BMP), which is hydrophobic, nonspecies-specific glycoprotein that has been extracted from bone and dentin matrix as well as from various bone tumors.[61, 86] Its presence is most convincingly demonstrated when the matrix is demineralized and sequentially extracted to remove any antigenic materials. The activity of BMP does not require viable graft cells, as it is a property of the bone matrix. Therefore, activity is present not only in fresh autografts and isografts but also in alloimplants that are preserved in a manner that does not destroy it. BMP activity has been demonstrated in frozen, freeze-dried, and decalcified, extracted alloimplants; autoclaving definitely destroys BMP activity.[55, 86]

These two modes of osteogenesis by bone grafts and implants illustrate the two current theories of the origin of bone cells in postfetal life. The first theory asserts that bone develops from pre-existing bone, particularly osteoprogenitor cells of the periosteum, endosteum, and marrow reticulum. The second theory addresses the problem of a source of osteoprogenitor cells and states that new osteoprogenitor cells are recruited by induction of residual mesenchymal cells in marrow reticulum endosteum, periosteum, and connective tissue. The first theory implies that the soft tissue bed is not important except as it affects bone blood supply. Critical importance is attributed to the soft tissues surrounding a graft by the second theory since they may be the source of new bone-forming cells. Osteoclasts and osteoclast precursors, on the other hand, are derived from bloodborne cells. Therefore, adequate vascularization is an absolute requirement for bone resorption and remodeling.

Mechanical Support

When placed in large defects from trauma or en bloc resection of neoplastic bone, bone grafts and implants act as weight-bearing space fillers or struts. Before the development of large, rigid metal implants, bone grafts had to provide their own stability and fixation in addition to maintaining the mechanical integrity of a bone or limb. Now, much of the weight-bearing function and all the stability can be supplied by rigid internal fixation. Thus, the bone graft or implant bears some weight and functions as classically described as "a trellis, or scaffold, for the ingrowth of new host bone."[18]

The three-dimensional process of ingrowth of sprouting capillaries, perivascular tissue, and osteoprogenitor cells from the recipient bed into the structure of an implant or graft is termed *osteoconduction*. Osteoconduction may result from osteoinduction, e.g., in a fresh cortical autograft, or it may occur without active participation of the implant, as is the case in porous ceramic or mineral apatite implants. It is important to note that osteoconduction is not random; indeed, it follows an ordered, predictable spatial pattern. *Creeping substitution* is an older term, coined before the development of ceramic and metal prostheses, that describes the gradual resorption of the graft or implant and replacement of it by new host bone. The theoretical end-point of creeping substitution is complete disappearance of the graft or implant and concurrent deposition and remodeling of host bone. The terms *osteoconduction* and *remodeling* are used in preference to creeping substitution in this chapter.

INCORPORATION OF BONE GRAFTS/IMPLANTS

There are recognized phases in the incorporation of bone grafts, just as there are in fracture healing.[59, 65, 91] The word *incorporation* is preferable to *healing* when discussing grafts, since the processes of new host bone formation on graft surfaces and remodeling of new host and old graft bone may never be completely resolved. The graft may function quite normally and be as biomechanically strong as normal host bone but still consist of 80 per cent dead bone. Therefore, it is very difficult to determine an end-point where one can call a graft "healed" even though it is adequately incorporated.

Radiology, histology, bone scintigraphy, and biomechanical testing are commonly used to measure and evaluate the incorporation of bone grafts. One must be careful when evaluating scintiscans, because even a thin layer of osteoblasts and new bone on the surface of an otherwise dead cortical graft will give a positive scintiscan.[6] A positive scan, when performed in the first week following implantation of a vascularized graft, does indicate microvascular patency and the probability that the osteocytes and osteoblasts are alive. Radiology is extremely helpful in evaluating the incorporation of cancellous autografts clinically; it is less helpful with large alloimplants of cortical bone because the denseness of the cortical implant makes subtle changes more difficult to see. Since the radiographic appearance and biomechanical strength of the graft reflect the cellular events taking place, the histological incorporation process is described and related to results of other methods of evaluation.

Cancellous Autografts

Phase I: Inflammation. Inflammatory changes occur within minutes to hours of the surgical procedure, and many of the cells die, particularly osteocytes in trabecular lacunae. As multiple vascular buds infiltrate the transplant bed, lymphocytes, plasma cells, and mononuclear cells appear throughout the area. By the second week the inflammatory process subsides, fibrous granulation tissue becomes increasingly dominant in the area, and osteoclastic activity increases.[13] Phase I lasts up to one week in cancellous autografts.

Phases II and III: Vascularization and Osteoinduction. Vascularization of cancellous grafts can occur as early as two days after implantation under favorable circumstances.[71] Because cancellous bone is quite porous, host vessels, osteoblasts, and osteoblast precursors can easily infiltrate the graft from the periphery toward the center. As osteoclast precursors are bloodborne, the ingrowth of host vessels marks the beginning of graft resorption.

During this phase of graft incorporation, the host immune system becomes sensitized to donor antigens. Autografts do not elicit an immune response,

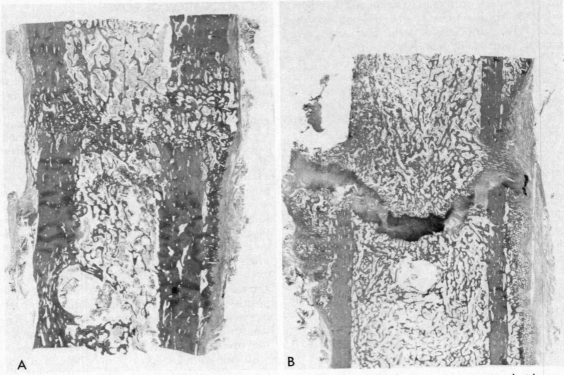

Figure 156–1. The effect of cancellous bone grafts on gap healing in femoral diaphyses. The femurs were osteotomized with an oscillating bone saw, a 3-mm wafer of bone was removed, and the bones were stabilized with 4.5-mm broad DC plates. *A,* A femur in which the 3-mm gap was packed with cancellous autograft. At six weeks postoperatively, the gap is bridged by bone tissue and remodeling is evident. *B,* When the gap is left empty, the space fills with fibrous connective tissue, cartilage, or fibrocartilage (the dark tissue). These tissues may eventually mineralize and be replaced with osseous tissue, but the bone is unstable much longer than when a cancellous bone graft is inserted.

but allografts or alloimplants may be sufficiently immunogenic to stimulate a humoral and cellular response that slows or even blocks subsequent phases of incorporation. Vascularization of cancellous autografts is usually complete by two weeks.

Phase IV: Osteoconduction. As the vascular invasion of the cancellous graft proceeds, primitive mesenchymal cells differentiate into osteogenic cells. Osteoblasts are seen lining the edges of dead trabeculae and depositing a seam of osteoid that eventually surrounds a central core of dead bone. Thus, radiographically an initial increase in the radiodensity of the transplanted area occurs. Subsequently, the graft is remodeled, i.e., the new host bone and entrapped cores of necrotic bone are gradually resorbed by osteoclasts. At this point, a decrease in the overall density of the cancellous transplant is noted. Concurrently, hematopoietic marrow elements accumulate within the transplanted bone. Because necrosis of bone does not alter its mechanical strength,[29] the cancellous graft is first strengthened by the addition of new bone. As remodeling proceeds, the mechanical strength of the transplanted area returns to normal.[13] The period of osteoconduction and remodeling may last up to several months in a cancellous autograft; it may persist for years in large alloimplants (Fig. 156–1).

Phase V: Mechanical. The final phase of bone graft incorporation rarely occurs in cancellous autografts

because usually they are completely resorbed and replaced by viable new bone.[13] During this phase of incorporation, nonviable, nonresorbed grafted material remains and functions in a mechanical, weight-bearing, or stress-transmitting fashion. The percentage of the graft or implant that remains in original form is variable but may approach 90 per cent in humans.[86] It should be noted that grafts are remodeled in response to the same mechanical stimuli (i.e., Wolff's law) as normal skeletal bone.[53] A graft placed subcutaneously or as an onlay graft is often completely resorbed with little or no new bone apposition[6] because the graft is not mechanically stressed. Conversely, when a graft is placed as a weight-bearing strut in a long bone segmental defect, it is remodeled similarly to the normal segment that it replaced, both spatially and temporally.

Cortical Autografts

Inflammatory changes noted after implantation of a cortical autograft do not vary significantly from those noted after placement of cancellous autologous bone. However, the rate of revascularization of cortical autografts is markedly slower than that of cancellous autografts. Generally, the cortical graft is not penetrated by blood vessels until the sixth day. Complete revascularization usually occurs within one to two months, or at least twice the time span required for cancellous transplants.[13] This delay in complete revascularization may be attributed to the structure of cortical bone, since vascular penetration of the transplant is primarily the result of peripheral osteoclastic resorption and vascular infiltration of Volkmann's and haversian canals.[29] Rapid vascular penetration may be enhanced by drilling holes (500/μ in diameter) in cortical autografts.[12] Holes of this size do not weaken the bone and may enhance early vascular ingrowth and new bone formation. However, at 24 weeks after grafting no significant difference in incorporation between cortical autografts with and without holes is seen.

A second major difference between the incorporation of cortical and cancellous autografts is that repair of cortical grafts is first initiated by osteoclasts[29] rather than by osteoblasts. Resorption of cortical bone at two weeks after transplantation was found to be significantly greater than that of normal bone, to increase until the sixth week, and to gradually decline to nearly normal levels by the end of one year.[18, 29] Radiographically, an increase in lucency is noted, and the graft is significantly weaker than normal bone. This mechanical weakness first becomes measurable at six weeks after transplantation and persists at least six months in canine segmental fibular autografts. New bone formation proceeds slowly, and the strength of the transplant returns to normal by one year,[29] even though 40 per cent of the necrotic graft bone remains. The radiographic appearance may not correlate well with actual mechanical strength, which complicates the clinical decision of metal implant removal. Additionally, while resorption proceeds independently of the general metabolic state, apposition of new bone is influenced by the anabolic state of the animal, by drugs such as methotrexate and doxorubicin (Adriamycin), and by radiation therapy.[16, 29, 32] Grafts of animals treated with those drugs or radiation demonstrate significantly less new bone formation while resorption continues normally, compared with untreated controls. These parallel processes result in grafts that are significantly weaker than control untreated grafts.[70]

As mentioned previously, the fifth, or mechanical, phase of bone graft incorporation is predominantly a feature of cortical grafts and implants. Although resorption is more active in cortical grafts than in the rest of the skeleton for up to one year, the osteoconductive remodeling process does not continue until all the grafted bone is removed and replaced by new host bone, as in cancellous grafts. Necrotic haversian canals are enlarged by osteoclasts; in fact, resorption consistently involves only osteonal systems and does not remove interstitial lamellae. These unreplaced necrotic lamellae account for the graft matrix that remains at eight weeks postoperatively. Because dead bone matrix is as strong as live bone matrix, this mixture of graft interstitial lamellae and new host osteons is as strong as control segments of bone.[29] The mechanical weakness noted during early phases

of graft incorporation, therefore, is related directly to the porosity that occurs during remodeling. It is not known whether necrotic interstitial lamellae are ever completely removed.

Vascularized Grafts

Vascularized grafts are not commonly used in veterinary clinical practice because of the technical difficulty of microvascular anastomoses and because of the expensive equipment required for microsurgery. However, some experimental work has been done that clarifies the techniques and incorporation of vascularized bone autografts in the dog.[6, 26, 37, 79] When the vessels are successfully anastomosed and the graft suffers only transient, intraoperative ischemia, over 90 per cent of osteocytes survive the transplantation procedure.[26] Graft-host union occurs quickly,[26, 37] and resorption followed by osteoconduction and remodeling, as consistently observed in free cortical grafts, is not seen.[26] Correct microvascular techniques as well as rigid internal fixation are very important for successful incorporation of vascularized grafts.[37] Successful transplantation of vascularized rib grafts into segmental femoral defects[26] and of vascularized entire knee joints[37] has been achieved in dogs. Because the vascular tree of the graft is anastomosed directly to that of the recipient, vascularized allografts and implants are probably more immunogenic than are nonvascularized allografts. As will be discussed later, sensitization of the donor is predominantly a response to recipient cell surface histocompatibility antigens (see Chapter 15, Transplantation Immunology). Recipients are exposed to more living donor cells, particularly endothelial and marrow cells, with vascularized grafts, and examples of acute rejection have been seen.[37]

Osteochondral Grafts

Two major types of osteochondral grafts are used: very thin, so-called shell grafts (articular cartilage plus 2 to 8 mm of subchondral bone)[54] and massive grafts that may include the entire metaphysis, epiphysis, and articular cartilage of a long bone.[57, 69] Shell grafts are generally used for joint resurfacing in the treatment of trauma or arthritis. Shell autografts are incorporated quickly and completely when fixation is adequate. The subchondral bone retains its supportive function throughout replacement so no distortion of the articular surface occurs.[54] Shell allografts, on the other hand, are subject to late pannus formation, and humoral antibodies to donor antigens have been identified.[74] Massive osteochondral grafts are almost always frozen alloimplants and are used in limb salvage procedures following en bloc tumor excision[57, 69] or massive trauma.[43] Although experimental massive autografts function quite well,[20] both experimental and clinical massive alloimplants show late complications, including subchondral bone collapse, cartilage erosion and fibrillation, luxations, and fractures of the grafts.[20, 69, 80] Originally it was thought that cartilage was not antigenic,[57] but recent work has demonstrated that chondrocytes do display histocompatibility antigens[72] and that components of cartilage matrix can stimulate a humoral and cellular immune response in dogs receiving osteochondral allografts.[93, 94] Because the appearance of antibodies and cells that are specific for cartilage matrix components corresponds temporally with destructive pannus formation by the synovium, it is now thought that the immune response is very important in long-term cartilage allograft survival and function.[93, 94]

Factors Affecting Incorporation of Bone Grafts and Implants

The factors that affect the incorporation of bone grafts and implants can be divided into two categories: those resulting from the surgical technique and those related to graft and implant immunogenicity and method of preservation.

Surgical Technique

The first and foremost requirement for the successful incorporation of any graft is absolute *stability*. Small cancellous autografts may be osteogenic enough for their cells to divide, to produce new bone, and eventually to stabilize themselves by callus formation,[5] but cortical grafts of any type fail when inadequately fixed.[46, 53, 77, 81] Small vascular buds are unable to penetrate the cortex and begin resorption of haversian systems because of the trauma of persistent movement. Without this invasion of vessels, no new bone can be formed, and sequestration almost invariably results. This principle has been proved experimentally in dogs,[53, 77] and veterinary clinical reports confirm the absolute necessity of rigid internal fixation with large cortical grafts.[46, 81]

Postoperative infection is also catastrophic and usually requires graft removal or even amputation for resolution.[46, 57, 69] For this reason it is inadvisable to insert a large alloimplant in a contaminated or previously operated site.[46] Cancellous autograft, however, may be used to great advantage in the treatment of osteomyelitis,[68, 84] provided certain guidelines are followed (see later section, Indications for Bone Grafts/Implants).

Graft/Implant Immunogenicity and Methods of Preservation

Differences in incorporation are noted in fresh allografts compared with fresh autografts and also in alloimplants preserved by various methods, even under optimal conditions of sterility and stability. Because osteocytes, chondrocytes, and marrow cells display histocompatibility antigens,[72] and humoral and cellular immune responses to donor histocompatibility antigens have been noted experimentally and clinically,[27, 34, 35, 41, 63, 87] the immune response is thought to modulate graft/implant revascularization and remodeling. Recent work has demonstrated that matching for histocompatibility antigens favorably affects incorporation of fresh and frozen canine allografts.[10, 83] Before the advent of tissue antigen matching, it was noted that fresh allografts were incorporated slowly or not at all, and many methods of preservation were developed to reduce the antigenicity of the graft and to provide a convenient means of storage.[18]

Fresh Cancellous and Cortical Allografts

The early phase of inflammation following implantation of fresh allografts is similar to that seen following implantation of autografts. However, beginning with the second week and continuing up to two months, lymphocytes are the major cell type present.[8] The most noticeable differences between the incorporation of autografts and allografts are the *rate* and pattern of revascularization.[36] Although the initial ingrowth of new host vessels may occur quite rapidly, these vessels are quickly surrounded by inflammatory cells, become occluded, and undergo hyaline degeneration.[8, 13, 18, 42] Subsequently, progressive necrosis of graft cells occurs. Owing to the impaired revascularization of bone allografts, the remodeling of both cortical and cancellous bone is delayed.[18] Once the allograft undergoes necrosis as a result of vascular insufficiency, a second phase of osteogenesis may be initiated by the host approximately four weeks after transplantation.[13, 42]

This second phase of osteogenesis in allografts is not as successful as osteogenesis in autografts and results in only a little remodeling and osteoconduction.[8, 9, 19] Cortical allografts remain significantly weaker than cortical autografts at least six months after transplantation.[13] However, after one year sufficient osteoconduction has occurred for allografts and autografts to be biomechanically and structurally similar, although more unremodeled, necrotic bone is noted in allografts.[18, 42] Variations in this pattern have been noted, ranging from absolute rejection with fibrous tissue encapsulation to incorporation only slightly slower than that of autografts.[28] These variations in host-allograft interaction are probably due to differences in graft immunogenicity and host responsiveness (see Chapter 15, Transplantation Immunology).

Primarily because of graft immunogenicity and the ensuing slowness or lack of incorporation, fresh allografts are only marginally satisfactory,[13, 21] and preserved alloimplants are preferred by most surgeons. Any method of preservation results in death of cells; however, some preserved alloimplants are still immunogenic, probably owing to intact antigens present on the surface of necrotic cells. Ideally, a method of preservation preserves the implant's ability to stimulate osteogenesis while eliminating its antigenicity. Many of the methods that adequately reduce the immunogenicity also destroy the ability of the implant to induce new bone formation; in fact, revascularization and accompanying resorption are often markedly impaired. Sterility is of primary concern with any method of preservation because of the catastrophic effects of infection on implant incorporation.

Boiled, Autoclaved, Deproteinized, and Merthiolated Alloimplants

Although these methods remove most of the immunogenicity of alloimplants, they also remove any capacity for osteoinduction.[18, 76] Treated bone is resistant to revascularization and remodeling by the host. Because of these experimental observations as well as extremely poor clinical results, these methods of preservation are rarely used.[13] Occasionally, following an operating room mishap, autologous bone is autoclaved and reinserted in a fracture site. It should be remembered that this process has turned an autograft into a functional alloimplant by denaturing the bone proteins. Although probably not antigenic, the autoimplant is very slowly revascularized and remodeled and requires absolute stability for a much longer period of time than the usual fresh fracture. There have been reports of successful clinical use of autoclaved segments of neoplastic and traumatized bone.[18, 24]

Decalcified Bone

Bone decalcified by hydrochloric acid retains its osteoinductive capacity, probably because of the persistence of BMP.[18] This bone has little strength and cannot be used as a weight-bearing strut. Reports conflict regarding its revascularization and remodeling.[18] Although probably preferable to boiling, autoclaving, deproteinizing, and merthiolation, decalcification as a means of implant preservation has largely been replaced by freezing and freeze-drying.

Frozen Alloimplants

Frozen alloimplants are less immunogenic than fresh allografts[34] and retain the ability to induce osteogenesis.[18] Although revascularization and remodeling are delayed compared with fresh autografts, resorption and osteoconduction occur more rapidly and completely in frozen implants than in fresh allografts.[42] When stable, even massive frozen alloimplants are incorporated well and have been clinically satisfactory in cats and humans.[45, 57] Less favorable results have been noted in dogs, probably because of inadequate fixation.[46]

Freeze-Dried Alloimplants

The freeze-drying process does not hinder implant incorporation, as freeze-dried autologous bone is repaired similarly to fresh autologous bone.[17] Experimental studies indicate that the antigenicity of freeze-dried alloimplants is minimal.[34] However, the use of freeze-dried alloimplants, although more successful than fresh allografts, results in significantly increased nonunions compared with autografts.[17] Revascularization and remodeling occur similarly to frozen alloimplants. Freeze-drying alters the mechanical properties of the bone, resulting in microfractures and brittleness. Therefore, implants must be carefully handled and protected with internal fixation devices.[13] Long-term complications of freeze-dried alloimplants are similar to those of frozen alloimplants and include fatigue fractures, nonunion or delayed graft-host union, and occasionally complete implant resorption.[13, 21]

Xenoimplants

Xenoimplants, usually of processed calf bone, were popular about 20 years ago.[56] The implants generally were deproteinized and freeze-dried or chemically treated.[18] Extremely slow resorption and osteoconduction have been observed following implantation of these materials, and they are now rarely used. Some nonosseous materials are currently being tested for use as bone implants. These materials, e.g., certain ceramics and coral skeletons, are similar in structure to cancellous bone. Osteoconduction, but not osteoinduction, occurs, and osteoclastic resorption and remodeling of these materials have been documented.[38, 47] They are not antigenic and, when combined with fresh autogenous cancellous bone as a source of osteogenesis, may be a good alternative to alloimplants.

Immunosuppression

An alternative to selecting an alloimplant that is minimally immunogenic is to choose an allograft that is maximally osteogenic (e.g., fresh allograft) and to suppress the immune response of the recipient. Azathioprine and cyclosporin A are the drugs most commonly used for this purpose. Normal autograft incorporation in dogs is not inhibited by 4 mg/kg/day of azathioprine for 21 days, followed by 2 mg/kg/day for six months.[14] Indeed, both short-term (six weeks) and long-term (six months) administration of azathioprine enhanced fresh cortical allograft incorporation in dogs.[1, 14, 15] Even fresh vascularized allogenic osteochondral grafts, which are highly antigenic, benefited from a combination of antilymphocyte serum, azathioprine, and prednisolone.[37] The side effects of azathioprine include delayed wound healing of skin, absolute lymphopenia, increased susceptibility to infection, and even death.[1, 14]

Summary

Fresh autologous cancellous bone is incorporated the most rapidly of any graft; it contributes to osteogenesis both by survival of graft cells and by induction of new bone formation at the graft site. Fresh autogenous cortical bone is incorporated more slowly because of its dense structure; osteoclasts must carve openings through necrotic haversian systems to allow revascularization. Fresh allogeneic bone is subject to attack by the immune system of the recipient; thus, its course of incorporation is less predictable but is certainly slower and less complete than that of autografts. Preserved alloimplants are useful when they retain some osteoinductive capacity while being minimally immunogenic. Xenoimplants and some of the preserved alloimplants are not very biologically acceptable, and they are poorly incorporated. Ceramics and coral skeletons may be adequate osteoconductors but are currently experimental. Certain immunosuppressive drugs enhance the incorporation of immunogenic allografts and implants by abrogating the immune response of the recipient without inhibiting new bone formation.

INDICATIONS FOR BONE GRAFTS/IMPLANTS

If rapid formation of large amounts of new bone is required, e.g., for an arthrodesis or for defects in a reconstructed comminuted fracture, cancellous autografts are clearly superior to allografts of any kind. When the graft functions primarily as a weight-bearing strut and can be stabilized with internal fixation for a relatively long period, allografts are an acceptable alternative to autologous bone. A frozen cortical alloimplant will *never* be incorporated when placed in an infected bed and inadequately stabilized. It would be far better to apply external fixation, treat the infection vigorously, and consider a delayed grafting procedure.

In general, there are two principal indications for bone grafts: to enhance healing and to replace bone lost through trauma or surgical resection.[49, 66] These indications are not mutually exclusive: in a severely comminuted fracture, both characteristics may be desirable. Specific clinical indications are listed next.

Enhancement of Healing

Comminuted or Retarded Fractures. All comminuted fractures benefit from a graft of autologous cancellous bone. Many comminuted fractures have avascular fragments that have a tendency to be resorbed. Additionally, it is not always possible to achieve stable internal fixation. Thus, the early and vigorous production of new bone originating from and stimulated by fresh autologous cancellous bone is extremely helpful.[49, 66] The mechanical stability provided by this early callus may prevent fatigue and eventual failure of the metal implant. Even simple fractures of bones known to be slow to heal (e.g., the distal radius in small breed dogs) benefit from the osteogenesis provided by a cancellous autograft (Figs. 156–2 and 156–3).

Arthrodesis

When an arthrodesis is performed, for whatever reason, it is of utmost importance to achieve a stable

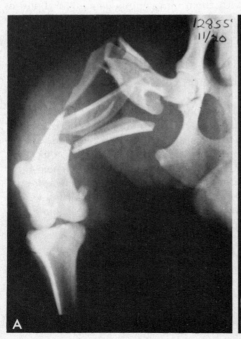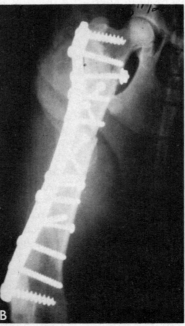

Figure 156–2. A, This preoperative radiograph demonstrates potentially avascular fragments in this comminuted femoral fracture. *B*, Uncomplicated healing was achieved in ten months following reconstruction and stabilization with interfragmentary lag screws and a neutralization plate. Large amounts of fresh autogenous cancellous bone were packed around the fracture surfaces. When the dog was in lateral recumbency for the femoral repair, both tibias and the ipsilateral humerus were accessible for graft harvest. (Courtesy of Dr. R. Bruce Hohn.)

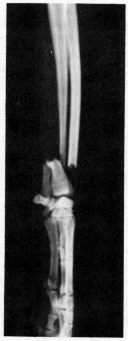

Figure 156–3. This distal radial fracture in a 5-kg dog was treated by external coaptation, resulting in a nonunion. An autogenous cancellous graft and internal fixation would probably have provided sufficient stability and osteogenic stimulus to successfully unite this slowly healing fracture.

bony union of the joint surfaces as quickly as possible. For a successful arthrodesis, the surgeon must (1) achieve rigid internal fixation, which is usually supplemented with temporary external fixation; (2) fuse the joint in a functional anatomical position; (3) remove *all* cartilage; and (4) implant a fresh autologous cancellous or corticocancellous bone graft.[62] The usefulness of autogenous cancellous and corticocancellous bone has been confirmed by numerous clinical reports.[62, 66, 88] and by an experimental study.[51] When carpi were stabilized with rigid internal fixation, significantly more new bone formation and bone remodeling were seen in grafted than nongrafted joint spaces.[51] The autografts were well incorporated by eight weeks after surgery. This early production of new bone with accompanying increase in mechanical stability may permit early removal of external coaptation devices.

Nonunions

Although the majority of nonunions following fractures of long bones in dogs are proliferative and are adequately treated by rigid internal fixation with compression if possible,[78] avascular and infected nonunions profit greatly from internal fixation augmented by an autologous cancellous bone graft. Avascular nonunions often occur in the distal radius or ulna of small breeds and in other bones with poor blood supply.[66, 88] Sclerotic bone ends are curetted to bleeding bone, if possible, and an abundance of fresh

autologous cancellous bone is packed into the nonunion site to enhance osteogenesis. This principle has been confirmed experimentally: fresh autologous grafts stimulated renewed osteogenesis in delayed union.[75]

Cancellous autografts may also be used to advantage in the treatment of infected nonunions.[60, 88] The nonunion site is debrided, sequestra are removed, and open irrigation drainage with an appropriate antibiotic solution is performed if possible.[60] When healthy granulation tissue forms and a minimum of purulent exudate is present, internal fixation and bone grafting may be carried out. Rigid fixation is an absolute requirement. Only fresh autogenous cancellous bone is useful in treating infected nonunions or other bone infections, as all other grafts and implants will sequestrate.

Contaminated and Infected Fractures; Osteomyelitis

Cancellous autografts are very important in the adequate treatment of open, contaminated fresh fractures.[64] They have great potential for revascularization and may be applied in any area at the initial debridement and stabilization, provided the surrounding soft tissues are viable and adequately vascularized. External fixation devices or plates and screws are recommended for these fractures because intramedullary pins tend to introduce the contaminated present on the ends of the bones deep into the marrow cavity, producing an osteomyelitis that can be difficult to treat.[64] The graft is not covered with skin or muscle and may be protected with a sterile petroleum jelly gauze dressing, followed by a bandage. If the graft fails, it is resorbed or expelled through the wound; sequestration is not usually a problem. If the soft tissue bed is poorly vascularized or inadequate, delayed grafting is preferable to immediate grafting. The wound should be debrided, protected, and left to granulate for approximately 14 days. When the bed of the wound is filled with healthy granulation tissue, the granulation tissue may be trimmed back around the bone and the graft inserted. Sterile petroleum jelly gauze and a dressing should be applied. Although the graft may initially appear to be dead, vascularization occurs in several weeks. If sufficient contraction and epithelialization of the skin do not occur, skin may be grafted over the revascularized bone graft.[64]

Cancellous autografts may also be extremely useful in the treatment of chronic osteomyelitis.[48, 68, 84] Chronic bone infections often result in large areas of avascular bone and dense scar tissue, which can be impenetrable barriers to antibiotics administered parenterally. However, when all sequestra, avascular bone, and scar tissue are removed, a large cavity results that is slow to fill with new bone and is easily reinfected.[68] A one-stage procedure is recommended: adequate debridement and lavage of the infected tissue followed by implantation of large amounts of cancellous autologous bone.[84] Appropriate antibiotics are given during and after surgery. Stability is extremely important in the healing of osteomyelitis. If the bone is rigidly fixed, implants may be left *in situ,* otherwise the implant should be removed and another method of fixation chosen.[73]

In all procedures involving the implantation of fresh cancellous autologous bone into an infected or contaminated bed, care is taken to avoid contamination of the donor site. The surgeon should drape the donor sites separately, reglove, and use a separate, clean set of surgical instruments. Alternately, the bone graft may be collected before approaching the infected site and stored in blood-soaked sponges, as described under Harvesting and Handling of Grafts/Implants.

Bone Loss

Relatively large segments of bone may be lost through trauma or surgical excision of tumors, cysts, or shattered fracture fragments. When the defect is not segmental and when the bone retains sufficient mechanical strength for weight-bearing, the defect may be packed with autogenous cancellous bone—e.g., curettage and grafting of a Brodie's abscess.[52] Large segmental defects require internal or external fixation and a cortical graft. Cancellous grafts are used in humans to fill relatively large segmental defects.[22]

However, since veterinary patients do not protect their limbs after surgery and quickly return to full weight-bearing, a graft/implant that can act as a weight-bearing strut and provide stability should be used. Otherwise, implant fatigue and failure may occur due to cyclic loading (walking, running, and so on).

Autologous rib grafts, together with plate fixation, have been used to repair comminuted fractures in dogs.[90] This technique requires two consecutive surgical procedures with the accompanying morbidity, and most surgeons prefer to use alloimplants to replace shattered diaphyseal bone.[44-46, 89] They think that allograft implantation significantly shortens surgery time, and that, in some cases, the only alternative to an allograft is amputation because of the impossibility of reconstruction. The bones most commonly repaired with an allograft are the femur, humerus, and tibia.[45] Allograft replacement of extremely comminuted diaphyseal segments is very successful in cats[44, 45, 89] but less so in dogs.[45] The surgical procedure, while not more difficult than a standard osteosynthesis, requires extreme attention to detail.[46] Adequate stability *must* be achieved, the wound must be free of infection, and maximal host-implant contact at the interface is desirable.[46] Several clinical[11, 81] and experimental[4, 25] reports have emphasized the importance of packing the implant-host interface and the alloimplant marrow cavity, if possible, with profuse amounts of cancellous autologous

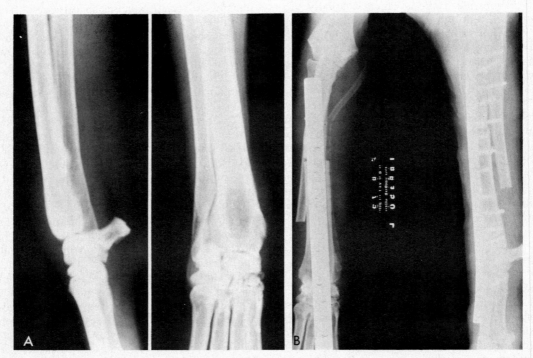

Figure 156–4. The entire distal radius and ulna were removed en bloc and replaced with a frozen alloimplant in this six-year-old St. Bernard with osteosarcoma. *A,* Although the neoplasm did not look extremely aggressive preoperatively, it had broken through the radial periosteum and involved the distal ulna. *B,* Postoperatively, note the 4.5 DC plate, which provides excellent stability, and the fenestrated continuous suction drain, which minimized fluid accumulation at the surgical site. The proximal graft-host interface and all carpal articular surfaces were packed with fresh cancellous autologous bone. The limb was further supported by a fiber glass cast for four weeks, and the dog was able to walk on the limb from the second postoperative day.

bone. This cancellous autograft stimulates host revascularization and osteogenesis and enhances incorporation of the large, dead alloimplant.

Occasionally, a highly comminuted fracture involves the joint surface, creating a very difficult clinical problem. These animals have usually been subjected to a joint arthrodesis or limb amputation when adequate reconstruction of the joint surface was not possible. Although somewhat experimental, preserved or fresh osteochondral alloimplants/grafts may be used to replace the destroyed fragment and retain joint function.[43] Careful attention should be paid to graft-host joint surface congruity and asepsis. Although articles in the veterinary[43] and human[57] literature report good short-term clinical results with this technique, long-term results are unknown. Recent experimental work indicates that a late immune response to cartilage matrix antigens may occur, with accompanying pannus formation and cartilage destruction.[93, 94]

Osteochondral or cortical alloimplants are also used to fill defects following en bloc tumor excision[57, 69] (Fig. 156–4). Distal radial osteosarcoma in giant breed dogs is quite common. Very large dogs have difficulty rising and walking following limb amputation. For these dogs, limb salvage may be appropriate. Great care should be taken preoperatively to assess the extent of the tumor locally and systemically. If the dog is free of metastases, and vital nerves and blood vessels are intact, the distal half of the radius (and ulna, if necessary) may be removed and replaced with a preserved alloimplant stabilized by a 4.5-mm broad dynamic compression plate. A pancarpal arthrodesis is usually necessary for limb function, since it is difficult to reconstruct the carpal ligaments. Dogs walk quite comfortably on the operated limb within one week of surgery. Long-term results of this technique are not available because the dogs usually die of metastases of the original osteosarcoma from 6 to 18 months after surgery.

Alloimplants have also been used to correct malunions. For example, when the pelvic canal is narrowed following pelvic malunion fracture, a symphysiotomy may be performed, the cut edges gently separated, and the space filled with an alloimplant.[30] The same principle could be applied to long bone malunion fractures, which require bone stock to fill surgically created defects.

HARVESTING AND HANDLING OF GRAFTS/IMPLANTS

Certain principles of graft handling must be followed to ensure optimum osteogenesis and incorporation at the recipient site and minimum morbidity at the donor site.

The first set of rules is designed to promote maximal survival of cells on the surface of the graft.[5] A key consideration is the selection of a donor site with a large population of surface cells. The most commonly selected sites in dogs are the proximal tibia, humerus, and femur for fresh cancellous bone and the iliac crest or rib for fresh corticocancellous bone. Once an appropriate site has been selected, the surgeon must harvest the graft with minimum trauma.[3]

Oscillating bone saws should be avoided when harvesting cancellous or corticocancellous grafts. Their use is associated with a marked temperature rise in adjacent bone, cell death, and retarded osteogenesis.[3, 50] In one experiment in rats, radial diaphyseal segmental osteotomies produced with oscillating saws became nonunions, whereas the same segmental fractures produced with bone-cutting forceps healed well.[50] If the use of power tools is unavoidable, they should be cooled with saline lavage during use, the edges kept well sharpened, and excessive speeds avoided (1500 rpm maximum).[3]

Large drill bits can be used to open the cortex for collection of cancellous bone. If a larger opening is needed, the hole should be lengthened along the longitudinal axis of the bone, keeping the corners rounded. This technique mechanically weakens the donor bone the least.[23] A square hole cut with an oscillating saw is undesirable because it not only has edges of dead bone from thermal necrosis but also weakens the bone significantly.[23]

Once the bone graft has been removed, numerous precautions must be taken to prevent the death of surface cells. Exposure of the graft to air for 30 minutes kills a significant number of cells.[5] Immersion in saline inhibits osteogenesis, and exposure of the grafts to antibiotic powders is absolutely contraindicated.[39] Irrigation of the recipient bed before graft placement with dilute solutions of bacitracin (25 to 50 units/ml) and polymyxin B sulfate (25 to 50 μg/ml) is permissible.[40] The use of antibiotic solutions after graft implantation is controversial and is probably best avoided. The optimum technique is to harvest the graft immediately before use and to transfer the graft directly into the recipient bed. If this is not possible because of risk of contamination of the donor site with bacteria or tumor cells, it is best to wrap the graft in a moistened, blood-soaked sponge. The graft can be placed in a metal bowl, covered with additional saline-soaked sponges, and held for three to four hours if necessary. If the graft is held for a short time in a blood-soaked sponge on the instrument table, it is wise to attach a large forceps to the sponge, so it is not inadvertently discarded.

Attention must also be paid to the recipient bed. Asepsis, hemostasis, and atraumatic technique are crucial. Additionally, several key steps need to be taken to promote effective diffusion of nutrients. First, prevent the interposition of dead space, hematoma, or necrotic tissue between the graft and the bed. Second, place cancellous portions of the graft next to cancellous portions of the bed. Third, do not pack the graft so tightly that diffusion is impossible.

Fourth, the importance of stable fixation of the grafted area has already been mentioned but cannot be overemphasized.

The recipient bed may also be affected by previous treatment; e.g., after radiation therapy vascularization is usually poor and excessive amounts of fibrous connective tissue may be present. Cancellous autografts have been used successfully in previously irradiated tissue,[58] but cortical grafts/implants are not recommended. Systemic factors such as chemotherapy, corticosteroid therapy, malnutrition, and debility affect incorporation.

Bone Graft Collection

Autografts

The medial aspect of the proximal tibia and the anterolateral aspect of the proximal humerus are easy to approach surgically and yield large amounts of cancellous bone.[49, 67, 92] The proximal femur is slightly more difficult to approach, and, in general, less cancellous bone is available from that site than from the other two.

Corticocancellous bone may be collected from the iliac crest or a rib.[79, 88, 90] Iliac crest bone is especially helpful when fusing joints, because the flat pieces may be wedged into the joint spaces to help stabilize the joint. Autogenous rib grafts require a moderately complicated collection procedure and are useful in segmental defects and in the repair of comminuted fractures. The ninth or tenth ribs are the easiest to harvest because there is little overlying muscle. The anterior ribs are straighter but are more difficult to approach. Cortical bone may be collected from any long bone of a suitable donor.

Allografts/Alloimplants

Potential donors are screened carefully for pre-existing bacterial, viral, metabolic, or neoplastic disease. If the entire length of the donor bone is to be implanted, the donor bone should not contain open epiphyseal growth plates, which may slip during the incorporation process. Osteochondral tissues may be removed up to 24 hours after death, and they remain biologically useful if the cadaver has been properly refrigerated.[33]

Aseptic technique is critical in implant collection unless some method of sterilization (irradiation, ethylene oxide) is used. Touch swabs or tissue blocks of the harvested bone (outer surface and medullary cavity) and donor site are cultured for aerobic and anaerobic organisms. Bones are double-wrapped in sterile plastic wrap for freezing. A slice of bone adjacent to the graft may be packaged similarly to be thawed and cultured just prior to implantation of the preserved graft. Pathogens, as well as tissue, are preserved by freezing and freeze-drying. An infection rate of 7 per cent or less has been reported in human alloimplant recipients, about twice the incidence of infection of patients receiving fresh cancellous autografts.[85] All care is exercised to prevent contamination of the graft during harvesting and storage. If an individual bone culture is positive, that graft is discarded. If 25 per cent of cultures from a given donor are positive, all tissue harvested from that donor is discarded.[33] Although the use of antibiotic solutions during harvest or storage is not recommended, the implant may be thawed or reconstituted in a dilute antibiotic solution (e.g., penicillin, polymyxin, bacitracin), and a brief perioperative regimen of broad spectrum systemic antibiotic administration is prudent.

The chosen method of storage dictates handling and packaging of grafts. If fresh implantation is desired, allografts may be held in a humidified atmosphere at 37°C in tissue culture medium supplemented with 20 per cent autologous serum for 24 to 48 hours. If stored, each packaged graft should be radiographed and marked with the name of the bone (indicating right or left), donor identification, date of harvest, and any additional pertinent information. The recommended temperature for storage of frozen grafts is −70°C, although −20°C has been used satisfactorily. Autolysis may occur at warmer temperatures (−10°C), since bone does not freeze at these temperatures. However, successful use of alloimplants stored in conventional freezers (−10°C) has been reported.[45] The period of safe storage by freezing is unknown; the current recommendation is not longer than two years. Frozen implants should be thawed quickly in warm, physiologic solutions just before use. Chondrocyte viability is important in maintaining the integrity of transplanted hyaline cartilage and should be protected when implants are frozen. The articular surface is immersed in 10% sterile glycerol for 30 minutes; the graft implant is refrigerated for 18 hours, then frozen. This technique results in 40 per cent chondrocyte viability when the implants are quickly thawed.[31]

Bone to be freeze-dried is held at −70°C until the results of the bacterial cultures are known. If the cultures are negative, the tissue is freeze-dried to approximately two to five per cent residual moisture in a vacuum of 5 to 10 microns and stored at −70°C or at room temperature in a vacuum.[85] This procedure requires approximately two to three days for a 5-cm segment of canine cortical bone.* Freeze-dried tissues theoretically may be held indefinitely. They are extremely brittle and require reconstitution with water or saline before use. The period required to return the biomechanical properties of freeze-dried bone toward normal depends on the size and shape of the graft.[31] Segments of long bone inadequately reconstituted crack while being drilled, and 18 to 24 hours of reconstitution may be needed to avoid these problems.*[31]

---

*Personal communication from Charles J. Schena, 1983.

The method of preparing chemosterilized bone is described by Urist,[86] and methods of irradiation, deproteinization, merthiolate preservation, and autoclaving of bone are discussed by Burwell and others.[18, 24]

In summary, bone grafts/implants may be implanted fresh or in a variety of preserved forms. The clinical problem guides the choice of graft type; the equipment available, the desired biological activity, and the preference of the surgeon determine the choice of preservation. Bone grafts/implants, particularly fresh autogenous cancellous bone, are not used as often as they could and should be in modern orthopedics, often simply because the surgeon does not think of it. However, the osteogenic activity contributed by a bone graft augments the technical expertise of the surgeon, and the combination results in enhanced healing of fractures, osteomyelitis, and delayed unions and nonunions, and in the salvage of limbs previously amputated.

1. Adeyanju, B. J., Butler, H. C., and Leipold, H. W.: Healing of cortical bone grafts in the dog—The role of azathioprine. Vet. Surg. 11:52, 1982.
2. Albee, F. H.: *Bone Graft Surgery*. W. B. Saunders, Philadelphia, 1915.
3. Albrektsson, T.: The healing of autologous bone grafts after varying degrees of surgical trauma. J. Bone Joint Surg. 62B:403, 1980.
4. Bacher, J. D., and Schmidt, R. E.: Effects of autogenous bone on healing of homogenous cortical bone grafts. J. Small Anim. Pract. 21:235, 1980.
5. Bassett, C. A. L.: Clinical implications of cell function in bone grafting. Clin. Orthop. Rel. Res. 87:49, 1972.
6. Berggren, A., Weiland, A. J., and Ostrup, L.: Bone scintigraphy in evaluating the viability of composite bone grafts revascularized by microvascular anastamoses, conventional autogenous bone grafts, and free non-revascularized periosteal grafts. J. Bone Joint Surg. 64A:799, 1982.
7. Bonfiglio, M.: Repair of bone-transplant fractures. J. Bone Joint Surg. 40A:446, 1958.
8. Bonfiglio, M., and Jeter, W. S.: Immunological responses to bone. Clin. Orthop. Rel. Res. 87:19, 1972.
9. Bonfiglio, M., Jeter, W. S., and Smith, C. L.: The immune concept: Its relation to bone transplantation. Ann. NY Acad. Sci. 59:417, 1955.
10. Bos, G., Goldberg, V. M., Powell, A. E., Heiple, K. M., and Zika, J. M.: The effect of histocompatibility matching on canine frozen bone allografts. J. Bone Joint Surg. 65A:89, 1983.
11. Brown, R. H., and Townsend, G. B.: Segmental defects in open fractures of long bones. Med. Ann. (D.C.) 39:555, 1970.
12. Burchardt, H., Busbee, G. A., and Enneking, W. F.: Repair of experimental autologous grafts of cortical bone. J. Bone Joint Surg. 57A:814, 1975.
13. Burchardt, H., and Enneking, W. F.: Transplantation of bone. Surg. Clin. North Am. 58:403, 1978.
14. Burchardt, H., Glowczewskie, F. P., and Enneking, W. F.: Allogeneic segmental fibular transplants in azathioprine-immunosuppressed dogs. J. Bone Joint Surg. 59A:881, 1977.
15. Burchardt, H., Glowczewskie, F. P., and Enneking, W. F.: Short-term immunosuppression with fresh segmental fibular allografts in dogs. J. Bone Joint Surg. 63A:411, 1981.
16. Burchardt, H., Glowczewskie, F. P., and Enneking, W. F.: The effect of Adriamycin and methotrexate on the repair of segmental cortical autografts in dogs. J. Bone Joint Surg. 65A:103, 1983.
17. Burchardt, H., Jones, H., Glowczewskie, F., Rudner, C., and Enneking, W. F.: Freeze-dried allogeneic segmental cortical bone grafts in dogs. J. Bone Joint Surg. 60A:1082, 1978.
18. Burwell, R. G.: The fate of bone grafts. In Apley, A. G. (ed.): *Recent Advances in Orthopaedics*. Williams & Wilkins, Baltimore, 1969, pp. 115–207.
19. Burwell, R. G.: Studies in the transplantation of bone. V. The capacity of fresh and treated homografts of bone to evoke transplantation immunity. J. Bone Joint Surg. 45B:386, 1963.
20. Campbell, C. J.: Homotransplantation of a half or whole joint. Clin. Orthop. Rel. Res. 87:146, 1972.
21. Carnesale, P. L., and Spankus, J. D.: A clinical comparative study of autogenous and homogenous bone grafts. J. Bone Joint Surg. 41A:887, 1957.
22. Chapman, M. W.: Closed intramedullary bone-grafting and nailing of segmental defects of the femur. J. Bone Joint Surg. 63A:1004, 1980.
23. Clark, C. R., Morgan, C., Sonstegard, D. A., et al.: The effect of biopsy-hole shape and size on bone strength. J. Bone Joint Surg. 59A:213, 1977.
24. Coupland, B. R.: Experimental bone grafting in the canine: The use of autoclaved autogenous normal tibial bone. Can. Vet. J. 10:170, 1969.
25. Desch, J. P., Butler, H. C., Guffy, M. M., et al.: Combination of a cortical allograft with a cancellous autograft in the canine tibia. Vet. Surg. 11:84, 1982.
26. Doi, K., Tominaga, S., and Shibata, T.: Bone grafts with microvascular anastomoses of vascular pedicles. J. Bone Joint Surg. 59A:809–815, 1977.
27. Elves, M. W.: Studies of the behavior of allogeneic cancellous bone grafts in inbred rats. Transplantation 19:416, 1975.
28. Enneking, W. F.: Histological investigation of bone transplants in immunologically prepared animals. J. Bone Joint Surg. 39A:597, 1957.
29. Enneking, W. F., Burchardt, H., Puhl, J. J., et al.: Physical and biological aspects of repair in dog cortical bone transplants. J. Bone Joint Surg. 57A:232, 1975.
30. Evans, I.: Use of an allogeneic bone graft to enlarge the pelvic outlet in a cat. Vet. Med./Small Anim. Clin. 75:218, 1980.
31. Friedlaender, G. E.: Current concepts review. Bone banking. J. Bone Joint Surg. 64A:307, 1983.
32. Friedlaender, G. E., Goodman, A., Hausman, M., and Troiano, N.: The effects of methotrexate and radiation therapy on histologic aspects of fracture healing. Trans. Orthop. Res. Soc. 8:224, 1983.
33. Friedlaender, G. E., and Mankin, H. J.: Bone banking: Current methods and suggested guidelines. In AAOS: *Instructional Course Lectures*, Vol. 30. C. V. Mosby, St. Louis, 1982, pp. 36–55.
34. Friedlaender, G. E., Strong, D. M., and Sell, K. W.: Studies on the antigenicity of bone. I. Freeze-dried and deep-frozen bone allografts in rabbits. J. Bone Joint Surg. 58A:854, 1976.
35. Friedlaender, G. E., Strong, D. M., and Sell, K. W.: Donor graft–specific HL-A antibodies following freeze-dried bone allografts. Trans. Orthop. Res. Soc. 2:91, 1977.
36. Goldberg, V. M., and Lance, E. M.: Revascularization and accretion in transplantation. J. Bone Joint Surg. 54A:807, 1972.
37. Goldberg, V. M., Porter, B. B., and Lance, E. M.: Transplantation of the canine knee joint on a vascular pedicle. J. Bone Joint Surg. 62A:414, 1980.
38. Goldstrom, G. L., Roberts, J. M., and Mears, D. C.: Replacement of canine segmental bone defects with tricalcium phosphate ceramic implants. Trans. Orthop. Res. Soc. 8:235, 1983.
39. Gray, J. C., and Elves, M. W.: Early osteogenesis in compact bone isografts: A quantitative study of the contributions of the different graft cells. Calcif. Tissue Int. 29:225, 1979.
40. Gray, J. C., and Elves, M. W.: Osteogenesis in bone grafts after short-term storage and topical antibiotic treatment. J. Bone Joint Surg. 63B:441, 1981.
41. Halloran, P. F., Ziv, I., Lee, E. H., et al.: Orthotopic bone transplantation in mice. Transplantation 27:414, 1979.
42. Heiple, K. G., Chase, S. W., and Herndon, C. H.: A

comparative study of the healing process following different types of bone transplantation. J. Bone Joint Surg. 45A:1593, 1963.

43. Helphrey, M. L., and Stevenson, S.: Osteoarticular allogeneic bone grafting in dogs. Vet. Surg. 9:83, 1980.

44. Henricksen, P.: Entire segment bone transplant in a cat. J. Am. Vet. Med. Assoc. 174:826, 1979.

45. Henry, W. B., and Wadsworth, P. L.: Diaphyseal allografts in the repair of long bone fractures. J. Am. Anim. Hosp. Assoc. 17:525, 1981.

46. Henry, W. B., and Wadsworth, P. L.: Retrospective analysis of failures in the repair of severely comminuted long bone fractures using large diaphyseal allografts. J. Am. Anim. Hosp. Assoc. 17:535, 1981.

47. Holmes, R. E., Tencer, A. F., Carmichael, T. W., and Mooney, V.: Mechanical properties of synthetic hydroxy-apatite for cancellous bone grafting. Trans. Orthop. Res. Soc. 8:67, 1983.

48. Hulse, D. A.: Use of a cancellous bone graft in the repair of a delayed union fracture complicated by osteomyelitis. J. Am. Anim. Hosp. Assoc. 9:378, 1973.

49. Hulse, D. A.: Pathophysiology of autologous cancellous bone grafts. Comp. Cont. Ed. 2:136, 1980.

50. Jacobs, R. L., and Ray, R. D.: The effect of heat on bone healing. Arch. Surg. 104:687, 1972.

51. Johnson, K. A., and Bellenger, C. R.: The effects of autologous bone grafting on bone healing after carpal arthrodesis in the dog. Vet. Rec. 107:126, 1980.

52. Knecht, C. D., Slusher, R., and Cawley, A. J.: Treatment of Brodie's abscess by means of bone autograft. J. Am. Vet. Med. Assoc. 158:492, 1971.

53. Kushner, A.: Evaluation of Wolff's law of bone formation. J. Bone Joint Surg. 22:589, 1940.

54. Lane, J. M., Brighton, C. T., Ottens, H. R., and Lipton, M.: Joint resurfacing in the rabbit using an autologous osteochondral graft. J. Bone Joint Surg. 59A:218, 1977.

55. Lindholm, T. S., and Urist, M. R.: A quantitative analysis of new bone formation by induction in composite grafts of bone marrow and bone matrix. Clin. Orthop. Rel. Res. 150:288, 1980.

56. Maniziano, C. F., and Mattheou, C.: Heterogenous bone grafts. Mod. Vet. Prac. 65:65, 1965.

57. Mankin, H. J., Fogelson, F. S., Trasher, A. Z., et al.: Massive resection and allograft transplantation in the treatment of malignant bone tumors. N. Engl. J. Med. 294:1247, 1976.

58. Marciani, R. D., and Trodahl, J. N.: Cancellous-marrow bone grafts in irradiated tissue. Oral Surg. 42:431, 1976.

59. McKibbin, B.: The biology of fracture healing in long bones. J. Bone Joint Surg. 60B:150, 1978.

60. Meyer, S., Weiland, A. J., and Willenegger, H.: The treatment of infected non-union of fractures of long bones. J. Bone Joint Surg. 57A:836, 1975.

61. Mitzutani, H., and Urist, M. R.: The nature of bone morphogenetic protein (BMP) fractions derived from bovine bone matrix gelatin. Clin. Orthop. Rel. Res. 171:213, 1982.

62. Moore, R. W., and Withrow, S. J.: Arthrodesis. Comp. Cont. Ed. 3:319, 1981.

63. Muscolo, D. L., and Kawai, S.: Bone transplantation antigens. Cellular and humoral immune response studies. Int. Orthop. 1:5, 1977.

64. Nunamaker, D. M.: Treatment of open fractures in small animals. Comp. Cont. Ed. 1:66, 1979.

65. Olds, R.: Bone grafting. In Bojrab, M. J. (ed.): Pathophysiology of Small Animal Surgery. Lea & Febiger, Philadelphia, 1981, pp. 534–541.

66. Olds, R. B., DeAngelis, M., Sinibaldi, K., et al.: Autogenous cancellous bone grafting in problem orthopaedic cases. J. Am. Anim. Hosp. Assoc. 9:430, 1973.

67. Olds, R. B., Sinibaldi, K., DeAngelis, M., et al.: Autogenous cancellous bone grafting in small animals. J. Am. Anim. Hosp. Assoc. 9:454, 1973.

68. de Oliveira, J. C.: Bone grafts and chronic osteomyelitis. J. Bone Joint Surg. 53B:672, 1971.

69. Parrish, F. F.: Allograft replacement of all or part of the end of a long bone following excision of a tumor: Report of twenty-one cases. J. Bone Joint Surg. 55A:1, 1973.

70. Pelker, R. R., Friedlaender, G., Markham, T., Hausman, M., Doganis, A. C., and Panjabi, H.: Effects of Adriamycin and methotrexate on fracture healing biomechanics. Trans. Orthop. Res. Soc. 8:186, 1983.

71. Ray, R. D.: Vascularization of bone grafts and implants. Clin. Orthop. Rel. Res. 87:43, 1972.

72. Richards, R. R., Langer, F., Halloran, P., et al.: The antigenic profile of the mouse skeletal system. Trans. Orthop. Res. Soc. 4:59, 1979.

73. Rittmann, W. W., and Perren, S. M.: Cortical Bone Healing after Internal Fixation and Infection. Springer Verlag, New York, 1974.

74. Rodrigo, J. J., Sakovich, L., Travis, C., and Smith, G.: Osteocartilaginous allografts as compared with autografts in the treatment of knee joint osteocartilaginous defects in dogs. Clin. Orthop. Rel. Res. 134:342, 1978.

75. Rokkanen, P., Paatsama, S., and Sittnikow, K.: Subcortical cancellous bone grafting (Phemister-Charnley) in the treatment of delayed union. Injury 2:185, 1971.

76. Ross, G. E.: Effect of diethylstilbestrol, prednisolone, and isoniazid on the healing rate of bone defects filled with certain bone grafting materials. Am. J. Vet. Res. 27:1745, 1966.

77. Sauer, H. D., and Schoettle, H.: The stability of osteosyntheses bridging defects. Arch. Orthop. Traum. Surg. 95:27, 1979.

78. Schenk, R. K., Muller, J., and Willenegger, H.: Experimentell-histologisher Beitrag zur Entstehung und Behandlung von Pseudarthrosen. Hefte Unfallh. 94:15, 1967.

79. Schlenker, J. D., Indresano, A. T., Raine, T., et al.: A new flap in the dog containing a vascularized rib graft—the latissimus dorsi myosteocutaneous flap. J. Surg. Res. 29:172, 1980.

80. Seligman, G. M., George, E., Yablon, I., Nutik, G., and Cruess, R. L.: Transplantation of whole knee joints in the dog. Clin. Orthop. Rel. Res. 87:332, 1972.

81. Sinibaldi, K.: Manuscript in preparation, 1984.

82. Smith, R. T.: The mechanism of graft rejection. Clin. Orthop. Rel. Res. 87:15, 1972.

83. Stevenson, S., Hohn, R. B., and Templeton, J. W.: Effects of tissue antigen matching on the healing of fresh cancellous bone allografts in dogs. Am. J. Vet. Res. 44:202, 1983.

84. Sudmann, E.: Treatment of chronic osteomyelitis by free grafts of cancellous autologous bone tissue. Acta Orthop. Scand. 50:145, 1979.

85. Tomford, W. W., Starkwether, R. J., and Goldman, M. H.: A study of the clinical incidence of infection in the use of banked allograft bone. J. Bone Joint Surg. 63A:244, 1981.

86. Urist, M. R.: Bone transplantation. In Urist, M. R. (ed.): Fundamental and Clinical Bone Physiology. J. B. Lippincott, Philadelphia, 1980, pp. 331–368.

87. Urovitz, E. P., Langer, F., Gross, A. E., et al.: Cell-mediated immunity in patients following joint allografting. Trans. Orthop. Res. Soc. 1:132, 1976.

88. Vaughn, L. C.: The use of bone autografts in canine orthopaedic surgery. J. Small Anim. Pract. 13:455, 1972.

89. Wadsworth, P. L., and Henry, W. B.: Entire segment cortical bone transplant. J. Am. Anim. Hosp. Assoc. 12:741, 1976.

90. Walker, R. G.: Rib grafts in the repair of comminuted fractures in the dog. Vet. Rec. 79:350, 1966.

91. White, A. A., Panjabi, M. M., and Southwick, W. O.: The four biomechanical stages of fracture repair. J. Bone Joint Surg. 59A:188, 1977.

92. Whittick, W.: Bone transplantation. In Bojrab, M. J. (ed.): Current Techniques in Small Animal Surgery. Lea & Febiger, Philadelphia, 1974, pp. 554–562.

93. Yablon, I. G., Cooperband, S., and Covall, D.: Matrix antigens in allografts. I. The humoral response. Clin. Orthop. Rel. Res. 168:243, 1982.

94. Yablon, I. G., Cooperband, S., and Covall, D.: Matrix antigens in allografts. II. The cell-mediated response. Clin. Orthop. Rel. Res. 172:277, 1983.

Chapter 157

Orthopedics of the Forelimb

Scapula

Robert B. Parker

GENERAL CONSIDERATIONS

Although the scapula is infrequently fractured, its anatomical location is very important. The scapula is a relatively flat, thin bone that acts as a support for the entire thoracic limb. Important osseous landmarks include the body, with associated supraspinatus and infraspinatus fossae; the spine, with its prominent distal acromion process; and the articular glenoid cavity, with the supraglenoid tuberosity and scapular neck (Fig. 157–1). Important soft tissue landmarks include the suprascapular nerve and the following muscles: serratus ventralis, trapezius, omotransversarius, infraspinatus, supraspinatus, teres minor, and spinous and acromial heads of the deltoideus.

Because of the scapula's anatomical location, sufficient trauma to produce a scapular fracture can easily produce concomitant injury. It is important to fully assess each patient for cervical and rib fractures, shoulder luxations, thoracic trauma (pneumothorax and pulmonary injury), brachial plexus trauma, and suprascapular nerve trauma.

Proper radiographic positioning is essential to fully evaluate the extent of scapular injury. General anesthesia or heavy sedation is required for patient comfort and cooperation. Posteroanterior (PA) and mediolateral (ML) views are the minimum requirement for a complete study. When the patient is positioned for the PA view, the sagittal plane of the thorax should be rotated approximately 30 degrees away from the affected limb (Fig. 157–2) to help prevent confusing overlap of bony densities. The mediolateral view is obtained with the patient in lateral recumbency with the affected leg adjacent to the film. The scapula should be extended approximately 45 degrees, placing it over the caudal cervical area and preventing superimposition of the sternum and ribs.

Fractures of the scapula can be classified according to their location as follows: (1) fractures of the scapular body and spine, including the acromion process; (2) fractures of the scapular neck; and (3) fractures involving the glenoid cavity, including fractures of the supraglenoid tuberosity.

FRACTURES OF THE SCAPULAR BODY

Because of protection afforded by the thorax and lateral supporting musculature, fractures of the scapular body are often minimally displaced. Frequently, a mid-body transverse fracture occurs with minimal medial displacement of the distal segment (Fig. 157–3). This fracture occurs as a result of direct trauma and can occur with variable clinical signs. Pain with minimal crepitus can be elicited over the scapula, and an incongruity of the scapular spine may be palpated. These fractures are best treated for three to four weeks by rest, scapular support bandages, or Velpeau slings. The prognosis for full function is excellent.

Comminuted fractures of the scapular body with minor displacement can be treated by either closed

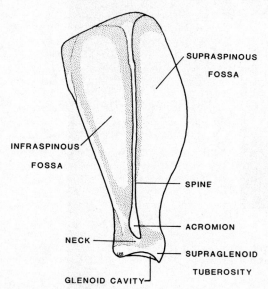

Figure 157–1. The canine scapula.

SUPRASPINOUS FOSSA

INFRASPINOUS FOSSA

SPINE

ACROMION

NECK

SUPRAGLENOID TUBEROSITY

GLENOID CAVITY

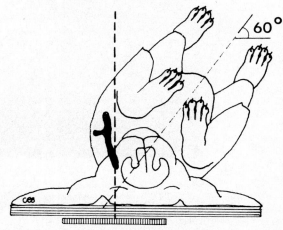

Figure 157–2. Rotation of the sagittal plane 30° to obtain a proper posteroanterior radiograph.

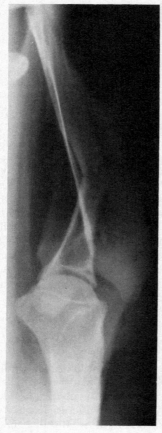

Figure 157–3. Posteroanterior radiograph of a minimally displaced scapular body fracture treated with a Velpeau sling.

or open methods. Because the blood supply to the scapula is extensive, healing of scapular fractures is generally excellent. Open reduction and internal fixation are indicated for scapular body fractures exhibiting severe instability or displacement (Fig. 157–4). Frequently, the distal fragment overrides medially and proximally, with the fracture site of the proximal fragment in the shoulder joint area (Fig. 157–5). Healing in this position could result in limited shoulder function.

The scapular body is approached through a lateral incision over the scapular spine. Incision of the deep fascia over the spine allows cranial retraction of the trapezius and omotransversarius muscles and caudal retraction of the spinous portion of the deltoideus muscle. The supraspinatus and infraspinatus muscles are elevated from the spine and body and are retracted.

After reduction, stabilization can be achieved with wire, small bone plates, or small fixation pins. Depending on the size of the animal, 18- to 22-gauge wire can be used as twisted "wire sutures" through preplaced holes in each fragment (Fig. 157–6). Depending on stability, stabilization may be supplemented with a scapular support bandage or a Velpeau sling.

Bone plates and screws can also be used to stabilize scapular body fractures. Because the scapular body is thin, the plate can be wedged into the angle formed by the body and spine. The resulting oblique direction of the screws allows slightly more bone purchase in the thicker bone at the base of the spine (see Fig.

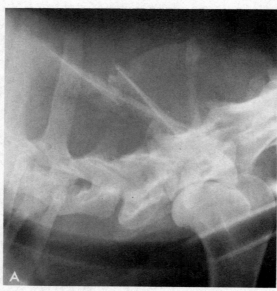

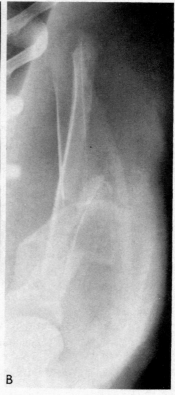

Figure 157–4. Preoperative (A and B) and postoperative (C and D) views of a comminuted scapular fracture with marked instability treated with a combination of a bone plate, wire sutures, and K-wires.

Illustration continued on opposite page

B

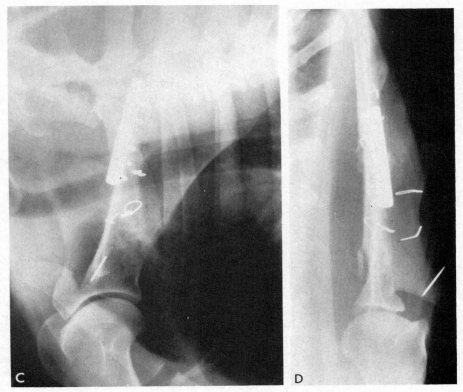

Figure 157–4. See legend on opposite page.

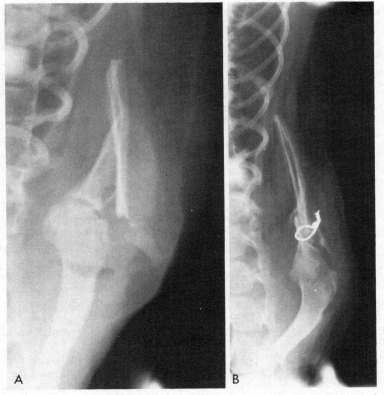

Figure 157–5. Preoperative (*A*) and postoperative (*B*) radiographs of a scapular body fracture with proximal medial displacement treated with a single wire suture and supported in a Velpeau sling.

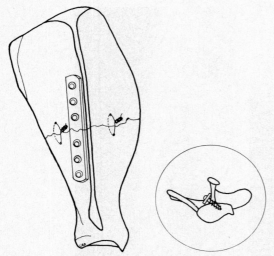

Figure 157–6. Wire and plate fixation of a scapular body fracture. *Inset* illustrates oblique screw position.

157–6). Plates can also be placed directly on the spine to provide stability to scapular body fractures (Fig. 157–7). Plastic (polyvinylidine fluoride) plates have been used for stabilization of comminuted scapular body fractures. Although they provide less rigid fixation than stainless steel plates, their ease in modification and conformability to bone have been cited as desirable features.[1]

Regardless of technique used, the surgeon should exercise care to prevent iatrogenic trauma to the brachial plexus and thorax from pins and drill bits.

FRACTURES OF THE ACROMION

Although infrequently encountered as a primary fracture, nonunion of the acromion process may occur

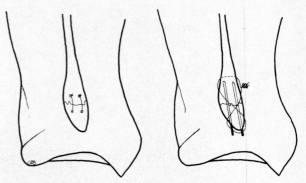

Figure 157–8. Fractured acromion repaired with either wire sutures or a pin and tension band.

secondary to inadequate repair of an acromion osteotomy following a lateral approach to the shoulder. The affected animal generally has a weight-bearing lameness with pain on palpation of the acromial process. The acromion serves as the origin of the acromial head of the deltoideus muscle; therefore, constant muscle pull distracts the fragment, and internal fixation is recommended.

The acromion is approached through a lateral incision centered over the acromial process. Incision of the deep fascia of the spine allows caudal retraction of the spinous head of the deltoideus muscle. The distal fracture fragment is ventrally displaced and is found attached to the origin of the acromial head of the deltoideus muscle. After reduction, fixation can be achieved with twisted stainless steel "wire sutures" or a small pin and tension band (Fig. 157–8). The distal fragment may be too small to accommodate two drill holes for the wire sutures; therefore, a small pin and tension band may be more appropriate.

If fixation is secure, postoperative bandages or slings are not necessary, and the prognosis for a full functional recovery is excellent.

FRACTURES OF THE SCAPULAR NECK, GLENOID, AND SUPRAGLENOID TUBEROSITY

Fractures in this area are frequently severely displaced and may involve the articular surface of the glenoid. Affected patients are presented with a non–weight-bearing lameness, and pain and crepitus are palpable upon manipulation of the shoulder joint. Because these fractures are usually severely displaced and are in close proximity to the shoulder joint, open reduction and internal fixation are indicated to prevent exuberant callus formation and possible limited shoulder function. Articular involvement is also an indication for open anatomical reduction and rigid fixation.

Surgical approach to the scapular neck and glenoid requires an appreciation of the regional surgical anatomy and a willingness to expose as much as necessary to reduce these often difficult fractures. A lateral approach to the shoulder is performed by osteotomy

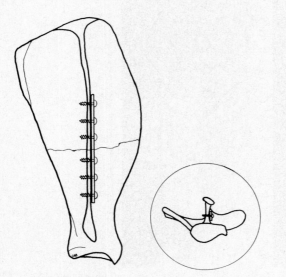

Figure 157–7. Plate application to the scapular spine for stabilization of a scapular body fracture.

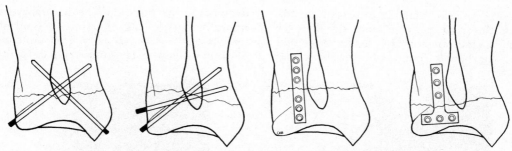

Figure 157–9. Various methods for stabilization of scapular neck fractures.

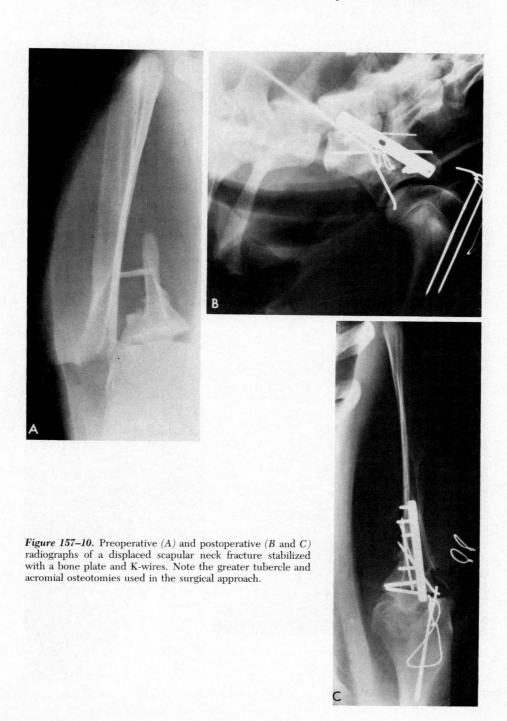

Figure 157–10. Preoperative *(A)* and postoperative *(B* and *C)* radiographs of a displaced scapular neck fracture stabilized with a bone plate and K-wires. Note the greater tubercle and acromial osteotomies used in the surgical approach.

of the acromion process. Starting proximally at the midportion of the spine and continuing distally over the lateral midshaft of the humerus, a curved incision is made over the shoulder joint. After incision of the deep fascia over the spine, the omotransversarius and trapezius muscles and the spinous head of the deltoideus muscles are retracted. The acromion is osteotomized to allow distal retraction of the acromial head

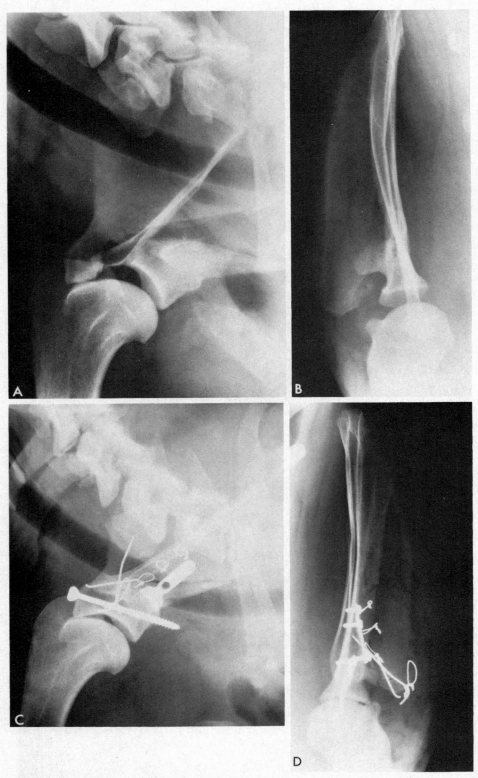

Figure 157–11. Preoperative *(A and B)* and postoperative *(C and D)* radiographs of an intra-articular scapular neck fracture stabilized with an interfragmentary lag screw and a small bone plate.

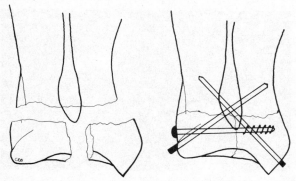

Figure 157–12. A T fracture of the scapular neck repaired with an interfragmentary lag screw and two crossed pins.

of the deltoideus muscle. Sufficient bone should remain attached to the muscle to allow subsequent fixation to the spine. The supraspinatus and infraspinatus muscles are retracted to expose the neck area, or more commonly, either one or both of these muscles are freed from their humeral insertions to allow maximum retraction. Lateral and posterior exposure is gained by infraspinatus or teres minor tenotomy. To allow proximal retraction of the supraspinatus muscle, the greater tubercle of the humerus is osteotomized. In all cases care should be taken to identify and protect the suprascapular nerve. After reduction and fixation are complete, closure is begun in layers. The greater tubercle osteotomy, if performed, is repaired with a pin and tension band. The infraspinatus and teres minor tenotomies are repaired

with either a horizontal mattress or Bunnell-Mayer suture pattern of nonabsorbable suture material. The acromial osteotomy is fixed with a pin and tension band, and the remainder of the closure is routine.

Stabilization of scapular neck fractures can be difficult. After reduction, initial stability can be maintained with a small Steinmann pin or K-wire inserted in the supraglenoid tuberosity and driven obliquely across the fracture site (Fig. 157–9). The scapula thins proximally, and care should be exercised to prevent pin penetration of the medial cortex. A second crosspin can be introduced from the posterior aspect across the fracture site. Excellent stability in this area can also be achieved with small bone plates (Fig. 157–10).

Fractures involving the articular surface can be particularly challenging, and the principles of anatomical reduction with rigid internal compression fixation should be followed if a satisfactory clinical result is desired (Fig. 157–11). With a T fracture of the scapular neck and the articular surface, the articular fragments are initially reduced and secured with a lag screw. The resulting two-piece fracture is now managed as described for scapular neck fractures (Fig. 157–12). Avulsion fractures of the supraglenoid tuberosity are displaced by the pull of the biceps brachii muscle (Fig. 157–13). After exposure and anatomical reduction, these fractures are stabilized with a lag screw or a pin and tension band (Fig. 157–14).

If stable fixation has been achieved, early limited weight-bearing or passive range-of-motion exercises

Figure 157–13. Preoperative *(A)* and postoperative *(B)* radiographs of a fractured supraglenoid tuberosity repaired with an interfragmentary lag screw and an antirotational pin. Note the greater tubercle and acromion osteotomies.

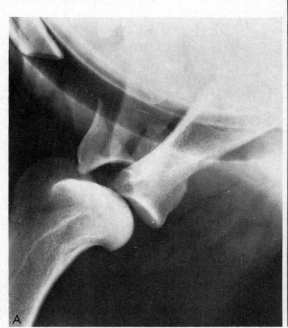
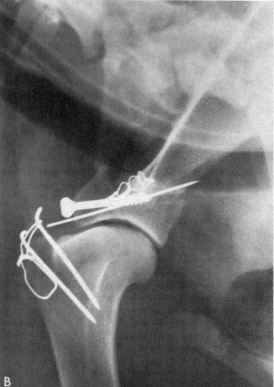

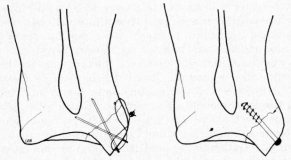

Figure 157–14. A supraglenoid tuberosity fracture repaired with a pin and tension band or an interfragmentary lag screw.

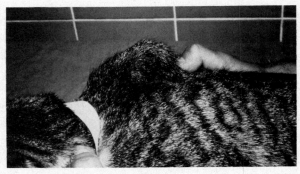

Figure 157–15. Clinical appearance of a cat with a scapular dislocation.

are encouraged. If necessary a scapular support bandage may be applied for ten to 14 days.

SCAPULAR DISLOCATION

The serratus ventralis muscle is a large muscle mass that covers the caudal half of the lateral thoracic wall and inserts on the proximal medial aspect of the scapula. It acts as the major muscular support for the scapula and thoracic limb. Occasionally, rupture of this muscle can occur secondary to trauma. The resulting clinical signs are dramatic, and there is a marked upward displacement of the scapula (Fig. 157–15). If the distal limb is adducted, the proximal scapula displaces laterally. Affected animals generally are not in pain but do have the characteristic gait abnormality.

Surgical repair is necessary for a functional and cosmetic result. Primary suture repair of the muscle and wire support are effective methods of repair.

To approach the medial aspect of the scapula, a longitudinal skin incision is made over the dorsal aspect of the bone. The trapezius insertion is elevated from its cranial and caudal attachments on the spine of the scapula. Proximal retraction of the trapezius exposes the insertion of the rhomboideus muscle on the dorsal aspect of the scapula. After the rhomboideus is divided, the medial scapula and serratus ventralis muscle are identified. After debridement, the serratus is united by a series of chromic gut sutures. The resulting scar tissue union is usually sufficient to support weight bearing.

A wire suture from the caudal margin of the scapula around the fifth rib can be used as primary repair or as a supplement to soft tissue repair. After the scapula is replaced in its normal position, a skin incision is made caudal to the scapular spine. The caudal margin of the scapula is palpated, and a small portion of the teres major muscle is elevated. The fifth rib is palpated, and a small portion is subperiosteally isolated. A loop of 20-gauge stainless steel wire is passed around the rib, care being taken not to enter the thorax. The free ends are passed through holes drilled through the caudal scapula and are twisted on the lateral surface.

A Velpeau sling, a shoulder spica coaptation splint, or a scapular bandage should be used for approximately three weeks.

1. Caywood, D., Wallace, L. J., and Johnson, G. R.: The use of a plastic plate for repair of a comminuted scapular body fracture in a dog. J. Am. Anim. Hosp. Assoc. *13*:176, 1977.
2. Ticer, J. W.: *Radiographic Technique in Small Animal Practice*. W. B. Saunders, Philadelphia, 1975.

Luxation of the Scapulohumeral Joint

P. B. Vasseur and C. R. Gregory

Scapulohumeral luxation in dogs and cats results from disruption of the supporting elements of the joint. The condition occurs infrequently in dogs and very rarely in cats.[1,2,5,13] Because of the paucity of information about shoulder luxations in cats, this section refers exclusively to the canine condition.

The majority of scapulohumeral luxations are either medial or lateral; cranial and caudal types have been described but occur much less often.[5,8,10,13] Although trauma is the predominant cause, small dogs may develop medial luxation in association with erosion of the glenoid labrum and capsular laxity, the cause of which is not known.[15]

ANATOMY

The scapulohumeral joint is supported by its joint capsule and associated glenohumeral ligaments and by the numerous muscles and tendons that span the

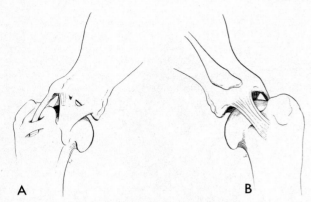

Figure 157–16. *A*, Medial glenohumeral ligament. *B*, Lateral glenohumeral ligament. (Redrawn with permission from Christensen, G. C., and Evans, H. E.: *Miller's Anatomy of the Dog.* 2nd ed. W. B. Saunders, Philadelphia, 1979.)

articulation. The joint capsule attaches to the scapula immediately proximal to the glenoid labrum and forms a loose sleeve that is especially voluminous caudally; it attaches to the humerus several millimeters distal to the articular surface of the humeral head. A portion of the capsule encloses the origin of the biceps brachii tendon and extends distally (approximately 2 cm) into the intertubercular groove. Medially, the capsule is attached to the tendons of the subscapularis and coracobrachialis muscles. Laterally, it attaches to the tendons of the infraspinatus and teres minor.

The glenohumeral ligaments are collateral supporting structures on the deep surface of the medial and lateral joint capsule (Fig. 157–16). Both ligaments invaginate into the joint cavity and are enveloped by synovial membrane. The medial ligament consists of cranial and caudal components; the lateral ligament is a solitary band wider at its origin and becoming narrower at its insertion on the humerus.

The muscles and tendons that cross the joint maintain stability; however, their individual functions and complex interactions relative to shoulder joint motion have yet to be adequately defined.

LATERAL SHOULDER LUXATION

Lateral luxation of the shoulder is generally associated with trauma, and large breeds are most often affected.[10,15] The mechanism of luxation has not been thoroughly defined;[19] however, it has been demonstrated experimentally that luxation cannot occur without severance of the infraspinatus tendon and the lateral surface of the joint capsule with its associated glenohumeral ligament.[16] These findings have been confirmed by observation of luxated joints during surgery.[15]

Clinical signs and physical examination are sufficient for diagnosis. The affected leg is carried in flexion with the foot rotated internally. Pain is elicited upon extension of the shoulder, and the greater tubercle of the humerus may be palpated lateral to

its normal position. A complete neurological examination is essential to detect brachial plexus or peripheral nerve deficits.

Radiographs of the shoulder are necessary to confirm the diagnosis and to detect fractures or excessive wearing of the glenoid labrum. If the luxation is intermittent, stress radiographs may be required to demonstrate the instability.

Conservative Management

Conservative management of acute lateral luxation consists of closed manual reduction and cage rest or reduction and placement of the limb in a non–weight-bearing sling or spica splint for two to three weeks. After induction of general anesthesia, the limb is placed in extension, and the head of the humerus is pressed medially while counterpressure is applied to the neck of the scapula.

If the reduction appears stable, cage confinement for seven to ten days may be adequate to prevent recurrence of the luxation. An unstable reduction requires that the limb be placed in some form of coaptation; a non–weight-bearing sling or spica splint may be used, depending on the temperament of the patient and the personal preference of the surgeon.[12]

Surgical Technique

Indications for surgical intervention in dogs with lateral shoulder luxation are recurrent luxation and fracture-luxations in which the fracture involves an articular surface.

The first surgical procedure for correction of lateral shoulder luxation in dogs was a modification of a technique used in humans,[1] using a Teflon band passed through drill holes in the proximal humerus and scapular spine. A similar technique using a strip of skin was described by Vaughn.[18] Denny[7] advocated the use of a large nylon mattress suture through the neck of the scapula and humeral neck to create strong medial and lateral collateral ligaments. Reefing of the joint capsule alone as a method for improving joint stability has also been described.[11]

Adapting another human technique, Hohn and colleagues[10] described the use of the biceps brachii tendon to stabilize lateral shoulder luxation. The skin incision is placed over the craniolateral joint surface. It extends distally, just medial to the midline of the humerus, and ends at the midshaft.[10,14] After incision and retraction of the subcutaneous tissue with the skin, the brachiocephalic muscle is identified and retracted medially following a fascial incision along its lateral margin. The superficial pectoral muscle is freed from the humerus from its proximal border distally to the distal communicating vein, which crosses the muscle. The deep pectoral is similarly incised to free its entire insertion.

Following elevation and retraction of the pectoral

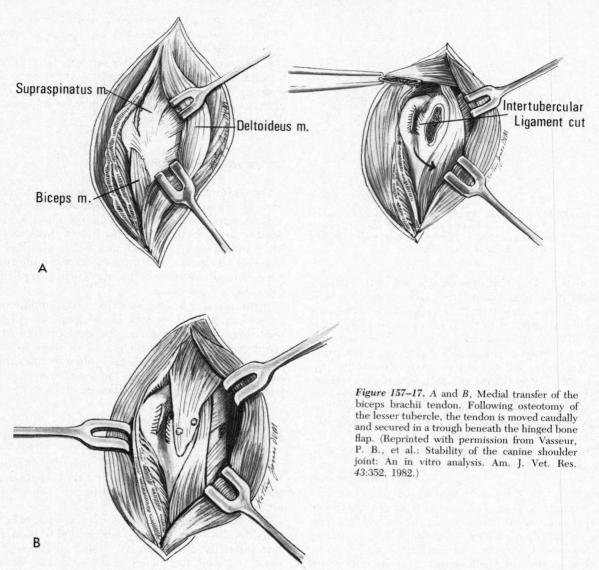

Supraspinatus m.

Deltoideus m.

Biceps m.

A

Intertubercular
Ligament cut

B

Figure 157–17. A and B, Medial transfer of the biceps brachii tendon. Following osteotomy of the lesser tubercle, the tendon is moved caudally and secured in a trough beneath the hinged bone flap. (Reprinted with permission from Vasseur, P. B., et al.: Stability of the canine shoulder joint: An in vitro analysis. Am. J. Vet. Res. 43:352, 1982.)

muscles, the fascial attachments between the deep pectoral and supraspinatus muscles are divided sufficiently to allow retraction of the supraspinatus. The transverse humeral ligament is incised and the biceps tendon freed from surrounding fascia and the joint capsule.

The greater tubercle is cut to reflect the tendinous insertion of the supraspinatus, and the joint capsule is incised dorsally to fully expose the tendon of the biceps brachii. The tendon is translocated to the lateral side of the cut greater tubercle (Fig. 157–17). The tendon may be placed in a preformed groove in the lateral humeral surface and anchored with staples, if necessary, to maintain its position. The greater tubercle is reattached with a screw or two Kirschner wires, and the dorsal joint capsule is closed with absorbable suture material. The superficial and deep pectoral muscles are sutured to the fascia of the deltoid muscle. The remaining fascial layers, subcutaneous tissues, and skin are closed separately. Cage rest is recommended for seven to ten days.

Six of seven dogs with lateral luxations corrected by means of the biceps tendon translocation procedure regained normal use of the limb.[15] Hohn and colleagues[10] described four dogs in their original report of the technique, all of which regained complete function.

Although concern has been expressed that alteration of the location of the biceps brachii tendon would negatively influence joint motion and potentially cause degenerative changes, *in vivo* experiments and clinical results support its use.[4,15,16,17]

MEDIAL SHOULDER LUXATION

Medial shoulder luxation may be associated with trauma; however, certain breeds have a tendency toward shoulder joint instability, especially on the medial side. In some dogs the problem may be bilateral.

Medial luxation occurs in small and toy

breds.[5,9,10,15] Luxation cannot occur until there is sufficient laxity or tearing of the subscapularis muscle and medial joint capsule with its associated glenohumeral ligament.[16]

The acutely affected limb is carried in flexion with the foot rotated outward. Pain is associated with extension of the shoulder, and the greater tubercle may be palpated medial to its normal position. Dogs with chronic luxation may not demonstrate pain. Often the luxation can be easily reduced and again dislocated simply by manipulation. A thorough neurological examination is essential.

Radiographs, as in the case of acute lateral luxation, should be made to confirm the diagnosis and to check for fractures of the glenoid or proximal humerus. In recurrent medial luxation, special note should be made of the degree of wear of the glenoid labrum. Severe bony erosion denotes chronically lax supporting structures and a guarded prognosis. Stress radiographs may be needed to document the instability.

Conservative Management

Conservative care of acute medial luxation consists of reduction and cage rest or reduction and placement of the limb in a Velpeau-type sling for two to three weeks. This type of sling distracts the humeral head laterally.

Unstable reductions and fractures involving the articular surfaces require surgical intervention. Recurrent luxations may not respond well to surgical treatment if severe instability or secondary joint changes exist. Judgment must be made in these cases on the basis of age, general health, and severity of disability.

Surgical Technique

In 1968, Ball[3] modified the procedure described by Vaughn for lateral luxation to stabilize medial luxation in a dog, utilizing a nylon prosthesis. Hohn and co-workers[10] described a tendon translocation similar to that used for lateral luxation.

In the Hohn procedure, the initial approach, with retraction of the pectoral muscles, is identical to that used for lateral luxation. The leg is rotated outward, and the subscapularis muscle is elevated and detached from the lesser tubercle. The tendon of the coracobrachialis muscle lies craniomedially and is retracted with the subscapularis. Tissues over the intertubercular groove and the transverse humeral ligament are transected, and the dorsal joint capsule surrounding the biceps brachii tendon is incised to allow mobilization of the tendon.

A crescent osteotomy is made in the lesser tubercle, with the bottom of the crescent following the contour of the humeral head. The flap of bone is elevated, with the hinged portion being craniodorsal. A small amount of cancellous bone is curetted from beneath the flap, the luxation is reduced, and the tendon is fitted into the groove beneath the bone flap (Fig. 157–18). The flap is secured with two Kirschner wires.

The medial joint capsule is reefed with heavy chromic suture. The subscapularis is advanced and tightened near the insertion of the deep pectoral with mattress sutures. Both pectoral muscles are attached to the deltoid and deep brachial fascia. The brachiocephalic muscle is sutured to the brachial fascia, and the subcutaneous and skin layers are closed separately. The leg is placed in a Velpeau-type sling for two weeks.

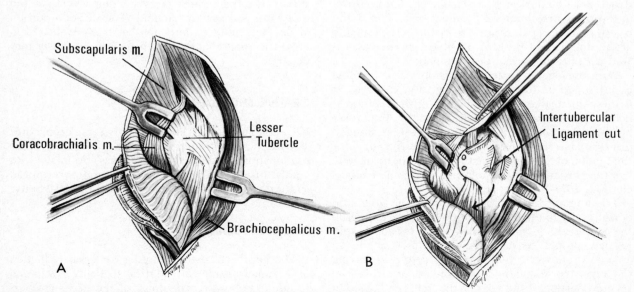

Figure 157–18. *A*, Lateral transfer of the biceps brachii tendon. Following osteotomy of the greater tubercle, the biceps tendon is freed and moved laterally. *B*, The greater tubercle is then replaced and held by small pins or a bone screw. (Reprinted with permission from Vasseur, P. B., et al.: Stability of the canine shoulder joint: An in vitro analysis. Am. J. Vet. Res. *43*:352, 1982.)

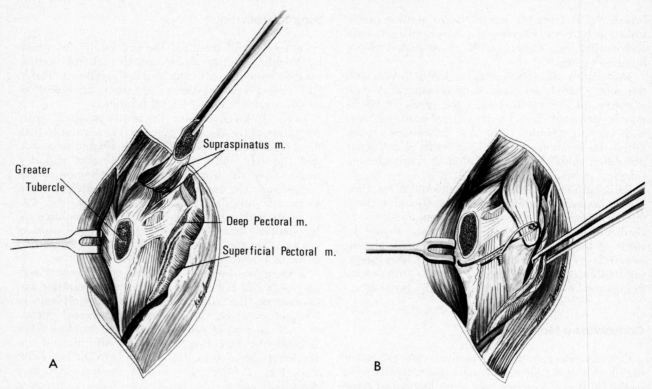

Greater
Tubercle

Supraspinatus m.

Deep Pectoral m.

Superficial Pectoral m.

A

B

Figure 157–19. A, Osteotomy of the proximal greater tubercle allows mobilization of a portion of the supraspinatus muscle. B, The bone fragment is moved to the area of the lesser tubercle and stabilized using a tension band apparatus. (Reprinted with permission from Vasseur, P. B., et al.: Stability of the canine shoulder joint: An in vitro analysis. Am. J. Vet. Res. *43*:352, 1982.)

Transfer of a portion of the supraspinatus insertion and reefing of the medial joint capsule have been advocated for luxations when damage has occurred to the biceps brachii tendon or tendon transfer has been unsuccessful.[4]

The approach to the joint is identical to that for a biceps brachii tendon translocation. The medial joint structures are imbricated, and if damage has occurred to the transverse humeral ligament or tendon of the biceps brachii, repair is made to maintain the function of the muscle and prevent possible lameness associated with loss of normal biceps function.

With the leg in an extended position, an osteotome is positioned on the crest of the greater tubercle. It is directed so that the medial line of the incision is parallel to the humeral border of the transverse humeral ligament, and the lateral line is positioned just cranial to the infraspinatus tendon. The cut splits the tendon of the supraspinatus so that approximately half remains attached to the remaining greater tubercle (Fig. 157–19).

The tendon of the supraspinatus is carefully split dorsally only to the extent that the free end can reach the area of the lesser tubercle. If the tendon is split too far, proper tension cannot be maintained. An area on the lesser tubercle is prepared by removing the outer cortex with an osteotome or drill. The severed portion of the greater tubercle is attached to the prepared site with two Kirschner wires. A hole is drilled in the humeral crest just distal to the

osteotomy site. A tension band wire is placed through the hole, then around the pins, and tightened. Following routine closure, the leg is immobilized in a Velpeau-type sling for two to three weeks.

In evaluating medial translocation of the biceps tendon, one survey reported satisfactory results in 11 of 12 dogs,[15] another in 10 of 11 dogs.[10] In the latter survey, the one unsatisfactory outcome was attributed to a worn and shallow glenoid. Transfer of a portion of the supraspinatus insertion has been evaluated in only two dogs, both of which had a satisfactory outcome.[4]

CRANIAL SHOULDER LUXATION

Cranial luxation of the shoulder is a rare occurrence associated with trauma.[6] Physical and radiographic examinations confirm the diagnosis. Animals with cranial luxation described in the literature required surgical intervention for correction of the instability.

Surgical Technique

The approach to the shoulder for open reduction of a cranial luxation is identical to that for a lateral luxation. Following osteotomy of the greater tubercle, a groove is made in the osteotomy site deep enough to accommodate the tendon of the biceps brachii. The tendon is mobilized by incising the transverse humeral ligament and the dorsal joint capsule and is placed in the groove beneath the greater tubercle. The joint capsule is closed and the greater tubercle is fixed in place with two Kirschner wires or bone screws. The remaining closure is routine. The limb is placed in a spica splint for ten to 14 days.

CAUDAL LUXATION

Caudolateral or caudodistal luxation is rare. Imbrication or reefing of the joint capsule works well in affected animals.[13]

An approach is made to the caudolateral region of the shoulder joint, and the joint capsule is imbricated with mattress or Lembert sutures of heavy chromic gut. The limb is supported in a non–weight-bearing sling for ten to 14 days.

Salvage Techniques

Dogs with chronic luxations may develop excessive wear of the glenoid labrum, and it may not be possible to reconstruct the glenoid–humeral head mechanism. Severe articular fractures or gunshot wounds resulting in luxation of the shoulder may not be amenable to routine surgical treatment. The traditional therapy in these situations has been arthrodesis, a procedure that is difficult to perform and generally requires bone plating equipment.

Alternative procedures include excision arthroplasty of the humeral head, resection of the glenoid, and temporary transarticular fixation. Piermattei[13] reported satisfactory results in four dogs of resection of the glenoid but gave a guarded prognosis and recommended the procedure as a salvage procedure only. Other techniques require more evaluation before recommendations can be made.

1. Alexander, J. E.: Open reduction and fixation of shoulder luxation. Small Anim. Clin. 2:379, 1962.
2. Alexander, J. W.: Orthopedic conditions of the forelimb. Am. Anim. Hosp. Assoc. Proc. 48:311, 1981.
3. Ball, D. C.: A case of medial luxation of the canine shoulder joint and its surgical correction. Vet. Rec. 83:195, 1968.
4. Craig, E., Hohn, R. B., and Anderson, W. D.: Surgical stabilization of traumatic medial shoulder dislocation. J. Am. Anim. Hosp. Assoc. 16:93, 1980.
5. DeAngelis, M. P.: Luxations of the shoulder joint. In Bojrab, M. J. (ed.): Current Techniques in Small Animal Surgery. Lea & Febiger, Philadelphia, 1975.
6. DeAngelis, M. P., and Swartz, A.: Surgical correction of cranial dislocation of the scapulohumeral joint in a dog. J. Am. Vet. Med. Assoc. 156:435, 1970.
7. Denny, H. R.: A guide to canine orthopedic surgery. Blackwell Scientific Publications, Oxford, 1980.
8. Dingwall, J. S., and Flipo, J.: Joints of the forelimb. In Archibald, J. (ed.): Canine Surgery. American Veterinary Publications, Inc., Santa Barbara, 1974.
9. Hinko, P. J.: Recurrent shoulder luxation. Canine Pract. 4:46, 1977.
10. Hohn, R. B., Rosen, H., Bohning, R. M., et al.: Surgical stabilization of recurrent shoulder luxation. Vet. Clin. North Am. 1:537, 1971.
11. Lippincott, C. L.: Reefing of the shoulder joint. A technique to surgically restore the integrity of a luxated scapulohumeral articulation in the dog. Vet. Med. Small Anim. Clin. 66:695, 1971.
12. Northway, R. B.: Joint immobilization in small animals. Mod. Vet. Pract. 56:191, 1975.
13. Piermattei, D. L.: Orthopedic conditions of the shoulder region. Am. Anim. Hosp. Assoc. Proc. 47:363, 1980.
14. Piermattei, D. L., and Greeley, R. G.: An Atlas of Surgical Approaches to the Bones of the Dog and Cat. W. B. Saunders Co., Philadelphia, 1979.
15. Vasseur, P. B.: Clinical results of surgical correction of shoulder luxation in dogs. J. Am. Vet. Med. Assoc. 182:503, 1983.
16. Vasseur, P. B., Moore, D., and Brown, S. A.: Stability of the canine shoulder joint: An in vitro analysis. Am. J. Vet. Res. 43:352, 1982.
17. Vasseur, P. B., Pool, R. R., and Klein, K.: Effects of tendon transfer on the canine scapulohumeral joint: An experimental study. Am. J. Vet. Res. 44:811, 1983.
18. Vaughn, L. C.: Dislocation of the shoulder joint in the dog and cat. J. Small Anim. Pract. 8:45, 1967.
19. Wadsworth, P. L.: Biomechanics of the luxation of joints. In Bojrab, M. J. (ed.): Pathophysiology in Small Animal Surgery. Lea & Febiger, Philadelphia, 1981.

Humeral Fractures

Jeffrey L. Berzon

Anatomically, the humerus is a structure changing in size, shape, diameter, and cortical thickness. It is one of the major weight-bearing bones. A heavy muscular architecture guards the humerus both medially and laterally over most of its length, making it a difficult structure to expose surgically. The muscles on the proximal and craniolateral aspects of the shaft act to adduct and internally rotate the limb, whereas the muscles on the caudomedial aspect abduct and externally rotate it.[13] The major blood supply to the limb passes down from the axilla on the medial aspect with the motor and sensory nerve supply to the medial antebrachium and flexors of the lower limb (brachial artery and vein, median artery and vein, and median and ulnar nerve). The radial nerve passes along the lateral midshaft border below the deltoid musculature, slightly cranial and medial to the biceps muscle group. Here, it is highly susceptible to injury owing to its location and must always be carefully evaluated prior to consideration of any surgical repair. Often a patient with humeral fracture carries the affected limb with the elbow dropped and with the paw resting on its dorsal surface because of a weakening of the extension apparatus (pseudoparalysis).[13]

Differentiation of a radial nerve paresis/paralysis must be made by performing a thorough neurological evaluation and establishing the presence of intact pain sensation (conscious perception of pain to toe pinch). To document complete denervation, a nerve conduction velocity and electromyogram can be obtained but are not valid if carried out before five days post-injury. Additionally, because the humerus lies over the cranial aspect of the thorax, careful auscultation, often combined with radiographic evaluation, is necessary to eliminate concomitant trauma such as pneumothorax, hemothorax, pulmonary hemorrhage, myocardial bruising, or rib fracture.

Humeral fractures were originally treated with cage rest and then by a variety of external coaptation splints.[10] The need to immobilize the joint above and below the fracture to minimize movement was soon recognized. More elaborate splints, such as full spicas, and the Shroeder-Thomas splint, were devised. Internal fixation, consisting of intramedullary pinning by both open and closed methods, began to evolve. With time and sophistication of surgical and aseptic technique, a variety of fixation methods allowed more accurate means of anatomical reconstruction (intramedullary pinning with wiring, plates and screws, Kirschner-Ehmer splint, etc.). Irrespective of what repair is used, early ambulation is always paramount, as well as daily physiotherapy to ensure a good range of joint motion. Physical size (e.g., overweight dog, giant breed), function, activity level (e.g., guard dog) of the patient, type and extent of injury, and experience of the surgeon all affect the repair technique chosen. If the stability of internal fixation is questionable, external coaptation may be combined but almost always sacrifices some degree of motion and encourages ankylosis ("fracture disease").

In the following pages, each area of the humerus is discussed along with individualized surgical approaches, techniques, and anatomy.

SURGICAL METHODS

Closed Reduction

Open or closed intramedullary pin fixation is the most conventional and most widely used means of repair for humeral fractures. Closed reduction requires general anesthesia, aseptic technique, and a knowledge of anatomical landmarks. Criteria for closed pinning include one or all of the following: (1) simple, two-piece fracture, (2) actively growing animals (animals younger than 12 weeks heal much faster, and reduction can be 50 to 60 per cent), and (3) experience of the operator. Contraindications for closed repair are multiple fragment injuries, joint and periarticular involvement, and rotationally unstable fractures.

The pin selected is usually determined by the humeral body diameter and area of involvement. The

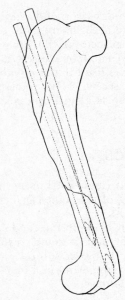

Figure 157–20. Multiple pins of the same diameter are seated distally to fill the canal and ensure rotational stability. (Reprinted with permission from Rudy, R.: Management of limb fractures in small animals. Vet. Clin. North Am. 5:223, 1975.)

largest pin that can be advanced easily into the medulla of the body is generally chosen for axial stability. Traction on the limb, by manual extension or an extender, is often necessary to fatigue the muscles around the fracture site for reduction. Muscle relaxants can also be used, depending on the degree of contraction and the time elapsed since injury. The entry site is via a small incision on the craniolateral aspect of the greater tubercle. Fractures are easier to reduce with the elbow in full extension. When a handchuck is used, a small amount of the pin (3 to 5 cm) should be exposed to avoid bending the pin. The pin is directed parallel to the humeral body and toward the lateral epicondyle, and seated as distally as possible into the subchondral bone in the trochlea (medial portion) or just above the supracondylar foramen. When paired pins are used, they are of equal diameter (Fig. 157–20). After each pin is placed, the elbow should be flexed and extended to check for crepitus from impingement. Radiographs can be taken prior to cutting the pin to check for proper placement and reduction. Greater than 50 to 60 per cent contact between fracture ends is considered acceptable with this technique. The proximal ends are then bent over with a vise-like grip or pin bender to "hook" the ends prior to cutting, as with a Rush pin, and to eliminate pin irritation. If the pin diameter is too large to bend, the cut end should be filed smooth.

Open Reduction (Intramedullary Fixation)

When open repair techniques are chosen, pins are passed retrograde from the proximal fracture end toward the craniolateral aspect of the humerus. The

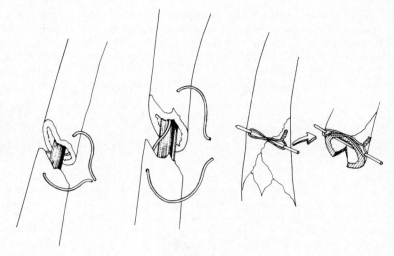

Figure 157–21. Patterns of interfragmentary wire placement. The hemi-cerclage may encircle the intramedullary pin. The small pin and figure-of-eight wire are used to secure small, unstable fragments. (Reprinted with permission from Rudy, R.: Management of limb fractures in small animals. Vet. Clin. North Am. 5:223, 1975.)

fracture is reduced manually or with bone-holding forceps, and the pins are advanced distally. All smaller fragments are wired into place prior to final reduction to reduce the injury into two major pieces. If rotational instability is present, one of the following techniques can be used to neutralize the movement: hemi-cerclage wires with or without incorporation of the intramedullary pin, figure-of-eight tension band wiring, full cerclage, or a Kirschner-Ehmer apparatus (half, full, or penetrating) (Fig. 157–21). Generally, 18- or 20-gauge stainless steel, orthopedic wire is selected for dogs, and 20- or 22-gauge for cats.

Plate Fixation

Plate fixation requires more elaborate equipment and a general understanding of plating techniques. Generally, plates are used under compression or neutralization or as a buttress, which is technically a neutralization plate with a cortical defect.[9] Compression plating involves rigid reduction of the two fragments by loading the plate with a tension device or plates with eccentrically designed holes (e.g., DCP plate). This method is generally used to repair transverse or short oblique fractures. Direct, primary bony union takes place without visible periosteal or endosteal callus.[9] Ideally, a minimum of six cortices should be penetrated above and below the fracture site with all plating procedures. The neutralization principle is used with multiple piece (comminuted) injuries in which the major fragments are "neutralized" following reduction of smaller fragments with interfragmentary compression (lag screws). Buttress plating is achieved when comminuted fractures are reduced in neutralization and cortical defects still exist. These defects, as well as other highly comminuted injuries, should *always* be packed with autogenous, cancellous bone grafts to provide fresh osteogenitor cells to the fracture interface and accelerate early bone remodelling.[3,9,12,13]

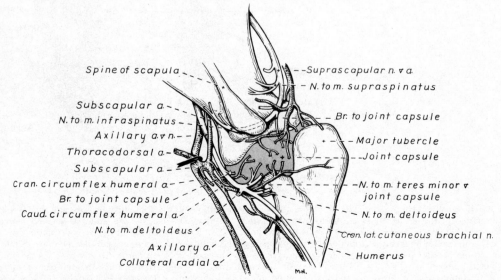

Figure 157–22. The neurovascular anatomy on the cranial, lateral, and caudal aspects of the right shoulder joint (all musculature is removed). (Reprinted with permission from Evans, H. E., and Christensen, G. C. (eds.): *Miller's Anatomy of the Dog.* 2nd ed. W. B. Saunders, Philadelphia, 1979.)

The tension side of the humerus is cranial and should ideally be selected for plate application.[14] It is preferable to plate the lateral surface for body fractures and the lateral, medial, or caudal surface for more distal injuries.[2,14] The plate should be contoured with a plate bender, using a template, or by assessing a radiograph of the opposite, uninjured limb. The size of the plate selected depends on the anatomical area of involvement, type of fracture, and activity level. Ideally, all plates should be removed at the time of radiographic union, but many are left in place with no long-term complications.

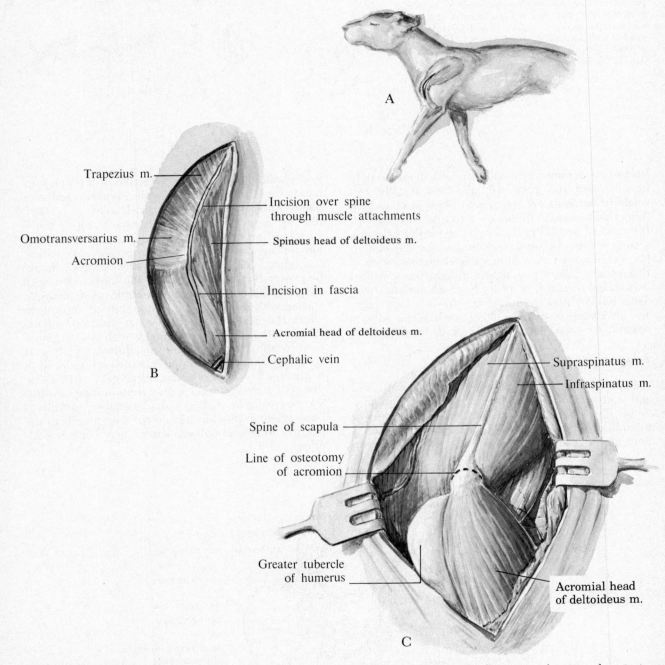

Figure 157–23. A, The curved incision begins at the middle of the scapula and follows the spine distally, crossing the joint and continuing over the lateral surface of the humerus to the midpoint of the shaft. B, The skin margins are undermined and retracted after the subcutaneous fascia and fat are incised in the same line as the skin incision. An incision is made in the deep fascia directly over the spine of the scapula and is deepened to free the origin of the spinous part of the deltoid and the omotransversarius muscles and the insertion of the trapezius muscle on the spine. The incision is continued distally through the deep fascia directly over the acromial part of the deltoid and is halted before it reaches the omobrachial vein. The incised fascia is undermined and retracted from the acromial part of the dentoid. C, The omotransversarius and trapezius are undermined and allowed to retract cranially. The division between the two parts of the deltoid muscle is developed by blunt dissection to allow freeing of the spinous part of the muscle and its caudal retraction with the deep fascia.

Illustration continued on opposite page

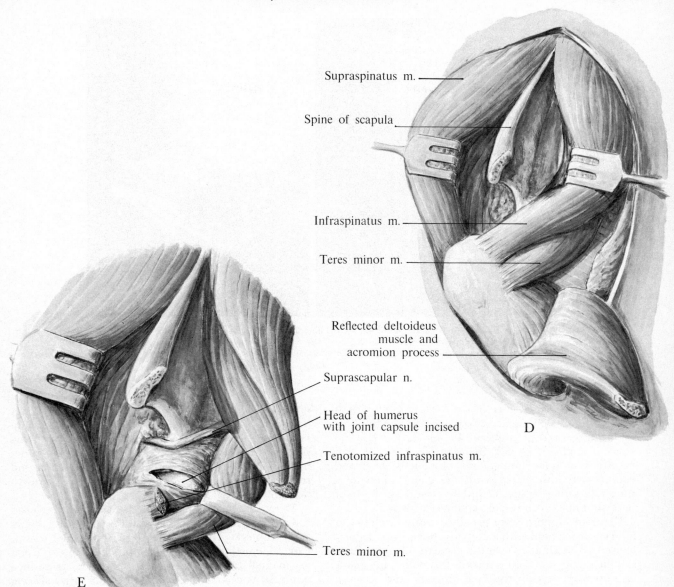

Figure 157–23 *Continued. D*, The supraspinatus and infraspinatus muscles are bluntly elevated from the spine and body of the scapula sufficiently to allow their retraction as shown. The surgeon should note the positon of the suprascapular nerve and avoid this structure during the elevation and retraction of the infraspinatus. *E*, Exposure of the joint requires tenotomy of the infraspinatus muscle. This cut is made near the muscle's insertion on the humerus, with enough stump being left to receive one or two sutures. In some cases it may be necessary to treat the teres minor muscle in a like manner, thus allowing greater exposure of the ventrolateral aspect of the joint capsule. (Reprinted with permission from Piermattei, D. L., and Greeley, R. G.: *An Atlas of Surgical Approaches to the Bones of the Dog and Cat.* W. B. Saunders, Philadelphia, 1979.)

FRACTURES OF THE PROXIMAL THIRD OF THE HUMERUS

Articular Surface Injuries

Fractures involving the articular surface of the humeral head are relatively uncommon. The affected limb is carried with the shoulder and elbow dropped and the paw resting on its dorsal surface (as in a brachial plexus or radial nerve injury), as with all humeral injuries.

The shoulder is protected by strong muscular support, and *full* surgical exposure of the articular surface is quite difficult. As with any injury disturbing the congruence of the joint surface, open reduction and fixation are always indicated, and exact alignment is imperative to ensure restoration of a smooth, gliding surface. If the joint surface has been irreparably damaged, surgical fusion (arthrodesis) should be considered as an alternative or salvage procedure.

Surgical exposure is through a craniolateral approach (Figs. 157–22 and 157–23). Additional exposure can be gained by osteotomizing the acromium or tenotomizing the infraspinatus and teres minor muscles if more caudal exposure is required (Fig. 157–23D and E). These fractures demand "compres-

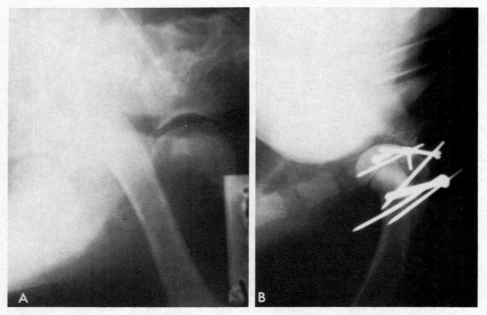

Figure 157–24. A, The right shoulder joint of an eight-month-old Labrador cross discloses a comminuted articular injury with a Salter I physeal separation. *B,* A lateral postoperative film shows repair of the articular surface with two large Kirschner wires (.0625-in.) and three lag screws (all screwheads countersunk so they are below the articular surface), and the Salter injury was repaired with one screw and three Steinmann pins.

sion" fixation using lag screws (or self-tapping screws as long as the proximal hole is overdrilled to allow for compression) or multiple Kirschner wires at divergent angles (Fig. 157–24). Any large defects can be filled with an autogenous cancellous graft and compressed into place to fill the gap. Following a thorough saline lavage, complete closure of the joint is recommended to reduce seroma formation.

External support is not usually required unless the injury is associated with a body fracture. Early return to weight-bearing and gentle, passive physiotherapy should begin soon after repair. Physiotherapy plays an important role in the final outcome and ensures the best functional results. Gentle extension and internal/external rotation with the elbow extended encourage restoration of muscle tone around the shoulder. Analgesics can be used, as well as hot packs and DMSO, to reduce discomfort. Restricted exercise, consisting of slow, controlled leash walking, is advised to encourage early limb usage. The later development of secondary degenerative osteoarthritis is always possible, depending on the amount of articular damage incurred at the time of injury.

Proximal Growth Plate (Salter I and II) Injuries

The proximal growth plate is a relatively common site for fracture cleavage in actively growing animals. Physeal or epiphyseal plate fractures are classified by the Salter system to clarify the site of involvement and predict the outcome. A Salter I injury is one in which the fracture line extends directly through the

epiphyseal plate and parallel to the joint surface. A Salter II injury is directed along the physis and includes a small portion of the metaphysis with the physeal fragment. Both injuries carry a good prognosis if repaired early with accurate reduction and rarely lead to premature physeal arrest or any growth deformities (Fig. 157–25).[1,13]

Many of these injuries can be treated by closed reduction if the fracture is fresh (less than five hours since injury). The patient is placed under deep, general anesthesia, and the limb is held in extension via manual traction or with an extender, to reduce muscular contraction. Muscle relaxants or paralyzing agents can be used to assist reduction. Once acceptable alignment is obtained, one or several small pins are advanced through the craniolateral aspect of the greater tubercle at a 30-degree angle into the distal segment for fixation. Postreduction lateral and craniocaudal radiographs are taken to check for alignment. If reduction is difficult or markedly unstable, the area can be opened and approached through a lateral skin incision (see Fig. 157–22). Intramedullary pins, half or full Kirschner-Ehmer apparatus, several smaller pins, or Rush pins can be used for immobilization. Plates, screws, and tension wires should not cross the epiphyseal plate, because compression of the plate may lead to physeal arrest and may affect bone length, width, and maturation (Fig. 157–26). One important suggestion is always to evaluate the supraglenoid tubercle of the scapula in growing dogs (origin of the biceps brachialis muscle) with proximal fractures to ensure that the apophyseal segment has not been avulsed. Healing time for epiphyseal injuries is shorter (4 to 6 weeks) owing to their proximity to the

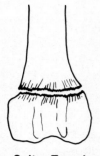 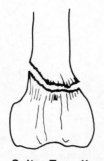 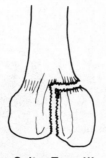 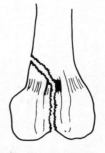 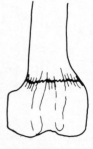

Salter Type I
Fracture line directed along physis (slipped epiphysis)

Salter Type II
Fracture line directed along physis and into the metaphysis

Salter Type III
Fracture line along physis and through epiphyseal plate into joint

Salter Type IV
Fracture line across physis, metaphysis and through epiphysis

Salter Type V
Compression or crushing injury to the epiphyseal plate without displacement

Figure 157–25. Classification of epiphyseal (physeal) plate fractures. (Reprinted with permission from Berzon, J. L.: The classification and management of epiphyseal plate fractures. J. Am. Anim. Hosp. Assoc. 16:651, 1980.)

growth zone. Pins should be removed at the time of radiographic union.

Proximal Body Injuries

The proximal body can be approached through a craniolateral skin incision (Fig. 157–27). The cranial aspect of the proximal body of the humerus has a convex surface with a large diameter and follows a sigmoid curve. Distally, the surface becomes more concave.[14] Lateral and medial full surgical exposure is difficult because of the large surrounding muscle mass (Fig. 157–28). Body fractures can be described as: transverse, short or long oblique, spiral, segmental (free central segment), or comminuted. Most of these injuries can be repaired with simple intramedullary pinning, stack pinning, pin and wire fixation (hemi-cerclage, figure-of-eight tension wire, etc.), use of Kirschner-Ehmer apparatus (half or full), or

plate fixation. The technique used depends on the equipment available, size of the patient (e.g., large, active dogs do best with rigid plate fixation), type of fracture (transverse vs. comminuted) and cost. Rotational stability is imperative when pinning techniques are used. Hemi-cerclage, half or full Kirschner-Ehmer apparatus, and cerclage (when the obliquity of the fracture is greater than twice the diameter) can be used (Figs. 157–29 and 157–30).[2,12] If cerclage wires are used, small grooves can be made in the cortical surface to keep the wires from sliding or migrating distally, as they may because of the rapid change in humeral diameter. Single cerclage wires are avoided to alleviate a fulcrum effect. Care is always taken to avoid placing the wires in or near the fracture lines. When intramedullary pins are used, the ends should be seated distally in the trochlea of the medial portion of the condyle. It is important to mention here that anatomically speaking, the shaft is called the body and the entire distal end of the

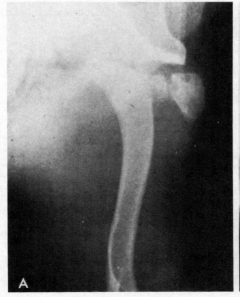 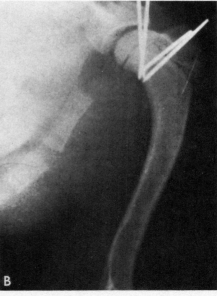

Figure 157–26. A, A physeal fracture (Salter I) with separation of the greater tubercle. *B,* Reduction of both fragments with two sets of paired Steinmann pins. (Courtesy of Dr. R. Dueland.)

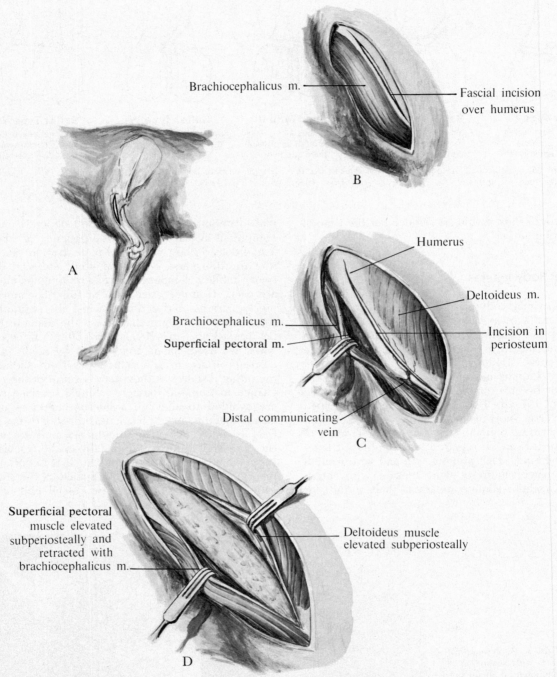

Brachiocephalicus m.

Fascial incision
over humerus

B

A

Humerus

Deltoideus m.

Brachiocephalicus m.

Superficial pectoral m.

Incision in
periosteum

Distal communicating
vein

C

Superficial pectoral
muscle elevated
subperiosteally and
retracted with
brachiocephalicus m.

Deltoideus muscle
elevated subperiosteally

D

Figure 157–27. *A,* The skin incision is made slightly lateral to the cranial midline of the bone and extends from the greater tubercle of the humerus proximally to a point near the midshaft of the bone. *B,* Following the undermining and retraction of the skin, an incision is made through the deep fascia along the caudal border of the brachiocephalicus muscle. *C,* The brachiocephalicus can be retracted cranially following blunt dissection between muscle and bone. An incision is made through the periosteum between the cranial border of the deltoideus muscle and the deep pectoral muscle. Several branches of the cephalic vein are severed by this incision and must be ligated. *D,* Exposure of the body is accomplished by the subperiosteal elevation of the deep pectoral and deltoideus muscles. This elevation usually includes a portion of the origin of the lateral head of the triceps, which lies under the deltoideus. (Reprinted with permission from Piermattei, D. L., and Greeley, R. G.: *An Atlas of Surgical Approaches to the Bones of the Dog and Cat.* W. B. Saunders, Philadelphia, 1979.)

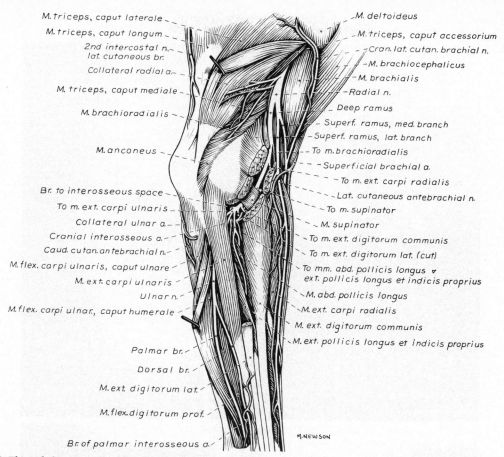

Figure 157–28. The radial nerve and its anatomical relationship to the surrounding lateral musculature. (Reprinted with permission from Evans, H. E., and Christensen, G. C. (eds.): *Miller's Anatomy of the Dog.* 2nd ed. Philadelphia, W. B. Saunders, 1979.)

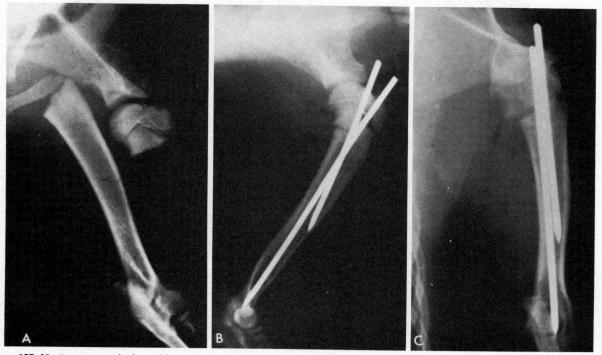

Figure 157–29. *A*, A proximal, short oblique body fracture just below the physis. *B*, Two intramedullary pins have been used to reduce the fracture and ensure rotational stability. *C*, Craniocaudal view showing 90 per cent reduction. (Courtesy of Dr. R. Dueland.)

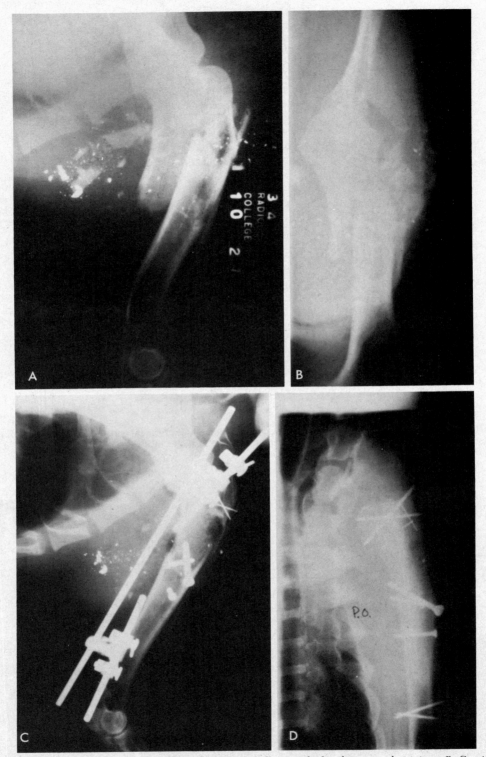

Figure 157–30. A, A highly comminuted, proximal body fracture secondary to a high-velocity gunshot injury. B, Craniocaudal view. C, Repair of the injury with multiple lag screws and small pins used to imobilize the larger fragments. The axial support is maintained with a full Kirschner-Ehmer apparatus. The small cortical defects and fracture site was packed with an autogenous cancellous bone graft. D, Craniocaudal view. (Courtesy of Dr. D. Aron.)

humerus is the condyle. There are no medial or lateral condyles, but there are medial and lateral epicondyles, and the lateral articular surface is called the capitulum and the medial surface the trochlea.[4,7,8]

When open reduction is performed, normograde or retrograde insertion of the distal pins is acceptable. Stability of these injuries can usually be completed with single or multiple pins combined with additional

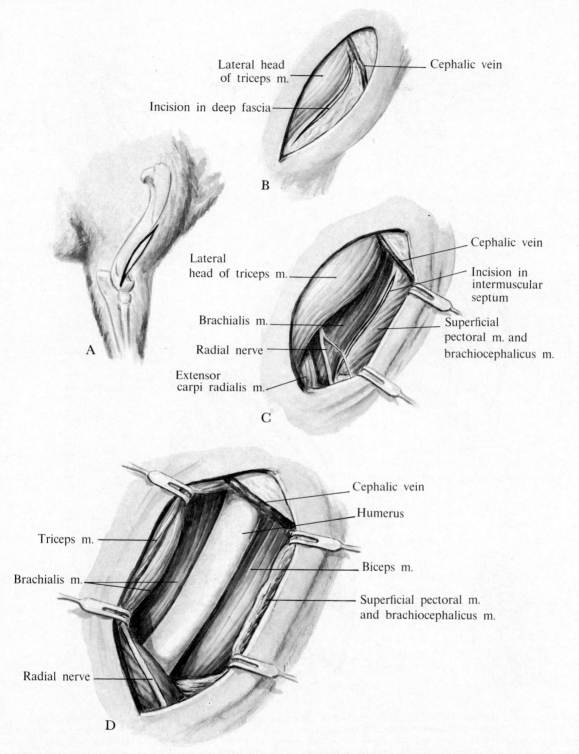

Figure 157–31. *A,* The craniolateral border of the humerus is the guide for this incision, which commences at the midshaft and ends at the lateral epicondyle. *B,* The skin margins are mobilized and retracted. Subcutaneous fascia and fat are incised in the same line as the skin, with the cephalic vein, which will cross the proximal end of the incision, being avoided. The deep fascia of the brachium is incised along the cranial border of the triceps. The incision curves caudally, parallel to the cephalic vein, to allow mobilization of the vein. The radial nerve must be protected when the distal end of this incision is opened. *C,* The deep fascia is undermined to allow cranial retraction of the cephalic vein and exposure of the radial nerve. An incision is made in the intermuscular septum between the brachialis and the brachiocephalicus muscle. *D,* The brachiocephalicus muscle and the distal portions of the superficial pectoral muscle are elevated at their insertions on the humerus to allow cranial retraction. The brachialis is freed from the bone by blunt dissection and is retracted caudally with the triceps and the radial nerve. To obtain better exposure of the distal portion of the bone, the lateral head of the triceps muscle can be retracted caudally, and the brachialis muscle and radial nerve retracted caudally. (Reprinted with permission from Piermattei, D. L., and Greeley, R. G.: *An Atlas of Surgical Approaches to the Bones of the Dog and Cat.* W. B. Saunders, Philadelphia, 1979.)

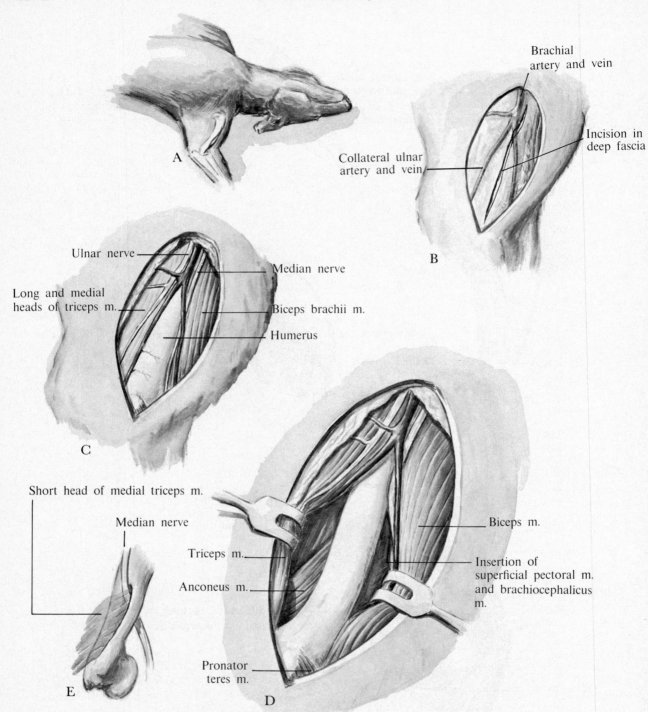

Figure 157–32. *A,* The skin incision extends from the medial epicondyle proximally along the cranial border of the humerus to the midbody of the bone. *B,* The skin is undermined and the subcutaneous fat is elevated sufficiently to allow visualization of the brachial and collateral ulnar vessels. The ulnar and medial nerves that accompany these vessels are not yet visible; they lie slightly deeper. An incision is made in the deep fascia directly over the distal shaft of the humerus and between the blood vessels. It may be necessary to continue the incision proximally over the vessels. *C,* Blunt dissection of the subfascial fat exposes the underlying structures. The manner in which the brachial vessels and the medial nerve are mobilized depends on the area of the bone that is to be exposed. The method illustrated here is used when the extreme distal portion of the bone is involved. If the proximal portion of the exposed area is of more interest, these vessels and nerves may be freed and retracted caudally with the triceps and the collateral ulnar vessels. The biceps and triceps muscles are elevated from the body of the bone. The periosteal branches of blood vessels are ligated as required. Subperiosteal elevation of a portion of the insertion of the superficial pectoral and branchiocephalicus muscles is necessary to expose fully the cranial surface of the bone. *E,* The cat shows a marked difference from the dog in this area. Note the supracondylar foramen in the bone through which the brachial artery and median nerve pass. Note also the short head of the medial triceps running caudal to the medial condyle and inserting on the medial side of the olecranon. The ulnar nerve passes under this muscle. (Reprinted with permission from Piermattei, D. L., and Greeley, R. G.: *An Atlas of Surgical Approaches to the Bones of the Dog and Cat.* W. B. Saunders, Philadelphia, 1979.)

wire stabilization (e.g., hemi-cerclage). Bending the pins at the area of the greater tubercle prior to cutting minimizes subcutaneous pin irritation, seroma formation, and pin migration. Large rods or nails can also be used following appropriate reaming procedures but require experience and familiarity with equipment. Plate fixation is also difficult owing to the contour of the proximal humerus. Specially designed plates such as buttress head, T plates, spoon plates, and cobra head plates afford excellent reduction and allow for multiple screw placement in the proximal segment. Absolutely accurate alignment is not always necessary here because the metaphyseal blood supply is rich and the surrounding muscle mass assists in holding the fracture in reduction. These injuries can be impacted (distal into proximal) if multiple cortical defects exist and precise anatomical reduction is not attainable.

MIDBODY HUMERAL FRACTURES

The general philosophy discussed in regard to proximal body injuries applies to midbody fractures. The associated soft tissue injuries must always be carefully evaluated prior to repair. The radial nerve crosses and branches from behind the brachialis muscle as it passes from medial to lateral over the musculospiral groove of the distal humerus. In this location, severe bruising (neurapraxia) or separation (neurotmesis) can occur, with severe injuries to the arm. Proper identification during open surgical reduction is imperative to avoid inadvertent injury. Traction is achieved by placing a Penrose drain around the nerve and gently moving it as needed. Anatomy of the radial nerve is depicted in Figure 157–28.

This area can be approached either laterally or medially (Fig. 157–31). The medial approach offers less muscular barriers but involves an extensive neurovascular network (Figs. 157–32 and 157–33). The medial aspect of the body has less curvature than the angulated lateral and cranial surfaces, eliminating the need for elaborate plate contouring.[14]

The method of repair depends upon the nature of the injury. Comminuted injuries are often complicated, with small voids in the cortical surface. These should be packed generously with autogenous, cancellous bone grafts following repair. Grafts are obtained from the iliac crest or proximal humerus.

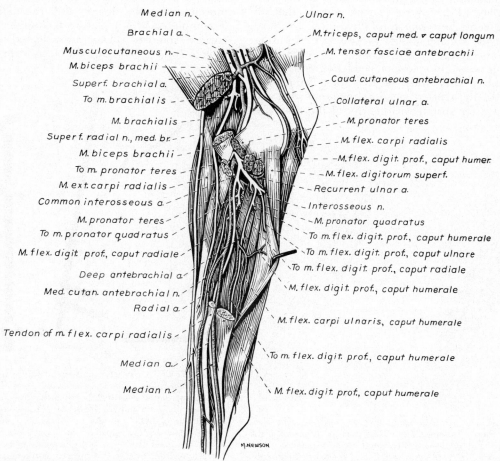

Figure 157–33. Medial aspect of the distal right forearm depicting the neurovascular supply. (Reprinted with permission from Evans, H. E., and Christensen, G. C. (eds.): *Miller's Anatomy of the Dog.* 2nd ed. W. B. Saunders, Philadelphia, 1979.)

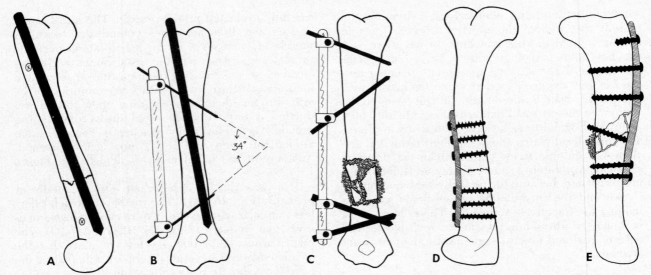

Figure 157–34. *A* and *B*, A transverse fracture repaired with one intramedullary pin and a half Kirschner-Ehmer apparatus. (Note the angle of K-E pins and that they penetrate both cortices.) *C*, A comminuted fracture repaired with an autogenous cancellous bone graft and a full Kirschner-Ehmer apparatus. *D*, A transverse fracture plated cranially under compression. (Transverse and oblique fractures can be compressed to encourage primary bone healing.) *E*, A comminuted fracture plated under neutralization (this plate neutralized the fragments in position) with a cancellous graft. (Reprinted with permission from Braden, T.: Surgical correction of humeral fractures. *In* Bojrab, M. (ed.): *Current Techniques in Small Animal Surgery.* Lea & Febiger, Philadelphia, 1975.)

Packing with grafts offers an early osteogenic effect for bone induction, supplying osteoblasts to the fracture interface. Principles of repair dictate that all minor fragments be reduced to a two-piece fracture. Several of the smaller pieces are prewired (tension band, hemi-cerclage) or lag screwed (interfragmentary compression) prior to final reduction with plate, intramedullary pins, rods, or Kirschner-Ehmer apparatus. Totally avulsed smaller fragments that are not required for structural integrity of the shaft are

discarded. This void can be packed with a cancellous graft or a muscular pedicle graft (transposition of a muscle across the defect) after the definitive repair is complete. When plating techniques are chosen, narrow (standard) plates are selected for repair, although broad plates should be used in larger (more

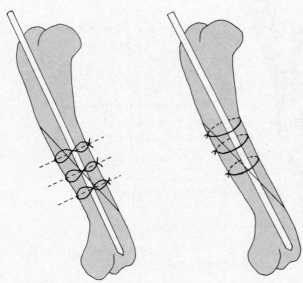

Figure 157–35. This pair of drawings depicts two wiring techniques that can be used with long oblique shaft fractures (figure-of-eight tension wire and cerclage). (Reprinted with permission from Braden, T.: Surgical correction of humeral fractures. *In* Bojrab, M. (ed.): *Current Techniques in Small Animal Surgery.* Lea & Febiger, Philadelphia, 1975.)

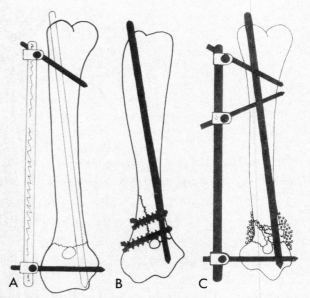

Figure 157–36. *A*, A distal transverse fracture repaired with one intramedullary pin, seated in the trochlea, and a half Kirschner-Ehmer apparatus. *B*, A distal oblique fracture repaired with one intramedullary pin and two lag screws. (Hemi-cerclage or tension band figure-of-eights can also be used.) *C*, A distal comminuted supracondylar fracture repaired with a three-pin Kirschner-Ehmer splint, intramedullary pin, and cancellous graft. (Reprinted with permission from Braden, T.: Surgical correction of humeral fractures. *In* Bojrab, M. (ed.): *Current Techniques in Small Animal Surgery.* Lea & Febiger, Philadelphia, 1975.)

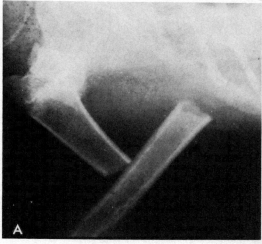

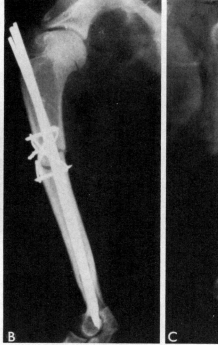

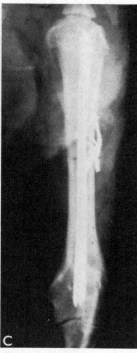

Figure 157–37. *A,* A transverse midbody fracture. *B,* Repair of the injury with two intramedullary pins and several tension band wires. *C,* Craniocaudal view.

than 35 to 40 kg), more active patients. Most plates are applied laterally but can be placed cranially (on the tension side) or medially where the shaft is relatively uniform and has minimal curvature.

Combination fixation techniques (e.g., full or half Kirschner-Ehmer with pin and wire fixation) as well as more rigid forms of neutralization plating can be considered for comminuted injuries (Figs. 157–34 to 157–36). Badly comminuted midbody injuries are also repaired using segmental allografts and compression plating to allow for "creeping substitution." With such an allograft, four to ten months are required for complete incorporation and remodelling. It is also acceptable to discard several or all of the cortical fragments and impact or remodel the fracture ends (like a rabbit joint) to allow for more stable reduction; a reduction of 1 to 2 cm in length is cosmetically and functionally acceptable. Several examples of these

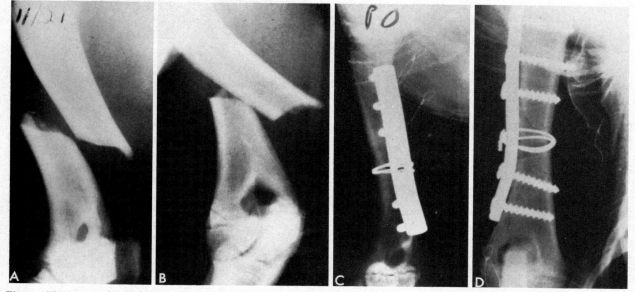

Figure 157–38. *A,* A short, oblique midbody fracture. *B,* Craniocaudal view. *C,* A plate has been used to compress the fracture line. A cerclage wire is used over an open screw hole for additional support and technically is only a hemi-cerclage wire. *D,* The contoured plate on the lateral surface. (Courtesy of Dr. R. Dueland.)

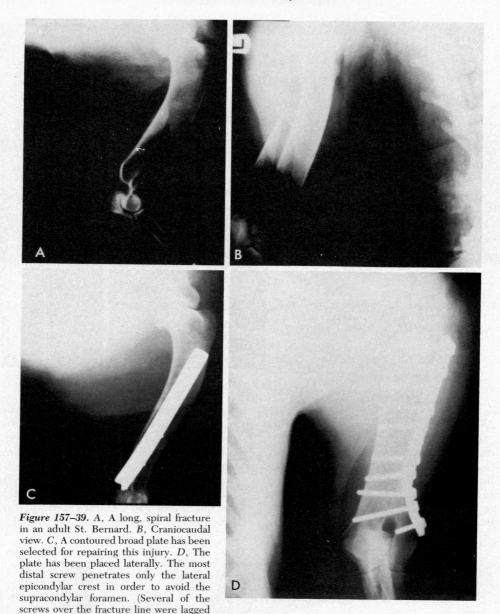

Figure 157–39. *A*, A long, spiral fracture in an adult St. Bernard. *B*, Craniocaudal view. *C*, A contoured broad plate has been selected for repairing this injury. *D*, The plate has been placed laterally. The most distal screw penetrates only the lateral epicondylar crest in order to avoid the supracondylar foramen. (Several of the screws over the fracture line were lagged directly through the plate.)

injuries and their repair are illustrated (Figs. 157–37 to 157–39).

FRACTURES OF THE DISTAL THIRD OF THE HUMERUS

Body Fractures

The distal third of the humeral body is narrow and flattened craniocaudally. Pin and wire fixation is the most common means of repair, and Rush pinning and plate fixation are also well accepted. Kirschner-Ehmer apparatus (half or full) can be used for additional or primary fixation (see Fig. 157–36). Some surgeons use the Kirschner-Ehmer apparatus (proximal pins in humeral body above the fracture line and distal pins in the radius/ulna) to span the elbow joint to minimize movement and have found minimal long-term inter-

ference with elbow motion. If this technique or any other external coaptation device is used, the elbow must be placed at a normal, functional standing angle (155 to 165 degrees) in case ankylosis (fracture disease) develops secondarily. It is also important to impress upon the owners the type of postoperative care required with a Kirschner-Ehmer device.

The distal lateral (most practical) or medial approach is used and can be combined with a triceps tenotomy or transolecranon osteotomy if additional exposure is required (see Figs. 157–31 and 157–32).[11,14] With intramedullary pin fixation, it is recommended that the pins span the entire length of the humeral body to ensure good axial stability. This principle often limits the number of pins that can be used, because the internal diameter of the distal medullary body is one-half to one-third of the proximal portion.[6,7]

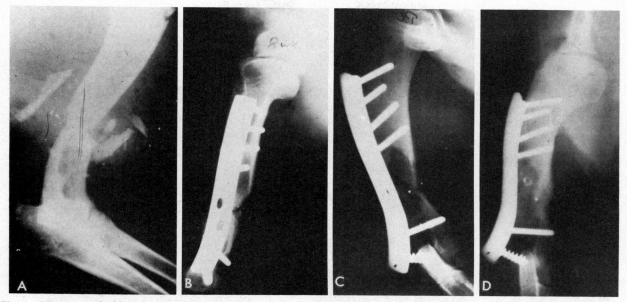

Figure 157–40. A, A highly comminuted, compound distal body fracture secondary to a high-velocity gunshot injury. B, Repair with a large contoured broad plate. Two holes had to be left open over a long cortical defect (buttress plate) that was grafted with cancellous bone. (This area was regrafted three weeks later.) C, Craniocaudal view. D, Craniocaudal view 20 weeks later. The defect is totally filled with cortical bone. (Courtesy of Dr. R. Dueland.)

Paired intramedullary pins used here should be of a small enough diameter to allow for the "bowing" required to advance them. Pins can be passed out proximally and then seated distally following reduction. In some instances, the pins can be passed out distally through the trochlea (medial), by the medial epicondyle, and then advanced proximally following reduction. Additional fixation (hemi-cerclage, cerclage) can be used if the fracture is rotationally unstable or to secure smaller fragments.

Plate contouring of the lateral diaphysis is difficult but gives excellent stability when correctly applied. Caudal or medial application can also be used. Neutralization or compression principles can be used, depending on the type of fracture, e.g., for transverse or short oblique fracture, compression is used; for a comminuted fracture, multiple lag screws and a neutralization plate are used. Several examples of injuries to this area and their repairs are illustrated in Figures 157–40 and 157–141. Occasionally, the distal physis is fractured, necessitating internal reduction and repair (Fig. 157–42). Postoperative physiotherapy is stressed to restore and maintain joint motion. It has been our experience that excessive callus formation occurs with injuries here, and limitation of elbow movement can occur secondarily. Careful attention must be paid to the location of the median nerve passing through the supratrochlear foramen in the cat in order to avoid injury.

Distal Humeral Condylar Fractures

The elbow joint consists of three articular surfaces (humeroradioulnar joint). Fracture of the lateral part of the humeral condyle (capitulum) is seen in actively growing animals (Salter IV fracture) and adult animals. Salter IV fractures are intra-articular injuries in which the split is directed parallel to the long axis of the bone and proceeds up through the physis and metaphysis (see Fig. 157–25).

The capitulum is the major (90–95%) weight–bearing surface (bears 90 to 95 per cent of weight), owing to its articulation with the proximal surface of the radial head. As forces are directed upward through the radius on weight-bearing, they go directly through the capitulum. Jumping from heights distributes large amounts of force through the condyle, resulting in "shear" fractures. Fractures of the trochlea (medial portion of the condyle) are extremely infrequent because of its less frequent weight-bearing position. The conformation of the humerus is such that the capitulum sits off the midline of the central axis of the body, predisposing itself to injury, whereas the trochlea is larger and acts as a base for the continuation of the diaphysis.[6] For this reason, intramedullary pins used in repairing the humerus are seated directly into the trochlea.

Formerly, closed reduction was performed for these injuries, with the use of a condyle clamp and placement of pins or a transcondylar screw across the fracture gap. This technique can be quite accurate, depending upon the expertise and experience of the surgeon performing the procedure. It is generally recommended that open reduction be performed to expose the articular surface and assess reduction.

A lateral approach to the elbow joint is the approach of choice and is a direct and easy route for exposure (Fig. 157–43). Additional exposure can be gained by a partial or complete triceps tenotomy. Transolecranon osteotomies are used in adult patients

Text continued on page 2082

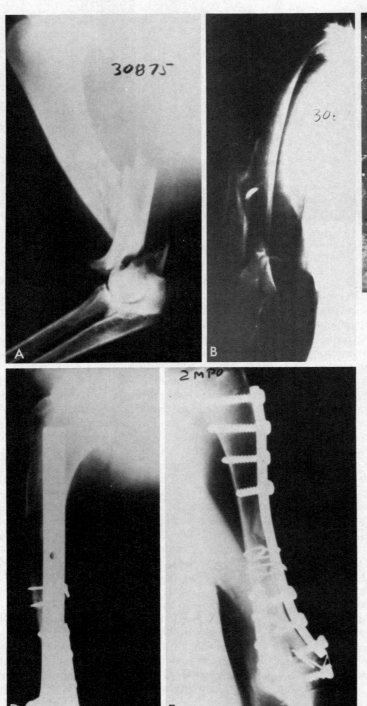

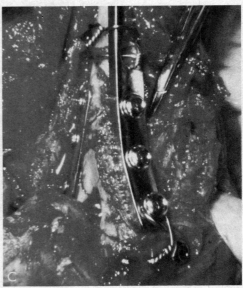

Figure 157–41. A, A distal, segmental supracon-dylar fracture. *B,* Craniocaudal view. *C,* One larger, lateral bone plate and one smaller, cau-domedial bone plate have been used to repair this injury. Several hemi-cerclage wires have been used over the plate for additional support. *D,* Lateral view. *E,* Craniocaudal view showing the contoured plate extending the entire length of the body. (Courtesy of Dr. R. Dueland.)

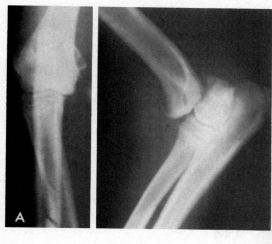

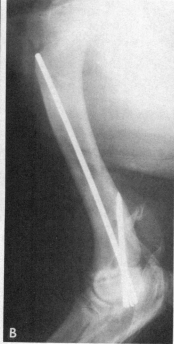

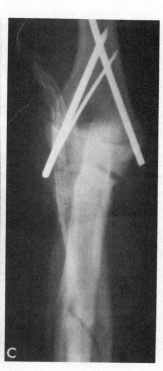

Figure 157–42. *A*, A distal Salter I humeral fracture in a seven-month-old dog. *B*, The injury has been repaired with multiple pins, with the medial pin spanning the entire length of the body. *C*, Craniocaudal view shows anatomical reduction.

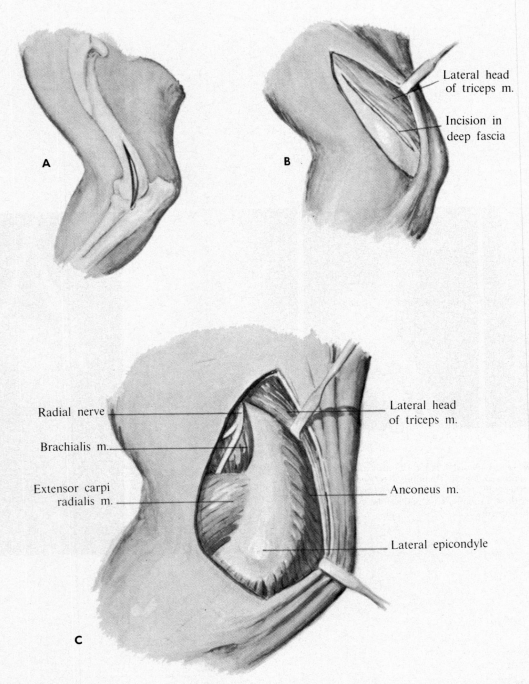

Figure 157–43. A, The skin incision extends along the lower fourth of the humerus and crosses the joint to end distally on the ulna. The incision passes over or slightly caudal to the lateral epicondyle. The subcutaneous fascia is incised on the same line. B, As the skin and subcutaneous fascia are retracted, the deep brachial fascia and the lateral head of the triceps muscle are exposed. An incision is made through the deep fascia near the cranial border of the triceps. C, Bluntly undermining the triceps allows it to be retracted caudolaterally so that the condylar part of the humerus is exposed.

Illustration continued on opposite page

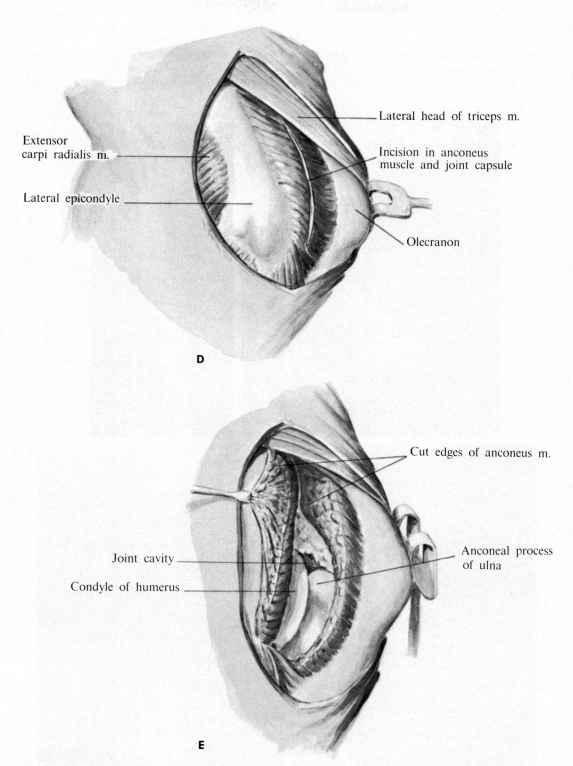

Extensor
carpi radialis m.

Lateral epicondyle

Lateral head of triceps m.

Incision in anconeus
muscle and joint capsule

Olecranon

D

Cut edges of anconeus m.

Joint cavity

Condyle of humerus

Anconeal process
of ulna

E

Figure 157–43 Continued. D, With the lateral head of the triceps sufficiently undermined to allow its free caudal retraction, an incision is made through the anconeus muscle and the adherent joint capsule. The incision is made parallel to the humerus and midway between the humeral condyle and the olecranon. *E,* Reflection of the incised muscle exposes the joint space. Extreme flexion of the joint provides the best view of the interior of the joint. (Reprinted with permission from Piermattei, D. L., and Greeley, R. G.: *An Atlas of Surgical Approaches to the Bones of the Dog and Cat.* W. B. Saunders, Philadelphia, 1979.)

but are avoided in actively growing patients because of possible interference with the growth zone of the proximal ulnar apophysis.

Transcondylar lag screw fixation is the repair technique of choice. Multiple small pins are used in the younger (four to eight weeks) animal owing to their rapid healing time (three to four weeks) and in the smaller (less than 5 kg) animal (Fig. 157–44). During drilling from the lateral surface of the condyle, the proximal drill hole is made slightly cranial and ventral to the palpable epicondyle (Fig. 147–45), in order to place the hole directly through the center of the condyle. If a screw were placed directly across the epicondyles, it would emerge in the caudal articular

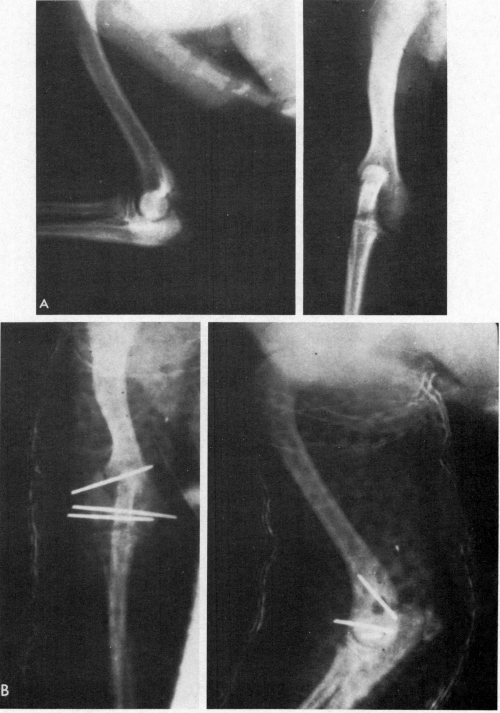

Figure 157–44. *A*, A capitular (or lateral aspect of the condyle) (Salter IV) fracture in an eight-week-old (4-kg) dog. *B*, Repair of the fracture with paired transcondylar Kirschner wires (0.625 in.) and one lateral epicondylar pin.

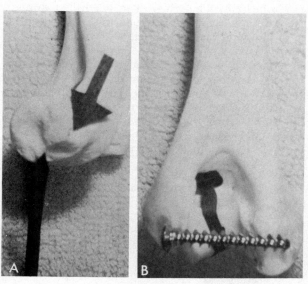

Figure 157–45

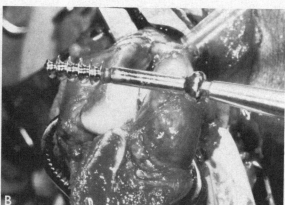

Figure 157–46

Figure 157–45. *A, Short arrow* depicts the palpable lateral epicondyle. The *long, thin arrow* shows the proper area to drill (cranial and slightly ventral). *B,* Craniocaudal view of humerus showing proper screw alignment (*black line* represents fracture line). (Courtesy of Dr. R. Dueland.)

Figure 157–46. Repair of a capitular fracture with a partially threaded, cancellous screw and one additional lateral pin. (Courtesy of Dr. R. Dueland.)

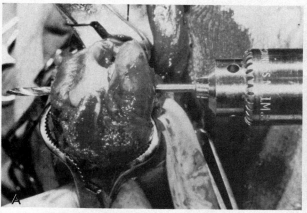

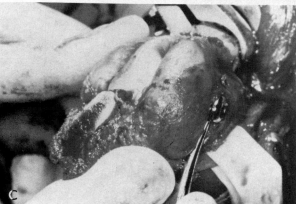

Figure 157–47. *A,* A caudal view of a capitular fracture held in reduction with bone-holding forceps while the transcondylar screw hole is drilled, medial to lateral (a transolecranon approach). The ulnar nerve is retracted with a Penrose drain medially. *B,* A partially threaded, cancellous screw is chosen. *C,* After the distal cortex is tapped, the screw is firmly seated and the repair is complete. (Usually the screw is seated lateral to medial.)

space because the axis of the screw would be off-center. The proximal hole in the lateral side of the condyle represents the "pilot" or guide hole and is over-drilled when cortical screws are used so that the screw threads gain purchase in only the medial segment and compress the fracture line. For example, with a 2.7-mm cortical screw, the lateral hole in the condyle is 2.7 mm and the medial hole in the condyle is 2.0 mm, so a 2.7-mm tap should be used.[9] A partially non-threaded cancellous screw does not require over-drilling because the non-threaded portion passes through the lateral segment without purchase (Fig. 157–46). Prior to screw placement, the segment is reduced and held in place manually or with bone-holding forceps or a towel clamp (Fig. 157–47). Careful attention must be paid to avoid any damage to the articular surface during reduction. A (.0625-inch) Kirschner wire can be drilled through the epicondylar area to maintain the reduction prior to drilling and placing the lag screw. Often, the K-wire is left in place with the screw as long as the wire does not emerge from the articular surface (Fig. 157–48). Another technique for drilling the pilot hole and ensuring central placement is to drill the hole from the intercondylar fracture surface out through the lateral side of the condyle from medial to lateral. The condyle is reduced and held in reduction while the hole is continued across into the medial aspect

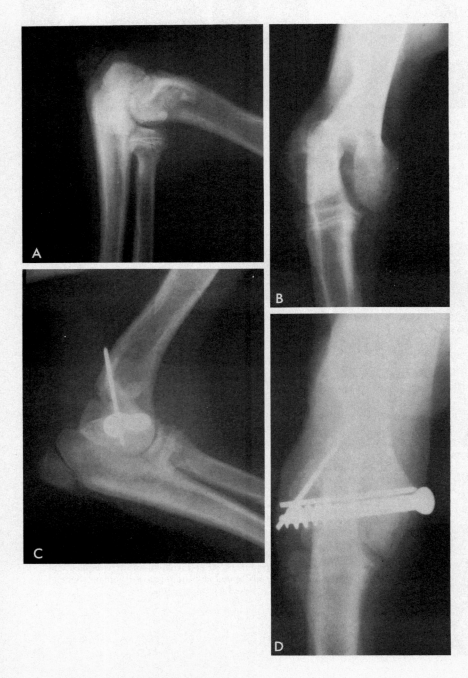

Figure 157–48. A, Mild displacement of the condylar articular surface. B, A lateral condyle fracture. C, Screw and pin repair. D, The transcondylar pin has been left in place with the screw and a lateral epicondylar pin. (Courtesy of Dr. E. Trotter.)

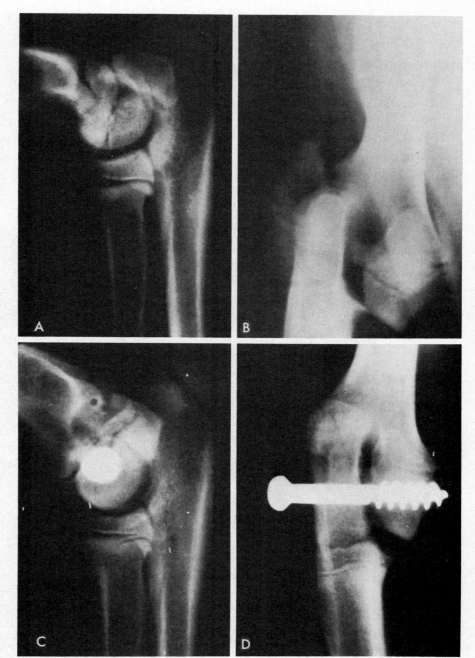

Figure 157–49. *A,* Mild dorsal displacement of the lateral aspect of the condyle. *B,* A "classic" capitular fracture (Salter IV). *C,* Restoration of a smoother articular surface with accurate cancellous screw placement. *D,* Proper screw placement with mild alteration of the medial aspect of the capitular articular surface. (Courtesy of Dr. R. Dueland.)

of the condyle and completed with tapping and screw placement. Visual inspection of the joint and a thorough lavage to remove fragments and debris should be conducted prior to closure. The elbow is flexed and extended to assess stability and to check for crepitus.

A modified Robert-Jones dressing is placed on the limb to control swelling and minimize pain. This bandage is removed at 12 to 24 hours to allow gentle, passive physiotherapy consisting of 25 to 35 flexion-extensions three to four times daily. Examples of these injuries and their repair are illustrated in Figures 157–49 to 157–51.

T and Y Humeral Condyle Fractures

T fracture and *Y fracture* are terms used to describe fracture involvement of the distal humeral body and condyle. These injuries consist of an intracondylar plus a supracondylar component. The T or Y indicates that the fracture line is through the condyle, separating the two sides of the condyle, and continues out through the medial epicondyle and lateral epicondylar crest, resulting in a T (transverse) or Y (oblique) configuration.

Often these injuries have a comminuted supracondylar component, which renders repair difficult. Ra-

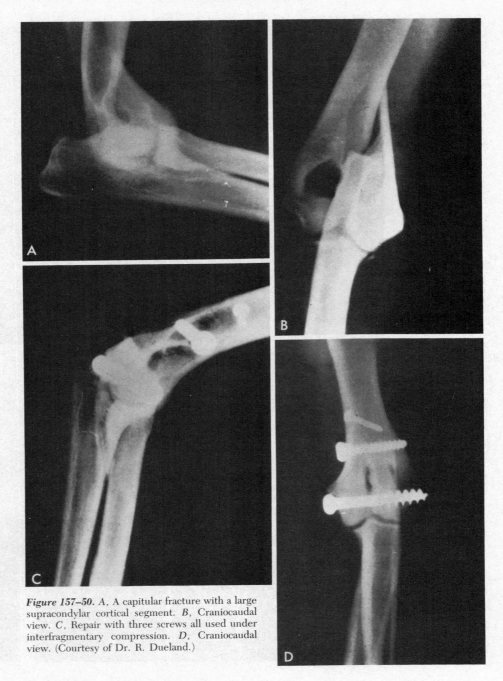

Figure 157–50. A, A capitular fracture with a large supracondylar cortical segment. B, Craniocaudal view. C, Repair with three screws all used under interfragmentary compression. D, Craniocaudal view. (Courtesy of Dr. R. Dueland.)

dial nerve function should always be evaluated prior to repair, as with any humeral injury.

The surgical exposure is via a lateral skin incision that extends over the distal humeral body and elbow joint (see Figs. 157–31 and 157–43). A triceps tenotomy or transolecranon osteotomy is used for full exposure (Fig. 157–52). The anconeus muscle is elevated from its caudolateral attachment on the distal body and is reflected distally. Careful attention should be paid to the presence of the radial nerve and its sensorimotor branches laterally under the triceps muscles and of the ulnar and median nerve medially to avoid injury (see Figs. 157–28 and 157–33). Retraction of these structures is carried out by

passing Penrose tubing. Care should be taken to leave as much of the extraperiosteal muscular attachments to the fracture segments as possible, in order to preserve a good cortical blood supply. On the other hand, full mobility of these segments often necessitates a considerable amount of elevation to obtain accurate reduction.

The key in handling T and Y injuries is to repair the articular portion first, ensuring that the joint surface is accurately reduced and making the injury a two-piece fracture. A transcondylar lag screw is placed across the condyle as discussed for injuries to the lateral aspect of the condyle. It is my preference to drill the pilot hole in the lateral epicondyle from

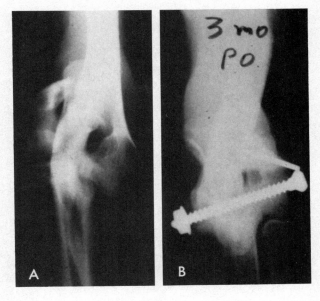

Figure 157–51. *A,* A capitular fracture in a 15-month-old bassett hound. *B,* This injury has been repaired by a transcondylar screw and washer with one lateral epicondylar pin. (Washers are used when the bone is extremely soft or if the distal, tapped hole strips out.) (Courtesy of Dr. R. Dueland.)

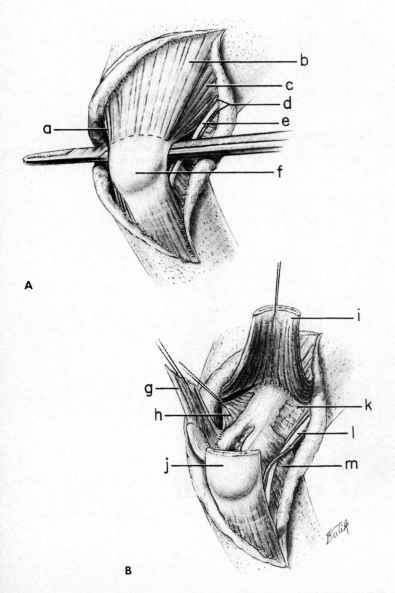

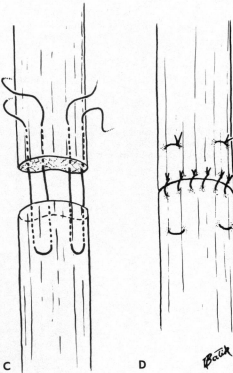

Figure 157–52. *A,* Surgical exposure of superficial structures: lateral head of triceps brachii *(a),* long head of triceps brachii *(b),* medial head of triceps brachii *(c),* collateral ulnar vessels *(d),* ulnar nerve *(e),* and olecranon *(f). Dotted line* indicates incision line. *B,* Deep exposure: reflected anconeus muscle *(g),* extensor carpi radialis *(h),* reflected triceps brachii *(i),* distal stump of triceps tendon *(j),* median nerve (deep) *(k),* ulnar nerve *(l),* and medial epicondyle *(m).* Distal end of humerus exposed, with the trochlea and capitulum accessible. *C* and *D,* Placement of horizontal mattress sutures in triceps tendon; mattress and interrupted sutures completed for closure of tendon. (Reprinted with permission from Dueland, R.: Triceps tenotomy approach for distal fractures of the canine humerus. J. Am. Vet. Met. Assoc. *165:*85, 1974.)

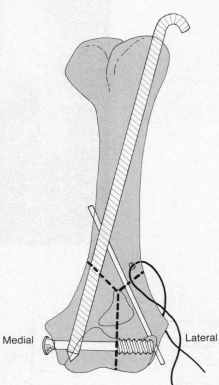

Medial   Lateral

Figure 157–53. A caudal view of a right humeral Y fracture has been repaired with one large intramedullary pin seated in the trochlea (medial portion of the condyle), a transcondylar screw (partially threaded, cancellous screw), and a small lateral Steinmann pin extending up the lateal epicondylar crest into the proximal, medial humeral cortex with an additional figure-of-eight tension wire.

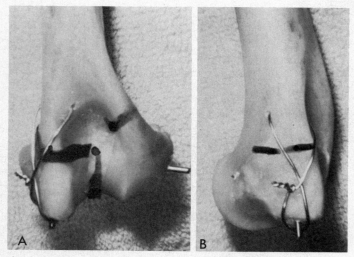

Figure 157–54. A, The figure-of-eight wiring technique used with lateral condyle injuries for repair of Y or T fractures. B, Completed stabilization with the wire extending above the fracture line in order to achieve compression.

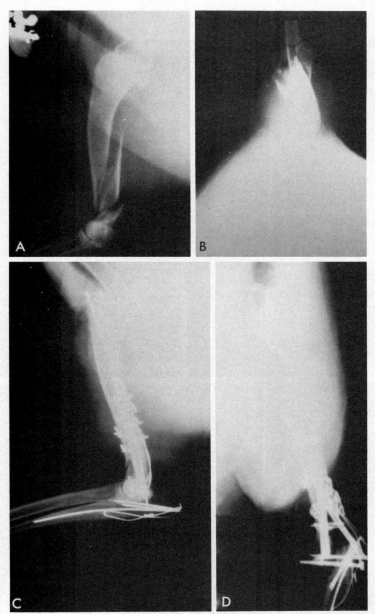

Figure 157–55. *A*, A distal, segmental supracondylar T fracture. *B*, Craniocaudal view. *C*, This injury has been repaired with multiple intramedullary pins extending the entire length of the body with multiple tension wires and a transcondylar screw (approached via a transolecranon osteotomy). *D*, Craniocaudal view. (Courtesy of Dr. E. Trotter.)

the fracture surface laterally through the lateral epicondyle to ensure central screw placement. The condylar (distal) segment is ready for approximation to the proximal shaft, and a multitude of techniques are used, including intramedullary pin and wire fixation, lateral or medial surface bone plating, and caudal plate fixation. Pin and wire fixation is carried out by passing the pins retrograde from the fracture end of the proximal portion up through the body so that they emerge from the greater tubercle (aiming from the medial aspect of the distal body and heading craniolaterally out proximally). The fracture is reduced and held in place with bone-holding forceps. These pins are seated distally in the medial side of the condyle, avoiding the transcondylar screw. Tension band wiring or hemi-cerclage is used when needed to cross the fracture segment and neutralize rotational instability. Another small pin and tension

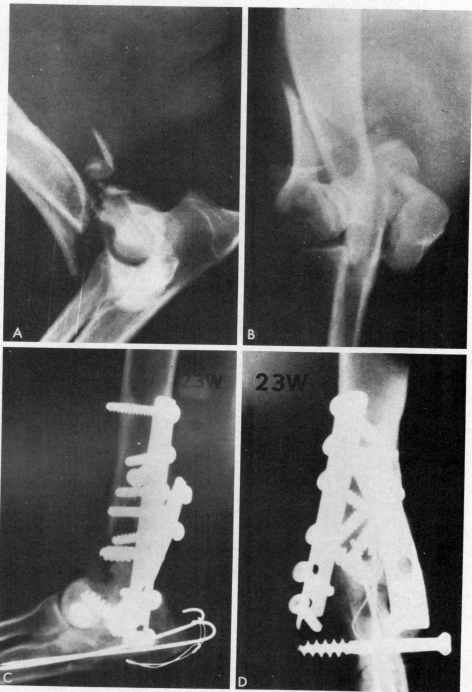

Figure 157–56. A, Lateral view of a highly comminuted distal Y fracture. B, Craniocaudal view. C, This injury was approached via a transolecranon osteotomy and repaired with a transcondylar screw and two caudal neutralization plates. D, Craniocaudal view. (Courtesy of Dr. R. Dueland.)

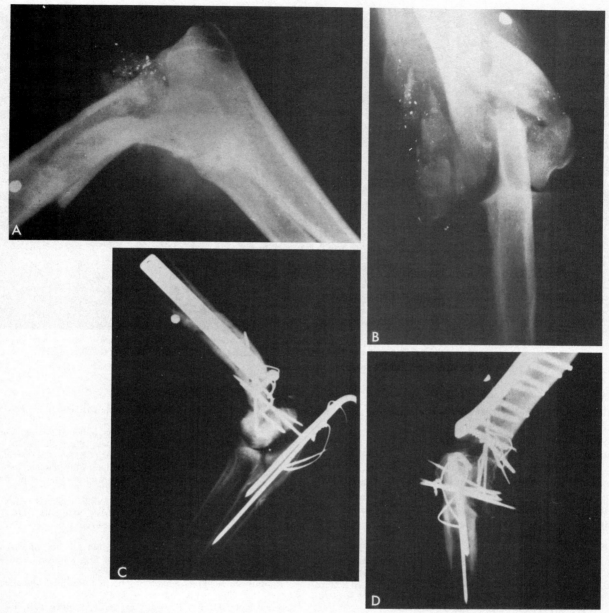

Figure 157–57. *A*, An intra-articular gunshot injury sustained to the left elbow joint with fragmentation of the condylar surface. *B*, Craniocaudal view. *C*, Partial restoration of the articular surface with multiple pins, lag screws, and lateral plate fixation approached via a transolecranon osteotomy. *D*, Craniocaudal view. (This patient had limited motion with 50 per cent limb usage.)

wire can be used, with the pin entered up the lateral portion of the condyle through the lateral epicondylar crest and exiting medially above the fracture site, for added support (Fig. 157–53).

Multiple fragments should be wired or screwed in place and secured prior to intramedullary reduction. Wires or screws used to secure fragments must not interfere with primary axial repair (Figs. 157–54 and 157–55). Plate fixation can be used in many positions. The more conventional lateral placement is commonly employed, but medial and caudal placements also have merit (Figs. 157–55 to 157–57). In lateral placement, the plate occasionally must extend distally below the epicondyle, necessitating placement of

screws that may cross the supracondylar foramen. To obtain this secured distal cortical purchase, the anconeal process (of the ulna) must be removed. Its removal rarely leads to serious clinical reduction of elbow motion. Placement of multiple pins and lag screws at divergent angles can also be used as a primary means of fixation (Fig. 157–58) but is generally not suggested in dogs over 15 kg.

Following repair, the elbow is tested for range of motion. Closure of the anconeus muscle is affected by the limitation of motion created. Often this muscle is loosely resutured so that motion is not sacrificed. The triceps tenotomy or trans-olecranon osteotomy is replaced, and closure is routine. A modified Rob-

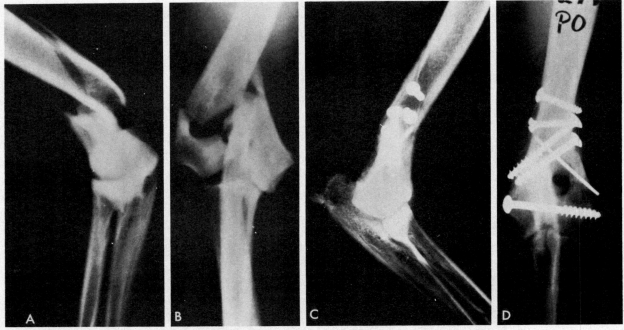

Figure 157–58. *A,* A comminuted Y fracture. *B,* Craniocaudal view. *C,* Lateral postoperative view at two months shows good healing following reduction with multiple lag screws used at divergent angles. *D,* Craniocaudal view. (Courtesy of Dr. R. Dueland.)

ert-Jones dressing is placed on the limb for 12 to 24 hours and removed so that physiotherapy may be given. Restriction of exercise to slow leash walking for at least one month is recommended. After a month, radiographs are taken to evaluate fracture healing. Intramedullary pins should be removed at the time of bony union, but small wires, pins, plates, and screws are often left in place with no long-term consequences.

1. American College of Surgeons: *Early Care of the Injured Patient.* 3rd ed. W. B. Saunders, Philadelphia, 1982.
2. Brader, T.: Surgical correction of humeral fractures. *In* Bojrab, M. J. (ed.): *Current Techniques in Small Animal Surgery.* Lea & Febiger, Philadelphia, 1975.
3. Bunker, W. O.: Fractures of the humerus. *In* Archibald, J. (ed.): *Canine Surgery.* American Veterinary Publications, Wheaton, Il, 1971.
4. deLahunta, A.: Personal communication, 1984.
5. Dingwall, J. S.: Management of elbow fractures in the dog. Mod. Vet. Pract., Feb., 1970, p. 37.
6. Evans, H. E., and Christensen, G. C. (eds.): *Miller's Anatomy of the Dog.* 2nd ed. W. B. Saunders, Philadelphia, 1979.
7. Evans, H., and deLahunta, A.: *Miller's Guide to the Dissection of the Dog.* 2nd ed. W. B. Saunders, Philadelphia, 1980.
8. McCurnin, D. M.: Surgery of the canine elbow joint. Vet. Med./Small Anim. Clin., July, 1976.
9. Miller, M. E., Allgöwer, M., and Willenegger, H.: *Manual of Internal Fixation.* Springer-Verlag, New York, 1969.
10. O'Connor, J. J.: *Dollar's Veterinary Surgery.* Bailliere, Tindall and Cox, London, 1938.
11. Piermattei, D. L., and Greeley, R. G.: *An Atlas of Surgical Approaches to the Bones of the Dog and Cat.* 2nd ed. W. B. Saunders, Philadelphia, 1979.
12. Rudy, R. R.: Management of limb fractures in small animals. Vet. Clin. North Am. 5:197, 1975.
13. Sabiston, D. C., Jr. (ed.): *Davis-Christopher Textbook of Surgery.* 12th ed. W. B. Saunders, Philadelphia, 1981.
14. Zaslow, I., and Hanssen, P. L.: Medial approach to bone plating in repair of humeral-shaft fractures. Vet Med./Small Anim. Clin., Nov., 1976, p. 1569.

Elbow Luxation

Richard G. Johnson and Nancy L. Hampel

Luxation of the elbow refers to displacement of one or more of the three bones that compose the joint. The result is malalignment of the articular surfaces with subsequent dysfunction. Typically, elbow luxation is caudolateral. Uncomplicated dislocation or luxation of the elbow joint is uncommon in quadrupeds, occurring less frequently than coxofemoral joint luxation by a factor of ten. The anatomy, including the humeral condyles, anconeal process of the ulna, joint capsule, and periarticular ligamentous structures, makes the elbow an inherently stable joint. Fracture of the humeral condyles, ulna, or radius is more common and can occur concomitantly with luxation. The disorder can be congenital or acquired, acute or chronic. Effective management is based on sound knowledge of the anatomy, pathogenesis, and modes of therapy.

Anatomy

The elbow is a compound synovial joint classified as a ginglymus, or hinge joint, permitting flexion and extension with a limited degree of rotation. It is composed of three distinct articulations: humeroradial (radiocapitular) joint, humeroulnar (olecranontrochlear) joint, and proximal radioulnar joint.

The trochlear notch of the olecranon articulates with the conical trochlea of the humerus and acts as a primary stabilizer, restricting movement of the joint to a sagittal plane. Additionally, with 90 degrees of flexion or less, an interlocking effect is created by the projection of the anconeal process into the olecranon fossa. This effect becomes important as a means of stabilizing the joint following reduction. The capitular depression of the radius articulates with the lateral condyle (capitulum) of the humerus and transmits the majority (80 per cent) of weight supported by the limb. The proximal radioulnar joint allows rotation of the antebrachium—up to 90 degrees of supination in the quadruped.

The joint has collateral ligament support that strongly resists lateral and varus movements. The lateral (ulnar) collateral ligament originates proximally at the lateral epicondyle and, after blending with the annular ligament, divides distally into two crura. The cranial crus inserts on the proximal radius and the caudal crus on the ulna.

The smaller radial collateral ligament originates at the medial humeral epicondyle, crosses the annular ligament, and also divides into two crura. The cranial crus inserts at the radial tuberosity, and the caudal crus passes into the interosseous space where it inserts primarily to the ulna with fewer fibers to the radius.

The annular ligament, a thin transverse band, forms a ring around the proximal radius in which the articular circumference of the radius turns when the antebrachium is rotated. The oblique ligament attaches proximally to the supratrochlear foramen, crosses the flexor surface of the joint, and blends into the radial collateral ligament and proximal medial radius (Fig. 157–59).[6]

CONGENITAL ELBOW LUXATION

Congenital elbow luxation accounts for 17 to 20 per cent of nonfracture elbow lameness in the dog. Small breeds such as Pekingese, English bulldog, Shetland sheepdog, dachshund, basset hound, and Yorkshire terrier are more commonly affected.[4] A possible hereditary basis of congenital elbow luxation has been suggested because of (1) the high incidence of bilateral involvement,[1,4,8,12,14] (2) multiple animals in a litter being affected,[1] and (3) multiple soft tissue and skeletal anomalies occurring in some animals.[8] The development of the early joint cavity and the shape of the joint surfaces are under genetic control. Bingel and Riser[1] have hypothesized that the condition occurs as a result of a failure at the embryonic stage of formation of the intra-articular ligaments, leading to agenesis or hypoplasia of the weaker medial collateral and small annular ligaments, which in turn permits rotation of the proximal ulna and subluxation or luxation of the radial head, the ulna, or both. It is unclear whether all the changes associated with congenital elbow luxation are primary defects or secondary changes due to incongruent joint surface articulation and abnormal weight-bearing. Examples of probable secondary changes include blunted anconeal process, deviated olecranon, delayed or premature ossification of one or more physis, and hypertrophied lateral collateral ligament.

Physical Findings

The condition is usually recognized by the owner when the pup is three to six weeks of age and may involve one or both forelimbs. Physical findings include a marked instability and varying degrees of deformity of the limb with pronation of the forearm (40 to 45 degrees) (Fig. 157–60). There is usually a non–weight-bearing lameness, with disuse atrophy of the affected limb. The animal cannot fully extend the elbow. Pain at rest is not a consistent finding; however, upon manipulation, pain becomes evident. The joint crepitates only if degenerative joint disease is advanced.

Radiographic Findings

Radiographic findings usually reveal gross abnormalities consistent with the physical examination.

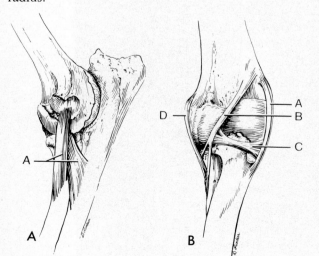

Figure 157–59. Lateral (A) and anteroposterior (B) views of the elbow joint. a, Lateral collateral ligament; b, oblique ligament; (c), annular ligament; d, medial collateral ligament.

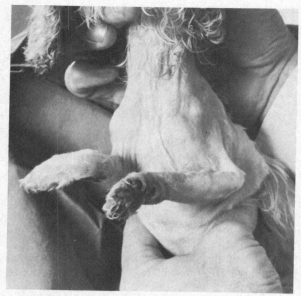

Figure 157–60. Congenital elbow luxation in a puppy. Flexion and pronation are characteristic. (Reprinted with permission from Milton, J. L.: Congenital elbow luxation in the dog. J. Am. Vet. Med. Assoc. 157:572, 1979.)

Humeral malarticulation with both the radius and ulna or ulnar surface alone is present. The anteroposterior view of the elbow exhibits a lateral view of the ulna (Fig. 157–61A). A lateral radiograph of the joint reveals a lateral view of the humerus and an anteroposterior view of the ulna (Fig. 157–61B).

Hypoplasia or aplasia of the coronoid process, anconeal process, humeral condyles, and radial notch or remodeling of the humeral trochlea may be evident. Additionally, cranial bowing of the distal radial or humeral diaphysis with physeal disorders may be observed. The fourth ulnar growth center, the olecranon apophysis, may also be distorted owing to the abnormal pull of the triceps muscle group.

Treatment

The primary objective of surgery should be restoration of function to the limb and not necessarily complete reconstruction of the joint, especially in cases of severe deformation. Two methods, open reduction and closed reduction, are currently being utilized, the choice being based on the age of the animal and the degree of pathological changes in both bone and soft tissue structures. Generally, closed reduction is indicated in dogs less than four months of age with minimal bone deformity, provided that manual reduction can be accomplished. Surgical correction should be reserved for those animals with chronic dislocation and severe limb deformity.

Closed Reduction

Manual reduction of the elbow joint is accomplished (see section on closed reduction of traumatic elbow luxation). The limb is clipped from carpus to

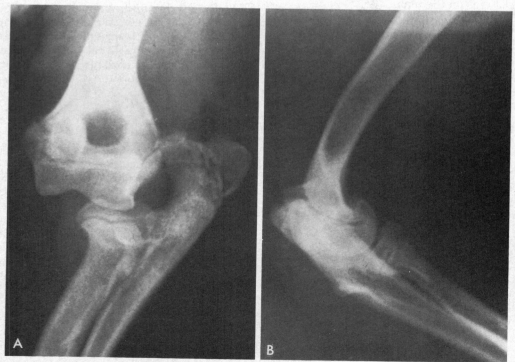

Figure 157–61. Typical radiographic appearance of congenital elbow luxation. A, Anteroposterior view. Note hypoplasia of the medial condyle, remodeling of trochlear notch, and malformation of radial head. B, Lateral view. The ulna is malpositioned. (Reprinted with permission from Milton, J. L.: Congenital elbow luxation in the dog. J. Am. Vet. Med. Assoc. 157:572, 1979.)

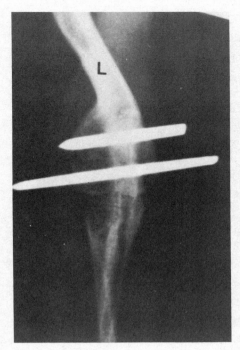

Figure 157–62. Postreduction radiograph with Steinmann pins placed transversely through the ulna and humerus. (Reprinted with permission from Milton, J. L.: Congenital elbow luxation in the dog. J. Am. Vet. Med. Assoc. *157*:572, 1979.)

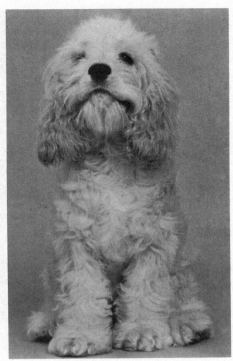

Figure 157–64. Long-term (four-year observation time) result of external reduction. (Reprinted with permission from Milton, J. L.: Congenital elbow luxation in the dog. J. Am. Vet. Med. Assoc. *157*:572, 1979.)

shoulder and surgically prepared. Small Steinmann pins are placed transversely and completely through the condyles of the humerus and olecranon of the ulna (Fig. 157–62). Reduction is maintained by placement of a heavy elastic band from the medial aspect of the proximal pin to the lateral aspect of the distal pin. The band exerts a caudomedial force on the proximal ulna. A protective padded metal splint is placed under the elastic band to lower the chances of tissue necrosis (Fig. 157–63). Postoperative care

includes elastic band replacement as needed and prevention or treatment of soft tissue trauma. The elastic band remains in place for ten to 14 days. Following removal of the pins, continued support is maintained for three to six weeks. Slow return to function has yielded good long-term results with this method of repair in selected cases (Fig. 157–64).

Open Reduction

Numerous surgical procedures have been used to achieve and maintain reduction and stabilization of the elbow joint. Specific procedures or a combination of procedures should be used to attain this result; they are as follows: (1) lateral capsulorrhaphy, (2) lateral desmotomy, (3) rotational reduction of the ulna, (4) transposition of the olecranon, (5) fixation of the proximal ulna to the radius, (6) reconstruction of the trochlea and trochlear notch, (7) partial removal of the anconeus process, and (8) application of prosthetic collateral ligaments.

Exposure may be obtained by a lateral approach through the anconeus muscle or by osteotomy of the olecranon process, the latter offering a more extensive exposure and release of the triceps pull.[13] It must be emphasized that an animal that has the ability to support weight and walk may not benefit from surgical correction, i.e., repair may not be indicated in all cases of congenital elbow luxation.

Postoperatively, external support should be maintained with a spica splint for ten to 14 days. Restricted

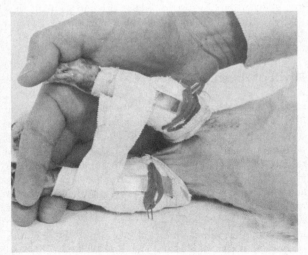

Figure 157–63. Rubber bands are placed to maintain reduction. The soft tissue is protected by metal splints and soft padded bandage. (Reprinted with permission from Milton, J. L.: Congenital elbow luxation in the dog. J. Am. Vet. Med. Assoc. *157*:572, 1979.)

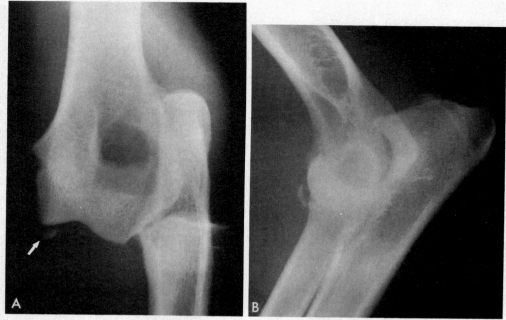

Figure 157–65. Radiographic appearance of traumatic elbow luxation. *A*, Anteroposterior view. Avulsion fracture of the proximal humeroradial ligament *(arrow). B*, Lateral view. Normal joint space is not visualized.

exercise in conjunction with physical therapy for two to four weeks following bandage removal is recommended.

If the preceding treatment modes are likely to fail, arthrodesis of the joint may be indicated. The articular cartilage is removed, the bone ends are aligned in normal anatomical position, and stabilization is achieved, preferably under compression (bone plating).[2]

TRAUMATIC ELBOW LUXATION

The majority of traumatic injuries sustained in the elbow region result in fracture rather than luxation

alone, because of previously described innate stability of the joint. There is, however, little soft tissue mass protecting the joint, and in some studies traumatic elbow luxation occurred more frequently than shoulder luxation.[5,9] The force most commonly required to produce luxation may be indirect (rotational). Rupture of the radial, ulnar, and oblique ligaments occurs. A direct medial thrust against the distal lateral humerus while the elbow is in flexion and a direct posterior thrust against the proximal cranial radius while the elbow is in extension are less common causes of luxation. A direct cranial blow to the posterior ulna can also displace the radial head cranially, but this injury is usually accompanied by a Monteggia fracture.[3]

Physical Findings

The clinical presentation is specific for traumatic elbow luxation, and the diagnosis can be made without difficulty. The non–weight-bearing lameness is sudden in onset and is accompanied by mild to moderate soft tissue swelling. The affected limb is in slight flexion with the elbow adducted and the forearm and paw rotated medially and abducted. Pain is noted on palpation, as well as a greatly reduced range of motion. Crepitation is commonly absent with acute luxation. The radial head is prominent lateral and posterior to the humerus. The medial humeral condyle is easily palpable, but the lateral condyle is indistinct. Radial nerve damage is not commonly reported with traumatic luxation, but the limb should be thoroughly evaluated for neurological deficits.

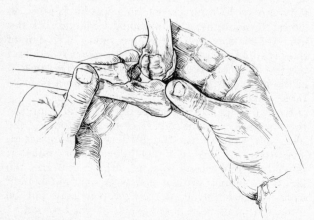

Figure 157–66. A method of closed reduction. Digital pressure is used to reduce the luxation while the joint is in flexion.

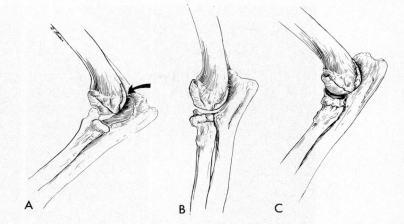

Figure 157–67. Second method of closed reduction. *A*, The limb is flexed and the proximal ulna is rotated inward to engage the anconeal process on the lateral condylar ridge *(arrow)*. *B*, The limb is extended and twisted to replace the trochlear notch into the trochlea. *C*, The limb is flexed and the joint is reduced.

Radiographic Findings

Radiological evaluation precedes repair to determine the presence of other injuries, including avulsion fracture and fracture in the region of the joint. Both lateral and anteroposterior views should be taken. The lateral projection may show the humeral condyles overlying the radial head with an irregular (either wide or absent) joint space. Displacement is apparent on the anteroposterior projection (Fig. 157–65).

Treatment

The prognosis for recent traumatic dislocation is good, but difficulty may be encountered in cases that have remained untreated a week or more. As with congenital luxation, the two general modes of repair are open reduction and closed reduction.

Closed Reduction

Most (95 per cent) recent uncomplicated luxations can be reduced externally without surgical invasion of the joint. Because of the associated pain and muscle spasm, general anesthesia with good muscle relaxation is required. The patient is placed in lateral recumbency with the affected limb. One of two methods of external reduction can be used. The first involves flexing the elbow to its greatest extent (ideally 45 degrees) and applying direct digital pressure to the radial head and olecranon to move them medially and to the medial humeral condyle to displace it laterally (Fig. 157–66). The second method uses the anconeal process as a lever against the ridge of the lateral condyle. The elbow is again flexed, the antebrachium is abducted, and the ulna is rotated inward. This maneuver should allow the anconeal process to engage the condylar ridge medial to the lateral epicondyle. The limb is extended and the trochlear notch is replaced into the trochlea (Fig. 157–67). Both methods require identification of the palpable anatomical landmarks, including the medial epicondyle, radial head, and olecranon. If muscle spasm is severe, attempts at reduction may not be successful. Spasm can be overcome with use of an extender for 20 minutes or longer. Manual reduction proceeds as previously described after the apparatus is removed. After reduction is accomplished, the joint is examined for instability. A spica splint is applied for two weeks, and activity is restricted for six weeks to minimize flexion of the joint. Physical therapy including passive range-of-motion exercises should begin after bandage removal.

Open Reduction

If the reduced elbow joint is unstable and readily redislocates or if closed reduction was not achieved, open reduction and stabilization is indicated. The limb is clipped and surgically prepared from the carpus to the proximal scapula.

A lateral approach to the elbow joint through the anconeus muscle is employed for exposure.[13] Once the joint is opened, a blunt instrument can be used to lever the bones into normal alignment. The instrument is placed between the medial aspect of the radial head and the lateral humeral condyle. With the elbow fully flexed, the condyles are levelled proximally and laterally (Fig. 157–68). The joint is examined for instability after reduction. If gross instability is present, one or both collateral ligaments

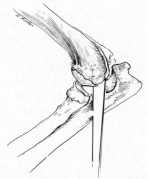

Figure 157–68. Open reduction of luxation. Lever placed between radial head and lateral condyle.

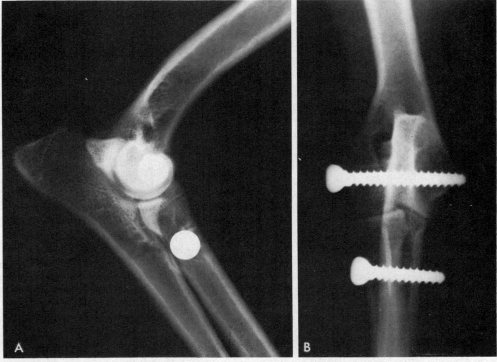

Figure 157–69. Postoperative placement of apparatus for instability due to collateral ligament rupture. *A,* Lateral view. *B,* Anteroposterior view.

have been damaged and must be reestablished. Rupture of the annular and oblique ligaments is difficult to repair, and reconstruction is unnecessary if the collateral ligaments are intact. If greater exposure to the medial aspect of the joint is needed for collateral ligament reconstruction, an olecranon osteotomy may be performed.[13] Two reconstructive procedures are described. The first uses a prosthetic material, and the second involves suturing the remaining torn ligament. In the first procedure, one screw is placed from lateral to medial (for reconstruction of the lateral ligament) through the humeral condyles and one screw through the radial head. A figure-of-eight suture is passed around the screw heads to simulate collateral ligament support. A nonabsorbable suture material of sufficient size is used. Our preference is Polydek*, No. 5 for large dogs and No. 2 for small dogs (Fig. 157–69). The second technique requires identification of the torn ligament ends and uniting of the ends with sutures.[4] If the ligament damage consists of an avulsion fracture at the ligament's origin, reduction and stabilization of the fragment may be achieved by use of a lag screw or pin and tension band wire. If the avulsion is associated with the insertion or the fragment is too small for stabilization, the first procedure described is recommended.

Postoperatively, a spica splint is used for two weeks, followed by a soft padded bandage for two weeks to lend support and restrict flexion. Exercise is strictly limited for six weeks. Passive range-of-motion exercises are begun after the splint has been removed. Removal of any internal fixation device may be necessary in 16 weeks or later.

1. Bingel, S. A., and Riser, W. H.: Congenital elbow luxation in the dog. J. Small Anim. Pract. *18*:445, 1977.
2. Bojrab, M. J. (ed.): *Current Techniques in Small Animal Surgery.* Lea & Febiger, Philadelphia, 1975.
3. Bojrab, M. J. (ed.): *Pathophysiology in Small Animal Surgery.* Lea & Febiger, Philadelphia, 1981.
4. Campbell, J. R.: Nonfracture injuries to the canine elbow. Am. Vet. Med. Assoc. *155*:735, 1969.
5. Campbell, J. R.: Luxation and ligamentous injuries of the elbow of the dog. Vet. Clin. N. Am. *1*:429, 1971.
6. Evans, H. E., and Christensen, G. C. (eds.): *Miller's Anatomy of the Dog.* 2nd ed. W. B. Saunders, Philadelphia, 1979.
7. Flipo, J.: Treatment of dislocations of the canine elbow. Mod. Vet. Pract. *45*:46, 1964.
8. Fox, M. W.: Polyarthrodysplasia in the dog. J. Am. Vet. Med. Assoc. *145*:1204, 1964.
9. Frankel, V. H., and Nordin, M. (eds.): *Basic Biomechanics of the Skeletal System.* Lea & Febiger, Philadelphia,
10. Leighton, R. L.: Personal communication, 1977.
11. Milton, J. L., et al.: Congenital elbow luxation in the dog. J. Am. Vet. Med. Assoc. *175*:572, 1979.
12. Pass, M. A., and Ferguson, J. G.: Elbow dislocation in the dog. J. Small Anim. Pract. *12*:327, 1971.
13. Piermattei, D. L., and Greeley, R. G.: *An Atlas of Surgical Approaches to the Bones of the Dog and Cat.* W. B. Saunders, Philadelphia, 1979.
14. Stevens, D. R., and Sande, R. D.: An elbow dysplasia syndrome in the dog. J. Am. Vet. Med. Assoc. *165*:1065, 1974.

*Polydek, Deknatel, Queens Village, NY.

Erick L. Egger

FRACTURES

Fractures of the radius and ulna represent 17 to 18 per cent of all fractures in the cat and dog.[22] The relatively high incidence of delayed unions, nonunions, joint stiffness, and even growth deformities after such fractures indicates the potential complexity of treating them.

Fractures of the Olecranon

The olecranon is the proximal extremity of the ulna that serves as the lever for the triceps, the powerful extensor muscles of the elbow. Consequently, complete fractures of the olecranon result in severe proximal displacement of the fragment away from the ulna (Fig. 157–70). Because external coaptation is unable to control the distractive pull of the triceps, open reduction and internal fixation are indicated for such fractures. Olecranon fractures can be limited to the bone of the olecranon or may extend into the elbow joint through the trochlear (semilunar) notch. In general, such fractures are exposed via a caudal approach in which subperiosteal elevation of the flexor carpi ulnaris and extensor carpi ulnaris muscles exposes the olecranon and ulnar shaft.[23] If the fracture is articular, the anconeus muscle and the joint capsules can also be incised to expose the interior of the joint.[23] Placing the elbow in extension to eliminate the pull of the triceps muscle facilitates fracture reduction. If the fracture extends into the joint, perfect reduction of the articular component is necessary to avoid the development of secondary arthri-

tis. The fracture can be fixed in several ways. The tension band wire technique uses monofilament orthopedic wire. Two Kirschner wires or Steinmann pins up to 3/32 inch (2.4 mm) in diameter are used to reduce the fracture and prevent rotation. The pins should be placed roughly parallel and should be oriented medially and laterally. They are started on the proximal tip of the olecranon and driven across the fracture to penetrate the cranial cortex of the ulnar shaft distal to the trochlear notch (Fig. 157–71A). A transverse hole large enough to accept the 18-gauge (20-gauge in very small dogs or cats) orthopedic wire is made from medial to lateral in the caudal ulna, approximately the same distance distal to the fracture as the length of the olecranon fragment. A single tightening twist is made in the center of a 25-cm length of the wire. One end is passed through the hole in the ulna (Fig. 157–71B). The center of the wire crosses behind the caudal ulna, and the opposite end is threaded under the triceps tendon around the cranial aspect of the pins. The free ends of the wire are twisted together to form a figure-of-eight (Fig. 157–71C). The two twists are alternately tightened until both wires are taut and the caudal part of the fracture is compressed. The extra wire is cut off, leaving three to four twists. The ends are carefully bent over with a slight tightening motion to lie flat on the bone. The ends of the pins are bent over, cut off, and rotated cranially over the wire. They are countersunk into the triceps tendon to avoid damage to the overlying soft tissues (Fig. 157–71D). A properly placed tension band wire is extremely strong and usually requires no postoperative support. The pins and wire are usually left in place, but they can be removed if desired or if they become loose.

A lag screw can be used to stabilize an olecranon fracture (Fig. 157–72). However, the ulnar shaft in many patients is very narrow, making hole drilling and screw placement difficult. Furthermore, the screw threads do not penetrate cortical bone but grip the inner walls of the medullary cavity and cancellous bone. Consequently, a cancellous screw should be used. Finally, the mechanical pull of the muscles is at a right angle to the screw shaft, predisposing to cycling stresses and failure of the screw (particularly if perfect reduction and compression of the fracture are not achieved.) Exercise restriction is advised until the fracture heals.

Comminuted olecranon fractures can be stabilized by applying a plate along the caudal ulnar shaft. In this location, the plate acts both as a tension band to resist the pull of the triceps and as a buttress to resist fracture collapse. The plate can be contoured to partially hook over the proximal end of the olecranon (Fig. 157–73). The proximal fragment must be large enough to accept two screws, and care must be taken to avoid placing screws through the articular surface

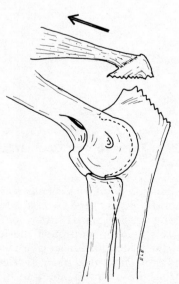

Figure 157–70. Olecranon fracture with the pull of the triceps muscle resulting in severe displacement.

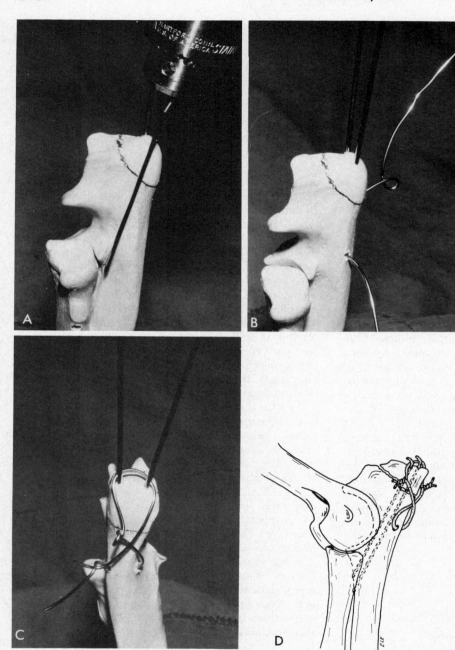

Figure 157–71. Pin and tension band repair of olecranon fractures. *A*, Pin placement. *B*, Wire passage. *C*, Twisting the wire to form a figure-of-eight. *D*, Completed pin and tension band repair.

of the trochlear notch. Postoperative management depends on the stability of the repair. If a good tension band effect is achieved, no additional support is needed. If bony defects persist after surgery, limitation of exercise or even a non–weight-bearing sling may be in order. Such a sling that still retains motion of the joint is a carpal flexion bandage (Fig. 157–74). This bandage prevents the animal from placing the limb on the floor and can be left on for several weeks to allow early fracture healing. In any case, passive range-of-motion exercises should be used to maintain elbow motion.

Proximal Ulnar Fracture with Luxation of the Radial Head

This combination of injuries is known as a Monteggia fracture in humans.[28] It was first described as a result of a blow on the palmar surface of the forearm as the arm was held up to protect the head during medieval battles. The radial head is usually displaced cranially and proximally. The ulnar fracture can occur anywhere from the trochlear notch to the midshaft. The proximal annular ligament may rupture or may remain intact. In either situation, swelling, muscle

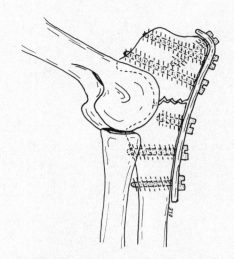

Figure 157–72. Lag screw fixation for olecranon fractures.

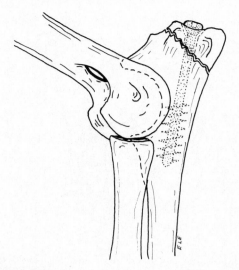

Figure 157–73. Bone plate fixation for olecranon fractures.

spasm, and fibrous proliferation dictate early treatment. A caudal approach to the ulna, as earlier described, is often adequate if the radial head can be manually reduced.[23] If the radial head cannot be relocated, owing to either fibrous tissue in the joint or muscle contraction and overriding, a craniolateral approach can be used.[30] This approach allows debridement of the joint and levering of the radial head back into place.

If the proximal annular ligament remains intact, as is often the case when the ulnar fracture occurs at the base or into the trochlear notch, the relationship of the radial head and the ulnar shaft remains normal (Fig. 157–75). Reduction of the ulnar fracture occurs only with reduction of the radial head luxation. Stable fixation of the ulnar fracture with pins and tension band wire or bone screws and plate, as previously described, also stabilizes the radial head.

When the ligament has been ruptured, the radial head separates from the proximal ulnar shaft. Rupture occurs when the ulnar fracture is distal to the annular ligament (Fig. 157–76). Treatment requires not only reduction and stabilization of the fracture but also approximation and fixation of the normal radial and ulnar relationship. In certain cases, the ligament ends can be identified and sutured primarily (Fig. 157–77). More often, additional implants are needed.

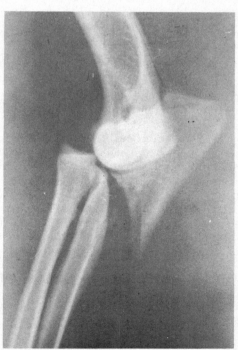

Figure 157–75. Monteggia fracture in which the proximal annular ligament remained intact, maintaining the normal relationship of the ulnar shaft and the radial head.

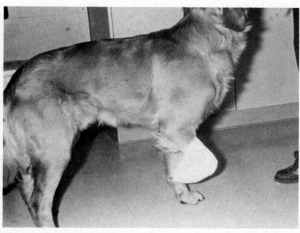

Figure 157–74. A carpal flexion bandage, which prevents weight-bearing but allows shoulder and elbow joint motion.

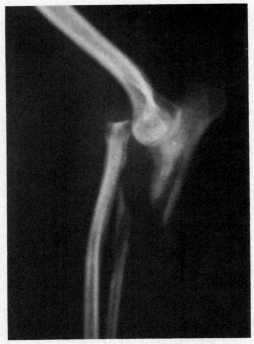

Figure 157–76. Monteggia fracture in which the ulnar fracture is distal to the proximal annular ligament and the ligament has ruptured. Note the separation of the radial head and the ulnar shaft.

Interfragmentary orthopedic wire can be applied (Fig. 157–78). Bone screws can be used either in interfragmentary lag fashion or by extending the fixation screws used in plating the ulnar fracture into the radius (Fig. 157–79). A postoperative compressive (Robert-Jones) bandage is often used for several days to control swelling, but early range-of-motion exercises are necessary to avoid elbow stiffness.

Fractures of the Radial Head

A fracture of the radial head is unusual. The anatomy of the elbow joint predisposes to fractures of the lateral humeral condyle, sparing the radius.[11] However, when fractures of the head do occur, they usually involve the articular surface. This situation demands meticulous reduction and stable internal fixation to prevent secondary arthritis and avoid joint stiffness. The fracture is approached through a lateral skin incision. Deep exposure depends on the location and extent of the fracture. Craniolateral exposure is obtained by incision of the origin and by distal medial retraction of the common digital extensor muscle.[30] Lateral exposure is obtained by osteotomy of the lateral humeral epicondyle followed by distal reflection of the collateral ligament and extensor tendons.[23] Caudolateral exposure is obtained by incision of the origin and by caudal distal retraction of the ulnaris lateralis and anconeus muscles.[23] Once the fracture is exposed and reduced, stabilization can take one of two forms.

The ideal method is an intrafragmentary lag compression screw. Splitting of the fragment can be

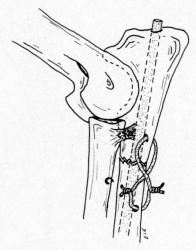

Figure 157–77. Primary suture repair of the proximal annular ligament and intramedullary pin fixation of the ulnar fracture for treatment of a Monteggia fracture.

avoided by countersinking the bone under the screw head. A Steinmann pin or Kirschner wire may be needed to control rotation of the fragment around the screw (Fig. 157–80). If screws are unavailable or too large for fixation without splitting the fragment, stabilization can be achieved with multiple Kirschner wires placed at divergent angles. Maximum reduction and compression of the fracture should be accomplished with bone-holding clamps, because driving the K-wires does not improve reduction. A minimum of two, and preferably three or more, K-wires should be placed at maximally divergent angles to prevent the fragment from rotating or sliding along the wire (Fig. 157–81). The K-wires are usually driven from the smaller fragment into the larger. The K-wires must be driven until they penetrate the far cortex to prevent loosening and migration, which would result

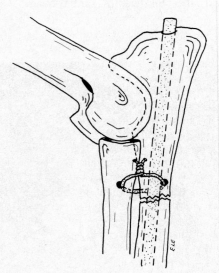

Figure 157–78. Interfragmentary wire stabilization of the radius and ulna and intramedullary pin fixation of the ulnar fracture for treatment of a Monteggia fracture.

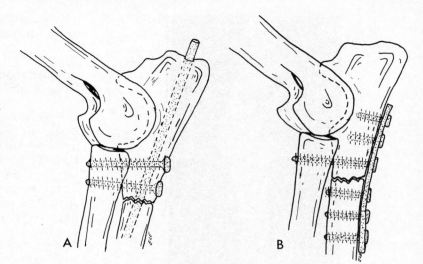

Figure 157–79. *A,* Interfragmentary lag screw stabilization of the radius and ulna and intramedullary pin fixation of the ulnar fracture for treatment of a Monteggia fracture. *B,* Extending the fixation screws of the ulnar plate into the radius.

in loss of fracture fixation. Closure is achieved by suturing the incised tendon origins or reattaching the humeral epicondyle with a lag screw or with pins and tension band wire. As with trochlear fractures, a delay in weight-bearing may be desired, depending on the stabilization obtained.

If the fracture is chronic with severe articular damage or is not reducible owing to severe comminution, a salvage procedure may be necessary. Resection of the radial head has been described as treatment for lateral luxation of the radial head secondary to growth deformities in small dogs.[7] It has also been cited as a potential method of treating radial head fractures.[24] Care should be taken to protect the radial nerve, and imposition of a free autogenous fat graft into the resection site seems to improve clinical results.[8] In larger, more athletic dogs, an elbow arthrodesis, as described elsewhere

in this text, would probably provide more stable results.[8]

Fracture and Separation of the Proximal Radial Physis

A fracture through the hypertrophied cartilaginous region of the proximal radial physeal plate is uncommon in young growing dogs (Fig. 157–82). It may be associated with lateral elbow luxation in some cases.[2] Closed reduction followed by immobilization in extension with a splint for seven to ten days may be possible, particularly with elbow luxation that can be reduced. Open reduction through a craniolateral approach should be performed if closed reduction is unsuccessful.[30] The radial head can be fixed in place with one or two Kirschner wires started at the

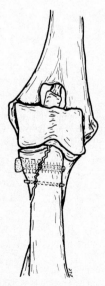

Figure 157–80. Lag screw and antirotational interfragmentary pin fixation of a radial head fracture.

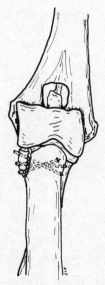

Figure 157–81. Divergent Kirschner wire fixation of a radial head fracture.

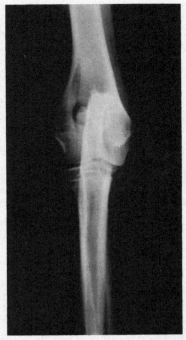

Figure 157–82. A fracture separation of the proximal radial physis.

articular edge and driven distally through the growth plate into the metaphysis (Fig. 157–83). If the animal is actively growing, the Kirschner wires should be placed as perpendicular to the physis as possible to avoid impeding growth. The K-wires are usually removed in two to three weeks, after healing occurs. The owner should be warned of possible premature physeal closure, and the animal should be periodi-

cally monitored for signs as described under "Premature Radial Physical Closure."

Isolated Fractures of Either the Radial or Ulnar Shafts

Isolated fractures of the radial or ulnar shafts with persistent continuity of the other bone occurs frequently, particularly in nonvehicular injuries such as horse kicks, bite wounds, and low-velocity gunshot injuries.[22] Because severe displacement of the fragments rarely occurs, two views with good-quality radiographs are often needed for diagnosis (Fig. 157–84). Treatment with a cast or splint is satisfactory in nearly all cases. The possibility that a synostosis (fusion) may develop between the radius and ulna with secondary elbow malarticulation should be considered in the young growing animal (see "Synostosis of the Radius and Ulna in the Growing Dog").

Shaft Fractures of Both the Radius and Ulna

Closed reduction by manipulation can often be achieved with simple, transverse, or mildly oblique fractures. This procedure is facilitated by early treatment (within 24 to 48 hours) and complete muscle relaxation with adequate anesthesia. Reduction can often be achieved by accentuating the fracture angle and apposing the fracture ends. Straightening the fracture angle then "toggles" the ends together to complete reduction (Fig. 157–85). Adequate reduction consists of at least 50 per cent fracture end contact on the *worse* of two standard (craniocaudal

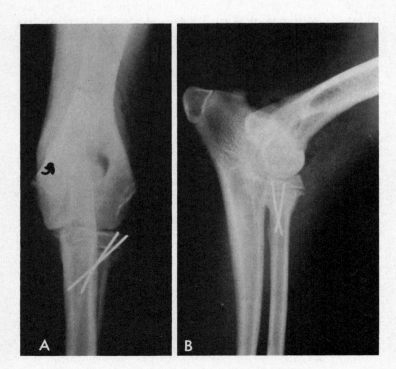

Figure 157–83. A and *B*, Fixation of a fracture separation of the proximal radial physis with two transphyseal Kirschner wires.

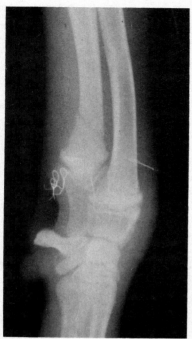

Figure 157–84. A minimally displaced ulnar fracture and intact radius.

and lateromedial) radiographic views (Fig. 157–86). Although some cranial or caudal angulation is acceptable, valgus or varus (lateral or medial) angulation should be carefully avoided because it can result in secondary arthritis from abnormal weight-bearing. The reduced fracture can be stabilized with a cast or Thomas splint. For antebrachial fractures, the cast needs to extend from the toes proximally to midway between the elbow and the point of the shoulder. It can often be cut down distal to the elbow in four to six weeks after early fracture consolidation, to allow elbow motion and better leg use. The cast should be kept dry and monitored daily by the owner for swelling, chewing, and abrasions. Initially, weekly office visits are suggested. The Thomas splint can be an effective means of coapting certain antebrachial fractures if properly applied. Thomas splints commonly hold the limb with the joints in excessive extension. Also, the splint makes patient ambulation difficult, and secondary decubital sores and abrasions are common. Primary treatment of antebrachial fractures with posterior or lateral splintage, either handmade or preformed (Mason Metasplint), is usually not sufficiently stable and should be discouraged.

External coaptation does not permit full motion of

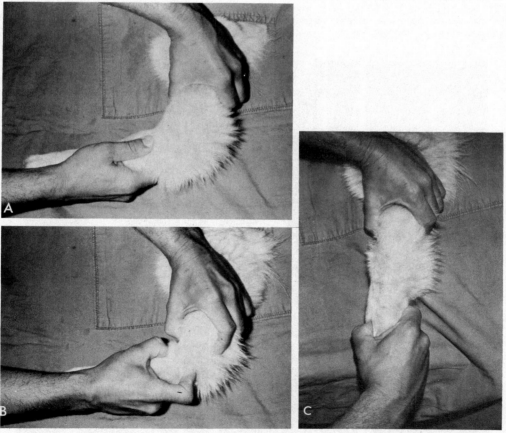

Figure 157–85. Closed reduction of a radius and ulnar fracture. *A,* Accentuating the fracture angle. *B,* Digitally apposing the fracture ends. *C,* Straightening the limb (toggling) to complete reduction.

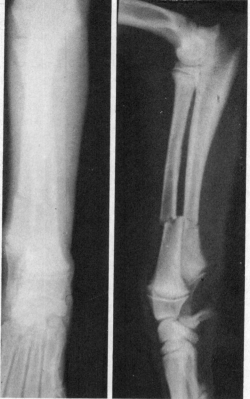

Figure 157–86. There must be at least 50 per cent cortical end contact in both craniocaudal and lateral medial planes for adequate closed reduction of a radius and ulnar fracture.

the thoracic limb joints. It usually precludes full weight-bearing, resulting in significant disuse muscle atrophy and joint stiffness. Sometimes, such treatment totally prevents weight-bearing, possibly resulting in atrophic nonunion. For these reasons, many clinicians treat antebrachial fractures with other means.[5,33]

External skeletal fixation can be employed as an effective means of stabilizing many antebrachial fractures following either closed or open reduction. If open reduction is required, it is limited to just a few centimeters in length through an anterior approach. The skin is incised just medial to the saphenous vein, and the extensor muscles are retracted laterally.[23] The specific configuration to be used depends on the inherent stability and location of the fracture.[10] Relatively stable, simple fractures can be treated with type 1 half-pin splintage applied to the cranial or medial aspect of the radius (Fig. 157–87). An unstable comminuted or open fracture with large defects is best treated with a quadrilateral frame or type II full-pin splintage. The latter method offers maximum resistance to fracture collapse.[10] The quadrilateral frame configuration allows pin fixation in two planes. Consequently, it can be used on very short fragments where other forms of fixation would not be stable (Fig. 157–88). External skeletal fixation is usually applied primarily to the radius, although the pins can be driven or applied primarily to the ulna if needed for fixation (Fig. 157–89). As in other methods of fixation, if open reduction of a comminuted fracture

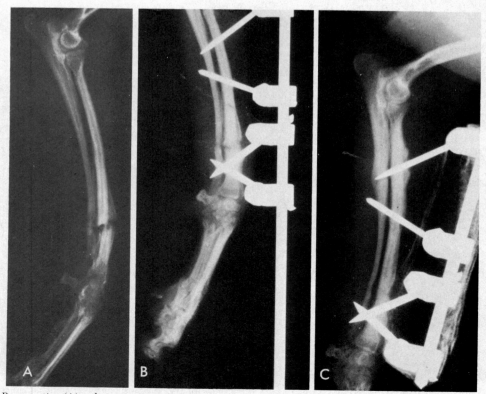

Figure 157–87. Preoperative (A) and postoperative (B) radiographs of a simple transverse radius and ulnar fracture fixed with a four-pin single bar configuration of external skeletal fixation after closed reduction. C, Eight weeks after surgery, the fracture has healed.

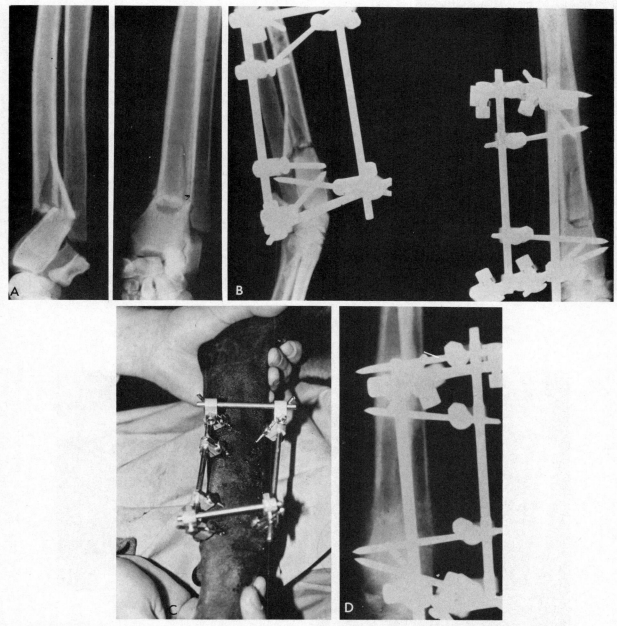

Figure 157–88. *A*, A distal radius and ulna fracture. *B*, Fixation with a quadrilateral frame. *C*, The quadrilateral frame in place. *D*, The healed fracture 11 weeks after surgery.

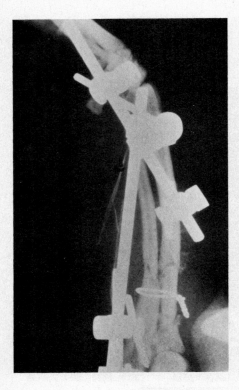

Figure 157–89. A radius and ulna fracture in which an iatrogenic fracture of the proximal radial fragment forced placement of the proximal pins into the ulna. (Courtesy of Dr. C. E. Blass.)

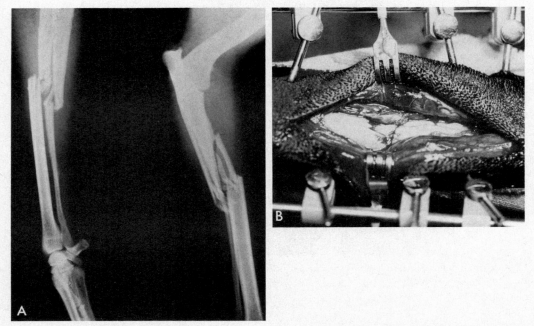

Figure 157–90. A, A severely comminuted radius and ulna fracture. *B,* Persistent fissures and defects after limited open reduction and external skeletal fixation.

Illustration continued on opposite page

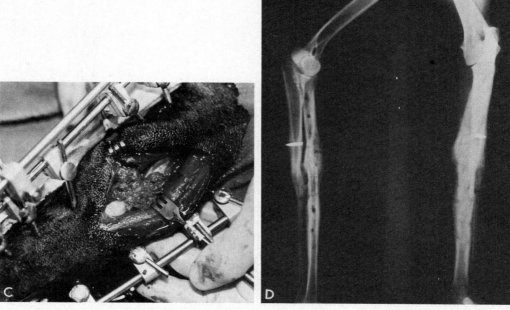

Figure 157–90 Continued. *C*, Packing of the defect with cancellous bone graft to stimulate rapid callus formation. *D*, The healed fracture at the time of fixation removal 14 weeks after surgery.

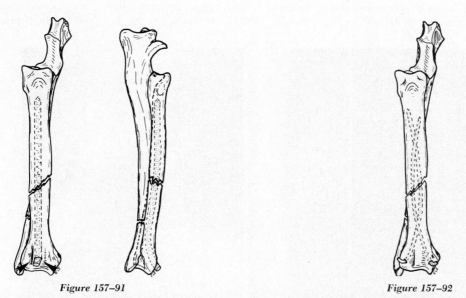

Figure 157–91   Figure 157–92

Figure 157–91. Fixation of a radius and ulna fracture with a single intramedullary pin. The pin should be driven retrograde from a point just proximal to the articular cartilage between the extensor carpi radialis and the common digital extensor tendons *(arrows)*.

Figure 157–92. Fixation of a fractured radius and ulna with two flexible Rush pins.

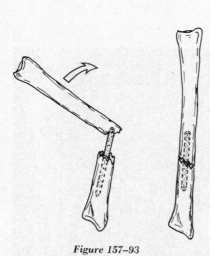

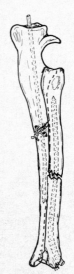

Figure 157–93

Figure 157–94

Figure 157–93. Fixation of a fractured radius by the buried pin technique. A small Kirschner wire is seated in the distal fragment and cut off, leaving approximately three millimeters protruding. The cut end is introduced into the medullary cavity of the proximal fragment, and the fracture is toggled into reduction.

Figure 157–94. Fixation of the ulnar fracture by either an intramedullary pin or an interfragmentary wire to control rotation around the intramedullary pin placed in the radial fracture.

leaves defects, a cancellous graft from the greater humeral tubercle should be used to stimulate early callus formation (Fig. 157–90).

Intramedullary pinning of radial fractures is usually accomplished via open reduction through an anterior approach.[23] The pin size should be selected to fill approximately three-fourths of the medullary canal. The pin is inserted in a normograde fashion, starting on the dorsal surface just proximal to the articular cartilage between the extensor carpi radialis and the common digital extensor tendons (Fig. 157–91). Retrograde placement of the pin results in damage to the cartilage and should be avoided. The distal end of the pin should be bent cranially to avoid interference with the antebrachial carpal joint. The oval cross-section of the medullary cavity limits the size of a single intramedullary pin in large dogs. However, two flexible pins can be used in Rush pin fashion to

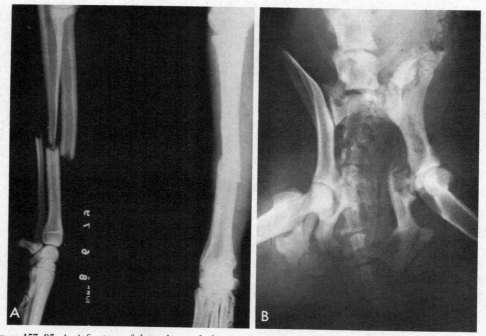

Figure 157–95. *A,* A fracture of the radius and ulna in a large dog. *B,* The pelvic fractures in the same animal.

Illustration continued on opposite page

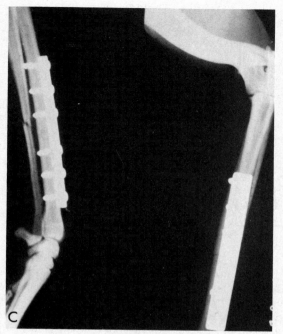

Figure 157–95 Continued. *C,* Plate fixation of the radial fracture allowing early use of the leg.

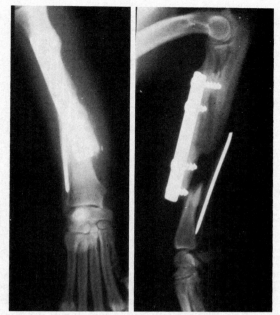

Figure 157–96. Fracture of the radius at the distal end of a plate applied three years earlier for a previous fracture.

improve fixation (Fig. 157–92). Intramedullary pins are commonly removed in two to four months, after the fracture heals.

In very small dogs, the distal radius is virtually solid bone with no distinct medullary cavity. Before intramedullary pinning, an artificial medullary canal may need to be drilled out from the fracture site. The buried pin is another method to manage these radial fractures in small dogs.[12] A small-diameter Kirschner wire is driven into the distal fragment until it is well seated. The K-wire is cut off with approximately 3 mm protruding from the distal fragment. This end is then introduced into the proximal fragment, and the fracture is toggled into reduction (Fig. 157–93). Because this method does not provide total angular stability, the bone should be supported with coaptation or external skeletal fixation until early healing is evident.

A single intramedullary pin in the radius may not totally prevent rotational motion, and supplemental fixation may be necessary. External coaptation or external skeletal fixation splint can be used for three to four weeks until the callus matures sufficiently. The ulna can also be stabilized either by a intramedullary pin driven normograde down from the olecranon or by an intrafragmentary wire applied through a separate caudal approach (Fig. 157–94).[18] Interfragmentary or cerclage wires may be employed to help stabilize long oblique fractures. However, passing the wires between the radius and ulna can be difficult, and the wires should not encompass both bones, because they would loosen.

Shaft fractures of the radius can be treated with bone screws and plates using the principles described

elsewhere. Plating offers very stable fixation that allows immediate weight-bearing. It is particularly useful in managing cases of trauma with multiple limb injuries (Fig. 157–95) and in managing distal radial and ulnar fractures in small dogs.[5] Such frac-

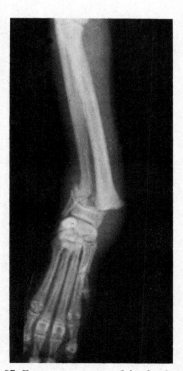

Figure 157–97. Fracture separation of the distal radial physis.

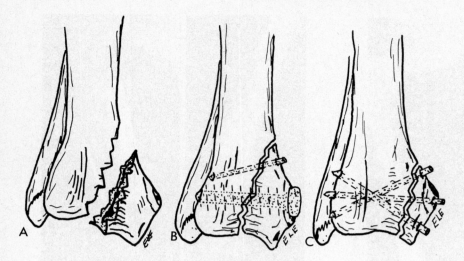

Figure 157–98. A distal radial articular fracture *(A)* fixed with a leg screw and antirotational cross pin *(B)* and multiple divergent Kirschner wires *(C)*.

tures commonly develop into atrophic nonunions if treated with coaptation or other methods that do not encourage normal weight-bearing.[5,33] Likewise, plating can be used to treat a nonunion once it develops. The plate is applied to the cranial surface of the radius through a cranial approach to the antebrachium.[23] The fracture is compressed to achieve maximum stability either by applying tension on the plate or by using interfragmentary screws. Any remaining defects are packed with cancellous bone from the greater tubercle of the humerus. In treatment of a nonunion, avascular sclerotic bone is resected, the fracture ends of the medullary cavity are opened to allow vascular ingrowth, and a copious cancellous bone graft is added to induce callus formation. A compressive bandage may be needed for several days after operation to control swelling. Because leg use is often normal within days, the owner is carefully instructed to restrict the dog's activity until the fracture heals.

Plate removal should be considered after the fracture heals and before stress protection from the plate weakens the bone, approximately five to 14 months after fixation in mature dogs.[1] Occasionally, weakening results in fracture of the bone at the end of the plate due to the "stress riser" effect (Fig. 157–96). Permanently implanted plates can become cold-sensitive, resulting in self-induced dermatitis, and can serve as a nidus for chronic infection and drainage.

Fracture Separation of the Distal Radial Physis

Fracture separations of the distal radial physis (Fig. 157–97), much like proximal physeal separations, can often be treated by closed reduction and external coaptation. If open reduction is needed, stabilization with a single small pin or Kirschner wire placed perpendicular to the physis, as previously described for intramedullary pinning of radial shaft fractures, is usually adequate. A posterior splint may be applied for ten to 14 days to protect the incision and control rotation. The pin should be removed in three to four weeks. As with proximal physeal injuries, the owner

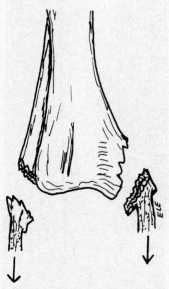

Figure 157–99. Avulsion fractures of the radial or ulnar styloid processes from traction by the corresponding collateral ligaments.

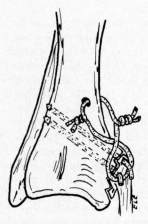

Figure 157–100. Fixation of a radial styloid avulsion fracture with two pins and a tension band wire.

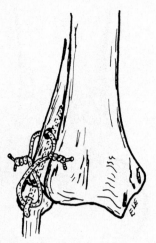

Figure 157–101. Fixation of an ulnar styloid avulsion fracture with a single pin and a tension band wire.

is advised of the possibility of premature physeal closure and secondary growth deformity.

Fractures of the Distal Radius and Ulna

A major fracture into the radial articular surface can be treated with an interfragmentary lag screw or multiple divergent Kirschner wires, as previously described for radial head fractures (Fig. 157–98).

Avulsion fracture of either the radial or ulnar styloid processes results from pull on the corresponding collateral ligament (Fig. 157–99). Consequently, such a fracture must be accurately reduced and stabilized so that normal antebrachial carpal joint stability may be regained. The pin and tension band wire technique, as described for olecranon avulsions, works well for an avulsion fracture. For radial avulsions, the pins are most stable when driven from the

fragment across the medullary cavity into the far cortex. After the figure-of-eight wire is placed, the pins are cut, bent, and buried in the collateral ligament (Fig. 157–100). For an ulnar avulsion, a single pin is normally used to stabilize the fracture and hook the tension band wire (Fig. 157–101). Postoperative bandaging may be used to protect the incision, and exercise is restricted until the fracture heals. Pins and wires should be removed if they become loose or irritate the soft tissues after the fracture heals.

GROWTH ABNORMALITIES OF THE ANTEBRACHIUM

Deformities of the foreleg can occur for various reasons. Fracture malunion, ligamentous injury with subsequent joint instability, and growth disturbances should be considered. The two-bone system of the antebrachium is predisposed to deformity caused by continual growth of one bone after premature growth cessation of its fellow. The bones normally grow in length by endochondral ossification.[6] A layer of chondroblastic germinal cells adjacent to the epiphysis forms the base of the physis or growth plate. The germinal cell layer continuously produces cartilage. As new cartilage is produced, the older cartilage is "pushed" toward the metaphysis. The chondrocytes in the cartilage progressively mature, palisade, and hypertrophy as they get further from the germinal cell layer. Finally, the cartilage calcifies as the chondrocytes degenerate. Chondroclasts and osteoblasts carried on invading metaphyseal capillary beds then replace the cartilage with bone (Fig. 157–102). The most common cause of premature growth cessation is traumatic injury to one of the physeal plates,[3] although inheritable and nutritional[19] causes have been described.

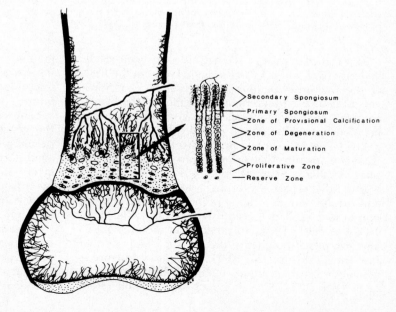

Figure 157–102. Diagram of the physis, which produces longitudinal growth through the process of endochondral ossification. (Reprinted with permission from Vet. Surg. *13*:172, 1984.)

Secondary Spongiosum
Primary Spongiosum
Zone of Provisional Calcification
Zone of Degeneration
Zone of Maturation
Proliferative Zone
Reserve Zone

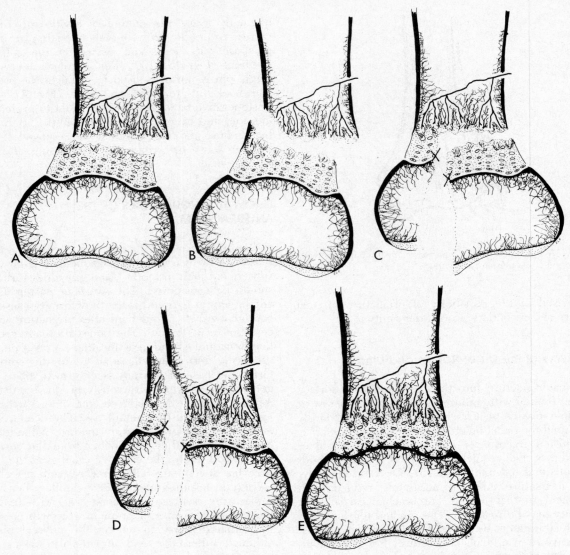

Figure 157–103. A, A Salter I fracture occurs transversely through the region of cartilage hypertrophy and degeneration. B, A Salter II fracture occurs transversely through the hypertrophied cartilage and extends into the metaphysis. C, A Salter III fracture occurs transversely through the hypertrophied cartilage and extends through the germinal cell layer into the epiphysis. D, A Salter IV fracture occurs longitudinally from the metaphysis through the physis and epiphysis into the joint. E, A Salter V fracture crushes the chondroblastic cell layer. (Reprinted with permission from Vet. Surg. *13*:172, 1984.)

Traumatic injuries to the physis have been classified into five groups by Salter and Harris on the basis of the fracture's anatomic configuration.[27] A transverse fracture through the weak region of the hypertrophied and degenerating cartilage, which is being invaded by capillaries and chondroclasts, is called a Salter I fracture (slipped epiphysis) (Fig. 157–103A). A similar fracture that extends into the metaphyseal bone is called a Salter II fracture (Fig. 157–103B). A fracture that is partially through the ossifying cartilage and extends through the germinal cell layer into the epiphysis is called a Salter III fracture (Fig. 157–103C). A Salter IV fracture begins in the metaphysis and extends through the physis and epiphysis and into the joint (Fig. 157–103D). A Salter V fracture is actually a crushing injury to the chondroblastic cell layer (Fig. 157–103E); it is not apparent on radio-

graphic examination and often occurs with other injuries or Salter fractures. Consequently, Salter V fractures are frequently not diagnosed at the time of injury.

Salter and Harris found that fractures that damage the germinal cell layer have a higher incidence of premature growth cessation (closures).[27] The damaged germinal cell layer stops producing new cartilage. However, the existing cartilage proceeds to hypertrophy, to ossify, and to be remodelled into bone. Consequently, the Salter V crushing injury has a high incidence of premature closure.

More recent studies have found that the prognosis for future normal growth is also affected by the severity of fracture displacement.[16] The displacement is related to damage to the vascular supply of the germinal cell layer. If sufficient vascular damage occurs, cartilage production ceases and premature physeal closure ensues.

Growth deformities of the antebrachium can result from injury to any one of three physes: distal ulnar, distal radial, or proximal radial. Each of these injuries is a specific set of resultant deformities, which are discussed independently. Not all of the changes associated with each physeal closure are seen in every clinical case. In general, angular deformities are seen more in the longer-limbed dogs, and more severe joint malarticulations in shorter-limbed dogs. The age of the animal at time of premature closure also affects the exact changes seen, perhaps because of the variation in stiffness of the bone with age and the duration of altered growth until maturity. Animals with growth deformity usually have a history of increasing limb angulation or relative limb shortening three to four weeks after forelimb injury of which, occasionally, the owners are unaware. Lameness is not common early in the disease. It usually occurs only after joint malarticulation results in significant arthritis or after angular deformity causes the dog to walk off the pads, with secondary ulcer formation.

Premature Closure of the Distal Ulnar Physis

The incidence of premature closure or fusion resulting in growth deformities is greatest in the distal ulnar growth plate of the dog,[17] apparently owing to the conical configuration of the distal ulnar physis. Although a transverse force applied to a simple physis such as the radial physis results in a Salter I fracture through the hypertrophied cartilage (Fig. 157–104), any significant transverse force applied to the ulna results in compression of one side of the cone (Fig. 157–105). This compression causes damage to the germinal layer of chondroblasts (Salter V fracture), cessation of cartilage production, and premature closure, as previously described.

The resulting growth deformities are particularly severe because the distal ulnar physis contributes 75 to 85 per cent of ulnar longitudinal growth (Fig. 157–106). The characteristic deformities reflect the two-bone anatomy of the forelimb. The ulna extends from

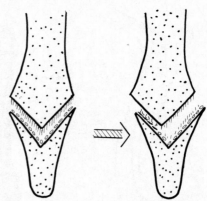

Figure 157–105. A shear force resulting in a Salter V fracture of the distal ulnar physis.

a medial position at the elbow obliquely across the long axis of the forelimb to a lateral position at the carpus and slightly caudal to the radius. Once the physis has fused, ulnar growth ceases, and the ulna behaves like a retarding strap twisted around the radius. As the radius continues to grow, it bows away from the ulna. This process results in three deformities of the radius: lateral deviation (valgus), anterior bowing (curvus), and external rotation (supination) (Fig. 157–107). This discrepancy in growth also results in caudolateral subluxation of the radial carpal joint, causing stretching of the medial soft tissue supporting structures. The radial head may also push the humeral condyles out of the trochlear notch of the ulna. Abnormal articulations resulting in irreversible degenerative osteoarthritis in the antebrachial carpal joint or the elbow are common. The net result of the retarding strap effect of the ulna and the radial deformities is shortening of leg length (Fig. 157–108). The appropriate treatment for antebrachial deformi-

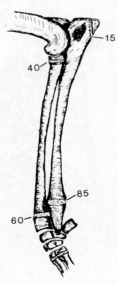

Figure 157–106. The relative contributions of the physes to the longitudinal growth of the radius and ulna.

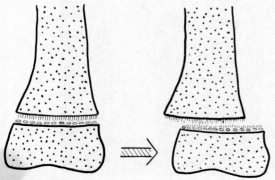

Figure 157–104. A shear force resulting in a Salter I fracture of the distal radial physis.

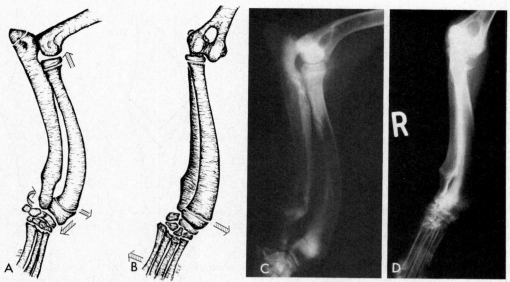

Figure 157–107. A to D, Valgus, anterior curvus, and external rotational deformities that occur following premature closure of the distal ulnar physis and continued radial growth.

ties due to premature ulnar closure depends on the age and remaining growth potential of the patient.

Dynamic Treatment of Immature Ulnar Physeal Closure

Animals in which a significant amount of radial growth potential remains (usually less than five to six months of age) should be treated with a dynamic technique that relieves the restraining effect of the ulna and allows the radius to continue to grow. This results not only in lengthening of the limb but also in partial spontaneous correction of the existing deformity.[19] The correction phenomenon has been attributed to accelerated physeal growth on the concave side of the bone once the retarding strap is removed.[13] The simplest of the dynamic techniques is a segmental ulnar ostectomy, which can easily be done through a caudal approach to the ulna as previously described.[23] Approximately 1 to 2 cm of the ulnar shaft and its periosteum is removed. If the dog is approaching completion of longitudinal bone

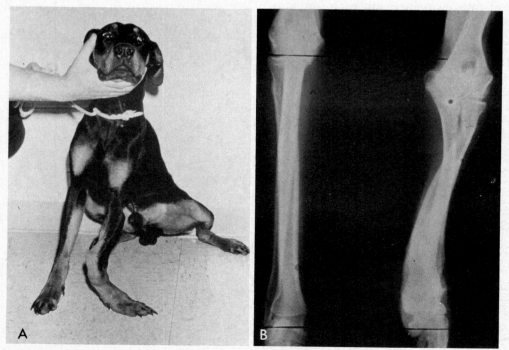

Figure 157–108. A and B, The absolute and functional relative shortening of leg length caused by premature closure of the distal ulnar physis.

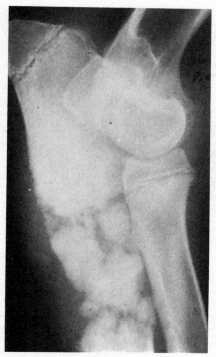

Figure 157–109. Radiograph taken three weeks after an ostectomy of the ulna performed for treatment of a prematurely closed distal ulnar physis. The restraining band effect of the ulna has re-formed, and the ostectomy must be repeated to prevent deformity. (Courtesy of Dr. S. G. Stoll.)

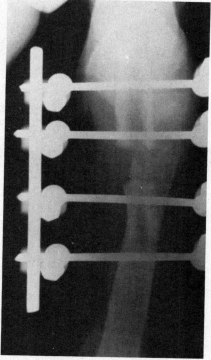

Figure 157–110. Radiograph taken after ulnar ostectomy and application of a type II full-pin splint to continuously spread the ulnectomy gap during radial growth.

growth, the procedure gives satisfactory results. However, if the dog is young (less than four to five months), the ulna frequently reunites prior to cessation of radial longitudinal growth, and repeated ostectomies are required to prevent progression of the deformities (Fig. 157–109).[19]

Distraction of the cut ends of the ulna with an external skeletal fixation device (Charnley, Stader, or Kirschner apparatus) lengthens the interval between ostectomies.[14,25] A full-pin type II splint should be applied (Fig. 157–110), as described in Chapter 153. The apparatus is extended three times a week until radial growth ceases.

In ulnar styloid transposition, the distal tip of the ulna is fused to the distal radial epiphysis after distal segmental ulnectomy.[9] This method retains carpal stability while preventing the reformation of a restraining ulnar band. A lateral approach to the distal ulna between the lateral digital extensor and the extensor carpi ulnaris tendons is used.[23] An oscillating bone saw is used to remove the distal third of the ulna to the level of the radial physis. The remaining ulna is trimmed to tilt over and lie flush against the radial epiphysis. The styloid can be fixed to the radius with either an interfragmentary bone screw or multiple divergent Kirschner wires (Fig. 157–111). The limb is placed in a compressive bandage for three to five days after surgery and then is given cast support for three weeks.

A technique has recently been described for preventing reformation of a restraining ulnar band by implanting a free autogenous fat graft into the ulnectomy site.[4] The interposed fat apparently prevents bone union by acting as a barrier to vascular invasion and secondary osteoblastic proliferation.[32] An ample quantity of fat is carefully harvested from a separate incision over the gluteal region. This fat is placed in a 2-cm defect created in the distal ulna and perios-

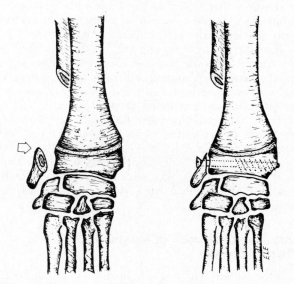

Figure 157–111. An ulnar styloid transposition following a segmental ulnectomy for treatment of premature distal ulnar physeal closure. (Reprinted with permission from Egger, E. L., and Stoll, S. G.: Ulnar styloid transposition as an experimental treatment for premature closure of the distal ulnar physis. J. Am. Anim. Hosp. Assoc. 14:690, 1978.)

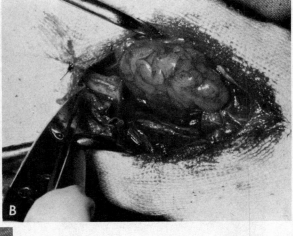

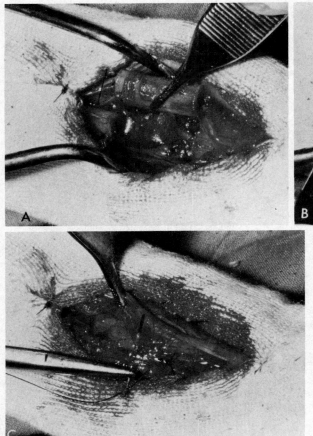

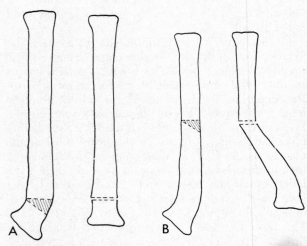

Figure 157–112. Autogenous fat graft for prevention of reformation of a restraining ulnar band. *A,* A segment of the distal ulna and periosteum is resected. *B,* An ample quantity of fat from the gluteal region is placed in the defect. *C,* The antebrachial fascia is sutured together to hold the fat in place.

teum (Fig. 157–112). The graft is one piece and is carefully handled to avoid trauma. The deep antebrachial fascia is sutured together over the fat to hold it in position. Bandaging of the limb with a posterior splint is suggested to minimize motion at the ostectomy site while the graft is being revascularized.[4]

The attainment of normal leg length, avoidance of permanent articular damage, and completeness of spontaneous straightening with any of the previous techniques depend on both the severity of the deformity and the remaining growth potential of the radius. Consequently, early diagnosis and dynamic treatment of premature ulnar closure offer the best prognosis for normal leg length, straightness, and joint function. Any angular deformity or joint malarticulation remaining after cessation of radial growth can be treated with a corrective osteotomy, as described later.

Definitive Correction of Mature Ulnar Physeal Closure

If the patient has stopped growing, definitive treatment is indicated, consisting of two components if needed. The first component is a corrective osteotomy of the angular and rotational deformities, which can be accomplished in a number of ways. Whichever technique is used for angular deformity, the correc-

tion is performed at the point of greatest curvature, in order to achieve the desired articular alignment with the best overall straightening (Fig. 157–113A). An angular correction at another point in the limb yields an S-shaped antebrachium (Fig. 157–113B).

Oblique osteotomies stabilized with external skel-

Figure 157–113. *A,* Location of a corrective osteotomy at the point of greatest deformity to achieve maximum correction. *B,* An S-shaped antebrachium from locating a corrective osteotomy at a point other than that of greatest deformity.

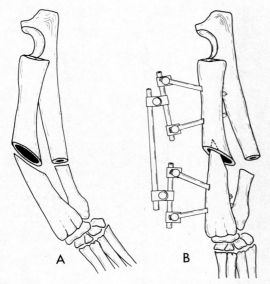

Figure 157–114. A, A 45-degree oblique osteotomy of the radius and ulna. B, Impaction of the proximal fragment into the medullary cavity of the distal, correction of the deformities, and application of a type I double-clamp external skeletal fixation following an oblique osteotomy.

etal fixation result in some restoration of leg length, can be applied to short and irregular fragments, and allow significant adjustment of alignment after surgery.[26]

The thoracic limb is prepared and draped so the elbow, carpus, and paw can be palpated and manipulated during surgery. Two fixation pins are placed into the radius proximal to the proposed osteotomy site, and two others are placed distal to the site from lateral to medial in half-pin fashion (see Chapter 153). The lateral surface of the ulnar shaft is approached through a small longitudinal incision.[23] The bone is

cut with an oscillating saw or osteotome, and the incision is closed. The cranial surface of the radius is approached through a separate longitudinal incision.[23] A 45-degree oblique osteotomy is performed (Fig. 157–114A). A double-clamp configuration of external skeletal fixation, using clamps and rods, is loosely attached to the fixation pins. The distal point of the proximal radial fragment is driven into the medullary cavity of the distal fragment (Fig. 157–114B). The cranial bowing, valgus curve, and particularly the external rotation are manually corrected and checked by flexing the elbow and antebrachial carpal joints. The connecting clamps are tightened, and the second skin incision is closed.

In a modified technique, the most proximal and distal fixation pins are driven in full-pin fashion from lateral to medial, parallel to the elbow and antebrachial carpal joints, respectively. The ulnar and radial osteotomies are performed as described. The appropriate connecting clamps and bars necessary for a type II full-pin splint are loosely attached to the fixation pins. The osteotomy is reduced, and the deformity corrected. The connecting clamps on the proximal and distal fixation pins are tightened (Fig. 157–115A). The intermediate pins are driven as either half pins or full pins through the remaining open connecting clamps (Fig. 157–115B). The clamps are tightened, and the incisions closed. The external skeletal fixation apparatus is removed when the osteotomy has healed.

Cuneiform wedge ostectomies provide a wide flat surface for fragment contact, which contributes significantly to stability and consequently to bone healing.[26] Although a wedge ostectomy does not increase the anatomical limb length, correction of the valgus deformity increases the functional length of the limb. The cuneiform ostectomy is a wedge with an angle in both the craniocaudal plane and the mediolateral

Figure 157–115. A, In a modified technique, the radius and ulna have been cut, the proximal and distal fixation pins have been placed, and appropriate clamps and connecting bars loosely attached to the pins. B, The deformities have been corrected and the osteotomy stabilized with a modified type II full-pin splint. (Courtesy of Dr. D. L. Piermattei.)

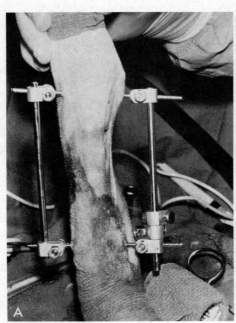
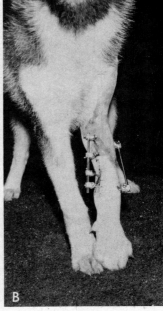

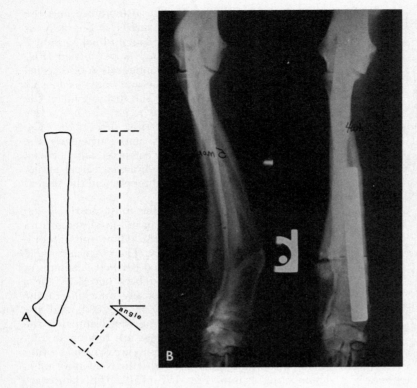

A

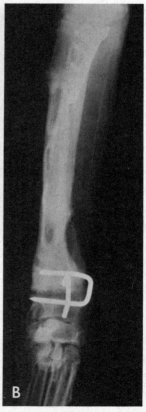

Figure 157–116. A, The appropriate angle for correcting deformities with a wedge ostectomy. *B,* The ostectomy can be stabilized with a bone plate and screws if the proximal and distal fragments are adequate in length. (*B* courtesy of Dr. S. G. Stoll.)

plane. The angle of these wedges can be determined by drawing perpendicular lines to the long axis of the proximal and distal fragments (Fig. 157–116A). Exsanguination of the limb with a sterile elastic wrapping and a tourniquet applied above the elbow reduces hemorrhage and improves surgical visibility. However, the use of a tourniquet results in significantly increased postoperative swelling. The calcu-

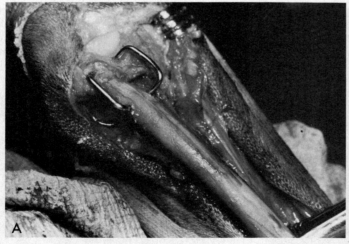

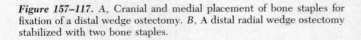

Figure 157–117. A, Cranial and medial placement of bone staples for fixation of a distal wedge ostectomy. *B,* A distal radial wedge ostectomy stabilized with two bone staples.

lated angles must be translated into a single three-dimensional wedge, which is created by performing two ostectomies that intersect at the caudolateral cortex of the radius. The ulna must also be cut to remove its restraining effect. The resected radial wedge is closed to reduce the angular deformities. The external rotation must also be corrected by internal rotation of the distal fragment and manus. If the fragments are adequate in length, the osteotomy can be stabilized with a bone plate and screws (Fig. 157–116B).[19] Distal ostectomies that result in very short distal fragments can be fixed with two bone staples.[29] The staples are handmade from appropriate sized (1/16- to 1/8-inch) Steinmann pins. Holes for the staple legs are created with the same size or a slightly smaller Steinmann pin. The staples are driven with a mallet or squeezed into place with a clamp. One staple is placed from cranial to caudal and one from medial to lateral (Fig. 157–117). Postoperative swelling is controlled with a compressive bandage. Because staples do not provide rigid stabilization, the limb is supported in a short cast until healing occurs (usually four to six weeks). External skeletal fixation can also be used to stabilize very short fragments, particularly when oriented in a two-plane configuration such as a quadrilateral frame.

The second component in treating a mature deformity is repositioning of the elbow articular components.[19] Because the affected limb is already shortened, lengthening the ulna is more appropriate than shortening the radius. A caudal approach is made to the shaft of the ulna and the trochlear notch.[23] The elbow joint should be examined for fibrosis and osseous proliferation, which are resected or remodelled. A transverse ulnar osteotomy is performed just distal to the elbow joint. The ulna is moved into place by spreading the osteotomy with a heavy periosteal elevator or self-retaining retractor. The ulna is fixed in position, if needed, with external skeletal fixation, a bone plate and screws, or transfixing screws placed from the proximal ulna to radial head (Fig. 157–118). An autogenous cancellous bone graft may be used to help induce bony healing. Early postoperative elbow joint motion, necessary for elbow mobility and articular remodelling, should be encouraged.

Premature Radial Physeal Closure

Either the proximal or the distal radial physis can prematurely cease growing, causing antebrachial abnormalities.[3] A premature closure of the proximal radial physis with continued ulnar growth results in malarticulation of the elbow joint characterized by widening of the radial–humeral joint space and the humeral–anconeal joint space (Fig. 157–119).[21] Severe malformation of the articular components with secondary arthritis rapidly develops. In some cases, decreased longitudinal growth results in shortening of the limb compared with the normal limb.

The abnormalities that result from premature closure of the distal radial physis can be quite variable.[3] If ulnar growth continues, the elbow malarticulation described for proximal closures very commonly occurs. If a complete symmetrical premature closure of the physis occurs, the limb may remain straight and may develop a widening radial–carpal joint space (Fig. 157–120A), or a caudal bow of both the radius

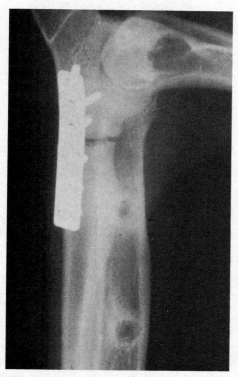

Figure 157–118. Postoperative radiograph in which the ulnar osteotomy has been spread and fixed with a bone plate and screws to improve elbow articulation.

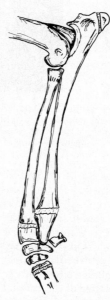

Figure 157–119. Elbow malarticulation from premature closure of the proximal radial physis.

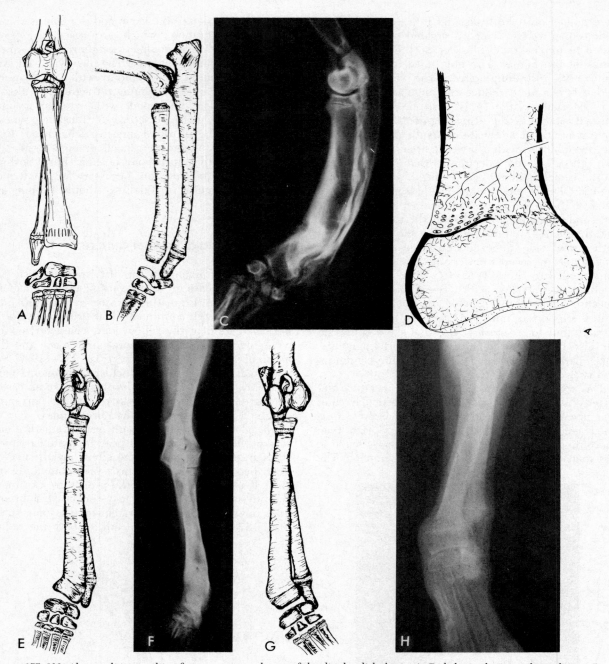

Figure 157–120. Abnormalities resulting from premature closure of the distal radial physis. *A*, Radial carpal joint malarticulation. *B* and *C*, Caudal radial and ulnar bowing. *D*, An angular deformity from asymmetrical premature closure of a physis and continued growth of the remaining portion. *E* and *F*, Varus angular deformity from premature closure of the medial side of the distal radial physis. *G* and *H*, Valgus deformity from premature closure of the lateral side of the distal radial physis.

and ulna may develop (Fig. 157–120*B* and *C*). More commonly, the physeal closure is asymmetrical, with bony bridging on one side of the physis and continued growth of the opposite side (Fig. 157–120*D*). Premature closure of the lateral side of the physis causes valgus angular deformity and external rotation characteristic of premature distal ulnar physeal closure, with which it is often concurrent (Fig. 157–120*E* and *F*). Premature closure of the medial side of the physis results in a varus angular deformity and, occasionally, inward rotation of the manus (Fig. 157–120*G* and *H*).

Treatment of Immature Radial Physeal Closure

Dynamic treatment of radial growth deformities prior to closure of the distal ulnar and remaining radial growth plate has three objectives: to maintain realignment of the elbow articular components, to develop maximum antebrachial length, and to correct or prevent angular deformities. With complete symmetrical or advanced asymmetrical physeal closures, these objectives are accomplished through progres-

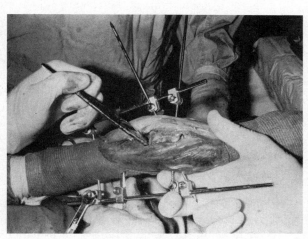

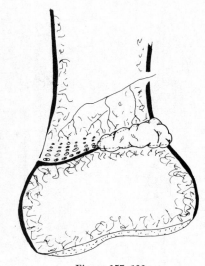

Figure 157–121   *Figure 157–122*

Figure 157–121. Spreading of the radial osteotomy to the limits of the surrounding soft tissues in the treatment of an immature distal radial physeal closure.

Figure 157–122. Treatment of an asymmetrical premature closure by bony resection and implantation of an autogenous fat graft.

sive spreading of a radial osteotomy.[20,25] An external skeletal fixation system (Charnley, Stader, or Kirschner apparatus) is utilized. Either full-pin or half-pin splintage can be employed, but a full-pin system remains stable longer. After the appropriate fixation pins are placed, the radius is cut through a cranial approach,[23] preferably at the point of greatest curvature. The fixation device is completed, and the osteotomy is spread to the limits of the surrounding soft tissues (Fig. 157–121). Complete reduction of elbow malarticulation and angular deformity is not immediately necessary. These corrections are continued as the apparatus is spread on an every other day basis while ulnar growth continues. Excessive spreading tension should not be put on the fixation at any one time, because the bones are soft and the fixation pins can cut through them. The leg should be examined frequently by radiograph so that elbow re-

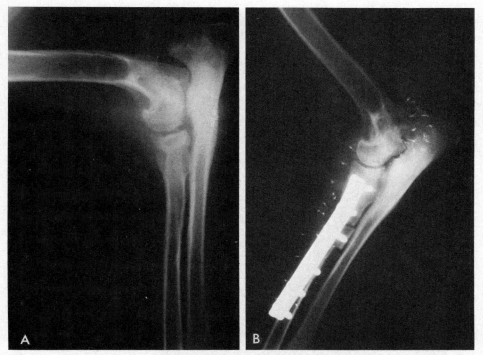

Figure 157–123. Preoperative *(A)* and postoperative *(B)* radiographs of the elbow malarticulation associated with premature radial physeal closure that was treated by imposition of a cortical allograft into a radial ostectomy and fixation with a bone plate and screws.

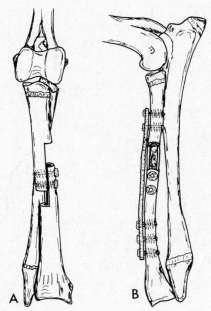

Figure 157–124. Elbow malarticulation associated with premature radial physeal closure treated with a step radial osteotomy stabilized with interfragmentary lag screws (A) and a neutralization plate (B).

duction and ulnar physeal status can be evaluated. The fixation device may have to be replaced if extended spreading is required for more than six to eight weeks. After the external skeletal fixation device is removed, external support should be applied for several weeks while the radius strengthens.

Early asymmetrical closure of the distal radial physis has recently been treated by resection of the osseous bridge and imposition of an autogenous fat graft.[31] The margins of the osseous bridge are determined by palpation with a 25-gauge needle. The bone bridge is resected with a curette, and the defect is packed with a fat graft obtained from the flank (Fig. 157–122). The graft should be held in place by suturing of the adjacent soft tissues over the area. Significant remaining angular deformities may need to be treated with corrective osteotomy.

Definitive Treatment of Premature Radial Physeal Closure

Definitive treatment of premature radial physeal closures will realign elbow articular components and straighten angular deformities.[20] The elbow is realigned by spreading a transverse osteotomy of the radius. Exploration of the elbow joint may be needed to resect excessive fibrous tissue and remodel osseous malformation and proliferation. A cortical allograft is placed into the osteotomy, which is then stabilized with either external skeletal fixation or a bone plate and screws (Fig. 157–123). Alternatively, a stair-step radial osteotomy may be performed.[31] After distraction of the osteotomy and realignment of the elbow articular components, the osteotomy is fixed with interfragmentary lag screws and further supported with a neutralization plate (Fig. 157–124). Correction of angular deformities usually requires a separate procedure in the distal antebrachium at the point of greatest curvature. Either an oblique osteotomy or a wedge ostectomy, as previously described, can be utilized.

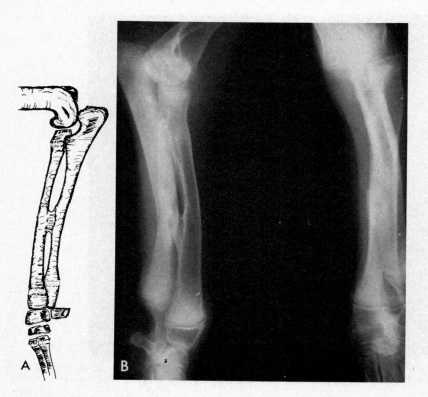

Figure 157–125. A and B, Elbow malarticulation secondary to synostosis of the radius and ulna.

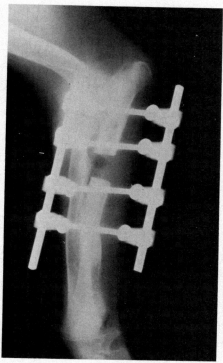

Figure 157–126. Articular alignment following ulnar osteotomy and spreading with a type II full-pin splint.

Synostosis of the Radius and Ulna in the Growing Dog

Synostosis of the radius and ulna is not a disease of the physeal growth plate, but a restriction in the relative proximal movement of the ulnar shaft that normally occurs during growth.[3] This movement reflects the virtually total contribution to ulnar length by the distal ulnar physis; the contributions of the proximal and distal radial growth plates to radial length are nearly equal. When ulnar shaft movement is restricted, a relative overgrowth of the proximal radius, with proximal displacement of the humeral condyles and deformation of the trochlear notch, occurs (Fig. 157–125). Significant shortening, angular deformity, or antebrachial carpal joint alterations usually do not occur. Apparently, the strong pull of the distal ulnar growth through the radioulnar ligament stimulates additional growth from the distal radial physis.[3] Synostosis of the radius and ulna is usually associated with a bridging callus following imperfect reduction of a fracture of the radius or ulna. Improper fixation of both bones by internal fixation devices such as fixation pins or bone screws during treatment of fractures can also restrict normal movement.

Treatment of synostosis is removal of the restricting element and realignment of the elbow joint. Transfixing pins or screws are removed. Bridging callus can be resected, and the defect can be filled with an autogenous fat graft to prevent reformation. An osteotomy of the ulna proximal to the synostosis, as previously described, is usually necessary to realign the elbow. The defect (1) may be implanted with an autogenous fat graft if the animal is still growing or (2) may be spread and fixed in position with external skeletal fixation or a bone plate and screws if the animal is mature (Fig. 157–126).

1. Brinker, W. O., et al.: Removal of bone plates in small animals. J. Am. Anim. Hosp. Assoc. *11*:577, 1975.
2. Brinker, W. O., Piermattei, D. L., and Flo, G. L.: *Handbook of Small Animal Orthopedics and Fracture Treatment.* W. B. Saunders, Philadelphia, 1983.
3. Carrig, C. B., and Wortman, J. A.: Acquired dysplasias of the canine radius and ulna. Comp. Cont. Ed. *3*:557, 1981.
4. Craig, E.: Autogenous fat grafts to prevent recurrence following surgical correction of growth deformities of the radius and ulna in the dog. Vet. Surg. *10*:69, 1981.
5. DeAngelis, M. P., et al.: Repair of fractures of the radius and ulna in small dogs. J. Am. Anim. Hosp. Assoc. *9*:436, 1973.
6. deKlerr, V. S.: Development of bone. *In* Sumner-Smith, G. (ed.): *Bone in Clinical Orthopaedics.* W. B. Saunders, Philadelphia, 1982.
7. Dieterich, H. F.: Repair of a lateral radial head luxation by radial head ostectomy. Vet. Med./Small Anim. Clin. *68*:671, 1973.
8. Dieterich, H. F.: Personal communication, 1983.
9. Egger, E. L., and Stoll, S. G.: Ulnar styloid transposition as an experimental treatment for premature closure of the distal ulnar physis. J. Am. Anim. Hosp. Assoc. *14*:690, 1977.
10. Egger, E. L.: Static strength evaluation of six external skeletal fixation configurations. Vet. Surg. *12*:130, 1983.
11. Evans, H. E., and Christensen, G. C. (eds.): *Miller's Anatomy of the Dog.* W. B. Saunders, Philadelphia, 1979.
12. Hoefle, W. D.: Fractures of radius and ulna. *In: Orthopedic Surgery Notes.* Iowa State University, 1978.
13. Karaharju, E. O., Ryoppy, S. A., and Makinen, R. J.: Remodeling by asymmetrical epiphyseal growth. J. Bone Jt. Surg. *58B*:122, 1976.
14. Knecht, C. D., and Bloomberg, M. S.: Distraction with an external fixation clamp (Charnley apparatus) to maintain length in premature physeal closure. J. Am. Anim. Hosp. Assoc. *16*:873, 1980.
15. Lau, R. E.: Inherited premature closure of the distal ulnar physis. J. Am. Anim. Hosp. Assoc. *14*:690, 1978.
16. Lombardo, S. J., and Harvey, J. P.: Fractures of the distal femoral epiphyses; factors influencing prognosis: a review of thirty-four cases. J. Bone Jt. Surg. *59A*:742, 1977.
17. Marretta, S. A., and Schrader, S. C.: Physeal injuries in the dog: a review of 135 cases. J. Am. Vet. Med. Assoc. *182*:708, 1983.
18. Neal, T. M.: Fractures of the radius and ulna. *In* Bojrab, M. J. (ed.): *Current Techniques in Small Animal Surgery.* Lea & Febiger, Philadelphia, 1975.
19. Newton, C. D.: Surgical management of distal ulnar physeal growth disturbances in dogs. J. Am. Vet. Med. Assoc. *164*:479, 1974.
20. Newton, C. D., Nunamaker, D. M., and Dickenson, C. R.: Surgical management of radial physeal growth disturbances in dogs. J. Am. Vet. Med. Assoc. *167*:1011, 1975.
21. O'Brien, T. R., Morgan, J. P., and Suter, P. F.: Epiphyseal plate injury in the dog: a radiographic study of growth disturbance in the forelimb. J. Small Anim. Pract. *12*:19, 1971.
22. Phillips, I. R.: A survey of bone fractures in the dog and cat. J. Small Anim. Pract. *20*:661, 1979.
23. Piermattei, D. L., and Greeley, R. G.: *An Atlas of Surgical Approaches to the Bones of the Dog and Cat.* W. B. Saunders, Philadelphia, 1979.
24. Putnam, R. W., and Archibald, J.: Excision of canine radial head. Mod. Vet. Pract. *49*:32, 1968.
25. Robertson, J. J.: Application of a modified Kirschner device in the distraction mode as a prevention of antebrachial

deformities in early physeal closure. J. Am. Anim. Hosp. Assoc *19*:345, 1983.

26. Rudy, R. L.: Corrective osteotomy for angular deformities. Vet. Clin. North Am. *1*:549, 1971.

27. Salter, R. B., and Harris, W. R.: Injuries involving the epiphyseal plate. J. Bone Jt. Surg. *45A*:587, 1963.

28. Sisk, T. D.: Fractures. *In* Edmonson. A. S., and Crenshaw, A. H. (eds.): *Campbell's Operative Orthopedics.* 6th ed. C. V. Mosby, St. Louis, 1980.

29. Stoll, S. G.: Personal communication, 1976.

30. Turner, T. M., and Hohn, R. B.: Craniolateral approach to the canine elbow for repair of condylar fractures or joint exploration. J. Am. Vet. Med. Assoc. *176*:1264, 1980.

31. Vandewater, A., and Olmstead, M. L.: Premature closure of the distal radial physis in the dog: a review of eleven cases. Vet. Surg. *12*:7, 1983.

32. Vandewater, A., Olmstead, M. L., and Stevenson, S.: Partial ulnar ostectomy with free autogenous fat grafting for treatment of radius curvus in the dog. Vet. Surg. *11*:92, 1982.

33. Veterinary Orthopedic Society: Fracture Documentation Study. 5th Annual Conference, Snowmass, Colorado, 1978.

Carpus and Digits

Robert W. Moore

ANATOMY OF THE FOREPAW

The forepaw is composed of the carpus, metacarpus, phalanges, and associated sesamoids. The carpus includes the carpal bones and sesamoids. There are seven carpal bones arranged in two transverse rows, plus a small medial sesamoid.[5] The radial, ulnar, and accessory carpal bones are found in the proximal row, and the first, second, third, and fourth carpal bones lie from medial to lateral in the distal row (Fig. 157–127).

The radial carpal bone, located on the medial side of the proximal row, is the largest carpal bone. It articulates proximally with the radius and distally with all four distal carpal bones. The ulnar carpal bone lies laterally in the proximal row and is slightly smaller. It articulates with both the radius and ulna proximally, with the fourth and fifth metacarpals distally, and with the accessory carpal on the palmar side. The accessory carpal bone articulates with only the ulnar carpal bone. A single sesamoid bone is located in the tendon of insertion of the abductor pollicis longus muscle near the proximal end of the first metacarpal.

The five metacarpal bones are numbered I to V from medial to lateral. The proximal end of each bone is the base and the distal end is the head. Metacarpals II to V are weight-bearing. Metacarpal

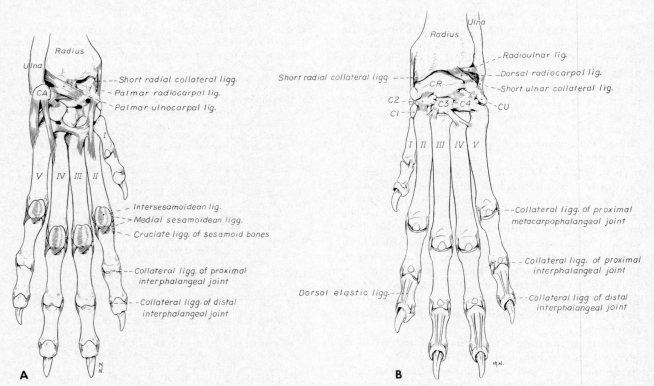

A

B

Figure 157–127. A, Palmar aspect of the carpus. B, Dorsal aspect of the carpus. *CR*, radial carpal; *CU*, ulnar carpal; *C1–C4*, first to fourth carpals; *CA*, accessory carpals; *I* to *V*, metacarpals. (Reprinted with permission from Evans, H. E., and Christensen, G. C. (eds.): *Miller's Anatomy of the Dog.* 2nd ed. W. B. Saunders, Philadelphia, 1979.)

I is smaller and has only two phalanges and no sesamoid bones. Metacarpals II to V have two sesamoids each on the palmar side and bear three phalanges. The middle part of the walls of each metacarpal is extremely dense, and the ends are thinner. Metacarpals II to V have distal epiphyses during development, but metacarpal I has only a proximal epiphysis.

The carpal joints act together to permit flexion and extension with a minimal amount of medial and lateral movement. The antebrachiocarpal joint (proximal or radiocarpal) is located between the distal radius and ulna and the proximal row of carpal bones. The middle carpal joint occurs between the two rows of carpal bones. The carpometacarpal joints are located between the distal row of carpal bones and the proximal ends of the metacarpal bones. The greatest amount of movement occurs in the antebrachiocarpal and middle carpal joints. Intercarpal and carpometacarpal joint surfaces permit very little movement.

No long collateral ligaments span all three points. Support to the carpus is provided by increased thickness in the joint capsule on the dorsal and palmar surfaces. Two separate layers of collagenous tissue can be found with tendons in between. The superficial layer is a thickened modification of the deep carpal fascia. The deep layer is the fibrous layer of the joint capsule. As these layers pass medially and laterally, they combine to form short collateral ligaments.

The transverse palmar carpal ligament attaches laterally to the accessory carpal bone and medially to the styloid process of the radius, radial carpal, and first carpal bones. This ligament is very well-developed in the dog and provides support proximally on the palmar side of the carpus (Fig. 157–128). The palmar carpal fibrocartilage crosses the palmar side of the carpal bones and attaches to all except the accessory carpal bone. Distally, it attaches to the proximal parts of metacarpals III, IV, and V and serves as the origin for the small intrinsic muscles of the digits. Short collateral ligaments extend both medially and laterally across the radiocarpal joint (see Fig. 157–127). The short radial collateral ligament

has straight and oblique portions originating from the styloid process and inserting on the most medial surface and the palmar medial surface of the radial carpal bone, respectively. The short ulnar collateral ligament extends from the ulnar styloid to the ulnar carpal bone. Multiple smaller ligaments attach the carpal bones to each other and the metacarpals (see Fig. 157–127). The palmar accessory carpometacarpal ligaments arise from the free end of the accessory carpal and attach to metacarpals IV and V. The radial carpometacarpal ligament also arises from the radial carpal bone and attaches on metacarpals II and III.

The flexor carpi radialis muscle inserts on the proximal palmar surfaces, and the extensor carpi radialis muscle inserts on the dorsal area of the bases, of metacarpals II and III. The adductor digiti quinti muscle inserts distally on metacarpals IV and V. The flexor carpi ulnaris muscle inserts on the accessory carpal bone. The abductor pollicis longus inserts on the proximal medial part of metacarpal I, and the extensor pollicis longus inserts distally on the same bone. The reader is referred to canine anatomy texts for additional description of anatomy of the carpus and digits.[5]

PHYSICAL EXAMINATION

Evaluation of any orthopedic problem begins with a careful history obtained from the client. The duration and cause of the injury should be determined along with the future potential use of the animal. For example, if an animal is presented with an open fracture or luxation involving the forepaw, early treatment including surgery may prevent contamination from turning into infection. In this case, the duration of injury is very important. Another example is that an injury that would cause no significant problem for a house dog might cause a chronic low-grade lameness in a working or hunting dog. In the latter example, the future use of the animal is important in determining whether surgery is required.

Physical examination begins by observation of the

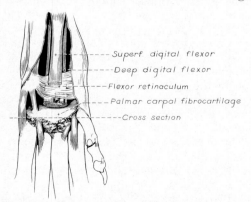

Figure 157–128. Palmar carpal ligaments and fibrocartilage. (Reprinted with permission from Evans, H. E., and Christensen, G. C. (eds.): *Miller's Anatomy of the Dog.* 2nd ed. W. B. Saunders, Philadelphia, 1979.)

Superf. digital flexor
Deep digital flexor
Flexor retinaculum
Palmar carpal fibrocartilage
Cross section

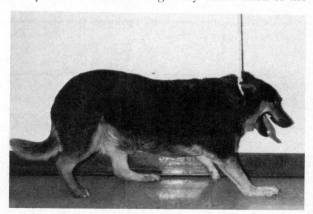

Figure 157–129. Hyperextension injury to the carpus resulting in palmigrade walking. Injury had resulted from jumping over a wall one month prior to presentation.

animal when standing and moving. Palmigrade walking ("dropped carpus") may be seen with a hyperextensional injury (Fig. 157–129). If the patient is bearing weight on the foot, ambulation should be encouraged to determine the severity of lameness and to rule out problems in other limbs. Often with carpal hyperextensional injuries, the patient bears slight weight on the affected leg or legs and shifts weight to the rear limbs. Acute injuries to one limb tend to be carried, with slight increases in weight-bearing in those patients presented several days after the injury. Other causes of lameness include paronychitis, interdigital dermatitis, penetrating foreign bodies such as foxtails, bite wounds, lacerated tendons, sprains, and strains. The location and severity of swelling and tenderness should be noted.

A thorough neurological examination must be performed to determine function in the affected limb. Radial nerve paralysis results in dorsal cutaneous sensory deficits and a decreased ability to place the foot palmigrade. Ulnar nerve paralysis is usually asymptomatic except for loss of cutaneous sensation on the lateral palmar aspect of the paw. However, carpal hyperextension and degenerative joint disease have been reported with ulnar nerve injuries.[12]

If septic or immune-mediated arthritis is suspected, joint paracentesis should be performed, synovial fluid analyzed, and hematologic tests performed. Other joints should be examined carefully for signs of pain or discomfort. In immune-mediated diseases, degenerative changes are usually most severe in the carpal and tarsal joints.[13] The non-erosive types of immune-mediated disease often exhibit only minimal radiographic changes, making the diagnosis even more difficult. Septic arthritis is more commonly caused by blood-borne infections than by organisms in penetrating wounds.[13] Larger breeds such as Great Danes, St. Bernards, and German shepherds are most often affected, with *Staphylococcus* and *Streptococcus* being the two most common organisms. Mycoplasmal and fungal infections are relatively uncommon.[13]

Primary neoplasms of the joint must also be considered but are relatively uncommon. Malignant synovioma and hemangiopericytoma have both been described. Lameness may precede radiographic changes by several weeks.[13]

RADIOGRAPHIC EXAMINATION

In most animals, sedation is required for good-quality radiographs of the carpus and digits. High-detail screens are indicated for demonstration of subtle changes. Craniocaudal and lateral radiographs are first taken of both the affected and the nonaffected limbs for comparison. However, carpal ligament injuries often cannot be seen until stress radiographs are taken. With the patient sedated, a gauze sling or plastic rod is used to hyperextend and flex the carpus (Fig. 157–130). Varus and valgus stress films are

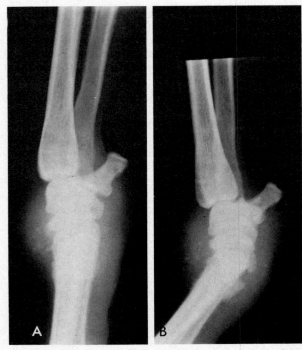

Figure 157–130. *A,* Lateral radiograph of carpus. Note soft tissue swelling and periarticular changes. *B,* Stress radiograph of same carpus, showing instability to involve only the carpometacarpal joint.

taken in the same manner. Differentiation of the joint or joints involved is important in determining whether surgery is necessary and which procedure is most appropriate. Oblique radiographs are occasionally needed to demonstrate smaller, nondisplaced fractures of the carpal bones.

PATHOPHYSIOLOGY

Trauma is the most common cause of lameness associated with the carpus and digits. Injuries due to jumping from automobiles or buildings result in carpal and metacarpal fractures or hyperextension of the joints from tearing of supportive ligaments and fibrocartilage. Slocum and Devine[19] categorized ligamentous tears in three groups: *Category 1* injuries involve the radiocarpal joint with rupture of the short radial collateral (oblique), palmar radiocarpal, and palmar ulnar carpal ligaments and allow palmar subluxation of the radial carpal bone (Fig. 157–131*A*). *Category 2* injuries involve the palmar accessory carpometacarpal ligaments and the short intercarpal ligament between the accessory and ulnar carpal bones; hyperextension of the radiocarpal joint with proximal displacement of the accessory carpal bone is seen (Fig. 157–131*B*). Only the flexor carpi radialis muscle is left intact to support the flexion of the carpus, because the pull of the flexor carpi ulnaris muscle is ineffective as it inserts on the accessory carpal bone. *Category 3* injuries involve the ligaments of the middle carpal and carpometacarpal joints

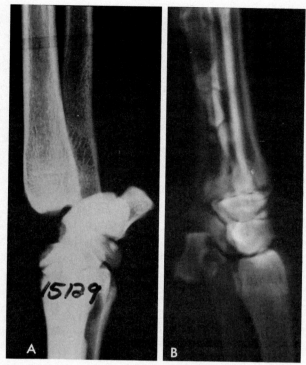

Figure 157–131. *A,* Instability of the radiocarpal joint with subluxation of the radial carpal bone. *B,* Hyperextension injury to the radiocarpal joint with proximal displacement of the accessory carpal bone. (*B* courtesy of Dr. R. B. Olds.)

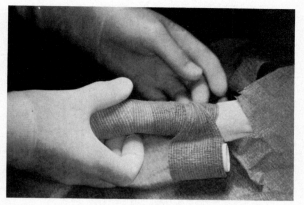

Figure 157–132. Vet Wrap* bandage applied to exsanguinate the forepaw prior to surgery.

and the overlying supportive joint capsule and fibrocartilage (Fig. 157–130*B*). Slocum and Devine[19] noted that all three categories of injury were more likely to occur in the large, heavy dog with a well-sloped manus. Gambardella and Griffiths[7] also reported a higher incidence in large breeds.

Gunshot, degloving, and shearing wounds are particularly devastating to the carpus owing to loss of soft tissue coverage, contamination of joints, and loss of collateral ligament support. Gunshot injuries pose additional problems because of poisoning of the cartilage cells from intra-articular lead, which results in chondrolysis, hypertrophic arthritis, and periarticular fibrosis.[16,17]

SURGICAL APPROACH TO THE CARPUS

Hair is clipped from the toes to just above the elbow and from a graft donor site such as the wing of the ilium or proximal humerus. The patient is placed on the table in sternal recumbency, and the leg is prepared and draped routinely. Because of the vascularity of the carpus and the dissection required to expose the joints, blood loss can be significant and may make exposure difficult. Exsanguination of the limb with a sterile Esmarch or Vet Wrap* tourniquet reduces blood loss and time spent with otherwise unnecessary hemostasis (Fig. 157–132). The Vet

*Vet Wrap, 3M Products, St. Paul, MN.

Wrap bandage may be wrapped on itself in a tight band at the elbow to provide a tourniquet and to reduce vascular return to the leg. Broad-based pressure cuff tourniquets can be left on for up to an hour without causing damage. Narrow Nye tourniquets, however, cause pressure necrosis and nerve damage directly under the tourniquet and are a poor second choice. The Vet Wrap is left in place to cover the toes and nails and is cut only where the incision is anticipated to be made.

The skin incision for the approach to the distal radius and antebrachiocarpal joint is made from the dorsal midline and extends from the junction of the cephalic and accessory cephalic veins to the middle of the carpus (Fig. 157–133). The accessory cephalic vein is retracted medially as the subcutaneous fascia is incised just lateral to the vein. Closure is facilitated if enough fascia is left lateral to the vein to permit suturing. The tendons of the extensor carpi radialis muscle and common digital extensor muscle are exposed, and the deep fascia is incised between the two. Over the radiocarpal joint, the joint capsule is incised at the same time as the deep fascia. The synovium must be incised separately over the other carpal joints following periosteal elevation of the deep fascia.[15]

The accessory carpal bone is approached laterally with an incision extending from the accessory carpal bone to the proximolateral end of metacarpal V. The abductor digiti quinti muscle and palmar transverse carpal ligament are identified (Fig. 157–134), and an incision is made along the cranial border of the muscle and through the ligament proximally. The muscle is dissected and retracted caudally, and the free end of the accessory carpal is exposed. The ligament must be sutured during closure.[15]

As an alternative, the carpus may be approached from a palmar direction. This approach is more difficult because of the increased number of nervous, vascular, and tendinous structures that must be dissected and elevated. The animal is placed in lateral recumbency with the affected leg down. The skin incision extends from the distal end of the radius on the medial side to midway between the base of the

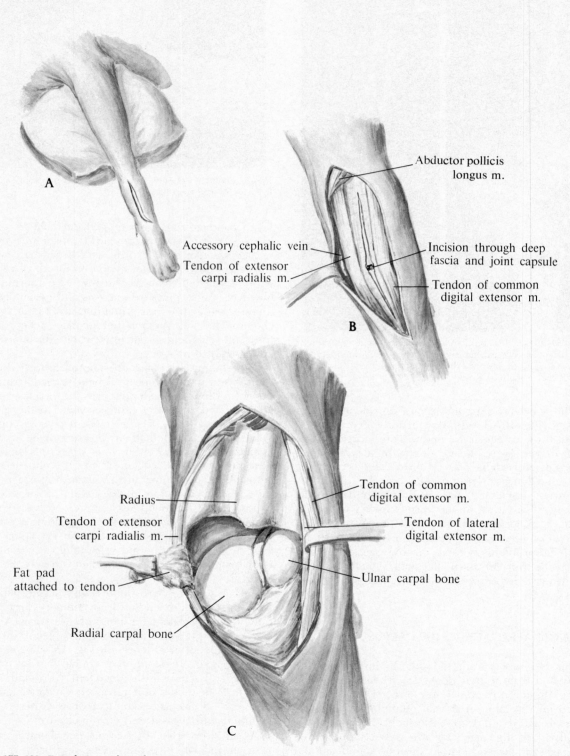

A

B

Abductor pollicis
longus m.

Accessory cephalic vein

Tendon of extensor
carpi radialis m.

Incision through deep
fascia and joint capsule

Tendon of common
digital extensor m.

Radius

Tendon of extensor
carpi radialis m.

Fat pad
attached to tendon

Radial carpal bone

Tendon of common
digital extensor m.

Tendon of lateral
digital extensor m.

Ulnar carpal bone

C

Figure 157–133. Dorsal approach to the carpus. (Reprinted with permission from Piermattei, D. L., and Greeley, R. G.: *An Atlas of Surgical Approaches to the Bones of the Dog and Cat.* W. B. Saunders, Philadelphia, 1979.)

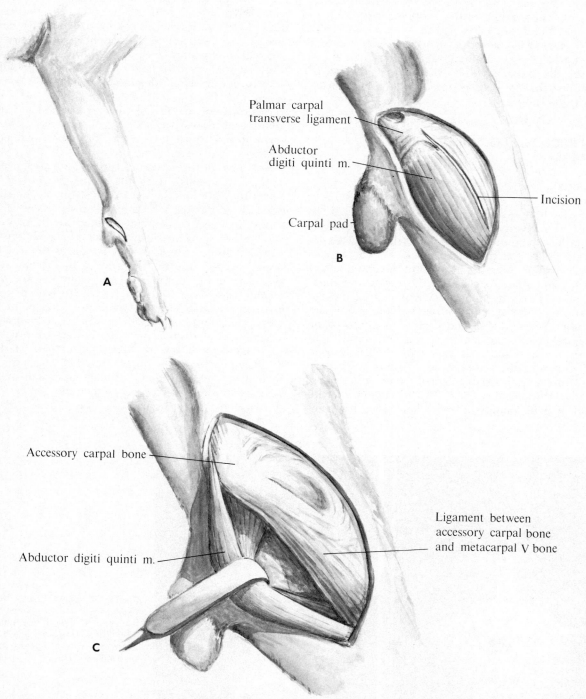

Figure 157–134. Approach to the accessory carpal bone. (Reprinted with permission from Piermattei, D. L., and Greeley, R. G.: *An Atlas of Surgical Approaches to the Bones of the Dog and Cat.* W. B. Saunders, Philadelphia, 1979.)

first digit and the carpal pad and along the medial side of the metacarpus. The cephalic vein is exposed and retracted medially. Deep sharp dissection is continued through the antebrachial fascia and periosteum on the radius and the transverse palmar carpal ligament. The tendons of the deep flexor to the first digit and the flexor carpi radialis muscle are transected. Aggressive periosteal elevation permits lateral retraction of the remaining flexor tendon bundle and exposes the articular surfaces. The primary use of this approach is for palmar surface plating for pancarpal arthrodesis.[2]

CONDITIONS OF THE CARPUS AND METACARPUS

Fractures

Because almost all fractures involving bones of the carpus also involve one or more joints, secondary osteoarthritis and degenerative joint disease are common sequelae and must be considered when treatment is chosen. Fractures involving the antebrachiocarpal joint either may be on the radial and ulnar side or may involve their respective carpal bones. Fractures of the articular surface of the radius are uncommon (see "Radius and Ulna"). Fractures of the ulnar styloid process may be seen with or without ligamentous instability. Repair is needed with instability or severe displacement (see "Radius and Ulna").

Fractures of the radial carpal bone occur infrequently. The dorsal surface is usually involved, with a slab of bone being sheared when abnormal compressive forces are applied through the carpus (Fig. 157–135B). Lameness may be severe acutely but partial weight-bearing may occur in more chronic cases. Displacement is usually minimal and diagnosis may be difficult. High-detail radiographs in oblique views often help with the diagnosis. In chronic cases, osteophytes and other signs of degenerative joint disease may be present. Treatment involves surgical removal of smaller pieces, stabilization with lag screws and K-wires for larger pieces (Fig. 157–135B), or arthrodesis when degenerative joint disease is severe.

Fractures involving the ulnar, intermediate, and first to fourth carpal bones are very rare. When encountered, most are in the form of small chip fractures, which should be removed.

Fractures of the accessory carpal bone are uncommon in all breeds except the racing greyhound, in which they are found almost exclusively on the right side. Three distinct fracture categories are possible. In the first, in the racing greyhound, small fractures may be found on the distal dorsal surface within the synovial lining. Swelling and lameness are usually severe. Early surgical removal of the fragment is necessary to prevent degenerative joint disease. The second category is midshaft transverse fractures not involving a joint surface, which are seen in racing greyhounds and occasionally secondary to trauma in large dogs. If displacement is minimal, coaptation splintage in a flexed position is effective. Marked displacement requires open reduction with pin and wire or lag screw fixation. Splintage in flexion should be used postoperatively to protect the repair. The third category is an avulsion of the palmar surface.

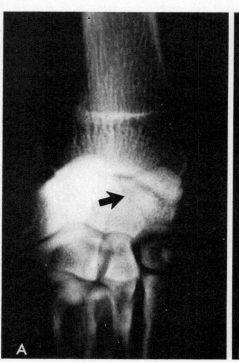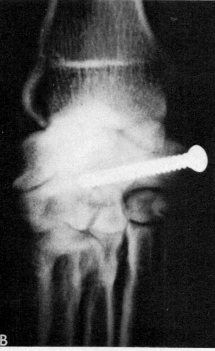

Figure 157–135. A, Fracture of the radial carpal bone in a racing greyhound. B, Fracture repair utilizing a cortical screw placed in lag fashion to compress the fracture (Courtesy of Dr. J. Dee.)

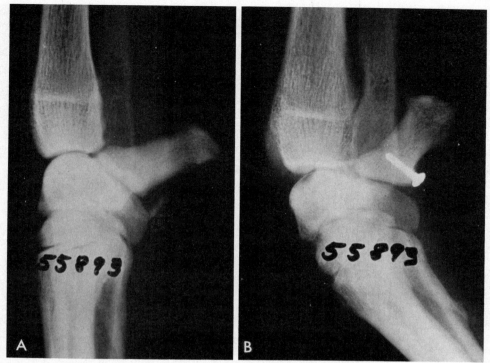

Figure 157–136. A, Avulsion fracture of the palmar surface of the accessory carpal bone. B, Fracture reduction and stabilization with a cortical screw placed in lag fashion. (Courtesy of Dr. D. Piermattei.)

Pain is marked on extension of the carpus. Surgical excision or stabilization is indicated, because splintage yields poor results in most cases (Fig. 157–136).

Fractures of metacarpal bones are seen more commonly than carpal bone fractures. Basilar fractures are seen most commonly in metacarpals II and V and can render the carpometacarpal joint unstable. The leg is carried at first, but some weight-bearing may occur in more chronic cases and may lead to progressive varus and valgus deformities. If displacement is minimal, external support by cast or coaptation splint may be adequate in cats and small dogs. Open reduction and repair with K-wires followed by a cast can be performed for large dogs or animals working heavily.

Midshaft metacarpal fractures may involve one or all metacarpal bones. If one of the primary weight-bearing metacarpals (III or IV) remains intact, a cast or splint is usually adequate. If all four are fractured, internal repair with intramedullary pins inserted normograde in metacarpals III and IV from the dorsal surface of the metacarpophalangeal joint and cerclage wire can be used for stabilization. The pins are inserted with the metacarpophalangeal joint flexed, the fractures are reduced, pins are seated in the bases of the metacarpal bones, and the distal ends of the pins are bent away from the joints and cut short. A flexional coaptation splint is used postoperatively to provide support. Finger plates may also be used in giant breeds.

Distal intra-articular fractures are difficult to repair but fortunately are only rarely encountered. Prognosis is guarded for full return to soundness if metacarpal III or IV is involved. Small chips should be excised. Arthrodesis or amputation of the digit may be performed for pain relief if degenerative joint disease occurs. External support is often satisfactory if only metacarpal II or V is involved.

Luxations

Ligament and joint capsule injuries result in partial or total luxations of the carpus. The most common injury is the result of application of hyperextension forces to the carpus, which causes medial and palmar surface tears. Total luxations are uncommon and usually are associated with severe skin and soft tissue injuries around the carpus (Fig. 157–137). The possibility of an open, contaminated joint should be considered. Arthrodesis may be required to regain function. If an open luxation of the carpus is seen within the first six to eight hours of injury, repair and stabilization may be undertaken early, and the chances of infection reduced.[3]

Hyperextension injuries most commonly affect the middle carpal and carpometacarpal joints.[7,14] Splinting may be attempted initially and is occasionally successful in smaller breeds. Flexional splintage of approximately 30 degrees apposes torn ligaments and fibrocartilage on the palmar surface. Splints should be maintained for at least ten weeks if they are used. Splintage is not successful in chronic cases and should be used only until internal stabilization is performed.

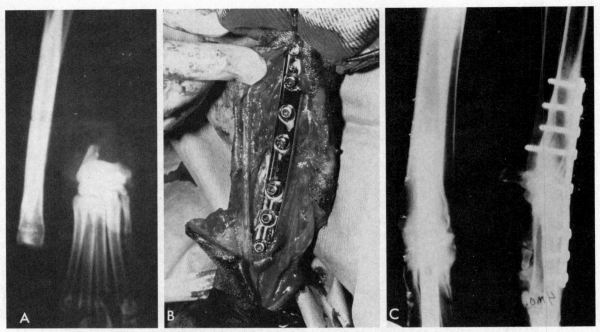

Figure 157–137. *A*, Total luxation of the radiocarpal joint with extensive soft tissue destruction in a dog that had been hit by a care. *B*, Following initial debridement, a pancarpal arthrodesis was performed. *C*, A four-month postoperative radiograph shows complete fusion of the carpus. Function in the leg was excellent.

Arthrodesis may still be performed if splintage fails. Dorsal ligament tears can usually be treated by straight splints if they are applied soon after injury. If degenerative joint disease is present with dorsal ligament injuries, arthrodesis can be used for pain relief.

When specific palmar ligament injuries can be identified, internal repair of affected ligaments combined with external splintage can have excellent results.[4] Repair may include autogenous tissue grafts, wire, or synthetic braided suture in place of torn ligaments or in combination with the suturing together of torn ligament ends. The flexor carpi radialis tendon can be used as an autogenous graft to repair either a torn short radial collateral ligament or palmar radial carpometacarpal ligaments (Fig. 157–138). The palmar accessory carpometacarpal ligaments can be repaired using either the ulnaris lateralis tendon or the caudal antebrachial fascia (Fig. 157–139). Combinations of screw and wire fixation can also be used to maintain normal position during healing (Fig. 157–140). External support for six weeks is needed with autogenous tissue repair and for approximately two to three weeks with wire reconstruction. With these repairs, normal motion is maintained in the joints.[4]

Many techniques have been described for the arthrodesis of the carpus, and results are generally good.[1,2,6,7,9,11,12,14,19] Most early joint fusions were of the panarthrodesis type in which all three joints were fused. Newer techniques have been described by which selective arthrodesis is performed.[7,11,14,19]

The basic principles of joint fusion, as previously described, must be rigidly followed. In one technique, a standard dorsal incision is used for the approach. All articular cartilage is removed from the joint surfaces using a high-speed drill, rongeur, or bone rasp. A corticocancellous bone graft from the wing of the ilium or proximal humerus is packed into the void left from burring the articular cartilage.

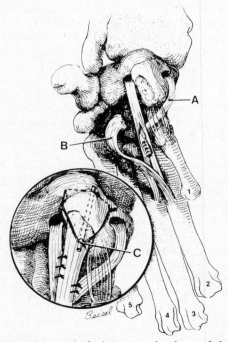

Figure 157–138. A method of repairing the short radial collateral ligament utilizing autogenous tissue. The flexor carpi radialis muscle tendon (*B*). Technique by Dr. T. Earley. (Reprinted with permission from Earley, T.: Canine carpal ligament injuries. Vet. Clin. North Am. 8:183, 1978.)

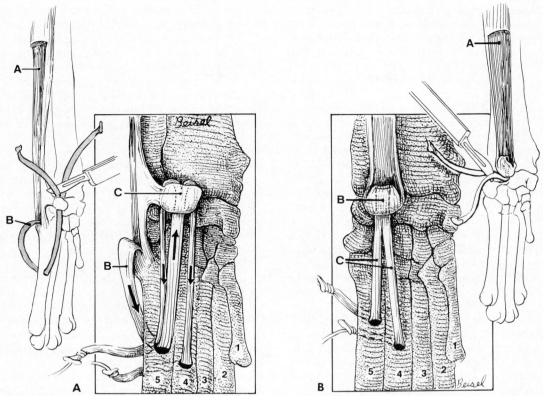

Figure 157–139. *A*, Repair of the palmar accessory carpometacarpal ligament using a one-half thickness of the ulnaris lateralis *(A)*. Accessory carpal bone *(C)*. Technique by Dr. T. Earley. *B*, Repair of the palmar accessory carpometacarpal ligament using a strip of the caudal antebrachial fascia *(A)*. Fascia is passed through holes in the metacarpals *(C)*. (Reprinted with permission from Earley, T.: Canine carpal ligament injuries. Vet. Clin. North Am. 8:183, 1978.)

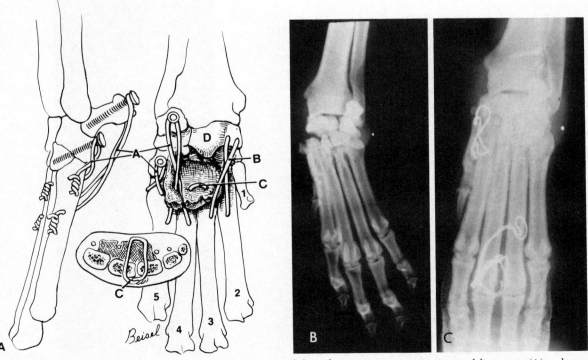

Figure 157–140. *A*, Multiple wire and screw repair for support of the palmar accessory carpometacarpal ligaments *(A)*, palmar radial carpometacarpal ligament *(B)*, and palmar carpal fibrocartilage *(C)*. Technique by Dr. T. Earley. *B*, Medial collateral ligament tear of the carpometacarpal and intercarpal joints. *C*, Repair utilizing wire reconstruction. (Courtesy of Dr. D. Piermattei.) (*A* reprinted with permission from Earley, T.: Canine carpal ligament injuries. Vet. Clin. North Am. 8:183, 1978.)

Rigid internal fixation is usually achieved with a straight bone plate. It is often advantageous to level the anterior cortex of the radius in order to enhance bone-plate seating and to contour the plate with five degrees of extension in order to promote improved placement of the toes without significant loss of bone length.[11,12] Screws are placed in the radius (three screws), radial carpal bone (one screw when possible), and third metacarpal bone (two to three screws) (see Fig. 157–137C). Care should be taken during removal of the articular surfaces not to remove so much bone as to prevent screw purchase into the smaller bones like the radial carpal bone. Compression should be achieved whenever possible. However, if rigid fixation is achieved with or without compression, successful arthrodesis can be expected. The subcutaneous tissues and skin are closed with simple interrupted sutures. Tissue closure over the plate may leave tension on the incision. In one series of 55 dogs with pancarpal arthrodesis, 97 per cent of the dogs had improved gaits, 75 per cent being totally normal.[12]

Panarthrodesis may also be performed with palmar surface plating.[2] Palmar surface plating is biomechanically superior to dorsal surface plating, because in the former, the plate is on the tension side of the bone. An implant failure rate of 33 per cent was reported in one series, and it was concluded that the inherent biomechanical weakness of dorsal surface plating was the most important factor in failure.[10] In palmar surface plating, screws are placed in the same bones as in dorsal surface plating. Other advantages of this technique are the improved coverage of the implant by the deep antebrachial and carpal fibrocartilage and fascia and the tensionless skin closure. The primary disadvantage is the increased time for exposure required by deep dissection.

Panarthrodesis can also be achieved with Steinmann pins that are driven normograde from just distal to the base of the metacarpal bones, cross through the radial carpal bone, and exit in the opposite cortex of the radius. This technique would generally be used for smaller breeds or when plating equipment is not available.[11]

An alternative means of panarthrodesis involves using perforating transfixation pins (Kirschner-Ehmer apparatus) placed proximally in the radius and distally in the metacarpals.[1,8,17] The limiting factor is the size of pin that can pass through the metacarpals. Usually a four-pin splint is used, with the first and fourth pins perforating both cortices and the opposite bar, and the second and third pins passing through both cortices but not connecting with the opposite bar. Pins can pass through only two of the metacarpals owing to the normal dorsal arch of the metacarpals relative to one another. The surgeon may choose to pass the pin through metacarpals II and V or III and IV. This technique is particularly useful for road injuries with extensive soft tissue involvement. Stabilization of the joint is achieved without placement of metallic implant in the affected area. Soft tissue management is facilitated, and the chance of subsequent osteomyelitis and draining tracts is reduced.

Hyperextension injuries to the middle carpal or carpometacarpal joints are indications for fusion of both joints. However, fusion of the radiocarpal joint can and should be avoided if that joint is not involved. Because partial carpal fusion permits close to normal flexibility in the carpus, many surgeons have advocated its use.[7,14,19] Several techniques are available and are reported to have good results. All utilize removal of joint cartilage and placement of autogenous cancellous bone. One technique involves the placement of small Steinmann pins driven normograde from metacarpals III and IV into the radial carpal bone. The pins originate either from slots drilled into the distal anterior cortex of metacarpals III and IV or from the distal end of the respective metacarpal bones just dorsal to the edge of the articular cartilage (Fig. 157–141). The pins are driven in Rush pin fashion while the joints are kept reduced in an extreme flexed position. The distal end of the pins are bent upward and turned toward the bone to prevent soft tissue and articular cartilage trauma.

Partial carpal arthrodesis may also be performed using a T plate contoured to fit on metacarpal III and the radial carpal bone. Usually, two screws can be placed in the radial carpal bone and two to three in metacarpal III. Care must be taken that the proximal end of the plate does not overlap the radiocarpal joint.

Fusion of the middle carpal and carpometacarpal

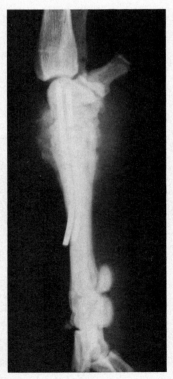

Figure 157–141. Repair of carpometacarpal instability (see Fig. 157–131A) with intramedullary pins inserted in dorsal slots in the metacarpal bones.

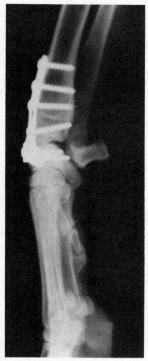

Figure 157–142. Repair of radiocarpal joint instability using a T plate.

joints can also be achieved without metallic implantation.[7] A cancellous graft is placed in and around the joints following removal of the joint cartilage. The leg is maintained in a cast or splint for three months or until healing is complete. The developers of this method report good success with large and small dogs and even have performed bilateral procedures simultaneously. They advocated grafting without internal fixation for only the middle carpal and carpometacarpal joints. However, other authors have reported successful fusion of the radiocarpal joint using wedge

grafts from the wing of the ilium without metallic implantation and with only external support.[6,9] It is obvious that the importance of grafting cannot be overemphasized.

The radiocarpal joint can also be fused alone using a small T plate for internal stabilization (Fig. 157–142).[11] Subsequent instability of the carpometacarpal joint has been reported following fusion of the radiocarpal joint alone in large dogs.[18]

Postoperative swelling is not uncommon. Lymphatic and venous drainage is often disrupted during dissection of soft tissues. Any interruption in the flow of the accessory cephalic vein significantly increases postoperative swelling. The leg should be maintained in a padded bandage supported by a spoon splint until swelling subsides and should then be in a cast for six to eight weeks or until radiographic healing is complete.

CONDITIONS OF THE PHALANGES

Fractures of the phalanges are relatively common but cause few problems. The third phalanx is only rarely fractured. Most fractures occur in the shaft of the first or second phalanx and are treated by external splintage. In large breeds, an articular surface fracture requires internal reduction with pins or small screws. Degenerative joint disease may still occur, necessitating amputation of the digit. The articular surface and condyles of the proximal bone should be removed by rongeur to reduce chances of continued lameness.

Occasionally, interphalangeal luxations are seen. Acute luxations may be reduced, and the joint capsule and ligaments may be sutured. Most chronic luxations require amputation, as described previously.

Osteomyelitis is commonly found in the third phalanx subsequent to some penetrating injury or paronychitis (Fig. 157–143). If antibiotic therapy fails, amputation may be performed for pain relief. The third and fourth phalanges are primary in weight-bearing function, but either one may be amputated even in large breeds with an excellent prognosis for full return to soundness.

SESAMOID FRACTURES

Sesamoid fractures are rarely seen and sometimes difficult to diagnose. It is often necessary to radiograph the opposite limb for comparison for a definitive diagnosis. Fractures of the second and seventh sesamoids are the most common. Chronic low-grade lameness is usually seen as a result of synovitis. Surgical excision is usually required for pain relief. An incision is made on the appropriate side of the central pad, the digital flexor tendons are retracted to the side, and the supporting suspensory ligament is incised to expose the sesamoid. Small fragments should be removed. Prognosis is good, even if the entire sesamoid is removed.

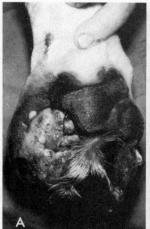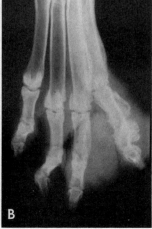

Figure 157–143. *A*, Infection in the digit started from a small penetrating wound. *B*, Bone reaction and infection involves both the second and third digits. Amputation of the second digit was performed.

1. Bjorling, D. E., and Toombs, J. P.: Transarticular application of the Kirschner-Ehmer splint. Vet. Surg. 1:34, 1982.
2. Chambers, J. N., and Bjorling, D. E.: Palmar surface plating for arthrodesis of the canine carpus. J. Am. Anim. Hosp. Assoc. 18:875, 1982.
3. Clawson, R. S., and McKay, D. W.: Arthrodesis in the presence of infection. Clin. Orthop. 114:209, 1976.
4. Earley, T.: Canine carpal ligament injuries. Vet. Clin. North Am. 8:183, 1978.
5. Evans, H. E., and Christensen, G. C.: *Miller's Anatomy of the Dog*. 2nd ed. W. B. Saunders, Philadelphia, 1979.
6. Frost, W. W., and Lumb, W. V.: Radiocarpal arthrodesis: a surgical approach to brachial paralysis. J. Am. Vet. Med. Assoc. 145:1073, 1966.
7. Gambardella, P. C., and Griffiths, R. C.: Treatment of hyperextension injuries of the canine carpus. Comp. Cont. Ed. 4:127, 1982.
8. Hurov, L.: Lateral deviation of the canine forepaw. Vet. Med./Small Anim. Clin. 131, 1963.
9. Hurov, L. I., Lumb, W. V., Hankes, G. H., and Smith, K. W.: Wedge grafting of the canine carpus. J. Am. Vet. Med. Assoc. 148:260, 1966.
10. Johnson, K. A.: Carpal arthrodesis in dogs. Aust. Vet. J. 56:565, 1980.
11. Moore, R. W., and Withrow, S. J.: Arthrodesis. Comp. Cont. Ed. 3:319, 1981.
12. Parker, R. B., Brown, S. G., and Wind, A. P.: Pancarpal arthrodesis in the dog: a review of 45 cases. Vet. Surg. 10:35, 1981.
13. Pedersen, N. C., and Pool, R.: Canine joint disease. Vet. Clin. North Am. 8:465, 1978.
14. Piermattei, D. L.: Arthrodesis of the middle carpal and carpometacarpal joint in the dog. *In: Proceedings*, Vet. Orth. Soc., 1981.
15. Piermattei, D. L., and Greeley, R. G.: *An Atlas of Surgical Approaches to the Bones of the Dog and Cat*. W. B. Saunders, Philadelphia, 1979.
16. Redano, V. T., and Abdinoor, D.: Management of intra- and extra-articular extremity gunshot wounds. J. Am. Anim. Hosp. Assoc. 13:577, 1977.
17. Renegar, W. R., and Stoll, S. G.: Gunshot wounds involving the canine carpus: surgical management. J. Am. Anim. Hosp. Assoc. 16:233, 1980.
18. Sexton, R. L., and Hurov, L. I.: Repair of carpometacarpal instability after radiocarpal arthrodesis in the dog. J. Am. Vet. Med. Assoc. 172:1186, 1978.
19. Slocum, B., and Devine, T.: Partial carpal fusion in the dog. J. Am. Vet. Med. Assoc. 180:1204, 1982.

Chapter **158**

Pelvic Fractures

C. W. Betts

Fractures of the pelvis result from trauma but differ considerably in the degree of osseous and soft tissue damage. Rarely, a pathological fracture may occur secondarily to a bone tumor of the pelvis. The majority of fractures occur from vehicular injuries, and many dogs sustain significant damage to other areas as well. Other causes of pelvic fracture include dog fights, gunshot wounds, and blunt trauma. Approximately 25 per cent of all fractures that occur involve the pelvis.[2] The majority of pelvic fractures are multiple because of the boxlike configuration of the pelvis and the short, strong musculotendinous support of the osseous structures. In a review of 299 dogs with a fractured pelvis, ilial fractures instituted 18.2 per cent of the total number of fractures; pelvic fractures, 28.2 per cent; acetabular fractures, 14.6 per cent; ischial fractures, 23.1 per cent; and sacroiliac dislocations, 15.9 per cent.[40] Because of the tendency toward multiple fractures and the degree of trauma necessary to fracture the pelvis or cause a fracture-dislocation, adjacent soft tissue and surrounding organ systems must be carefully evaluated.

In human pelvic fractures, unrelenting extraperitoneal hemorrhage is the primary cause of death and is second only to skull fracture as the most common fatal injury to bone.[10] Pelvic fracture–related iliac or femoral vessel disruption has been associated with a mortality rate as high as 75 per cent.[28] Postmortem dissection and injection studies of hypogastric arteries following fatal pelvic fractures in humans have demonstrated that multiple lacerations of small and medium-sized arteries and veins occur, giving rise to persistent hemorrhage.[15] Because of multiple injured vessels and the rich arterial collateralization of the pelvic retroperitoneum, standard methods of hemostasis are difficult to achieve and often ineffective.[10, 24, 27, 28, 36] In addition to hemorrage from intrapelvic vessels, rupture of the urinary bladder and avulsion of the membranous urethra in males are of significant concern.[9, 36] In one study, genitourinary injuries occurred in 30.5 per cent of 282 people with pelvic fractures.[38] Injury to the genitourinary organs should be suspected in a patient with pelvic fracture if the patient has hematuria, is unable to void, or has a bloody urethral discharge. Injury to the urinary bladder may occur by perforation or by sudden compression, which may result in rupture because of a rapid rise in intravesicular pressure.[38] Rupture of the urethra is more common in male dogs than in female dogs.[40] Spontaneous, pressure-elicited micturition occurs more readily in the female because of the short, wide pelvic urethra, in contrast to the longer, more narrow penile urethra of the male. Ureteral avulsion and urinary bladder rupture occur with about equal frequency in males and females.[29a]

Open fractures of the pelvis in humans are associated with a high mortality rate.[24] The presence of a laceration in proximity to a pelvic fracture is indicative of an open fracture despite the fact that the laceration may not always provide direct acesss to the fracture site. Lacerations in the perineum and perianal area also indicate an open fracture and

Acknowledgment: Felicia J. Paras, B. S., A. M. I., North Carolina State University; Professor Dr. Ultitze Matis, Chirurgie Univesity Tierklinik.

probable fecal contamination of the fracture hematoma.[19] Infection in the retroperitoneal hematoma resulting in subsequent septicemia is the most common cause of late death following pelvic fracture in humans.[10]

In addition to direct injury or perforation, the compressive force transmitted to the pelvic viscera may cause injuries of the urinary bladder, perineal urethra, rectum, lumbosacral nerve roots, and hypogastric vessels. The rectal wall is less susceptible to rupture or tearing than the perineal skin from compression forces, but when it occurs the tear frequently is just inside the anus, where the rectum is fixed and less distensible.[1] The rectum may also be injured by compression against the sacral promontory and by perforation of intruding bony edges. Sensory and motor functions in the extremity may be lost either by lumbosacral nerve root avulsions or by sciatic nerve injury from acetabular fracture.[32] Sciatic nerve injury was recorded in two of 45 dogs with pelvic fracture.[21] Severe pelvic trauma instigates one to check for adjacent soft tissue damage, but it also portends possible multiple organ injury. Traumatic rupture of the diaphragm, spleen, or liver as well as severe contusion of the kidneys is seen with pelvic injuries. Because of the tremendous transfer of kinetic energy with a deceleration injury from impact trauma, major injury to other organ systems and body structures is common. In a study of 604 patients with pelvic fractures, an average index of 3.1 concomitant injuries were sustained by the 71 patients that died, compared with an average of 1.0 for the survivors.[27]

Although the history is usually straightforward, it is important to inquire whether the dog had urinated shortly before being hit. Perforation or laceration is still a concern, but rupture from vesicle pressure changes is unlikely. If the dog did not urinate before the accident, or the owner is unsure of the circumstances, one should ask whether the dog has urinated since the injury. The ability to urinate does not preclude bladder or urethral damage, but the voiding of a normal amount of clear urine is not compatible with serious injury to the urinary tract.

Dogs often support their weight and even walk despite a major pelvic fracture, especially if it is bilateral. With unilateral fractures, the hind limb on the affected side may be carried. The owner should be asked whether the dog has been able to support weight on all four limbs, or just three, or has refused to stand. By the time the dog is brought to the veterinarian, it may be reluctant to support weight because of musculoskeletal pain, so an accurate history is important. If immediate soft tissue repair is needed, one should ascertain when the dog has eaten last, to minimize complications with anesthesia.

PHYSICAL EXAMINATION

Patients that have sustained trauma of sufficient magnitude to fracture the bones of the pelvic girdle are exposed to a high risk of associated injuries.[6, 38] The necessity of performing a thorough physical examination cannot be overemphasized. In 26 patients in whom pelvic fracture was the primary cause of death, 93 per cent were in shock or had clinical evidence of hypovolemia at the time of admission; 18 patients (69 per cent) exsanguinated from their pelvic fractures shortly after hospital admission (mean, nine hours).[27]

An immediate assessment of vital signs must be done when the dog is brought in within minutes or a few hours of injury. This matter is of more concern for the practitioner than for the referral institution, because the majority of animals have been stabilized by the time of referral. Unless the dog is in imminent danger of dying, a systematic physical examination starting at the head should be done. The color of the mucous membranes and capillary refill time should be noted. The eyes and cranial nerves should be evaluated for signs of cranial trauma. Nystagmus and anisocoria are readily detected, and Horner's syndrome may be present in the event that low cervical trauma has occurred. The mandible and maxilla should be palpated for fractures and the oral cavity checked for lacerations, hard or soft palate injury, fractured teeth, and the malocclusion seen with temporomandibular luxations. The cervical spine should be carefully palpated and manipulated. The heart and lungs are auscultated for any evidence of diaphragmatic hernia, pneumothorax, or pulmonary contusion. The strength and character of the femoral pulse should be evaluated simultaneously with auscultation of the heart, to evaluate blood pressure subjectively and to rule out a pulse deficit that could indicate traumatic myocarditis. The front limbs are checked for evidence of long bone fracture or joint luxations. The rib cage and thoracolumbar spine are palpated for fractures or displacement. One should gently palpate the abdomen to assess for evidence of a urine-filled bladder, but the bladder should not be compressed, because contusion or small tears may be present. One should determine whether pain or tenderness is elicited by palpation of the kidneys and sublumbar area; pain may be elicited with renal or ureteral trauma and bruising of or hemorrhage into the sublumbar muscles and retroperitoneal space. The abdomen is carefully ballotted for evidence of fluid accumulation. Prior to palpation of the pelvis, the hindlimbs are carefully checked for fractures or joint luxations. The downside limb should be checked again when the dog is turned. The stifle should always be assessed for drawer motion, collateral stability, and traumatic patella luxation. The patellar reflex, withdrawal reflex, and reflex, and pain sensation should always be evaluated and the response documented.

Extensive palpation and manipulation of the pelvis are not necessary, because diagnostic radiographs will be taken. Pelvic asymmetry can be determined by comparative palpation of the iliac crests, greater trochanters, and ischial tuberosities. The relative positions of these three bony prominences to one another in the os coxae may also provide diagnostic information. These prominences normally form a shallow √ with the long arm of the √ between the iliac crest and the greater trochanter and the short arm between the greater trochanter and the ischial tuberosity. A greater trochanter which is difficult-to-palpate that seems medially displaced, with crepitus, decreased rotation, and pain elicited by manipulation, indicates an impacted acetabular fracture. Dorsal and cranial displacement of the greater trochanter would be associated with a coexisting craniodorsal hip luxation, whereas dorsal displacement alone is more compatible with a tentative diagnosis of a femoral neck fracture, capital physeal separation, or combination of femoral head or neck fracture and avulsion of the greater trochanter. Cranial displacement of the iliac crest occurs with sacroiliac separations and sacral fractures. Instability of the sacroiliac joint(s) can often be detected by applying medial and caudal pressure. A fracture of the iliac shaft with cranial displacement of the caudal segment shortens the distance between the iliac crest and the greater trochanter. An isolated ischial fracture may shorten the distance between the ischial tuberosity and the greater trochanter and may facilitate hyperextension of the stifle by effectively lengthening the hamstrings, but withdrawal may be impaired. The upper limb is carefully elevated, and the groin area is inspected for lacerations and bruising. Severe bruising and inability to palpate the ventral abdominal wall occur with rupture of the prepubic tendon or avulsion fracture of the pubis. These patients should be checked carefully for inguinal and femoral ring hernias.

Lastly, a rectal examination is gently done. If this procedure is unusually painful for the animal, a sacral or coccygeal fracture should be suspected. Blood on the examining gloved finger is presumptive evidence of rectal injury. During rectal palpation of the male dog, the prostate should be sought; if it is not palpable, a tear in the pelvic urethra may be assumed.[19] If perineal lacerations are present, they should be closely inspected but not deeply probed for fear of stimulating recurrence of bleeding.

If there is evidence of genitourinary damage, the injury is confirmed by radiography. A retrograde urethrogram is done prior to catheterization of the bladder. If the urethra is lacerated or separated, catheterization may introduce infection into the pelvic hematoma, may add to the trauma of the injured urethra, and may fail to reveal an incomplete urethral injury. If the urethra is intact, a cystogram is done, including a post-evacuation film. Intravenous pyelography is used to evaluate the upper urinary tracts.[38] If the urinary system is intact but there is blood in the urine, a urinalysis is indicated.

Once the general examination is over, the animal should be carefully raised to a standing position. The majority of the weight on the rear limbs should be borne by the examiner. Conscious proprioception should be evaluated, but musculoskeletal pain may render the test useless. The single most important criterion is the presence of pain sensation in the distal extremity, acknowledged by cerebral recognition. Femoral and sciatic responses should be checked. The absence of sensation in the lateral digits indicates sciatic injury from nerve root avulsion, sacroiliac luxation, acetabular fracture, or a proximal third femoral fracture. Anesthesia of the medial digit and inability to lock the stifle in extension are evidence of a femoral nerve injury and possibly a lower lumbar fracture.

A complete data base is obtained for any dog that has sustained major pelvic fractures. Documented death from hemorrhage is seldom seen in dogs with pelvic fractures at referral institutions. It is doubtful that such dogs are referred, and dogs that die of trauma seldom undergo necropsy. However, pelvic fracture patients that require abdominal exploration for associated injuries usually have evidence of extensive sublumbar extravasation and retroperitoneal hemorrhage with occasional free blood in the abdominal cavity. A complete blood count is done to establish a baseline for therapy and monitoring. Serum chemistry measurements are needed to assess and monitor major organ injury and response; and levels of electrolytes, especially potassium, are measured because of often massive amount of muscle bruising and possible renal damage. If there is leakage of urine into the abdominal cavity, renal function is reduce in proportion to the amount of urine reabsorbed.[38]

A frequently overlooked, easily monitered parameter is urine production. In addition to measurement of renal output in severe trauma cases, serial urinalyses may be beneficial. Specific gravity, protein level, and presence or absence of blood often provide critical information.

Radiographic examination should be performed after a thorough history has been obtained, a physical examination has been done, and the laboratory samples for the data base have been taken. Most dogs experience minimal discomfort when radiographed in lateral recumbency. It may be necessary to permit the dog to lie on its back with the hips and stifles flexed and the limbs abducted in a frogleg position in order to obtain a ventrodorsal view. If necessary, a lateral decubital view with a horizontal beam can be used to assess the upper hemipelvis. Thoracic and abdominal radiographs are taken at this time if the need is justified. If the dog is in severe pain and difficult to position, it is better to wait until the dog has been stabilized and can be sedated or anesthetized to take diagnostic radiographs.

ASSESSMENT

Pelvic fractures are treated so as to decrease both the morbidity associated with multiple injuries and the length of hospitalization. The choice of surgical intervention or conservative therapy is based on experience and radiographic interpretation. Surgical repair is considered when (1) there is a marked decrease in the diameter of the pelvic canal, (2) displacing fractures involve the acetabulum, (3) a series of fractures result in instablity of the hip joint, and (4) there is marked displacement of the bone fragments.[4]

A useful classification scheme is employed in human pelvic fractures. A type I fracture is comminuted and involves three or more of the six major pelvic components (rami/ischium, symphysis, ilium, acetabulum, sacrum, sacroiliac joints); these unstable fractures are associated with extensive blood loss and soft tissue injury. Type II fractures include diametric fractures (Malgaigne or segmental), acetabular fractures, and "open book" fractues, which involve the pubic symphysis and at least one caudal element (sacroiliac joints, body or ala of the sacrum); all type II fractures are unstable. Type III fractures are stable and are associated with less soft tissue injury and mortality.[24, 36] Type I and type II fractures in the veterinary patient require surgical intervention, because traction is not feasible. Type III fractures in humans and dogs respond well to a conservative approach.

One must keep postural influence on muscle pull and bony displacement in mind when assessing radiographs taken soon after trauma, particularly if the dog is anesthetized. Encroachment on the pelvic canal by a segmental fracture of the ilium and ischium is much more pronounced when the limbs are abducted for the ventrodorsal view. When evaluating the lateral view of an acetabular fracture, one should consider that films taken with the involved hip flexed show a wider fracture gap and more ventral displacement of the ischial tuberosity than films taken with the hip in a neutral or extended position. Radiographs of acetabular fractures that are difficult to interpret can be enhanced by linear tomography.

TREATMENT PLAN

Conservative Therapy

A conservative course of action is taken for animals with little or no displacement of the fracture segments, an intact acetabulum, and essentially intact continuity of the pelvic ring.[3] The sturdy pelvic girdle provides an effective muscular sling for minimally displaced fractures. The abundant soft tissue cover also assures adequate blood supply. Conservatively treated pelvic fractures almost always heal. Unfortunately, the majority of pelvic fractures are treated conservatively because of the tired old axiom that "the fractures will heal and your dog will be a functional pet." If one critically assesses these dogs months and years after injury, many are not functioning as well as expected. The fractures have healed, but dogs with segmental fractures now have obstipation and, less frequently, dysuria. If pelvic encroachment becomes established, breeding females may experience dystocia or may need cesarean section. Dogs with cranially displaced ilial shaft fractures or sacroiliac luxations may have a noticeable gait abnormality that is unacceptable for a performance animal. The dogs that had significantly displaced acetabular fractures, especially with an impacted femoral head, frequently developed severe coxofemoral osteoarthritis. When such dogs are subjected to a femoral head and neck excision for the impaction fracture, the results are usually disastrous, with virtual fusion resulting. However, patients correctly selected for conservative management do well.

A successful conservative regimen consists of confinement, comfortable quarters, restricted and supervised exercise, and attention to hydration, alimentation, urination, and defecation. A padded area with easy access to water and food should be provided. Because of musculoskeletal pain from the fracture, the dog lies continuously on its good side and may develop decubital ulcers. Hydrotherapy is beneficial to relieve the aches and pains from bruised muscles and healing areas. It is also important to keep the dog clean.

A simple rehabilitation program should be initiated to keep the owner involved in the pet's care and aware of its progress. Warm compresses, flexion and extension exercises, and early, assisted ambulation decrease the convalescent period.

Some simple supportive measures can be taken to reduce motion at the fracture site and the chances of additional trauma. The easiest to provide is firm footing to prevent slipping and abduction injuries. A simple tape hobble around the hocks restricts mobility and prevents severe abduction:adduction positions independent of the opposite limb. A bandage roll can be taped between the stifles and the hocks hobbled in slight adduction to maintain lateral leverage on fractures that displace medially. Animals bound in this fashion need close supervision and nursing care. Because daily digital levering of medially displaced segments is ineffectual, painful for the animal, and potentially dangerous (iatrogenic rectal laceration), it is not recommended.

The animal with a minimally displaced unilateral acetabular fracture with an intact contralateral hemipelvis is a candidate for a non–weight-bearing sling. A figure-of-eight (Ehmer) sling is not necessary, because a neutral position of the hip is preferred. Also, the Ehmer sling must be put on very carefully, because pressure sores are not uncommon over the cranial aspect of the thigh and the caudal metatarsus owing to the amount of tension necessary to internally rotate the hip. The sling is maintained for 10 to 14 days, the toes are checked carefully for swelling during this time, and the dog is gradually returned to normal activity over two to three weeks.

Because of soft tissue injuries, renal function should be monitored and assisted if necessary. Water intake may be limited because of reluctance to move around, and urination may be difficult because of inability to posture and because of house training habits.

For the same reasons, constipation may develop, necessitating enemas, laxatives, or suppositories.

Surgical Therapy

The criteria generally accepted for prompt surgical intervention are, as previously mentioned under "Assessment": (1) marked decrease in the size of the pelvic canal; (2) fracture of the acetabulum (displacement of articular surfaces) (see Fig. 158–10); (3) instability of the hip (fracture of the ilium, ischium, and pubis on the same side; segmental or Malgaigne fracture); and (4) unilateral or bilateral instability, particularly if accompanied by coxofemoral dislocation or other limb fractures) (see Fig. 158–3).[4]

Early operative management of pelvic fractures in dogs was performed with intramedullary pins, wire sutures, and the Kirschner fixation splint.[7, 18] External fixators are gaining new popularity for treatment of pelvic fractures in humans.[20, 34] Until recently, most human pelvic fractures were treated by pelvic slings, bed rest, skeletal traction, or internal fixation. The prolonged hospitalization required led to pulmonary and urological problems, with long-term complications from residual pelvic deformity, leg length discrepancy, and sacroiliac pain. Open reduction with internal fixation was associated with major bleeding and limited success even in the hands of experienced surgeons. The combination of external fixators, primarily the Hoffman apparatus, and the Swiss system of internal fixation has markedly improved the results of pelvic surgery in humans.[34, 35]

Fortunately, the pelvic anatomy of the dog is more suitable for application of plates and screws. The external fixators, excluding the Kirschner device, are cost-prohibitive for veterinary surgery. Pin and wire fixation does work, often well, but the highest percentage of success comes from the use of bone plates and screws.[4, 8]

The priorities necessary for the successful management of traumatized patients is described by the A to F scheme: A, airway management; B, blood and fluid replacement; C, central nervous system management; D, digestive or gastrointestinal management; E, excretory or genitourinary management; and F, fracture management. Early fracture management is encouraged. Concomitant pelvic stabilization may reduce damage to the lumbosacral plexus, reduce venous bleeding, and prevent further genitourinary trauma.[34] Because of the extent of soft tissue injury pre-existing in animals with multiple fractures, surgical and anesthetic risks are increased. It is incumbent on the surgeon to select the area for initial repair that will provide the most benefit to the patient if further surgery must be delayed. Surgical repair should be attempted as soon as feasible for the condition of the animal, preferably within four days of injury.[4] Each additional day considerably increases the effort and iatrogenic trauma necessary for repair.

After eight or nine days, reduction of major ilial shaft fractures in large dogs is almost impossible. Postoperative morbidity is higher in trauma patients also, and every effort should be made to decrease length of hospitalization.

Ilial Fractures

Ilial fractures are one of the more commonly encountered pelvic fractures. The basic tenets of internal fixation apply, namely, anatomical reduction, stable fixation, and early return to function. The majority are oblique ilial shaft fractures with retention of the sacroiliac joint by the cranial segment. Occasionally, the cranial and ventral aspect of the cranial segment is also fractured, with ventral displacement from the pull of the sartorius and tensor fascia muscles. The caudal segment encompasses the acetabulum. If there is an accompanying fracture of the pubis and ischium, the fracture is classified as a segmental or Malgaigne fracture. Because these fractures often result from car accidents, the shearing force generated in a cranial direction may result in extreme cranial displacement of the caudal segment. Such fractures are very difficult to reduce after four to five days, especially if injuries are bilateral. The caudal segment more commonly is depressed medially, increasing the likelihood of sciatic or sacral nerve injury. Also, if the fracture is not repaired, the resulting callus further compromises the size of the pelvic canal. Because the free segment includes the coxofemoral joint, motion will occur at the fracture site with weight-bearing, which prolongs post-trauma pain, delays healing, and stimulates callus formation.

If surgery is ill-advised because of associated multiorgan injury or is not a feasible economic alternative, conservative measures can be taken. Confinement to a small area is essential. Food and water should be readily accessible, and a padded area should be provided for the animal to rest on. If there are concomitant adductor muscle and pubic symphysis injuries, a simple tape hobble will prevent further abduction injury. Segmental fractures with medial displacement may be gently manipulated and somewhat reduced per rectum with the animal under general or epidural anesthesia.[30] The reduction can be maintained to an acceptable degree by placing a roll of cotton or foam rubber proximally between the thighs and taping the stifles together to provide leverage against the roll, providing a fulcrum effect. This support is maintained for eight to ten days to assure early collagen deposition and some strength to the initial fibrous tissue support. An animal supported in this manner needs frequent nursing care, which usually requires hospitalization or a conscientious, capable owner. Urine and fecal soilage and pressure sores are the main problems. Metabolism cages or expanded metal racks facilitate keeping the animal clean. If possible, sling support should be provided twice a day for extended periods. Because of established behavior habits, many dogs are reluctant to void inside. This reluctance is further complicated by inability to stand. Daily monitoring of urination and defecation should be done and appropriate assistance provided when necessary. Activity should be restricted and supervised for three weeks more after the roll is removed. Tape hobbles should be used for one or two weeks after the roll is removed in dogs with segmental fractures.

With long oblique fractures of the ilial shaft, satisfactory results can be obtained by pinning from dorsal to ventral at right angles to the fracture site. Large pins cannot be used because of the concavity of the cranial half of the ilium and the narrow lateral-to-medial medullary cavity. For more transverse ilial shaft fractures, a leverage pinning technique can be used by starting the pins on the medial aspect of the iliac crest, placing them antegrade to the level of the acetabulum without invading the joint. The sacroiliac joint provides a stable fulcrum against which to lever the caudal segment to prevent medial displacement. Placing intramedullary pins is facilitated by a power drill and insertion of the pin in a prestressed manner. Bowing the pin with slight leverage against the drill allows the point of the pin to follow the bow, and a straight pin can be made to follow the curvature of the bone (Fig. 158–1). Two to three pins should be used to provide additional stability against bending forces with transverse ilial shaft fractures (Fig. 158–2) and to counteract the shearing forces that predominate with oblique fractures.

The prevailing preference among veterinary orthopedic surgeons is bone plate and screw fixation for iliac fractures.[4, 5, 8, 26, 33] Occasionally, long oblique fractures in large dogs can be rigidly fixed with two lag screws, but plate application is usually necessary (Fig. 158–3). One lag screw is insufficient unless

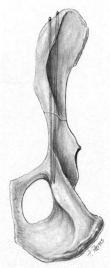

Figure 158–2. Leverage pinning has been used to repair a relatively transverse ilial shaft fracture.

combined with plate fixation. The latter provides maximum stability (Fig. 158–4).

The lateral approach to the ilium is recommended over the dorsal approach (Fig 158–5). It provides access through muscle separation and subperiosteal elevation rather than transection of muscle.[4, 5, 14, 22] The incision extends from the iliac crest to the greater trochanter at the level of the dorsal neck of the femur. Once the subcutaneous tissue and superficial fascia latae muscles are exposed, careful dissection is necessary to separate the aponeurotic junction between the two muscles while retracting the middle gluteal muscle dorsally. The aponeurosis is followed along the ventral margin of the ilium and then dorsally along the cranial margin of the iliac crest between the middle gluteal and sartorius muscles. If necessary, the middle gluteal muscle can be entirely elevated from all but the dorsum of the ilium. The deep gluteal muscle is elevated as necessary from the caudal segment. Once adequate exposure is achieved, reduction requires a combination of levering, traction, and rotation.[4] Kern or Lewin bone-holding forceps or a large towel clamp applied to the crest of the ilium provides a handle for cranial traction. Lewin or Vulsellum bone holding forceps are applied to the greater trochanter, great care being taken to avoid the sciatic nerve (Fig. 158–6), to aid in caudal retraction of the acetabular component of segmental fractures. An intramedullary pin can also be placed normograde into the femur and the affixed Jacobs chuck used for a handle on the caudal segment. When the ischial component is continuous with the acetabulum, caudal retraction is gained by securing a grasp on the ischial tuberosity with Lewin or Kern forceps. A Steinmann pin placed in a ventral-to-dorsal plane can also be used as a point of purchase for caudal traction on the ischium. Simultaneous elevation and leverage are utilized with traction to gain reduction. Self-retaining retractors (Gelpis,

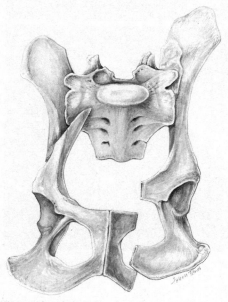

Figure 158–1. The ilial and ischial fractures have resulted in instability of the hip joint. The opposite hemipelvis is unstable because of the cranial sacroiliac displacement.

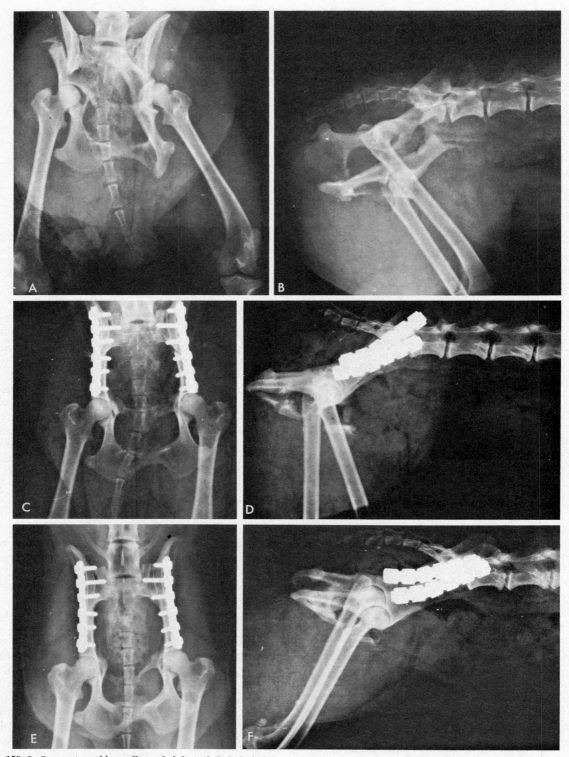

Figure 158–3. Seven-year-old poodle with bilateral ilial shaft fractures. This case demonstrates the versatility of ASIF reconstruction plates. *A* and *B*, Preoperative ventrodorsal and lateral views. *C* and *D*, Postoperative ventrodorsal and lateral views. *E* and *F*, Ventrodorsal and lateral views taken ten months after operation. (Courtesy of Dr. Ulrike Matis.)

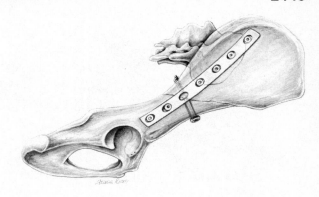

Figure 158–4. An oblique ilial shaft fracture has been maximally stabilized with an interfragmentary lag screw and a dynamic compression plate.

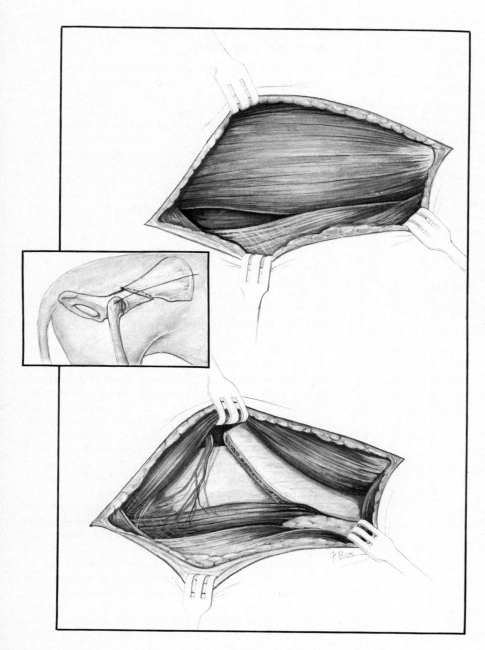

Figure 158–5. The lateral approach using a gluteal roll-up method is advocated for ilial shaft fractures.

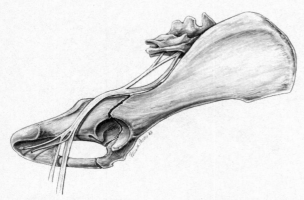

Figure 158–6. The sciatic nerve courses just caudal to the acetabulum.

Weitlaner, pediatric Beckman's) are beneficial to aid in freeing the surgeon's and assistant's hands while maintaining adequate exposure. Once reduction is achieved in long oblique fractures, application of self-retaining forceps (Kern, Speed-lock, Verbrugge) from dorsal to ventral across the segments will maintain reduction during plate application. An awareness of the proximity of the sciatic nerve to the medial aspect of the body of the ilium during placement of bone clamps is essential (see Fig. 158–6).

The use of the dynamic compression plating system is recommended for maximum stability. The plate should be contoured in excess of the normal concavity of the ilium to assure as wide a pelvic canal as possible. Anatomic reduction is desirable, but stable fixation and restoration of the normal pelvic canal diameter are higher priorities. The plate is affixed to the caudal segment first to enable the surgeon to take advantage of the stable cranial segment for levering the caudal segment laterally (Fig. 158–7). If

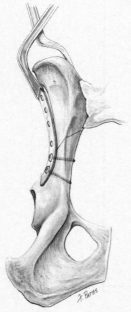

Figure 158–7. The plate is secured first to the caudal segment, then to the cranial segment.

the plate is secured to the cranial segment first, the caudal segment has to be help up to the overcontoured plate; this maneuver is difficult because it is the mobile segment. Finger plates and 2.7-mm and 3.5-mm dynamic compression plates are routinely used, depending on the size of the animal.

Closure is routine, and postoperative care is minimal. A non–weight-bearing sling is not necessary. Standard wound management is followed, and exercise is limited and supervised for three to four weeks after operation, after which normal exercise is gradually resumed. Follow-up radiographs are taken four to six weeks after operation to evaluate fracture healing.

Acetabular Fractures

Few acetabular fractures can be handled satisfactorily by conservative methods. Minimally displaced fractures, especially of the caudal third of the dome, can be managed by confining the dog for three or four weeks. Preferably, a moderate non–weight-bearing sling should be used in conjunction with the confinement to minimize motion at the fracture site. The sling should maintain the hip joint in a neutral position, and no attempt should be made to internally rotate or flex the hip as with the Ehmer sling. The sling is maintained for ten to 14 days to ensure early healing of soft tissue and initial callus. The sling is removed, physical therapy is initiated, and supervised activity is started. The owner should be advised that some degree of coxarthrosis will develop.

Open reduction is indicated for acetabular fractures of the cranial and middle thirds of the articular surface. The majority of weight-bearing occurs on the cranial two-thirds of the acetabulum. Fractures of the caudal third of the acetabulum are seldom repaired unless the caudal segment is a significant component of the overall pelvic injury.

Open reduction and fixation of acetabular fractures is one of the true orthopedic challenges. An understanding of the "personality" of the fracture will aid in deciding whether open repair should be attempted. The personality of the patient, the personality of the health care team, and the personality of the fracture are intertwined and directly affect the operative decision. The personality of the patient includes age, general medical condition, associated injuries, activity level, and the future performance expectations of the owner. The personality of the health care team is determined by the ability and experience of the surgeon, adequate facilities and instrumentation, an understanding of plating principles, and the ability to manage the trauma patient in a prioritized manner. The factors that influence the prognosis determine the personality of the fracture. The prognosis depends on the type of fracture, the amount of damage to the weight-bearing surface, the degree of persistent displacement or incongruity of the articular surface, and the presence or absence of other pelvic fractures.[35] Whenever dislocation or instability of the fracture segments is present, surgical repair is advised to decrease the severity and extent of the predictable osteoarthritis that will inevitably develop. Crepitus is usually felt when the hip is manipulated.[4] Regardless of the plan, the priority sequence should always be: the patient first, the limb second, and the fracture third. With concomitant limb injury, more important fractures may preempt definitive repair of the acetabular fracture. An attempt should always be made to first repair the fracture that will afford the patient the most benefit.

Acetabular fractures have been classified into four groups according to the course of the transacetabular fracture line.[16, 17] The majority of fractures fit into one of the following four groups: cranial, central, caudal, and comminuted (Fig. 158–8). Central transacetabular fractures occur most commonly with comminuted transacetabular second in frequency.[17] Tomograms are helpful in determining articular surface involvement of comminuted fractures and aid the surgeon in determining the feasibility of operative repair.

The principles and goals of articular surgery are: anatomic reduction of the articular surfaces, rigid reduction, and early return to full function. These principles must be adhered to for successful results with repair of acetabular fractures. To achieve them, good exposure to the fracture site and the ability to maneuver the fragments while protecting soft tissue structures are imperative. Most surgeons prefer the dorsal approach by trochanteric osteotomy (Fig. 158–9).[3, 16, 17, 22, 39] A muscle separation technique that provides exposure to the dorsal acetabular rim through caudal retraction of the superficial gluteal muscle, cranial retraction of the middle gluteal muscle, and elevation of the deep gluteal muscle has been described.[37] The advantages of this technique are less tissue trauma and decreased operative time. Additional exposure for caudal acetabular fractures can be obtained by incision of the conjoined insertion of the internal obturator and gemelli muscles. The insertions of the external obturator and quadratus femoris muscles are left intact. The gemelli muscles are elevated subperiosteally with the internal obturator muscle. Opening the bursa under the internal obturator muscle accomplishes maximal utilization of the external rotators as a physiological retractor for the sciatic nerve. Elevation of the internal rotators exposes the cranial half of the ischium. Reduction of the cranially displaced ischial component of an acetabular fracture is facilitated by a Z-plasty release of the sacrotuberous ligament.[31] The approach selected should provide adequate exposure for that particular fracture while minimizing soft tissue trauma, especially to the sciatic nerve.

Reduction can be difficult because of limited access to the fracture fragments for application of bone clamps. Cranial traction can be obtained by grasping the iliac crest with a Lewin forceps or towel forceps. Caudal retraction of the caudal segment can be accomplished by securing the ischial tuberosity with a Lewin forceps or towel forceps or by placing a Steinman pin through the ischial tuberosity from ventral to dorsal and then using the Jacobs chuck as a handle. With additional dissection, Kern bone-holding forceps can be applied to the caudal ischium, improving the surgeon's ability to apply medial and lateral leverage and rotation. If the cranial ischium is exposed, bone forceps can be placed just cranial and caudal to the acetabulum, but extreme care must be used not to stretch or compress the sciatic nerve excessively. When the femoral head is impacted through the medial acetabulum, lateral traction on the proximal femur is necessary. The greater trochanter can be grasped with Lewin bone forceps or Vulsellum bone clamps, or a Steinman pin can be placed antegrade into the proximal femur with the Jacobs chuck used as a handle for lateral leverage. Reduction forceps can also be placed on the distal portion of the dome cranially by spanning the greater trochanter. Once reduction is achieved, temporary reduction may be possible by placing Kirschner wires across the fracture. A lag screw is used as a compo-

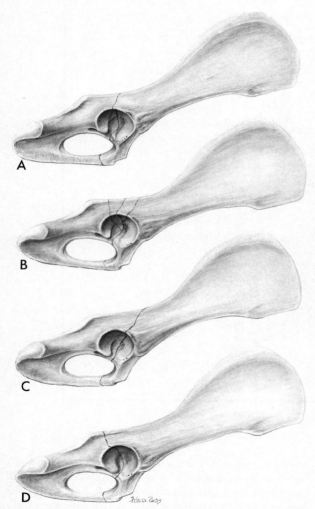

Figure 158–8. Acetabular fractures: *A*, central; *B*, comminuted; *C*, cranial; *D*, caudal.

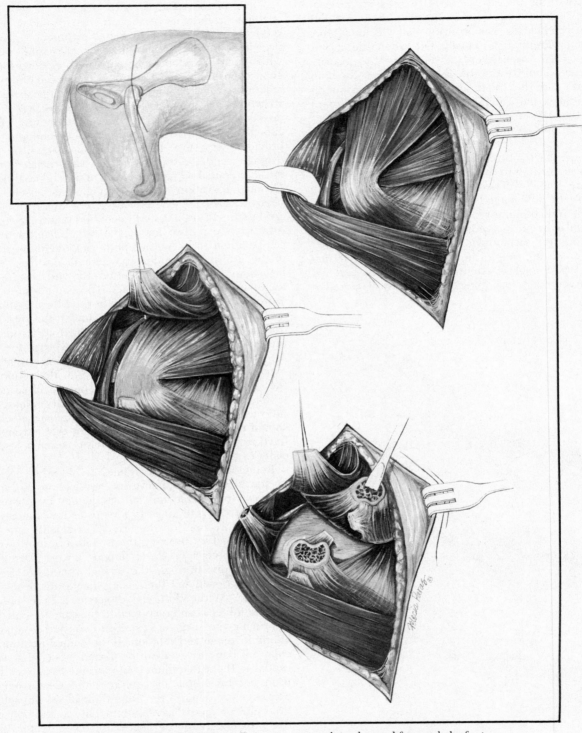

Figure 158–9. The trochanteric osteotomy approach is advocated for acetabular fractures.

nent of the final fixation whenever the fracture is sufficiently oblique.

Plate and screw fixation consistently yields the best results. Pins are difficult to place in acetabular fractures and may not provide stable fixation. Also, pins may loosen prior to fracture healing.[3] Interlocking

stable fragments can be fixed with bone screws and orthopedic wire used as a tension band.[3, 13] Multiple pin fixation or screw and wire fixation as a tension band can be incorporated with methyl methacrylate bone cement instead of plating.[25] However, the introduction of the ASIF small fragment set marked

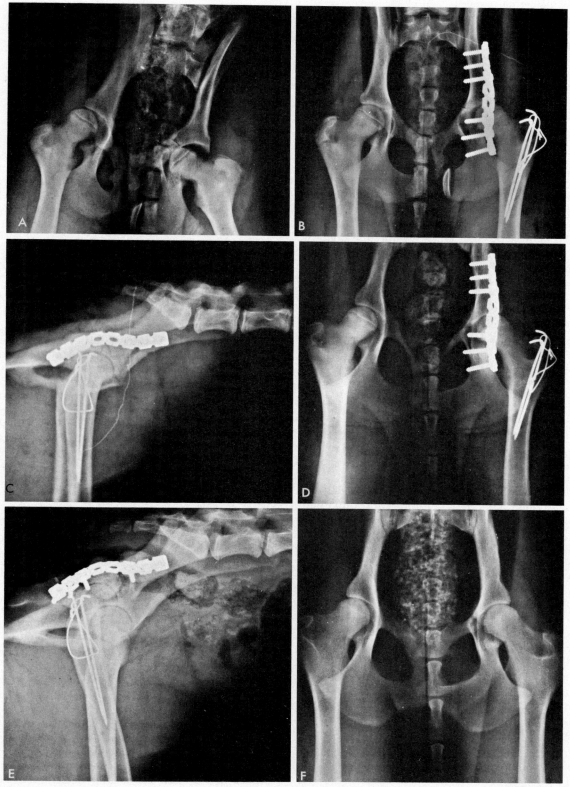

Figure 158–10. Acetabular fracture in a six-month-old German shepherd–type mixed-breed dog, that was repaired using an ASIF reconstruction plate. *A,* Preoperative ventrodorsal view. *B* and *C,* Postoperative ventrodorsal and lateral views. *D* and *E,* Ventrodorsal and lateral views taken ten weeks after operation. *F,* Ventrodorsal view taken two years after operation. (Courtesy of Dr. Ulrike Matis.)

the turning point in repair of acetabular fractures.[11] The fingerplates are readily adaptable to the contours of the dog acetabulum, and the surgeon's versatility is enhanced by the ability to select either a straight, L-shaped, or T-shaped finger plate. Although seldom used, the smaller mini-plates provide a means of secure fixation for fractures in animals too small for the finger plates. With ASIF reconstruction plates, contouring of acetabular plates has been markedly simplified (Fig. 158–10). Also, a precontoured horseshoe-shaped acetabular plate is available. For large and giant breed dogs, the 2.7-mm and 3.5-mm dynamic compression plates may be more appropriate. Because the plate is applied to the tension side of the acetabulum, a small plate is strong enough for weight-bearing forces unless there is a defect that would subject the plate to cyclic bending stress with weight-bearing. Thus, it is avisable to inspect the articular side of the fracture as well as the dome to avoid a fracture gap at the articular surface from undercontouring of the plate. Fibrin, clots, and bone fragments or debris should also be removed from the joint. If anatomic reduction is not possible, the surgeon should err on the caudal fragment. Because weight-bearing occurs primarily on the cranial two-thirds of the dome, congruency between the femoral head and the cranial articular surface is imperative. The tendency is for a slight dorsal disparity between the caudal and cranial segments at the level of the cartilaginous labrum. This tendency results from an inability to rotate the caudal segment laterally and ventrally.

Wound closure should proceed sequentially to assure re-establishment of tissue planes and a stable hip joint. The limb is usually placed in a non–weight-bearing sling for ten to 14 days after operation, unless additional injuries make this impractical. Close confinement and supervised exercise are important. After the sling is removed, relative confinement and leash walks only are continued for two weeks longer. During the first 24 to 48 hours after operation, loss of sensation is a consequence of excessive sciatic nerve retraction. Urination is monitored, because walking and posturing are difficult with the operated limb in a sling. An occasional dog needs catheterization or bladder expression. The sling must be kept clean and dry to avoid unnecessary sling changes. If the toes of the operated limb are excessively swollen, the sling has to be adjusted or changed. A slight amount of swelling is not unusual and can be relieved by massaging the foot and getting the dog up frequently. Postoperative radiographs are taken to assess fracture healing at four to six weeks after operation. Range of motion, crepitus, and elicitable pain should also be noted.

Ischial Fractures

Isolated ischial fractures are uncommon and seldom need operative repair. When ischial fractures accompany other pelvic fractures, stabilization and

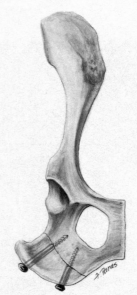

Figure 158–11. A substantial fracture of the ischium has been repaired with lag screws.

reduction of the major fragments usually result in acceptable reduction and stabilization of the ischial fracture.[3] When the ischial fragment is large and isolated from the rest of the pelvis, the resulting instability justifies correction. Conservative therapy consists of confinement and a non-weight-bearing sling in a neutral position. Flexion of the hip causes caudal and distal displacement of the ischial fragment because of the pull on the origin of the hamstring muscles. The loss of caudal stability may cause problems such as hyperextension of the stifle and delayed healing of the fracture if the dog is allowed to bear weight and walk.

The caudal approach to the hip and cranial ischium is used.[3, 22, 31] Fixation is achieved by an intramedullary pin, wire sutures, or small bone plates. Fractures of the ischial tuberosity can be repaired with bone screws (Fig. 158–11).

Sacroiliac Joint Fracture-Luxation

Unilateral separation of the sacroiliac joint is much more common than bilateral luxation.[3, 23, 29] Because of the geometry of the pelvis, unilateral displacement cannot occur without associated fractures or a pelvic symphyseal separation. Surgery is indicated for fractures with marked instability, pain, or bilateral instability.[3, 12]

A dorsal approach to the iliac crest is made, with ventral reflection of the middle gluteal muscle and medial retraction of the sacrospinalis to gain access to the sacroiliac joint. The separation on the medial aspect of the ilium has usually been established by the tissue separation that occurs at the time of displacement. The cranial gluteal artery, vein, and nerve are avoided where they pass from medial to lateral over the caudodorsal iliac spine to enter the middle gluteal muscle. The articular surface of the ilium is just ventral to the caudal half of the dorsal iliac crest. A diagonal from the dorsal iliac spine to the ventral iliac spine also bisects the body of the sacrum. Reduction is accomplished by caudal displacement of the ilium, which can be facilitated by having the anesthetist hold the forelimbs. Bone-holding forceps can be applied to the cranial iliac crest, but lateral leverage on the greater trochanter or ischial tuberosity should also be attempted to overcome the associated medial displacement of the caudal portion of the hemipelvis. When the ilium is reduced, visual access to the sacroiliac joint is limited. A mosquito hemostat can be used to indirectly palpate the reduction. Preplacement of a vertical Kirschner wire in the sacral wing and the dorsal iliac crest at the midpoints of the respective articulations provides a reference point for reduction. Temporary reduction can be maintained with a Kirschner wire. For small dogs and cats, the Kirschner wire is left in place after fixation is secured with a single lag screw to provide two-point fixation and eliminate rotational forces. In larger dogs, two lag screws are preferable. The angle of drilling should be about 20 degrees from dorsal to ventral, in order to gain purchase in the body of the sacrum and to direct the screw below the vertebral foramen. Prior to drilling, an estimated safe depth for drilling should be obtained by checking the ventrodorsal radiograph to prevent inadvertent entry into the spinal canal during placement of the lag screws. If the opposite hemipelvis or sacroiliac joint is intact, a transilial bolt can be placed to decrease shearing forces and subsequent pullout of the lag screws (Fig. 158–12).[3] The transilial bolt is indicated for markedly overweight dogs, in impacted fractures of the sacrum, and in some bilateral fractures. An alternative to the transilial bolt for unilateral hemipelvis displacement is wiring of the pelvic

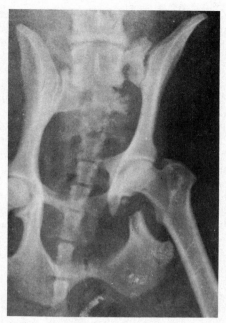

Figure 158–13. A sacral fracture is seen. Animals with these injuries must be carefully evaluated for neurological damage.

symphysis after the sacroiliac luxation is reduced and stabilized.

Sacral fractures are, fortunately, less frequent. Exposure and reduction are more difficult. It is critical to place the lag screws in the sacral body to have sufficient fixation (Fig. 158–13). A common mistake with fixation of sacroiliac luxations is securing the ilium into the body of L7. If the fixation is stable and no neurological damage occurs, reoperation is not worthwhile.

After operation the dog is in much less pain and is rehabilitated more quickly. Exercise should be limited to decrease mechanical force on the screws and to permit a strong soft tissue repair as bone to bone union does not occur. A significant number of sacroiliac luxations repaired with lag screw fixation alone become displaced again after surgery. The displacement occurs slowly, and the owner may not be aware of it. Exercise should be limited for four to six weeks to decrease the chances of this complication. The dog should be observed for any indication of sciatic nerve dysfunction after operation, because the sciatic nerve passes just ventral to the lateral aspect of the body of the sacrum. Sacral nerve injuries may be reflected by abnormal urination or defecation.

Pubic Fractures and Pelvic Symphyseal Separation

Pubic fractures commonly occur with other pelvic fractures. Stabilization of the major segments usually provides adequate reduction and stability for the pubic fractures. When a concurrent sacroiliac luxation is present, the animal has considerable difficulty adducting the legs.[4] Hobbles should be used for ten to 14 days to prevent abduction injuries and disrup-

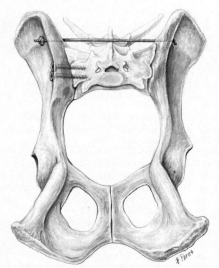

Figure 158–12. A transilial bolt has been placed to augment the lag screw fixation of the sacroiliac luxation.

tion of early soft tissue healing. Damage to the genitourinary system may result from pubic bone fracture or separation-displacement of the pelvic symphysis. Marked cranial displacement of the pubic brim indicates an avulsion fracture of the prepubic tendon. In these cases, the inguinal and groin area is usually severely bruised. Caudal ventral hernias are common with this particular injury.

Surgical repair is effected by wiring the fragments together. Exposure is gained through an open approach to the ventral surface of the pelvic symphysis. This can be combined with a caudal celiotomy for repair of prepubic tendon injuries or other caudal abdomen injuries. The obturator nerve should be avoided in fractures involving the obturator foramen. Malleable retractors can be placed under bone fragments during drilling, to protect underlying soft tissue structures. Maximum stability can be achieved with finger plating if fragment size is large enough. Double plating of pubic symphyseal fractures is recommended in humans who have sustained a wide "open-book" type of symphyseal diastasis.[34]

COMPLICATIONS ASSOCIATED WITH PELVIC FRACTURES

Major complications may arise during conservative or operative management of animals with pelvic fractures. These problems arise from associated soft tissue or multi-organ trauma. The importance of thorough history and physical examination cannot be overemphasized. Serial monitoring of vital functions for several days is equally important. Traumatic myocarditis may not appear for 48 to 72 hours after trauma. Because of the strong muscular support of the pelvis, surgical intervention is needed within two to four days of injury. Reduction, especially in large dogs, becomes increasingly difficult with each passing day. Unfortunately, pulse deficits, a ruptured bladder, and occasionally a diaphragmatic hernia may not be diagnosed initially.

Operative complications include hemorrhage and possible nerve trauma. One must take care when using power drills and bone taps to avoid penetration or laceration of adjacent structures, including the sciatic nerve, cranial and caudal gluteal arteries, urethra, and rectum.

Postoperative complications comprise inadequate reduction, implant failure, sciatic nerve damage, and, rarely, osteomyelitis. Non-union seldom occurs, but malunion from conservative treatment or inadequate surgical reduction can result in obstipation, dysuria, and dystocia.

ADVANTAGES OF PELVIC FRACTURE REPAIR

Dogs with repaired pelvic fractures are rehabilitated and convalesce much better and more rapidly than those conservatively managed. Musculoskeletal function is better in operated dogs than in dogs with similar injuries that are managed conservatively. Clients are generally pleased with the results, and hospitalization and nursing care are less than required for conservative treatment. An important factor is the reduced morbidity from concomitant injuries and associated complications such as pressure sores, pulmonary problems in recumbent animals, and urine or fecal soilage. Postoperatively, an animal that has minor musculoskeletal discomfort is much easier to treat and more responsive to therapy than one with major fractures that is functionally recumbent.

1. Berman, A. T., and Tom, L.: Traumatic separation of the pubic symphysis with associated fatal rectal tear: a case report and analysis of mechanism of injury. J. Trauma 14:1060, 1974.
2. Brinker, W. O.: Fractures of the pelvis. In Archibald, J. (ed.): Canine Surgery. 2nd ed. American Veterinary Publications, Santa Barbara, 1974.
3. Brinker, W. O.: The pelvis. In Bojrab, M. J. (ed.): Current Techniques in Small Animal Surgery. Lea & Febiger, Philadelphia, 1975.
4. Brinker, W. O., Piermattei, D. L., and Flo, G. L.: Fractures of the pelvis. In: Handbook of Small Animal Orthopedics and Fracture Treatment. W. B. Saunders, Philadelphia, 1983.
5. Brown, S. G., and Biggart, J. F.: Plate fixation of ilial fractures in the dog. J. Am. Vet. Med. Assoc. 167:472, 1975.
6. Bryan, W. J., and Tullos, H. S.: Pediatric pelvic fractures: a review of 52 patients. J. Trauma 19:799, 1979.
7. Clark, J. H.: Repairing pelvic fractures. Mod. Vet. Pract. 31–36, 1967.
8. Denny, H. R.: Pelvic fractures in the dog: a review of 123 cases. J. Small Anim. Pract. 19:151, 1978.
9. Diokno, A.: Late genitourinary tract complications associated with severe pelvic injury. Surg. Gynecol. Obstet. 150:150, 1980.
10. Flint, L. M., Jr., Brown, A., Richardson, J. D., and Polk, A. C.: Definitive control of bleeding from severe pelvic fractures. Ann. Surg. 189:709, 1979.
11. Heim, U., and Pfeiffer, K. M.: Small Fragment Set Manual Technique: Recommended by the ASIF Group. Springer-Verlag, New York, 1974.
12. Herron, M. R.: Sacroiliac luxations: methods of closed repair. Feline Pract. 46–49, 1976.
13. Herron, M. R.: Screw-wire fixation of acetabular fractures. Canine Pract. 48–50, 1977.
14. Hohn, B. H., and James, J. M.: Lateral approach to the canine ilium. J. Am. Anim. Hosp. Assoc. 2:111, 1966.
15. Huittenen, V., and Slatis, P.: Postmortem angiography and dissection of the hypogastric artery in pelvic fractures. Surgery 73:454, 1973.
16. Hulse, D. A., and Root, C. R.: Management of acetabular fractures: long term evaluation. Comp. Cont. Ed. 2:189, 1980.
17. Hulse, D. A.: Acetabular Fractures. In Bojrab. M. J. (ed.): Current Techniques in Small Animal Surgery. 2nd ed. Lea & Febiger, Philadelphia, 1983.
18. Leighton, R. L.: Surgical treatment of some pelvic fractures, J. Am. Vet. Med. Assoc. 153:1739, 1968.
19. Maull, K. I., Sachatello, C. R., and Ernst, C. B.: The deep perineal laceration—an injury frequently associated with open pelvic fractures: a need for aggressive surgical management. J. Trauma 17:685, 1977.
20. Mears, D. C., and Fu, F.: External fixation in pelvic fractures. Orthop. Clin. North Am. 11:465, 1980.
21. Phillips, I. R.: A survey of bone fractures in the dog and cat. J. Small Anim. Pract. 20:661, 1979.
22. Piermattei, D. L., Greely, R. G.: An Atlas of Surgical approaches to the Bones of the Dog and Cat. 2nd ed. W. B. Saunders, Philadelphia, 1979.

23. Pond, M. J.: Sacroiliac luxation. *In* Bojrab. M. J. (ed.): *Current Techniques in Small Animal Surgery.* Lea & Febiger, Philadelphia, 1975.
24. Raffa, J., and Christenson, N. M.: compound fractures of the pelvis. Am. J. Surg. *132*:282, 1976.
25. Renegar, W. R., and Griffeth, R. C.: The use of methyl methacrylate bone cement in the repair of acetabular fractures. J. Am. Anim. Hosp. Assoc. *13*:582, 1977.
26. Robins, G. M., Dingwall, J. S., and Sumner-Smith, G.: The plating of pelvic fractures in the dog. Vet. Rec. *93*:550, 1973.
27. Rothenberger, D. A., Fischer, R. P., and Perry, J. F., Jr.: Major vascular injuries secondary to pelvic fractures: an unsolved clinical problem. Am. J. Surg. *136*:660, 1978.
28. Rothenberger, D. A., Fischer, R. P., Strate, R.G. et al.: The mortality associated with pelvic fractures. Surgery *84*:356, 1978.
29. Ryan, W. W.: Sacroiliac luxation. *In* Bojrab, M. J., (ed.): *Curent Techniques in Small Animal Surgery.* 2nd ed. Lea & Febiger, Philadelphia, 1983.
29a. Selcer, B. A.: Urinary tract trauma associated with pelvic trauma. J. Am. Anim. Hosp. Assoc. *18*:785, 1982.
30. Singleton, W. B.: Limb fractures in the dog and cat. V: Fractures of the hind limb. J. Small Anim. Pract. 7:163, 1966.
31. Slocumb, B., and Hohn, R. B.: A surgical approach to the caudal aspect of the acetabulum and the body of the ischium in the dog. J. Am. Vet. Med. Assoc. *167*:65, 1975.
32. Stone, H. H., Rutledge, B. A., and Martin, J. D., Jr.: Massive crushing pelvic injuries. Am. Surg. *34*:869, 1968.
33. Tarvin, G. B.: Management of pelvic fractures. *In* Bojrab, M. J. (ed.): *Current Techniques in Small Animal Surgery.* 2nd ed. Lea & Febiger, Philadelphia, 1983.
34. Tile, M.: Pelvic fractures: operative versus nonoperative treatment. Orthop. Clin. North Amer. *11*:423, 1980.
35. Tile, M.: Fractures of the acetabulum. Orthop. Clin. North Am. *11*:481, 1980.
36. Trunkey, D. D., Chapman, M. W., Lim, R. C., Jr., et. al.: Management of pelvic fractures in blunt trauma injury. J. Trauma *14*:912, 1974.
37. Wadsworth, P. L., and Henry, W. B.: Dorsal surgical approach to acetabular fractures in the dog. J. Am. Vet. Med. Assoc. *165*:908, 1974.
38. Weems, W. L.: Management of genitourinary injury in patients with pelvic fractures. Ann. Surg. *189*:717, 1979.
39. Wheaton, L. G., Hohn, R. B., and Harrison, J. W.: Surgical treatment of acetabular fractures in the dog. J. Am. Vet. Med. Assoc. *162*:385, 1973.
40. Wingfield, W. E.: Lower urinary tract injuries associated with pelvic trauma. Canine Pract. 25–28, 1974.

Chapter **159** # Orthopedics of the Hindlimb

The Hip Joint

J. Hauptman

This chapter deals with the diseases and treatments of the hip joint, exclusive of fractures.

FUNCTIONAL ANATOMY OF THE COXOFEMORAL JOINT

The hip joint is a ball-and-socket joint that allows a wide range of motion, primarily flexion, and extension.[64] It is enclosed by a joint capsule that extends from the acetabulum to the neck of the femur (Fig. 159–1). The hip joint capsule does not have definite ligaments. The ligament of the head of the femur runs from the fovea capitis of the femur to the acetabular fossa (see Fig. 159–1). The capsule and the ligament of the femoral head add stability to the hip joint.[87]

Many muscles act on and about the hip joint to effect the functions of flexion, extension, abduction, adduction, and internal and external rotation (Figs. 159–2 to 159–4). The muscles of extension of the hip are the most numerous and well developed, and they are most essential for locomotion and weight-bearing. These muscles include the gluteal muscle group (superficial, middle and deep gluteals) and thigh muscle group (biceps femoris, semitendinosus, semimembranosus, gracilis, and adductor). The gracilis and adductor muscles, along with the pectineus muscle, also act on the hip joint to adduct the femur.

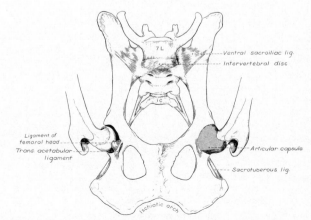

Figure 159–1. Ligaments of pelvis, ventral aspect. The joint capsule and ligament of the head of the femur (round ligament) are demonstrated. (Reproduced with permission from Evans, H. E., and Christensen, G. C.: *Miller's Anatomy of the Dog*, 2nd ed. W. B. Saunders, Philadelphia, 1979.)

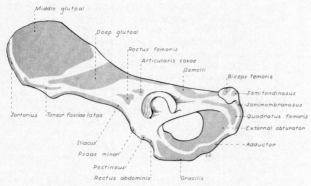

Figure 159–2. Left os coxae, showing areas of muscle attachment, lateral aspect. (Reproduced with permission from Evans, H. E., and Christensen, G. C.: *Miller's Anatomy of the Dog*, 2nd ed. W. B. Saunders, Philadelphia, 1979.)

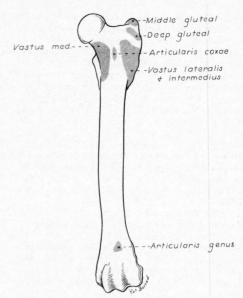

Figure 159–4. Left femur, showing areas of muscle attachments, cranial aspect. (Reproduced with permission from Evans, H. E., and Christensen, G. C.: *Miller's Anatomy of the Dog*, 2nd ed. W. B. Saunders, Philadelphia, 1979.)

The gluteal muscle group, in addition to extending the hip joint, rotates the hip joint internally and abducts the femur. External rotation of the hip is effected by a group of muscles (internal obturator, gemelli, external obturator, quadratus femoris, and iliopsoas). The quadratus femoris inserts on the caudal aspect of the femur, whereas the internal and external obturator and gemelli insert in the trochanteric fossa. The iliopsoas originates from the ventral lumbar vertebrae and ilium and inserts on the second, or lesser, trochanter. In addition to internally rotating the hip joint, the iliopsoas also flexes it. Other flexors of the hip joint include the sartorius and tensor fascia lata muscles. The small capsularis coxae muscle is both a flexor and internal rotator.

The vascular supply to the dog's hip joint is extensive and anastomotic (Fig. 159–5).[53,81] From most to least important, this supply comprises the lateral circumflex femoral, medial circumflex femoral, caudal gluteal, cranial gluteal, and iliolumbar arteries. The

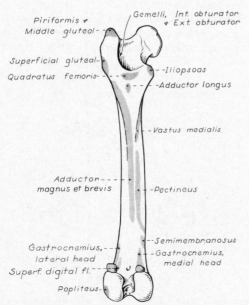

Figure 159–3. Left femur, showing areas of muscle attachment, caudal aspect. (Reproduced with permission from Evans, H. E., and Christensen, G. C.: *Miller's Anatomy of the Dog*, 2nd ed. W. B. Saunders, Philadelphia, 1979.)

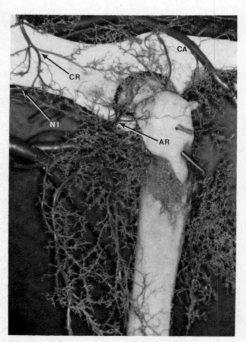

Figure 159–5. Left hemipelvis and proximal femur, lateral view. NI = nutrient artery of the ilium, CR = cranial gluteal artery, CA = caudal gluteal artery, AR = ascending ramus of the lateral circumflex artery. (Reproduced with permission from Kaderly, R. E., Anderson, W. D., and Anderson, B. G.: Extraosseous vascular supply to the mature dog's coxofemoral joint. Am. J. Vet. Res. 43:1208, 1982.)

lateral circumflex femoral artery originates from the femoral artery. It approaches the hip joint from its cranioventral aspect and ramifies in capsular arteries on the dorsal and cranial aspects of the hip joint. The medial femoral circumflex originates from the deep femoral artery. It approaches the hip joint from its ventral aspect and ramifies in capsular arteries that supply primarily the caudal and ventral aspects of the hip joint. These capsular arteries combine with lesser contributions from the caudal gluteal artery, caudodorsally, to form an arterial ring about the femoral neck. This arterial ring permits anastomosis between the aforementioned vessels.

The arterial ring gives rise to superior (dorsal) and inferior (ventral) epiphyseal arteries that enter the femoral head at the edge of the articular cartilage and anastomose in the center of the femoral head.[81] Similarly, the arterial ring yields superior, inferior, and anterior metaphyseal arteries that enter the femoral neck and anastomose with terminal branches of the nutrient artery of the shaft of the femur. Vessels have been observed in the ligament of the head of the femur.[7,26,81] They make a small contribution to the blood supply of the head of the femur.[7,81]

The acetabular side of the hip joint receives its blood supply from the iliolumbar, cranial gluteal, and caudal gluteal arteries.[53] The iliolumbar artery yields the nutrient artery of the ilium. The cranial gluteal artery supplies the craniodorsal aspects of the acetabulum and anastomoses with the lateral circumflex

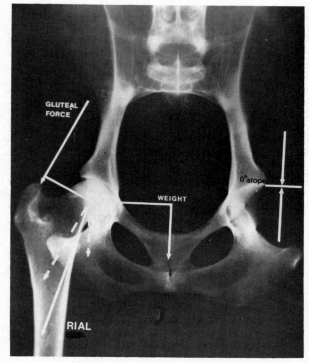

Figure 159–7. Radiograph of pelvis in approximate weight-bearing position. The acetabulum has 0° slope, perpendicular to an upward femoral force. The summation of the weight vector and gluteal force vector results in an intra-articular load that exceeds body weight.

femoral. The caudal gluteal supplies the caudodorsal acetabulum and continues to complete the arterial ring around the femoral neck.

Biomechanically, the femur meets the pelvis in a manner allowing maximal stability and range of motion (Fig. 159–6). The acetabulum is a deep socket that covers the femoral head. Coverage of the femoral head may be subjectively assessed on the ventrodorsal radiograph and by measuring the acetabular angle of Wiberg (Norberg-Olsson angle)[97] or the Rhodes-Jenny acetabular index.[79] The Wiberg angle, formed by the center of the femoral head, the outer lip of the acetabulum, and a perpendicular to the long axis of the body, should exceed 105 degrees (see Fig. 159–6).[71,95] The acetabulum should have a craniodorsal roof that is perpendicular to an upward femoral force (Fig. 159–7). If the acetabular roof slants the femoral head is more easily subluxated. Additional forces must be generated by the abductor muscle group or joint capsule to maintain the femoral head in the acetabulum. Total hip joint load is increased with sloping of the acetabular roof (Fig. 159–8). Thickening of subchondral acetabular bone is termed the acetabular sourcil (see Fig. 159–6).[72] The acetabular sourcil is thickest on the craniodorsal aspect of the acetabulum and indicates the area of greatest intra-articular stress.[72] The fact that the greatest intra-articular stress is craniodorsal, and not dorsal, is important in understanding the biomechanics of the

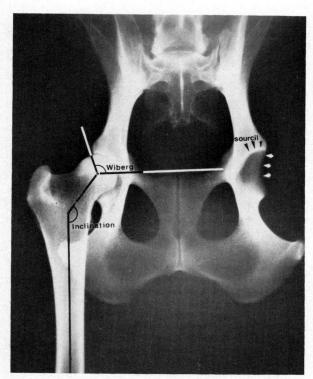

Figure 159–6. Ventrodorsal radiograph of a normal pelvis demonstrating the angle of Wiberg, the angle of inclination, the acetabular sourcil, and the depth of the acetabulum (white arrows).

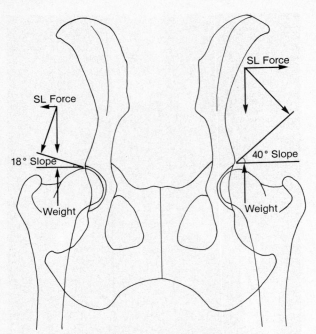

Figure 159–8. Schematic diagram of pelvis with acetabular slopes of 18 and 40°. The subluxation force and total hip joint load increase proportionally to the degree of acetabular slope.

hip joint. In addition, the normal acetabulum has a posterior tilt, or retroversion of five to ten degrees (Fig. 159–9).

The femur also has important biomechanical con-

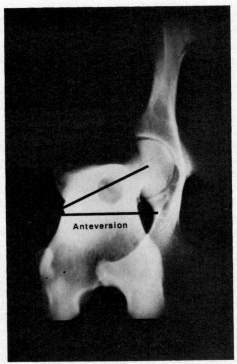

Figure 159–9. The normal angle of anteversion. This angle is observed in the transverse plane, sighting down the shaft of the femur.

figuration. The femoral neck-shaft angle has two components. The angle of inclination is the angle observed in the frontal (dorsal) plane (see Fig. 159–6). The normal angle is 146 degrees.[36,83] It is related to technique of measurement, positioning, and anteversion angle; it is not related to age, sex, or breed.[35,36] The angle of anteversion is the angle observed in the transverse plane (see Fig. 159–9). The normal angle, measured radiographically, is 27 degrees.[67] It may be measured by sighting down the shaft of the femur[67] (see Fig. 159–9) or by using trigonometry and two radiographic views (see Fig. 159–38).[5,83] The length of the femoral neck and position of the greater trochanter, relative to the femoral head, are also important.[72] The proximal tip of the greater trochanter should be approximately level with, or only slightly distal to, the most proximal part of the femoral head (see Fig. 159–6). This distance is termed the articulotrochanteric distance.[34]

The intra-articular hip joint stress is 4.4 times the load placed on the leg in the normal standing dog.[2] The axis of the center of gravity of the dog is medial to the hip joint. Consequently, the weight-bearing load placed on the hip has a torque with a lever arm equal to the distance from the center of gravity to the center of the head of the femur (see Fig. 159–7). This torque must be counterbalanced by an opposite but equal torque generated by the abductor muscles (gluteals) with a lever arm that is perpendicular to the gluteal muscle vector and extends to the center of the head of the femur. The summation of the weight (loading force) and abductor muscle force results in an intra-articular load that exceeds body weight.[2,65,72,77] The intra-articular load vector is oriented along the trabecular stress lines in the proximal femur (see Fig. 159–6). Critical factors that determine abductor muscle force and intra-articular load in the standing dog are: angle of inclination of the femoral neck, length of the femoral neck, position of the greater trochanter, and distance of the femoral head from the center of gravity. In the running quadruped, the majority of intra-articular forces are oriented cranially in a horizontal plane, as opposed to the vertically oriented forces in the standing animal.[77] This fact is re-emphasized by observing the thickened acetabular sourcil craniodorsally (see Fig. 159–6). Consequently, the angle of anteversion, or cranial angulation of the femoral head and neck, assumes great importance. The biomechanics of the anteversion angle are not as well-defined as the biomechanics of the angle of inclination; excessive anteversion angles result in increased intra-articular forces.[77]

Intra-articular hip joint forces markedly exceed weight load placed on the hip. This stress increases with increased angle of inclination, increased angle of anteversion, short femoral neck, and distal or medial displacement of the greater trochanter. In addition, intra-articular stresses are greater if the distance from the femoral head to the center of gravity increases. Such an increase frequently occurs clinically with femoral head subluxation.

SURGICAL APPROACHES TO THE HIP JOINT

It is imperative that the surgeon be able to approach the hip joint in a manner that combines maximal exposure with minimal time and trauma. There are four main approaches to the hip joint: cranial, dorsal, ventral, and caudal. The cranial and the dorsal approaches are most commonly used.

Cranial Approach

The cranial approach to the hip joint is commonly performed. It is highly recommended for excision arthroplasties and is commonly performed for hip luxation, fractures of the femoral head and neck, total hip replacement, and femoral osteotomies. It is a most versatile approach, because it can be enlarged into an approach to the shaft of the femur or wing of the ilium, or into the dorsal approach to the hip.

A skin incision is made, centered over a point just anterior to the greater trochanter and extending about a third of the distance down the shaft of the femur. The incision is continued through the subcutaneous tissue. The superficial biceps fascia is identified and incised in the same direction, for the length of the skin incision, along the anterior border of the biceps femoris muscle (Fig. 159–10). The biceps femoris muscle is retracted posteriorly and the fascia anteriorly, exposing the tensor fascia lata muscle anteriorly, the superficial gluteal muscle superficial to the greater trochanter, and fascia lata overlying the quadriceps muscle group (Fig. 159–11). The fascia lata is incised in a ventrodorsal direction, and the incision is continued dorsally between the tensor fascia lata muscle and superficial gluteal muscle. In some animals, the superficial biceps fascia and fascia lata may be incised as one layer.

Retraction of these incised layers reveals a triangle

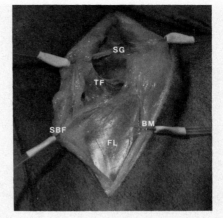

Figure 159–11. The superficial biceps fascia (SBF) and biceps muscle (BM) are retracted to expose the tensor fascia lata muscle (TF), superficial gluteal muscle (SG), and fascia lata (FL).

bounded by the middle and deep gluteal muscles dorsally, the vastus lateralis muscle laterally, and the rectus femoris muscle anteriorly (Fig. 159–12). The femoral head and neck and the acetabulum can be palpated. Dorsal retraction of the gluteal muscles aids in identification of the hip joint (Fig. 159–13). After the hip joint is identified, an incision is made in the craniodorsal joint capsule medially from the rim of the acetabulum and laterally along the femoral neck to the proximal shaft of the femur. Retraction of the incised joint capsule reveals the femoral head, neck, and acetabulum. The capsularis coxae muscle is cut with the incision in the joint capsule.

Exposure to the hip joint may be enhanced if necessary. The cranial half of the tendon of insertion of the deep gluteal muscle may be incised. Caudodorsal retraction of the gluteal muscles exposes the dorsal aspect of the joint capsule of the hip, which may be further incised. Exposure may be enhanced cranioventrally by periosteally elevating the origins

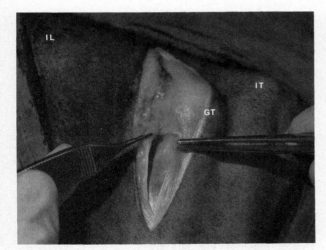

Figure 159–10. Cranial approach to the left hip. The superficial biceps fascia is incised. IL = Ilium, GT = greater trochanter, IT = ischemic tuberosity.

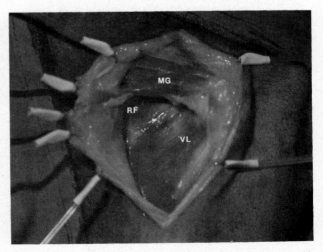

Figure 159–12. Retraction of the superficial biceps fascia and biceps muscle reveals a triangle bounded by the middle (MG) and deep gluteal, vastus lateralis (VL), and rectus femoris (RF) muscles.

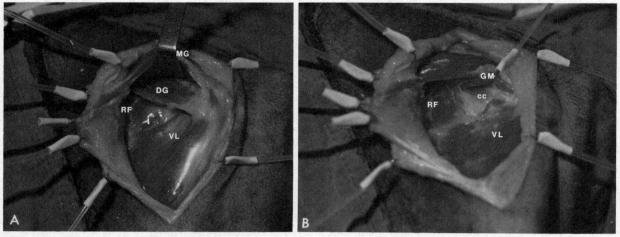

Figure 159–13. A, Dorsal retraction of the middle gluteal muscle (MG) exposes the deep gluteal muscle (DG). *B,* Dorsal retraction of the gluteal muscles (GM) aids identification of the capsularis coxae muscle (cc) and hip joint.

of the vastus medialis, intermedius, and lateralis muscles from the cranial aspect of the proximal femur (Fig. 159–14). Elevation of these muscles allows exposure of the entire cranial aspect of the proximal femur and femoral head and neck.

The joint capsule is closed with interrupted sutures, which may be of absorbable or nonreactive nonabsorbable material. The fascial layers are closed with a continuous absorbable suture. The subcutaneous and skin layers are closed with continuous sutures.

The cranial approach to the hip is particularly versatile because it may be continued into a dorsal approach to allow complete exposure of the dorsal hip joint. The approach may further be continued into a lateral approach to the ilium by dorsal retraction of the gluteal muscles or a lateral approach to the femur.

Dorsal Approach

The dorsal approach allows maximum exposure of the hip joint. It is useful for fractures of the posterior shaft of the ilium, acetabulum, ischium, and femoral head and as well as for neck, hip dislocations, pelvic osteotomies, and total hip replacement.

A curved skin incision is made, beginning craniodorsal to the greater trochanter, continuing posterior to the greater trochanter at its midpoint, and ending just cranial to the midshaft of the femur. The incision is continued through the subcutaneous tissues (Fig. 159–15). The biceps femoris muscle and superficial fascia are identified. The fascia is incised along the cranial border of the biceps muscle from the midshaft of the femur to the extent of the incision dorsally. The incision is continued through the fascia lata and between the tensor fascia lata and superficial gluteal muscles, as with the cranial approach. The biceps muscle is retracted posteriorly and the fascia ante-

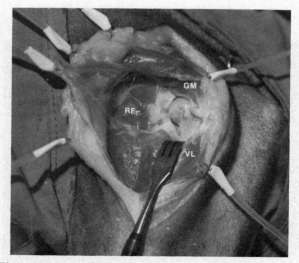

Figure 159–14. An incision has been made in the craniodorsal joint capsule from the rim of the acetabulum along the neck of the femur. Periosteal elevation of the vastus lateralis (VL), medialis, and intermedius muscles exposes the cranial aspect of the proximal femur.

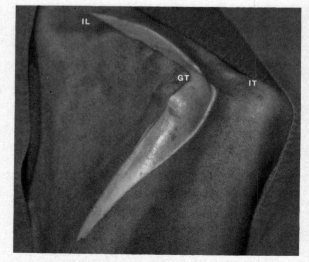

Figure 159–15. Dorsal approach to the left hip, skin incision. IL = Ilium, GT = greater trochanter, IT = ischiatic tuberosity.

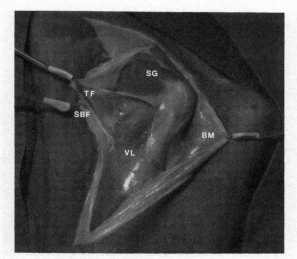

Figure 159–16. The incision is continued through the superficial biceps fascia (SBF) and fascia lata, as with the cranial approach. Retraction of the biceps muscle (BM), tensor fascia lata muscle (TF), and SBF exposes the vastus lateralis (VL) and superficial gluteal muscle (SG).

riorly (Fig. 159–16). Retraction may be maintained with self-retaining retractors. The sciatic nerve is identified. It lies just deep to the biceps muscle, approximately two centimeters posterior to the femur

in an average size dog. Proximally, this nerve lies just superficial to the internal obturator and gemelli muscles and continues proximally to lie between the middle and deep gluteal muscles (Fig. 159–17).

The superficial gluteal muscle is identified, and its distal tendon is incised near its insertion on the third trochanter. The superficial gluteal muscle is reflected dorsally, and the middle and deep gluteal muscles are identified (Fig. 159–18). After the tendon of insertion of the deep gluteal muscle is identified, a Gigli wire is easily passed between the deep gluteal muscle and the femoral neck with a hemostat. The sciatic nerve is again identified. The surgeon then performs the osteotomy, sawing with the Gigli wire from medial to lateral, in a distal to lateral direction at an angle of approximately 45 degrees. The osteotomy should end laterally, near the third trochanter (Fig. 159–19). The greater trochanter, with its attached middle and deep gluteal muscles, is reflected dorsally so that the dorsal hip joint may be identified.

A Gigli wire is used to osteotomize the greater trochanter for two reasons. First, the Gigli wire is placed between the femoral neck and deep gluteal muscle, assuring that the osteotomy is correct. Second, the sawing action of the Gigli wire results in hemostasis of the cut ends of bone. Alternative methods of transecting the greater trochanter include use of an osteotome or an oscillating saw. Possible dis-

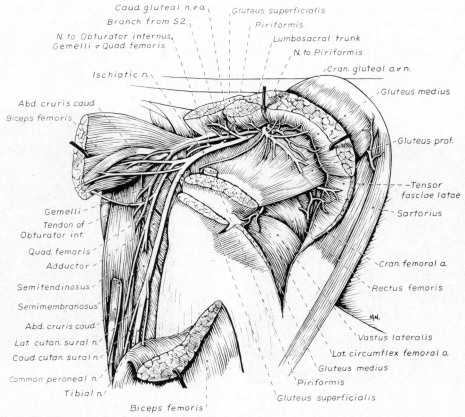

Figure 159–17. Nerves, arteries, and muscles of the right hip, lateral aspect. The course of the sciatic (ischiatic) nerve and its relation to surrounding structures are demonstrated. (Reproduced with permission from Evans, H. E., and Christensen, G. C.: *Miller's Anatomy of the Dog*, 2nd ed. W. B. Saunders, Philadelphia, 1979.)

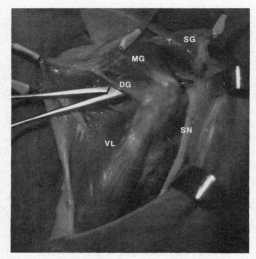

Figure 159–18. A hemostat has been passed between the deep gluteal muscle (DG) and the femoral neck. The superficial gluteal muscle (SG) has been dorsally reflected and the sciatic nerve (SN) identified.

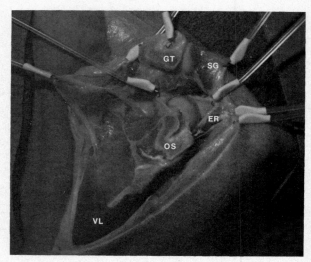

Figure 159–20. The dorsal joint capsule has been incised from the rim of the acetabulum to the neck of the femur. The external rotators (ER) have been incised at their insertions in the trochanteric fossa and caudally reflected. The greater trochanter (GT) and superficial gluteal muscle (SG) are reflected dorsally. OS = osteotomy, VL = vastus lateralis.

advantages of the osteotome or saw include a less precise osteotomy and more bleeding.

Exposure of the dorsal hip joint may be enhanced by cutting the insertions of the internal obturator and gemelli muscles near their insertions in the trochanteric fossa. Caudodorsal retraction of these muscles increases caudal exposure (Fig. 159–20). Resuturing of these muscles is not absolutely required at the time of closure. However, mattress sutures of a nonabsorbable suture material are usually placed. As with the cranial approach, the dorsal approach may

also be continued into a lateral approach to the ilium or femur.

Closure is begun by suturing the joint capsule as indicated. The greater trochanter is reattached with a tension band. The proximal femur is exposed at a point two to three centimeters distal to the osteotomy site. Exposure is attained by reflecting the vastus lateralis muscle anteriorly and the adductor muscle posteriorly. Exposure is maintained by means of curved forceps placed between the muscle and bone and retracted medially (Fig. 159–21). A hole is drilled

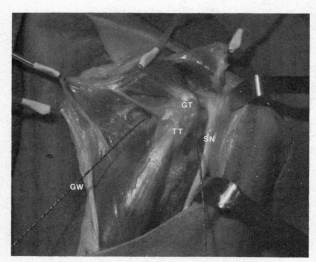

Figure 159–19. The Gigli wire (GW) is in place between the deep gluteal muscle and femoral neck. The osteotomy is performed, ending laterally near the third trochanter (TT). The sciatic nerve (SN) is preserved.

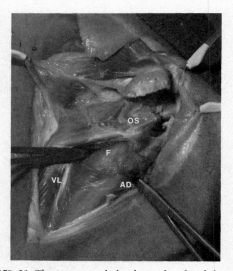

Figure 159–21. The joint capsule has been closed and the external rotators resutured. The femur (F) has been exposed 2 to 3 cm distal to the osteotomy (OS). Exposure of the femur is maintained by curved hemostats retracting the vastus lateralis (VL) cranially and adductor (AD) caudally. A caudal-cranial hole is drilled through the femur at this point for placement of the tension band wire.

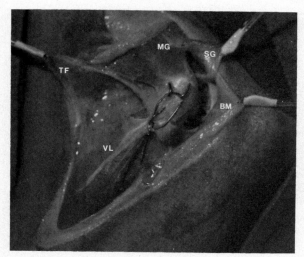

Figure 159–22. The greater trochanter has been fixed to the proximal femur by two pins and a tension band. MG = Middle gluteal, SG = superficial gluteal, BM = biceps muscle, VL = vastus lateralis, TF = tensor fascia lata muscle.

in a caudal to ventral direction through the femur, and an 18-gauge wire is passed through the hole. The greater trochanter is replaced on the osteotomy site and reattached with two pins (⅛-inch for large dogs, K-wire for small dogs). The pins are bent laterally 90 degrees at their points of insertion on the greater trochanter. The wire is passed on the lateral aspect of the femur, in a figure-of-eight pattern, and around the pins. The pins are rotated 180 degrees so that the proximal bent ends of the pins are now pointing medially. The wire is tightened in a tension band fashion (Fig. 159–22).

The superficial gluteal muscle is reattached to the third trochanter by means of nonabsorbable suture. The tensor fascia lata muscle is reattached to the superficial gluteal muscle and fascia lata by means of a continuous absorbable suture. The biceps femoris muscle is sutured to the superficial fascia with a continuous absorbable suture. The subcutaneous tissues and skin are closed routinely.

Ventral Approach

Because the ventral approach to the hip joint allows limited exposure, it is useful only for excision arthroplasty.

The animal is positioned in dorsal recumbency with the hind legs abducted. The iliopectineal eminence of the pubic bone and the pectineus muscle are palpated. A straight skin incision, centered over the hip joint, is made in a medial to lateral direction. The incision is continued through the subcutaneous tissues to the pectineus muscle. The origin of the pectineus muscle on the iliopectineal eminence is identified. Bleeding is minimized by incising the fibrous tissue origin of the pectineus muscle with a scalpel. The femoral artery and vein lie immediately

anterior to the pectineus muscle at this point. They must be identified, and scalpel incision of the origin of the pectineus must be in a cranial to caudal direction to further protect these vessels. Alternatively, the belly of the pectineus muscle may be incised. The pectineus muscle is reflected distally to expose the deep femoral vessels, the iliopsoas muscle craniolaterally, and the adductor muscle caudally. The adductor muscle is retracted caudally, and the iliopsoas muscle and deep gluteal vessels are retracted craniolaterally to expose the ventral hip joint. A craniocaudal incision is made in the joint capsule to expose the femoral head and neck and acetabulum. The iliopsoas muscle may, alternatively, be retracted caudomedially to maximize exposure.

There is no need to close the incised joint capsule or to reattach the pectineus muscle. Closure consists of routine subcutaneous and skin sutures.

Caudal Approach

The caudal approach allows limited exposure of the dorsal acetabulum, cranial ischium, and hip joint. It has been used to repair fractures and luxations of this area.

A curved skin incision is made, centered just posterior to the greater trochanter. The incision is continued through the subcutaneous tissue so that the biceps femoris muscle and superficial fascia can be identified. The fascia is incised along the cranial border of the biceps, just as in the cranial and dorsal approaches. The biceps is retracted posteriorly and the sciatic nerve is identified. The femur is rotated internally, and the gluteal muscles are retracted anteriorly. Dissection of loose fat and areolar tissue aids identification of gluteal muscles, internal obturator tendon, and gemelli muscles. The internal obturator and gemelli muscles are incised near their insertions in the trochanteric fossa. Caudal reflection of these muscles protects the sciatic nerve and exposes the joint capsule.

The internal obturator and gemelli muscles are reattached with a mattress suture. The biceps and fascia are sutured with a continuous suture. The subcutaneous tissue and skin are closed routinely.

HIP DISLOCATION

Dislocation of the hip joint is the most common luxation.[28,43] Most often, the dislocation is secondary to trauma. It may also occur infrequently because of hip dysplasia or as a postoperative complication of total hip replacement. The traumatically dislocated femoral head is most frequently displaced anterodorsal to the acetabulum. The relatively strong pull of the gluteal musculature accounts for this displacement. The dislocated femoral head will infrequently be ventral to the acetabulum, trapped in the obturator foramen, and, rarely, posterior to the acetabu-

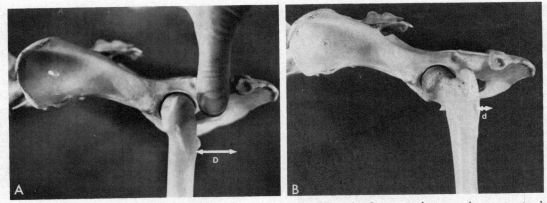

Figure 159–23. A, To test the integrity of the hip joint, the thumb is placed in the depression between the greater trochanter and ischiatic tuberosity (D). B, With external rotation of the femur, the distance between the greater trochanter and ischiatic tuberosity is decreased (d) and the thumb is forced out of the depression.

lum. Medial, or intrapelvic, luxations are always associated with fracture of the acetabulum and are classified and treated as acetabular fractures.

Dislocation of the hip may be evident on physical examination. The animal may allow the leg to bear some weight, and the toes are mildly rotated externally. The external rotation of the leg is due to the anterodorsal displacement and external rotation of the proximal femur. The leg is palpated for other abnormalities, with special attention to the hip. The greater trochanter may be identified and palpated in all but very obese dogs with anterodorsal hip luxation. The greater trochanter is dorsally displaced relative to the other trochanter and to the ilium and ischium. This assessment is best made with the animal stand-ing. The orientation of the greater trochanter to the ischium and the other greater trochanter is a sensitive indicator of hip joint congruity (see Fig. 159–25A). Congruity of the hip joint may be further assessed by placing the thumb between the greater trochanter and ischium. External rotation of the leg always displaces the thumb from between the ischium and greater trochanter of the dog with a normal hip (Fig. 159–23). If the thumb is not displaced, the integrity of the hip joint has been violated by fracture or luxation. Hind leg length may also be compared, although it is the least reliable of the three assessments.

Investigation for abnormalities of other systems should be made in the animal with a traumatically

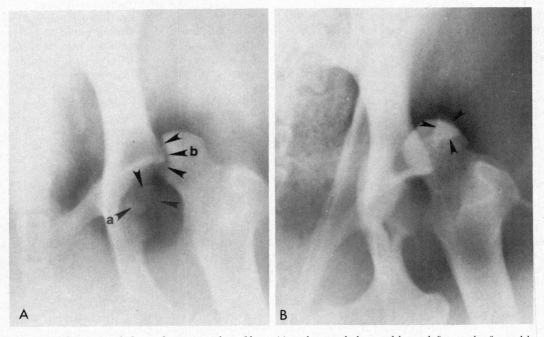

Figure 159–24. A, Hip luxation with femur fracture. A chip of bone (a) in the acetabulum and bony deficit in the femoral head (b) can be seen. B, Hip luxation with acetabular fracture. A chip of bone from the dorsal acetabulum can be seen (arrows).

dislocated hip. In addition, radiography of the hip should always be performed.

Specifically, hip dysplasia and acetabular or femoral head fractures should be sought. Hip dysplasia is associated with altered conformation of the femoral head or acetabulum that may be mild to severe. If the femoral head is misshapen or the acetabulum is shallow, the congruity of the ball-and-socket joint is less than optimal. Stability of the hip joint is therefore impaired. Reduction of a coxofemoral luxation with severe hip dysplasia is not recommended. Overall prognosis of dogs with mild to moderate dysplasia should include arthritis and reluxation.

The radiograph should also be inspected for fractures (Fig. 159–24). If acetabular or femoral fractures are present, closed reduction is not recommended; instead, open reduction with fracture fixation and hip relocation are performed. In one series of hip dislocations in the dog, an 84 per cent success rate was reported; of the failures (16 per cent), two-thirds were associated with either fractures or acetabular dysplasia.[22] It is interesting to observe that the remaining third of the failures were in the miniature poodle. This breed has a propensity for hip luxation and recurrence of luxation.[22,33]

Stability of the hip joint is a function of joint capsule, round ligament of the head of the femur, and surrounding muscles. In addition, femoral neck shaft angles are important.[2,77] The importance of these angles (inclination and anteversion) in the pathogenesis of hip luxation is ill-defined. Because trauma is the primary cause, hip angles are probably insignificant. In one study, the angle of inclination of the femoral head and neck in luxated hips was normal.[33] A similar determination of the angle of anteversion has not been made. The importance of the angle of anteversion in hip dislocation after total hip replacement is better defined. Special care is taken in the implantation of a total hip prosthesis to avoid an excessive anteversion angle and the instability associated with it.[69]

Treatment

The type of definitive treatment of coxofemoral luxation is a function of species, size, other disease, and economics. Reduction and fixation of coxofemoral luxations in the cat are usually not done. Because cats do so well with an excision arthroplasty, this surgical procedure is often performed, in the interests of time and money, as the original definitive treatment. Alternatively, treatment in the cat may be as described for the dog. If surgery is not elected because of financial constraints or other disease, the luxated femoral head may be left to form a false-fibrous joint in its luxated position. Many cats so treated recover fully without surgery.

If severe hip dysplasia is present in a dog with hip luxation, reduction is not recommended. It is preferable to perform an excision arthroplasty or total hip replacement, depending on the size of the dog, economics, and the surgeon's preference. With associated fractures of the femoral head or acetabulum, the fracture should be fixed as outlined in other chapters. The luxation is repaired via an open approach.

Treatment of the luxated hip is via a closed or open approach. Closed reduction of the recently luxated hip is attempted following radiographic examination. Closed reduction is attempted as soon as possible after the injury, depending on the patient's health.

Closed Reduction

The animal is positioned in lateral recumbency with the affected leg uppermost (Fig. 159–25A). A towel or strap is placed over the flank and under the involved leg and tail so that traction on the pelvis may be applied by an assistant as necessary; this arrangement is especially useful in larger dogs. For a left hip luxation, the stifle area is grasped with the right hand as the operator stands ventral to the animal. The left hand is placed on the pelvis with thumb or index finger on the greater trochanter to aid reduction. The affected leg is rotated externally to a moderate degree, abducted, and pulled distally so that the femoral head lies at the acetabulum (Fig. 159–25B). The femur is rotated internally and adducted to a normal position (Fig. 159–25C and D). Preferably, a "pop" is heard as the femoral head firmly seats into its acetabulum. The hip is palpated and put through its full range of motion. Proper reduction should be confirmed by palpation and postoperative radiographs. Postoperatively, the leg is placed in an Ehmer sling or figure-of-eight flexion bandage to prohibit weight-bearing for seven days. Exercise is restricted to walking for two weeks longer.

Unfortunately, the luxated femoral head does not always firmly seat in its acetabulum. If hip conformation is good, improper seating is most likely due to blood clots or tissue debris in the acetabulum or to an inverted joint capsule. The hip is put through its full range of motion while medial pressure is applied to the greater trochanter to expel clotted blood. If this maneuver does not obtain firmer seating, the hip may be reluxated to evert the joint capsule, and another attempt made at closed reduction. If this second attempt is unsuccessful, open reduction is indicated.

If the luxated head seats into the acetabulum without interposed soft tissue, and joint laxity and a tendency to reluxate are still present, more support may be required. In addition to the flexion bandage and exercise restriction, a Devita pin may be inserted, as described later, to provide additional dorsal support to the hip and lessen the likelihood of reluxation.[23] Open reduction and stabilization are recommended: (1) if the luxated head does not seat well in the acetabulum, or interposed soft tissue is suspected; (2) if a hip has reluxated after closed reduction; (3) if

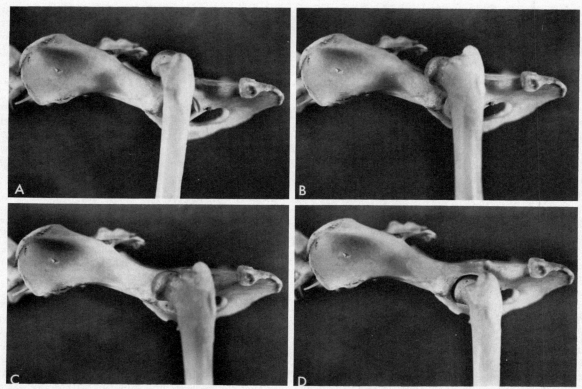

Figure 159–25. *A*, Hip dislocation: the animal is in lateral recumbency with the affected leg uppermost. Note the relationship of the greater trochanter, wing of the ilium, and ischiatic tuberosity. *B*, Reduction of the dislocated hip. The femur is externally rotated, abducted, and pulled distally. *C*, When the femur has been pulled distally so that the femoral head lies at the level of the acetabulum, it is internally rotated to reduce the luxated femoral head into the acetabulum. *D*, The reduced hip dislocation. Note the relationship of the greater trochanter, wing of the ilium, and ischiatic tuberosity.

the hip has been chronically luxated; or (4) if fractures are present.

Devita Pinning

The Devita pin is an intramedullary pin that is placed so that it lies ventral to the lateral aspect of the ischium and dorsal to the femoral head and neck and is embedded into the bone of the wing of the ilium.[23] The pin is inserted through a stab incision in the skin just ventral to the ischiatic tuberosity. The pin is advanced anteriorly, slowly, with a rotating motion. The sciatic nerve is in the path of the pin and will not be speared if the pin is advanced slowly with rotation. The pin is advanced to the femoral neck, and the neck is "palpated" with the tip of the pin. The pin is further advanced anteriorly so that it lies just dorsal to the femoral head and neck and lateral to the dorsal acetabular lip, through the gluteal musculature and into the wing of the ilium (Fig. 159–26). The pin is cut just below the skin and is removed in two to four weeks.

The major complication of Devita pinning is pin migration, which may be serious. Use of a threaded pin in the wing of the ilium may reduce the likelihood of migration. Alternatively, an additional pin may be placed in the ischium at an angle to the Devita pin

and connected to the Devita pin with a Kirschner apparatus to prevent migration.[74]

Open Reduction

Open reduction of coxofemoral luxation may be via the described anterior or dorsal approach. The critical facets of open reduction are that the acetabulum must be cleaned of debris and the joint capsule must be

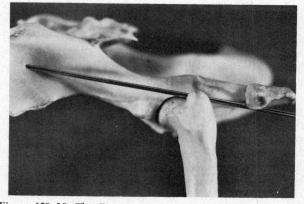

Figure 159–26. The Devita pin, properly placed dorsal to the femoral head/neck, lateral to the dorsal rim of the acetabulum.

sutured. The acetabulum is identified, and any inverted joint capsule is everted. Debris in the acetabulum, such as blood clot, or fibrous tissue, is removed as necessary. Remnants of the round ligament of the head of the femur are removed from the acetabulum and head of the femur. The head of the femur is anatomically replaced into the cleaned and smooth acetabulum. Any tear or incision of the joint capsule is securely sutured with nonabsorbable suture in a simple interrupted, horizontal mattress, or cross-mattress pattern.

In some cases, portions of the fibrous joint capsule cannot be sutured or the joint capsule is avulsed from its acetabular or femoral insertion. In such cases, every attempt should be made to reestablish a joint capsule. Secure suture bites may be taken of: tendon of insertion of internal obturator muscle, origin of vastus lateralis muscles, periosteal origin of deep gluteal muscle on dorsal acetabulum, and fibrous joint capsule. Sutures are placed as necessary to reestablish a joint capsule. If the dorsal acetabulum

has been stripped of joint capsule and the periosteal origin of gluteal muscle, screws or pins may be placed in bony tissue to secure sutures. Similarly, on the femoral side, holes may be drilled from anterior to posterior through the interconnecting ridge of bone, between the femoral head and greater trochanter, to secure sutures.

Closure of the approach to the hip is as previously described. Postoperatively, the leg is placed in a flexion bandage for one week, and exercise is restricted for two weeks longer.

Open Reduction with Relocation of the Greater Trochanter

Open reduction, through the dorsal approach with relocation of the greater trochanter, is highly recommended for luxations that are chronic or recurrent or are unstable after closed reduction.[1,22,33] The primary advantage of using the dorsal approach, is that it allows maximum exposure of the hip joint. The

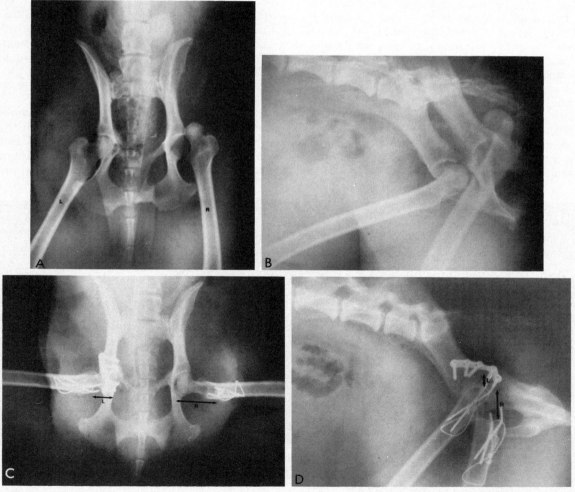

Figure 159–27. A, Hip luxation (R) and fractured acetabulum (L). Preoperative ventrodorsal radiograph. B, Hip luxation and fractured acetabulum. Preoperative lateral radiograph. C, Postoperative ventrodorsal radiograph. Both hips were exposed by the dorsal approach. The greater trochanter was distally relocated on the side of the hip dislocation (R). Note the increased articulotrochanteric distance. D, Postoperative lateral radiograph. Though desirable, a postoperative flexion sling could not be used on the leg with the hip dislocation.

joint capsule may be securely sutured on the anterior, dorsal, and posterior aspects of the joint, as necessary. If joint capsule has been torn from the acetabulum or femur, these bony structures are adequately exposed for placement of screws, pins, or drill holes. The closure of this approach is secure and allows relocation of the greater trochanter in a posterodistal location. Such a relocation increases gluteal muscle tension, abducts and internally rotates the femur (only temporarily until muscle elongation occurs), and firmly seats the femoral head in the acetabulum. This procedure temporarily decreases the angles of inclination and anteversion by abduction and internal rotation, and increases intra-articular hip force, rendering the joint more stable until healing occurs.

Following routine surgical preparation of the dog in lateral recumbency, the previously described dorsal approach to the hip joint is made. The proximal femur is grasped with bone-holding forceps and manipulated to allow identification of the acetabulum. The acetabulum is cleaned of all debris, including blood clot, fibrous tissue, and ligamentous remains. The joint is flushed with sterile saline. The smooth hyaline cartilage of the acetabulum should be apparent. Ligamentous remnants are removed from the head of the femur. The luxation is reduced. The joint capsule is securely sutured with nonabsorbable suture, as described for open reduction. This approach facilitates maximum joint capsule closure.

The surgical site is lavaged and closure is begun. The hind leg is held in abduction by padding or an assistant. The greater trochanter is repositioned approximately one to two centimeters (in an average dog) distal and slightly posterior to its original site. The greater trochanter is fixed in this position by two small pins and a tension band wire (Fig. 159–27).

In the routine fixation of the osteotomized greater trochanter, the pins may be placed closer to the axis of the shaft of the femur. With the laterally relocated greater trochanter, the pins are necessarily placed less parallel to this axis. Recognition of this fact is necessary to prevent the pins from passing beyond the medial cortex of the femur into soft tissue. Some surgeons prefer to make a distal "bed" for the osteotomized greater trochanter. This procedure is unnecessary, because rigid fixation of this fracture allows healing.

Postoperatively, the operated leg is in up to 20 degrees of abduction and mild internal rotation, which return to normal over one or two weeks. A non–weight-bearing flexion sling is placed on the leg for one week, unless the surgeon is very confident of closure or other conditions do not allow a sling to be used (Fig. 159–27D). Exercise is restricted for three weeks.

Open Reduction with Pin Fixation

Open reduction with transarticular pin fixation has been recommended for the management of hip luxations.[8,30,41] This technique ensures that the femoral head remains in the acetabulum. Problems with the technique include bending, breakage, or migration of the pin and perforation of the rectum. The procedure is reserved for those cases in which the joint capsule is severely damaged and closure is not secure.[1]

The animal is positioned in lateral recumbency, and either a dorsal or an anterior approach is made to the hip joint. The luxation is identified, and the joint cleaned. A 1-mm to $5/32$-inch pin,[8,30,41] is inserted from the lateral aspect of the femur, passed through

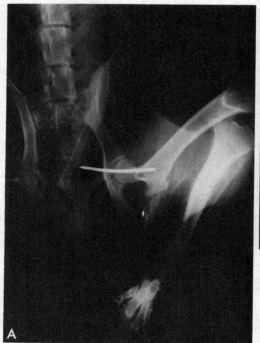

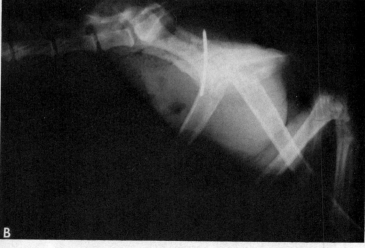

Figure 159–28. A, Ventrodorsal radiograph. The transarticular pin is bent and migrating. B, Lateral radiograph. The leg was maintained in a flexion sling, as can be seen from the position of the distal extremity on the radiograph.

the femoral neck, and made to exit at the fovea capitis of the head of the femur. The luxation is reduced, and the pin is driven through the acetabular fossa of the acetabulum until it passes beyond the medial cortex of the acetabulum. Care is taken not to penetrate the rectum. The pin is bent 90 degrees on the lateral aspect of the femur to aid removal. Closure is routine.

Postoperatively, the leg is placed in a flexion bandage and exercise is absolutely restricted to walking for two weeks. Ten to fourteen days post-operatively, the pin, bandage, and sutures are removed. The most likely complication encountered with this technique is breaking or bending of the pin due to intra-articular shear forces (Fig. 159–28). If a pin breaks, it must be retrieved. A perineal incision is made over the ischium. Cranial dissection, ventral to the internal obturator muscle, is made until the medial acetabulum and pin are encountered and the pin is removed.[41] A bent pin is removed through the lateral approach.

HIP DYSPLASIA

Hip dysplasia (abnormal development of the hip) is a common disorder of the hip joints of dogs (see

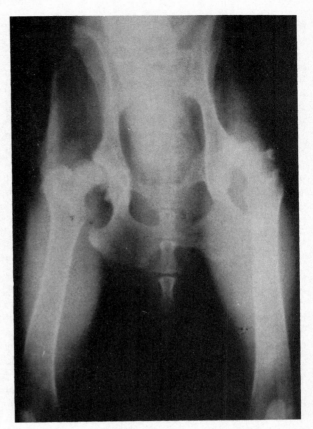

Figure 159–30. Hip dysplasia, degenerative joint disease. Note subluxation, exostoses, and remodelling of the femur and acetabulum.

also Chapter 165). It has a multifactorial etiology, at least part genetic[39] and part nutritional.[38,54] Most likely, a number of different diseases of the hip result in a "dysplastic hip." This endproduct can be clinically characterized in broad terms. Radiographically, the affected hip of a young dog exhibits varying degrees of subluxation, shallowness of the acetabulum, sloping of the acetabular roof, and joint incongruity (Fig. 159–29). With aging, joint incongruity and remodelling become prominent, and degenerative joint disease (osteoarthrosis) is evident (Fig. 159–30).

There have been many different treatments for disorder. The evaluation of the effectiveness of any therapy for hip dysplasia is compounded by two problems. First, the severity of radiographic signs of disease does not necessarily correlate with the severity of clinical signs of disease.[95] Second, the dysplastic dog seems to be most prone to clinical signs when it is young, with hip subluxation and related pain, and to degenerative joint disease (osteoarthrosis) when it is old. The young dog may have a recovery from the clinical signs of hip dysplasia without therapy.[27,80,92] Therefore, the severity and significance of dysplastic disease may be difficult to measure, and the ultimate response to therapy of the young dog may be difficult to evaluate.

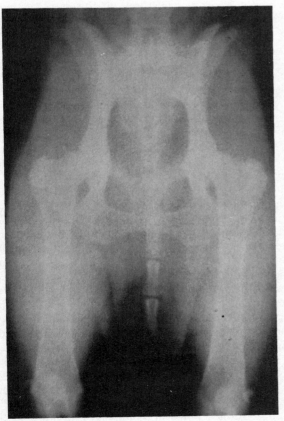

Figure 159–29. Hip dysplasia in a young dog. Note the shallow acetabulum, the sloping of acetabular roof, and the positioning.

Treatment

Therapy may be conservative or surgical. Conservative therapy includes weight loss and medical treatment. Given the nature of hip joint biomechanics, and the fact that hip joint load is approximately four times the load placed on the joint, the benefit of weight loss is obvious. Reduction of weight should be a high priority that is recommended in both the young dog with subluxation and the old dog with osteoarthrosis. Nutritional recommendations should include reduction and maintenance of body weight with a good, name-brand dog food. Overnutrition, in the form of high protein, vitamin, and mineral supplementation, and overfeeding are not recommended.

Medical therapy includes the use of analgesics. Aspirin has been established as effective for the relief of joint pain. A dose of 25 mg/kg is recommended for the dog.[12] Therefore, three 5-grain aspirin tablets may be given to a 35-kg (75-lb) dog twice a day; frequency may be increased to three times a day if necessary. Signs of toxicity are vomiting and gastrointestinal bleeding resulting in black stools. Other effective analgesic therapy includes meclofenamic acid (Arquel)[80] and phenylbutazone (Butazolidin).

Surgical therapy includes many procedures. Total hip prostheses replace the dysplastic articulation. Pelvic and femoral osteotomies reorient it. Excision arthroplasties remove it. Pectinotomy is a muscle release operation that relieves pain but does not affect the development of the dysplastic joint. These procedures are discussed in detail later.

The young dog with subluxation, pain, and the absence of osteoarthritic changes is a candidate for excision arthroplasty, osteotomy, or pectinotomy. The decision to perform one of these procedures is, in large part, a matter of surgeon's preference. Firm guidelines have not been established to determine the surgical procedure that an individual dog should receive. Weight reduction to a lean mass is always recommended.

Ventrodorsal pelvic radiographs should be obtained of the young dysplastic dog (see Fig. 159–29).[96] Hip joint conformation is assessed, revealing varying degrees of subluxation and poor conformation of the acetabulum or femur. Acetabular conformation is examined by looking at the acetabular roof and coverage of the femoral head. The acetabular index of Wiberg assists in this determination. If a shallow acetabulum is present, with poor coverage of the femoral head and sloping acetabular roof, consideration should be given to a pelvic osteotomy.

Femoral conformation should be examined for neck-shaft angles, relation of the greater trochanter to the femoral head, and femoral neck length. If proximal femoral dysplasia is present, especially if acetabular dysplasia is absent, consideration should be given to femoral osteotomy.

Alternatively, pectinotomy or excision arthroplasty may be performed. Excision arthroplasty is a salvage procedure. It is best performed on a smaller dog with severely debilitating dysplasia, in which only one surgical procedure is possible. An advantage of pectinotomy is that excision arthroplasty may always be performed at a later date. Pectinotomy often relieves the clinical signs of dysplasia, though it does not influence the progression of the disease.[14,15] Owing to the fact that part of the etiology of hip dysplasia is genetic, neutering should be discussed.

The older dysplastic dog has degenerative joint disease. Osteophytes and remodelling of the femur and acetabulum are present. Weight reduction to a lean mass and analgesics are always indicated in these dogs. If conservative methods fail to relieve the clinical signs of arthritis due to hip dysplasia, surgery is indicated. Procedures have included pectinotomy and femoral osteotomy; such procedures may result in relief of pain, but their effect is expected to be temporary. Recommended surgical procedures are excision arthroplasty and total hip replacement, which are discussed later.

EXCISION ARTHROPLASTY

Excision arthroplasty is the surgical removal of the femoral head and neck with formation of a false-fibrous joint. The procedure is common as a salvage operation for end-stage diseases of the hip joint, including: aseptic necrosis of the femoral head, chronic hip luxations not responsive to other forms of therapy, debilitating degenerative joint disease not responsive to conservative therapy, septic arthritis,[85] and fractures of the femoral or acetabular component of the hip in which fixation is either not possible or not desired. Excellent results can be expected from excision arthroplasty in the cat.[9] Therefore, this procedure is frequently performed in cats with fractures of the hip joint, whereas definitive repair is more frequently performed in the dog.

Excellent results from excision arthroplasty are expected in the cat, and good results are expected in the dog. A correctly performed excision arthroplasty should result in a pain-free joint. A false-fibrous joint forms as early as two weeks after operation.[25] The fibrous joint that results has a smaller range of motion and less stability than the normal ball-and-socket hip joint. Motion of the leg is therefore not normal, and varying degrees of lameness may be expected. Because the induced changes in hip mobility are unimportant in the majority of household pets, excision arthroplasty results in good to excellent functional results approximately 80 per cent of the time.[9,21,24,29,46,75]

Favorable results of excision arthroplasty are also weight-dependent. Although many large dogs do well with excision arthroplasty, the overall success rate has been found to be less than for smaller dogs.[21,24,29] Other studies, however, found no difference in the success rate of excision arthroplasties between large and small breeds.[9,75] This procedure may also be successfully performed in humans, cows, and horses.[37,60,82] Excision arthroplasty is a good surgical salvage procedure for diseases of the hip. The decision to perform an excision arthroplasty should be based on surgical condition, size and expected use of the animal, and economic constraints.

Surgical Technique

Cranial Approach

The cranial approach to the hip joint is recommended. If the femoral head is luxated, identification of the femoral head and neck is facilitated. If the femoral head is not luxated, the hip joint capsule is incised from the acetabulum along the femoral neck to its lateral-most aspect. The joint capsule, along with the vastus muscles, is elevated from the cranial aspect of the proximal femur to allow complete exposure of the femoral neck. The round ligament of the head of the femur is severed by scalpel, periosteal elevator, or heavy curved scissors. The femoral head is luxated and the femur is externally rotated 90 degrees (Fig. 159–31). Complete elevation of the vastus muscles and joint capsule and 90-degree external rotation of the femur are important in exposure of the complete femoral neck. The femoral head and neck are excised by osteotome, oscillating saw, Gigli wire, or bone cutters. Bone cutters are preferred in small dogs and cats because of their ease of use. If an osteotome is used, its point is placed at the junction of the femoral neck and shaft distally, and the osteotomy is made from distal to proximal (see Fig. 159–31). The osteotome is not directed from proximal to distal because this direction is less precise

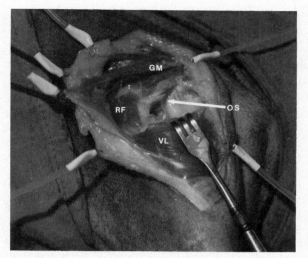

Figure 159–32. The femoral head and neck have been excised. Note the smooth continuity and lack of bony spurs between the osteotomy (OS) and the medial shaft of the femur. GM = gluteal muscles, RF = rectus femoris, VL = vastus lateralis.

and may result in continuation of the osteotomy being beyond the neck of the femur and down the shaft.

Regardless of the means by which the femoral head and neck are removed, the osteotomy must be continuous with the shaft of the femur (Fig. 159–32). The osteotomy must be smooth and there must not be any bony spurs, which occur most commonly distally, at the junction of the osteotomy and femoral shaft, and posteriorly. If bony spurs are palpated they are removed, and the osteotomy is made smooth with rongeurs or bone rasp.

Once a smooth osteotomy is attained, the wound is flushed with sterile saline. The joint capsule is not closed. The wound is closed as described in the cranial approach. In my experience with the anterior approach, stability of the pseudarthrosis is derived from the external rotators of the hip and ventral joint capsule. The integrity of these structures is therefore preserved.

Postoperative Care

Postoperative exercise is encouraged. The animal should begin bearing weight on the leg one to seven days postoperatively, depending upon any original trauma and the animal's nature. Motion of the false hip joint aids formation of a fibrous joint with a good range of motion. If motion is restricted for any reason, the fibrous joint forms with a decreased range of motion and less desirable results.

Cats are allowed normal, unrestricted exercise postoperatively with suture removal in seven to ten days. Dogs are encouraged to use the operated leg on leash walks. Running and jumping are restricted for the first three postoperative weeks. If the animal does not use the leg, and painful bony spurs are not present, physical therapy and swimming should be

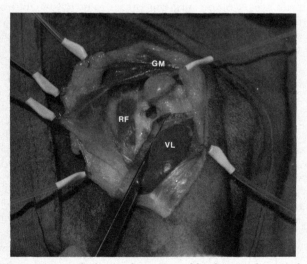

Figure 159–31. The hip has been exposed by the cranial approach (see Fig. 159–14), the ligament of the head of the femur cut, the femoral head luxated, and the femur externally rotated 90°. Note the position and direction of the osteotome.

encouraged. If bony spurs are present, the operation should be performed again.

Alternative Approaches

Excision arthroplasty may be performed through a ventral approach.[21] The ventral joint capsule is incised to allow identification of the junction of the femoral neck and shaft. An osteotome is placed at this point and held at a slight angle from parallel to the femoral shaft, and the osteotomy is performed. The direction and positioning of the osteotome are important. If the femur is held in abduction and the osteotome is directed perpendicular to the surgery table, the entire proximal femur may be osteotomized. This must be avoided by correct direction of the osteotome. Also, the osteotome must be positioned at the junction of the femoral neck and shaft. It is easier, with this approach, to leave in a portion of the femoral neck (distal bony spur). Palpation of the osteotomy site and postoperative radiographs are recommended. Closure is routine. The dorsal (trochanteric osteotomy or gluteal tenotomy) and caudal approaches to the hip joint are not recommended for excision arthroplasty.

Muscle flaps, interposed between the acetabulum and femoral osteotomy, have been recommended in two versions of excision arthroplasty.[9,57] Both procedures use the anterior approach. In one, a flap of deep gluteal muscle is brought across the osteotomy site and sutured to the area of insertion of the iliopsoas muscle on the femur.[9] In the other, a flap of biceps femoris muscle is wrapped around the proximal femur to interpose muscle in the ostectomy site.[57] It is unproven that excision arthroplasty with a muscle flap is superior to a properly performed conventional excision arthroplasty. However, there do not appear to be any contraindications to its use. Regardless of the technique preferred, correct osteotomy of the femoral head and neck with no bony spurs must be attained.

OSTEOTOMIES OF THE HIP

Osteotomies around the hip joint are being performed with increasing frequency in veterinary surgery. They may be divided into three groups: (1) pelvic osteotomy, (2) varisation femoral osteotomy, and (3) derotational femoral osteotomy. The purpose of pelvic osteotomy is to re-orient the acetabulum in order to increase coverage of the femoral head, which previously had inadequate coverage and subluxation (Fig. 159–33). The purpose of femoral osteotomy is to redirect the femoral head and neck into a biomechanically more favorable position. The varisation osteotomy puts the femoral head and neck in a more varus position (decreased angle of inclination). The derotational osteotomy corrects excessive anteversion angles. The varisation and derotational osteotomies may be done together.

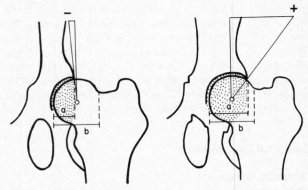

Figure 159–33. Measurement of the acetabular coverage of the femoral head before (left) and after (right) pelvic osteotomy. The center of head to edge of acetabulum angle (Wiberg) has been converted from a negative to a positive value, and dorsal femoral head coverage has been improved. (Reproduced with permission from Schrader, S. C.: Triple osteotomy of the pelvis as a treatment for canine hip dysplasia. J. Am. Vet. Med. Assoc. *178*:39, 1981.)

These procedures have a sound basis in light of the functional anatomy of the hip joint. They are not, however, in common use in veterinary practice at this time. They require technical proficiency in surgery and internal fixation of fractures.

Pelvic Osteotomy

Pelvic osteotomy combines an osteotomy of the ilium with an osteotomy of the ischium and pubis to reposition the acetabulum.[11,42,47,84,89] The degree of acetabular coverage of the femoral head is assessed on the preoperative ventrodorsal radiograph (see Figs. 159–6, 159–8, and 159–33). Correct acetabular repositioning increases coverage to the extent that subluxation of the femoral head does not occur postoperatively.[84] The exact technique is a matter of preference. Some surgeons prefer to osteotomize the pubis,[84,89] whereas others do not.[11,42,47] The osteotomy of the ischium may be made just caudal to the acetabulum[84] or posterior through the ramus of the ischium.[11,42,47] The osteotomy of the ilium may be transverse or stepwise. It is fixed by means of screw and wire[11,42,47,84,89] or bone plate.[86]

The dog is positioned in lateral recumbency with the affected hip up and is draped to allow approach to the ilium and pubis.[89] The ventral pubis is exposed, and the ischium and pubis are cut at the medial aspect of the obturator foramen. The wound is packed with a moist towel.

The ilium and hip joint are exposed via the cranial or dorsal approach. The shaft of the ilium is cut and the hip joint is rotated to obtain greater coverage of the femoral head (see Fig. 159–33). The hip joint is evaluated for stability, and the osteotomized ilium is fixed by bone plate.

An arthrotomy is performed, allowing inspection of the femoral head and acetabulum, documentation of pathological changes, and joint lavage. If the joint capsule is lax, redundant capsule is resected and a firm capsular closure is attained to further hip joint stability.[47] The ischial and pubic osteotomies may be fixed with wire. The surgical wounds are lavaged, and closure is routine. If the dorsal approach is used, the greater trochanter is reattached normally, although others have recommended reattachment in a more posterodistal location.[47,84] Distal relocation of the greater trochanter increases intra-articular hip forces. Such an increase may be advantageous in the short term, but in the dysplastic dog, it may not be advantageous in the long term owing to altered hip biomechanics.

Postoperatively, the angle of Wiberg (see Fig. 159-33) is increased and subluxation of the hip is not present.[84] The leg is placed in a non–weight-bearing sling for two weeks. Depending on the status of the other hip and age of the dog, the same procedure may be performed on the second hip three to six weeks after the first.

This procedure is indicated in large breed dogs five to ten months of age with subluxation of the femoral head and acetabular dysplasia (sloping and shallowness of the acetabular roof) and without secondary osteoarthritic changes. Short-term success of pelvic osteotomy appears encouraging.[47,84,86] Long-term success and progression of hip dysplasia are not well documented.

Varisation Femoral Osteotomy

In this procedure, an intertrochanteric osteotomy, with removal of a wedge-shaped piece of bone, is performed. Removal of this wedge and fixation of the resulting fracture result in varus deviation of the femoral head and neck (Fig. 159–34). The angle of inclination has been decreased. In addition, and probably more important, the greater trochanter is elevated relative to the femoral head. This biomechanical re-orientation of forces should result in a more stable hip and decreased intra-articular forces. Varisation femoral osteotomy has been recommended in young dogs suffering from hip dysplasia and subluxation, to relieve clinical signs and delay the onset of osteoarthrosis, and in older dogs with osteoarthrosis, to relieve pain.[78]

An additional feature of this technique is that the osteotomy is identical to the intertrochanteric osteotomy required to correct excessive anteversion (derotational osteotomy); therefore, anteversion may be corrected at the same time. The primary disadvantage of varisation osteotomy is that it does not correct acetabular dysplasia, which is frequently present in young dysplastic dogs. Short-term success has been good, in that the procedure subjectively delays the onset or progression of osteoarthrosis and adds to stability of the hip joint.[78] However, as with pelvic osteotomy, long-term success and progression of hip dysplasia are not well documented.

This procedure has been recommended in both humans[72] and dogs[78] with osteoarthrosis of the hip joint. It appears to be most appropriate in the young

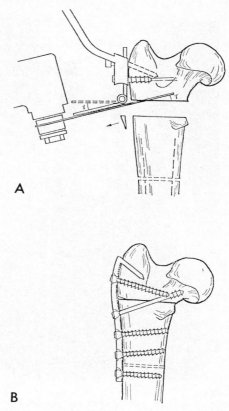

A

B

Figure 159–34. Technique of varus osteotomy. *A,* A wedge of bone is removed. *B,* Fixation is by screws and plate. Note the varus deviation of the head and neck and dorsal displacement of the greater trochanter. (Reproduced with permission from Prieur, W. D.: Double hook plate for intertrochanteric osteotomy in dogs. Synthes Bulletin, Veterinary Bone Surgery, No. 1, Synthes Ltd.)

dog with subluxation and femoral dysplasia and without acetabular dysplasia. The reasons that varisation osteotomy appears to work are multiple. Primarily, it should result in a more stable ball-and-socket articulation. Also, it changes the "wear" points of the femoral head and acetabulum; this re-orientation of pressure may aid in the relief of pain. Finally, it has been subjectively observed in humans with osteoarthritis that relief of pain occurs after various operations about the hip, including muscle decompression, division, or release, osteotomy, and drilling of holes into bone about the hip.[63,98] Symptoms of osteoarthritis of the first carpometacarpal joint in humans have been relieved by osteotomy.[99]

The surgical technique of intertrochanteric osteotomy has been described.[76] The femur is approached laterally. The superficial gluteal muscle is cut at its insertion on the third trochanter and reflected. The vastus lateralis is elevated, and the proximal femur exposed. A femoral osteotomy, from lateral to medial is made just proximal to the second trochanter on the medial aspect of the femur (see Fig. 159–34). A wedge of bone is removed from the proximal femur. A bone plate fixes the proximal segment to the distal segment and stabilizes the osteotomy. Excessive anteversion angles of the femoral head and neck may be corrected by internally rotating the proximal fe-

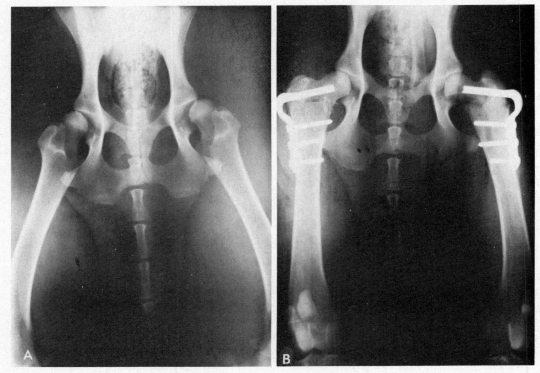

Figure 159–35. A, Ventrodorsal pelvic radiograph of a 10-month-old St. Bernard with coxofemoral subluxation. B, Ventrodorsal radiograph after derotational osteotomy of the right hip. The left hip had been operated on seven weeks earlier. (Reproduced with permission from Nunamaker, D. M.: Surgical correction of large femoral anteversion angles in the dog. J. Am. Vet. Med. Assoc. *165*:1061, 1974.)

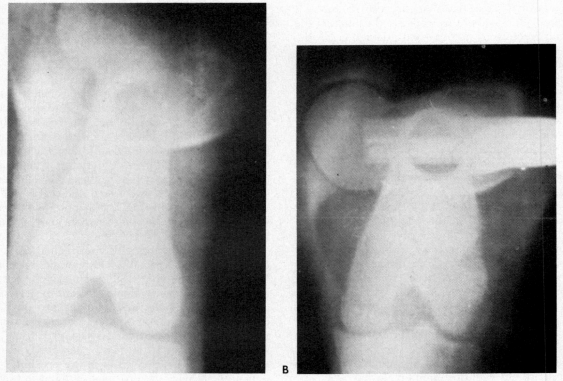

Figure 159–36. A, Preoperative anteversion of the left femur of the dog in Figure 159–35, showing 55° anteversion, with cranial subluxation of the femur. B, Postoperative view showing 0° anteversion, with complete reduction of the femoral head into the acetabulum. (Reproduced with permission from Nunamaker, D. M.: Surgical correction of large femoral anteversion angles in the dog. J. Am. Vet. Med. Assoc. *165*:1061, 1974.)

mur relative to the distal femur prior to plate fixation. Special instruments have been developed to facilitate this operation.[76] After fixation of the osteotomy, the surgical site is lavaged and closed routinely in layers.

Derotational Femoral Osteotomy

Large femoral anteversion angles are associated with hip disease in large breed dogs.[66] Clinical signs included hip pain, instability, and subluxation, hindlimb weakness, and gait irregularity. Palpation of the hip joint reveals that the femoral head slides out of the acetabulum on external rotation of the femur and that the hip may be inwardly rotated more than normal. A properly indicated and performed derotational osteotomy should relieve these signs.

Radiographically, the affected hips show subluxation with minimal or no abnormality of the femoral heads or acetabula.[66] If severe abnormality (degenerative joint disease, shallow acetabulum, flattened femoral head) is present, derotational femoral osteotomy is not indicated, because the results are poorer in such a situation.[66] On the ventrodorsal radiograph, the femoral head and neck have a valgus deformity (Fig. 159–35A). This appearance, not a true increase in the angle of inclination, is due to an increase in the angle of anteversion.[36] If one observes valgus

deformity of the femoral head and neck on the ventrodorsal radiograph, anteversion angles should always be assessed. This assessment may be made by direct measurement of the angle on a radiographic view that is directed down the shaft of the femur (see Figs. 159–9, 159–36, and 159–38C)[67] or by assessing the angle on a true lateral view of the femur. The degree of angulation of the femoral head and neck can be assessed on the true lateral view. This angle may also be calculated using trigonometry and measurements made on the true lateral and ventrodorsal radiographs (Fig. 159–37).[5,83]

Derotational femoral osteotomy is the same as varisation osteotomy. The principal difference is that a wedge of bone is not removed from the intertrochanteric osteotomy unless varisation is desired. The degrees of correction may be assessed by placing Kirschner wires in the proximal and distal fragments or by scoring the bone at the osteotomy site, proximally and distally, prior to the osteotomy. The excessive anteversion angle is corrected to an angle of zero to five degrees.[66] This degree of derotation is assessed according to the orientation of the Kirschner wires or scorings on the bone and the resulting hip stability. Fixation of the osteotomy is done by plate. Postoperatively, radiographs are obtained to assess the anteversion angle and reduction of the femoral head (see Figs. 159–35 and 159–36). For one month postoperatively, exercise is restricted to walking.

Excessive anteversion angles may also be caused iatrogenically. In the fixation of diaphyseal femoral fractures, consideration should be given to rotational instability and fixation in relation to the anteversion angle of the femoral head and neck. Following a

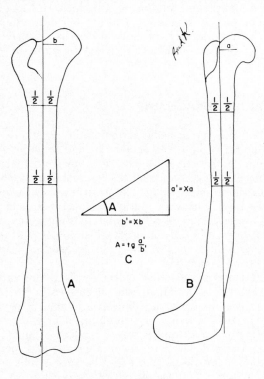

RIGHT TRIANGLE METHOD

Figure 159–37. Calculation of anteversion angle by trigonometry. *A,* The distance "b" is measured on the ventrodorsal view. *B,* The distance "a" is measured on the true lateral view. *C,* The anteversion angle equals tangent a/b. (Reproduced with permission from Bardet, J. F., Rudy, R. L., and Hohn, R. B.: Measurement of femoral torsion in dogs using a biplanar method. Vet. Surg. *12*:1, 1983.)

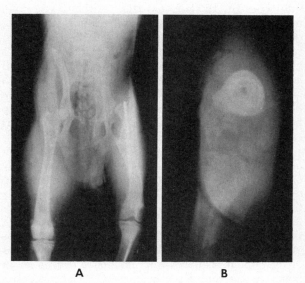

A   **B**

Figure 159–38. Excessive anteversion angle produced iatrogenically with pin fixation of a femoral fracture. *A,* Ventrodorsal radiograph. Note the subluxation and the appearance of a valgus deformity due to an excessive anteversion angle, not an altered angle of inclination. *B,* Anteversion radiograph. The anteversion angle is 55°.

diaphyseal femoral fracture, the proximal fragment rests in external rotation, owing to the strong pull of the external rotators. If the fracture is fixed in this abnormal position, disease results. Experimentally, osteoarthritis developed as early as ten weeks after a 25-degree increase in anteversion was produced by femoral osteotomy.[4]

As with spontaneous excessive anteversion, iatrogenic anteversion results in femoral head subluxation and valgus deformity (Fig. 159–38A). The anteversion angle is assessed by direct measurement or by taking a lateral radiograph. Depending on clinical signs, use, age, and size of the animal, and economic constraints, corrective femoral osteotomy is indicated.

PECTINOTOMY

The pectineus muscle was first implicated in hip dysplasia in 1968. It was proposed that puppies with lax coxofemoral joints and tensed pectineus muscles were prone to hip dysplasia.[3] Since that time, there have been a number of reports dealing with the pectineus muscle and canine hip dysplasia.[10,13,17,31,48,49,50,51,59] The pectineus muscle of two-month-old German shepherd pups has been examined; the pups were later determined to be healthy or dysplastic at two years of age.[52] It was shown that the total number of type I and type II myofibers did not differ in dysplastic and normal dogs. However, the type I and type II muscle fibers were smaller than normal (hypotrophy), and there were smaller myofiber and larger nonmyofiber components to the pectineus muscles of dysplastic dogs.[52] Hypotrophied canine pectineus muscles have been studied further, and myofiber types I and II have been subdivided into types IA, IB, IIA, and IIC.[16] Although the total number of myofiber types is not less in the hypotrophied pectineus muscle, the number of myofiber type IIA is decreased, the number of type IIC is increased, and the numbers of types IA and IB remain unchanged. It was proposed that there is a fault in differentiation of type IIC and IIA muscle fibers.[16] It has not been established if the relationship between the pectineus muscle and hip dysplasia is causal or merely associative.[52]

Regardless of the association between the pectineus muscle and hip dysplasia, pectineal myectomy or tenotomy has no effect on the development of hip dysplasia.[14,15] Even though pectinotomy does not alter the natural course of hip dysplasia, it does seem, at least temporarily, to relieve the pain associated with the dysplastic hip.[61,92,94] The reason for this remains elusive. It is known that in humans with osteoarthritis of the hip, procedures that cut bone, drill holes in bone, or cut muscles relieve pain.[63,96] The relief of pain after cutting of a muscle may be related to relief of muscle spasm or to a reduction in intra-articular stress forces. Many dysplastic puppies recover with

age and without treatment.[27,79,92] The surgical transection in pectinotomy may be at its tendon of origin,[94] at its tendon of insertion,[3,14,40,94] or in the muscle belly.[10,95] All[15,92] or portions of[31] the pectineus muscle have been removed. The site of pectinotomy is a matter of personal preference and may be performed at any level.

The dog is positioned in dorsal recumbency with the hind legs abducted. The pectineus muscle is taut and easily palpated. The skin incision is made directly over the muscle. The femoral artery, vein, and saphenous nerve lie immediately cranial to the pectineus muscle and give rise to a neurovascular bundle that crosses the medial surface of the myotendinous junction of the pectineus muscle.[40] These structures should be identified and preserved. If the pectinotomy is performed proximally, the iliopectineal eminence, proximal tendon of origin of the pectineus muscle, prepubic tendon, and femoral artery and vein are identified. The tendon of origin is elevated from bone with a scalpel, cutting from cranial to caudal, with special care taken to preserve the prepubic tendon, femoral vessels, and underlying deep femoral vessels. If the pectinotomy/pectinectomy is performed more distally, the pectineus muscle and tendon are isolated by blunt dissection, with care taken to preserve the femoral vessels and neurovascular bundle, and are incised with a scalpel. The entire muscle and tendon must be incised. Cut ends are completely separated. Closure is routine in layers. Postoperatively, no special care is required. If relief from pain is achieved, it may be immediate or delayed.[92,94]

TOTAL HIP REPLACEMENT

Total hip replacement refers to the prosthetic replacement of both the acetabular and femoral components of the hip joint. The acetabular prosthesis is high-density polyethylene; the femoral component is a cobalt-chromium alloy. The prostheses are secured to the host bone with methyl methacrylate cement. This replacement is differentiated from resurfacing techniques, whereby an artificial surface is placed on existing bone stock,[88,90] and from procedures that do not utilize cement.[58]

Total hip replacement is frequently performed in humans[93,100] with a high rate of success.[18,20,73] Total hip replacement was introduced into veterinary surgery in 1957, when a prosthetic hip joint was evaluated for probable application in humans.[32] Since that time, there have been a number of attempts to develop a prosthesis that could be successfully used in the dog.[6,19,44,45] In the 1970s, a prosthesis* was developed for the dog that has been successfully used for total hip replacement (Fig. 159–39).[56,70]

---

*Richards Canine II Total Hip System, Richards Manufacturing Co., Memphis, TN.

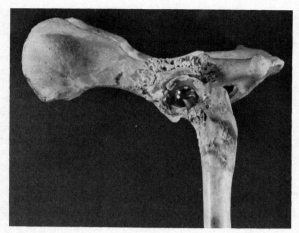

Figure 159–39. Pelvis with total hip prosthesis implanted. Severe exostoses around the acetabulum are due to a chronically luxated, unreduced hip.

Indications

The primary indication for implantation of a total hip prosthesis is disabling hip dysplasia (see Fig. 159–30). Other, less frequently encountered indications, in order of frequency, include: primary osteoarthritis unrelated to hip dysplasia; chronic non-reducible coxofemoral luxations, failed excision arthroplasties, severe fractures, non-unions or malunions of the femoral head, neck, or acetabulum; and avascular necrosis of the femoral head.[70] These indications are basically the same as those for the performance of an excision arthroplasty. The decision to perform either an excision arthroplasty or a total hip replacement is a function of the surgeon, client, and patient. The surgeon must be properly trained in the performance of total hip replacement and dedicated to asepsis and exacting surgical technique.[68,69] The client must be willing to make a large financial investment with a good probability of success and the possibility of total failure. The patient must be large enough to make excision arthroplasty a less desirable method.

Contraindications

Contraindications for the performance of a total hip replacement include neurological dysfunction, systemic or local infection, neoplasia, disease other than in the hip joint, and skeletal immaturity. The most likely neurological dysfunction encountered in a dog that would otherwise be a candidate for total hip replacement is degenerative myelopathy. Degenerative myelopathy is a disease of aged German shepherds that results in hindlimb paresis and proprioceptive deficits that progress to hindlimb paralysis.[45] These dogs may also have hip dysplasia. In no way, however, should the neurological and gait abnormalities be attributed to the dysplastic hips. A neurological examination must be performed.[45] If neurological abnormalities are identified and degen-

erative myelopathy is diagnosed, surgery is contraindicated. The dog with systemic or local infection (pyoderma, abscess, etc.) is not a candidate for total hip replacement. The importance of asepsis cannot be overemphasized. The prosthesis must be free of bacteria that may occur at operation or hematogenously from an infected site elsewhere in the body. Infection must be avoided; otherwise failure occurs.[70] Total hip prostheses are not suitable for replacement of a neoplastic joint, nor should they be implanted in dogs with other disease (e.g., renal failure, ruptured cruciate). Finally, the dog must be skeletally mature. The physeal growth plates must be closed and the cortical bone matured into hard, compact bone. In summary, total hip replacement is contraindicated if the patient is other than a mature dog that is healthy in all respects except for the hip disease.

Preoperative Preparation

Preoperatively, a history, physical examination, and laboratory and radiographic evaluations are obtained. The dog is given a bath one day prior to operation. Anesthesia on the day of operation is routine according to recommended standards. Prophylactic antibiotics are indicated, and are limited to an intraoperative dose.[91] Sodium cephalothin (25 mg/kg) is given intravenously at the time of induction. The entire leg from the hock to beyond the dorsal and ventral midlines is clipped of hair. The patient is positioned with the pelvis in exact lateral recumbency, and a hanging leg preparation is performed.[69]

Surgical Technique

The hip joint is exposed by the dorsal or the anterior approach. Exposure by the anterior approach is enhanced by tenotomy and dorsal retraction of the cranial half of the tendon of insertion of the deep gluteal muscle. The vastus muscles are elevated from the cranial aspect of the proximal femur. The joint capsule is incised from medial (acetabulum) to lateral (femoral), and distally along the cranial margin of the femur (see Fig. 159–14). The ligament of the head of the femur is incised, the femoral head luxated, and the femur externally rotated exactly 90 degrees (see Fig. 159–31). The femoral head and neck are cut at the appropriate angle to accept the femoral prosthesis, which must also be oriented in zero anteversion (Fig. 159–40). The acetabulum is reamed with an appropriate-sized reamer to the level of the medial cortex of the acetabular pelvis. Acetabular reaming must be done to this level to obtain appropriate seating of the acetabular cup, but not beyond into the pelvic cavity. Cancellous bone is removed from the ischium and ilium to create anchor holes for the cemented prosthetic acetabulum (Fig. 159–41). The femoral shaft is prepared to accept the femoral prosthesis (Fig. 159–42). Special instruments for this and

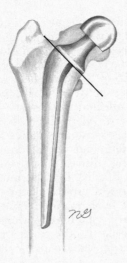

Figure 159–40. The prosthesis is aligned with the long axis of the femoral shaft. The angle and position of the osteotomy are determined by the base of the prosthetic collar. (Reproduced with permission from Olmstead, M. L., Hohn, R. B., and Turner, T. M.: Technique for canine total hip replacement. Vet. Surg. *10*:44, 1981.)

other parts of the procedure are required.* A "relief hole" (3.2-mm) is drilled in the femoral shaft one-third the distance from the proximal end.

The acetabular cup is implanted. The polymethyl methacrylate cement is prepared.[69] One gram of sodium cephalothin powder is mixed with 30 grams of powdered polymer and the liquid monomer is mixed with the powdered polymer. Methyl methacrylate changes from a sticky, to doughy, to cement consistency. It is in the acetabulum while in a doughy consistency. The acetabular prosthesis is seated in the acetabular bed. Exact positioning of the acetabular prosthesis is vital to the success of the procedure and is attained by the correct use of special instruments (Fig. 159–43).[69]

Polymethyl methacrylate cement is prepared as before. The proximal femur is filled with cement. The femoral prosthesis is inserted so that it correctly apposes the femoral osteotomy site and rests in zero anteversion (see Fig. 159–40). Once the polymethyl methacrylate has hardened, the femoral prosthesis is placed into the prosthetic acetabular cup. The surgical site is lavaged with saline, and the joint capsule is securely closed with nonabsorbable suture material. The remainder of the closure is routine.

Postoperative Care

Postoperatively, exercise is restricted to walking for one month. If the other hip is diseased, total replacement of it is recommended only when there are severe clinical signs associated with the diseased hip unresponsive to conservative therapy, when there

---

*Richards Canine II Total Hip System, Richards Manufacturing Co., Memphis, TN.

is good to excellent function of the prosthetic hip, and at least two months have elapsed since the first total hip replacement.

The overall success rate of total hip replacement is very good. Of 221 total hip replacements in 190 dogs with a one-month to five-year follow-up, 91 per cent had good to excellent function.[70] One or more complications occurred in 20 per cent of cases; 59 per cent of those complications were resolved with a good to excellent end result, and 41 per cent (9 per cent of the total) ultimately had fair to poor function.

Complications

A number of complications may occur with total hip replacement. They are minimized if the surgeon is skilled at the surgical procedure and exercises care and exacting technique preoperatively, operatively, and postoperatively. Complications include: dislocation of the femoral prosthesis, osteomyelitis, loose acetabular component, femoral fracture, and sciatic neuropraxia.[70]

Dislocation is the most common complication. Its occurrence is minimized by proper positioning of the acetabular component, avoiding excessive anteversion of femoral component, and tightly closing the joint capsule. Dislocation occurs most frequently

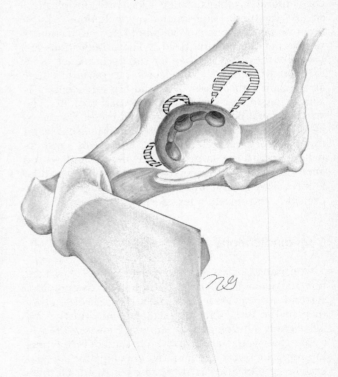

Figure 159–41. Three anchor holes for the polymethyl-methacrylate are created in the acetabular bed. The clear area indicates the original drill holes in the pelvis. A curette can be used to widen the deep portion of these holes, creating a narrowing effect at the opening. This makes it more difficult for the cement to loosen. The holes may be interconnected by a trough. (Reproduced with permission from Olmstead, M. L., Hohn, R. B., and Turner, T. M.: Technique for canine total hip replacement. Vet. Surg. *10*:44, 1981.)

Figure 159–42. *A*, A drill is used to start the hole in the intramedullary canal of the femur. *B*, The fluted reamer is used to widen the opening in the canal. *C*, The femoral rasp is used to achieve the final shape and depth in the reaming process. (Reproduced with permission from Olmstead, M. L., Hohn, R. B., and Turner, T. M.: Technique for canine total hip replacement. Vet Surg. *10*:44, 1981.)

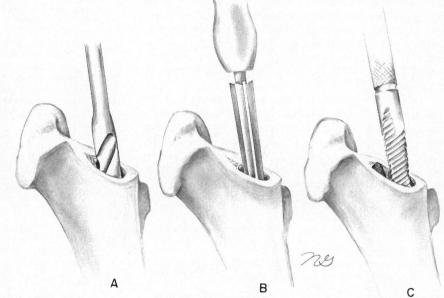

A   B   C

within one month after surgery and usually responds to corrective surgery.[70]

Infection with osteomyelitis is the most devastating complication and ultimately accounts for the majority of failures.[70] Infection is best prevented, but it may still occur operatively or late postoperatively because of hematogenous spread. Removal of the infected prosthesis is indicated, creating an excision arthroplasty.

Loosening of a noninfected acetabular cup may occur because of progressive resorption of bone at the bone-cement interface.[70] Corrective surgery is

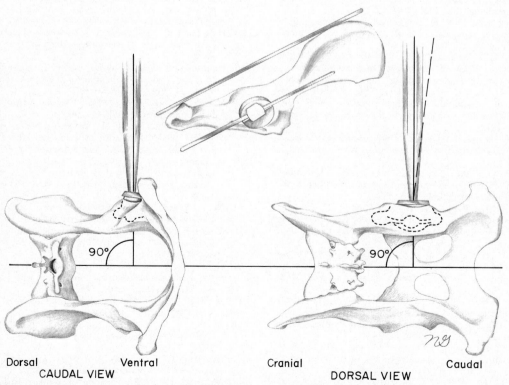

Dorsal   Ventral   Cranial   Caudal
CAUDAL VIEW   DORSAL VIEW

Figure 159–43. The cross bar of the acetabular positioner is held parallel to a line that runs from the cranial dorsal iliac spine to the ischiatic tuberosity. The main shaft of the positioner is aligned perpendicular to the median sagittal plane in a dorsal-to-ventral relationship. It is aligned either perpendicular or tilted slightly toward the ischium in the cranial-to-caudal relationship. (Reproduced with permission from Olmstead, M. L., Hohn, R. B., and Turner, T. M.: Technique for canine total hip replacement. Vet Surg. *10*:44, 1981.)

indicated. Femoral fractures occur infrequently and may be related to intraoperative technique or postoperative trauma. Sciatic neuropraxia occurs because of excessive intraoperative traction on tissues or nerve contact with cement during its exothermic reaction prior to hardening, resulting in a temporary nonfunctional limb. Function returns to normal in one to four months.[70]

Total hip replacement is a viable alternative for the large dog with debilitating hip disease. Results may exceed 90 per cent with a follow-up of up to five years. Results beyond that time are not known in the dog. These results are limited to surgeon who implants the prosthesis with exacting care, technique, and appropriate indications.

1. Alexander, J. W.: Coxofemoral luxations in the dog. Comp. Cont. Ed. 4:575, 1982.
2. Arnoczky, S. P., and Torzilli, P. A.: Biomechanical analysis of forces acting about the canine hip. Am. J. Vet. Res. 42:1581, 1981.
3. Bardens, J. W., and Hardwick, H.: New observations on the diagnosis and cause of hip dysplasia. Vet. Med./Small Anim. Clin. 63:238, 1968.
4. Bardet, J. F.: Femoral torsion and experimental midshaft femoral rotational osteotomies in dogs. Master's thesis, Ohio State University, Columbus, 1981.
5. Bardet, J. F., Rudy, R. L., and Hohn, R. B.: Measurement of femoral torsion in dogs using a biplanar method. Vet. Surg. 12:1, 1983.
6. Bartel, D. L., Dueland, R. T., and Quentin, J. A.: Biomechanical considerations in the design of a total hip prosthesis. J. Am. Anim. Hosp. Assoc. 11:553, 1975.
7. Bassett, F. H., Wilson, J. W., Allen, B. L., and Azuma, H.: Normal vascular anatomy of the head of the femur in puppies with emphasis on the inferior retinacular vessels. J. Bone Jt. Surg., 51A:1139, 1969.
8. Bennett, D., and Duff, S. R.: Transarticular pinning as a treatment for hip luxation in the dog and cat. J. Small Anim. Pract. 21:373, 1980.
9. Berzon, J. L., Howard, P. E., Covell, S. J., et al.: A retrospective study of the efficacy of femoral head and neck excisions in 94 dogs and cats. Vet. Surg. 9:88, 1980.
10. Bowen, J. M., Lewis, R. E., Kneller, S. K., et al.: Progression of hip dysplasia in German shepherd dogs after unilateral pectineal myotomy. J. Am. Vet. Med. Assoc. 161:899, 1972.
11. Brinker, W. O.: Corrective osteotomy procedures for treatment of canine hip dysplasia. Vet. Clin. North Am. 1:467, 1971.
12. Brinker, W. O., Piermattei, D. L., and Flo, G. L.: Handbook of Small Animal Orthopedics and Fracture Treatment. W. B. Saunders, Philadelphia, 1983.
13. Cardinet, G. H., Fedde, M. R., and Tunnell, G. L.: Correlations of histochemical and physiologic properties in normal and hypotrophic pectineus muscles of the dog. Lab. Invest. 27:32, 1972.
14. Cardinet, G. H., Guffy, M. M., and Wallace, L. J.: Canine hip dysplasia: effects of pectineal tenotomy on the coxofemoral joints of German shepherd dogs. Am. Vet. Med. Assoc. 164:591, 1974.
15. Cardinet, G. H., Guffy, M. M., and Wallace, L. J.: Canine hip dysplasia: effects of pectineal myectomy on the coxofemoral joints of greyhound and German shepherd dogs. Am. Vet. Med. Assoc. 165:529, 1974.
16. Cardinet, G. H., Leong, C. L., and Means, P. S.: Myofiber differentiation in normal and hypotrophied canine pectineal muscles. Muscle Nerve, 5:665, 1982.
17. Cardinet, G. H., Wallace, L. J., and Fedde, M. R.: Developmental myopathy in the canine with type II muscle fiber hypotrophy. Arch. Neurol. 21:620, 1969.
18. Carlsson, A. S.: 351 total hip replacements according to Charnley. Acta Orthop. Scand. 53:339, 1981.
19. Creed, J. E., Lumb, W. V., and Smith, K. W.: Stainless steel-vinylidene fluoride resin complete hip prosthesis—evaluation in the dog. Am. J. Vet. Res. 32:757, 1971.
20. Cupic, Z.: Long-term follow-up of Charnley arthroplasty of the hip. Clin. Orthop. Rel. Res. 141:28, 1979.
21. DeAngelis, M., and Hohn, R. B.: The ventral approach to excision arthroplasty of the femoral head. Am. Vet. Med. Assoc. 152:135, 1968.
22. DeAngelis, M., and Prata, R.: Surgical Repair of Coxofemoral Luxation in the Dog. Am. Anim. Hosp. Assoc. 9:175, 1973.
23. Devita, J.: A method of pinning for chronic dislocation of the hip joint. Proc. 89th Ann. Am. Vet. Med. Assoc., p. 191, 1952.
24. Duff, R., and Campbell, J. R.: Long term results of excision arthroplasty of the canine hip. Vet. Rec. 101:181, 1977.
25. Duff, R., and Campbell, J. R.: Effects of experimental excision arthroplasty of the hip joint. Res. Vet. Sci. 24:174, 1978.
26. Fitzgerald, T. C.: Blood supply of the head of the canine femur. Vet. Med. 56:389, 1961.
27. Flo, G. L.: Lameness and disfigurement in the dog. Master's thesis, Michigan State University Press, Lansing, 1978.
28. Fry, P. D.: Observations on the surgical treatment of hip dislocation in the dog and cat. J. Small Anim. Pract. 15:661, 1974.
29. Gendreau, C., and Cawley, A. J.: Excision of the femoral head and neck: the long-term results of 35 operations. Am. Anim. Hosp. Assoc. 13:605, 1977.
30. Gendreau, C., and Rouse, G. P.: Surgical management of the hip. Proc. Ann. Mtg. Am. Anim. Hosp. Assoc. 42:393, 1975.
31. Giardina, J. F., and MacCarthy, A. W.: Salvaging the predysplastic puppy for use as a working dog. Vet. Med./Small Anim. Clin. 67:785, 1972.
32. Gorman, H. A.: A new prosthetic hip joint. Milit. Med. 121:91, 1957.
33. Hammer, D. L.: Recurrent coxofemoral luxations in fifteen dogs and one cat. Am. Vet. Med. Assoc. 177:1018, 1980.
34. Hauptman, J., and Butler, H. C.: Effect of osteotomy of the greater trochanter with tension band fixation on femoral conformation in beagle dogs. Vet. Surg. 8:13, 1979.
35. Hauptman, J., and Butler, H. C.: Measurements of femoral neck-shaft angle in the growing beagle. Vet. Surg. 9:39, 1980.
36. Hauptman, J., Prieur, W. D., Butler, H. C., and Guffy, M. M.: The angle of inclination of the canine femoral head and neck. Vet. Surg. 8:74, 1979.
37. Haw, C. S., and Gray, D. H.: Excision arthroplasty of the hip. Bone Jt. Surg. 58B:44, 1976.
38. Hedhammar, A., Wu, F-M., Krook, L., et al.: Overnutrition and skeletal disease. An experimental study in growing Great Dane dogs. Corn. Vet. 64(Suppl. 5), 1974.
39. Hedhammer, A., Olsson, S-E., Andersson, S-A., et al.: Canine hip dysplasia: study of heritability in 401 litters of German shepherd dogs. Am. Vet. Med. Assoc. 174:1012, 1979.
40. Henry, J. E.: A modified technique for pectineal tendonectomy in the dog. Am. Vet. Med. Assoc. 163:465, 1973.
41. Henry, W. B.: Transarticular K wires for fixation of traumatic hip luxations. Abstract, 10th Ann. Conf. Vet. Orthop. Society, 1983.
42. Henry, W. B., and Wadsworth, P. L.: Pelvic osteotomy in the treatment of subluxation associated with hip dysplasia. Am. Anim. Hosp. Assoc. 11:636, 1975.
43. Herron, M. R.: Coxofemoral luxations in small animals. J. Vet. Orthop. 1:30, 1979.
44. Hoefle, W. D.: A surgical procedure for prosthetic total hip replacement in the dog. J. Am. Anim. Hosp. Assoc. 10:269, 1974.
45. Hoerlein, B. F.: Canine Neurology, Diagnosis and Treatment. W.B. Saunders, Philadelphia, 1978.
46. Hofmeyr, C. F. B.: Excision arthroplasty for canine hip lesions. Mod. Vet. Pract. 47:56, 1966.
47. Hohn, R. B., and Janes, J. M.: Pelvic osteotomy in the treatment of canine hip dysplasia. Clin. Orthop. Rel. Res. 62:70, 1969.

48. Ihemelandu, E. C.: Analysis of pectineal myofiber populations and their relationships to canine hip dysplasia. Diss. Abst. Int. *38B*:4586, 1978.

49. Ihemelandu, E. C.: Genesis of fibre type predominance in canine pectineus muscle hypotrophy. Br. Vet. J. *136*:357, 1980.

50. Ihemelandu, E. C.: Loss of type I fibres in canine pectineus muscle hypotrophy. Acta Anat. *107*:66, 1980.

51. Ihemelandu, E. C., and Cardinet, G. H.: Differences in pectineal muscles of normal and dysplastic German shepherd dogs. Anat. Rec. *187*:610, 1977.

52. Ihemelandu, E. C., Cardinet, G. H., Guffy, M. M., and Wallace, L. J.: Canine hip dysplasia: differences in pectineal muscles of healthy and dysplastic German shepherd dogs when two months old. Am. J. Vet. Res. *44*:411, 1983.

53. Kaderly, R. E., Anderson, W. D., And Anderson, B. G.: Extraosseus vascular supply to the mature dog's coxofemoral joint. Am. J. Vet. Res. *43*:1208, 1982.

54. Kasstrom, H.: Nutrition, weight gain and development of hip dysplasia. Acta Radiol. (Stockh.) [Suppl.] *344*:135, 1975.

55. Leidhott, J. D., and Gorman, H. A.: Teflon hip prosthesis in dogs. Bone Jt. Surg. *47A*:1414, 1965.

56. Lewis, R. H., and Jones, J. P.: A clinical study of canine total hip arthroplasty. Vet. Surg. *9*:20, 1980.

57. Lippincott, C. L.: Improvement of excision arthroplasty of the femoral head and neck utilizing a biceps femoris muscle sling. Am. Anim. Hosp. Assoc. *17*:668, 1981.

58. Lord, G. A., Hardy, J. R., and Kummer, F. J.: An uncemented total hip replacement: experimental study and review of 300 Madreporique arthroplasties. Clin. Orthop. Rel. Res. *141*:2, 1979.

59. Lust, G., Craig, P. H., Ross, G. E., and Geary, J. C.: Studies on pectineus muscles in canine hip dysplasia. Cornell Vet. *62*:628, 1972.

60. Mackay-Smith, M. P.: Management of fracture and luxation of the femoral head in two ponies. Am. Vet. Med. Assoc. *145*:248, 1964.

61. Marcellot, J. P., and Berigaud, R.: Interet de la myetomie du muscle pectine dans le traitement de la dysplasie de la hanche chez le chien: analyse de trente et un cas. Point Veterinaire *9*:87, 1979.

62. Mayer, P. J.: Current concepts of the biomechanics of the hip. Orthop. Rev. *7*:67, 1978.

63. Mercer, W., and Duthie, R. B.: *Orthopedic Surgery.* Williams & Wilkins, Baltimore, 1964.

64. Miller, M. E.: *Anatomy of the Dog.* W.B. Saunders, Philadelphia, 1964.

65. Morris, J. M.: Biomechanical aspects of the hip joint. Orthop. Clin. North Am. *2*:33, 1971.

66. Nunamaker, D. M.: Surgical correction of large femoral anteversion angles in the dog. Am. Vet. Med. Assoc. *165*:1061, 1974.

67. Nunamaker, D. M., Biery, D. N., and Newton, C. D.: Femoral neck anteversion in the dog: its radiographic measurement. J. Am. Vet. Radiol. Soc. *14*:45, 1973.

68. Olmstead, M. L., and Hohn, R. B.: Ergebnisse mit der Hufttotalprothese bei 103 klinischen Fallen an der Ohio State University. Kleintier-Praxis, *25*:407, 1980.

69. Olmstead, M. L., Hohn, R. B., and Turner, T. M.: Technique for canine total hip replacement. Vet. Surg. *10*:44, 1981.

70. Olmstead, M. L., Hohn, R. B., and Turner, T. M.: A five year study of 221 consecutive clinical total hip replacements in the dog. J. Am. Vet. Med. Assoc. *183*:91, 1983.

71. Olsson, S-E.: Roentgen examination of the hip joints of German shepherd dogs. Adv. Small Anim. Pract. *3*:117, 1962.

72. Pauwels, F.: *Biomechanics of the Normal and Diseased Hip.* Springer-Verlag, New York, 1976.

73. Pellici, P. M., Salvati, E. A., and Robinson, H. J.: Mechanical failures in total hip replacement requiring reoperation. Bone Jt. Surg. *61A*:28, 1979.

74. Pettit, G. D.: Coxofemoral luxation. Vet. Clin. North Am. *1*:519, 1971.

75. Piermattei, D. L.: Femoral head ostectomy in the dog: indications, technique, and results in ten cases. Anim. Hosp. *1*:180, 1965.

76. Prieur, W. D.: Double hook plate for intertrochanteric osteotomy in dogs. Synthes Bulletin, Veterinary Bone Surgery No. 1, Synthes LTD., 1900.

77. Prieur, W. D.: Coxarthrosis in the dog. I: Normal and abnormal biomechanics of the hip joint. Vet. Surg. *9*:145, 1980.

78. Prieur, W. D., and Scartazzini, R.: Die Grundlagen und Ergebnisse der intertrochanteren Varisationsosteotomie bei Huftdysplasie. Kleintier-Praxis *25*:393, 1980.

79. Rhodes, W. H., and Jenny, J.: A canine acetabular index. J. Am. Vet. Med. Assoc. *137*:97, 1960.

80. Riser, W. H., and Newton, C. D.: Canine hip dysplasia as a disease. *In* Bojrab, M.J. ed.: *Pathophysiology in Small Animal Surgery.* Lea & Febiger, Philadelphia, 1981.

81. Rivera, L. A., Abdelbaki, Y. Z., Titkemeyer, C. W., and Hulse, D. A.: Arterial supply to the canine hip joint. J. Vet. Orthop. *1*:20, 1979.

82. Sahu, S., and Saxena, O. P.: Excision arthroplasty of the hip in bovines; a report of two cases. Indian Vet. J. *53*:294, 1976.

83. Schawalder, P., and Sterchi, H. P.: Der Centrum-Collum-Diaphyseniwinkel (CCD) und der Antetorsionswinkel (AT) beim Hund. Kleintier-Praxis, *26*:151, 1981.

84. Schrader, S. C.: Triple osteotomy of the pelvis as a treatment for canine hip dysplasia. Am. Vet. Med. Assoc. *178*:39, 1981.

85. Schrader, S. C.: Septic arthritis and osteomyelitis of the hip in six mature dogs. Am. Vet. Med. Assoc. *181*:894, 1982.

86. Slocum, B.: Pelvic osteotomy: a review of 62 cases. Abstract, 10th Ann. Conf. Vet. Orthop. Soc., 1983.

87. Smith, W. S., Coleman, C. R., Olix, M. L., and Slager, R. F.: Etiology of congenital dislocation of the hip. Bone Jt. Surg. *45A*:491, 1963.

88. Steinberg, M. E.: Evolution and development of surface replacement arthroplasty. Orthop. Clin. North Am. *13*:661, 1982.

89. Tarvin, G. B.: Corrective osteotomies for treatment of selected hip joint disorders. *In* Bojrab, M.J. (ed.): *Current Techniques in Small Animal Surgery.* Vol. II. Lea & Febiger, Philadelphia, 1983.

90. Thomas, B. J., and Amstutz, H. C.: Revision surgery for failed surface arthroplasty of the hip. Clin. Orthop. Rel. Res. *170*:42, 1982.

91. Van Scoy, R. E.: Prophylactic use of antimicrobial agents. Mayo Clin. Proc. *52*:701, 1977.

92. Vaughan, L. C., Jones, D. G. C., and Lane, J. G.: Pectineus muscle resection as a treatment for hip dysplasia in dogs. Vet. Rec. *96*:145, 1975.

93. Walker, P. S.: Biomechanics of joints. *In* Resnick, D., and Niwayama, G., (eds.) *Diagnosis of Bone and Joint Disorders.* W. B. Saunders, Philadelphia, 1981.

94. Wallace, L. J.: Pectineus tendonectomy or tenotomy for treating clinical canine hip dysplasia. Vet. Clin. North Am. *1*:455, 1971.

95. Whittick, W. G.: *Canine Orthopedics.* Lea & Febiger, Philadelphia, 1974.

96. Whittington, K. (Chrmn.): Report of Panel on Canine Hip Dysplasia. Am. Vet. Med. Assoc. *139*:791, 1961.

97. Wiberg, G.: Shelf operation in congenital dysplasia of the acetabulum and in subluxation and dislocation of the hip. J. Bone Jt. Surg. *35A*:65, 1953.

98. Wilson, J. N.: The place of surgery in the treatment of osteoarthritis. *In* Ali, S.Y. (ed.): *Proceedings of the Symposium; Normal and Osteoarthrotic Articular Cartilage.* 1973.

99. Wilson, J. N., and Bossley, C. J.: Osteotomy in the treatment of osteoarthritis of the first carpometacarpal joint. J. Bone Jt. Surg. *65B*:179, 1983.

100. Wilson, P. D., Salvati, E. A., Hughes, P. W., et al.: Total prosthetic replacement of the hip. J. Cont. Educ. Orthop. *6*:23, 1978.

J. L. Milton and M. E. Newman

The femur has the highest incidence of fracture, surgical treatment, nonunion, and osteomyelitis in our experience. Because of the proximity of the femur to the trunk, the heavy surrounding musculature, and the complexity of many fractures, adequate alignment and stabilization are often difficult, if not impossible, to achieve by external fixation. Of 2,116 fractures treated at our clinic over a five-year period, 26 per cent involved the femur; internal fixation was recommended as the treatment of choice in nearly all cases. The high incidence of internal fixation as the preferred treatment is reflected in recent studies that report the femur as the most common site of nonunion and osteomyelitis.[6,7,37] These studies demonstrate present inadequacies in commonly used methods of repair and frequency of error in surgical judgment, especially in respect to surgical treatment of complicated femoral fractures.[18]

ANATOMICAL CONSIDERATIONS

Structural Features

The femur consists of a cylindrical shaft and flared, irregularly shaped proximal and distal extremities that absorb the stresses of weight-bearing and muscle contraction and provide a wide range of motion to the limb (Figs. 159–44 and 159–45).

The *proximal end* of the femur is composed of the greater, lesser, and third trochanters and the femoral head and neck. The nearly hemispherical head appears tilted in a dorsocaudal direction on the end of the neck. Its articular surface of hyaline cartilage is supported by dense trabecular bone. A crater-like depression, the fovea capitus, positioned slightly ventral to the central axis, marks the attachment of the

ligament of the head of the femur (ligamentum teres or round ligament). In immature animals, the capital physis is dome-shaped and creates a cup-like depression in the head. The dorsal half of the head is thicker than the ventral portion, with the thickest section located dorsocentrally.

The femoral neck projects obliquely from the shaft in a dorsomedial and slightly cranial direction. The angle of inclination (neck-shaft angle) is approximately 135 to 145 degrees, and the anteversion angle is zero to 40 degrees, with 30 to 35 degrees most commonly reported. These angles vary with the method of determination and the age, size, and conformation of the dog.[2,16,31] The neck is strengthened dorsocranially by a ridge of bone that extends between the head and greater trochanter and ventrally by a thickened continuation of cortical bone from the shaft (calcar). The core of trabecular bone increases progressively in density toward the physis and femoral head. The femoral neck is covered by the fibrous layer of the joint capsule or fibrous periosteum, which possesses little osteogenic potential.

The trochanters are tractional epiphyses and serve as muscle attachments. The lever-arm effect from the greater trochanter and gluteal muscles is important in normal movement, stability, and development of the hip joint. The trochanteric fossa is visible caudally, positioned between the femoral neck and greater trochanter, and is the site of attachment of the external rotator muscles.

The tubular *shaft* (diaphysis, body) is slightly bowed cranially and is narrowest (isthmus) near its middle. The central two-thirds is fairly uniform in diameter and is composed almost entirely of cortical bone with little trabecular support. The adductor muscle attaches along the caudal surface; the remainder of the shaft is free of muscle attachment and is

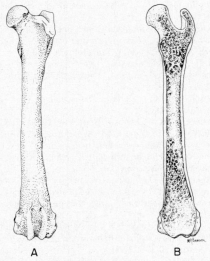

Figure 159–44. *A*, Cranial view of femur. *B*, Frontal section. Note structure and conformation.

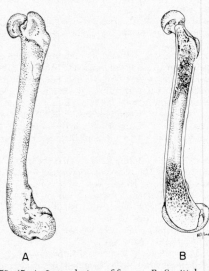

Figure 159–45. *A*, Lateral view of femur. *B*, Sagittal section. Note structure and conformation.

covered by a thin layer of periosteum. The osteons (haversian systems) have a slight spiral pattern and frequently branch.

Proximally and distally, the shaft flares to form the metaphyses; the cortical bone thins, especially cranially, and trabecular bone progressively increases in density. Weight-bearing forces transmitted between the medially positioned femoral head and neck and the caudally positioned condyles create compression forces along the medioproximal and caudodistal shaft and tension forces cranially and laterally. The cranial surface of the *distal metaphysis* is covered by the fibrous layer of the joint capsule (fibrous periosteum), which possesses little osteogenic capacity.

The distal *physis* has an irregular W shape and interdigitates with the epiphysis. The *epiphysis* is composed of a trochlea and two condyles. The comma-shaped condyles extend caudal to the shaft. The cruciate ligaments attach in the intercondylar fossa, and the collateral ligaments attach to the epicondyles. The popliteus and long digital extensor muscles attach within the joint capsule to the cranial and lateral aspect of the lateral condyle, respectively. The gastrocnemius muscle, with its medial and lateral sesamoid bones, originates from the caudal aspect of the condyles and metaphysis.

Blood Supply

The blood supply to the canine *femoral head* (capital epiphysis) (Fig. 159–46) is derived primarily from the lateral and medial circumflex femoral arteries with limited contribution from the caudal gluteal artery.[19,32] The terminology used in describing specific branches of these vessels coincides with human nomenclature and may be confusing. Branches of these vessels ascend the femoral neck (ascending cervical) in the joint capsule, cross the physis, and enter the head adjacent to the articular cartilage (epiphyseal vessels). The core of the femoral neck is supplied by intraosseous branches of these extraosseous ascending cervical vessels and by ascending branches of the nutrient artery. In the immature animal, the capital femoral epiphysis totally depends on the extraosseous ascending cervical arteries for its blood supply, because of the physeal barrier and absence of epiphyseal penetration by vessels of the ligament of the head of the femur.

Fractures of the femoral head and neck may cause complete disruption of this unidirectional blood supply to the peripheral or femoral head segment. Concurrent stripping of the joint capsule from the neck may predispose segments of the neck to avascular necrosis and resorption. However, with proper treatment, these devitalized areas of trabecular bone are rapidly revascularized and remodeled, so that substantial osseous resorption and deformity rarely occur in the dog.[17].

The blood supply to the *shaft* is similar to that in other long bones, with the major contribution from the nutrient artery. In normal mature animals, the periosteal blood flow is minimal and is most evident along the linea aspera, where the adductor muscle fascia attaches. Cortical blood flow is predominantly centrifugal, from medullary to periosteal vessels. An elaborate system of collateral circulation is established by anastomosis among the nutrient, periosteal, and metaphyseal-epiphyseal vessels. However, local blood supply to the dense cortical bone of the shaft through the haversian canals is rather limited, and experimental studies have shown that following destruction of the periosteal and nutrient arterial systems, the metaphyseal-epiphyseal vessels are not capable of maintaining the viability of the middle or central portion of the shaft.[30,39] Most occurrences of nonunion and osteomyelitis with sequestration of the femur involve the central one-third of the femoral shaft.

Sufficient collateral circulation to the *distal metaphysis* and *epiphysis* exists that substantial avascularity following trauma is not a problem.

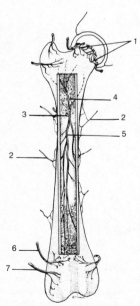

Figure 159–46. Blood supply to the femur, cranial view. *1,* Ascending cervical aa.; *2,* periosteal aa.; *3,* nutrient a.; *4,* ascending branch; *5,* descending branch; *6,* distal metaphyseal a.; *7,* distal epiphyseal a.

Growth

Longitudinal growth of the femur occurs from the proximal and distal physes (Fig. 159–47A). As osseous and muscle development occur, the proximal end forms two epiphyses and physes, the femoral head and the greater trochanter. Although all studies agree that most of the longitudinal growth occurs at the distal physis, the exact percentage reported varies from 60 to 75 per cent.[31,39] Both the physis of the greater trochanter and the femoral head contribute the remainder.

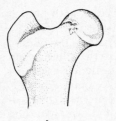
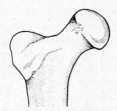
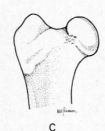

A   B   C

Figure 159–47. Development of proximal femur. *A,* Normal. *B,* Premature closure of trochanteric physis. *C,* Premature closure of capital physis.

Physeal fractures of the distal femur frequently produce premature closure, but the reduction in femoral length rarely presents a clinical problem. Experimental studies on fusion or retardation in growth of the physis of the femoral head or the greater trochanter have produced proximal deformity but little alteration in total length of the femur.[39] Apparently, growth of the distal physis is accelerated to compensate. Deformities reported from premature closure of the trochanteric physis (Fig. 159–47*B*) include shortened trochanter, coxa valga, elongated femoral neck, and narrow femoral neck.[10,41] However, a recent study in beagles demonstrated that these changes were insignificant with respect to normal function of the limb.[15] Deformities following premature closure of the capital physis (Fig. 159–47*C*) include shortened femoral neck, coxa vara, and elongated greater trochanter.[41] Substantial deformity of the femoral head and neck may cause significant malformation of the hip. Unfortunately, the long-term effect of any of these abnormalities has not been studied (Fig. 159–47).

The time of physeal closure is quite variable, with reported ages ranging from six to 14 months.[31,39] Riser[31] studied femoral growth in greyhounds and reported radiographic evidence of closure of the femoral physes between ten and 14 months. He observed that the most rapid growth period was between three and five months, and that 80 per cent of the growth occurred by five months, with 95 per cent by seven months.[31] Sumner-Smith[39] studied the times of physeal closure in a number of breeds and found that the femoral physes close between six and nine months.

FRACTURES OF THE PROXIMAL FEMUR

The rather complex anatomical classification of proximal femoral fractures in human orthopedics has been adapted to veterinary medicine, with division into femoral head and neck, trochanteric, and subtrochanteric fractures (Fig. 159–48).[9,34] Femoral head and neck fractures have been classified as intracapsular (medial) and extracapsular (lateral) and further divided into epiphyseal, physeal, subcapital, transcervical, and basilar. The classification of intracapsular and extracapsular has been used for years in veterinary medicine for establishing a prognosis based upon correlation of fracture location to disruption of blood supply and avascular necrosis of the femoral head. However, avascular necrosis of the femoral head has not been a real problem in veterinary medicine with fractures treated properly by internal fixation, and in this respect, these divisions serve little purpose. The extensive subdivision of neck fractures is not used here because most are treated by similar surgical techniques regardless of their location. A prognosis for any fracture is more accurately based upon a number of factors, including age, animal size, type of fracture, extent of soft tissue damage, and accuracy of treatment.

In this discussion, proximal femoral fractures are divided into four general groups: femoral head and neck, greater trochanter, subtrochanteric, and multiple. Intertrochanteric fractures are included with femoral neck and subtrochanteric fractures. Femoral head and neck fractures are further divided into epiphyseal, physeal, and femoral neck.

Femoral Head and Neck Fractures

In the majority of femoral head and neck fractures, open reduction and internal fixation are required to

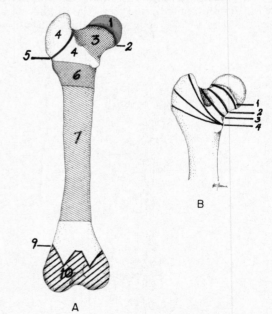

Figure 159–48. *A,* Anatomical classification of femoral fractures. *1,* Capital epiphyseal (femoral head); *2,* capital (proximal) physeal; *3,* femoral neck; *4,* trochanteric and intertrochanteric; *5,* trochanteric physis; *6,* subtrochanteric; *7,* diaphyseal or shaft; *8,* distal metaphyseal (supracondylar); *9,* distal physeal; *10,* distal epiphyseal. *B,* Anatomical classification of femoral neck fractures including intertrochanteric fractures. *1,* Subcapital; *2,* transcervical; *3,* basilar; *4,* intertrochanteric.

achieve the alignment and stabilization necessary for bone healing and return of normal joint function. Regardless of the location of the fracture, treatment involves similar surgical approaches, techniques of fixation, and regimens of aftercare.

The craniolateral approach to the hip provides adequate exposure of the femoral head and acetabulum.[28] Additional exposure of the joint and femoral neck can be obtained by tenotomy of the deep gluteal muscle, reflection of the origin of the vastus lateralis muscle from the neck and greater trochanter, and trochanteric osteotomy (Gorman).

Alignment and stabilization of the fracture are maintained by multiple K-wires, compression screw fixation, or a combination of the two. Excision arthroplasty should be considered a salvage procedure and limited to those fractures that are irreparable or have degenerative changes. Hip prosthesis may be a viable alternative to excision arthroplasty, especially in larger dogs.

Postoperatively, activity should be restricted by cage confinement and leash exercise for at least three weeks. Osseous union should occur between three and six weeks. A gradual return to normal activity is instituted after radiographic examination demonstrates adequate healing. Early immobilization of the limb with a flexion or figure-of-eight bandage for seven to 14 days is optional.

The prognosis is generally good in animals that are treated early with accurate alignment and rigid stabilization. Fracture segments are rapidly revascularized and remodeled. Avascular necrosis is not a problem.

Capital Epiphyseal Fractures

Avulsion fractures of the femoral head occur frequently with coxofemoral luxations (Fig. 159–49A). Coxofemoral luxation occurs predominantly in mature animals after trauma (see "Coxofemoral Luxations").

In most cases the small, predominantly cartilaginous segment is simply excised with the round ligament prior to reduction of the femoral head. Rarely, the avulsed segment is large with substantial subchondral bone. In these cases, a major defect is produced in the femoral head, and additional treatment considerations include internal fixation and excision arthroplasty.

Multiple small (.035- to .045-inch) K-wires are used for fixation (Fig. 159–49B). The pins are inserted in an antegrade or retrograde fashion. With the antegrade technique, the pins are driven from the articular surface into the head and through the neck, cut adjacent to the articular cartilage, and retracted laterally from the neck into the subchondral bone. The free or protruding ends of the pins are cut adjacent to the neck or greater trochanter, and the joint capsule and surgical wound are closed. The limb is immobilized with a flexion or figure-of-eight bandage for seven to ten days postoperatively.

The literature is void of case reports and our experience is too limited to accurately define a prognosis. With proper treatment and postoperative care, the prognosis should be favorable.

Capital Physeal Fractures

The physis is the weak point of the immature skeleton, and trauma frequently results in fracture at this site rather than dislocation. Physeal fractures are the most common fracture of the proximal femur and are observed in animals between four and 11 months of age, with the highest incidence between six and eight months. Most are Salter-Harris type I.

For a number of years, veterinary orthopedics lived with the myth that the dog, like the human, was prone to avascular necrosis following capital physeal

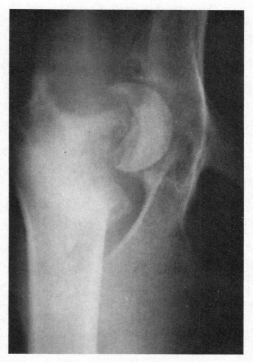

Figure 159–50. Chronic untreated capital physeal fracture shows gross resorption of the ventral portion of the femoral neck, little change in the osseous structure of the femoral head, and remodelling and degeneration of the acetabulum.

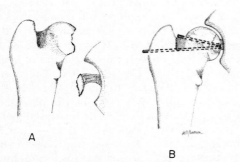

A

B

Figure 159–49. A, Coxofemoral luxation with avulsion fracture of the capital epiphysis. *B,* Stabilization with two Kirschner wires.

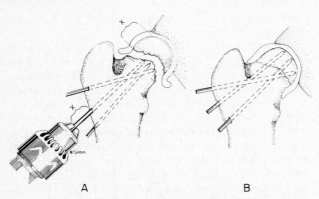

Figure 159–51. Capital physeal fracture treated with multiple Kirschner wires. *A*, Kirschner wires (.062-inch) were inserted in an antegrade fashion to the fracture site. *B*, The fracture was reduced and the K-wires were seated into the subchondral bone.

fractures, regardless of the method of treatment. Disruption of the ascending cervical vessels following a physeal fracture produces avascularity to portions of the femoral head (epiphysis) and neck. Without adequate treatment, the femoral head and neck eventually undergo extensive necrosis and resorption (Fig. 159–50). With proper treatment, however, revascularization rapidly develops, and remodeling and healing readily ensue. Avascular necrosis and resorption are not common with correctly used internal fixation technique—multiple K-wires or a compression screw. The common practice of routinely treating this fracture by excision arthroplasty should be discontinued.

Surgery should not be delayed, since remodeling of the neck produces an incongruent and unstable reduction. Multiple K-wires are most frequently used to stabilize this small epiphyseal segment and offer a simple, comparatively atraumatic technique (Fig. 159–51). Compression screw fixation provides a rigid fixation that promotes revascularization. However, compression of the physis in an actively growing animal may promote premature closure and deformity of the proximal femur.

At least two K-wires or Steinmann pins, .062 to 5/64 (.078) inch, are inserted through the neck and into the femoral head. Retrograde and antegrade techniques of pin placement have been described. Specific steps in the procedure vary with the surgeon's preference.

With the antegrade technique, the pins are inserted from the lateral aspect of the proximal femur into the neck to the level of the fracture. Pin placement is examined at the fracture site, the fracture is reduced, and the pins are driven into subchondral bone of the femoral head. Examination of pin placement at the fracture site is optional, and reduction of the femoral head may precede insertion of the pins. The angle of pin placement varies from parallel to the central axis of the neck to perpendicular to the shaft. The pins should be directed into different segments of the head. It is important to remember that the dorsocentral portion of the head is thickest.

With the retrograde technique, the pins are drilled laterally through the femoral neck from the fracture to emerge along the lateral aspect of the proximal femur. The pins are retracted to the level of the fracture, the fracture is reduced, and the pins are seated into the head. The articular surface of the head is checked for pin penetration by subluxation of the head and visual inspection or by movement of the joint.

The technique of compression screw fixation is described under femoral neck fractures. With capital physeal fractures, the glide hole is drilled through the greater trochanter and femoral neck (near segment) prior to reduction of the fracture.

The prognosis is good for a return to normal function but guarded for normal development of the femoral head and neck. Factors that influence the prognosis include remaining growth potential, type of fracture, degree of fracture displacement (soft tissue damage), and technique and accuracy of treatment. Premature closure of the physis is usually observed within three weeks and, in animals with significant growth potential, may cause shortened femoral neck, deformed femoral head, and eventual degenerative changes in the hip.

Femoral Neck Fractures

Fractures of the femoral neck (subcapital, transcervical, basilar) occur predominantly in mature animals. Most fractures are basilar and are frequently observed with subtrochanteric and trochanteric fractures. Intertrochanteric fractures that are similar to basilar fractures are treated in the same manner as femoral neck fractures (see Fig. 159–48B).

Compression or lag screw techniques and multiple K-wires or Steinmann pins have been used for internal fixation (Fig. 159–52A). Compression screw fixation offers the most rigid stabilization and is principally indicated in large dogs. Multiple K-wires or pins provide satisfactory fixation, especially in small and medium-sized animals.

Specific steps in the compression screw technique may vary according to the surgeon's preference and type of screw used, but the end result—thread purchase in only the far fragment (head) with a glide hole in the near fragment—is common to all techniques.

Reduction of the fracture prior to drilling of the screw hole aids in positioning and aiming the drill in respect to the femoral neck and head. Once reduced, the fracture is stabilized with one or two K-wires (.062-inch) placed eccentrically through the neck and into the head (Fig. 159–52B). To ensure proper direction of the drill, a small pilot hole can be drilled and enlarged after evaluation of placement, a C-shaped drill guide can be used, or a guide pin can be placed adjacent to the femoral neck and head. The thread hole is drilled from the third trochanter through the central core of the neck and into the

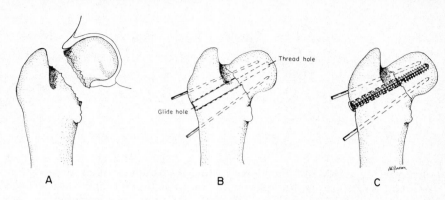

Figure 159–52. A, Femoral neck fracture treated with a compression screw (technique) and Kirschner wires. B, The fracture is stabilized with one or two K-wires and a glide hole and thread hole are created. C, Compression is provided by insertion of the screw.

subchondral bone of the head. The drilling depth can be evaluated by measurements taken from a parallel course along the exposed cranial aspect of the head, neck, and greater trochanter. For a fully threaded screw, a glide hole is created in the outer (near) segment by enlarging the channel to the diameter of the screw. The length of the hole is measured with a depth gauge, and two millimeters are subtracted from the measurement to allow for compression at the fracture and sinking of the screw head (Fig. 159–52C). The thread hole in the far segment (head) is tapped for a non–self-tapping screw, and the screw is inserted.

An alternative technique involves drilling the glide hole first (antegrade or retrograde), followed by reduction of the fracture, stabilization with K-wires, and drilling of the thread hole through the appropriate drill guide inserted in the glide hole.

The technique for insertion of multiple K-wires or Steinmann pins is similar to that described previously for physeal fractures. The fracture is usually reduced prior to antegrade insertion of the pins. Immobilization of the limb postoperatively with a flexion bandage is optional but is usually not employed. Activity is restricted by cage confinement and leash exercise for three to six weeks.

Fractures of the Greater Trochanter

Fractures of the greater trochanter are not common and occur most frequently at the trochanteric physis in immature animals in conjunction with capital physeal fractures. Fractures of the greater trochanter in mature animals may occur with fractures of the femoral neck or dislocations of the hip.

The avulsed greater trochanter is subject to tractional and shearing forces from the middle gluteal muscle and compression forces from the vastus lateralis muscle. Although fixation with a compression screw or multiple pins and a tension band wire is usually recommended, interfragmentary compression is not always required to provide adequate stabilization in this broad-based angular fracture of trabecular bone.

A lateral approach to the proximal femur provides surgical exposure. The vastus lateralis muscle may be transected from its origin on the greater trochanter to facilitate exposure of the fracture. Fractures in immature animals are treated satisfactorily with multiple K-wires or Steinmann pins directed diagonally into the medial cortex of the proximal diaphysis. Tension band wire is optional but should be used for additional stabilization when needed and without fear

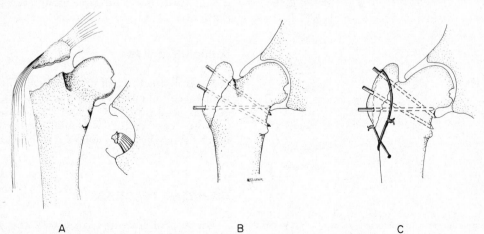

Figure 159–53. A, Fracture of the greater trochanter with coxofemoral luxation and avulsion of a fragment of the femoral head. B, Following reduction of the femoral head, the greater trochanter is fixed with three Kirschner wires. C, Tension band wiring may be used for additional support.

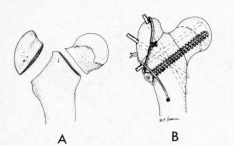
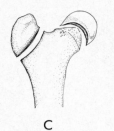
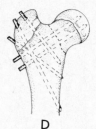

A   B   C   D

Figure 159–54. A and *C,* Fracture of the greater trochanter and femoral neck or capital physis. *B,* Treated with multiple pins, tension band wiring, and a compression screw. *D,* Treated with multiple pins.

of producing substantial functional disturbance from premature closure of the physis in an immature animal (Figs. 159–53 and 159–54). In mature animals, interfragmentary compression with a bone screw or multiple pins and tension band wire is recommended.

Subtrochanteric Fractures

Subtrochanteric fractures are not common and are most often observed with multiple fractures of the proximal femur. Repair of such fractures can be difficult because of the frequent presence of comminution, involvement of the femoral neck, the comparatively short proximal segment, and the large medullary canal and tapered contour of the subtrochanteric area. Certain intertrochanteric fractures are treated like subtrochanteric fractures.

A lateral approach to the proximal femur exposes the fracture.[28] The origin of the vastus lateralis is reflected to increase exposure. Surgical treatments include bone plating and intramedullary fixation techniques (Fig. 159–55).

Bone plating techniques (compression, neutralization, buttress) are technically more complicated but offer greater immobilization of the fracture. Bone plates are especially indicated in large dogs and for comminuted fractures. The plate must be contoured to the greater trochanter so that adequate numbers of screws can be anchored into the short proximal segment. Screw purchase can be increased by placing the plate so that one screw is inserted into the central core of the femoral neck and by bending the proximal end of the plate over the greater trochanter so that the most proximal screw can be directed distally and medially into the base of the femoral neck.

Commonly used intramedullary fixation techniques include use of a single Steinmann pin, use of multiple pins, and Rush pinning. Intramedullary fixation has more application in simple transverse, oblique, and spiral fractures, especially in small and medium-sized animals. In this metaphyseal fracture, involving a short proximal segment with a comparatively large medullary canal, a single intramedullary pin provides little resistance against rotational, compression, and shear forces. Multiple intramedullary pins and Rush pins provide more stable fixations. Rush pin principles can be effectively used with multiple Steinmann pins. Supplemental fixation with cerclage and hemicerclage wire or external pin splints is often indicated.

Activity is restricted by cage confinement and leash exercise for three to six weeks. Periodic radiographic examinations are used to evaluate the healing process, which is usually complete between six and 12 weeks. The Steinmann pins are removed following union; Rush pins and bone plates are not removed routinely.

Multiple Fractures

Multiple fractures of the proximal femur, involving various combinations of femoral neck, greater trochanter, and proximal metaphyseal (subtrochanteric) fractures, are treated by combining the various techniques described for each of the individual fractures (see Figs. 159–54 and 159–55).

DIAPHYSEAL FRACTURES

Diaphyseal fractures constitute the greatest percentage of femoral fractures. The tubular shape and cortical structure of the shaft provide the necessary strength for absorbing and transferring the tremendous forces of weight-bearing and muscle contraction.

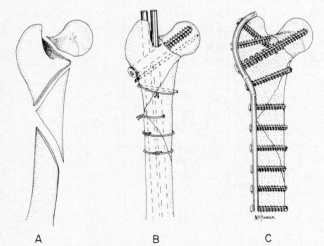

A   B   C

Figure 159–55. A, A comminuted fracture of the proximal femur involving the subtrochanteric area and femoral neck. *B,* Repaired by compression screw fixation of the neck fracture, axial alignment with multiple pins, and fragment stabilization with cerclage and hemicerclage wiring and a transcortical pin. *C,* Repaired by bone plating (neutralization technique). The plate is positioned so that a screw can be inserted properly into the neck.

The high energy absorbed by the bone necessary to create a fracture often produces explosive, comminuted-type fractures. Diaphyseal fractures are noted for complexity of comminution and difficulty of repair. Extensive soft tissue damage and loss of periosteal and medullary blood supply predispose this cortical area to problems associated with inadequate revascularization—nonunion and osteomyelitis. Three general groups of fractures occur: transverse, oblique-spiral, and comminuted. Compound fractures are rare because of the heavy surrounding musculature. The type of fracture is important in considering the forces that must be neutralized by the internal fixation device: a transverse fracture involves rotational and bending forces; oblique fractures, shearing, bending, and rotational forces; and comminuted fractures, compression, rotational, and bending forces. Internal fixation techniques that have been used in the treatment of femoral shaft fractures include bone plating (compression, neutralization, and buttress techniques) and intramedullary fixation (with single Steinmann pin, multiple pins, Rush pins, and Kuntscher nail). The proximity of the femur to the body and the heavy musculature of the thigh make alignment and stabilization of the fracture difficult, if not impossible, to achieve by external fixation.

Although Kirschner half-pin splints have been recommended as a method for treating femoral fractures, the strength of fixation is not as great as with plates and intramedullary devices. The use of such splints as primary fixation must be viewed cautiously. However, they offer much needed supplemental support to intramedullary fixation techniques in the treatment of femoral fractures.

Bone plating techniques offer rigid stabilization of the fracture against all forces that act on the bone. They are indicated for treatment of any diaphyseal fracture of the femur. Their use is limited primarily by the cost of treatment and by the required equipment and skills for application. Bone plating techniques are especially indicated in mature dogs weighing more than 20 to 25 kg. The plate is applied to the lateral or craniolateral (tension) side of the shaft, and accepted techniques and principles of application are followed. Interfragmentary fixation with compression screws, cerclage wires, and transcortical pins can be used in comminuted fractures. The independent use of bone screws in treatment of femoral shaft fractures should be questioned because of inadequate strength of fixation.

The most common method of intramedullary fixation is a single Steinmann pin inserted in a retrograde fashion. Internal fixation with a single, smooth, round rod will not stabilize a fracture against all forces that act on the bone. Intramedullary pins provide longitudinal (axial) alignment and resist bending and, to some degree, shearing forces. Single pins are ineffective in stabilizing diaphyseal fractures against rotation (torsion) and compression. For this reason, this technique has its greatest application in immature dogs with good osteogenic capacity; in small to medium-sized dogs with comparatively small bones and low body weight; for oblique and spiral fractures in which fixation can be supplemented by wiring techniques; and for certain transverse fractures whose opposing surfaces interdigitate to provide rotational stability. Pin size and seating are important factors in achieving maximum stability. Pin size is determined by the degree of fixation sought from the pin. The more the pin fills the medullary canal and binds the inner cortex, the more accurate the anatomical alignment and the greater the resistance to rotation and shear. As a general rule, a single pin should comfortably fill the medullary canal at the isthmus (narrowest point). Stabilization from a small pin can be maximized by directing the pin obliquely through the medullary canal so that it rests against and binds the caudal aspect of the shaft—in effect, applying the Rush pin principle by using a straight pin in a curved bone.

Ideally, the pin should be seated in the subchondral bone of the condyles. Cranial bowing of the femur predisposes to shallow seating of the pin in the cranial metaphyseal area near the trochlea. Pins that do not completely fill the medullary canal can be directed obliquely so that seating is in the caudomedial aspect of the distal segment. Over-reduction of the distal segment aids proper seating of the pin but may create malalignment and instability at the fracture.

Multiple pins, Rush pins, and Küntscher nails provide greater stability than a single pin but involve more complicated techniques of application. Multiple pins are commonly used in diaphyseal fractures of the femur, especially in transverse and comminuted fractures in large dogs. Stabilization against rotation is increased, but compression forces are not neutralized and should be of concern with comminuted fractures. The medullary blood supply is disturbed, but vascular spaces are preserved between and around the pins.

Rush pins and Küntscher nails are similar in application to multiple pins, but are not commonly used in the treatment of diaphyseal fractures of the femur. However, the Küntscher nail provides the most rigid intramedullary fixation.

Supplemental fixation with wiring techniques and Kirschner external pin splints are frequently used to increase stabilization following intramedullary fixation. Cerclage and hemi-cerclage wirings are used with oblique, spiral, and comminuted fractures; their independent use in these femoral fractures should be discouraged because of questionable strength of fixation. The Kirschner device is used with transverse and comminuted fractures to prevent rotation and collapse of the fracture.

Transverse Fractures

Transverse fractures can be treated by compression plating or by various intramedullary fixation tech-

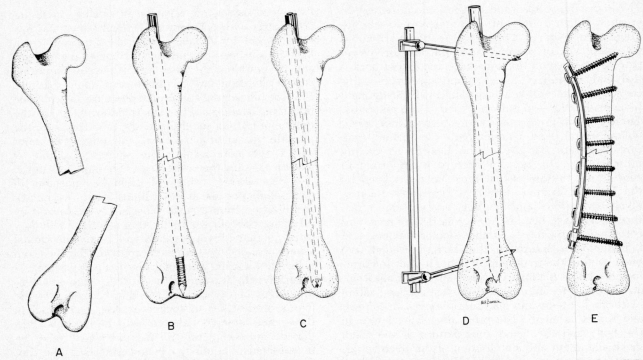

B   C   D   E

A

Figure 159–56. *A,* A transverse midshaft fracture. Treated with a single intramedullary pin *(B),* multiple pinning (pins placed parallel) *(C),* intramedullary pin and a two-pin, half-pin splint *(D),* and a bone plate (compression technique) *(E).*

niques (Fig. 159–56). Compression plating provides a rigid fixation by abutting the fragments and eliminating or decreasing the fracture gap. The plate is under minimal stress, because forces can be transferred directly from one bone segment to the other, and plate failure, in these cases, is rare.

Intramedullary fixation with a single Steinmann pin does not eliminate the detrimental forces of torsion or rotation. Complete filling of the medullary canal with the pin and accurate alignment of the fragment so that the opposing surfaces interdigitate increase stabilization. Supplemental fixation with a Kirschner 2-pin, half-pin splint or a figure-of-eight wiring technique is often indicated. Multiple pins, Rush pins, and Küntscher nails provide more rigid fixation and are especially indicated in large dogs.

In small immature animals under six months of age with good osteogenic capacity, closed reduction and blind pinning may be used successfully. Reduction and stabilization achieved by this technique are adequate for bone healing but are usually not as good as those that can be achieved by open reduction.

Oblique and Spiral Fractures

Oblique and spiral fractures of the femur can be satisfactorily repaired with a number of techniques (Fig. 159–57). Intramedullary fixation combined with cerclage and hemi-cerclage wirings provides good alignment and stabilization (Fig. 159–57B). Pin size and filling of the medullary canal with the device are not critical in these fractures, because axial stabili-

zation from the pin(s) is supplemented by wiring techniques. The uniform tubular shaft is conducive to various wiring techniques.

Compression screws, used in conjunction with a

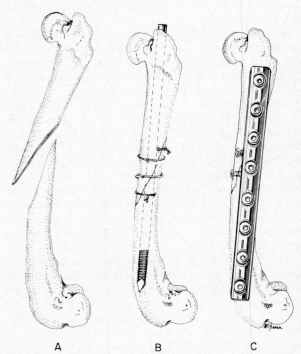

A   B   C

Figure 159–57. *A,* An oblique diaphyseal fracture. *B,* Repaired with intramedullary pinning and hemicerclage and cerclage wiring and *(C),* a bone plate and compression screws (neutralization plating).

bone plate (neutralization plating), provide rigid fixation by interfragmentary compression and accurate alignment with minimal fracture gap (Fig. 159–57C). The plate and screws are under minimal stress, and complications are not common. The independent use of compression screws has been advocated with certain spiral fractures. However, the use of this technique in a bone such as the femur should be questioned because of inadequate strength of fixation.

Comminuted Fractures

Comminuted fractures of the femoral shaft are often presented with small fragments that are especially difficult to align accurately and stabilize completely. These complicated fractures require sophisticated repair techniques capable of resisting compression, bending, and rotation (Fig. 159–58). Rebuilding of the fractures so that all fragments are accurately aligned and gaps are eliminated is often impossible. Malalignment and substantial osseous defects decrease fixation and shift stresses from the bone to the appliance, predisposing to failure. Nonunion and osteomyelitis have their highest incidence in these fractures.

Intramedullary fixation supplemented with wiring techniques is commonly used to treat comminuted fractures of the femur (Fig. 159–58B). Compression forces on the fracture are not completely neutralized and tend to cause collapse and loss of fixation. Stabilization can be increased by using multiple pins or a Kuntscher nail. Additional fixation with a Kirschner two-pin, half-pin splint provides support against compression and rotation.

Bone plating with interfragmentary compression screws (neutralization or buttress plating) provides the most stable reduction and is especially indicated in medium, large, and giant breeds (Fig. 159–58C and D). With small fragments, cerclage wire may be used instead of screws for alignment and stabilization. When cortical defects exist or the fracture cannot be completely rebuilt with compression screws or wire, the plate buttresses the fracture area and absorbs the stresses of weight-bearing. Substantial gap formation opposite the plate allows compression and bending movement and predisposes the plate and screws to loosening or failure.

Because of the comparatively high percentage of complications associated with internal fixation of comminuted femoral shaft fractures, special consideration should be given to surgical technique, strength of appliance, and postoperative care. Bone grafts should be used when fracture gaps and osseous defects exist.

DISTAL FEMORAL FRACTURES

Fractures of the distal femur can be classified as metaphyseal, physeal, or epiphyseal. The predominantly trabecular bone in this area of the femur possesses a rich blood supply and excellent osteogenic potential, which support the healing response. Contrarily, substantial obstacles to rigid fixation and rapid bone healing are the proximity of the fracture to the stifle, the short distal fracture segment, the large proximal medullary canal, the tapered diameter of the metaphysis, and the outer layer of articular cartilage or thin cortical bone.

The distal extremity of the femur is surgically exposed by a lateral approach to the femoral shaft and stifle.[28] Medial displacement of the quadriceps and patella facilitates exposure of the condyles. Various bone plating and intramedullary fixation techniques are used. Intramedullary fixation techniques

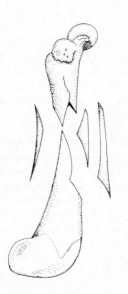 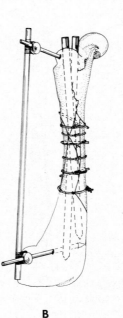 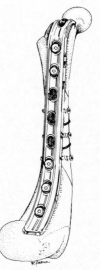 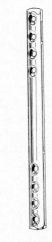

Figure 159–58. A, A comminuted diaphyseal fracture. B, Repaired with multiple intramedullary pins, cerclage wiring, transcortical pins, and a two-pin, half-pin splint. C, Repaired with a bone plate (buttress technique) with fragment alignment by compression screws and cerclage wiring. D, Plates without screw slots over the fracture area offer greater strength.

      A   B   C   D

are more adaptable to physeal and epiphyseal fractures with a short distal segment and articular involvement.

Postoperatively, use of the limb is controlled by cage confinement and leash walks for three to six weeks. Rigid immobilization with a splint or cast should be avoided, because early use of the leg is important in the normal development of the joint and surrounding musculature. Every attempt should be made to satisfactorily stabilize the fracture internally so that early function is returned and restricted joint movement is avoided. Normal joint development and bone growth are of particular concern in physeal fractures of immature animals.

The prognosis for return to normal function is good following accurate alignment and satisfactory stabilization. Physeal fractures in immature animals with substantial growth potential, comminuted fractures, and fractures that involve the articular surface have more guarded prognoses.

Metaphyseal Fractures

Transverse and comminuted fractures are the most common fractures at this junctional area between the (cortical) diaphysis and (cancellous) epiphysis. Comminuted fractures can be especially difficult to treat because of the factors previously listed. The femoropatellar joint capsule covers the cranial aspect of the metaphysis and is disrupted by the fracture.

Bone plating (compression, neutralization, buttress) produces the most stable reduction and is the preferred treatment for large dogs and comminuted fractures (Fig. 159–59C). The use of a bone plate may be limited by the length of the short distal

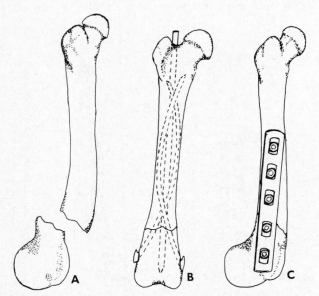

Figure 159–59. A, Transverse fracture of the distal metaphysis. B, Repaired with Rush pins and an intramedullary pin. C, Repaired with a compression plating technique.

segment in respect to adequate screw fixation. Cancellous bone screws may be needed to increase holding power in the cancellous bone of the metaphyseal-epiphyseal area.

Intramedullary fixation techniques using a single Steinmann pin, multiple pins, and Rush pins have been used successfully (Fig. 159–59B). However, stabilization may be inadequate with these intramedullary techniques because of the morphology of the bone and the type of fracture. The large medullary canal and short distal segment make stabilization with a single Steinmann pin difficult. Multiple Rush pins or Steinmann pins, used according to Rush pin principles, provide greater fixation and are usually preferred over a single pin. Over-reduction of the short distal segment facilitates seating of the pin in the condyles, but the resultant malalignment at the fracture may decrease stabilization. Simple metaphyseal fractures, in the supracondylar region, can be repaired with any of the techniques described for Salter type I or II fractures of the physis.

Additional fixation is often needed and can be provided with Kirschner two-pin, half-pin splints, compression screws, or various wiring techniques. The type of fracture dictates the method of supplemental fixation.

Physeal Fractures

Physeal fractures occur in immature animals between three and 11 months of age, with the greatest incidence between five and eight months. Most physeal fractures in the dog are Salter type II and those in the cat are Salter type I. Salter types III and IV are rare in both species. Type V compression fractures may occur in conjunction with any of the other physeal fractures and retard growth. The degree of retardation is related to the age of the animal, the method of treatment, and the amount of trauma to the physis (type of fracture) and surrounding tissue.

Various methods of treatment have been described, including flexion bandages, Schroeder-Thomas splints, Kirschner external pin splints, single intramedullary pins, double intramedullary pins, Rush pins, cross-pins, bone plates, bone screws, staples, and orthopedic wire (Fig. 159–60). Interference with growth is a consideration in the selection of the method of repair. However, its importance has probably been overemphasized, because premature closure of the physis commonly occurs as a result of the initial trauma regardless of the method of treatment, and most physeal fractures occur in dogs more than five months of age who have already achieved over 90 per cent of their skeletal growth. The method of treatment should provide adequate stabilization but, in dogs under five months of age, should not mechanically bridge the physis. The morphology of the metaphyseal-epiphyseal junction—protuberances from the metaphyseal segment and corresponding

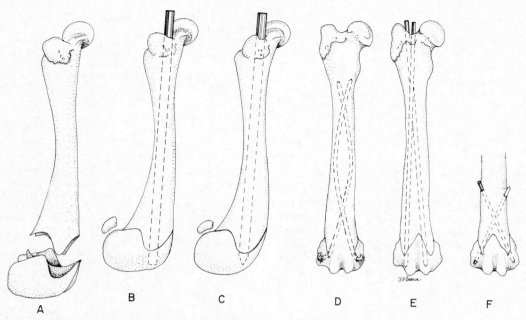

Figure 159–60. A, Distal physeal fracture. Treated by intramedullary pinning (antegrade) *(B)*, retrograde intramedullary pinning *(C)*, Rush pinning *(D)*, double pinning *(E)*, and cross-pinning *(F)*.

fossae in the epiphyseal segment—contributes to stabilization following reduction of the fracture.

Salter-Harris Type I and Type II Fractures:

A single intramedullary pin interferes minimally with bone growth and provides adequate stabilization of the fractures whose opposing surfaces interlock following anatomical reduction. This technique is especially indicated in dogs three to four months of age with substantial growth potential. In large dogs, however, fixation of the fracture using single pin fixation may be inadequate to allow early use of the limb.

The small nonthreaded Steinmann pin is placed longitudinally into the proximal and distal segments with either a retrograde or an antegrade technique. The pin does not fill the medullary canal. It is directed along the caudal aspect of the shaft so that maximum seating occurs in the epiphyseal segment. Retrograde insertion avoids damage to the articular cartilage but may require over-reduction of the epiphyseal segment to assure good seating. Antegrade insertion through the trochlea damages articular cartilage but provides binding of the blunted pin throughout its length in the epiphyseal segment. Either technique can be used with satisfactory results.

Double pins, Rush pins and cross-pins provide more than one point of fixation, thereby increasing stabilization and making their application especially indicated in large dogs. With the double-pinning technique, the pins are inserted retrograde so that they are seated in the medial and lateral condyle. Pin protrusion from the trochanteric fossa facilitates removal following healing. Rush pins are inserted from the medial and lateral epicondylar area into the metaphyseal segment. Steinmann pins may be used in a similar fashion. The pins are inserted at approximately a 30-degree angle to the long axis of the bone and should intersect above the fracture. Cross-pins are inserted in a similar fashion but should penetrate cortical bone of the metaphyseal segment. These small, nonthreaded pins are directed at opposing angles and should intersect or cross above the fracture. Stabilization can be increased by increasing the number of pins. Rush pins and cross-pins are not removed routinely.

Salter-Harris Type III and Type IV (Intercondylar) Fractures

Intercondylar fractures rarely occur. Following such a fracture, the collateral and cruciate ligaments remain attached and maintain some degree of intercondylar alignment, and poor-quality radiographs may fail to demonstrate the intercondylar fracture. Fractures in the supracondylar area that involve the trochlea or occur below the area of the physis should be suspected of having an intercondylar component.

Simple intercondylar fractures most often involve the medial condyle. Multiple Kirschner wires, compression screws, and various combinations of the two have been used for fixation. Multiple pins are most indicated in immature animals and small dogs and cats. The rigid fixation provided by compression screws is desirable in the articular fractures (Fig. 159–61A and B).

Comminuted intercondylar (T-Y) fractures are treated by fixation and compression of the condyles

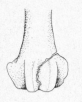 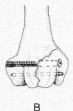 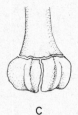 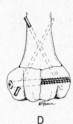

A   B   C   D

Figure 159–61. *A*, Simple intercondylar fracture. *B*, Treated with a compression screw and Kirschner wire. *C*, A comminuted intercondylar fracture ("T-Y", supracondylar-intercondylar). *D*, Repaired with a compression screw and cross-pins.

with a compression screw or Kirschner wire, and stabilization of the repaired epiphyseal segment to the metaphysis is provided by Rush pins, double pins or cross-pins (Fig. 159–61*C* and *D*). Fragmentation of the articular cartilage frequently occurs with intercondylar fractures. Small cartilage fragments are discarded. Large fragments with a subchondral bone component are reduced and fixed with .035- to .045-inch Kirschner wires. The ends of the wires are seated into subchondral bone.

Epiphyseal Fractures

Isolated fractures of the epiphysis occur with ligament and tendon injuries. Ruptures of the cranial cruciate and collateral ligaments and popliteus and long digital extensor tendons may produce avulsion fractures of the epiphysis. Further information on these injuries is provided in the appropriate sections on tendon and ligament injuries.

1. Archibald, J.: *Canine Surgery.* 2nd ed. American Veterinary Publications, Santa Barbara, 1974.
2. Bardet, J. F., Rudy, R. L., and Hohn, R. B.: Measurement of femoral torsion in dogs using a biplanar method. Vet. Surg. *12*:1, 1983.
3. Black, A. P., and Withrow, S. J.: Changes in the proximal femur and coxofemoral joint following intramedullary pinning of diaphyseal fractures in young dogs. Vet. Surg. 8:19, 1979.
4. Calandruccio, R. A., and Anderson, W. E.: Post-fracture avascular necrosis of the femoral head: correlation of experimental and clinical studies. Clin. Orthop. *152*:49, 1980.
5. Carr, C. R., and Wingo, C. H.: Fractures of the femoral diaphysis. J. Bone Jt. Surg. *55A*:690, 1973.
6. Caywood, D. D., Wallace, L. J., and Braden, T. D.: Osteomyelitis in the dog: a review of 67 cases. J. Am. Vet. Med. Assoc. 8:943, 1978.
7. Cechner, P. E., Knecht, C. D., Chaffee, V. W., and Robinson, W. C.: Fracture repair failure in the dog: a review in 20 dogs. J. Am. Anim. Hosp. Assoc. *13*:613, 1977.
8. Crock, H. V.: An atlas of the arterial supply of the head and neck of the femur in man. Clin. Orthop. *12*:17, 1980.
9. Daly, W. R.: Femoral head and neck fractures in the dog and cat: a review of 115 cases. Vet. Surg. 7:29, 1978.
10. Ewald, F. C., and Hirohashi, K.: Effect of distal transfer of the greater trochanter in growing animals. J. Bone Jt. Surg. *55A*:1064, 1973.
11. Frey, A.J., and Olds, R.: A new technique for repair of comminuted diaphyseal fractures. Vet. Surg. *10*:51, 1981.
12. Gambardella, P. C.: Full cerclage wires for fixation of long bone fractures. Comp. Cont. Ed. *11*:665, 1980.
13. Gilmore, D. R.: Application of the lag screw. Comp. Cont. Ed. 5:217, 1983.
14. Grauer, G. F., Banks, W. J., Ellison, G. W., and Rouse, G. P.: Incidence and mechanisms of distal femoral physeal fractures in the dog and cat. J. Am. Anim. Hosp. Assoc. *17*:579, 1981.
15. Hauptman, J., and Butler, H. C.: Effect of osteotomy of the greater trochanter with tension band fixation on femoral conformation in beagle dogs. Vet. Surg. 8:13, 1979.
16. Hauptman, J., Prieur, W. D., Butler, H. C., and Guffy, M. M.: The angle of inclination of the canine femoral head and neck. Vet. Surg. 8:74, 1979.
17. Hulse, D. H., Abdelbaki, Y. Z., and Wilson, J.: Revascularization of femoral capital physeal fractures following surgical fixation. J. Vet. Orthop. 2:50, 1981.
18. Hunt, J. M., Aitken, M. L., Denny, H. R., and Gibbs, C.: The complications of diaphyseal fractures in dogs: a review of 100 cases. J. Small Anim. Pract. *21*:103, 1980.
19. Kaderly, R. E., Anderson, W. D., and Anderson, B. G.: Extraosseous vascular supply to the mature dog's coxofemoral joint. Am. J. Vet. Res. *43*:1208, 1982.
20. Kagan, K. G.: Multiple intramedullary pin fixation of the femur of dogs and cats. J. Am. Vet. Med. Assoc. *182*:1251, 1983.
21. Lee, R.: Proximal femoral epiphyseal separation in the dog. J. Small Anim. Pract. *11*:669, 1976.
22. Lombardo, S. J., and Harvey, J. P.: Fractures of the distal femoral epiphyses. J. Bone Jt. Surg. *59A*:742, 1977.
23. Milton, J. L., Horne, R. D., and Goldstein, G. M.: Cross-pinning: a simple technique for treatment of certain metaphyseal and physeal fractures of the long bones. J. Am. Anim. Hosp. Assoc. *16*:891, 1980.
24. Morrissy, R.: Hip fractures in children. Clin. Orthop. *152*:202, 1980.
25. O'Brien, E. T., and Fahey, J. J.: Remodeling of the femoral neck after in situ pinning for slipped capital femoral epiphysis. J. Bone Jt. Surg. *59A*:62, 1977.
26. Olerud, S.: Operative treatment of supracondylar-condylar fractures of the femur. J. Bone Jt. Surg. *54A*:1015, 1972.
27. Phillips, I. R.: A survey of bone fractures in the dog. and cat. J. Small Anim. Pract. *20*:661, 1979.
28. Piermattei, D. L., and Greeley, R. G.: *An Atlas of Surgical Approaches to the Bones of the Dog and Cat.* 2nd ed. W. B. Saunders, Philadelphia, 1979.
29. Renegar, W. R., Leeds, E. B., and Olds, R. B.: The use of the Kirschner-Ehmer splint in clinical orthopedics. Comp. Cont. Ed. 4:381, 1982.
30. Rhinelander, F. W., and Wilson, J. W.: The blood supply of developing mature and healing bone. *In* Sumner-Smith, G. (ed.): *Bone in Clinical Orthopedics*, W. B. Saunders, Philadelphia, 1982.
31. Riser, W. H.: Growth and development of the normal canine pelvis, hip joints and femurs from birth to maturity: a radiographic study. J. Vet. Radiol. Soc. 2:24, 1973.
32. Rivera, L. A., Abdelbaki, Y. Z., and Hulse, D. A.: Arterial supply to the canine hip joint. J. Vet. Orthop. *1*:20, 1979.
33. Salter, R. B., and Harris, W. R.: Injuries involving the epiphyseal plate. J. Bone Jt. Surg. *45A*:587, 1963.
34. Schultz, R. J.: *The Language of Fractures.* Williams & Wilkins, Baltimore, 1972.
35. Shelbourne, K. D., and Brueckmann, F. R.: Rush-pin fixation of supracondylar and intercondylar fractures of the femur. J. Bone Jt. Surg. *64A*:161, 1982.
36. Shires, P. K., and Hulse, D. A.: Internal fixation of physeal fractures using the distal femur as an example. Comp. Cont. Ed. *11*:854, 1980.
37. Smith, C. W., Schiller, A. G., Smith, A. R., and Dorner, J.

L.: Osteomyelitis in the dog: a retrospective study. J. Am. Anim. Hosp. Assoc. *14*:589, 1978.

38. Stone, E. A., Betts, C. W., and Rowland, G. N.: Effect of Rush pins on the distal femoral growth plate of young dogs. Am. J. Vet. Res. *42*:261, 1981.

39. Sumner-Smith, G.: Observations on epiphyseal fusion of the canine appendicular skeleton. J. Small Anim. Pract. 7:303, 1966.

40. Toridis, T. G.: Stress analysis of the femur. J. Biomechanics 2:163, 1969.

41. Weissman, S. L., Tadmor, A., Khermosh, O., et al.: Growth of the upper end of the femur: experimental investigation in the rabbit. Acta Orthop. Scand. 45:225, 1974.

The Stifle Joint

Donald A. Hulse and Peter K. Shires

The joint is a complex diarthrodial joint that allows axial movement as well as flexion and extension (Figs. 159–62 and 159–63). The joint components are the femorotibial articulation and the femoropatellar articulation. The main part of the joint is formed by the large roller-like condyles of the femur and the flattened tibial plateaus. Two fibrocartilage discs, lateral and medial menisci, are interposed between the articulating surfaces of the femur and tibia to account for incongruencies between the two surfaces. The femoropatellar joint is formed by the articulating surfaces of the femoral trochlea and the patella. This joint is interdependent with the femoral-tibial joint and provides the mechanical efficiency necessary for flexion and extension of the femorotibial joint. Four primary ligaments provide stability during movement of the stifle joint. The anterior cruciate and posterior cruciate ligaments, within the joint, provide anteroposterior and rotary stability. The medial and lateral collateral ligaments, closely associated with the joint capsule, provide varovalgus and rotary stability.

Standing dogs have a normal stifle angle of 130 to 140 degrees. The normal range of motion is 110 degrees, from 40 degrees of flexion to 150 degrees in full extension. To comfortably carry weight in a partially flexed stance at all times, the extensor mechanism of the stifle joint is extremely well developed. The main extensors of the stifle are the four muscles of the quadriceps group.[29] A minor extensor of the stifle, the long digital extensor muscle, originates from the lateral femoral condyle and is significant as a landmark and as a structure to avoid when

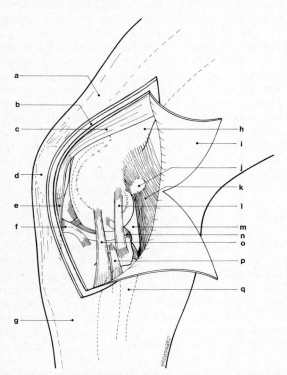

Figure 159–62. Craniolateral left hind limb. The biceps femoris (*i*) is split for diagrammatic purposes. *a*, rectus femoris; *b*, retinaculum; *c*, vastus lateralis; *d*, patella; *e*, patellar tendon; *f*, intermeniscal ligament; *g*, tibia; *h*, femur; *j*, lateral fabella; *k*, head of gastrocnemius; *l*, lateral collateral ligament; *m*, posterior joint capsule; *n*, popliteal tendon; *o*, long digital tensor tendon; *p*, fibularis longus; *q*, fibula.

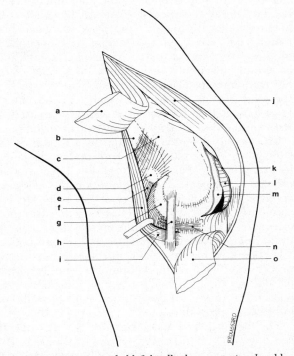

Figure 159–63. Craniomedial left hindlimb. *a*, sartorius; *b*, adductor; *c*, femur; *d*, medial fascius; *e*, medial head of gastrocnemius; *f*, semimembranosus; *g*, posterior joint capsule; *h*, medial collateral ligament; *i*, tendon of semimembranosus; *j*, vastus medialis; *k*, capsule; *l*, synovium; *m*, medial femoral trochlea; *n*, medial meniscus; *o*, sartorius.

making a lateral, parapatellar approach to the stifle joint.

The vastus lateralis, medialis, and intermedius and the rectus femoris muscles, which constitute the quadriceps muscle group, insert on the tibial tuberosity via the quadriceps tendon, which includes the patella. Portions of the very strong tendon (also called the straight patellar tendon), are used in a number of anterior cruciate repair techniques.[3,6] Realignment of the quadriceps unit is used for correction of patellar luxations, and the tendon is also used as an anchor in many imbrication and plication techniques.

The patellar tendon is extra-articular and receives its blood supply proximally from muscular branches of the deep femoral artery and distally from the infrapatella fat pat and the tibia. Rupture of the tendon, or its tibial attachment, results in an inability to extend the stifle. While movement of the stifle depends on free movement of the patella, removal of this sesamoid bone causes a 3 fold reduction in the moments of force the quadriceps apply during extension. Adhesions or fusion of the patella or quadriceps unit to the distal femur effectively prevents movement of the stifle joint.[9] The quadriceps tendon receives additional support from the fascia lata and the biceps femoris fascia laterally and from the sartorius fascia medially. This cradle of fascial tissue helps to support the stifle, a quality used in several reconstruction techniques.

Deep to this fascial plane lies the fibrous joint capsule (retinaculum), which is a tough layer of connective tissue surrounding the joint and on which lie the lateral and medial collateral ligaments, the femoropatellar ligaments, the femorofabellar ligaments, and, caudally, the tendon of the popliteal muscle. This layer of tissue has clinical significance in chronic instability, in which a thickening of the fibrous joint capsule develops and helps to stabilize the joint but also restricts normal joint movement. Plication of this fibrous joint capsule is used to stabilize the injured joint in some repair techniques.

The popliteal muscle unit acts as a rotator of the stifle joint. The tendon and its insertion on the lateral femoral condyle has been surgically transposed to provide a dynamic replacement for the posterior cruciate ligament. The flexors of the stifle are less closely associated with the joint than the extensors or rotators. The gastrocnemius muscle inserts on the distal femur through the fabellae and is used both as a landmark and as an anchor in some reconstructive procedures. The semimembranosus muscle inserts on the proximal medial tibia and must be partly incised to expose the posterior joint capsule for imbrication procedures.

The fibrous joint capsule supports the synoviocytic layer, which is the true synovial membrane.[57] This layer is normally one to three cells thick and lines the joint space, forming numerous villi. The two cell types present in the synovial membrane serve a phagocytic (type A) and secretory (type B) function. The synovia produced by type B cells contain a high proportion of glycoproteins, which coat the cartilage to lubricate the joint surfaces. Hyaluronic acid serves as a tissue lubricant below the cartilage surface. Subsequent to even a simple arthrotomy incision, the synoviocytic layer hypertrophies and becomes hyperplastic. More chronic conditions, like rheumatoid arthritis and instability secondary to cruciate ligament rupture, precipitate the same initial reaction, which rapidly progresses to include inflammatory cell proliferation, nodule formation, vascular infiltration, villus formation, and perivascular cuffing. The progressive reduction in the number and function efficiency of the type B cells results in osteoarthritic changes owing to poor nutrition and poor lubrication of the articular cartilage cells. When the fibrous joint capsule is used for stabilization procedures, care should be taken not to compromise or irritate the underlying synovial membrane to prevent iatrogenic postoperative osteoarthritic changes.

STABILIZING MECHANISMS

The normal stifle joint has a number of basic movements: flexion, extension, varus angulation, valgus angulation, anteroposterior movement, and axial rotation. These movements or degrees of freedom are controlled by the primary and secondary restraints. With flexion and extension of the stifle joint, there is a posterior rolling and sliding movement of the femoral condyles relative to the tibial plateau. Conversely, as the joint is extended, there is an anterior movement of the femoral condyles relative to the tibial plateau. The primary restraints for this normal degree of movement are the anterior and posterior cruciate ligaments. The anterior cruciate ligament primarily functions to prevent forward displacement of the tibia relative to the femur (anterior drawer movement), whereas the posterior cruciate ligament prevents backward movement of the tibia relative to the femur (posterior drawer). Injury to the anterior or posterior cruciate ligament results in an abnormal movement between the femur and tibia during flexion and extension. The secondary restraints for abnormal anteroposterior movement of the femur and tibia during flexion and extension are the fibrous joint capsule, the lateral and medial menisci, the lateral and medial collateral ligaments, dynamic muscular forces, and the normal geometrical shape of the femoral and tibial articulating surfaces. Each of these secondary restraints helps stabilize the femorotibial joint against abnormal anteroposterior movement during flexion and extension of the stifle joint. However, the secondary restraints are generally not effective in preventing abnormal drawer movement and may be damaged themselves when called upon to function as primary restraints against excessive anteroposterior movement. An example would be the high incidence of meniscal tears associated with anterior cruciate ligament injury. The medial meniscus functions as a stabilizer against excessive anterior drawer movement, becoming wedged between the femoral condyle and tibial plateau. This action commonly results in a bucket-handle tear of the medial meniscus.

As the stifle is flexed, the lateral collateral ligament begins to relax, allowing posterior displacement of the lateral femoral condyle on the tibial plateau. This process results in an internal rotation of the tibia relative to the femur. The axial movement of the tibia is reversed with extension as the lateral collateral ligament begins to tighten, causing a forward displacement of the lateral femoral condyle on the tibial plateau. The primary restraints against abnormal axial rotation are the medial and lateral collateral ligaments as well as the anterior and posterior cruciate ligaments. When the stifle joint is in extension, the collateral ligaments restrain the tibia against abnormal axial movement. With flexion of the stifle joint, the cruciate ligaments restrain the joint from abnormal internal axial movement, and the medial collateral ligament restrains the joint from abnormal external axial movement. The anterior and posterior cruciate ligaments are able to provide axial stability because of their spatial orientation within the joint. The cruciate ligaments twist about each other as the stifle is flexed, limiting internal axial rotation. With injury of one of the primary axial stabilizers, the examiner elicits excessive rotational movement of the tibia relative to the femur. As an example, with anterior cruciate ligament injury, when the joint is flexed, abnormal internal rotation of the tibia is found. The secondary restraints to abnormal axial movement are the menisci, fibrous joint capsule, dynamic muscle forces, and normal geometry of the articulating surfaces. The secondary restraints are not able to counter abnormal axial movement effectively when primary restraints are injured. Subjecting the secondary restraints to these abnormal forces often results in their injury. Meniscal tears and fibrillation of the articular surfaces are often sequelae to abnormal axial movement following injury of the anterior cruciate ligament.

The primary restraints against abnormal varovalgus angulation are the medial and lateral collateral ligaments and the fibrous joint capsule. Injury to the medial or lateral restraints gives rise to excessive varus or valgus angulation.

ANTERIOR CRUCIATE LIGAMENT RUPTURE

Clinical Signs

Typically two clinical syndromes are recognized.[3] The acute syndrome is seen in the active dog, generally young and fit, as a sudden onset of non–weight-bearing lameness during strenuous exercise. The knee may develop an effusion, and capsular distension can be palpated or seen. The dog remains non–weight-bearing for at least a week and then starts to use the leg more and more with time, until it is functionally sound. When the leg is stressed or overworked or after sudden weather changes, lameness may recur. With developing age, lameness may return as chronic osteoarthritis of the stifle. At any time during the post-injury stage, the dog may become acutely lame again, usually during exercise but sometimes for no apparent reason. A clicking or popping sound may be heard or felt during stifle movement; it is frequently related to secondary meniscal injury in the unstable joint.

The chronic syndrome is generally seen in older, overweight dogs or dogs with long-standing stifle deformities. Poodles have been over-represented in retrospective studies, perhaps because of a high incidence of patellar luxation in the breed. These animals are usually non–weight-bearing or partially weight-bearing for a much longer time than those with the acute syndrome. Frequently, the other hind leg becomes affected, and bilateral hind leg lameness results. Meniscal injury as a result of stifle instability is also seen in this group. Joint effusion is not a consistent finding.

The excessive internal rotation of the tibia after any anterior cruciate ligament rupture precipitates a "toe in, hock out" stance on the affected side. Pain is not a significant finding on palpation, but manipulation of the stifle in acute injuries induces protective muscular tensing and anxious reactions.

The clinical signs of anterior cruciate ligament rupture are not diagnostic unless an anterior drawer sign is elicited in the injured stifle. Because chronic fibrous tissue development secondary to the instability tends to stabilize the joint, and because muscular tensing obscures signs of joint instability, failure to elicit the anterior drawer sign in an awake dog does not eliminate a diagnosis of anterior cruciate ligament rupture.

Diagnosis

Elicitation of the anterior drawer sign is regarded as diagnostic for anterior cruciate ligament rupture. The best technique to determine anterior drawer movement in the stifle should test continuity of this ligament only and should be minimally affected by other influences. Isolated posterior cruciate ligament rupture can easily be mistaken for anterior ligament rupture if the examiner is not acutely aware of the normal relative positions of the femur and tibia.

To test for the drawer sign, the examiner should stand behind the recumbent patient. The animal should be relaxed and calm, and the leg to be examined should be uppermost. For the anterior drawer test, the distal femur is stabilized by placement of the middle finger on the medial femoral condyle, the index finger lightly on the patella, and the thumb on the lateral femoral condyle. The left hand is used for the right stifle, and *vice versa*. The tibia is secured by placement of the thumb of the other hand behind the proximal fibula, the index

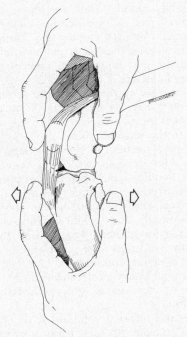

Figure 159–64. The proper positioning of the examiner's hands when performing an anterior drawer test.

finger on the tibial crest, and the middle, ring, and little fingers on the proximal medial tibia (Fig. 159–64).

The femur is held immobile and the proximal tibia is moved anteriorly and posteriorly. This maneuver is repeated with the stifle in full extension, in a neutral standing position (140 degrees of flexion), and in full flexion. Anterior drawer should also be tested while internal and external rotation is applied to the tibia. Care must be taken not to inhibit stifle movement by grasping the quadriceps muscles in the hand holding the femur.

Movement should be recorded as measurement in millimeters. Normal anterior drawer measurements have been estimated; however, it would probably be more appropriate for each clinician to establish a set of "normal" values from his or her own experience or to use the patient's other leg for purposes of comparison.

As mentioned previously, a negative result in the awake patient does not rule out the diagnosis of anterior cruciate ligament rupture. Some form of tranquilization, muscle relaxation, or anesthesia is necessary to eliminate voluntary stabilization of the stifle joint by the animal. Even in the normal dog, the anterior drawer movement is more distinct when the dog is tranquilized (1 to 3 mm *versus* 0 to 2 mm). Accurate diagnosis is ultimately based on experience, supporting the inclusion of this maneuver as part of the routine orthopedic examination in every lameness case.

Evaluation of the recorded movement is primarily of value in cases of partial rupture and cases in which other ligamentous damage is suspected. If a stifle

shows increased anterior drawer movement in the flexed position, minimal movement in the 140-degree position, and no anterior drawer movement in the extended position, the diagnosis is partial rupture of the anteromedial band of the anterior cruciate ligament. Internal rotation of the tibia tightens the stifle by twisting the intact cruciate ligaments together. If one cruciate is ruptured, tightening will not occur, and any instability present in the straight position will not be reduced in the internal rotation position. External rotation should not affect the anterior drawer movement, but it does demonstrate the status of the collateral ligaments.[3]

During all manipulations of the stifle, the clinician should be feeling for crepitance, clicking, popping, or "giving way." All of these signs are associated with meniscal injuries.

An additional diagnostic test for anterior cruciate ligament rupture or, more correctly, anterior tibial subluxation, is the tibial compression test. Standing in the same position behind the dog and using the same hand as described for the anterior drawer test, the examiner holds the distal femur between the thumb and middle finger with the index finger placed on the proximal tibial cest. The dog's foot is held in the other hand, and the hock joint is flexed and extended while the tibial crest is pressed posteriorly. With anterior cruciate ligament rupture, the tibia "subluxes" forward when the gastrocnemius muscle is tensed (in hock flexion). This subluxation can be seen or felt and is diagnostic of anterior cruciate ligament rupture (Fig. 159–65).

Additional diagnostic tests include radiographic evaluation of the stifle joint. If stress lateral views are taken with the tibia forward on the femoral condyles, radiographic confirmation of anterior ligament rupture may be obtained (Fig. 159–66). Clinical evaluation is, however, less costly and more consistent. Radiographs allow evaluation of the osteoarthri-

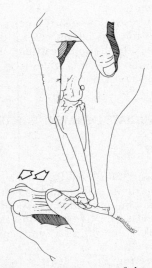

Figure 159–65. The proper positioning of the examiner's hands when performing the tibial compression test.

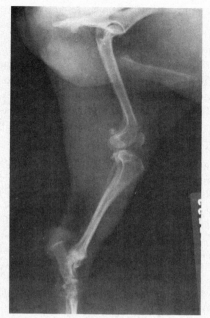

Figure 159–66. Lateral radiograph of the stifle joint of a dog showing the forward (anterior) displacement of the tibia relative to the femur with anterior cruciate ligament injury.

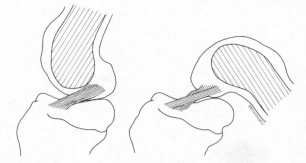

Figure 159–67. The tautness of the anteromedial and posterolateral bands of the anterior cruciate ligament at flexion (left) and extension (right). Note that with flexion, the posterolateral band becomes spiraled and slightly lax.

tic changes present in the joint, thereby aiding in prognostication to the client before therapeutic advice is offered.

Joint fluid evaluation provides information about the degree and type of effusion present. An inflammatory, nonseptic type of effusion can be expected in most cases of anterior cruciate ligament rupture. The degree of hemorrhage present can be a rough indication of the acuteness of the injury. Many clinicians suggest that the risk of contamination involved is not worth the information received by sampling the stifle joint with a ruptured anterior cruciate ligament. The technique is useful to rule out septic arthritis in selected cases.

Pathophysiology

The canine anterior cruciate ligament has two main parts, the anterior medial band and the posterior lateral part.[6] These two segments blend together, and the ligament is probably best visualized as being made up of hundreds of separate strands, each of which has its own point of origin and insertion and is most taut in a certain stifle position of flexion and rotation (Fig. 159–67). The ligament originates in a fossa on the posterior aspect of the medial side of the lateral femoral condyle and runs cranially, medially, and distally between the condyles of the femur to insert on the cranial intercondyloid area of the tibia. The precise distribution of the numerous collagen fibers of the ligament ensures continuous joint congruity throughout the normal rocking, sliding, and rotation movements of the stifle during motion.

The canine stifle joint is usually in a partially to fully flexed position. During all phases of stifle flexion, the anterior cruciate ligament is responsible for preventing the tibia from sliding forward on the femoral condyles. When the gastrocnemius muscle contracts, the proximal tibia would slide forward if the anterior cruciate were absent. Internal rotation of the tibia is also prevented by the anterior cruciate ligament, a function that is accentuated in flexion because the anterior and posterior cruciate ligaments twist around each other and tighten during flexion. This check to internal rotation of the tibia is necessary because of the conformation of the femoral condyles. During flexion, the lateral collateral ligament is relaxed, allowing the tibia to rotate internally if the anterior cruciate ligament were absent. A third function of the anterior cruciate ligament is to prevent hyperextension of the stifle joint.

The anterior cruciate works with the other stifle ligaments, surrounding tendons, muscles, and fascial planes to control the movement of the stifle joint. Multiple ligamentous injuries occur frequently and modify the clinical signs seen in specific cases.

An isolated injury to the anterior cruciate ligament in a healthy dog is usually associated with hyperextension of the stifle or with a sudden movement on a flexed, weight-bearing stifle. Hyperextension injuries occur when a running animal abruptly fixes the tibia (steps into a hole) while the rest of its body continues forward (Fig. 159–68). The primary check against hyperextension is the anterior cruciate ligament, which is also the first to rupture. Because normally this ligament can withstand 59.4 N per kg of body weight,[1] this type of injury is usually associated with overexuberant activity or with an automobile injury. The posterior cruciate ligament is the secondary restraint against hyperextension, so it may be injured concomitantly.

When the stifle is flexed 20 to 50 degrees, the cruciate ligaments twist on each other and become taut. If the tibia is forcibly rotated internally, or more commonly, if the animal rotates its body (and femur) externally, the anterior cruciate is stretched over the medial femoral condyle and is subject to crushing

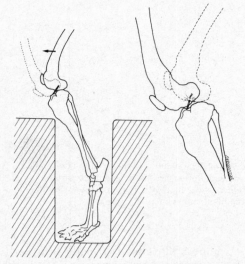

Figure 159–68. Trauma resulting in hyperextension of the stifle joint can result in a rupture of the anterior cruciate ligament.

against the intercondylar prominence of the tibia (Fig. 159–69). Injury in this situation is particularly common in an animal with insufficient muscle tone to help support the stifle during such a stressful movement. Lack of training or fatigue contributes to anterior cruciate ligament rupture by this means.

Whatever the cause, traumatic rupture of the anterior cruciate ligament results in immediate pain, intra-articular hemorrhage, and effusion. Non–weight-bearing lameness and pain-induced yelping

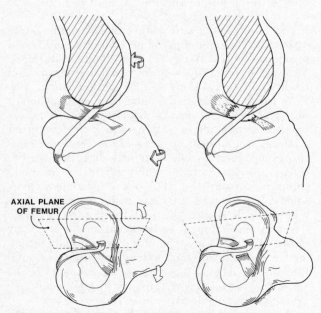

AXIAL PLANE OF FEMUR

Figure 159–69. The mechanism of injury to the anterior cruciate ligament with internal rotation of the tibia. The anterior cruciate ligament is stretched over the medial condyle of the femur and is subject to crushing against the intercondylar prominence of the tibia.

usually accompany the injury. Distension of the joint soon limits joint laxity and stops the hemorrhage. During the non–weight-bearing phase of injury, damage to the intra-articular structures is limited to the anterior cruciate ligament and to the superficial cartilage cells, which rely on weight-bearing to assist in distribution of oxygen and nutrient from the synovial fluid into the cartilage. Provided no stresses are applied, these superficial cells can survive and regenerate when the joint is returned to normal function and fluid content.

The ends of the ruptured anterior cruciate ligament retract and fan out ("mop-end" appearance). Leukocyte infiltration is moderate in the ruptured ligament ends. Over a period of months the free ends of ligament are removed, presumably through collagenase activity. Sometimes the free ends adhere to another part of the joint, revascularize, and survive as a continuous structure.

In the unstabilized stifle with a ruptured anterior cruciate ligament, focal areas of roughening and occasional small clefts are found on the articular surface within one week of injury.[67] The lesions progress, resulting in deep clefts by seven weeks and erosion by 16 weeks. Osteophyte development begins in the periarticular areas three days after transection of the ligament, and osteophytes are evident macroscopically by two weeks and radiographically by five weeks.[35]

The synovial membrane of dogs with transected anterior cruciate ligaments showed an acute, nonsuppurative inflammatory response with intimal thickening evident one week after injury that progressed in severity for up to 13 weeks, when apparent regression was noted.[57] The early cartilage changes may be the result of enzyme and collagenase release by the inflammatory cells in the reactive synovial membrane, and not *vice versa* as previously thought.

Over a longer period, transection of this ligament resulted in atrophy of the quadriceps muscles, a five- to ten-degree extension deficit in the stifle, joint capsule thickening, and progressive osteophyte formation around the articular margins. Lameness was less evident as time progressed and was not observed at all 19 to 21 months after ligament transection.[62] The menisci are invariably damaged after clinical[34, 66, 84] or experimental[62] separation of the ligament. Clinical lameness is often associated with meniscal injury in the chronically ruptured anterior cruciate ligament.

There is no doubt that clinical rupture of the anterior cruciate ligament in dogs produces a series of events related to instability of the stifle. These pathological changes lead, in most instances, to lameness. Other animals return to an apparently sound functional status unless a secondary injury supervenes, precipitated by chronic instability, or until chronic degenerative joint disease progresses to the point of functional interference and pain-related lameness.

Treatment of Anterior Cruciate Ligament Rupture

Conservative Treatment

The diminishing signs of lameness in many clinically affected dogs has led to a conservative therapeutic approach by some veterinarians.[77] It is suggested that the majority of small dogs will recover to satisfactory function after two months of enforced rest. Large and working dogs apparently do not show the same recovery after rest.

Conservative therapy may also be considered when severe degenerative joint disease is already present at the time of initial diagnosis, as may occur in chronic injuries or in concurrent joint disease such as rheumatoid arthritis or systemic lupus erythematosus. Because the prognosis is less favorable in these cases, nonsurgical management may be justified.

Rest is defined as close confinement for four to eight weeks with only short walks on the lead allowed. Arthritic pain that develops in these dogs is treated with phenylbutazone at the initial dose of 200 to 600 mg per day in two or three doses for four days, followed by a reduced dose of 100 mg per day for ten days.[77] Aspirin at a dose of 10 mg per kg every 12 hours for two or three days is equally effective in reducing pain.

Any dog that shows persistent lameness after eight weeks of strict rest is considered a surgical candidate. Most veterinary surgeons currently recommend surgical exploration and stabilization immediately on diagnosis of persistent lameness, in order to prevent secondary joint damage.

Surgical Treatment

Many surgical techniques have been described for the repair, replacement and augmentation of the anterior cruciate ligament.[52] A description of all these techniques is not possible. No single technique has been proven to be clearly more effective than any other in the few, objective studies with long-term follow-up that have been reported. By describing a few of the more commonly used procedures, we hope to assist the uncommitted surgeon in a rational choice of procedure suited to his or her personal experience.

All the described techniques have a common initial approach. The injured leg is clipped and prepared for sterile surgery. The stifle area is draped to isolate the lateral or medial aspect of the leg from the proximal tibia to the mid-femur region. A lateral or medial, parapatellar incision is made from the distal one-third of the femur to the tibial crest (Fig. 159–70). In techniques requiring a fascia lata graft, the incision should be extended proximally to the lateral mid-femur or proximal femur. Skin drapes are recommended—plastic, towel, or stockinette.

If a fascial graft is required, it is isolated at this stage. A lateral or medial parapatellar arthrotomy is made by incising the fibrous and membranous joint

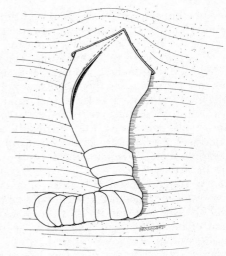

Figure 159–70. The proper placement of the skin incision for exposure of the stifle joint.

capsule lateral or medial to the vastus lateralis or medialis muscle, freeing the patella and the patellar tendon to the proximal tibia. The patella is luxated medially or laterally, and the stifle joint is examined for articular erosions, osteophytes, and ligamentous and meniscal injuries.

Unless a primary repair is to be attempted, the remnants of the ruptured anterior cruciate ligament are carefully excised using a small (No. 11 or 15 Bard-Parker) blade. Removal of all of the osteophytes using a No. 10 blade has been recommended,[81] but they grow back, even in the stabilized joint.[36] If an osteophyte is interfering with normal joint movement, it should be removed. Eburnated bone exposed by cartilage erosion should be fenestrated with multiple small drill holes to allow fibrocartilaginous ingrowth from the subchondral cancellous bone.

Particular attention should be paid to examining

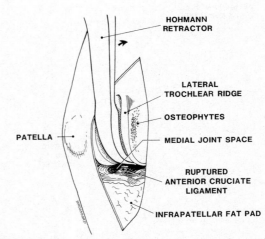

Figure 159–71. Positioning of a Hohmann retractor for visualization of the posteromedial compartment of the stifle joint during examination of the menisci for injury.

the medial compartment of the joint and the caudal, medial meniscus. A Hohmann retractor increases the visibility of the posterior medial compartment (Fig. 159–71).[45] A portion of the infrapatellar fat pad may be excised,[81] but this maneuver increases hemorrhage and possibly compromises the vascular supply of the fascial graft. Injured meniscal tissue is removed (see "Meniscal Injury"). The joint is lavaged thoroughly to remove all debris. At this stage, the surgical technique of preference is performed to repair, stabilize, supplement, or replace the ruptured anterior cruciate ligament.

Primary Repair. Primary repair of a ruptured anterior cruciate ligament is generally applied to proximal or distal avulsion injuries. The incidence of this type of injury is about 5 per cent in humans[88] and in one study was 6 per cent in dogs.[78]

If a large enough fragment of bone is avulsed, a compression screw, wire, or tension band fixation technique can be used to secure the bone fragment (Fig. 159–72). Tibial avulsions are more common than femoral avulsions in dogs. With rigid fixation and primary bone healing, a rapid and complete recovery can be expected once healing is complete.

Primary repair has also been advocated in humans for proximal or distal ligament ruptures not involving bone.[64] The technique requires that several multiloop sutures be placed in the free end of the ligament and secured through holes drilled in the bone at the point of attachment (Fig. 159–73). The different parts of the ligament are reattached in their normal anatom-

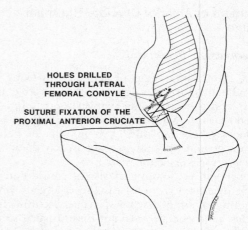

HOLES DRILLED THROUGH LATERAL FEMORAL CONDYLE

SUTURE FIXATION OF THE PROXIMAL ANTERIOR CRUCIATE

Figure 159–73. Primary suture repair of an anterior cruciate ligament injury in which the failure was at the bone-ligament junction. Sutures are preplaced in the ligament and are then secured to the bone by passing the suture ends through predrilled holes positioned at the failure site.

ical positions. The technique is applicable to acute injuries only; it has resulted in a very high (95 per cent) return to normal, high-performance athletic function.[64] The technique has not been evaluated in dogs.

Primary repair in other types of injury to the anterior cruciate ligament has proved singularly unsuccessful. The most commonly encountered "mop end," mid-substance rupture does not hold sutures well and often resorbs completely rather than healing.[30, 33, 63, 70]

Augmentation of Primary Repair. Augmentation of a primary repair procedure is recommended[30] and has been tested in dogs.[14] The proximal rupture was sutured as described for primary repair. The medial one-third of the patellar tendon and a fragment of patella were sutured to the medial aspect of the lateral femoral condyle to augment the primary repair. The strength of the repair was considerably better than that of primary repair alone, although still only half of the normal strength had returned eight months after operation. All repairs healed with no reabsorption.

Augmentation may be used to supplement reconstructive procedures.[16] Synthetic and natural materials have been used both intra- and extra-articularly.[14, 70] The principal objective of augmentation is to provide immediate, short-term protection to the primary procedure, be it reconstruction or repair. At this time, no definite recommendations can be made about augmentation.

Extracapsular Stabilization. In 1966, Childers[15] described an extracapsular technique that involved the use of Lembert sutures to stabilize the stifle joint by tightening the lateral retinaculum. The sutures were placed in the fibrous tissue and were not anchored to any osseous structures. A few years later, McCurnin and associates[65] and Pearson and co-workers[74] improved on the technique by reposition-

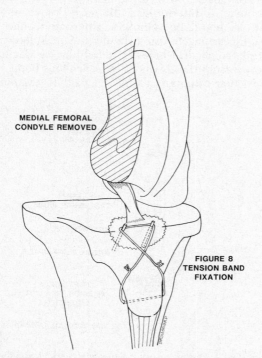

MEDIAL FEMORAL CONDYLE REMOVED

FIGURE 8 TENSION BAND FIXATION

Figure 159–72. Primary repair with a tension band of an anterior cruciate ligament injury in which the bony insertion of the ligament avulsed from the tibial plateau.

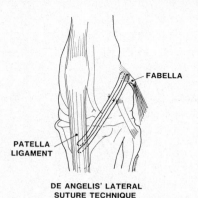

FABELLA

PATELLA
LIGAMENT

DE ANGELIS' LATERAL
SUTURE TECHNIQUE

Figure 159–74. Extracapsular reconstruction of anterior cruciate ligament insufficiency using nonabsorbable suture placed through the femorofabellar ligament and patella tendon.

ing and increasing the number of the Lembert sutures and by adding medial imbrication sutures for added support.

At about the same time, DeAngelis and Lau[21] modified the technique to increase the holding power of the lateral sutures. By anchoring the two lateral imbrication sutures in the heavy fascia caudal and proximal to the lateral fabella and by securing the distal end of the suture in the straight patella tendon, they achieved a more reliable support with one or two sutures (Fig. 159–74).

A similar approach was described more recently by Gambardella and colleagues,[34] using three lateral sutures through the straight patellar tendon. The most proximal suture was secured around the lateral fabella. The other two were passed around the lateral collateral ligament (Fig. 159–75).

Probably the most commonly used imbrication technique was described by Flo.[31] After an exploratory arthrotomy through a medial parapatellar approach, both medial and lateral fabellae are exposed by soft tissue retraction. Medially, the sartorius mus-

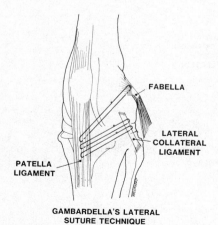

FABELLA

LATERAL
COLLATERAL
LIGAMENT

PATELLA
LIGAMENT

GAMBARDELLA'S LATERAL
SUTURE TECHNIQUE

Figure 159–75. Extracapsular reconstruction of anterior cruciate ligament insufficiency using nonabsorbable suture placed through the femorofabellar ligament and lateral collateral ligament to the patella tendon.

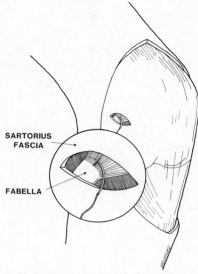

SARTORIUS
FASCIA

FABELLA

Figure 159–76. Medial view of Flo's extracapsular reconstruction for anterior cruciate ligament insufficiency passing nonabsorbable suture through the medial femorofabellar ligament and a predrilled hole in the tibial tubercle.

cle is separated from fascia over the fabella to expose this sesamoid bone in the gastrocnemius muscle insertion (Fig. 159–76). A needle threaded with heavy nonabsorbable suture material (Vetafil, Tevdek) is passed between the fabella and the femur.

Laterally, the biceps femoris muscle fascia is incised over the lateral fabella, and a double strand of suture is passed between the sesamoid and the femur (Fig. 159–77A). A hole is drilled horizontally through the cranial tibial tubercle. One arm of the medial suture and one arm of the lateral suture are passed through the hole (see Fig. 159–79).

With the stifle in 40 degrees of flexion, the tibia is pushed caudally and rotated externally while the lateral suture and then the medial suture are tied tightly. The remaining lateral fabellar suture is passed through the fascia lateral to the patella and is tied with the leg at the normal standing angle (Fig. 159–77B). Routine fascial and skin closure is used. The postoperative care of the imbrication suture technique is similar to that of, and is discussed at the end of the section on, intra-articular reconstruction techniques.

Two other extracapsular support techniques have been described.[40, 79] The first is a procedure in which the tendon of the long digital extensor muscle is left attached at its origin on the lateral femoral condyle and secured in a groove on the proximal tibia, creating a ligament that binds the tibia to the femur and prevents medial rotation and the anterior drawer sign.

In a later publication, the extensor digitorum longus tendon operation was superseded by posterior capsulorrhaphy techniques. The capsulorrhaphy requires an anterior medial arthrotomy for joint inspection and lavage; the arthrotomy is closed before the lateral, posterior joint pouch is exposed. The biceps

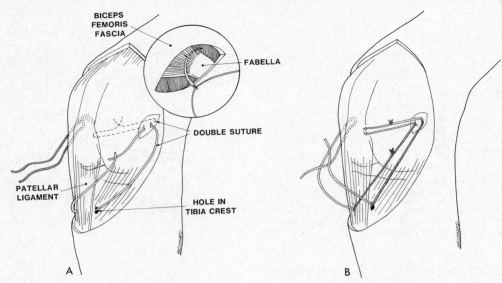

Figure 159–77. *A* and *B*, Lateral view of Flo's extracapsular reconstruction for anterior cruciate ligament insufficiency. One suture is placed through the femorofabellar ligament and a predrilled hole in the tibial tubercle while a second suture is tied between the lateral parapatellar fibrocartilage and femorofabellar ligament.

muscle is freed from the distal fascia lata and elevated to expose the gastrocnemius and flexor hallucis muscle origins. The gastrocnemius is separated from the flexor hallucis and retracted caudally to expose the joint capsule (Fig. 159–78). The joint capsule is incised caudally from the lateral collateral ligament to the intercondylar space. The arthrotomy is closed with two mattress sutures while the joint is held in flexion and external rotation. This procedure is generally supplemented by one or two support sutures through the lateral collateral ligament and around the lateral fabella. Closure includes plication of the biceps tendon and fascia lata to the patellar tendon, patella, and quadriceps insertion while the stifle is held in extension.

Additional support is supplied by a posterior medial capulorraphy in joints with severe subluxation.

The posterior medial joint capsule is exposed by retracting the posterior sartorius muscle caudally, incising the distal tendinous insertion of the semimembranosus muscle, and retracting the gastrocnemius muscle. The popliteal vessels are retracted to allow incision and closure of the joint capsule with three mattress sutures. An additional suture may be placed circumferentially from the posterior joint capsule to the medial collateral ligament (Fig. 159–79). All sutures are tightened with the limb in flexion. The semimembranous muscle is attached to the medial collateral ligament, and the remaining fascia is closed routinely.

All of the described extra-articular stabilization techniques require the implantation of heavy, nonabsorbable synthetic suture material. Stainless steel wire was used but fractured because of cyclic stresses

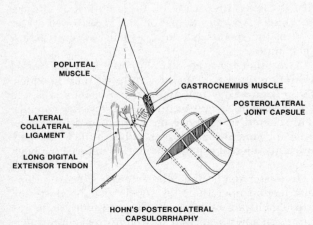

HOHN'S POSTEROLATERAL CAPSULORRHAPHY

Figure 159–78. Extracapsular reconstruction of anterior cruciate ligament insufficiency using nonabsorbable suture to imbricate the posterolateral joint capsule.

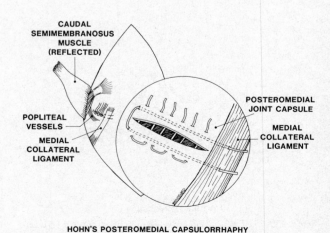

HOHN'S POSTEROMEDIAL CAPSULORRHAPHY

Figure 159–79. Extracapsular reconstruction of anterior cruciate ligament insufficiency using nonabsorbable suture to imbricate the posteromedial joint capsule.

induced by stifle movement. Suture reaction has been reported in 10 per cent of all dogs in which a coated, multifilament polyamide (Vetafil) was used.[25] Bacterial infection, associated primarily with less experienced surgeons, was regarded as the main cause of the reactions.[26] A similar reaction to a braided multifilament polyester fiber suture has been observed by other surgeons.

All the extracapsular techniques rely on periarticular fibrosis to provide long-term support for the stifle joint and hence to prevent the secondary disease associated with instability. A consistently high (60 to 95 per cent) clinical success rate has been reported in the few long-term follow-up studies published. Most authors regard these techniques as being particularly well suited to smaller dogs. Osteoarthritis, present before surgical repair, is generally slowed but not altogether stopped.

In summary, the extracapsular stabilization techniques are generally technically undemanding, require no special instrumentation to perform, and produce gratifying clinical results, especially in the lighter (smaller) breeds.

Intracapsular Reconstruction. Since 1917, when Hey Groves[38] first described a fascia lata pedicle graft technique to replace the ruptured anterior cruciate ligament in man, many modifications of the procedure have been developed. Originally, Paatsama[72] modified the Hey Groves technique for dogs and then improved on the procedure.[73] Eleven years later, Rudy[81] offered some additional improvements. The following description is a combination of all these modifications, which has now come to be regarded as the classic "Paatsama" technique and which forms the basis for most comparative studies involving new techniques.

A lateral parapatellar approach is made from the

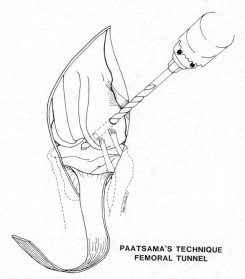

Figure 159–81. Predrilling a hole through the lateral femoral condyle for future passage of the fascia lata graft.

greater trochanter to below the tibial tuberosity. The fascia lata graft is prepared by incising along the cranial edge of the biceps femoris muscle from the tensor fascia lata muscle proximally to the level of the tibial tuberosity distally. A second incision is made parallel, and about 2.5 cm (in small dogs, only 1 cm) cranial, to the first (Fig. 159–80). The pedicle is freed proximally and dissected from the vastus lateralis muscle and the fibrous joint capsule to leave a broad base attached to the craniolateral tibia. A lateral arthrotomy, with intra-articular inspection, debridement, and lavage, is performed as previously described.

The biceps femoris and vastus lateralis muscles are separated to expose the lateral fabella. A muscular branch of the deep femoral artery may be double-ligated and transected to facilitate exposure. A femoral tunnel is drilled through the lateral femoral condyle to penetrate intra-articularly at the site of origin of the anterior cruciate ligament on the medial aspect of the lateral femoral condyle. The drill may be started from the lateral femoral condyle between the lateral collateral ligament and the fabella (Fig. 159–81), or a drill guide may be used to position the tunnel correctly.[10] The hole on the lateral femoral condyle should be at the pivotal point of the arc formed by the fascial strip throughout flexion and extension.

With the stifle in full flexion, a second tunnel is drilled from the tibial plateau, starting between the cranial meniscal attachments, passing under the intermeniscal ligament, and emerging from the proximal tibia just distal to the medial tibial condyle (Fig. 159–82).

A wire loop is passed from the joint through the femoral tunnel to pull the fascial strip through. The strip is similarly drawn from the joint through the tibial tunnel. The joint is thoroughly lavaged to

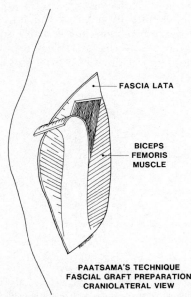

- FASCIA LATA

BICEPS FEMORIS MUSCLE

PAATSAMA'S TECHNIQUE
FASCIAL GRAFT PREPARATION
CRANIOLATERAL VIEW

Figure 159–80. Isolation of a fascia lata graft for intracapsular reconstruction of anterior cruciate ligament insufficiency.

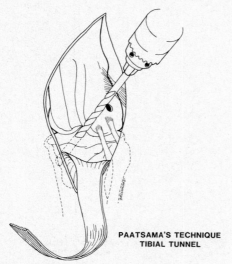

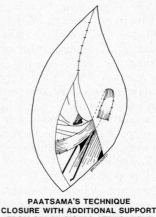

**PAATSAMA'S TECHNIQUE
TIBIAL TUNNEL**

**PAATSAMA'S TECHNIQUE
CLOSURE WITH ADDITIONAL SUPPORT
FROM GRAFT/BICEPS ATTACHMENT**

Figure 159–82. Predrilling a hole through the insertion site of the anterior cruciate ligament on the tibial plateau for future passage of the anterior cruciate ligament graft.

Figure 159–85. The free end of the fascial graft is sutured back on itself providing a complete circle of fascia around the tibia.

remove all bone chips, and the patella is replaced in the trochlea. With the joint in a normal standing position, the strip is pulled tightly over the tibial crest and secured to the tibial periosteum with several 2-0 nylon sutures (Fig. 159–83).

A strand of heavy, nonabsorbable suture material or wire is passed between the lateral fabella and the femur. The suture is passed through a small hole drilled in the proximal tibial crest and tied tightly to help anchor the tibia to the femur (Fig. 159–84).

The joint capsule is closed with fine nylon sutures, and the defect in the fascia lata is closed with 2-0

nylon in an interrupted pattern. Closure of the fascial defect tightens or imbricates the fascia on the lateral side of the joint. The free end of the fascial graft is sutured to its pedicle of origin on the lateral side of the tibia, passed through the distal biceps femoris muscle, and sutured back on itself, providing a complete circle of fascia around the tibia and the lateral femoral condyle (Fig. 159–85).[81]

Skin has been used instead of fascia with good results,[55,92–94] as have several synthetic materials.[13,22,46,51,82,86,90,92] Despite many successful results, no material has proved sufficiently superior to fascia lata to warrant the expense and problems associated with implanting a foreign substance intra-articularly. As a result, until a suitable substance is discovered, fascia lata remains the most commonly used ligament substitute in the repair of the anterior cruciate ligament.

Dickinson and Nunamaker[23] expressed concern about the possibility of shearing the intra-articular fascia because the two bone tunnels are close together where the graft crosses the joint. They recommended that only the femoral tunnel be drilled and that the

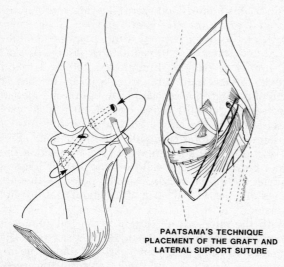

Figure 159–83   Figure 159–84

**PAATSAMA'S TECHNIQUE
PLACEMENT OF THE GRAFT AND
LATERAL SUPPORT SUTURE**

Figure 159–83. Passage of the fascial graft through the predrilled holes in the femur and tibia. The graft is secured by suturing to the periosteum of the tibial tubercle.

Figure 159–84. The intracapsular reconstruction may be supported by an extracapsular suture placed from the femorofabellar ligament and a predrilled hole through the tibial tubercle.

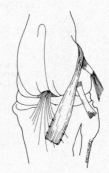

**DICKINSONS'S TECHNIQUE
CRANIOLATERAL VIEW**

Figure 159–86. Intracapsular reconstruction of anterior cruciate ligament insufficiency. Here, the fascial graft is only placed through a femoral tunnel. The free end of the graft is then sutured back onto itself.

fascial graft be pulled into the joint from the tibia through a lateral arthrotomy. Suturing the distal end of the graft back to itself and to the fibrous joint capsule forms a sling around the lateral femoral condyle, attached to the proximal tibia by the fascial pedicle (Fig. 159–86). This arrangement was found to effectively stabilize the joint, and a viable "ligament" was found in the joint three years after surgery.[23]

Several techniques using part of the patellar tendon to replace the ruptured ligament have been described. Because this tendon is biomechanically the strongest available fibrous tissue in the immediate area, it is a suitable substitute. At least two veterinary procedures have developed since a biomechanical awareness was applied to the evaluation of anterior cruciate ligament reconstruction techniques.

"Over-the-Top" Procedure. The "over-the-top" procedure described by Amoczky,[801] was developed as a modification of two human procedures.[47,48,59] The skin incision extends from the anteromedial mid-shaft femur over the patellar tendon to the anterolateral aspect of the proximal tibia. The patellar tendon is incised longitudinally to isolate the medial third of the tendon from the tibial tubercle over the patella and proximolaterally to incorporate the fascia lata. A pie-shaped wedge of patella is osteotomized from the dorsal surface of the patella to be included in the tendon graft; the articular surface of the patella is not penetrated (Fig. 159–87).

The graft is freed proximally from the biceps femoris muscle and dissected free down to the tibial tubercle. Blood vessels to the graft from the infrapatellar fat pad must be left intact. The joint is examined, debrided, and lavaged through the medial arthrotomy. The patella and quadriceps muscle are retracted laterally to expose the lateral fabella. An incision is made vertically in the fibrous tissue be-

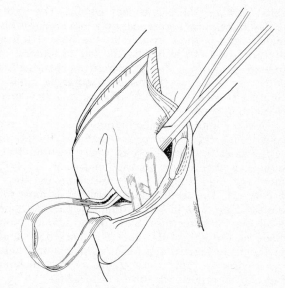

Figure 159–88. The graft is passed through the joint using the "over the top" maneuver.

tween the femur and the fabella. With the joint kept in full flexion, curved hemostatic forceps are passed through the incision and over the top of the lateral femoral condyle into the intercondylar notch. The forceps are kept close to the bone until the posterior joint capsule is penetrated. The forceps are manipulated until the tips are visible in the intercondylar space (Fig. 159–88).

The ends of a 3-0 stainless steel suture that secures the free end of the graft in a Bunnell pattern are grasped in the forceps. Using the suture, the surgeon pulls the graft through the posterior joint capsule and over the top of the lateral femoral condyle so that it

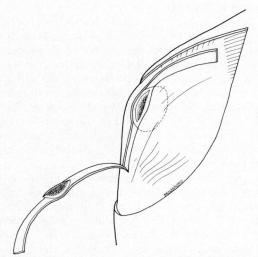

Figure 159–87. Intracapsular reconstruction of anterior cruciate ligament insufficiency using the medial third of the patella tendon in the tissue graft.

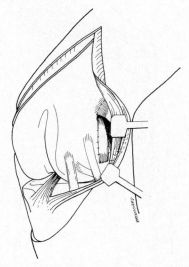

Figure 159–89. The graft is secured to the lateral femoral condyle by suturing the graft to the femorofabellar ligament and periosteum.

exits between the femur and fabella. The graft is pulled tight, until anterior drawer movement is eliminated, and is then sutured to the periosteum and fibrous tissue of the fabella and lateral femoral condyle (Fig. 159–89). The arthrotomy incision is closed, with care taken not to luxate the patella medially. Routine closure is used for the fascia, subcutaneous tissue, and skin.

This technique is recommended as being more consistently reliable in correct anatomical positioning of the graft through the joint than the tunnel techniques. Furthermore, abrasion and wear of the ligament on rough tunnel edges are eliminated by this procedure. The technique is regarded as most suitable for large dogs in which sufficient patellar bone is available for osteotomy and the additional biomechanical strength of the graft is needed for stability in the stifle joint. Long-term biomechanical follow-up reports are not yet available for this technique but clinical reports are most encouraging.

"Under-and-Over" Technique. A similar technique was first described by Hulse and colleagues[44] and evaluated a few years later.[84] The "under-and-over" technique retains the anatomical alignment found in the "over-the-top" procedure but does not require a bone wedge to be resected from the patella.

A lateral parapatellar approach is made from the mid-femur to the proximal tibia. The lateral third of the patellar tendon is isolated from the remainder of the tendon and from the lateral aspect of the patella by a longitudinal incision. The incision is continued proximally up to the fascia lata muscle. A parallel incision is made down the cranial border of the biceps

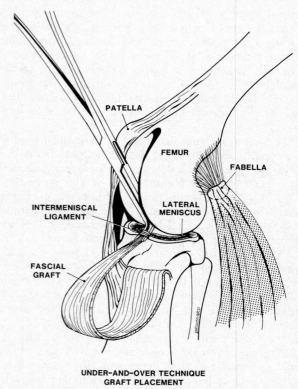

UNDER-AND-OVER TECHNIQUE GRAFT PLACEMENT

Figure 159–91. Right-angle forceps are passed beneath the intermeniscal ligament to grasp the free end of the graft. The forceps are withdrawn to pull the graft into the joint beneath the intermeniscal ligament.

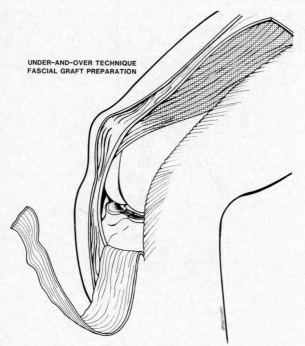

UNDER-AND-OVER TECHNIQUE FASCIAL GRAFT PREPARATION

Figure 159–90. Isolation of the lateral third of the patella tendon and fascia lata for intracapsular reconstruction of anterior cruciate ligament insufficiency.

(2.5 cm caudal and parallel to the first) over the lateral joint capsule to the proximal tibia. Consistent width must be maintained throughout the full length of the graft. Graft width varies with the size of the dog. The graft is freed proximally and reflected off the underlying muscle and joint capsule, down to the tibia. The blood supply to the patellar tendon and the fascia from the infrapatellar fat pad is not disturbed (Fig. 159–90).

A lateral arthrotomy allows inspection, debridement, and lavage of the joint. The biceps femoris and vastus lateralis muscles are separated to expose the lateral fabella and to allow medial luxation of the patella. Right-angled forceps (Mixter gallbladder forceps) are passed from the joint, under the intermeniscal ligament, through the fat pad, and lateral to the tibial tubercle. The free end of the graft is grasped in the forceps and drawn through the fat pad, under the intermeniscal ligament, and into the joint without being twisted (Fig. 159–91).

To pass the graft "over the top" of the lateral femoral condyle, slightly curved bile duct forceps (Monihan gall duct forceps) are maneuvered from the fabella in between the femoral condyles, keeping close to the lateral femoral condyle. The posterior joint capsule is penetrated lateral to the posterior cruciate ligament, and the ends of the forceps are observed in the intercondylar space. The free end of the graft is grasped with the forceps and pulled

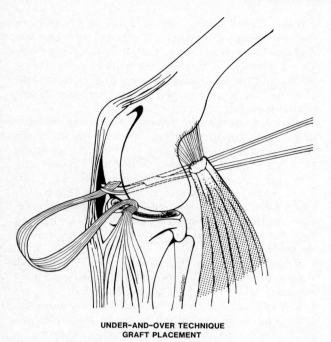

**UNDER-AND-OVER TECHNIQUE
GRAFT PLACEMENT**

Figure 159–92. Curved forceps are used to penetrate the posterior joint capsule to grasp the free end of the graft. The graft is then pulled through the posterior joint capsule to complete the over-the-top maneuver.

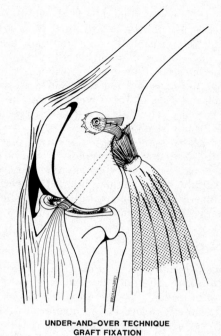

**UNDER-AND-OVER TECHNIQUE
GRAFT FIXATION**

Figure 159–94. The free end of the graft is secured to the femoral condyle using a spiked washer and screw. The graft may also be sutured to the femorofabellar ligament as it passes deep to the latter.

through the joint without being twisted (Fig. 159–92). A small longitudinal incision is made in the fibrous tissue between the fabella and the femur, and the graft is pulled through the incision with the curved forceps (Fig. 159–93).

A 5-mm wide strip of periosteum is elevated from

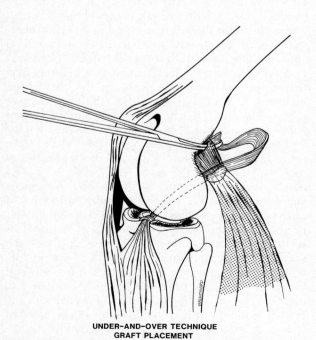

**UNDER-AND-OVER TECHNIQUE
GRAFT PLACEMENT**

Figure 159–93. The free end of the graft is passed beneath the femorofabellar ligament.

the lateral femoral metaphysis between the graft and the proximal trochlea groove. A 3.2-mm (2.0-mm in small dogs) hole is drilled through the femoral metaphysis from lateral to medial. The hole is measured and tapped, and a 4.5-mm ASIF (3.5-mm in small dogs) cortical screw is threaded through a 12.5-mm ASIF (8.5-mm in small dogs) spiked washer and started in the hole. The fascial graft is looped around the screw shaft, under the spiked washer, and is pulled tight while the screw is tightened down (Fig. 159–94). If ASIF equipment is not available, the fascial graft is secured as described for the "over-the-top" technique.

The free end of the graft is sutured to itself around the screw and to the perifabellar fascia (Fig. 159–94). The joint capsule is closed with fine nylon sutures, the fascia with 2-0 nylon interrupted sutures, and subcutaneous and skin layers by standard techniques.

A follow-up study of clinical cases showed the "under-and-over" technique to be equally effective to any other technique over a three-year period in clinical evaluations.[84] An experimental study showed that the biomechanical strength of the substitute continued to improve from eight weeks to six months after implantation (the end of the study).[12,43]

Comparison of Techniques. Many of the intracapsular reconstructive procedures involve capsular imbrication during closure; some argue that imbrication alone is the reason for postoperative stability. On the other hand, the protagonists of reconstruction suggest that extracapsular techniques are temporary, whereas reconstruction is more physiological in the long term. Many other arguments have been raised for and against the many "modified" techniques used throughout the world. Until one is conclusively shown to be consistently superior to all the others, in everyone's hands, the choice of technique continues to be based on "personal experience." Generally speaking, the extracapsular techniques are reserved for smaller dogs and the "over-the-top" procedure for larger dogs. The "under-and-over" procedure is suitable for any size dog.

Other grafts and synthetic materials have been used with these newer techniques,[39,50] but no obvious advantage can be assigned to any one material. The use of supplemental augmentation, to speed up the return of normal biomechanical values to the graft, is currently under investigation.

Postoperative Care

Collagen healing, even under ideal conditions, is slow. Minimal inherent strength is found until six weeks after repair. Within the confines of a joint space, healing is delayed even further. Unrestrained early stress on a primary repair therefore relies totally on the suture material for strength for at least six weeks. Because of this, six weeks of cast immobilization have been favored for primary repair of the anterior cruciate ligament in humans.

Immobilization itself leads to cartilage degeneration,[80] pannus formation,[28] and weakening of the ligament structure.[68] Piper and Whiteside[75] recently suggested that immobilization is contraindicated after primary repair. They found fewer degenerative changes, more strength, and less laxity in joints mobilized for six weeks after surgery than in those treated with cast fixation. However, the anterior drawer sign was slightly more prominent in mobilized dogs than in immobilized dogs.

Reconstructive procedures are based on the assumption that autogenous fibrous tissue will invade and add to the substitute ligament until a functional strength is attained. Wolff's law dictates that such a response is in proportion to the stress applied. Immobilization reduces the stress and, presumably, the response. However, the substitute most commonly used, fascia lata, does not have the biomechanical strength of a normal anterior cruciate ligament, and if unduly stressed after the replacement process, it will fail.

Caught between the disastrous results of either extreme, a clinician must strive for a middle-of-the-road approach. Ideally, the substitute (or primary repair) should be minimally stressed initially, with slow progressive increases in the stress over a long period. No precise information is available on the specific requirements of postoperative stress on the canine anterior cruciate ligament during healing. On the basis of clinical evaluations, we recommend the following protocol:

A padded, coaptation bandage is applied to the operated rear leg to restrict movement to all but a few degrees of flexion. The leg is kept in extension initially. This bandage (or replacements) is kept on the leg for four weeks. As activity and painless movement increase during the postoperative period, the dog will use the leg more and more, hence weakening the bandage and promoting more flexion. Confinement to a cage, playpen, or crate during this period is mandatory.

After four weeks, the bandage is removed, and the dog is kept confined for another four weeks. Eight weeks postoperatively, a controlled exercise program is initiated. Leash walking is begun with one city block and progressed to one mile daily over two weeks. During this time, swimming is highly recommended as a non–weight-bearing exercise to redevelop the muscle mass. A half hour of swimming daily is sufficient; it is split into shorter periods, depending on the dog.

Twelve weeks postoperatively, return to normal function, including short periods of unrestricted play, running, and training, is allowed. The owners are reminded that they have to start training from the beginning again, assuming that the dog is totally unfit. No competitive events should be entered for at least six months after operation. The screw and washer used in the "under-and-over" technique, are removed six months after the operation.

MENISCAL INJURY

Clinical Signs

The majority of meniscal injuries in the dog are associated with anterior cruciate ligament injury. A variable degree of limb disuse is present with the instability associated with anterior cruciate ligament insufficiency. Whether or not meniscal injury accentuates this limb dysfunction in the dog is controversial. One study showed that meniscal injury has no clinical effect on limb disuse in the dog.[76] However, I agree with others[32] that certain types of meniscal tears accentuate lameness. Although the body of the meniscus is avascular and without nerve endings,[69] the mechanical intereference of a sliding bucket handle tear may result in "locking" or a "giving way" feeling as it does in humans. A palpable "click" when the stifle is flexed and extended is suggestive of meniscal injury in the dog. Again, this is usually noted with anterior cruciate ligament insufficiency and occurs when the femoral condyles slide forward as the stifle is extended. When a bucket handle tear of the posterior body of the medial meniscus is present, the medial femoral condyle displaces the section of torn meniscus forward. The hypermobile section of torn meniscus is still attached laterally and medially to the main body of the meniscus and can be displaced only a few millimeters forward with the medial femoral condyle. At the limit of this forward excursion, the medial femoral condyle continues forward and the hypermobile section of torn meniscus snaps posteriorly, creating the palpable "click" within the joint. It is not uncommon for the examiner or client to hear the "click" when the patient is walking or when the stifle is palpated.

Diagnosis

An audible or palpable "click" with flexion and extension of the stifle joint suggests meniscal injury. Confirmation of a meniscus tear can be made only by observing it directly during arthrotomy or arthroscopy.

Arthroscopy for diagnosis and treatment of knee injuries in humans has become popular in the last decade. The technique in dogs[85] has not gained the same popularity. There is little doubt that as veterinary surgeons become more adept with the arthroscope, indications for its use in diagnostics and treatments of joint injuries will increase.

At present, the most accurate method of diagnosing a meniscal tear is by direct observation and inspection of both menisci at arthrotomy. The entire lateral meniscus and anterior body of the medial meniscus may be observed readily. However, observing the posterior body of the medial meniscus, where the majority of meniscal tears occur,[45] is very difficult. To aid inspection of the posterior body of the medial meniscus, the surgeon may use a levering maneuver with a small Hohmann retractor (see Fig. 159–71). The tip of the retractor is positioned on the midline just behind the caudal edge of the tibial plateau. The body of the retractor is levered against the nonarticular portion of the distal trochlea, forcing the tibia downward and forward. This manuever exposes the posterior body of the medial meniscus. To protect against possible damage to the articular cartilage, a moistened gauze sponge is placed between the retractor and the distal trochlea.

Anatomy

The menisci are semilumar discs of fibrocartilage interposed between the articulating surfaces of the femur and tibia (Fig. 159–95). Each is positioned in the joint with the open or concave side of the C facing the midline of the joint. The cross section of each meniscus is wedge-shaped, with a thin, almost transparent free edge positioned toward the midline of the tibial plateau. The peripheral margin of the meniscus is thick, being as much as 6 to 8 mm in large dogs and lies adjacent to and has attachments to the joint capsule. The menisci are held in place by six meniscal ligaments, which are often referred to as the meniscal horns. Each meniscus is also firmly attached to the femur and tibia through their attachments to the joint capsule.

Histologically, the collagen of the body and horns of the menisci differ. The collagen of the meniscal body is arranged in a herringbone pattern and no septa are present. The collagen in the horns is

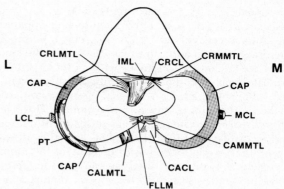

Figure 159–95. Overhead view of the tibial plateau. *CRLMTL* = cranial lateral meniscotibial ligament; *IML* = intermeniscal ligament; *CRCL* = cranial cruciate ligament; *CRMMTL* = cranial medial meniscotibial ligament; *CAP* = joint capsule attachment to the meniscus; *MCL* = medial collateral ligament; *CAMMTL* = caudal medial meniscotibial ligament; *CACL* = caudal cruciate ligament; *FLLM* = femoral ligament of the lateral meniscus; *CALMTL* = caudal lateral meniscotibial ligament; *PT* = popliteal tendon; *LCL* = lateral collateral ligament. (Reprinted with permission from Hulse, D. A., and Shires, P. K.: The meniscus: anatomy, function, and treatment. Comp. Cont. Ed. Pract. Vet. 5:765, 1983.)

organized into discrete longitudinal bundles separated by loose connective tissue septa. Also, the meniscal horns are richly supplied with blood vessels and nerves, whereas the body is almost completely devoid of nerves and vessels. Only the peripheral 10 to 15 per cent of the meniscal body is supplied by a rich synovial plexus arising from the joint capsule. The vessels are oriented in a circumferential pattern, with radial branches directed toward the free edge of the meniscus. However, they penetrate only the outer periphery of the meniscus. This capillary plexus is interrupted along the course of the popliteal tendon. A synovial vascular fringe extends onto the femoral and tibial articular surfaces, but these vessels apparently do not penetrate the meniscal stroma.[3] The central zone of the meniscal body is nourished by diffusion of synovial fluid.

Function and Normal Mechanics

The importance of the menisci is a matter of debate. Recent retrospective clinical studies in humans and experimental animals have shown that the menisci are important intra-articular structures. The importance of the menisci in the stifle joint is reflected by the number of functions attributed to them. Krause and associates[54] showed in dogs that the menisci perform a load-transmitting and energy-absorbing function in the stifle joint. They found that, in the dog, the menisci in the normal standing position transmit approximately 65 per cent of the weight-bearing load.

Seale and co-workers[83] studied the role of meniscectomy on knee stability in human cadavers and found that the menisci play an important role in both rotational stability and varovalgus stability. Levy and associates[56] used an *in vitro* knee-testing apparatus on human cadavers to study the effect of medial meniscectomy on anteroposterior motion of the knee. They concluded that in knees with an intact anterior cruciate ligament, the anterior tibial displacement is not sufficient to allow the medial meniscus to participate in restraining anterior movement. However, with a disrupted anterior cruciate ligament, the anterior displacement of the tibia (anterior drawer movement) wedges the posterior body of the medial meniscus between the tibial plateau and the femoral condyle. In this situation, the medial meniscus acts as a restraint to anterior movement.

Other functions attributed to the menisci include lubrication and prevention of synovial entrapment.[24] The menisci may increase the efficiency of joint lubrication by acting as space-filling buffers. This function is reflected by a 20 per cent rise in the coefficient of friction within the joint following meniscectomy.[58] Synovial entrapment between the articulating surface of the femur and tibia is painful owing to the pain receptors within the joint capsule. The joint capsule is firmly attached to the peripheral border of the meniscus, preventing impingement of the capsule between the articulating surfaces. With total meniscectomy, impingement of the capsule between the femur and tibia may occur with flexion and extension.

Mechanism of Injury

Meniscal injury is most commonly associated with ligament injury affecting the stifle joint in the dog. With the instability associated with anterior cruciate ligament injury, abnormal compressive, shearing, and rotational forces act on the meniscus. The most common meniscal injury is a bucket-handle tear of the posterior body of the medial meniscus (Fig. 159–96A). This type of meniscal tear is usually associated with an isolated anterior cruciate ligament tear. The resultant instability allows abnormal posterior displacement of the medial femoral condyle on the tibial plateau during flexion and extension. The medial meniscus is relatively immobile, and the posterior body becomes wedged between the femoral condyle and tibial plateau. This arrangement places abnormal compressive and shearing forces on the fibrocartilage of the meniscus, resulting in a tear through the substance of the posterior body.

The location of the tear in the posterior body varies from close to the free edge to a few millimeters from the peripheral capsular attachment. It is not uncommon for the surgeon to perceive a tear near the periphery as being a capsular tear with folding of the entire posterior body of the medial meniscus (Fig. 159–96B). However, a capsular tear is uncommon in our experience and is usually seen with multiple ligament injury secondary to severe trauma. With severe trauma, it is probable that the initial impact

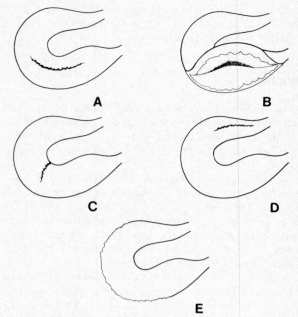

Figure 159–96. Locations of common meniscal tears. *A,* Bucket-handle tear of the caudal body of the medial meniscus. *B,* Peripheral capsular tear resulting in a forward folding of the caudal body of the medial meniscus. *C,* Transverse tear extending from the free edge toward the peripheral border. *D,* Cranial bucket-handle tear. *E,* Peripheral capsular tear along the entire border of the meniscus. (Reprinted with permission from Hulse, D. A., and Shires, P. K.: The meniscus: anatomy, function, and treatment. Comp. Cont. Ed. Pract. Vet. 5:765, 1983.)

separates the meniscotibial and meniscofemoral capsular attachments. Another mechanism for a capsular tear causing a folding of the entire posterior body of the medial meniscus may be femorotibial subluxation, which results from multiple ligament injury and places abnormal shearing forces on the capsular attachments. A less common type of injury is a transverse tear of the meniscus extending from the free edge toward the periphery of the meniscus (Fig. 159–96C). It usually involves the medial meniscus and is secondary to abnormal rotary forces due to anterior cruciate ligament injury. The abnormal displacement of the medial femoral condyle coupled with the internal rotational instability of the ligament injury places excessive torsional forces on the meniscus. The result is a transverse tear in the meniscus generally located more anterior than a bucket-handle tear. We have seen one case of a bucket-handle tear involving the anterior body of the medial meniscus in a patient with an isolated anterior cruciate ligament injury (Fig. 159–96D). The only explanation for this injury is that excessive compressive forces act on the meniscus during extension.

Hyperextension of the stifle has been reported as a cause of anterior cruciate ligament injury. The meniscal injury in this case may have occurred simultaneously with the ligament rupture. Rupture of the meniscofemoral and meniscotibial capsular attachments along the entire periphery of the lateral or medial meniscus is uncommon (Fig. 159–96C). It is associated with severe internal derangement of the stifle joint secondary to the patient's being struck by an automobile. Associated structures usually injured include: anterior or posterior cruciate ligament, one or both collateral ligaments, and the joint capsule. This meniscal injury occurs with the initial impact.

The lateral meniscus is not commonly injured with isolated anterior cruciate ligament insufficiency. The explanation for the low incidence of this injury is that the lateral meniscus is more mobile than the medial meniscus. The femoral ligament of the lateral meniscus, the action of the popliteal muscle, and limited posterior meniscotibial capsular attachment allow movement of the lateral meniscus with the lateral condyle of the femur, preventing wedging and keeping excessive forces from acting on the fibrocartilage of the lateral meniscus.

Treatment

Each meniscal injury must be assessed individually and in conjunction with other joint derangements before a type of treatment is selected. The methods of treatment for meniscal injuries include: (1) partial meniscectomy, (2) total meniscectomy, (3) primary repair, (4) vascular access channelization, and (5) conservative therapy.

Surgical Treatment

Partial Meniscectomy. A partial meniscectomy is the removal of a damaged section of the meniscus (Fig. 159–97). The advantages of using this technique are that (1) it is relatively quick and simple to perform and (2) normal meniscus is left *in situ* to protect the articular cartilage. The disadvantage of partial meniscectomy is that removing a section of meniscus where the cut edge does not communicate with the synovium results in little or no meniscal regeneration. Nevertheless, experimental partial meniscectomy produces less degenerative articular cartilage change than total meniscectomy.[18] Malcolm and Danile[60]

studied the effect of partial meniscectomy on contact stress between articular surfaces using force transducers. They found that with a normal lateral meniscus, 29 per cent of the total lateral load was transmitted between the femur and tibial plateau. When one-quarter of the meniscus was removed in a shape resembling a bucket-handle tear, there was a 45 per cent increase in contact stress. Total meniscectomy resulted in a 313 per cent increase in contact stress. They concluded that peripheral rim of meniscus left *in situ* was valuable in protecting the articular cartilage.

When a partial meniscectomy is performed, adequate exposure of the damaged section of meniscus is necessary. Exposure is facilitated by using the levering maneuver described previously and by suction. With adequate exposure, the surgeon may grasp the body of the section of meniscus to be excised. With a bucket-handle tear of the posterior body of the medial meniscus, the most medial attachment of the torn section is incised first, followed by the most lateral attachment. Care must be exercised not to mistakenly cut the posterior cruciate ligament. The normal articular cartilage must not be lacerated with the scalpel blade. Following excision of the torn section of meniscus, the remaining meniscus must be carefully inspected for additional tears.

Complete Meniscectomy. A complete meniscectomy is the removal of the entire meniscus (Fig. 159–98). The advantages of the technique are that (1) with complete removal, tears of the meniscus that are difficult to see are not inadvertently left *in situ* and (2) the meniscus is incised at the vascular capsular attachments, allowing access to pleuripotential cells necessary for regeneration. The disadvantages of complete meniscectomy are (1) the increase in contact stress on the articular cartilage, (2) the difficulty in incising the posterior capsular attachments of the meniscus, and (3) experimental demonstration of a greater degree of degenerative articular cartilage changes with total meniscectomy than with partial meniscectomy.

For a total meniscectomy, the anterior meniscotibial ligament is incised with a scalpel blade. The

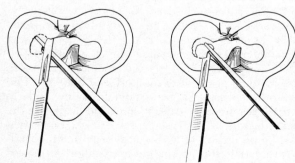

Figure 159–97. Partial meniscectomy. The torn meniscus is grasped with a forceps and the remaining attachments excised with a scalpel blade. (Reprinted with permission from Hulse, D. A., and Shires, P. K.: The meniscus: anatomy, function, and treatment. Comp. Cont. Ed. Pract. Vet. 5:765, 1983.)

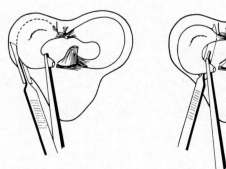

Figure 159–98. Incision of ligament and capsule attachments when performing a complete meniscectomy. (Reprinted with permission from Hulse, D. A., and Shires, P. K.: The meniscus: anatomy, function, and treatment. Comp. Cont. Ed. Pract. Vet. 5:765, 1983.)

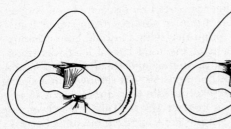

Figure 159–99. Primary repair, which is direct suturing of a torn peripheral meniscocapsular attachment. (Reprinted with permission from Hulse, D. A., and Shires, P. K.: The meniscus: anatomy, function, and treatment. Comp. Cont. Ed. Pract. Vet. 5:765, 1983.)

ligament is grasped with forceps, and an assistant retracts the meniscus medially. Sharp dissection is used to incise the capsular attachments to the periphery of the meniscus. The posterior meniscotibial ligament is cut, and the meniscus removed. If the lateral meniscus is being removed, its femoral ligament must be incised.

Primary Repair. Primary repair is direct suturing of the torn meniscus (Fig. 159–99). The advantage of this technique is that the meniscus is left *in situ*. The disadvantages of this technique are: (1) technical difficulty and (2) the possibility of poor healing. Direct suturing of meniscal injuries is generally reserved for peripheral capsular tears. However, Krackow and Vetter[53] studied direct suturing of vertical tears in the substance of the meniscus using adult mongrel dogs. Preliminary studies indicate that the repaired lacerations remain well approximated during the first three to six weeks. For repairing a peripheral capsular tear of the meniscus, simple interrupted sutures of non-absorbable suture are used. I prefer 3-0 or 4-0 nylon. This type of injury has been seen with multiple ligamentous and joint capsule damage. Knowledge of the normal capsular attachments of the involved meniscus and precise anatomical suturing are essential to ensure normal healing and function of the damaged meniscus.

Vascular Access Channelization. Vascular access channelization is the creation of a channel from the interstitium of the meniscus to the synovia (Fig. 159–100). The purpose of the channel is to allow a fibrovascular response, arising from the vascular synovia, access to the substance of the meniscus, where normally little or no healing capability is present. Arnoczky,[4] the first to develop and study vascular access channeling, was able to show healing of bucket-handle tears in the substance of the meniscus. We have studied vascular access channelization following removal of bucket-handle tears of the posterior body of the medial meniscus. Preliminary results show enhanced regeneration to fill the defect created by partial meniscectomy. The advantage of vascular access channelization is that either healing of meniscus tears or increased regeneration following partial meniscectomy allows improved protection for the articular cartilage. At present, the technique has no disadvantages, but the results are preliminary and more studies are necessary for an accurate long-term prognosis. The current technique for creation of a vascular access channel is quite simple. The surgeon uses a scalpel blade to make a cut through the meniscus from the edge of the torn meniscus posteriorly to the synovia.

Conservative Treatment

Conservative treatment of meniscal tears means leaving the torn section of the meniscus in place. Advocates of this method of treatment believe that a torn meniscus does not cause clinical symptoms nor result in long-term degenerative articular cartilage changes. Experimentally, Cox and Cordell[17] have studied various types of meniscal tears in dogs. They showed that in a stable joint, meniscal tears that were not free-floating or sliding between articular surfaces caused minimal or no degenerative changes. However, meniscal tears that did slide and become trapped between articular surfaces did result in severe degenerative changes of the articular cartilage. Excision of small transverse vertical tears in a stable joint may not be necessary.

Recommendations for Treatment of Meniscal Tears in the Dog

Bucket-Handle Tear of the Meniscus. This is the most common type of meniscal injury and is associated with anterior cruciate ligament insufficiency. The tear is always within the body of the meniscus, but its location in relation to the free edge varies. A partial meniscectomy leaving as much normal meniscus in place as possible is recommended. If more than 80 to 90 per cent of the posterior body must be removed, a vascular access channel may be made to increase regenerative capacity or to aid healing of the bucket-handle tear. Vascular access channelization must be used cautiously, because experimental studies evaluating this technique were short-term and used stable joints.

Peripheral Capsular Tear. Laceration of the meniscofemoral and meniscotibial capsular attachments is not common in my experience but has been associated with multiple ligament and capsular injuries.

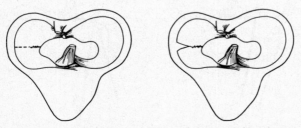

Figure 159–100. Creation of a vascular access channel. An incision is made from the edge of the transverse tear to the peripheral capsular attachment. (Reprinted with permission from Hulse, D. A., and Shires, P. K.: The meniscus: anatomy, function, and treatment. Comp. Cont. Ed. Pract. Vet. 5:765, 1983.)

The treatment of choice is primary suturing of the meniscofemoral and meniscotibial capsular attachments.

Transverse Tear of the Meniscal Body. This type of injury is uncommon. The tear is usually located in the posterior body of the medial meniscus, extending from the free edge toward the periphery. Treatment is directed toward removing any section of meniscus that is hypermobile and may interfere with mechanical function. A partial meniscectomy is done to remove this abnormal section of meniscus. This lesion heals in a stable joint if the tear communicates with the synovia.[35] Therefore, for a tear that does not reach the synovia, an incision from the tear in the meniscus to the synovia can be made to create a vascular access channel. By this means, the fibrovascular response has access to the lacerated meniscus, increasing the chances of the torn meniscus to heal. Because reports of vascular access channeling are preliminary, the technique should be used with caution.

POSTERIOR CRUCIATE LIGAMENT INJURY

Clinical Signs and Diagnosis

The patient with a ruptured posterior cruciate ligament usually has sustained a severe injury to the stifle joint. The most common cause is a high-velocity injury such as being struck by an automobile. With such an injury, multiple capsular, ligament, and meniscal injuries occur, resulting in marked instability of the stifle joint in all planes. The patient may have concurrent fractures or other soft tissue injuries and must be given a thorough physical examination. Stabilization of all vital parameters is necessary before treatment of stifle ligament injury is undertaken. The patient exhibits a non–weight-bearing lameness with pain on palpation of the stifle joint. With injury to the posterior cruciate ligament, the anterior cruciate ligament, one or both collateral ligaments, secondary joint capsule restraints, and one or both menisci are also commonly injured. Palpation of a stifle joint that sustained such a severe injury reveals marked anteroposterior as well as varovalgus instability. Crepitation and a "popping" sound can be elicited, owing to subluxation of the femorotibial articulation, and malalignment of the stifle joint can be observed.

Isolated rupture of the posterior cruciate ligament in the dog is rare. One group reported only one case of isolated injury to this ligament in over 500 cases of cruciate ligament rupture.[20] The one patient would not bear weight on its rear limb and exhibited pain, swelling and a posterior drawer sign. When palpating a joint for anterior-posterior instability, it may be hard to differentiate between isolated ruptures of the anterior and posterior cruciate ligaments because of the difficulty in determining the pre-injury neutral point. The examiner should palpate the stifle joint at 10, 35, and 90 degrees of flexion. With anterior cruciate ligament injury, instability is prominent at all planes of flexion-extension, but with posterior cruciate ligament injury, instability is more prominent at 90 degrees of flexion. This fact has been confirmed experimentally by Arnoczky and Marshall,[6] who found 8 mm of posterior drawer movement at 90 degrees of flexion and 2 mm of posterior drawer movement in extension after cutting the posterior cruciate ligament. Another method of differentiating isolated injuries of these two ligaments is to place the anesthetized patient in dorsal recumbency with the longitudinal axis of both femurs perpendicular to the table. The stifle joints are held flexed to 90 degrees, i.e., the longitudinal axis of the tibia parallel to the table, by the examiner's support of the foot. A comparison is made between the patellotibial crest relationships of the normal leg and the injured leg. The injured leg may reflect a "posterior sag," indicating an isolated posterior cruciate ligament injury. This comparison is commonly used in humans to distinguish anterior posterior ligament injury.[42] We have noted the "posterior sag" sign in cats who had posterior cruciate and medial collateral ligament injury, and we have observed posterior sag in one isolated posterior cruciate ligament injury in a dog.

Radiographs should be taken of the injured stifle joint to evaluate the osseous structures. Careful scrutiny of the origins and insertions of the cruciate ligaments and collateral ligaments may reveal small osseous densities associated with ligament-bone failure. Ligament and joint capsule failure may be diagnosed radiographically by demonstration of subluxation or joint space widening. Arthroscopy may be valuable to differentiate isolated posterior and anterior cruciate ligament injuries.

Anatomy and Function of the Posterior Cruciate Ligament

The posterior cruciate ligament originates from the lateral aspect of the medial femoral condyle (Figs. 159–101 and 159–102). The origin is elliptical, extending from a point just below the articular cartilage of the femoral trochlea posteriorly to the level of the medial epicondyle. The fibers of the ligament pass posteriorly and distally to insert on the medial side of the popliteal notch. The fibers are vertically oriented and pass medial to the joint midline. There is a slight spiral of the posterior cruciate ligament because of the orientation of the femoral and tibial attachments. The fibers of the ligament are divided into a anterior band, which is taut in flexion and loose in extension, and a small posterior band, which is loose in flexion and taut in extension. The primary function of the posterior cruciate ligament is as a primary restraint against posterior drawer movement, i.e., posterior displacement of the tibia relative to the femur. This function as a primary restraint against anteroposterior instability is a function of the anterior band and is most important with the stifle joint in

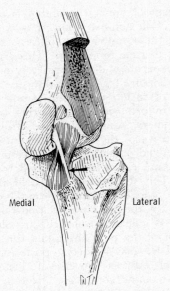

Figure 159–101. Posterior cruciate ligament in extension. Notice that only the posterior part (arrow) is taut. (Reprinted with permission from Arnoczky, S. P., and Marshall, J. L.: The cruciate ligaments of the canine stifle. An anatomical and functional analysis. Am. J. Vet. Res. 38:1807, 1977.)

flexion. The smaller posterior band of the ligament is taut in extension and helps against hyperextension. The cruciate ligaments are secondary restraints for rotational stability because they twist on themselves during flexion. An injury to the posterior cruciate ligament results in an increase in rotational instability. The degree of rotational instability is greater with internal rotation than with external rotation. Experimentally, isolated transection of the posterior cruciate ligament did not result in increased flexion or extension.[6]

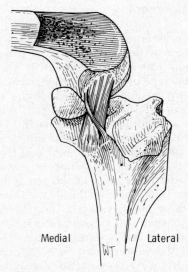

Figure 159–102. Posterior cruciate ligament in flexion. Notice that cranial bulk is taut, whereas posterior band is loose. (Reprinted with permission from Arnoczky, S. P., and Marshall, J. L.: The cruciate ligaments of the canine stifle. An anatomical and functional analysis. Am. J. Vet. Res. 38: 1807, 1977.)

Mechanism of Injury

Isolated posterior cruciate ligament injury is rare in the dog and cat. The type of trauma that results in this type of injury is a force directed against the anterior tibial surface close to the joint. Because the bulk of the posterior cruciate ligament acts as a primary restraint to posterior drawer movement during flexion, if the traumatic force occurs during flexion in an anterior-to-posterior direction, isolated rupture of the ligament may result. This mechanism is supported by the surgical findings in one case, in which an area of bruising and hemorrhage was apparent in the subcutaneous tissue on the anterior tibial crest.[20] The majority of posterior cruciate ligament injuries occur secondary to severe trauma directed at the stifle joint.

Most commonly, this type of trauma results from the dog's being struck by an automobile. In addition to the posterior cruciate ligament rupture, other primary restraints, including the anterior cruciate ligament and one or both collateral ligaments, are commonly injured. Severe injury to secondary restraints, e.g., the joint capsule and menisci, are also likely to be present. The result is subluxation or complete luxation of the stifle joint. A less severe injury has been seen in cats, in which the posterior cruciate ligament and the medial collateral ligament are injured but the anterior cruciate ligament is intact. The cats have also had joint capsule and medial meniscal injuries.

Treatment

Loss of the posterior cruciate ligament results in severe anteroposterior instability. Long-term instability causes degenerative arthritis and a variable degree of limb disuse. Because the degree of limb disuse is difficult to predict and may be marked, we recommend surgical stabilization of posterior cruciate ligament injury. As a rule, the patient will have sustained a severe injury, and all vital parameters must be stable before surgery is undertaken. Other ligaments and the joint capsule are likely to also be ruptured. The surgeon must be prepared to treat these other internal derangements of the stifle joint. The methods of treatment for posterior cruciate ligament injury can be divided into primary repair and secondary reconstructive procedures.

Primary Repair

Primary bone repair of the posterior cruciate ligament is reserved for those cases in which there is an avulsion fracture at the origin or insertion of the ligament. The patient is anesthetized, clipped, scrubbed, and draped for a lateral arthrotomy of the stifle joint. A parapatellar skin incision is made from 5 cm above the proximal pole of the patella to 3 cm below the tibial crest. The subcutaneous tissue is

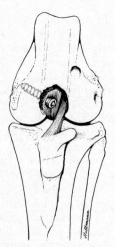

Figure 159–103. Compression screw fixation of an avulsion fracture of the femoral origin of the posterior cruciate ligament.

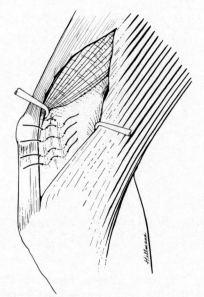

Figure 159–105. Primary suture repair of a posterior cruciate ligament injury at the femoral origin.

incised along the same line, and the skin edges are clipped to towels or a stockinette. A lateral parapatellar arthrotomy is made, the patella is luxated medially, and the internal structures of the joint are examined. The avulsion fracture is located at the femoral origin or tibial insertion of the ligament. If the bone fragment is large enough, it is reduced and stabilized with a compression screw (Fig. 159–103). If the bone fragment is too small to accommodate a screw, it is stabilized (Fig. 159–104). Two parallel drill holes .062 cm in diameter are drilled through the parent bone at the fracture site. Two corresponding holes are drilled through the bone fragment, and nonabsorbable suture is passed through the holes and ligament. The free ends of the suture are passed through the parallel drill holes, pulled taut, and tied to maintain tension. This arrangement secures the avulsion fragment, allows for bony union of the fragment to the femoral condyle, and returns the functional integrity of the posterior cruciate ligament.

If an avulsion fragment is too small to stabilize with fixation devices or if the failure through the ligament is at its origin or insertion, primary repair of the ligament with augmentation is the technique of choice (Fig. 159–105). The ligament end is debrided, and nonabsorbable suture is placed in the substance of the ligament using a Bunnell-Mayer pattern. The failure site at the popliteal notch or lateral surface of the medial femoral condyle is prepared by curettage to subchondral bone. Two parallel (.062-cm) drill holes are made through the bone at the failure site, and the free ends of the ligament suture are passed through the holes with the aid of preplaced wire loops. The suture is pulled taut, bringing the torn ligament into apposition with the bone, and then is tied at the point where the free ends exit from the

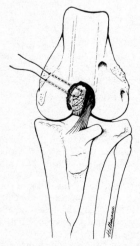

Figure 159–104. Suture fixation of an avulsion fracture of the femoral origin of the posterior cruciate ligament.

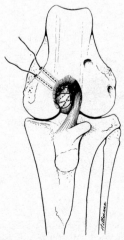

Figure 159–106. Extracapsular reconstruction of posterior cruciate ligament injury using imbrication sutures.

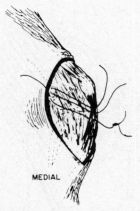

Figure 159–107. Medial imbrication. (Reprinted with permission from DeAngelis, M. P., and Betts, W. C.: Posterior cruciate ligament rupture. J. Am. Anim. Hosp. Assoc. 9:447, 1973.)

drill holes. Primary ligament repair should be augmented with a secondary reconstructive procedure.

Reconstruction of Posterior Cruciate Ligament Injury

Extracapsular Reconstruction

Imbrication of the Fibrous Joint Capsule (Fig. 159–106). A lateral parapatellar capsulotomy is performed to remove the remnants of the posterior cruciate ligament and to inspect the anterior cruciate ligament and the menisci. The capsulotomy is sutured with simple interrupted absorbable sutures. No. 2 polyester suture is used for the imbrication of the joint capsule. The sutures are preplaced from proximal to distal, with one pass of the suture through the fibrous joint capsule on each side of the arthrotomy line. The row of sutures is preplaced from 2 cm proximal to the patella distally to the level of the tibial crest. The sutures are tied, causing an imbrication, i.e., tucking of the fibrous joint capsule. A similar row of sutures may be placed through the medial fibrous joint capsule for additional stability. The principle of this technique is that the sutures give initial joint

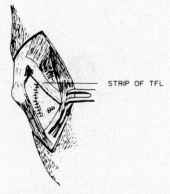

Figure 159–108. Correction of posterior lateral instability. TFL = tensor fascia lata. (Reprinted with permission from DeAngelis, M. P., and Betts, W. C.: Posterior cruciate ligament rupture. J. Am. Anim. Hosp. Assoc. 9:447, 1973.)

stability and the fibroblastic reaction in the capsule, from the surgical intervention and from the instability, gives later stability. This technique is adequate for small dogs and cats but is not applicable in medium, large, and giant dogs.

Medial Imbrication with Fascia Lata Transposition (Fig. 159–107 and 159–108). A lateral parapatellar capsulotomy is performed to remove the remnants of the posterior cruciate ligament and to inspect the anterior cruciate ligament as well as both menisci. The capsulotomy is sutured in a simple interrupted pattern. Two sutures of No. 2 polyester are placed on the medial side of the joint against the bone from the area of the medial fabellae and are anchored in the medial third of the patellar ligament just above its insertion on the tibia. Laterally, a 10-mm-wide section of fascia lata is freed proximally and transposed distally to create a reinforcing posterolateral ligament. The fascial strip is sutured to the deep fascia overlying the posterolateral femoral condyle and tibial plateau. If the anterior cruciate ligament is concurrently ruptured, the fascia lata may be used for its reconstruction.

Redirection of the Medial Collateral Ligament and Long Digital Extensor Tendon (Fig. 159–109). A

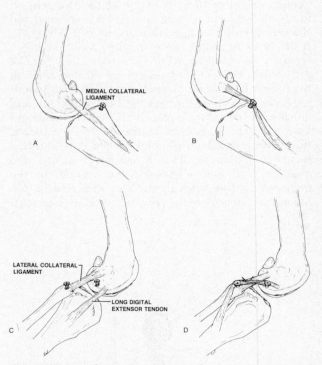

Figure 159–109. The current technique for treating a rupture of the caudal cruciate ligament. *A,* Placement of a bone screw in the caudomedial corner of the proximal tibia. *B,* Trapping the medial collateral ligament "behind" the bone screw. *C,* Placement of bone screws in the fibular head and midway between the long digital extensor origin and the proximal attachment of the lateral collateral ligament. *D,* Trapping the long digital extensor tendon "behind" the bone screws and stabilizing it with a figure-of-eight suture over the screw heads. (Reprinted with permission from Egger, E. L.: Caudal cruciate ligament injuries. *In* Bojrab, M. J. (ed.): *Current Techniques in Small Animal Surgery,* 2nd ed. Lea & Febiger, Philadelphia, 1983.)

lateral parapatellar capsular incision is made to inspect the internal structures of the joint and remove the remnants of the torn posterior cruciate ligament. The capsulotomy is sutured using standard methods. Stabilization is achieved through redirection of the medial collateral ligament and the long digital extensor tendon. The insertion of the caudal head of the sartorius muscle is incised and reflected posteriorly to expose the medial collateral ligament. The ligament is carefully undermined using sharp dissection and redirected anteroposteriorly. Redirection is accomplished by trapping the distal third of the ligament behind a bone screw and a spiked washer placed in the posterior medial corner of the tibial epiphysis. The long digital extensor tendon is redirected on the lateral aspect of the joint. The proximal portion of the muscle and tendon are dissected free from the synovial sheath and surrounding musculature as it crosses the joint. The dissection is carried distally for approximately one-third the length of the tibia. The tendon is retracted posteriorly and trapped in this position with a screw and a spiked washer placed in the head of the fibula.

Intracapsular Reconstruction of the Posterior Cruciate Ligament

Transposition of the Fascia Lata (Fig. 159–110). A 12 × 1 ½-cm section of fascia lata is freed proximally and left attached distally to the tibial plateau. The free end is brought beneath the lateral collateral ligament and continued posteriorly to penetrate the joint capsule just medial to the femoral ligament of the lateral meniscus. A 4.5-mm bone tunnel is drilled from the anteromedial aspect of the medial femoral condyle to the origin of the posterior collateral ligament on the lateral inner surface of the medial femoral condyle. The free end of the fascia lata graft is passed through the bone tunnel, pulled taut, and

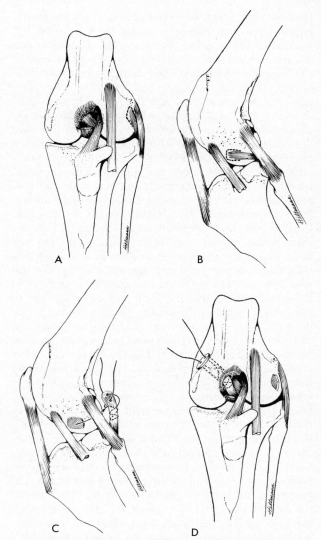

Figure 159–111. Frontal (A) and lateral (B) views of the stifle joint showing osteotomy of the origin of the popliteal tendon. C, Lateral view of the stifle joint showing suture placement and posterior transposition of the popliteal tendon with bone block. D, Frontal view of the stifle joint showing transposition of the popliteal tendon through the joint medial to the femoral ligament of the lateral meniscus and through a predrilled tunnel in the medial femoral condyle.

sutured to the periosteum. The joint capsule is sutured using simple interrupted sutures. Extracapsular reconstruction with sutures, as described previously, may be used for additional stability.

Transposition of the Popliteal Tendon. A lateral parapatellar capsulotomy is made to inspect the internal structures of the joint (Fig. 159–111). The remnants of the posterior cruciate ligament are excised, and a 4.5-mm drill bit is used to create a bone tunnel through the medial femoral condyle. The drill bit is positioned outside the medial femoral condyle and is directed from anteromedial to posterolateral, exiting on the lateral inner surface of the medial condyle at the center of the origin of the posterior cruciate ligament. The parapatellar incision through

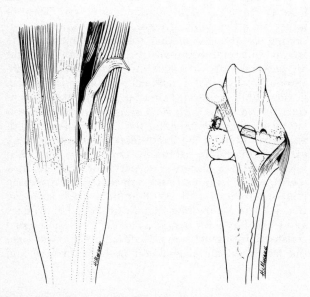

Figure 159–110. Isolation of fascia lata graft and posterior transposition for reconstruction of posterior cruciate ligament injury.

the fascia lata is extended posteriorly along the lateral femorotibial articulation. Caution must be used not to cut the fibular nerve inadvertently. The fascia lata is undermined and retracted posteriorly to expose the fibrous joint capsule, long digital extensor tendon, lateral collateral ligament, and lateral fabellae. The popliteal tendon inserts onto the lateral femoral condyle just proximal to the articular cartilage border and immediately posterior to the origin of the long digital extensor tendon. The popliteal tendon with a thin rectangular bone block (3 × 7 mm) is harvested with a small osteotome and mallet. The popliteal tendon is freed by carefully incising the capsular attachments and by passing the bone and tendon posteriorly beneath the lateral collateral ligament. Posterior to the lateral collateral ligament, there are distal meniscal reflections to the popliteal tendon that need to be carefully incised to allow further posterior reflection of the popliteal tendon. There are no meniscal reflections from the proximal surface of the meniscus to the popliteal tendon posterior to the lateral collateral ligament. To gain access to the posterolateral compartment of the stifle joint, the capsule is incised along the joint line posterior to the lateral collateral ligament and the incision is extended proximally to the lateral fabella. This incision exposes the large posterolateral capsular pouch and allows access to the posterolateral compartment of the stifle joint. Two or three .062-cm drill holes are placed in the 3 × 7 mm rectangular bone block harvested with the insertion of the popliteal tendon. No. 2 polyester suture is passed through the drill holes and interstitium of the popliteal tendon in a Bunnell-Mayer pattern. The free end of the popliteal tendon should penetrate the joint medial to the femoral ligament of the lateral meniscus. To accomplish this maneuver, the joint capsule reflection onto the proximal surface of the lateral meniscus must be incised. Held with curved hemostat, the free ends of the suture are brought to penetrate the posterior capsule and emerge within the joint. The free ends of the suture are used to pull the bone block and popliteal tendon into the joint. If difficulty is encountered at this point, larger hemostats are used to enlarge the opening through the posterior joint capsule. The free ends of the suture are passed through the previously created bone tunnel in the medial femoral condyle with wire loops. The suture is pulled taut, guiding the rectangular bone block and popliteal tendon into the bone tunnel. The free ends of the suture are passed through the eyes of a button and tied on the medial surface of the medial femoral condyle. Other capsular, ligamentous, or meniscal injuries are treated at this time. The posterolateral joint capsule is accurately sutured, as is the parapatellar capsulotomy. The soft tissues are closed using standard methods.

Postoperative Care

Immobilization of the limb in a modified Robert-Jones bandage is maintained for four weeks. This type of bandage allows minimal movement and stress but does not permit overextension or overflexion during the early postoperative period. The bandage must be checked weekly and changed with the patient under sedation, if necessary. Following bandage removal, enforced rest with supervised exercise on a leash only is begun. Passive flexion and extension of the hip, stifle, tarsal, and phalangeal joints helps maintain the normal range of motion during the convalescent period. Ten weeks postoperatively, supervised leash exercise may be increased and swimming therapy begun. Five months postoperatively, the patient may gradually return to normal activity. The animal must not be forced to engage in sporting activities until muscle function has regained preinjury status. This is extremely important to prevent injury to primary or secondary reconstructive procedures. The muscles surrounding the joint are important in dynamic stabilization of the stifle joint; if this support is not present, the surgical correction may fail.

Prognosis

For the patient with an isolated posterior cruciate ligament injury, the prognosis for good use of the limb following surgery is good to excellent. The patient that had multiple ligament injury and has undergone multiple reconstructive procedures for stabilization, the prognosis for good use of the limb is fair.

COLLATERAL LIGAMENT INJURY

Clinical Signs

The degree of instability resulting from collateral ligament injury is highly dependent on the extent of injury to other joint structures. Experimental sectioning of either the medial collateral ligament or the lateral collateral ligament results in only a slight increase in varus or valgus instability.[91] A moderate amount of external rotational instability is seen in flexion, and moderate internal rotary instability is seen in extension with sectioning of the medial collateral ligament. Sectioning the lateral collateral ligament results in a moderate increase in internal and external rotation in extension. Only when associated joint structures (anterior or posterior cruciate ligament) were sectioned did substantial increases in joint instability result. With trauma, such as being struck by an automobile, significant injury to primary and secondary joint restraints may occur. The medial collateral ligament is more commonly injured than the lateral collateral ligament in both the dog and

cat. With medial collateral ligament injury the anterior cruciate ligament, medial meniscus, and medial
joint capsule are often also injured. In the cat, we
have seen posterior cruciate ligament injury commonly associated with medial collateral ligament and
medial joint capsule injuries. The patient has a non–
weight-bearing lameness. On physical examination,
the stifle is swollen and painful. The patient should
be sedated so that ligamentous injury may be assessed
following stabilization of all vital parameters. In extension, marked valgus instability (medial restraint
injury) or marked varus instability (lateral restraint
injury) are noted. A patient with multiple ligament
injury has anteroposterior instability as well as increased rotational instability. With flexion and extension, a "popping" sound may be noted. It indicates
meniscal injury or femorotibial joint subluxation.

Diagnosis

The diagnosis of collateral ligament injury is based
on history and physical examination. Because the
stifle joint is painful and swollen, sedation is required
for accurate assessment of joint instability. The patient should not be sedated until all vital parameters
are stable for 12 hours. Thorough palpation of the
stifle joint in flexion, normal standing angle, and
extension with the tibia in neutral, internal, and
external positions should be performed. Radiographs
of the stifle joint are taken while the patient is under
sedation. Careful evaluation of the origins and insertions of the collateral and cruciate ligaments may
reveal small bone densities indicating ligament injury. Subluxation may be noted radiographically with
plain or stress radiographs.

Anatomy and Function of the Collateral Ligaments

Medial Collateral Ligament

The longitudinal fibers of the medial collateral
ligament originate from the medial femoral epicondyle (Fig. 159–112). From here the fibers are directed
distally across the joint space and tibial plateau to
insert over a large rectangular area of the proximal
tibia. As the ligament passes over the joint space, it
blends with the joint capsule and meniscotibial capsule attachment. Also, as the ligament passes over
the proximal tibial plateau, a fluid-filled bursa is
present. The ligament is taut during extension, but
with flexion it slides posteriorly, with the anterior
fibers remaining taut and the posterior fibers relaxing
slightly. The medial collateral ligament functions as
a primary restraint to valgus angulation when the
stifle joint is extended. In extension, it provides a
slight degree of internal rotary stability and a moderate degree of external rotary stability. With flexion

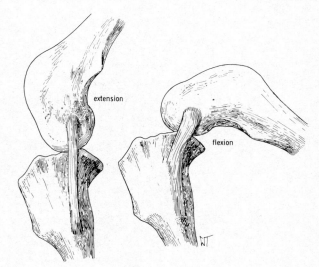

Figure 159–112. The medial collateral ligament in flexion and
extension. The cranial portion remains taut in flexion, whereas the
caudal portion becomes lax. (Reprinted with permission from
Vasseur, P., and Arnoczky, S.: Collateral ligaments of the canine
stifle joint: Anatomic and functional analysis. Am. J. Vet. Res.
142:1133, 1981.)

of the stifle joint, this ligament provides a moderate
degree of stability against external rotation and a
slight amount of valgus stability.

Lateral Collateral Ligament

The lateral collateral ligament originates from the
lateral epicondyle of the femoral condyle (Fig. 159–
113). The popliteal tendon passes deep to the ligament to insert slightly anterior to the epicondyle.
The ligament passes distally and caudally to insert on

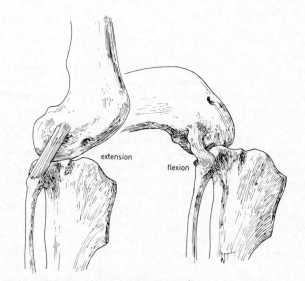

Figure 159–113. The lateral collateral ligament in flexion and
extension. Notice how the entire ligament loosens in flexion.
(Reprinted with permission from Vasseur, P., and Arnoczky, S.:
Collateral ligaments of the canine stifle joint: Anatomic and functional analysis. Am. J. Vet. Res. *142*:1133, 1981.)

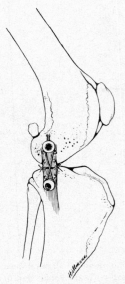

Figure 159–114. Primary repair of an interstitial tear of the medial collateral ligament. The primary repair is augmented with suture or carbon fiber placed around screws at the origin and insertion of the ligament.

the head of the fibula. It is taut in extension, acting as a primary restraint against varus angulation and a secondary restraint against internal and external rotation. During flexion, the lateral collateral ligament relaxes and allows the lateral femoral condyle to move posteriorly, resulting in internal rotation of the tibia. Conversely, as the stifle is extended, the ligament becomes tighter, causing forward excursion of the lateral femoral condyle and external tibial rotation.

Treatment of Injury

Primary repair or primary repair with augmentation is the procedure patient is likely to have sustained severe trauma to the stifle joint and to have concurrent ligamentous, meniscal, and joint capsule injury. Meticulous repair or reconstruction of associated injuries is necessary for optimum results.

The medial collateral ligament is exposed by posterior reflection of the fascial plane of the caudal sartorius muscle. The lateral collateral ligament is exposed with posterior reflection of the fascia lata and biceps femoris muscle. Accurate identification of the injured collateral ligament is difficult owing to swelling, hemorrhage, and joint capsule injury. Careful and meticulous identification of the ligament is necessary before primary repair is begun.

Surgical Techniques for Interstitial Failure. The torn ends of the ligament must be carefully isolated and debrided. Nonabsorbable 0 to 3-0 suture is placed in a Bunnell-Mayer or a vertical mattress (far-near-near-far) suture pattern. Care must be taken not to place excessive tension on the sutures, or the capillary blood supply will be inhibited. The primary

ligament repair is augmented by placing a screw in close proximity to the origin and a second screw near the insertion of the ligament (Fig. 159–114). Nonabsorbable suture or carbon fiber is passed around the screw heads in a figure-of-eight manner. The augmentation provides an internal splint while healing of the ligament occurs.

Surgical Technique for Ligament-Bone Failures. With this injury, the ligament is torn from its origin or insertion (Fig. 159–115). The ligament end is carefully isolated and debrided. It may be secured to the bone by suturing or with a polyacetyl spiked washer. With the suture technique, a Bunnell-Mayer pattern using nonabsorbable suture is preplaced in the ligament end (Fig. 159–116). Two parallel drill holes are made at the failure site, passing through the bone in a transverse plane. The suture ends are passed through the drill holes with wire loops and tied to each other (Fig. 159–117). With the spiked washer technique, the ligament end first is identified. A No. eleven blade is used to make a small longitudinal incision two millimeters from the ligament end. The screw is passed through the incision into the bone. As the screw is tightened, the polyacetyl spiked washer secures the ligament end to the bone (Fig. 159–118).

Surgical Technique for Ligament Bone Avulsion. With this type of failure, the ligament end has an associated piece of cancellous bone (Fig. 159–119). Stability is achieved by implant fixation of the section of bone to the parent bone. Fixation may be with K-wires, a compression screw, or orthopedic wire (Figs. 159–120 and 159–121).

PATELLAR LUXATION

Patellar luxation is one of the most common stifle joint abnormalities seen in small animal orthopedics. The luxation may be traumatic or congenital and medial or lateral. Congenital medial patellar luxation is more common in the toy and miniature breeds, such as miniature poodles, Yorkshire terriers, toy poodles, chihuahuas, Pomeranians, Pekingese and Boston terriers. Lateral patellar luxation occurs more frequently in the large breeds, such as St. Bernard, malamute, and Irish setter.

Anatomy and Function

The etiology and pathogenesis of medial patellar luxation have been attributed to many factors but remain controversial. When describing the abnormalities associated with this condition, one must first have a good understanding of the functional components of the extensor mechanism of the stifle joint (Fig. 159–122).

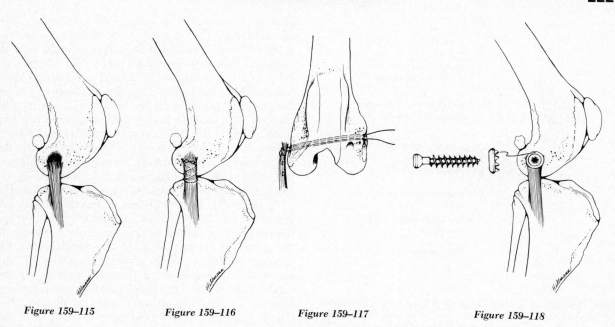

Figure 159–115   *Figure 159–116*   *Figure 159–117*   *Figure 159–118*

Figure 159–115. Medial view showing failure of the medial collateral ligament at its origin on the femur.

Figure 159–116. Medial view showing primary repair with suture placed in the ligament using a Bunnell-Mayer pattern.

Figure 159–117. Frontal view showing the free ends of the suture passed through parallel drill holes in the femur. The suture ends are tied to secure the ligament to the site of failure.

Figure 159–118. Medial view showing fixation of the medial collateral ligament to its femoral origin with a screw and washer.

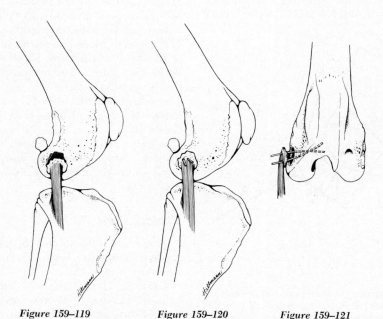

Figure 159–119   *Figure 159–120*   *Figure 159–121*

Figure 159–119. Medial view showing avulsion failure of the medial collateral ligament from its femoral origin.

Figure 159–120. Medial view showing reduction and stabilization of the bone fragment with diverging K-wires.

Figure 159–121. Frontal view showing placement of diverging K-wires for stabilization of the bone fragment. The fragment is not reduced for diagrammatic purposes.

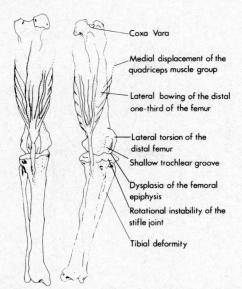

Figure 159–122. The normal alignment of the extensor mechanism and abnormalities associated with medial displacement of the extensor mechanism. (Reprinted with permission from Hulse, D. A.: Pathophysiology and management of medial patellar luxation in the dog. Vet. Med./Small Anim. Clin. 76:43, 1981.)

Medial Patellar Luxation

The extensor mechanism of the stifle joint is composed of the quadriceps muscle group, patella, trochlear groove, straight patellar ligament, and tibial tuberosity. The proper anatomical alignment, that is, a straight line of force, is necessary for anterior stability and efficiency of the extensor mechanism. The quadriceps muscle group is formed by the rectus

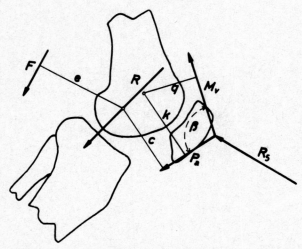

Figure 159–123. Forces acting on the knee projected in a sagittal plane. *F,* Force tending to flex the knee; P_a, force exerted by the patella tendon; M_v, force exerted by the quadriceps muscle; *R,* resultant of F and P_a; R_5, resultant of M_v and P_a; *e,* lever arm of force F; *q,* lever arm of force M_v; *k,* lever arm with which force P_a acts on the patella; *c,* lever arm with which force P_a acts on the tibia; β, angle formed by the lines of action of forces M_v and P_a. (Reprinted with permission from Maquet, P.: Mechanics of osteoarthritis of the patellofemoral joint. Clin. Orthop. *144*:70, 1979.)

femoris, vastus lateralis, vastus intermedius, and vastus medialis. The muscle group converges on the patella and continues distally as the straight patellar ligament. The vastus medialis and vastus lateralis are fixed to the patella by the lateral and medial parapatellar fibrocartilages. The fibrocartilages ride on the crests of the femoral trochlea and aid in patellar stability. The function of the quadriceps muscle group is extension of the stifle joint and tensing of the fascia cruris. In addition, the quadriceps, along with the entire extensor mechanism, aids in the stability of the stifle joint. The patella and trochlear groove are also important in the extensor mechanism and stability of the stifle. By articulating within the boundaries produced by the medial and lateral trochlear ridges, the patella contributes anterior and rotary stability to the joint. The articulation of the patella with the articular cartilage of the trochlear groove is also necessary for maintaining proper nutrition for the articular cartilage of the patella and trochlear groove. Absence of this articulation results in degenerative changes in the articular cartilage.

The patella is also an essential component of the functional mechanism of the extensor apparatus. The patella maintains even tension when the stifle is extended and also acts as a lever arm, increasing the mechanical advantage of the quadriceps muscle group. The single straight patellar ligament and the anatomical location of the tibial crest are important for the anterior stability and efficiency of the extensor mechanism. The patella is pulled upward and backward by the quadriceps muscle, which counters the downward and backward pull of the patellar ligament, as shown in Figure 159–123.[61] The resultant forces M_v (quadriceps muscle) and P_a (patellar ligament) act on the patella with lever arms *q* and *k*, respectively. The origin of these lever arms is the geometric center of the load-transmitting patellofemoral articular surfaces. The patella is compressed against the trochlea by the resultant force (R_5) of the forces M_v and P_a. The magnitude of forces M_v and P_a and most importantly, the angle *B* formed by the lines of action of these forces determine the magnitude of force R_5. The more acute the B angle, the greater the compressive force. Therefore, the degree of force normally increases during flexion and decreases during extension.

Clinical Signs

There are four grades of patellar luxation, with grade I being the least severe and grade IV being the most severe.[87]

Grade I. The patient with a grade I luxation rarely exhibits lameness. It may occasionally skip as the patella slips over the trochlear ridge, but this condition is usually diagnosed as an incidental finding on physical examination. Medial rotation of the tibia is near normal. Manual luxation of the patella may be accomplished, but the patella spontaneously reduces when pressure is released.

Grade II. The lameness varies from an occasional "skip" as the patella luxates to a continuous weight-bearing lameness. The patient is slightly bow-legged. There is some degree of tibial rotation, and slight angular and torsional deformities may be present. With palpation, the patella may luxate with flexion and extension. The patella generally reduces spontaneously or is easily replaced manually. A grade II luxation may progress to a grade III luxation with continued stretching of the lateral retinacular tissues.

Grade III. There is generally some degree of lameness varying from a slight weight-bearing lameness to an acute non–weight-bearing lameness. The patient with acute non–weight-bearing lameness has acutely sprained its stifle. Sometimes, grade III patellar luxation does not cause lameness and is detected during routine physical examination. Often, a patient with a grade III patellar luxation is moderately or severely bow-legged. There is a greater degree (30 to 60 degrees) of tibial rotation, and angular and torsional deformities are more apparent. One may notice a medial displacement of the quadriceps muscle group. On palpation, the patella is often luxated but may be replaced manually. However, after manual reduction, manipulation of the stifle results in reluxation of the patella.

Grade IV. This patient exhibits lameness and a conformational abnormality. The lameness may be a non–weight-bearing lameness, and if it is bilateral, the patient may walk balanced on its front legs. However, the patient usually bears weight with the limbs but cannot extend the stifle joint and "crawls" with the rear legs. Conformationally, the stifle is flexed with the foot turned toward the midline. The patella is permanently luxated and cannot be reduced. The patella is hypoplastic and articulates with the medial condyle of the femur. The angular and torsional deformities are marked.

Pathological Changes

The degree of pathological derangement depends on the grade of patella luxation, but 95 per cent of the patients with medial patellar luxation exhibit some type of structural abnormality.[81]

The following is a list of musculoskeletal abnormalities associated with medial patellar luxation in the dog (see Fig. 159–126): (1) Coxa vara, (2) Lateral torsion of the distal femur, (3) Medial displacement of the quadriceps muscle group, (4) Lateral bowing of the distal one-third of the femur, (5) dysplasia of the femoral epiphysis, (6) rotational instability of the stifle joint, (7) tibial deformities, and (8) degenerative joint disease.

Deformities range from mild soft tissue changes to marked skeletal abnormalities. At present, there is not enough clinical or experimental evidence to definitively establish a sequence of events leading to the musculoskeletal abnormalities. The severity of change is related to the age of the patient and the duration of luxation. The age of the dog is important,

because the angular and torsional abnormalities occur secondary to abnormal forces directed against the open physis. The duration of luxation is important in that the longer the abnormal forces are allowed to act on the physis, the greater the torsional and angular deformities. Hence the greater degree of deformity with grade IV luxations. Simply stated, if force increases on an active physis, growth retardation occurs. Conversely, if force decreases on an active physis, growth acceleration occurs. Also, if an abnormal force is directed perpendicular to an active physis, the physis grows away from the deforming force, resulting in a torsional deformity.[2] The articular cartilage functions as the growth plate for the femoral epiphysis and reacts to pressures in a similar manner. Increased pressure retards growth of the femoral epiphysis, and decreased pressure accelerates it.

The pathogenesis of the angular, torsional, and epiphyseal developmental abnormalities may be appreciated when one displaces the quadriceps muscle force medially. Many theories attempt to explain the sequence of events leading to a medial displacement of the quadriceps muscle force. The majority of authorities believe that the displacement relates to congenital hip abnormalities. For instance, coxa vara may cause a more lateral positioning of the limb, resulting in medial displacement of the quadriceps muscle force. Femoral capital retroversion and anteversion both have been discussed as the initiating cause of medial displacement of the quadriceps muscle force. Also, hypoplastic development of the vastus lateralis may alter the overall quadriceps muscle force by allowing a greater medial vector force produced by the vastus medialis. Whatever the initiating sequence, the medially directed quadriceps muscle force increases pressure on the medial aspect of the distal femoral physis and medial femoral epiphysis and decreases pressure on the lateral distal femoral physis and lateral femoral epiphysis, resulting in lateral bowing of the femur and femoral condylar dysplasia. Also, patellar luxation, the absence of the normal physiological pressure exerted by the patella on the trochlear groove results in a shallow trochlear groove.

Treatment of Medial Patellar Luxation

Surgical treatment for medial patellar luxation should be related to the pathogenesis. Marked skeletal deformities result from abnormal pressures exerted on an open physis. These deformities may occur rapidly, particularly in grade III or grade IV luxations. Therefore, one should not advise delay until the patient is older for surgical correction. The longer the abnormal forces are present, the greater the musculoskeletal deformities. The goal of surgical treatment is to realign the extensor apparatus in order to return the forces acting on the growth plates (physis and articular cartilage) to normal. A number of different techniques are described to stabilize patellar luxation in the dog. A combination of stabi-

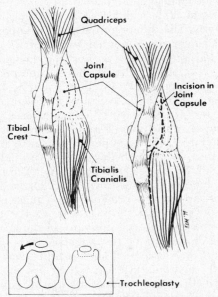

Figure 159–124. Incision for tibial crest transplant. The proper appearance of a trochleoplasty is shown in inset. (Reprinted with permission from Hulse, D. A.: Pathophysiology and management of medial patellar luxation in the dog. Vet. Med./Small Anim. Clin. 76:43, 1981.)

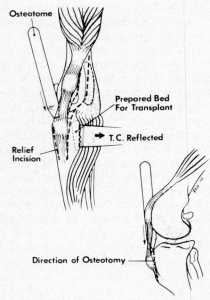

Figure 159–125. Osteotomy of the tibial crest. (Reprinted with permission from Hulse, D. A.: Pathophysiology and management of medial patellar luxation in the dog. Vet. Med./Small Anim. Clin. 76:43, 1981.)

lization techniques is usually necessary, and the greater the severity of the problem, the greater the number of techniques necessary to obtain optimum stability and function.

Tibial Crest Transposition. An anterolateral incision is made 5 cm proximal to the patella and extending distally 3 cm below the tibial crest (Fig. 159–124). The subcutaneous tissues are incised along the same line, and the skin edges clipped to the stockinette to reduce bacterial contamination. A parapatellar tendon incision is made through the fascia lata approximately 0.5 cm lateral to the patellar tendon. The incision is extended proximally and distally the length of the surgical wound. The tibialis cranialis muscle is reflected from its lateral origin on the tibial crest and the lateral tibial plateau. Care must be taken not to inadvertently sever the long digital extensor tendon. The tibialis cranialis muscle is retracted posteriorly from the proximal lateral aspect of the tibia. An incision through the fascia and periosteum on the *medial* aspect of the tibial crest is made as a relief incision to allow the tibial crest to be moved laterally. Blunt dissection is used to gain access to the underside of the patellar tendon. Next, an osteotome and mallet are used to perform the osteotomy of the tibial crest. The osteotomy should begin proximally, 3 to 5 mm caudal from the anterior point of the tibial crest, and extend distally (Fig. 159–125). The distal periosteal attachment is not transected. The degree of lateral transposition of the tibial crest is subjective but should be based on the realignment of the tibial crest with the trochlear groove to establish a straight line of pull for the

extensor mechanism of the stifle. Once the amount of transposition is decided, the site on the proximal lateral tibia is prepared by removing the thin layer of cortical bone to expose the cancellous surface. This may be accomplished with a power drill, rongeurs or a bone rasp. The tibial crest is moved laterally and stabilized with two Kirschner wires directed in a

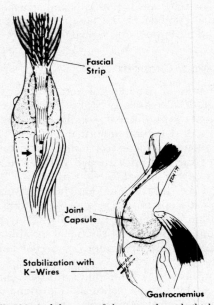

Figure 159–126. Stabilization of the transplanted tibial crest and incision in fascia lata to isolate a section for augmenting the lateral retinaculum. (Reprinted with permission from Hulse, D. A.: Pathophysiology and management of medial patellar luxation in the dog. Vet. Med./Small Anim. Clin. 76:43, 1981.)

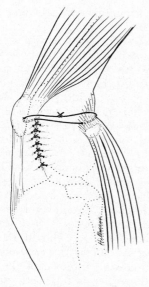

Figure 159–127. Lateral view showing placement of fabella-patellar suture and imbrication sutures for lateral retinacular reinforcement.

posteriorly and slightly proximal direction (Fig. 159–126).

Reinforcement of the Lateral Retinaculum. Reinforcement of the lateral retinaculum may be achieved by synthetic suture augmentation or autologous fascia lata transposition. Suture augmentation involves placement of the suture from the femorofabellar ligament to the lateral patellar fibrocartilage. The suture material should be nonabsorbable and have good tensile strength with minimal elongation and tissue reaction. Any of the polyester (Dacron) suture materials is acceptable. Lateral retinacular reinforcement may also be achieved with imbrication of the lateral fibrous joint capsule (Fig. 159–127). The suture should pass through the fibrous joint capsule only, to prevent exposure of the stifle joint to foreign material. Imbrication is accomplished by preplacing a row of interrupted Lembert inverting sutures in the fibrous joint capsule. The row of sutures extends from 1 cm proximal to the patella distally to the tibial crest. The lateral retinaculum may be reinforced by transposing autologous fascia lata (Fig. 159–128). A section of fascia lata the width of the patella and equal in length to twice the distance from the patella to the fabella is freed proximally and left attached to the superior pole of the patella. The biceps femoris muscle is reflected caudally to expose the fabella, lateral gastrocnemius muscle, and femorofabellar ligament. Sharp dissection is used to undermine the femorofabellar ligament. Curved hemostatic forceps are passed beneath the femorofabellar ligament, and the free end of the fascial strip is grasped and pulled beneath the ligament and back to its origin at the patella. The fascial strip is pulled taut to prevent medial patellar luxation and sutured to itself with 3-0 nylon using a simple interrupted pattern.

Medial Release. Medial release relieves contracture of the medial fibrous joint capsule and the muscular pull of the vastus medialis and sartorius muscles. A medial parapatellar incision is made with a scalpel through the medial fascia and the fibrous and synovial joint capsule. The incision is extended from the tibial crest proximally through the cranial belly of the sartorius muscle. The incision is left open. If the patient is severely bowlegged, so that

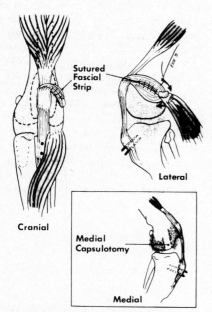

Figure 159–128. Augmentation of the lateral retinaculum with a section of fascia lata. Inset shows the incision through the medial joint capsule to relieve medial tension on the patella. (Reprinted with permission from Hulse. D. A.: Pathophysiology and management of medial patellar luxation in the dog. Vet. Med./Small Anim. Clin. 76:43, 1981.)

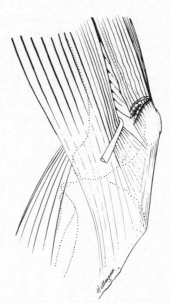

Figure 159–129. Medial view showing partial tendonotomy of the insertions of the cranial sartorius and vastus medialis to release medial force on the patella.

an abnormal angle of force is directed on the patella by the vastus medialis, the insertion of the vastus medialis on the superior pole of the patella may be incised. The insertion is reflected proximally and sutured to the vastus intermedius (Fig. 159–129).

Lateral Joint Capsule Reinforcement. Lateral capsulectomy is performed to reinforce the lateral joint capsule if it is lax and is giving no support to the lateral retinaculum. The amount of capsule removed is subjective but should be sufficient to produce slight lateral tension when the joint capsule is sutured. The capsule is sutured using a simple interrupted pattern. Lateral reinforcement of the joint capsule may also be accomplished with a row of imbrication sutures, as described previously.

Deepening of the Trochlear Groove. Increasing the depth of the trochlear groove may be necessary to restrain the patella within the confines of the medial and lateral trochlear ridges. Deepening of the trochlear groove may be accomplished by three methods. The most common procedure is trochleoplasty, which involves removal of the articular cartilage and subchondral bone to deepen the trochlear groove. Methods of deepening the trochlear groove are chondroplasty and trochlear wedge recession, whereby subchondral bone is removed but the articular cartilage is preserved.

Trochleoplasty. The joint capsule is incised and the patella luxated medially to expose the trochlear groove (see Fig. 159–124). The width of the articular surface of the patella is measured, and the measurement is used to determine the proper width of the trochleoplasty. The articular cartilage is removed with the aid of a power burr, rongeur, or bone file. The new groove should extend proximally to the articular cartilage margin and distally to the articular cartilage margin just above the intercondylar notch. The depth of the groove exposes cancellous bone and is deep enough to accommodate 50 per cent of the height of the patella. The newly formed medial and lateral trochlear ridges are parallel to each other and perpendicular to the bed of the new trochlear groove. On completion, the patella is reduced and the joint flexed and extended to assess the stability of the patella. The advantage of this technique is its ease and simplicity, but its disadvantage is that it destroys normal articular cartilage. The bed of the trochleo-

plasty fills with a combination of hyaline cartilage and fibrocartilage.

Chondroplasty. The joint capsule is incised and the patella luxated medially to expose the trochlear groove. The width of the articular surface of the patella is measured, and this measurement used to determine the proper width of the new trochlear bed. Two parallel incisions are made through the articular cartilage, extending proximally from the articular cartilage margin and distally to the articular cartilage margin at the intercondylar notch. The two incisions are joined proximally with a horizontal incision, and the articular cartilage is elevated from proximal to distal, creating a rectangular cartilage flap. Subchondral bone is removed from the trochlear bed to deepen the trochlear groove (Fig. 159–130). Enough subchondral bone should be removed to allow seating of at least 50 per cent of the height of the patella. Following removal of the subchondral bone, the cartilage flap is replaced, and the patella reduced. The stability of the patella is assessed by repeated flexion and extension of the joint. The advantage of this technique is that hyaline articular cartilage is maintained. The disadvantage is that creation of the cartilage flap is difficult in mature patients, in which flap is often thin and tears easily.

Trochlear Wedge Recession. This surgical technique was developed to deepen the femoral trochlear groove in order to restrain the patella while maintaining the hyaline articular cartilage of the trochlear surface.[89] Realignment of the quadriceps mechanism, reconstruction of ligamentous and retinacular patellar restraints, and modification of knee biomechanics may be necessary with trochlear wedge recession to provide optimum restraint of the patella within the trochlea (Fig. 159–131A). If an isoceles triangle is cut from the femoral trochlea, the free osteochondral wedge of bone and the V-shaped groove in the trochlea are similar triangles. However, owing to the cutting width of the blade (Kerf) the base and depth of the V groove differ from those of the free osteochondral wedge, resulting in a recessed V trochlear groove (Fig. 159–131B). The amount of recession is independent of the size of the wedge and may be predetermined using the following formula: $D = K/\sin \theta/2$, where D is the depth of the trochlear recession, K is the Kerf (width of the saw cut), and

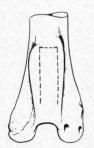 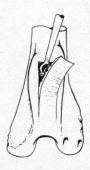 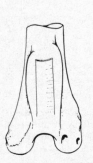 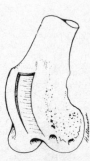

Figure 159–130. Frontal view chondroplasty showing elevation of cartilage and curettage of subchondral bone to deepen the trochlear groove.

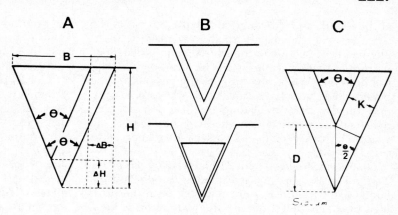

Figure 159–131. Wedge recession principle. *A*, Similar triangles have equal angles (θ) but vary in height (H) and base (B). *B*, A wedge cut from a solid will be recessed when replaced. *C*, The depth of recession (D) is proportional to the kerf (K) and apex angle (θ). D = K/(SIN (θ/2)). (Reprinted with permission from Slocum, B., Slocum, D., et al.: Wedge recession for treatment of recurrent luxation of the patella. Clin. Orthop. *164*:48, 1982.)

θ is the apex of the inverted isoceles triangle (Fig. 159–131*C*). Radiographs are used to determine the proper Kerf (width of the saw cut) to be used preoperatively. The initial osteochondral osteotomy is made so that the two oblique planes that form the free wedge intersect at the articular margin distally near the intercondylar notch and proximally at the dorsal edge of the trochlear articular cartilage.

The medial and lateral osteotomy line lies within the trochlear ridges, the widest point being halfway between the dorsal and ventral limits of the trochlea. When the osteotomy is completed, the surgeon can determine whether sufficient wedge recession is present. The wedge must be recessed to house at least 50 per cent of the patellar thickness. If the recession is not adequate, the saw blade may be used to widen and deepen the V groove. The free osteochondral wedge is replaced in its original position to obtain a recessed trochlear groove. The articular cartilage of the proximal trochlear surface is widened to allow efficient gliding of the patella as it enters the recessed trochlear surface. The stability of the osteochondral wedge is maintained by the compressive vector force of the quadriceps muscle mass and the patellar tendon. Also, the cohesiveness and friction between the bony trabeculae of the wedge and V groove are far greater than the shearing forces between the articular cartilage of the patella and trochlea. The advantage of a trochlear wedge recession is that the normal hyaline articular cartilage is preserved. The disadvantage is that the technique is technically demanding, particularly in small dogs.

Wedge Osteotomy of the Femur or Tibia. An immature patient with an active physis in which abnormal forces are continuously exerted across the growth plate may have severe torsional and angular skeletal deformities. If it is determined by physical examination and radiographic evaluation that the success of other stabilization procedures is in jeopardy if the skeletal deformities are not corrected, a wedge osteotomy of the femur and/or tibia should be performed. The site and correct angle of the osteotomy are determined from radiographs preoperatively. As a rule, the osteotomy should be performed at the point of maximum curvature, with the base of the osteotomy wedge on the convex side of the bone

and the apex of the osteotomy wedge on the concave side of the bone. If a torsional deformity exists, derotation of the osteotomy should be accomplished before the osteotomy site is stabilized.

Operative Procedure for Wedge Osteotomy of the Femur. A standard lateral approach to the distal femur is performed, and the point of maximal curvature identified. An assessment of the degree of torsional deformity is made before the femur is osteotomized. It is difficult to standardize absolute angle relationships between the femoral condyles and the longitudinal axis of the femur because of conformational differences between dogs. The extensor mechanism of the stifle must be aligned. In the frontal plane, the femoral condyles should be perpendicular to the longitudinal axis of the femur, and the trochlea should be in line with the longitudinal axis of the femur. The longitudinal axis of the quadriceps muscle mass must be taken into consideration during alignment of the trochlea. A degree of medial-to-lateral inclination may be necessary to restrain the patella. In the lateral plane, the trochlea lies at an average angle of 37 degrees to the longitudinal axis

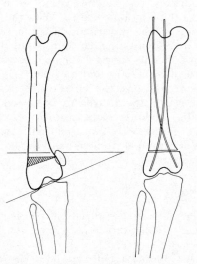

Figure 159–132. Diagrammatic representation of a wedge osteotomy of the femur to correct angular bowing secondary to medial patellar luxation.

of the femur, and the longitudinal axis intersects the trochlea near the distal articular cartilage margin. Slight over-reduction in the lateral plane is beneficial for proper seating of pins in the femoral condyle with stabilization. When the proper dimensions of the bone wedge have been calculated, the osteotomy is performed with an oscillating saw. The femoral condyles are positioned as described previously and stabilized with Steinmann pins or Kirschner wires (Fig. 159–132).

Operative Procedure for Wedge Osteotomy of the Tibia. The skin incision is extended distally and the lateral extensor muscles are reflected from the proximal tibia. The point of maximum curvature is identified, and the osteotomy is performed with an oscillating saw. The bone should be cut to allow the tibial plateau to align with the femoral condyles in both frontal and lateral planes. The tibial crest must be rotated to align with the trochlear groove in the frontal plane. The fibula must be osteotomized to accomplish derotation. Once the tibial plateau is aligned properly, it is stabilized with Steinmann pins or Kirschner wires.

Lateral Patellar Luxation

This condition, which has been referred to as "knock-knee" or genu valgum, is seen more frequently in large dogs. However, lateral patellar luxation is also seen in small dogs. The etiology and pathogenesis have been attributed to various factors but remain speculative. Most authorities believe that the original problem is in the coxofemoral joint.[71] Coxa valga is thought to cause positioning of the limb toward the midline, which would shift the line of force produced by the quadriceps muscles and body weight lateral to the longitudinal axis of the femoral trochlea. Another theory posits that increased femoral capital anteversion, which would also shift the force of the quadriceps muscle mass lateral to the longitudinal axis of the femoral trochlea. With the abnormal forces acting on the physis and articular cartilage of the femoral condyles, angular and torsional deformities are produced. There is medial bowing of the distal third of the femur and a disparity in condylar development. Because the force on the lateral condyle is increased, its growth rate is slowed, whereas the medial condyle develops normally or even at an accelerated rate. With the abnormal stresses, the medial retinaculum is stretched and the lateral retinaculum tightens.

Clinical Signs

There are four grades of lateral patellar luxation, with grade I being the least severe and grade IV being the most severe.

Grade I. Generally, gait is normal. The client may report that the patient occasionally skips when walking. On physical examination, the surgeon will note a hypermobile patella, i.e., the patella may easily be moved over or lateral to the trochlear ridge. The patella reduces itself if the lateral force exerted by the examiner is discontinued.

Grade II. The majority of patients with grade II luxation walk normally but exhibit an occasional limp. A small percentage have a continued weight-bearing lameness. On physical examination, flexion and extension of the limb results in lateral luxation of the patella. The examiner may force the patella laterally, but when the force is discontinued or the limb is flexed and extended, the patella reduces spontaneously. Slight angular and torsional deformities may be noted on radiographic evaluation.

Grade III. There is usually some degree of lameness. It is quite variable and may consist of an occasional skip or a continued weight-bearing lameness. Flexion and extension of the stifle readily elicit lateral luxation of the patella. The patella may be reduced manually, but it spontaneously luxates with flexion and extension of the stifle. Lateral displacement of the quadriceps muscle mass as well as a "knock-knee" conformation may be noted. Radiographic assessment shows varying degrees of angular and torsional deformities.

Grade IV. The patient shows marked lameness and conformational deformities, is unable to extend the stifle, carries most of the body weight with the front legs, is "knock-kneed," and has muscle atrophy of the rear limbs. On physical examination, the patella is located lateral to the trochlear ridge, is hypoplastic, and cannot be reduced. The quadriceps muscle mass is displaced laterally, and severe torsional and angular skeletal deformities are demonstrated radiographically.

Pathological Changes

Pathological changes vary, in relation to the grade of patellar luxation, from mild soft tissue alterations to marked skeletal deformities. The greater the permanency of luxation and the more active the physis, the more apparent the soft tissue and skeletal deformities.

Figure 159–133 represents an extreme degree of deformity, but 95 per cent of patients with lateral patellar luxation have one or more of these structural defects illustrated.

Treatment of Lateral Patellar Luxation

There are a number of techniques for stabilization of lateral patellar luxation in the dog. A combination of techniques is usually necessary to obtain optimum stability and function. The techniques for trochleoplasty, chondroplasty, and trochlear wedge recession are described in the section on treatment of medial patellar luxation. The technique for wedge osteotomy of the femur or tibia is the same as that described for medial patellar luxation, except that the base and apex of the osteotomy wedge are reversed.

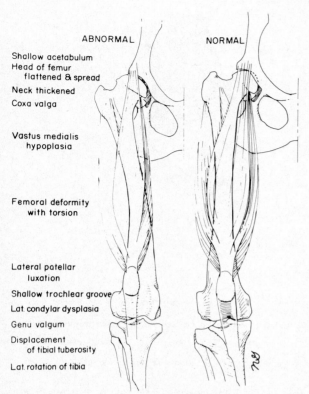

ABNORMAL   NORMAL

Shallow acetabulum
Head of femur
  flattened & spread
Neck thickened
Coxa valga

Vastus medialis
  hypoplasia

Femoral deformity
  with torsion

Lateral patellar
  luxation
Shallow trochlear groove
Lat. condylar dysplasia
Genu valgum
Displacement
  of tibial tuberosity
Lat. rotation of tibia

Figure 159–133. The abnormal anatomy associated with lateral patellar luxation is contrasted with a normal limb. (Reprinted with permission from Olmsted, M. L.: Lateral luxation of the patella. *In* Bojrab, M. (ed.): *Pathophysiology in Small Animal Surgery.* Lea & Febiger, Philadelphia, 1981.)

Tibial Crest Transposition. An anterolateral incision is made 5 cm proximal to the patella and extending distally 3 cm below the tibial crest. The subcutaneous tissues are incised along the same line, and the skin edges clipped to the stockinette to reduce bacterial contamination. A parapatellar incision is made through the fascia lata approximately 1 cm lateral to the patellar tendon. This incision is extended proximally and distally the length of the surgical wound. The tibialis cranialis muscle is reflected from its lateral origin on the tibial crest and the lateral tibial plateau. Care must be taken not to sever the long digital extensor tendon inadvertently. The tibialis cranialis muscle is retracted laterally to expose the proximal lateral metaphysis of the tibia. A parapatellar relief incision is made medially and extended 3 cm below the tibial crest. Blunt dissection is used to gain access to the underside of the patellar tendon. Once the tendon is undermined, an osteotome and mallet are used to perform the osteotomy of the tibial crest. The osteotomy should be directed proximal to distal, beginning 3 to 4 mm caudal to the most anterior point of the tibial crest. The distal periosteal attachment is not severed. The tibial crest is levered medially to align with the trochlea of the femur. The amount of medial transposition is subjective, but the extensor mechanism of the stifle should be aligned. Once the amount of medial transposition

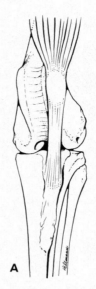

A

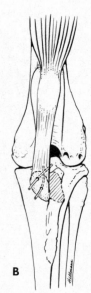

B

Figure 159–134. Lateral patellar luxation. *A*, Preoperative frontal view. *B*, Postoperative frontal view showing medial transposition of the tibial crest.

is decided, the site is prepared by removing the thin layer of cortical bone to expose the cancellous surface. The tibial crest is moved medially and stabilized with two Kirschner wires directed in a posterolateral direction (Fig. 159–134).

Reinforcement of the Medial Retinaculum. The medial retinaculum may be reinforced by synthetic suture fascia lata transposition. Sutures may be augmented by the placement of nonabsorbable suture from the medial femorofabellar ligament to the medial parapatellar fibrocartilage or by imbrication of

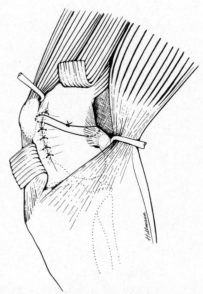

Figure 159–135. Medial view showing reinforcement of the medial retinaculum with a fabellar-patellar suture and imbrication of the fibrous joint capsule.

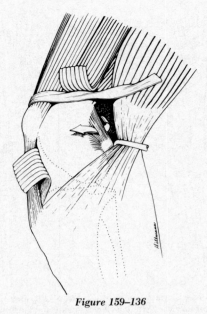

Figure 159–136

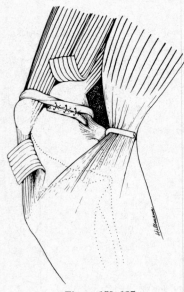

Figure 159–137

Figure 159–136. Medial view showing isolation of a section of fascia lata and exposure of the medial femorofabellar ligament for medial retinacular reinforcement.

Figure 159–137. Medial view showing transposition and suturing of the fascia lata for medial retinacular reinforcement.

the medial fibrous joint capsule (Fig. 159–135). The fascial plane of insertion for the cranial and caudal sartorius muscles is incised and retracted caudally to expose the fibrous joint capsule. A row of interrupted Lembert sutures is preplaced in the fibrous joint capsule, care being taken not to penetrate the joint cavity. The sutures are tied, causing a tightening of

the medial joint capsule. The row of sutures extends from 1 cm proximal to the patella distally to the tibial crest.

The medial retinaculum may be reinforced by transposing autologous fascia lata. A section of fascia lata, the width of the patella and equal in length to twice the distance from the patella to the medial

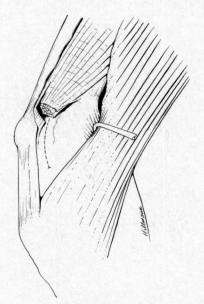

Figure 159–138

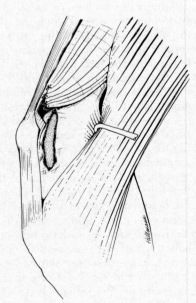

Figure 159–139

Figure 159–138. Lateral view showing release of the lateral retinaculum and vastus lateralis.

Figure 159–139. Lateral view showing the vastus lateralis sutured to the rectus femoris.

fabella, is freed proximally and left attached to the superior pole of the patella. The fascial plane of insertion for the cranial and caudal sartorius muscles is incised and reflected caudally to expose the fabella and medial head of the gastrocnemius muscle. The medial femorofabellar ligament is undermined and a pair of curved forceps passed beneath the ligament to grasp the free end of the fascial graft (Fig. 159–136). The fascial graft is pulled beneath the femoral-fabellar ligament and back to the patella. The fascial graft is pulled taut to prevent lateral patellar luxation and sutured to itself with simple interrupted nonabsorbable sutures (Fig. 159–137).

Lateral Release. A lateral release is performed to relieve lateral tension on the patella exerted by the contracted and thickened lateral retinaculum and lateral joint capsule. The biceps femoris muscle with the fascia lata is reflected caudally, and a parapatellar incision is made through the fibrous joint capsule and retinaculum. The incision may extend into the joint if necessary. In some patients, the vastus lateralis is displaced so that the force it exerts on the patella results in lateral subluxation or luxation. Release of the muscular force may be accomplished by incising the insertion of the vastus lateralis muscle on the superior pole of the patella (Fig. 159–138). The muscular insertion is reflected proximally and sutured to the rectus femoris muscle (Fig. 159–139).

Medial Joint Capsule Reinforcement. Medial capsulectomy is performed to remove the stretched and redundant medial joint capsule produced by lateral patellar luxation. The amount of joint capsule removed is subjective but should be enough to give slight medial tension when sutured. The joint capsule is sutured using a simple interrupted pattern.

PATELLAR FRACTURES

The patella is a sesamoid bone enveloped in the tendon of insertion of the quadriceps muscle group.

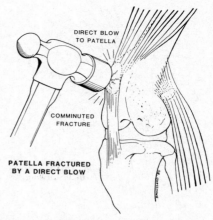

Figure 159–141. A direct blow to the patella may result in a severe fracture of the patella.

It serves as a fulcrum to concentrate the forces of muscular contraction onto the distal femur through the trochlear groove. Contact between the articular surface of the patella and the articular cartilage of the trochlea is intimate and essential for the correct nutrition of both components. Fracture of the patella compromises both the extensor mechanism of the stifle and the normal structure of the cartilage. Chondrolysis is a consequence of unrepaired patellar fracture leading eventually to osteoarthritis.

Patellar fractures occur by one of two mechanisms.[19] First, intense traction forces, propagated by powerful contractions of the quadriceps muscle group and compounded by gravity forces generated when the patient lands on its rear leg(s) during a fall, produce a transverse fracture of the patella (Fig. 159–140). Second, a direct forceful blow crushes the patella against the distal femur, producing a comminuted fracture (Fig. 159–141). Both of these fractures are uncommon in small animal practice.[7,11,19]

Clinical Signs

An acute onset of non–weight-bearing lameness associated with a fall or blow to the affected leg is typical of this condition. Palpation usually reveals localized pain and crepitation over the patella. A separation between fragments can often be palpated. Characteristically, the animal is not able to extend the leg fully or to support weight in extension. Radiographic confirmation is essential to determine the severity of the fracture. Temporary stabilization with an extension splint relieves much of the associated pain and should be used if any delay of surgical repair is likely.

Treatment

Retention of all or part of the patella is essential for functional repair.[7] The objectives of repair tech-

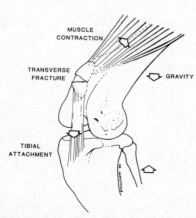

Figure 159–140. Muscular forces resulting in an indirect fracture of the patella.

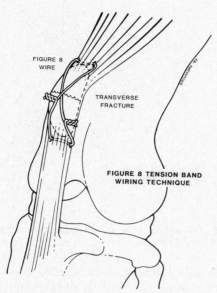

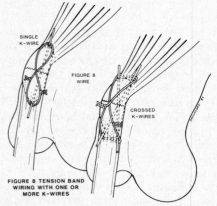

Figure 159–143. Stabilization of a transverse patellar fracture with K-wires and orthopedic wire. The K-wires are positioned in line with the longitudinal axis and the orthopedic wire is positioned around the K-wire ends.

Figure 159–142. Stabilization of a transverse patellar fracture with orthopedic wire. Note the position of the wire in the quadriceps tendon proximally and the patella tendon distally.

niques are to reestablish continuity of the articular surface, to preserve the integrity of the quadriceps extensor mechanism, and to provide stable fixation during bone healing. A number of techniques that fulfill these objectives have been described for transverse fractures.

In every case, the animal is prepared for sterile surgery of the stifle joint. A lateral parapatellar approach is used to enter the joint and examine the articular surface of the patella. All repair maneuvers are performed with the stifle in full extension to relieve tension on the patella tendon.

Figure-of-Eight Tension Band Wiring. Heavy (18-gauge) orthopedic wire is passed through the quadriceps tendon proximal and deep to the proximal pole of the patella. The free ends of wire cross diagonally over the cranial surface of the fractured patella, and one end is passed through the patellar tendon distal and deep to the distal pole of the patella.

The free ends of the wire are twisted together, and a loop of the other diagonal wire is twisted. The fracture is reduced in perfect alignment, and both twists are tightened to maintain reduction under compression (Fig. 159–142).

Figure-of-Eight Tension Band Wiring with Kirschner Wires. The fracture is reduced in alignment and clamped in position. One or two K-wires may be used. The K-wire is drilled through the length of the patella across the fracture line. The figure-of-eight orthopedic wire is positioned around and deep to the ends of the protruding K-wire and twisted tight, as described previously. If two K-wires are used, they may be placed parallel to each other or crossed (Fig. 159–143).

The advantage of additional K-wires is increased stability against rotation and shearing. The orthopedic wire's holding power is greater when it is anchored

by protruding pins and not just tendon tissue. In all of these techniques, the tension and bending forces applied to the patella during flexion are converted into compression forces by the tension band wire.

A similar technique using orthopedic wire in a square configuration around the patella does not have the mechanical advantage of wire support on the cranial aspect of the patella (Fig. 159–144).

Neutralization Wiring. This technique is of particular use with comminuted fractures of the patella. Small free fragments of the comminuted fracture are removed, and the articular surface of the patella is smoothed off with rongeurs. The remining bone is held in apposition with two or more horizontal mattress steel wire sutures through the patellar tendon. Simple interrupted wire sutures are placed in the torn fibrous tissue surrounding the fragmented patella. To allow healing, the tension forces are neutralized by placing a heavy (18-gauge) orthopedic

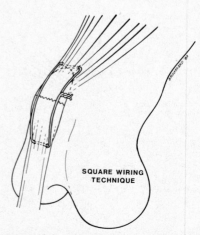

Figure 159–144. Stabilization of a transverse patellar fracture with orthopedic wire. The wire is positioned in the quadriceps tendon proximally and the patella tendon distally. The wire ends run parallel to each other over the anterior surface of the patella, resulting in the square wiring technique.

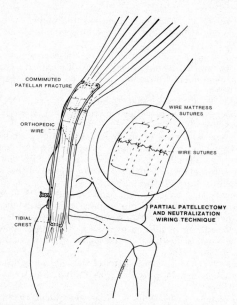

Figure 159–145. Stabilization of a comminuted patellar fracture with a partial patellectomy and neutralization wiring technique. Distraction forces are neutralized with orthopedic wire positioned in the quadriceps tendon proximally and the tibial crest distally in a rectangular pattern. Small fracture lines are additionally stabilized with orthopedic wire sutures.

wire suture through the tibial crest and the quadriceps tendon proximal to the fractured patella. This maneuver transfers the quadriceps pull directly to the tibia, avoiding the healing patella (Fig. 159–145). The wire invariably breaks after four weeks and should be removed.

Postoperative Care

In all cases the operated leg should be placed in a padded coaptation bandage to restrict flexion of the stifle. The bandage should be maintained for at least four weeks while bony union occurs. Following bandage removal, passive flexion exercises should be initiated and continued until a normal range of motion is regained.

Pins and wires can be removed once radiographic signs of complete healing are observed. Early removal results in separation under tension.

Prognosis

Simple transverse fractures carry an excellent prognosis, but comminution frequently results in progressive arthritis.

1. Alm, A., Ekstrom, H., Gillquist, J., and Stromberg, B.: The anterior cruciate ligament: a clinical and experimental study on tensile strength, morphology and replacement of patellar tendon. *Acta Chir. Scand.* (Suppl) 445, 1974.
2. Arkin, A. M.: The effects of pressure on epiphyseal growth: a mechanism of plasticity of growing bone. J. Bone Jt. Surg. *38A*:1056, 1956.
3. Arnoczky, S. P.: Surgery of the stifle—the cruciate ligaments (Part I). Comp. Cont. Ed. 2:106, 1980.
4. Arnoczky, S. P.: The microvasculature of the meniscus and its response to injury: an experimental study in the dog. Proc. Orthop. Res. Soc., 1981.
5. Arnoczky, S. P., Marshall, J. L., et. al.: Meniscal nutrition—an experimental study in the dog. Proc. Orthop. Res. Soc., 1980.
6. Arnoczky, S. P., and Marshall, J. L.: The cruciate ligaments of the canine stifle: an anatomical and functional analysis. Am. J. Vet. Res. *38*:1807, 1977.
7. Arnoczky, S. P., and Tarvin, G. B.: Patellar surgery. *In* Bojrab, M. J. (ed.): *Current Techniques in Small Animal Surgery.* 2nd ed. Lea & Febiger, Philadelphia, 1983.
8. Arnoczky, S. P., Tarvin, G. B., Marshall, J. L., and Saltzman, B.: The over-the-top procedure: a technique for anterior cruciate ligament substitution in the dog. J. Am. Anim. Hosp. Assoc. *15*:283, 1979.
9. Braund, K. G., Shires, P. K., and Mikeal, R. L.: Type I fiber atrophy in the vastus latralis muscle in dogs with femoral fractures treated by hyperextension. Vet. Pathol. *14*:165, 1980.
10. Brinker, W. O., Brown, R., and Keller, W. F.: A drill guide for use in repair of a ruptured anterior (lateral) cruciate ligament in the dog. Vet. Med./Sm. Anim. Clin. *60*:709, 1965.
11. Brinker, W. O., Piermattei, D. L., and Flo, G. L.: *Handbook of Small Animal Orthopedics and Fracture Treatment.* W. B. Saunders, Philadelphia, 1983.
12. Butler, D. L., Hulse, D. A., Kay, M. D., et al.: Biomechanics of anterior cruciate ligament reconstruction in the dog. II: Mechanical properties. Vet. Surg. (accepted for publication) 1983.
13. Butler, H. C.: Teflon as a prosthetic ligament in repair of ruptured anterior cruciate ligaments. Am. J. Vet. Res. *25*:55, 1964.
14. Cabaud, H. E., Feagin, J. A., and Rodkey, W. G.: Acute anterior cruciate ligament injury and augmented repair. Am. J. Sports Med. *8*:395, 1980.
15. Childers, H. E.: New methods for cruciate ligament repair. II: Repair by suture technique. Mod. Vet. Pract. *47*:59, 1966.
16. Clancy, W. G., Nelson, D. A., Reider, B., and Narechania, R. G.: Anterior cruciate ligament reconstruction using one-third of the patellar ligament, augmented by extra-articular tendon transfers. J. Bone Jt. Surg. *64A*:352, 1982.
17. Cox, J. S., and Cordell, L. D.: The degenerative effects of the medial meniscus tears in dog's knees. Clin. Orthop. *125*:237, 1977.
18. Cox, J. S., Nye, C. E., Shaefer, W., et al.: The degenerative effects of partial and total resection of the medial meniscus in dog's knees. Clin. Orthop. *109*:178, 1975.
19. DeAngelis, M.: Fractures of the appendicular and heterotrophic skeleton. *In* Bojrab, M. J. (ed.): *Pathophysiology in Small Animal Surgery.* Lea & Febiger, Philadelphia, 1981.
20. DeAngelis, M. P., and Betts, C. W.: Posterior cruciate ligament rupture. J. Am. Anim. Hosp. Assoc. *9*:447, 1973.
21. DeAngelis, M., and Lau, R. E.: A lateral retinacular imbrication technique for the surgical correction of anterior cruciate ligament rupture in the dog. J. Am. Vet. Med. Assoc. *157*:79, 1970.
22. Denny, H. R., and Goodship, A. E.: Replacement of the anterior cruciate ligament with carbon fibre in the dog. J. Sm. Anim. Pract. *21*:279, 1980.
23. Dickinson, C. R., and Nunamaker, D. M.: Repair of ruptured anterior cruciate ligament in the dog: experience of 101 cases, using a modified fascia strip technique. J. Am. Vet. Med. Assoc. *140*:827, 1977.
24. DiStefano, V. J.: Function, post-traumatic sequelae and current concepts of management of knee meniscus injuries: a review article. Clin. Orthop. *151*:143, 1980.
25. Dulisch, M. L.: Suture reaction following extra-articular stifle stabilization in the dog. Part I: A retrospective study of 161 stifles. J. Am. Anim. Hosp. Assoc. *17*:569, 1981.
26. Dulisch, M. L.: Suture reaction following extra-articular stabilization in the dog. Part II: A prospective study of 66 stifles. J. Am. Anim. Hosp. Assoc. *17*:572, 1981.
27. Egger, E. L., and Rigg, D. L.: Caudal cruciate ligament

injuries in the dog and cat: a review of pathophysiology, treatment and clinical experience. J. Vet. Surg. 1983.

28. Emmeking, W. F., and Horowitz, M.: The intraarticular effects of immobilization on the human knee. J. Bone Jt. Surg. *54A*:973, 1972.

29. Evans, H. E., and Christensen, G. C. (eds.): *Miller's Anatomy of the Dog.* 2nd ed. W. B. Saunders, 1979.

30. Feagin, J. A.: The syndrome of the torn anterior cruciate ligament. Orthop. Clin. North Am. *10*:81, 1979.

31. Flo, G. L.: Modification of the lateral retinacular imbrication technique for stabilizing cruciate ligament injuries. J. Am. Anim. Hosp. Assoc. *11*:570, 1975.

32. Flo, G. L., and DeYoung, D.: Meniscal injuries and medial meniscectomy in the canine stifle. J. Am. Anim. Hosp. Assoc. *14*:683, 1978.

33. Frank, C., Rademaker, F., Becker, K., and Edwards, G.: A computerized study of knee ligament injuries—the anterior cruciate; repaired vs. removed. Proc. 27th Annual Orthop. Res. Soc., Las Vegas, 1981.

34. Gambardella, P. C., Wallace, L. J., and Cassidy, F.: Lateral suture technique for management of anterior cruciate ligament rupture in dogs: a retrospective study. J. Am. Anim. Hosp. Assoc. *17*:33, 1981.

35. Gilbertson, E. M. M.: The development of periarticular osteophytes in experimentally induced osteoarthritis in the dog. Ann. Rheum. Dis. *34*:12, 1975.

36. Heffron, L. E., and Campbell, J. R.: Osteophyte information in the canine stifle joint following treatment for rupture of the cranial cruciate ligament. J. Small Anim. Pract. *20*:603, 1979.

37. Henderson, R. A., and Milton, J. L.: The tibial compression mechanism: a diagnostic aid in stifle injuries. J. Am. Anim. Hosp. *14*:474, 1978.

38. Hey Groves, E. W.: The classic operation for repair of the crucial ligaments. Clin. Orthop. Rel. Res. *147*:4, 1980.

39. Hinko, P. J.: The use of a prosthetic ligament in repair of the torn anterior cruciate ligament in the dog. J. Am. Anim. Hosp. Assoc. *17*:563, 1981.

40. Hohn, R. B., and Miller, J. M.: Surgical correction of the anterior cruciate ligament in the dog. J. Am. Vet. Med. Assoc. *150*:1133, 1967.

41. Hohn, R. B., and Newton, C. D.: Surgical repair of ligamentous structures of the stifle joint: *In Current Techniques in Small Animal Surgery.* Lea & Febiger, Philadelphia, 1975.

42. Hughston, J. C., and Degenhardt, T. C.: Reconstruction of the posterior cruciate ligament. Clin. Orthop. *164*:1982.

43. Hulse, D. A., Butler, D. L., Kay, M. D., et al.: Biomechanics of anterior cruciate ligament reconstruction in the dog. I. In vitro laxity testing. Vet. Surg. *12*:109, 1983.

44. Hulse, D. A., Michaelson, F., Johnson, C., and Adelbaki, Y. Z.: A technique for reconstruction of the anterior cruciate ligament in the dog: preliminary report. Vet. Surg. *9*:135, 1980.

45. Hulse, D. A., and Shires, P. K.: Observation of the posteromedial compartment of the stifle joint. J. Am. Anim. Hosp. Assoc. *17*:575, 1981.

46. James, S. L., Woods, G. W., Homsy, C. A., et al.: Cruciate ligament stents in reconstruction of the unstable knee. Clin. Orthop. Rel. Res. *143*:90, 1979.

47. Jones, K. G.: Reconstruction of the anterior cruciate ligament: a technique using the central third of the patellar ligament. J. Bone Jt. Surg. *45A*:925, 1963.

48. Jones, K. G.: Results of use of the central one-third of the patellar ligament to compensate for anterior cruciate ligament deficiency. Clin. Orthop. Rel. Res. *147*:39, 1980.

49. Kappakas, G., Brown, T., Goodman, M. A., et al.: Delayed surgical repair of ruptured ligaments. Clin. Orthop. *135*:281, 1978.

50. Kennedy, J. C.: Application of prosthetics to anterior cruciate ligament reconstruction and repair. Clin. Orthop. Rel. Res. *172*:125, 1983.

51. Kennedy, J. C., Roth, J. H., Mendenhall, H. V., and Sanford, J. B.: Intraarticular replacement of the anterior cruciate ligament-deficient knee. Am. J. Sports Med. 8:1, 1980.

52. Knecht, C. D.: Evolution of surgical techniques for cruciate ligament rupture in animals. J. Am. Anim. Hosp. Assoc. *12*:717, 1976.

53. Krackow, K. A., and Vetter, W. L.: Surgical reimplantation of the medial meniscus and repair of meniscal lacerations: an experimental study in dogs. Proc. Orthop. Res. Soc. 1980.

54. Krause, W. R., Pope, M. H., Johnson, R. J., et al.: Mechanical changes in the knee after meniscectomy. J. Bone Jt. Surg. *58A*:599, 1976.

55. Leighton, R. L.: Repair of ruptured anterior cruciate ligament with whole thickness skin. Sm. Anim. Clin. *1*:246, 1961.

56. Levy, M., Torzilli, P., and Warren, R.: The effect of medial meniscectomy on anterior-posterior motion of the knee. J. Bone Jt. Surg. *64A*:883, 1982.

57. Lipowitz, A. J., Wong, P. L., and Stevens, J. B.: Reaction of articular tissue of the dog to disease: the early changes of osteoarthritis. Proc. 29th Gaines Vet. Symp. 1979.

58. MacConail, M. A.: The movements of bone and joints. III: the synovial fluid and its assistants. J. Bone and Jt. Surg. *32B*:244, 1950.

59. Macintosh, D. L.: Acute tears of the anterior cruciate ligament: over-the-top repair. Acad. Orthop. Surgeons, Dallas, 1974.

60. Malcolm, L., and Danile, D.: The biomechanical rationale for partial meniscectomy. Unpublished report presented at International Arthroscopy Association Meeting, Philadelphia, 1980.

61. Maquet, P.: Mechanics of osteoarthritis of the patellofemoral joint. Clin. Orthop. *144*:70, 1979.

62. Marshall, J. L., and Olsson, S. E.: Instability of the knee: a long term experimental study in dogs. J. Bone Jt. Surg. *53A*:1561, 1971.

63. Marshall, J. L., and Rubin, R. M.: Knee ligament injuries—a diagnostic and therapeutic approach. Orthop. Clin. North Am. 8:641, 1977.

64. Marshall, J. L., Warren, R. F., and Wickiewiez, T. L.: Primary surgical treatment of anterior cruciate ligament lesions. Am. J. Sports Med. *10*:103, 1982.

65. McCurmin, D. M., Pearson, P. T., and Wass, W. M.: Clinical and pathologic evaluation of ruptured cranial cruciate ligament repair in the dog. Am. J. Vet. Res. *32*:1517, 1971.

66. McDaniel, W. J., and Dameron, T. B.: Untreated ruptures of the anterior cruciate ligament. J. Bone Jt. Surg. *62A*:696, 1980.

67. McDevitt, C., Gilbertson, E., and Muir, H.: An experimental model of osteoarthritis; early morphological and biochemical changes. J. Bone Jt. Surg. *59B*:24, 1977.

68. Noyes, F. R., Butler, D. L., Paulos, L. E., and Grood, E. S.: Intra-articular cruciate reconstruction. I: Perspectives on graft strength, vascularization and immediate motion after replacement. Clin. Orthop. Rel. Res. *172*:71, 1983.

69. O'Connor, B.: The histologic structure of dog knee menisci with comments on its possible significance. Am. J. Anat. *147*:407, 1977.

70. O'Donoghue, D. H., Frank, G. R., Jeter, G. L., et al.: Repair and reconstruction of the anterior cruciate ligament in dogs. J. Bone Jt. Surg. *53A*:710, 1971.

71. Olmsted, M. L.: Lateral luxation of the patella. *In* Bojrab, M. J. (ed.): *Pathophysiology in Small Animal Surgery.* Lea & Febiger, Philadelphia, 1981.

72. Paatsama, S.: Ligament injuries of the canine stifle joint: a clinical and experimental study. Thesis, Helsinki, 1952.

73. Paatsama, S.: Ein Weiterer Beitragzu Den Kniegelenksoperatonen Beim Humd. XVII World Vet. Cong., 1963.

74. Pearson, P. T., McCurmin, D. M., Carter, J. D., and Hoskins, J. D.: Lembert suture technique to surgically correct ruptured cruciate ligaments. J. Am. Anim. Hosp. Assoc. 7:1, 1971.

75. Piper, T. L., and Whiteside, L. A.: Early mobilization after knee ligament repair in dogs: an experimental study. Clin. Orthop. Rel. Res. *150*:277, 1980.

76. Pond, M. J.: Arguments in favor of barely performing a meniscectomy. Proc. Vet. Orthop. Soc., 1979.

77. Pond, M. J., and Campbell, J. R.: The canine stifle joint. I: Rupture of the anterior cruciate ligament. J. Small Anim. Pract. 13:1, 1972.

78. Reinke, J. D.: Cruciate ligament avulsion injury in the dog. J. Am. Anim. Hosp. Assoc. 18:254, 1982.

79. Roush, J. C., Hohn, R. B., and DeAngelis, M.: Evaluation of transplantation of the long digital extensor tendon for correction of anterior cruciate ligament rupture in dogs. J. Am. Vet. Med. Assoc. 156:309, 1970.

80. Roy, S.: Ultrastructure of articular cartilage in experimental immobilization. Ann. Rheum. Dis. 29:634, 1970.

81. Rudy, R. L.: Stifle joint Surgery. In: Archibald, J. (ed.): Canine Surgery. 2nd ed. American Veterinary Publications, Santa Barbara, 1974.

82. Scharling, M.: Replacement of the anterior cruciate ligament with a polyethylene prosthetic ligament. Acta Orthop. Scand. 52:575, 1981.

83. Seale, K. S., Haynes, D. W., et al.: The effect of meniscectomy on knee stability. Proc. Orthop. Res. Soc., 1981.

84. Shires, P. K., Hulse, D. A., and Liu, W.: The under-and-over fascial replacement technique for anterior cruciate ligament rupture in dogs. A retrospective study. J. Am. Anim. Hosp. Assoc. 20:69, 1983.

85. Siemering, G. H.: Arthroscopy of dogs. J. Am. Vet. Med. Assoc. 172:575, 1978.

86. Singleton, W. B.: Observations based upon the surgical repair of 106 cases of anterior cruciate ligament rupture. J. Small Anim. Pract. 10:269, 1969.

87. Singleton, W. B.: The surgical correction of stifle deformities in the dog. J. Small Anim. Pract. 10:59, 1969.

88. Sisk, T. D.: Traumatic affections of the joint. In Edmonson, A. S. (ed.): Campbell's Operative Orthopedics. 6th ed. C. V. Mosby, St. Louis, 1980.

89. Slocum, B., Slocum, D., Devine, T., and Boone, E.: Wedge recession for treatment of recurrent luxation of the patella. Clin. Orthop. 164:48, 1982.

90. Strande, A.: Replacement of the anterior cruciate ligament in the dog. J. Small Anim. Pract. 7:351, 1966.

91. Vasseur, P., and Arnoczky, S.: Collateral ligaments of the canine stifle joint: anatomic and functional analysis. Am. J. Vet. Res. 142:1133, 1981.

92. Vaughan, L. C.: A study of the replacement of the anterior cruciate ligament in the dog by fascia, skin and nylon. Vet. Rec. 75:537, 1963.

93. Vaughan, L. C., and Bowden, N. L. R.: The use of skin for the replacement of the anterior cruciate ligament in the dog: a review of thirty cases. J. Small Anim. Pract. 5:167, 1964.

94. Vaughan, L. C., and Scott, M. G. A. D.: An experimental study of the fate of autografts of whole-thickness skin used to replace the anterior cruciate ligament. Vet. Rec. 79:412, 1966.

Fractures of the Tibia and Fibula

Norman Gofton

Fractures of the tibia, like those of the other long bones, are conveniently divided into epiphyseal, metaphyseal, and diaphyseal fractures. Fractures of the epiphyses are often more demanding because of the small fragments of bone available for fixation, the need for accurate realignment when articular surfaces are involved, and the potential for degenerative joint disease when joint instability persists after avulsion fractures involving ligamentous insertions.

The small amount of soft tissue covering the tibia, particularly the distal tibia, provides little protection, accounting for the higher incidence of compound fractures of the tibia.[10] Similarly, when cast immobilization is employed and the fracture is inadequately reduced or the cast improperly applied, there is a greater potential for the skin to ulcerate and for a fracture to become compound beneath the cast. Closed reduction and pinning techniques are facilitated by reduced soft tissue coverage. The diaphysis of the tibia has a tendency to develop spiral fractures, especially in the chondrodysplastic breeds.

Fractures of the fibula are usually of little significance, with the exception of fractures of the lateral malleolus and proximal fibula. Instability or luxation of the tibiotarsal joint is associated with lateral malleolar fractures, necessitating rigid internal fixation. Instability of the stifle joint may be associated with proximal fibula fractures, because the lateral collateral ligament of the stifle joint attaches to the head of the fibula.

PREOPERATIVE CARE OF TIBIAL FRACTURES

Several considerations are important in the preoperative care of tibial injuries.

Compound fractures are more common in the tibia and require special care. Early treatment is essential to reduce the incidence of osteomyelitis. The wound should be inspected, thoroughly cleaned, and debrided of foreign material and devitalized tissue. If primary closure is indicated, it should be performed as soon as possible or a sterile dressing should be applied to the wound. The fracture may be stabilized at the time of wound debridement or may be delayed, according to the condition of the animal. Kirschner splints are particularly useful for treating compound fractures, because they avoid implantation of foreign materials in potentially infected wounds and permit access to the wound for cleaning.

Swelling of the limb is a common complication, especially when a fracture has been present for 24 to 48 hours. The application of a Robert-Jones bandage for 24 hours before operation reduces wound swelling or prevents its occurrence, greatly facilitating the procedure and in addition acting as a temporary splint

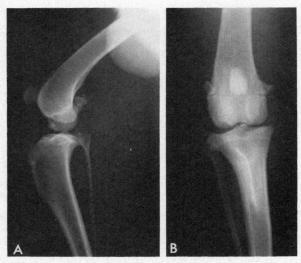

Figure 159–146. Lateral *(A)* and craniocaudal *(B)* radiographs of the stifle joint demonstrating an avulsion fracture associated with a cruciate ligament injury. The origin of the bone fragments is difficult to determine from the radiographs.

to protect the soft tissues and bone from further injury.

FRACTURES OF THE EPIPHYSES

Avulsion Fractures

Avulsion Fractures of the Proximal Epiphysis

Avulsion fractures may occasionally be observed in the proximal epiphysis. The insertion of the cruciate or collateral ligament may be affected.

Clinical Signs. There is usually a history of trauma, and the animal is reluctant to bear weight on the affected leg. Pain should be localized to the stifle joint on palpation. Joint swelling and hemarthrosis are present with intra-articular fractures.

Diagnosis. Radiographs revealing bone fragments within the stifle joint suggest a cruciate ligament avulsion (Fig. 159–146). It is often difficult to determine the origin of the bone fragments on the radiograph. The popliteal fabella often appears to be in the stifle joint on a craniocaudal radiograph. Its smooth outline and lateral location distinguish it from a fracture fragment.

Avulsion of the collateral ligaments is suggested by the presence of bone fragments in the region of the collateral ligaments. Additional craniocaudal radiographs taken while the medial and lateral collateral ligaments are individually stressed aids the diagnosis. Distraction of the fracture fragments and significant widening of the joint space should be detected.

Treatment. The method of treatment depends primarily on the size of the avulsed fragment of bone. A large fragment may be reattached with a lag screw or Kirschner wires. A small fragment associated with the cruciate ligament should be treated in the same manner as a cruciate ligament rupture, after the damaged ligament is debrided.

Small avulsion fractures of the insertions of the collateral ligaments are treated by employing one of the techniques of collateral ligament repair described earlier in this chapter.

Surgery. Whenever bone fragments are detected within the joint, an arthrotomy is indicated. Avulsion fractures associated with the tibial insertion of the cranial cruciate ligament are most readily approached through a medial parapatellar arthrotomy.

Fractures associated with the tibial insertions of the collateral ligaments are approached by direct incision over the affected collateral ligament. A large bone fragment can be reduced and retained with a lag screw or Kirschner wires and a figure-of-eight tension band wire.

Avulsion Fractures of the Distal Epiphysis

A fracture of the medial or lateral malleolus may be caused by avulsion of a collateral ligament. This

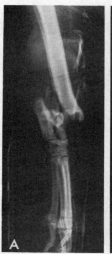
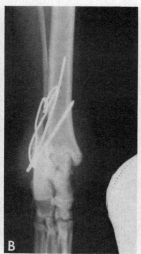
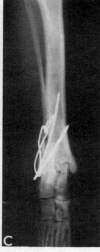

Figure 159–147. *A,* An avulsion fracture of the lateral malleolus with luxation of the tibiotarsal joint and angular deformity. *B,* A postoperative radiograph demonstrating the tension band technique. *C,* Healed fracture four weeks after surgery.

is a relatively common injury and requires early treatment to achieve good reduction and stabilization and to minimize the development of degenerative joint disease.

Clinical Signs. A severe or non–weight-bearing lameness is usually present. Palpation should localize the injury to the tibiotarsal joint. If the tibiotarsal joint is luxated, an angular or rotational deformity may be evident (Fig. 159–147).

Diagnosis. Radiographic examination is essential to the diagnosis. In most cases, the avulsed bone fragment is readily identified on the craniocaudal radiograph, although in some instances, the lesion may be less apparent. Craniocaudal radiographs taken while the medial and lateral collateral ligaments are alternately stressed will distract avulsed bone fragments and aid in the diagnosis.

Treatment. The preferred method of treatment depends on the size of the malleolar fragment. Open reduction and internal fixation is indicated, because the fracture is usually intra-articular and accurate reduction is necessary to minimize degenerative joint disease. Large fragments may be repaired with lag screws (Fig. 159–148).[9] Malleolar screws specifically designed for this purpose are available. Most malleolar fractures, even when the bone fragment is small, can be repaired using two Kirschner wires and a figure-of-eight tension band wire (see Figs. 159–150 and 159–151). The probability of splitting a small bone fragment is smaller with this technique, and the wires are readily applied with minimal equipment.

When the avulsed portions of the malleolus are too small to permit the use of Kirschner wires, one of the techniques for repair of a ruptured collateral ligament described earlier in this chapter should be employed.

Surgery. A curved skin incision is made directly over the malleolus. The soft tissues are carefully dissected from the malleolus with preservation of the collateral ligament. The tendons of the fibularis longus, fibularis brevis, and extensor digitorum lateralis muscles are located immediately caudal to the lateral malleolus and should be identified and preserved. The tendons of the tibialis caudalis and the flexor digitorum longus muscles are closely associated with

the caudal aspect of the medial malleolus and should also be preserved. The fracture line is identified. Incision of the joint capsule cranial and caudal to the malleolus may aid accurate realignment of the articular surface. Once realigned, the fracture is stabilized with two Kirschner wires and a figure-of-eight tension band wire. If a malleolar screw is used, a small Kirschner wire may be used to maintain reduction while the bone is drilled and tapped prior to insertion of the screw. A cortical bone screw may be used instead of a malleolar screw; however, it is then necessary to overdrill the malleolus to achieve a lag effect. This maneuver may be difficult and if not performed carefully may result in splitting of the bone fragment.

Avulsion Fractures of the Tibial Tuberosity

Avulsion of the tibial tuberosity may occur in the skeletally mature animal; however, it is uncommon. The clinical signs, diagnosis, and treatment are similar to those of a growth plate separation of the tibial crest and are discussed later.

Articular Fractures

Fractures of the proximal or distal epiphyses may occur as an extension of an oblique or longitudinal fracture of the diaphysis or metaphysis or may be confined to the epiphysis as with a Salter type III injury to the metaphyseal growth plate (Fig. 159–149).

Clinical Signs. The leg is usually carried, and pain and swelling should be localized to the affected joint. A hemarthrosis is present.

Diagnosis. Routine radiographs of the affected joint reveal fracture lines extending through the articular surface.

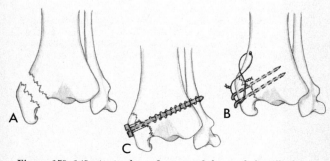

Figure 159–148. A, Avulsion fracture of the medial malleolus of the tibia. Repair using the tension band principle (B), and a malleolar screw (C).

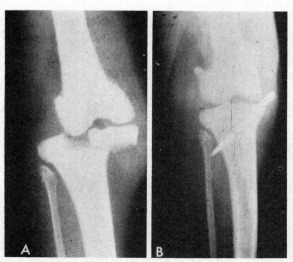

Figure 159–149. A, Salter type III fracture of the proximal tibial epiphysis. B, Repair with a single Steinmann pin.

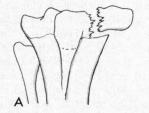 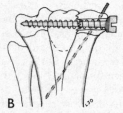

Figure 159–150. *A,* Salter type III fracture of the proximal epiphysis of the tibia. *B,* Fracture stabilized with a lag screw and Kirschner wire.

Treatment. The method of repair chosen depends on the type of fracture; however, because of the involvement of the articular surface, several factors are important. An arthrotomy of the affected joint should be performed to permit accurate reduction of the articular surfaces and the removal of debris and hematoma from the joint. Immobilization of the fragments is usually most adequately achieved with one or several lag screws (Fig. 159–150). It is important to avoid placing lag screws across the metaphyseal growth plate while growth potential remains.

GROWTH PLATE SEPARATION

There are five growth plates in the tibia and fibula: proximal and distal metaphyseal growth plates in the tibia and in the fibula and the growth plate associated with the tibial crest. The growth plates of the proximal tibia and fibula fuse between the ages of six and 11 months, whereas those of the distal tibia and fibula normally fuse between five and eight months.[11]

The most common injuries involve the proximal tibial metaphyseal growth plate and the distal tibial and fibular metaphyseal growth plates. As with other metaphyseal growth plates, the line of separation is usually through the zone of hypertrophied chondrocytes. Thus, the zone of dividing cartilage cells is on the epiphyseal side of the separation. Care must be observed, in handling the epiphysis, to remove hematoma and debris and realign the fracture. Excess damage to the dividing cartilage cells may initiate a partial or complete premature closure of the growth plate.

Premature closure is always a consideration in treatment of growth plate injuries, especially when considerable skeletal growth remains. Closure of the growth plate may be symmetrical, resulting in a short limb, or asymmetrical, resulting in shortening of the limb and a varus or valgus deformity (see Fig. 159–71).

Rush pins and crossed Steinmann pins are commonly used to repair epiphyseal separations. Both can initiate premature growth plate closure. Carefully placed crossed Steinmann pins are less likely to injure the growth plate.[2]

Proximal Tibial Growth Plate Separation

Separation of the proximal tibial growth plate is often caused by a lateral blow to the stifle joint that results in a lateral displacement of the epiphysis (Fig. 159–151). In the young animal, the epiphysis displaces before the collateral ligaments rupture. The fact that the growth plate of the proximal fibula may also be affected is significant, because the lateral collateral ligament attaches to the head of the fibula.

Clinical Signs. The affected leg is usually carried, and pain is localized to the stifle joint. An angular limb deformity may be apparent if the degree of displacement is sufficient.

Diagnosis. Lateral and medial displacements of the epiphysis are most obvious on the craniocaudal radiograph. A lateral radiograph should be taken because cranial and caudal displacements of the epiphysis occur and may not be obvious on the craniocaudal view.

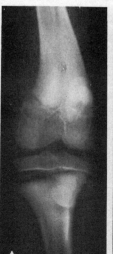 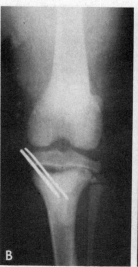 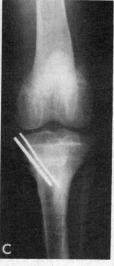

Figure 159–151. *A,* Separation of the proximal tibial metaphyseal growth plate. Note the greater displacement on the medial side. *B,* Parallel pin fixation of the fracture. *C,* Healed fracture four weeks after surgery.

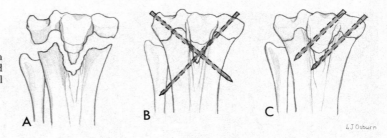

Figure 159–152. A, Proximal tibial metaphyseal growth plate separation. B, Technique for insertion of crossed Steinmann pins. C, Technique for insertion of parallel Steinmann pins.

Treatment. The injury may be treated by closed reduction followed by the application of a coaptation splint. Greater stability can be achieved with open reduction and pin fixation.

Cross-Pin Fixation. Bilateral approaches are made over the collateral ligaments, and the line of separation is identified. The hematoma and debris are removed, and the epiphysis is carefully reduced. Fixation is achieved by introducing pins into the epiphysis, in the region of the collateral ligaments, and directing them toward the opposite cortex of the tibial shaft (Fig. 159–152). Care should be taken during insertion of the pins to prevent interference with the articular surfaces of the tibia and femur. The pins are removed as soon as healing is apparent, in order to prevent injury to the metaphyseal growth plate.

Parallel Pin Fixation. Displacement of the proximal tibial epiphysis is often more marked on either the medial or the lateral side (see Fig. 159–154). In this case and when considerable growth potential remains, parallel pin fixation may be preferable, because premature closure of the growth plate is unlikely to be caused by this type of pin placement.

A skin incision is made over the collateral ligament on the side of greater displacement. After the hematoma and debris are removed and the displacement is reduced, a pin is inserted into the epiphysis in the region of the collateral ligament and directed into the tibial metaphysis. A second pin is then placed parallel to the first to add rotational stability (see Figs. 159–151 and 159–152).

Separation of the Growth Plate of the Tibial Crest

Injuries causing hyperflexion of the stifle joint may precipitate avulsion of the tibial crest in the immature animal.

Clinical Signs. The clinical signs are, usually, a reluctance to bear weight on the affected limb and swelling and pain in the region of the stifle joint.

Diagnosis. Proximal displacement of the tibial crest and patella should be apparent in a lateral radiograph (Figs. 159–153 and 159–154). Tibial crest avulsion may be incorrectly diagnosed, because the width and irregularity of the normal growth plate may be misinterpreted as a fracture. On a lateral radiograph with the joint in flexion, the fracture, if present, should be distracted, thus aiding the diagnosis. A lateral radiograph of the normal femorotibial joint permits a comparison of the growth plates.

Treatment. Surgical intervention is indicated, and several techniques are described.[1,5–7,14] The size of the bone fragment dictates the most appropriate technique.

A lateral parapatellar incision is made over the anterior aspect of the stifle joint and tibial crest. The fracture is located, and the hematoma and debris are removed. The fracture is reduced by extension of the joint. Use of two Kirschner wires and a figure-of-eight tension band wire is a simple and effective means of repair (Fig. 159–155; see Fig. 159–153). However, if the fragment is sufficiently large, a lag

Figure 159–153. A, Separation of the growth plate of the tibial crest. Note the proximal displacement of the tibial crest and the patella. B, Postoperative radiograph demonstrating treatment using the tension band technique.

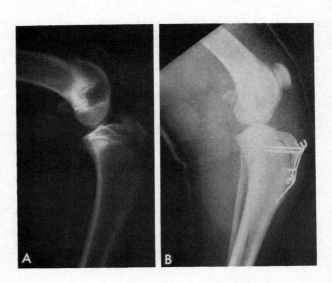

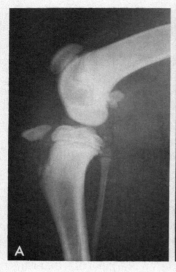
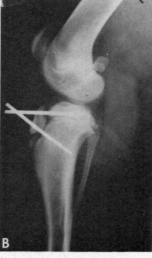
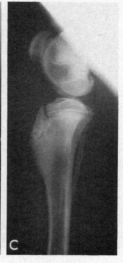

Figure 159–154. A, Separation of the growth plate of the tibial crest. Note the proximal displacement of the tibial crest and patella. *B,* Repair using crossed Steinmann pins. *C,* Healed fracture at the time of pin removal four weeks after surgery.

screw or two Steinmann pins may be employed (see Figs. 159–154 and 159–155). Whatever means of fixation is employed, it should be capable of withstanding the pull of the quadriceps muscles. Considerable tension can be generated in the quadriceps tendon, making the tension band principle or lag screw fixation a more mechanically stable technique.

When the bone fragment is small, screw or pin fixation may not be possible. Under these circum-stances, a Bunnell-Mayer suture can be placed in the patellar tendon and attached to the tibia through holes drilled in the tibial crest (Fig. 159–156).

Separation of the Distal Tibial and Fibular Growth Plates

Either epiphysis may be separated singly; how-ever, it is usual for both to be displaced. Separation of the distal metaphyseal growth plates is usually a result of a lateral or medial blow to the tibiotarsal joint.

Clinical Signs. A reluctance to use the limb, with pain and swelling that can be localized to the hock joint is the most common sign. With severe displace-ments, angular limb deformities may be apparent (Fig. 159–157).

Diagnosis. Craniocaudal and lateral radiographs should be taken. Because the displacement is most

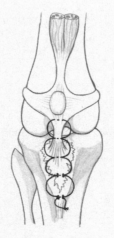
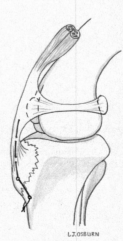

Figure 159–155. A, Separation of the growth plate of the tibial crest. Repair using the tension band principle *(B),* a lag screw *(C),* and crossed Steinmann pins *(D).*

Figure 159–156. Repair of an avulsion of the tibial crest using a Bunnell-Mayer suture. The tibial crest is anchored to the tibia by passing the suture through transverse holes drilled in the tibia.

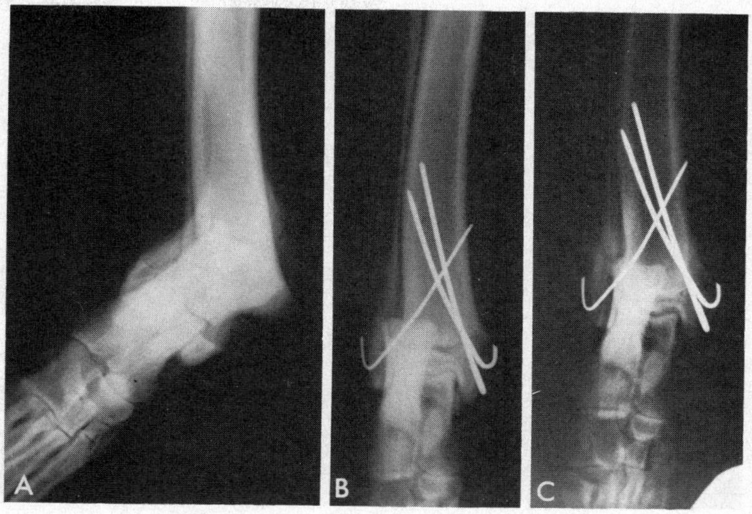

Figure 159–157. *A*, Salter type I separation of the distal metaphyseal growth plate of the tibia and fracture of the metaphysis of the fibula. *B*, Repair using crossed Kirschner wires. *C*, Healed fracture seven weeks after surgery.

often lateral or medial, the craniocaudal radiograph is usually most suitable.

Treatment. If a satisfactory reduction can be achieved, cast immobilization or a coaptation splint is an effective means of treatment. The separation, once reduced, has a degree of stability because of the interdigitations of the distal tibial epiphysis and metaphysis.

When a stable reduction cannot be achieved or external immobilization is undesirable, internal fixation is preferred.

Surgery. Rush pins or crossed Steinmann pins are very effective in stabilizing distal metaphyseal growth plate separations; however, the surgeon should always consider the potential for premature growth plate closure and should remove the implants as soon as healing is complete in order to minimize the possibility of growth arrest. Although a single transarticular intramedullary pin may also be employed, some joint damage is inevitable with this type of fixation, making the other techniques preferable.

Crossed Steinmann Pin or Rush Pin Fixation. Bilateral skin incisions are made over the malleoli, and the line of separation is carefully debrided. After reduction, the cross-pins are inserted into the medial and lateral malleoli and are directed toward the opposite cortex of the tibial shaft (Figs. 159–158 and 159–159; see Fig. 159–160).[12,13,14] When Rush pins are employed, the malleoli are predrilled prior to insertion of the pins. The holes are made at approximately 30-degree angles to the long axis of the tibia. The pins are positioned and alternately driven until fully inserted.

Transarticular Intramedullary Pin Fixation. After closed or open reduction of the fracture, a single intramedullary pin is passed through the fibular tarsal bone into the medullary canal of the tibia (see Fig. 159–158). This technique, though effective, is less desirable, because it reduces joint mobility. The transarticular pin should be large enough to fill the medullary canal of the tibia. If the pin is too small or is left too long, the shearing force may fatigue and

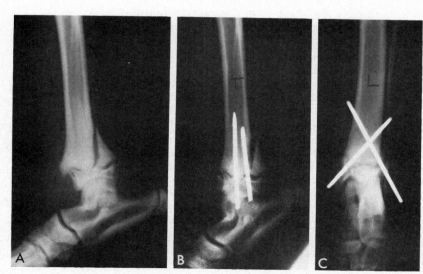

Figure 159–158. *A*, A Salter type II fracture of the distal metaphyseal growth plate of the tibia. *B* and *C*, Repair using crossed Steinmann pins.

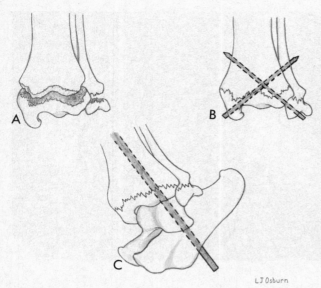

Figure 159–159. *A*, Separation of the distal metaphyseal growth plates of the tibia and fibula. Repair using crossed Steinmann pins *(B)* and a transarticular intramedullary pin *(C)*.

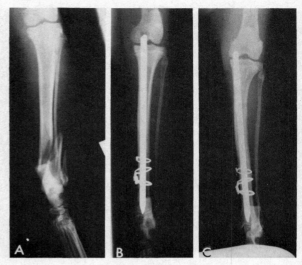

Figure 159–160. *A*, An oblique fracture of the distal metaphysis of the tibia and fibula. *B*, Repair using an intramedullary pin and full cerclage wires. *C*, Healed fracture eight weeks after surgery.

break the pin at the level of the tibiotarsal joint. The proximal fragment of the pin may cause considerable joint damage and is difficult to remove.

METAPHYSEAL FRACTURES

Metaphyseal fractures are most difficult to repair when close to a joint or severely comminuted. Stable internal fixation is preferable because it permits early ambulation, preventing the undesirable sequelae of periarticular fractures such as decreased range of joint motion and, in severe cases, fixation of the joint. Crossed Steinman pins, Rush pins, plates, and intramedullary pins are all applicable to metaphyseal fractures.

Comminuted fractures of the metaphysis are the most difficult to repair. To minimize loss of length and to achieve the most stable fixation, a buttress plate is the best method of fixation. A T plate can be applied to the proximal tibia, but application of a buttress plate to the distal tibia is difficult.

Intramedullary Pin Fixation. A simple fracture that is rotationally stable may be treated with a single intramedullary pin. The pin is introduced from the tibial plateau into the medullary cavity, as described for diaphyseal fractures of the tibia (Fig. 159–160). In low distal metaphyseal fractures, a transarticular pin must be placed through the hock joint to provide adequate stability. The pin may be introduced in a retrograde manner from the fracture site, through the tibiotarsal joint, or from the plantar aspect of the joint. Prior to introduction of the pin, the joint should be held in a functional position. Some loss of joint function occurs because of the presence of the pin in the joint, making this technique less desirable.

Crossed Steinmann Pin or Rush Pin Fixation. Either technique may be applied to simple transverse or short oblique fractures of the proximal or distal metaphysis. After open reduction of the fracture, the pins are introduced and directed across the fracture line to the opposite cortex of the tibia. In a distal tibia fracture, the pins are inserted in the medial and lateral malleoli, whereas in a proximal tibial fracture, the pins are inserted in the region of the collateral ligaments (Figs. 159–161 and 159–162). Holes must be predrilled to permit the introduction of Rush pins. The techniques are similar to those for proximal or distal metaphyseal growth plate separations.

Bone Plating. Bone plates are more difficult to

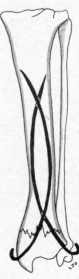

Figure 159–161. Rush pin fixation of a distal metaphyseal fracture of the tibia.

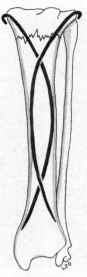

Figure 159–162. Rush pin fixation of a proximal metaphyseal fracture of the tibia.

employ in the treatment of fractures close to the joints. It is usually impossible to obtain sufficient points of screw fixation in the small fragment using conventional bone plates.

The breadth of the proximal tibia permits application of a T plate (see Fig. 159–172). It may be used as a buttress plate for comminuted fractures. A hook plate, developed for intertrochanteric osteotomy of the femur, has been applied to metaphyseal fractures of the long bones and can be applied to a proximal or distal tibial fracture. The two hooks and a screw can be positioned in a small fragment to provide stable fixation (see Fig. 159–171).

DIAPHYSEAL FRACTURES

All the conventional methods of fracture repair may be applied to fractures of the tibial diaphysis. External fixation in the form of a cast or coaptation splint is most satisfactory for fractures from the mid-tibia to distal tibia. If external fixation is employed for fractures of the proximal tibia, the cast or splint must extend proximal to the stifle joint to provide adequate stability.

Simple fractures of the diaphysis may be effectively treated with (1) an intramedullary pin, (2) a combination of cerclage or hemi-cerclage wire and an intramedullary pin, (3) plates, or (4) Kirschner splints.

Complex fractures of the diaphysis, in which there is significant comminution or loss of bone, are better treated with bone plates or Kirschner splints. Occasionally, when comminution of the bone is not severe, the fragments may be secured with a combination of cerclage wires and an intramedullary pin.

Spiral fractures of the tibia are relatively common. Two methods of treatment are particularly appropriate to spiral fractures and long oblique fractures:

multiple full-cerclage wires in conjunction with an intramedullary pin, and multiple interfragmentary lag screws in conjunction with a neutralization plate. Multiple cerclage wires or lag screws have been used successfully without the addition of an intramedullary pin or bone plate; however, the additional axial stability added by the pin or plate is advisable.[3]

Surgical Approach to the Diaphysis of the Tibia. A skin incision is made over the medial aspect of the tibia parallel to the long axis. The medial saphenous artery and vein and the saphenous nerve are identified as they cross the medial aspect of the tibia obliquely from the caudal aspect of the proximal tibia to the cranial aspect of the distal tibia. After these structures are identified and preserved, any remaining connective tissue is divided to expose the tibia.

An anterior approach to the tibial diaphysis has been described.[13] A skin incision is made along the anterior aspect of the tibia. The medial saphenous artery and vein are identified and retracted caudally, exposing the anterior and medial aspects of the tibial diaphysis.

Intramedullary Pinning. Intramedullary pins provide good axial stability but no rotational stability. When used alone to treat fractures, they are applied to rotationally stable fractures only.[12]

Retrograde introduction of a pin from the fracture site into the proximal tibia is inadvisable, because the surgeon has little control over the location at which the pin emerges in the femorotibial joint and because, if the pin is inappropriately placed, significant interference with joint function can occur (Fig. 159–163). The pin is introduced from the tibial plateau into the medullary cavity.

A small incision is made over the anterior medial aspect of the proximal tibia and femorotibial joint. The pin is introduced at a point midway between the

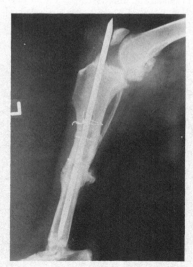

Figure 159–163. Tibial fracture treated with an intramedullary pin and full cerclage wire. The fracture has healed, but poor positioning of the pin has interfered with the patella and caused degenerative changes in the stifle joint.

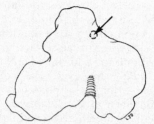

Figure 159–164. The tibial plateau. Site for introduction of an intramedullary pin (arrow).

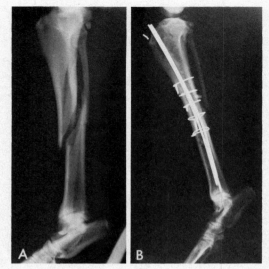

Figure 159–165. *A*, Spiral oblique fracture of the tibial diaphysis. *B*, Repair using stacked intramedullary pins and multiple full cerclage wires to add rotational stability.

tibial crest and the medial collateral ligament and is directed into the medullary canal (Fig. 159–164). Fractures that are rotationally stable and easily reduced can often be treated in this manner without surgical exposure of the fracture site. If closed reduction is difficult or if there is rotational instability, the fracture site should be exposed. A full or hemicerclage wire may be employed to add rotational stability (Fig. 159–165).

Kirschner Splinting. Kirschner splints may be applied to the tibia in three different configurations, all of which are suitable for the treatment of simple or complex fractures. They are as follows.

1. Pins are introduced in pairs above and below the fracture. The pairs of pins are joined with external bars, and the paired external bars are connected with a third bar that bridges the fracture (Fig. 159–166). This technique is less rigid than the other two methods but allows more adjustment for realignment of the fracture.
2. Pins are introduced in pairs above and below the fracture, and a single external bar is employed to bridge the fracture (Fig. 159–167A). The external bar and clamps are assembled, and the half-pins are introduced into the tibia through the clamps. The fracture should be reduced before the pins are placed. Some adjustment can be made to the reduction after the pins are placed, but not as easily as with the first technique.

3. Two connecting bars are used, one on either side of the tibia, to connect penetrating pins, which are placed in pairs above and below the fracture (Fig. 159–167B and C). The external bars and clamps are assembled, and the pins are introduced through the clamps into the tibia. The fracture is carefully reduced before application of the splint, because major adjustments to the reduction cannot be made once the pins are placed. This technique provides the most rigid fixation.

Bone Plating. Both simple and complex fractures of the tibial diaphysis may be treated using the plating techniques described elsewhere. Simple transverse fractures are ideally suited to compression plating (Fig. 159–168). Comminuted fractures are treated with interfragmentary compression in conjunction with a neutralization or compression plate (Fig. 159–169).

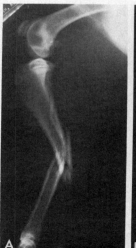
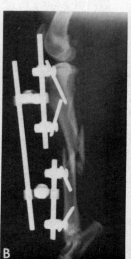
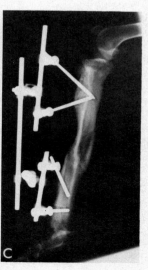

Figure 159–166. *A*, Comminuted fracture of the diaphysis of the tibia. *B*, The fracture has been stabilized with a Kirschner splint. *C*, Healed fracture ten weeks after surgery.

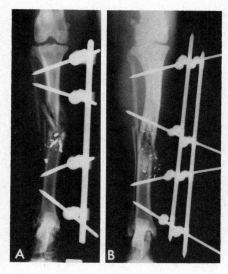

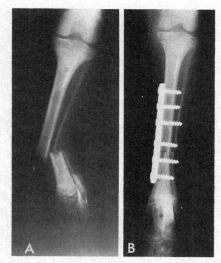

Figure 159–168. *A*, Transverse fracture of the tibia and fibula. *B*, Application of a compression plate.

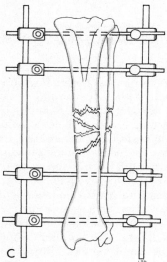

Figure 159–167. Alternative techniques for application of Kirschner splints. *A*, Single joining bar. *B*, Double joining bars both on the lateral side of the leg. *C*, Penetrating pins with joining bars medially and laterally.

CORRECTIVE OSTEOTOMY FOR ANGULAR TIBIAL DEFORMITY

Angular deformities of the tibia may develop because of asymmetric premature closure of either the proximal or the distal metaphyseal growth plate of the tibia.[12] Trauma is the most common cause of premature growth plate closure, but occasionally other musculoskeletal disorders may be responsible. Angular and rotational deformities may also occur after inadequate fracture stabilization. (Fig. 159–170).

The deformities are esthetically displeasing and may cause gait abnormalities and abnormal loading of adjacent joints. Major deformities warrant correction to prevent the development of degenerative joint disease, whereas mild deformities are usually of less significance and are corrected for cosmetic reasons.

Deformities are treated by corrective osteotomy. Simple rotational deformities are treated by trans-

Figure 159–169. *A* and *B*, Severely comminuted fracture of the tibia. *C*, Treatment using interfragmentary lag screws and a neutralization plate.

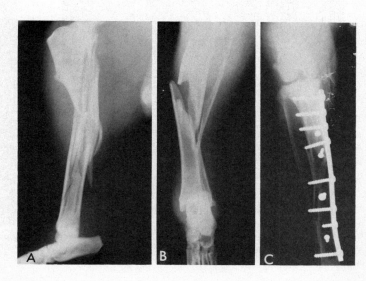

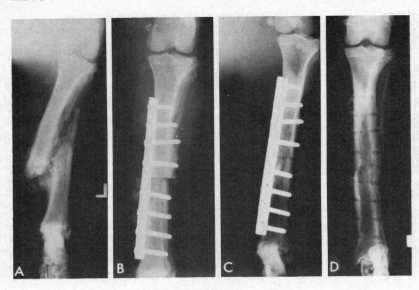

Figure 159–170. *A,* Inadequate reduction and stabilization of a tibial fracture leading to a malunion. *B,* Osteotomy, realignment, and stabilization of the fracture. Healed fracture nine months after surgery (*C*) and after plate removed (*D*).

verse osteotomy and derotation followed by stable fixation. Angular deformities require a wedge osteotomy, which is performed at the point of greatest curvature. Some loss in length of the limb is associated with this type of osteotomy, although in most cases the animal is able to compensate. Before the operation is begun, the size and location of the osteotomy should be carefully planned on the basis of radiographs. Stable fixation is necessary to prevent loss of alignment after reduction (Fig. 159–171). This is most easily achieved with a bone plate; however, with metaphyseal osteotomies, crossed Steinmann pins or Rush pins are suitable alternatives. In the proximal tibia, a T plate may be employed, whereas in the distal tibia, a hook plate is useful (Fig. 159–172).

POSTOPERATIVE CARE OF TIBIAL FRACTURES

Appropriate postoperative care differs according to the type and location of the fracture and the method of stabilization. After articular and periarticular fractures, rigid internal fixation followed by controlled early ambulation is most likely to achieve optimal return of function. The amount of exercise permitted during the healing period should be adjusted according to the strength of the repair and the healing process. Postoperative swelling or hematoma formation predisposes to wound infection and wound dehiscence. A Robert-Jones bandage applied at the completion of the operation is an effective means of reducing swelling in the hindlimb, especially below the stifle joint. Application of a Robert-Jones bandage

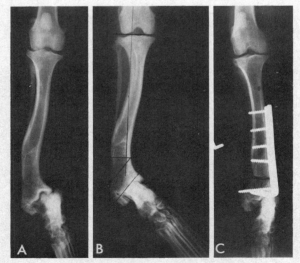

Figure 159–171. *A,* Varus deformity of the distal tibia. *B,* Determination of the size and location of the osteotomy from the radiograph. *C,* Completed osteotomy stabilized with a hook plate.

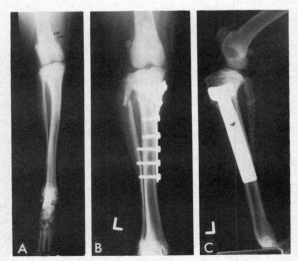

Figure 159–172. *A,* Angular deformity of the tibia. *B* and *C,* Proximal metaphyseal osteotomy stabilized with a "T" plate.

prior to casting or coaptation splinting often eliminates the need for a cast or splint change when significant swelling is present.

1. Dingwall, J. S.: A technique for repair of avulsion of the tibial tubercle in dogs. J. Small Anim. Pract. 12:665, 1971.
2. Goldstein, G.: The effect of cross pins and single pin implantation on the distal femoral growth plate. Paper presented to the 15th Annual General Meeting of the American College of Veterinary Surgeons, 1980.
3. Hinko, P. J.: Screw fixation of spiral tibial fractures: two case reports. J. Am. Anim. Hosp. Assoc. 10:69, 1974.
4. Leger, L., Sumner-Smith, G., Gofton, N., and Prieur, W. D.: A. O. hook plate fixation for metaphyseal fractures and corrective wedge osteotomies. J. Small Anim. Pract. 23:209, 1982.
5. Leighton, R. L.: Avulsion of the tibial tubercle. Vet. Med. Small Anim. Clin. 73:755, 1978.
6. Pettit, G. D., and Slatter, D. H.: Tension band wires for fixation of an avulsed canine tibial tuberosity. J. Am. Vet. Med. Assoc. 53:377, 1973.
7. Power, J. W.: Avulsion of the tibial tuberosity in the Greyhound. Aust. Vet. J. 52:491, 1976.
8. Ramadan, R. O., and Vaughan, L. C.: Disturbances in the growth of the tibia and femur in dogs. Vet. Rect. 104:433, 1979.
9. Sinibaldi, K. R.: Medial approach to the tarsus. J. Am. Anim. Hosp. Assoc. 15:77, 1979.
10. Smith, C. W., Schiller, A. G., Smith, A. R., and Dorner, J. L.: Osteomyelitis in the dog: a retrospective study. J. Am. Anim. Hosp. Assoc. 14:589, 1978.
11. Sumner-Smith, G.: Observations on epiphyseal fusion of the canine appendicular skeleton. J. Small Anim. Pract. 7:303, 1966.
12. Vincent, Z. D.: The repair of tibial fractures by intramedullary pinning. Vet. Rec. 64:64, 1952.
13. Wilson, J. W.: An anterior approach to the tibia. J. Am. Anim. Hosp. Assoc. 10:67, 1974.
14. Withrow, S. J.: Treatment of fractures of the tibial tuberosity in the dog. J. Am. Vet. Med. Assoc. 168:122, 1976.

Conditions of the Tarsus and Metatarsus

Gary W. Ellison

ANATOMY

The canine tarsus consists of seven bones arranged in three irregular rows that define four clinically important horizontal joints: the tarsocrural (hock), proximal intertarsal, distal intertarsal, and tarsometatarsal joints. (Fig. 159–173). The vertical joints between individual bones of the tarsus or intratarsal joints are very rigid.[16]

The tibial tarsal bone or talus is the only tarsal bone to articulate with the distal tibia and fibula, forming the tarsocrural joint. The trochlea of the talus is formed by a medial and lateral ridge that articulates with the sagittal grooves and intermediate ridge (cochlea) of the distal tibia. This arrangement allows primarily flexion and extension, although some rotation, translation, and medial lateral movement is present. The sides of the trochlea articulate with the medial (tibial) and lateral (fibular) malleoli, respectively.[16]

The fibular tarsal bone, or calcaneus, is divided into a proximal half or tuber calcis, to which the calcaneon tendon attaches, and a distal part, which articulates with the talus and the central and fourth tarsal bones. A flat medial process, the sustentaculum tali, provides a groove for passage of the flexor hallicus longus tendon on its plantar surface. The distal articulation of the calcaneus with the fourth tarsal bone (calcaneoquartal joint) joins the articulation of the talus with the central tarsal bone (talocalcaneoquartal joint), forming the proximal intertarsal joint. Some side movement as well as mild flexion and extension are possible, because the slightly convex distal ends of the tibial and fibular tarsals fit into the glenoids of the central and fourth tarsals.[16]

The central tarsal bone touches a'l of the other tarsal bones.[16] Distally, it articulates with the first, second, and third tarsal bones, forming the distal intertarsal joint on the medial aspect of the tarsus. Laterally, it articulates with the proximal half of the fourth tarsal.

The first, second, and third tarsal bones articulate primarily with the bases of metatarsals I to III, and the fourth tarsal with the bases of metatarsals IV to V, forming the tarsometatarsal joints.[16]

Metatarsal bone I is reduced in size and is sometimes fused with the first tarsal bone. Metatarsal bones II to V are similar in shape, with a proximal base, a shaft or body, and a distal head that articulates with its respective proximal phalanx.

The anatomy of the sesamoid bones and phalanges is similar to that of the carpus, with the exception of the first digit or "dewclaw." Some breeds (e.g., Great Pyrenees) are recognized by the American Kennel Club as normally possessing first digits on their hind paws. This variably shaped digit may be present in a rudimentary form, with a claw-bearing appendage attached by skin only to the medial tarsus. The proximal phalanx may be completely absent. Two claws of equal size are occasionally present, and complete duplication of the phalanges and metatarsal I, forming supernumerary digits, is sometimes encountered. When the dewclaw is lacking, a rudiment of metatarsal I is often seen as a flattened osseous

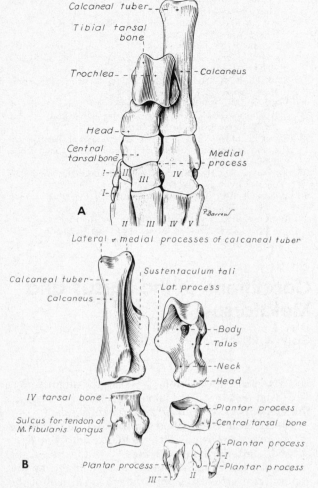

Figure 159–173. A and B, Bony anatomy of the canine tarsus. (Reprinted with permission from Evans, H. E., and Christensen, G. C.: *Miller's Anatomy of the Dog*, 2nd ed. W. B. Saunders, Philadelphia, 1979.)

plate lying in the fibrous tissue on the medial side of the tarsus.[16]

The tarsus, like the carpus, is supported by multiple soft tissue structures (Fig. 159–174). The medial or tibial collateral ligament is divided into a long segment and a short segment. The long superficial part runs from the medial malleolus and attaches distally on the first tarsal bone and metatarsals I and II. The short part of the ligament originates craniodistal to the long part and passes under it before dividing into a caudal part, which attaches on the tibial tarsal bone, and a longer, more cranial part, which attaches distally to the sustentaculum tali and first tarsal bone. The lateral or fibular collateral ligament is also divided into a long part and a short part. The long part passes from the lateral malleolus, attaching along its path to the fibular tarsal and fourth tarsal and ending on the base of the fifth metatarsal. The short part lies under and runs nearly at right angles to the long part, sending one band to the tuber calcis of the fibular tarsal and another band to the tibial tarsal bone.[16]

Dorsal ligamentous support is provided by many small intertarsal and tarsometatarsal ligaments. Proximal and distal transverse ligaments also exist. The proximal transverse ligament arises from the distal one-third of the tibia and forms a loop that holds the long digital extensor, extensor hallucis longus, and tibialis cranialis in place before blending distally with a proximal dorsal ligament that runs between the tibial tarsal and the third and fourth tarsal bones. The distal transverse ligament is a loop that surrounds the tendon of the long digital extensor.[16]

The plantar ligaments are heavier so that they can support tensile stresses placed on the joint. Several are prominent. Laterally and posteriorly, a strong ligament passes from the body of the fibular tarsal to the body of the fourth tarsal and the bases of meta-

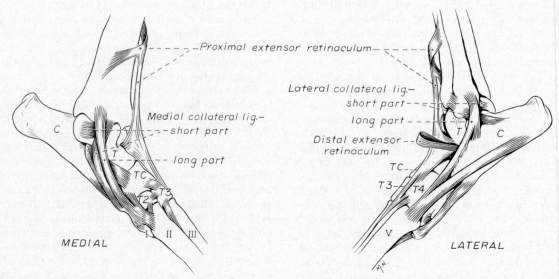

Figure 159–174. Ligaments of the canine tarsus. *C*, Calcaneus; *T*, talus; *T2, T3, T4*, second, third, and fourth tarsals, respectively; *TC*, central tarsal; *I* to *V*, metatarsals. (Reprinted with permission from Evans, H. E., and Christensen, G. C.: *Miller's Anatomy of the Dog*, 2nd ed. W. B. Saunders, Philadelphia, 1979.)

tarsals IV and V. Another conspicuous band leaves the caudolateral surface of the calcaneus and blends distally with the long portion of the fibular collateral ligament.[16] Medially, a strong band originates from the sustentaculum tali, passes over the central tarsal attaching to it, and then blends into the prominent tarsal fibrocartilage.

The fibrous part of the tarsal joint capsule extends from the distal articular cartilage of the tibia and fibula to the bases of the metatarsal bones. It has dorsal and plantar thickenings and fuses to the free surfaces of bones and ligaments as it passes over them.[16] On the plantar aspect of the tarsometatarsal joint, the fibrous joint capsule is especially thick and fuses with the plantar ligaments to form the plantar tarsal fibrocartilage. (see Fig. 159–174).[18]

The synovial layer of the joint capsule extends to the edges of articular cartilages. Three lateral and four medial joint sacs are present.[16]

DIAGNOSIS

Systematic examination and careful palpation of the individual tarsal joints are essential and often require sedation or general anesthesia. Palpation of the medial and lateral malleoli, fibular tarsal, and individual tarsal and metatarsal bones may indicate fractures. Joints are inspected for range of motion, crepitus, and swelling. It is essential to stress the joints in dorsoplantar, mediolateral, and rotary planes to evaluate them for ligament laxity, subluxation, or luxation.

In examination of the lateral collateral ligament, the tarsus is first flexed. In this position the long portion of the ligament is relaxed and the short segment is taut. The foot is twisted inward (inverted) on its longitudinal axis, and if opening of the joint occurs, rupture of the short portion of the collateral ligament is present. When the tarsus is extended, the long portion of the collateral is taut and the short portion relaxes. If the joint opens laterally when varus stress is applied to the tarsus, the long portion of the ligament is ruptured.

Rupture of the short portion of the medial collateral ligament is evident if the foot can be externally rotated (everted) while the tarsus is flexed. When the joint is extended, rupture of the long portion of the ligament is evident if a valgus stress opens the medial aspect of the tarsocrural joint.[18]

Ability to hyperextend the carpus indicates dorsal ligamentous injury and subluxation. Hyperflexion of the joint indicates tearing of the plantar ligaments or plantar fibrocartilage.

RADIOGRAPHY

Clinical findings suggest which type of injury is present and determine which radiographic views are necessary. When fractures are suspected, standard

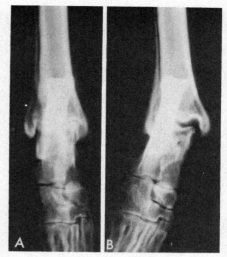

Figure 159–175. Nonstressed (A) and stressed (B) dorsoplanar views demonstrating a medial collateral ligament rupture and resulting valgus deformity of the hock.

lateral and dorsoplantar views are indicated. Compound injuries such as shear wounds should also be radiographed to diagnose inapparent fractures and luxations or to pinpoint radiographic foreign bodies.

In ligamentous laxity, clinical findings determine the proper stress view. A dorsoplantar view taken with medial tarsal pressure applied by a padded Plexiglas rod or wooden spoon creates a varus stress for evaluation of lateral collateral tear or a malleolar avulsion fracture. Conversely, lateral tarsal pressure stresses the joint medially (valgus) and will demonstrate medial collateral dysfunction (Fig. 159–175). Dorsal subluxations or luxations are delineated on the lateral view by hyperextension of the tarsus via dorsal digital pressure (Fig. 159–176A and B). Plantar subluxations are similarly demonstrated on the lateral views by hyperflexion of the tarsus through plantar digital pressure (Fig. 159–176C). If ligamentous damage is present, the stressed view demonstrates wedging, subluxation, or luxation that is often not apparent on the unstressed dorsoplantar or lateral view.

BIOMECHANICS OF TARSAL INJURIES

Luxations of the tarsus often involve the tarsocrural joint (tibiotarsal joint). Sufficient rotational force in either direction around the hock may cause luxation of this joint. Usually, a concurrent fracture of the medial or lateral malleolus is present. As the trochlea of the talus rotates out of joint, it may shear off the malleolus, or the pull of the collateral ligament may create an avulsion fracture. A direct blow to the medial or lateral aspect of the joint with the tarsus extended and bearing weight may also cause rupture of collateral ligaments or fracture of the malleoli (Fig. 159–177; see Fig. 159–175).[28]

Shearing injuries of the hock most often involve the medial aspect of the joint. In such an injury, the

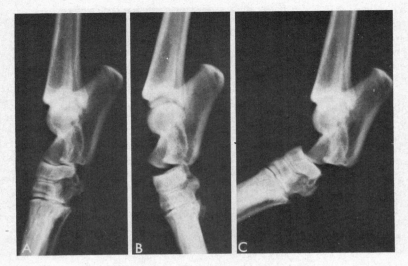

Figure 159–176. A, Nonstressed lateral view of a tarsus. *B,* A dorsal proximal intertarsal subluxation is demonstrated on the lateral view by applying dorsal digital pressure and hyperextending the joint. *C,* Plantar digital pressure demonstrates a plantar proximal intertarsal subluxation.

animal has been pushed or dragged along the road surface, causing the skin, collateral ligament, and often the malleolus to be ground off. The tarsocrural joint is rendered unstable and luxates easily during rotation.

Racing greyhounds commonly sustain damage to the central tarsal bone and associated structures of the right tarsus. As the dog races counterclockwise around the track, the lateral aspect of the right tarsus is placed under tension while the medial aspect undergoes compression and rotation. The central tarsal bone acts as a buttress or pivot that accumulates the greatest forces.[8] Compression fractures, which are often comminuted and subluxated, result. When the central tarsal bone fractures, there is a loss of cranial medial support, and the continued pull of the tendocalcaneus may cause the tibial tarsal bone to act as a fulcrum over which the fibular tarsal bone fractures. Associated nondisplaced fractures of the fourth tarsal have been noted.[8] It is also hypothesized that the plantar ligamentous support is placed under

extreme tension when the hock is flexed, and avulsion of the plantar ligaments from the base of the calcaneus results. The three main plantar ligaments may be involved, but the ligament most commonly torn is the one that originates on the body of the calcaneus and attaches to the fourth tarsal bone before inserting at the base of the fourth and fifth metatarsal bones.[14] If complete avulsion or tear of ligaments occurs, plantar proximal intertarsal, distal intertarsal, or tarsometatarsal subluxation occurs, and the patient walks plantigrade like a rabbit. If the joint is hyperextended, dorsal support is disrupted, and dorsal proximal intertarsal subluxation, distal intertarsal subluxation, or tarsometatarsal subluxation may result.

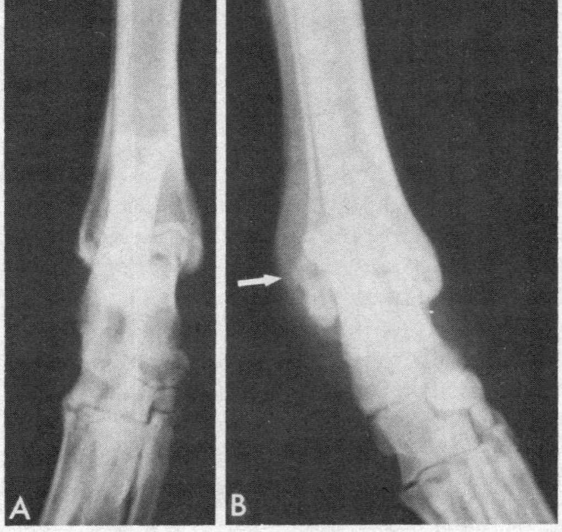

FRACTURES

Malleolar Fractures

Instability and sometimes complete luxation of the talocrural joint are features of a malleolar fracture. If swelling is severe and no joint crepitus is present, a malleolar fracture may be difficult to distinguish from a collateral ligament tear. Often, distraction of the fragments is minimal, and the fracture is most easily demonstrated on the stressed DP view (see Fig. 159–177).

Open reduction and fixation are indicated with malleolar fractures, because an unstable joint with secondary degenerative joint disease may result without this treatment. Usually, two small Steinmann pins or K-wires in conjunction with a figure-of-eight tension band wire of 20-gauge orthopedic wire facilitate fixation (Fig. 159–178). In animals under 10 kg, only a single 22-gauge K-wire may be possible. In giant breeds, interfragmentary compression with lag screws may be used.[24] The pins should be introduced near the tip of the malleolus, angled across the distal tibia, and seated into the opposite cortex (Fig. 159–179). A drill hole through the medial tibial cortex

Figure 159–177. A, This lateral malleolar fracture is not apparent on the dorsoplantar view. *B,* By placing varus stress on the joint, distraction of the fragments becomes evident (arrow).

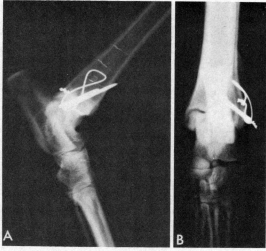

Figure 159–178. A and B, Fixation of the fracture in Figure 159–177 with two Steinmann pins and a figure-of-eight wire.

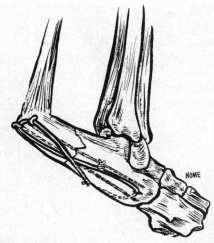

Figure 159–180. A transverse fracture of the tuber calcis is ideally repaired with two intramedullary pins to counteract rotation in conjunction with the figure-of-eight tension band wire.

should be placed 1.5 to 2.5 cm from the fracture line to accommodate the figure-of-eight wire. The K-wires may be bent to form hooks and tapped flush with the bone. Fixation of the lateral malleolus involves drilling the K-wires thru the fibula and lateral tibial cortex. The figure-of-eight wire is passed through a drill hole in the fibula or lateral tibial cortex much as described for the medial malleolus.

Postoperative care involves a soft Robert-Jones bandage to minimize swelling for five to ten days, followed by free weight-bearing on the limb. Follow-up radiographs may be taken at two- to three-week intervals until union is complete. Postoperative loosening of pins often necessitates their removal.

Fractures of the Fibular Tarsal Bone (Calcaneus)

The proposed biomechanics of these fractures has been previously described. External fixation alone is

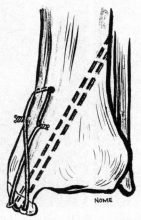

Figure 159–179. A medial malleolar fracture repair. A similar fixation is used after approach to the joint via a medial malleolar osteotomy.

inadequate because the strong pull of the tendocalcaneus causes distraction of the fragments, resulting in a plantigrade deviation of the limb. Definitive therapy involves open reduction, anatomic alignment and fixation with an intramedullary pin, or screw fixation accompanied by a figure-of-eight tension band wire.

Avulsion fractures of the calcaneus are usually transverse and often involve the proximal half of the fibular tarsal bone or tuber calcis. A lateral approach is made to the calcaneus, and the superficial digit flexor tendon is retracted medially to complete the exposure. Fixation is accomplished either by directing the pin retrograde from the proximal fragment out through the tip of the tuber calcis, by reducing the fracture and seating the pin distally, or by first reducing the fracture and passing the pin from the tip of the tuber calcis down the shaft of the calcaneus. In the patient over 10 kg, a second K-wire or intramedullary pin is ideal to prevent rotation (Fig. 159–180). Pins should be seated in the distal aspect of the calcaneus. The tension band wire is placed by drilling a transverse hole in the plantar surface of the distal fragment equidistant between the calcaneus and the tuber calcis and applying a figure-of-eight band of 20-gauge wire around the proximal pins (Fig. 159–181). Proximally, the wire must lie beneath the superficial digital flexor tendon. An alternate way of fixation involves drilling a separate hole in the tuber calcis for the proximal loop of the figure-of-eight wire (Fig. 159–182). If the fracture involves the distal half of the calcaneus or the calcaneoquartal joint, the pins are driven across the proximal intertarsal joint into the fourth tarsal bone, and the distal loop of the figure-of-eight wire engages the plantar process of the fourth tarsal bone. If degenerative joint disease is imminent, the surgeon may want to proceed with a calcaneoquartal arthrodesis.

Comminuted calcaneal fractures are difficult surgical problems. If the fragments are large and longi-

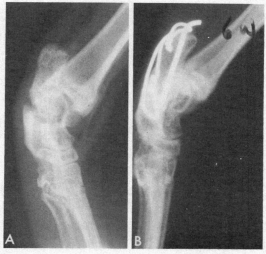

Figure 159–181. *A*, A transverse fracture of the calcaneus in a 5-kg poodle. *B*, Repair with a single intramedullary pin and figure-of-eight wire. In spite of poor distal pin placement the tension band wire counteracted tensile forces sufficiently to allow union at six weeks.

tudinally oriented, they may be immobilized with cerclage wire in conjunction with intramedullary pins and figure-of-eight tension wires. Often, the fragments are small and transversely oriented, necessitating bone plate fixation. Commonly, in highly comminuted calcaneal fractures, there are concurrent central tarsal fractures, and complete proximal intertarsal arthrodesis using a laterally placed bone plate, as described for arthrodesis, may be required.

Aftercare of simple calcaneal fractures involves a postoperative soft cotton bandage to reduce swelling

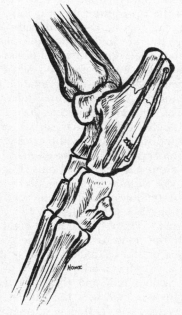

Figure 159–182. Alternate fixation involves drilling a separate hole for the proximal loop of the figure-of-eight wire. (Adapted with permission from Brinker, N. O., Piermattei, D. L., and Flo, G. L.: *Handbook of Small Animal Orthopedics and Fracture Treatment.* W. B. Saunders, Philadelphia, 1983.)

for five days, followed by restricted weight-bearing on the limb. Comminuted fractures may be supported in a splint or cast above the stifle. Follow-up radiographs are taken at 2- to 3-week intervals until union is complete. As with malleolar fractures, pin loosening or soft tissue irritation often necessitates pin removal.

Fractures of the Tibial Tarsal Bone (Talus)

These fractures are not common, and their repair is not well documented. In my experience, they often are caused by severe direct trauma to the hock and accompany other injuries. Fractures may involve the body (including the trochlea), neck, or head.[23] Oblique views are sometimes necessary for diagnosis of undisplaced fractures. Osteochondrosis of the medial talar condyle is well described and must not be confused with an articular fracture (see discussion of osteochondrosis).

If the fracture is nonarticular and relatively well aligned, immobilization with a circumferential cast above the stifle for five to six weeks may allow adequate healing. Displaced trochlear fractures involve the articular surface and necessitate open reduction and interfragmentary lag screw compression. Exposure of the fractures may be accomplished by osteotomy of the medial malleolus. (see Fig. 159–179). Fractures of the neck may be treated by cross-pinning or fixation with lag screws (Fig. 159–183 and 159–184). Fractures of the head of the talus may be fixed in similar fashion. If the fracture is comminuted and involves the talocalcaneocentral joint, a proximal intertarsal arthrodesis may be necessary. Postoperative support involves a lateral splint or circumferential cast for four to six weeks or until healing is complete. Prognosis is good for neck and head fractures and guarded for trochlear joint fractures, because of the potential for postoperative osteoarthritis.

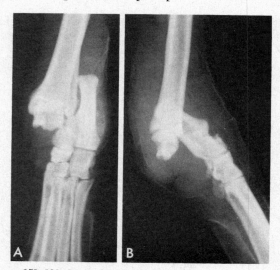

Figure 159–183. Dorsoplantar (*A*) and lateral (*B*) views of a neck fracture of the tibial tarsal in a 10-kg cocker spaniel. Severe lateral displacement of the distal fragment and rupture of the medial collateral ligament are evident.

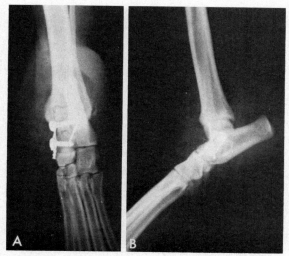

Figure 159–184. *Dorsoplantar (A) and lateral (B) views of the repair of the fracture in Figure 159–183. A 0.045-inch K-wire and two medial screws with a wire loop were used to stabilize the fracture. The medial collateral ligament was repaired with braided Dacron placed through a drill hole in the medial malleolus and looped around the proximal screw. A small avulsion fracture is evident from the lateral malleolus, but no instability was present.*

Fractures of the Central Tarsal Bone

Central tarsal fractures are seen primarily in the right hindfoot of racing greyhounds because they run counterclockwise.[17] Fractures of the left central tarsal bone are described in animals that move in a clockwise direction.[8] These fractures frequently show radiographic evidence of compression, subluxation, and comminution but are never compound. Five distinct types of fractures have been described, management and prognosis varying according to the location and the degree of severity.[10]

Dorsal slab fractures with no displacement can be managed via external fixation with a cast or lateral splint and reportedly have a good prognosis. Dorsal slab fractures with dorsal or proximal displacement are repaired via open reduction and fixation with a single lag screw. The surgical approach involves an incision directly over the bone with medial retraction of the tendon of the tibialis cranialis and lateral retraction of tendons of the extensor digitorum brevis and long digital extensor. The fragment is reduced with Vulsellum uterine forceps and overdrilled. A short 2.0- or 2.7-mm cortical screw directed into the main body of the central tarsal bone provides interfragmentary compression. The fixation is supported for three to four weeks in a splint or until union is complete. Prognosis is good if anatomic reduction is accomplished at operation.

Fractures in the sagittal plane often create a large medial fragment that may displace dorsally and require surgical fixation. Reduction may be accomplished by hyperextending, everting, and placing distal traction on the limb. The reduction is maintained with Vulsellum forceps, and fixation is performed with a lag screw placed in the medial to

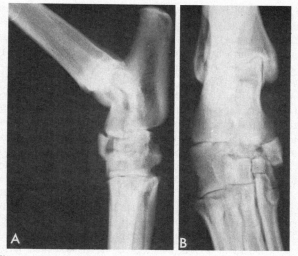

Figure 159–185. *Lateral dorsoplantar views of a comminuted central tarsal fracture with medial sagittal (A) and dorsal slab fragments (B). (Courtesy of D. L. Piermattei.)*

lateral direction and transfixing the large slab fracture to the fourth tarsal bone.

When the fracture involves a combination of the large medial fragment and a smaller dorsal slab fragment (Fig. 159–185), the medial fragment is reduced first, followed by the dorsal slab fragment. With both fragments held in reduction with two Vulsellum forceps, the medial fragment is fixed using a 3.5-mm cortical or 4.0-mm cancellous screw, which is started slightly proximal to the distal articulation of the central tarsal and lagged into the fourth tarsal bone. The dorsal slab is then lagged with a 2.0- or 2.7-mm screw placed a few millimeters proximal to the shaft of the first screw (Fig. 159–186).

Highly comminuted fractures with displacement carry the worst prognosis of all central tarsal fractures.

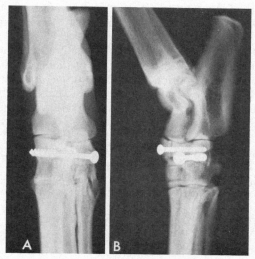

Figure 159–186. *Postoperative radiographs of the fracture in Figure 159–185. A, The medial fragment has been lagged into the body of the fourth tarsal with a cancellous screw. The dorsal slab fragment has been lagged with a smaller cortical screw. (Courtesy of D. L. Piermattei.)*

Collapse of the joint space occurs, and varus deviation of the tarsus may be observed. Closed manual reduction followed by external coaptation is the most common method of management. If joint collapse is severe, open reduction is performed, and a cortico-cancellous rib graft is inserted into the collapsed space as a buttress.[17] Plaster or fiber glass cast support may be necessary for eight to ten weeks. Complete replacement of the central tarsal bone with a prosthesis has also been described;[4,5,23] the technique has not found acceptance because of loosening of the implant and failure of the animal to return to winning form.

Luxations of the central tarsal bone may occur and may involve dorsomedial displacement of the bone. Although closed reduction can sometimes be done, the central tarsal bone usually does not remain in place, and internal fixation is necessary. In large dogs, the central tarsal is reduced and transferred to the fourth tarsal bone with a bone screw. In toy breeds, K-wire transfixation may be used.[10] The tarsus is supported in a splint for two to three weeks, and free weight-bearing is allowed.

Other Fractures of the Tarsus

Fractures of the first and second tarsals are extremely uncommon and may be seen only in conjunction with distal intertarsal or tarsometatarsal joint injuries.

Isolated third tarsal fractures or subluxations have been described in the racing greyhound but are not nearly as common as central tarsal luxations. A swelling may be present, or pain may be evident upon direct palpation of the third tarsal bone.

Compression fractures of the fourth tarsal bone may be seen in association with the more severe types of central tarsal fractures. As the craniomedial aspect of the tarsus collapses, the head of the talus is displaced distally, allowing the fourth tarsal bone to accumulate the remaining compressive forces. The fourth tarsal bone may subluxate laterally, shearing off the lateral aspect of the base of metatarsal V, or an avulsion fracture of its collateral ligament attachment may result from medial joint collapse.[8] Reports of management of these fractures are limited, but as with fractures of the central tarsal bone, external reduction and coaptation should be chosen if the fracture is either undisplaced or too comminuted for the fragments to be successfully immobilized surgically.

SUBLUXATIONS AND LUXATIONS

Tarsocrural Luxations

Tarsocrural luxations are often associated with malleolar fractures (see section on malleolar fractures) or

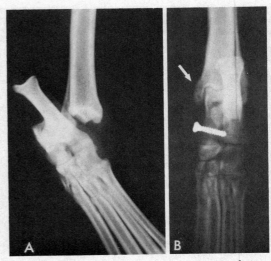

Figure 159–187. *A,* Complete luxation of the tarsocrural joint with rupture of the medial collateral ligament. Repair involved open reduction and direct approximation of the ligament ends. *B,* A nylon prosthesis anchored through a proximal osseous tunnel in the medial malleolus (arrow) and around a distal screw head served as support. The lateral collateral ligament remained intact.

rupture of both the collateral ligaments and joint capsule (Figs. 159–187 and 159–188). Subluxations often involve a rupture of a single collateral ligament, which is demonstrable on a stress radiograph. Occasionally for luxations that involve only the soft tissues, closed reduction and coaptation may be successful. However, most ligament tears require direct surgical repair.

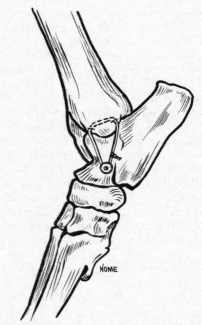

Figure 159–188. Medial collateral ligament prosthesis used in Figure 159–187B. Wire, braided polyester, or monofilament nylon is looped around the distal screw head and through the proximal osseous tunnel.

Collateral Ligament Repair

Three options are available for ruptured collateral ligament repair; direct suturing, reattachment of an avulsion fracture, and prosthetic replacement of the ligament.

Direct suturing of the ligament may be possible if the injury is fresh and the ligament ends are minimally frayed. A Bunnell or modified Kessler (locking loop) suture pattern of nonabsorbable nylon or polypropylene may be used to successfully approximate the ligament ends.[1,27] The fixation is often also used in conjunction with one of the prosthetic ligament replacements, which serves as support until the ligament heals.

Commonly, the collateral ligament avulses from its attachment on the malleolus. The long portion may be reattached by anchoring the avulsed portion of the ligament with a Bunnell or locking-loop stitch, which is passed through two drill holes in the distal malleolus (Fig. 159–189).[14] When the short portion of the collateral ligament is torn from its tibial attachment, it is often severely frayed, precluding either direct suturing or reattachment to the bone. Another alternative for fixation of avulsed collateral ligaments is reattachment with a screw and spiked washer.[22]

Prosthetic ligament replacement is used to support primary suturing of the ligament or when fraying or loss of the ligament ends prevents direct primary reconstruction. A number of prosthetic ligament re-

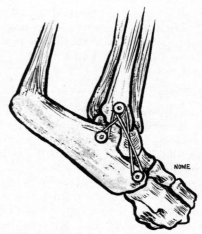

Figure 159–190. A three-screw technique for lateral collateral ligament replacement. This configuration replaces both the long and short parts of the collateral ligament. (Adapted with permission from Aron, D. M.: Prosthetic collateral ligament replacement of the talocrural joint—A proposed technique in the dog. Paper presented at the 9th Annual V.O.S. Conference, 1982.)

placements have been described. Orthopedic wire and synthetic materials such as monofilament nylon and braided polyesters have been most commonly used.[18–20] Medial collateral repair using two stainless steel screws and a figure-of-eight wire involves placing one screw proximal to the malleolus at the origin of the collateral ligament and the other at the center of the talus. In small dogs, the distal screw head may impinge on the malleolus in the flexed position, and excessive angling of the wire from the proximal to distal screw may cause the wire to slip off the distal screw head. The technique has been modified by drilling a dorsoplantar tunnel in the malleolus to anchor the proximal aspect of the prosthesis. Monofilament nylon or braided polyester suture is looped through the osseous tunnel and anchored around a distally placed screw or drill hole in the talus (see Fig. 159–188). This modification reduces the impingement of the prosthesis on the malleolus and lessens the chances that the prosthesis will slip from the screw head. Success rates for these procedures have varied owing to loosening or breakage of the prosthesis, which causes joint instability and resultant degenerative joint disease.

A recent report suggests that conventional techniques have not been more successful because the normal anatomy of the collaterals and biomechanics of the talocrural joint have not been reproduced more closely.[2] This study found that a three-screw technique allows functional replacement of both the long and short portions of the collateral ligaments (Fig. 159–190). Braided polyester suture material more closely approximated the normal biomechanics of the ligament than wire did. The major advantage of the technique is maintenance of stability without sacrificing range of motion.[3]

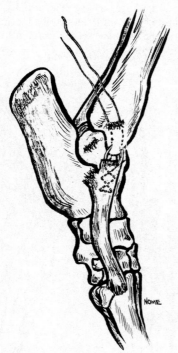

Figure 159–189. A modified Bunnell suture pattern anchors the long portion of the medial collateral ligament through two drill holes in the medial malleolus. (Adapted with permission from Early, T. D., and Dee, J. F.: Trauma to the carpus, tarsus, and phalanges of dogs and cats. Vet. Clin. North Am. 10:717, 1980.)

Postoperative care of collateral ligament repair involves a soft cotton wrap to reduce postoperative swelling, followed by four to five weeks of rigid immobilization in a splint or cast.

Shear Injuries

Shear wounds usually involve the medial aspect of the hock. Often, the medial malleolus and collateral ligament are completely ground off, leaving no medial support to the joint. These grossly contaminated wounds require aggressive surgical debridement, joint lavage, and bacterial culture prior to primary closure. Soft tissues are often devitalized, and skin defects may be severe, necessitating healing by second intention. If adequate debridement is possible, the wound may be closed over drains (Fig. 159–191). Immobilization of the joint may be accomplished with splints that require frequent changing. Immobilization of the joint may also be accomplished using transarticular Kirschner-Ehmer apparatus.[6,15] Two proximal pins are driven across the distal tibia, and two distal pins traverse the metatarsals. Single connecting bars placed medially and laterally represent a penetrating configuration (Fig. 159–192).

Screw and wire reconstruction of medial support may be attempted if wound contamination is minimal or as a secondary procedure following primary wound care. A screw is positioned in the center of an imaginary circle made by the medial condyle of the talus. The screw angles slightly proximally but does not pass out the lateral side. The proper location for the proximal screw in the tibia is located, by flexing and extending the joint, at a point where a pin and loop of wire are snug but not stressed through the complete range of motion (Fig. 159–193).

Aggressive postoperative antibiotic therapy is often critical to the success of shear wound injuries. The

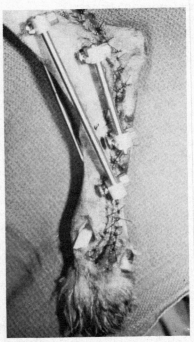

Figure 159–192. After aggressive surgical debridement, the wound is closed over drains and supported with a penetrating transarticular Kirschner-Ehmer apparatus.

development of septic arthritis or osteomyelitis often causes clinical failure in spite of a stable repair. The appropriate antibiotic, as determined by intraoperative bacterial culture and sensitivity testing is administered for at least two weeks and often prevents these unwanted complications.

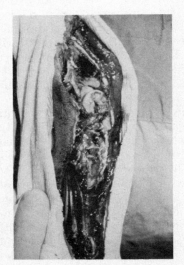

Figure 159–191. A severe shear wound of the medial hock. The medial malleolus and collateral support have been ground off, allowing luxations of the talocrural joint.

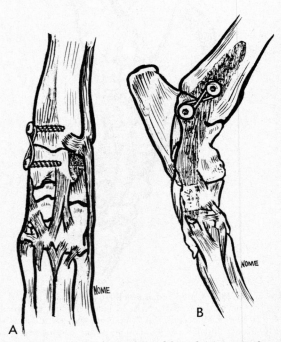

Figure 159–193. Dorsoplantar (A) and lateral (B) views of screw and wire fixation of a medial shear wound that has ground off the medial malleolus and collateral ligament.

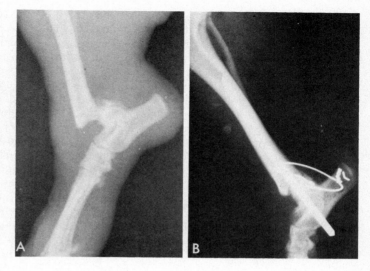

Figure 159–194. *A,* Lateral radiograph of a tarsocrural luxation in a 6-kg Lhasa apso with bimalleolar fractures. *B,* Five-week postoperative radiograph. A large transarticular pin and tension band wire were used because a fractured femur in the same limb precluded any external support and necessitated early weight-bearing. Bony ankylosis of the joint occurred, and the implants were removed after three months.

Transarticular Pin Fixation of Tarsocrural Luxations

In cats and small dogs under 7 kg, malleolar fractures and the supporting ligamentous structures are often too small to be reconstructed primarily (Fig. 159–194A). The use of a temporary transarticular pin can be used in conjunction with external splinting to facilitate healing of the soft tissue structures around the joint. A .064-inch Kirschner wire or larger Steinmann pin is introduced from the trochlear surface of the talus through the sustentaculum tali of the calcaneus and is withdrawn to be flush with the articular surface. After the luxation is reduced and the tarsocrural joint is placed in a functional position (135 degrees for dogs, 120 degrees for cats), the pin is passed across the joint and seated in the middle to proximal tibia. The tarsus is splinted for four weeks to prevent bending or breaking of the pin. The pin is removed at this time, and full weight-bearing is allowed.

If arthrodesis is desired, the cochlea of the distal tibia and trochlea of the talus may be debrided of articular cartilage and packed with cancellous graft. A wire loop extends thru a drill hole in the distal tibia and tuber calcis to overcome tensile forces (Fig. 159–194B). The tarsus is supported in a splint or circumferential cast for six to eight weeks or until union is complete. Full weight-bearing is allowed at this time. The pin is removed if it migrates or pain is evident.

Arthrodesis of the Tarsocrural (Hock) Joint

Indications for arthrodesis of the talocrural joint are irreparable soft tissue injuries, highly comminuted articular fractures and severe chronic degenerative joint disease.

The joint is approached through a medial incision via osteotomy of the medial malleolus.[15] The angle of arthrodesis is chosen (135 degrees for dogs, 120 degrees for cats), and the condyles of the talus and distal cochlea of the tibia are removed with an oscillating saw or osteotome. Two K-wires are used to stabilize the joint while a lag screw is applied. A hole is drilled beginning 2 to 3 cm above the medial malleolus through the talus and exiting from the base of the calcaneus. The angle of the drill hole is approximately 15 degrees to the long axis of the tibia. The tibial hole is overdrilled and the distal hole is tapped prior to compression of the tarsocrural joint with a screw (Fig. 159–195A). A cancellous bone graft is packed around the arthrodesis site to facilitate

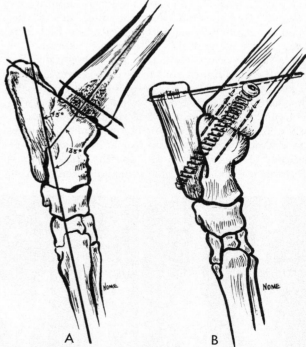

Figure 159–195. Technique for talocrural arthrodesis. *A,* After the appropriate angle is chosen, the articular surfaces of the talus and distal tibia are osteotomized and the reduction is maintained with two K-wires. The proximal hole in the distal tibia is overdrilled and the distal threads in the talus and calcaneus tapped prior to compressing the joint with the screw. *B,* A wire loop or small Steinmann pin between the distal tibia and calcaneus counteracts tensile forces.

healing. An additional pin or wire loop may be drilled from the distal tibia to the tuber calcis to counteract bending forces (Fig. 159–195B).

An alternative technique involves placement of the lag screw through the plantar surface of the tibial tarsal bone into the distal tibia. A Kirschner wire is placed before the hole for the screw is drilled, to maintain the joint at the proper angle and to serve as a guide for the parallel hole drilled for the screw. A cancellous screw whose threads will engage only the distal tibia, creating compression across the joint, is selected. If a cortical screw is used, the tibial tarsal bone is overdrilled prior to tapping of the distal tibia.

The arthrodesis is splinted for six to eight weeks or until union is complete.[13] Free weight-bearing is then allowed. Implant migration and associated pain may require pin removal at a later date.

Dorsal Proximal Intertarsal Subluxations

These injuries are caused by acute hyperextension of the tarsus that results in rupture of the dorsal joint capsule and small intertarsal ligaments. (see Fig. 159–176B). Subluxation of the talocalcaneocentral joint (joint between the talus and central tarsal bone) alone or simultaneous subluxation of the talocalcaneocentral joint and the calcaneoquartal joint (joint between the calcaneus and fourth tarsal bone) may be apparent (Fig. 159–196A). Dorsal soft tissue swelling may be evident, but usually no associated bony injuries are present. Pain is often minimal, and because the plantar ligamentous support is intact, the limb may bear weight without obvious deformity. Diagnosis is made by physical examination and radiography, because the joint opens dorsally when hyperextended.

Dorsal proximal intertarsal subluxations can usually be treated with closed reduction and coaptation with a circumferential cast or lateral splint for one month. If the instability remains or the initial injury requires stabilization, a calcaneoquartal arthrodesis with transfixation of the talus to the fourth tarsal bone is performed. A dorsal incision is made, extending from the head of the talus to the base of the metatarsal II. The tibialis cranialis tendon is retracted medially, and the long digital extensor laterally. A dorsal arthrotomy is performed, and the articular cartilage of the proximal intertarsal joint is removed down to bleeding subchondral bone. The joint space is packed with cancellous bone, the luxation is reduced, and a Steinmann pin (in larger dogs) or cancellous screw (cats and small dogs) is driven from the tuber calcis into the fourth tarsal bone. In larger dogs in which instability exists, another pin or screw is placed from medial to lateral in order to transfix the head of the talus to the distal portion of the fourth tarsal bone. Because plantar ligamentous support is intact, tensile forces are counteracted, and a tension band is not necessary unless collateral support is impaired (Fig. 159–196B). The joint is splinted for four to six weeks or until union is complete, and limited weight-bearing is allowed. Prognosis is good for full recovery.

Dorsal Distal Intertarsal and Dorsal Tarsometatarsal Subluxations

Dorsal distal intertarsal subluxations are rare and are always associated with a concomitant partial tarsometatarsal subluxation. The distal intertarsal joint involves only the medial aspect of the tarsal joint because of the lateral boundary presented by the fourth tarsal bone. Therefore, this subluxation is actually a distal intertarsal luxation on the medial aspect and a tarsometatarsal subluxation on the lateral aspect.

With a dorsal tarsometatarsal luxation, the bases of metatarsals II to V are luxated from their respective articulations on the second to fourth tarsal bones. The distal bony components are generally displaced dorsally and proximally, with plantar support kept intact (Fig. 159–197).

If the luxations are reducible, small dogs and cats may be managed by external coaptation for four weeks. In larger dogs, wiring between the central and second tarsal bones is needed, followed by ex-

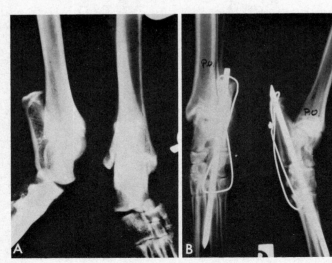

Figure 159–196. A, Dorsoplantar and lateral radiographs of a dorsal proximal intertarsal subluxation with a compression fracture of the head of the talus and rupture of collateral ligament between the fourth tarsal and calcaneus. B, Proximal intertarsal fixation using a pin and figure-of-eight wire technique.

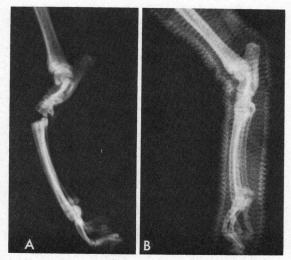

Figure 159–197. *A*, A dorsal tarsometatarsal luxation in a 4-kg domestic short-haired cat. *B*, Closed manual reduction was followed by three weeks of support in a fiber glass cast.

ternal support for four weeks.[24] If external support is unsuccessful, the area may be immobilized by driving a pin through the calcaneus and fourth tarsal bone and seating it distally in the base of the metatarsals. A second pin may be driven from the medial portion of the central tarsal through the fourth tarsal and seated in the base of the metatarsals. As with the dorsal proximal intertarsal subluxation, no figure-of-eight tension band is necessary if the plantar ligaments are intact. External splinting is used for four weeks.

Plantar Proximal Intertarsal Subluxations

Plantar proximal intertarsal luxations are caused by disruption of the plantar support apparatus. Simultaneous laxity of the talocalcaneocentral and the calcaneoquartal joint allows excessive dorsoflexion and subluxation of the joints. The severity of the injury may vary from mild plantigrade deviation of the hock to an injury so severe that the tarsus may actually contact the ground.[21]

These injuries have been described as both chronic progressive lesions and acute traumatic injuries. The Sheltland sheepdog and collie breeds are reportedly predisposed, with Shetland sheepdogs accounting for 50 per cent (22 of 44) and collies for 23 per cent (10 of 44) of the cases reported in one study.[7] Dogs from six to nine years of age were most commonly involved. In over half of these cases, no known trauma such as that caused by automobiles, jumping, or falls could be documented. In the majority, the lameness was not preceded by any appreciable activity.

Conversely, in the racing greyhound or athletic dog, excessive tensile stresses placed on the plantar support apparatus of the running animal are thought to break down the plantar ligamentous support causing an acute injury and lameness. Reportedly, the ligament that runs from the base of the calcaneus and

attaches to metatarsals IV and V is most commonly torn.[8,14] The ligament usually tears or bone is avulsed from the base of the calcaneus, and often a fracture can be seen radiographically. Moderate to severe lameness is present, and excessive dorsoflexion is evident at the proximal intertarsal joint during manipulation. Radiographic diagnosis is made by comparing stressed and unstressed lateral radiographs (see Fig. 159–176C). When plantigrade stress is applied to the toes, angulation of the tarsus at the proximal intertarsal joint is evident. The degree of subluxation varies from mild displacement to nearly complete luxation of the joint. Slipping of the anterior margins between the talus and central tarsal and calcaneus and fourth tarsal bones may be seen, as well as roughening and periosteal reaction near the base of the calcaneus.

Proximal intertarsal luxations are usually managed surgically. The extensive tensile forces placed on the joint during weight-bearing make closed reduction and coaptation unsuccessful and requiring surgical stabilization of the joint. Definitive treatment of this injury involves pin and figure-of-eight arthrodesis of the calcaneoquartal joint or plate arthrodesis of the complete proximal intertarsal joint. (See "Pin and Figure-of-Eight Arthrodesis" and "Plate Arthrodesis of the Proximal Intertarsal Joint.")

Plantar Distal Intertarsal and Plantar Tarsometatarsal Subluxations

As with dorsal distal intertarsal subluxations, plantar distal intertarsal subluxations are uncommon, having accounted for less than five per cent of all intertarsal subluxations in one study.[20] These injuries involve plantar displacement of the central tarsal from the first, second, and third tarsal bones on the medial aspect of the tarsus and plantar displacement of the fourth tarsal from metatarsals IV and V on the lateral aspect (Fig. 159–198). History and clinical signs are

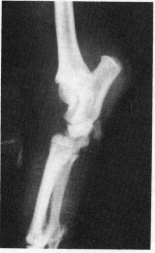

Figure 159–198. Lateral radiograph of a plantar distal intertarsal subluxation with associated avulsion fracture of the distal calcaneus.

similar to those described for proximal intertarsal subluxations.

Tarsometatarsal subluxations are much more common and are usually associated with trauma. Automobile accidents cause the majority of these injuries, but catching of the foot in a fence while jumping or in a door while running has also caused the injury.[7] The patient is usually presented with pain and swelling of the affected joint. Dorsiflexion of the tarsus reveals angulation at the tarsometatarsal joint. If the patient is weight-bearing, a plantigrade deviation of the tarsus is evident.

Management of plantar distal intertarsal and tarsometatarsal injuries is similar to that described for proximal intertarsal subluxations. The plantar ligamentous support is disrupted, and joint arthrodesis is necessary to counteract the tensile forces placed on the limb.

Pin and Figure-of-Eight Arthrodesis

A plantar incision is made extending from the tuber calcis distally to the base of metatarsal IV. The superficial digital flexor tendon is reflected medially, and a 2-mm hole is drilled from lateral to medial in the plantar tubercle of the fourth tarsal bone in order to house the distal part of the figure-of-eight wire. The intra-articular cartilage of the joint is removed with a Hall air drill or bone curette, and the space is packed with cancellous bone graft. With the joint in a normal reduced position, a Steinmann pin is inserted at the tuber calcis, down the medullary canal of the calcaneus, and across the joint and is seated

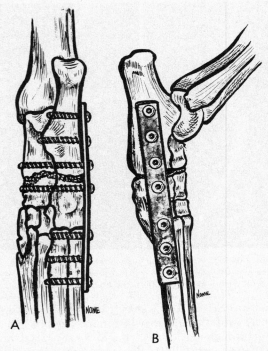

Figure 159–200. Plantar (A) and lateral (B) views of a proximal intertarsal arthrodesis using a laterally placed bone plate. (Adapted with permission from Brinker, N. O., Piermattei, D. L., and Flo, G. L.: *Handbook of Small Animal Orthopedics and Fracture Treatment.* W. B. Saunders, Philadelphia, 1983.)

into the distal aspect of the fourth tarsal bone. Another hole is drilled in the tuber calcis approximately 1 cm from its tip. Twenty-gauge orthopedic wire is passed through the proximal hole in a figure-of-eight pattern, and the medial and lateral strands are twisted (Fig. 195–199).

In plantar distal intertarsal or tarsometatarsal subluxation, the figure-of-eight wire must engage the bases of metatarsals II to V distally. After the tarsometatarsal joint is curetted and packed with cancellous graft, the Steinmann pin is driven down the calcaneus, through the fourth tarsal bone, and across the tarsometatarsal joint to engage the base of metatarsal IV (see Fig. 159–196).

Plate Arthrodesis of the Proximal Intertarsal Joint

The incision is extended from the tuber calcis to the distal third of metatarsal V on the lateral aspect of the tarsus. Articular cartilages of the talocalcaneocentral joint as well as the calcaneoquartal joint are burred away with a Hall air drill, and the joint is packed with cancellous bone graft. A plate is chosen that will allow placement of two to three screws in the calcaneus, one or two screws in the fourth tarsal, and two to three screws in metatarsal V. The lateral aspect of the fourth tarsal bone and the base of metatarsal V are removed with rongeurs, and the plate is contoured to the lateral aspect of the joint (Fig. 159–200). The distal screws engage metatarsal

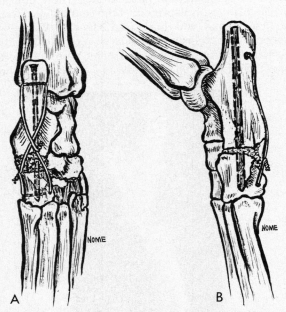

Figure 159–199. Plantar (A) and lateral (B) views of pin and figure-of-eight arthrodesis of the calcaneal quartal joint. (Adapted with permission from Brinker, N. O., Piermattei, D. L., and Flo, G. L.: *Handbook of Small Animal Orthopedics and Fracture Treatment.* W. B. Saunders, Philadelphia, 1983.)

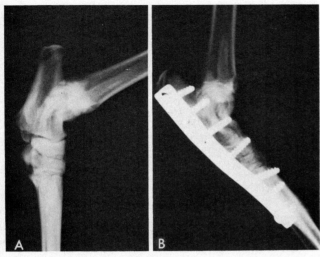

Figure 159–201. A, Lateral radiograph of a plantar proximal intertarsal subluxation in a 30-kg collie with associated chronic lameness. The case was treated with a proximal intertarsal arthrodesis with the bone plate positioned on the caudolateral aspect of the tarsus. The three distal screws are seated in metatarsal IV. B, Union is present eight weeks postoperatively.

IV and V, and the screws driven across the fourth tarsal should also engage the central tarsal.

If the technique is used for a tarsometatarsal or distal intertarsal subluxation, these joints are debrided of cartilage and filled with cancellous bone prior to plate fixation.

I have successfully used a modification of this technique in which the plate is applied to the caudolateral aspect of the tarsus, closely approximating the true tensile stresses on the joint. After joint curettage of the calcaneoquartal and talocalcaneoquartal joints, the plate is contoured to the plantar aspect of the calcaneus and fourth tarsal bone and is positioned beneath the superficial and deep flexor tendons. The distal screws engage metatarsal IV (Fig. 159–201).

Luxations of the Phalanges

See "Carpus and Digits" (Chapter 157).

Tendinous Injuries of the Tarsus

For injuries of the calcanean tendon, see Chapter 166.

For injuries of the flexor tendons, see "Carpus and Digits" (Chapter 157).

Displacement of the Superficial Digital Flexor Tendon

As the superficial digital flexor tendon glides over the calcaneal groove, it broadens like a cap and is supported by medial and lateral attachments to the tuber calcis.[14] Tears in either of these collateral insertions allow the tendon to luxate from the calcaneal groove toward the opposite side. Reportedly, laxity of the medial collateral support and lateral displacement of the superficial digital flexor tendon are seen most frequently.[25] Collies and Shetland sheepdogs are commonly affected, although age and sex predilections are not established. The condition has been surgically corrected in one limb only to recur in the opposite leg, indicating possible breed predisposition.

Although the exact mechanism of injury is unknown, owners have reported a popping sound at the time of insult.[12] Acute non–weight-bearing lameness may be present initially but usually diminishes with time. Persistent lameness is present in some dogs, whereas others walk normally and periodically carry the limb after the tendon luxates. Distension of the calcanean bursa is a consistent finding. Diagnosis is made by careful palpation. With the talocrural joint extended, the tendon can usually be reduced to its normal position in the calcaneal groove (Fig. 159–202A). As the joint is flexed, the tendon often displaces and remains in the luxated state (Fig. 159–202B). In the chronic injury, the tendon may remain permanently displaced.

Definitive repair of displaced superficial digital flexor tendons involves resuturing of the torn collateral fascia with nonabsorbable suture material.[9] External support alone is not recommended because of the difficulty in retaining reduction of the tendon. A curvilinear incision is made over the caudomedial aspect of the calcaneus for a lateral displacement. A caudolateral incision is made for a medial displacement. The incision is extended along the length of the calcaneus, and the superficial digital flexor tendon is separated from the other calcanean tendons (Fig.

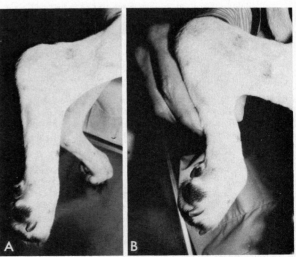

Figure 159–202. Lateral displacement of the superficial digital flexor tendon. A, When the talocrural joint is extended the tendon remains in the calcaneal groove. B, When the hock is flexed the tendon is displaced laterally. (Courtesy of Dr. Guy B. Tarvin.)

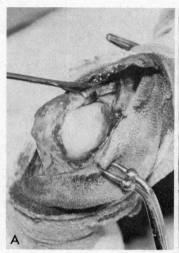
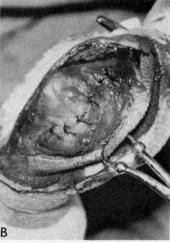

Figure 159–203. *A,* A medially displaced superficial digital flexor tendon. *B,* The peritendinous tissue has been sutured to lateral calcaneal fascia with single interrupted sutures of monofilament nylon.

159–203*A*). The tendon is positioned in the calcaneal groove, and redundant fibrous tissue opposite the displacement is excised. Collateral stability is established by suturing paratendinous tissue to fascia with simple interrupted suture of nylon, polypropylene, or wire (Fig. 159–203*B*). If the tendon is permanently displaced, a fascial release incision is required on the side of the displacement for reduction. After repair, the talocrural joint is flexed and extended to ensure that the tendon remains reduced. The stabilization is supported for two weeks in a splint, followed by restricted exercise for a month.

1. Aron, D. N.: A "new" tendon stitch. J. Am. Anim. Hosp. Assoc. *19*:587, 1981.
2. Aron, D. N., and Purington, T.: Collateral ligaments of the talocrural joint—an anatomic study. Presented at the 9th Winter Conference Veterinary Orthopedic Society, Park City, Utah, March, 1982.
3. Aron, D. N., Purington, T., and Rowland, G.: Prosthetic collateral ligament replacement of the talocrural joint—a proposed technique in the dog. Presented at the 9th Winter Conference, Veterinary Orthopedic Society, Park City, Utah, March, 1982.
4. Bateman, J. K.: Brahem hock in the greyhound: repair methods and the plastic scaphoid. Vet. Rec. *70*:621, 1958.
5. Bateman, J. K.: The racing greyhound. Vet. Rec. *72*:893, 1960.
6. Bjorling, D. E., and Toombs, J. P.: Transarticular application of the Kirschner Ehmer splint. Vet. Surg. *11*:34, 1982.
7. Campbell, J. R., Bennett, D., and Leer, R.: Intertarsal and tarsometatarsal subluxation in the dog. J. Small Anim. Pract. *17*:427, 1976.
8. Dee, J. F.: Fractures in the racing greyhound. *In* Bojrab, M. J. (ed.): *Pathophysiology in Small Animal Surgery.* Lea & Febiger, Philadelphia, 1981.
9. Dee, J. F.: Non-compound traumatic hock injuries. Proc. Am. Anim. Hosp. Assoc. Boston, Massachusetts, 1977.
10. Dee, J. F., Dee, J., and Piermattei, D.: Classification, management and repair of central tarsal fractures in the racing greyhound. J. Am. Anim. Hosp. Assoc. *12*:398, 1976.
11. Early, T. D.: Displacement of the superficial digital flexor tendon. Presented at the 9th Annual Conference of the Veterinary Orthopedic Society, Park City, Utah, March, 1982.
12. Early, T. D.: Personal communication, 1983.
13. Early, T. D.: Tibiotarsal arthrodesis. Abstract from the 5th Annual Meeting, Veterinary Orthopedic Society, Vail, Colorado, Feb., 1979.
14. Early, T. D., and Dee, J. F.: Trauma to the carpus, tarsus, and phalanges of dogs and cats. Vet. Clin. North Am.: Small Anim. Pract. *10*:717, 1980.
15. Ellison, G. W., and Tarvin, G. B.: Use of the Kirschner-Ehmer apparatus for selected juxtaarticular injuries in the dog and cat. Presented at the 9th Winter Conference, Veterinary Orthopedic Society, Park City, Utah, March, 1982.
16. Evans, H. E., and Christensen, G. C. (eds.): *Miller's Anatomy of the Dog.* 2nd ed. W. B. Saunders, Philadelphia, 1979.
17. Hickman, J.: Greyhound injuries. J. Sm. Anim. Pract. *16*:455, 1975.
18. Holt, P. E.: Collateral ligament prosthesis in the canine tarsus. Can. Pract. *6*:53, 1979.
19. Holt, P. E.: Ligamentous injuries to the canine hock. J. Small Anim. Pract. *15*:457, 1974.
20. Holt, P. E.: Treatment of tibio-tarsal instability in small animals. J. Small Anim. Pract. *18*:415, 1977.
21. Lawson, D. D.: Intertarsal subluxation in the dog. J. Small Anim. Pract. *1*:179, 1960.
22. Parker, R. B., and Schubert, T. A.: Repair of ligamentous joint injuries in three dogs using spiked washers. J. Am. Anim. Hosp. Assoc. *17*:45, 1981.
23. Pettit, G. D.: *Tarsal, Metatarsal and Phalangeal Joints in Canine Surgery.* American Veterinary Publications, Santa Barbara, 1974.
24. Piermattei, D. L.: Personal communication.
25. Reinke, J. D., and Kus, S. P.: Achilles mechanism injury in the dog. Comp. Cont. Ed. *4*:639, 1982.
26. Stoll, G., Sinibaldi, K. R., De Angelis, M. P., and Rosen, H.: A technique for tibiotarsal arthrodesis utilizing cancellous bone screws in small animals. J. Am. Anim. Hosp. Assoc. *11*:185, 1975.
27. Tomlinson, J., and Moore, R.: Locking loop tendon suture use in repair of five calcanean tendons. Vet. Surg. *3*:105, 1982.
28. Wadsworth, P. L.: Biomechanics of fractures, *In* Bojrab, M. J. (ed.): *Pathophysiology in Small Animal Surgery.* Lea & Febiger, Philadelphia, 1981.

Arthrodesis

Arnold S. Lesser

Arthrodesis is the removal of motion from a joint through the fusion of the opposing surfaces into a solid bony unit. It is usually performed as a salvage procedure to restore use to a painful or unstable joint that is not responsive to more conservative treatment. Arthrodesis is indicated when continued motion of the joint is counterproductive mechanically or physiologically and a less drastic, more anatomical repair is not possible.

There are alternatives to arthrodesis. Total joint replacement with a prosthesis is commonly used in human medicine but is still relatively new to veterinary clinical practice. Ablation such as a femoral head and neck excision arthroplasty can be used for the coxofemoral joint but rarely in other joints of the body. A third alternative is homogenous osteochondral joint replacement, in which both the bone and cartilaginous structures are transplanted to replace a diseased joint. This procedure is still in the experimental stages but, if perfected, holds some exciting prospects for joint surgery.

GENERAL INDICATIONS

Fusion of a joint is usually performed to relieve a painful condition due to instability or inflammatory disease. Instability induces pain because of the abnormal motion and stresses placed on the soft tissues and nerves surrounding the joint. This is relieved by rigid support provided by arthrodesis. Inflammation of a joint is termed arthritis. As a clinical entity arthritis is not a simple disease but one with various manifestations, subtypes, and causes. It is also the most common indication for arthrodesis. Arthritic pain is caused by abnormal wear on both hard and soft tissues, combined with the release of inflammatory products, proteolytic enzymes, prostaglandins, and other agents. Much of this pain is centered in the joint capsule and adjacent soft tissues. By obliterating the joint, arthrodesis arrests this process.

The most common indications for arthrodesis in veterinary medicine can be divided into three categories: traumatic, developmental, and congenital. Traumatic injuries to joints consist of both fractures and ligamentous disruptions with or without dislocation. They include fractures involving a joint surface in which a primary repair leads to chronic instability, degenerative joint disease, and pain. Examples include (1) shearing injuries and fracture dislocations of the hock or carpus with major bone and ligament loss and (2) severely comminuted condylar fractures of the distal humerus and femur, especially in miniature breeds. In either case it may be impossible to recreate a functional joint with a primary fracture repair. Postfracture osteomyelitis and malunions also fit into this category.

The major developmental diseases can be included under the heading "arthritis" and are further subdivided into primary or secondary degenerative joint disease, septic arthritis, and immune-mediated arthritis (rheumatoid or polyarthritis).

Congenital elbow luxations and stifle deformities that are not amenable to primary reconstruction are examples of congenital indications.

A fourth category is the use of arthrodesis to improve the mechanics of a limb rather than to relieve pain and instability—for example, arthrodesis of the carpus for radial nerve paralysis or the talocrural joint in conjunction with a muscle transfer for ischiatic paralysis.

GENERAL PROCEDURE

The actual surgical procedure, regardless of the joint, involves certain principles. Stability is of prime importance, even more so in arthrodesis than in fracture fixation, because the mechanical structures of a limb are designed to provide and maintain motion at this location. Therefore, the body is working against maintaining immobility at the fixation point. Factors to be overcome are the longer lever arm provided by both long bones adjacent to the joint and the anatomical arrangement of the muscles and tendons spanning the joint. For these reasons it is mechanically more difficult to provide a stable fixation. Therefore, the type of fixation and the surgical technique become more critical, and the use of compression, which provides more rigid fixation, is desirable. Plates, screws, cross-pins, tension band wire, and external pin splints used alone or in combination, plus external coaptation, are the common devices used to accomplish rigid fixation.

The articular cartilage should be removed down to bleeding subchondral bone to enhance bone contact and facilitate early union. Rasps, curettes, osteotomes, or an air drill or oscillating saw can be used for this purpose. If an angular or rotational deformity exists, it can be corrected at this time by removing a suitable amount of bone. It is also possible to contour the opposing surfaces to provide maximum bone-to-bone contact and enhance stability.

For added insurance, autogenous cancellous bone grafts should be used to shorten healing time and also to fill in small defects in the opposing surfaces.[3] Where added bone is required, cortical onlay or inlay grafts from the rib or ilium can also be used. Grafts provide osteoinduction, some viable osteoblasts, and a scaffold for ingrowth of new blood vessels via creeping substitution.

Normal angles for different joints have been reported, but the simplest method of determining the correct angle is to measure the opposite normal limb during weight-bearing. This angle may have to be adjusted if there will be shortening at the end of the procedure.[6] The more obtuse the angle (the straighter the limb), the longer the limb; conversely, the more acute the angle (more bend), the shorter the limb will be. Therefore, the surgeon can adjust the final length of the limb by varying the angle of the fused joint. If it is necessary to remove bone to fuse a joint like the stifle, the final angle should be more obtuse to make up for any shortening. The angle can be measured during surgery with a sterile goniometer, preplaced pins, or a prebent template.

GENERAL COMPLICATIONS

When a point of motion is obliterated via arthrodesis, increased stress is transferred to adjacent bones and joints. This is especially true in the carpus and vertebrae. The fusion of the antebrachiocarpal joint without fusion of the adjacent intercarpal joints results in degenerative joint disease of the latter. When performing arthrodesis on a midlimb joint, these stresses are transferred to the long bones themselves, increasing the risk of fracture, especially in large active dogs. The ends of plates and screw holes act as stress risers, further increasing the risk of fracture. Therefore, plates should be removed after fusion is complete and the limbs protected, or the patient's exercise should be restricted until the screw holes have filled in.

Other possible causes for failure are infection, insufficient fixation, or insufficient removal of carti-

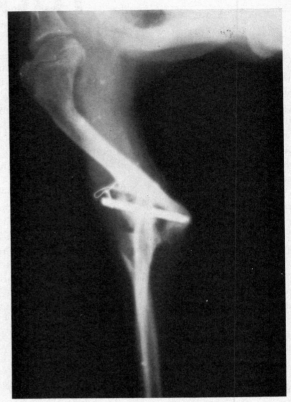

Figure 160–2. A comminuted lateral condylar fracture in a 2-kg Yorkshire terrier that collapsed after surgical repair. The resulting malunion with valgus deformity and subluxation warrants an arthrodesis.

lage. Any technical error such as poor plate placement or too small or too short a plate can also lead to a failed fusion.

ELBOW

Indications

The most common indication for arthrodesis of the elbow is degenerative joint disease, which in this joint usually occurs secondary to trauma, fractures and luxations, or developmental diseases such as ununited anconeal process, ununited coronoid process, osteochondritis dissecans, or premature closure of the distal radius or ulnar growth plates (Fig. 160–1).

Condylar fractures, especially comminuted Y or T fractures, can be difficult to treat and can lead to degenerative joint disease if the postoperative alignment or final healing is not perfect. This is particularly true in miniature breeds, in which there is very little bone stock to hold the implants (Fig. 160–2).

The elbow is also prone to loss of motion after any fracture through or adjacent to the joint, probably because of the three-bone configuration. When a joint loses motion, normal nutrition to the cartilage is adversely affected and degeneration can ensue, requiring fusion later on (Fig. 160–3).

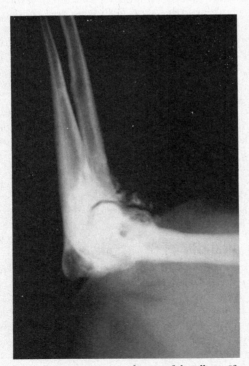

Figure 160–1. Degenerative joint disease of the elbow. If pain and disuse are unresponsive to medication, then an arthrodesis may be warranted.

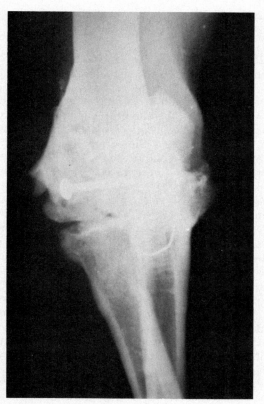

Figure 160–3. An old distal humeral fracture that has ankylosed. If the animal is in pain, an arthrodesis is indicated.

Congenital and traumatic fracture-luxations (Fig. 160–4) that cannot be stabilized while preserving motion are indications for arthrodesis, as are such general diseases as rheumatoid or septic arthritis.

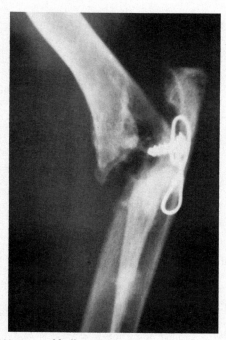

Figure 160–4. An old elbow fracture-luxation in which a primary repair to reestablish the elbow joint failed. There is now so much bone atrophy that only a fusion will produce a stable foreleg.

Procedure

Because of its configuration, the elbow is a difficult joint to fuse. In moderate and large breeds of dogs, affixing a plate along the caudal aspect of the humerus and ulna is the best method (Fig. 160–5). Fortunately, the caudal aspect of the elbow is the tension band side. However, the olecranon must be osteotomized to allow the plate to achieve good contact with both the humerus and the ulna. The angle at which the olecranon is osteotomized can be determined by continuing a line parallel to the caudal aspect of the humerus across the olecranon, with the joint held at the proposed angle (Fig. 160–6). This ensures better contact for the plate as it crosses the joint. The olecranon can be reattached to the ulna or humerus with a screw and tension band wire. An alternative method is to use the olecranon as graft material and suture the triceps tendon to tissue in the same area. Besides the olecranon osteotomy, it may be necessary to incise the lateral collateral ligaments and elevate the origins of the extensor muscles from the lateral humeral condyle to provide exposure for removal of the cartilage from the distal humerus, radial head, and coronoid process. These structures should be contoured to provide good areas of contact. The ulna nerve runs on the medial aspect of the elbow in this area and should be identified and protected.

The angle of the arthrodesis can be measured in surgery with the use of preplaced K-wires and a

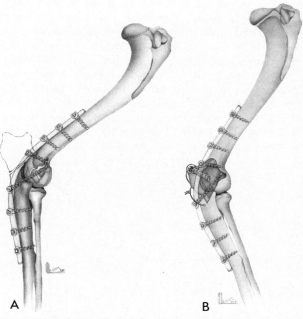

Figure 160–5. *A*, The plate is placed on the caudal aspect (tension side) of the elbow with a minimum of three screws in the humerus and three screws in the ulna. Screws crossing the arthrodesis should be placed under compression. *B*, The olecranon can be sacrificed as graft and the triceps sutured down or it can be attached to the humerus on either side of the plate with a screw and tension band wire.

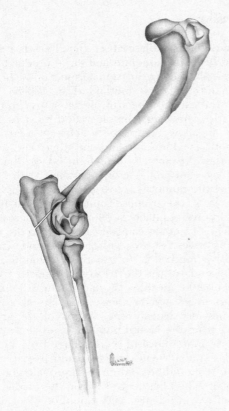

Figure 160–6. The olecranon is osteotomized at an angle parallel to the caudal aspect of the humerus to facilitate plate placement.

goniometer. The pins are placed at premeasured angles to the humerus and ulna, so they become parallel when these bones form the proper angle (Fig. 160–7). Another method is to x-ray one leg at the desired angle and prebend an old plate or plate template to the proper angle by comparing it with the x-ray. When the plate is placed on the bones, the joint will be at the measured angle. If the actual plate to be used is prebent, the holes may not line up optimally. The bones can then be maintained in this position with a pin through the ulna into the humerus. The angle of the fusion can be predetermined by measuring the opposite leg. The average

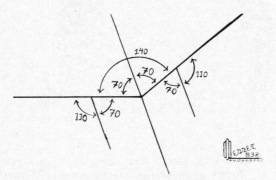

Figure 160–7. The surgeon can calculate the angle of arthrodesis at operation by placing pins at set angles in the humerus and ulna. If the angle of arthrodesis is 140°, placing the pins at 70° (one-half of 140°) to these bones with the angle facing the elbow will make the pins parallel when the elbow is at 140°.

angle of the elbow is approximately 130 to 150°. This angle may be increased to increase leg length or vice versa.

The triceps muscles can be elevated to allow placement of the plate on the caudal aspect of the humerus. The plate also sits nicely on the caudal aspect of the ulna. A minimum of three screws (six cortices) should be used in the humerus and ulna respectively, and one or more cancellous or compression screws can be placed across the fusion site for additional interfragmentary compression. A self-compressing plate with nine or ten holes is adequate for a 30- to 35-kg dog.

In cats or small dogs, other methods of fixation combining pins, screws, and wire can be used.[6] A screw can be placed under compression from the olecranon across the joint and up the humeral shaft (Fig. 160–8). In addition, a figure-of-eight wire should be placed from the olecranon to the humerus to oppose flexion of the elbow with weight-bearing. A triceps tenotomy is used for exposure. Cross-pins can be substituted for the screw, but then there are no compressive forces across the joint and any motion at the fusion site encourages migration of the pins. With these techniques, a full cast is necessary for added protection, and it should be left on until there is evidence of bone union. There is no reason why a small plate cannot be used in these cases, since it provides superior fixation. If the plate fixation is

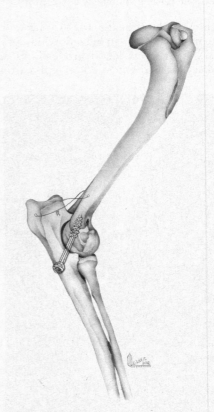

Figure 160–8. In small or toy breeds, a compression screw can be used to fuse the elbow with the assistance of a figure-of-eight wire. When possible, a plate should be used owing to the superior stability produced.

proper, only a padded bandage is necessary for a few weeks.

External pin splints such as a Kirschner-Ehmer apparatus can be used either as a secondary support for one of the above or as the primary fixation device. If used alone, a full splint should be applied using multiple external bars with the pins protruding through both sides of the limb. The protruding transosseous pins are connected, and one or two bars should be used to oppose flexion of the joint by connecting the proximal and distal pins. This method is not as adaptable in the elbow as in the tarsocrural joint because of the thicker muscles and the interference of the chest wall with the medial pins and bar.

Whenever there is any question of sufficient stability, an external cast or splint should be added, since there is no concern for loss of joint motion as there is for loss of fixation. The length of time casts and splints should remain in place depends on the quality of the internal fixation and the size and activity of the patient and should be decided on a case-by-case basis. If there is any question, the safest policy is to leave the external support on until there is radiographic evidence of healing. Six weeks is the average time.

Complications

Insufficient stability or infection is the most common cause of failure, especially if a plate is not used. If a plate is used on a large, active dog, fracture of the radius and ulna or humerus may occur at the end of the plate where a stress riser occurs because of the difference in the elasticity between the plate and bone. It is recommended that the plate be removed once fusion is complete.

CARPUS

Indications

The most frequent indications for arthrodesis of the carpus are fracture-luxations, especially old injuries (Fig. 160–9). Many of these luxations are no longer reducible, or if so are very unstable because of accompanying ligament damage. Casting alone is often insufficient—especially in larger breeds with hyperextension injuries, which may be incurred from falls or leaping from heights or moving vehicles. Other surgical reconstructive procedures have been reported, but arthrodesis is a viable alternative. The antebrachiocarpal joint may be spared or included in the arthrodesis, depending on the extent of the trauma. If the luxation or fracture is at the middle carpal or carpometacarpal joints only and the ligamentous structures of the accessory carpal bone are intact, it is possible to fuse these joints only, sparing the antebrachiocarpal joint.[2,7] However, if the antebrachiocarpal joint is fused, the other joints of the carpus must be included or secondary degenerative joint disease will develop in the latter, causing pain.

As in any joint, severe degenerative joint disease or other arthritic condition unresponsive to medication is an indication for fusion. Rheumatoid arthritis is especially prevalent in the carpal joint, and in advanced cases these joints become very unstable as a result of ligament damage (Fig. 160–10).

Affected dogs have similar clinical signs to hyperextension injuries but without any history of trauma. They are more frequent in the smaller breeds.

Another indication for carpal fusion is peripheral nerve damage. If the patient can support weight on the leg but lands on the dorsal surface of the paw, arthrodesis can improve this condition. However,

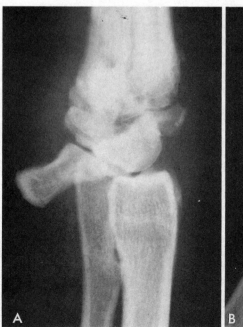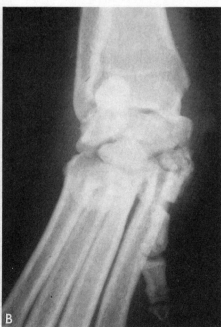

Figure 160–9. *A* and *B*, Multiple fractures of the carpal bones. If the ligamentous structures of the accessory carpal bone are also ruptured, a pancarpal arthrodesis is indicated. These animals are presented with hyperextension of the carpus.

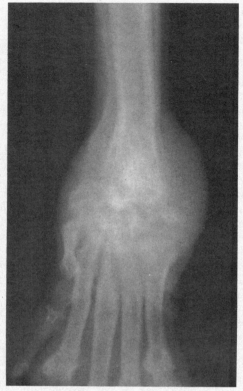

Figure 160–10. Rheumatoid arthritis in a miniature breed dog. There is often multiple joint involvement, and the disease is progressive so a successful arthrodesis may only be palliative.

most of these animals suffer from brachial plexus injuries and too many muscles are affected for arthrodesis to be helpful. In simple radial paralysis, other treatments are available but fusion can be considered.

Another situation requiring carpal fusion is nonunion of fractures of the radius and ulna in miniature breeds. Severe bone atrophy precludes simple handling of these cases. Fusion of the carpus provides adequate bone distal to the fracture to anchor plates or external pin splints in conjunction with cortical grafts. The other general indications mentioned earlier also apply to the carpal joint.

Procedure

In a pancarpal arthrodesis, all three joints—the antebrachiocarpal (radiocarpal), the middle carpal, and the carpometacarpal—are included. The common forms of fixation are external pin splints, cross-pins, and plates. The cartilage of all involved joints, including the middle carpal, must be removed. It is necessary to incise the carpal fascia, each individual capsule, and some of the short intercarpal ligaments to accomplish this. It is then also possible to pack all of these joints with cancellous bone graft. If crosspins are used, they should enter from the proximal third of the second or fifth metacarpal bone, cross the three joints, and exit from the radius or ulna, respectively. The pins should emerge proximal to the

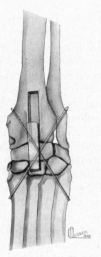

Figure 160–11. The use of crossed pins combined with an inlay graft formed from a slot in the distal radius and advanced into a bed cut into the carpal bones.

flare of the distal radius medially and exit from the ulna at the same level laterally (Fig. 160–11). Starting the pins proximally ensures a proper bite in these bones. The bone of the carpus is very hard, and power equipment is helpful in placing these pins. However, the dense bone may cause excessive heat production during pin insertion under power. This can lead to heat necrosis and early loosening of the pins. A superior procedure is the use of a plate. Most reports recommend placement of the plate on the cranial (dorsal) aspect of the radius and carpus. This placement allows the simplest approach but places the plate on the compression side rather than the tension side, where it belongs. An alternate approach for the placement of the plate on the palmar aspect has been reported (Fig. 160–12).[1]

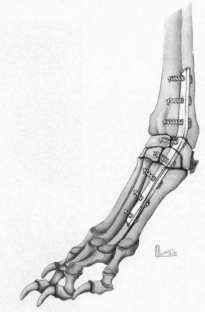

Figure 160–12. A plate placed on the caudal surface of the radius and palmar surface of the metacarpals places the plate on the tension side of the joint but requires a more difficult approach.

In this procedure, an Esmarch's bandage or tourniquet is recommended to control hemorrhage. A skin incision is made on the palmar aspect of the limb and joint, exposing the distal third of the radius and extending distocaudally midway between the base of the first digit and the carpal pad. The incision is continued distocranially along the medial side of the metacarpus. The cephalic vein is separated and retracted medially, and the dissection is continued down to the deep antebrachial and carpal fascia. The periosteum and deep fascia over the medial aspect of the radius are incised along with the transverse palmar carpal ligament. The tendons of the deep flexor to the first digit and the flexor carpi radialis are transected, and the incision is continued through the periosteum of the second metacarpal bone. The flexor tendon, and vascular and neural bundles are freed from the underlying bone subperiosteally and retracted laterally. This exposes the radius, carpal bones, and proximal two-thirds of the metacarpal bones. The cartilage is removed from the joint surfaces, and the plate is placed on the palmar aspect of the radius, carpal bones, and third metacarpal bones. Placing the joint in five degrees of extension is recommended. Any bony prominences interfering with placement of the plate should be removed with a rongeur or burr. Three screws should be placed in the radius, three in the third metacarpal bone, and one each in the radial and third carpal bones if possible.[1]

This procedure has the advantage of placing the plate on the tension side of the bones but does require a more difficult and time-consuming approach. The minimum surgical exposure time reported was 30 minutes.[1]

When the dorsal approach is used (Fig. 160–13),

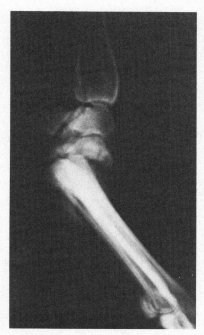

Figure 160–14. In this example the antebrachiocarpal joint and the ligaments of the accessory carpal bone are uninjured. Fusion of the carpometacarpal joints alone is sufficient.

the skin incision should expose the same area of the bones, but the only deeper structures encountered are the cephalic and accessory cephalic veins and the extensor tendons. The extensor carpi radialis can be transected, exposing the intercarpal and carpometacarpal joints for curettage. The tendon of the abductor pollicis longus can be transected or retracted. The following screws should be placed: three in the radius (six cortices), one in the radial carpal bone to pull this section up to the plate, and three more in the third or fourth metacarpal bone.[3] The plate can be bent to provide two to five degrees of extension or can be left straight. Both methods have been reported, and since there is still motion at the metacarpophalangeal joint, the foot can be flexed dorsally for proper placement.

A self-compressing dynamic compression plate has the advantage of providing compression between screw holes and therefore between the multiple joint surfaces. Plates also provide rigid support and are well tolerated for the prolonged healing periods required for fusions. Cross-pins and external pin splints require more postsurgical care. Therefore, as in the elbow, plates are the first choice in carpal arthrodesis. External pin splints are effective when there is extensive soft tissue damage.

If the antebrachiocarpal joint and its ligaments are not injured and the accessory carpal bone and its attached ligaments are intact, a partial arthrodesis can be performed. Injuries to the middle carpal or carpometacarpal joints and disruption of the palmar carpal fibrocartilage are common indications for this procedure (Fig. 160–14). A simplified procedure using cancellous bone graft and a cast alone with no internal fixation has been reported.[2] A T-plate ex-

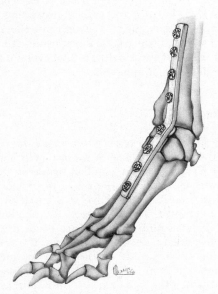

Figure 160–13. The preferred method of pancarpal arthrodesis is a plate with at least three to four screws in the radius, one in the radiocarpal bone, and three more in the third or fourth metacarpal bone. The carpus is placed in 0 to 5° of extension.

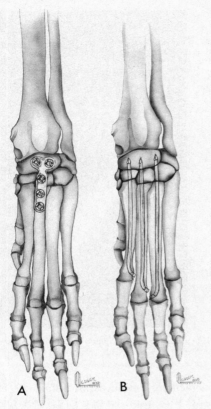

A   B

Figure 160–15. Partial carpal injuries can be treated by fusing the involved joints excluding the antebrachiocarpal joint. *A,* The use of a T-plate. *B,* Intramedullary pins placed through slots in the distal metacarpals and driven up into the radial and ulnar carpal bones. Three or four pins can be used, depending on the size of the patient.

tending from the proximal metacarpal II or III to the radial and ulnar carpal bones can be used, with the cross of the T being proximal. Two other procedures are acceptable: (1) cross-pins emerging from the carpal bones rather than the radius and (2) two or three pins driven up the second, third, and fourth metacarpal bones via the metacarpophalangeal joint and across the metacarpocarpal joint into the carpal bones (Fig. 160–15).

Cancellous bone is good insurance with any arthrodesis, but onlay or inlay grafts are especially suitable at the carpus. A rectangular section of ilium, rib, or distal radius can be placed in a slot formed across the antebrachiocarpal or intercarpal joints. Cortical grafts are especially suited to fusion of the carpus in atrophic nonunion of the radius and ulna in toy breeds. Sections of rib or ilium can be used to span the atrophied bone and carpal joint. The fixation is provided by two or three K-wires above and below the fracture, protruding from both sides of the leg and connected with bars or methyl methacrylate. The carpus is fused in these cases because there is not enough bone stock remaining on either side of the fracture in the radius and ulna.

Complications

Fusion of the antebrachiocarpal joint without fusion of the intercarpal or carpometacarpal joints leads to degenerative joint disease of the latter due to increased stress imposed on these structures. Failure of arthrodesis is commonly due to infection, incomplete cartilage removal, or technical error in size or placement of the implants. Plates in this area should be removed to prevent osteolysis of the carpal bones from stress protection. Also, cranially placed plates have very little soft tissue cover and may cause discomfort from temperature changes or proximity to the overlying skin.

STIFLE

Indications

Degenerative disease of the stifle is usually secondary to ligament injuries, the two most common of which are old, chronic anterior cruciate ruptures and severe, traumatic derangements (Fig. 160–16). In the latter, numerous structures are torn, and primary reconstructive procedures may be unsuccessful or excessive cartilage damage may require arthrodesis. With chronic cruciate tears, the degree of secondary degenerative joint disease determines whether primary repair or arthrodesis should be attempted. Compound fractures involving the stifle and accompanied by cartilage damage or bone and cartilage loss are another indication, along with other degenerative diseases (Fig. 160–17). Another indication unique to the stifle is "fracture disease" (Fig. 160–18). Although this disease can affect any joint, it is seen most commonly in the stifle and usually in young dogs treated for femoral fractures. The quadriceps is tied down to the callus, restricting motion of the stifle and leading to atrophy of the muscles and bones and fibroplasia of the capsule. All motion is eventually lost, and if the joint becomes painful, arthrodesis is recommended.

Procedure

In the stifle, it is necessary to remove the cruciates and both menisci along with the articular cartilage.[6] Excision of the straight patellar ligament from the tibial crest, along with removal of the fat pad, provides easy access to the above structures. If a plate is placed along the cranial aspect, the patella can be excised. If cross-pins or screws are used, the patella can be retained. Besides removing the cartilage, contouring of the ends of the tibia and femur is recommended to provide good bone contact. The angles at which the ends are cut are important, since they determine the final angle of fusion. Both angles are determined with a sterile goniometer or wires before the cuts are made. An oscillating saw works

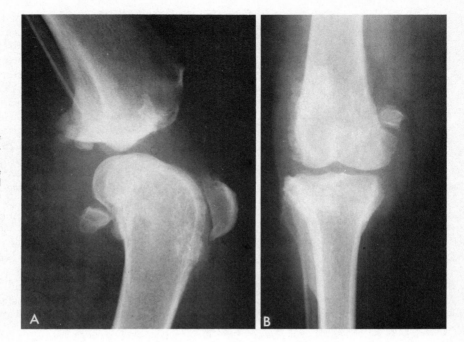

Figure 160–16. A and B, Degenerative joint disease of the stifle is often secondary to unrepaired ligamentous injuries, especially longstanding cranial cruciate tears. If there is significant pain and disuse unresponsive to medication, an arthrodesis is indicated.

better than curettes or a burr for this purpose. After the cuts are complete, a Steinmann pin is placed from the medial aspect of the tibia across the joint proximally and out the lateral femoral condyle. This pin holds the joint at the proper angle. If cross-pins or cross-screws are to be the method of fixation (small dogs or cats), then either a second pin is run from the medial femoral condyle to the lateral tibial cortex or a hole is drilled in the same manner and a screw

is placed from the tibia to the femur (distal to proximal). The flare of the tibial plateau laterally does not provide good holding for the threads. Either cancellous screws or overdrilling the first hole provides compression across the fusion. The first pin is then replaced by another compression screw (Figs. 160–19 and 160–20). If the pins are not replaced with

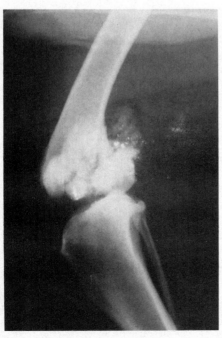

Figure 160–17. A gunshot wound causing severe comminution of the distal femur not amenable to a primary repair is a candidate for arthrodesis.

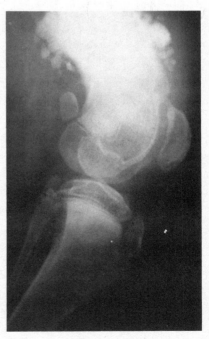

Figure 160–18. An untreated femoral fracture in a young dog leading to immobility of the stifle, atrophy of bone, and fibroplasia of the joint capsule. This limb was fixed in full extension and the dog could not place the leg properly. Arthrodesis at a normal angle plus fracture fixation would return this limb to function. Attempts at returning motion to these joints is often unrewarding.

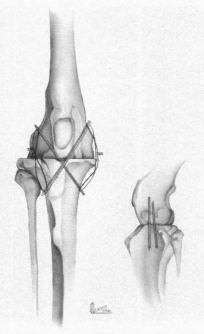

The use of a plate on the cranial aspect of the femur and tibia is the best method for larger dogs and smaller patients as well (Fig. 160–21). The patella is removed or transplanted to one side or the other. The quadriceps are elevated subperiosteally to allow placement of the plate on the cranial cortex of the femur, and the plate is contoured over the cranial aspect of the tibia. The tibial crest and tibial tuberosity are removed to provide a flat bed for better plate contact. At least three to four screws should be placed in the diaphysis of the femur and tibia respectively. Any screws between these should compress the opposing surfaces. A guide pin is used to hold the joint at the proper angle while the plate is attached. The joint is prepared in the manner discussed previously, and the bone from the excised tibial and humeral condyles can be ground up for graft and placed between the bone ends prior to compressing them.

The angle should be calculated from the opposite leg, the average angle being 125 to 150°. Since a significant amount of bone is removed, it is usually

Figure 160–19. If cross-pins are used to fuse the stifle an 18- or 20-gauge wire should be added around the pins to produce compression across the arthrodesis for added stability.

screws, it may be necessary to add figure-of-eight wire (18- or 20-gauge) over the ends of the pins medially and laterally to create added stability and compression. Casts, splints, or external pin splints should be used in addition to these methods for extra support until healing is evident.

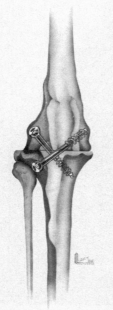

Figure 160–20. The stifle can be fused with two compression screws. It is important to start the screw that runs from the lateral aspect of the tibia to the medial condyle of the femur from distal to proximal. If the screw is run the opposite way, there is insufficient bone on the lateral aspect of the proximal tibia for the threads to engage.

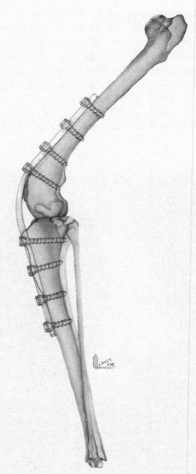

Figure 160–21. The favored method of arthrodesis of the stifle is a plate on the cranial aspect of the joint. The tibial crest and possibly part of the trochlea can be removed to improve the seating of the plate. The excised section of the tibial crest is shown overlapping the plate.

necessary to fuse the leg in a straighter angle to regain length.

External pin splints are adaptable to this joint, either alone or in combination with internal pins or screws. If used alone, more than two pins should be used above and below the joint, along with multiple bars, as shown previously. In humans, in whom the joint is fused at 180°, these splints are the most commonly used method of fixation. In dogs and cats, the standing angle of the stifle ranges from 125 to 150°. Therefore, compression can be applied across the joint, but extra bars must be placed to buttress against flexion. The problem with external pin splints in such instances is the inability to place a bar on the medial aspect of the femur for added strength.

Complications

Fusion of the stifle creates a very long lever arm and therefore excessive forces at the arthrodesis site. To overcome this, the plate must cover almost half of the femur and tibia. Too short a plate and poor bone contact are the most common causes of technical failure. This long lever arm creates a risk of fracture at the plate ends. Therefore, the plate should be removed eventually and the limb protected for 3 to 4 weeks longer.

HOCK

Indications

The tarsal joints are subject to traumatic injury as well as degenerative disease (Fig. 160–22). One of the most common traumatic injuries encountered in

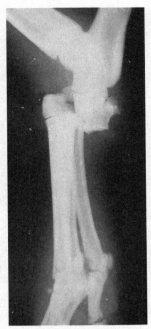

Figure 160–23. In this injury in which the talocrural joint is spared it is only necessary to fuse the joints involved.

this joint is the shearing fracture, which may occur when the leg has been dragged along the road by a car, causing significant loss of soft tissue and bone because of the grinding action of the pavement. The collateral ligaments and most of the malleolus are lost in these injuries, leaving the joint open with no soft tissue coverage or stability. The medial aspect is more frequently affected than the lateral. These wounds usually heal without active signs of infection, and often sufficient fibroplasia occurs to stabilize the joint without further surgery. However, if instability remains and simple replacement of the appropriate collateral ligament is insufficient, arthrodesis is indicated. It is usually adequate to fuse the talocrural joint alone. Severe fracture-luxations of the tarsocrural, middle tarsal, or tarsometatarsal joints also occur and can be treated with fusions of the involved joints alone (Fig. 160–23). Rupture of the plantar ligament also requires fusion of one or more of these latter joints.

Rupture of the calcaneal ligament not amenable to suture because of either severe trauma to the ligament or fragmentation of the calcaneus (Fig. 160–24) can be treated by fusion of the talocrural joint.

Rheumatoid or polyarthritis also commonly affects the hock, and, as with the carpus, arthrodesis can be used as a palliative treatment. Osteoarthritis or septic arthritis, if severe enough, can require arthrodesis. Degenerative joint disease from an osteochondritis dissecans lesion of the talus is one such situation.

A unique indication for fusion of the talocrural joint is its use in conjunction with muscle transfer for the treatment of ischiatic nerve paralysis. In this case, the fusion positions the foot properly and removes a

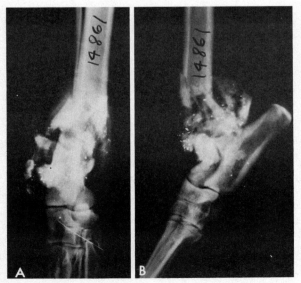

Figure 160–22. A and B, A severe intra-articular fracture of the hock, where a primary repair is not feasible. Gunshot wounds are often responsible for this type of injury, which requires arthrodesis.

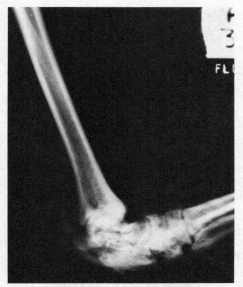

Figure 160–24. The collapse of the calcaneus due to osteomyelitis allowed avulsion of the calcaneal tendon. Since the lever arm of the fibular tarsal bone is gone, reattachment of the calcaneal tendon may not be effective. Arthrodesis of the talocrural joint would accomplish the same goal of relieving the plantograde stance of the animal.

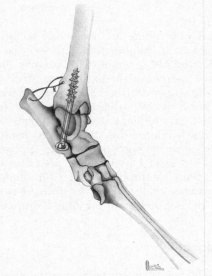

Figure 160–25. A screw can be placed from the fibular tarsal bone through the tibial tarsal bone up into the medullary canal of the tibia. Once the medullary canal becomes wider than the screw this placement is no longer viable. A figure-of-eight wire is placed for support and to prevent flexion of the hock during weight-bearing.

point of motion along the path of the transferred tendon.

Procedure

The simplest method of removing motion from the talocrural joint is driving a Steinmann's pin up through the sustentaculum tali of the fibular tarsal bone, through the tibial tarsal bone, and up the medullary cavity of the tibia. If the cartilage is not removed and the pin is removed within weeks, not months, this provides temporary support. If the pin is left *in situ* for months or years, fibroplasia of the capsule and surrounding tissues creates an ankylosed or fibrosed joint. If the cartilage is removed, true arthrodesis can occur; however, the pin does not create compression across the fusion site, and more efficient alternatives are available.

In small and medium-sized dogs and cats, a compression screw from the sustentaculum tali into the medullary cavity of the tibia provides stable fixation as long as the threads of the screw can obtain sufficient bone contact (Fig. 160–25).[8] Once the medulla is wider in diameter than the shaft of the screw, this technique will not suffice and the screw must be anchored in the cortex of the tibia. The screw can be placed in either direction, proximally from the medial malleolus of the tibia through the tibial tarsal bone and exiting from the fibular tarsal bone or vice versa (Fig. 160–26). In either case, it is recommended that the orthopedic wire (18 or 20 gauge) be passed from the calcaneus to the caudal cortex of the tibia to support the talocrural joint against flexion.[8] This helps prevent the screw from moving and should be used

whenever a screw is used alone. In addition, to facilitate screw placement, a small guide wire should be passed first to hold the joint in the proper alignment for drilling and tapping for the screw. The placement of this pin is critical so as not to interfere with the drill hole of the screw. This pin can be removed or left in place or replaced with a larger pin for additional stability.

Another technique is the use of a plate along the

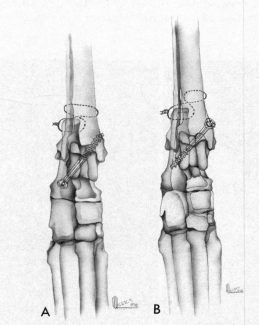

Figure 160–26 The screw can also be placed from the fibular tarsal bone to emerge from the medial malleolus (A) or the opposite, from proximal to distal (B). A wire is placed as shown in Figure 160–25.

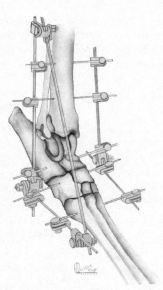

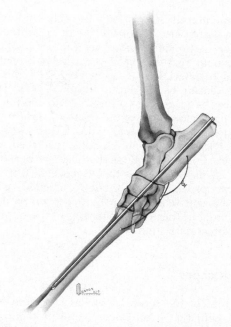

Figure 160–27. An external splint such as a Kirschner-Ehmer apparatus is well adapted for use in fusing the hock. Compression should be placed across the talocrural joint, and another bar (or bars) should be added to support against flexion.

cranial aspect of the tibia and tarsal bones. As in the carpus, this is not the tension side, so a cast or splint should be added even when the plate is used and always when a screw and wire are employed.

As mentioned earlier, external pin splints can be used as either the primary or secondary method of fixation. In the hock, it is best to place the pins through with bars both medially and laterally. A minimum of two pins should be placed in the tibia, one in the tibial tarsal bone and two more either in the middle tarsal bone and the metatarsals or both in the metatarsals.

The pins spanning the talocrural joint should be under compression, and bars should support the joint against flexion during weight-bearing (Fig. 160–27).

Figure 160–29. A partial luxation of either the fibular or tibial tarsotarsal or the tarsometatarsal joint can be treated with an intramedullary pin and tension band wire. The wire can extend from a hole drilled in the fibular tarsal bone as illustrated or alternately from around the proximal end of the pin before it crosses to enter the proximal metatarsals.

Crossed Steinmann's pins can be used in larger dogs. They are placed from the tibial tarsal and fibular tarsal bones across the joint to emerge from the lateral and medial cortex of the distal tibia, respectively. Care must be taken not to distract the joint surfaces while driving the two pins. On the contrary, it is beneficial to have an assistant place compressive forces across the joint as the pins are driven.

When removing the cartilage from the talocrural joint, it is especially important to produce two congruent surfaces. Use of a curette, burr, or miniature oscillating saw allows the surgeon to create a flat plateau on the trochlea of the tibial tarsal bone and a rectangular depression of the distal tibia. The latter is accomplished by removing the intermediate ridge of the distal tibial articular surface, along with the cartilage from the lateral aspect of the medial malleolus. These locking surfaces create a stable condition from which the fixation device can work (Fig. 160–28). Cancellous graft should be used to fill in gaps and will speed healing of the fusion.

The standing angle varies from 130 to 150 degrees for the hock of the average dog but does differ between individuals of different conformation. Therefore, measuring the opposite leg is still the safest method of determining the proper angle. The angle for cats has been reported to be 115 to 125 degrees.

When an injury involves just the intertarsal or tarsometatarsal joints (e.g., fractures or luxations), only the joints involved need be fused. One method involves placing a Steinmann's pin down the fibular tarsal bone, through the fourth tarsal bone, into the

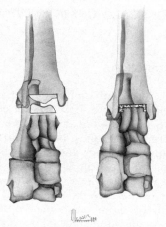

Figure 160–28. When the articular cartilage is being removed, it is advantageous to shape the opposing surfaces to produce the most stable configuration possible. In the talocrural joint two congruent rectangular surfaces can be shaped and filled with cancellous bone to create optimum bone-to-bone contact.

fourth metatarsal bone. This is reinforced with a figure-of-eight wire (18- or 20-gauge) extending from either (1) the proximal end of the pin or (2) a hole in the calcaneus or tuber calcis to a hole through the proximal metatarsal bones (Fig. 160–29). This wire acts as a tension band. With multiple disarticulations on a very large dog, an alternative technique is to place a plate along the caudal (plantar) surface of the fibular tarsal bone across to the fourth metatarsal bone. At least two screws should be placed in the metatarsal bone. A padded bandage rather than a cast or splint is often all that is necessary in these latter two procedures. Although cancellous graft is very important in fusion of the talocrural joint, it is not essential in these partial fusions of the intertarsal and tarsometatarsal joints.

Complications

Fracture of the screw or pin in talocrural fusions due to oscillation is of concern, and protection with a splint or cast along with the wire previously mentioned is recommended. Once the fusion is solid, the risk decreases, but the screw can be removed simply if desired. Insufficient removal of the cartilage in this joint and insufficient stability are the most common causes of failure.

1. Chambers, J. N., and Bjorling, D. E.: Palmar surface plating for arthrodesis of the canine carpus. J. Am. Anim. Hosp. Assoc. 18:875, 1982.
2. Gambardella, P. C., and Griffiths, R. C.: Treatment of hyperextension injuries of the canine carpus. Compend. Cont. Educ. 4:127, 1982.
3. Johnson, K. A.: Carpal arthrodesis in dogs. Aust. Vet. J. 56:515, 1980.
4. Johnson, K. A., and Bellenger, C. R.: The effects of autologous bone grafting on bone healing after carpal arthrodesis in the dog. Vet. Rec. 107:126, 1980.
5. Miller, M. E., Christensen, G. C., and Evans, H. E.: *Anatomy of the Dog.* W. B. Saunders, Philadelphia, 1964. pp. 231–261.
6. Olds, R. B.: Arthrodesis. *In* Bojrab, M. J. (ed.): *Current Techniques in Small Animal Surgery.* 1st ed. Lea and Febiger, Philadelphia, 1975. pp. 542–548.
7. Slocum, B.: Partial carpal fusion in the dog. J. Am. Vet. Med. Assoc. 180:1204, 1980.
8. Stoll, S. G., Sinibaldi, K. R., De Angelis, M. P., and Rosen, H.: A technique for tibiotarsal arthrodesis utilizing cancellous bone screws in small animals. J. Am. Anim. Hosp. Assoc. 11:185, 1975.

=== Chapter 161 ===

Amputations

Joseph P. Weigel

Of 780,407 dog and cat admissions in the American Veterinary Medical Data Program, 2,624 were admitted for amputation. Most of these were elective, e.g., claw amputation in the cat. There were 716 (0.09 per cent) admissions for major amputation of a limb. This figure may be low when compared with general practice, because the American Veterinary Medical Data Program surveys principally the clinics of veterinary colleges in the United States.

Indications for amputation include severe trauma, ischemic necrosis, and intractable orthopedic infection. Severe disability due to advanced arthritis, paralysis, or congenital deformity may result in the decision to amputate. Amputation is a primary surgical treatment for certain malignancies.

There are some philosophical considerations that a veterinary surgeon should consider when faced with amputation surgery. One should consider the adaptability of the animal to amputation and of the owner to the animal's disabled condition. The emotions and wishes of the owner must be respected, and the ultimate decision to amputate should be the owner's. The veterinarian is charged with the responsibility to adequately assess the patient's condition and to communicate that to the owner. Only then can the owner make a reasonable decision. Reported owners' responses to major amputation have been favorable.[4] Aside from the medical feasibility of amputation, the relationship between the owner and the animal must be handled with great sensitivity and concern.

GENERAL CONSIDERATIONS IN AMPUTATION SURGERY

Level of Amputation

In general, high limb amputation in small animal surgery is done, because limb prostheses are not an option. However, there are advantages and disadvantages to different techniques. In forelimb amputation, scapular removal is faster and easier than shoulder disarticulation. If the scapula is left in short-haired dogs, subsequent muscle atrophy allows the bony prominences of the scapula to be seen, creating an appearance that is cosmetically unacceptable to some owners. The single disadvantage for scapular disarticulation is the loss of protection to the chest wall that the scapula provides. In the rear limb, amputation at midthigh is more acceptable because the stump can protect the genitalia in the male and the procedure

OCTOBER							NOVEMBER							DECEMBER						
S	M	T	W	T	F	S	S	M	T	W	T	F	S	S	M	T	W	T	F	S
					1	2		1	2	3	4	5	6				1	2	3	4
3	4	5	6	7	8	9	7	8	9	10	11	12	13	5	6	7	8	9	10	11
10	11	12	13	14	15	16	14	15	16	17	18	19	20	12	13	14	15	16	17	18
17	18	19	20	21	22	23	21	22	23	24	25	26	27	19	20	21	22	23	24	25
24/31	25	26	27	28	29	30	28	29	30					26	27	28	29	30	31	

Hyperparathyroidism Secondary to Chronic Renal Failure in Cats

Hyperparathyroidism affects 84% of cats with chronic renal failure. The prevalence and severity of the hyperparathyroidism increase with the degree of renal dysfunction. Because an assay of parathyroid hormone is expensive and not widely available, several routine biochemical measurements were assessed as markers for the presence of renal secondary hyperparathyroidism. The most efficient screening test proved to be plasma phosphate concentration, which was specific but relatively insensitive.

The veterinarian should pay particular attention to calcium homeostasis in cats with compensated chronic renal failure. In these cats derangement of calcium homeostasis may be mild and possibly easier to correct. This may prevent parathyroid hyperplasia, which is impossible to reverse and has a major influence on basal nonsuppressible secretion of parathyroid hormone.

Barber PJ, Elliott J: Feline chronic renal failure: Calcium homeostasis in 80 cases diagnosed between 1992 and 1995. *J Small Anim Pract* 39:108, 1998.

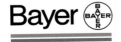

Tuesday   November 23 1999

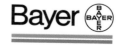

is less complicated and easier to perform than disarticulation at the hip. In either case, it is always advisable to perform the amputation where there is normal tissue and well proximal to neoplastic tissue; this principle alone may determine the level at which the limb is to be removed.

Amputation Through the Joint versus Amputation Through Bone

It is generally advisable to sever the limb through the shaft of the bone, allowing the bone to atrophy, remodel and diminish in size. If the limb is severed through the joint, the articular epiphysis remains intact without significant atrophy. The soft tissue will atrophy, leading to an inadequate coverage of the bone. The stump could be subjected to trauma, which may result in pain. When the limb is severed proximally, i.e., through the shoulder or hip joint, there is sufficient soft tissue and muscle to protect the bone. When the amputation is carried through the joint, there is generally no need to scrape the articular cartilage from the bone nor to strip out remaining synovial membrane.

Division of the Muscles

There is less hemorrhage when the muscle is severed at an insertion or lifted from the bone at an origin; however, it is not always feasible to preserve entire muscles. A surgeon should not hesitate to cut a major muscle through its belly with a scalpel. Indiscriminate division of large masses of muscle with electrosurgery may be deleterious if the proper setting is not used. Electroincision should not produce grossly visible coagulation of tissue.

Division of Vessels

Major arteries are double-ligated with nonabsorbable, inert ligature. The artery and vein should not be ligated together in order to avoid an arteriovenous fistula. The vein may be ligated with a single nonabsorbable ligature. The level of interruption in arterial supply should be planned so that the blood supply to the stump musculature is not significantly reduced. In general, the artery is ligated first to allow blood to drain from the limb through the vein before the flow is completely interrupted. This preserves vascular volume, electrolytes, and protein. With diseased limbs in which there is a possibility of disseminating the disease by surgical manipulation, it is advisable to ligate the vein first and the artery immediately afterward.

Division of the Nerves

There is little recorded clinical experience of the occurrence of neuromas after amputation in the small animal. The nerves should be placed under tension and severed as proximally as is feasible.

Closure of the Stump

Even though the basic techniques of closure are described here, the surgeon must plan the closure to meet the needs of individual patients. The lateral skin should cover the stump because it is thicker and more trauma-resistant. The hard tissues should be adequately covered with viable muscle. In closure of the deep tissues, fascia is sutured rather than muscle, and tension is kept to a minimum. Simple continuous or interrupted suture patterns may be used. Closure should be snug, not tight and restrictive to blood flow.

Seroma formation can be a sequel of amputation. Unless the operation and closure involves diseased or reactive tissue, seroma formation should not usually be a problem. Seromas are prevented by gentle technique, good hemostasis, secure closure of fascial planes, elimination of dead space, and avoidance of extensive subcutaneous dissection.

PHYSIOLOGICAL CONSIDERATIONS

Preoperative evaluation of the physiological status of the patient is important, particularly when a major amputation is planned. A complete hematology battery with a chemistry panel is advisable. When a limb is removed, a large amount of tissue with fluid, electrolytes, and red cells is lost. This loss becomes more important when the patient is in poor preoperative condition or the diseased limb has increased blood flow and inflammation. In neoplastic disease, chest radiographs to evaluate metastases are always advisable prior to amputation. Adequate hydration is required preoperatively, and intravenous fluid administration during the operation. Postoperative monitoring is essential to the recognition and treatment of impending shock. Conditions for the development of shock subsequent to a major amputation are present because of the large amount of tissue that is removed.

TECHNIQUES*

Foreleg Amputation by Shoulder Disarticulation[2]

The lateral skin incision is curved, starting in the region of the major tubercle of the humerus and extending caudodistally half of the length of the arm and then being redirected caudoproximally to end in the caudal point of the axillary space connecting the

*All anatomical references were taken from: Evans, H.E., and Christensen, G.C.: *Miller's Anatomy of the Dog*. 2nd ed. W. B. Saunders, Philadelphia, 1979.

cranial and caudal points of the lateral incision. The skin distal to the incision is dissected free of its subcutaneous attachments down to the elbow joint on both the lateral and medial sides. The cephalic vein is isolated from its fascial bed, ligated, and divided as it passes cranially under the cleidobrachialis muscle. The axillobrachial vein is a major branch of the cephalic vein that courses caudally over the lateral head of the triceps muscle and deep to the spinous portion of the deltoideus muscle. This vein is divided and ligated as it branches from the cephalic vein. The cleidobrachialis muscle is lifted from its insertion on the distal end of the humeral crest. The acromial portion of the deltoideus muscle is now lifted from its insertion on the deltoid tuberosity and reflected proximally. The brachial fascia is incised distally along the border of the lateral head of the triceps muscle down to the olecranon. To fully isolate the triceps tendon, the brachial fascia on the caudomedial surface of the leg is incised. This fascia is dissected parallel with the collateral ulnar vessels along the cranial border of the medial head of the triceps muscle. This incision is confined to the distal quarter of the arm and extends to the olecranon. The triceps tendon is fully isolated and transected just above the olecranon (Fig. 161–1).

Attention is now directed to the medial side of the leg. The superficial pectoral muscles are severed from their insertion on the crest of the major tubercle. The deep pectoral muscle is now visible and can be separated from its insertion on the minor and major tubercles of the humerus and the medial fascia of the brachium. The cutaneous trunci muscle, which runs medial to the vasculature and nerves, is severed and reflected distally to expose the main neurovascular structures. The cutaneous trunci muscle is continuous with the insertion of the latissimus dorsi muscle, which lies lateral to these neurovascular structures. The brachial artery is isolated, double-ligated, and divided between its deep brachial branch and the bicipital branch. The brachial vein is ligated and incised at the same level. The median and ulnar nerves are transected caudal to the brachial artery. The radial nerve is severed as it passes lateral to the brachial artery and into the accessory and medial heads of the triceps muscle. The musculocutaneous nerve is transected as it passes cranial to the nerves and vessels just described. The cranial circumflex humeral artery is divided as it branches from the proximal portion of the brachial artery. The severed vessels and nerves are retracted so that the combined insertion of the latissimus dorsi, teres major, and cutaneous trunci muscles can be lifted from the teres tubercle of the humerus. The fascia along the cranial border of the tensor fasciae antebrachii muscle is incised distally and retracted caudally. The division between the medial and accessory heads and the lateral and long heads of the triceps muscle is exposed. The triceps muscle is separated so that the medial and accessory heads are left with the amputated arm. The major portion of this division can be easily carried out by blunt dissection. The medial

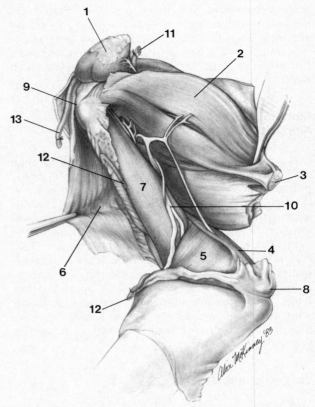

Figure 161–1. Lateral dissection of the foreleg. *1*, Deltoideus muscle (acromial portion); *2*, triceps muscle (lateral head); *3*, triceps tendon; *4*, anconeus muscle; *5*, extensor carpi radialis muscle; *6*, cleidobrachialis muscle; *7*, brachialis muscle; *8*, olecranon process of the ulna; *9*, major tubercle of the humerus; *10*, radial nerve; *11*, axillobrachial vein; *12*, cephalic vein; *13*, omobrachial vein.

and accessory heads are severed from the common tricipital tendon distally by sharp dissection.

The branches of the collateral ulnar artery supplying the distal portion of the triceps are severed as they enter the long head of the triceps. Branches of the radial nerve to the lateral and long heads are transected. The deep brachial artery is still intact and supplies the lateral and long heads of the triceps muscle. The axillobrachial vein is divided and ligated again as it terminates in the axillary vein (Fig. 161–2).

The final step in the dissection of the limb is carried out by the division of the muscles in close association with the joint. This dissection is started by severing the insertion of the supraspinatus muscle from the major tubercle of the humerus and is continued laterally around the joint. The joint capsule is incised along with the muscle. The tendon of the infraspinatus muscle is incised from its insertion just distal to the major tubercle. Then the insertion of the teres minor muscle is severed from the special eminence of the humeral crest just above the deltoid tuberosity. The aponeurosis of the lateral head of the triceps muscle is lifted from the humeral crest. The incision in the lateral joint capsule is continued

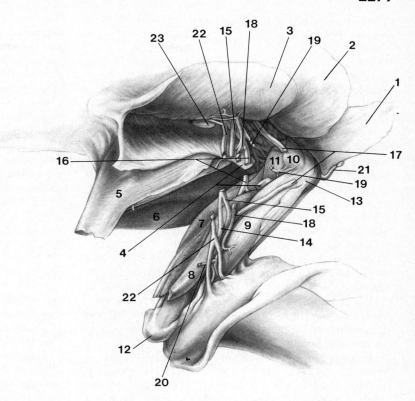

Figure 161–2. Medial dissection of the foreleg. *1*, Cleidobrachialis muscle; *2*, superficial pectoral muscle; *3*, deep pectoral muscle; *4*, combined insertion of the latissimus dorsi muscle, teres major muscle, and cutaneous trunci muscle; *5*, triceps muscle (long head); *6*, triceps muscle (lateral head); *7*, triceps muscle (accessory head); *8*, triceps muscle (medial head); *9*, biceps brachii muscle; *10*, subscapularis muscle; *11*, coracobrachialis muscle; *12*, olecranon process of the ulna; *13*, major tubercle of the humerus; *14*, ulnar nerve; *15*, median nerve; *16*, radial nerve; *17*, musculocutaneous nerve; *18*, brachial artery; *19*, cranial circumflex humeral artery; *20*, collateral ulnar artery; *21*, cephalic vein; *22*, brachial vein; *23*, axillary lymph node.

caudally and around the joint to the medial side, where the subscapularis muscle is severed from its insertion on the minor tubercle of the humerus. The medial incision is carried cranially, severing the tendon of origin of the coracobrachialis muscle. The last structure to be cut is the tendon of origin of the biceps brachii muscle as it crosses the cranial aspect of the joint (Fig. 161–3). The medial and accessory

heads of the triceps, brachialis, biceps brachii, and the coracobrachialis muscles are left with the humerus.

Closure of the stump is carried out by positioning the triceps tendon cranially and suturing the fascia of the triceps to the fascia of the superficial pectorals. The fascia of the supraspinatus and deltoid muscles is sutured to the fascia of the cleidobrachialis muscle.

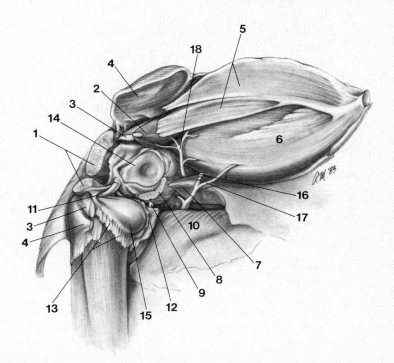

Figure 161–3. Dissection around the shoulder joint, lateral view. *1*, Supraspinatus muscle; *2*, teres minor muscle; *3*, infraspinatus muscle; *4*, deltoideus muscle (acromial portion); *5*, triceps muscle (lateral head); *6*, triceps muscle (long head); *7*, combined insertion of the latissimus dorsi muscle, teres minor muscle, and cutaneous trunci muscle; *8*, subscapularis muscle; *9*, tendon of the coracobrachialis muscle; *10*, deep pectoral muscle; *11*, partially severed tendon of origin of the biceps brachii muscle; *12*, tendon of insertion of the subscapularis muscle; *13*, joint capsule; *14*, glenoid cavity of the scapula; *15*, head of the humerus; *16*, brachial artery (reflected proximally); *17*, deep brachial artery; *18*, caudal circumflex humeral artery.

The subcutaneous tissue and skin are closed in a routine fashion.

Foreleg Amputation with Removal of the Scapula[1]

The skin incision is started several centimeters dorsal to the upper border of the scapula and continued in a straight line distally along the spine of the scapula to the shoulder joint. The next incision is carried circumferentially around the shoulder joint. It is started at the distal point of the first incision and runs cranial to the point of the shoulder, around the shoulder, and straight through the axillary space around the caudal aspect and to the lateral side, ending at its starting point. The skin on both sides of the straight incision is lifted by dissecting close to the deep muscle plane. It is advisable to leave as much of the subcutaneous tissue and cutaneous muscle with the skin as possible to facilitate suturing and closure of dead space, and to preserve vascular supply to the skin flaps.

During the skin incision, the cephalic vein is encountered. It is ligated and divided as it runs deep to the cleidobrachialis muscle. The origin of the omotransversarius muscle is severed from the distal part of the scapular spine and the omobrachial fascia.

The cervical part of the trapezius muscle can be separated from the spine of the scapula with the omotransversarius muscle. The incision along the spine of the scapula is continued in a proximal direction to the most dorsal point of the scapular spine, where the incision is turned distally for a short distance by cutting away the thoracic part of the trapezius muscle. The insertion of the rhomboideus muscle is separated from the dorsomedial border of the scapula. Caudally, the rhomboideus is in close association with the latissimus dorsi muscle and is separated by sharp dissection (Fig. 161–4). The origin of the serratus ventralis muscle (1.5 to 2 cm thick) is lifted from the facies serrata of the scapula. The scapula can now be partially abducted from the body. In the caudal aspect of the axillary space, the intermuscular fascia is bluntly dissected, exposing the latissimus dorsi, teres major, and cutaneous trunci muscles as they come together to insert on the teres tubercle of the humerus. The insertion of these muscles is severed proximal to the level where the teres major joins the common insertion. The thoracodorsal artery and vein are separately ligated and divided. The thoracodorsal nerve is also cut. The axillary lymph node or nodes can be seen lying along the dorsal border of the deep pectoral muscle. The specific vascular and nerve plexus of the arm can be discerned after blunt dissection of the surrounding loose fascia.

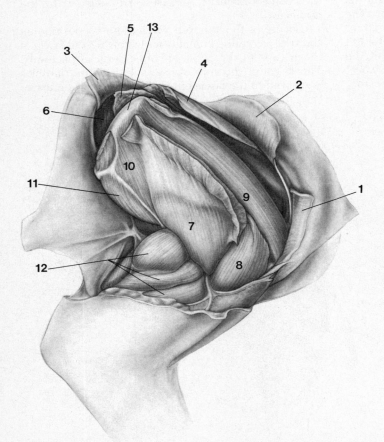

Figure 161–4. Lateral dissection of the foreleg. *1*, Omotransversarius muscle; *2*, trapezius muscle (pars cervicalis); *3*, trapezius muscle (pars thoracica); *4*, rhomboideus cervicis muscle; *5*, rhomboideus thoracis muscle; *6*, latissimus dorsi muscle; *7*, deltoideus muscle (spinous portion); *8*, deltoideus muscle (acromial portion); *9*, supraspinatus muscle; *10*, infraspinatus muscle; *11*, teres major muscle; *12*, triceps muscle; *13*, dorsal border of the scapula.

The scapula is now held in abduction, and the cranial border rotated medially. The axillary artery is isolated, double-ligated, and divided between the origin of the external and lateral thoracic arteries. The lateral thoracic artery is ligated and divided from the axillary artery. The brachial and axillary veins are individually ligated and divided. Transection of the brachial plexus is carried out in a caudal-to-cranial direction. The first nerve bundle to be severed contains the median and ulnar nerves. Transection of the radial nerve, then the axillary nerve, subscapular nerve, and the suprascapular nerve follows. The musculocutaneous nerve lies deep to these nerves and is transected before it enters the biceps brachii muscle. Branches of the superficial cervical artery, including the suprascapular artery, can be ligated and divided at this time. With the nerves and vessels divided, the scapula can be further abducted, exposing the ventral musculature (Fig. 161–5). The deep pectoral muscle is separated from its insertion on the major and minor tubercles of the humerus and the medial brachial fascia. The superficial pectorals are separated from the crest of the humerus. The last muscle, the cleidobrachialis, is severed through the distal third of its belly, and the amputation is complete (Fig. 161–6).

Closure is carried out by suturing the fascia of the deep pectoral muscle to the scalenus muscle. The fascia of the cleidobrachialis muscle is sutured to the fascia of the superfical pectorals. The fascia of the deep pectoral muscle is sutured to the ventral border of the latissimus dorsi muscle, and the fasciae of the trapezius and omotransversarius muscles are sutured to the dorsal border of the latissimus dorsi muscle. The skin and subcutaneous tissues are closed in a routine fashion.

Rear Leg Amputation at Midfemur[3]

The lateral skin incision is semicircular, starting in the flank, extending distally to the level of the patella, and ending at the tuber ischii. The medial skin incision, connecting the cranial and caudal points of the lateral incision, is also semicircular but extends only to midthigh. In the cranial lateral skin incision, a branch of the superficial circumflex iliac artery may be encountered. The skin distal to the incision on both sides of the thigh is reflected down to the level of the stifle joint. The caudal belly of the sartorius muscle is transected midway through the belly. The gracilis muscle is transected at the same level. The

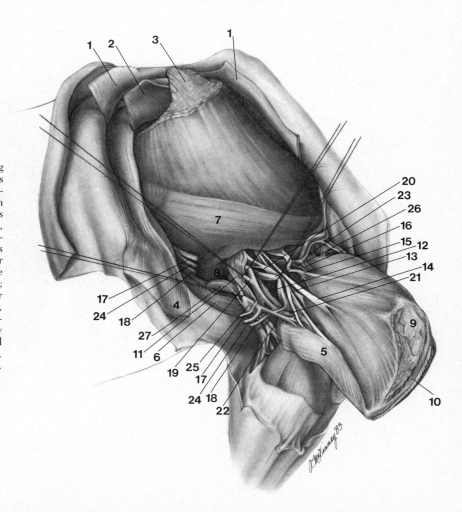

Figure 161–5. Dissection of the foreleg with the scapula abducted. *1*, Trapezius muscle; *2*, rhomboideus muscle; *3*, serratus ventralis muscle; *4*, severed insertion of the latissimus dorsi and cutaneous trunci muscle; *5*, teres major muscle; *6*, deep pectoral muscle; *7*, scaleneus muscle; *8*, rectus thoracis muscle; *9*, facies serrata of the scapula; *10*, dorsal border of the scapula; *11*, ulnar and median nerve trunk; *12*, radial nerve; *13*, axillary nerve; *14*, subscapular nerve; *15*, suprascapular nerve; *16*, musculocutaneous nerve; *17*, thoracodorsal nerve; *18*, thoracodorsal artery; *19*, lateral thoracic artery; *20*, axillary artery; *21*, subscapular artery; *22*, brachial artery; *23*, superficial cervical artery; *24*, thoracodorsal vein; *25*, brachial vein; *26*, axillary vein; *27*, axillary lymph node.

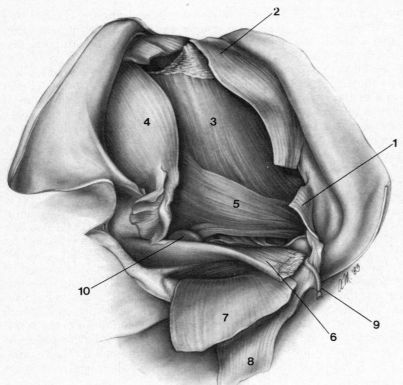

Figure 161–6. Final dissection of the forelimb. *1*, Omotransversarius muscle; *2*, trapezius muscle; *3*, serratus ventralis muscle; *4*, latissimus dorsi muscle; *5*, scaleneus muscle; *6*, deep pectoral muscle; *7*, transverse superficial pectoral muscle; *8*, descending superficial pectoral muscle; *9*, cephalic vein; *10*, axillary lymph node.

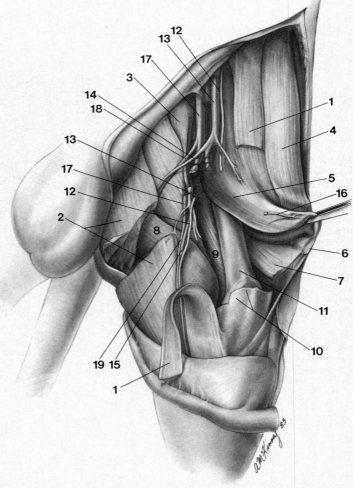

Figure 161–7. Medial dissection of the rear leg. *1*, Sartorius muscle (caudal belly); *2*, gracilis muscle; *3*, pectineus muscle; *4*, sartorius muscle (cranial belly); *5*, vastus medialis muscle; *6*, quadriceps tendon; *7*, vastus lateralis muscle; *8*, semimembranosus muscle; *9*, adductor magnus et brevis muscle; *10*, joint capsule (stifle); *11*, femur; *12*, saphenous nerve; *13*, femoral artery; *14*, proximal caudal femoral artery; *15*, saphenous artery; *16*, descending genicular artery; *17*, femoral vein; *18*, proximal caudal femoral vein; *19*, saphenous vein.

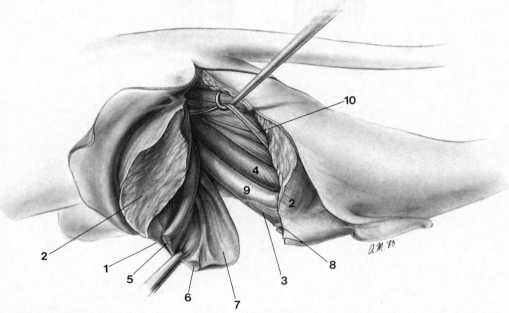

Figure 161–8. Lateral dissection of rear leg. *1*, Fascia lata and aponeurosis of the biceps femoris muscle; *2*, biceps femoris muscle; *3*, articularis genus muscle; *4*, adductor magnus et brevis muscle; *5*, vastus lateralis muscle; *6*, quadriceps tendon; *7*, vastus medialis muscle; *8*, joint capsule (stifle); *9*, femur; *10*, sciatic nerve.

fascia over the femoral artery and vein is dissected free. The saphenous nerve, which is closely associated with the femoral artery, is isolated and divided. The artery is double-ligated and divided between the proximal caudal femoral artery and the saphenous artery. The femoral vein is ligated at the same level. The vascular stumps are retracted, and the musculotendinous portion of the pectineus muscle is transected down to the bone. Before the quadriceps muscle group is transected, the descending genicular artery is ligated and separated from the femoral artery. The cranial belly of the sartorius muscle and the quadriceps muscle group are transected just proximal to the patella (Fig. 161–7).

Lateral dissection of the leg is started by incising the aponeurosis of the biceps femoris muscle, the fascia lata, and the belly of the biceps femoris muscle parallel to the lateral skin incision. A branch of the distal caudal femoral artery or a muscular branch directly from the femoral artery to the biceps femoris muscle may be encountered. The articularis genis muscle is not included with the quadriceps dissection. The biceps femoris muscle is retracted dorsally, and the sciatic nerve trunk is isolated and severed at the greater trochanter (Fig. 161–8).

The remaining muscles are transected at midthigh. These include the abductor cruris caudalis, then the semitendinosus, the two bellies of the semimembra-

Figure 161–9. Final dissection of rear leg. *1*, Biceps femoris muscle; *2*, vastus lateralis muscle; *3*, vastus medialis muscle; *4*, quadriceps tendon; *5*, adductor magnus et brevis muscle; *6*, gracilis muscle; *7*, semimembranosus muscle; *8*, semitendinosus muscle; *9*, abductor cruris caudalis muscle; *10*, femur.

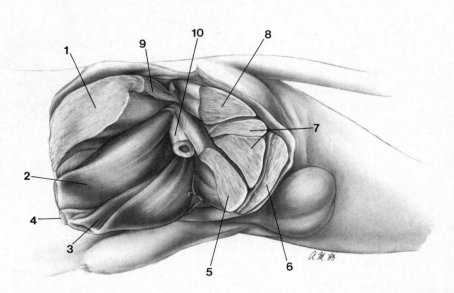

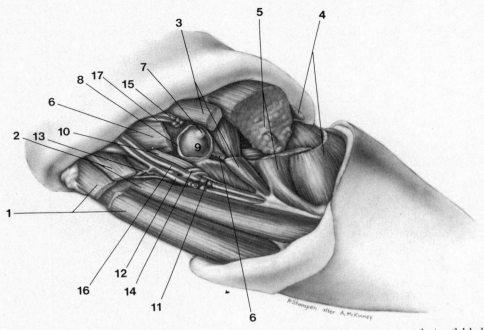

Figure 161–10. Medial dissection of the pelvic limb. *1*, Sartorius muscle (cranial belly); *2*, Sartorius muscle (caudal belly); *3*, pectineus muscle; *4*, gracilis muscle; *5*, adductor magnus et brevis muscle; *6*, iliopsoas muscle; *7*, ligament of the head of the femur; *8*, joint capsule (hip); *9*, head of the femur; *10*, femoral nerve; *11*, saphenous nerve; *12*, femoral artery; *13*, superficial circumflex iliac artery; *14*, lateral circumflex femoral artery; *15*, medial circumflex femoral artery; *16*, femoral vein; *17*, medial circumflex femoral vein.

nosus, and lastly the adductor magnus et brevis. After the adductor muscle is partially lifted from the shaft of the bone, the femur is cut at the junction of its middle and proximal thirds (Fig. 161–9).

Closure is carried out by bringing the distal end of the quadriceps muscle group caudally and suturing it to the adductor muscle. The biceps femoris muscle is brought medially and sutured to the gracilis mus-

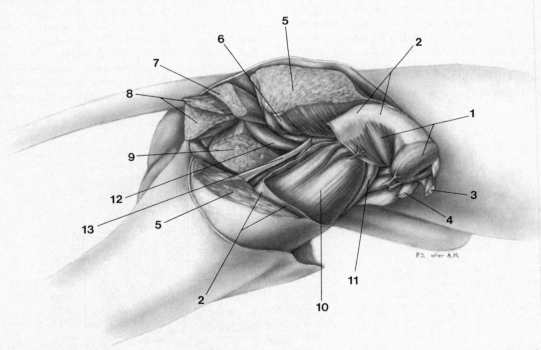

Figure 161–11. Lateral dissection of the pelvic limb. *1*, Tensor fasciae latae muscle; *2*, fascia lata; *3*, sartorius muscle (cranial belly); *4*, sartorius muscle (caudal belly); *5*, biceps femoris muscle; *6*, abductor cruris caudalis muscle; *7*, semitendinosus muscle; *8*, semimembranosus muscle; *9*, adductor magnus et brevis muscle; *10*, vastus lateralis muscle; *11*, rectus femoris muscle; *12*, quadratus femoris muscle; *13*, sciatic nerve.

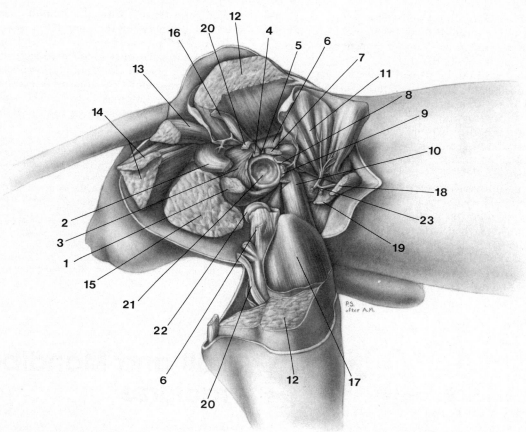

Figure 161–12. Final dissection of the pelvic limb. *1*, adductor longus muscle; *2*, quadratus femoris muscle; *3*, external obturator muscle; *4*, internal obturator muscle; *5*, gemelli muscle; *6*, superficial gluteal muscle; *7*, middle gluteal muscle; *8*, deep gluteal muscle; *9*, articularis coxae muscle; *10*, partially severed origin of the rectus femoris muscle; *11*, tensor fasciae latae muscle; *12*, biceps femoris muscle; *13*, semitendinosus muscle; *14*, semimembranosus muscle; *15*, adductor magnus et brevis muscle; *16*, abductor cruris caudalis muscle; *17*, vastus lateralis muscle; *18*, sartorius muscle (cranial belly); *19*, sartorius muscle (caudal belly); *20*, sciatic nerve; *21*, acetabulum; *22*, head of the femur; *23*, superficial circumflex iliac artery.

cle. The caudal sartorius muscle is sutured to the fascia lata. The skin and subcutaneous tissues are sutured in a routine manner.

Amputation of the Pelvic Limb by Disarticulation of the Hip[3]

The lateral skin incision is semicircular, starting in the flank, extending to midthigh, and ending at the tuber ischii. By passing just distal to the inguinal fold, the medial skin incision parallels the fold connecting the cranial and caudal points of the lateral skin incision. The skin distal to the incision is reflected to facilitate anatomical identification. The dissection is begun on the medial side by exposing the femoral artery and vein as they leave the vascular lacunae. The femoral artery is double-ligated and divided proximal to the origin of the lateral circumflex femoral artery and vein. The femoral vein is divided and ligated at the same level. The superficial circumflex iliac artery should also be ligated. Both the cranial and caudal bellies of the sartorius muscle are transected approximately 2 cm from their origin on the

iliac crest and ventral spines of the ilium. The pectineus, gracilis, and adductor magnus et brevis muscles are cut at the same level. The medial circumflex femoral artery and vein is ligated and divided as it passes lateral to the pectineus muscle. The iliopsoas muscle is now exposed and can be lifted from its insertion on the trochanter minor of the femur. The iliopsoas muscle may be retracted cranially, exposing the saphenous and femoral nerves, which are now severed. The medial joint capsule is incised cranial to caudal, and the ligament of the head of the femur is transected (Fig. 161–10).

The dissection of the lateral side is begun by transecting the tensor fascia latae muscle at the junction of the proximal and middle thirds of the thigh. This incision is carried through the biceps femoris muscle. The abductor cruris caudalis muscle is cut with the biceps femoris. The surgeon should return to the cranial aspect of the leg, incise the fascia lata, and lift it from the shaft of the femur to expose the greater trochanter. The biceps femoris muscle and tensor fasciae latae muscles are retracted dorsally, exposing the semitendinosus and semimembranosus muscles, which are now transected in the proximal third of the thigh. The sciatic nerve is exposed and severed distal to the branches supplying the semimembranosus, semitendinosus, and biceps femoris muscles (Fig. 161–11).

The hip can now be placed in flexion and abduction, exposing the quadratus femoris muscle, which is lifted from its insertion just proximal to the trochanter tertius of the femur. With the leg in the same position, the external rotators are severed as they enter the trochanteric fossa. The rotators include the internal obturator, external obturator, and gemelli muscles. The hip can be abducted and flexed with some internal rotation, and the gluteal muscles transected. The superficial gluteal muscle is transected first, followed by the medial gluteal and piriformis muscles. The last muscle to be cut from the trochanter is the deep gluteal. The dorsal joint capsule and articularis coxae muscle are transected, completely freeing the femur from the joint cavity of the acetabulum. The rectus femoris muscle is re-

moved from its origin on the iliopubic eminence of the ilium, completing the amputation (Fig. 161–12).

Closure is accomplished by suturing the fascia of the biceps femoris muscle to the gracilis muscle and, if necessary, also to the semimembranosus or semitendinosus muscles. The tensor fascia latae can be sutured to the iliopsoas muscle. The subcutaneous tissue and skin are closed in a routine fashion.

1. Borzio, F.: Amputation of the foreleg of the dog. *In* Bojrab, M. J.(ed.). *Current Techniques in Small Animal Surgery.* Lea & Febiger, Philadelphia, 1975.
2. Leighton, R.L.: Amputation of the foreleg of the dog. *In* Bojrab, M. J.(ed.). *Current Techniques in Small Animal Surgery.* Lea & Febiger, Philadelphia, 1975.
3. Slocum, B.: Amputation of the canine pelvic limb. *In* Bojrab, M. J.(ed.): *Current Techniques in Small Animal Surgery.* Lea & Febiger, Phildelphia, 1975.
4. Withrow, S. J., and Hirsch V. M.: Owner response to amputation of a pet's leg. Vet. Med/Small Anim. Clin. 74:332, 1979.

Chapter **162** # Skull and Mandibular Fractures

Mary L. Dulisch

PREOPERATIVE DIAGNOSIS AND MANAGEMENT

The most common causes of skull and mandibular fractures are automobile accidents and falls from heights. Clinically, the animal may have severe injuries to both the bony structures and soft tissues or subtle conformational deformities. Any animal presented with bleeding from the mouth or ears or subconjunctival hemorrhage should be thoroughly examined for related fractures.

The initial management depends on the clinical signs. Any animal with a traumatic injury should be given a thorough physical examination, evaluated for shock, and treated appropriately. In addition, all such animals should have a thoracic radiograph taken. Many patients with maxillary injuries breathe via the mouth. They do well if allowed to rest and not stressed. Oxygen cage therapy may be beneficial. If the patient has severe respiratory distress, a tracheostomy should be performed.

Once the animal's cardiovascular and respiratory systems are stable, the fractures can be further assessed and repaired if necessary. If the patient is younger than five years of age and was healthy prior to the trauma, total solids and packed cell volume are evaluated. For older animals, a complete blood count and chemistry profile are assessed prior to

anesthesia. Once the animal is anesthetized, skull and mandibular radiographs are taken to determine the bony damage.

ANESTHESIA

Although the preanesthetic medication and induction technique are based on the preoperative data, all animals requiring fracture repair should be intubated endotracheally. The technique must allow access to the fractures and ensure that normal dental occlusion is maintained. If the endotracheal tube interferes with fracture alignment or prevents evaluation of occlusion, it should be temporarily removed. This problem can be avoided with a tracheostomy or intubation by a pharyngotomy. With the latter technique, the animal is intubated normally. After being surgically prepared, an incision is made in the piriform fossa, posterior to the tongue and laterorostral to the hyoid apparatus. After the endotracheal tube adapter is removed and the cuff is deflated, a hemostat is passed through the skin incision, which grasps the end of the tube in the mouth and pulls the tube through the incision. The adapter is replaced and the animal is reconnected to the anesthetic system. The cuff tubing still exits from the mouth; however, it is small in diameter and does not

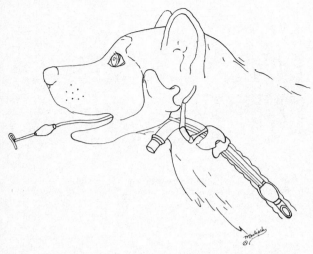

Figure 162–1. Endotracheal pharyngostomy allows manipulation of the fracture and evaluation of dental occlusion without interference from the endotracheal tube.

interfere with surgery (Fig. 162–1). Postoperatively, the adapter is again removed and the technique reversed. A pharyngostomy tube can be placed through this incision if one is required during the postoperative period.[8]

SKULL FRACTURES

Surgical fractures of the skull can be divided into depression fractures, maxillary fractures, hard palate separations, and zygomatic arch fractures. Soft tissue injuries associated with these fractures can be severe and may be life-threatening.

Depression Fractures

Depression fractures of the skull and cranium may require emergency surgery if the fragments penetrate the brain or if the animal has deteriorating neurological signs despite vigorous medical management. The bony fragments must be elevated carefully to prevent further damage to the brain. Burr holes ½ to 1 cm from the fracture site allow the introduction of a small elevator, which can be used to lift the fragments from beneath. Any loose fragments are discarded. The dura may be opened to drain hematomas, achieve hemostasis, and thoroughly irrigate the area to decrease the chance of brain abscesses or encephalitis.[6, 22] In the dog, the temporal muscles provide sufficient padding so that the bony defects do not need reconstruction. Concurrent medical therapy for brain trauma is essential in these cases before, during, and after surgery.

Depression fractures of the frontal bones require surgical intervention; however, these usually are not emergencies. Fragments of the zygomatic process of the frontal bone that are markedly displaced ventrally

should be removed or stabilized as soon as possible so that the eye is not pierced. Small fragments can be discarded, and all sharp edges should be removed with rongeurs. Large pieces can be wired together using 22- to 24-gauge stainless steel wire. If large bony defects leave the eye unprotected, synthetic mesh can be used to reconstruct the area. Fragments in the frontal sinus are removed, and the sinus is lavaged to decrease the chance of bacterial or fungal infections, bone sequestra, and nonhealing wounds.[22] Reconstruction of the sinus roof is usually not necessary; however, small polyethylene tubing placed in the sinus and exiting through the skin will help prevent subcutaneous emphysema in the postoperative period.

Maxillary Fractures

Maxillary fractures need to be repaired if there is conformational deformity with malocclusion or depressed fragments in the nasal cavity. Stabilization may be attained with muzzling, wires, interdental wiring, or pins. If maxillary fractures are minimally displaced but dental malocclusion is present, realignment under anesthesia is necessary. A tape muzzle may be sufficient support to maintain the alignment. The muzzle can also be used as an adjunct to other fixation methods.

Further treatment is needed if there are depressed fracture fragments involving the dorsum of the nasal cavity. As in frontal sinus fractures, failure to remove pieces of avulsed bone can lead to bone sequestra and chronic sinusitis. A dorsal midline incision is made and the soft tissues are reflected laterally until the bone fragments are exposed. Small fragments are discarded, whereas larger ones can be secured to the maxilla with 22- to 24-gauge stainless steel hemicerclage wires. Holes for the wires can be made with 0.035- or 0.045-inch Kirschner wires or an air drill. If the rostral part of the maxilla is transected from the rest of the skull, multiple wires crossing the fracture line perpendicularly help achieve stabilization and alignment. Fascial and subcutaneous tissues are closed to give as tight a seal as possible, and the skin is apposed. A tape muzzle is used for added support in the first two to three weeks.

Severely comminuted fractures may be impossible to wire together. In these animals orthodontic wiring can be used to prevent malocclusion during the healing process. Stout's multiple-loop orthodontic wiring technique requires that both arcades of incisors be intact. Eyelets are formed by passing 20-gauge stainless steel wire between the teeth in a continuous manner. The eyelets of the upper arcade are then wired to those of the lower arcade (Fig. 162–2). During the postsurgical period, the wires may need to be tightened with the animal anesthetized. Alimentation is maintained with a pharyngostomy tube for three weeks. Sufficient callous forms within this time so that the wires can be removed. A

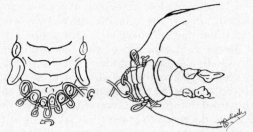

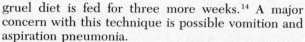

Figure 162–2. Stout's multiple loop orthodontic wiring can be used to align severely comminuted fractures and prevent malocclusion.

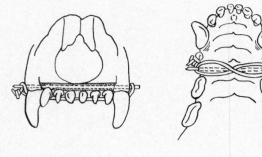

Figure 162–4. Apposition of a hard palate separation using a pin. Further compression is achieved with a figure-of-eight wire.

gruel diet is fed for three more weeks.[14] A major concern with this technique is possible vomition and aspiration pneumonia.

A second stabilization technique utilizes external pin splints. There are many variations of this technique. Two Steinmann pins or Kirschner wires are placed into each fragment, and the pins are bridged by metal rods and clamps, a metal bar and wires with an acrylic bridge molded over them, or an acrylic bridge alone.[2, 21] The advantage of the easily molded acrylic splint is that many and multiple size pins can be used in any configuration. Because normal alimentation is possible, the chance of regurgitation and aspiration is reduced. Two major disadvantages are possible pin tract infections (although their occurrence is low) and the apparatus catching on objects and pulling off.[21]

Avulsion fractures of the maxilla involving the dental arcade are best stabilized with pins and figure-of-eight wires. First, 0.062-inch pins are placed from the fragment to the maxilla. Then, to prevent pin migration, figure-of-eight wires of 20-gauge stainless steel bridge the pins (Fig. 162–3).

Hard Palate Separations

Animals with hard palate separations may need surgical intervention to prevent food from accumulating in the nasal cavity. The oral mucosa can migrate and seal defects less than 2 mm wide. With wider defects inversion of the oral mucosal surface can produce a fistula. Healing can be expedited by suturing the mucosa together with a pliable, nonabsorbable suture such as 3–0 or 2–0 Dacron or silk using a simple interrupted pattern. If the defect is wider, the hard palate can be re-apposed by placing medial pressure on the lateral aspects of the maxilla. Apposition is maintained by inserting a 1/16- or 3/32-inch Steinmann pin across the hard palate, alternating from one lateral side to the other, avoiding the teeth roots. If compression is needed, a 20-gauge, figure-eight wire incorporating the pin ends can pass ventral to the hard palate. The soft tissue is sutured as previously described (Fig. 162–4).

A second technique utilizes wire only. A strand of 20-gauge wire is passed through a drill hole through the lateral cortex of the maxilla directly above the hard palate, exits on the opposite side of the maxilla through another hole, and then passes back ventrally between the hard palate and mucosa. The two ends are brought together and twisted (Fig. 162–5).

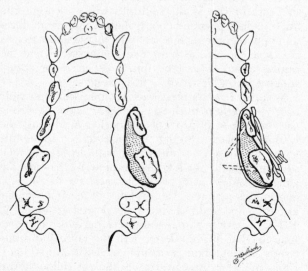

Figure 162–3. Avulsion fractures can be stabilized with diverging pins and figure-of-eight wire.

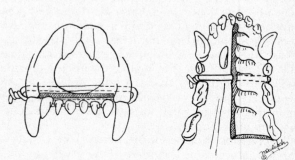

Figure 162–5. Apposition of a hard palate using 20-gauge wire passed through two lateral holes in the maxilla above the hard palate and ventrally between the hard palate and mucosa.

Zygomatic Arch Fractures

Nondisplaced zygomatic arch fractures do not need stabilization and heal well on their own. Medially displaced fragments, however, may interfere with the globe or the ability of the animal to open and close its mouth. Surgical stabilization is best achieved with 20-gauge stainless steel cerclage wiring of the pieces to the intact part of the arch. To expose the arch, a longitudinal skin incision is made directly over the arch and the platysma muscle is incised on the same line. The palpebral nerve and transverse facial artery and vein should be avoided in the caudal aspect of the arch.[17] If the arch is so comminuted and displaced that re-alignment and stabilization are not possible, the pieces should be removed. A plastic plate* can be secured to both intact ends of the arch to bridge the gap.[25]

TEMPOROMANDIBULAR LUXATIONS AND FRACTURES

On physical examination, the luxated mandible is displaced rostral and dorsal. Usually the temporomandibular luxation can be reduced by closed reduction with the animal anesthetized. A soft wooden dowel or pencil is placed at the level of the last molars. The mouth is closed by placing downward pressure on the maxilla, and the mandible is forced backward. After reduction, a tape muzzle limits opening of the mouth and helps prevent reluxation.

Interarcade wiring is another technique for preventing reluxation. It is essential that a pharyngostomy tube be placed prior to the wiring. On both sides of the skull and mandible, the gingiva are elevated from the fourth upper premolar and the first lower molar. Drill holes, perpendicular to the long axis of the teeth, are made from the buccal to the lingual surface between the tooth roots at the level of the root and tooth body. For a 15- to 20-kg dog, 20-gauge stainless steel wire is passed through the holes as illustrated (Fig. 162–6). Once all wires are placed, the animal is allowed to recover. As the swallowing reflex returns, the endotracheal tube is removed and the wires tightened. The twist should be at the level of the lower hole, and once the twist

---

*Lubra Plate, Lubra Co., Fort Collins, CO.

is tight, the end is bent proximally. This technique is rapid and inexpensive, and no pyoderma results from wire irritation. Complications such as wire breaking or stretching, aspiration pneumonia, and hyperthermia due to inability to pant are possible. Also, postoperative management of the pharyngostomy tube must be maintained for several weeks.[11]

If manual reduction is not successful, open reduction is necessary. The skin incision follows the ventral border of the zygomatic arch and continues caudally over the area of the temporomandibular joint. The platysma muscle is incised and reflected. An incision is made in the periosteum at the origin of the masseter muscle, and the muscle is reflected ventrally to expose the joint capsule. Care is taken to avoid the transverse facial artery and vein and the masseteric nerve. A wide incision of the joint capsule exposes the joint. Any fibrin and debris are removed by suction, and the joint is reduced. The joint capsule is closed with an absorbable suture, and the masseter muscle and fascia are sutured to fascia on the zygomatic arch. The platysma, subcutaneous tissue, and skin are closed in a routine manner.[17]

If severe comminution or ankylosis is present, the temporal condyle may be resected to establish a false joint. A gigli wire or air drill and osteotome can be used to excise the condyle, being careful to preserve the soft tissues. If severe comminution is present, the fragments and condyle are removed. Biomechanically, the jaw is altered and contraction of the ipsilateral masseter muscle causes the mandible to shift toward the opposite side and some malocclusion to occur. There is also the potential of osteoarthritis developing in the remaining temporomandibular joint.[12]

MANDIBULAR SYMPHYSEAL SEPARATION

Symphyseal separations may occur alone or in combination with other facial fractures. The symphyseal separation should be repaired last. Many techniques have been described for the stabilization. If the incisors are intact, Stout's orthodontic wiring as described can be used. If the mandible is large enough, compression of the symphysis can be obtained with a lag screw. The separation is first held in reduction with bone-holding forceps. After an incision is made in the buccal mucosa caudal to the canines, a drill hole that avoids teeth roots is made

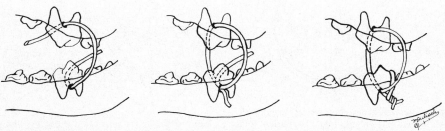

Figure 162–6. Interarcade wiring can be used to prevent reluxation of temporomandibular luxations.

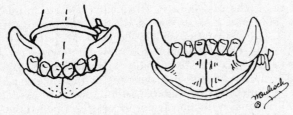

Figure 162–7. Mandibular symphyseal separation stabilized with an encompassing wire twisted lateral to the oral mucosa.

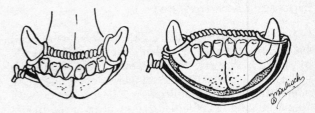

Figure 162–9. Mandibular symphyseal separation stabilized with an interdental encompassing wiring technique.

across the symphysis and through the opposite cortex. The hole is tapped and either a lag screw can be inserted or, after the proximal hole is overdrilled, a cortical screw is used to achieve compression. Rapid healing takes place owing to rigid stability, and there is an early return to normal feeding. The implant is usually well tolerated. Disadvantages of this technique include the need for special equipment and the potential of food entering the drill hole once the screw is removed.[7, 26]

Mandibular symphyseal separations can also be stabilized by various wire techniques. A wire passer can be introduced through the buccal mucosa caudal to the canines and positioned ventral to the mandible, staying close to the border of the mandible. Twenty-gauge wire is passed to encompass the mandible. The wire is twisted at the side and the end bent down (Fig. 162–7).[13] A variation of this technique introduces the wire passer from a skin incision ventral to the symphysis. The wire again encompasses the jaw close to the bone, penetrates the mucosa on the opposite side, and exits through the same skin incision. The strands are tightened ventrally to bury the wire (Fig. 162–8).[9]

In a third technique using 28-gauge wire, a loop is made around the left canine and the wire is twisted. The right canine is encompassed by the strands, which are again twisted several turns. One strand is passed under the mandible to the left side, threaded through the left canine loop, returned under the mandible to the right side, and twisted to the other strand (Fig. 162–9).[10]

Transmandibular Pin

A transmandibular pin can stabilize symphyseal separations. A 0.062-inch Kirschner wire or 1/16- to

3/32-inch Steinmann pin is inserted across the symphysis, starting on the lateral aspect of the mandible behind the canine tooth, and exits through the opposite side of the mandible. If sufficient stability is not achieved, a figure-eight of 20-gauge wire can be placed on the lingual surface of the mandible with the loops around the pin ends (Fig. 162–10).

FRACTURES OF THE BODY OF THE MANDIBLE

Intraoral Fixation

Acrylic Splints

Intraoral acrylic splints can be used to stabilize mandibular fractures anterior to the fourth premolar after open reduction and wiring are performed. First a cast is made from an impression tray, and an acrylic splint is made from the cast. The splint is formed for the lingual surface of the teeth and is held in place with 24- to 28-gauge circummandibular wires. The splints remain in place for four to six weeks (Fig. 162–11).[19]

Pin Splint

Unilateral mandibular fractures can be splinted with a U-shaped, 1/16- to 3/32-inch pin. A hole, ½ inch below and posterior to the last molar, is made in both mandibles on the lingual side using a pin the same diameter as the splint. The splint's ends are inserted into the holes so the U is on the floor of the mouth between the tongue and lingual surface. Small holes can be made in the mandible and near the incisors to further anchor the splint with cerclage (Fig. 162–12).[1]

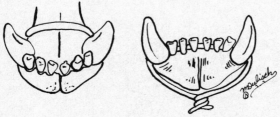

Figure 162–8. Mandibular symphyseal separation stabilized with an encompassing wire twisted ventrally so that it is buried subcutaneously.

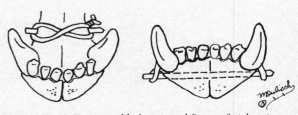

Figure 162–10. Transmandibular pin and figure-of-eight wire used to stabilize a symphyseal separation.

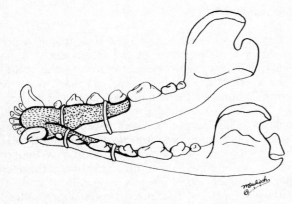

Figure 162–11. Intraoral splint to supplement stabilization of mandibular fractures anterior to the fourth premolar.

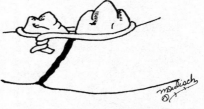

Figure 162–13. Interdental wiring should be as low on the teeth as possible to help prevent slipping.

Interdental Wiring

Interdental wiring can be used as the sole fixation in simple, nondisplaced fractures of the mandible or as an adjunct technique. The two teeth rostral and caudal to the fracture line are encircled with a 20- to 21-gauge cerclage wire. The wire should be as low on the teeth as possible to prevent slippage (Fig. 162–13).[20] In bilateral fractures just caudal to the canines, a figure-eight of 18-gauge wire can be used. Better anchorage of the wires is achieved in these cases if the wire is passed through drill holes just rostral to the canine and caudal to the first premolar (Fig. 162–14).[5]

External Fixation

There are many techniques for external splintage; however, all utilize rods or pins protruding from the bone and a connecting apparatus. These techniques are easy and rapid to apply, do not disturb the fragments or their blood supply, and allow movement of the temporomandibular joints so that joint stiffness is prevented. The splints are usually well tolerated by the patient and allow for normal alimentation, although a gruel is recommended initially. The techniques are versatile and can be used for comminuted fractures with or without large bony gaps, delayed or nonunion fractures, and fractures with associated infections.

The Kirschner-Ehmer splint is the best known. Two pins in the rostral and caudal fragments are necessary. The pins in each fragment should be placed 35 to 45° to each other. Both cortices are pentrated so that the pin is just protruding through the far cortex. The four pins are then connected with cross bars. A second manner of application is to insert the most rostral and caudal pins and then connect them with a bar with two extra clamps through which the second and third pins are inserted. This method gives more stability, since fewer bars and clamps are used, and it is less expensive (Fig. 162–15).[3]

Variations of the Kirschner-Ehmer splint use dental acrylics to bridge the pins rather than bars and clamps. For bilateral mandibular fractures, the pins are inserted perpendicular to the mandible and penetrate both sides. The pins are bridged with acrylic bars placed on each side or with one bar that curves rostral to the mandible. The acrylic should be placed

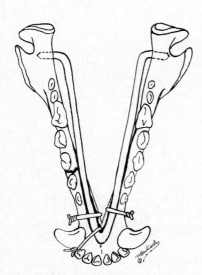

Figure 162–12. Pin splint used to stabilize a unilateral mandibular fracture.

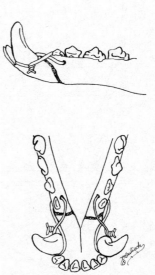

Figure 162–14. Stabilization of bilateral fractures caudal to the canines and rostral to the first premolar using figure-of-eight wire.

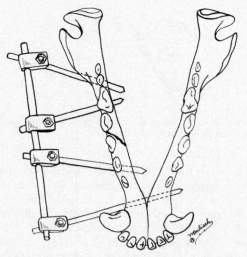

Figure 162–15. Kirschner-Ehmer pin splint technique to stabilize mandibular fractures. Two pins are placed in each fragment 35 to 45° to each other.

at least 1 cm from the skin surface to prevent irritation (Fig. 162–16).[18]

A biphase external splint has been described that involves the application of special Vitallium bone screws into the mandible. Two screws are needed on both sides of the fracture site, and the screw's collar must rest on the cortical bone at the ventral border. External clamps and rods are used to facilitate reduction and temporary fixation until an acrylic bar is placed on the screws. Once the acrylic has polymerized and is rigid, the clamps and rods are removed. If there is generalized bone disease, this technique cannot be used. The technique is also more costly than the pin techniques, and the screws may loosen.[23]

Internal Fixation

For internal fixation, the ventral approach is preferred because exposure of the fragments is unobstructed by the teeth and both sides of the mandibular cortices are exposed. The approach does not further traumatize the oral mucosa, and ventral drainage is easily established if postoperative fluid accumulates. The incision is made over the mandible itself, or, if bilateral fractures are present, both sides can be exposed from a midline incision. When repairing comminuted mandibular fractures, the most caudal or least accessible one is stabilized first. To achieve adequate stabilization, a combination of techniques may be needed.

Wire Stabilization

Although the use of hemicerclage wires is the simplest method of internal fixation, some basic principles must be followed for successful repair. For adequate strength, 18- to 20-gauge stainless steel wire should be used to avoid any unnecessary bending. A guide loop may help to prevent bending or kinking. All wires should be tightened with even tension and adequate tightness so that wire move-

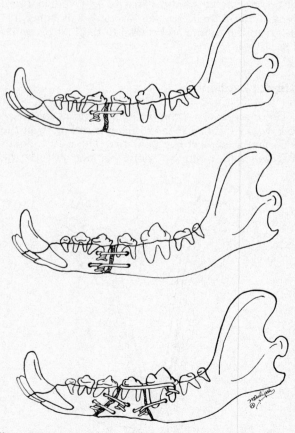

Figure 162–17. Mandibular wires should be placed perpendicular to the fracture line. If one wire near the alveolar border does not give adequate stabilization, a second parallel wire or interdental wiring can be used.

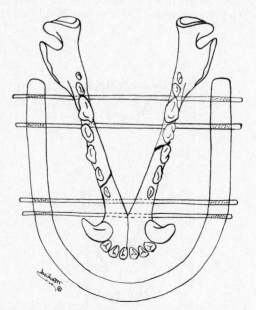

Figure 162–16. Dental acrylics rather than bars and clamps can be used to bridge transmandibular pins.

ment and bone absorption do not occur. Ideally, fixations should be applied to the tension band side, which for the mandible is at the alveolar border.[2] Therefore, the wires should be placed as close to the alveolar border as possible, but teeth roots are avoided. Holes for the wire can be made with 0.045- to 0.062-inch Kirschner wire or with an air drill. To further prevent deviation of the mandible's dorsal margin, interdental wiring can be used. For transverse fractures, the wires are placed perpendicular to the fracture. If one wire does not stabilize a fracture, a second parallel wire should be used. A separate wire is also used for each fracture line (Fig. 162–17). In oblique fractures, two wires perpendicular to each other and each crossing the fracture line help prevent sliding of the fragments (Fig. 162–18). Another option is to place one wire from medial to lateral and a second wire from rostral to caudal.[20]

Intramedullary Pin

Intramedullary pinning can be used in unilateral or bilateral mandibular fractures. The ideal fractures for this technique are oblique or transverse fractures of the body from the second premolar to the first molar. Depending on the size of the animal, a 0.035-inch Kirschner wire to a 9/64-inch Steinmann pin can be used. The pin is introduced into the mandibular

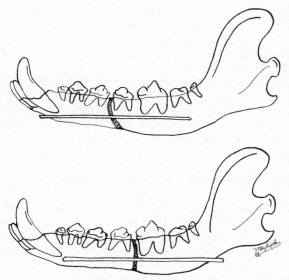

Figure 162–19. Intramedullary pins inserted rostrally should stop at the level of the first molar. Intramedullary pins inserted caudally can be seated at the level of the canine and need not penetrate the rostral cortex.

canal of the rostral fragment from the fracture site and directed craniad so the pin penetrates the cortex ventral to the root of the canine tooth. The fracture is reduced and the pin seated caudally at the point where the mandibular canal curves at the level of the first molar. It is also possible to reduce the fracture first and then normograde the pin from caudal to rostral or vice versa (Fig. 162–19).[4]

Plate Stabilization

Adherence to the technical principles of plate application is as important for mandibular fractures as for other fractures. Plates provide rigid stability

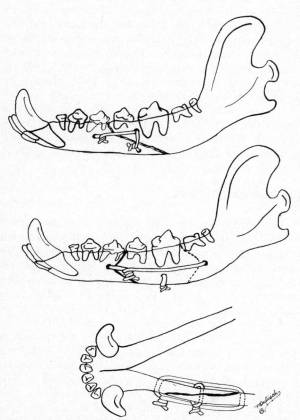

Figure 162–18. Oblique fractures. Two perpendicular wires that cross the fracture line will prevent sliding, as will one encompassing wire medial to lateral and another rostral to caudal.

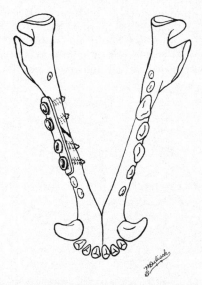

Figure 162–20. Mandibular plating. There should be a minimum of four cortices rostral and caudal to the fracture penetrated.

and rapid return to function. They are particularly useful in complicated and bilateral fractures. When applying a bone plate, perfect occlusion, not perfect fracture alignment, is the goal. Although the tension side of the mandible is near the alveolar border, a bone plate is applied along the ventral mandibular border to avoid teeth roots and the mandibular nerve in the medullary canal. Compression of the fragments is desired, and penetration of four cortices rostral and caudal to the fracture is essential (Fig. 162–20).[2]

FRACTURES OF THE RAMUS OF THE MANDIBLE

Fractures caudal to the body of the mandible are more difficult to stabilize owing to the thinness of the cortical bone. In many instances, the fractures heal well with muzzling. If there is much displacement, the fractures can be stabilized with either cerclage wire, using the same principles as those for fractures of the body of the mandible, or mini or finger plates.

Another technique provides continuous antagonism of the distracting muscle forces on the mandible to maintain dental occlusion during the healing period. A screw is placed into the maxilla on each side just above the ventral surface of the hard palate and just caudal to the roots of the upper canine teeth. A screw is also placed into the mandible on each side in an area to achieve anatomical dental alignment. The two screws on each side are connected with elastic bands placed over the screw heads. Tension can be varied by using multiple bands or loops of a band. Breakage of the bands is the major complication of this technique (Fig. 162–21).[15]

SOFT TISSUE REPAIR AND DENTAL FRACTURES

After the fractures have been stabilized, soft tissue and dental injuries need to be treated. Because food particles can become trapped in large mucosal lacerations, the mucosa should be sutured with 3–0 chromic catgut in either a continuous or simple interrupted pattern. Small defects do not need to be

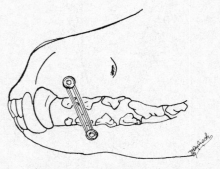

Figure 162–21. Dental occlusion can be maintained for caudal mandibular fractures by using a continuous antagonism technique consisting of two screws and elastic bands.

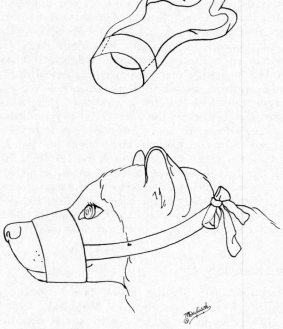

Figure 162–22. Tape muzzles are useful as a primary method of support or as an adjunct to internal fixation.

sutured, as the mucosa contracts and rapidly restores the surface integrity.[16] Avulsions of the lower lip are re-attached with 3–0 or 2–0 nylon horizontal mattress sutures that pass through the skin and incorporate the canines and incisors. If the mucosa is sutured closed, ventral drainage is established with a Penrose drain. Teeth that are split and loose should be removed. If the teeth have chips or cracks but are not loose, it is better to remove them after the fractures are healed so that the stabilization is not stressed. If a tooth's pulp cavity is exposed, either a root canal can be done or the tooth is extracted later.

POSTOPERATIVE CARE

As a primary method of support or as an adjunct to fixation, the tape muzzle can be invaluable in preventing an animal from overusing the jaw or chewing on objects. A muzzle may also be used for highly comminuted or ventral ramus fractures if the opposite side is intact, thus acting as a splint. The animal's mouth should be held shut while ½- to 2-inch tape, sticky side up, is placed around the muzzle. If the animal is to be fed per os, a 1-cm gap is allowed. If nutrition is supplied through a pharyngostomy tube, the mouth is completely taped closed. A second piece of tape is either secured to the encompassing piece of tape, passed around the ears and back of the head, and secured to the opposite side, or two tape strands are secured to the circle and the strands tied behind the head. A layer of tape, sticky side down, is then placed over the first encircling tape. The muzzle is left on for two to eight weeks, depending on its function. An Elizabethan collar will keep the animal from removing the muzzle (Fig. 162–22).

Although the muzzle has advantages such as ease and economy of application, nondisruption of the bone fragment's blood supply, and a decreased infection rate, stability is less than that seen with other techniques and soft tissues may contract and develop fibrous adhesions from the immobilization. Dermatitis, full thickness skin necrosis, and loosening of the muzzle can occur if the owner is not giving adequate home care. An animal may also become hyperthermic from the inability to pant.[24]

If the mouth is wired closed or if the animal refuses to eat, a pharyngostomy tube is used to supply nutrition. If the mouth is taped with a 1-cm gap, a dog food gruel is fed. After internal fixation or external splintage, a gruel is fed for the first few days, followed by a soft diet. Because fractures of the maxilla produce an opening into the nasal cavity and mandibular fractures often have concomitant mucosal injuries, patient management should include antibacterial therapy for five to ten days.

1. Barchfeld, W. P.: A mandibular splint for a dog. J. Am. Vet. Med. Assoc. 133:209, 1958.
2. Brinker, W. O.: Fractures of the upper and lower jaw. In Small Animal Fractures, 3rd rev. Continuing Education Service, Michigan State University, 1978.
3. Brinker, W. O., and Flo, G.: Principles and application of external skeletal fixation. Vet. Clin. North Am. 5:197, 1975.
4. Cechner, P. E.: Malocclusion in the dog caused by intramedullary pin fixation of mandibular fractures: two case reports. J. Am. Anim. Hosp. Assoc. 16:79, 1980.
5. Chaffee, V. W.: A technique for fixation of bilateral mandibular fractures caudal to the canine teeth in the dog. Vet. Med./Small Anim. Clin. 73:907, 1978.
6. Gage, E. D.: Surgical correction for fractures involving the nasal and frontal sinuses. Vet. Med./Small Anim. Clin. 65:1070, 1970.
7. Garruba, C. N., Jr., and Robertson, R. D.: Lag screw repair of feline mandibular symphyseal fracture. Vet. Med./Small Anim. Clin. 74:1752, 1979.
8. Hartsfield, S., Gendreau, C., et al.: Endotracheal intubation by pharyngotomy. J. Am. Anim. Hosp. Assoc. 13:29, 1979.
9. Hinko, P. J.: Reduction and fixation of symphyseal fractures of the mandible. J. Am. Anim. Hosp. Assoc. 12:98, 1976.
10. Kitto, H. W.: A technique of mandibular fixation in cat symphyseal fractures. Vet. Rec. 91:591, 1972.
11. Lantz, G.: Interarcade wiring as a method of fixation for selected mandibular injuries. J. Am. Anim. Hosp. Assoc. 17:599, 1981.
12. Lantz, G., Cantwell, H. D., et al.: Unilateral mandibular condylectomy: experimental and clinical results. J. Am. Anim. Hosp. Assoc. 18:883, 1982.
13. Lieberman, L. L.: Open reduction of fractures of the mandible of dogs and cats. J. Am. Vet. Med. Assoc. 132:334, 1958.
14. Merkley, D. F., and Brinker, W. O.: Facial reconstruction following massive bilateral maxillary fracture in the dog. J. Am. Anim. Hosp. Assoc. 12:831, 1976.
15. Nibley, W.: Treatment of caudal mandibular fractures: a preliminary report. J. Am. Anim. Hosp. Assoc. 17:555, 1981.
16. Peacock, E. E., and Van Winkle, W.: Wound Repair, 2nd ed. W. B. Saunders, Philadelphia, 1976.
17. Piermattei, D. L., and Greeley, R. G.: An Atlas of Surgical Approaches to the Bones of the Dog and Cat, 2nd ed. W. B. Saunders, Philadelphia, 1979.
18. Robins, G. M., and Read, R. A.: The use of a transfixation splint to stabilize a bilateral mandibular fracture in a dog. J. Small Anim. Pract. 22:759, 1981.
19. Ross, D. L.: Anterior mandibular fracture fixation. In Bojrab, M. J. (ed.): Current Techniques in Small Animal Surgery. Lea & Febiger, Philadelphia, 1975.
20. Rudy, R. L.: Fractures of the maxilla and mandible. In Bojrab, M. J. (ed.): Current Techniques in Small Animal Surgery. Lea & Febiger, Philadelphia, 1975.
21. Stambaugh, J. E., and Nunamaker, D. M.: External skeletal fixation of comminuted maxillary fractures in dogs. Vet. Surg. 11:72, 1982.
22. Turner, A. S.: Surgical management of depression fractures of the equine skull. Vet. Surg. 8:29, 1979.
23. Weigel, J. P., Dorn, A. S., et al.: The use of the biphase external fixation splint for repair of canine mandibular fractures. J. Am. Anim. Hosp. Assoc. 17:547, 1981.
24. Withrow, S. J.: Taping of the mandible in treatment of mandibular fractures. J. Am. Anim. Hosp. Assoc. 17:27, 1981.
25. Withrow, S. J., and Doige, C. E.: En bloc resection of a juxtacortical and three intra-osseous osteosarcomas of the zygomatic arch in dogs. J. Am. Anim. Hosp. Assoc. 16:867, 1980.
26. Wolff, E. F.: Use of a cortical screw in repair of fractured mandibular symphysis in the cat. Vet. Med./Small Anim. Clin. 69:859, 1974.

Chapter **163** # Degenerative Joint Disease

Steven P. Arnoczky and Alan J. Lipowitz

Degenerative joint disease (DJD) is a chronic noninflammatory disorder of moveable joints characterized by articular cartilage degeneration, marginal osteophyte formation, and relative degenerative and proliferative joint changes.[4,23,24] The disease affects many species of animals, including humans, and has been observed in fossil dinosaur skeletons dating from 200 million years ago.[23] The terminology for this disorder is varied and often confusing, and at least 50 terms have been used to describe it. Although osteoarthritis is the most popular term, it is inaccurate in that it implies an inflammatory process

pertrophic arthritis, senescent arthritis, and osteoarthrosis are other terms that have been used, but degenerative joint disease is the most accurate description of the underlying pathological process.[23]

Pathogenesis of Degenerative Joint Disease

Degenerative joint disease classically has been divided into primary and secondary etiologies.[4,8,13,19,22–24,28–30] In primary DJD, the degeneration of the articular cartilage is the initial change and appears to be intrinsic in origin. In secondary DJD, alterations of the articular tissues are a consequence of abnormal mechanical stresses acting on the joints. Although primary and secondary DJD are discussed as separate entities, the DJD observed in animals actually may be an interaction of the two.

PRIMARY DEGENERATIVE JOINT DISEASE

Primary or idiopathic DJD has been related to changes originating within the cartilage itself. These changes may be associated with the aging process, but the exact mechanism is not known.

Many investigators consider that primary DJD is the result of the constant "wear and tear" on the joints throughout life, and that the joints that bear the most stress are the most vulnerable.[9,19] A study in dogs lent support to this theory by demonstrating a high incidence of DJD in the hip and shoulder joints of Huskies used for pulling sleds.[2] Conversely, others have shown that the occasional use of the unloaded, noncontact areas of the joint during some extreme range of movement causes the initial damage to the joint.[7] From these studies, it is reasonable to assume that the initial damage to the joint cartilage can occur in both weight-bearing and nonweight-bearing areas of the joint cartilage.[19]

It has been postulated that following initial trauma to the joint surface, the synovial fluid, which contains a hyaluronidase enzyme, gains access to the matrix through a break in the surface layer of the cartilage and begins to break down the chondroitin chains of mucopolysaccharides.[3] Additional stress on the cartilage produces more cracks and fissures and allows more synovial fluid to seep through; thus, the process continues. It has been further proposed that the chondrocytes themselves may release lysosomal hydrolases which degrade either the protein or the polysaccharide portion of the proteoglycan, and a vicious cycle of degeneration ensues.[5]

Other theories for the pathogenesis of primary DJD are based on histologic studies of normal and degenerated joints.[23] One study has shown that with cartilage disruption and matrix depletion the mature chondrocyte reverts to a more primitive and metabolically active cell capable of matrix repair.[13] It is not certain whether this response is an attempt by the cell to compensate for the loss of matrix or whether the cell change is primary and in some way related to the initiation of the disease process. Another theory suggests that the inability of vascular tissue and mesenchymal cells from the bone marrow to gain access to the cartilage following closure of the epiphyseal plate limits the potential for repair of cartilage defects, thus permitting further cartilage degeneration to occur.[22]

SECONDARY DEGENERATIVE JOINT DISEASE

Secondary DJD occurs in response to interference with the normal mechanical properties of the joint. Most of the DJD observed in small animals is secondary to some demonstrable mechanical stress.[4,11,19,31] The mechanical stress may be of the various kinds and degrees incurred by abnormal conformation, congenital or adaptational deformities of the skeleton, abnormal locomotion, or trauma. The most common causes of secondary DJD in the dog are hip dysplasia, Legg-Perthés disease, osteochondritis dissecans, chronic patellar dislocations, elbow dysplasia, trauma, and joint instability secondary to ligamentous insufficiency.[4,19] In these instances, the normal biomechanics of the joint are altered, and the resultant pathological motion produces changes in that articular cartilage as well as in other joint structures.

It is usually easy to trace the underlying cause of secondary DJD as long as the changes are moderate. In more advanced cases it is often impossible to tell whether the DJD is primary or secondary.[19]

Pathology

On gross examination, normal articular cartilage is white, translucent, and smooth. With early degenerative changes, the cartilage is likely to become yellowish, opaque, and less elastic than normal. The articular cartilage shows local areas of softening (chondromalacia) and roughening. Chondromalacia is the earliest sign of degeneration and is attributed to a decrease in sulfated mucopolysaccharides in the ground substance of the cartilage.[11,13,23,28,29] The softened cartilage is mechanically inadequate to support the collagen framework, the complex structure of which begins to break down.[23,27] There is a dehiscence of cartilage along the planes of the collagen fibers, and the articular surfaces show irregular depressions, pits, and fibrillations. Fibrillation is the term applied to the exposure of the collagen framework through the loss of ground substance.[28,29]

Histologically, the softened cartilage demonstrates clustering, or "clones," of cartilage cells. Some pathologists regard this as a response to the dehiscence of tissue, either as an abortive repair phenomenon or as a consequence of the increased access of the synovial fluid.[29] The cells begin to show mucoid

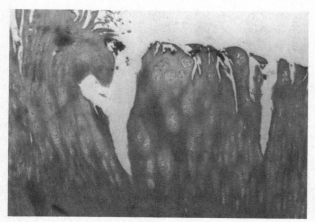

Figure 163–1. Fibrillated articular cartilage illustrating the clefts within the matrix and the "clones" of chondrocytes. (H & E, ×40)

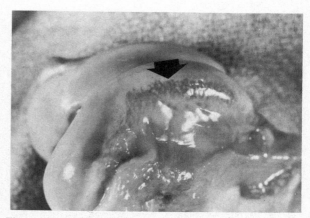

Figure 163–3. The medial femoral condyle of a dog three weeks after resection of the anterior cruciate ligament. Note the area of hyperemia at the attachment of the synovial membrane (arrow).

degeneration,[3] and a loss of metachromasia is evident[22,29] (Fig. 163–1).

As fibrillation progresses, the cartilage may fragment and erode, a result of erosion of the fibrillar cartilage in those areas where it comes into functional contact with apposing articular surfaces. Erosion may continue until all cartilage is worn away and the subchondral bone is exposed (Fig. 163–2). The subchondral bone becomes sclerotic from mechanical pressure or the effect of synovial fluid, a process called eburnation,[19,22] and looks like polished ivory. With increasingly severe degeneration, changes occur in the marginal joint tissues. The synovial membrane shows a proliferation of the surface cells, an increase in vascularity, and a gradual fibrosis of the subsynovial tissue. [1,22] The fibrous portion of the joint capsule becomes thick and sclerotic.

Formation of Periarticular Osteophytes

In secondary DJD associated with instability, proliferative changes occur in the periarticular areas of the joint. These changes always begin in the periarticular region of the joint at the attachments of the

synovial membrane[14] (Fig. 163–3). The initial change is a fibrous hypertrophy, which eventually forms cartilage and immature bone (Fig. 163–4). As growth of the osteophyte continues, the cortex is penetrated by vessels, and communication with the underlying bone marrow cavity is established (Fig. 163–5). It is not certain whether osteophytes in all forms of DJD exhibit this histogenesis. However, it is thought that once a joint is subjected to repeated abnormal motion, the osteophytes develop in this manner. These periarticular changes are not correlated with articular cartilage changes and often develop in the presence of normal articular cartilage.[14]

In long-term (two-year) studies of knee instability in the dog secondary to anterior cruciate ligament resection, it was found that there were minimal changes in the articular cartilage despite large periarticular osteophyte formation, proliferative thickening of the joint capsule, and degeneration of the menisci.[15] Periarticular osteophytes, therefore, are a primary sign of instability and are not necessarily

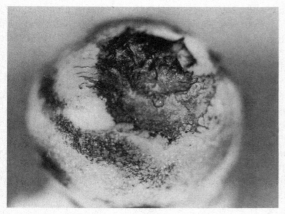

Figure 163–2. Femoral head of a dog. The cartilage surface has been painted with India ink to illustrate areas of fissuring, pitting, and cartilage erosion.

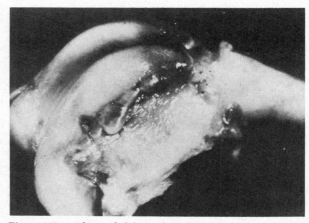

Figure 163–4. The medial femoral condyle of a dog three months after resection of the anterior cruciate ligament. Note the periarticular osteophyte formation. (Reprinted with permission from Arnoczky, S. P., and Marshall, J. L.: Degenerative joint disease. In Bojrab, M. J. (ed.): Pathophysiology of Small Animal Surgery. Lea and Febiger, Philadelphia, 1981.)

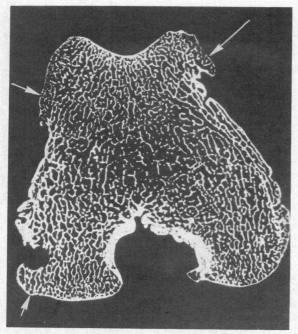

Figure 163–5. Microradiograph of mature osteophytes *(arrows)* with communication of its marrow spaces with those of the preexisting bone. (Reprinted with permission from Arnoczky, S. P., and Marshall, J. L.: Degenerative joint disease. *In* Bojrab, M. J. (ed.): *Pathophysiology of Small Animal Surgery.* Lea & Febiger, Philadelphia, 1981.)

associated with articular cartilage degeneration. Along with the hypertrophied joint capsule, the osteophytes may represent part of a stabilization process because, as the joint eventually becomes stable, the osteophytes mature and cease growth.[15] The osteophytes may break loose and become free bodies in the joint ("joint mice").

Clinical Presentation

Primary degenerative joint disease is an insidious, progressive condition which most commonly affects older animals; secondary degenerative joint disease may be more acute in onset and occurs in the young or old patient. Once the pathological transformation begins, however, the general signs and symptoms are similar.

Animals affected with degenerative joint disease are usually presented with a history of lameness or gait abnormality. This may range from the subtle, such as difficulty in climbing stairs, jumping, and so on, to the obvious, such as a pronounced limp or nonweight-bearing lameness.

Since the majority of the cases of DJD that occur in small animals are the result of another condition, the primary etiology must be diagnosed and treated to curtail the degenerative processes that are occurring in the affected joint. A carefully taken history and a thorough physical examination are necessary in evaluating lameness. The patient's breed and age are combined with information from the history and physical examination and are central in reducing the list of differential diagnoses.

Physical examination should include all body systems, especially the nervous system, and not be confined solely to the apparently affected limb. Examination of the limb should include palpation of the musculature and joints; a comparison should be made with the opposite normal limb. The affected joint(s) should be manipulated gently through their full range of motion, and the vibratory sensations of crepitus should be noted if present. Crepitation usually indicates articular cartilage wear or periarticular changes (osteophyte formation, capsular thickening, and so on). Ligamentous and tendinous structures should be assessed for integrity and laxity. Again, this should be done throughout the range of motion.

Joint enlargement is most frequent in the more chronic cases and varies with periarticular changes. In chronic anterior cruciate ligament insufficiency, the soft tissue fibrosis that occurs over the medial condyle and collateral ligament is pathognomonic for this condition.

Excessive joint effusion is not a prominent feature of degenerative joint disease, although slight increases in joint fluid volume are not uncommon. In chronic cases the effusion is usually moderate and may not be readily detectable by palpation.

Radiographic Evaluation

Once the affected joint or joints have been determined, radiographs are taken to indicate the relative degree of the degenerative changes. It is important to obtain good quality radiographs of the joints in at least two standard views. Patient positioning is important, and sedation or anesthesia may be required.

The characteristic radiographic features of degenerative joint disease include subchondral bony sclerosis, subchondral cyst formation, joint space narrowing, and periarticular osteophyte formation.[16]

Subchondral bony sclerosis is most commonly seen in chronic cases of DJD. It appears as a homogeneous, radiodense area beneath the articular surface of the affected joint (Fig. 163–6). This increased density may reflect an increased stress on the subchondral bone, which was normally shared by the articular cartilage.

Subchondral cysts are not true cysts as they lack a definitive capsule but rather are fluid- or mucus-filled spaces in the subchondral bone. These spaces usually result from microfractures of the subchondral trabeculae in response to increased mechanical stresses. As fractures increase, the trabecular spaces coalesce, and a cystlike space is formed. Radiographically, these cysts appear as rounded, lucent areas surrounded by a thin layer of sclerotic subchondral bone (Fig. 163–7).

While joint space narrowing is a fairly consistent radiographic finding in chronic DJD, the interpreta-

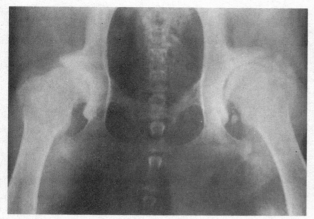

Figure 163–6. Ventrodorsal radiograph of a canine pelvis illustrating the radiographic changes associated with degenerative joint disease: subchondral bony sclerosis, joint space narrowing, and periarticular osteophyte formation.

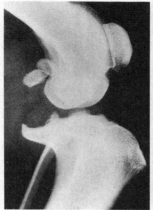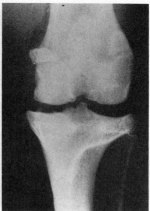

Figure 163–8. Stifle joint of a dog six months after transection of the anterior cruciate ligament. Note the osteophytes at the joint margins and in the intercondylar notch.

tion of this narrowing must be done with care. Joint space narrowing with chronic DJD occurs because of the loss of significant amounts of articular cartilage. This allows the more radiodense subchondral bone to come in closer contact, giving the appearance of a narrow joint space (Fig. 163–6). The radiographic appearance of the joint space, however, is also affected by patient positioning (weight-bearing vs. non-weight-bearing) at the time of the radiograph, joint effusion, and the integrity of the ligamentous structures of the affected joints. A true assessment of joint space width is best made from radiographs of the joint during weight-bearing. However, this may not be practical.

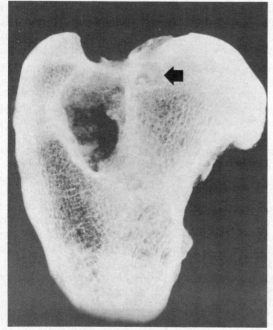

Figure 163–7. Proximal femur specimen illustrating a subchondral bone cyst *(arrow)*.

Osteophyte formation is most commonly seen in chronic cases of DJD. As noted, osteophytes appear as periarticular spurs or outgrowths of bone arising from the margins of the articular surface (Fig. 163–8).

Clinical Laboratory Findings

No specific diagnostic laboratory abnormalities are associated with DJD. Complete blood counts and serum chemistries are usually within normal limits unless other conditions exist.

In both acutely and chronically affected joints, synovial fluid analysis may demonstrate an increase in volume (often 10 to 20 times normal) and a decrease in viscosity caused by a fall in the concentration of hyaluronic acid.[22] The total amount of mucopolysaccharide in the joint, however, is not decreased.[22] The total cell count of the synovial fluid is also increased in both acute and chronic DJD. The total cell count rarely rises above 500 cells per mm^3 in chronic DJD and contains 70 to 80 per cent lymphocytes and an average of 5 per cent neutrophils. The total protein content of the fluid also increases.[22] Synovial fluid changes are a result of inflammation of the synovial membrane and consequent increased blood flow and capillary permeability.[22]

Treatment of Degenerative Joint Disease

The goals in the treatment of degenerative joint disease are to alleviate patient discomfort, prevent further degenerative joint changes from occurring, and restore the affected joint(s) to as near normal and painfree function as possible.

Because most DJD in small animals is the result of another condition, the primary etiology must first be diagnosed and treated to halt or minimize the degenerative processes which occur in the affected joint(s). This includes such procedures as joint stabilization in cruciate ligament rupture, removal of a loose body as in ununited anconeal process or osteochondritis dissecans, and correction of abnormal joint mechanics as in patellar or shoulder luxations. While such procedures may eliminate the inciting etiology, degenerative joint disease is not a condition that can be completely cured in the sense of returning the patient to normal. In chronic cases in which degenerative changes are already present, some residual abnormality may remain in the affected joint(s) even after surgical correction of the inciting etiology. This abnormality often continually produces difficulties for the animal. Thus, the treatment of degenerative joint disease must also include medical methods to alleviate patient discomfort.

Medical treatment of degenerative joint disease is symptomatic and nonspecific; basically it consists of rest, physical therapy, and drug therapy. Rest and physical therapy are employed to initially decrease inflammation of the affected joint and to strengthen the supporting structures of the joint. Pharmacological therapy includes a wide variety of compounds and medicaments, each with essentially the same purpose: to reduce inflammation and act as an analgesic.

Rest, especially in the acute stages of DJD when joint effusion is present and the inflammatory process is at its peak, is very important. Once joint effusion has subsided and the analgesic anti-inflammatory medications have been given, controlled exercise is advisable. Stressful activity should be kept to a minimum and the animal's tolerance to activity judged carefully. Walking the animal on a leash several times a day for short distances is advisable initially. As the patient responds to this and if there are no untoward effects, such as a reluctance to walk, stiffness or soreness several hours following the activity, or changes in gait patterns, longer walks should be undertaken. More strenuous activities can be introduced as the patient gains strength.

In obese patients, weight reduction should be encouraged. The increased sedentary nature of animals with degenerative joint disease, however, makes this task even more difficult. The owners should be made aware of the stresses placed on the joints by increased weight and a program of weight reduction instituted.

Drug Therapy

No drugs or combination of drugs will consistently prevent or reverse the pathological changes of degenerative joint disease. Drugs are administered primarily as analgesics and anti-inflammatory agents for the symptomatic relief of clinical signs.

Aspirin. Acetylsalicylic acid (aspirin) is an analgesic and anti-inflammatory as well as antipyretic agent and is the basic drug for the treatment of degenerative joint disease. It is a nonsteroidal anti-inflammatory agent (NSAIA). When used with care it can be quite effective and relatively free of side effects. Aspirin affects a wide variety of metabolic processes and enzyme systems. Mild-to-moderate peripheral pain is relieved by the ability of aspirin to block the effect of inflammatory mediators, such as bradykinin, on pain endings.[6] In contrast to the opiates, aspirin acts as an analgesic peripherally rather than centrally. The action of aspirin as an anti-inflammatory agent is due to its ability to inhibit prostaglandin synthesis.[26]

As with any drug, sufficient dosages must be taken to obtain adequate effects. A dose of 25 mg/kg three times daily is given initially and the therapeutic results observed.[6,26,32] If the desired effects have not been obtained in four to five days, the dosage may be increased slightly. Dosages reaching 50 mg/kg may produce emesis.[32] Vomiting can occur at lower doses as well and may be prevented by administering the drug with food. Patients with gastric intolerance to plain aspirin may tolerate it well when taken with oral antacids such as magnesium-aluminum hydroxide.

At therapeutic levels, aspirin is virtually free of serious side effects. Gross overdoses may produce hyperthermia, severe acid-base and electrolyte disturbances, renal hemorrhage, convulsions, and coma.[6] Treatment for such acute and severe problems includes gastric lavage to remove any unabsorbed drug, urine alkalinization with sodium bicarbonate to enhance renal excretion of salicylate, and peritoneal dialysis to remove salicylates from plasma.[6]

Less life-threatening toxic manifestations include skin eruptions, edema, gastrointestinal bleeding and ulceration, hypoprothrombinemia, vomiting, and deafness. In the dog, the most common of these are vomiting and melena. Withholding medication alleviates these problems.[6]

Phenylbutazone. This agent has been used with a good deal of success in the symptomatic treatment of chronic DJD. It is quite valuable in some animals that are unresponsive to aspirin therapy. Because of the bone marrow depression it may cause, phenylbutazone has not been as widely used in humans as it has in animals. When properly administered and monitored, it can be a most valuable drug for the symptomatic treatment of degenerative joint disease in the dog.

Phenylbutazone is a nonsteroidal anti-inflammatory drug with a mechanism of action similar to that of aspirin.[26] It is given in doses of 1.0 mg/kg of body weight three times daily. Bone marrow depression may be the most serious of its side effects, and animals on long-term therapy with the drug should be evaluated periodically with hemograms. Peptic ulcers, malaise, pruritus, rashes, and renal dysfunction are among human side effects.[12]

Other Nonsteroidal Anti-Inflammatory Agents (NSAIA). These agents are similar in their action to aspirin. They are anti-inflammatory, analgesic, and antipyretic and act by the inhibition of prostaglandin synthesis or release. These drugs include fenoprofen, ibuprofen, indomethacin, mefenamic acid, naproxen, oxyphenylbutazone, sulindac, and tolmetin.[18] While these drugs have gained great popularity in the treatment of human DJD because of a lower incidence of side effects, few data show that any of these compounds are superior to aspirin in effectiveness when the object of therapy is an immediate anti-inflammatory effect. Many of these drugs have not been identified for use in animals, although ibuprofen and indomethacin have been suggested for the treatment of DJD in the dog. Ibuprofen is given orally in a total dose of 15 mg/kg of body weight divided three times daily, and indomethacin is given in an oral dose of 1.0 to 1.25 mg/kg of body weight divided two to three times daily.[21] Both drugs, however, may cause gastrointestinal problems with prolonged use.

Steroids. Corticosteroids are potent anti-inflammatory agents which may be beneficial in some animals with degenerative joint disease. They should not be considered the agent of choice in the treatment of DJD but can be reserved for those cases unresponsive to the previously mentioned agents. Steroids are most commonly administered orally or parenterally in low doses and for short periods of time. Prednisolone may be given parenterally at a dose of 1 to 2 mg/kg followed by an oral maintenance dose of 0.5 to 1 mg/kg once daily. The lowest possible maintenance dose should be established, such as alternate day or every third day administration of 0.5 to 1.0 mg/kg.[12]

Steroids have been used with nonsteroidal anti-inflammatory drugs. Aspirin and corticosteroids are administered concomitantly in the doses previously mentioned.[12] Each subsequent day, decreasing doses are administered so that by the fifth or sixth day steroids are no longer given and the aspirin is being administered in low maintenance doses.[12] Although some patients respond to this regime, they may be prone to gastrointestinal hemorrhage.[10]

Intra-articular injection of steroids has been used in both humans and animals for the treatment of degenerative joint disease. Effects of the drug last for varying periods and are often repeated on an "as needed" basis. The beneficial effects derived from intra-articular steroid administration may be due to the absorption and systemic distribution of the drug.[17] The practice of intra-articular steroid injection, however, is not without complications. Postinjection flare, a synovitis induced by steroid crystals, may occur. In addition, the injected joint may be more susceptible to infection. Experiments in animals and clinical observations in humans have shown that intra-articular steroids have a deleterious effect on articular cartilage already damaged by disease.[17] Thus we do not advocate the use of intra-articular steroids for the treatment of DJD in small animals.

As noted previously, the degenerative changes in a joint are not totally reversible, and the animal (or owner) must learn to "live within the limits" of these debilitated joints. Most animals voluntarily limit activity or "guard" the joint in response to the pain and discomfort of degenerative joint disease, so owners should be cautioned that the analgesia euphoria associated with medications may encourage the animal to be more active. Such overactivity could further compromise the debilitated joint, resulting in increased degenerative changes as well as increased discomfort once the medication wears off. Thus, the policy of rest and limited exercise should be stressed during medical therapy of degenerative joint disease.

Surgical Treatment

As noted, surgical correction of the inciting cause of degenerative joint disease may limit or halt the progression of the degenerative changes. In some cases, however, the degenerative changes are so advanced that surgical correction of the initial problem or medical therapy or both are not sufficient to return the joint to painfree function. In these joints salvage procedures such as arthrodesis, excision arthroplasty, or total joint replacement may be the only alternative. The reader is directed to these chapters for specific indications and techniques.

1. Arnoczky, S. P., and Marshall, J. L.: Degenerative joint disease. *In* Bojrab, M. J. (ed.): *Pathophysiology in Small Animal Surgery.* Lea & Febiger, Philadelphia, 1981.
2. Bellars, A. R. M., and Godsal, M. F.: Veterinary studies on the British Antarctic Survey's sledge dogs. II. Occupational osteoarthritis. Br. Antarctic Survey Bull. *22*:15, 1969.
3. Bollet, A. J.: An essay on the biology of osteoarthritis. Arthritis Rheum. *12*:152, 1969.
4. Brown, S. G.: Skeletal diseases. *In* Ettinger, S. J.: *Textbook of Veterinary Internal Medicine.* W. B. Saunders, Philadelphia, 1975.
5. Chrisman, O. D.: Biochemical aspects of degenerative joint disease. Clin. Orthop. *64*:77, 1969.
6. Davis, L. E.: Clinical pharmacology of salicylates. J. Am. Vet. Med. Assoc. *176*:65, 1980.
7. Goodfellow, J., and Bullough, P. G.: The pattern of aging of the articular cartilage of the elbow. J. Bone Jt. Surg. *49B*:175, 1967.
8. Jaffe, H. L.: *Metabolic, Degenerative, and Inflammatory Diseases of Bones and Joints.* Lea & Febiger, Philadelphia, 1972.
9. Jubb, K. V. F., and Kennedy, P. C.: *Pathology of Domestic Animals.* 2nd ed. Vol. 1. Academic Press, New York, 1970.
10. Kantor, T. G.: Anti-inflammatory and analgesic drugs. *In* Katz, W. A. (ed.): *Rheumatic Diseases.* J. B. Lippincott, Philadelphia, 1977.
11. Leonard, E. F.: *Orthopedic Surgery of the Dog and Cat.* W. B. Saunders, Philadelphia, 1971.
12. Lipowitz, A. J.: Degenerative joint disease. *In* Newton, C. D., and Nunamaker, D. M. (eds.): *Textbook of Small Animal Orthopaedics.* J. B. Lippincott, Philadelphia, in press.
13. Mankin, H. J.: Biochemical and metabolic aspects of osteoarthritis. Orthop. Clin. North Am. *2*:1, 1971.
14. Marshall, J. L.: Periarticular osteophytes: Initiation and formation in the knee of the dog. Clin. Orthop. *62*:37, 1967.
15. Marshall, J. L., and Olsson, S. E.: Instability of the knee. J. Bone Jt. Surg. *55A*:1561, 1971.
16. Morgan, J. P.: *Radiology in Veterinary Orthopaedics.* Lea & Febiger, Philadelphia, 1972.
17. Moskowitz, R. W.: Treatment of osteoarthritis. *In* McCarty, D. J. (ed.): *Arthritis and Allied Conditions.* Lea & Febiger, Philadelphia, 1979.
18. Nickander, R., McMahon, F. G., and Ridolfo, A. S.: Nonsteroidal anti-inflammatory agents. Ann. Rev. Pharmacol. Toxicol. *19*:469, 1979.

19. Olsson, S. E.: Degenerative joint disease. A review with special reference to the dog. J. Small Anim. Prac. 12:333, 1971.
20. Owens, J. M., and Ackerman, N.: Roentgenology of arthritis. Vet. Clin. North Am. 8:453, 1978.
21. Pedersen, N. C., and Pool, R.: Canine joint disease. Vet. Clin. North Am. 8:465, 1978.
22. Pond, M. J.: Normal joint tissues and their reaction to injury. Vet. Clin. North Am. 1:523, 1971.
23. Rodman, G. P. (ed.): Primer on the rheumatic diseases. J. Am. Med. Assoc. 224(Suppl.):78, 1973.
24. Rudy, R. L., Hohn, R. B., and Harrison, J. W.: Rheumatoid and Osteoarthritis in the Dog. Twenty-second Annual Gaines Veterinary Symposium, 27, 1972.
25. Rydell, N. W., Butler, J., and Balazs, E. A.: Hyaluronic acid in synovial fluid. VI. Effect of intra-articular injection of hyaluronic acid on the clinical symptoms of arthritis in track horses. Acta Vet. Scand. 11:139, 1970.

26. Short, C. R., and Beadle, R. E.: Pharmacology of antiarthritic drugs. Vet. Clin. North Am. 8:401, 1978.
27. Sledge, C. B.: Structure, development, and function of joints. Orthop. Clin. North Am. 6:619, 1975.
28. Sokoloff, L.: The Biology of Degenerative Joint Disease. University of Chicago Press, Chicago, 1969.
29. Sokoloff, L.: Pathology and pathogenesis of osteoarthritis. In McCarty, D. J., and Hollander, J. L. (eds.): Arthritis and Allied Conditions: A Textbook of Rheumatology. Lea and Febiger, Philadelphia, 1979.
30. Turek, S.: Orthopaedics: Principles and Their Application. 3rd ed. J. B. Lippincott, Philadelphia, 1977.
31. Whittick, W. G.: Canine Orthopaedics. Lea & Febiger, Philadelphia, 1974.
32. Yeary, R. A., and Brant, R. J.: Aspirin dosages for the dog. J. Am. Vet. Med. Assoc. 167:63, 1975.

Chapter **164**

Immune-Mediated Articular Disease

Alan J. Lipowitz

Immune-mediated articular diseases of the dog are inflammatory, purulent, and nonseptic in nature.[28] Two distinct clinical types have been recognized: the erosive type that is usually evidenced by loss of joint surfaces and articular cartilage destruction and the nonerosive type in which articular cartilage is usually not affected grossly.[25,27] The erosive type is similar to human rheumatoid arthritis and is far less common than the nonerosive type. Nonerosive immune-mediated articular disease of the dog is much more common than the erosive type and is frequently associated with systemic lupus erythematosus. Early signs of each condition may be similar.

Immune complexes are integral to the pathogenesis of both types of immune arthritis in the dog. In the erosive type the complexes are frequently called rheumatoid factors. These immune adherent units are composed of altered host IgG that serves as antigen, host IgM produced in response to the antigenic IgG, and complement. In the nonerosive type host cellular nuclear material becomes antigenic, stimulating antinuclear antibody production. The deposition and phagocytosis of these complexes within certain body tissues is responsible for the lesions in each condition.

Nonerosive Immune-Mediated Articular Disease

This type of articular disease in the dog is most commonly associated with systemic lupus erythematosus (SLE). Occasionally it has been reported in dogs without systemic lupus erythematosus that have inflammatory conditions such as bacterial endocarditis, pyometra, dirofilariasis, chronic otitis, and fungal infections.[27] In these situations one or more joints may be affected although the articular involvement is a small part of the syndrome. The infection is confirmed by culture or histologic examination of the primary lesions. Organisms are usually not identified in the synovial fluid or synovial membrane of affected joints.

The articular component may be due to the deposition of immune complexes in synovial tissues and their subsequent phagocytosis, resulting in synovitis and joint effusion. The immune complexes are most likely composed of antigenic substances originating from the invading organisms and antibodies produced by the host. Treatment is directed at the primary problem; joint involvement subsides with time as the primary problem is brought under control.

Systemic Lupus Erythematosus (SLE)

Systemic lupus erythematosus affects many organ systems. Polyarthritis, dermatitis, myositis, glomerulonephritis, and anemia are frequent manifestations of the disease. Additional findings include oral ulcerations, petechial hemorrhage, pleuritis, myocarditis, pneumonitis, pericarditis, intermittent fever, and generalized lymphadenopathy.[4,6,33] Every affected animal does not exhibit all these findings. Polyarthritis and dermatitis (although not necessarily concomitant) are most frequently found.

The etiology of SLE is unknown. Though confirmation is lacking, there is a strong suspicion that certain viruses are prominent in the pathogenesis.[33] In addition, certain individuals appear more prone to SLE than others; in humans there may be a familial tendency to develop the disease.[37] However, specific genetic predisposition has not been confirmed. Extensive genetic and breeding studies in a colony of dogs with SLE have failed to confirm any conventional genetic mechanisms by which the disease may be transmitted.[12] Although the specific causes of SLE remain unknown, present evidence indicates the importance of genetics, immunoregulatory defects, viral infections, and other factors in disease development.[33]

Incidence

The dog with SLE may have a variety of clinical signs. Almost any body system may be involved. Age at the time of presentation ranges from 2 months to 12 years.[6,33] Collies, Shetland sheepdogs, and beagles are more commonly affected than other breeds; German shepherds and poodles are also more prone to the condition.[33] Males and females are nearly equally affected although different retrospective studies favor one sex or the other.[4,6,33]

Patients are most frequently seen because of polyarthritis or dermatitis or both. Concomitant joint and skin involvement is quite variable. Other common findings include anemia, proteinuria, and fever. Less frequently, oral ulcers, pleuritis, myocarditis, myositis, and thrombocytopenia are noted.[4,6,33]

Clinical Presentation, General Features, and Pathology

Signs are often episodic in nature. The first abnormalities noted by the owner are depression, anorexia, and a reluctance to move about. Fever often accompanies these episodes, each lasting for several days. Spontaneous remission is followed by recurrence varying from days to months.

Musculoskeletal Involvement

Polyarthritis occurs in over 60 per cent of the affected animals.[4,6] In the majority two or more joints are noticeably affected. These animals move about reluctantly, taking short, purposeful steps. In the acute condition affected joints may be warm compared with nonaffected joints, may be enlarged owing to joint capsule effusion, and may be painful when palpated. Periarticular soft tissue swelling may also be present.

In chronic cases periarticular enlargement is due to soft tissue fibrosis, and affected joints usually are not painful on palpation. Range of motion may be decreased by joint effusion or enlargement of periarticular tissue. In some cases joint laxity may be noted. Periarticular or intra-articular ligaments may be weakened by the inflammatory processes of the disease, resulting in joint instability. Hindleg lameness

with an anterior draw sign in the stifle caused by a ruptured or weakened anterior cruciate ligament is common. Secondary osteoarthritis may also develop in the SLE-affected joint as a result of ligamentous injury and joint laxity.

Myositis has been reported as an accompanying feature of SLE.[4] While not as frequently encountered as polyarthritis, the inflammatory involvement of muscle should not be overlooked, especially in the rare patient that has difficulty walking but does not have joint involvement. Histologically, lymphocytes and plasma cells are found in the perimysium and perivascular areas of affected muscle.[4]

Common radiographic features of the active stages of SLE include joint capsule distension and periarticular soft tissue swelling (Fig. 164–1). In chronic cases, increased periarticular soft tissue fibrosis produces increased densities about the affected joints. Periosteal reactivity may be seen at the bony attachments of ligaments and joint capsule. Also, changes of secondary osteoarthritis may be found in chronic cases, particularly in those in which ligamentous damage has occurred.[4,27]

SLE is a nonerosive, immune-mediated disease, and, unlike rheumatoid arthritis, there is little or no loss of articular cartilage. The striking histological feature of affected joints is found in the synovial membrane. Synoviocytic proliferation and fibrous villous synovitis are typical. Increased numbers of plasma cells, monocytes, and neutrophils are found infiltrating the subsynoviocytic layers (Fig. 164–2). These cells are scattered throughout the tissue and also may be found in small aggregates, particularly around vessels in the deeper regions of the subsynoviocytic tissues. Pannus formation and destruction

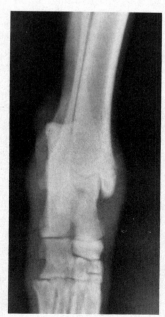

Figure 164–1. Systemic lupus erythematosus. Joint capsule distension and periarticular soft tissue swelling in the tibiotarsal joint of a one-year-old springer spaniel.

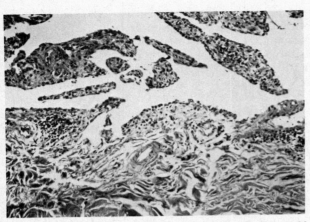

Figure 164–2. Synovial membrane from the stifle of a six-year-old Labrador retriever with ruptured anterior cruciate ligament and SLE. Note the villous hypertrophy, increased subsynovial vascularity, and plasma cell and lymphocyte infiltration of the synoviocytic and subsynoviocytic layers.

of articular cartilage are not prominent, although increased vascularity and villous hypertrophy are noted.[27] Changes associated with secondary osteoarthritis also may be found, including periosteal new bone formation and fibrosis of periarticular soft tissue.

Synovial fluid from an affected joint is usually increased in volume and decreased in viscosity, with a mucin clot test rating of fair to poor. Cells in the fluid reflect the inflammatory, purulent, nonseptic nature of the joint involvement. White cell counts greater than 5,000 per mm³ are usually found but may range up to several thousand. Neutrophils are the predominant cell type. Lymphocytes, monocytes, and macrophages are also present (Fig. 164–3). On occasion, DNA material has been seen in phagocytic cells, and typical LE cells also have been identified.[28]

Skin and Mucocutaneous Lesions

Lesions of the skin, mucous membranes, and mucocutaneous areas are almost as prevalent as the

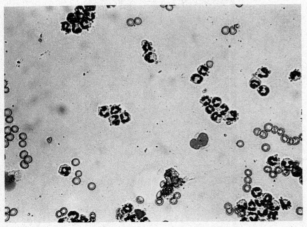

Figure 164–3. Synovial fluid from an affected joint of a dog with SLE. Mature neutrophils are the predominant cells. Mononuclear phagocytes are frequently seen as well.

occurrence of polyarthritis. Skin lesions and articular involvement do not necessarily occur in the same patient at the same time.

A variety of lesions may occur.[4,33] The most common is a seborrhea-like syndrome affecting the face, ears, and limbs, accompanied by erythema, crusting or scaling, alopecia, and pruritus. In other patients ulcers may be found at the mucocutaneous junctions of the oral commissures, anus, or vulva. Ulcers also may be found on the skin of the ventral abdomen, on distal limbs, and on the footpads. Oral ulcers may also occur.

The skin and mucous membrane lesions are associated with immune complex deposition. Complement components (C_3) and immunoglobulins (IgA, IgM) have been found by direct immunofluorescent staining in the basement membrane zone, in walls of small dermal vessels, and in intracellular spaces of the epithelium.[30,31,33]

Common histological findings of skin and mucosal biopsies include hydropic degeneration of the basal cell layer and mononuclear cell infiltration of periadnexal areas. Other findings may include focal thickening of the basement membrane zone, subepidermal vascular degeneration, pigmentary incontinence, and dyskeratosis.[7,33]

Renal Involvement

Nearly 50 per cent of SLE-affected dogs have proteinuria;[4,6,27,33] 30 to 1,000 mg/dl of urine have been reported.[27] Renal lesions include increased mesangial matrix, hyaline droplet formation in renal tubules, and infiltration of renal interstitium by mononuclear cells.[6] While involvement of other organ systems in an SLE patient may be more dramatic, one of the most common causes of death in dogs with SLE is renal failure.[33]

Hematological Involvement

Hemolytic anemia and thrombocytopenia are two components of classic canine SLE.[33] Autoimmune hemolytic anemia may occur, but chronic nonregenerative anemia is probably more common.[4,6,33] Approximately 50 per cent of SLE-affected dogs have anemia; 10 to 20 per cent may have hemolytic anemia; even fewer are Coombs'-positive.

Petechi may be found in SLE patients that are thrombocytopenic. They may occur on the mucous membranes of the mouth, vagina, or prepuce and in the skin.[4,6,33] Thrombocytopenia occurs in approximately 10 per cent of SLE-affected dogs. Circulating antiplatelet antibodies are probably responsible for the decreased number of platelets.[6,30,31,33]

Neutrophilia is a common finding.[3,6,18,33] Leukopenia has been reported but is unusual. Increased white blood cell counts may be a response to secondary bacterial infection or to the generalized inflammation of SLE.

Miscellaneous Organ Involvement [4,6,30,33]

Respiratory disease, manifested as pneumonia, interstitial pneumonitis, or pleuritis, may be found in a small number of cases. Myocarditis caused by ischemic necrosis of cardiac muscle fibers secondary to vasculitis is another infrequent finding. Clinically significant cardiac dysrhythmias may result from the myocardial necrosis.

Meningitis and myelitis resulting in central nervous system signs are rare but have been reported. Histological changes in the spleen and liver are known but are not severe enough to result in clinical signs.

Diagnosis

The variety of clinical signs make diagnosis difficult. Criteria have been established for the diagnosis of human[37] and canine[4,6,30,31,33] SLE. These include various clinical manifestations frequently found in SLE patients. The diagnostic criteria serve mainly to identify and classify patients with a particular set of signs and symptoms. This is valuable in the study of groups of patients, such as in comparing responses to different therapies in a similarly affected group of individuals. However, the clinician should not establish a diagnosis based on a list and lose sight of the patient and its problems. As more knowledge is gained regarding the pathogenesis, pathophysiology, and clinical expression, diagnostic criteria of SLE will continue to change.

Criteria for the diagnosis of canine SLE proposed by different groups are quite similar.[4,6,30,31,33] Each includes dermatological lesions typical of SLE: polyarthritis, hemolytic anemia, thrombocytopenia, protein-losing glomerulonephropathy, and the presence of antinuclear antibodies and lupus erythematosus cells. While no laboratory test is specific for a particular disease, according to the proposed diagnostic criteria, the presence of antinuclear antibodies or LE cells is almost mandatory if a diagnosis of SLE is to be made. While both have been reported in patients without SLE, when coupled with the signs typical of the disease a diagnosis of SLE can usually be made with confidence. Table 164–1 presents the most frequently cited criteria for canine SLE diagnosis.[4,6,30,31,33]

LE cells are polymorphonuclear phagocytes, primarily neutrophils, that have engulfed antibody-coated nuclear material of other cells. Nuclear material of damaged or ruptured leukocytes is exposed and is immunologically recognized as foreign protein. The antibody produced in response to this foreign protein is called an LE factor. An immune complex, called an LE body, is formed when the LE factor (antibody) combines with the foreign protein (antigen). Phagocytic cells that have engulfed the LE body are called LE cells. The formation of LE cells, termed the LE phenomenon, is a laboratory reaction and rarely occurs *in vivo*. LE factor cannot penetrate living cells.

TABLE 164–1.   Criteria for Diagnosis of Canine Systemic Lupus Erythematosus

Criterion	Clinical Expression
Dermatological disorders	Alopecia, erythema, scaling, crusting, ulceration; mucocutaneous involvement, ulceration; oral ulcers; petechiae
Arthritis	Nonseptic inflammatory nonerosive arthritis; swelling, tenderness, effusion usually involving two or more joints
Renal disorders	Proteinuria; renal casts; azotemia
Hematological disorders	Anemia; hemolytic anemia; thrombocytopenia
Immunological disorders	Positive LE cell preparation
Antinuclear antibody	Presence of antinuclear antibody by immunofluorescence or other reliable methods at any point in time in the absence of drugs that may produce "drug-induced lupus" syndrome
Serositis, myositis, myocarditis	Pleuritis, pericarditis, myocardial involvement documented by auscultation or ECG; generalized muscle involvement

The pathogenic mechanisms of disease activity in SLE are related to the phagocytosis of immune complexes deposited in various tissues. Autoantibodies and host nuclear material make up these immune complexes.[35] These antinuclear antibodies are formed in response to a variety of antigens. In dogs with SLE, antibodies to native, double-stranded DNA, heat-denatured single-stranded DNA, and antibodies to nonhistone nuclear protein have been detected.[12,18] However, false positives regarding double-stranded native DNA may occur because dogs possess a nonantibody anionic protein that nonspecifically binds DNA.[30,33] Each of the different types of antinuclear antibody are not present in every patient with SLE. However, there is good correlation between the clinical expression of the disease and the type of antinuclear antibody present.

Antinuclear antibodies are identified by indirect immunofluorescence and by measuring serum titers. Antinuclear antibodies are not species specific, and any test source of nuclear material may be used; the antiserum used must be species specific and polyvalent.[30,33] In testing for fluorescent antinuclear bodies, patient serum is reacted with specially prepared tissue sections—frequently mouse or rat liver—and the reactivity of the serum antinuclear antibody with the nuclear material of the tissue section is noted via fluorescent microscopy. Various patterns of nuclear fluorescence are characteristic of different antinuclear antibodies. Human and canine patients with SLE frequently exhibit a peripheral (rim) or homogeneous (diffuse) staining pattern.[30,33] Nuclear rim staining is produced by antibodies to native DNA and histones; a homogeneous pattern is produced by antibody to histones; a speckled pattern of nuclear staining is produced by the antibodies to nonhistone nuclear antigens.[18]

In 20 dogs with SLE and polyarthritis, proteinuria was transient or absent in 15. Antinuclear antibody staining in these dogs resulted in a speckled pattern. The remaining five dogs, each of which had persistent proteinuria, also had a homogeneous fluorescent staining pattern.[18] Many lists of diagnostic criteria for SLE emphasize the importance of antinuclear antibodies and LE cells in establishing a diagnosis. Unfortunately, there is no standardized, universally accepted test for antinuclear antibodies.[6,33] Results may vary considerably from one laboratory to another, making comparisons extremely difficult.

The lupus band test is a direct immunofluorescent technique for detecting immunoglobulins or complement components deposited at the dermal-epidermal junction in SLE patients. In a very limited number of dogs with SLE, 90 per cent had positive results; the immune components detected consisted of IgM or, more commonly, IgA. The complement component most frequently detected was C_3.[33] A positive lupus band test has also been found in dogs with discoid lupus erythematosus.[34]

Treatment

There is no known cure for SLE; the best that can be accomplished is to control the disease medically. In some well-controlled cases, long-term drugfree remissions may occur.

Long-term follow-up on the treatment and progress of a large number of canine SLE patients is not yet available. Approximately 40 per cent of dogs treated with glucocorticoids respond favorably.[4,27,33] Prednisolone (1.5 to 3.0 mg/kg) is given initially. After a favorable response, alternate-day drug administration may be begun. If the favorable response is maintained, prednisolone is discontinued. Return of signs necessitates further medication.

Patients refractory to prednisolone or those that develop adverse reactions to the drug (pancreatitis, diabetes mellitus, Cushing's syndrome, behavioral abnormalities) may respond to cyclophosphamide or azathioprine.[23,24,26] These drugs may be given in combination with reduced dosages of prednisolone or by themselves. Cyclophosphamide is given orally at 1.5 to 2.5 mg/kg of body weight for four consecutive days of each week; dogs weighing 10 kg and less receive 2.5 mg/kg; 10- to 25-kg dogs receive 2.0 mg/kg; and dogs weighing more than 25 kg receive 1.5 mg/kg. Azathioprine is given orally at 2.0 mg/kg daily. White blood cell counts are monitored weekly for the first several months of therapy; if the count falls below 7,000 per mm^3 the cytotoxic drug dosages are reduced by one-half. If remission occurs, azathioprine is discontinued first. Cyclophosphamide is discontinued after three consecutive months of remission. Some

dogs may require low doses of prednisolone after the cytotoxic agents have been discontinued.

Side effects of cytotoxic agents include vomiting, bloody diarrhea, salivation, changes in body temperature, anorexia, weight loss, and hematuria.[13] Administration of cytotoxic agents should stop if any of these signs develop. Therapy may be resumed at lower dosages after symptomatic treatment for the adverse reactions has been completed.

Erosive, Immune-Mediated Articular Disease

Great similarities exist between erosive, immune-mediated arthritis in dogs and rheumatoid arthritis in humans.[20,25] Clinical signs and findings, radiographic appearance, and pathological changes of affected tissues are nearly identical. To date, investigations of human rheumatoid arthritis have not determined its cause. Likewise, the etiology of rheumatoid arthritis in dogs is unknown. Infectious agents have been suspected, but extensive, repeated investigations have not identified an organism or organisms responsible for the disease. Streptococcal and mycobacterium infections in rabbits and mycoplasm and erysipelothrix infections in mammals and birds produce articular tissue changes nearly identical to those of rheumatoid arthritis. Experimental erysipelothrix infections in dogs have been used as a model for the study of rheumatoid arthritis.[44]

Despite these extensive studies, an infectious agent responsible for the disease has not been recovered from individuals with naturally occurring rheumatoid arthritis. Failure to isolate an infectious agent from a naturally affected individual does not necessarily eliminate the participation of the organism in the disease process. In experimental mycoplasma or erysipelothrix infections, the organisms can be recovered from affected articular tissues early in the disease process; when chronic synovitis is well established, the organisms can no longer be isolated. In addition, nonbiodegradable bacterial cell wall components can sustain chronic joint inflammation.[44] Replicating viruses and alteration of host cellular nuclear material by viral genomes have been suggested as possible causes of rheumatoid arthritis.[44] Cellular alterations suggesting viral activity have been found in the synoviocytes of dogs with erosive, immune-mediated joint disease by electron microscopy.[30,31] These changes also have been seen in tissues from dogs affected with neoplasia and known viral infections. Also, certain viral infections of other mammals and some birds produce a chronic synovitis closely resembling rheumatoid arthritis. To date, isolation or identification of viruses in the tissues of canine or human rheumatoid arthritis has not occurred.

Autoimmune components are significant factors in the initiation, development, and perpetuation of the erosive disease process. Inflammatory reactions accompanying the phagocytosis of immune complexes are responsible for the liberation of substances that cause destruction of articular cartilage and perpetuation of joint disease. These immune complexes are formed between structurally altered host IgG and IgM antibody produced in response to the altered IgG. Complement is also a component of the immune complex.

Rheumatoid factor is found in approximately 20 to 25 per cent of the dogs affected with erosive, immune articular disease.[26] In one study, 7 per cent (3 of 45) of normal dogs tested had significant titers of rheumatoid factor.[20] Rheumatoid factor also may be found in dogs with other autoimmune diseases, such as systemic lupus erythematosus. In a recent report, rheumatoid factor was found in 17 of 50 dogs (34 per cent) with keratoconjunctivitis sicca.[10]

Immune complexes other than those involving rheumatoid factors are found in joints affected by erosive articular disease.[29] Cartilage components and especially collagen are known stimulators of antibody production. During the destruction of articular cartilage, molecules of collagen and proteoglycan are altered and then immunologically perceived as foreign. Antibodies are produced, and immune complexes form. Phagocytosis occurs, releasing substances that cause further cartilage destruction and exposure of altered collagen. This is a self-perpetuating, self-destructive, autoimmune cycle. Indeed, this may be the mechanism in rheumatoid arthritis by which the ongoing destruction of articular tissues occurs.[29]

Proteases, enzymes, and other substances responsible for the destruction of the joint are produced by the affected synovial tissues.[2,9,42] The collagenases responsible for articular cartilage collagen breakdown are produced by polymorphonuclear leukocytes found in great numbers in the synovial fluid of affected joints and by fibroblasts in the synovial tissues. Prostaglandins, also released by activated synovial fibroblasts, are primarily responsible for resorption of subchondral bone.[3,19] It is now believed that these substances promote destruction of bone by aiding in the removal of its mineralized portions. Collagenases responsible for the degradation of bone collagen are effective only after the mineralized portion of bone has been removed.

Incidence and Clinical Presentation

Erosive, immune-mediated articular disease is an uncommon condition occurring primarily in small or toy breeds. Affected animals range in age from eight months to nine years, with an average age of onset of four years.[20,25]

Early clinical signs include a shifting lameness with swelling of the periarticular soft tissue. Very early in the course of the disease the lameness may involve only one joint, with barely noticeable joint capsule distension. As the condition progresses other joints become involved. Other clinical signs include anor-

exia, depression, pyrexia, and reluctance to move about. These signs, along with lameness and joint capsule distension, frequently wax and wane, lasting for several days only to subside.[20,25]

The condition is progressive; over a period of weeks to months the signs return; the time between clinical episodes decreases and the duration of each clinical episode increases. The continuous erosion of articular cartilage and damage to periarticular structures eventually leads to severe destruction of the articular surfaces, rupture of ligaments, and angular deformities. These deformities are more frequent in the carpal and tarsal joints; some have progressed to complete joint luxation. Lymphadenopathy, splenomegaly, anemia, and muscle atrophy are extra-articular or visceral manifestations of the condition.

Clinical Laboratory Findings

Hemograms are often normal or more commonly reflect a generalized inflammatory condition. In some cases a mild normochromic, normocytic anemia may be present. Leukocytosis, usually as a neutrophilia, is common, with counts rarely exceeding 30,000 per mm^3.[13,20,25] Other significant laboratory findings include a negative Coomb's test, increases in gamma-2 globulin and fibrinogen, and an increase in serum levels of total hemolytic complement.[20,24,25,40]

The common method of testing for serum rheumatoid factor involves coating particles (latex beads or sheep red blood cells) with antigen and agglutinating the particles with serial dilutions of serum suspected to contain rheumatoid factor. Rheumatoid factor is present in comparatively low titer in about 25 per cent of cases.[26] Results of rheumatoid factor tests must be interpreted in light of the type of assay system used.

Systems using human IgG to coat the particles are less specific and less sensitive for rheumatoid factor in dogs than systems using canine, IgG-coated particles.[13,41] Also, sheep erythrocytes coated with sub-agglutinating doses of rabbit or canine antisheep serum may detect a different rheumatoid factor than canine IgG-coated latex particles.[41]

Radiographic Findings

The earliest radiographic findings of erosive immune arthritis are nonspecific and include periarticular soft tissue swelling and joint capsule distension.[1,22] The joint space may be wider than normal because of effusion. Joint space width must be interpreted in light of the position of the patient and the amount of traction on the affected joint when the radiograph was made. Joint space width is best evaluated when the patient is fully weight-bearing on the affected joint.

Later radiographic findings include loss of articular cartilage and subchondral bone, leading to a collapse of the joint and the radiographic appearance of a narrowed joint space; luxation, subluxation, and ankylosis of the affected joint; periarticular soft tissue mineralization; soft tissue atrophy; and changes characteristic of secondary degenerative joint disease[1,22,24] (Fig. 164–4). Osteoporosis of juxta-articular bone also has been reported as an early radiographic bony change associated with erosive immune arthritis.[20,25] It is not seen until weeks or months following the onset of the disease. Lucent cystlike areas are frequently found in the subchondral bone.

Osteophytes and subchondral bony sclerosis are frequent in secondary degenerative joint disease. Angular deformity, particularly of the carpal, tarsal, and interphalangeal joints, may occur owing to loss of normal joint surface architecture and destruction of ligamentous support.[1,20,25]

Diagnostic Criteria

As in systemic lupus erythematosus, diagnostic criteria have been established for rheumatoid arthritis.[30] These criteria are clinical manifestations that make a diagnosis increasingly likely. In addition, an exclusion list is also used when evaluating rheumatoid arthritis patients.[30] Regardless of how many criteria for rheumatoid arthritis a patient may have, if one of the features on the list of exclusions is demonstrated,

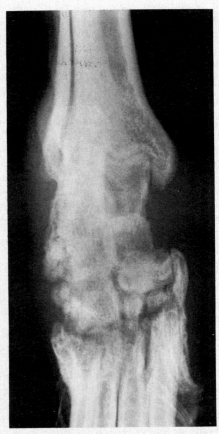

Figure 164–4. Rheumatoid arthritis. Severe destruction of articular surfaces and subchondral bone is readily apparent. (Reprinted with permission from Resnick, D., and Niwayama, G.: *Diagnosis of Bone and Joint Disorders*. W. B. Saunders, Philadelphia, 1981.)

TABLE 164–2. Diagnostic Criteria for Human Rheumatoid Arthritis by the American Rheumatism Association*

Morning stiffness
Joint pain or tenderness on motion
Swelling of a joint
Swelling of a second joint
Symmetrical joint swelling
Subcutaneous nodules
Positive rheumatoid factor test
Roentgenographic changes typical of RA
Poor synovial fluid mucin precipitate
Positive synovial biopsy
Positive nodule biopsy

*Patients with seven or more criteria are defined as having "classic" rheumatoid arthritis; five or six as having "definite" rheumatoid arthritis; three or four as "probable" rheumatoid arthritis.

a diagnosis of rheumatoid arthritis should not be made. In the absence of knowledge of pathogenesis, these criteria (both the diagnostic list and the exclusion list) are useful in grouping similar patients for study. Table 164–2 presents the 11 criteria established by the American Rheumatism Association for the diagnosis of human rheumatoid arthritis; Table 164–3 presents the list of exclusions. A recent analysis of these criteria has shown their clinical applicability and relevance in establishing a diagnosis of human rheumatoid arthritis.[17]

Canine rheumatoid arthritis is not diagnosed frequently. Many cases reported have used human diagnostic criteria. Although the condition appears to be identical in humans and dogs, the etiology is not known. Until it is, it may be best to utilize the terms

TABLE 164–3. Exclusion Precluding Diagnosis of Human Rheumatoid Arthritis

Typical rash of systemic lupus erythematosus
High concentration of lupus erythematosus cells
Histological evidence of periarteritis nodosa
Weakness of neck, trunk, and pharyngeal muscles or persistent muscle swelling or dermatomyositis
Definite scleroderma
Clinical picture characteristic of rheumatic fever
Clinical picture characteristic of gouty arthritis
Tophi
Clinical picture characteristic of infectious arthritis
Tubercule bacilli in joints or histological evidence of joint tuberculosis
Clinical picture characteristic of Reiter's syndrome
Clinical picture characteristic of shoulder-hand syndrome
Clinical picture characteristic of hypertrophic osteoarthropathy
Clinical picture characteristic of neuroarthropathy
Homogentisic acid in urine
Histological evidence of sarcoid
Multiple myeloma
Characteristic skin lesions of erythema nodosum
Leukemia or lymphoma
Agammaglobulinemia

"erosive" and "nonerosive" when discussing immune-mediated joint diseases of the dog and keep in mind the lists of diagnostic criteria and exclusions when comparing these conditions to similar human diseases.

Pathology of Erosive, Immune-Articular Disease

The characteristic pathological changes are first seen in the synovial membrane and then in the articular cartilage. Early lesions are not well documented because of the lack of sample material. Present evidence indicates that changes first appear in the synovial membrane and then the articular cartilage; subchondral bone, ligaments, and tendons are secondarily affected.[20,25]

The degree of inflammation in the synovial tissue varies with the severity and duration of the condition. The characteristic lesion in the synovial membrane is a villous, finger-like projection of fibrovascular proliferative granulation tissue (called pannus) that advances across the articular cartilage of affected joints (Fig. 164–5). The cells of this invasive front of tissue produce proteases, enzymes, and other substances responsible for destruction of the joint.[8,39] In some cases, pannus extends beneath the articular cartilage, causing subchondral bony destruction. Joint surface collapse results from loss of the underlying supportive structures.

Significant changes in the synovial membrane include increased thickness of the synoviocytic layer, hypertrophy of individual synoviocytes with an accompanying change in their shape and axial orientation, infiltration of the subsynoviocytic areas with plasma cells, lymphocytes, and small blood vessels, perivascular accumulation of inflammatory cells in the subsynovium, and occasional fibroblasts and hemosiderin-laden macrophages, also in the subsynovial region.[20,25]

Treatment

Erosive, immune-mediated joint disease of dogs, like human rheumatoid arthritis, is a chronic, lifelong disease for which there is no known cure. The goals of therapy are to relieve patient discomfort, prevent further joint destruction, and preserve joint function.

It is important that the pet owner be made aware of the chronicity of the condition and its variable, unpredictable course. In addition to drug therapy, controlled exercise and physiotherapy to prevent muscle atrophy and contracture are prominently featured in treatment. Each patient is carefully observed, and an exercise program is tailored to its abilities and response to therapy. Overweight animals must be placed on a weight-reducing diet. Caloric requirements are calculated based on the ideal weight of the patient and its expected activities.

Aspirin is the preferred drug for initial therapy. It is relatively free of side effects and is the least expensive drug available for the treatment of rheumatoid arthritis. It must be given in sufficient doses for sufficient time before a decision is made to abandon it. Oral aspirin, 25 mg/kg body weight three times per day, maintains a plasma concentration sufficient to produce anti-inflammatory effects.[2] Aspirin compounds, even those that are buffered, should always be given with food. Salicylates containing magnesium-aluminum hydroxide may be given to patients experiencing gastric upset from aspirin.

It may take up to two weeks to observe benefits from aspirin; dosages may be increased within five to seven days if the desired effects have not been achieved. Dosages approaching 50 mg/kg frequently produce vomiting.[43] Drug dosages may be decreased after relief of clinical signs has been maintained for two weeks. The amount being given is usually reduced by one-half while maintaining the three times per day schedule. Reducing the aspirin dosage by half every two weeks can be continued as long as clinical remission is maintained.

Aspirin therapy is not successful in all dogs. Some are refractive to the drug regardless of the dosage administered. However, before other drugs are substituted, it must be determined whether the aspirin has been given at the proper dose for a sufficient length of time. A difficulty in home therapy is convincing the pet owner that such seemingly large dosages of aspirin are needed and that the drug must be given as directed for the prescribed length of time.

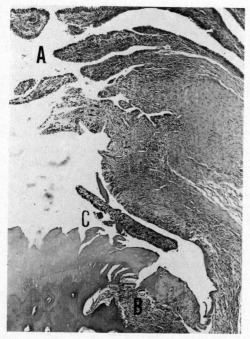

Figure 164–5. Joint margin from a dog with rheumatoid-like arthritis. Note the villous hypertrophy (A), destruction of the subchondral bone by granulation tissue arising from the inflamed synovium (B), and fibrillation of the articular cartilage (C). (Reprinted with permission from Resnick, D., and Niwayama, G.: *Diagnosis of Bone and Joint Disorders.* W. B. Saunders, Philadelphia, 1981.)

Other drugs, or drug combinations, may benefit those patients not responding to aspirin. Many non-steroidal anti-inflammatory drugs are presently available. They exert their effect by inhibiting either synthesis or release of prostaglandins. To date, data regarding the comparative efficacy in the dog between aspirin and these compounds are not available.

Glucocorticoids have been used successfully in those dogs with erosive, immune articular disease that have not responded to aspirin.[20] They may be given initially when the patient is so debilitated by disease that rapid relief is mandatory. Prednisolone is given parenterally at a dose of 1 to 2 mg/kg of body weight bid; this is followed by oral administration of 0.5 to 1.0 mg/kg bid. Favorable response may be evident within 24 to 48 hours after therapy has begun. Once control of disease signs has been established for a minimum of five to seven days, the amount of drug being given may be reduced. The dosage is reduced by half while the same frequency of administration is maintained.

Aspirin may be beneficial after the initial inflammatory episode has been controlled by glucocorticoids. Decreasing doses of glucocorticoids with increasing doses of aspirin may then be effective in patients originally refractive to aspirin alone. Patients receiving both aspirin and glucocorticoids must be carefully monitored for gastrointestinal disturbances, such as vomiting or melena. All drugs must be withheld if disturbances occur.

Glucocorticoids in combination with cytotoxic drugs have been used as the preferred treatment in dogs with erosive, immune-mediated arthritis.[23,26] The advantage of this treatment is that it is usually effective in those not responding to aspirin or glucocorticoids. The disadvantage is the potential side effects of vomiting, salivation, diarrhea, hematuria, and so on. Not all patients receiving these drugs develop side effects, but if they do, drug administration should cease immediately.

Cyclophosphamide has been helpful in bringing about early remission, but it should not be administered for longer than four months to avoid sterile hemorrhagic cystitis. Thiopurines such as azathioprine and 6-mercaptopurine can be substituted for cyclophosphamide. They may also be used to induce remission but frequently take longer than does cyclophosphamide.

Cytotoxic agents and glucocorticoid combinations for the treatment of rheumatoid arthritis may be used as follows:[23,26] cyclophosphamide is given orally at 1.5 to 2.5 mg/kg for four consecutive days each week. Dogs weighing 10 kg or less receive 2.5 mg/kg, those 10 to 35 kg receive 2.0 mg/kg, and dogs weighing more than 35 kg receive 1.5 mg/kg. Prednisolone is given at 1 to 2 mg/kg bid; larger dogs receive a lower dose. Azathioprine is given orally at 2.0 mg/kg daily for two to three weeks, then at this dose but on alternate days. If progress has been made at the end of this time, prednisolone and azathioprine may be given on alternate days.

Remission usually occurs within 16 weeks;[23,26] the cytotoxic drugs are discontinued after one month of sustained complete remission. Prednisolone is continued, and after another month of remission the dose may be reduced by half, or alternate day therapy may be instituted.

Complete blood counts are done weekly on all animals receiving cytotoxic drugs.[23,26] If the white blood count falls below 7,000 cells/mm^3 the dosages are decreased by one-fourth; below 4,000 cells/mm^3 the drugs are discontinued for one week and then started again at half the previous dose.

Chrysotherapy, the use of gold compounds, has been used with success in humans suffering from rheumatoid arthritis refractory to other drugs.[5,45] To date, gold salts have been used in a limited number of dogs with erosive, immune-mediated joint disease.[21,32] Results, however, have been encouraging. Gold sodium thiomalate may be given intramuscularly once a week at 1 mg/kg of body weight.

Even in remission dogs may still have abnormal joint motion and function due to secondary degenerative joint disease or ligamentous changes. One must be able to differentiate between the immune component of the condition and the secondary changes so that unnecessarily prolonged immunosuppresive therapy need not occur. Septic arthritis, although rare, has been a complication of immunosuppresive therapy.[26] Careful physical examination of the patient and the involved joints and analysis of synovial fluid from affected as well as nonaffected joints may help in differentiating continued immune-mediated disease from secondary degenerative joint disease.[26]

Synovectomy is a routine procedure for human rheumatoid arthritis. Indications include persistent synovitis, minimal but progressive radiographic changes, and consistent, unremitting pain.[11] Because not every patient benefits from synovectomy, patients are carefully selected on the basis of the degree of joint destruction, success of previous medical therapy, and presence of joint pain. Success, as judged by reduction in pain and increase in joint use and range of motion, has been quite good in carefully selected human patients.[36] Synovectomy for erosive, immune-mediated disease of the dog has not been described.

Arthrodesis has been recommended in humans and dogs affected with severe joint destruction associated with uncontrollable pain.[36,38] The procedure may restore some function to a limb rendered useless because of severe joint disease.

1. Biery, D. N., and Newton, C. D.: Radiographic appearance of rheumatoid arthritis in the dog. J. Am. Anim. Hosp. Assoc. 11:607, 1975.
2. David, L. E.: Clinical pharmacology of salicylates. J. Am. Vet. Med. Assoc. 176:65, 1980.
3. Dayer, J. M., Robinson, D. R., and Krane, S. M.: Prostaglandin production by rheumatoid synovial cells. J. Exp. Med. 145:1399, 1977.

4. Drazner, F. H.: Systemic lupus erythematosus in the dog. Compend. Cont. Ed. 2:243, 1980.

5. Ehrlich, G. E.: Remittive pharmacological agents. *In* Katz, W. A. (ed.): *Rheumatic Diseases.* J. B. Lippincott, Philadelphia, 1977.

6. Grindem, C. B., and Johnson, K. H.: Systemic lupus erythematosus; Literature review and report of 42 new canine cases. J. Am. Anim. Hosp. Assoc. 19:489, 1983.

7. Halliwell, R. E. W.: Autoimmune skin diseases. *In* Kirk, R. W. (ed): *Current Veterinary Therapy VII.* W. B. Saunders, Philadelphia, 1980.

8. Harris, E. D., Jr.: Recent insights into the pathogenesis of the proliferative lesions in rheumatoid arthritis. Arthritis Rheum. 19:68, 1976.

9. Harris, E. D., Jr.: Role of collagenases in joint destruction. *In* Sokoloff, L. (ed.): *The Joints and Synovial Fluid.* Vol. I. Academic Press, New York, 1978.

10. Kaswan, R. L., Martin, C. L., and Dawe, D. L.: Rheumatoid factor determination in 50 dogs with keratoconjunctivitis sicca. J. Am. Vet. Med. Assoc. 183:1073, 1983.

11. Kauffman, M. S.: Arthritis surgery. *In* Katz, W. A. (ed.): *Rheumatic Diseases.* J. B. Lippincott, Philadelphia, 1977.

12. Lewis, R. M., and Schwartz, R. S.: Canine systemic lupus erythematosus: Genetic analysis of an established breeding colony. J. Exp. Med. 134:417, 1971.

13. Lipowitz, A. J., and Newton, C. D.: Laboratory parameters of rheumatoid arthritis of the dog: A review. J. Am. Anim. Hosp. Assoc. 11:600, 1975.

14. Madewell, B. R.: Adverse effects of chemotherapy. *In* Kirk, R. W. (ed.): *Current Veterinary Therapy VIII.* W. B. Saunders, Philadelphia, 1983.

15. Mannick, M.: Rheumatoid factors. *In* McCarty, D. J. (ed.): *Arthritis and Allied Conditions.* 9th ed. Lea & Febiger, Philadelphia, 1979.

16. McMillan, R. M., Fahey, J. V., Brinkerhoff, C. E., and Harris, E. D., Jr.: Secretion of inflammatory mediators from synovial fibroblasts: Dissociation of collagenase and prostaglandin release. *In* Samuelson, B., Ramwell, P. W., and Padetti, R. (eds.): *Advances in Prostaglandin and Thromboxane Research.* Raven Press, New York, 1980.

17. Mitchell, D. M., and Frien, J. F.: An analysis of the American Rheumatism Association criteria for rheumatoid arthritis. Arthritis Rheum. 25:481, 1982.

18. Monier, J. C., Dardenne, M., Rigal, D., et al.: Clinical and laboratory features of canine lupus syndrome. Arthritis Rheum. 23:294, 1980.

19. Newcombe, D. S., and Ishikawa, Y.: The effect of anti-inflammatory agents on human synovial fibroblast prostaglandin synthetase. Prostaglandins 12:849, 1976.

20. Newton, C. D., Lipowitz, A. J., Halliwell, R. E., et al.: Rheumatoid arthritis in dogs. J. Am. Vet. Med. Assoc. 168:113, 1976.

21. Newton, C. D., Schumacher, H. R., and Halliwell, R. E. W.: Gold salt therapy for rheumatoid arthritis in dogs. J. Am. Vet. Med. Assoc. 174:1308, 1979.

22. Owens, J. M., and Ackerman, N.: Roentgenology of arthritis. Vet. Clin. North Am. 8:453, 1978.

23. Pedersen, N. C.: Therapy of immune-mediated diseases. *In* Kirk, R. W. (ed.): *Current Veterinary Therapy VIII.* W. B. Saunders, Philadelphia, 1983.

24. Pedersen, N. C., and Pool, R.: Canine joint disease. Vet. Clin. North Am. 8:465, 1978.

25. Pedersen, N. C., Pool, R., Castles, J. J., and Weisner, K.: Noninfectious canine arthritis: Rheumatoid arthritis. J. Am. Vet. Med. Assoc. 169:295, 1976.

26. Pedersen, N. C., Pool, R., and Morgan, J. P.: Joint diseases of dogs and cats. *In* Ettinger, S. J. (ed.): *Textbook of Veterinary Internal Medicine; Diseases of the Dog and Cat.* 2nd ed. W. B. Saunders, Philadelphia, 1983.

27. Pedersen, N. C., Weisner, K., Castles, J. J., et al.: Noninfectious canine arthritis: The inflammatory nonerosive arthritides. J. Am. Vet. Med. Assoc. 169:304, 1976.

28. Perman, V.: Synovial fluid. *In* Kaneko, J. (ed.): *Clinical Biochemistry of Domestic Animals.* 3rd ed., Academic Press, New York, 1980.

29. Poole, A. R., Golds, E. E., and Champion, B. R.: The immunopathology of inflammatory arthritis: Some new insights. Surg. Clin. North Am. 61:353, 1981.

30. Primer on the Rheumatic Diseases. 7th ed. Arthritis Foundation, Atlanta, GA, 1973.

31. Schumacher, H. R., Newton, C. D., Holliwell, R. E. W.: Synovial pathologic changes in spontaneous canine rheumatoid-like arthritis. Arthritis Rheum. 23:412, 1980.

32. Scott, D. W.: Chrysotherapy (gold therapy). *In* Kirk, R. W. (ed.): *Current Veterinary Therapy VIII.* W. B. Saunders, Philadelphia, 1983.

33. Scott, D. W., Walton, D. K., Manning, T. O., et al.: Canine lupus erythematosus. I: Systemic lupus erythematosus. J. Am. Anim. Hosp. Assoc. 19:461, 1983.

34. Scott, D. W., Walton, D. K., Manning, T. O., et al.: Canine lupus erythematosus. II: Discoid lupus erythematosus. J. Am. Anim. Hosp. Assoc. 19:481, 1983.

35. Shull, R. M., Miller, H. A., and Chilina, A. R.: Investigation of the nature and specificity of antinuclear antibody in dogs. Am. J. Vet. Res. 44:2004, 1983.

36. Sledge, C. B.: Correction of arthritic deformities in the lower extremity and spine. *In* McCarthy, D. J. (ed.): *Arthritis and Allied Conditions.* 9th ed. Lea & Febiger, Philadelphia, 1979.

37. Tan, E. M., Cohen, A. S., Fries, J. F., et al.: The 1982 revised criteria for the classification of systemic lupus erythematosus. Arthritis Rheum. 25:1271, 1982.

38. Turner, T., and Lipowitz, A. J.: Arthrodesis. *In* Bojrab, M. J. (ed.): *Current Techniques in Small Animal Surgery.* 2nd ed. Lea & Febiger, Philadelphia, 1983.

39. Weissman, G., Smolen, J. E., and Korchak, H. M.: Release of inflammatory mediators from stimulated neutrophils. N. Engl. J. Med. 303:27, 1980.

40. Wolfe, J. H., and Halliwell, R. E. W.: Total hemolytic complement values in normal and diseased dog populations. Vet. Immunol. Immunopathol. 1:287, 1980.

41. Wood, D. D., Hurvitz, A. I., and Schultz, R. D.: A latex test for canine rheumatoid factor. Vet. Immunol. Immunopathol. 1:103, 1980.

42. Wooley, D. E., Brinkerhoff, C. E., Mainardi, C. L., et al.: Collagenase production by rheumatoid synovial cells: Morphological and immunohistochemical studies of the dendritic cell. Ann. Rheum. Dis. 38:262, 1979.

43. Yeary, R. A., and Brant, R. J.: Aspirin dosages for the dog. J. Am. Vet. Med. Assoc. 167:63, 1975.

44. Zvaifler, N. J.: Etiology and pathogenesis of rheumatoid arthritis. *In* McCarty, D. J. (ed.): *Arthritis and Allied Conditions.* 9th ed. Lea & Febiger, Philadelphia, 1979.

45. Zvaifler, N. J.: Gold and antimalarial therapy. *In* McCarty, D. J. (ed.): *Arthritis and Allied Conditions.* 9th ed. Lea & Febiger, Philadelphia, 1979.

Chapter 165

Orthopedic Diseases

J. W. Alexander

CRANIOMANDIBULAR OSTEOPATHY
(Mandibular Periostitis, Craniomandibular Hyperostosis, Lion's Jaw)

Canine craniomandibular osteopathy is a noninflammatory, nonneoplastic proliferative bone disease that usually occurs in the third to sixth month of life. The syndrome has a predilection for bones of endochondral origin and most commonly affects the occipital bones, bulla tympanica of the temporal bone, and the mandibular rami.[56] Lesions are most often bilateral and symmetrical.

Craniomandibular osteopathy has been documented most often in the Scottish terrier and West Highland white terrier.[64] It has also been reported in the Boston terrier,[64] Cairn terrier,[64] Labrador retriever,[35,77] Great Dane,[13] Doberman pinscher,[79] and boxer.[66]

Most dogs are presented because of pain associated with opening the mouth. Other frequently reported clinical signs include depression, excessive salivation, intermittent fever episodes, and bilateral firm swellings of the mandible.

A suspected diagnosis of craniomandibular osteopathy can usually be confirmed by radiographic evaluation of the involved areas. The typical dense proliferative osseous lesions are readily seen on lateral and ventrodorsal radiographs of the skull (Fig. 165–1). They project from the periosteal surfaces of the involved bones. The angular processes of the mandible and bullae may fuse and mechanically obstruct the motion of the jaw or lead to complete bony fusion of the temporomandibular joints.

The etiology of this syndrome is unknown. The occurrence of craniomandibular osteopathy in a few breeds of dogs and in littermates has suggested a genetic basis.

The prognosis in any individual case depends on which bones are involved and to what degree. At times only the mandibles are affected, and in a few instances the involvement may be so limited that the disease may go undetected unless radiographs are taken. In other dogs the occlusal surface of the teeth cannot be separated or can be spread only a few millimeters owing to extensive involvement of the temporomandibular joints. Bony fusion of the temporomandibular joint makes it almost impossible for the dog to grasp and masticate food. Although the condition is not in itself fatal, extensive involvement may necessitate euthanasia (Fig. 165–2). The disease is often self-limiting, and with skeletal maturity the abnormal bone growth ceases, often regresses, and may recede completely.

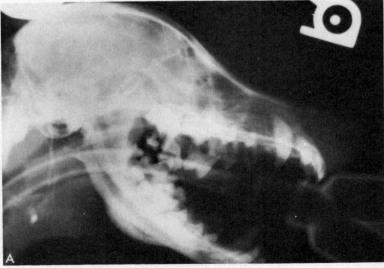

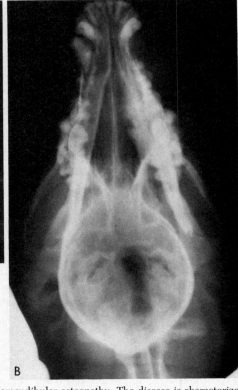

Figure 165–1. Lateral *(A)* and ventrodorsal *(B)* skull radiographs of a dog with craniomandibular osteopathy. The disease is characterized by dense proliferative osseous lesions on the mandibles.

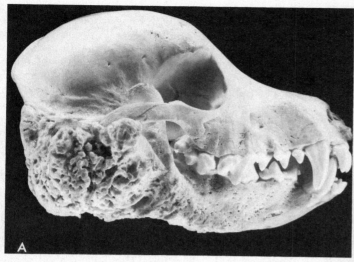

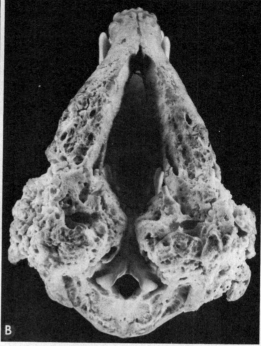

Figure 165–2. *A* and *B,* Skull from a dog with craniomandibular osteopathy. The dog was unable to open its mouth owing to a bony fusion of the temporomandibular joints.

HYPERTROPHIC OSTEODYSTROPHY (Canine Scurvy, Moller-Barlow's Disease, Osteodystrophy I, Osteodystrophy II, Metaphyseal Osteopathy)

Hypertrophic osteodystrophy is a disease of the skeletal system that affects young, rapidly growing, large and giant breeds of dogs. It has been reported in a variety of breeds including the Great Dane,[2,25,46,62] boxer,[25,35,46,69] collie,[25,35] Irish setter,[25,69] Labrador retriever,[46,78] German shepherd[25,78] greyhound,[78] Weimaraner,[25] German pointer,[25] golden retriever,[25] borzoi,[25] Irish wolfhound,[46] and basset hound.[25] The syndrome is usually first manifested when the dog is between three and seven months of age. It is characterized by warm painful swellings of the metaphyseal areas of the long bones where endochondral osteogenesis is most active. The distal radius, distal ulna, and distal tibia are the most commonly affected skeletal sites; however, the mandible, metacarpal bones, costochondral junction, and other long bones can be involved.

The clinical signs of hypertrophic osteodystrophy vary tremendously. Dogs most commonly are presented because of visible, hypersensitive enlargement in the metaphyseal areas of the affected bones (Fig. 165–3). The disease may be accompanied by variable pyrexia. Many individual animals are depressed, anorexic, and reluctant to stand or move. Involved sites are warm and tender on palpation.

A tentative diagnosis of hypertrophic osteodystrophy can be confirmed by radiographic examination of the involved areas. In the acute state, the radiographic picture is dominated by sclerosis of the metaphysis, in which there are areas of radiolucency often coalescing to a linear area of low density parallel to the growth plate (Fig. 165–4). This radiolucent area is near, but not in contact with, the growth plate. In a very early lesion a dense line may be seen next to the epiphyseal plate. In the more advanced stages of the disease, radiographs demonstrate excessive enlargement of the metaphyses and beaded

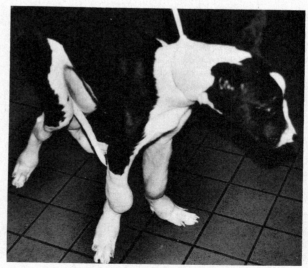

Figure 165–3. Great Dane with hypertrophic osteodystrophy. Note the gross enlargements of the distal forelimb.

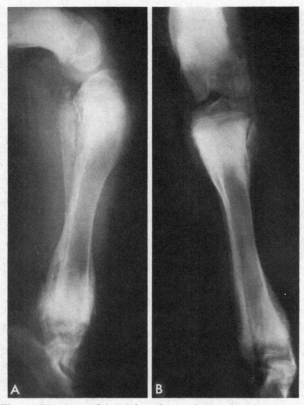

Figure 165–4. Lateral *(A)* and caudocranial *(B)* radiographs of the tibia in a dog with hypertrophic osteodystrophy. The radiograph demonstrates sclerosis and enlargement of the metaphyses. Areas of periosteal hemorrhage have become mineralized and appear as radiopaque depositions of bone surrounding the proximal and distal metaphyses.

radiopaque deposition of bone surrounding areas in the soft tissue outside the periosteum.[62] In areas where bone growth is not normally as rapid (i.e., proximal radius and proximal tibia), the metaphysis can be extremely radiopaque.

The etiology of canine hypertrophic osteodystrophy is a controversial subject. The disease has been compared both clinically and radiographically to human scurvy, and some investigators have incriminated hypovitaminosis C as the underlying cause of canine hypertrophic osteodystrophy.[46] However, the evidence that vitamin C deficiency may be in some way involved with this syndrome is somewhat circumstantial. Vitamin C is generally regarded as required only in the diets of primates and guinea pigs. In dogs, the body levels of ascorbic acid are not dependent on dietary intake, as this vitamin is synthesized by the liver and intestines. In some dogs with hypertrophic osteodystrophy, decreased plasma and urinary ascorbic acid levels tend to add support to the hypovitaminosis C theory.[25,35,46,78] Other investigators have attempted to explain marginally low ascorbic acid levels based on the notion that dogs with hypertrophic osteodystrophy are under stress and have decreased food intake. The response to vitamin C therapy in humans with scurvy is a dra-

matic one; however, this has by no means always been the case in dogs with hypertrophic osteodystrophy. In one recent study investigators concluded that ascorbic acid treatment was contraindicated, as it tended to aggravate the osseous lesions.[74] Overnutrition and subsequent mineral overloading have been implicated as possible etiological factors in hypertrophic osteodystrophy. Skeletal lesions similar to those seen in clinical cases of hypertrophic osteodystrophy have been experimentally produced by feeding a free choice diet high in protein, calories, and calcium.[31,74]

Although the majority of reports in the veterinary literature have concerned unrelated individuals, one study related the manifestations of hypertrophic osteodystrophy in four Weimaraner littermates and in a fifth dog that was the daughter of one of these.[25]

Failure to define the etiology of hypertrophic osteodystrophy has hampered the development of specific treatment regimens. It is difficult to evaluate the true value of a given management method, as spontaneous remission and exacerbations are a part of the natural history of this disease. Spontaneous improvement can easily be mistaken for a drug or management effect. I feel that affected dogs should be managed by (1) correction of any dietary imbalances, (2) administration of analgesics such as aspirin or phenylbutazone to control pain, and (3) supportive therapy as needed. This last-named treatment may include parenteral fluids in cases of dehydration, forced feeding in cases of anorexia, and antibiotic therapy should secondary infection complicate the primary disease process.

The prognosis for dogs with hypertrophic osteodystrophy must be guarded. Although many dogs recover spontaneously, others develop permanent bony changes and subsequent physical deformities. Unfortunately, in many dogs treatment does not appear to influence the eventual outcome.

MULTIPLE CARTILAGINOUS EXOSTOSIS (Hereditary Multiple Exostosis, Diaphyseal Aclasis)

Multiple cartilaginous exostosis is a condition in which multiple partially ossified excrescences arise from the cortical surfaces, forming tubular extensions roughly transverse to the long axis of the bone involved. The syndrome has been reported in the dog,[16,20,21,23,24,51,52,57,58] horse,[27,47,67] cat,[11,55,61] and man.[1,37]

Bony protuberances may arise in any bone formed by endochondral ossification. The lesions are a cylinder of cortical bone surrounding a core of cancellous tissue that is covered with a layer of cartilage. The cancellous bone communicates with that of the host bone and frequently supports hematopoietic marrow. The cartilaginous portion is comparable to the physis of a long bone, except that it has no osseous nucleus and acts both as an epiphyseal and articular plate.[1]

The bony portion is covered with an extension of periosteum from the normal cortical bone, and the cartilage cap is covered with perichondrium.[1]

In dogs, the vertebrae, ribs, and long bones are the most frequently reported locations of the exostoses. The outgrowths are most frequently found in the metaphyseal portion of the bone, where they are progressively replaced by the underlying bone. The exostosis ceases growing at the same time that other epiphyseal plates close. Growth after the animal matures is highly suggestive of malignant transformation.

In man, multiple cartilaginous exostosis is a hereditary disease characterized by autosomal dominance with about one-half of the affected parents' offspring showing manifestations.[1] There is evidence suggesting that multiple cartilaginous exostosis may be hereditary in the dog[16,24] and the horse.[47,67]

Many divergent theories have been offered to explain the pathogenic mechanism in the development of multiple cartilaginous exostosis in man. The most widely accepted theory was proposed by Virchow, who suggested that the exostoses are derived from cartilaginous growth plates.[36] According to this theory, a small portion of cartilage may become separated from the lateral aspect of the epiphyseal plate, turn at right angles, turn shaftward, and thereby establish an exostosis.

The clinical features of multiple cartilaginous exostosis are dependent on the location of the exostoses. In general, significant signs do not occur in the newborn but usually become detected during active bone growth. If the lesion is not large and fails to cause any clinical disability, it may remain unnoticed until adulthood; in some instances it may never be observed. The animal may be presented simply for a firm hard swelling on the involved bone. Pain or disability develops only when adjacent structures are compressed and mechanically distorted by the exostoses. The bony growth can cause pressure on tendons that must slide over them. They can compress vessels and interfere with blood supply or cause pain secondary to pressure on adjacent nerves. Occasionally, neurological signs may be the presenting complaint (ataxia, paralysis, and so on), as vertebral exostoses can cause spinal cord compression.

Any animal suspected of having multiple cartilaginous exostosis should have a radiographic skeletal survey. The exostotic growths may involve any bone except the skull. The lesions are characterized as radiopaque osseous densities of variable size interspersed with large radiolucent areas of hyaline cartilage (Fig. 165–5). The lesions usually involve the metaphyses and vary in size and shape. To confirm a tentative diagnosis of multiple cartilaginous exostosis, a biopsy should be obtained from any suspicious area.

The prognosis of the osteochondromas is usually favorable. The growth of the lesion apparently begins at an early age and continues until the nearest epiphyseal center ossifies, i.e., its growth period is the same as that of the host bone.[1] In man it is estimated

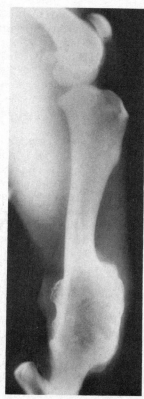

Figure 165–5. Lateral radiograph of the tibia from a dog with multiple cartilaginous exostosis. The lesions usually involve the metaphyses and are variable in size and shape.

that a secondary chondrosarcoma develops as a complication in about 5 to 25 per cent of cases of multiple cartilaginous exostosis.[36] Most commonly secondary chondrosarcomas in man involve the region of the pelvic or shoulder girdles. These patients are usually mature adults; however, malignant transformation of the exostoses have been reported in young adults.[36] Several instances of malignant transformation of the exostoses to either chondrosarcoma[5,21] or osteosarcoma[51] have been reported. In general, continued growth of the osteochondroma after maturity or re-activation of growth is highly suggestive of neoplastic transformation.

Treatment of multiple cartilaginous exostosis depends on the location of the lesion and the resulting clinical disability, if any. In many cases, no treatment is necessary; however, at times the exostosis may need to be removed to relieve pain or loss of function or for cosmetic purposes.

PANOSTEITIS (Enostosis, Eosinophilic Panosteitis, Juvenile Osteomyelitis)

Panosteitis is a disease of unknown etiology that causes pain and lameness in young growing dogs, primarily of the large and giant breeds. The syndrome has been reported in a variety of breeds including the German shepherd,[8,14,18,75] St. Bernard,[8,18] Airedale terrier,[8,18] German short-haired pointer,[8,18] Doberman pinscher,[8,18] Great Dane,[8] and Irish setter.[8] In addition to these large breed dogs, the disease has also been documented in basset hounds[8,28] and a miniature schnauzer.[8] The disease is seen more often in males than females (4:1) between the ages of 5 and 11 months.

Clinically, panosteitis is characterized by a sudden onset of a weight-bearing lameness without history of recent trauma. Often lesions resolve in one bone and re-appear in another, resulting in histories of shifting leg lameness. It is not unusual for affected animals to go through periods of normal gait only to have the lameness re-appear in a different limb. Deep palpation of the affected long bone shaft often elicits pain.

Panosteitis is due to the formation of bone within the medullary cavity. Pathological studies have revealed that during the course of the disease endosteal and periosteal bone is formed in a rather haphazard manner.[39] Bone formation in one long bone may slow down while speeding up in another.[39] The exact source of pain is still not clear.

Suspected cases can usually be confirmed by radiographic evaluation of the involved sites. The disease most commonly affects the diaphyses of the long bones—humerus, radius, ulna, femur, and tibia. The earliest radiographic evidence is poorly marginated areas of increased density and accentuation of the trabecular pattern within the medullary cavity.[75] The lesions, initially focal or multifocal, commonly are first present in the area of the nutrient foramen.[22] This is followed by progressive mottling and eventual opacification.[8] The bone cortices may be thickened and indistinct in affected sites.[75] Shortly after the intramedullary changes are observable, a linear, homogeneous periosteal proliferation possessing smooth margins and density less than that of the cortical bone can be seen. With prolonged severity, the periosteal new bone becomes thicker and more dense.[6] As the disease progresses, the intramedullary bone increases in density and may even obliterate the trabecular pattern in focal areas (Fig. 165–6). In the resolution phase, the sclerotic areas gradually decrease in size and density, but radiographic signs may persist for several months after cessation of lameness.[75]

There is no relationship between the severity of the radiographic changes and the resulting clinical signs.[8] After a bone has passed through the entire lesion cycle, it is unlikely that it will be affected again.[8] However, lameness may return to the same limb should a different bone become involved with the disease process.

In most cases, treatment is only necessary to relieve pain, as the disease is self-limiting. In one study involving 100 dogs, aspirin was most effective.[8]

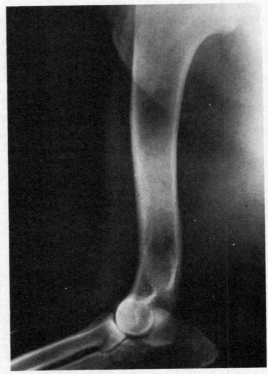

Figure 165–6. Lateral radiograph of the humerus from a dog with panosteitis. Note areas of increased density within the medullary cavity.

AGENESIS OF THE RADIUS (Radial Agenesis)

Although several congenital limb deformities have been reported in animals, agenesis of the radius appears to be the most common.[44,60,73] This syndrome is seen more frequently in cats than in dogs.

The etiology of radial agenesis is unknown. In man, it is often considered inheritable.[50] A dysplastic factor arising during the first few weeks of fetal life has been incriminated. In one report of radial agenesis in a kitten, a repeat mating of the kitten's parents produced eight kittens, three of which had radial agenesis.[73]

Affected animals are usually presented within a few days to weeks post partum owing to abnormal limb configuration. The most striking finding on physical examination is a medial deviation of the lower forearm (Fig. 165–7). The syndrome may be present bilaterally or unilaterally. Radiographic evaluation readily confirms a suspect diagnosis of radial agenesis. Complete or partial absence of the radius is readily observable (Fig. 165–8).

Treatment is usually impractical, with the exception of amputation in unilateral cases. Prior to amputation, a thorough physical examination and possible radiographic skeletal survey should be performed to rule out any other concurrent congenital abnormalities. Affected animals should not be used for breeding.

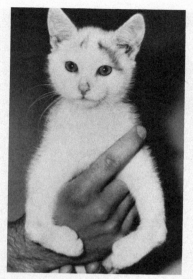

Figure 165–7. A cat with bilateral agenesis of the radius. Note medial deviation of the lower forelimbs.

OSTEOCHONDRITIS DISSECANS

Osteochondritis dissecans is a syndrome of the immature joint characterized by localized separation of articular cartilage and subchondral bone that may lead to the formation of a cartilage flap or ossicle. Although osteochondritis dissecans has been seen most frequently in the proximal humerus, it has also been reported with some frequency in the distal humerus, distal femur, and tibial tarsal bone.

The cause of osteochondritis dissecans is unknown. Several theories have been proposed, including hypercalcitonism associated with overnutrition,[31] trauma to immature cartilage,[15,19] hormonal disturbances,[53] and osteonecrosis.[76]

The natural course of osteochondritis dissecans, which is intimately related to the history of the lesion itself, is variable. Free-floating "joint mice," partially detached chondrosseous fragments, and intact, essentially asymptomatic defects are seen. It is not uncommon for the lesion to be bilateral; however, the clinical signs, radiographic findings, and course of the syndrome in one limb may differ from those of the contralateral limb.

Shoulder Joint

Osteochondritis dissecans of the shoulder joint is a lesion of the proximal humeral epiphysis. It affects primarily young, large and giant breed dogs between the ages of 4 and 12 months. Males are two to five times more likely to be affected than females.[70]

The most common presenting sign is a variable degree of lameness of one or both front limbs. Physical examination reveals pain or crepitation upon flexion and extension of the shoulder joint.

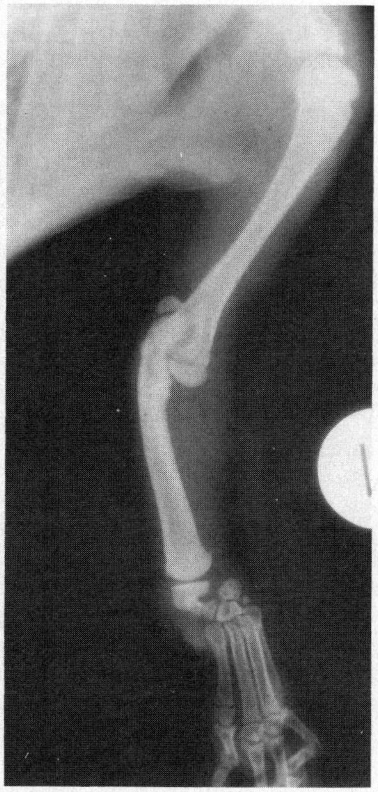

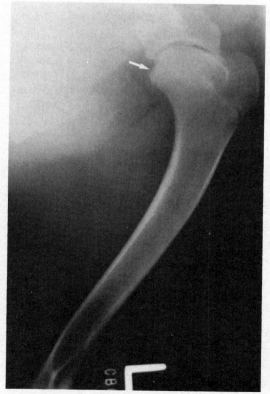

Figure 165–8. Radiograph of the cat in Figure 165–7 demonstrating agenesis of the radius.

Figure 165–9. Lateral radiograph of the humeral head showing the characteristic osteochondral defect *(arrow)* of osteochondritis dissecans.

A tentative diagnosis of osteochondritis dissecans of the humeral head can be confirmed by radiographic examination of the affected shoulder. The characteristic osteochondral defect is usually evident on the central portion of the caudal third of the articular surface of the humeral head (Fig. 165–9). Both shoulders should be radiographed, as a significant number of dogs have bilateral lesions.

Although it is possible that the loose cartilage flap may break off and subsequently lead to a resolution of the lameness, this phenomenon is the exception rather than the rule. In dogs showing pain and lameness, surgical intervention is indicated to relieve the immediate clinical signs and to prevent the development of degenerative joint disease.

Although several surgical approaches to the shoulder joint have been described, I prefer the technique originally described by Hohn.[33] The dog is positioned in lateral recumbency, and a craniolateral curved skin incision is made from the midpoint of the scapular spine to the midhumeral shaft (Fig. 165–10). The subcutaneous fat is incised in the same line as the initial skin incision. The underlying branches of the cephalic vein, the two bellies of the deltoideus muscle, and the omotransversarius muscle can now be identified (Fig. 165–11). Using a periosteal elevator, the insertion of the acromial head of the deltoideus muscle is elevated subperiosteally off the humerus and retracted in a caudal direction. This retraction will expose the underlying tendons of insertion of the infraspinatus muscle (Fig. 165–12). The infraspinatus tendon is transected close to its insertion on the humerus. Care must be taken to leave sufficient infraspinatus tendon on the humerus to allow re-attachment at the time of closure (Fig. 165–13). To make retrieval of the severed infraspinatus muscle easier at closure, the muscle and its associated tendon can be "tagged" with a suture prior to severing the tendinous insertion. The capsule of the shoulder joint is now exposed and incised along the line of curvature of the humeral head so as to allow adequate capsular

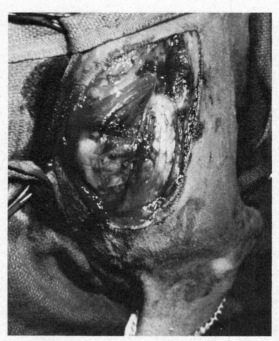

Figure 165–11. Exposure of the underlying muscles following dissection of the subcutaneous tissues during a lateral approach to the shoulder.

tissue on both sides of the incision for closure. Once the joint is opened, the lesion on the humeral head can be seen by internally rotating the humerus and dislocating the humeral head laterally (Fig. 165–14). The loose cartilage flap is removed and the flap bed curetted to bleeding subchondral bone (Fig. 165–15). Initially, granulation tissue and, ultimately, fibrocar-

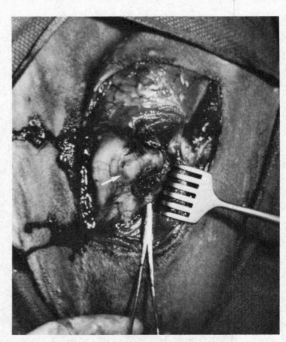

Figure 165–12. Retraction of the acromial head of the deltoideus muscle, which allows exposure of the infraspinatus tendon proximally (*arrow*) and the teres minor tendon distally (under hemostat).

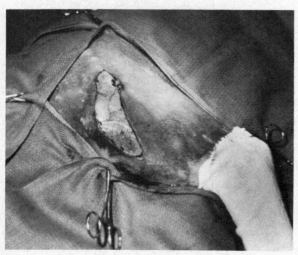

Figure 165–10. Location of the initial skin incision for a lateral approach to the shoulder joint.

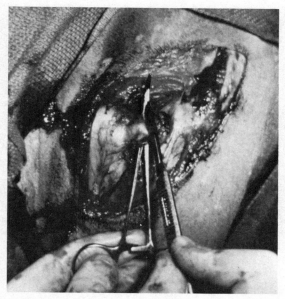

Figure 165–13. Tenotomy of the infraspinatus muscle tendon.

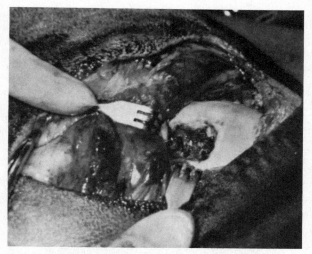

Figure 165–15. Appearance of the cartilage flap bed following curettage in a dog with osteochondritis dissecans of the shoulder.

tilage fill the curetted defect in the articular surface. The joint is thoroughly irrigated, and any floating "joint mice" or bony ossicles attached to the joint capsule are removed.

Closure is accomplished by suturing the joint capsule with an absorbable suture in a simple continuous pattern. The tendon of the infraspinatus muscle is re-attached to its insertion on the humerus with a nonabsorbable suture using a horizontal mattress pattern. The subcutaneous tissue and skin are closed in a routine manner. Postoperatively, the patient's activity is restricted to leash exercise for two to three weeks.

Elbow Joint

Osteochondritis dissecans of the canine elbow occurs on the medial humeral condyle. The syndrome

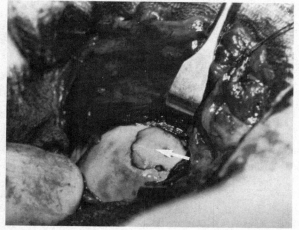

Figure 165–14. Osteochondritis dissecans of the humeral head (*arrow*).

has been reported as an isolated lesion and in combination with ununited coronoid process.[81] Osteochondritis dissecans of the elbow joint is seen most often in growing large and giant breeds of dogs of both sexes.

Dogs with this syndrome are presented to the clinician because of lameness of the involved limb. Pain and crepitation upon flexion and extension of the elbow joint are the most common clinical findings. Craniocaudal radiographs of the elbow reveal a saucer-shaped defect surrounded by a sclerotic zone in the articular cartilage of the medial condyle of the humerus (Fig. 165–16).

The treatment for osteochondritis dissecans of the elbow is the same as that for osteochondritis dissecans of the shoulder—osteochondroplasty by removal of the cartilage flap and curettage of the remaining cartilage defect.

To approach the medial aspect of the elbow joint, a medial skin incision is made from midhumerus to midradius and ulna, with the medial humeral epicondyle as the midpoint (Fig. 165–17). Following dissection of the subcutaneous tissue, the pronator teres and flexor carpi radialis muscles are identified at their tendon of origin on the medial humeral epicondyle (Fig. 165–18). Both muscles are isolated by blunt dissection and are individually transected close to their origin. Care should be taken to leave sufficient tendon on both the epicondyle and the muscle bellies to allow a strong closure. The median artery and nerve lie deep to the pronator teres muscle and should be identified at the time of this muscle's transection (Fig. 165–19). An incision is then made through the medial collateral ligament and the underlying joint capsule parallel to the joint space. To expose the articular surface of the medial condyle of the humerus, the forearm is rotated laterally and pulled distally (Fig. 165–20). The loose cartilage flap is removed, and the cartilage crater is curetted to bleeding subchondral bone. Prior to closure the joint is lavaged with saline. Closure is accomplished by

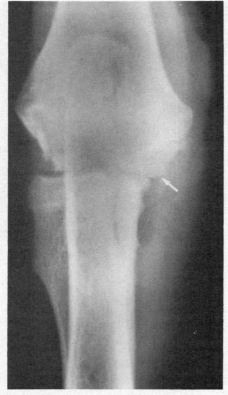

Figure 165–16. Caudocranial radiograph of the elbow showing the typical osteochondral defect *(arrow)* associated with osteochondritis dissecans of the distal humerus.

suturing the flexor carpi radialis and pronator teres muscles back to their respective tendons of origin. The remainder of the closure is routine.

Postoperatively, the limb is placed in a Robert-Jones bandage for three to five days, and activity is restricted to leash exercise for two to three weeks.

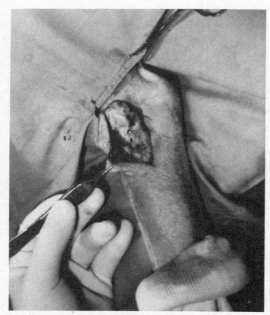

Figure 165–17. Initial skin incision for performing a medial approach to the elbow joint.

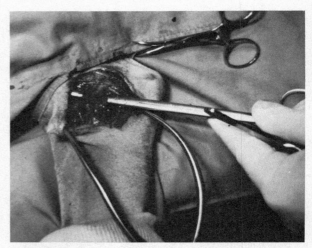

Figure 165–18. Tendons of origin of the pronator teres muscle and the flexor carpi radialis muscle.

Femoro-tibial Joint

Although osteochondritis dissecans of the femoro-tibial joint has been reported in both the lateral and medial femoral condyles, the most common site is the medial aspect of the weight-bearing surface of the lateral femoral condyle. The disease is usually seen in large or giant breeds of dogs between the ages of three and nine months.[4]

The dog is usually presented because of a weight-bearing lameness of the involved limb. Physical examination usually reveals discomfort and, in long-standing cases, crepitation upon flexion and extension of the joint. A craniocaudal radiograph demonstrates a radiolucent area on the distal end of the affected condyle (Fig. 165–21).

Treatment consists of performing a standard stifle arthrotomy with removal of the offending osteochon-

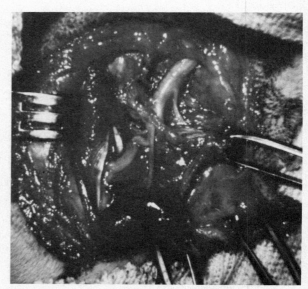

Figure 165–19. Location of the median artery and nerve, which are exposed following transection of the pronator teres muscle's tendon of origin.

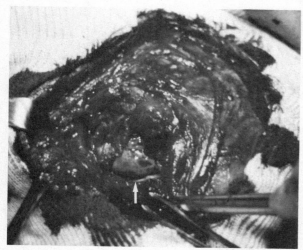

Figure 165–20. Exposure of the medial humeral condyle (*arrow*) following a medial approach to the elbow joint.

dral flap and any free-floating "joint mice." Postoperatively, the limb is supported in a Robert-Jones bandage for two weeks.

Tibiotarsal Joint

Osteochondritis dissecans of the tibiotarsal joint affects the tibial tarsal bone, primarily the medial

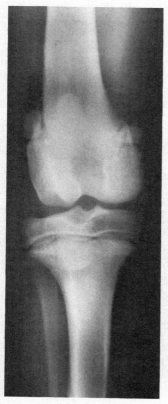

Figure 165–21. A caudocranial radiograph of the stifle showing an osteochondral defect of the lateral femoral condyle associated with osteochondritis dissecans of the femorotibial joint.

ridge of the trochlea. Most dogs are presented because of a weight-bearing lameness. The clinical signs usually develop between the ages of four and eight months, affect primarily large or giant breeds, and, although both sexes have been reported to have this syndrome, is seen most frequently in males. The syndrome most commonly occurs bilaterally.

Physical examination reveals moderate joint distension, especially on the medial aspect of the tarsus, and pain or crepitation upon flexion and extension of the tibiotarsal joint. Marked hyperextension of the hock is a common conformational fault associated with osteochondritis dissecans of this joint (Fig. 165–22). Radiographic findings include joint distension, a radiolucent bony defect on the medial ridge of the talus, the presence of variably sized mineralized joint bodies, and evidence of remodeling of the distal tibia and lateral medial malleolus (Fig. 165–23).

The treatment of osteochondritis dissecans of the tibiotarsal joint consists primarily of removal of the osteochondral flap, exposure accomplished through a caudomedial approach. With the dog in lateral recumbency and the affected leg down, an incision is made, following the angle of the hock, just caudal to the medial malleolus of the tibia. The superficial branch of the tibial nerve, the plantar branch of the saphenous artery, the superficial plantar metatarsal vein, and the deep digital flexor tendon should be identified and retracted caudally toward the tuber calcaneus. The joint capsule is then incised in a longitudinal direction and the joint flexed to expose the affected trochlear ridge (Fig. 165–24). A medial malleolar osteotomy has been described for increased exposure.[68]

The surgical treatment of osteochondritis of the hock differs from that of osteochondritis of other joints. There is some clinical evidence to suggest that curettage of the bed following removal of the cartilage

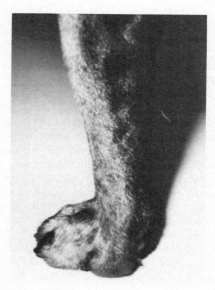

Figure 165–22. Photograph of a dog with osteochondritis dissecans of the tibiotarsal joint. Note hyperextension of the tarsus.

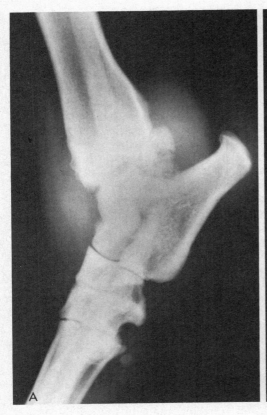
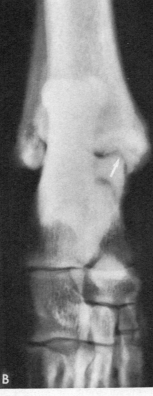

Figure 165–23. Lateral *(A)* and caudocranial *(B)* radiographs of the tarsal joint of a dog with osteochondritis dissecans of the hock. Radiographic findings include joint distension, a radiolucent bony defect associated with the medial ridge of the talus *(arrow)*, and variably sized mineralized joint bodies.

flap is contraindicated. In one study it was noted that in those cases that were curetted down to subchondral bone, there was a greater incidence of degenerative joint disease.[65] The investigators concluded that this postoperative complication was due to increased joint instability secondary to a flattening of the medial trochlear ridge of the tibial tarsal bone following curettage of the flap bed.

Postoperatively, the tarsal joint is supported with a soft bandage for the first seven to ten postoperative days and exercise is restricted to a leash for three weeks.

UNUNITED ANCONEAL PROCESS (Elbow Dysplasia)

Ununited anconeal process is a syndrome of young, giant and large breeds of dogs that results from failure of the fourth ossification center to unite with the ulna.[72] As a result there is a separation of the anconeal process from the diaphysis of the ulna, which results in weight-bearing lameness and secondary degenerative joint disease. Ununited anconeal process has been reported in numerous breeds, with the highest reported incidence in the German shepherd,[17] St. Bernard, and basset hound.[29]

Although the most common sign of ununited anconeal process is a forelimb lameness, which may be shifting in nature if the lesion is bilateral, the clinical presentation can be somewhat variable. In addition to the lameness, clinical signs may include (1) disten-

sion of the joint capsule, (2) crepitation, (3) disuse atrophy of the limb, and (4) lateral deviation of the elbow when standing or walking.[72] Physical examination reveals pain and crepitation upon flexion and extension of the elbow joint.

A tentative diagnosis of ununited anconeal process can be confirmed by radiographic examination of the involved elbow joint. As mentioned previously, the anconeal process in large dogs develops from a sep-

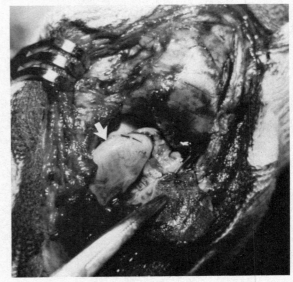

Figure 165–24. Osteochondritis dissecans of the tibiotarsal joint. The osteochondral flap *(arrow)* is associated with the medial ridge of the tibiotarsal bone.

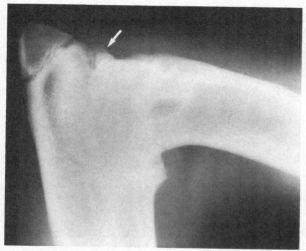

Figure 165–25. Lateral radiograph of a dog with an ununited anconeal process. The anconeal process *(arrow)* has failed to unite with the ulna.

arate center of ossification. This center appears at 93 ± 11 days and unites with the ulnar diaphysis at 124 ± 17 days.[17] For this reason the diagnosis of ununited anconeal process can be confirmed radiographically after the dog is between 16 and 22 weeks of age. The radiographic findings are an anconeal process that is not fused to the ulna (Fig. 165–25) and distorsion of the anconeal process with secondary degenerative joint disease in longer-standing cases.

Although re-attachment of the anconeal process with a bone screw has been described,[32,59] I prefer surgical removal of the offending bone fragment. The anconeal process can be readily removed by employing a lateral approach to the elbow joint. A skin incision is made slightly caudal to the lateral humeral epicondyle and the underlying anconeus muscle identified (Fig. 165–26). A stab incision which will also penetrate the underlying joint capsule, is made through the anconeus muscle. By lengthening the incision the anconeal process can be identified (Fig.

165–27) and removed. Fibrous connective tissue may actually attach the anconeal process to the ulna; however, gentle pressure will readily break this connection down. Closure is accomplished by suturing the anconeus muscle and underlying joint capsule in one layer with absorbable sutures. The subcutaneous tissue and skin are then closed in separate layers. Postoperatively, the limb is placed in a soft bandage for five days and exercise is restricted to a leash for three weeks.

The etiology of ununited anconeal process is unknown. The prevalence in the German shepherd breed suggests a genetic predisposition.[17] Another theory suggests that ununited anconeal process may be a form of osteochondrosis, with characteristic fissures between the cartilage and bone.[48]

FRAGMENTED CORONOID PROCESS (Ununited Coronoid Process, Elbow Dysplasia)

Fragmented or ununited medial coronoid process of the ulna should be considered in the differential diagnosis of elbow lameness in young, actively growing dogs of the large and giant breeds. The syndrome has been most commonly reported in the Newfoundland, St. Bernard, German shepherd, and golden retriever.[7] Fragmented coronoid process can occur as an isolated lesion and in conjunction with osteochondritis dissecans of the distal medial humeral condyle. The clinical signs and radiological findings associated with these two lesions are almost the same, and some investigators have suggested that the osteochondral lesion on the medial humeral condyle represents an "erosion" secondary to the fragmented coronoid process.[49]

The clinical signs of fragmented coronoid process are those of a weight-bearing lameness. In bilateral

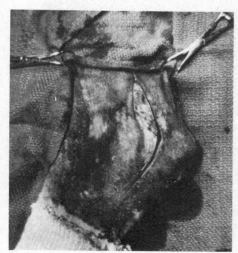

Figure 165–26. Initial skin incision for making a lateral approach to the elbow joint.

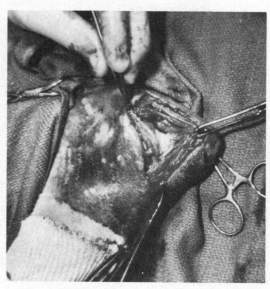

Figure 165–27. Exposure of the anconeal process.

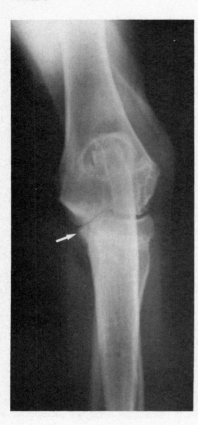

Figure 165–28. Caudocranial view of the elbow joint of a dog with a fragmented coronoid process *(arrow)*.

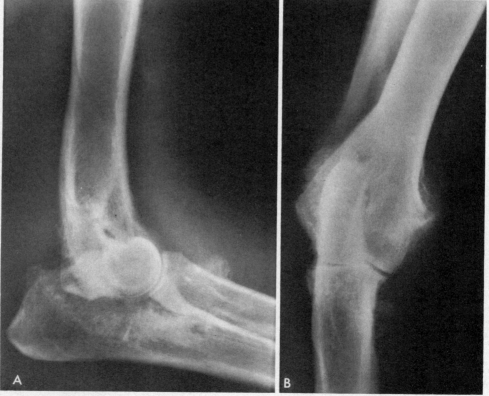

Figure 165–29. Lateral *(A)* and caudocranial *(B)* radiographs of a dog with a chronic case of fragmented coronoid process. Note extensive degenerative disease.

cases the lameness may have a "shifting" nature. Pain and crepitation can usually be elicited upon flexion and extension of the elbow joint.

Radiographic findings in cases of fragmented coronoid process may be somewhat equivocal, although at times the fragmented process can be seen (Fig. 165–28). This is not a consistent finding, as the coronoid process is often superimposed by the radial head. The most common radiographic findings are those of early osteophyte formation on the proximal surface of the anconeal process, the lateral and medial humeral epicondyles, the anterior rim of the humeral articular surface, and the anterior, medial, and lateral rims of the radial articular surface[7] (Fig. 165–29).

Confirmation of fragmented coronoid process often requires an arthrotomy using the medial approach to the elbow joint described for osteochondritis dissecans of the medial humeral condyle. Therapy consists of surgical removal of the fragmented portion of the coronoid process. Variable results can be expected following surgical removal depending on the degree of degenerative joint disease present at the time of surgical intervention. Postoperative care is the same as that for ununited anconeal process.

HYPERTROPHIC OSTEOARTHROPATHY
(Hypertrophic Pulmonary Osteoarthropathy)

Hypertrophic osteoarthropathy is a quadrilateral syndrome of the extremities in which periosteal bone proliferation occurs in the limbs as a sequel to a primary lesion elsewhere in the body. The inciting disease process is most commonly located within the thoracic cavity but can be elsewhere.

The term *hypertrophic osteoarthropathy* is a misnomer. Although the deposition of periarticular collagenous tissue causes the joints to appear swollen, postmortem studies have shown that the articulations are essentially normal.[10]

In the dog and cat hypertrophic osteoarthropathy is most often associated with primary and secondary (metastatic) pulmonary neoplasms; however, the disease has been reported secondary to pneumonia,[80] pulmonary abscesses, subacute bacterial endocarditis, dirofilariasis, bronchiectasis, and *Spirocerca lupi* granulomas.[10] The majority of cases seen in the absence of pulmonary lesions have involved rhabdomyosarcomas of the urinary bladder.[9]

With this syndrome there is an initial increase in peripheral blood flow in the distal half of the extremities. This increased blood flow is followed by formation of excessive amounts of highly vascular connective tissue and subsequent periosteal bone formation.[80] The most popular theory to explain this increased blood flow involves a neural mechanism. According to this theory, a nervous reflex, mediated by the vagus or intercostal nerves, is initiated by conditions that cause pleural irritation. This nervous reflex involves afferent fibers originating in the thorax and efferent pathways, either nervous or humeral, leading to an increased peripheral limb blood flow and subsequent connective tissue and periosteal changes.[34]

The animal with hypertrophic osteoarthropathy is usually presented with a history of sudden or gradual lameness of all four limbs. Early in the course of the disease the affected extremities are painful, warm, pulsatile, and swollen distally. As the condition becomes more chronic, pain is less evident and the animal walks with a more stiff and stilted gait.

The diagnosis can be confirmed by radiographic evaluation of the affected limbs. Periosteal proliferation and new bone formation with accompanying soft tissue swellings are very obvious and are most often bilaterally symmetrical. The periosteal new bone first appears along the shafts of the metacarpal and metatarsal bones (Fig. 165–30). This new bone starts out distally on the shafts of the long bones and spreads proximally. The periosteal proliferations usually run parallel to the length of the bone and can be seen along areas of musculotendinous insertions. The radiographic changes are often seen as far proximally as the humerus and femur (Fig. 165–31).

The diagnosis of hypertrophic osteoarthropathy should be considered in any patient who is suffering from a lameness involving all four limbs with radiographic findings of a bilaterally symmetrical periostitis of the metacarpals, metatarsals, and long bones.

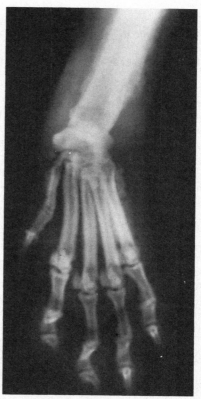

Figure 165–30. Craniocaudal radiograph of the metacarpal bones of a dog with hypertrophic osteoarthropathy showing the characteristic lesions of periosteal new bone formation.

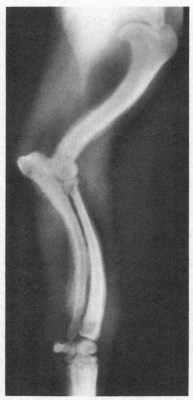

Figure 165–31. Lateral radiograph of the forelimb of a dog with hypertrophic osteoarthropathy showing extensive periosteal new bone formation.

These findings further suggest a radiographic survey of the thoracic cavity to identify the primary lesion.

The treatment of hypertrophic osteoarthropathy is aimed at elimination of the primary cause. Surgical resection of the primary lung lesion results in decreased peripheral blood flow and gradual regression of the clinical signs with eventual resolution of the periostitis. It is interesting to note that in both man and animals cervical vagotomy, which interrupts both efferent cholinergic and afferent nervous impulses, produces a prompt reduction in peripheral blood flow and a subsequent resolution of clinical signs.[34,80] The vagotomy should be performed in the cervical area or high in the mediastinum, as the nerve fibers concerned leave the affected lung lobe near the bronchus and join the vagal trunk in the anterior mediastinum. This therapy is feasible only in cases of unilateral pulmonary involvement, as bilateral vagotomy is impractical.

Unfortunately, the most common cause of hypertrophic osteoarthropathy in the dog is metastatic neoplasia, and treatment is often impossible.

LEGG-CALVÉ-PERTHES-LIKE DISEASE (Perthes Disease, Avascular Necrosis of the Femoral Head, Coxa Plana)

Legg-Calvé-Perthes disease is an ischemic necrosis of the femoral head in young dogs of small and miniature breeds. The syndrome has been seen most frequently in dogs between the ages of 4 and 11 months that weigh less than 10 kg. The syndrome can occur bilaterally but most commonly affects only one femoral head. There is apparently no sex predilection.

The etiology of Legg-Calvé-Perthes disease is unknown. The initial event appears to be an ischemic necrosis of an otherwise normal bone and marrow tissue of the femoral capital epiphysis.[42] Continued growth of the deeper layers of the articular cartilage with failure of the ossific nucleus to grow results in an increase in thickness of the articular cartilage. Continued weight-bearing leads to trabecular fragmentation, deformity, and cavitation. Concurrent with this stage of deformation is the beginning of vascular invasion with hyperemia of the metaphysis and the soft tissues of the joint. Highly vascular granulation tissue then penetrates the growth plate and rapidly results in revascularization and replacement of the dead tissue by the process of "creeping substitution."[42] This vascular invasion occurs at the same time as the natural closure of the growth plate. The revascularized head remains deformed, and there is associated osteophytic proliferation around the femoral neck and acetabular rim. Several causes have been suggested to explain the apparent circulatory disturbance to the femoral head including infection, trauma, toxemia, and hormonal, metabolic, and genetic factors.[71]

The primary clinical sign associated with Legg-Calvé-Perthes disease is the sudden onset of a leg-carrying lameness. In those cases with bilateral involvement, the client may complain of a shifting rear limb lameness. Physical examination reveals pain, crepitation, and a reduced range of motion in the affected hip.

The tentative diagnosis can be confirmed by radiographic evaluation of the affected coxofemoral joint. A variety of changes affecting the proximal femoral metaphysis, epiphysis, and acetabulum have been described, including[41] the following (Fig. 165–32):

1. Flattening or irregularity of the articular surface of the femoral head,
2. Irregular radiographic density of the femoral epiphyseal and metaphyseal regions,
3. An apparent shortening and increase in width of the femoral neck in the metaphyseal area, and
4. An increase in the width of the apparent joint space.

The treatment for Legg-Calvé-Perthes disease is femoral head and neck excision. The technique for this procedure is described elsewhere.

HIP DYSPLASIA

Canine hip dysplasia is the most common skeletal developmental defect in dogs. Simply defined, it is a subluxation (laxity, instability) of the femoral head in relationship to the acetabulum. Unlike hip dysplasia

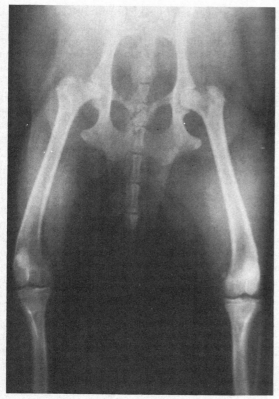

Figure 165–32. Ventrodorsal radiograph of the hip joints of a dog showing the typical lesions of Legg-Calvé-Perthes disease.

in man, canine hip dysplasia is not a congenital condition. Its main development takes place within the first six months of life.[30]

The frequency of incidence and severity of this syndrome are influenced by a number of factors. Canine hip dysplasia has been referred to as "an example of a biomechanical disease representing a disparity between primary muscle mass and too rapid growth of the skeleton. There is a lag or failure of the muscles to develop and reach maturity at the same rate as the skeleton. This allows a major joint such as the hip, that depends on muscle power for stability, to pull apart and thus trigger a series of events that end in hip dysplasia and degenerative joint disease."[63]

There is little question that canine hip dysplasia is a quantitatively inherited trait, and a heritability rate of 0.25 has been reported for German shepherd dogs.[43] When breeding animals or their parents and littermates have hip dysplasia, the risk of the condition developing in the progeny increases.[30] The degree of hip dysplasia in littermates can vary from those with normal hips to those that are severely affected. This is explained by the notion that the genetic pattern of hip dysplasia is "multifactorial" or "polygenetic."[38]

Nutrition, as it affects growth rate, has been thoroughly studied. Rapid weight gain can induce hip dysplasia in progeny of phenotypically normal parents;[45] however, dietary restriction alone cannot pre-

vent the development of this syndrome in progeny whose parents have moderate to severe hip dysplasia.

Since the heritability rate of canine hip dysplasia is 0.25, management conditions influence the expression of the condition or phenotype. The hip joint phenotype that an individual dog has is the result of its genotype interacting synergistically with environmental conditions.[45]

The clinical signs exhibited by the dysplastic dog can be quite variable, ranging from no apparent symptoms to pronounced lameness and disability. Symptoms can be seen as early as four weeks of age but generally are not detected, except in severe cases, until after six months of age. The dysplastic dog can exhibit one or more of the following clinical signs:

1. Weight-bearing lameness that may be more apparent after prolonged exercise,
2. Waddling or swaying gait,
3. Morning stiffness,
4. Difficulty in rising,
5. Reluctance to move,
6. Change in temperament, or
7. Leg-carrying lameness.

Physical examination reveals pain or crepitation upon manipulation of the coxofemoral joints. The dog may have very poorly developed musculature in the hind quarters.

Radiographic examination of the coxofemoral joints is necessary to confirm the diagnosis of canine hip dysplasia. Radiography of the canine hip to demonstrate the presence or absence of dysplastic changes requires a ventrodorsal view, with the rear limbs extended and the femurs rotated inward and parallel both to one another and to the table top. Radiographs should be assessed to determine (1) the shape and depth of the acetabulum, (2) the shape, contour, and position of the femoral head, and (3) the presence of any degenerative joint disease. The basic radiographic change in canine hip dysplasia is a subluxation of the femoral head in relationship to the acetabulum (Fig. 165–33).

Depending on the degree of subluxation, the dysplastic condition of the patient may be classified as mild, moderate, or severe. The treatment of canine hip dysplasia can be medical, surgical, or a combination of both. Although there is no "cure" for hip dysplasia, appropriate therapy and management can help patients live "within their joints."

Medical or conservative therapy involves enforced (cage) rest during periods in which the dog is experiencing discomfort. Mild analgesics such as salicylates (aspirin) in adequate doses (25 mg/kg q8h) can be helpful in relieving the arthritic pain secondary to hip joint laxity. Anti-inflammatory drugs (corticosteroids) should be used when other medications have failed and then only with extreme caution.

The surgical approach to hip dysplasia is covered elsewhere.

In recent years an attempt has been made to try and eliminate or at least reduce the incidence of

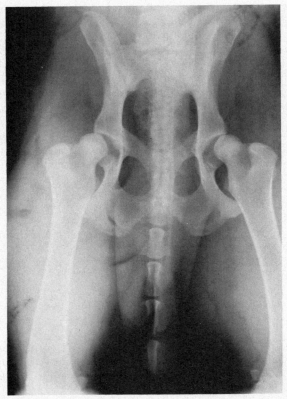

Figure 165–33. Ventrodorsal radiograph of the hip joints of a dog showing the classic radiographic signs of canine hip dysplasia.

canine hip dysplasia by radiographic evaluation of prospective parents. Although these efforts have met with some success, the accuracy of identifying canine hip dysplasia genotype by analyzing phenotype is not great.[54] Selection for breeding based on individual normal hip radiographs (phenotype) has limited success in reducing the incidence of this syndrome. However, selection based on family performance or progeny testing can rapidly and significantly reduce the incidence of canine hip dysplasia, as this method greatly improves the accuracy of identifying individuals of superior genotypes.[54]

METABOLIC BONE DISEASES

Hyperparathyroid Bone Disease

Increased secretion of parathyroid hormone results in generalized bone disease. Primary hyperparathyroidism (caused by a parathyroid adenoma, carcinoma, or hyperplasia) and secondary hyperparathyroidism (occurring as a result of hypocalcemia due to any cause, e.g., chronic renal disease or nutritional imbalance) both result in bone disease.[40] In the former instance, the changes are those resulting from parathyroid hormone action alone, whereas in the latter other features may be present in addition to those of hyperparathyroidism.

All actions of parathyroid hormone are either directly or indirectly involved with maintaining the serum calcium concentration. The abnormalities seen with hyperparathyroidism can be predicted from understanding the primary actions of parathyroid hormone. Those actions are[26] (1) to increase the efflux of calcium from bone; (2) to indirectly increase the intestinal calcium absorption; (3) to increase the tubular re-absorption of calcium from the kidney; (4) to increase the renal phosphate excretion by decreasing the renal tubular re-absorption of phosphate; and (5) to stimulate the bone remodeling system with an increase in the number of activation centers. The resultant biochemical changes are an increase in plasma calcium, a decrease in plasma phosphate, and an increase in urinary phosphate excretion.[26] The stimulation of the bone remodeling system results primarily in an increase in the number of activation centers, with the rate of bone formation and resorption within any one remodeling center being affected only minimally. The sum total of effects of parathyroid hormone depends on the relative rates of osteoblastic and osteoclastic activity. In general, osteoclastic activity predominates[40] and there is an increase in the total number of "bites" taken out of the bone at any one time, with an increase in the amount of bone that is missing at any one time.[26]

The changes seen in secondary hyperparathyroidism are complicated by the effects of the primary disease in addition to those biochemical and pathological changes associated with an increase in parathyroid hormone.

In general, primary hyperparathyroidism is rare in small animals and is usually associated with a parathyroid neoplasm. The most common abnormalities associated with increased parathyroid hormone secretion are secondary to nutritional imbalances and renal disease. These syndromes are discussed in detail elsewhere[12] and are only superficially discussed here.

Renal secondary hyperparathyroidism is a result of the inability of the kidneys to eliminate phosphate normally. The resulting hyperphosphatemia stimulates increased parathyroid hormone secretion, which leads to increased resorption of bone. Renal secondary hyperparathyroidism is most often a disease of older animals with advanced kidney disease but can be seen in younger animals in association with congenital renal disease. Clinically the skeletal changes associated with bone resorption are often confined to the jaws and skull. Increased resorption of alveolar bone can be detected through radiographic studies of the involved areas.

Nutritional secondary hyperparathyroidism is most commonly the result of feeding young animals a predominantly meat diet. Skeletal flesh, heart, liver, and kidney are very low in calcium content and have an imbalanced calcium-phosphorus ratio. These low calcium–high phosphorus food products lead to hypocalcemia, which serves as a stimulus for parathyroid overactivity. Affected animals suffer from increased bone resorption and resulting generalized osteitis fibrosa in young animals and osteoporosis in adults. Clinical signs are related to bone pain and pathological fractures in growing animals. In adults, periodontal disease with loss of alveolar bone is a prominent feature of this syndrome. Radiographically there is a generalized decrease in bone density with a loss of fine trabeculation and a thinning of the cortices. In young animals, the lamina dura dentis may become invisible around the deciduous teeth. Treatment of this syndrome primarily involves dietary corrections and supplementation with calcium.

Rickets and Osteomalacia

Osteomalacia is a disorder characterized by impaired mineralization of newly formed osteoid tissue.[40] Consequently, the bones are soft and cannot bear mechanical stress adequately. This leads to bending and deformity of the bones. Osteomalacia occurs in adults in whom bone growth at the epiphyseal plate has ceased.

Rickets is a disease characterized by impaired mineralization of cartilage in the growth plate, leading to arrest in the formation of the primary spongiosa during enchondral ossification.[26] Rickets occurs prior to the closure of the epiphyseal plate and therefore affects only growing animals.

Both rickets and osteomalacia are the result of inadequate plasma levels of vitamin D. This vitamin, through its active metabolite 1,25-dihydroxy-vitamin D, enhances the absorption of calcium and phosphate by the intestine and plays an important role in the maintenance of the normal plasma levels of these ions.[40]

Rickets and osteomalacia are extremely rare in the dog and cat. It is important that they not be confused with more common skeletal disorders.

1. Aegerter, E., and Kirkpatrick, T. A.: *Orthopedic Disease*. W. B. Saunders, Philadelphia, 1968.
2. Alexander, J. W.: Hypertrophic osteodystrophy. Canine Pract. *5*:48, 1978.
3. Alexander, J. W., and Kallfelz, F. A.: A case of craniomandibular osteopathy in a Labrador retriever. Vet. Med./Small Anim. Clin. *70*:560, 1975.
4. Alexander, J. W., Richardson, D. C., and Selcer, B. A.: Osteochondritis dissecans of the elbow, stifle, and hock—a review. J. Am. Anim. Hosp. Assoc. *17*:51, 1981.
5. Banks, W. C., and Bridges, C. H.: Multiple cartilaginous exostoses in a dog. J. Am. Vet. Med. Assoc. *129*:131, 1956.
6. Barrett, R. B., Schall, W. B., and Lewis, R. E.: Clinical and radiographic features of canine eosinophic panosteitis. J. Am. Anim. Hosp. Assoc. *4*:94, 1968.
7. Berzon, J. L, and Quick, C. B.: Fragmented coronoid process: Anatomical, clinical, and radiographic considerations with case analyses. J. Am. Anim. Hosp. Assoc. *16*:241, 1980.
8. Bohnig, R. H., Suter, P. F., Hohn, R. B., et al.: Clinical and radiographic survey of canine panosteitis. J. Am. Vet. Med. Assoc. *156*:870, 1970.
9. Brody, R. S.: Hypertrophic osteoarthropathy in the dog: A clinico-pathologic survey of 60 cases. J. Am. Vet. Med. Assoc. *159*:1242, 1971.
10. Brody, R. S.: Hypertrophic osteoarthropathy. *In* Kirk, R. W. (ed.): *Current Veterinary Therapy V.* W. B. Saunders, Philadelphia, 1974.
11. Brown, R. J., Trevethan, W. P., and Henry, V. L.: Multiple osteochondroma in a Siamese cat. J. Am. Vet. Med. Assoc. *160*:433, 1972.
12. Brown, S. G.: Skeletal diseases. *In* Ettinger, S. J. (ed.): *Textbook of Veterinary Internal Medicine.* W. B. Saunders, Philadelphia, 1975.
13. Burk, R. L., and Broadhurst, J. J.: Craniomandibular osteopathy in a Great Dane. J. Am. Vet. Med. Assoc. *169*:635, 1976.
14. Burt, J. K., and Wilson, G. P.: A study of eosinophilic panosteitis (enostosis) in German shepherd dogs. Acta Radiol. (Suppl. *319*):7, 1972.
15. Carrig, C. B., and Morgan, J. P.: Microcirculation of the humeral head in the immature dog. J. Am. Vet. Radiol. Soc. *25*:28, 1974.
16. Chester, D. K.: Multiple cartilaginous exostoses in two generations of dogs. J. Am. Vet. Med. Assoc. *159*:895, 1971.
17. Corley, E. A., Sutherland, T. M., and Carlson, W. D.: Genetic aspects of canine elbow dysplasia. J. Am. Vet. Med. Assoc. *153*:543, 1968.
18. Cotter, S. M., Griffiths, R. C., and Leav, I.: Enostosis of Young Dogs. J. Am. Vet. Med. Assoc. *153*:401, 1968.
19. Craig, P. H., and Riser, W. H.: Osteochondritis dissecans in the proximal humerus of the dog. J. Am. Vet. Radiol. Soc. *6*:40, 1965.
20. Dingwall, J. S., Pass, D. A., Pennock, P. W., et al.: Case report, multiple cartilaginous exostoses in a dog. Can. Vet. J. *11*:114, 1970.
21. Doige, C. E., Pharr, J. W., and Withrow, S. J.: Chondrosarcoma arising in multiple cartilaginous exostoses in a dog. J. Am. Anim. Hosp. Assoc. *14*:605, 1978.
22. Evers, W. H.: Enostosis in a dog. J. Am. Vet. Med. Assoc. *154*:799, 1969.
23. Gambardella, P. C., Osborne, C. A., and Stevens, J. B.: Multiple cartilaginous exostoses in the dog. J. Am. Vet. Med. Assoc. *166*:761, 1975.
24. Gee, B. R., and Doige, C. E.: Multiple cartilaginous exostoses in a litter of dogs. J. Am. Vet. Med. Assoc. *156*:53, 1970.
25. Grondalen, J.: Metaphyseal osteopathy (hypertrophic osteodystrophy) in growing dogs. A clinical study. J. Small Anim. Pract. *17*:721, 1976.
26. Grubb, S. A., and Talmage, R. V.: Metabolic bone diseases. *In* Wilson, F. C. (ed.): *The Musculoskeletal System, Basic Processes and Disorders.* J. B. Lippincott, Philadelphia, 1983.
27. Hanselka, D. V., and Thompson, R. B.: Equine multiple cartilaginous exostoses. Vet. Med./Small Anim. Clin. *69*:979, 1974.
28. Hardy, W. D., and Stockman, W. S.: Clinico-pathologic conference. J. Am. Vet. Med. Assoc. *154*:1600, 1969.
29. Hayes, H. M., Selby, L. A., Wilson, G. P., et al.: Epidemiologic observations of canine elbow disease (emphasis on dysplasia). J. Am. Anim. Hosp. Assoc. *15*:449, 1979.
30. Hedhammar, O., Olsson, S. E., Andersson, S. O., et al.: Canine hip dysplasia: Study of heritability in 401 litters of German shepherd dogs. J. Am. Vet. Med. Assoc. *174*:1012, 1979.
31. Hedhammer, O., Wu, F. M., Krook, L., et al.: Overnutrition and skeletal disease. An experimental study in growing Great Danes. Cornell Vet. *64*:1, 1974.
32. Herron, M. R.: Ununited anconeal process. *In* Bojrab, M. J. (ed.): *Current Techniques in Small Animal Surgery.* Lea & Febiger, Philadelphia, 1981.
33. Hohn, R. B.: Osteochondritis dissecans of the humeral head. J. Am. Vet. Med. Assoc. *163*:69, 1973.
34. Holling, H. E., Danielson, G. K., Hamilton, R. W., et al.: Hypertrophic pulmonary osteoarthropathy. J. Thorac. Cardiovasc. Surg. *46*:310, 1963.
35. Holmes, J. R.: Suspected skeletal scurvy in the dog. Vet. Rec. *74*:801, 1962.
36. Huvos, A. G.: *Bone Tumors*. W. B. Saunders, Philadelphia, 1979.

37. Jaffe, H. L.: *Tumor and Tumorous Conditions of Bones and Joints.* Lea & Febiger, Philadelphia, 1964.

38. Jessen, C. R., and Spurrell, F. A.: The heritability of canine hip dysplasia. Proc. Symp. Hip Dysplasia, 1973, pp. 53–61.

39. Kasstrom, H., Olsson, S. E., and Suter, P. F.: Panosteitis in the dog: A radiographic scintimetric and trifluorchrome investigation. Acta Radiol. (Suppl. *319*):15, 1972.

40. Kumar, R., and Riggs, L.: Pathologic bone physiology. *In* Urist, M. R. (ed.): *Fundamental and Clinical Bone Physiology.* J. B. Lippincott, Philadelphia, 1980.

41. Lee, R.: A Study of the radiographic and histological changes occurring in Legg-Calvé-Perthes disease (LCP) in the dog. J. Small Anim. Pract. *11*:621, 1970.

42. Lee, R.: Legg-Perthes disease in the dog: Histological and associated radiological changes. J. Am. Vet. Rad. Soc. *XV*:24, 1974.

43. Leighton, E. A., Linn, J. M., and Willham, R. L.: A genetic study of canine hip dysplasia. Am. J. Vet. Res. *38*:241, 1977.

44. Lewis, R. E., and Van Sickle, D. C.: Congenital hemimelia (agenesis) of the radius in a dog and a cat. J. Am. Vet. Med. Assoc. *156*:1892, 1970.

45. Lust, G., Farrell, P. W., and Sheffy, B. E.: II. An improved procedure for genetic selection against hip dysplasia in dogs. Cornell Vet. *68*:41, 1978.

46. Meier, H., Clark, S. T., Schnelle, G. B., and Will, D. H.: Hypertrophic osteodystrophy associated with disturbance of vitamin C synthesis in dogs. J. Am. Vet. Med. Assoc. *130*:483, 1957.

47. Morgan, J. P., Carlson, W. D., and Adams, O. R.: Hereditary multiple exostoses in the horse. J. Am. Vet. Med. Assoc. *140*:1320, 1962.

48. Olsson, S. E.: Osteochondrosis—a growing problem to dog breeders. Gaines Progress:1, 1976.

49. Olsson, S. E.: Osteochondrosis in the dog. *In* Kirk, R. W. (ed.): *Current Veterinary Therapy VI.* W. B. Saunders, Philadelphia, 1977.

50. O'Rahilly, R.: An analysis of cases of radial hemimelia. Arch. Pathol. *44*:28, 1974.

51. Owen, L. N., and Bostock, D. E.: Multiple cartilaginous exostoses with development of a metastasizing osteosarcoma in a Shetland sheepdog. J. Small Anim. Pract. *12*:507, 1971.

52. Owen, L. N., and Nielsen, S. W.: Multiple cartilaginous exostoses (diaphyseal aclasis) in a Yorkshire terrier. J. Small Anim. Pract. *9*:519, 1968.

53. Paatsama, S., Rokkanen, P., Jussila, J., et al.: Somatotropin, thyrotropin, and corticotropin hormone-induced changes in the cartilages and bones of the shoulder and knee joint in young dogs. J. Small Anim. Pract. *12*:595, 1971.

54. Pharr, J. W.: Canine hip dysplasia. Vet. Clin. North Am. *8*:309, 1978.

55. Pool, R. R., and Carrig, C. B.: Multiple cartilaginous exostoses in a cat. Vet. Pathol. *9*:350, 1972.

56. Pool, R. R., and Leighton, R. L.: Craniomandibular osteopathy in a dog. J. Am. Vet. Med. Assoc. *154*:657, 1969.

57. Power, J. W.: Osteochondromatosis in the racing greyhound. J. Small Anim. Pract. *16*:803, 1975.

58. Prata, R. G., Stoll, S. G., and Zaki, F. A.: Spinal cord compression caused by osteocartilaginous exostoses of the spine in two dogs. J. Am. Vet. Med. Assoc. *166*:371, 1975.

59. Pritchard, D. L.: Anconeal process pseudoarthrosis: Treated by lag-screw fixation. Canine Pract. *6*:18, 1976.

60. Richardson, D. C.: Radial agenesis. J. Vet. Orthop. *1*:39, 1979.

61. Riddle, W. E., and Leighton, R. L.: Osteochondromatosis in a cat. J. Am. Vet. Med. Assoc. *156*:1428, 1970.

62. Riser, W. H.: Radiographic differential diagnosis of skeletal diseases of young dogs. J. Am. Vet. Rad. Soc. *5*:15, 1964.

63. Riser, W. H.: Canine hip dysplasia: Cause and control. J. Am. Vet. Med. Assoc. *165*:360, 1974.

64. Riser, W. H., Parker, L. J., and Shiver, J. F.: Canine craniomandibular osteopathy. J. Am. Vet. Rad. Soc. *8*:23, 1967.

65. Rosenblum, G., Rogins, G. M., and Carlisle, C. H.: Osteochondritis dissecans of the tibiotarsal joint in the dog. J. Small Anim. Pract. *19*:759, 1978.

66. Schulz, S.: A case of craniomandibular osteopathy in a boxer. J. Small Anim. Pract. *19*:747, 1978.

67. Shupe, J. L., Olson, E. E., Sharma, R. P., et al.: Multiple exostoses in horses. Mod. Vet. Pract. *51*:34, 1970.

68. Sinibaldi, K. R.: Medical approach to the tarsus. J. Am. Anim. Hosp. Assoc. *15*:77, 1979.

69. Sinibaldi, K. R.: Hypertrophic osteodystrophy. *In* Bojrab, M. J. (ed.): *Pathophysiology in Small Animal Surgery.* Lea & Febiger, Philadelphia, 1981.

70. Smith, C. W., and Stavater, J. L.: Osteochondritis of the canine shoulder joint. A review of 35 cases. J. Am. Anim. Hosp. Assoc. *11*:658, 1975.

71. Smith, K. W.: Legg-Perthes disease. Vet. Clin. North Am. *1*:479, 1971.

72. Stevens, D. R., and Sande, R. D.: An elbow dysplasia syndrome in the dog. J. Am. Vet. Med. Assoc. *165*:1065, 1974.

73. Swalley, J., and Swalley, M.: Agenesis of the radius in a kitten. Feline Pract. *8*:25, 1978.

74. Teare, J. A., Krook, L., Kallfelz, F. A., et al.: Ascorbic acid deficiency and hypertrophic osteodystrophy in the dog: A rebuttal. Cornell Vet. *69*:384, 1979.

75. Turnier, J. C., and Silverman, S.: A case study of canine panosteitis: Comparison of radiographic and radioisotopic studies. Am. J. Vet. Res. *39*:1550, 1978.

76. Vaughan, L. C., and Jones, D. G. C.: Osteochondritis dissecans of the head of the humerus in dogs. J. Small Anim. Pract. *9*:283, 1968.

77. Watkins, J. D., and Bradley, R.: Craniomandibular osteopathy in a Labrador puppy. Vet. Rec. *79*:262, 1966.

78. Watson, A. D. J., Blair, R. C., Farrow, B. R. H., et al.: Hypertrophic osteodystrophy in the dog. Austr. Vet. J. *49*:433, 1973.

79. Watson, A. D. J., Huxtable, C. R. R., and Farrow, B. R. H.: Craniomandibular osteopathy in Doberman Pinschers. J. Small Anim. Pract. *16*:11, 1975.

80. Watson, A. D. J., and Porges, W. L.: Regressing hypertrophic osteopathy in a dog following unilateral vagotomy. Vet. Rec. *14*:240, 1973.

81. Wolfe, D. A.: Surgical correction of osteochondritis dissecans of the medical humeral condyle and ununited coronoid process in a dog. Vet. Med./Small Anim. Clin. *71*:1554, 1976.

Chapter 166

Muscles and Tendons

Mark Bloomberg

Injuries to muscles and tendons of small animals present a diagnostic challenge. Such injuries are often masked by more severe skeletal injuries such as fractures of bones or dislocations of joints. Unless the musculotendinous insult is severe enough to be disabling or is presented in the acute stages, the animal may show minimal clinical signs, making a specific diagnosis challenging. The majority of musculotendinous injuries do not require surgical intervention; instead, careful postdiagnostic management, including physical therapy, topical medication, and gradual return to training or normal activity, is necessary.

Injuries to muscles and tendons may be separate entities or a combination of trauma to the musculotendinous unit either at its origin or insertion. Injuries to muscle and tendons are divided into: (1) muscle belly, (2) musculotendinous junction, (3) tendon, and (4) tendon at its origin or insertion. The basic principles of healing, injury, and surgical repair are discussed and these principles applied to specific muscle and tendon injuries.

SKELETAL MUSCLE

Injuries to skeletal muscles in small animals are not as dramatic as tendon injuries.[16] Bruised (contused) or partially ruptured muscles are common. A physical examination, complemented by a thorough history and detailed palpation of the animals' musculature, is necessary to pinpoint the damaged muscles. This is in contrast to severe muscle or musculotendinous ruptures or tears which are unusual yet more easily diagnosed in their acute stages because of dramatic clinical signs.

Lameness at a walk caused by isolated muscle injuries may not persist past 24 hours after the initial injury. If lameness persists for longer than 24 hours, additional injuries should be suspected.[16] Though the animal may be sound at a walk, the effects of muscle injury may be more readily discernible at a faster gait. This is an important diagnostic fact when examining racing or working animals.

Anatomy

In mammals, skeletal muscles comprise approximately one-third to one-half the total body weight.[19] A skeletal or striated muscle fiber is made up of long, cylindrical fibers formed into bundles. Collections of these bundles form the muscle as a whole. The significance of any injury to muscle relates to changes in the individual fibers. Each muscle fiber is surrounded by connective tissue, which supports each individual fiber (endomysium), fiber bundle (perimysium), and the entire muscle (epimysium).[24] All these connective tissue sheaths communicate with each other. The fibrous connective tissue septa contain blood vessels and nerve fibers, bind and integrate the action of the individual fibers, and simultaneously allow freedom of motion between individual muscle components and muscles.[35] A muscle fiber is composed of individual myofibrils, the basic unit of muscle. Many myofibrils lie within the sarcolemmal sheath. The myofibrils are connected by the sarcoplasm containing the retinaculum, which provides the connecting link for transmission of impulses from the sarcolemmal sheath to the myofibril.

Skeletal muscles are attached by connective tissue to bone or cartilage. These connective tissue attachments may be cordlike tendon or a flat aponeurosis. Some muscles have no tendons or aponeurosis but attach directly to periosteum via fleshy attachments. The proximal fixed portion of muscle is its origin, and the immovable distal point of attachment is its insertion. The expanded fleshy part of a muscle is its belly; the origin is the head; and minor insertions are called slips.[19]

The contraction of muscle is initiated by a nerve impulse travelling through a motor nerve fiber (axon) to the muscle fiber or cells. Each axon serves several muscle fibers. Neuromuscular units are known as motor units. The more motor units per muscle fiber, the greater the precision of movement of the muscle. The more muscle fibers, the stronger the muscle.[19]

Healing of Skeletal Muscle

The sarcolemmal or muscle nucleus is the basic unit of the muscle fiber. Muscle cells do regenerate. All myofibrils have the capability of regenerating if they are not strangulated by extensive fibrous tissue.[41] Healing between muscle ends by fibrous protein synthesis is not as desirable as regeneration of myofibrils. If the sarcolemmal nuclei are destroyed, regeneration does not take place. If they survive, their reaction to injury is rapid and effective. If the endomysial support of the fibers is not destroyed, the new fibers replace degenerated ones, and long stretches of muscle may be reconstructed. If the endomysial tube has been destroyed, the growing bud becomes a multinucleated club which may be successful in sprouting branches, depending upon the amount of obstruction by fibrous tissue or hemorrhage. Undifferentiated cells lying adjacent to muscle fibers may form myoblasts and contribute to muscle regeneration.[41]

Muscle Injuries

Minor injuries to muscles can be divided into contusions, strains, and lacerations. Contusions frequently accompany traumatic injury. Unless the contusion is massive, treatment is usually unnecessary. A massive contusion results in excessive inflammation and edema owing to hematoma formation that can result in marked muscle dysfunction requiring treatment. Treatments for muscle contusions depend on whether the injury is acute (less than 24 hours since injury) or chronic. Initial first aid therapy consists of immobilization, cold, and elevation. After 24 hours, therapy consists of warm water compresses or baths, regional compressive wraps, protective bandaging, and immobilization.[20] Additional therapy may include topical DMSO applied locally two to three times daily during the recovery period.[38] The systemic administration of antibiotics should be reserved for massive contusions that have resulted in muscle necrosis. Nonsteroidal anti-inflammatory drugs are preferred over systemic corticosteroids.

A strained muscle is the result of overstretching or overuse of any part of the muscle-tendon unit causing structural alterations and signs of inflammation, such as pain and lameness.[20] An accurate history relating a particular activity to the onset of pain or lameness may be helpful in diagnosing the injury. The treatment of muscle strains is similar to that of muscle contusions. Therapy is immobilization of the affected muscle and enforced rest. Topical or systemic administration of nonsteroidal anti-inflammatory agents along with hydrotherapy hastens return of function of the injured muscle.

The treatment of muscle lacerations depends on whether the injury is acute or chronic or if there is potential for a loss of function because of fibrous healing. Before conservative therapy or surgical repair of a lacerated muscle, the basic principles of the treatment of open wounds should be followed. Wounds should be irrigated with copious amounts of fluid and adequately debrided. Sutures should be placed in the muscle sheaths rather than the muscle fibers themselves if the fibrous sheath has sufficient strength to hold sutures. Synthetic, monofilament, nonabsorbable sutures placed in an interrupted horizontal mattress pattern are preferred because of the minimal amount of adhesion formation (Fig. 166–1A). If the muscle sheath has been severely damaged or if it is necessary to reappose a deeply lacerated muscle belly, muscle fibers can be apposed with interrupted horizontal mattress sutures placed deep into the muscle bellies and reinforced with rubber tubing or buttons to prevent sutures from pulling out (Fig. 166–1)[8,12,35]

Occasionally transecting a muscle belly may give better surgical exposure for application of an internal fixation device, e.g., transection of the teres minor for approach to the shoulder joint or the brachialis muscle of the forelimb to better expose the distal humerus. Transection of a muscle can be avoided by adequate mobilization, subperiosteal elevation, tenotomy, or osteotomy of its origin or insertion. If a muscle must be incised, it should be parallel to the muscle fibers as in a grid incision, to avoid postop-

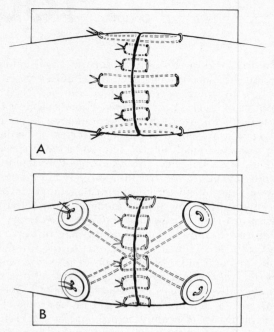

Figure 166–1. Suture techniques for anastomosis of muscle. *A,* Interrupted horizontal mattress sutures placed deep and superficial in an attempt to penetrate any available fascial sheaths within the muscle. *B,* Interrupted horizontal mattress sutures have been bolstered by the addition of button tension sutures. (Modified from Milton, J. L., and Henderson, R. A.: Muscles and tendons. In Bojrab, M. J. (ed.): *Current Techniques in Small Animal Surgery.* 2nd ed. Lea & Febiger, Philadelphia, 1983.)

erative complications affecting use of the limb.[8] If transection of the muscle is performed, subsequent repair should follow the guidelines described under treatment of muscle rupture.

Muscle Rupture

Rupture of muscle may be partial or complete. It most often occurs in younger animals, compared with tendon rupture in older animals. The cause of muscle rupture is a powerful active contraction of a flexor motor unit at the same time that forced passive extension occurs.[41] Muscle is a highly differentiated tissue that is more resistant to trauma than is tendon. Complete ruptures are unusual in small animals, except for the diaphragm and abdominal muscles.[8] Muscle ruptures have been reported more frequently in the racing greyhound as a result of strenuous athletic activity. Such injuries include ruptures of the gracilis, triceps, and gastrocnemius muscles.[16,24,55] Rupture of the serratus ventralis occurs in cats and dogs.[26,35] Muscle ruptures secondary to joint dislocations and fractures can result in rupture of adjacent musculature.[35]

It is often difficult to differentiate between a partial or complete muscle rupture. Muscular injuries may show signs of local tenderness, subcutaneous ecchymosis, swelling, and lameness. Chronic injuries may show lameness and muscular atrophy. A higher percentage of muscle ruptures occur at the musculotendinous junction rather than through the fleshy belly.[8]

Incomplete ruptures usually do not require operative repair. The acutely injured muscle may be initially treated with immobilization, cold packs, and elevation. Immobilization with a modified Robert-Jones dressing for two to three weeks, followed by two or three more weeks of restricted activity, may be all that is necessary. Immobilization prevents excessive movement and further separation of the torn muscle to allow optimal muscle cell regeneration and minimize scar tissue formation.

If complete or partial rupture of a muscle is difficult to determine, the damaged muscle can be explored through a small skin incision. It is better to make an early diagnosis of a muscle rupture and repair it rather than attempt resection of scar tissue at a later date.

Complete rupture of a muscle, either midsubstance (belly) or musculotendinous, resulting in loss of function or a crippling injury, is an indication for reparative surgery. The clinical signs of a ruptured muscle vary with the severity of the muscle damage and the significance of the particular muscle injured. An animal with a ruptured muscle initially shows acute onset of lameness or altered gait and localized signs of inflammation. In addition, there may be a palpable gap or discontinuity between the ends of the muscle belly, accompanied by hematoma formation. The loss of integrity of the muscle belly is often termed "dropped muscle" (Fig. 166–2).[16,35] Diagnosis of the ruptured muscle by palpation may be difficult if the muscle sheath remains intact.

Delay in surgical repair of a ruptured muscle permits extensive fibrous protein synthesis in and around the muscle ends.[41] New connective tissue forms rapidly between the severed muscle bellies, resulting in a fibrous scar. If the muscle heals in a shortened position the range of motion is decreased. With physical therapy and active and passive movement, scar tissue can remodel and elongate but not

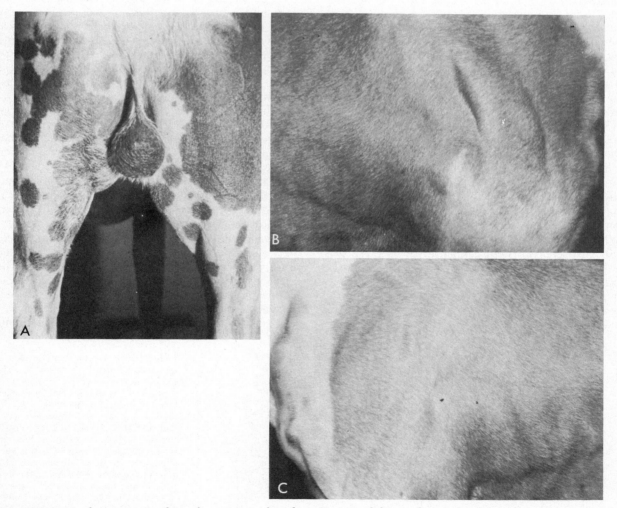

Figure 166–2. Muscle ruptures involving the racing greyhound. *A,* Rupture of the gracilis muscle of the right rear leg. Note the tremendous disparity in size of the medial thigh due to swelling and hematoma formation. *B,* Ruptured or "dropped" long head of the triceps muscle involving the right front leg. Note the swelling in the area of the triceps muscle and the depressed area caudal to it. Contrast this to the dog's normal left front leg (*C*). (Courtesy of J. Dee and L. Dee, Hollywood Animal Hospital, Hollywood, Florida.)

without a serious loss of power. "Dropped muscles" or complete ruptures in the racing greyhound are often treated conservatively, yielding unsatisfactory results.[35]

Ultimately primary muscle repair is the goal of treatment. If secondary repair is performed, the old scar tissue must be excised using precise debridement and coaptation of unscarred muscle fibers. Even in primary repair severely damaged or devitalized muscle and connective tissue should be debrided to minimize fibrous scarring and promote regeneration of muscle fibers.[41]

Surgical Repair of Ruptured Muscle. Care should be taken in the handling of healthy and damaged muscles. The surgical approach to muscles is made through tissue planes. Muscles are surrounded by fascial sheaths and loose areolar tissue connecting different muscle groups by an intermuscular septum. Muscles should be retracted gently to avoid iatrogenic fiber rupture and should be kept moist with sterile saline or lactated Ringer's solution. If additional exposure is needed the skin incision should be lengthened. If muscles need to be separated further, their origins or insertions should be carefully freed by sharp dissection, osteotomy, or subperiosteal elevation. It is much better to elevate the periosteum with the muscle attached. This allows return of periosteum to its original position when the muscle is replaced. Because of the vascular connection of muscle to periosteum the periosteum heals much faster if this connection is left intact.

Severed muscles should be reattached as soon as possible after the diagnosis is made, by an anatomical alignment of the muscle ends with an end-to-end anastomosis. The tension on muscles is longitudinal, thus paralleling the muscle fibers. These longitudinal forces, combined with the inherent weak suture-holding power of muscle, contribute to sutures pulling out when tension is applied to aligned muscle segments. The severed muscle ends should be carefully inspected for deep fascial layers as these may provide holding power for sutures. Muscles may be uni-, bi- or multipennate, which means there are one or more tendons running alongside or invading the muscle.[19] These tendons also provide solid tissue for sutures.

The ends of the ruptured muscle, after thorough debridement, may be approximated using large horizontal mattress sutures of a nonabsorbable, nonreactive suture material such as nylon, polypropylene, or polyester fiber. These sutures are tightened until the muscle edges are together. Muscle should be handled gently with traction sutures, muscle hooks, or fine tooth forceps. To help prevent sutures from pulling out through the tissue the suture material can be tied over stents, buttons, fascia, or rubber tubing to relieve tension. These can be used alone or in conjunction with intramuscular sutures (Fig. 166–1).[8,12,35] Once the edges of the muscle are apposed, the muscle sheath at the anastamotic site is sutured circumferentially with horizontal mattress sutures of a nonabsorbable material smaller than the intramuscular sutures. In some cases, such as with small muscles or flat, sheetlike muscles, two buttons or stents used as tension absorbers are sufficient.

Postoperatively, it is important that the affected muscle be immobilized for two to three weeks, followed by gradual return to activity and physical therapy after four to six weeks. The prognosis for complete return of function for working or racing dogs remains guarded.[16] With or without surgical intervention, postoperative sequelae such as atrophy, fibrosis, and varying degrees of dysfunction may result from muscle injuries. Surgical resection of scar tissue (cording) followed by muscle-to-muscle anastomosis may restore function if combined with physical therapy.[30] Muscle can be freed from surrounding adhesions to restore function. Scarred muscle that severely restricts joint motion can be excised if that particular muscle is not essential to normal function of the limb.[35]

As stated, musculotendinous rupture is more common than rupture of the muscle belly. The musculotendinous rupture may be less traumatic in its physical appearance because of the decreased amount of hemorrhage and hematoma function. There is less pain and swelling with this type of injury and often it may be a chronic injury.[16] The severity of the rupture and the function of the involved muscle determine the clinical signs and treatment needed. Diagnosis of a musculotendinous rupture may be more difficult because the separation of the segments

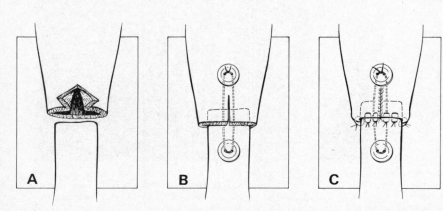

Figure 166–3. Anastomosis of muscle at musculotendinous junction. *A,* The muscle has been slit for two to three centimeters, creating a bed for implantation of the end of the tendon. *B,* The tendon end has been implanted in the bed and secured with button tension sutures. *C,* Following implantation, the fascial sheath of the muscle has been sutured to the paratenon of the tendon with simple interrupted horizontal mattress sutures of nonabsorbable material. (Modified from Braden, T. D.: Tendon and muscles. *In* Bojrab, M. J. (ed.): *Current Techniques in Small Animal Surgery.* 2nd ed. Lea & Febiger, Philadelphia, 1983.)

is usually not palpable for the rupture occurs over a broad area and portions of the tendon and muscle sheath may remain intact. There will be signs of inflammation over the damaged area in acute injuries. A diagnosis of a musculotendinous rupture is supported by conformational changes and lameness caused by loss of muscle function.[35]

If the rupture is complete, immediate surgical repair is indicated. When the muscle and tendon are of similar size, the ends can be approximated as described for muscle tears. It is important to locate any fascial tissues deep in the muscle that may provide firm attachments for sutures. If a disparity exists in size of the tendon and muscle, the tendon can be implanted into the end of the muscle for 2 to 3 cm (Fig. 164–3),[8] by slitting the muscle for 2 to 3 cm halfway through its depth. A bed is prepared in the muscle elevating the edges of the muscle incision. Approximately 1 cm of tendon is laid in the muscular bed and the muscle flaps laid over the tendon. The tension can be taken off the anastomosis using a two polypropylene button tension technique.[8,12] The end of the tendon is attached further using horizontal mattress sutures running from muscle to tendon to muscle. The muscle sheath is sutured to the paratenon with similar suture and suture patterns.

Postoperative care is as for repair of muscles but differs in that immobilization is extended to three to four weeks, followed by restricted activity for an additional three to four weeks.

SPECIFIC MUSCLE INJURIES

Rupture of the Serratus Ventralis Muscle

Trauma to the forelimb may result in rupture of all or part of the serratus ventralis muscle and in upward displacement of the scapula.[26,35] Diagnosis and treatment of this condition are described in Chapter 157.

Rupture of the Gracilis Muscle

Rupture of the gracilis muscle is an injury more commonly seen in the racing greyhound and may be referred to as "dropped muscle."[12,16,21,25] It has also been reported in the foxhound and German shepherd.[30]

The gracilis muscle is a sheetlike muscle on the medial surface of the thigh. It arises from the pelvic symphysis and inserts along the entire length of the tibial crest. At its insertion it sends a part of its crural fascia as a reinforcing band to the calcanean tendon. The caudal part of the gracilis muscle is the portion that attaches to the tuber calcis.[19] The caudal part of the gracilis is an important extensor of the tarsus and may rupture in racing greyhounds.[21] There are also attachments to the tendon of the semimembranosus muscle. The function of the gracilis muscle is adduction of the thigh and extension of the hip. The signs of the injury are a distinct hind leg lameness resulting

from an inability to extend the stifle. The lameness is noted immediately after injury. The ruptured muscle is characterized by a hematoma on the medial surface of the thigh (see Fig. 166–2A), which may become fibrous and cordlike (termed "cording" in the racing greyhound) if not surgically repaired in the acute stages.

If this condition is diagnosed immediately after injury, surgical intervention is necessary. This consists of a small skin incision over the medial thigh and reattachment of the muscle ends, or, if it is a musculotendinous tear, attachment of the tendon of origin to its insertion with interrupted horizontal mattress sutures of a monofilament nonabsorbable suture material, such as nylon or polypropylene.

If this condition remains undiagnosed or untreated, a fibrous scar or "cording" develops on the caudomedial midthigh. This muscle fibrosis may result in a contracture of the rear leg, resulting in a distinct rear leg lameness because of inability to extend the stifle. Surgical release of the contracture is the treatment of choice. The procedure consists of horizontal sectioning of the caudal edge of the band of scar tissue or excision of the entire muscle. Partial resection of the fibrous tissue bands may result in recurrence of the contracture. It is best to remove the entire muscle and fibrotic tissue, followed by physical therapy to ensure complete range of motion of the stifle joint.[30]

Rupture of the Long Head of the Triceps

This is an injury primarily described in the racing greyhound (see Fig. 166–2B and C), although it has been described in two dogs in connection with intratendon steroid injections.[15] As with any muscle tear or rupture, a cold compress, ice pack, or cold spray should be applied to the area soon after injury. The application of cold reduces edema, swelling, pain, and hematoma formation.[16] Ideally, prompt surgical intervention is indicated to reattach the fleshy ends of the belly of the long head of the triceps, as described earlier. It is important to manage the surgical repair with bandage immobilization for two weeks, followed by gradual return to activity. Dogs with this injury will heal with rest and moderate exercise (to prevent adhesions). They may return to racing but will drop one or two grades at the track.[16]

Rupture of the Achilles Mechanism

The Achilles mechanism is composed of five muscles which have three tendinous components forming the common calcanean or Achilles tendon (Fig. 166–4A). The gastrocnemius muscle arises by distinct medial and lateral heads from the supracondylar tuberosities of the femur. At the point of origin there is a sesamoid bone or fabella within each muscle head. The medial and lateral heads fuse distally to form a large tendon that inserts on the tuber calcanei. The tendon of the gastrocnemius is the major com-

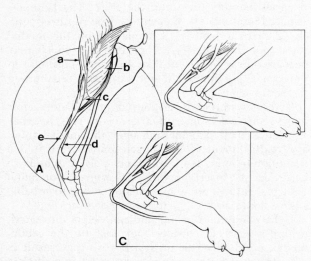

Figure 166–4. Rupture of the gastrocnemius tendon and common tendon of the biceps femoris, gracilis, and semi-tendinosus muscles. *A,* Lateral view of Achilles mechanism: *a,* semi-tendinosus muscle; *b,* gastrocnemius muscle; *c,* superficial digital flexor muscle; *d,* tendon of the gastrocnemius muscle; *e,* common tendon of the biceps femoris muscle, gracilis muscle, and semi-tendinosus muscle. *B,* Note hyperflexion of the hock with complete rupture of the common calcanean tendon. *C,* Upon weightbearing, the hock not only drops, but the digits flex, indicating the superficial digital flexor tendon is intact *(arrow)*. (Modified from Reinke, J. D., and Kus, S. P.: Achilles mechanism injury in the dog. Comp. Cont. Ed. 8:639, 1982.)

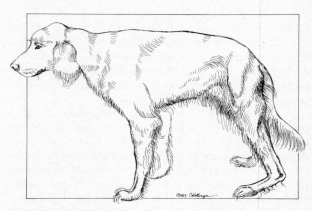

Figure 166–5. Rupture of the Achilles mechanism is demonstrated by this dog, showing tarsal hyperflexion and stifle hyperextension of the left rear leg. Damage to only the superficial digital flexor may also result in a plantigrade posture of the paw.

ponent of the common calcanean tendon. The other two tendinous components are formed by the tendon of the superficial digital flexor muscle and a common tendon of the biceps femoris, gracilis, and semitendinosus muscles. The primary function of the Achilles mechanism is to extend the tibial-tarsal joint while flexing the stifle and digits.[19]

Muscular or musculotendinous rupture of the Achilles mechanism is a disease primarily of mature dogs of the working and racing breeds.[6–9,12,35,36,48–50,52,55,57,59] A typical history includes trauma resulting when the animal jumps and lands on its rear legs. There has been a report of rupture caused by parasitic disease of the gastrocnemius muscles.[40] The condition may be bilateral and manifests itself by tarsal hyperflexion and stifle hyperextension owing to inability to extend the tarsus (Fig. 166–5), the degree of which depends on the severity and completeness of the disruption. A diagnosis of Achilles mechanism injury is based on postural changes and flaccidity of the calcanean tendon. A complete musculotendinous separation can mimic a separation of the tendon structure itself. Careful palpation of the gastrocnemius muscle and calcanean tendon reveals inflammatory changes near the musculotendinous junction. A thorough orthopedic examination should be followed by radiographic evaluation of the stifle and hock. Standing or stress radiographs assist in the diagnosis of musculotendinous injury, as it has been shown that all three musculotendinous units must be disrupted before excessive tarsal hyperflexion is present.[47,48]

The origin of the lateral or medial head of the gastrocnemius muscle may avulse or tear from trauma to the stifle in hyperextension.[14,48] This may result in plantigrade postural changes in the hock accompanied by palpable pain and swelling in the caudal distal femur. Extension of the stifle may result in discomfort. Radiographic evaluation of the stifle reveals distal displacement of the fabella (Fig. 166–6). If the position of one or both fabellae is in question, it is best to compare their location with those of the opposite stifle. It is important to note that the superficial digital flexor muscle is also avulsed if the lateral fabella is displaced.

This is a surgically treatable condition requiring reattachment of the head of the gastrocnemius muscle, especially if clinical signs are severe. The surgical approach to the head of the gastrocnemius muscle is made through a parapatellar skin incision, depending on whether the avulsion is of the lateral or medial head. The incision may extend from the distal one-third of the femur to the tibial tuberosity. After undermining the subcutaneous tissues, further dissection depends upon whether a lateral or medial approach was chosen. Laterally the biceps femoris muscle is separated from the vastus lateralis muscle and retracted caudally. Medially the insertion of the caudal head of the sartorius muscle is incised and retracted caudally. In either instance, the underlying capsular tissue is incised to expose the respective supracondylar area of the femur. The torn heads of the gastrocnemius muscle and superficial digital flexor muscle can be found with careful dissection. A fabella should be palpable in the head of the gastrocnemius muscle. If possible, the torn muscle is reattached using nylon or polypropylene in a mattress, figure-of-eight, or alternative pattern (Fig. 166–7). This involves drilling a hole in the distal femur 2 to 3 cm proximal to the origin of the head of the gastrocnemius muscle. An 18- or 20-gauge stainless steel wire is passed through this hole and either through or around the avulsed fabellae and tied on itself. Placement of the stifle in slight flexion aids in

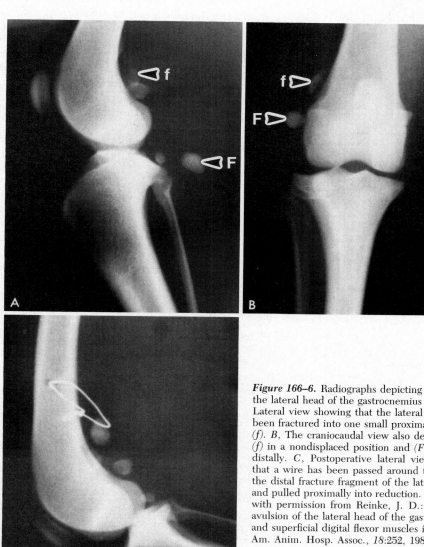

Figure 166–6. Radiographs depicting avulsion of the lateral head of the gastrocnemius muscle. *A,* Lateral view showing that the lateral fabella has been fractured into one small proximal fragment *(f)*. *B,* The craniocaudal view also demonstrates *(f)* in a nondisplaced position and *(F)* displaced distally. *C,* Postoperative lateral view showing that a wire has been passed around the base of the distal fracture fragment of the lateral fabella and pulled proximally into reduction. (Reprinted with permission from Reinke, J. D.: Traumatic avulsion of the lateral head of the gastrocnemius and superficial digital flexor muscles in a dog. J. Am. Anim. Hosp. Assoc., *18:*252, 1982.)

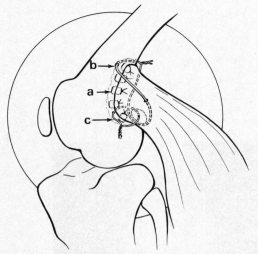

Figure 166–7. Depiction of various methods of repair of an avulsion of the head of the gastrocnemius muscle. The muscle may be reattached by primary suture of the tendinous tissue of origin (*a*), figure-of-eight wire suture around the fabella and through drill hole in distal femur (*b*, see also Figure 166–6C), wire suture through caudodistal femur and the fabella (*c*), or any combination of these methods.

reducing the avulsed muscle. Postoperatively, the leg is placed in a full leg cast or Schroeder-Thomas splint, with the stifle in slight flexion, for two to three weeks. After removal of the external coaptation,

exercise should be restricted for an additional two to three weeks.

Acute cases of musculotendinous rupture of the Achilles mechanism are treated surgically by apposition of the muscle-tendon junction. It is important to prevent stress on the anastomotic site by rigid immobilization of the tarsus and the stifle. An injury such as this can be conservatively treated successfully as long as the stifle is placed in partial flexion and the tarsus in partial extension, best accomplished with a Schroeder-Thomas splint or full leg cast.[35,36] More rigid stabilization can be combined with surgical repair of the musculotendinous rupture. The musculotendinous junction is approached through a skin incision directly over the caudal aspect of the middle third of the tibia. The proximal muscle and tendon are anastomosed, as described earlier (Fig. 166–8). Rigid internal fixation can be accomplished by a number of methods, including the insertion of a bone screw[6–8] or intramedullary pin[10] from the tuber calcanei to the distal tibia or with external pin splintage spanning the tibial tarsal joint (Fig. 166–9).[22] The size of the bone screw depends on the size of the animal. A self-tapping lag screw is used. This prevents soft tissues caudal to the distal tibia from getting caught in the bone tap and allows for adjustment of the degree of extension of the tarsus. Any of these internal fixation devices should be supplemented with casts, splints, or coaptation bandages. The external support is removed in four to six weeks and the internal fixation between six and eight weeks.

If an injury to the musculotendinous junction of the Achilles mechanism is not recognized or treated during the acute phase, the animal may be presented

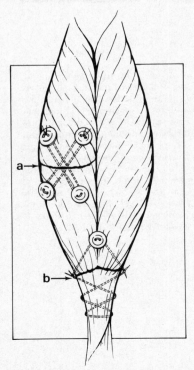

Figure 166–8. *a*, Surgical repair of a rupture of the muscle belly of the gastrocnemius using tension button technique. *b*, Musculotendinous rupture of the distal end of the gastrocnemius muscle repaired with button tension technique and Bunnell-Mayer suture pattern. (Modified from Reinke, J. D., and Kus, S. P.: Achilles mechanism injury in the dog. Comp. Cont. Ed. 8:639, 1982.)

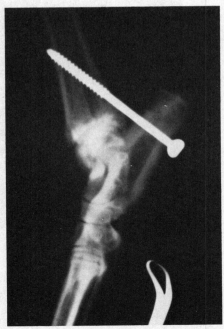

Figure 166–9. Lateral radiograph illustrating internal fixation of the tibiotarsal joint at a 135-degree angle to relieve tension on the anastomotic site.

with a chronic injury or one that has failed with conservative treatment. Chronic injuries can be treated by shortening the calcanean tendon to re-establish function of the gastrocnemius and superficial digital flexor muscles. The tendon can be shortened by doubling over, plication, or resection of a portion of the tendon.[8,12,35] Resection of the fibrous scar at the musculotendinous junction is extremely traumatic and unnecessary and results in a weaker repair. The tarsus should be stabilized as described previously. Postoperative care is identical to that of musculotendinous anastomosis.

Rupture of the belly or fleshy portion of the gastrocnemius muscle is unusual.[36,40] Although in one report the muscle healed spontaneously, it had been immobilized for four weeks in a Schroeder-Thomas splint.[36]

Rupture of the superficial digital flexor at its musculotendinous junction has been reported.[9,48] The clinical signs and treatment are identical to avulsion of the head of the gastrocnemius muscle.[35]

Other specific muscles that may be ruptured in working or racing animals include the tensor fascia latae, rhomboideus thoracis, origin of the infraspinatus, origin of the pectorals, insertion of the biceps brachii, sartorius, origin of the pectineus, and origin of the external abdominal oblique and longissimus muscles.[16,35]

Muscle Atrophy

Atrophy of muscle may be due to disuse or denervation. Interference with venous drainage, arterial blood supply, or nerve supply results in degenerative changes in muscles. These changes may be due to insults of the muscle and its surrounding tissue from trauma or fracture disease.

The most common and striking cause of muscle degeneration in small animals is denervation. Atrophy following denervation is a reversion of muscle to the status of fetal muscle fiber. This type of atrophy is much more rapid than disuse atrophy. Muscle atrophy due to denervation may be associated with injury to the spinal cord or peripheral nerves.[12]

Muscle Contractures and Fibrosis

Muscle contractures, whether occurring from skeletal muscle fibrosis caused by trauma or from congenital factors, are due to damage to muscle fibers, nerves, and blood vessels. These changes, which result in fibrosis, adhesions, and contracture, are irreversible and often result in lameness ranging from minor changes in gait to complete loss of limb function.[35] The causes of muscle damage may be: (1) circulatory insufficiency from arterial or venous obstruction, i.e., Volkmann's contracture and subfascial hematoma, (2) response to parasitic or protozoan infections or autoimmune diseases, such as dirofilariasis, toxoplasmosis, and eosinophilic myositis, and (3) the end result of injuries, fractures, and misman-

agement of orthopedic problems.[30] Muscle contractures resulting in clinical lameness include those of the quadriceps, infraspinatus, and gracilis muscles. The pectineus muscle may have characteristics of contracture associated with hip dysplasia.[35]

Infraspinatus Muscle Contracture

Contracture of the infraspinatus muscle has been described primarily in hunting dogs.[27,42,55] The animal shows pain in the shoulder during or soon after exercise.[42] There may be a history of trauma with acute onset of lameness that gradually subsides.[35] Although the lameness may decrease, it is accompanied by a characteristic gait that demonstrates persistent outward rotation, adduction of the elbow, and abduction of the distal limb with a carpal flip (Fig. 166–10). This deformity develops two to four weeks after the initial injury, as a result of the contracture of the infraspinatus muscle. There is also a limited range of motion of the shoulder and abduction of the elbow. Disuse atrophy of the shoulder may develop when surgical treatment is delayed. It is usually unilateral but I have seen it bilaterally in a Labrador retriever.

The exact cause is unknown, but it appears to be a primary muscle disorder rather than neurological in origin. Histologically affected tissues show degeneration and atrophy of skeletal muscle with fibrous tissue replacement.[42] This correlates with the theory that an injury causes incomplete rupture of the infraspinatus muscle, leading to fibrosis and contracture.

Surgical treatment consists of a caudal lateral ap-

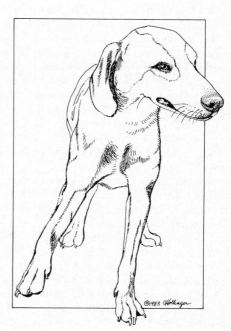

Figure 166–10. Infraspinatus muscle contracture involving the right front leg of a dog. Note the characteristic adduction of the limb at the elbow, abduction of the distal limb, and outward rotation of the antibrachium.

proach to the affected shoulder joint.[43] The affected infraspinatus muscle appears fibrotic, with atrophy of the belly of the muscle. Blunt and sharp dissection is used to free the musculotendinous area of the scarred, fibrotic muscle from where it crosses the scapulohumeral joint. Once the fibrous tissue is freed from the joint capsule, it is incised. This incision may be in the tendon or musculotendinous capsular portion of the infraspinatus. A distinct popping noise may be heard when the fibrous tissue is severed, and immediately the forelimb should be more easily adducted. It is important that all evidence of fibrous contracture is incised and that the range of motion of the shoulder joint is improved. The myectomy or tenectomy provides correction of the deformity and restores normal function. Postoperatively the animal should be allowed restricted exercise for one to two weeks. The affected front leg is not immobilized following surgery.

Quadriceps Muscle Contracture

Contracture of the quadriceps groups of muscles has been recognized in human and veterinary medicine for many years.[12,30,35,41,55] It has been documented with distal femoral fractures of young, actively growing dogs. It is most often associated with inadequate fracture repair, osteomyelitis, or overzealous handling of tissues surrounding the femur in conjunction with prolonged immobilization in extension due to external splints or disuse of the limb.[55] Congenital quadriceps contracture has been described in puppies.[12,35,49] Not all the muscles of the quadriceps group may be affected.[30] The joint stiffness develops initially as a result of adhesions between the quadriceps muscle and the distal femur. With time, the affected leg is held in marked extension to such an extent that the knee may be bent backward in a position of genu recurvatum (Fig. 166–11). As a result the hock is extended. The affected leg essentially becomes a "walking stick" for the animal with little use in locomotion. The cranial thigh becomes atrophied, taut, and cordlike and essentially tied to the femur. As the condition becomes chronic the pathologic changes become more complex; degenerative changes and fibrosis occur periarticularly and intraarticularly.

Numerous surgical procedures are advocated for treatment of quadriceps contracture[12,30,35,55] by restoring motion to the stifle joint through any combination of the following mechanisms: (1) breaking down of adhesions between the quadriceps muscle group and distal femur, (2) loosening of adhesions in and around the femorotibial joint, (3) lengthening of the quadriceps mechanism, and (4) releasing of the restrictive action of adjacent extensors of the stifle, such as the sartorius and tensor fascia lata muscles.[35] Whatever surgical procedure is chosen, the prognosis remains guarded for complete return of function of the stifle joint. Because of the tendency for adhesions to reform postoperatively, it is critical that the surgeon impart

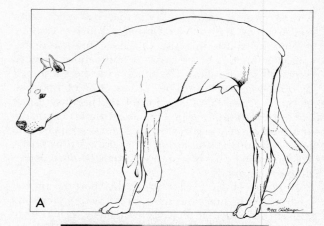

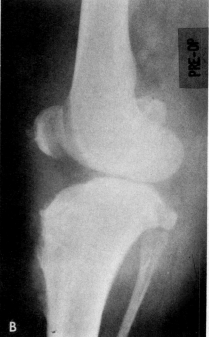

Figure 166–11. A, Quadriceps muscle contracture illustrated by the hyperextension (genu recurvatum) of this dog's left rear leg. B, Lateral radiographic projection of the stifle of a dog with quadriceps contracture following open reduction of a proximal diaphyseal femoral fracture. Note degree of hyperextension and bony proliferation in and around the stifle.

to the owner the necessity for good postoperative physical therapy.

Surgical procedures described for release of the contracture include partial quadriceps myotomy,[30] "Z" myoplasty,[35] and freeing of adhesions and implantation of ophthalmic Gelfoam between the quadriceps and the distal femur to prevent recurrence of adhesions.[60] The treatment varies with the severity of the contracture and often incorporates a combination of surgical techniques.

A lateral approach to the stifle and femur is made through a generous skin incision.[43] The quadriceps adhesions are freed from the femur. This may require removal of excessive bony callus from the distal femur after previous fracture repair. The quadriceps muscle group is a cordlike fibrotic structure. The incision is extended into the stifle joint capsule to free patellar adhesions and improve joint flexibility. It may be necessary to perform a medial arthrotomy and carry the incision proximally along the caudal border of the vastus medialis. Once the quadriceps muscle group has been freed from the distal femur, the patella should be luxated medially to allow for forcible flexion of the stifle. Manipulation of the stifle joint is continued with the patella turned to its normal position. Care should be taken, when forcibly flexing the stifle in immature animals, not to avulse the tibial tuberosity or proximal tibial physis. If adequate range of motion (20 to 40° flexion) cannot be restored, various lengthening procedures should be performed—such as the "Z" plasty or a sliding myoplasty.

The "Z" myoplasty is performed by isolating the cordlike bands of the quadriceps group and being sure all adhesions between the distal femur and the muscles have been freed. The "Z" incision is made in the fibrotic muscle to include any medial or lateral bands. The stifle is then flexed as much as possible. The "Z" transected muscles are sutured together with a monofilament nonabsorbable suture, with the quadriceps muscle lengthened enough to allow the knee to be flexed in at least a functional standing angle.

An alternative and equally successful procedure is the sliding myoplasty.[35] The surgical approach and exposure are the same as for the "Z" myoplasty. In this technique restrictive muscles are incised and lengthened. The first step is to incise the cranial belly of the sartorius near its insertion on the patella. Likewise the rectus femoris is isolated and transected near the patella, avoiding the neighboring femoral nerve and cranial femoral artery. The vastus group is isolated as a unit and elevated from the origin on the proximal femur. The stifle is then flexed through a range of motion, allowing the vastus to slide beside the rectus femoris. As in the previous procedure the stifle is flexed until it reaches a functional angle. The vastus group of muscles is sutured to the rectus femoris and cranial belly of the sartorius with simple interrupted or horizontal mattress sutures of a monofilament nonabsorbable suture material.

Postoperatively, regardless of the surgical procedure utilized, the stifle is kept in flexion with either a figure-of-eight bandage, Gordy Robinson sling, or external pin splintage for four to five days. The external support should be removed on day 5 or 6 and forcible passive flexion and extension performed. The first postoperative manipulation of the stifle may be best accomplished while the animal is under general anesthesia or heavy sedation. The external support is not reapplied, but the stifle is subjected to passive extension and flexion exercises two to three times per day thereafter. Exercise is encouraged and when the dog can bear weight on the limb with it held in slight flexion, passive physical therapy is discontinued.

The surgical procedure is a success if it returns the animal to 50 to 75 per cent use of the affected limb. If the outcome of the surgical treatment of quadriceps contracture is unsatisfactory, the alternatives include arthrodesis of the stifle and amputation of the affected limb.

Myositis Ossificans

This condition occurs in similar locations in humans and animals. Myositis ossificans is classified as generalized, progressive, or localized and has been reported as having a predilection for the muscles around the hip joints.[32,37] The pathogenesis is unclear, but it may be related to trauma resulting in hematoma formation that organizes and undergoes calcification. The lesions may involve tissues other than muscle and may be inflammatory.[32] The animal may exhibit chronic lameness with subsequent muscle atrophy, possible neurological deficits, and pain after exercise. Calcification usually occurs two to four weeks after trauma. Radiographically, the lesion may be a well-defined calcified mass with a central transparency (Fig. 166–12). Histologically, the lesions consist of

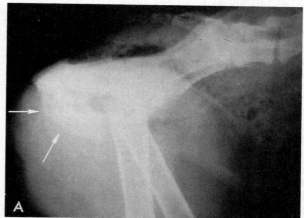

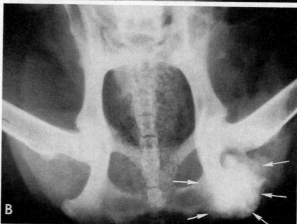

Figure 166–12. Lateral *(A)* and ventral *(B)* dorsal views of the pelvis of an adult Doberman pinscher, depicting a well-defined calcified mass typical for myositis ossificans involving the ischial tuberosity *(arrows)*. Surgical excision of the calcified tissue resulted in recovery with no recurrence. (Courtesy of Dr. Robert Parker, University of Florida, Gainesville, Florida.)

zonal proliferation of cellular fibrous tissue, osteoid tissue, and immature bone. Although attempts have been made to link myositis ossificans with neoplastic changes, the presence of neoplastic changes may be due to either a chronic inflammatory insult or a biological potential for malignancy.[44]

Muscle Biopsy

It may be necessary from time to time to evaluate muscle tissue histopathologically to differentiate neurological, neoplastic, parasitic, or other degenerative disease processes. The sample of muscle tissue should be isolated between two stay sutures, excised, and stretched by wedging the sutures in clefts made in a wooden tongue depressor. This prevents contracture and damage to the myofibrils. The tissue sample should be wrapped in a moist saline sponge. The sample is fixed immediately in solutions such as glutaraldehyde or paraformaldehyde, or frozen in liquid nitrogen.[35]

Tumors of Muscle[8]

See Chapter 184.

TENDONS

Anatomy

Tendons are dense, irregular, collagenous tissues composed of fibroblasts, parallel collagen fibers embedded in a ground substance, and extracellular fluid.[18] The fibroblasts or tenocytes are the only cells in tendons. The collagen fibers are arranged in fascicles, or bundles, which are surrounded by a woven mesh of loose areolar connective tissue termed endotenon. The endotenon permits some longitudinal movement of the collagen bundles and carries all the blood vessels, lymphatic vessels, and nerves. The entire tendon is covered by another fine connective tissue sheath called the epitenon, which is continuous on its undersurface with the endotenon. In like fashion the epitenon is continuous on its outside surface with the paratenon. The paratenon covers and separates other tendons from each other and facilitates free gliding of the tendon. In areas of local pressure on the tendon the paratenon forms a tendon synovial sheath.

The vascular supply to tendons enters at three major locations. The proximal third of the tendon is supplied by vessels entering at the musculotendinous junction. The middle third of the tendon is supplied by extrinsic vessels passing longitudinally in the paratenon or synovial sheath. The distal third of the tendon is supplied by vessels entering at the osseous tendon insertion. The vessels within the tendon running between the fascicles or tendon bundles (intrinsic vessels) supply the collagen bundles and anastomose freely with each other and the extrinsic vessels.[13]

The vascularity of tendons depends on their loca-tion. Paratenon-covered tendons are more vascular than synovial-sheathed tendons. The degree of vascularity plays an important role in healing.[18]

Tendon Healing

An important factor is whether a tendon will heal without formation of adhesions to adjacent tissues, resulting in decreased gliding function. Tendon injuries are often accompanied by injury to surrounding soft tissues or bone. Consequently, their healing does not take place in an isolated environment. The adhesions that develop are part of the healing process, resulting in the tendon and its surrounding tissues healing according to the principles of "one wound—one scar."[41] The healing process of tendons can be divided into paratenon-covered tendons and sheathed tendons. This division is necessary because of the greater role the paratenon and its extrinsic blood supply play in healing than does the intrinsic blood supply of the sheathed tendons. The cells of the mature tendon are spindle-shaped tenocytes which have little capacity for reproduction or production of collagen.[8] Thus, primary healing of isolated tendon units is even more affected with damage to the intrinsic blood supply.

Healing in a paratenon-covered tendon depends less on intrinsic blood supply, as undifferentiated fibroblasts and capillary buds from the paratenon invade the damaged area between the tendon ends. The fibroblasts synthesize collagen. As the ground substance increases outside the fibroblast, the collagen polymerizes into fibrils. Within the first week of injury the healing tissue becomes visible as thin wavy fibers deposited randomly in and around the tendon wound. During the second week of healing the vascular reaction reaches its peak, as do fibroblastic proliferation and collagen production. During the third and fourth week the collagen fibers near the tendon ends become more longitudinally oriented. The collagen fibers in the center of the healing wound remain unorganized and perpendicular to the lines of stress.[41]

The final stage of tendon healing involves the secondary remodelling that takes place. There is a reduction in mass as the collagen remodels and the tensile strength increases owing to the high degree of organization along the lines of stress. The collagenization continues until about 20 weeks, at which time there is little histological difference between scar tissue and tendon. As movement and function return, the adhesions are weakened and remodelled.[18,34,41]

Controversy remains over the exact physiology of healing of sheathed tendons. The "one wound—one scar" theory does not apply if healing recurs without adhesions. If the primary intrinsic blood supply is not damaged, then primary union between tendon ends does occur. If the trauma, however, damages the blood supply and tendon sheath, resulting in an inflammatory wound healing process as seen in paratenon-covered tendons, then "one wound—one scar" healing results with adhesion formation.[18] Although under ideal conditions sheathed tendons do have the capability of primary repair, more commonly the laceration involves tendon and tendon sheath, resulting in adhesion formation.

The importance of adhesions in tendon surgery depends upon the necessity for restoration of gliding function. The prevention of adhesions is paramount in human hand surgery but less so in small animals. Thus the factors that are essential in minimizing adhesions may be of less importance in veterinary surgery. Although various techniques have been described to minimize adhesion formation, such as synthetic cuffs around the anastomotic site, they have resulted in retardation of the healing process. A more practical approach to minimizing adhesion formation is to use proper surgical technique and postoperative care.

The return of sufficient tensile strength may be more important than gliding function in veterinary surgery.[18] Postoperative care must be based on the proper suture techniques, postoperative immobilization, and gradual return to activity. During the first four to five days following surgical repair, the tendon ends soften, resulting in loss of holding power. During the following two weeks the strength of the repair gradually increases during the initial fibroplasia and collagen stages, at which time the strength is primarily due to the suture material. The suture pattern may be more important than the suture material.[53] Immobilization of the tendon repair site during the first three weeks postoperatively is critical to prevent increases in separation of the tendon ends with resulting invasion of excessive scar tissue and decreased tensile strength. Thus it appears that the ideal postoperative immobilization period is two to three weeks, followed by three weeks of restricted activity, then gradual return to normal activity.[8]

General Principles of Tendon Surgery

As with any surgical procedure, the basic principles of asepsis and atraumatic handling of tissues should be followed. The goal is to minimize adhesion formation (tenodesis) and restore as much gliding function as possible. An essential part of tendon surgery is careful and meticulous planning of the surgical procedure. Skin incisions should not be made directly over the tendon but rather parallel to the proposed surgical site or curved over the tendon so the healing skin wound does not adhere to the tendon repair (tenorrhaphy) site. Maintenance of hemostasis must be complete and may be accomplished by pressure from moist sponges, electrocautery used in moderation, or a tourniquet. Tourniquets work well on the distal extremities of animals.

Prior to application of an elastic or pneumatic tourniquet, an Esmarch's bandage should be applied to the leg from the tips of the toes to above the point of tourniquet application. Incising through the Esmarch's bandage and leaving the proximal portion intact allows it to act as a tourniquet. An Esmarch's bandage can be made with elastic bandage material or flat rubber tubing (bicycle tire inner tube). Careful planning of the surgical procedure and arrangement of all surgical equipment and materials in advance minimizes the time required for the tourniquet to be in place. The time of ischemia should not exceed 1 to 1.5 hours unless accompanied by local hypothermia or periods of tourniquet release for 10 to 15 minutes.

To minimize adhesions, all tissues should be handled as gently as possible. The tissues should be kept moist with sterile saline. The tendon segments should be handled by the gloved fingers of the surgeon, by straight needles placed through the tendon, or by skin hooks. If the ends of the tendon must be grasped by forceps for traction or suture placement, the traumatized end of the tendon should be excised after the sutures have been secured.[8,11,12] The end results are best when the tendon ends are most nearly perfectly united.

Although the suture material and pattern for tendon surgery may vary based on the preference of the surgeon, the shape of the tendon, and the particular technique utilized, basic principles must always be followed.[2,8,11,12,34,47,51,53] The suture material should be inert, strong, easy to pass through tissues, and nonabsorbable.

Such suture materials include stainless steel wire, braided polyester fiber, monofilament nylon, and polypropylene. Although stainless steel wire has maximum knot security, it can be difficult to work with and breaks with fatigue. Polyester fiber is a multifilament suture requiring many knots for security, thus decreasing its desirability. Monofilament nylon and polypropylene are the most desirable sutures for repair of tendons. The size of the material depends upon the size of the tendon; thus the largest size that will comfortably pass through the tendon should be used.[8] The suture pattern chosen should provide adequate holding power in the tissues. The most commonly used suture patterns described in veterinary surgery have been the horizontal mattress, Bunnell, and Bunnell-Mayer (Fig. 166–13).[8,12] Two more recently described suture techniques, the locking loop (Kessler-Mason-Allen) and the modified Kessler are favored because they are less constrictive to the intrinsic blood supply and provide greater tensile strength than do Bunnell sutures (Fig. 166–14).[2,52]

Surgical Repair of Severed Tendons

The majority of tendon injuries in small animals are related to lacerations rather than to rupture. Unless the injury has been chronic and tendon segments have severely contracted or the injury has devitalized large segments of tendon, primary end-to-end tenorrhaphy is the best method for restoration. Sound surgical judgment must be used prior to surgical treatment of a lacerated tendon. The repair should be performed with minimal delay in those wounds that have minimal trauma and contamination.

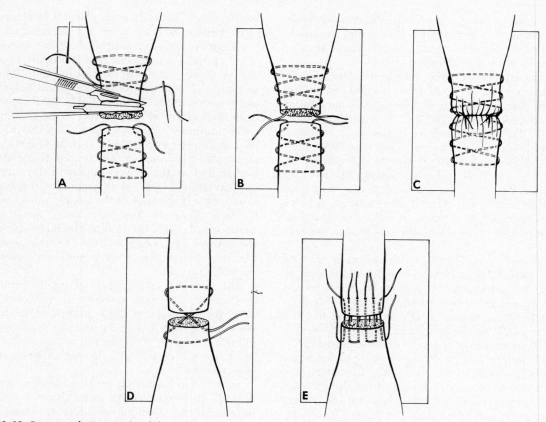

Figure 166–13. Suture techniques utilized for end-to-end anastomosis. *A, B,* and *C,* Bunnell-Mayer technique. *D,* Bunnell technique. *E,* Interrupted horizontal mattress suture technique.

If the four to six hour period for primary closure has passed or if contamination is severe, then an alternate approach should be taken. This period for primary closure can be extended with thorough debridement and copious lavage if trauma and contamination are minimal and there appear to be adequate soft tissues and blood supply surrounding the surgical site.

If primary anastomosis of the tendon ends is undertaken, the wound must be thoroughly cleaned and debrided and tendon stumps exposed. When tendons are cut, the proximal segment retracts as muscles contract. If the proximal stump cannot be located in the wound, further enlargement of the wound can be avoided by making a small incision proximal to the site of injury. The proximal tendon stump can be located through this wound; then, by placing a suture through the end of the tendon, it can be carried subcutaneously along the tendon bed to emerge at the surgical site for reattachment.[12] Traction can be maintained on the tendon segments by the placement of straight needles transversely through the tendon proximal and distal to the proposed suture pattern.

If too much time has elapsed since the injury, the tissue is infected or grossly contaminated, or the surrounding soft tissues are too severely traumatized to afford adequate blood supply, repair should be delayed. The wound is thoroughly debrided and a small piece of colored suture material placed in the ends of the tendon stumps. The leg is immobilized to reduce separation of the tendon segments. These sutures act as markers so that following healing of the wound and resolution of the infection, secondary tendon repair may be attempted.[12,41] Successful repair of tendon lacerations in an infected wound has been reported but is not encouraged because of the possibility of wound breakdown and excessive adhesion formation.[6]

The particular technique and suture pattern should provide accurate anatomical apposition of the tendon segments and adequate strength for repair. No one suture pattern is satisfactory in all instances. In small animals the end-to-end pattern is used because it maintains the original length and diameter of the tendon while being simple to perform. Techniques such as the overlapping side-to-side or fish mouth provide a stronger anastomosis but require longer tendon lengths (Fig. 166–15). Round or semiround tendons of 2 cm or more in length should be anastomosed by the Bunnel-Mayer or locking loop (modified Kessler) suture patterns. The tendon end is grasped with a skin hook or by a straight needle passed transversely through it. The Bunnel-Mayer pattern is started transversely across the tendon as tendons have the majority of their holding power transversely oriented. The largest suture that can be buried in the tendon is used on a double-armed straight needle configuration. The needle enters the

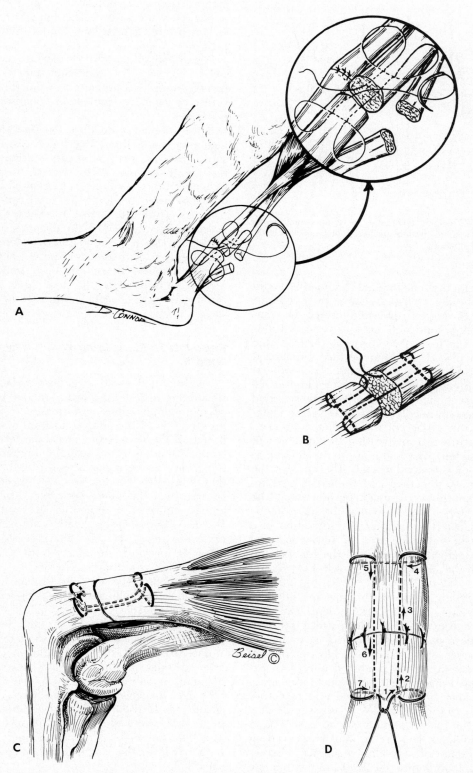

Figure 166–14. A and B, Locking loop (Kessler-Mason-Allen) suture technique. C and D, Modified Kessler suture. These two suture patterns can be used for end-to-end tendon anastomosis. It is important that the transverse segment of either suture pattern passes just superficial to the two longitudinal segments of the suture (D). (A and B reprinted with permission from Tomlinson, J. and Moore, R.: Locking loop tendon suture use in repair of five calcanean tendons. Vet. Surg. 3:105, 1982. C and D reprinted with permission from Aron, D. N.: A "new" tendon stitch. J. Am. Anim. Hosp. Assoc., 17:587, 1981.)

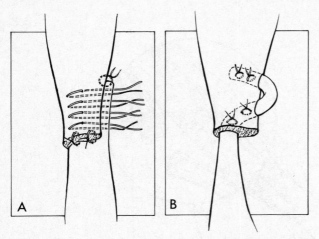

Figure 166–15. Overlapping techniques for tendon anastomosis may be used when there is adequate length of tendon ends. *A*, Side-to-side. *B*, Fishmouth.

tendon 2 cm from the tendon end. The needle should penetrate the tendon transversely and then re-enter at an angle of 45 degrees, pointing toward the traumatized end. A second oblique bite is placed at a right angle to the first. Two corresponding oblique bites are then placed. The end of the traumatized tendon is excised with a scalpel and the needle is inserted and brought out through the middle of the tendon's cross-section. The same procedure is carried out with the second needle. Very little suture material is left on the surface of the tendon, with both ends of the suture material exiting through the cut end of the tendon. The same suture technique is used on the opposite tendon end. The ends of the tendon are drawn together and the knots tied securely with four throws. Enough tension should be placed on the tendon ends so that the anastomotic site appears pleated to prevent the formation of a gap during healing. The knots in the suture material should fall beneath the cut edge of the tendon, out of contact with the surface (see Fig. 166–13A, B, and C).

Another excellent suture technique for round or semiround tendons is the locking loop (Kessler-Mason-Allen) and modified Kessler pattern (see Fig. 166–14).[2,52] These two suture patterns have the advantages of preservation of intrinsic blood supply of the tendon, gap formation produced only with extreme load, rapid placement, and reduction in adhesions.[52] The same principles of selection of suture materials apply to this pattern. A curved needle may be used, and the tendon stumps can be as short as 1 cm. In the modified Kessler the knot is secured on the outside of one of the tendon segments, whereas in the locking loop suture the knot falls within the tendon substance at the anastomotic site (Fig. 166–14B and D). If the tendon sutures are placed so that the suture patterns in the proximal and distal stumps are mirror images of each other, the tendon ends will be anatomically apposed with minimal buckling. It is

critical that the transverse portion of the suture pattern passes superficial to the two longitudinal segments of the suture. This forms a loop of suture locking around a bundle of tendon fibers (Fig. 166–14D).

Regardless of the suture pattern used, the next step is to close the paratenon with a single interrupted, simple continuous, or horizontal mattress suture of a fine, monofilament nonabsorbable suture material.

If the tendon stumps are too short for the above techniques, the Bunnel technique is an alternative suture pattern, with a simple, continuous suture in the paratenon placed 45 degrees to the tendon.[8] Other suture patterns are better suited for short, flat, or aponeurotic tendons. An interrupted horizontal mattress suture may be used as well as the buttonhole overlapping suture. The disadvantages of this latter suture are that it requires excessive tendon length, a small portion of tendon is exposed, sutures are not buried, and the area of repair is bulky. Since the tendon ends overlap, this technique is contraindicated where a tendon passes through a synovial sheath.

Repair of Tendons Lying Within a Synovial Sheath

Tendons that serve as gliding surfaces should be repaired to restore the gliding function by minimizing or eliminating adhesion formation.[12,41] In animals, preservation of the gliding function of extensors and flexors of the carpus and tarsus and occasionally the bicipital tendon of the scapulohumeral joint is most important. Following anastomosis of the severed tendon ends, the tendon synovial sheath should be sutured over the anastomotic site with fine monofilament, nonreactive, nonabsorbable suture material. If reconstruction of the sheath is not possible because of severe tissue damage, alternate steps should be taken to prevent fibroblasts from penetrating the surgical site, resulting in adhesions.

Construction of a new sheath can be performed, using an arterial allograft or polyethylene tubing as a cuff (Fig. 166–16). Following repair of the tendon the artery or tubing is placed around the anastomotic site. The cuff should be long enough to cover the surface over which the tendon glides. The wall of the artery or edges of the tubing are sutured with monofilament, nonabsorbable suture material to form a tube over the anastomosed area. This type of artificial sheath should also be used if a laceration has occurred in an area where there is a common tendon sheath. The cuff should be wrapped around the lacerated tendon within the confines of the common tendon sheath.[12]

Tendon Lengthening and Shortening

Tendon Lengthening. This may be indicated when there has been contracture of a tendon or muscle

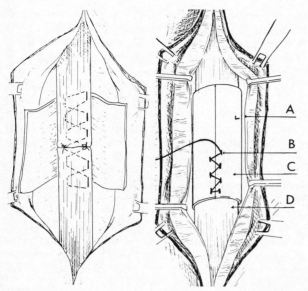

Figure 166–16. *Left*, a tendon anastomosis with an arterial cuff in place prior to suturing. *Right*, the arterial cuff surrounds the tendon. *A*, fascia around tendon; *B*, simple continuous suture of arterial silk; *C*, arterial graft; *D*, tendon. (Reprinted with permission from Butler, H. C.: Tendon, muscle and fascia. *In* Archibald, J. (ed.): *Canine Surgery*. 2nd. ed. American Veterinary Publications, Santa Barbara, 1974.)

tendon unit with resulting chronic lameness or a conformation defect. In young, actively growing dogs, contracture or laxity of a muscle-tendon unit may be due to parasitism, malnutrition, dietary imbalances, or improper environment.[35] These animals may have

buckling or dropping of the carpus or tarsus. Initial treatment is aimed at correction of the initial cause. Mild cases may be treated with splints or support bandages. Surgical intervention is necessary only in severe cases.

Prior to determining whether a tendon-lengthening procedure is necessary, the status of the muscle-tendon unit should be assessed. If the function of the muscle can be sacrificed, a simple tenotomy or tenectomy can be performed as in the treatment of infraspinatus muscle contracture.[35] When the function of the muscle must be preserved, then the tendon should be lengthened. This lengthening can be performed on the muscle belly or the tendon, but lengthening the tendon is less difficult and has fewer complications. The most common technique for lengthening a tendon is the "Z" tenotomy (Fig. 166–17A and B). This involves a half-section splitting of the tendon. An enlongated "Z" incision is made in the tendon, first by splitting it longitudinally and then by incising the ends of the incision in opposite directions. The split ends of the tendon are separated the desired distance but left overlapping so that the anastomosis is a side-to-side rather than an end-to-end repair. This provides for stronger, more rapid healing. The tendon ends are apposed with an interrupted horizontal mattress suture pattern, followed by closure of the paratenon in a simple continuous pattern. Other methods of tendon lengthening include the oblique splitting and gliding, accordion, and Lange techniques (Fig. 166–17C, D, and E).[8,12,50]

Specific clinical indications for tendon lengthening

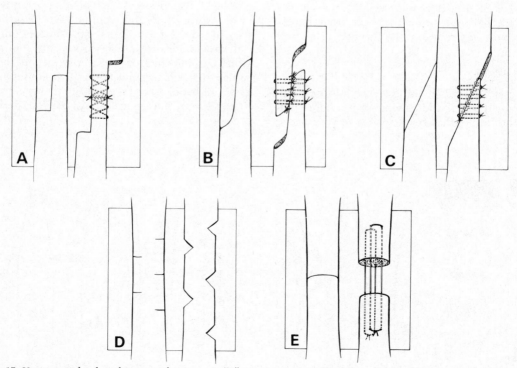

Figure 166–17. Various tendon lengthening techniques: *A*, "Z" tenotomy. *B*, Modification of the "Z" tenotomy. *C*, Oblique section and gliding. *D*, Accordion partial tenotomy. *E*, Lange method. (Modified from Butler, H. C.: Tendon, muscle and fascia. *In* Archibald, J. (ed.): *Canine Surgery*. 2nd ed. American Veterinary Publications, Santa Barbara, 1974.)

include quadriceps, Achilles (common calcanean) tendon, superficial and deep flexor, and flexor carpi ulnaris tendon contractures.[12]

Tendon Shortening. The most common indication for tendon shortening involves the improper healing of tendons following injury, especially if they have healed while the joint is hyperextended or hyperflexed. In addition, excessive strain during growth may cause breakdown of supporting structures, causing a tendon to stretch. An Achilles mechanism injury may result in improper healing of the gastrocnemius muscle-tendon junction or tendon itself, resulting in excessive tendon length and hyperflexion of the tarsus. Also, a similar situation can arise with improper healing of the superficial and deep flexor tendons of the forelimb.[12]

A tendon can be shortened by a number of methods, but the technique chosen should not involve a tenotomy because of the morbidity of anastomotic breakdown (Fig. 166–18D). Hoffa's method of tendon shortening is easy and reliable but less applicable in tendons that are thickened and scarred (Fig. 166–18A).[8] If the sutures loosen prematurely the tendon may lengthen again. A tendon can also be shortened by doubling-over the tendon on itself and using horizontal mattress sutures to secure the overlap (Fig. 166–18B). Tenotomy techniques for shortening tendons include the "Z" tenotomy, in which an area of the "Z" incision is excised, or a simple tenectomy of a transverse section of the tendon followed by an end-to-end anastomosis (Fig. 166–18C).

Regardless of the tenoplasty technique used to shorten or lengthen a tendon, postoperative care involves internal or external immobilization of the limb until gradual return to activity can be initiated, following return of strength to the tendon.

Tendon Grafting

Tendon grafts are rarely indicated or performed in small animal surgery.[35] Indications for a tendon graft are when the tendon has been so severely damaged that tenorrhaphy is impossible or when generalized tenodesis is present and tendolysis is not possible.[8] Regardless of the type of graft, survival of a tendon graft depends on adequate nutrition.[18] Although both autografts and allografts have been described in humans, their use in animals is limited by availability. Tendons harvested from outside tendon sheaths that have a paratenon covering are more vascular than those from within tendon sheaths. This increased vascularity may promote healing but also results in more adhesions.

An excellent source of donor tissue to replace a portion of tendon in small animals is the tensor fascia lata.[8,9] After harvesting an adequate length of fascia lata it is rolled into a tubelike structure and anastomosed to the tendon ends using a Bunnell-Mayer or Bunnell suture pattern. Postoperative management of tendon grafts is similar to that of any tenorrhaphy procedure, except that the period of immobilization should be extended by three weeks.[9]

Many tendon graft techniques are described in humans and research animals: composite grafts, vascular and avascular grafts, and tendon grafts attached to bone.[18]

Carbon Fiber Implants

Recently filamentous carbon fiber implants have been described for replacement of tendon and ligamentous defects. Many experimental and limited clinical trials have demonstrated that the carbon fibers act as a biological scaffold for the growth of fibroblasts and subsequent deposition of collagen.[1,28,54] The braided carbon fiber strands may be either sutured to the tendon ends or attached by weaving the carbon fibers into the tendon. Specific indications for use of a carbon fiber implant are situations in which there is a defect in the tendon rather than in an end-to-end anastomosis. Carbon fiber implants have been used to repair the deep digital flexor tendon, calcanean tendon, and anterior cruciate ligament.[1,17,28,54,56,57]

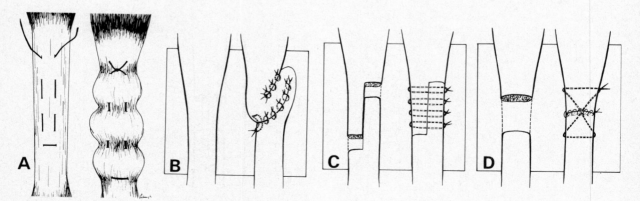

Figure 166–18. Tendons may be shortened using the following techniques. A, Hoffa's method. B, Doubling over. C, "Z" tenectomy. D, Segmental tenectomy. (Modified from Butler, H. C.: Tendon, muscle and fascia. In Archibald, J. (ed.): *Canine Surgery.* 2nd ed. American Veterinary Publications, Santa Barbara, 1974.)

Carbon fiber implants are available from commercial or industrial sources or as prepared ligament substitutes from medical supply companies. If industrial carbon fibers are used, the sizing on the fibers must first be removed by dipping the fibers in methylethyl ketone and letting them air dry. Filamentous carbon fibers can be gas or steam sterilized. One should be cautious in handling the carbon fiber filaments as they are very brittle and irritating to the skin. Numerous investigators have demonstrated that coating the carbon fiber implants with various polymers has improved handling properties and decreased the fragmentation of filaments in the soft tissues, limiting migration of the carbon fibers in the lymphatic system.[1] As use of filamentous carbon fiber implants is still in the investigative phase, their unlimited clinical application is not possible.

Tendolysis

Surgical release of tendon adhesions (tenodesis) is termed tendolysis. The presence of tendon adhesions is of little concern in small animals unless it involves a gliding tendon such as the digital flexors or has resulted in severe contracture. The critical factor is the extent of the tenodesis rather than the tissues attached.[8] To restore a soft tissue layer between the movable and immovable scar, fascia, fat, or subcutaneous tissue can be used as a layer. If such tissues are not available, paratenon can be used. Although tendolysis following superficial burns, severe contusions, closed fractures, and soft tissue injury results in a high success rate, the same does not hold true for tendolysis following tendon repair.[8]

Following trauma to soft tissues or bones, adhesions of tendons to these structures during the healing process may occur, especially if the paratenon remains unanastomosed or there is no soft tissue to incorporate between immovable and movable scar.[8] This is an indication for a paratenon transplant. The best source of paratenon in small animals is the calcanean tendon. The paratenon is carefully harvested from around the calcanean tendon and kept from contracting and adhering to itself by means of stay sutures placed at the corners of the transplant. The paratenon transplant should be sutured to any existing paratenon and not to the tendon. If paratenon is not available to suture to, loose fascia around the muscle and tendon junction is used. A fine monofilament nonabsorbable suture is used for the attachment of the transplant.

Surgical Tenotomies

As mentioned earlier in this chapter in the discussion of myectomies, it may be necessary to perform a tenotomy for a surgical approach to a bone or joint. This usually involves short, flat tendons whose function is duplicated by surrounding muscles.[35] Tenotomies may be indicated for exposure of the scapulohumeral, tibial tarsal, coxofemoral, and elbow joints.[14] The tenotomies should be repaired using horizontal mattress, Bunnell or locking-loop suture patterns and a monofilament nonabsorbable suture material.

If surgical exposure of the origin or insertion of the tendon can be as readily accomplished, an osteotomy is the preferred method because of the more secure reattachment of the osteotomy with screws or pins and tension band wire. An osteotomy usually heals faster with less postoperative immobilization than does a tenotomy.

SPECIFIC TENDON INJURIES

Severed Digital Flexor Tendons

Severance of the digital extensor and flexor tendons of small animals commonly accompanies laceration of the skin. Trauma to the digital extensor tendons is of less concern because of the many anastomoses after they branch from the main tendon (Fig. 166–19). If function following trauma to the digital extensors or flexors is normal, surgical intervention is not warranted. If loss of function is noted at a later date, a secondary repair can be performed.[8,55]

More commonly the lacerations occur on the plantar surface of the carpus and tarsus, resulting in severance of all or part of the superficial and deep digital flexor tendons.[5,8,35,55] The superficial and deep digital flexor tendons insert on the proximal end of P_2 and P_3, respectively (Fig. 166–20). The function of these tendons is to maintain the toes in proper position in relation to the digital and metacarpal or metatarsal pads. The flexor action of these tendons is maintained by the lubrication provided by the synovial sheaths and annular ligaments, which function as pulleys to change direction of the tendon. Because of the duplicity of the digital flexor tendons, sever-

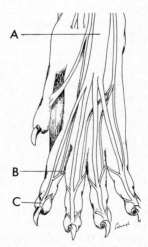

Figure 166–19. Cranial view of the carpus of the dog. Note that the common digital extensor tendon (A) has numerous anastomotic sites (B) prior to its final insertion on P3 (C). (Reprinted with permission from Butler, H. C.: Tendon, muscle and fascia. In Archibald, J. (ed.): American Veterinary Publications, Santa Barbara, 1974.)

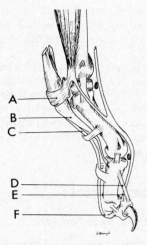

Figure 166–20. Lateral view of the tendons of the digit. *A*, Palmar annular ligament; *B*, superficial digital flexor; *C*, deep digital flexor; *D*, dorsal elastic ligament; *E*, insertion of the common digital extensor tendon; *F*, insertion of the deep digital flexor tendon. (Reprinted with permission from Butler, H. C.: Tendon, muscle and fascia. *In* Archibald, J. (ed.): *Canine Surgery.* American Veterinary Publications, Santa Barbara, 1974.)

ance of the superficial digital flexor alone may have little effect on posture whereas severance of the deep digital flexor results in flattening of one or more digits.[55]

The most common location of severance of the digital flexor tendons is above and below the metatarsal and metacarpal pads.[35] The injured animal is often presented with profuse hemorrhage and accompanying soft tissue damage. By having the dog stand on the affected leg or by pushing its foot hard against the palm of the hand, any change in posture of the digits can be detected.[55] The metacarpal or metatarsal pads may be excoriated if a chronic postural defect has been attributed to previous digital flexor tendon injury.

The site of the laceration as well as the direction and size of the wound may be helpful in determining which structures have been damaged. If the cut is across the back of the metatarsus and metacarpus, both digital flexors may be severed. If the wound is small, only a portion of the digital flexors may be damaged. If the wound is extremely deep, the muscles beneath the tendons may also be severed.

If postural defects, such as flattening of one or more digits or elevation of the toes, are present, surgical exploration is indicated. Since the deep digital flexor tendon is of primary importance in posture of the toe, injuries to the superficial and deep digital flexor tendons in the metacarpal and metatarsal area and deep digital flexor in the area of the digit require surgical treatment.

Surgical exposure of the digital flexors in the metacarpal and metatarsal areas is not difficult. A tourniquet enhances the exposure and results in less tissue trauma. Tendon ends should be anastomosed as described under tendon repair. Adequate soft tissues are available to cover the surgical repair.

Lacerations of the deep digital flexor tendon near the phalanges may damage annular ligaments and synovial sheaths. Exposure of the tendon ends is much more difficult as they may retract into the synovial sheaths beneath the annular ligament and superficial digital flexor tendon. The thick footpads and short ends of the severed tendons may require the annular ligament to be excised to expose the proximal segment if flexion and milking of the proximal tissue does not expose the tendon end.[35] Following tenorrhaphy, any damaged annular ligaments or synovial sheaths should be sutured. The smaller the breed of dog or cat, the more difficult is the identification and reattachment of the tendon ends. Postoperative management is similar to that of other tendon injuries in that the metacarpus or metatarsus is immobilized for at least three weeks, with the addition of placing it in a flexion bandage, splint, or cast.

Chronic injuries are more difficult to treat in that the soft tissues on the plantar surface of the foot may be traumatized. Identification of the tendon segments is made difficult by the fibrous scar tissue in the wound. The tendon ends can be reattached as described earlier, but often large defects remain. These defects in the digital flexor tendons can be filled with tendon grafts, fascial grafts, or carbon fibers, but the prognosis for return to normal posture is guarded.[35]

Severed Achilles Mechanism (Common Calcanean Tendon)

The Achilles mechanism is composed of five muscles having three tendinous components which combine to form the common calcanean (Achilles or tendocalcaneus) tendon.[47] The function of the Achilles mechanism is to extend the tibiotarsal joint. In addition, this group of muscles and tendons flex the stifle and digits. The main component of the common calcanean tendon is the gastrocnemius tendon. The remaining two tendons are formed by the superficial digital flexor and the common tendon of the biceps femoris, gracilis, and semitendinosus muscles.[19]

The major cause of rupture of the common calcanean tendon is direct trauma, usually by a sharp object. The skin wound may be small, horizontal, and anywhere proximal to the tuber calcanei.[55] Damage to the muscle bellies of the gastrocnemius muscle or separation at the musculotendinous junction has been covered earlier in this chapter.[6–9,12,35,36,48,50,52,55,57,59]

Clinical signs of injury include tarsal hyperflexion and stifle hyperextension. If the superficial digital flexor is severed, the paw becomes more plantigrade than normal (see Fig. 166–5). Diagnosis is aided by having the animal bear weight on the leg. These postural changes along with flaccidity of the tendon upon flexion of the hock confirm the diagnosis. If the superficial digital flexor tendon remains intact, the animal assumes a dropped hock posture with flexion of the digits. Thorough palpation of the Achilles

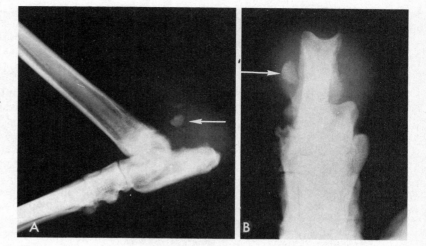

Figure 166–21. Lateral *(A)* and skyline *(B)* views of the tarsus of a dog with a chronic avulsion of the calcanean tendon. Note the avulsed bone fragment *(arrows)* and hyperflexed tibiotarsal joint *(A)*.

tendon mechanism is indicated to locate the site of injury. If no skin wound is present avulsion of the tendon from the proximal calcaneus, with or without a piece of bone, should be suspected. Radiographs of the stifle and tarsus should always be taken, along with stress films if indicated (Fig. 166–21).[47]

Surgical repair of the severed calcanean tendon should occur as soon after injury as possible. Restoration of gliding function is not of extreme importance. As a result surgical correction can be undertaken in open, contaminated wounds if proper debridement is practiced.[6] The calcanean tendon is approached through a dorsal lateral skin incision that may incorporate the previous skin wound. After thorough debridement of the wound a primary tenorrhaphy is performed on each of the three tendon components. A Bunnell-Mayer or locking loop (Kessler) suture pattern may be used (see Fig. 166–14). The suture is as large as the tendon will allow and consists of nonabsorbable monofilament material. Following anastomosis of the tendon ends the paratenon is closed over the surgical repair. This is followed by subcutaneous tissue and skin closure.

It is common to find the calcanean tendon avulsed from the tuber calcaneus (Fig. 166–22). The tendon is reattached by first placing the suture in the proximal tendon and drilling two holes in the tuber calcaneus. The two ends of the suture are passed through the drill holes, the tendon approximated to its insertion, and the suture tied. The soft tissues surrounding the calcaneus are sutured to the tendon of insertion with simple interrupted sutures. This helps prevent the sliding of the tendon to one side of the tuber calcaneus (Fig. 166–22).

Avulsion of a piece of the calcaneus (epiphysis in immature animals) may occur along with the tendon (Fig. 166–23). In this instance the piece of bone along with its tendon of insertion is reattached using a bone screw or pin and tension band wire.

As in chronic injuries, primary end-to-end tenorrhaphy may not be possible because of tendon retraction or tendon damage. Defects in the common

calcanean tendon have been repaired with tensor fascia lata,[9] transposition of the deep digital flexor,[33] and carbon fiber implants.[57]

Postoperatively the hock is immobilized for three to four weeks in a splint or cast in a semiextended position, followed by three weeks of limited activity in a modified Robert-Jones dressing. In large or obese dogs, additional internal immobilization of the tibiotarsal joint can be accomplished by an 18-gauge stainless steel wire placed in a figure-of-eight between the tuber calcaneus and the distal caudal tibia. Another method of internal immobilization is placement of a bone screw between the tuber calcanei and the distal tibia, with the tibiotarsal joint at a functional angle (135°) (see Fig. 166–9). Any internal immobilization device should be removed approximately six weeks after surgery.[6,8]

The prognosis for functional recovery is good in all except very large dogs. Unsatisfactory hyperflexion

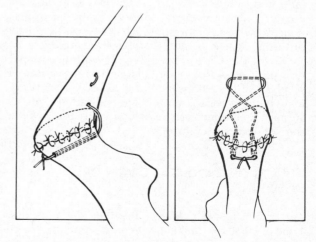

Figure 166–22. Repair of an avulsion of the calcanean tendon from the tuber calcaneus. A Bunnell suture has been woven through the tendon and then continued through two drill holes in the calcaneus and tied to itself. Sutures should be placed in the paratendinous tissue to enhance collateral stability of the tendon.

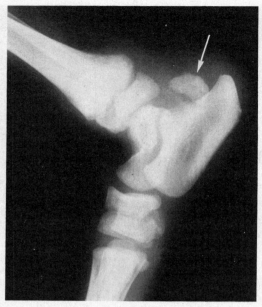

Figure 166–23. Avulsion of the calcaneal epiphysis in a young dog. Note displacement of epiphysis *(arrow).* (Courtesy of Dr. Steven M. Fox, University of Florida, Gainesville, Florida.)

of the hock may result because of failure to immobilize the tibiotarsal joint properly or too early a return to normal activity.[55]

Displacement of the superficial digital flexor tendon has been described as a separate clinical entity.[3,5,48] Diagnosis and treatment of this condition is discussed in the chapter on surgical diseases of the tarsus.

Tendon Transposition or Relocation

Transposition or relocation of a tendon is carried out to alter the function of a muscle—for example, transpose a flexor muscle onto an extensor muscle in the case of nerve paralysis. Such relocations are also indicated to stabilize a joint, such as relocation of the greater trochanter in the surgical treatment of luxation of the coxofemoral joint or transposition of the sartorius muscle for stabilization of the stifle.

One of the more rewarding surgical procedures is transposition of the tendon of a flexor muscle to treat paralysis of the extensors of the carpus (radial nerve) and tarsus (peroneal nerve). The indications for such surgical techniques are described in greater detail in the veterinary literature.[4,31]

INJURIES OF TENDONS AT ORIGIN OR INSERTION

It is common for injuries to occur at the tendon-bone or cartilage junction, where the tendon of origin or insertion blends with the periosteum and collagen fibers of the bone or cartilage. Collagen fibers of the tendon that blend with the bony substance are termed Sharpey's fibers.[24] The extrinsic vascular supply of the tendon is continuous with that of the periosteum at the tendon-bone junction.[35]

Since most tendons insert or originate near the metaphyseal region of long bones, there is a rich vascular supply that promotes healing. These injuries consist of avulsion of the origin or insertion, often accompanied by a piece of bone (avulsion fracture). The prognosis for successful healing of such injuries is very good, based on the rich vascular supply of the metaphyseal region of the bone and the fact that this type of injury is more common in immature animals.[35] The repair of injuries at tendon-bone junctions must be based on sound biomechanical principles. Many of the injuries occur at traction epiphyses, which result in delayed healing and malunions because of constant motion and muscle contraction.

Three basic types of tendon-bone injuries occur: (1) separation of tendon from bone, (2) avulsion fractures, and (3) avulsion of a small piece of bone with the tendon.[35] Once a diagnosis has been made, there should be no delay in surgical correction.

The repair of tendon separations involves the basic principles discussed earlier of the reattachment of tendon separations with short segments. If little tissue remains adjacent to the bone, a drill hole can be placed at the site of tendon insertion or origin and a horizontal mattress, Bunnell, or modified Kessler suture used to reattach the avulsed segment. The suture material of choice should be nonabsorbable and monofilament, such as stainless steel or nylon. If a small fragment of bone has been avulsed with the tendon, it can either be discarded or left with the tendon. If the bone segment is large enough, the suture can pass through it or it can be secured with Kirschner wires or a small bone screw.

Traction epiphyses are common sites of avulsion fractures, especially in young, large dogs. The sites include the greater trochanter, tibial tuberosity, greater tubercle of the humerus, tuber calcanei, and supraglenoid tubercle. The medial malleolus of the tibia, distal fibular epiphysis, distal ulnar epiphysis, and proximal ulnar epiphysis (olecranon) may also be affected with similar disorders. Although the cause may be traumatic, the injuries are usually not severe and may be overlooked initially until presented as a chronic injury. Avulsions of tendons and fractures involving the pressure epiphyses usually involve a superficial layer of bone and cartilage.[35] Such injuries involve the long digital extensor and popliteus tendon.

These injuries are frequently near the metaphysis and are closely associated with the joints. Besides having a detectable lameness, the injured animal may resist manipulation and palpation of the joint nearest the site of injury. Radiographs should be taken to confirm the presence of a tendon separation and are especially helpful in detecting the abnormal location of a sesamoid bone or epiphysis. Displacement of the avulsed bony segment may be subtle; therefore, radiographs of the opposite limb should be taken for comparison.

SPECIFIC TENDON AVULSION INJURIES

Avulsion of the Tendon of Origin of the Long Digital Extensor

The long digital extensor muscle is located on the proximal cranial tibia. It is partially covered by the cranial tibial muscle medially and peroneus longus muscle laterally. The tendon of origin arises from the extensor fossa of the lateral condyle of the femur and passes distally through the muscular groove on the craniolateral aspect of the tibia to blend with its muscle belly. The tendon inserts on the extensor process of the third phalanges of digits 2, 3, 4, and 5. The long digital extensor muscle functions to extend the digits and flex the tarsus.[19]

This injury has been described primarily in immature, large dogs.[3,10,29,35,39,45,55] The injured animal has a weight-bearing lameness and pain on manipulation of the affected stifle. Some lateral soft tissue swelling may be noticed. Clinically this condition should not be confused with a ruptured or avulsed anterior cruciate ligament or osteochondrosis of the femoral condyles. Radiographs of the affected stifle reveal an avulsed segment of bone and cartilage near the extensor fossa of the lateral femoral condyle. The lateral radiographic view best demonstrates the lesion (Fig. 166–24). If the animal is very immature the avulsed segment may consist primarily of cartilage and may not be visible radiographically. In either case, the diagnosis is confirmed by exploratory arthrotomy.

The surgical treatment of choice is reattachment of the avulsed piece of bone to its origin on the lateral femoral condyle. The surgical approach is a lateral approach to the stifle.[43] The avulsed segment of bone and tendon should be reattached using a bone screw(s). Use of a spiked washer with the bone screw will assist in securing the soft tissues surrounding the bone fragment.

In some cases the avulsed portion of bone is too small for screw fixation. In addition, chronic injuries may not allow positioning of the avulsed bony segment in the extensor fossa. In such cases, the bone fragment may be left in place or excised and a fresh bed prepared on the lateral femoral condyle. The avulsed segment can be wired or stapled in place. If no bone remains in the avulsed tendon it can be sutured to the joint capsule near its point of penetration.

Postoperatively, fixation should be protected for two weeks by placing the affected limb in a Schroeder-Thomas splint, full length cast, or modified Robert-Jones dressing. The animal is gradually returned

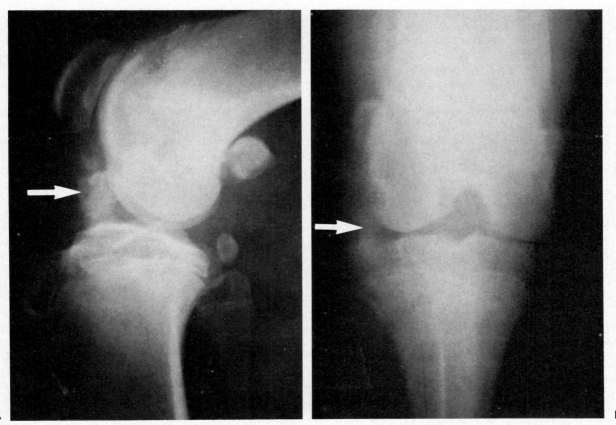

A B

Figure 166–24. Lateral (*A*) and craniocaudal (*B*) views of the stifle of a seven-month-old Great Dane. Note a calcified density present in the anterolateral aspect of the stifle joint (*arrow*). (Reprinted with permission from Lammerding, J. J., et al.: Avulsion fracture of the origin of the extensor digitorium longus muscle in three dogs. J. Am. Anim. Hosp. Assoc., *12*:764, 1976.)

to normal activity over a three to four week period following removal of the external support. The prognosis for return of function of the affected limb is excellent.

Avulsion of the Greater Trochanter

This injury is described in the chapter on injuries of the femur. It is important to note that avulsion of the greater trochanter may occur by itself. In dogs less than six months of age it commonly accompanies Salter fractures of the capital epiphysis.

Avulsion of the Origin of the Popliteus Muscle

The popliteus muscle is covered by the gastrocnemius muscle and superficial digital flexor muscle as it lies in the lateral joint capsule of the stifle and proximal tibia. It arises by a long tendon from the lateral femoral condyle just medial to the lateral collateral ligament of the stifle. Its tendon contains a sesamoid bone. The tendon continues caudally and lateral to the lateral meniscal cartilage to its muscle belly on the caudal aspect of the proximal tibia. The tendon inserts on the proximal third of the caudal surface of the tibia. The function of the popliteus muscle is to flex the stifle and inwardly rotate the leg.[19]

This injury has been reported twice, and both injuries were chronic in nature.[35,46] The clinical signs are similar to those of other stifle injuries, such as avulsion of the long digital extensor tendon. The diagnosis is confirmed by radiographs of the affected stifle which reveal distal displacement of the popliteal sesamoid bone that may also be accompanied by a bone fragment positioned caudal to the point of attachment of the popliteus tendon (Fig. 166–25).[35]

The treatment of choice involves surgical reattachment of the avulsed tendon. The approach is made through the lateral surface of the stifle.[43] Reflection of the biceps femoris muscle caudally reveals the lateral collateral ligament, joint capsule, popliteus tendon, and lateral head of the gastrocnemius muscle. Reattachment of the avulsed tendon and its accompanying bone fragment is accomplished with a small cortical bone screw with or without a spiked screw washer (Fig. 166–26).

Postoperative care is similar to that for an avulsed long digital extensor tendon.

Avulsion of the Head of the Lateral or Medial Gastrocnemius Muscle

This injury has been reported in the fox terrier,[14] Alsatian,[55] and Labrador retriever.[35] The gastrocnemius muscles are the main component of the common calcanean tendon. The lateral and medial heads of the gastrocnemius muscle originate from the lateral and medial supracondylar tuberosities, respectively, of the femur. Each head of the gastrocnemius muscle has a sesamoid located in its tendon of origin.[19] These sesamoids are commonly referred to as fabellae. The gastrocnemius muscle inserts on the tuber calcanei and extends the tarsus and flexes the stifle. The lateral and medial fabellae articulate with the femoral condyles and are bound to them by ligamentous tissue.

Clinical diagnosis of this condition is based on an animal exhibiting hyperflexion of the hock with weight bearing. Radiographs of the affected stifle reveal distal displacement of the fabella. Surgical repair of the avulsion is the treatment of choice and is described in a previous section discussing rupture of the common calcanean tendon.

Postoperative care consists of immobilization of the affected stifle for two to three weeks in a Schroeder-Thomas splint, full leg cast, or modified Robert-Jones dressing. After removal of the external support the animal should be gradually returned to normal activity over the next three to four weeks. Prognosis for return to normal activity is excellent if the initial repair remains stable.

Avulsion of the Origin of Biceps Tendon

The biceps brachii muscle is a long muscle lying on the cranial surface of the humerus. Its tendon of origin arises on the supraglenoid tuberosity, and the muscle completely spans the humerus to insert on the proximal ends of the radius and ulna. The transverse humeral ligament holds the tendon of origin in the intertubercular groove by spanning the greater and lesser tubercles. The function of the biceps brachii muscle is to flex the elbow and extend the shoulder.[19]

This condition has been described primarily in large dogs of 4 to 8 months of age.[35] The clinical signs include a weight-bearing lameness and pain or discomfort upon flexion and extension of the shoulder. Treatment of choice involves surgical reduction of the tendon and accompanying avulsed piece of bone (Fig. 166–27). The scapulohumeral joint is exposed through a craniomedial approach.[43] Lateral retraction of the supraspinatus muscle reveals the avulsed tubercle of the scapula. Care should be taken to avoid damage to the suprascapular nerve. The tendon of origin and the tubercle are aligned after placing the scapulohumeral joint in extension. The tubercle is attached to the glenoid of the scapula with a pin and tension band wire or small bone screw.

Postoperative care consists of external bandaging of the affected front limb, with the shoulder extended and the elbow flexed. The external support is removed at the end of two weeks, and the animal's activity is restricted to leash exercise only for the next three to four weeks. The prognosis for return to normal function is excellent only if the avulsed portion of bone has been securely fastened. In my experience, any fixation other than with a bone screw or pin and tension band wire will fail.

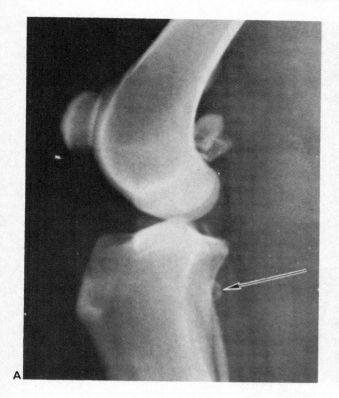

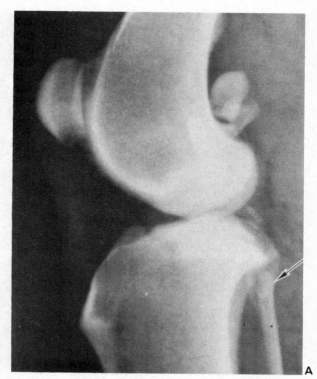

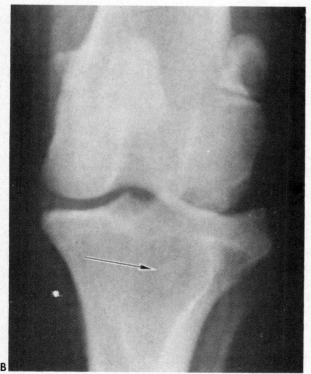

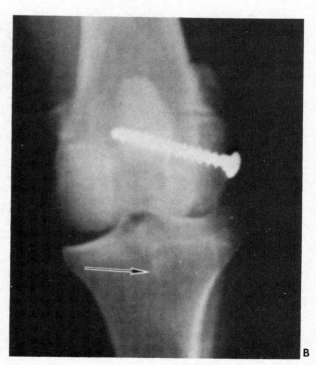

Figure 166–25. Lateral *(A)* and craniocaudal *(B)* radiographs of the stifle showing distal displacement of the sesamoid bone of the popliteal tendon *(arrow).* (Reprinted with permission from Pond, M. J., and Losonsky, J. M.: Avulsion of the popliteus muscle in the dog: a case report. J. Am. Anim. Hosp. Assoc. 12:60, 1976.)

Figure 166–26. Lateral *(A)* and craniocaudal *(B)* radiographs of the stifle shown in Fig. 166–25, taken immediately postoperatively. A bone screw has been placed in the lateral condyle of the femur. The arrow points to the sesamoid bone, which is located more proximally than noted preoperatively. (Reprinted with permission from Pond, M. J., and Losonsky, J. M.: Avulsion of the popliteus muscle in the dog: a case report. J. Am. Anim. Hosp. Assoc., *12*:60, 1976.)

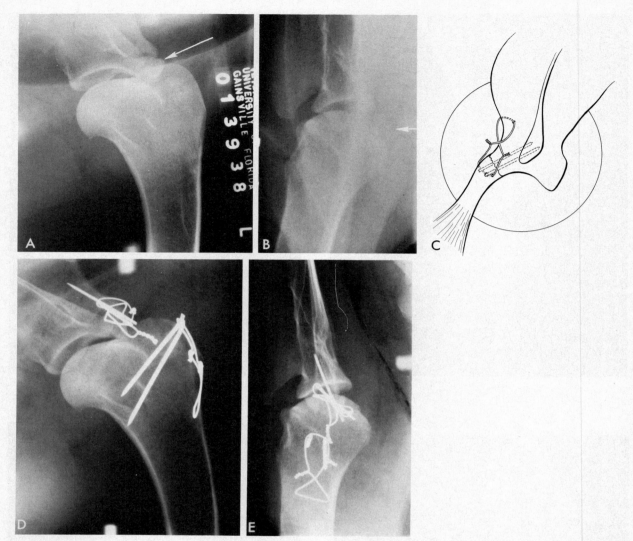

Figure 166–27. *A* and *B*, Lateral and craniocaudal radiographs of the scapulohumeral joint of a mature Doberman pinscher. The *arrow* points to the accompanying avulsion of the supraglenoid tubercle with the origin of the biceps brachii muscle. *C*, Repair technique for avulsion of the origin of the biceps brachii muscle utilizing pin and tension band wire. *D* and *E*, Lateral and craniocaudal radiographs taken postoperatively depict repair of the avulsion with a pin and tension band wire technique. Note that surgical exposure was enhanced following osteotomy of the greater tubercle of the humerus. The osteotomy was also repaired with a pin and tension band wire.

Avulsion of the Gastrocnemius Tendon from the Tuber Calcanei

This condition has been described earlier in this chapter in conjunction with rupture of the common calcanean tendon. It should be noted that physeal fractures of the tuber calcanei may result in medial displacement of the tuber calcanei, which is prevented from displacing proximally by the plantar ligament. In such instances suturing of the lateral supportive fascia is adequate to maintain reduction (see Fig. 166–22).[35]

Unusual Tendon Avulsions

Numerous other injuries involving the avulsion of tendons of origin or insertion have been described, but their occurrence is extremely rare. The treatment of these conditions follows the basic principles of the more common injuries discussed in this section and is aimed at restoring the normal anatomy. Such unusual tendon avulsions include (1) avulsion of the medial epicondyle of the humerus;[55] (2) rupture or avulsion of the triceps tendon from the olecranon;[15] (3) insertion of the biceps brachii muscle and brachialis tendons from the proximal ulna;[35] and (4) insertion of the extensor carpi radialis tendon from the proximal metaphysis of metacarpals II and III.[35]

Tendon Displacement

The displacement of a tendon from its normal position can impair limb function and result in clinical lameness. The cause of such displacement is usually traumatic, but it frequently goes unnoticed in the acute stages.

Displacement of the Tendon of Origin of the Long Digital Extensor

Two cases of caudal displacement of the long digital extensor have been described.[3,55] Both were in young animals exhibiting severe chronic lameness.[55] Upon flexion and extension of the stifle, the tendon of origin could be felt to snap out of the muscular groove on the craniolateral aspect of the proximal tibia.[35,55] Surgical treatment involved the creation of a stainless steel wire or staple roof over the muscular groove in the tibia to prevent displacement of the tendon.[3]

Displacement of the Superficial Digital Flexor Tendon

Medial displacement of the tendon of the superficial digital flexor of the rear limb is described in the chapter on the tarsus and digits.[5,35,47,48,58]

Displacement of the Tendon of Origin of the Biceps Brachii

Medial displacement of the tendon of origin of the biceps brachii muscle has been reported in a border collie,[3] miniature poodle,[35] and a greyhound.[23] The biceps tendon is held in the intertubercular groove by the transverse humeral ligament extending from the greater to the lesser tubercle of the humerus.

The lameness is usually weight bearing and chronic. Manipulation of the shoulder joint reveals pain and discomfort. Careful palpation over the cranial medial aspect of the joint shows medial slipping of the biceps tendon during flexion. On extension of the shoulder the tendon often returns to its normal location. Extension of the elbow with the shoulder partially flexed may also produce slipping of the tendon.[3]

The biceps tendon is approached through a craniomedial skin incision over the shoulder.[43] With the shoulder in extension the biceps tendon is replaced into the groove. If the groove is shallow it can be enlarged or deepened with a bone curette or rongeurs. Any remnants of the synovial sheath are sutured over the tendon with a nonabsorbable monofilament suture material. Additional fixation in the form of mattress sutures, wire staples, or a bone plate can be placed over the groove between the greater and lesser tubercles, forming a lid over the tendon.[3,23,33]

Postoperative care consists of strict confinement with no exercise for two weeks. No external support to the limb is necessary. This is followed by three to four weeks of leash exercise only. The animal is then gradually returned to normal activity. The greyhound cited earlier returned to successful competitive racing four months after surgical treatment.[23]

1. Alexander, H., Parsons, J. R., Strauchler, J. D., et al.: Canine patellar tendon replacement with a polylactic acid polymer-filamentous carbon degrading scaffold to form new tissue. Orthop. Rev. 10:44, 1981.
2. Aron, D. N.: A "new" tendon stitch. J. Am. Anim. Hosp. Assoc. 17:587, 1981.
3. Bennett, D., and Campbell, J. R.: Unusual soft tissue orthopaedic problems in the dog. J. Small Anim. Pract. 20:27, 1979.
4. Bennett, D., and Vaughn, L. C.: The use of muscle relocation techniques in the treatment of peripheral nerve injuries in dogs and cats. J. Small Anim. Pract. 17:99, 1976.
5. Bernard, M. A.: Superficial digital flexor tendon injury in the dog. Can. Vet. J. 18:105, 1977.
6. Bloomberg, M. S., Hough, J. D., and Howard, D. R.: Repair of severed Achilles tendon in a dog: A case report. J. Am. Anim. Hosp. Assoc. 12:841, 1976.
7. Braden, T. D.: Musculotendinous rupture of the Achilles apparatus and repair using internal fixation only. Vet. Med. Small Anim. Clin. 69:729, 1974.
8. Braden, T. D.: Tendons and muscles. In Bojrab, M. J. (ed.): Current Techniques in Small Animal Surgery. Lea & Febiger, Philadelphia, 1975, p. 342.
9. Braden, T. D.: Fascia lata transplants for repair of chronic Achilles tendon defects. J. Am. Anim. Hosp. Assoc. 12:800, 1976.
10. Brinker, W. D., Piermattei, D. L., and Flo, G. L.: Handbook of Small Animal Orthopedics and Fracture Treatment. W. B. Saunders, Philadelphia, 1983.
11. Bunnell, S.: Primary repair of several tendons: The use of stainless steel wire. Am. J. Surg. 47:502, 1940.
12. Butler, H. C.: Tendon, muscle, and fascia. In: Canine Surgery. 2nd Archibald ed. American Veterinary Publications, Inc., Santa Barbara, 1974, p. 933.
13. Caplan, H. S., Hunter, J. M., and Merklin, R. J.: Intrinsic vascularization of tendons. In American Academy of Orthopaedic Surgeons: Symposium on Tendon Surgery in the Hand. C. V. Mosby, St. Louis, 1975, p. 48.
14. Chaffee, V. W., and Knecht, D. C.: Avulsion of the medial head of the gastrocnemius in the dog. Vet. Med. Small Anim. Clin. 70:929, 1975.
15. Davies, J. V., and Clayton-Jones, D. G.: Triceps tendon rupture in the dog following corticosteroid injection. J. Small Anim. Pract. 23:779, 1982.
16. Dee, J. F., Dee, L. G., and Eaton-Wells, R. D.: Injuries of high performance dogs. In Whittick, W. G. (ed.): Canine Orthopedics. 2nd ed. Lea & Febiger, Philadelphia, in press.
17. Denny, H. R., and Goodship, A. E.: Replacement of the anterior cruciate ligament with carbon fiber in the dog. J. Small Anim. Pract. 21:279, 1980.
18. Early, T. D.: Tendon disorders. In Bojrab, M. J. (ed.): Pathophysiology of Small Animal Surgery. Lea & Febiger, Philadelphia, 1981, p. 851.
19. Evans, H. E., and Christensen, G. C.: Miller's Anatomy of the Dog. 2nd ed. W. B. Saunders, Philadelphia, 1979.
20. Farrow, C. S.: Sprain, strain and contusion. Vet. Clin. North Am. 8:169, 1979.
21. Frandson, R. D., and Davis, R. W.: "Dropped muscle" in the racing greyhound. J. Am. Vet. Med. Assoc. 126:468, 1955.
22. Gleeson, L. N.: Treatment of traumatic lesions of tendo-Achilles by joint fixation with a Stader splint. Vet. Med. 41:442, 1946.
23. Goring, R. L., Parker, R. B., and Dee, L.: Medial displacement of the tendon of origin of the biceps brachii muscle in the racing greyhound. J. Am. Anim. Hosp. Assoc., in press.
24. Ham, A. W.: Histology. 8th ed. J. B. Lippincott, Philadelphia, 1980.
25. Hichman, J.: Greyhound injuries. J. Small Anim. Pract. 16:455, 1975.
26. Hoerlein, B. F., Evans, L. E., and Davis, J. M.: Upward luxation of the canine scapula: A case report. J. Am. Vet. Med. Assoc. 136:258, 1960.
27. Hufford, T., Olmstead, M. L., and Butler, H. C.: Contracture of the infraspinatus muscle and surgical correction in two dogs. J. Am. Anim. Hosp. Assoc. 11:613, 1975.

28. Jenkins, D. H. R., Forester, D. W., McKibbon, B., et al.: Induction of tendon and ligament formation by carbon implants. J. Bone Joint Surg. *59B*:53, 1977.

29. Lammerding, J. J., Noser, G. A., Brinker, W. O., and Carrig, C. B.: Avulsion fracture of the origin of the extensor digitorum longis muscle in 3 dogs. J. Am. Anim. Hosp. Assoc. *11*:613, 1975.

30. Leighton, R. L.: Muscle contractures in the limbs of dogs and cats. Vet. Surg. 3:132, 1981.

31. Lesser, A. S., and Soliman, S. S.: Experimental evaluation of tendon transfer for the treatment of sciatic nerve paralysis in the dog. Vet. Surg. 9:72, 1980.

32. Liu, S. K.: A condition resembling human localized myositis ossificans in two dogs. J. Small Anim. Pract. *17*:371, 1976.

33. Malnati, G. A.: Deep digital flexor tendon transposition for rupture of the calcanean tendon in a dog. J. Am. Anim. Hosp. Assoc. *17*:451, 1981.

34. Mason, M. L., and Allen, H. S.: The rate of healing of tendon. An experimental study of tensile strength. Ann. Surg. *113*:424, 1941.

35. Milton, J. L., and Henderson, P. A.: Surgery of muscles and tendons. *In* Bojrab, M. J. (ed.): *Current Techniques in Small Animal Surgery*. 2nd ed. Lea & Febiger, Philadelphia, 1983, p. 495.

36. Mitchell, M.: Spontaneous repair of a ruptured gastrocnemius muscle in a dog. J. Am. Anim. Hosp. Assoc. *16*:513, 1980.

37. Moore, R. W., Rouse, G. P., Piermattei, D. L., and Ferguson, H. R.: Fibrotic myopathy of the semimembranosus muscle in four dogs. Vet. Surg. *10*:169, 1981.

38. O'Brien, T. J.: The use of DMSO in traumatic musculoskeletal injuries in racing greyhounds. Anim. Hosp. *1*:272, 1965.

39. Olmstead, M. L., and Butler, H. C.: Surgical correction of avulsion of the origin of the long digital extensor muscle in the dog: A case report. Vet. Med. Small Anim. Clin. *71*:608, 1976.

40. Parker, R. B., and Cardinet, G. H.: Myotendinous rupture of the Achilles mechanism associated with parasitic myositis. J. Am. Anim. Hosp. Assoc. *20*:115, 1984.

41. Peacock, E. E., and Van Winkle, W. V.: *Surgery and Biology of Wound Repair*. 2nd ed. W. B. Saunders, Philadelphia, 1976.

42. Pettit, G. D., Chatburn, C. C., Hegreberg, G. A., and Meyers, K. M.: Studies on the pathophysiology of infraspinatus muscle contracture in the dog. Vet. Surg. 7:8, 1978.

43. Piermattei, D. L., and Greeley, R. G.: *An Atlas of Surgical Approaches to the Bones of the Dog and Cat*. 2nd ed. W. B. Saunders, Philadelphia, 1979.

44. Pollock, S., Franklin, G. A., and Wagner, B. M.: Clinical significance of trauma, myositis ossificans, and malignant mesenchymoma in the dog: Report of an unusual case. J. Am. Anim. Hosp. Assoc. *14*:237, 1978.

45. Pond, M. J.: Avulsion of the extensor digitorum longus muscle in the dog. A report of four cases. Small Anim. Pract. *14*:785, 1973.

46. Pond, M. J., and Lasonsky, J. E.: Avulsion of the popliteus muscle in the dog: A case report. J. Am. Anim. Hosp. Assoc. *12*:60, 1976.

47. Reinke, J. D., and Kus, S. P.: Achilles mechanism injury in the dog. Comp. Cont. Ed. 8:639, 1982.

48. Reinke, J. D., Kus, S. P., and Owens, J. M.: Traumatic avulsion of the lateral head of the gastrocnemius and superficial digital flexor muscles in a dog. J. Am. Anim. Hosp. Assoc. *18*:252, 1982.

49. Rudy, R. L.: Stifle joint. *In*: Canine Surgery. 2nd Archibald ed. American Veterinary Publications, Inc., Santa Barbara, 1974, p. 1156.

50. Smith, K. W.: Achilles tendon surgery for correction of hyperextension of the hock joint. J. Am. Anim. Hosp. Assoc. *12*:848, 1976.

51. Srugi, S., and Adamson, J. E.: A comparative study of tendon suture material in dogs. Plast. Reconstruct. Surg. *50*:31, 1972.

52. Tomlinson, J., and Moore, R.: Locking loop tendon suture use in repair of five calcanean tendons. Vet. Surg. *11*:105, 1982.

53. Urbaniak, J. R., Cahill, J. O., and Mortenson, R. A.: Tendon suturing methods: Analysis of tensile strength. *In*: American Academy of Orthopedic Surgeons: *Symposium on Tendon Surgery of the Hand*. C. V. Mosby, St. Louis, 1975, p. 70.

54. Valdez, H., Coy, C. H., and Swanson, T.: Flexible carbon fiber for repair of gastrocnemius and superficial digital flexor tendons in a heifer and gastrocnemius tendon in a foal. J. Am. Vet. Med. Assoc. *181*:154, 1982.

55. Vaughn, L. C.: Muscle and tendon injuries in dogs. J. Small Anim. Pract. *20*:711, 1979.

56. Vaughn, L. C.: Tendon injuries in dogs. Calif. Vet. *34*:15, 1980.

57. Vaughn, L. C., and Edwards, G. B.: The use of carbon fibers (Grafil) for tendon repair in animals. Vet. Rec. *102*:287, 1978.

58. Vaughn, L. C., and Faull, W. B.: Correction of a luxated superficial digital flexor tendon in a greyhound. Vet. Rec. 67:335, 1955.

59. Vierheller, R. C.: Surgical repair of severed tendons and ligaments in the dog. Mod. Vet. Pract. *53*:35, 1972.

60. Wright, J. R.: Correction of quadriceps contractures. Calif. Vet. *34*:7, 1980.

Section **XIX**

Oncology

Dennis D. Caywood
Section Editor

Chapter 167

Biology of Neoplastic Diseases

Ralph C. Richardson and Glenn S. Elliott

Spontaneous tumors seldom behave exactly the same from patient to patient; therefore, understanding basic concepts relating to tumors allows veterinarians deeper insight into the behavior of a specific tumor in an individual animal. Epidemiological studies have helped define the prevalence of tumors and possible relationships in the environment causing neoplastic disease. Basic research has allowed greater understanding of tumor growth at the cellular and subcellular levels. Clinical research has defined many tumor effects on the host and is beginning to identify methods of predicting behavior and therapeutic responsiveness of tumors in dogs and cats. Histopathologists and clinical pathologists have provided tumor diagnostic aids that are accurate and clinically useful. By integrating this knowledge, veterinarians may become better diagnosticians, therapists, and researchers.

PREVALENCE/INCIDENCE OF TUMORS IN DOGS AND CATS

Incidence is a frequently misused term in veterinary medicine. It is defined as the rate at which a certain event occurs or the number of new cases of a specific disease occurring during a period of time.[12] It is often used synonymously with the term incidence rate, which is the frequency of a disease per unit of population per unit of time and is usually reported as cases per 100,000 population at risk over one year's time.[70] The most accurate source of extensive veterinary data for incidence rate is the California Animal Neoplasia Registry, established in 1961.[13,14] Even here, reports come from an estimated population base and should be regarded as estimated annual incidence rate.

Most reports of the "incidence" of tumors in dogs and cats have been from collections of cases without regard to the population bases from which they were drawn. Necropsy and biopsy reports compiled at various centers have been the major source of data.

Reports from sources that lack a population or time reference should be presented as prevalence data. Prevalence is the proportion of affected individuals in a series.[70] Many small prevalence series are reported in the veterinary literature; however, the most extensive series come from the Veterinary Medical Data Program established in 1964.[54] In this program, all neoplasms diagnosed at participating veterinary colleges in the United States and Canada are evaluated in comparison with the population of that particular animal species at the same college. Although some bias from referral patterns and investigator interest may be present, these data provide a good overview of tumor distribution within a species. They fail to provide adequate data to compare information gathered in one species with that of another (e.g., dog or cat versus humans).

The skin is the most common site for tumors in dogs (Table 167–1), and the hemic and lymphatic systems are most frequent in cats (Table 167–2). Dogs have the widest spectrum of all tumor types observed in domestic animals, and both dogs and cats have an increasing tumor risk with age. In studies in which animal population sampling has been conducted, the estimated annual incidence rates for malignant neoplasms at all sites have been reported as 381.2 per 100,000 dogs and 155.8 per 100,000 cats.[14] Certain dog breeds are at unusually high risk for malignant tumor development (Table 167–3). The mammary gland is the most frequent site involved with malignant neoplasia in dogs (Table 167–4). Distribution of malignant feline tumors is given in Table 167–5.

Breed, size, and color are important in determining the prevalence of tumors in dogs and cats. Dark-colored dogs develop malignant melanoma more often than lightly pigmented breeds, and white cats

TABLE 167–1. Distribution of Primary Canine Tumors by Anatomical Site*

Site	Prevalence (Per Cent)	Malignancy (Per Cent)
Skin	28.1	20
Mammary	12.2	46
Digestive	9.6	33
Hemic and lymphatic	7.4	95

*Modified from Priester, W. A., and Mantel, N.: Occurrence of tumors in domestic animals. Data from 12 United States and Canadian colleges of veterinary medicine. J. Natl. Cancer Inst. 47:1333, 1971.

Note: 6,009 tumors studied.

TABLE 167–2. Distribution of Primary Feline Tumors by Anatomic Site*

Site	Prevalence (Per Cent)	Malignancy (Per Cent)
Hemic and lymphatic	34.8	97
Skin	17.6	41
Buccal cavity	7.6	68
Digestive system	7.2	75

*Modified from Priester, W. A., and Mantel, N.: Occurrence of tumors in domestic animals. Data from 12 United States and Canadian colleges of veterinary medicine. J. Natl. Cancer Inst. 47:1333, 1971.

Note: 488 tumors studied.

TABLE 167–3. Dog Breeds at Unusually High Tumor Risk*

Breed†	Sites at Significant Risk for Malignant Tumor	Malignant Tumor Type at Significant Risk
Boxer	Skin, bone and joint, hematopoietic/lymphatic system, testis	Adenocarcinoma (mammary, thyroid, or perianal), lymphoma, angiosarcoma, mast cell tumor
Saint Bernard	Bone and joint, hematopoietic/lymphatic system, oral cavity	Lymphoma, fibrosarcoma, osteosarcoma
Airedale terrier	Nasal cavity, hematopoietic/lymphatic system	Adenocarcinoma (mammary, thyroid, or perianal), lymphoma
Scottish terrier	Skin, nasal cavity, hematopoietic/lymphatic system	Adenocarcinoma (mammary, thyroid, or perianal), squamous cell carcinoma, malignant melanoma, lymphoma
Basset hound	Skin, hematopoietic/lymphatic system	Squamous cell carcinoma, lymphoma, fibrosarcoma, mast cell tumor
Weimaraner	Skin, hematopoietic/lymphatic system, oral cavity	Adenocarcinoma (mammary, thyroid, or perianal), squamous cell carcinoma, mast cell tumor
Great Dane	Bone and joint	Angiosarcoma, fibrosarcoma, osteosarcoma
Golden retriever	Skin, bone and joint, hematopoietic/lymphatic system, oral cavity	Angiosarcoma, fibrosarcoma, osteosarcoma, mast cell tumor
Doberman pinscher	Bone and joint, hematopoietic/lymphatic system	Malignant melanoma, fibrosarcoma, osteosarcoma
Bulldog	Skin, hematopoietic/lymphatic system	Lymphoma, mast cell tumor
German short-haired pointer	Skin, mammary gland, oral cavity	Adenocarcinoma (mammary, thyroid, or perianal), malignant melanoma
Pointer	Mammary gland	Adenocarcinoma (mammary, thyroid, or perianal), angiosarcoma, fibrosarcoma, mast cell tumor
English setter	Mammary gland, hematopoietic/lymphatic system	Adenocarcinoma (mammary, thyroid, or perianal), malignant mixed mammary, angiosarcoma, fibrosarcoma
Irish setter	Bone and joint	Fibrosarcoma, osteosarcoma
Labrador retriever	Mammary gland, bone and joint, hematopoietic/lymphatic system	Adenocarcinoma (mammary, thyroid, or perianal), lymphoma, fibrosarcoma, osteosarcoma, mast cell tumor
Afghan hound	—	—
German shepherd	Bone and joint, hematopoietic/lymphatic system, testis	Angiosarcoma, fibrosarcoma, osteosarcoma

*Modified from Priester, W. A., and McKay, F. W.: The occurrence of tumors in domestic animals. Natl. Cancer Inst. Monogr. 54, 1980.

†Other studies[23] cite the cocker spaniel, Boston terrier, and wire-haired fox terrier as breeds at risk. Breeds listed are in order of prevalence (boxer > German shepherd).

TABLE 167–4. Distribution of Malignant Canine Tumors by Anatomical Site*

Site	Incidence Rate of Malignant Tumors (per 100,000)
Mammary gland	105.0
Skin (other than melanoma)	90.4
Connective tissue	35.8
Cutaneous malignant melanoma	25.0
Hemic and lymphatic	21.7

*Modified from Dorn, C. R., et al.: Survey of animal neoplasms in Alameda and Contra Costa Counties, California. II. Cancer morbidity in dogs and cats from Alameda County. J. Natl. Cancer Inst. 4:307, 1968.

TABLE 167–5. Distribution of Malignant Feline Tumors by Anatomical Site*

Site	Incidence Rate of Malignant Tumors (per 100,000)
Hemic and lymphatic	43.8
Skin (other than melanoma)	34.7
Connective tissue	17.0
Mammary gland	12.8
Buccal cavity	11.6

*Modified from Dorn, C. R., et al.: Survey of animal neoplasms in Alameda and Contra Costa Counties, California. II. Cancer morbidity in dogs and cats from Alameda County. J. Natl. Cancer Inst. 40:307, 1968.

risk development of squamous cell carcinomas of the ears and face. Giant breed dogs risk developing osteogenic sarcomas. Brachycephalic dogs are more prone to develop mast cell tumors than are mesocephalic and dolichocephalic dogs.

Tumor prevalence is also influenced by sex. Male dogs have a 2.4 times greater relative risk of developing malignant neoplasia of the buccal cavity than do female dogs.[14] Perianal gland tumors are almost exclusively confined to male dogs. Male cats have a 2.3 times greater risk of developing lymphosarcoma than do female cats.[14] Neutering of female dogs and cats significantly lowers the development of mammary cancer when compared with the intact animals.[14] Intact female dogs or cats have approximately a seven-fold higher relative risk of mammary cancer than do animals neutered at a young age.

ETIOLOGY OF SPONTANEOUS TUMORS IN DOGS AND CATS

The causative factors of cancer in dogs and cats are not fully known, but possible causes have been provided through epidemiological studies (Table 167–6), and some known causes have been demonstrated by testing specific etiological "agents" (Table 167–7). Multiple predisposing factors may sometimes be required before a specific etiological agent can transform normal cells into a tumor.

Oncogenic Viruses. Oncogenic RNA viruses (oncornaviruses) are of major importance as a cause of the leukemia-sarcoma complex in cats as well as nonneoplastic feline diseases. They replicate best in rapidly dividing cells (e.g., myeloid and lymphoid cells). Feline leukemia virus (FeLV) is the most widespread of the oncornaviruses and acts on the host cell by using an enzyme called RNA-dependent DNA polymerase, or reverse transcriptase, which can make DNA copies from the viral RNA. The virally specified DNA is incorporated into the host cat's cellular DNA (genes), and cells may be transformed from normal to neoplastic.[24] Neoplastic disorders most frequently encountered are malignant lymphoma, erythroleukemia, and myeloproliferative diseases. Transmission is horizontal (contagious) and may also be *in utero*. Multicentric fibrosarcomas develop when FeLV acts as a helper virus in the presence of another oncornavirus, the feline sarcoma virus (FeSV).[68] There is constant concern that oncornaviruses such as the FeLV or FeSV could be responsible for some human tumors. No proof of human disease has been demonstrated; however, oncogenicity has been demonstrated experimentally in the dog, rat, rabbit, pig, sheep, and monkey.[24] In addition to the FeLV and FeSV, the avian sarcoma virus (ASV) causes neoplasia in dogs and cats.[24,59] Because cross-species induction of neoplasia exists with these viruses, it is only reasonable to treat hosts bearing the virus with discretion and minimize animal-animal or animal-human exposure.

Another group of viruses causing tumors in dogs are the oncogenic DNA viruses. Canine oral papillomavirus causes multiple wartlike masses on the mucous membranes and tongues of dogs when direct inoculation into or contact with mucous membranes occurs. A papovavirus may be associated with cutaneous papillomas in the dog,[24] but confirming evidence is not available.

Irradiation. Ultraviolet (UV) irradiation from sunlight is the only significant form of radiation causing spontaneous cancer in domestic animals. The white cat and possibly the collie and Shetland sheepdog are susceptible to UV light–induced squamous cell carcinoma.[15, 25] The white cat develops erythema of the ear tips, which may progress to chronic inflammation and later to squamous cell carcinoma. There is a 13.4 times greater relative risk of developing sun-exposed site (ears and nose) squamous cell carcinoma compared with oral squamous cell carcinoma.[15] Hypopigmented areas posterior to the planum nasale in dogs may be susceptible to tumor induction, and the pathogenesis is similar to that in the white cat.[24] A high prevalence of solar-induced hemangiomas and hemangiosarcomas of the nonpigmented temporal limbus has been observed in beagles housed at high altitude.[25] The prevalence of UV-induced neoplasia in dogs does not appear nearly as great as for cats.

TABLE 167–6. Possible Causes of Tumors of Dogs and Cats*

General Etiological Factor	Specific Etiological Factor	Species	Tumor Produced
Heredity	Genes	Dog (boxer)	Numerous
	Genes (coat color)	Cat (white)	Squamous cell carcinoma
Hormones	Estrogen	Dog and cat	Mammary tumors
	Testosterone	Dog	Perianal adenoma
Congenital factor	Abnormal embryogenesis	Dog	Embryonal nephroma
	FeLV *in utero*	Cat	Malignant lymphoma
Trauma	Fractures, internal metallic fixation of bones	Dog and cat	Fibrosarcomas and osteosarcomas
	Epiphyseal plate trauma	Dog (giant breed)	Osteosarcoma
Nutrition	Dietary carcinogens	Dog and cat	Intestinal tumors

*Modified from Hardy, W. D.: The etiology of canine and feline tumors. J. Am. Anim. Hosp. Assoc. *12*:313, 1976.

TABLE 167–7. Known Causes of Tumors of Dogs and Cats*

General Etiological Factor	Specific Etiological Agent	Species	Tumor Produced

Viruses	Oncornaviruses (RNA)
	  FeLV
	  FeSV
		Cat	Lymphosarcoma
			Fibrosarcoma (multicentric)

	ASV	Dog and cat	Neurogenic tumors[59]
	Papovaviruses (DNA) canine oral papilloma virus	Dog	Oral papillomas
Irradiation	UV irradiation	Cat (white) Dog (collie)	Squamous cell carcinoma (ear) Squamous cell carcinoma (nose) Hemangioma[25] Hemangiosarcoma[25]
	Beta radiation (strontium 90)	Dog	Myelogenous leukemia Osteosarcoma Reticulum cell sarcoma Lymphosarcoma
Parasites	*Spirocerca lupi*	Dog	Esophageal osteosarcoma and fibrosarcoma
Transplantation	Intact tumor cells	Dog	Canine transmissible venereal tumor
Carcinogens	Chemicals	Dog and cat	Tonsillar carcinomas Lung tumors Bladder tumors Skin tumors Myeloid tumors
	Drugs	Dog and cat	Lymphosarcoma

*Modified from Hardy, W. D.: The etiology of canine and feline tumors. J. Am. Anim. Hosp. Assoc. *12*:313, 1976.

X-irradiation and radioactive isotopes (beta and gamma emitters) can cause experimental neoplasia in dogs and cats;[24] however, no evidence of induction of spontaneous tumors by these methods has been documented.

Hormones. Development of mammary tumors in dogs and cats appears to depend on the influence of ovarian hormones. Bitches neutered prior to any demonstration of estrus (usually less than six months of age) have a 200-fold less risk of mammary tumor development than do intact bitches or bitches having gone through five or more estrous cycles.[60] Cats show the same protective effect except that queens neutered after more than one estrous cycle are at the same risk as intact queens.[44] No influence on risk is caused by pregnancy, pseudopregnancy, estrous regularity, parity, or fecundity in the dog.[6,60] Neutering after cancer diagnosis does not alter survival.[60] It is not known whether neutering at the time of cancer diagnosis decreases the development of additional primary tumors. Estrogen and progestin receptor concentrations can be assayed in dog and cat mammary tumors following mastectomy.[33,55] Early studies with an antiestrogen drug (tamoxifen*) failed to alter the behavior of metastatic malignant mammary tumors in the dog;[58] however, as further knowledge is gained regarding the hormonal influence of neoplastic

tissue, such information may be used to prolong survival and alter the behavior of canine and feline mammary tumors.

Testosterone levels influence the development of perianal gland tumors. Females and castrated male dogs seldom develop perianal adenomas, and intact male dogs with tumor frequently demonstrate remission of disease following castration.[75]

Other tumors that may be related to hormonal influence include those of the gonads, adrenal glands, prostate, and thyroid glands.[24] Because of this, care should be taken whenever exogenous hormones are administered, particularly on a long-term basis.

Trauma. A simple injury is probably not significant as a cause of cancer, but chronic irritation, repeated trauma, or trauma with concurrent tumor-stimulating factors may result in tumor growth. Osteogenic sarcoma, canine and feline fibrosarcoma, and mammary tumors may be associated with traumatic incidences.[24,65] Osteogenic sarcomas commonly occur in the metaphyseal regions of the radius and ulna of giant breed dogs. Repeated trauma associated with weight-bearing stresses to growth plates may be partially responsible for tumor growth.[24,65] Bone pinning and plating has been associated with bone tumor development,[24,65] but only anecdotal reports are found. Fibrosarcoma in a dog[24] and in cats[69] has followed single traumatic incidences with rapid tumor development at the site of trauma. Mammary tumors

*Nolvadex, Stuart Pharmaceuticals, Wilmington, DE.

occur most frequently in the caudal mammary glands and may be associated with repeated trauma to the more pendulous glands.[56]

Parasites. In the southern United States and in warm countries where *Spirocerca lupi* is endemic, tumors of the esophagus, stomach, and aorta have been found, and a direct association between the parasites and the tumor has been made. The exact mechanism of carcinogenesis is unknown; however, the parasite is routinely found within the tumor tissue. Esophageal tumors comprise the majority of the induced tumors, of which 66 per cent are osteosarcomas and 34 per cent are fibrosarcomas.[1] They are associated with local tumor infiltration and disseminate primarily to the lungs.[1] Bile duct carcinomas in dogs and cats have been caused by the liver fluke, *Clonorchis sinensis*.[44] The parasite is found primarily in Hong Kong, and infestation may be induced by feeding animals raw fish containing clonorchid cysts.

Transplantation. The canine transmissible venereal tumor (TVT)[57] is the only tumor passed by intact cells from dog to dog without the aid of viral or carcinogenic factors. The usual mode of transmission is by coitus, and lesions are seen most frequently on the penis or in the vagina. Orogenital contact allows cellular implantation in the oral cavity and nose. Whole-cell suspensions injected subcutaneously can form a tumor and be used as an experimental model for comparative oncology studies. The cells divide and grow and may even metastasize, but the host's own cells are not transformed to tumor. The tumors are immunologically active as antibodies are directed against the tumor cells, and remission may occur. This phenomenon is most frequently observed in experimentally transmitted tumors.

Congenital Origin. Embryonal nephromas appear occasionally in dogs and may be detected in puppies less than six months of age. An abnormality of embryogenesis is the probable cause of the tumor.

Heredity. Tumors are not heritable, but predisposition to tumor development is. Cats with white coats exposed to UV light are predisposed to squamous cell carcinoma of the nose and ears. Heredity of coat color, therefore, predisposes to cancer. Brachycephalic dogs are more prone to develop mast cell tumors than are other breeds. Some factor (e.g., chronic hypoxia?) may therefore predispose to mast cell tumor development. Intense inbreeding may have allowed tumor-causing genes (oncogenes) to inadvertently be selected and passed to offspring.[24]

Carcinogens. Spontaneous dog and cat neoplasms induced by chemical carcinogens are almost impossible to document. Excellent data generated experimentally clearly demonstrate that many tumors may be induced by intensive carcinogenic stimulation. Tonsillar squamous cell carcinoma and malignant mesothelioma are the only spontaneous tumors with significant epidemiological evidence indicating that they are induced by chemical carcinogens. Dogs living in urban areas and therefore exposed to more chemical wastes in the atmosphere have more tonsil-

lar carcinomas than do dogs in rural areas.[44] Dogs exposed to asbestos fibers develop malignant mesothelioma at a significantly greater rate than those not exposed.[22a]

TUMOR CELL GROWTH

A tumor is an abnormal swelling of tissue, the growth of which exceeds and is uncoordinated with the growth of the normal tissues, that persists in the same excessive manner after cessation of the stimuli that evoked the change and has no physiological use.[12] Benign tumors are usually slow growing, circumscribed, or encapsulated and do not metastasize. They grow by expansion and usually have an adequate blood supply. Mitotic figures are rare, and cells are well differentiated. When completely removed, they do not recur. Malignant tumors, on the other hand, usually grow rapidly, infiltrate surrounding tissues, and frequently metastasize or recur at the local site after removal. Mitotic figures are common, and the cells are anaplastic. Invasion of vessels and other structures is common and the blood supply is usually adequate, but rapid growth may allow a necrotic center to form. They are progressive and frequently result in death of the host. The invasive and metastatic properties of malignant cells resulting in organ failure cause death.

It is not fully understood whether tumors develop from a mutation of a single cell or from many transformed cells. There is growing acceptance of the theory that tumors develop as a clone from a single cell of origin termed a *stem cell*. From such a cell, sequential selection of further mutant subpopulations may occur. With time, most mutant subpopulations die, but a few sublines may be suited for survival and grow as a tumor. These aggressive sublines may demonstrate genetic variability, allowing advanced malignancies to have highly individualistic karyotypes and biological behavior.[47] This may account for variability in treatment response between patients or within the treatment course of a single patient. Therapy effective against a certain population of transformed cells may be effective only as long as that particular population is present. It is possible that, from the initially responsive population, a new subgroup may develop that is totally unresponsive to the original therapy—thus the clinically observed phenomena of drug resistance and relapse of disease despite ongoing therapy.

Tumors that reach clinically detectable size represent the late stages of malignant growth.[2] A clinically detectable tumor (1 cm^3) composed of cells 10 μ in diameter would contain approximately 1×10^9 (1 billion) cells. If the tumor had started as a stem cell and had grown by geometric progression (exponential growth) and if all daughter cells from the parent cells had survived, 30 doublings would have been required before the tumor was detected. A further ten doublings would produce approximately 1 kg of cancer tissue. Tumors of this size are seldom compatible with life. At least half of this growth would have occurred prior to the earliest possible clinical diagnosis. If tumor doubling time of observed metastatic lung lesions is used to estimate the duration of tumor presence in lungs of dogs with osteogenic sarcoma, it has been shown that metastasis often occurs prior to the detection of the primary tumor. If tumor doubling time ranges from 7 to 20 days[2] and if the average tumor doubling time is 8 days, 240 days of metastatic tumor presence would be required before detection (at time preceding the onset of clinical signs of the primary tumor).

Exponential growth probably does not occur in tumors, since many cells may not survive. Rapid growth and good survival may be present in the early stages of tumor growth when optimal tumor cell nutrition and lack of crowding are present, but tumor doubling time probably increases as tumors enlarge.

TUMOR INVASION AND METASTASIS

Criteria to predict the behavior of malignancy are frequently sought. Local invasion and metastasis are the best clinical criteria of malignancy available. Local invasion of histologically malignant tumor without metastasis (infiltration) occurs in several tumor types in dogs and cats. These tumor cells may actually invade blood vessels, but metastasis does not frequently develop because of several possible factors (e.g., cohesiveness of the cells, rate of tumor growth, degree of necrosis, amount of connective tissue surrounding the tumor). Examples of such tumors include carcinoma of the adrenal cortex, thyroid carcinomas, pheochromocytomas, hepatomas, and chemoreceptor tumors. Tumors that have a high metastatic rate include malignant melanomas and osteogenic sarcomas. There are no good criteria to predict invasion versus metastasis of a tumor. The only criteria that predict the behavior of several tumor types are tumor size and rate of growth. As potentially metastatic tumors increase in size, their probability of metastasis increases.

Tumor metastasis involves several major steps: (1) invasion of cells from the primary tumor into surrounding tissue, including blood and lymph vessels, (2) release of embolic tumor cells into the circulation, (3) arrest of emboli in capillary beds of distant organs, (4) invasion of cells from the embolic focus, infiltration into the surrounding tissue, and multiplication, and (5) angiogenesis.[19] Tumor invasion at the primary site may occur by increased pressure and destruction of host stroma, decreased cohesiveness of neoplastic cells, and increased mobility of the cells. A major biochemical prerequisite of an invasive tumor is its ability to form and secrete high levels of proteolytic enzymes that disrupt host stroma and facilitate invasion. Actively growing tumors may cause a local inflammatory response, generating chemotaxis for leukocytes that contain large amounts of proteolytic enzymes. Proteolytic enzymes may cause further destruction of normal tissues and enhance invasion. After invasion has occurred, tumors may metastasize by direct extension or transplantation or through the lymphatics or blood stream.

Metastasis by *direct extension* is simply an extension of local tumor invasion. As an invasive tumor expands, it may spread to any adjacent organ. Soft tissues are invaded most easily. Some barriers to direct extension occasionally exist (e.g., joint spaces, fascial planes).

Spread by *transplantation* occurs in body cavities. The term *transcoelomic migration* may be used to describe this spread. Ovarian carcinomas are the best example of this. Malignant cells exfoliated from the primary tumor may seed any serosal surface of the abdomen and grow. Migration of malignant cells around major vessels passing through the diaphragm allows implantation onto the serosal surfaces of the pleural space. Metastasis beyond these sites is seldom seen.

Spread by the *lymphatic system* is the most common method of metastasis from many carcinomas. Lymphatic spread denotes the infiltration of a draining lymph node by tumor cells.[19] Initially, tumor emboli may invade thin-walled lymphatic vessels, follow lymphatic flow, and grow in the first lymph node they encounter. They may even bypass the first set of nodes and grow farther along the lymphatic chain. Affected lymph nodes become enlarged, firm, and sometimes fixed.

Spread by the *hematogenous route* occurs following invasion into thin-walled veins. Arteries are relatively resistant to tumor invasion. Emboli of tumor cells are probably released early in the course of primary tumor development and transported to many parts of the body via the blood stream. The lung is a favored site for hematogenous metastasis, since it receives and "filters" all venous return for the body before it returns to the heart. The liver, another reticuloendothelial organ receiving a large amount of venous blood, is also predisposed to hematogenous metastasis. Sarcomas have a greater tendency to metastasize hematogenously than do carcinomas. The observation of tumor emboli in the blood stream does not constitute metastasis, but if large numbers of malignant cells are found in the blood, there is a correlation with clinical duration, size, and necrosis of the tumor.[19] Large clumps of embolic tumor cells are more likely to cause metastasis than small clumps.[47] Before metastasis can develop, the circulating tumor cells must survive the turbulence of the blood stream, evade possible host defense mechanisms, attach firmly to the endothelium of distant small vessels (capillaries), and gain entrance to extravascular spaces by invasion.[19]

During primary tumor or metastatic focus development, the host's immune response to the tumor may play a dual role.[19] In the early course of the development of cancer or with weakly antigenic tumors, cell-mediated responses might directly stimulate rather than inhibit tumor growth. The tumor might be inhibited at a later stage of growth when the immune response becomes stronger or if the tumor is highly antigenic. Small numbers of sensitized immune lymphocytes aid successful spread of neoplasms, whereas high numbers of the same immune cells dramatically reduce metastasis. Low numbers of sensitized lymphocytes may cause tumor cell clumping and thus easier adhesion in the capillary beds, leading to metastasis, but high numbers of immune-stimulated lymphocytes may cause death of tumor cells.

CLINICAL STAGING

Clinical staging determines the extent of disease in living animals. For spontaneous tumors in dogs and cats it serves two purposes: (1) groups of animals may be matched for study, and (2) the clinician may use the information to plan treatment. A third purpose may develop after enough data have been gathered and reported using consistent staging methods. Accurate prognostic criteria based on clinical presentation may become available. In group studies of animals, particularly for therapeutic trials, it is important to compare animals with minimal disease with other animals with minimal disease and not with animals with extensive disease so that bias is not introduced into the study. Additionally, if an animal is to be treated for cancer, the extent of disease must be known to avoid inappropriate therapy. A simple differentiation of local disease versus systemic disease is of the utmost importance. Therapy with curative intent must be adequately planned. It makes no sense to attempt cure through some method of local therapy (e.g., surgery, radiation, cryotherapy) in an animal with extensive disease. Local disease generally requires local therapy, and widespread cancer requires systemic therapy (e.g., chemotherapy, immunotherapy). An exception to this is local palliation of one portion of widespread disease.

In veterinary medicine, the standard for clinical staging is the TNM system[50] (T = tumor; N = regional lymph node; M = distant metastasis) developed through the World Health Organization. Appropriate assignment of TNM classification is conducted only after histological confirmation of a primary tumor and may include histological, cytological, radiographic, and physical findings.

Size of the primary tumor is designated from T0 to T4. A small tumor is designated T1, and T4 designates a large tumor. Size variations are given for each particular tumor type. The symbol T0 means no evidence of tumor.

The term N0 suggests no regional lymph node involvement and N1 that regional lymph nodes are positive for metastatic disease. A few select tumor types carry an N2 or N3 designation. The staging of animals with a primary tumor and enlarged regional lymph nodes sometimes creates a dilemma. Are the lymph nodes positive for metastasis or not? Lymph nodes become enlarged, firm, and sometimes fixed following tumor invasion. Normal lymph nodes are freely movable and frequently not palpable. Enlarged, soft nodes may be reactive to tumor inflammation, superficial infection, or antigenic stimulation of the host. To solve the dilemma, all enlarged regional nodes should be examined cytologically by fine needle aspiration if possible. Observation of tumor cells in fine needle aspirates from enlarged lymph nodes confirms metastasis. These nodes should be removed and submitted for histopathological examination at the time of primary tumor resection if surgical therapy is attempted. Firm or fixed nodes cytologically negative for tumor cells should be removed at the time of primary tumor resection and submitted for histopathological evaluation before confirming staging. Soft and enlarged nodes free of cytological evidence of cancer should be left in place and observed closely for any change suggesting tumor involvement. Non-neoplastic nodes may act as immunological barriers to further tumor spread and should be left in place whenever possible.

Distant metastasis is described by the terms M0 or M1. Radiographic findings provide the evidence used most frequently to establish distant metastasis.

Once the TNM classification has been completed, most tumors are assigned a "clinical stage," designated from I to IV. Clinical stage I defines local disease with no metastasis. Clinical stages II, III, and IV designate degrees of metastasis, with stage IV being the most severe. The functional capacity of the patient is often designated with the clinical stage. The letter (a) following a clinical stage means the

TABLE 167–8. Paraneoplastic Syndromes Associated with Topic Hormone Production by Endocrine Tumors in Dogs and Cats

Syndrome	Neoplasms	Reference
Hyperadrenocorticism	Adrenal tumors	7
	Pituitary tumors	7
Hypercalcemia	Parathyroid tumors	7,16,32,36,76
Hyperestrogenism	Sertoli cell tumors	17,43,72
Hypertension	Pheochromocytoma	70
Hyperthyroidism	Thyroid tumors	70
Hypoglycemia	Pancreatic islet cell adenocarcinoma	70
Zollinger-Ellison syndrome	Pancreatic non-β islet cell tumors	7,22,43,72

TABLE 167–9. Paraneoplastic Syndromes Associated with Ectopic Hormones or Production of Biochemical Substances in Dogs and Cats

Syndrome	Neoplasms	Reference
Anemia	Various	7,37,43,72
Anorexia/cachexia	Various	10,43,72
Coagulation abnormalities	Hemangiosarcoma	20,31
	Mastocytoma	43,70,72
	Nasal adenocarcinoma	52
	Various (see also monoclonal gammopathy and hyperviscosity)	18,20,38,72
Erythrocytosis (secondary polycythemia)	Renal tumors	51,61
Fever	Various	43,72
Glomerulonephritis	Various	48
	Mastocytoma	70
Histaminosis	Mastocytoma	7,43,72
Hypercalcemia	Metastatic adenocarcinoma of undetermined origin	29,78
	Epidermoid carcinoma of the lung	46
	Fibrosarcoma	7,36
	Interstitial cell tumor	7,36,72
	Lymphosarcoma/lymphocytic leukemia	11,16,36,43,49,72,77
	Mammary adenocarcinoma	36,43,72
	Myeloma	34,72
	Myeloproliferative disease	79
	Pancreatic carcinoma (exocrine)	72,73
	Perianal tumors	16,26,41,43,72,77
Hypertrophic osteopathy	Primary and metastatic lung tumors	5,7,39,43,72
	Atypical nephroblastoma	9
	Renal papillary adenoma (cat)	45
	Embryonal rhabdomyosarcoma of the urinary bladder	5,7,21,43,72
Hyperviscosity syndrome	Polycythemia vera (see also monoclonal gammopathy)	40,51,72
Hypoglycemia	Hepatic tumors	66,67,72
	Lymphocytic leukemia	7,11,43,72
Leukocytosis	Pulmonary adenocarcinoma	71
	Lymphosarcoma	7
	Various	43,72
Monoclonal gammopathy (hyperviscosity syndrome, coagulation abnormalities, nephrotoxicity)	Lymphosarcoma/lymphocytic leukemia	3,7,34,35,43,72,74
	Macroglobulinemia	7,27,34
	Myeloma	4,7,34,43,62,63,72
Myasthenia gravis	Thymoma	30,72
Neuromyopathy	Bile duct carcinoma	8
	Intestinal adenocarcinoma	8
	Lymphosarcoma	8
	Pancreatic adenocarcinoma	8
	Prostatic adenocarcinoma	8
	Metastatic anaplastic pulmonary carcinoma	64
	Seminoma/perianal gland adenoma	8

patient is without systemic signs, whereas (b) means systemic signs are present.

The system of clinical staging is not perfect, but it is a logical beginning. The support of numerous veterinarians willing to report their findings in a consistent manner is required to provide information necessary to accurately describe and optimally care for animals with spontaneous neoplasia.

INDIRECT EFFECTS ON THE HOST

Neoplasia in dogs and cats can produce signs and symptoms directly related to invasion or obstruction by the tumor or its metastases. Tumors also produce signs and symptoms at a distance from the tumor or its metastases. These remote effects are referred to as *paraneoplastic syndromes*. Any effect not caused directly by the tumor or its metastases is a paraneoplastic effect.[42] Paraneoplasia includes *topic hormone production* by cells of endocrine tumors, *ectopic hormone production* by cells of nonendocrine tumors, and production of various *biochemical substances* by cancer cells.[42] Recent studies in humans indicate that production of topic hormones, ectopic hormones, or other biochemical substances is a universal feature of neoplasms.[28] These substances do not always cause signs, because of either insufficient quantities or lack of biological activity.[28] The reason that tumor cells produce these products is unknown. The most common explanation is simple derepression of genes. Differentiated somatic cells carry genetic information for all the potential cell phenotypes of the body, although most of the information is repressed during development. According to this theory, the genes of neoplastic cells are derepressed and capable of coding for substances produced by any cell of the body.[28]

Examples of hormone production by endocrine tumors (topic production) include adrenocorticotropin (ACTH) production by pituitary tumors, cortisol from adrenal tumors, insulin from functional pancreatic islet cell tumors, and many others (Table 167–8). Tumor cells arising from nonendocrine tissue may produce ectopic hormones, hormone precursors, prostaglandins, immunoglobulins, enzymes, immune complexes, antigens that provoke immune responses, biologically inactive products that block receptors, and many unknown substances[42] (Table 167–9).

Paraneoplastic syndromes are important for many reasons. They may be the first indication of neoplasia, creating signs that allow early diagnosis. The paraneoplastic syndrome itself may be more debilitating or immediately life-threatening than the tumor from which it arose. Paraneoplasia can also be used as a marker for tumor recurrence or to monitor response to the therapy.[42]

1. Baily, W. J.: Parasites and cancer: Sarcoma in dogs associated with *Spirocerca lupi*. Ann. N.Y. Acad. Sci. *108*:890, 1963.
2. Bech-Nielsen, S., et al.: The use of tumor doubling time in veterinary clinical oncology. J. Am. Vet. Radiol. Soc. *17*:113, 1976.
3. Braund, K. G., Everett, R. M., and Albert, R. A.: Neurologic manifestations of IgM gammopathy associated with lymphocytic leukemia in a dog. J. Am. Vet. Med. Assoc. *172*:1407, 1978.
4. Braund, K. G., Everett, R. M., Bartels, S. E., and DeBuysscher, E.: Neurologic complications of IgA multiple myeloma associated with cryoglobulinemia in a dog. J. Am. Vet. Med. Assoc. *174*:1321, 1979.
5. Brodey, R. S.: Hypertrophic osteoarthropathy in the dog: A clinicopathologic survey of 60 cases. J. Am. Vet. Med. Assoc. *159*:1242, 1971.
6. Brodey, R. S., et al.: The relationship of estrous irregularity, pseudopregnancy and pregnancy to the development of canine mammary neoplasms. J. Am. Vet. Med. Assoc. *149*:1047, 1966.
7. Brown, N. O.: Paraneoplastic syndromes of humans, dogs and cats. J. Am. Anim. Hosp. Assoc. *17*:911, 1981.
8. Cardinet, G. H., and Holliday, T. A.: Neuromuscular diseases of domestic animals: A summary of muscle biopsies from 159 cases. Ann. N.Y. Acad. Sci. *317*:290, 1979.
9. Caywood, D. D., Osborne, C. A., Stevens, J. B., et al.: Hypertrophic osteoarthropathy associated with an atypical nephroblastoma in a dog. J. Am. Anim. Hosp. Assoc. *16*:855, 1980.
10. Crow, S. E.: Cancer cachexia. Comp. Cont. Educ. *3*:681, 1981.
11. DeSchepper, J., VanDerStock, J., and DeRick, A.: Hypercalcaemia and hypoglycaemia in a case of lymphatic leukaemia in the dog. Vet. Rec. *94*:602, 1974.
12. *Dorland's Illustrated Medical Dictionary*, 24th ed. W. B. Saunders, Philadelphia, 1965.
13. Dorn, C. R., et al.: Survey of animal neoplasms in Alameda and Contra Costa Counties, California. I: Methodology and description of cases. J. Natl. Cancer Inst. *40*:295, 1968.
14. Dorn, C. R., et al.: Survey of animal neoplasms in Alameda and Contra Costa Counties, California. II. Cancer morbidity in dogs and cats from Alameda County. J. Natl. Cancer Inst. *40*:307, 1968.
15. Dorn, C. R., et al.: Sunlight exposure and risk of developing cutaneous and oral squamous cell carcinomas in white cats. J. Natl. Cancer Inst. *46*:1073, 1971.
16. Drazner, F. H.: Hypercalcemia in the dog and cat. J. Am. Vet. Med. Assoc. *178*:1252, 1981.
17. Edwards, D. F.: Bone marrow hypoplasia in a feminized dog with a Sertoli cell tumor. J. Am. Vet. Med. Assoc. *178*:494, 1981.
18. Feldman, B. F., Madewell, B. R., and O'Neill, S.: Disseminated intravascular coagulation: Antithrombin, plasminogen and coagulation abnormalities in 41 dogs. J. Am. Vet. Med. Assoc. *179*:151, 1981.
19. Fidler, I. J.: General concepts of tumor metastasis in the dog and cat. J. Am. Anim. Hosp. Assoc. *12*:374, 1976.
20. Greene, C. E.: Disseminated intravascular coagulation in the dog: A review. J. Am. Anim. Hosp. Assoc. *11*:674, 1975.
21. Halliwell, W. H., and Ackerman, N.: Botryoid rhabdomyosarcoma of the urinary bladder and hypertrophic osteoarthropathy in a young dog. J. Am. Vet. Med. Assoc. *165*:911, 1974.
22. Happe, R. P., VanDer Gaag, I., Lamers, C. B. H. W., et al.: Zollinger-Ellison syndrome in three dogs. Vet. Pathol. *17*:177, 1980.
22a. Harbison, M. L., and Godeski, J. J.: Malignant mesothelioma in urban dogs. Vet. Pathol. *20*:531, 1983.
23. Hardy, W. D.: General concepts of canine and feline tumors. J. Am. Anim. Hosp. Assoc. *12*:295, 1976.
24. Hardy, W. D.: The etiology of canine and feline tumors. J. Am. Anim. Hosp. Assoc. *12*:313, 1976.
25. Hargis, A. M.: A review of solar-induced lesions in domestic animals. Comp. Cont. Educ. *3*:287, 1981.
26. Hause, W. R., Stevenson, S., Meuten, D. J., et al.: Pseudohyperparathyroidism associated with adenocarcinomas of anal sac origin in four dogs. J. Am. Anim. Hosp. Assoc. *17*:373, 1981.
27. Hurvitz, A. I., MacEwen, E. G., Middaugh, C. R., et al.: Monoclonal cryoglobulinemia with macroglobulinemia in a dog. J. Am. Vet. Med. Assoc. *170*:511, 1977.
28. Imura, H.: Ectopic hormone production viewed as an abnormality in regulation of gene expression. Adv. Cancer Res. *33*:39, 1980.
29. Johnson, J. T.: Pseudohyperparathyroidism associated with metastatic adenocarcinoma of undetermined origin in the dog. J. Am. Vet. Med. Assoc. *173*:82, 1978.
30. Kelly, M. J.: Myasthenia gravis—A receptor disease. Comp. Cont. Ed. *3*:544, 1981.
31. Legendre, A. J., and Krehbiel, J. D.: Disseminated intravascular coagulation in a dog with hemothorax and hemangiosarcoma. J. Am. Vet. Med. Assoc. *171*:1070, 1977.

32. Legendre, A. M., Merkley, D. F., Carry, C. B., et al.: Primary hyperparathyroidism in a dog. J. Am. Vet. Med. Assoc. 168:694, 1976.

33. MacEwen, E. G., et al.: Estrogen receptors in canine mammary tumors. Cancer Res. 42:2255, 1982.

34. MacEwen, E. G., and Hurvitz, A. I.: Diagnosis and management of monoclonal gammopathies. Vet. Clin. North Am. 7:119, 1977.

35. MacEwen, E. G., Hurvitz, A. I., and Hayes, A.: Hyperviscosity syndrome associated with lymphocytic leukemia in three dogs. J. Am. Vet. Med. Assoc. 170:1309, 1977.

36. MacEwen, E. G., and Siegel, S. D.: Hypercalcemia: A paraneoplastic disease. Vet. Clin. North Am. 7:187, 1977.

37. Madewell, B. R., and Feldman, B. F.: Characterization of anemias associated with neoplasia in small animals. J. Am. Vet. Med. Assoc. 176:419, 1980.

38. Madewell, B. R., Feldman, B. F., and O'Neill, S.: Coagulation abnormalities in dogs with neoplasia. Thromb. Haemost. 44:35, 1980.

39. Madewell, B. R., Nyland, T. G., and Weigel, J. E.: Regression of hypertrophic osteopathy following pneumonectomy in a dog. J. Am. Vet. Med. Assoc. 172:818, 1978.

40. McGrath, C. J.: Polycythemia vera in dogs. J. Am. Vet. Med. Assoc. 164:1117, 1974.

41. Meuten, D. J., Capen, C. C., Kociba, G. J., et al.: Hypercalcemia of malignancy. Hypercalcemia associated with an adenocarcinoma of the apocrine glands of the anal sac. Am. J. Pathol. 108:366, 1982.

42. Minna, J. D., and Bunn, P. A.: Paraneoplastic syndromes. In DeVita, V. T., Hellman, S., and Rosenberg, S. A. (eds.): Cancer: Principles and Practice of Oncology. J. B. Lippincott, Philadelphia, 1982.

43. Morrison, W. B.: Paraneoplastic syndromes of the dog. J. Am. Vet. Med. Assoc. 175:559, 1979.

44. Moulton, J. E. (ed.): Tumors in Domestic Animals, 2nd ed. University of California Press, Berkeley, 1978.

45. Nafe, L. A., Herron, A. J., and Burk, R. L.: Hypertrophic osteopathy in a cat associated with renal papillary adenoma. J. Am. Anim. Hosp. Assoc. 17:659, 1981.

46. Nafe, L. A., Patnaik, A. K., and Lyman, R.: Hypercalcemia associated with epidermoid carcinoma in a dog. J. Am. Vet. Med. Assoc. 176:1253, 1980.

47. Nowell, P. C.: The clonal evolution of tumor cell populations. Science 194:23, 1976.

48. Osborne, C. A., Hammer, R. F., Stevens, J. B., et al.: Immunologic aspects of glomerular disease in the dog and cat. Gaines Veterinary Symposium 26:15, 1976.

49. Osborne, C. A., and Stevens, J. B.: Pseudohyperparathyroidism in the dog. J. Am. Vet. Med. Assoc. 162:125, 1973.

50. Owen, L. N. (ed.): TNM Classification of Tumors in Domestic Animals, 1st ed. World Health Organization, Geneva, 1980.

51. Peterson, M. E., and Randolph, J. F.: Diagnosis of canine primary polycythemia and management with hydroxyurea. J. Am. Vet. Med. Assoc. 180:415, 1982.

52. Prasse, K. W., Hoskins, J. D., Glock, R. D., et al.: Factor V deficiency and thrombocytopenia in a dog with adenocarcinoma. J. Am. Vet. Med. Assoc. 160:204, 1972.

53. Priester, W. A., and Mantel, N.: Occurrence of tumors in domestic animals. Data from 12 United States and Canadian colleges of veterinary medicine. J. Natl. Cancer Inst. 47:1333, 1971.

54. Priester, W. A., and McKay, F. W.: The Occurrence of Tumors in Domestic Animals. Natl. Cancer Inst. Monogr. 54, 1980.

55. Raynaud, J. P., et al.: Spontaneous canine mammary tumors: A model for human endocrine therapy. J. Steroid Biochem. 15:201, 1981.

56. Richardson, R. C.: Mammary tumors in animals. In Hoogstraten, B., and McDivitt, R. W. (eds.): Breast Cancer. CRC Press, Inc., Boca Raton, 1981, pp. 27–38.

57. Richardson, R. C.: Canine transmissible venereal tumor. Comp. Cont. Ed. 3:951, 1981.

58. Richardson, R. C., and Bottoms, G. D.: Tamoxifen therapy in seven dogs with malignant mammary tumors. Unpublished data, 1981.

59. Saleman, M., et al.: Transplantable canine glioma model for use in experimental neuro-oncology. J. Neurosurg. 11:372, 1982.

60. Schneider, R., et al.: Factors influencing canine mammary cancer development and postsurgical survival. J. Natl. Cancer Inst. 43:1249, 1969.

61. Scott, R. C., and Patnaik, A. K.: Renal carcinoma with secondary polycythemia in the dog. J. Am. Anim. Hosp. Assoc. 8:275, 1972.

62. Shepard, V. J., Dodds-Laffin, W. J., and Laffin, R. M.: Gamma A myeloma in a dog with defective hemostasis. J. Am. Vet. Med. Assoc. 160:1121, 1972.

63. Shull, R. M., Osborne, C. A., Barrett, R. E., et al.: Serum hyperviscosity syndrome associated with IGA multiple myeloma in two dogs. J. Am. Anim. Hosp. Assoc. 14:58, 1978.

64. Sorjonen, D. C., Braund, K. G., and Hoff, E. J.: Paraplegia and subclinical neuromyopathy associated with a primary lung tumor in a dog. J. Am. Vet. Med. Assoc. 180:1209, 1982.

65. Stevenson, S., et al.: Fracture-associated sarcoma in the dog. J. Am. Vet. Med. Assoc. 180:1189, 1982.

66. Strombeck, D. R.: Clinicopathologic features of primary and metastatic neoplastic disease of the liver in dogs. J. Am. Vet. Med. Assoc. 173:267, 1978.

67. Strombeck, D. R., Krum, S., Meyer, D., et al.: Hypoglycemia and hypoinsulinemia associated with hepatoma in a dog. J. Am. Vet. Med. Assoc. 169:811, 1976.

68. Theilen, G. H.: Feline leukemia–sarcoma disease complex. Proceedings for Clinical Oncology, 10th Annual Veterinary Surgical Forum, 1982, pp. 46–51.

69. Theilen, G. H.: Personal communication. 10th Annual Veterinary Surgical Forum, 1982.

70. Theilen, G. H., and Madewell, B. R. (eds.): Veterinary Cancer Medicine. Lea & Febiger, Philadelphia, 1979.

71. Tomlinson, J. M., Jennings, B., Wendt, J. B., et al.: Adenocarcinoma of the lung with secondary pericardial effusion and leukemoid response in a dog. J. Am. Vet. Med. Assoc. 163:257, 1973.

72. Weller, R. E.: Paraneoplastic disorders in companion animals. Comp. Cont. Ed. 4:423, 1982.

73. Weller, R. E., Pool, R. R., and Hornof, W. J.: Paraneoplasia and hypercalcemia. Calif. Vet. 7:25, 1980.

74. Williams, D. A., and Goldschmidt, M. H.: Hyperviscosity syndrome with IgM monoclonal gammopathy and hepatic plasmacytoid lymphosarcoma in a cat. J. Small Anim. Pract. 23:311, 1982.

75. Wilson, G. P., and Hayes, H. M.: Castration for treatment of perianal gland neoplasms in the dog. J. Am. Vet. Med. Assoc. 174:1301, 1979.

76. Wilson, J. W., Harris, S. G., Moore, W. D., et al.: Primary hyperparathyroidism in a dog. J. Am. Vet. Med. Assoc. 164:942, 1974.

77. Yarrigton, J. T., Hoffman, W. E., Macy, D., et al.: Morphologic characteristics of the parathyroid and thyroid glands and serum immunoreactive parathyroid hormone in dogs with pseudohyperparathyroidism. Am. J. Vet. Res. 42:271, 1981.

78. Zenoble, R. D., Crowell, W. A., and Rowland, G. N.: Adenocarcinoma and hypercalcemia in a dog. Vet. Pathol. 16:122, 1979.

79. Zenoble, R. D., and Rowland, G. N.: Hypercalcemia and proliferative myelosclerotic bone reaction associated with feline leukovirus infection in a cat. J. Am. Vet. Med. Assoc. 175:591, 1979.

Chapter 168

Biopsy: Techniques, Cytology, and Histopathology

Ralph C. Richardson and Wolfgang Janas

The purpose of a biopsy is to obtain tissue or other material for diagnosis and to provide information for planning therapy. If the biopsy is to provide this information, proper technique must be used to obtain an adequate sample. Biopsies may be as simple as collection and analysis of accumulated fluid or as complex as removing tissue for evaluation during involved surgical procedures aimed at excising a lesion. In general, it is prudent to evaluate any tissue cytologically prior to initiating a more invasive procedure. Following cytological examination, tissue is submitted for histopathological evaluation for definitive diagnosis. Incisional or excisional biopsy may be used, but the latter is preferable.

Risk to the patient in biopsy procedures should be avoided. Hemorrhage is the most serious complication.[3] Clotting tests and correction of abnormalities should be conducted prior to biopsy. A clotting abnormality is an absolute contraindication for biopsy of most organs and tissues; with the exception of a bone marrow biopsy. A second contraindication is improper or damaged equipment.[3] This may preclude procurement of an adequate sample, and repeated attempts to obtain a sample compound the risk of complications. Lastly, the person performing the biopsy should be familiar with the procedure.[3] Study and practice are essential before attempting biopsy techniques on patients. This enhances procurement of adequate specimens and minimizes the risk of postbiopsy complications. Although risk may be present, it must be kept in perspective. The value of the information obtained through the biopsy often outweighs the potential negative aspects of the biopsy procedure.

FINE NEEDLE ASPIRATION

One of the quickest and easiest biopsy techniques is needle aspiration. Cells are removed from a lesion with a 22- or 25-gauge needle using negative pressure created with a syringe. The needle size depends on the location and accessibility of the lesion. The most direct path to the lesion should be chosen. It is not necessary to extensively prepare the area if a dermal, subcutaneous, or submucosal mass is to be aspirated, since this technique is no more invasive than an injection. Alcohol swabbing of the skin and parting of hair facilitates collection from superficial masses without complications. If intrathoracic or intra-abdominal masses are to be aspirated, a small area should be clipped and prepared as for surgery. If the lesion is palpable, it should be localized and stabilized with one hand while the other hand guides the needle, with syringe attached, through the skin into the lesion.

Negative pressure should be created by drawing back on the plunger, and using a jabbing motion, the needle should be passed through several tangents of the lesion. The movement of the needle should be rapid to prevent dilution of the sample with peripheral blood. The needle should not leave the lesion during the negative pressure phase and draw cells from surrounding tissues or pass completely through the lesion and pull air through the needle into the syringe. Negative pressure is released before removing the needle from the lesion. The sample may appear in the barrel of the syringe but is usually present in the lumen of the needle. After detaching the needle, the syringe should be filled with air and the air used to force the needle contents onto several glass slides or into an appropriate container.

Once the sample is collected, processing depends on the testing procedure. If material is to be submitted for bacterial culture, it is transferred to an appropriate culture medium. Fluids of low viscosity are prepared for microscopic examination by using a conventional blood smear technique. Viscous fluids are prepared by a "squash" technique, in which a drop of the sample is placed on a glass slide.[10] A second glass slide is placed on top of the sample. The sample spreads between the two slides. Downward pressure on the top slide is usually not necessary. More viscous fluids require gentle pressure, but excessive pressure is avoided to prevent alteration of microscopic structure of the sample by causing disruption or destruction of the cells. The cohesive effect of the fluids causes the slides to cling together. The slides are drawn apart by sliding the top slide away from the bottom slide, leaving a smear of cells and fluid in a monolayer. Slides prepared in such a manner are ready for staining.

FLUID SPECIMEN PREPARATION

Abnormal accumulations of body fluid should be collected aseptically. The first portion of the sample is saved for evaluation. Because of rapid *in vitro* alteration of cytological features of body fluids, at least four to six direct smears should be made immediately. An additional quantity of fluid should be placed into suitable culture media for bacterial examination, if required. When possible, 5 ml is placed into a container without anticoagulant for chemical tests, and another 5 ml into a container with anticoagulant (EDTA) for cell counts and concentration techniques.

Abdominocentesis

Abdominocentesis is indicated when there is evidence of abnormal fluid accumulation in the peritoneal cavity.[10,12] Caution is exercised in thrombocytopenic animals because hemorrhage through the biopsy site may occur. Care is also taken to prevent penetration of abdominal viscera. Abdominocentesis is generally done with the animal in a standing position. The biopsy site is to the right of and anterior to the umbilicus, away from the spleen and other major viscera. The area is clipped and prepared as for surgery. Local anesthesia is optional, but most animals do not require it. A 12-ml syringe and a 19-gauge, 7/8 inch Butterfly infusion set* are used. The needle is introduced into the peritoneal cavity with the bevel toward the parietal peritoneum, preventing the omentum from obstructing the lumen. Gentle negative pressure is applied as the needle penetrates the abdominal wall, and fluid is obtained just as the needle penetrates the peritoneum. If no fluid is obtained, the syringe is disconnected, 1 to 2 ml of air or sterile saline is blown through the needle to clear any possible blockage, and negative pressure is reapplied. If no fluid is obtained following this procedure, all four quadrants of the abdomen should be sampled.

Thoracentesis

Thoracentesis is used to sample abnormal fluid accumulations in the pleural space.[10,11] Again, care should be exercised in thrombocytopenic animals. Movement of the needle is minimized to prevent laceration of the lung. Thoracentesis is done with the animal in a standing position, if possible. The site depends on radiographic findings identifying the location of the fluid. The area should be clipped and prepared as for surgery. Local anesthesia is optional. A 12- to 60-ml syringe, three-way valve, and Butterfly infusion set with attached plastic tubing allow manipulation of the syringe and three-way valve independent of the needle. An intravenous catheter may also be used in place of the infusion set. The needle is introduced into the pleural space with the bevel toward the parietal pleura, preventing the lung parenchyma from obstructing the lumen. Gentle negative pressure should be applied as the needle penetrates the thoracic wall. As the fluid is withdrawn from the chest, negative pressure is maintained within the thorax. Excessive patient movement or violent coughing may necessitate needle withdrawal.

*Abbott Hospitals, Inc., North Chicago, IL.

The slight pneumothorax that occasionally results from thoracentesis usually does not cause serious problems.

Transtracheal Aspiration

Transtracheal aspiration is used to obtain samples from the bifurcation of the trachea or one of the mainstem bronchi.[10] The aspiration is performed through the cricothyroid ligament, which is palpated as a small notch within the larynx. The site is clipped and prepared for surgery. Local anesthesia is administered to prevent excessive struggling during the procedure. A long, indwelling intravenous catheter capable of sliding through a needle is used. It must be long enough to reach the tracheal bifurcation. The needle is introduced through the cricothyroid ligament into the trachea. The catheter is gently threaded into the trachea and the needle withdrawn. The animal usually coughs during this process. Sterile saline (3 to 10 ml) is injected into the trachea and negative pressure is applied. Air, mucus, and some fluid are drawn into the syringe. The syringe (12 to 30 ml) may be disconnected, the excess air expelled, and the aspiration repeated several times.

Cerebrospinal Fluid Collection

See Chapter 88.

SKIN BIOPSY

Biopsy of the skin is the most frequent of all biopsy procedures.[1] In many cases there are multiple lesions, and selecting the proper one is important. The histological features are more likely to be diagnostic if the site has clinically diagnostic features. In general, a lesion should be selected that is typical, not subjected to trauma, not encrusted, and not altered by treatment. The best biopsy is from a fully developed lesion, but if different stages of development are observed, multiple samples should be taken. Older lesions may have degenerating, necrotic centers and should be avoided.

One of the quickest and easiest skin biopsy procedures is the *fine needle aspirate*, discussed previously. Fine needle aspiration is most appropriately used as a method of detecting neoplasia. It may also be used to obtain culture material.

A second method is to perform a *skin scraping*. A scalpel blade, mineral oil, and glass slides with coverslips are required. One or two drops of mineral oil are placed on a slide. The scalpel blade is dipped into the oil and the selected site scraped. The skin is held flat and taut or folded and squeezed. The scraping should contain material from the deep as well as well as the superficial layers of the skin, so scraping must be deep enough to cause slight bleeding. The scrapings and mineral oil are spread on a glass slide and covered for examination.

Direct impression smears can be made of any lesion that contains exudate or exfoliating material. To make the smears, the area should be clear of debris, and excessive fluid or contaminating exudate is blotted. A glass slide is pressed firmly against the lesion, transferring cells to the slide. Alternatives are to scrape the lesion with a scalpel blade or to collect the exudate on a cotton-tipped applicator premoistened with saline and transfer the material to a glass slide.

A piece of tissue can be removed by *punch biopsy*. Most skin biopsy specimens can be taken with a cutaneous punch. Scalpel biopsies are rarely required. Both the lesion and adjacent normal tissues should be obtained. While it is possible to obtain both by sampling the periphery of the lesion, there is a possibility that one portion may be missed. If only one sample is submitted, the pathologist should be aware that normal and abnormal tissues are represented in the sample. It is a good practice to submit multiple samples, one from the lesion and lesion edge and one from the adjacent normal tissues.

The biopsy site should be clipped and prepared according to the test desired. Only a light alcohol swabbing should be done if the sample is to be submitted for histopathological examination. Vigorous surgical scrubbing may destroy the underlying microscopic structure; however, if the sample is submitted for bacterial culture, a vigorous surgical scrub is indicated to remove surface contaminants.

Manual restraint and local anesthesia should suffice for a skin biopsy. Some dogs may require sedation. The local anesthetic agent should not be injected directly into the biopsy site because this may cause artifacts. It should be injected in a ring around the lesion and into the deep subcutaneous area. It is also a good idea to avoid using epinephrine in conjunction with local anesthesia. While it aids in controlling local hemorrhage during the procedure, the site may bleed once the effects of the epinephrine have worn off.

The only special equipment needed is a cutaneous punch. Either a Keyes skin punch* or disposable Baker's biopsy punch† in 4- to 8-mm sizes is available. Optional equipment is a Walsh pressure ring,* which stabilizes the skin and helps control local hemorrhage (Fig. 168–1). To perform the biopsy, the punch is placed on the biopsy site and drilled into the tissue with a rotary motion and moderate pressure. When the punch reaches the desired depth, generally to the subcutaneous fat, the instrument is withdrawn, the specimen is gently lifted from the skin, and the base is cut with scissors or a scalpel blade. Digital pressure generally controls hemorrhage. One or two sutures may be used or the wound may be left to heal without suturing. The sample should be blotted to remove excess blood. Direct impressions for cy-

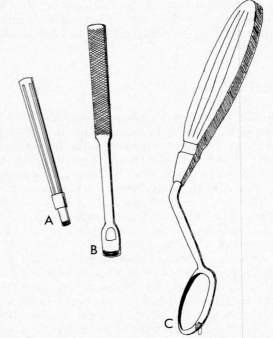

Figure 168–1. *A*, Baker's biopsy punch. *B*, Keyes skin punch. *C*, Walsh pressure ring.

tological examination can be made with the tissue sample by gently touching it to a glass slide, or scrapings can be prepared if the sample is of a fibrous nature. The tissue sample is placed into a container of suitable fixative for further evaluation.

Excisional biopsy yields a larger and deeper specimen. This is most often done on lesions that are small and easily removed. With this approach, diagnosis and treatment are performed in one procedure. Excision utilizing electrocutting and cautery is discouraged because adjacent cells may be coagulated.

BONE MARROW BIOPSY

Any unexplained abnormality in the peripheral blood and the possibility of neoplastic infiltration are indications for a bone marrow biopsy.[7] Although biopsies performed on thrombocytopenic animals may result in slight postbiopsy hemorrhage, thrombocytopenia is not an absolute contraindication to bone marrow biopsy, and hemorrhage usually can be controlled by digital pressure.

Bone marrow aspiration for cytological examination is most frequently used in veterinary medicine. A number of needles are available (15 to 18 gauge, 1 to 1.5 inches), and all provide satisfactory results. The Illinois sternal needle*(Fig. 168–2) has a stylet screwed into the needle, preventing accidental dislodging during insertion and also aiding removal of the stylet for aspiration. An ample hub and guard

*V. Mueller Co., Chicago, IL.
†Chester A. Baker Laboratories, Inc., Miami, FL.

*V. Mueller Co., Chicago, IL.

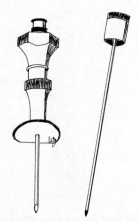

Figure 168–2. Illinois sternal needle with stylet.

provide a good handle as it is augered through dense cortical bone. It is available in a 15 gauge, 1-inch adult size and an 18 gauge, 1 inch pediatric size for smaller animals. The length is sometimes a disadvantage, but with the number of sites available this is rarely a major problem.

The most common sites for bone marrow sampling include (1) the wing of the ilium, dorsally or laterally, (2) the greater tubercle of the proximal humerus, and (3) the trochanteric fossa of the proximal femur. Since the character of samples obtained from active marrow sites is similar regardless of location, selection of a specific site is not important. The biopsy site should be clipped and prepared as for surgery. Local anesthesia of the periosteum accompanied by manual restraint permits an adequate procedure. For injecting the local anesthetic, a 22-gauge needle of the same length as the biopsy needle is used. This serves as a probe to determine whether the biopsy needle can reach the chosen site and also provides a mental picture of the site in relation to the landmarks used. A small amount of local anesthetic agent (0.25 to 0.5 ml) is injected into the periosteum in a circle approximately 1 cm in diameter. A small incision with a

#11 scalpel blade aids passage of the biopsy needle through the skin.

The most common approach to the *ilium* is from the *dorsocranial aspect*. The disadvantages of the approach are that it is a curved surface, making initial seating of the needle difficult, and it is relatively narrow so that it is important to advance the needle parallel to the two sides of the ilium. An advantage is that the depth of penetration is not crucial. The animal may be in sternal or lateral recumbency. The biopsy site is located at the widest portion of the wing of the ilium, 1 to 2 cm caudal to the crest (Fig. 168–3). The skin is held tightly, with the thumb and index finger pushing downward over the lateral and medial aspects of the wing. The needle, with stylet in place, is pushed through the skin and overlying muscle onto the bone. With gentle pressure, the needle is rotated to create a small notch on the surface of the bone. Moderate pressure is applied and the needle is firmly seated into the bone. Once solidly seated, the bevel of the needle is usually in the marrow cavity. The stylet is removed and a 12-ml syringe attached. Vigorous negative pressure is applied. Aspiration usually causes transient pain by stimulating sensory nerve endings in the marrow cavity. This response generally indicates that the tip of the needle is in the marrow cavity. As soon as red marrow appears in the hub of the syringe, negative pressure is released. It is essential to discontinue aspiration as soon as the marrow appears in the syringe to minimize dilution of the sample with peripheral blood.

After aspiration, the syringe is removed, leaving the needle in the bone. Small drops of the marrow are expelled onto glass slides and smeared using the "squash" technique previously described. These smears must be made as soon as possible after the marrow is aspirated. The sample will clot within 10 to 30 seconds because the speed of clotting is increased by the release of thromboplastin from damaged cells. If too large a drop is expelled onto the slide, it is difficult to make a good monolayer smear.

Figure 168–3. *A,* Dorsal approach to the ilium. *B,* lateral approach to the ilium. Arrow indicates the crest of the ilium, dots indicate respective biopsy sites. Note relation of the needle to the marrow cavity.

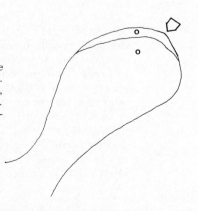
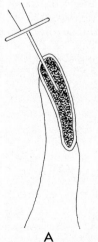
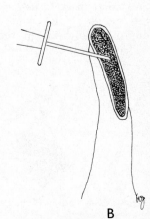

A   B

If this occurs, standing the slide on end and allowing the sample to run down the slide will permit pulling another slide across only one portion, making a good smear. Bone marrow material that remains following slide preparation may be allowed to clot and the clot placed into a container of suitable fixative for histopathological examination. If an adequate sample is to be procured, the pain response on aspiration should be observed, the smear should be a good monolayer with a nicely feathered edge, and there should be fat globules in the smear. If these criteria are met, the needle may be removed from the patient. Before submitting them for evaluation, representative slides can be stained and examined microscopically. If marrow particles and megakaryocytes can be identified, the sample is generally adequate for evaluation. If not, another biopsy may be indicated.

An alternative approach to the *ilium* is from the *lateral aspect*. The disadvantage of this approach is that it is a relatively narrow site, making depth of penetration crucial. It offers the advantage of a relatively large and flat surface, making initial seating of the needle easier. Positioning, preparation, and anesthesia of the site are as previously described. The biopsy site is located 1 to 2 cm caudal to the crest of the ilium and 0.5 to 1 cm ventral on the lateral surface (Fig. 168–3). With this approach, the needle is advanced into the bone until it is *just* solidly seated. This places the bevel of the needle in the marrow cavity. The most common problem is to advance the needle too far so that the lumen of the needle becomes occluded by the opposite cortex. If no marrow is aspirated, the needle can be slightly withdrawn with a slow and careful rotating motion, with negative pressure still maintained. An aspirate can be obtained as the lumen is pulled into the marrow cavity.

In an obese animal, the wing of the ilium may not be readily accessible. A good alternative site is the *greater tubercle* of the *proximal humerus*. The disadvantages of this approach are that it is a curved surface, making initial seating difficult, and it is in close proximity to the animal's mouth. The animal is placed in lateral recumbency and the foreleg held flexed. A small flat area is found on the anterolateral aspect of the greater tubercle (Fig. 168–4). One hand is used to palpate and stabilize the humerus while the needle is inserted. The needle is started at approximately 45° in relation to the shaft of the

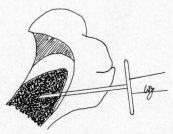

Figure 168–4. Position of the needle in the greater tubercle of the proximal humerus.

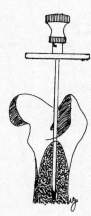

Figure 168–5. Position of the needle in the trochanteric fossa of the proximal femur.

humerus, and a small notch is made with gentle pressure. Once the needle is started into the bone, it is rotated more in line with the shaft (approximately 30°) and advanced until solidly seated in the bone. Detection of decreased resistance to advancement of the needle may indicate that the needle has passed through the cortical bone and entered the marrow cavity.

The *trochanteric fossa* at the proximal end of the *femur* is the site of choice in cats and small dogs. A 1-inch needle is generally sufficient; however, in larger animals a needle 1.5 or more inches may be necessary. This is a relatively easy site to enter, and there is no problem with depth of penetration. The animal is placed in lateral recumbency and the site prepared and anesthetized as previously described. The greater trochanter is palpated while the leg is manipulated. The point of insertion is just medial to the greater trochanter and parallel to the shaft of the femur (Fig. 168–5). One hand is used to stabilize and palpate the femur while the needle is inserted. Detection of decreased resistance to advancement of the needle may indicate that the needle has passed through the cortical bone into the marrow cavity.

A *bone marrow core* can be taken from any of the sites used in bone marrow aspiration. These cores are usually taken with a Jamshidi biopsy needle* (Fig. 168–6). The Jamshidi needle has a uniform tubular configuration except for the distal tip, which tapers like a cone. The tip is beveled and has a sharp cutting edge. The tip of the Jamshidi needle allows the core sample to expand in the shaft, preventing compression of the sample and facilitating removal of the core from the bone. The proximal end has an adapter for a syringe, which permits its use as an aspiration needle as well.

To obtain a biopsy sample with a Jamshidi needle, the needle is seated, with stylet in place, into the cortical bone. The stylet is removed and the needle slowly advanced 1 to 2 cm, using a rotating motion. Depth can be gauged by positioning the thumb at a

---

*Kormed, Inc., Minneapolis, MN.

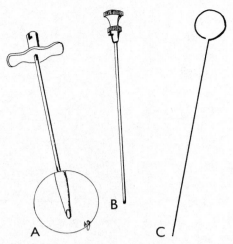

Figure 168–6. A, Jamshidi biopsy needle illustrating conical shape of the tip. *B,* Stylet. *C,* Wire probe used to push sample out of the needle.

point 1 to 2 cm from the skin on the shaft of the needle or by inserting the stylet and observing its displacement. After the needle has been advanced to an appropriate depth, the needle is rotated 360° in one direction several times to twist the core loose at its base. The needle and bone core are removed from the bone. The core is gently pushed out of the needle with a wire probe by inserting it through the distal cutting end. The core should not be pushed from the hub end because of the conical tip. The sample can be placed between two glass slides and gently rolled back and forth for cytological examination. The core can then be placed into a container of suitable fixative for histopathological examination.

BONE BIOPSY

A large core of bone may be removed using a Michele trephine* (Fig. 168–7). Power-driven trephines are available, but these are not recommended for good biopsy samples because the heat associated with the high speed burns the specimen. Hand-driven trephines give some indication of bone density and strength. Core size can vary from 3/16 to 5/16 inch, depending on the size of the bone involved. This technique requires general anesthesia and normal clotting parameters. The lesion is first located radiographically, and the area to be sampled is determined. The site is clipped and prepared as for surgery. Generally an incision of the skin and underlying musculature to accommodate the trephine is necessary. The trephine, with stylet in place, is inserted through the skin incision and advanced through the muscle to the bone. The stylet is removed and the trephine is advanced into the bone to an appropriate depth, using a rotating motion. The depth can be gauged by using the calibrations on the

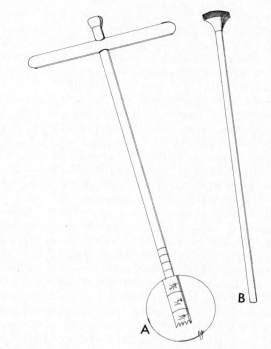

Figure 168–7. A, Michele trephine illustrating cutting saw-toothed tip. *B,* Stylet.

shaft of the trephine or by inserting the stylet and observing its displacement. The trephine is rotated 360° in one direction several times and rocked back and forth to break the core loose at its base. The trephine and core samples are removed from the bone and the sample gently expelled by means of the stylet. Since there is no mechanism to hold the sample in the end of the trephine, occasionally it may be difficult to remove the core from the bone. Holding a thumb over the proximal end of the trephine and creating a vacuum or applying lateral torque during withdrawal may be helpful.

The sample is placed between two glass slides and gently rolled back and forth to prepare it for cytological examination. The core can then be placed into a container of suitable fixative for histopathological examination. Often there will be postbiopsy hemorrhage. Packing the biopsy site with Bone Wax* or Gelfoam† aids control. The skin requires suturing, and a pressure dressing may be needed for a short time.

LYMPH NODE BIOPSY

Local or generalized lymph node enlargement is an indication for lymph node biopsy.[8] Prior to biopsy, lymph nodes should be carefully palpated. In addition to specific areas of involvement, the consistency of the nodes should be evaluated. Soft and fluctuant nodes may indicate significant suppuration or necro-

*V. Mueller Co., Chicago, IL.

*Ethicon, Inc., Somerville, NJ.
†The Upjohn Co., Kalamazoo, MI.

sis. Abnormally firm or fixed nodes may contain neoplastic or inflammatory elements. Nodes involved in an acute inflammatory process may be quite painful, whereas nodes affected with chronic inflammatory or neoplastic disorders usually are not painful. Several methods of biopsy are available.

Fine needle aspiration is the quickest and easiest procedure for biopsy of lymph nodes. It can be performed on nodes of any size provided they can be adequately localized and stabilized by palpation. Deeper lymph nodes can be reached with the aid of radiography. Lymph nodes can be wholly removed by *surgical excision*. While this provides the best possible specimen for examination, the need for general anesthesia and the time required to excise a lymph node explain the infrequency of this method. In lieu of excision, a specimen can be obtained using a *needle punch biopsy* technique. This can be used on the same lymph nodes accessible to aspiration. The disadvantages of a needle punch biopsy are the small amount of tissue procured, lack of direct observation for needle placement, and the chance of missing a focal lesion. The most commonly used instrument for this method is the Tru-Cut disposable biopsy needle* (Fig. 168–8).

The Tru-Cut needle biopsy technique must be well understood to obtain the best results[3, 13] Local anesthesia is generally sufficient, but general anesthesia may be necessary for restraint and pain control if deep tissues are biopsied. The area over the biopsy site is clipped and prepared as for surgery. A small incision facilitates passage of the needle through the skin. The Tru-Cut needle is introduced through the skin to the lymph node capsule with the obturator specimen rod fully retracted within the outer cannula. If the node is large enough and in a relatively safe area, a thrusting technique may be used. After the capsule is penetrated, the outer cannula is kept stationary and the obturator specimen rod is thrust into the lymph node by pushing forward on its handle section. If the node is smaller than the specimen notch or in a risky location, the thrusting technique should not be used. The capsule should be penetrated and the needle advanced through the lymph node to the distal extent of the node. While the obturator specimen rod is kept stationary, the outer cannula is slowly drawn back to the proximal edge, with care not to pull it out of the capsule. In either case, without moving the obturator specimen rod, the outer cannula is advanced forward over the specimen

*Travenol Laboratories, Inc., Deerfield, IL.

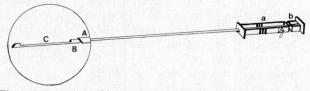

Figure 168–8. Disposable Tru-cut biopsy needle. *A*, Outer cannula with plastic handle section *(a)*. *B*, Obturator-specimen rod with plastic handle section *(b)*. *C*, Specimen notch.

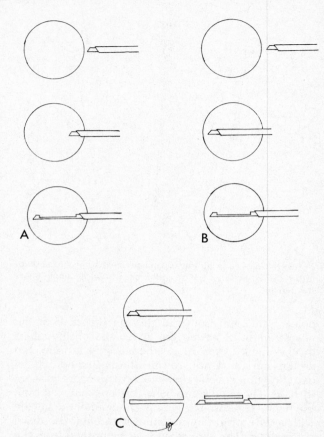

Figure 168–9. Tru-cut penetration methods. *A*, In larger lesions, penetrate capsule and then thrust obturator-specimen rod forward. *B*, In smaller lesions, penetrate through capsule to far edge of lesion and pull back outer cannula to near edge. *C*, Cut specimen and remove.

notch with a quick thrust to cut and trap the biopsy specimen in the specimen notch. The needle is withdrawn from the body with the specimen (Fig. 168–9).

The tissue sample can be gently teased out of the specimen notch with a sterile hypodermic needle and fixed. If desired, direct impressions can be made for cytological examination. The tissue can be placed on a glass slide, and another slide can be gently touched to the tissue. A hypodermic needle or fine-toothed forceps also may be used to lift and move the tissue around. In any case, great care must be taken in handling the tissue. It is generally best to obtain multiple samples if cytological and histopathological specimens are to be prepared. Hemorrhage is usually the only postbiopsy complication and can be minimized by applying digital pressure and possibly a pressure dressing to the area.

PROSTATIC BIOPSY

Evaluation of an enlarged prostate gland may be done by examining cellular material from it. The easiest method of obtaining such material is to perform a *prostatic massage*. The animal is placed in lateral recumbency, and the penis is extruded and cleansed. A polyethylene urinary catheter is passed through the urethra to the prostate. The tip of the catheter can be palpated per rectum as it approaches the base of the prostate. While an assistant applies gentle negative pressure with a 12-ml syringe, the prostate is vigorously massaged per rectum. Fluid may flow into the syringe, or only a small amount of material may be drawn into the tip of the catheter. Following massage and aspiration, negative pressure is released and the catheter withdrawn. Some of the material can be put onto glass slides for direct smears. Some should be saved for bacterial culture. If a large amount of fluid is obtained, it can be placed in a sterile container for centrifugation to concentrate cells for examination.

Fine needle aspiration through the abdominal wall or the colonic wall or transperineally (beside the colon) can provide cells or fluid from the prostate. To perform the transabdominal approach, the prostate must be easily palpable through the abdominal wall. The area of entry should be prepared as for surgery, and a large syringe with a three-way valve should be available if large amounts of fluid are obtained (e.g., prostatic cyst). If the prostate is not palpable per abdomen, the transrectal approach may be used. Care should be taken to clear the colon of fecal matter prior to aspiration. If adequate samples cannot be obtained by either of these techniques, a long needle may be passed through the skin lateral to the anus and alongside the colon into the prostate.

After carefully evaluating material obtained by one of the cytological methods just described, a tissue *core biopsy* may be required. This may be obtained by using a Tru-Cut biopsy needle. Any of the routes of fine needle aspiration may be used. Local anesthesia for the transperineal approach is required, and sedation is sometimes needed for fractious animals. If a prostatic cyst or infection is suspected, percutaneous biopsy should not be performed. Complications of biopsy include hemorrhage, infection and urethral fistula.

LIVER BIOPSY

Liver biopsy has many indications and contraindications. Indications include abnormal laboratory values, abnormal liver size (either hepatomegaly or microhepatica), assessment of hepatic disease, detection of etiology of ascites, hepatodynia (pain on liver palpation), and biochemical evaluation of liver tissue.[4] General contraindications include bleeding disorders, marked anemia, and extrahepatic cholestasis.[4] Percutaneous liver biopsy contraindications are hepatic abscess, vascular tumors, infection along the biopsy pathway, ascites, pleuritis, and hepatic cysts.[4] Complications of liver biopsy include hemorrhage, intrahepatic hematoma, and arteriovenous (AV) fistula.[4]

Percutaneous liver biopsy may result in puncture of adjacent organs, puncture of the gallbladder, biliary fistulae, bile peritonitis, pneumothorax, hemothorax, or transfer of ascitic fluid to the thorax.[4] Prior to biopsy, clotting tests (e.g., activated clotting time [ACT], platelet count) and abdominal radiographs are made. The patient is fasted to assure an empty stomach. A small portion of a high-fat meal may be given 30 minutes prior to biopsy to decrease gallbladder size.

Biopsy techniques include percutaneous methods (Menghini* or Tru-Cut), keyhole approaches, or direction via either laparoscopy or laparotomy. *Percutaneous liver biopsy* has the advantage of being able to obtain samples rapidly under local anesthesia, and it can provide serial biopsies with a minimum of invasion. It is safe, easy, and inexpensive and affords good owner compliance. Its main disadvantage is that sampling error may be encountered with focal lesions since the liver cannot be seen. *Keyhole* access to the liver is an accurate and safe procedure and allows palpation of parts of the liver. It frequently requires general anesthesia for adequate restraint and suturing. *Laparoscopy* and *laparotomy* allow observation of the liver, but both methods require general anesthesia. Equipment expense is significant in these methods, but laparotomy may allow excisional biopsy of focal lesions.

Percutaneous liver biopsy by the transthoracic and transabdominal approaches is the most frequently used method. Many techniques have been described: the following are effective and simple.

Transthoracic liver biopsy using the Menghini needle (Fig. 168–10) can be done with the animal standing or in dorsal recumbency. In the standing

*Becton-Dickinson, Rutherford, NJ.

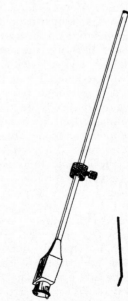

Figure 168–10. Menghini needle with biopsy stop in position on shaft. Wire tissue stop is inserted into lumen from proximal end of needle to prevent sample from being pulled into the syringe.

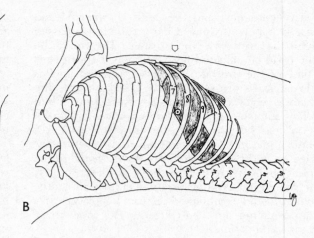

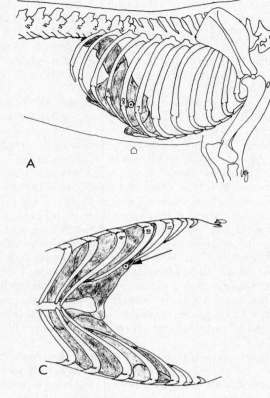

Figure 168–11. A, Transthoracic percutaneous biopsy site in the standing position. Enter above the xiphoid cartilage at the right costochondral junction (arrow). B, Transthoracic percutaneous biopsy site in dorsal recumbency. Enter at the level of the xiphoid cartilage on the right side midway between the vertebrae and sternebrae (arrow). C, Transabdominal percutaneous biopsy site in right lateral recumbency. Enter below the costochondral junction of the tenth or eleventh rib and direct the biopsy needle toward the right scapulohumeral joint (arrow).

position, an area over the right costochondral junction at the xiphoid cartilage is prepared for surgery (Fig. 168–11A). A local anesthetic agent is infiltrated into the site. After incising the skin with a #11 scalpel blade, the Menghini needle, with tissue stop in place and attached to a 12-ml syringe, is placed against the subcutaneous tissues. The biopsy stop is set to an appropriate depth, depending on the size and obesity of the animal. Strong negative pressure (approximately 6 ml) is applied, and a quick thrust-pause-withdraw motion, directed parallel to the table, is used. A total elapsed time of 1 to 1.5 seconds is all that is necessary. If a tissue core is obtained, negative pressure will be maintained in the syringe. If a core of tissue is not obtained in the needle, air fills the syringe as it leaves the body. If tissue is not obtained after two attempts, the animal should be placed in dorsal recumbency and an area midway between the vertebrae and sternebrae at the level of the xiphoid prepared (Fig. 168–11B). The liver lobes lie against the diaphragm because of gravity, and the same thrust-pause-withdraw technique should be used.

If no tissue is obtained via the suction technique with the Menghini needle, a biopsy using the Tru-Cut needle should be attempted. The *transabdominal* approach is well suited for the Tru-Cut needle. The animal is placed in right lateral recumbency and an area at the costochondral junction of the tenth or eleventh rib is prepared (Fig. 168–11C). After infil-

tration of local anesthetic and incision of the skin with a #11 scalpel blade, a Tru-Cut biopsy needle is directed toward the right scapulohumeral joint. As the liver is encountered, some resistance is usually transmitted through the needle. One of the cutting techniques previously described may then be used. If no tissue is obtained after two attempts with the Tru-Cut needle, biopsy via laparoscopy or laparotomy is indicated. Tissue obtained by any method may be examined cytologically and fixed.

The major complication following percutaneous liver biopsy of animals properly evaluated for clotting functions is gallbladder puncture and bile peritonitis. When this complication develops, animals may demonstrate an acutely painful abdomen and signs of shock. Appropriate shock therapy and cage rest allow most animals to recover within 24 hours with no complications. If adequate patient preparation is done and proper prebiopsy considerations taken, complications are infrequent.

GASTROINTESTINAL BIOPSY

In animals requiring evaluation of the gastrointestinal system, significant data can be obtained with noninvasive biopsy techniques by the oral and anal routes. Techniques for the stomach, small intestine, colon, and rectum are described.

Biopsy of the *stomach* can best be conducted with a fiberoptic endoscope and biopsy channel. The animal must be fasted and anesthetized. Observation of the gastric mucosa can be conducted and portions biopsied. Multiple biopsy specimens are taken and labelled. Cytological and histopathological studies can be made from the samples collected.

The *stomach* and *small intestine* can also be sampled with a biopsy capsule that has a wire or suction-activated knife. The knife is used to cut folds of mucosa that have been drawn into the capsule by negative pressure. The biopsy sites are chosen blindly, and delay in passing through the pylorus may occur, but the procedure has the advantage of being conducted in the awake animal.

Biopsy of the *colon* and *rectum* may be conducted via the fiberoptic endoscope or rigid proctoscope. Preparation of the animal for colonoscopic examination is essential. A 24- to 36-hour fast is preferred. A warm water enema 16 to 18 hours and again 2 hours before the procedure allows adequate observation of the lower intestinal tract. General anesthesia is usually required for complete fiberoptic examination and biopsy of the proximal colon. The distal colon and rectum can be seen by either a fiberoptic colonoscope, a rigid colonoscope, or a proctoscope in the awake or mildly sedated animal. Pain does not occur during mucosal biopsy of the colon or rectum, but, if the mesenteric attachments of the colon are stretched during examination, discomfort will be demonstrated unless the animal is anesthetized.

Observation and biopsy of the lower intestinal tract are aided by insufflation of the examined area and positioning in right lateral recumbency. To most accurately assess the colon with the fiberoptic colonoscope, the lumen is viewed as the scope is passed into the animal. Insufflation and washing are done as the instrument is advanced. Mucosal biopsy specimens may be obtained through the biopsy channel as the endoscope is withdrawn. If the rigid colonoscope is used, it is advanced to the maximum length possible, and insufflation, viewing, and biopsy are

conducted as it is withdrawn. A uterine biopsy forceps is frequently used to obtain tissue, but care must be taken to prevent perforation of the colon since the punch is capable of penetrating mucosa, submucosa, muscularis, and serosa.

A fold of mucosa should be manipulated into the end of the colonoscope, and the jaws of the biopsy instrument should be only slightly opened to prevent deep penetration. Small pinching forceps that pass through fiberoptic viewing instruments do not penetrate deeply. Ideally, mucosa and submucosa only should be obtained. All obvious lesions should be biopsied. If no lesions are seen, multiple biopsy samples (at least three) should be taken at different distances from the anus. All specimens obtained should be examined cytologically and submitted for histopathological examination.

KIDNEY BIOPSY

Biopsy of the kidney is indicated to establish a specific diagnosis and to predict the probable course of a disease.[5] Proteinuria, abnormal renal shape, or clarification of laboratory findings frequently indicates biopsy. The Tru-Cut biopsy needle is used most often. Fine needle aspiration should be conducted as a first step in abnormally shaped kidneys. Percutaneous fine needle aspiration and cytological examination can be safely conducted in all animals except those with bleeding tendencies. Tru-Cut biopsy is contraindicated in animals with bleeding tendencies, pyelonephritis, hydronephrosis, or extreme azotemia (BUN > 150 mg/dl).

The usual approach to core biopsy of the canine kidney is through a small keyhole incision made just caudal to the last rib. Immobilization of the kidney and passage of the Tru-Cut biopsy needle through a tangent of the renal cortex, being careful to protect the renal artery and vein, allow a representative sample. A similar biopsy may be performed in cats

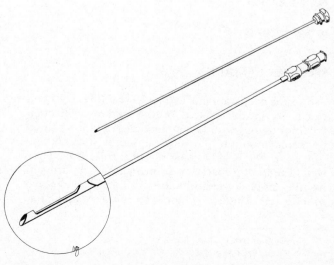

Figure 168–12. Lee biopsy needle. Note the combination cutting (notch) and suction (lumen) features.

by a blind percutaneous technique, since the feline kidneys are often very easily palpated and immobilized against the abdominal wall. Hemorrhage is the most significant complication following renal biopsy. Microscopic and occasionally gross hematuria for one to three days following biopsy may be observed. If hemorrhage is severe, blood transfusions may be warranted, but such occasions are rare. Usually, careful observation and possibly fluid diuresis are all that are required following biopsy.

PERCUTANEOUS LUNG BIOPSY

Fine needle aspiration, Lee biopsy needles,* and Tru-Cut needles provide adequate tissue to diagnose most lung lesions. Based on radiographic and sometimes fluoroscopic imaging, cells or tissue may be obtained from affected areas of the lung. Fine needle aspiration and Tru-Cut techniques have been previously described. Tru-Cut techniques should be used for solid masses in the thorax; the Lee biopsy needle, which combines aspirating action with cutting action, may be used in aerated lung tissue without severe complications. The Lee needle is similar to the Tru-Cut needle but is smaller and has suction capabilities through the inner cutting needle (Fig. 168–12).

After placing the needle, negative pressure is applied, and the inner needle is withdrawn while the outer cannula is held steady, thus severing the tissue and drawing it into the suction device (e.g., 50-ml syringe or Gomco vacuum†). The outer cannula may be withdrawn and the process repeated, thus allowing numerous samples to be collected across the biopsied area. Complications may include pneumothorax and hemoptysis. The procedure should not be conducted if gross blood is aspirated. If hemoptysis develops, the animal should be restrained with the biopsied side down. Close observation for dyspnea should be maintained for 12 to 24 hours following all lung biopsies.

NASAL BIOPSY

See Chapter 185.

SPECIMEN HANDLING

Specific preparation of cytological samples has been discussed in the course of the various collection techniques; however, some general principles should be kept in mind.[2] Cytological samples should be processed as quickly as possible after collection. They should not be prepared near or mailed with formalin fixative. Even formalin fumes will fix cells and leave routine stains ineffective for cytological examination.

A histopathological sample should be placed into an appropriate fixative to prevent autolysis and bacterial contamination and to preserve its architecture. The most commonly used fixative is 10% buffered formalin. Fixative must be used in the specified concentrations and in a 10:1 volume:tissue ratio.

Ideally, specimens should be no larger than 1 cm in any dimension. Larger specimens, encapsulated specimens, or those composed of fibrous connective tissue will fix poorly. To allow proper fixation, such specimens should be lanced or transected. Small specimens (e.g., Tru-Cut samples) may miss focal lesions. Multiple samples from various sites and depths can help minimize this. Each sample should be kept separate and the biopsy location noted. Tissues should be handled very gently so that the architecture is not disrupted. Tissues should not be crushed or torn while removing them. and should be cut with a sharp blade rather than scissors to prevent crushing. If the specimen is soft and friable, fixing it for 15 to 30 minutes facilitates cutting. If immediate fixation is not possible (e.g., during surgery), the tissue should be prevented from drying by covering it with saline-soaked gauze.

PATHOLOGY OF NEOPLASMS—CYTOLOGY AND HISTOPATHOLOGY

The pathological diagnosis of malignancy is often accepted by the clinician as infallible truth, but recognition of cell type is not always an easy task for the pathologist or cytologist. In one center* where all previously biopsied tumors are submitted for a tissue or cytological review (second opinion) before any therapy is instituted, approximately 5 per cent of the diagnoses are changed to a significantly different finding (e.g., malignant to benign neoplasia). When cells are well differentiated and normal tissue is at the edge of the sample, identification is usually easy. When growth is rapid or normal tissues are not present, cellular differentiation may not be possible, or differences of opinion may exist. If the clinical impression, cytological findings, and histopathological diagnosis fail to agree, the clinician should ask for a second opinion or repeat the biopsy to obtain a more representative sample.

Routine diagnostic procedures, such as history, physical examination, radiography, and laboratory testing for hematological, biochemical, and urine abnormalities, are essential parts of the prebiopsy approach to a patient suspected of having cancer. In addition, cytological examination has become standard. Cytological examination does not replace biopsy or histopathological study, but it has become as much a part of cancer diagnosis in veterinary medicine as the "Pap smear" in human cervical and uterine cancer. When possible, cells should be obtained for

---

*Unique Industries, Memphis, TN.
†Gomco Surgical Manufacturing Corp., Buffalo, NY.

*Purdue Comparative Oncology Program, Purdue University, West Lafayette, IN.

evaluation before more invasive procedures are conducted.

The cytological criteria of malignancy are well described[6,9] and follow the same guidelines established for humans in whom the Papanicolaou stain is used. Nuclear, cytoplasmic, and structural criteria are evaluated. Such features as variation of nuclear size and nuclear/cytoplasmic ratio, irregular and thickened nuclear membranes, number and shape of nucleoli, chromatin clumping, abnormal mitotic figures, and cytoplasmic staining are features of malignant cells. Although histopathological examination is the best way to evaluate structure, cells obtained by fine needle aspiration may maintain some semblance of their tissue origin (e.g., clusters resembling tubular or acinar patterns). Most samples do not maintain a structural component. A few tumors known as "discrete cell neoplasms" are amenable to cytological diagnosis. Cytological study of discrete cell neoplasms (e.g., mast cell tumors, transmissible venereal tumors, and malignant lymphomas) may be of more diagnostic value than histopathological examinations. In general, when cytological examination is used, recognition of the presence or absence of neoplasia is adequate to help plan therapy.

Histopathological study and an accurate history and description of the biopsied lesion provide a definitive diagnosis in most cases of cancer. If cancer therapy of any type is to be applied, histopathological diagnosis is mandatory, based on evaluation of accurately biopsied tissue.

Differentiation of benign tumors from malignant tumors is of utmost importance to the animal owner and veterinarian alike, but the line that demarcates benign from malignant is ill-defined. The ultimate behavior of the tumor (e.g., metastasis, death of the host due to invasion, and so on) clearly demonstrates its true nature. The pathologist can only evaluate and predict. Fortunately, morphological and differential characteristics are generally good predictors for most neoplasms. Consult standard pathology texts for a complete discussion of the histopathological criteria of malignancy.

Lastly, the relationship with the pathologist is a particularly important one. Communication and cooperation are essential to a sound diagnosis. The pathologist strives to render a definitive diagnosis, but this can be very difficult in some cases. If a diagnosis is incompatible with the clinical presentation, it is essential that this inconsistency be discussed. Special attention should be given to the pathologist's descriptive terminology and not merely the "bottom line" diagnosis.

1. Allen, S, K., and McKeever, P J.: Skin biopsy techniques. Vet. Clin. North Am. 4:269, 1974.
2. Histopathology Hints and Helps. Veterinary Reference Laboratory, Inc., Newsletter, Vol. 3, No. 5, Sept./Oct., 1979.
3. Osborne, C. A.: General principles of biopsy. Vet. Clin. North Am. 4:213, 1974.
4. Osborne, C. A., Hardy, R. M., Stevens, J. B., and Perman, V.: Liver biopsy. Vet. Clin. North Am. 4:333, 1974.
5. Osborne, C. A., Stevens, J. B., and Perman, V.: Kidney biopsy. Vet. Clin. North Am. 4:351, 1974.
6. Perman, V., Alsaker, R. D., and Riis, R. C.: Cytology of the dog and cat. Monograph, Am. Anim. Hosp. Assoc., 1979.
7. Perman, V., Osborne, C. A., and Stevens, J. B.: Bone marrow biopsy. Vet. Clin. North Am. 4:293, 1974.
8. Perman, V., Stevens, J. B., Alsaker, R. D., and Osborne, C. A.: Lymph node biopsy. Vet. Clin. North Am. 4:281, 1974.
9. Rebar, A. H.: Handbook of Veterinary Cytology. Ralston Purina Co., St. Louis, 1978.
10. Richardson, R. C., and Rebar, A. H.: Collection techniques in veterinary cytology. In Rebar, A. H. (ed.): Handbook of Veterinary Cytology. Ralston Purina Co., St. Louis, 1978, pp. 2–14.
11. Schall, W. D.: Thoracentesis. Vet. Clin. North Am. 4:395, 1974.
12. Scott, R. C., Wilkins, R. J., and Green, R. W.: Abdominal paracentesis and cystocentesis. Vet. Clin. North Am. 4:413, 1974.
13. Withrow, S. J., and Lowes, N.: Biopsy techniques for use in small animal oncology. Proceedings Oncology Short Course, Colorado State University, 1981.

Chapter **169** # Surgical Therapy

Stephen H. Levine and Dennis D. Caywood

For decades, the treatment of neoplasia rested in the hands of surgeons. If the neoplasm could be completely removed, then a cure was considered possible. If the neoplasm was widespread and complete removal was not feasible, then it was considered inoperable.

As our understanding of neoplasia has evolved, so has the role of surgery in its management. A neoplasm can no longer be simply looked upon as an entity separate from its host, requiring removal before it spreads. The dynamic and complex interrelationships that occur between the neoplasm and patient have produced newer, more effective treatment regimens, and have helped to explain past failures.[5]

A neoplasm is a struggle between the intrinsic forces within the tumor promoting its growth and the host's immune resistance. It is the balance between these opposing forces that determines whether a tumor will survive or be destroyed by the host's responses.

Undetectable metastasis is the major cause of failure of surgical treatment of neoplasia. Indeed, in most instances the neoplasm is systemic by the time it is diagnosed.[5]

ROLE OF SURGERY IN ONCOLOGIC THERAPY

Although many tumors are amenable to surgical therapy alone, the surgeon is a member of a much larger team that considers all aspects of patient/tumor interactions. There are several indications for surgery in the overall management of tumor patients. These indications include definitive procedures, palliative procedures, exploratory procedures, combination therapies, and surgery as immunotherapy.

Definitive Procedures

There are still many neoplasms for which surgery is a definitive procedure. If surgery alone is to be curative, the neoplasm must be localized to a nonvital organ or region and amenable to total removal. Examples in the dog include tumors of the skin, mammary glands, and genitalia. A few surgical procedures prevent the formation of neoplasms. For example, it has been shown that an ovariohysterectomy performed on a bitch before two years of age decreases the frequency of mammary neoplasms.[4, 18]

Palliative Procedures

The veterinary surgeon is often called upon to provide relief for a patient through local reduction of a tumor mass in spite of local invasion or metastasis. For example, many fibrosarcomas are slow growing and recur locally.[1, 3, 8, 10, 17, 19] Repeated removal of such masses may ameliorate the clinical signs and allow the animal to live a fairly comfortable existence for several months to years. Amputation of a limb with osteosarcoma may also be included in this category. Although it is generally recognized that amputation will not increase survival time even in conjunction with other treatment modalities, removal of a limb may reduce the pain and problems associated with the local disease, and make the patient more comfortable for several months. However, the vast majority of these dogs die or are euthanized within eight months regardless of treatment.[6]

Exploratory Procedures

Surgery is often a valuable aid in establishing a diagnosis and prognosis for various neoplastic conditions. Exploratory celiotomy, or thoracotomy is often used to confirm or rule out a suspicion of neoplasia based on history, physical exam, laboratory data, and radiographs. Direct visual examination with palpation is sometimes the only way to further define a mass observed radiographically or palpated transabdominally. In addition, the extent of the tumor and the visual presence of metastasis in other sites can aid as a prognostic tool or can indicate other therapy. Biopsy specimens are often taken during an exploratory procedure for microscopic examination.

Combination Therapies

The multidisciplinary approach to the management of neoplasia provides the newest and most expanding role for the veterinary surgeon. The treatment of neoplasia is no longer the province of a single discipline. It is insignificant which discipline effects a cure but rather whether a cure or prolonged survival can be obtained.[5] The surgeon may become a member of a multidisciplinary team that includes immunologists, radiologists, pathologists, pharmacologists, and biochemists. The surgeon's role in decreasing the tumor load is an extremely important aspect of a multidisciplinary approach. Established metastasis is the most common cause of failure of surgical therapy. The most effective treatments require maximum reduction of the tumor cell mass by surgery or radiation therapy. Surgical removal often results in improved immunocompetence.[5, 15] In addition, residual microfoci of tumor cells are more sensitive to chemotherapy and immunotherapy than the primary tumor because metastases have a better blood supply and a more rapid rate of cell turnover.[15]

Surgery as Immunotherapy

Cancer surgery is perhaps the most frequently used form of immunotherapy.[15] There is evidence that a host's immune defenses can be limited by a growing neoplasm. Certain neoplasms are able to evade an immune attack by producing specific and nonspecific immunosuppression of the cancer patient. Growing neoplasms constantly shed soluble tumor-associated antigens into the blood, which circulate alone or as antigen-antibody complexes. These serum antigens inhibit the lymphocyte-mediated destruction of tumor cells *in vitro* and may play a similar role *in vivo*.[15]

In addition to blocking of tumor-specific antigens, a growing neoplasm often causes a nonspecific generalized immune suppression of the patient. Humoral factors produced by or in response to the neoplasm can be found in the sera of patients and may cause general immune depression.[13] The extent of immunosuppression correlates with the stage of disease and size of tumor burden. This immunosuppression is reversed by removal of the growing neoplasm. Therefore, any therapeutic maneuver that lowers tumor mass may reverse both specific and nonspecific immunosuppression and alter the immune balance in favor of the patient. In this respect, surgery is immunotherapy because it effectively decreases the cancer cell mass and increases the patient's immune competency.

PREOPERATIVE CONSIDERATIONS

Patient Status

The selection of patients for surgery depends on a number of factors. Besides overall patient status, the surgeon must consider the neoplasm's biological behavior, location, and extent. Curability is not always the prime consideration. Often, surgery will extend and improve the quality of life without eliminating the disease.

Complete and objective evaluations of each patient are necessary prior to the consideration and initiation of any treatment. The majority of patients with neoplasms are older animals. In addition to their tumor, these patients are more likely to have other systemic or metabolic disorders, which may be related to the neoplasm. Therefore, a thorough history and physical examination are essential, as well as a complete blood count, electrocardiogram, and laboratory assessment of renal and hepatic function.

It is important to attempt to define the boundaries of the tumor to determine whether the neoplasm is localized, invasive, or metastatic. Regional lymph nodes are carefully evaluated for evidence of metastasis. Bone in close proximity to a growing neoplasm is radiographed for evidence of invasion. Most patients should have thoracic radiographs, especially if the neoplasm has a tendency toward pulmonary metastasis. Pulmonary metastases are often undetected on radiographic examination if their cross-sectional diameter is less than that of the major pulmonary vessels.[5] Therefore, a "negative" chest radiograph does not ensure the absence of metastases. In addition, the evaluation of thoracic radiographs is a valuable aid in the assessment of the patient's cardiopulmonary status.

Diagnosis and Prognosis

Once the diagnosis of neoplasia has been made, the clinician is faced with the decision whether or not to surgically intervene. There are many factors to be considered before recommending surgery. The surgeon must consider the tumor type, presence or absence of metastatic disease, the location of the neoplasm, the appearance and function of the pet after surgery, and a myriad of owner considerations, including the cost and the client's emotional well-being and wishes.

The majority of the skin tumors in the dog are benign.[4, 5, 20] The routine practice of hospitalization and surgical removal of small subcutaneous lipomas and papillomas in older dogs is questionable. These are almost never malignant, and unless they are very

TABLE 169–1.   TNM Clinical Staging* of Canine Mammary Tumors

T—Primary Tumor

T_0	No evidence of tumor (use for rechecks after surgical removal of 1° tumor)
T_1	Tumor less than 1 cm maximum diameter (a) not fixed (b) fixed to skin (c) fixed to muscle
T_2	Tumor 1 to 3 cm maximum diameter (a) not fixed (b) fixed to skin (c) fixed to muscle
T_3	Tumor greater than 3 cm maximum diameter

N—Regional Lymph Nodes (RLN)

N_0	No RLN involved
N_1	Ipsilateral RLN involved (a) not fixed (b) fixed
N_2	Bilateral RLN involved (a) not fixed (b) fixed

M—Distant Metastasis

M_0	No evidence of distant metastasis
M_1	Distant metastasis (distant nodes included)

*Approved by World Health Organization, Geneva, April 1978.

large, inhibit mobility, cause pain, or are cosmetically displeasing to the owner, the potential benefit from such surgery may be overshadowed by the potential risks to the patient.

Owners frequently request information on survival rates of animals afflicted with various neoplasms. Unfortunately, this information is now available for only a few types of cancer.

In order to standardize the classification and aggressiveness of various neoplasms, staging systems have been designed.[11] The objectives of a classification (staging) system for cancer are (1) to aid the clinician in planning treatment, (2) to indicate prognosis, (3) to assist in the evaluation of results, (4) to facilitate the exchange of information between treatment centers, and (5) to assist in the continued investigation of neoplasia.

The most widely accepted staging system is the TNM system (T, tumor; N, regional lymph node; M, distant metastasis).[11] An example of the complete TNM system for mammary gland neoplasia is shown in Table 169–1. A tumor classified as $T_1N_0M_0$ is small and noninvasive. A $T_3N_2M_1$ is a large, locally invasive tumor with distant metastases.

SURGICAL MANAGEMENT

Anesthesia

The anesthetic management of cancer patients is essentially the same as that for any aged or debilitated patient. Neoplasms in certain locations may be amenable to epidural or regional nerve blocks, provided the clinician is thoroughly familiar with the techniques. Local infiltration anesthesia should be avoided in most tumor resections, especially for neoplasms known to be malignant or of questionable pathogenicity. Local anesthetics may greatly distort the architecture of the tumor and increase the difficulty of microscopic interpretation. In addition, some experimental studies suggest that local anesthesia potentiates metastasis.[16]

Experimental and clinical studies have shown that general anesthesia and surgery have a suppressive effect on a patient's immune competence.[7, 14] This may be a significant factor in patients who may already be in a state of immunodepression as a result of their neoplasm.

Surgical Technique

Sound general surgical techniques are applicable to all forms of surgery for neoplasia. Specific considerations apply to patients with neoplasia.

A wide area around the lesion is prepared for surgery should a much larger incision than originally planned be needed. This provides a wide exposure at the surgical site aiding excision of the tumor with minimal manipulation and trauma.

Aseptic surgical technique is an important aspect in all forms of surgery, and it is particularly important in cancer surgery. Patients are often debilitated and immunosuppressed, increasing the likelihood of infection. Therefore, to minimize the chances of surgically induced infections, strict aseptic techniques must be maintained. The preoperative prophylactic use of antibiotics may be considered.

Tissue Handling

Minimal and gentle handling of neoplastic tissues is imperative. Excessive surgical trauma may result in exfoliation of tumor cells into the wound and systemic circulation.[4, 5, 15, 20] This applies to preoperative as well as operative periods. Excessive manipulation of a neoplasm or even simple injection with saline results in a tremendous increase in the shedding of cells and clumps of cells by the neoplasm. These clumps of cells are most likely to survive and grow as metastatic foci.[15]

Ligation of the venous vascular supply of the tumor early in the surgical procedure may minimize exfoliation of cells during surgery and prevent the release of cells into the systemic circulation.

Once a tumor has been removed, flushing of the wound with sterile physiological saline may wash away exfoliated cells and help prevent recurrence. There is debate concerning flushing within body cavities because of difficulty in recovering all of the fluid and the possibility of dissemination.[9] However, the potential risks of flushing body cavities are probably outweighed by the beneficial diluting effects of such flushing.

Margins

It is generally accepted that the best opportunity for a surgical cure of neoplasia is at the first surgery. Therefore, a wide margin of normal tissue must be excised to ensure total removal of the neoplasm. The scalpel should pass through normal tissues both on the surface and around the tumor. Margins of at least 1 cm should suffice in all but the most highly malignant neoplasms. Fortunately for the veterinary surgeon, there is usually enough loose skin in animals to allow easy closure of surgical wounds. However, in certain sites it may be impossible to close the defect, but it is still imperative to include normal wide margins. It is far better to leave the wound open to heal by granulation or to perform later plastic and reconstructive procedures than to risk leaving tumor cells behind, with subsequent regrowth of the neoplasm.

Histological examination of the normal margins is necessary to determine the presence of microscopic invasion of the normal tissue, which might necessitate a second, wider surgical resection.

En Bloc Resections

An en bloc resection is removal of the primary tumor, intervening lymphatics, and regional lymph node in continuity. If a regional lymph node in close proximity to the primary neoplasm appears to be involved in a neoplastic process, en bloc resection is indicated. Independent removal of the primary tumor and lymph node through separate incisions could leave tumor cells behind in communicating lymphatics.

The practice of routine lymph node removal in conjunction with excisional biopsies of tumors is contraindicated because lymph nodes are much more than mechanical filters designed to remove foreign agents. Recent evidence indicates that the regional lymph nodes respond to tumor-specific antigens and are the body's first line of immune defense.[12] Random removal of the lymph nodes may actually impair the host's defense mechanisms and shorten the patient's survival time.

Although controversial, it is generally recommended that only those regional nodes that appear to be clinically affected be removed. However, this determination is often very difficult for even the most experienced surgeons. A regional lymph node may appear enlarged for many reasons other than metastatic invasion by neoplasm. Lymph nodes may be enlarged due to hyperplasia secondary to tumor-antigen stimulation or to hemorrhage or infection within the tumor. Obviously if the lymph node is enlarged because it is producing stimulated lymphocytes it should not be excised, since it is one of the body's defense mechanisms. If however the lymph node is enlarged due to tumor infiltration, it should be removed. It is probably best to remove those nodes that definitely appear neoplastic along with those that are questionable in appearance.

POSTOPERATIVE MANAGEMENT

Many neoplasms can be removed by routine surgical methods without the need for any significant or specific postoperative management. However, some forms require special medical therapy on a short-term or permanent basis.

Many surgeons, depending on the surgical procedure employed, routinely administer antibiotics to a patient during the postoperative period. In addition, certain surgical procedures require special postoperative medical management. For example, surgical resection of a functional pancreatic beta cell adenocarcinoma may result in functional diabetes for a variable length of time. A patient with this surgically induced diabetes requires closely monitoring of blood glucose and may ultimately need insulin therapy. Surgical management of thyroid neoplasms in both the dog and cat may also require replacement therapy. Removal of thyroid neoplasms may require prolonged treatment with thyroid hormone replacements and calcium supplementation if the parathyroids were also included in the resection. Special diets and stool softeners may be indicated in various gastrointestinal-colonic resections. Some patients may need pharyngostomy tubes, gastrostomy tubes, thoracic drains, and so on that require close supervision and maintenance postoperatively.

The surgeon's job is not over once the surgical procedure has been completed. Each case is unique and may have specific postoperative management problems that are as important as the surgical procedure itself. The finest surgical techniques do not reduce the need for sound patient management.

Combination Therapy

A combined interdisciplinary approach (surgical management chemotherapy, immunotherapy, radiotherapy, and so on) increases survival rates and improves palliation in many forms of neoplasia. Although adjuvant therapy may be started before surgery, other phases of combination therapy are often implemented in the immediate postoperative period. There are many factors to consider before initiating therapy, including (1) Will this neoplasm respond better to immediate postoperative radiation therapy, or should it be delayed until some healing has occurred? and (2) If chemotherapy or immunotherapy is employed, should it be initiated before, during, or after the operation? A plan must be clearly laid out before any action is taken with the multidisciplinary approach.

Patient Follow-Up

The type of neoplasm dictates the intensity of postoperative follow-up. Patients with highly malignant tumors should be re-evaluated frequently. Weekly evaluations may be necessary immediately following surgery. Later in the postoperative course monthly examinations may be adequate. A thorough physical exam should be performed at each visit, including palpation of the original surgical site for evidence of local recurrence and the regional lymph nodes for metastasis.

A repeat examination may include thoracic radiography of neoplasms that have the potential for pulmonary metastases. In addition, certain neoplasms warrant abdominal radiography to assess mesenteric or sublumbar lymph nodes. Other patients may be followed with laboratory evaluations of hepatic or renal function as an aid in detecting metastases.

Careful repeat examinations are not only important to individual patient care but also for comparison and evaluation of various treatment regimens. In addition, it allows continued development of rational clinical protocols and establishment of more accurate prognoses.

Finally, knowledge obtained from necropsies on patients dying from tumor recurrence, euthanasia, or totally unrelated circumstances provides information on the neoplasm's biological behavior and the efficacy of various surgical procedures.

CONCLUSIONS

The treatment of neoplasia is no longer totally within the realm of the surgeon. The complete management of patients demands a concerted, combined effort by clinicians in various specialties. The surgeon must develop an understanding of the biological behavior of each neoplasm encountered to appreciate the newer and expanding indications for surgery in therapy. The proper execution of a diagnostic and therapeutic plan for each neoplasm must encompass a comprehensive presurgical, surgical, and postsurgical evaluation. Finally, additional experimental data and clinical experience will allow a more accurate diagnosis and prognosis as well as a clearer appreciation and understanding of newer treatment protocols.

1. Abbas, J. S., Holyoke, E. D., Moore, R., and Karakousis, C. P.: The surgical treatment and outcome of soft-tissue sarcoma. Arch. Surg. *116*:765, 1981.
2. Aust, V. B.: Oncology. *In* Schwartz, S. I. (ed.): *Principles of Surgery*. McGraw Hill, New York, pp. 249–258.
3. Bostock, D. E., and Dye, M. T.: Prognosis after surgical excision of fibrosarcomas in cats. J. Am. Vet. Med. Assoc. *175*:727, 1979.
4. Brodey, R. S.: Surgical treatment of cancer in the dog. J. Am. Vet. Med. Assoc. *166*:494, 1975.
5. Brodey, R. S.: Surgery. *In* Theilen, G. H., and Madewell, B.

R. (eds.): *Veterinary Cancer Medicine.* Lea & Febiger, Philadelphia, 1979, pp. 67–79.

6. Brodey, R. S., and Abt, D. A.: Results of surgical treatment in 65 dogs with osteosarcoma. J. Am. Vet. Med. Assoc. *168*:1032, 1976.

7. Bruce, D. L., and Wingard, D. W.: Anesthesia and the immune response. Anesthesiology *34*:271, 1971.

8. Castro, E. B., Hajdu, S. I., and Fortner, J. G.: Surgical therapy of fibrosarcomas of extremities. Arch. Surg. *107*:284, 1973.

9. Committee on Professional Education of UICC: *Clinical Oncology.* Springer-Verlag, Berlin, 1973, p. 73.

10. Devereux, D. F., Wilson, R. E., Corson, J. M., Antman, K. H., and Greenberger, J. S.: Surgical treatment of low grade soft tissue sarcomas. Am. J. Surg. *143*:490, 1982.

11. Engstrom, P. F.: The impact of cancer staging on cancer management in the community hospital. *In* Sutnick, A. I., and Engstrom, P. F. (eds.): *Oncologic Medicine.* University Park Press, Baltimore, 1976, pp. 125–139.

12. Fisher, B., and Fisher, E. R.: Studies concerning the regional lymph node in cancer. I. Initiation of immunity. Cancer *27*:1001, 1971.

13. Harvey, H. J.: General principles of veterinary oncologic surgery. J. Am. Anim. Hosp. Assoc. *12*:335, 1976.

14. Lee, Y. T. N.: Effect of anesthesia and surgery on immunity. J. Surg. Oncol. *9*:425, 1977.

15. Morton, D. L., and Wells, S. A.: Immunobiology of neoplastic disease. *In* Sabiston, D. C. (ed.): *Textbook of Surgery.* W. B. Saunders, Philadelphia, 1977, pp. 583–622.

16. Peyton, W. T.: Danger in the use of local filtration anesthesia in operations upon malignant tumors. Ann. Surg. *11*:453, 1940.

17. Rosenberg, S. A., et al.: Prospective randomized evaluation of the role of limb sparing surgery, radiation therapy, and adjuvant chemoimmunotherapy in the treatment of adult soft-tissue sarcomas. Surgery *84*:62, 1978.

18. Schneider, R., Dorn, C. R., and Taylor, D. O. N.: Factors influencing canine mammary cancer development and postsurgical survival. J. Nat. Cancer Inst. *43*:1249, 1969.

19. Suit, M. D., Russell, W. D., and Martin, R. G.: Management of patients with sarcoma of soft tissue in an extremity. Cancer *31*:1247, 1973.

20. Withrow, S. J.: Surgical management of cancer. Vet. Clin. North Am. 7:13, 1977.

Chapter **170**

Radiation Therapy

Gary R. Johnston and Daniel A. Feeney

Ionizing radiation alone or in combination with other modalities has achieved increased acceptance as a treatment for neoplasia throughout the veterinary profession. Radiotherapeutic equipment necessary to effectively treat tumors is found in most veterinary teaching institutions. Increased interest by veterinary radiologists trained in the subspeciality of radiation therapy has resulted in development of consistent radiotherapy protocols for many spontaneous neoplasms. Also, the demands by companion animal owners for an aggressive approach to tumor management have influenced interest in radiation therapy.

The purpose of this chapter is to outline the basic principles of radiation therapy, the techniques of radiotherapy, its application to specific tumors, and the availability of radiotherapy within veterinary institutions.

PRINCIPLES OF RADIATION THERAPY

Radiobiology

Radiobiology is the study of the interaction between ionizing radiation and living matter. Radiation therapy is the administration of ionizing radiation and its absorption by normal or neoplastic tissue. Therapeutic forms of ionizing radiation include x-ray, gamma-ray, electrons, neutrons, and other charged particles that deposit their energy randomly within matter in discrete clusters of ionization.[9, 18, 27, 43] This deposited energy is greater than the chemical binding energies of the molecules within the tissues. Ionization of the molecule results in ejection of orbital electrons that can lead to chemical changes within the vicinity of the ionization and eventually damage biologically important intracellular molecules. The density of local ionization is dependent on the absorber and the velocity and charge of the ionizing radiation.[18, 27] Charged particles (electrons and protons) have a lower velocity and a greater charge than electromagnetic radiation (x-rays and gamma-rays) and ionize more densely but dissipate their energy over a shorter tract for equivalent energy.

The conversion of kinetic energy to biological damage by ionization within the cell can result from direct interaction between the ionizing photon or particle and the critical molecule or may occur indirectly by the interaction of chemically reactive products formed by ionization and their subsequent absorption by nearby molecules.[9, 18, 27, 43] The indirect mechanisms for producing biological damage predominate, and the most frequently involved molecule is water. Ionization of water results in the production of reactive radicals, which can fix radiation damage and result in irreversible chemical bonds. Considerable evidence indicates that nuclear DNA is the cellular target, damage to which is responsible for cell death.[9, 18, 27, 43] Ionizing radiation produces a variety of reversible and irreversible lesions in the DNA molecule, including single- and double-strand breaks and alterations within the nucleic acid bases.

All mammalian cells, whether normal or neoplastic, proliferate by mitosis. Since cell division is cyclical, it is frequently depicted as a circle (Fig. 170–1).[27, 40] The total circumference of the circle represents the cell cycle time (T_c), which varies considerably between cell types. The cell cycle is subdivided into

Figure 170–1. All dividing mammalian cells, whether normal or neoplastic, can be symbolized by a circle, which represents cell division. Neoplastic cells have three nondividing stages. The proliferating phase is represented by those cells that are actively dividing in the cell cycle. G_0 cells are nondividing cells that have left the proliferating phase to remain in a quiescent phase. They may re-enter the cell cycle when appropriately stimulated or may lose their reproductive capability and die. Cells in the proliferative phase may die without progression into G_0 or may lose their reproductive capacity and die within weeks to months. (Reproduced by permission from Mendelsohn, M. L., and Dethlefsen, L. A.: Tumor growth and cellular kinetics in the proliferation and spread of neoplastic cell. *In* Moss., W. T., Brand, W. N., and Battifora, H.: *Radiation Oncology Rationale, Technique, Results.* C. V. Mosby Co., St. Louis, 1979, p. 16.)

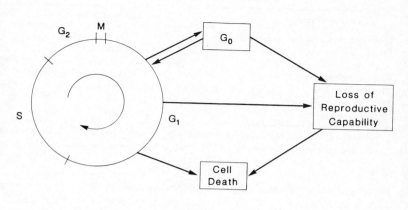

periods of mitosis (M) and interphase. Interphase is further subdivided into G_1 S, and G_2 phases, depending on the presence of DNA synthesis. G_0 cells are nondividing cells that have left the cell cycle. These cells may die without dividing or may remain in a quiescent phase without dying. With an appropriate stimulus the quiescent G_0 cells may re-enter the cycle. Cells may leave the cycle, lose their reproductive capability, and die later. The sensitivity of a cell to the effects of radiation depends on its position within the cell cycle at the time of irradiation. Cells in the late S phase are more radioresistant, whereas those in the M and G_2 phases are the most radiosensitive. Two mechanisms of radiation induced–cell death are recognized: mitotic cell death and interphase death.[27, 40, 43] Mitotic cell death occurs with moderate but lethal doses of radiation and results in the ultimate failure of cells to pass through mitosis after having completed one or more relatively normal mitoses. Alternately, in more sensitive cells or cells receiving large doses of radiation, a cell may degenerate in interphase and fail to reach its first mitosis.

Radiosensitivity, Radioresponsiveness, and Radiocurability

The law of Bergonié and Tribondeau relates the radiosensitivity of cells to their mitotic rate, further reproductive capabilities, and degree of differentiation and specialization.[5] These criteria have been utilized to categorize mammalian cells on the basis of their relative radiosensitivity (Table 170–1).[9, 27, 45] Cells with a high mitotic rate and no differentiation between divisions are termed *vegetative intermitotic cells* (e.g., the basilar layer of the epidermis) and are highly radiosensitive. Cells that do not divide and are highly differentiated and specialized are termed *fixed postmitotic cells* and are radioresistant. Examples include nervous tissue and skeletal muscle cells.

Radiosensitivity is also influenced by other factors unrelated to the cell's mitotic activity and degree of differentiation. Tumor size, cell type, patient condition, and presence of infection influence radiosensitivity. Radiosensitivity can be defined as the ability of radiation to biologically damage cells in normal or neoplastic tissue.[40]

Radioresponsiveness has frequently been equated with radiosensitivity. However, radioresponsiveness refers to the time required for visible structural or functional changes to occur and is measured by the rate at which the clinical manifestations of radiation injury take place.[40]

Radiocurability is the ability of ionizing radiation to reduce the number of malignant cells below a critical level so that no further clinical manifestations of their presence occur during the remaining lifetime of the patient.[40] Radiocurability in man is recognized if no tumor regrowth occurs within five years of radiotherapy treatment. In companion animals, radiocurability is accepted if no tumor regrowth occurs within two years of treatment. A tumor that shrinks

TABLE 170–1.   Categories of Mammalian Cell Radiosensitivity*

Cell Type	Example	Radiosensitivity
Vegetative intermitotic cells	Intestinal crypt cells, germinal layer of the epidermis	High
Differentiating intermitotic cells	Myelocytes, erythroblasts	Moderate to high
Multipotential connective tissue cells	Fibroblasts, endothelial cells	Moderate
Reverting postmitotic cells	Hepatocytes, renal tubular cells, smooth muscle cells	Moderate to low
Fixed postmitotic cells	Nerve cells, skeletal muscle erythrocytes	Low

*Modified with permission from Rubin, P., and Casarett, G. D.: *Clinical Radiation Pathology.* W. B. Saunders Co., Philadelphia, 1968, p. 6.

TABLE 170–2.   Radiotherapy for Companion Animal Neoplasms*

Tumor Type	Radiosensitivity	Responsiveness	Curability
Canine transmissible venereal tumors	High	Rapid	Excellent
Perianal adenomas	High	Rapid	Excellent
Squamous cell carcinoma	Variable†	Moderate to rapid	Fair to good
Fibrosarcomas	Low to moderate†	Slow	Poor to fair
Mast cell tumors	Moderate	Moderate to slow	Good to fair
Melanocarcinomas	Low	Slow	Poor to none
Osteosarcoma	Low	Slow	Poor to none

*Based on the authors' clinical experience in radiotherapy of companion animal neoplasms.
†Biologic behavior following radiotherapy varies with location on the patient and species.[29, 54, 56]

rapidly following irradiation is radioresponsive. A tumor that shrinks very slowly is considered nonradioresponsive. Either tumor may be radiocurable. Failure to decrease the size of a tumor during or shortly following radiotherapy does not constitute a radiotherapy failure provided no tumor regrowth and subsequent metastases occur. Connective tissue tumors such as fibrosarcomas respond much slower (if at all) than epithelial tumors. The application of the terminology to spontaneous tumors of companion animals is described in Table 170–2.

Principles of Radiation Therapy

Intracellular damage resulting from irradiation may cause cell death or recovery. The purpose of multiple external beam treatments is to use the varied characteristics of normal and neoplastic cells to promote proliferation of normal cells and mitotic cell death of tumor cells. Four factors, termed the "4 Rs" of radiotherapy, are involved in designing radiotherapy protocols.[18, 66]

Repair of sublethal injury is possible to a greater degree in normal cells than in neoplastic cells. This advantage is increased by dividing the total dose into a number of smaller doses (fractionation), since neoplastic cells may not have had sufficient time or the capability to repair sublethal injury before a subsequent dose is administered.

Repopulation by regeneration of stem cells may differ between normal and neoplastic cells. In normal tissues, restoration to pre-irradiation patterns of cell differentiation and rate of mitosis is a complex process under homeostatic control. The ability of neoplastic cells to regenerate and repopulate relative to normal tissues under external homeostatic control is believed to occur at a slower rate. If normal tissues have a more rapid regrowth relative to tumor tissues post irradiation, these tissues would be less responsive to the effects of fractionated radiotherapy treatments.

Redistribution of cells within the cell cycle is another possible advantage of fractionated radiotherapy. Cells surviving a dose of radiation tend to synchronize in resistant phases of the cell cycle. However, the rate at which individual cells progress through the cell cycle varies considerably, resulting in a phase difference between cells and decreasing the probability that surviving cells will be in a resistant phase at the time of the next radiation fraction.

Reoxygenation of hypoxic cells is a result of several complex processes. Tumors greater than 150 to 200 μ in size are composed of a relatively radiosensitive, oxygenated population and a more radioresistant, hypoxic population.[27] The presence of hypoxic radioresistant cells may contribute to post irradiation recurrence. Oxygenated cells are more sensitive to radiation than hypoxic cells and are selectively killed during fractionated treatment. A reduced population of oxygenated cells following radiation reduces the separation of hypoxic cells from blood vessels and results in more effective oxygen diffusion. In addition, decreased tissue pressure within the tumor following radiation because of reduced number of tumor cells re-opens compressed blood vessels and increases vascular flow in areas of previous hypoxia. The net effect of re-oxygenation is increased sensitivity of previously hypoxic cells to subsequent dose fractions.

Radiobiological Basis of Radiation Therapy and Tissue Tolerance

The response of normal tissue in an irradiated field is the limiting factor in the planning of radiotherapy.[18, 21, 22, 24, 40, 50, 57] If only tumoricidal doses are considered, any tumor can be controlled by an appropriate dose of ionizing radiation. The radiotherapist's ultimate goal is to cure without normal tissue complications. However, the risk must be evaluated for each patient. Although tumor control is the major objective for radiotherapists, the risk of major, potentially life-threatening complications may require the use of a radiation dose that minimizes the risk of complications yet decreases the probability of tumor control. If the complications encountered can be managed medically or surgically, a protocol that uses a maximum dose of radiation to increase the probability of tumor control may be chosen. The concept of tissue tolerance and the acceptable level of complications vary between institutions and radiotherapists. Tolerance doses have been derived from clinical and experimental data for a variety of tissues.[16, 44] In human radiotherapy a minimum tissue tolerance dose (TD 5/5) results in no more than a 5 per cent complication rate within five years.[44, 46] The maximum tissue tolerance dose (TD 50/5) results in no more than a 50 per cent severe complication rate within five years of treatment.[44, 46] Similar definitions for companion animals have not been determined.

Normal Tissue Reaction to Ionizing Radiation

Radiation injury depends on the relative radiosensitivity of the tissues receiving the radiation. Concurrent infection, trauma, or other diseases may influence the degree of tissue injury by radiation. Of primary consideration in radiation injury is turnover of parenchymal cells and its relationship to microcirculation.[44, 45] Also, the radiosensitivity of the parenchymal tissue relative to stromal tissues is important in determining acute and chronic effects of radiotherapy injury.[44] Rapidly renewing parenchymal tissues, such as the basilar layer of the epidermis, are vegetative intermitotic cells.[44] These cells are highly radiosensitive compared with more radioresistant vascular and stromal tissues. Moderate radiation doses may destroy the more radiosensitive basilar layer of the epidermis with minimal damage to the more radioresistant vascular and stromal elements. However, the ability of vegetative intermitotic cells to regenerate and repopulate following irradiation depends on their survival and the integrity of supporting vascular and stromal structures. Large doses of irradiation may cause necrosis of the more radiosensitive parenchymal tissues resulting in regeneration and repopulation only to be followed by chronic progressive injury mediated by vascular damage and interstitial fibrosis ("increased histohematic connective tissue barrier").[44, 45] The end result of the vascular injury may be ischemia and necrosis even if more radiosensitive parenchymal tissues have repopulated to pre-irradiation levels.

A major problem of clinical radiotherapy is that acute radiotherapy changes do not predict later chronic changes. In slow, non-renewing cell systems such as the brain and spinal cord, heart, liver, and kidneys, minimal or no acute functional change may be recognized following moderate to high doses of irradiation. Later vascular changes may not be encountered for several months. Accurate prediction of late radiotherapy injury is tenuous even if the acute manifestations are well recognized.

METHODS OF RADIOTHERAPY

External Beam Radiotherapy (Teletherapy)

External beam radiotherapy uses a source of ionizing radiation separated at a distance from the patient. The primary beam of radiation is limited by collimation to expose only a specified area of the patient. The sources of external beam radiotherapy currently available in veterinary institutions include orthovoltage x-ray, cobalt-60 (^{60}Co), cesium-137 (^{137}Cs), and linear accelerators.

Orthovoltage Radiotherapy

Orthovoltage radiotherapy uses x-rays with a low-to-medium energy range of 150 to 400 kVp.[47] The quality of radiation produced by orthovoltage x-ray is further described by its halfvalue layer (HVL). The HVL is defined as the amount of absorber required to reduce the intensity of the primary beam by one-half. The HVL for orthovoltage x-ray beams ranges from 4 mm of aluminum to 4 mm of copper.

Orthovoltage x-ray therapy has many limitations when compared with higher energy x-rays and gamma-rays in the megavoltage range (in excess of 1.0 MeV). The ability to penetrate tissue and achieve an adequate depth dose is one limitation of orthovoltage radiotherapy compared with megavoltage radiotherapy. With orthovoltage radiotherapy the skin dose exponentially decreases with increasing depth beneath the skin surface. With megavoltage radiotherapy the maximum dose is below the skin surface, thus achieving a degree of "skin sparing." This is a major limitation of orthovoltage, since the dose the skin can tolerate may be too small to allow tumoricidal doses for deep tumors. Another disadvantage of orthovoltage radiotherapy is the disparity of dose distribution between soft tissue and bone in the same field. A primary x-ray beam with a HVL of 2 mm of copper delivers a dose to bone that may be 1.5 times greater than the dose in soft tissue. This can result in doses greater than the tolerated dose for bone if tumoricidal doses to soft tissue were in the range of 4500 to 5000 rads. With megavoltage radiotherapy, no differential absorption occurs between bone and soft tissue. Although major limitations exist with orthovoltage radiotherapy, it is the most commonly used method in veterinary institutions in North America. Its major advantages are its simplicity, low cost, and reduced requirements for environmental shielding compared with those for megavoltage equipment.

Supervoltage (Megavoltage) Radiotherapy

Supervoltage (megavoltage) teletherapy uses x-rays, gamma rays, or electrons in an energy range in excess of 500 KeV.[47] Cobalt-60 (^{60}Co), cesium-137 (^{137}Cs), x-rays, and electron teletherapy units are limited to a few veterinary institutions. Both gamma-rays and x-rays are forms of electromagnetic radiation. However, they differ in their origin. Gamma rays originate from spontaneous nuclear decay of a radioactive isotope, and x-rays originate from an event outside the nucleus. Cobalt-60 (^{60}Co) has an average gamma ray energy of 1.25 MeV, a half-life of 5.3

years, and a HVL of 12 mm of lead. Cesium-137 (^{137}Cs) has a gamma ray energy of 0.66 MeV, a half-life of 30 years, and a HVL of 6.6 mm of lead. Cesium-137 gamma emissions are intermediate in energy between orthovoltage (400 KeV [0.400 MeV]) and megavoltage ^{60}Co emissions (1.25 MeV). The greater energy of ^{137}Cs radiation provides a higher percentage depth dose penetration in the tissues than orthovoltage radiation. Because of its lower energy, less shielding is required than that for ^{60}Co. The major disadvantage of ^{137}Cs is its low specific activity (disintegrations per second) and therefore low radiation output, its lower percentage depth dose, and its minimal if any skin sparing effect compared with ^{60}Co. Although ^{137}Cs has advantages over orthovoltage radiotherapy, the added advantages of depth dose penetration, skin sparing and uniform dose distribution for soft tissue and bone, and ease of maintenance (compared with linear accelerators) make ^{60}Co the method of choice for radiotherapy. High-energy x-ray and electron beam therapy from linear accelerators in the energy range of 4 to 35 MeV are receiving increased acceptance in human radiotherapy centers. At present, only one veterinary institution has linear accelerator capability.

Interstitial Brachytherapy

With interstitial brachytherapy, a radioisotope sealed in a metallic container, usually a seed, needle, or applicator, is placed in or on the patient.[24, 28] Radiation is administered in one prolonged dose over minutes, hours, or days. The sources may subsequently be removed depending on the physical half-life of the isotope. The primary advantage of brachytherapy is that the sources are placed in the tumor, providing maximum tumor dose while minimizing the dose to surrounding normal tissues. The disadvantages of brachytherapy include (1) exposure to the personnel involved in placing the sources, (2) the necessary isolation facilities required for hospitalization of the patient to prevent environmental contamination with lost sources, and (3) unnecessary exposure to the client.

Interstitial brachytherapy differs from teletherapy in that organ tolerance depends on the volume of tissue implanted. The tolerance dose decreases as the size of the volume implant increases.[28] Implant volumes of less than 10 cm^3 can tolerate higher doses than implant volumes in excess of 200 cm^3. Consequently, implant volumes less than 5 cm in diameter are more suitable for implant therapy. The radioactive isotopes currently available to the veterinary radiotherapist include cobalt-60 (^{60}Co), cesium-137 (^{137}Cs), gold-198 (^{198}Au), iridium-192 (^{192}Ir), and iodine-125 (^{125}I).[28, 63] The most important factor in selecting a therepeutic radionuclide is its half-life. Radiation quality, radiation safety, availability, and economy are also considered when selecting a radionuclide.

Systemic Radiotherapy

The internal use of radionuclides resembles interstitial brachytherapy except that the radioactive source is submicroscopic. The radionuclides can be administered orally, intravenously, or into the peritoneal or pleural space. Their localization into normal or neoplastic tissue depends on the chemical characteristics of the radionuclide. The application of systemic radiotherapy is limited to selected neoplastic diseases that cannot be adequately treated by teletherapy, chemotherapy, surgery, or other treatment methods. Iodine-131 has been utilized for the treatment of metastatic thyroid carcinoma in man and animals.[30, 38, 42, 47] Phosphorus-32 (^{32}P) is currently used for the treatment of polycythemia vera and the palliative treatment of chronic leukemia and metastatic cancers to bone.[47] Phosphorus-32 (^{32}P) and gold-198 (^{198}Au) are used for the palliative treatment of malignant pleural and peritoneal effusions.[47] The disadvantages of systemic radiotherapy are similar to those seen with brachytherapy: the patient becomes radioactive, and the environment is contaminated. Urine and feces must be handled as radioactive waste. Patients receiving systemic radiotherapy must be monitored during confinement to ensure that the level of radioactivity is safe for the general human population before the patient can be released. Systemic radiotherapy is currently limited to institutions with confinement facilities.

SEQUENCE OF RADIOTHERAPY IN COMBINATION WITH SURGERY

Surgery and radiotherapy are the major potentially curative methods available for veterinary tumor treatment. Surgery and irradiation may be used in several combinations. Surgery may be used to salvage early radiotherapy failures but is considered less effective in late radiotherapy failure.[18, 40] Radiotherapy may be used in surgical failures but is considered less effective because gross recurrence and distant metastasis usually have already occurred.[18, 40] Surgery and radiotherapy may be used to treat different areas. For example, surgical resection of tonsillar carcinomas with regional irradiation of the lymph nodes has been reported in dogs.[35] Surgery and irradiation may be used in a combined treatment protocol to treat the same area. Surgical failures occur because all microscopic disease is not removed, even with radical resection. Radiation failure occurs because of the inability of the exponential cell-killing characteristics of ionizing radiation to reduce the tumor cell burden below a level that can be managed by the patient's immune system. This is especially important in the treatment of large masses, since the incidence of recurrence increases with increasing tumor size.[18, 40] Clinical data indicate that 5000 rads given over five weeks eliminates microscopic neoplastic disease in 90 per cent of human patients.[18] It is logical to assume that surgery and radiotherapy can be complementary, surgery removing the gross mass and irradiation eliminating microscopic foci. Irradiation may be preoperative, intraoperative, or postoperative.[18, 25, 40]

Preoperative Radiotherapy

The arguments in favor of preoperative radiotherapy include the following: rendering a locally diffuse tumor removable, decreasing the extent of surgical resection of normal tissues, and rendering nonviable any malignant cells that may be inadvertently implanted surgically in the wound or circulatory system.[17] Radical surgical resection has been associated with distant metastasis in human clinical studies.[17, 18, 40] The argument against preoperative radiotherapy concerns impaired wound healing, which is directly proportional to the radiation dose.[17, 18, 40] Tumor shrinkage from preoperative radiotherapy may cause the client to refuse or delay curative resection or the surgeon to perform less radical resection.[17, 18, 40] Clinical and experimental data on increased cure rates for preoperative compared with those for postoperative radiotherapy are inconclusive. The optimum dose of preoperative radiotherapy varies with the tumor cell type and location. In man, the total dose of preoperative radiotherapy is from 2000 rads in 8 treatments to 5000 rads in 20 treatments.[40] The interval between preoperative radiotherapy and surgery is usually three to six weeks.[40] However, a 24- to 48-hour interval between the two procedures has been reported.[18] Preoperative radiotherapy is of benefit in neoplasms with a high incidence of postoperative recurrence.

Intraoperative Radiotherapy

Radiotherapy during surgery has received increased recognition in man. Accurate beam collimation to encompass the tumor and the ability to displace sensitive organs outside the radiation field are the major advantages of such therapy. The major disadvantage is the expense of a combined radiotherapy and surgical facility. When less than optimum facilities exist, anesthetized patients must be moved to a nonsterile area for radiation of the open surgical field. The risk of introducing pathogens under these circumstances is considerable. The trend in human radiotherapy centers is to design special operating rooms in the radiotherapy area. Single doses of 1000 to 3000 rads of orthovoltage x-rays or electrons (from linear accelerators) are currently used in human radiotherapy centers.[25] Application to veterinary radiotherapy is limited because of the expense.

In general, radiotherapy during surgery should be reserved for diffuse neoplasms that are not responsive to postoperative, fractionated, external beam, megavoltage radiation or interstitial brachytherapy. Principles of radiotherapy and clinical experience of normal tissue tolerance suggest that the risk of long-term complications increases with a smaller number of higher-dose fractions for a specified total dose.[54] Large single doses of radiotherapy may result in fibrosis, stricture formation, loss of function, and necrosis. The decision to employ this method of treatment must take into account the organs involved, the probability of long-term survival (long enough for complications to occur), the quality of life after treatment, and the therapeutic advantage over more conventional approaches.

Postoperative Radiotherapy

The primary indication for postoperative radiotherapy is a local neoplasm that cannot be completely removed. When the inaccuracies of assessing tumor involvement have been clarified by surgery, radiotherapy can be better adjusted.[17, 18] A higher total dose of irradiation can be given compared with preoperative or intraoperative radiotherapy.[17, 18] Surgical resection and healing are favored in the irradiated field compared with preoperative or intraoperative radiotherapy. There are several disadvantages of postoperative radiotherapy: (1) distant metastases may be produced by the surgical procedure, (2) surgery may decrease vascularity and predispose to tissue hypoxia, and (3) tumor proliferation may occur before irradiation is initiated if surgical healing is prolonged. Veterinary radiotherapists often elect to have the tumor reduced in size by surgery, followed by radiotherapy immediately or three to four weeks postoperatively. It has been suggested that, if irradiation is not begun immediately after surgery, it should be delayed about three weeks to permit tissue healing and decrease the likelihood of radiation-induced dehiscence.[55, 62] However, this philosophy is controversial. The decision to combine surgery and radiotherapy follows careful consideration of the cell type, extent of local invasion, and physical characteristics of the tumor.

RADIATION COMBINED WITH NONSURGICAL TREATMENT

The presence of hypoxic cells in a solid tumor is a major consideration in radiotherapy because of their relative radioresistance compared with that of both normal and neoplastic oxygenated cells. Several methods have been investigated to overcome hypoxia and increase the therapeutic effect. These include the use of hyperthermia, substances that increase sensitivity to radiation, and chemical protectants. Attempts to improve the therapeutic ratio in clinical radiotherapy have also employed the sequential or simultaneous use of chemotherapy in combination with surgery and radiation.[39]

Hyperthermia (see also Chapter 174)

Hyperthermia uses heat at temperatures of 40°C or greater to treat tumors. Hyperthermia may be used as a primary treatment method or may be combined with radiotherapy or chemotherapy. The therapeutic effects of hyperthermia have been observed in cell cultures and in spontaneous tumors in companion animals.[8, 11, 23, 32, 36, 37, 59] Cell death by heat alone begins at 42 to 43°C (tissue temperature). The lethal intracellular effects of heat are the result of rupture of plasma membranes, disruption of mitochondria, clumping of nuclear chromatin, and focal cytoplasmic swelling.[37, 52] These effects are both time- and temperature-dependent. In mice with implanted tumors, the destructive effects of heat began at 42°C.[13] For each degree rise in temperature above 42°C, the time required to produce the same biological effects was halved.[13] Results using hyperthermia alone for squamous cell carcinomas with tissue temperatures varing from 43 to 44.5°C for 30 minutes have been encouraging, with complete regression of the tumor in several patients.[23, 37] Clinical hyperthermia in combination with either interstitial brachytherapy or teletherapy has been utilized in human and veterinary radiotherapy. Encouraging results for squamous cell carcinomas and fibrosarcomas using combined hyperthermia and radiotherapy have been reported in dogs and cats.[8, 37] The results using hyperthermia and radiotherapy for canine osteosarcomas are less encouraging.[34]

The application of hyperthermia may be local or systemic. Radiofrequency (RF), microwave, ultrasound, and water immersion or whole-body chambers are currently used for heating tissue.

No definite evidence exists that tumor cells are more sensitive to heat than normal tissues. The local tumor environment which is considered to play an important role in hyperthermic killing of tumor cells, is substantially different from that of normal tissue.[52] The tumor's microenvironment consists of areas of necrosis, hypoxia, and reduced pH. The primitive vascularity of tumors reduces their ability to dissipate heat. The net result is that the tumor tissue has a higher temperature than the normal surrounding tissues. The decreased pH found in a tumor and the reduced nutrition of the tumor cells may also increase their sensitivity to high temperatures. Hypoxic cells found in a tumor are more resistant to radiation than oxygenated cells but are more sensitive to heat than oxygenated cells.[14]

The rationale for combining hyperthermia and radiotherapy is based on their synergistic effects. Results in clinical trials using hyperthermia either alone or in combination with other methods are encouraging. However, protocols for specific tumors are either incomplete or still under investigation. The use of hyperthermia and radiotherapy is limited to educational or research institutions. However, the use of heat alone by localized radiofrequency instruments has been reported in the treatment of localized tumors in veterinary practice.[26]

Hypoxic Cell Sensitizers

Chemical sensitizers are compounds that selectively increase the sensitivity of hypoxic tumor cells to radiation without altering the response of oxygenated cells. Nitroheterocyclic compounds with affinity for electrons sensitize hypoxic cells to radiation.[2, 41] Radiosensitizers may have a similar mechanism of action to oxygen on cells by promoting effects of radiation within cells.[1, 41] Hypoxia protects cells against the effects of radiation by a factor of 2.5 to 3.0 compared with well-oxygenated cells. With adequate concentrations of radiosensitizers in vitro, this level of protection encountered by hypoxic cells is reduced, and may approach the level of sensitivity shown by oxygenated cells.[2, 48, 49]

Nitromidazoles are compounds that have displayed encouraging radiosensitizing properties in in vitro and in vivo investigations in animal tumors. Metronidazole and misonidazole are radiosensitizers that have been extensively investigated. Misonidazole has been used extensively in clinical trials in man.[3, 7] Nausea, vomiting, and neurotoxicity are reported complications of multiple-dose regimens with misonidazole.[3, 7] To limit neurotoxicity to an acceptable clinical level in man, the total dose of misonidazole recommended is 10.5 to 15.0 gm/m^2.[64] This reduces the number of doses (of radiation and therapeutic cell sensitizers) that can be administered to between 4 and 10 (less than the 20 to 40 doses that would be administered with a conventional multifractionated radiotherapy protocol).

Radiation sensitizers are promising compounds that may enhance radiocurability of tumors. The use of misonidazole and irradiation for the treatment of fibrosarcomas in dogs has been reported.[12] However, no statistical difference was found in survival rates between those dogs treated with radiation alone and those treated with radiation and misonidazole.

Agents that Protect Against Radiation

Oxidation of biological molecules by free radicals produced from irradiation of intracellular water is an accepted cause of radiation injury. These molecules may be DNA or associated proteins. Certain sulfhydryl compounds, such as cysteamine and cystine, are recognized for their protective capacities when present during irradiation. Depletion of sulfhydryl compounds is reported to increase cellular radiosensitivity.[61, 67] The addition of exogenous sulfhydryl compounds protects aerated cells yet only provides minimal protection to hypoxic cells.[61, 67] It is likely that these compounds are scavengers of or competitors for the oxidative effects of the radiation-induced free radicals, thus permitting repair of sublethal diseases. If normal tissues can be protected, total radiation doses could be increased, resulting in greater tumor control without increased damage to normal tissue. Several sulfhydryl compounds have been developed that provide protection *in vitro* and *in vivo*. WR2721 is reported to protect normal aerated tissues without protecting the hypoxic tumor cells.[58, 60, 61, 67] WR2721 and radiation have been used experimentally for the treatment of spontaneous tumors in dogs.[58] Dogs treated with WR2721 and radiation had milder dermatitis than dogs treated with radiation alone.[58] Longer tumor regression and reduced damage to normal tissues were obtained in dogs with spontaneous neoplasms treated with WR2721 and radiation.[52]* More clinical trials are necessary to determine the therapeutic gain obtained with radioprotectants and radiation in spontaneous neoplasms of companion animals. Their use in combination with radiation, radiosensitizers, and hyperthermia require further investigation.

Chemotherapy

The combination of chemotherapy and radiation has received little attention by veterinarians, although considerable attention has been given to combined chemotherapy and radiation for human adult and pediatric neoplasms.[18] Increased therapeutic ratios are obtained in large mediastinal masses of Hodgkin's disease when chemotherapy is utilized to shrink the tumor mass so the radiotherapist can reduce the field size and irradiate less lung tissue and a smaller tumor mass.

Better therapeutic results have been obtained using combined chemotherapy and radiation in lung cancer[15] and in head and neck tumors in man.[65] Combinations have been recommended in the treatment of pediatric Wilm's tumor, Hodgkin's disease,

rhabdomyosarcoma, and leukemia of the central nervous system.[18] In dogs and cats, combined radiation therapy and chemotherapy has received less emphasis. Radiation therapy, testosterone, and menadiol sodium diphosphate were used in the unsuccessful treatment of an undifferentiated mammary carcinoma in an 11-year-old female pointer.[51] Menadiol sodium diphosphate, a synthetic vitamine K preparation, has been used as an early radiosensitizer but is reported to have little activity. Its use with radiation for spontaneous tumors in dogs has been reported.[51] Surgery or radiotherapy followed by chemotherapy was recommended for the treatment of canine osteosarcoma.[6]

Chemotherapeutic agents such as antibiotics, alkylating agents, and antimetabolites may be used with radiation therapy to prevent metastasis during irradiation of the primary tumor.[18] These compounds act as apparent sensitizers and appear to potentiate the effects of radiation.[27] In reality, they do not increase the lethal effects of radiation but probably add to the effect of radiation.[27] The early and late effects of chemotherapeutic drugs are well known. The severity of complications encountered when radiation and chemotherapy are simultaneously combined may produce unacceptable complications, which would be more severe if either had been used alone.[39] The toxicity of each compound and its potential effect if used in conjunction with radiation should be considered. The toxicity of commonly used chemotherapy agents combined with radiation is listed in Table 170–3. Additional investigations using radiation therapy and chemotherapy are needed to determine if increased survival rates occur compared with treatment by either irradiation or chemotherapy alone. Currently, no recommendations based on results are available for use as guidelines to reduce dosage when radiation and cytotoxic drugs are used simultaneously. Until proved otherwise, it is probably safer and possibly more efficacious to use these methods sequentially rather than simultaneously in clinical practice and to use them at currently recommended doses (see Chapter 172).

*Section editor's note: WR2721 is not approved for use in dogs by the United States Food and Drug Administration.

TABLE 170–3. Major Toxic Effects of Drugs Commonly Used in Conjunction with Radiotherapy*

Complication	Vincristine	Actinomycin D	Cyclophosphamide	Adriamycin	High-Dose Methotrexate
Leukopenia	−	+	+ +	+ + +	+ + +
Thrombocytopenia	−	+ + +	+	+	+ +
Neurotoxicity	+ +	−	−	−	−
Cardiotoxicity	−	−	+	+ + +	−
Cystitis	−	−	+ + +	−	−
Mucositis	−	+ +	−	+ +	+ + +
GI toxicity	+ +	+ +	+ +	+ +	−
Cellulitis (local)	+ +	+ +	−	+ +	−
Erythema	−	+ +	−	−	+
Hepatotoxicity	−	−	−	−	+ + +

*Reprinted with permission from Suton, W. W., and Chan, R. C.: Irradiation and chemotherapy in pediatric tumors. *In* Fletcher, G. H.: *Textbook of Radiotherapy.* Lea & Febiger, Philadelphia, 1980, p. 639.
Notes: Increasing number of " + " signs indicates increasing severity and frequency of complication.
Complications represented by (+) are for combined protocols of chemotherapeutic agents and radiation.

APPLICATIONS

Evaluation Before Radiotherapy

Evaluation before radiotherapy is critical and directly influences the decision to accept a patient for radiotherapy. The minimum data base for each patient should include a physical examination, complete blood count (CBC), urinalysis, serum chemistry profile, thoracic radiographs (and abdominal radiographs if the neoplasm is caudal to the diaphragm), radiographs of the primary tumor if near osseous structures, and a biopsy. If lymphadenopathy is encountered, a biopsy should be obtained to determine if inflammatory or metastatic disease is present. Thoracic radiographs may indicate if metastases are present in addition to assessing the cardiopulmonary system. Abdominal radiographs are recommended with tumors of the perineum, anus, and hind legs to evaluate abdominal lymph nodes. A serum chemistry profile will determine if hepatic or renal insufficiency exists concurrently. Patients with these insufficiencies would be considered poor anesthetic risks and may have a decreased life expectancy.

A biopsy is a prerequisite to radiotherapy and provides a histological diagnosis and an aid in determining the prognosis. However, the biopsy technique may influence the accuracy of the diagnosis. Fine-needle biopsies should not be considered definitive except in mast cell tumors because of the "hit or miss" nature of the technique. In addition, cell distortion may preclude an accurate histological diagnosis. An excisional biopsy is recommended because it provides the veterinary pathologist with an adequate nontraumatized sample. If excisional biopsy is not appropriate, a trephined core or wedge biopsy should be obtained. (see Chapter 168). A qualified *veterinary* histopathologist should evaluate tissue samples for histological diagnosis, degree of malignancy, and completeness of an excisional biopsy.

Patient Selection

Radiation therapy is not a panacea for all neoplasms, nor should it be considered a "last ditch effort" when all other therapies have failed to control the tumor. A practitioner may be reluctant to refer a patient because of age and life expectancy. However, the physical examination should determine the general health of the patient. An older patient in good physical condition is a potential candidate for radiotherapy. The data from the evaluation determine if concurrent disease exists, which may preclude radiation therapy. Neoplasms such as lymphosarcoma, lymphoblastic leukemia, systemic mast cell sarcomas, and metastatic neoplasms should be treated with chemotherapy. In general, the physical characteristic of a tumor determines treatment. Superficial neoplasms that are not locally invasive should be surgically resected. Superficial tumors that are localized but invasive may be effectively treated by radiation. Frequently, surgical resection followed by irradiation is appropriate for tumor therapy. Surgical resection is recommended even in invasive tumors to reduce the size of the tumor mass, because tumor volume adversely affects radiocurability. The greater the number of cells, the greater the total dose required to cure the tumor. Since normal tissue tolerance is the factor that limits dose in radiotherapy, adequate tumoricidal doses may not be obtained in large tumor masses if the normal tissues are treated to the tolerance level.

Selection of Radiotherapy

The selection of a radiotherapy regimen for an individual case depends on the location and physical characteristics of the tumor and the availability of radiotherapy facilities. Cobalt-60 or ^{137}Cs needles, ^{125}I and ^{198}Au seeds, and ^{181}Ir ribbons or wire can be used for localized superficial tumors that cannot be surgically resected. However, brachytherapy requires special facilities for housing the patient. Some older patients in good physical condition may not tolerate hospitalization and may be treated as outpatients with either orthovoltage or telecobalt therapy.

Brachytherapy using a ^{90}Sr applicator is suitable for the treatment of superficial inflammatory and neoplastic lesions of the cornea. Strontium-90 is a beta emitter. These particles have a small range of penetration before attenuation by tissues. Fifty per cent of beta radiation is attenuated by 1 mm of soft tissue.[47] Doses in the range of 8000 to 10,000 rads (cGy*) given as one fraction are usually employed, except in benign lesions.[24]

Superficial lesions up to 5 mm in depth can be effectively treated utilizing low-energy x-rays. An orthovoltage x-ray unit operated at 150 kVp and 15 mA may have an effective photon energy of 47 KeV and a half value layer (HVL) of approximately 6.5 mm of aluminum. Fifteen per cent of the x-ray photons are attenuated within the first 5 mm of tissue and 50 per cent within the first 2 cm of tissue.[10] Low-energy x-ray photons can be used for superficial tumors over the abdomen when the underlying intestine can be protected. However, these low-energy x-rays should not be used to treat superficial lesions directly over bone. Low-energy x-rays are disproportionally absorbed by bone. Radiation doses in excess of bone tolerance may occur if therapeutic doses between 3,500 and 4,500 rads are used to treat the soft tissues of the tumor.

For the treatment of deep tumors, high-energy orthovoltage x-ray may be used. An orthovoltage x-ray unit operated at 250 kVp and 15 mA with appropriate added filtration has an effective photon energy of 100 to 140 KeV and a HVL between 1.5 and 4.0

---

*1 antiGray (cGy) = 0.01 gray = 1 rad. 1 gray (Gy) = 100 rads.

mm of copper, providing a 50 per cent dose at 3 to 6 cm depth depending on the field size.[10] High-energy orthovoltage x-rays can be used for the treatment of tumors 3 to 4 cm in depth. The main limitation at these depths is the excessive surface dose, which can be avoided in some patients by using multiple treatment portals. High-energy orthovoltage x-ray also delivers a higher dose to bone than to soft tissue.

High-energy gamma rays from ^{60}Co have an average energy of 1.25 MeV. Photon and electrons from supervoltage linear accelerators may be in excess of 2 MeV. These megavoltage radiotherapy units have the advantage of delivering tumoricidal doses to deep-seated tumors yet sparing skin because the maximum dose is several millimeters below the skin surface. Bone and soft tissue attenuate radiation similarly with megavoltage radiation; consequently, a more even distribution of dose is obtained. Supervoltage and megavoltage radiation are currently limited by availability. With increasing interest in radiation therapy, it is anticipated that the availability of supervoltage radiation will increase within veterinary institutions.

Cure versus Palliation

The ultimate goal in radiation therapy is to deliver a tumoricidal dose with an acceptable degree of complications. With large nonresectable tumors, radiotherapy may be used as a palliative treatment. Tumoricidal doses of 4000 to 4,500 rads may produce unacceptable complications, and doses of 2,500 to 3,500 rads may be necessary to reduce the size of the tumor. Single-fraction treatments during surgery

TABLE 170–4. Probability of Cure for Neoplasms With Multimodality Therapy Using Radiotherapy*†

| Tumor | Probability of Cure (%)‡ | | | | | Reference |
	0–29	30–49	50–69	70–89	90–100	
Perianal gland adenoma			RS, RC	R(2), RS(2), RSCCh	R, RS(2)	20, 22, 24, 26, 55, 57
Perianal gland adenocarcinoma	R, RS	RS, RSC	R, RS, RSCCh	RS(2)		20, 22, 24, 57
Squamous cell carcinoma (excluding nasal)		R(2), RSC	R(4), RS(4), RC, RSChH	R, RS, RSCH		19, 20–24, 26, 35, 37, 50, 51, 55, 57, 58
Adenocarcinoma (excluding nasal)	RSC	R	R, RSC		R	20–23, 37, 50, 51, 57, 58
Tooth: germ neoplasms			R, RS	R(5), RS	R, RS	26, 33, 37, 58
Fibrosarcoma (see references)	RS, RSI	R	R(4), RSChH	RH		8, 12, 20–22, 26, 29, 37, 50, 51, 53, 55, 57, 58
Malignant melanoma	RSI	RS, RSCCh	RS			26, 37, 50, 51, 55, 58
Chondrosarcoma	R		R, RSC, RSH			
Intranasal adenocarcinoma	RS		R	R		
Intranasal neoplasms (mostly epithelial origin)	R, RS	RS	R, RS, RSC	RS		55, 56, 58
Transmissible venereal tumor					R(3)	24, 54, 55
Mast cell tumors	RS, RCh	RS	R(2), RS(2), RSC	RSC		4, 20, 22–24, 37, 50, 55
Hemangiopericytoma	RH		RS	RS		55
Osteosarcoma	RI					34, 50, 51

*Reprinted with permission from Feeney, D. A., and Johnston, G. R.: Radiation therapy: Applications and availability. *In* Kirk, R. W. (ed.): *Current Veterinary Therapy VIII.* W. B. Saunders, Philadelphia, 1983, pp. 428–434.

†Based on a survey of the veterinary institutions listed in Table 107–5 and the veterinary literature. Cure defined as a two-year survival, no continued growth, and no subsequent metastases.

‡Number in parentheses indicates number of institutions responding using that therapeutic mode. No number indicates one (1) institution responding using that method.

Notes: Each abbreviation represents a response by an institution and the mode(s) of therapy utilized. Data in this table do not take into account size, local invasion, etc. These criteria may vary among institutions when tumors are selected for treatment.

R	=	radiotherapy alone
RH	=	radiotherapy + hyperthermia
RS	=	radiotherapy + surgery (includes castration, if applicable)
RC	=	radiotherapy + cryosurgery
RCh	=	radiotherapy + chemotherapy
RI	=	radiotherapy + immunotherapy
RSC	=	radiotherapy + surgery + chemotherapy
RSH	=	radiotherapy + surgery + hyperthermia
RSI	=	radiotherapy + surgery + immunotherapy
RSCCh	=	radiotherapy + surgery + cryosurgery + chemotherapy
RSCH	=	radiotherapy + surgery + cryosurgery + hyperthermia
RSChH	=	radiotherapy + surgery + chemotherapy + hyperthermia

TABLE 170–5. Availability of Radiotherapy Facilities in North American and Australian Veterinary Institutions

Institution	Location	External Beam Therapy				Brachytherapy				Miscellaneous	
		Ortho-voltage	Cesium-137	Cobalt-60	Linear Accelerator	Inter-stitial	Intra-cavitary	Plieso-therapy	Systemic Isotopes	Other	No Radiation Therapy
United States											
Animal Medical Center	New York, NY										X
Angel, Memorial Hospital	Boston, MA										X
Auburn University School of Vet. Med.	Auburn, AL	X		X							
University of California-Davis, School of Vet. Med.	Davis, CA	X		X		^{137}Cs, ^{125}I, ^{192}Ir	^{196}Au	^{137}Cs, ^{90}Sr	^{131}I		
Colorado State University, College of Vet. Med.	Fort Collins, CO			X	6 MeV			^{90}Sr			
Cornell University, New York State College of Vet. Med.	Ithaca, NY		X					^{90}Sr	^{131}I		
University of Florida, College of Vet. Med.	Gainesville, FL										X
University of Georgia, College of Vet. Med.	Athens, GA	X						^{90}Sr			
University of Illinois, College of Vet. Med.	Urbana, IL	X						^{90}Sr	^{131}I		
Iowa State University, College of Vet. Med.	Ames, IA	X						^{90}Sr			
Kansas State University, College of Vet. Med.	Manhattan, KS	X				^{137}Cs		^{90}Sr			
Louisiana State University, School of Vet. Med.	Baton Rouge, LA	X				^{137}Cs		^{90}Sr			
Michigan State University, College of Vet. Med.	East Lansing, MI	X						^{90}Sr*			
University of Minnesota, College of Vet. Med.	St. Paul, MN	X				^{222}Rn		^{90}Sr	^{131}I*		
Mississippi State University, College of Vet. Med.	Starkeville, MS										X

								Neutrons (cyclotron produced)
University of Missouri-Columbia, College of Vet. Med.	Columbia, MO	X	†	^{137}Cs	^{32}P	^{137}Cs, ^{90}Sr	^{131}I, ^{32}P	
Ohio State University, College of Vet. Med.	Columbus, OH	X	X	^{198}Au, ^{192}Ir, ^{222}Rn		^{90}Sr	^{131}I	
Oklahoma State University, College of Vet. Med.	Stillwater, OK	X				^{90}Sr		
University of Pennsylvania, School of Vet. Med.	Philadelphia, PA	X	‡			^{90}Sr		
Purdue University, School of Vet. Med.	West Lafayette, IN	X		^{222}Rn		^{90}Sr		
University of Tennessee, College of Vet. Med.	Knoxville, TN	X	X	^{125}I, ^{222}Rn		^{90}Sr	^{131}I	
Texas A&M University, College of Vet. Med.	College Station, TX	X	X	^{198}Au, ^{137}Cs	^{198}Au, ^{32}P	^{137}Cs, ^{90}Sr	^{131}I, ^{32}P	
Tufts University, School of Vet. Med.	Boston, MA							X
Tuskegee Institute, School of Vet. Med.	Tuskegee, AL							N/R
Virginia-Maryland Regional College of Vet. Med.	Blacksburg, VA							X
Washington State University, College of Vet. Med.	Pullman, WA	X		^{137}Cs		^{90}Sr		
Yale University School of Medicine, Section of Comparative Medicine	New Haven, CT	X						
Canada								
Ontario Veterinary College, University of Guelph	Guelph, ON, Canada	X						
University of Saskatchewan, Western College of Vet. Med.	Saskatoon, SK, Canada					^{90}Sr		
Australia								
Murdoch University School of Vet. Studies	Perth, Western Australia	X		^{198}Au		^{90}Sr		
School of Vet. Science, University of Sydney	Sydney, New South Wales					^{90}Sr		
School of Vet. Science, University of Melbourne	Melbourne, Victoria					^{90}Sr		
School of Vet. Science, University of Queensland	Brisbane, Queensland					^{90}Sr		

*Soon to be available.

†Available and *routinely used* at a *local* hospital or medical school.

‡In process of development: date of availability uncertain.

N/R No response. (Modified with permission from Feeney, D. A., and Johnston, G. R.: Radiation therapy: Applications and availability. *In* Kirk, R. W. (ed.): *Current Veterinary Therapy VIII.* W. B. Saunders, Philadelphia, 1983.)

for locally diffuse tumors are palliative. Clients may wish to treat the primary site of a metastatic tumor if the quality of life for the patient can be temporarily improved.

Specific Application to Selected Tumors

The tumors most frequently treated by radiotherapy are listed in Table 170–4. The probability of cure and the choice of therapy were obtained from the veterinary literature.[4, 19, 20, 29, 33, 53, 54, 56] Most veterinary radiotherapists treat malignant neoplasms by delivering a total dose of 4000 to 5000 rads in ten fractions at a rate of three fractions per week. These doses result in acceptable complication rates. Benign tumors and other benign lesions such as lick granulomas and rodent ulcers are treated with a total dose of 600 to 2,400 rads given in one to four fractions.

FAILURE OF RADIOTHERAPY AND COMPLICATIONS

Failure of radiotherapy results from an inadequate field size to cover the primary tumor site and failure to detect regional or distant metastases. Careful evaluation before therapy may detect regional lymph node involvement. Examination of an excisional biopsy by a qualified veterinary histopathologist may determine if the tumor extends beyond the edge of the resected sample. Failure of radiotherapy may also result from the inherent resistance of the tumor because of hypoxic cells or because adequate lethal doses could not be delivered without exceeding normal tissue tolerance.

Complications of radiation therapy are primarily limited to the site of irradiation. Nausea and vomiting are not encountered unless the abdominal viscera are irradiated directly or unless during the course of treating periabdominal neoplasms sufficient doses are given to these organs. Complications of radiotherapy indicate that the radiation dose exceeded the tolerance of normal tissues in the field. Necrosis is the most common sequela if tissue or organ tolerance is exceeded. Tissue or organ atrophy and fibrosis may be the end result of radiotherapy depending on the dose (total and per fraction) and schedule and specific tissue and size of the irradiated field.

Since the surface dose is usually greater than the maximum tumor dose with orthovoltage radiotherapy, the most common sites for injury are the skin and mucous membranes. Epilation, depigmentation, and moist desquamation are the most frequently encountered complications.[31] It is important that these complications be explained to the client prior to radiotherapy. Epilation is encountered with surface skin doses in excess of 500 rads. Epilation is often a temporary complication of radiotherapy. The hair frequently grows back but may be a different color and less dense. Moist desquamation is encountered with orthovoltage radiotherapy when surface doses range from 4000 to 5000 rads. These doses are encountered with conventional ten-fraction protocols in which tumor doses range from 3,500 to 4,500 rads. Moist desquamation is a result of injury to the germinal layer of the epidermis. Sloughing of the epidermis results in a thin desquamated epithelium and hyperemia and vascular injury result in a serous exudate. Moist desquamation occurs around the seventh fraction of a ten-fraction protocol and reaches its peak intensity at 10 to 14 days after therapy. This reaction usually subsides in two to three weeks after therapy. The owner should be instructed to keep the area clean and free of encrusted debris and prevent the animal from mutilating the area. Inflammation of mucous membranes occurs in treatment of oral tumors, and its pathogenesis is similar to that of moist dermatitis.

Radiation-induced bone necrosis may occur after orthovoltage radiotherapy. It is important that the absorbed dose in both bone and soft tissues in an orthovoltage-treated field be calculated to avoid overtreatment of bone.

GENERAL AVAILABILITY OF RADIATION THERAPY

Radiotherapy facilities in veterinary institutions are listed in Table 170–5.

1. Adams, G. E.: Hypoxia-mediated drugs for radiation and chemotherapy. Cancer 48:696, 1981.
2. Adams, G. E., Flockhart, I. R., Smithen, C. E., Stratford, I. J., Wardman, P., and Watts, N. E.: Electron-affinic sensitizers VII: A correlation between structures. 1: Electron reduction potentials and efficiencies of some nitromidazoles as hypoxic cell radiosensitizers. Radiat. Res. 67:9, 1976.
3. Adams, G. E., Fowler, J. F., and Wardman, P.: Hypoxic cell sensitizers in radiobiology and radiotherapy. Br. J. Cancer 37(Suppl. III):1, 1978.
4. Allan, G. S., and Gillette, E. L.: Response of canine mast cell tumors to radiation. J. Nat. Cancer Inst. 63:691, 1979.
5. Bergonié, J., and Tribondeau, L.: Interprétation de queiques resultats de la radiotherapie et assae de fixation d'une technique rationale. CR Acad. Sci. 143:983, 1906.
6. Bostock, D. E., and Owen, L. N.: Chemotherapy of canine and feline neoplasms. J. Small Anim. Pract. 13:357, 1972.
7. Brady, L. W. (ed.): Radiation sensitizers: Their use in the clinical management of cancer. In: Cancer Management, Vol. 5. Masson Publishing USA, New York, 1980.
8. Brewer, W. G., and Turrel, J. M.: Radiotherapy and hyperthermia in the treatment of fibrosarcomas in the dog. J. Am. Vet. Med. Assoc. 181:146, 1982.
9. Casarett, A. P.: Radiation Biology. Prentice-Hall, Inc., Englewood Cliffs, NJ, 1968, pp. 7–30, 57–89, 159–170.
10. Cohen, M., Jones, D. E. A., and Greene, D.: Central axis depth dose data for use in radiotherapy. Br. J. Radiol. (Suppl.) 11:1, 1972.
11. Connor, W. G., McKelvie, D. H., Miller, R. C., and Boone, M. L. M.: Localized current field heating as an adjunct to radiation therapy. I. The use of LCF hyperthermia and irradiation in the treatment of spontaneous animal tumors. Radiat. Environ. Biophys. 17:219, 1980.

12. Creasey, W. A., Phil, D., and Thrall, D. E.: Pharmacokinetic and antitumor studies with radiosensitizers misonidazole in dogs with spontaneous fibrosarcomas. Am. J. Vet. Res. 43:1015, 1982.

13. Crile, G.: The effects of heat and radiation on cancers implanted on the feet of mice. Cancer Res. 23:372, 1963.

14. Dritschilo, A., and Piro, A. J.: Therapeutic implications of heat as related to radiation therapy. Semin. Oncol. 8:83, 1981.

15. Eagen, R. T.: What the radiation oncologist should know about chemotherapy and the treatment of lung cancer. Paper presented at Current Concepts in Radiation Therapy, University of Minnesota, Minneapolis, 1982.

16. Ellis, F.: Tolerance of normal tissues and tumors to radiation. Front. Radiat. Ther. Oncol. 12:101, 1978.

17. Fletcher, G. H.: Combination of irradiation and surgery. Int. Adv. Surg. Oncol. 2:55, 1979.

18. Fletcher, G. H.: Textbook of Radiotherapy, 3rd ed. Lea & Febiger, Philadelphia, 1980, pp. 103–180, 219–224, 637–661.

19. Gavin, P. R.: Radiation response to oral squamous cell carcinoma in the dog. Vet. Radiol. 20:81, 1979.

20. Gillette, E. L.: Radiation therapy of canine and feline tumors. J. Am. Anim. Hosp. Assoc. 12:359, 1976.

21. Gillette, E. L.: Radiation therapy. In Kirk, R. W. (ed.): Current Veterinary Therapy VII. W.B. Saunders, Philadelphia, 1977, pp. 479–482.

22. Gillette, E. L.: Radiotherapy. In Theilen, G. H., and Madewell, B. R. (eds.): Veterinary Cancer Medicine. Lea & Febiger, Philadelphia, 1979, pp. 85–94.

23. Gillette, E. L.: Large animal studies of hyperthermia and irradiation. Cancer Res. 39:2242, 1979.

24. Gillette, E. L., and Carlson, W. B.: Radiation therapy. In Carlsons Veterinary Radiology, 3rd ed. Lea & Febiger, Philadelphia, 1977, pp. 477–489.

25. Goldson, A. L.: Past, present and prospects of intraoperative radiotherapy (IOR). Semin. Oncol. 8:59, 1981.

26. Grier, R. L., Brewer, W. G., and Theilen, G. H.: Hyperthermic treatment of superficial tumors in cats and dogs. J. Am. Vet. Med. Assoc. 177:227, 1980.

27. Hall, E. J.: Radiobiology for the Radiologist, 2nd ed. Harper & Row, Hagerstown, MD, 1978, pp. 27, 31–62, 81–92, 95–110, 113–128, 171–194, 195–202.

28. Hilaris, B. S.: Handbook of Interstitial Brachytherapy. Publishing Sciences Group, Inc., Acton, MA, 1975, pp. 1–24, 25–43, 61–85.

29. Hilmas, D. E., and Gillette, E. L.: Radiotherapy of spontaneous fibrous connective-tissue sarcomas in animals. J. Natl. Cancer Inst. 56:365, 1976.

30. Johns, H. E., and Cunningham, J. R.: The Physics of Radiology, 3rd ed. Charles C Thomas, Springfield, IL, 1978, pp. 532–579.

31. Johnston, G. R., and Feeney, D. A.: Radiotherapy of the extremities: tissue tolerance and complications. Vet. Radiol., accepted for publication, 1983.

32. Kveld, R. S., and Boone, M. L. M.: Prospects of hyperthermia in human cancer therapy. Part I: Hyperthermia effects in man and spontaneous animal tumors. Radiology 123:489, 1977.

33. Langham, R. F., Mostosky, U. V., and Shirmer, R. G.: X-ray therapy of selected odontogenic neoplasms in the dog. J. Am. Vet. Med. Assoc. 170:820, 1977.

34. Lord, P. F., Kapp, D. S., and Morrow, D.: Increased skeletal metastasis of spontaneous canine osteosarcoma after fractionated systemic hyperthermia and local X-irradiation. Cancer Res. 41:4331, 1981.

35. MacMillan, R., Withrow, S. J., and Gillette, E. L.: Surgery and regional irradiation for treatment of canine tonsillar squamous cell carcinomas: Retrospective review of eight cases. J. Am. Anim. Hosp. Assoc. 18:311, 1982.

36. Marmor, J. B., Pounds, D., Hahn, N., and Hahn, G. M.: Treatment of spontaneous tumors in dogs and cats by hyperthermia induced by ultrasound. Int. J. Radiat. Oncol. Biol. Phys. 4:967, 1978.

37. Miller, R. C., Connor, W. G., Heusinkveld, R. C., and Boone, M. L. M.: Prospects for hyperthermia in human cancer therapy. Radiol. 123:489, 1977.

38. Mitchell, M., Hurov, L. I., and Troy, G. C.: Canine thyroid carcinomas: Clinical occurrence, staging by means of scintiscans and therapy of 15 cases. Vet. Surg. 8:112, 1979.

39. Moore, J. V.: Timing and dose in experimental combinations of cytotoxic drugs and radiation. Appl. Radiol. 11:113, 1982.

40. Moss, W. T., Brand, W. N., and Battifora, H.: Radiation Oncology: Rational, Technique, Results, 5th ed. C. V. Mosby, St. Louis, 1979, pp. 1–36, 37–51.

41. Phillips, T. L.: Sensitizers and protectors in clinical oncology. Semin. Oncol. 8:65, 1981.

42. Riknberk, A.: Iodine Metabolism and Thyroid Disease in the Dog. Drukkerij Elinkwijh, Utrecht, 1971.

43. Ritter, M. A.: The radiobiology of mammalian cells. Semin. Oncol. 8:3, 1981.

44. Rubin, P.: The radiographic expression of radiotherapeutic injury: An overview. Semin. Roentgenol. 9:5, 1974.

45. Rubin, P., and Casarett, G. W.: Clinical Radiation Pathology. W.B. Saunders, Philadelphia, 1968, pp. 1–61.

46. Rubin, P., and Casarett, G.: A direction for clinical radiation pathology. The tolerance dose. Front. Radiat. Ther. Oncol. 6:1, 1972.

47. Selmon, J.: The Basic Physics of Radiation Therapy, 2nd ed. Charles C Thomas, Springfield, IL, 1976, pp. 120–172, 311–318, 472–533.

48. Sheldon, P. W., Foster, J. L., and Fowler, J. F.: Radiosensitization of C3H mouse mammary tumors by a 2-nitromedazole drug. Br. J. Cancer 30:560, 1975.

49. Sheldon, P. W., Foster, J. L., and Fowler, J. F.: Radiosensitization of C3H mouse mammary tumors using fractionated dose of x-rays with the drug Ro-07-0582. Br. J. Radiol. 49:76, 1975.

50. Silver, I. A.: Use of radiotherapy for the treatment of malignant neoplasms. J. Small Anim. Pract. 13:351, 1972.

51. Silver, I. A., and Carter, D. B.: Radiotherapy and chemotherapy for domestic animals. II. Treatment of malignant tumors in dogs and cats. Acta Radiol. 2:457, 1964.

52. Suit, H. D.: Hyperthermic effects on animal tissues. Radiology 123:483, 1977.

53. Thrall, D. E.: Orthovoltage radiotherapy of oral fibrosarcomas in dogs. J. Am. Vet. Med. Assoc. 179:159, 1981.

54. Thrall, D. E.: Orthovoltage radiotherapy of canine transmissible venereal tumor. Vet. Radiol. 23:217, 1982.

55. Thrall, D. E.: Principles of radiation therapy in cancer. In Ettinger, S. J. (ed.): Textbook of Veterinary Internal Medicine, 2nd ed. W. B. Saunders, Philadelphia, 1982, pp. 393–405.

56. Thrall, D. E., and Adams, W. M.: Radiotherapy of squamous cell carcinomas of the canine nasal plane. Vet. Radiol. 23:193, 1982.

57. Thrall, D. E., and Biery, D. N.: Principles and application of radiation therapy. Vet. Clin. North Am. 7:35, 1977.

58. Thrall, D. E., Biery, D. N., and Girardi, A. J.: Evaluation of radiation of WR-2721 in dogs with spontaneous tumors. In Brady, L. W. (ed.): Cancer Management, Vol. 5. Masson Publishing USA, New York, 1980, pp. 343–347.

59. Thrall, D. E., Gerweck, L. E., Gillette, E. L., and Dewey, W. C.: Response to cell in vitro and tissues in vivo to hyperthermia and x-irradiation. Adv. Radiat. Biol. 6:211, 1976.

60. Utley, J. F., Phillips, T. L., and Kane, L. J.: Protection of normal tissues by WR2721 during fractionated radiotherapy. Int. J. Radiat. Oncol. Biol. Phys. 1:699, 1976.

61. Utley, J. F., Phillips, T. L., Kane, L. J., Wharam, M. D., and Wara, W. M.: Differential radioprotection of enoxic and hypoxic mouse mammary tumors by a thiophosphate compound. Radiology 110:213, 1980.

62. Vikram, B.: Importance of the time interval between surgery and postoperative radiation therapy in the combined management of head and neck cancer. Int. J. Radiat. Oncol. Biol. Phys. 5:1837, 1979.

63. Walker, M. A.: A review of permanent interstitial implant

radiotherapy using Radon-22 and Iodine-125. Vet. Radiol. 23:223, 1982.

64. Wasserman, T. H.: Hypoxic cell radiosensitizers—present and future. Radiol. Oncol. Biol. Phy. 7:849, 1981.

65. Weaver, A., Loh, J. J. K., Vandenberg, H., Powers, W., Fleming, S., Mathog, R., and Muhyi, A.: Combined mo-

dality therapy for advanced head and neck cancer. Am. J. Surg. 140:549, 1980.

66. Withers, H. R.: The four R's of radiotherapy. Adv. Radiat. Ther. 5:241, 1975.

67. Yuhas, J. M.: Improvement of lung tumor radiotherapy through differential chemoprotection of normal and tumor tissue. J. Natl. Cancer Inst. 48:1255, 1972.

Chapter **171**

Immunotherapy

Steven J. Susaneck

Immunotherapy of neoplasia is the use of any or all components of an animal's immune system to control, damage, or destroy malignant cells. Although theoretically, immunotherapy should be an effective method of treatment, it's application is still in the early stages of development.

TUMOR IMMUNOLOGY

Immunotherapy is just one part of the complex field of tumor immunology, the subject of a great deal of research and controversy for many years. Researchers and clinicians have long recognized the effect of the immune system on tumor growth, development, metastasis, and regression. As early as the 1900s certain tumors were observed to regress when patients developed bacterial infections.[17] In spite of some sporadic, early, and dramatic regressions, interest in immunotherapy soon diminished because of few consistent favorable results and advances in chemotherapy, radiotherapy, and surgery.

Interest in immunotherapy re-appeared in the mid 1950s with the demonstration of tumor-specific antigens in chemically induced neoplasms in inbred mice.[11] Subsequently, tumor-specific transplantation antigens were demonstrated in tumors induced by viruses, chemical carcinogens, and certain spontaneous animal neoplasms.

With the discovery of tumor-specific transplantation antigens in experimental animals, it was assumed that similar antigens would be found in spontaneous tumors in man and animals. Much controversy still exists regarding the presence of specific antigens on spontaneous human and canine tumors. Morton has reported the existence of tumor-specific transplantation antigens in Burkitt's lymphoma, malignant melanoma, nephroblastoma, skeletal and soft tissue sarcomas, and colonic neoplasms in man.[16] However, some researchers question the existence of tumor-specific antigens.[18]

Regardless of whether tumor-specific antigens can

be demonstrated in spontaneous tumors, there are many clinical observations that suggest that the immune system has a significant effect on tumor behavior. These observations include the following:

1. An increased incidence of malignant disease in human patients with congenital immunodeficiency diseases such as ataxia telangiectasia and the Wiskott-Aldrich syndrome.[7,8]

2. A higher incidence of neoplasia (about 12.6 percent, or 25 times the expected incidence) in human transplantation patients that have been deliberately immunosuppressed.

3. The demonstration of "blocking factors" (thought to be antigen-antibody complexes) that inhibit the ability of lymphocytes to destroy cancer cells *in vitro*.[11]

4. Spontaneous regression of tumors.

5. Regression of metastases after resection of a primary tumor.

6. Failure of circulating tumor cells to metastasize.

7. Infiltration of tumors by mononuclear cells.

8. Increased tumor incidence with age.

EVASION OF IMMUNOLOGICAL SURVEILLANCE BY TUMORS

If spontaneous tumors do contain tumor-specific antigens, why are these tumors able to develop in an animal with a normal immune system? Several mechanisms have been postulated to explain the escape of tumors from immunological destruction.

Tumors In Privileged Sites. Tumors may proliferate in areas of the body that are not reached by affected cells of the immune system (e.g., central nervous system, eye).

Antigenic Modulation. Loss of or change in antigenicity may enable a tumor to escape immunological recognition.

Blocking Factors. Blocking factors may include "blocking" antibodies, soluble tumor-associated antigens, or immune complexes. The production of blocking factors early in the course of a neoplasm could result in masking of all surface antigens and blocking of the afferent arm of the immune response. In dogs with osteosarcoma, levels of blocking factors have been found to be high before surgery, to regress after amputation, and to rise again with recurrence.[13]

Overwhelming the Immune System. Rapidly growing tumors may overwhelm the immune system's ability to control tumor growth. Normal human defenses can control about 10^8 tumor cells before being overwhelmed.[22]

IMMUNOLOGICAL DESTRUCTION OF TUMOR CELLS

The immune system's response to tumor cells is highly complex. Components utilized in an immune response against neoplasia include natural killer cells (NK cells, null cells), sensitized lymphocytes, activated macrophages, and antibodies. The interaction of these various components is intricate and involves a series of feedback mechanisms associated with the generation of suppressor thymus-derived lymphocytes (T cells) and macrophages.[2,26] In addition to the immunological response to the tumor, the tumor itself may produce soluble factors, including antigen-antibody complexes that may interfere with the body's response to the tumor. Although each element of the immune system may react differently to the presence of tumor, it is likely that ultimate tumor rejection involves multiple effective mechanisms.

Thymus-Derived Lymphocytes

Thymus-derived lymphocytes (T cells) are a heterologous population of cells of different functions, including helper T cells, which assist bursa-derived lymphocytes (B cells) in antibody synthesis in response to certain antigens; suppressor T cells, which act to suppress immune responses; and killer T cells, which are involved in the recognition and destruction of tumor cells.

Natural Killer Cells

Natural killer (NK) cells are a distinct population of cells whose lineage has not been completely worked out. Some investigators feel that NK cells are of T cell lineage, whereas others feel that they arise from neither T nor B cells. It has been recently proposed that NK cells play an important part in the host defense against neoplastic cells.[23]

Macrophages

Macrophages have been shown to be an important component of host defense against tumors. Activated macrophages both kill tumor cells and inhibit their multiplication. Many of the biological agents used in nonspecific stimulation of the immune system act through activation of macrophages, causing them to kill tumor cells. In addition, macrophages can be activated by lymphokines released from sensitized T cells.

Antibodies

There are two mechanisms by which antibodies can cause tumor cell death. The first mechanism is complement-dependent cell lysis, which involves the activation of the complement pathway following antibody interaction with tumor antigen on the cell surface. The second mechanism is antibody-dependent cell-mediated cytotoxicity (ADCC), which involves the interaction of affected cells with tumor cells coated with the Fc portion of IgG antibody. The effector cells are thought to include granulocytes, macrophages, and killer T cells. Although the exact mechanism of cell lysis is not known, ADCC may not be augmented by complement and may require close contact between affected and target cells. ADCC can be blocked by "blocking" antibodies and immune complexes that bind to the Fc portion of the specific IgG.

ACTIVE SPECIFIC IMMUNOTHERAPY

Active specific immunotherapy is based on the premise that tumor cells contain antigens recognizable by the host as foreign; as such, the host can mount an immune response against them. This basic assumption has been the subject of controversy for many years. Since the first discovery of tumor-specific transplantation antigens, researchers have attempted to document the presence of these antigens on spontaneous tumors. If spontaneous tumors contain tumor-specific antigens as do experimentally produced tumors and if these antigens can be incorporated into a vaccine, this form of therapy may have a place in the treatment of neoplasia.

Few specific antigens have been isolated from spontaneous tumors. Most research with tumor vaccines has been done using modified or killed preparations of whole cells. Radiation is the most widely used method of modifying tumor cells. In studies of experimental tumor systems, chemically altered cells offered greater antigenicity than irradiated cells. In addition to radiation, cell treatments that produce vaccines involve the use of mitomycin-C (a cytotoxic drug), poorly antigenic sulfhydryl blocking agents, lipophylic agents, neuraminidase (removes sialic acid from the cell wall), and viral oncolysis.

It is beyond the scope of this chapter to discuss all of the technical problems involved in the production of tumor vaccines. There are many variables and procedures that may influence the ultimate effectiveness of a vaccine.[10,20,21] One significant problem is that experimentally produced tumors are often heterogeneous with respect to drug sensitivity, metastatic capacity, and immunogenicity. Therefore, it is possible to produce a vaccine against a tumor that is immunologically different from the metastatic lesions in the patient being treated.

There have been some encouraging results using tumor vaccines in the treatment of residual disease in experimental tumor models,[9] and some favorable results using tumor vaccines in the treatment of human lung cancer, breast cancer,[1] renal cancer,[15] and melanoma have been achieved. In initial studies, dogs treated for lymphosarcoma with acetoacetylated, soluble, tumor-associated antigens plus Freund's complete adjuvant showed longer remission and survival times than those receiving only chemotherapy.[3,5] The active ingredient in the tumor vaccine was probably Freund's complete adjuvant and not modified or nonmodified lymphoma cells, resulting in nonspecific immunostimulation.[25] Specific active immunotherapy may be more effective when used in combination with nonspecific active therapy. This may be due to an increase in the number of immunocytes available because of nonspecific stimulation.

Presently there are many studies in progress using tumor vaccines. Much work still needs to be done in the areas of isolation and purification of tumor-specific antigens before this method will be useful for the treatment of neoplasia. It must be stressed that the tumor mass must first be reduced before specific immunotherapy can be expected to be effective.

PASSIVE IMMUNOTHERAPY

In passive immunotherapy, mediators of immunity are administered to the tumor patient. Since tumor destruction by the immune system may involve both the humoral and cell-mediated systems, passive trials of immunotherapy have incorporated elements of both systems, including immune lymphocytes, specific antibodies, complement, transfer factor, and "immune" RNA preparations.

The transfer of immune lymphocytes has been generally successful in clinical situations, but there are many technical problems associated with the technique. Experimental studies reveal that as many as 300 lymphocytes are needed to kill one tumor cell. Rejection of the transferred lymphoid cells is a common problem in man, and for this reason the technique has not been feasible for therapy in either man or animals.[16]

Passive immunotherapy using immune sera is useful in treating tumors in experimental animals, dogs, cats, and man. In dogs and cats, responses have resulted from the use of sera from normal animals to treat animals with lymphosarcoma. It is believed that antibody directed toward antigens on the leukemic cell membrane is present, but because of a deficiency in the level of complement or a component of complement, lysis of tumor cells cannot occur.[13] Of 44 cats with lymphosarcoma treated with blood or plasma from healthy cats, 100 per cent regression was obtained in 50 per cent of the cats, whereas 25 per cent of the cats showed partial regression and 25 per cent showed no response. In 19 dogs with lymphosarcoma treated with whole blood or plasma, some regressions were noted. Of five dogs treated with whole blood, one showed complete remission and four showed partial remission. Of ten dogs treated with high doses of fresh plasma (20 ml/kg body weight), two showed complete remission, four showed partial response, and four showed no response. None of the four dogs treated with low-dose (6 mg/kg) fresh plasma responded.[14] Although some efficacy has been shown with this method, there are many technical problems associated with implementing it: (1) large amounts of normal blood or plasma are necessary (15 to 20 ml/kg); (2) the type of anticoagulant is critical; and (3) the blood must be given within four hours of collection. Until the specific antileukemic factor can be isolated and purified, it is doubtful that this type of therapy would be useful clinically.

A newer adaptation of passive immunotherapy could use monoclonal antibodies, which are antibodies with a high degree of specificity for a particular antigen. Monoclonal antibodies are produced by the chemical fusing of an antibody-producing T cell with a myeloma plasma cell. The resulting hybrid cell can be maintained in vitro and can produce an antibody to one particular antigen. Recently, monoclonal antibodies against certain human tumor cells have been manufactured. Although monoclonal antibodies are generally not tumoricidal, they may serve as vehicles to deliver other antineoplastic agents. In addition, monoclonal antibodies may serve as valuable tools in the diagnosis of metastatic tumors by attaching radioactive labels to mark metastasis.

Immunoabsorption therapy is another modification of passive immunotherapy. Immunoabsorption involves the removal of certain immune modulators (antigen-antibody complexes, suppressor T cells) from a tumor patient's sera. In dogs with mammary gland carcinomas, five of ten dogs showed a reduction in the size of their tumors when their plasma was perfused through chambers bearing *Staphylococcus aureus* Cowan strain 1 as an immunoadsorbent.[12]

NONSPECIFIC IMMUNOTHERAPY

The principle behind nonspecific immunotherapy is that certain substances stimulate the immune system to be nonspecifically tumoricidal. The exact mechanism of this nonspecific stimulation is not completely understood, although it is known that these compounds can stimulate T cells, NK cells, and macrophages to tumoricidal activity.

Nonspecific immunotherapy was first recognized at the turn of the century when Dr. Bradford Coley observed that a thrice recurrent inoperable sarcoma completely regressed after the patient suffered two episodes of erysipelas. From these observations, Coley attempted to treat other patients with mixtures of different bacteria in various proportions. Although some positive results were observed, this treatment was generally unimpressive.

One of Coley's most widely used preparations, known as mixed bacterial vaccine (MBV), is a combination of *Streptococcus pyogenes* (10^8 to 10^9 organisms/ml) and *Serratia marcescens* protein content (2.5 mg/ml). MBV can be administered intramuscularly or intralesionally. The major side effects of MBV are fever (39.9 to 40.5° C), chills, nausea, and vomiting. An overdose can lead to endotoxic shock and death. In one study, MBV was given to 200 animals with many different histological tumor types in varying stages. When used alone in advanced cancer patients, MBV does not appear to be an effective antitumor agent.[13] Studies using MBV and surgery for the treatment of oral melanoma in dogs showed no significant difference between those treated with MBV and surgery and those treated with surgery alone.[14]

Another biological immunostimulator is bacillus Calmette Guérin (BCG), an attenuated strain of *Mycobacterium bovis* developed by Calmette and Guérin for use as a vaccine against human tuberculosis. BCG is a potent stimulator of the reticuloendothelial system, and since stimulation of this system is associated with prevention of tumor growth, BCG became the prototype of biological immunostimulators.

Methods of administration of BCG include intralesional injection, intravenous injection, scarification on the skin, intralymphatic injection, oral administration, intrapleural injection, and intravesicular instillation. Side effects include fever, chills, local necrosis at the site of injection, and granulomatous lesions in the lung and liver.

In man, BCG is most effective in the treatment of localized cutaneous melanoma when injected intralesionally. In addition, BCG is of some benefit in the treatment of acute lymphoblastic leukemia in children and in myelogenous leukemia when combined with chemotherapy.

In dogs, BCG has been used in the treatment of osteosarcoma in association with surgery. These studies indicate that there may be some effect on osteosarcomas, but only a small number of dogs were used in the study.[19] Of six dogs treated with BCG and surgery, four lived approximately one year after amputation and two had no radiographic evidence of metastasis after a year. Owen and Bostock demonstrated that intravenous BCG delayed the onset of metastasis but did not influence local recurrence in canine mammary gland tumors.[19] Theilen and Madewell have had disappointing results with intralesional use of BCG for the treatment of skin and oropharyngeal tumors in dogs in preliminary uncontrolled studies at the University of California Veterinary Medical Teaching Hospital.[24] Excellent results have been obtained with BCG in the treatment of equine periorbital fibrosarcoma ("sarcoid").

In experimental conditions, BCG is effective in preventing the development of metastasis. In dogs and humans, BCG stimulates pulmonary macrophages to kill tumor cells *in vitro*. The mechanism of action is postulated to be stimulation of monocytes and NK cells to become tumoricidal through the release of lymphokines from sensitized lymphocytes.

The problem in evaluating the effectiveness of BCG is that its effectiveness depends on a number of factors: (1) the strain of BCG; (2) how the BCG was cultured and prepared; (3) the ratio of viable to nonviable cells; (4) the route of administration; (5) the histological type of tumor; and (6) the size of the tumor. As with all forms of immunotherapy, BCG seems to be most effective when the tumor is small. Recently, attempts to identify the portion of the organism responsible for antitumor activity have been made. Portions used include methanol extraction residue (MER) and water-soluble adjuvant (WSA), disrupted cell walls attached to oil droplets and a complex of mycolic and arabinogal actane-mucopeptide from cell walls. In dog studies using MER, the results among cases were variable but the overall effect was no better than those of surgery alone.

Corynebacterium parvum is a third biological immunostimulator. It is a formal in-killed bacterial preparation that is shown to have stimulatory effects on the reticuloendothelial system. *C. parvum* increases the activity of macrophages and B lymphocytes but temporarily depresses T cell function. This killed bacterial preparation can be given intravenously or intralesionally. Side effects, such as pseudoleukopenia, fever, and bleeding disorders, have been reported.

In man, positive responses with *C. parvum* have been demonstrated with oat cell carcinomas, various sarcomas, metastatic breast cancer, and melanomas. In veterinary medicine, the use of *C. parvum* has been associated with some favorable but nonconclusive results in the treatment of metastatic melanoma. In addition to the three biological immunostimulators discussed, many more exist and are under investigation. Table 171–1 contains a partial list of these compounds.

Interferon

Interferon refers to a family of glycoproteins synthesized by many types of animal cells. Since their discovery in 1957, interferons have shown promise for their possible development into potent nontoxic antiviral drugs and in the late 1960s began to receive a great deal of attention as an antitumor drug.

Interferon is considered a biological immunostimulator because it augments lymphocyte cytotoxicity *in vitro* and *in vivo* and increases macrophage activity. Interferon has antitumor effects that are mediated in part, by the immune system. Interferon's major

TABLE 171–1. Agents Used to Stimulate Nonspecific Immunotherapy

Agent	Proposed Mechanism of Action
Biological Modulators	
Mixed bacterial vaccine (MBV)	Stimulates macrophages and T lymphocytes
	Affords endotoxicity
Bacillus Calmette Guérin (BCG)	Stimulates macrophages and lymphocytes
	Increases delayed hypersensitivity reaction
Corynebacterium parvum and *C. granulosum*	Stimulates macrophages and increases phagocytosis
	Inhibits T-cells
Vaccinia virus	Delayed-type hypersensitivity (bystander effect)
	Viral oncolysis
Freund's adjuvant	Causes slow release of antigen
	Induces local chronic inflammation
	Stimulates antibody-dependent cell-mediated cytotoxicity
Lipopolysaccharides (LPS) and polysaccharides	Activates alternate pathway for complement
Chemical Immunostimulators	
Levamisole	Immune modulator
	Normalizes T cell function
Dinitrochlorobenzene (DNCB)	Stimulates local delayed hypersensitivity reaction
Polyadenylic-polyuridylic acid	Activates macrophages
(Poly A:U)	Augments antibody production
	Induces interferon
Muramyl dipeptide (MDP)	Stimulates macrophages
Azimexon	Stimulates delayed hypersensitivity reactions
Tuftsin	Enhances antibody-dependent cellular toxicity
	Stimulates macrophages too by cytostatic effect

antitumor effect is probably mediated primarily by NK cell stimulation. Presently, many studies are under way to evaluate interferon as an antitumor agent.

Chemical Adjuvants

Owing to inherent problems with biological immunostimulants, chemical immunostimulants have been developed. The best known of these are drugs of the imidothiazole class (e.g., levamisole and thiabendazole). Levamisole is a phenylimidazothiazole developed as an anthelmintic and subsequently shown to have immune potentiating properties. Levamisole increases phagocytosis, stimulates lymphoblast transformation, and increases delayed hypersensitivity reactions, primarily in circumstances in which these functions are depressed. Levamisole does not, however, appear to directly affect tumor cell growth *in vitro*. In two dogs with recurrent nodules after a mastectomy, complete regression was observed with levamisole alone.[14] In a study using levamisole and surgery in the treatment of feline mammary tumor, there was no significant difference in either the survival patterns or the disease-free remission patterns of the levamisole and placebo groups.[14]

Within the past few years a new chemical immunostimulant has been developed. The new compound, *N*-acetylmuramyl-*L*-ala-*D* isoglutamine (MDP), is a ubiquitous constituent of bacterial cell walls. MDP stimulates both T cells and macrophages to kill tumor cells *in vitro*. *In vivo* tests with mice indicate that MDP may be most effective in the treatment of metastatic cancer. There are many advantages of MDP over the biological immunostimulators. It is nontoxic and nonimmunogenic and can be synthesized with a great degree of purity. At the present time, the only studies using MDP have been done in mice and rats. Toxicity studies using encapsulated liposome and free MDP have been performed in dogs, and both have been shown to be relatively nontoxic. Studies are currently under way to determine the toxicity of MDP in man.

CONCLUSION

Although attempts at immunotherapy have been made since the turn of the century, scientific evaluation of immunotherapy as a mode of treating neoplasia is still in its infancy. It is only with the advent of newer technology in the past few years that tumor immunity has been better understood and adapted to therapy. To evaluate immunotherapy, controlled studies with standardized treatments are needed. Immunotherapy, if used under the right conditions, may offer a valuable adjuvant in the treatment of neoplasia. The conditions for optimal application of immunotherapy include (1) treatment of residual lesions once the primary tumor burden has been removed; (2) the combination of immunotherapy with other modes of therapy; and (3) an immune system capable of responding to stimulation.

1. Adler, A., Stein, J. A., Goldborg, A. J., Levy, E., Inbor, M., Altboim, I., Teva, Z., and Czernobilsky, B.: Active specific immunotherapy of Stage III breast cancer. Cancer Immunol. Immunother. *10*:45, 1980.

2. Benjamini, E., Rennick, D. M., and Sell, S.: Tumor immunology. *In* Stites, D. P. (ed.): *Basic and Clinical Immunology.* Lange Medical Publications, Los Altos, CA, 1982 pp. 223–249.

3. Benjamini, E., Theilen, G., Torten, M., Fong, S., Crow, S., and Henness, A. M.: Tumor vaccines for immunotherapy of canine lymphosarcoma. Ann. NY Acad. Sci. 227:305, 1976.

4. Bostock, D. E., and Gorman, N. T.: Intravenous BCG therapy of mammary carcinoma in bitches after surgical excision of the primary tumor. Eur. J. Cancer 14: 879, 1978.

5. Crow, S. E., Theilen, G. H., Benjamini, E., Torten, M., Henness, A. M., and Buhles, W.: Chemoimmunotherapy for canine lymphosarcoma. Cancer 40:2102, 1977.

6. Fiedler, I. J.: Tumor heterogenicity and the biology of cancer invasion and metastasis. Cancer Res. 38:2651, 1978.

7. Gatti, R. A., and Good, R. A.: Occurrence of malignancy in immunodeficiency disease: A clinical review. Cancer 28: 89, 1971.

8. Good, R. A.: The immunologic deficiencies in man. Birth Def. 4:17, 1968.

9. Hanna, M. G., Jr., and Peters, L. C.: Immunotherapy of established micrometastasis with BCG tumor cell vaccine. Cancer Res. 38:204, 1978.

10. Hanna, M. G., Jr., Peters, L. C., and Brandhorst, J. S.: Active specific immunotherapy of residual micrometastasis: conditions of vaccine preparation and regimen. *In* Crispin, R. G. (ed),: *Tumor Progression.* Elsevier-North Holland, Inc., New York, 1980, pp. 59–80.

11. Hellstrom, I., Sjogren, H. O., Warner, G., and Hellstrom, K. E.: Blocking of cell mediated tumor immunity by sera from patients with growing neoplasms. Int. J. Cancer 7:226, 1971.

12. Holohan, T. V., Phillips, T. M., Bowles, C., and Deisseroth, A.: Regression of canine mammary carcinoma after immunoadsorption therapy. Cancer Res. 43:3663, 1982.

13. MacEwen, E. G.: An immunologic approach to the treatment of cancer. Vet. Clin. North Am. 7:65, 1977.

14. MacEwen, E. G.: Progress report: A summary of work currently in progress in the Donaldson-Atwood Cancer Clinic. New York, 1979.

15. McCune, G. S., Schapira, D. V., and Intenshaw, E. G.: Specific immunotherapy of advanced renal carcinoma: Evidence of the polyclonality of metastases. Cancer 47:1984, 1981.

16. Morton, D. L.: Immunotherapy of cancer: Present status and future potential. Cancer 30:1647, 1972.

17. Nauts, H. C., Fowler, G. A., and Bogatko, F. H.: A review of the influence of bacterial infection and bacterial products (Coley's toxins) on malignant tumors in man. Acta Med. Scand. 276(Suppl.):5, 1953.

18. Old, L. J.: Cancer immunology: The search for specificity — B.H.S. Clowes Memorial lecture. Cancer Res. 41:361, 1981.

19. Owen, L. N., and Bostock, D. E.: Effects of intravenous BCG in normal dogs and in dogs with spontaneous osteosarcoma. Eur. J. Cancer 10:775, 1974.

20. Peters, L. C., Brandhorst, J. S., and Hann, M. G.: Preparation of immunotherapeutic autologous tumor cell vaccines from solid tumors. Cancer Res. 39:1353, 1979.

21. Peters, L. C., and Hanna, M. G.: Active specific immunotherapy of established micrometastases: Effect of cryopreservation procedures on tumor cell immunogenicity in guinea pigs. J. Natl. Cancer Inst. 64:1, 1980.

22. Southam, C. M.: Evidence for cancer specific antigens in man. Prog. Exp. Tumor Res. 9:1, 1967.

23. Talmadge, J. E., Meyers, K. M., Prieur, D. J., and Starkey, J. R.: Role of natural killer cells in tumor cell growth and metastasis. C57BL/6 normal and beige mice. J. Natl. Cancer Inst. 65:929, 1980.

24. Theilen, G. H., and Madewell, B. R.: Immunotherapy. *In* Theilen, G. H., and Madewell, B. R. (eds.); *Veterinary Cancer Medicine* Lea & Febiger, Philadelphia, 1979, pp. 113–118.

25. Weller, R. E., Theilen, G. H., Madewell, B. R., et al.: Chemoimmunotherapy for canine lymphosarcoma: A prospective evaluation of specific and nonspecific immunomodulation. Am. J. Vet. Res. 41:516, 1980.

26. Woodruff, M.: *The Interaction of Cancer and the Host: Its Therapeutic Significance.* Grune & Stratton, New York, 1980.

Chapter **172** Chemotherapy

Robert C. Rosenthal

Chemotherapy is an increasingly important treatment for malignant disease. Over 100 years ago, the antineoplastic effect of potassium arsenate was noted. The modern use of chemotherapy dates from the 1940s in both human and veterinary medicine.[19,28] In the past four decades, numerous agents have been introduced, and more than 50 (including hormones) are considered useful in human medicine.[7] The number of agents used in veterinary medicine is smaller. Antineoplastic drugs act in a number of different ways, but the biological and pharmacological principles underlining their rational use apply to all sound chemotherapeutic protocols.

Chemotherapy may be employed with a number of goals in mind. Ultimately, the goal of chemotherapy is to cure the disease, but whether this occurs in veterinary medicine is debatable.[28] Although it is possible that transmissible venereal tumor may be "cured" with various chemotherapeutic approaches alone,[4] the high rate of spontaneous remission of this tumor makes this difficult to evaluate.[28] Even if a total cure is not obtainable by chemotherapy alone, there are other benefits from its use. Chemotherapy may help control generalized rapidly progressive disease not amenable to surgery or irradiation or may help increase the disease-free interval after such initial therapy. It may help prevent spread of the neoplasm by controlling early metastases that are proliferating rapidly and have a relatively small likelihood of containing resistant cells. Chemotherapy may also benefit the patient by symptomatic relief of related problems and temporary restoration of deteriorated function.[19,28]

Traditionally, surgery has been the treatment of

choice for neoplasia. In some cases, radiation therapy is another effective mode of treatment for localized disease. Neither of these approaches, however, is able to deal with systemic or undetected metastatic disease. Metastatic disease is the primary cause of death in patients with neoplasia regardless of the mode of therapy.[13] Clearly, the more effective the chemotherapy in controlling the distant spread of the disease, the longer the comfortable survival of the patient. An understanding of the basic principles of chemotherapy can help provide a basis for sensible, effective chemotherapy and prolonged survival.

BIOLOGICAL BASIS OF CHEMOTHERAPY

There are three aspects of cell kinetics that must be considered when discussing the biological basis of chemotherapy: cell cycle,[22,28] growth classes of tissues,[45] and Gompertzian growth of tumors.[40]

Both normal and neoplastic cells proceed through the cell cycle in orderly progression from mitosis to mitosis. There are four phases of the cell cycle (Fig. 172–1). Mitosis (m) marks the beginning of the cell cycle. Cell division in mammalian cells takes an average of 30 to 90 minutes. The G_1 (gap 1) phase is the period of greatest temporal variability. Days to weeks may be involved in this period of RNA and protein synthesis, depending on the tissue type. From G_1, cells may enter a G_0 phase, which is a resting, nonproliferating state. Cells may remain in G_0 for long periods or return to G_1 and proceed in the cell cycle. The period of DNA synthesis (S phase) follows G_1 and generally lasts about two hours. This is followed by the G_2 (gap 2) phase, another period of RNA and protein synthesis, which generally lasts about six to eight hours. Various chemotherapeutic agents affect the cell cycle at various points. A knowledge of the cell cycle is fundamental to the establishment of a sensible chemotherapeutic plan.

Tissues do not all behave in the same manner

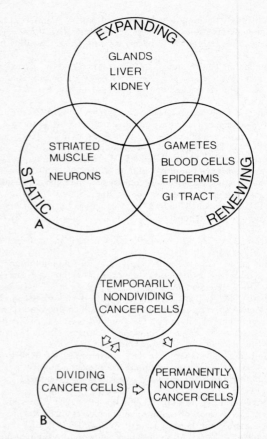

Figure 172–2. A, Interrelationships of the tissue growth classes of normal cells. B, Interrelationships of neoplastic cells regarding proliferative capability.

regarding their growth and renewal characteristics. Tissues may be grouped as static, expanding, or renewing (Fig. 172–2A).[28] This classification separates highly differentiated tissues (static tissues such as nerves or striated muscle) that do not undergo mitosis from those with the capacity for mitosis. Tissues in the expanding group (organs and glands) can undergo mitosis with the proper stimulus. The renewing tissues are those with mitotically active cell populations and include leukocytes, erythrocytes, mucosa, epidermis, and gametes. This group of tissues with short half-lives is precisely the group of tissues most susceptible to the drug effects intended to kill neoplastic cells.[28]

Just as tissues can be grouped, cells within tissues can also be categorized. A cell may have stem cell potential, may be maturing, or may be functional. A stem cell is an undifferentiated cell found in tissue undergoing renewal. Stem cells can synthesize DNA and divide. One daughter cell remains a stem cell, whereas the other differentiates more fully.[33] Stem cells respond to stimuli such as hormones or possibly to chemical feedback from mature cells, which may stimulate or inhibit division. The loss of mature cells may cause the stem cell compartment to become more active. Neoplastic cells may be dividing, temporarily nondividing, or permanently nondividing.

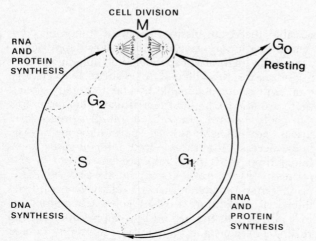

Figure 172–1. The cell cycle. See text for description of events and importance to chemotherapy.

The interrelationships of these three groups is shown in Figure 172–2B. In malignant neoplastic tissue, only a small proportion of the cells are differentiated. The remainder are dividing or retain the capacity to do so. In normal tissues, only a small proportion of the cells are dividing.[45]

In both normal and neoplastic cell populations, there are relatively more dividing cells in a small population and relatively fewer dividing cells in a large population. There is, then, a relationship between size and growth rate. Gompertzian growth refers to a growth pattern exhibiting increased doubling time and decreased growth fraction as a function of time.[19] The increase in doubling time is related to both the decreased proportion of proliferating cells and the increased cell loss from exfoliation, metastasis, and cell death. It is evident that the cytoreductive effects of surgery or radiation therapy can induce a renewed level of proliferative activity within a tumor and render the tumor more susceptible to chemotherapeutic attack as its constituent cells proceed around the cell cycle.

The emergence of resistance is related to the mutation rate of the genetically unstable neoplastic cells and to the tumor mass. The larger the number of tumor cells (tumor mass), the greater the number and proportion of resistant clones. Once such clones emerge, clinical resistance develops relatively rapidly; approximately 1.8 logs of growth (6 doublings) are required to go from a 95 per cent chance of no resistant cells to a less than 5 per cent chance of no resistant cells. Thus, there is a greater probability of success in treating micrometastatic disease or a small mass than a large tumor burden.[13a]

PHARMACOLOGICAL FACTORS IN CHEMOTHERAPY

To affect a tumor, the chemotherapeutic agent must reach the site of action. Its effectiveness is measured in terms of its concentration and exposure time at the site. The effective contact time, the product of drug concentration multiplied by drug exposure time, is affected by a number of important factors.[19] Route of administration and absorption may influence the efficacy of an administered drug. Chemotherapeutic agents may be administered orally, subcutaneously, intravenously, or intramuscularly for systemic effect. Local effect may be obtained by topical administration or introduction of the drug into the pleural cavity, peritoneal cavity, urinary bladder, or cerebrospinal fluid. All the drugs, however, cannot be given by every route. Proper selection of route of administration can help maximize efficacy and ease of administration. Biotransformation of the drug also needs to be considered. Prednisone is frequently included in chemotherapies but needs to be converted to prednisolone by the liver before it becomes an active drug. Cyclophosphamide is likewise metabolized by the liver to an active form and is therefore effective orally or parenterally but not when locally instilled.

Distribution of a drug partially determines its effectiveness. If the drug does not reach the tumor, its exposure will be nil and the neoplastic cells will be unaffected. The blood-brain barrier represents such a problem in distribution. Most chemotherapeutic agents will not gain access to the brain. Prednisone will enter the brain and is considered a potentially effective chemotherapeutic agent for brain tumors. The effect of tumors on the integrity of the blood-brain barrier is still open to question. Drugs normally excluded from the brain may enter the cancer-afflicted brain.

Once a drug has been properly administered, adequately absorbed, and biologically transformed into an active form as necessary, there are other pharmacological factors to be considered. Drug resistance, interactions, and toxicities all may affect the usefulness of a therapeutic agent. It is not unusual for the first trial of a drug to be beneficial and later trials to be much less so. Resistance to a drug may develop by several means. Such acquired resistance by the tumor may occur owing to decreased activation or increased deactivation of the drug, reducing its effective contact time. Resistance may also be related to impermeability of the tumor cell to the drug, shifts in enzyme specificity, increased repair of cytological lesions, or bypassing of inhibited reactions with alternate biochemical pathways.[19]

Patients may be receiving multiple drug therapy, including therapies directed at problems other than the tumor. The chemotherapeutic protocol itself may call for multiple drugs given simultaneously or sequentially. The potential for drug interaction is great. Such possibly harmful interactions may either decrease the effectiveness of a drug to nonbeneficial levels or increase its toxicity. Interactions may occur on several levels including direct chemical or physical interactions, interference with intestinal absorption, and altered renal excretion. Altered plasma transport mechanisms or altered receptor sites on the cell may cause drug interactions. In addition, some factors of cell resistance mentioned earlier may alter drug levels and lead to interactions.[19]

Chemotherapy treads a narrow path between efficacy and toxicity. In fact, chemotherapeutic protocols are most often limited not by the level of tumor cell killing but by toxicities to the patient. Recalling one of the biological bases for chemotherapy, i.e., that the proliferating neoplastic cells can be attacked most effectively as they pass around the cell cycle, will help explain some of the more commonly noted toxicities related to rapidly renewing cell classes. The most commonly encountered problems relate to gastrointestinal toxicity, bone marrow suppression, and immunosuppression.[19,27] Vomiting and anorexia may be noted as the gastrointestinal epithelium is affected. Although this problem is usually not life-threatening, it can be detrimental to the patient. Antiemetics may or may not be helpful. Other gastrointestinal toxicities seen less frequently include diarrhea, stomatitis, esophagitis, and peptic ulcer.[17]

Bone marrow toxicity leading to leukopenia and immune suppression affecting both humoral and cell-mediated immunity are two very serious problems associated with chemotherapy. Bone marrow toxicity may affect all the cellular components of the blood. Anemia and thrombocytopenia can be life-threatening, but leukopenia and the associated risk of infection are the primary and more common problems. Different chemotherapeutic agents cause different patterns of myelosuppression; some are more profound and persistent than others. Chemotherapy may need to be postponed until acceptable white blood cell numbers are again seen in the peripheral blood. Recommended leukocyte levels at which to postpone therapy vary.[19,22,33] One such guideline is 4,000 total white blood cells with at least 2,500 granulocytes. As veterinary chemotherapists use more intensive protocols in the future, these guidelines will almost certainly be amended to reflect both the acceptance of more myelosuppression (to gain an increased likelihood of cure) and improved methods of dealing with myelosuppression. Generally, chemotherapy can be re-instituted in one to two weeks based on a return to normal white blood cell parameters. When resuming chemotherapy, it is best to decrease the amount of the offending drug by 25 per cent.

The problems of immunosuppression tie in closely with bone marrow toxicity and myelosuppression. There is great variation in the amount of immunosuppression encountered with chemotherapy, and the clinician must be constantly aware of its dangers. The combination of reduced nonspecific immunity (myelosuppression) and impaired humoral and cell-mediated immunity can render the patient prone to serious, life-threatening infection with little or no means of defense. Fortunately, immunosuppression associated with chemotherapy usually does not last long beyond the time of drug administration. Nonetheless, chemotherapies should include as few immunosuppressive drugs as feasible without compromising the treatment.

Less common toxicities involve other body systems. Hemorrhagic cystitis associated with cyclophosphamide is a well-known complication that limits the prolonged use of that drug.[11] The bladder is not the only susceptible organ of the genitourinary system. The kidney is subject to damage from methotrexate, streptozotocin, *L*-asparaginase, and other chemotherapeutic agents. Sterility in males and congenital malformations are also possible complications. Skin reactions and alopecia are less frequent in veterinary medicine than in human medicine but do occur.[10] Clipped hair may not regrow or may regrow a different color. Wire-haired and curly-coated breeds seem more likely to develop alopecia. Cats may be more likely to have problems with alopecia

than dogs. The lung, liver, heart, and central nervous system are all subject to toxicity from various chemotherapeutic agents, although these manifestations are seen far less often than the others.

The list of possible complications of chemotherapy is long. It is ironic that anticancer drugs themselves may be mutagenic. Their increased use may reveal this to be a more serious problem than is currently appreciated.

A final pharmacological factor influencing chemotherapy, as it influences any drug usage, is excretion. Most antineoplastic drugs are excreted by the kidneys or liver; if these organs are not functioning adequately to rid the body of the drug, rapid accumulation may result in severe, perhaps unmanageable, toxicity. The amount of drug given or the dosage interval may need to be adjusted to compensate for impaired excretion.[1]

It is clear that just as the biological principles underlying chemotherapy intertwine, so do the pharmacological principles. The effects of administration, absorption, distribution, and biotransformation cannot be separated from those of drug interactions, resistance, toxicity, and excretion. They are all important in management by chemotherapy; it is equally important that the clinician understand what can realistically be expected of a chemotherapeutic protocol. This understanding will lay the groundwork for reasonable guidelines for chemotherapy.

Although patients may benefit from the use of a single chemotherapeutic drug, more often there are advantages to the use of multiple drugs in combination. Chemotherapeutic drugs kill a constant fraction of the tumor cells present independent of the total number of cells, and the fraction killed by one drug is independent of that killed by another. Drugs can be used in combination to specifically attack different portions of the cell cycle. Drugs can be chosen that have different major toxicities, thus limiting toxicity of any one type and allowing each drug to be used in a full dose. It is toxicity and not the ability to kill cancer cells that limits the ability to administer chemotherapy. Combination chemotherapy also helps avoid the problems of both inherent drug resistance and the emergence of resistant subpopulations due to acquired resistance.[9] Intermittent treatment schedules allow intensive attack on the neoplasm and a rest period for recovery of normal cells before the next treatment.[8] In theory, there should be added benefit from intensifying the chemotherapeutic attack when very small numbers of neoplastic cells remain. At the biochemical level, combinations may act by sequential, concurrent, or complementary inhibition,[19] and it may be possible to design protocols based on these drug interactions. However, it appears that, to date, the most successful combined regimens have been empirical in nature, employing drugs known to be individually active against the tumor.[8] There are many unanswered questions concerning not only the best combinations for any particular cancer but also how best to schedule chemotherapy in relation to surgery, radiotherapy, immunotherapy, and hyperthermia. A few principles of combination chemotherapy follow.

1. Use drugs known to be effective as single agents.
2. Use drugs with different mechanisms of action.
3. Use drugs with different toxicities.
4. Use an intermittent treatment schedule.

GUIDELINES FOR CHEMOTHERAPY

To use the principles of chemotherapy previously discussed safely and effectively, the clinician must satisfy certain guidelines.[9,23] A thorough history and physical examination along with an appropriate data base are necessary for chemotherapy. In all cases, a histological diagnosis of malignancy is imperative. An understanding of the biological behavior of the tumor aids in both prognosis and the selection of drugs with a known effect against the tumor. The clinician must also understand the drugs and their toxicities, which are often a limiting factor in chemotherapy. Toxic levels of drugs vary among species, and human dosages cannot always be adopted without modification. Safe dosage schedules for the species being treated should be used. Monitoring the toxicities associated with the treatment and evaluation of patient response follow hand in hand. Both are important to the proper management of chemotherapy. Monitoring toxicity to alter or limit treatment is needed for the well-being of the patient. The patient should be evaluated to judge the effect of the treatment on the disease as well as the recovery of the patient. No chemotherapy should be undertaken without the full understanding and cooperation of the owner concerning the goals of the therapy as well as the costs and the necessary commitment to regular follow up. Certainly not all owners will elect chemotherapy; some will opt for no therapy and some for euthanasia. Chemotherapy can, however, help extend the patient's happy, comfortable life in many instances. This is the primary consideration in offering chemotherapy as a realistic alternative in the management of neoplasia.

DRUGS USED IN CHEMOTHERAPY

Chemotherapeutic agents can be placed into broad classifications that help make them more easily understood, yet each drug has its own characteristics and peculiarities. A brief classification with comments on the mechanisms, indications, and toxicities of selected drugs (Table 172–1) should help the clinician provide effective, rational chemotherapy. Note that doses are expressed as mg per meter squared (body surface area) rather than mg per kg. This is a physiologically more accurate method of determining dosages of chemotherapeutic drugs.[20] Weight in grams is converted to body surface area in meters squared by a fractional exponential function

$$m^2 = \frac{Km \times W^{2/3}}{10^4}$$

where m^2 is the body surface area in square meters, W is the body weight in grams, and Km is a species-specific constant (10.1 for dogs, 10.0 for cats). Table 172–2 is a conversion table for dogs. The table is also applicable to domestic cats but is not appropriate for larger nondomestic cats.

Alkylating Agents

Alkylating agents are compounds that substitute an alkyl radical ($R–CH_2–CH_2^+$) for a hydrogen atom on some organic compounds. Alkylation causes breaks in the DNA molecule and crosslinking of the twin strands of DNA. This interferes with the DNA replication and RNA transcription.[18,28] There are five classes of alkylating agents: (1) nitrogen mustard derivatives: mechlorethamine, cyclophosphamide, chlorambucil, and melphalan; (2) ethenimine derivatives: triethylenethiophosphoramide; (3) alkyl sulfonates: busulfan; (4) triazene derivatives: dacarbazine; and (5) nitrosoureas: carmustine, lomustine and semustine. Most of these compounds contain more than one alkylating group and are considered polyfunctional alkylating agents. Dacarbazine and the nitrosoureas seem to have other mechanisms of cytotoxicity in addition to alkylating activity.[18] The alkylating agents are cell cycle phase nonspecific drugs. With the exception of dacarbazine and the nitrosoureas, resistance to one alkylating agent implies resistance to the others.

Cyclophosphamide is the most widely used alkylating agent in veterinary medicine. It has been employed for lymphoreticular neoplasia, various sarcomas and carcinomas, mast cell tumors, and transmissible venereal tumors both as a single agent and in combination with other drugs.[22,28] Cyclophosphamide requires activation to its active metabolite 4-hydroxycyclophosphamide by the liver microsomal mixed-function oxidase system and thus must be given by oral or intravenous routes. Its major dose-limiting toxicities are hematological and gastrointestinal. Leukopenia may be most severe within a week or two of administration, with recovery usually following within ten days. Anemia and thrombocytopenia are less common.[7,18]

A unique and important toxicity associated with cyclophosphamide is sterile hemorrhagic cystitis. Active metabolites of cyclophosphamide cause mucosal ulceration, necrosis of smooth muscle and small arteries, and hemorrhage and edema in the urinary bladder. The renal pelves may also be affected. The patient may show signs of hematuria, pollakiuria, and stranguria.[11] Early recognition of signs, diuresis, and

TABLE 172–1. Chemotherapeutic Agents Used in Veterinary Medicine

Name	Brand Name (Manufacturer)	Cell Cycle Specificity*	Possible Indications	Suggested Dosages	Toxicity
ALKYLATING AGENTS					
Cyclophosphamide	Cytoxan (Mead Johnson)	CCNS	Lymphoreticular neoplasms, mammary and lung carcinomas, miscellaneous sarcomas	50 mg/m² PO or IV four days per week	Leukopenia, anemia, thrombocytopenia (less common), nausea, vomiting, sterile hemorrhagic cystitis
Chlorambucil	Leukeran (Burroughs Wellcome)	CCNS	Lymphoreticular neoplasms, chronic lymphocyte leukemia	2 mg/m² PO two to four days per week	Mild leukopenia, thrombocytopenia, anemia, nausea, vomiting (not common)
Nitrogen mustard	Mustragen (Merck Sharp & Dohme)	CCNS	Lymphoreticular neoplasms	5 mg/m² IV	Leukopenia, thrombocytopenia, nausea, vomiting, anorexia
Triethylenethio-phosphoramide	Thio-TEPA (Lederle)	CCNS	Various carcinomas and sarcomas	9 mg/m² as a single dose or divided over two to four days (60 mg in 60 ml water for bladder instillation, 30 minutes per week)	Leukopenia, thrombocytopenia, anemia
Busulfan	Myleran (Burroughs Wellcome)	CCNS	Granulocytic leukemias, myeloproliferative disorders	3 to 4 mg/m² PO daily	Leukopenia, thrombocytopenia, anemia
Melphalan	Alkeran (Burroughs Wellcome)	CCNS	Multiple myeloma, monoclonal gammopathies, lymphoreticular neoplasms	1.5 mg/m² PO for seven to ten days, repeat cycle	Leukopenia, thrombocytopenia, anemia, anorexia, nausea, vomiting
Dacarbazine	DTIC (Dome Laboratories)	CCNS	Malignant melanoma, various sarcomas	200 mg/m² IV for five days every three weeks	Leukopenia, thrombocytopenia, anemia, nausea, vomiting, diarrhea (often decreases with later cycles)

Drug	Trade name (Manufacturer)	Class	Indications	Dose	Toxicity
Lomustine	CeeNU (Bristol)	CCNS	Various carcinomas, lymphosarcoma	100 mg/m² PO every six weeks	Leukopenia, thrombocytopenia (both develop in three to six weeks), nausea, vomiting (transient)
ANTIMETABOLITES					
Methotrexate	Methotrexate (Lederle)	S	Lymphoreticular neoplasms, myeloproliferative disorders, various carcinomas and sarcomas	2.5 mg/m² PO daily	Leukopenia, thrombocytopenia, anemia, stomatitis, diarrhea, hepatopathy, renal tubular necrosis
6-Mercaptopurine	Purinethol (Burroughs Wellcome)	S	Lymphosarcoma, acute lymphocytic leukemia, granulocytic leukemia	50 mg/m² PO daily until response or toxicity	Leukopenia, nausea, vomiting, hepatopathy
5-Fluorouracil	Fluorouracil (Roche Laboratories)	S	Various carcinomas and sarcomas	200 mg/m² IV weekly	Leukopenia, thrombocytopenia, anemia, anorexia, nausea, vomiting, diarrhea, stomatitis
	Efudex Cream (Roche Laboratories)		Cutaneous tumors	Apply twice daily for two to four weeks	
Cytosine arabinoside	Cytosar-U (Upjohn)	S	Lymphosarcoma, myeloproliferative disorders	100 mg/m² SQ or IV drip for four days	Leukopenia, thrombocytopenia, anemia, nausea, vomiting, anorexia
PLANT ALKALOIDS					
Vincristine	Oncovin (Eli Lilly)	M	Transmissible venereal tumor, lymphosarcoma	0.5 mg/m² IV weekly	Peripheral neuropathy, paresthesia, constipation
Vinblastine	Velban (Eli Lilly)	M	Lymphosarcoma, various carcinomas	2.5 mg/m² IV weekly	Leukopenia, nausea, vomiting
ANTIBIOTICS					
Doxorubicin	Adriamycin (Adria Laboratories)	CCNS	Lymphosarcoma, osteogenic sarcoma, various carcinomas and sarcomas	30 mg/m² IV every three weeks (do not exceed 240 mg/m² total)	Leukopenia, thrombocytopenia, nausea, vomiting, cardiac toxicity, reactions during administration

Table continued on following page

TABLE 172–1. Chemotherapeutic Agents Used in Veterinary Medicine *Continued*

Name	Brand Name (Manufacturer)	Cell Cycle Specificity*	Possible Indications	Suggested Dosages	Toxicity
ANTIBIOTICS *Continued*					
Actinomycin D	Cosmegen (Merck Sharp & Dohme)	CCNS	Lymphosarcoma, various carcinomas and sarcomas	1.5 mg/m² IV weekly	Thrombocytopenia, leukopenia, stomatitis, proctitis, nausea, vomiting
Bleomycin	Blenoxane (Bristol Laboratories)	CCNS (G_1, S, and M)	Squamous cell carcinomas, other carcinomas	10 mg/m² IV or SQ for three to nine days, then 10 mg/m² IV weekly (do not exceed 200 mg/m² total)	Allergic reactions following administration, pulmonary fibrosis
HORMONES					
Prednisolone		NA	Lymphoreticular neoplasms, mast cell tumors, CNS tumors	Vary widely depending on indication: 60 mg/m² PO daily to 20 mg/m² PO every 48 hours	Hyperadrenocorticism, secondary adrenocortical insufficiency
Diethylstilbestrol		NA	Perianal adenomas, prostatic neoplasms (adjunctively)	1.1 mg/kg IM once (do not administer more than 25 mg) or 1 mg PO every 72 hours	Bone marrow toxicity, feminization
MISCELLANEOUS					
L-Asparaginase	Elspar (Merck Sharp & Dohme)	NA	Lymphoreticular neoplasma	20,000 units per m² IP weekly	Anaphylaxis, leukopenia
o, p-DDD	Lysodren (Calbiochem)	NA	Adrenocortical tumors	50 mg/kg PO daily to effect, then 50 mg/kg PO every 7 to 14 days PRN	Adrenocortical insufficiency

*Notes: CCNS = cell cycle phase nonspecific; S = S phase specific; M = M-phase specific; NA = not applicable.

TABLE 172–2. Conversion Table of Weight in Kilograms to Body Surface Area in Square Meters for Dogs

kg	m²	kg	m²
0.5	0.06	26.0	0.88
1.0	0.10	27.0	0.90
2.0	0.15	28.0	0.92
3.0	0.20	29.0	0.96
4.0	0.25	30.0	0.96
5.0	0.29	31.0	0.99
6.0	0.33	32.0	1.01
7.0	0.36	33.0	1.03
8.0	0.40	34.0	1.05
9.0	0.43	35.0	1.07
10.0	0.46	36.0	1.09
11.0	0.49	37.0	1.11
12.0	0.52	38.0	1.13
13.0	0.55	39.0	1.15
14.0	0.58	40.0	1.17
15.0	0.60	41.0	1.19
16.0	0.63	42.0	1.21
17.0	0.66	43.0	1.23
18.0	0.69	44.0	1.25
19.0	0.71	45.0	1.26
20.0	0.74	46.0	1.28
21.0	0.76	47.0	1.30
22.0	0.78	48.0	1.32
23.0	0.81	49.0	1.34
24.0	0.83	50.0	1.36
25.0	0.85		

cessation of cyclophosphamide administration help limit the problem in most cases. Some cases may be persistent and require more aggressive therapy, such as the instillation of a 1% formalin solution into the bladder.[43] Measures helpful in avoiding cyclophosphamide-associated sterile hemorrhagic cystitis include (1) not administering cyclophosphamide to a patient with concurrent cystitis or hematuria; (2) administering the daily dose in the morning and providing free access to fresh water at all times as well as ample opprtunity to urinate; and (3) being certain the patient urinates before the owners retire for the night. Gastrointestinal and dermatological toxicities may sometimes be seen and may require dosage adjustment.

Chlorambucil is often used in chemotherapy of canine lymphosarcoma as a replacement for cyclophosphamide, either in maintenance regimens or when myelosuppression or sterile hemorrhagic cystitis has been a problem. Although chlorambucil acts more slowly than cyclophosphamide and seems to have less myelosuppressive toxicity, regular monitoring of white blood cell parameters is warranted. Triethylenethiophosphoramide has been used in the therapy of mammary, prostatic, and other carcinomas. Because it can be given by the intracavitary as well as intravenous route, triethylenethiophosphoramide has also been employed in the therapy of transitional cell carcinoma of the urinary bladder, ovarian carcinoma, and malignant pleural effusions. Melphalan appears to be most useful in multiple myeloma but has also been of some use in lymphoreticular neoplasia, mammary and lung carcinomas, and osteogenic sarcoma.[22,28]

Antimetabolites

The antimetabolites are structural analogues of normal metabolites required for cell function and replication. They damage cells by interacting with cell enzymes (1) by substituting for a metabolite needed in a key molecule, rendering it functionally abnormal; (2) by competing successfully with a normal metabolite for the catalytic site of a key enzyme; or (3) by competing with a normal metabolite that acts at an enzyme regulatory site to alter the catalytic rate of a key enzyme.[18]

The antimetabolites are S phase–specific drugs. They are highly schedule dependent, and many questions remain unanswered regarding their best use.[7,18]

Methotrexate acts in S phase to inhibit dihydrofolate reductase competitively and interferes with both DNA and RNA synthesis.[18,28] This folic acid antagonist has been used in the therapy of lymphoreticular neoplasms and myeloproliferative disorders as well as metastatic transitional cell tumor, transmissible venereal tumor, Sertoli cell tumor, and osteogenic sarcoma.[22,28] Methotrexate toxicity to the bone marrow and gastrointestinal tract can be severe; with high-dose regimens, appropriately timed "rescue" may be achieved by administering citrovorum factor (folinic acid), the specific antidote. More commonly in veterinary medicine, methotrexate is given in a low-dose regimen that is far less toxic and does not require "rescue." [28]

The purine analogue 6-mercaptopurine (6-MP) interferes with purine synthesis and interconversion and has been used in the therapy of lymphocytic and granulocytic leukemias.[28] Useful pyrimidine analogues include 5-fluorouracil and cytosine arabinoside. 5-Fluorouracil inhibits thimidylate synthetase and interferes with DNA synthesis. It also blocks uracil phosphatase and inhibits utilization of preformed uracil in RNA.[18] 5-Fluorouracil has been used in the therapy of various carcinomas. Its major toxicities are hematological and gastrointestinal[7,28] It should not be used in cats because of severe neurotoxicity. Cytosine arabinoside blocks DNA synthesis by inhibiting DNA polymerase, blocking conversion of cytodine to dioxycytodine. In addition to this S phase action, cytosine arabinoside also blocks the progression of cells from G_1 to S.[7] Administration by the subcutaneous route or by slow intravenous drip over a prolonged period may thus be beneficial in the recruitment and synchronization of neoplastic cells. Myelosuppression is the major dose-limiting toxicity, although gastrointestinal signs ranging from anorexia to vomiting may be observed.[7]

Plant Alkaloids

Vincristine and vinblastine are alkaloids extracted from the periwinkle plant, *Vinca rosea*.[35] They act specifically in M phase by binding with the microtubular protein tubulin and blocking mitosis by interfering with chromosomal separation in metaphase. Although vincristine and vinblastine share a common mechanism of action, resistance to one does not imply resistance to the other.[18] They also have different major toxicities. Vincristine affects the nervous system. Paresthesia, loss of deep tendon reflexes, and sensory neuropathy are more easily assessed in human patients than animal patients. Lymphoid hypoplasia and constipation are more frequent veterinary complications.[35] Vinblastine toxicity is primarily hematological. Myelosuppression may be a severe problem.[7] Both drugs have been used in the treatment of lymphoreticular neoplasms. Vincristine is the treatment of choice for transmissible venereal tumor and has been used for various sarcomas and carcinomas.[4,22,38] Vinblastine has been used in the treatment of carcinomas and mast cell tumors.[22,28]

Antibiotics

The antitumor antibiotics, like the plant alkaloids, are natural products. They are derived from various strains of the soil fungus *Streptomyces*. They are cytotoxic, cell cycle phase nonspecific drugs, that damage DNA by binding (intercalating) DNA and inhibiting DNA or RNA synthesis.[18] Doxorubicin has been the most frequently used member of this class of cytotoxic drugs in veterinary medicine. It has important hematological, gastrointestinal, and cardiac toxicities. Although signs of gastrointestinal upset, vomiting, and diarrhea can usually be managed symptomatically and supportively, myelosuppression may be a dose-limiting problem in the short term.[7] Cumulative cardiac toxicity results in a dose-related cardiomyopathy. All patients receiving doxorubicin should have initial chest radiographs and an electrocardiogram. An electrocardiogram should precede each treatment, and therapy should be discontinued if abnormalities such as decreased size of QRS complexes, premature ventricular contractions, or any arrhythmias develop. Dosages should be reduced if hepatic damage develops. Doxorubicin must be administered slowly through a free-flowing intravenous line. Patient restlessness, facial swelling, or head shaking may signal excessively rapid administration. If these signs are seen, administration should be stopped temporarily and started at a slower rate when signs abate. Pretreatment with antihistamines may help avoid some of these complications. Despite its apparently numerous drawbacks, doxorubicin has had wide application in the treatment of canine lymphosarcoma as both a first line and a salvage drug. It has also been used for various carcinomas and sarcomas with limited success.[22,28]

Bleomycin has had limited use in squamous cell carcinoma of animal patients. Although it is not a myelosuppressive drug, pulmonary fibrosis may be a lethal complication in some patients.[28]

Hormones

The potential for hormonal intervention in neoplasia is great. Unlike other chemotherapeutic agents, hormones are not primarily cytotoxic drugs and are therefore less toxic to the patient. Hormonal agents are more selective than cytotoxic drugs in their actions.[36] Peptide hormones interact with cell membrane–bound nucleotide cyclase systems such as those that convert adenosine triphosphate (ATP) to cyclic adenosine monophosphate (cAMP). cAMP acts as a "second messenger" to deliver and amplify regulatory signals to intracellular sites. Steroid hormones enter the cells and bind to a specific receptor protein. "Transformation" ("activation") of this newly formed complex allows it to pass the nuclear membranes, where it binds to DNA. This binding alters the transcription of the cell's messenger RNA, resulting in synthesis of new protein. Steroid-induced increases in free fatty acids may cause dissolution of the nuclear membrane, leading to cell death.[7,23,29]

Adrenal corticosteroids have important clinical uses in the therapy of lymphosarcoma and mast cell tumors and may be of benefit in the therapy of central nervous system neoplasms because of their ability to cross the blood-brain barrier. Their beneficial actions in other solid tumors probably relate more to anti-inflammatory effects than to direct antitumor effects.

Sex hormones have been used in the treatment of hormone-dependent tumors of mammary, prostatic, or perianal gland origin. Hormonal therapy may be supplemental or ablative. With increasing availability of estrogen receptor analysis, rational hormonal therapy of mammary gland tumors will become likely.[36] Currently, antiestrogenic therapy remains experimental. Hormones also have a valuable role as replacement therapy following ablative surgery, in the management of some metastatic problems, and in dealing with paraneoplastic syndromes such as hypercalcemia and anemia.[36]

Miscellaneous Agents

A number of other drugs that do not easily fall into any of the previously mentioned categories have also been used to treat animal cancers.

L-Asparaginase is an enzyme preparation derived from a variety of bacteria. By hydrolyzing asparagine to aspartic acid and ammonia, L-asparaginase deprives neoplastic cells that lack the ability to synthesize L-asparagine of extracellular sources, thereby rapidly inhibiting protein synthesis. L-Asparaginase acts against cells in G_1.[7,18] It has been used in the therapy of canine lymphoreticular neoplasms.[28] Anaphylaxis has been the most dangerous side effect. Other toxicities include gastrointestinal disturbances, hepatotoxicity, hemorrhagic pancreatitis, and coagulation defects.[7]

The cell cycle nonspecific drug o,p-DDD directly suppresses both normal and neoplastic adrenocortical cells.[7] With proper management, o,p-DDD may be beneficial in patients with inoperable adrenocortical carcinoma as well as patients with adrenocortical hyperplasia secondary to a pituitary neoplasm.[18] In addition to careful monitoring for impending hypoadrenocorticism, the clinician must be aware of toxic manifestations including vomiting, diarrhea, and depression.[7] Aminoglutethimide inhibits the enzymatic conversion of cholesterol to pregnenolone and blocks adrenal steroidogenesis. It may find use in the treatment of adrenal tumors, ectopic ACTH-secreting tumors, and adrenocortical hyperplasia. Reported toxicities include a macular pruritic rash, which appears early in treatment and may regress spontaneously, and central nervous system disturbances including lethargy, ataxia, and nystagmus.[7]

Streptozotocin is a cell cycle phase nonspecific antibiotic derived from *Streptomyces achromogenes*. It is able to inhibit DNA synthesis, NAD, NADH, and enzymes important in gluconeogenesis.[18] Streptozotocin has been suggested for use in the treatment of islet cell carcinoma but has generally been deemed too toxic for use in the dog.[28]

Platinum complexes have been shown to have tumoricidal activity; *cis*-dichlorodiammineplatinum is a cell cycle phase nonspecific drug that inhibits DNA synthesis and has some alkylating activity. It has been used in human medicine for testicular, ovarian, and bladder carcinoma. It causes nausea and vomiting, which may be severe and prolonged. Renal insufficiency is usually the dose-limiting toxicity, but myelosuppression may also be a problem.[18] Its routine use in veterinary medicine is not warranted at this time.

Of the drugs available to treat cancer, it is not clear that the best use of any single drug—let alone the best drug combination or multimodality therapy—has been clearly established for any neoplasm. An understanding of the drugs available for use and their mechanisms, indications, and toxicities will help the clinician provide rational chemotherapy.

PREDICTORS OF CHEMOTHERAPEUTIC RESPONSE

It is evident from the foregoing discussion that, although much information is available regarding biological and pharmacological bases for chemotherapy and the drugs themselves, successful chemotherapy protocols are often empirical in nature. However, chemotherapeutic agents are not chosen at random. The development of a new drug involves a rigorous, stringent process. Each new drug must undergo preclinical toxicity studies before entering Phase I, II, and III clinical trials and becoming available for general use.[25] Even this protocol for drug development does not assure clinical success for any tumor type and certainly not for any individual case. There is great interest and value in developing a predictive test for chemotherapeutic response similar to culture and sensitivity testing for bacterial diseases. There are several intriguing possibilities. Biochemical tests to assess enzyme levels in neoplastic cells may be of some value in predicting responsiveness to cytosine arabinoside, 5-fluorouracil, 6-mercaptopurine, and L-asparaginase,[24] but these tests are currently of no real significance to the practitioner.

The cloning of tumor cells in soft agar is already an important research tool, and drug sensitivity as measured by stem cell assay may also have clinical application.[14,38,39] A positive predictive ability of about 65 per cent and a negative predictive ability of about 90 per cent are encouraging.[6] A limited number of canine mammary gland tumors have been successfully cloned and tested for drug sensitivity on an experimental basis.[37] The rate at which neoplastic cells take up tridiated thymidine has also been used to predict response to chemotherapy.[5,31] Techniques to grow tumor xenografts in the subrenal capsule of normal mice may prove to be valuable predictors of chemotherapeutic response.[3] Comparisons of various predictive techniques of cell killing indicate that clonogenic assays are the most efficient predictors of response available.[2,34] However, practical problems, such as low plating efficiency, adequate identification of colonies, and *in vitro* pharmacology, will delay the adoption of clonogenic assays as a routine procedure.[41] Such assays may ultimately have their greatest value as screening tests for new drugs and as a staging procedure to detect malignant cells in bone marrow.[42]

Estrogen receptor analysis has been a significant predictor of response in human breast cancer.[6] Estrogen receptors have been identified in mammary carcinomas of cats[15] and in several types of mammary tumors of dogs,[16,30] but no clear strategy for hormonal intervention in mammary neoplasia in veterinary medicine has yet been defined.

Nonetheless, the clinician may be able to prognose with some accuracy on several bases. A histological diagnosis provides a beginning.[22] With that information in hand, knowledge of the biological behavior of the tumor helps predict response. The larger the tumor burden, the greater the number of residual tumor cells and resistant tumor cells that will remain after first-order kinetic tumor cell kill. Larger tumors are also more likely to have more profound metabolic effects on the host that are likely to limit its ability to tolerate chemotherapy.[26] Note that these factors are consistent with the principles and guidelines for therapy previously discussed. The distribution of metastases may also affect response. However, rapidly growing tumors should theoretically be more amenable to chemotherapeutic intervention with S phase–specific drugs.[26] To some extent, clinical parameters are quantitated by staging the tumor. Staging is a technique of describing the extent of a neoplastic process in terms of the primary tumor, lymph node involvement, and metastatic spread at a given time. Staging protocols are available for animal tumors,[32] and their expanded use will undoubtedly contribute valuable information.[44]

CONCLUSION

Chemotherapy has progressed tremendously in the past 40 years but is still in its infancy in veterinary medicine. An understanding of the biological and pharmacological principles underlying chemotherapy, the chemotherapeutic agents, and the potentials and limitations of drug therapy will enhance the delivery of appropriate therapy. The near future will present promising new therapeutic and prognostic options for a very vexing problem for the clinician.

1. Bennett, W. M., et al.: Guidelines for drug therapy in renal failure. Ann. Intern. Med.86:754, 1977.
2. Bhuyan, B. K., Loughman, B. E., Fraser, T. J., et al.: Comparison of different methods of determining cell viability after exposure to cytotoxic compounds. Exp. Cell Res. 97:275, 1976.
3. Bogden, A. E., Cobb, W. R., Le Page, D., et al.: Chemotherapy responsiveness of human tumors as first transplant generation xenographs in the normal mouse. Cancer 48:10, 1981.
4. Brown, N. O., MacEwen, E. G., and Calvert, C.: Follow-up on chemotherapy of venereal tumors. J. Am. Vet. Med. Assoc. 177:676, 1980.
5. Burns, C. P., Armentrout, S. A. and Stjernholm, R. L.: Prediction of the response of patients with acute nonlymphocytic leukemia to cytosine arabinoside (NSC-63878) therapy. Cancer Chemother. Rep. 56:527, 1972.
6. Carter, S. K.: Predictors of response and their clinical evaluation. Cancer Chemother. Pharmacol. 7:1, 1981.
7. Carter, S. K., and Livingston, R. B.: Drugs available to treat cancer. In Carter, S. K., Glatstein, E., and Livingston, R. B. (eds.): Principles of Cancer Treatment. McGraw-Hill, New York, 1981.
8. Carter, S. K., and Livingston, R. B.: Principles of cancer chemotherapy. In Carter, S. K,., Glatstein, E., and Livingston, R. B. (eds): Principles of Cancer Treatment. McGraw-Hill, New York, 1981.
9. Chabner, B. A.: The role of drugs in cancer treatment. In Chabner, B. A. (ed).,: Pharmacologic Principles of Cancer Treatment. W. B. Saunders, Philadelphia, 1982.
10. Conroy, J. D.: The etiology and pathogenesis of alopecia. Comp. Cont. Ed. 1:806, 1979.
11. Crow, S. E., Theilen, G. H., et al.: Cyclophosphamide-induced cystitis in the dog and cat. J. Am. Vet. Med. Assoc. 171:259, 1977.
12. DeVita, V. T.: Principles of cancer therapy. In Thorn, G. W., et al. (eds.): Harrison's Principles of Internal Medicine, 8th ed. McGraw-Hill, New York, 1977.
13. Fidler, I. J.: General concepts of tumor metastasis in the dog and cat. J. Am. Anim. Hosp. Assoc. 12:374, 1976.
13a. Goldie, J. H., and Coldman, A. J.: A mathematical model for relating the drug sensitivity of tumors to their spontaneous mutation rate. Can. Trt. Rep. 63:1727, 1979.
14. Hamburger, A. W., and Salmon, S. E.: Primary bioassay of human tumor stem cells. Science 197:461, 1977.
15. Hamilton, J. M., Else, R. W., and Forshaw, P.: Oestrogen receptors in feline mammary carcinomas. Vet. Rec. 99:477, 1976.
16. Hamilton, J. M., Else, R. W., and Forshaw, P.: Oestrogen receptors in canine mammary tumors. Vet. Rec. 101:258,1977.
17. Harris, J. B.: Nausea, vomiting and cancer treatment. CA 28:194, 1977.
18. Haskell, C. M.: Drugs used in cancer chemotherapy. In Haskell, C. M. (ed.): Cancer Treatment, W. B. Saunders, Philadelphia, 1980.
19. Haskell, C. M.: Principles of cancer chemotherapy. In Haskell, C. M. (ed.): Cancer Treatment, W. B. Saunders, Philadelphia, 1980.
20. Henness, A. M., Theilen, G. H., Madewell, B. R., et al.: Use of drugs based on square meters of body surface area. J. Am Vet. Med. Assoc. 171:1076, 1977.
21. Hess, P. W.: Cancer chemotherapy. In Kirk, R. W. (ed.): Current Veterinary Therapy VI. W. B. Saunders, Philadelphia, 1977.
22. Hess, P. W.: Principles of cancer chemotherapy. Vet. Clin. North Am. 7:21, 1977.
23. Hess, P. W., MacEwen, E. G., and McClelland, A. J.: Chemotherapy of canine and feline tumors. J. Am. Anim. Hosp. Assoc. 12:350, 1976.
24. Kessel, D., and Hall, T. C.: Biochemical predictive tests. In Holland, J. E., and Frei, E., III (eds.): Cancer Medicine, 2nd ed. Lea & Febiger, Philadelphia, 1982.
25. Livingston, R. B., and Carter, S. K.: Experimental design and clinical trials: clinical perspectives. In Carter, S. K., Glatstein, E., and Livingston, R. B. (eds): Principles of Cancer Treatment. McGraw-Hill, New York, 1981.
26. Lokich, J. J.: Predicting tumor response to cytotoxic therapy. Hosp. Prac. 15:74, 1980.
27. MacEwen, E. G.: Cancer chemotherapy. In Kirk, R. W. (ed.): Current Veterinary Therapy VII. W. B. Saunders, Philadelphia, 1980.
28. Madewell, B. R., and Theilen, G. H.: Chemotherapy. In Theilen, G. H., and Madewell, B. R. (eds.): Veterinary Cancer Medicine. Lea & Febiger, Philadelphia, 1979.

29. Meyers, F. H., Jawetz, E., and Goldfein, A.: The adrenocortical steroids. *In* Meyers, F. H., Jawetz, E., and Goldfein, A. (eds.): *Review of Medical Pharmacology*, 6th ed. CA, Lange Medical Publications, Los Altos, 1978.
30. Monson, B. S., Malbica, J. O., and Hubben, K.: Determination of estrogen receptors in canine mammary tumors. Am. J. Vet. Res. 38:1937, 1977.
31. Murphy, W. K., Livingston, R. B., Riuz, V. G., et al.: Serial labeling index determination as a predictor of response on human solid tumors. Cancer Res. 35:1438, 1975.
32. Owen, L. N. (ed). *T.N.M. Classification of Tumors in Domestic Animals*. W.H.O., Geneva, 1981.
33. Pierce, G. B., and Fennell, R. H., Jr.: Pathology. *In* Holland, J. F., and Frei, E., III (eds.): *Cancer Medicine*, 2nd ed. Lea & Febiger, Philadelphia, 1982.
34. Roper, P. R., and Drewinko, B.: Comparison of *in vitro* methods to determine drug-induced cell lethality. Cancer Res. 36:2182, 1976.
35. Rosenthal, R. C.: Clinical applications of *vinca* alkaloids. J. Am. Vet. Med. Assoc. 179:1084, 1981.
36. Rosenthal, R. C.: Hormones in cancer therapy. Vet. Clin. North Am. 12:67, 1982.
37. Rosenthal, R. C., and Leinen, J.: Unpublished data, 1982.
38. Salmon, S. E. (ed.): *Cloning of Human Tumor Stem Cells*. Alan R. Liss, Inc., New York, 1981.
39. Salmon, S. E., Hamburger, A. W., Soehnlen, B., et al.: Quantitation of differential sensitivity of human tumor stem cells to anticancer drugs. N. Engl. J. Med. 298:1321, 1978.
40. Schabel, F. M.: The use of tumor growth kinetics in planning "curative" chemotherapy of advanced solid tumors. Cancer Res. 29:2384, 1969.
41. Selby, P., Buick, R. N., and Tannock, I.: A critical appraisal of the "human tumor stem-cell assay." N. Engl. J. Med. 308:129, 1983.
42. Von Hoff, D. D.: "Send this patient's tumor for culture and sensitivity." N. Engl. J. Med. 308:154, 1983.
43. Weller, R. E.: Intravesical instillation of dilute formation for treatment of cyclophosphamide-induced hemorrhagic cystitis in two dogs. J. Am. Vet. Med. Assoc. 172:1206, 1978.
44. Weller, R. E., Theilen, G. H., and Madewell, B. R.: Chemotherapeutic responses in dogs with lymphosarcoma and hypercalcemia. J. Am. Vet. Med. Assoc. 181:891, 1982.
45. Yoxall, A. T., and Hind, J. E. R. (eds.): Veterinary applications of the pharmacology of neoplasia. *In Pharmacological Basis of Small Animal Medicine*. Blackwell Scientific Publications, London, 1975.

Chapter **173** Cryosurgery

William D. Liska

Cryosurgery (Greek *kryos* = cold) may be defined as the surgical use of freezing temperatures. With neoplastic disease, the desired effect in most situations is the tissue necrosis that results from freezing. Occasionally cold temperatures are used to manipulate tissues that have adhered to frozen metallic probes. Conventional surgery and electrosurgery are often performed concurrently with but are not necessary parts of cryosurgery. As with any technique, cryosurgery has definite advantages, disadvantages, indications, and contraindications. A thorough understanding of the basic principles and proper technique is very important. Cryosurgery is most commonly used when dealing with anorectal, oral, dermatological, or ophthalmological surgical disease. Neoplasia is the most common specific indication.

DEVELOPMENT

Modern cryosurgery requires sustained freezing temperatures. The earliest clinical reports of the use of cryosurgery in the management of neoplastic disease are from the mid 1800s. Ice and brine solutions were applied to human breast and skin tumors by James Arnott in London. He was probably frustrated by inadequate equipment and an inability to reach adequately low temperatures. In the late 1800s, devices using ether and air evaporation, dry ice, and liquified air kept the interest in cryosurgery alive but were still not very practical.

Liquid nitrogen production led to modern cryosurgery. Initially in the mid 1900s, cotton swabs were dipped in liquid nitrogen and placed on the lesion to be frozen. Fairly reliable results were obtained for small superficial lesions. Cooper and Lee developed a cryosurgery machine in New York in 1961.[60] Liquid nitrogen was circulated through a hollow metal probe tip. The probe was applied to the basal ganglion in the thalamus to produce selectively localized necrosis in the treatment of Parkinson's disease. Their neurosurgical technique has been greatly expanded with present day technology. Today computerized scanners with a three-coordinate system can guide probe tips mechanically to deep CNS lesions and tumors that are inaccessible by conventional means.

A considerable amount of clinical, experimental, and technical cryosurgical literature has been published since the early 1960s.[16] Superspecialties have been developed in cryobiology, cryopreservation, and cryodestruction, and the clinical application of cryosurgery is now commonplace.

Cryosurgery first appeared in the veterinary literature in the early 1970s with reports from England published by Borthwick,[2] Lane and Burch,[39,40] and Robbins and Lane.[49] In the mid 1970s, general cryosurgical articles were published in the United States by Withrow, Greiner, and Liska[19,55] and Goldstein and Hess.[17,18] Since then, general and specific information has been published dealing with both companion[19,36,48,51,52,55,58] and food animals.[10,11,14,34,38]

CRYOBIOLOGY

Cryobiology, the study of life at subfreezing temperatures, is divided into two categories—cryonecrosis and cryopreservation.[1,12] Both of these opposing disciplines are important to veterinary medicine. For years, it has been possible to preserve cells such as sperm *in vitro* for long periods at very low temperatures. Tissue and organ preservation for future transplantation is feasible and of clinical interest. Organ preservation is particularly difficult, because different tissue types exist in the same structure.[35]

Cryosurgeons and oncologists use the principles of cryonecrosis to destroy tissue. Making logical decisions about equipment and case selection, technique, and aftercare of the patient is easier if the basic concepts of cryonecrosis are understood. Cell death during cryonecrosis occurs as the result of direct and indirect injury.

Direct Injury

Cell death from freezing is a direct result of ice crystal formation, intracellular fluid and electrolyte disturbances, denaturation of cell membranes, and thermal shock. These factors act dynamically to cause overwhelming cellular pathology.[33,50]

Intracellular and extracellular water forms ice crystals when tissue freezes. The intracellular crystals rupture cell membranes and organelles, disrupting their function. In addition, the formation of ice crystals essentially dehydrates the cells, causing severe intracellular hyperosmolarity. Metabolic enzyme systems and membrane homeostatic mechanisms are adversely affected by the lethal toxic concentrations of electrolytes.

The rate at which tissue is frozen and allowed to thaw affects how lethal the freezing will be. Intracellular dehydration becomes more severe with rapid freezing than with slow freezing. However, rapid freezing results in the formation of small ice crystals, which are physically less disruptive than large ice crystals. These small crystals convert into large crystals (recrystalization) if the tissue is allowed to thaw slowly. Therefore, in clinical use, the most practical approach for maximal cellular destruction is to freeze the tissue as rapidly as possible and allow it to thaw slowly (rapid freeze–slow thaw cycle). Mitochondria are particularly susceptible to rapid freezing compared with slow freezing.

Rapid freezing is best achieved by using a potent cryogen, e.g., liquid nitrogen. In a clinical setting, the surgeon need not worry about freezing too fast. Slow thawing means nothing more than allowing ice crystals in the frozen tissue to melt from warming by ambient temperatures and adjacent blood circulation. Tissue and cell water content determines susceptibility to freezing and ice crystal formation. Cells with high water content are more susceptible than dehydrated tissue. This is advantageous, since plump and well-hydrated neoplastic cells are often targets. Freezing denatures cellular lipoprotein complexes. This has a profound effect on cellular homeostasis. Cell membrane permeability is altered, lysosomal enzymes are released, and energy production is inadequate.

Cryoshock is probably the least important direct effect. Enzyme systems and active transport mechanisms are most efficient at normal body temperatures. Even small alterations in body temperature are known for their potential adverse consequences unless performed and reversed under a well-monitored controlled setting. Cryoshock is the result of ultrasevere local hypothermia. No effort is made to reverse the process; therefore, it contributes to cell death. Some cell types, such as spermatozoa, are not sensitive to cryoshock.

Indirect Injury

Vascular stasis develops in the frozen tissue secondary to destruction caused by freezing. The greatest destruction occurs at the capillary level. Thrombosis and infarction are the results of endothelial damage, erythrocyte clumping, alterations in permeability, platelet aggregation, and activation of the clotting mechanism. The resultant ischemia leads to anoxia and death. Vascular collapse is complete in approximately 20 minutes postoperatively.

CRYOGENS

The cryogen is the gas or liquid used to extract heat from the tissue to be frozen. Special instrumentation[5] is necessary to contain the cryogen and to apply it to the lesion. A large number of substances[5,33] could be chosen as cryogens, but few have practical use. Ideally, a cryogen is nonflammable, nontoxic, noncorrosive to metal, easily handled and stored, and inexpensive and has a very low boiling point. A comparison of cryogen temperatures is listed in Table 173–1.

Liquid nitrogen is the best cryogen for general use in veterinary medicine. It is colorless, odorless, nontoxic, and very cold ($-196°C$). By itself it adds little to the overall cost of the procedure. It is available through most medical, welding, and industrial gas sources. For economy, it should be purchased in bulk volume (over 20 liters) and stored in a pressur-

TABLE 173–1. Potential Cryogens for Cryosurgery

Cryogen	Temperature
Freon	$-60°C$ or warmer
Carbon dioxide (dry ice)	$-78°C$
Nitrous oxide	$-89°C$
Liquid nitrogen	$-196°C$

ized dewar. Boiling and rapid loss to the atmosphere occur if it is stored in an unpressurized container. The liquid nitrogen, as with other cryogens, need not be sterile.

Nitrous oxide has several advantages over liquid nitrogen: it is readily available, is easily stored, and has equipment available for its application. The biggest disadvantage is that it is not as cold ($-89°C$) as liquid nitrogen ($-196°C$). Because of this temperature difference, only small neoplasms can be managed with nitrous oxide cryosurgery. Other disadvantages include use limited to probes only (spray has limited use) and combustibility. In addition, surgical suite ventilation must be considered if large amounts of nitrous oxide are used.

Freon is used primarily in disposable units for lens extraction. The moist lens adheres to the frozen probe tip and is removed.

Carbon dioxide is not recommended as a cryogen. It is not as cold as nitrous oxide. Its maximum cooling capability is inadequate except for all but the smallest lesions.

EQUIPMENT

Cryosurgery Machines

Cryosurgery machines are available from several manufactures.[5] The choice of machine is extremely important. Cost is obviously a factor in the selection. The machine should be versatile for use in a small animal practice. It must be capable of freezing both small and large lesions. This is best accomplished by a liquid nitrogen machine that can both spray and probe freeze. If the machine is to have a unique function, e.g., use on small lesions only, liquid nitrogen and nitrous oxide units should be considered. Other factors to consider when purchasing a cryosurgery machine include the following:

1. Cryogen storage capability—The machine can function simultaneously as an operating unit and a pressurized storage dewar.

2. Cryogen transfer—The need to transfer the cryogen from a storage dewar to the operating machine may be inconvenient and time-consuming and may occur at an inopportune time during the procedure. This is a definite disadvantage that is difficult to anticipate until the machine is purchased and put into use.

3. Spray freeze control—The liquid nitrogen spray should be easily controlled when the machine is functioning properly. The surgeon should have fine control over the volume of spray, which should be a fine mist that is uniform from one moment to the next. The mist should not splutter from the spray orifice and should not contain large droplets that fall short of the target lesion.

4. Probe tip variety—A variety of sizes and designs for various applications should be available.

5. Machine freezing—Poorly designed machines are affected by humidity. Ice can accumulate in cryogen lines, around spray orifices, and in moving parts. If this occurs, the machine will function improperly.

Tissue Temperature Monitors

Tissue temperature monitoring equipment is used to ensure freezing to the desired degree and temperature. Temperature monitoring is indispensable when dealing with neoplasms with adjacent vital structures (e.g., nerves, tendons, bone, large vessels). Monitoring equipment generally consists of thermocouple needles attached to a pyrometer. The inserted needles rest at the junction of healthy and pathological tissues. The temperature reading on the pyrometer is the tissue temperature in contact with the tip of the needle. Cryosurgery machines are available with built-in monitors.

TECHNIQUE

Restraint

The patient must be immobile during the procedure. Since variable degrees of pain may be elicited, analgesia must be provided. Local anesthesia is adequate for small superficial lesions. In cooperative patients with large lesions, local anesthesia with tranquilization may be adequate, but general anesthesia is usually necessary.

Preparation of the Surgery Site

Strict aseptic technique is not necessary for lesions that have surface drainage postoperatively. However, the hair should be clipped and the skin prepared in a routine fashion. Strict asepsis must be maintained for deep lesions without drainage.

Biopsies for histopathological diagnosis are procured prior to cryosurgery. Freezing disrupts tissue architecture such that interpretation is difficult even if the specimens are procured immediately after cryosurgery.

Large lesions are often best managed by a combination of electrosurgery and cryosurgery. An electrocutting and electrocoagulating instrument is initially used to reduce the size of the mass and control hemorrhage. Cryosurgery is performed to freeze the bed of the lesion. When the bulk of the mass is removed, there is a smaller mass to freeze and slough.

Insulators are used to protect normal tissue when spray freezing. They are not a substitute for good technique or a poorly operating machine. Liquid nitrogen droplets may fall on tissue other than the lesion being frozen. Vaseline or styrofoam (thickness of coffee cups) can be used to protect the tissue by directing excess liquid nitrogen away from the patient. A thick layer of Vaseline must be used, or the styrofoam must be in close contact with the skin. Vaseline and styrofoam work well together. One should not rely totally on insulators. Tissue temperature monitors and constant inspection of lesions by the surgeon are still necessary.

Probe Freezing

Cryosurgery probes are metallic attachments through which the cryogen flows. They become a heat sink as the cryogen extracts heat from the metal. The tips are available in a large variety of sizes and shapes for different uses. Probe freezing is the safest method of cryosurgery. The surgeon should be adept at probe freezing before he attempts spray freezing. Cryoprobes can be gas sterilized for freezing deep internal structures.

The probe should be at room temperature when applied to a lesion. The machine is switched on to start probe cooling. When the probe reaches 0°C, the tissue adjacent to the probe freezes and adheres to it. This bond is useful to manipulate a lesion and lift it away from deep structures to be spared.

Good cryoadhesion occurs if the tissue is moist. Contact with or insertion into a biopsy site is often the most practical way to place the probe. When freezing a dry skin surface, scarification of the skin over the lesion improves adhesion owing to the presence of blood and serum. Cryoadhesion is poor if the probe is already frozen when applied to the lesion. Likewise, cryoadhesion is poor if the lesion is being frozen during the second freeze-thaw cycle and the tissue has not yet completely thawed.

When cryoadhesion is achieved, freezing is allowed to proceed until the entire mass is frozen to the desired temperature. The cryoprobe is allowed to thaw spontaneously. Once above 0°C, the probe detaches from the tissue. No attempt should be made to detach the probe from the tissue prior to thawing. Prethaw detachment unnecessarily traumatizes tissues and can bend or break probes owing to the tight adhesion. On some models, the probe tips can be detached from the operating mechanism of the machine. If multiple probe tips are available, the surgeon can freeze another lesion while the initial probes and lesions are thawing. Other machines have heaters in the probes for early detachment. Both machine options decrease overall surgery time.

Spray Freezing

Spray freezing is performed by applying liquid nitrogen directly to a lesion. The mist is emitted from an orifice in the operating arm of the machine. If the orifice is held 1 to 5 mm from a large lesion, a small, thin pool of liquid nitrogen accumulates on the surface. The periphery of the pool boils and vaporizes into the atmosphere or may drip from the edge of the lesion. If dripping occurs, it should go onto the floor or into a container or should be aspirated into a suction system. It should not contact healthy tissue.

The spray method rapidly freezes tissue to the lowest temperatures possible. The surgeon must carefully monitor tissue temperature at the periphery of the lesion. Otherwise, inadvertent freezes are likely to occur. Large masses are best spray frozen. Spray freezing is not limited to large lesions; small superficial lesions can be frozen just as readily.

OPTIMUM CONDITIONS FOR CELL DEATH

Regardless of the cryogen used, equipment available, tissue involved, and method of application (probe or spray), several conditions should be met to ensure cell death. Each of the following principles should be considered in every case.

1. The tissue should be frozen rapidly and allowed to thaw slowly.

2. Tissue should be frozen to −20°C or colder. The cell is unlikely to survive under clinical circumstances beyond this point. It should be emphasized that a temperature of −20°C or *colder* be reached. Cell types and tissues are being discovered that may require even colder temperatures for consistent death.

3. To rule out any possibility that cells might survive at −20°C, the tissue should be frozen twice, i.e., two freeze-thaw cycles. This means that the lesion is frozen, allowed to thaw, and is frozen again. Thaw time averages two to three times the initial freezing period. The tissue need not be maintained at −20°C for a set period of time. Once −20°C is reached, the tissue is allowed to thaw.

4. Tissue temperature should be accurately monitored at the predetermined edge of the tumor so that tumor ablation will be complete with minimal disruption to adjacent vital structures. Without a tissue temperature monitor, the surgeon can only subjec-

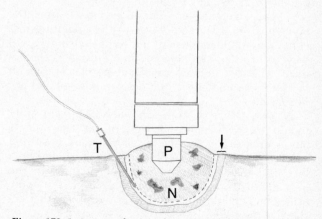

Figure 173–1. A cryoprobe (*P*) is being used. The entire neoplasm (*N*) is frozen to −20° C or colder. The zone of tissue (arrow) frozen at 0 to −20° C will survive. A thermocouple needle (*T*) is in place to accurately assess tissue temperature.

tively evaluate the amount of tissue he is destroying. A sharp line of demarcation is visible between the white discolored frozen tissue and unfrozen tissue. The frozen tissue is hard, and its edge is easily palpated. The mass may be movable, but as freezing progresses the mass will become fixed if it freezes to deep immovable structures. Appearance, palpation, and fixation, however, only indicate when tissue temperature is 0°C or colder. The zone of tissue at the periphery of the frozen mass that is frozen between 0°C and −20°C survives. The surgeon's "senses" cannot detect the width of this zone. If it is important to accurately control what will or will not die, tissue temperature monitors must be used (Fig. 173–1).

WOUND HEALING AFTER CRYOSURGERY

Wound healing after cryosurgery is similar to wound healing after any injury.[6,9] The gross and microscopic tissue alterations caused by cryosurgery are consistent from one tissue to the next. A summary of the events taking place during cryosurgery and the postoperative appearance are presented here. The sequence of events seen after thawing to 0°C is illustrated in Fig. 173–2.

The initial ischemia lasts less than one minute. While the tissue is frozen, there is no blood flow. As soon as the tissue thaws, arterial blood enters and venous blood flows out. The vascular system functions very briefly. Hyperemia and edema soon follow ischemia. If the epithelial surface of the tumor is penetrated, capillary hemorrhage occurs. The hemorrhage is minor and easily controlled. Digital pressure or mattress or purse-string sutures are effective hemostatic aids. Contrary to some reports, freezing in itself, is not a hemostatic aid. In fact, vasodilation due to altered sympathetic tone may actually briefly increase hemorrhage until vascular collapse is complete.[60] If the epithelium is intact, the lesion appears edematous and erythematous and weeps serum from the surface. The stage of hyperemia and edema lasts 6 to 12 hours. Near the end of this stage, the lesion appears dark purple.

The lesion then becomes necrotic and sloughing begins. The necrotic area resembles an infarct with a sharply delineated border. The slough may be

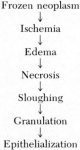

Frozen neoplasm
↓
Ischemia
↓
Edema
↓
Necrosis
↓
Sloughing
↓
Granulation
↓
Epithelialization

Figure 173–2. Wounds progress in stages from cryosurgery to a healed surface.

complete as early as the fifth day if the patient aggressively licks the lesion. More typically, the detachment occurs between the tenth and twelfth day. If the patient does not lick the lesion and tough fibrous tissue is present, the mass may not detach until the fifteenth day or later. Small lesions (less than 1 cm in diameter) have a hard, dry eschar. Most lesions greater than 2.5 cm in diameter are soft and moist. They discolor from purple to a gray or yellow-green "gangrenous-appearing" mass. Detachment of the mass is gradual. Hemorrhage will not occur at the time of detachment unless the patient licks the area excessively.

A bed of granulation tissue proliferates under the necrotic tissue. When sloughing is complete, a crater of pink, vascular, immature granulation tissue remains. Maturation of the granulation tissue progresses to the stage of fibroplasia and contracture. The connective tissue becomes firm, dense, and less vascular with minimal inflammatory response.

Epithelium covers the wound by advancing from the periphery of the granulation bed to the center. Activation of this process is evident microscopically 24 to 48 hours postoperatively. The epithelialization rate is directly proportional to the size of the initial mass. Epithelium covers the surface in 20 to 22 days under normal circumstances if the initial mass is 2 to 3 cm in diameter. Small lesions may heal in as few as 12 days. Wound licking is of no consequence except during epithelialization; during this stage, licking disrupts the thin layers of epithelium and delays healing. Licking is usually of minimal clinical significance. The exceptions are healing wounds on the distal extremities (especially distal to the carpus or tarsus), where chronic ulcerated pyogranulomas may form. Therefore, restraint devices, such as Elizabethan collars, should be considered if excessive licking or wound mutilation is anticipated or encountered.

The healed wound is a slightly thickened scar that is devoid of pigmentation and adnexal structures. Epidermis at the periphery of the initial cryosurgery site undergoes first and second degree frostbite. Deep layers of epithelium and adnexal structures survive, but melanocytes are destroyed. In the zone where hair follicles survive, white hair may grow permanently ("freeze branding"). Epidermal pigmentation usually returns in three to six months.

Wound healing of organs and deep structures such as kidney,[3,26] liver,[25] spleen,[27] brain,[28] myocardium,[7] intraocular structures,[4] bone,[44,45] and hypophysis[16] have been studied. Repair progresses as an area of aseptic necrosis in the respective tissues.

Controversy exists when comparing healing and degree of fibrosis resulting from electrosurgical necrosis and cryonecrosis. Arguments by advocates of each technique have been based on empirical results. A microscopic and cell kinetic study[24] was conducted using radioisotope-labelled fibroblasts. The study indicated that fibroblast proliferation is most active and similar in both types of lesions between the second

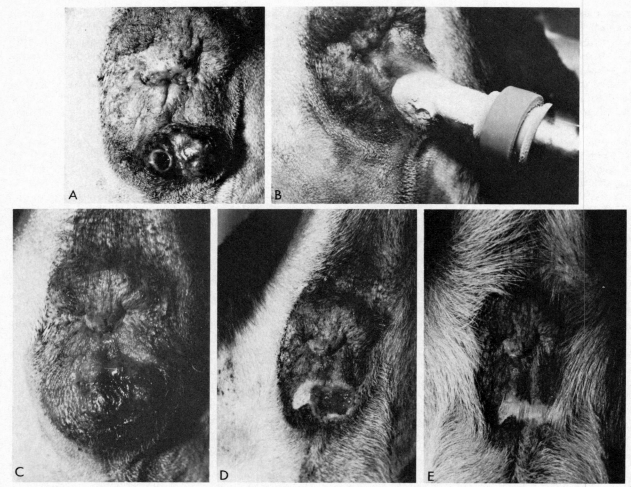

Figure 173–3. *A*, A perianal adenoma. *B*, Frozen with cryoprobe. *C*, One day postoperatively. *D*, Fourteen days postoperatively. *E*, Six months postoperatively.

and third postoperative days. However, two weeks after cryosurgery the numbers of radioactive, labelled fibroblasts return to near normal. This corresponds to rapid healing with minimal fibrosis after cryosurgery. Comparatively, four weeks after thermal necrosis, the numbers of labelled fibroblasts are still increased by a factor of ten. Carbonized material is still present, which may be the reason for the longer and more intense granulomatous response. The leukocytic reaction is also prolonged in thermal lesions compared with cryolesions. Thermosurgical tissue lesions thus exhibit delayed healing in comparison to cryosurgical wounds.

IMMUNE RESPONSE

The immune system is stimulated after a cryosurgical lesion is created.[29,47] This is potentially beneficial to the cancer patient if released tumor antigens stimulate antibody production. Cell-mediated and humoral immunity are both involved. An anamnestic response is observed experimentally with a repeated sequence of freezing. The degree of immune stimulation is greater after cryosurgery than after cold

scalpel excision or electrocoagulation of a tumor because cell membranes and tumor-specific antigens are able to escape from frozen tumors through the still intact vasculature.[29,47] When lesions are excised, intact cells escape. Thermal necrosis is more destructive to the vascular network than cryosurgery, making escape of antigens less likely. Also, the greater degree of protein denaturation after thermal necrosis compared with cryosurgery may lead to decreased immunostimulation.

The immune response has not yet been proved great enough to alter survival time in patients with metastasis or tumor recurrence. At present, the response can only be considered a potential adjuvant to conventional cancer therapy. Cryosurgery may have a greater immune-stimulating affect on some tumor types than on others.

SPECIFIC INDICATIONS

Anorectal Lesions

Perianal gland adenomas are readily ablated cryosurgically (Fig. 173–3).[41,43] Regardless of their location, they may be probe or spray frozen. An incisional biopsy is taken from the center of a tumor. A probe tip is inserted in the center of each mass at the biopsy site. After the tumor thaws (after the second freeze-thaw cycle) and the probe is removed, a purse-string suture is placed around the site to minimize hemorrhage.

Castration is performed in addition to cryosurgery. About 50 per cent of dogs with perianal gland adenomas also have interstitial cell tumors. Castration by itself is recommended as the initial treatment phase for patients with severe 360° multiple ulcerated perianal adenomas. Hypertrophied perianal glands atrophy within four weeks. The discrete neoplasms remaining are then frozen individually. Recurrences

are seen, but the incidence is less than 10 per cent. Adenomas may re-appear at the surgery site or as separate tumors in the perianal area. These recurring tumors are slow growing and are treated successfully by additional surgery.

Perianal gland adenocarcinomas are much less responsive to cryosurgery and castration than perianal adenomas. They are much more invasive. Therefore, the cryosurgery must be more aggressive. Surgery is only palliative in some instances. Recurrence rates are high, and metastasis to the iliac lymph nodes is common.

Other neoplastic anorectal diseases that may be treated cryosurgically include rectal polyps and rectal adenocarcinomas. Proliferative adenocarcinomas that

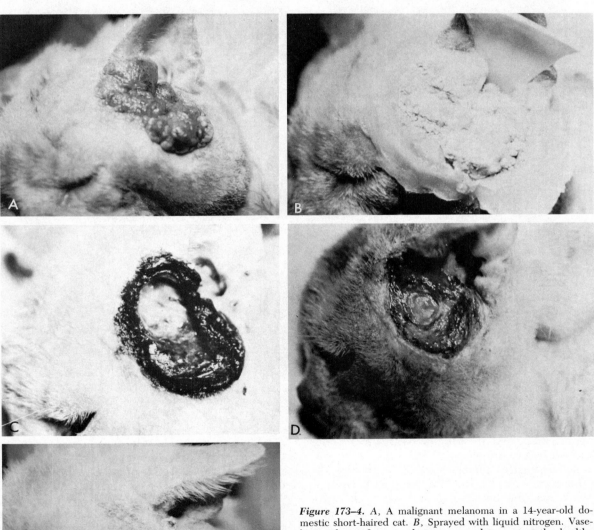

Figure 173–4. A, A malignant melanoma in a 14-year-old domestic short-haired cat. *B*, Sprayed with liquid nitrogen. Vaseline and styrofoam insulation are used to protect the healthy skin and ear. *C*, Eight days postoperatively. *D*, Fourteen days postoperatively. *E*, Six weeks postoperatively.

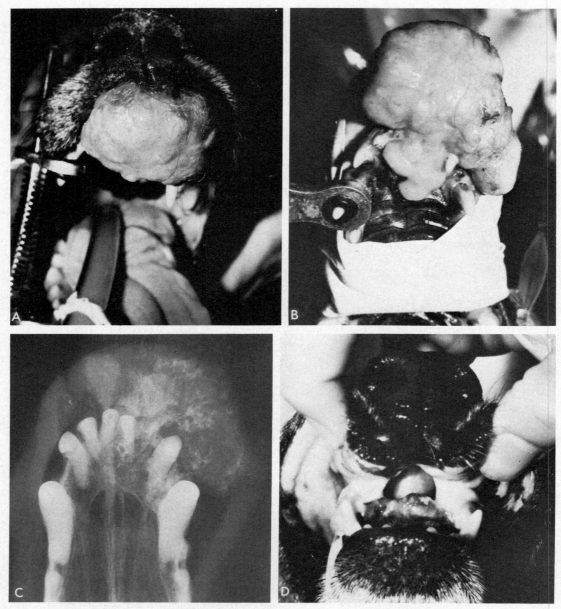

Figure 173–5. *A* and *B*, Gross and *(C)* radiographic appearance of an adamantinoma in a ten-year-old akita. Cryosurgery was performed twice. Dead bone was removed once. *D*, Seven months after the original surgery, the patient has no evidence of disease.

do not extend beyond the submucosa are much better candidates for cryosurgery than infiltrative adenocarcinomas. The latter tumors have often invaded the muscularis mucosa by the time of diagnosis. Cryosurgery may be considered at best as palliative therapy for these tumors. Rectal polyps are readily frozen *in situ*, with good prognosis. Superficial anal inflammation and problems associated with anal sac disease should not be treated with cryosurgery. Perianal fistulae may be treated cryosurgically.[40,42]

Skin Lesions

Skin and subcutaneous tissues are the most common sites for neoplasia in domestic animals. Fortu-

nately, a majority of the neoplasms are benign. Cryosurgery is just one of many treatment methods. Cure rates are inversely proportional to the degree of malignancy.[37,53,54]

Benign neoplasms, as with other modes of therapy, have very high cure rates. Sebaceous adenomas, papillomas, trichoepitheliomas, histiocytomas, basal cell tumors, hidradenomas, and benign melanomas are all good cryosurgery candidates.

Malignant tumors must be treated aggressively. Therapy may be curative, but palliation is sometimes the primary objective. Malignant melanomas (Fig. 173–4), squamous cell carcinomas, fibrosarcomas, malignant adnexal tumors, neurofibromas, and neoplasms of vascular origin may all be approached cryosurgically. Precautions should be taken when treating mast cell tumors. Cryosurgery of mast cell tumors may be complicated by massive degranulation of the mast cells. Histamine, other vasoactive amines, and heparin are released. Edema and erythema are excessive postoperatively, and uncontrollable hemorrhage may occur. Premedication with antihistamine and protamine is used to antagonize the excessive release of histamine and heparin, respectively. Mast cell tumors greater than 1 cm in diameter should be treated by means other than cryosurgery.

Oral Tumors

Benign tumors treated cryosurgically include oral papilloma, hemangioma, and epulis.[8] The most common malignant oral tumors treated are malignant melanoma, squamous cell carcinoma, adamantinoma (Fig. 173–5), and fibrosarcoma.[22] Other tumors seen but rarely treated cryosurgically include osteosarcoma, hemangiosarcoma, and adenocarcinoma.

Benign tumors have the expected high cure rates.[8] The malignant tumors are often incurable regardless of the mode of therapy.[23] Oral cryosurgery has some advantages over conventional surgery. It is quick and easy, hemorrhage is minimal, and bone is left intact. Palliative relief of pain is evident within 24 hours, and additional pain is not created by the surgery.

Three disadvantages must be considered: (1) edema around tumors in the pharynx or on the tongue may obstruct airways or hinder ingestion; (2) halitosis due to tumor necrosis will be present; and (3) removal of dead bone at the cryosurgery site may be necessary four to six weeks postoperatively.

Ophthalmic Lesions

Cryosurgery is performed by ophthalmologists for both extraocular and intraocular diseases.[4,30,46] Palpebral neoplasms can be frozen and still maintain eyelid function (Fig. 173–6). The cure rate in one study was 91 per cent.[30,31] Cryosurgery is very effective for bovine ocular squamous cell carcinomas.[10,11]

Miscellaneous Lesions

New indications for cryosurgery will continue to be recognized in the future. Descriptions of its use for bone tumors,[44,45,56] nasal tumors,[57] prostate disease,[16] brain lesions,[16] and metastatic pulmonary tumors[16] have been reported. Both positive and negative findings have been described. Long-term results must be evaluated for many specific disease entities before success or failure can be determined.

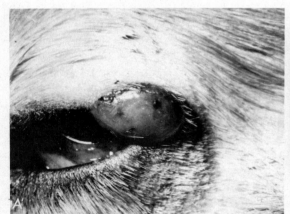
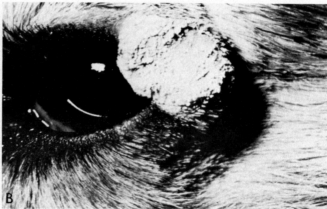
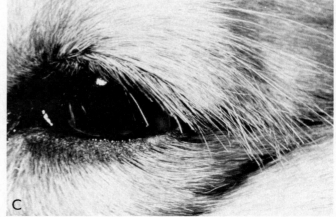

Figure 173–6. A, A palpebral neoplasm. B, Frozen. C, Sixty days after cryosurgery. (Courtesy of S. J. Withrow.)

AFTERCARE

Postoperative care is the same as that for any wound that is to heal by secondary intention. The use of topical antiseptics is necessary only if the wound is moist. Antibiotics are used prophylactically for debilitated patients or those with accompanying diseases. Wounds on the extremities are protected with wound dressings or devices to prevent licking. The licking of wounds on the torso is rarely of any consequence.

The client should be advised of how the healing process will proceed and that an odor may be present. Wounds should be rechecked on a regular basis until healing is complete. Adjunctive cancer therapy should proceed as indicated. Biopsy specimens should be procured to assess therapy, and additional surgery should be performed if indicated.

COMPLICATIONS

Complications are most commonly related to overzealous freezing, resulting in unwanted necrosis of healthy adjacent vital structures. These complications can be avoided if the basic cryosurgical principles are followed and proper precautions are taken. Tissue temperature monitoring is the most important precaution to avoid problems.[15]

Embolization of air or vapor from liquid nitrogen into the venous system and to the right heart has been reported.[21] The complication was associated with oral tumor cryosurgery. Embolization is most likely to occur when cryogen is sprayed into a highly vascular area, such as cancellous bone.

Swelling will be present during the immediate postoperative period. The swelling is inconsequential unless it secondarily disrupts the function of adjacent structures. Vasodilation that occurs immediately postoperatively at the surgery site can potentiate capillary hemorrhage from the biopsy site. Suture closure or compression bandages readily control the hemorrhage if it occurs. Hemorrhage will not occur during wound healing unless the patient mutilates the surgery site. Infection rates are comparable to those after conventional surgery. Septicemia is extremely rare. The scar and the hair that regrows around the periphery of a surgery site may be white, perhaps constituting an unacceptable cosmetic appearance.

1. Ablin, R. J.: *Handbook of Cryosurgery.* Marcel Dekker, Inc., New York, 1980.
2. Borthwick, R.: Cryosurgery in veterinary practice: A preliminary report. Vet. Rec. 86:683, 1970.
3. Breining, H., et al.: The parenchymal reaction of kidney after local freezing. Urol. Res. 2:29, 1974.
4. Brightman, A. H., et al.: Cryosurgery for the treatment of canine glaucoma. J. Am. Anim. Hosp. Assoc. 18:319, 1982.
5. Bryne, M. D.: Cryosurgical instrumentation. Vet. Clin. North Am. 10:771, 1980.
6. Bushby, P. A., Hoff, E. S., and Hankes, G. H.: Microscopic tissue alterations following cryosurgery of the canine skin. J. Am. Vet. Med. Assoc. 173:177, 1978.
7. Camm, J., et al.: The successful cryosurgical treatment of paroxysmal ventricular tachycardia. Chest 75:621, 1979.
8. Chapin, M. E.: Cryosurgery of benign oral lesions. J. Dermatol. Surg. Oncol. 3:428, 1977.
9. Elton, R. F.: The course of events following cryosurgery. J. Dermatol. Surg. Oncol. 3:448, 1977.
10. Farris, H. E.: Cryosurgical treatment of bovine ocular squamous cell carcinoma. Vet. Clin. North Am. 10:861, 1980.
11. Farris, H. E., and Fraunfelder, F. T.: Cryosurgical treatment of ocular squamous cell carcinoma of cattle. J. Am. Vet. Med. Assoc. 168:213, 1976.
12. Farrant, J., and Walter, C. A.: The cryobiological basis for cryosurgery. J. Dermatol. Surg. Oncol. 3:403, 1977.
13. Fraunfelder, F. T., Farris, H. E., and Wallace, T. R.: Cryosurgery for ocular and periocular lesions. J. Dermatol. Surg. Oncol. 3:422, 1977.
14. Fretz, P. B., and Barber, S. M.: Prospective analysis of cryosurgery as the sole treatment for equine sarcoids. Vet. Clin. North Am. 10:847, 1980.
15. Fretz, P. B., and Holmberg, D. L.: Sequelae to cryosurgery. Vet. Clin. North Am. 10:869, 1980.
16. Gage, A. A.: *American College of Cryosurgery 1979 Newsletter–December.* Clinton, CT, 1979.
17. Goldstein, R. S., and Hess, P. W.: Cryosurgical treatment of cancer. Vet. Clin. North Am. 7:51, 1977.
18. Goldstein, R. S., and Hess, P. W.: Cryosurgery of canine and feline tumors. J. Am. Anim. Hosp. Assoc. 12:340, 1976.
19. Greiner, T. P.: Cryosurgery. Proc. 43rd Ann. Mtg. Am. Anim. Hosp. Assoc. 1976, pp. 395–399.
20. Greiner, T. P., Liska, W. D., and Withrow, S. J.: Cryosurgery. Vet. Clin. North Am. 5:565, 1975.
21. Harvey, H. J.: Fatal air embolization associated with cryosurgery in two dogs. J. Am. Vet. Med. Assoc. 173:175, 1978.
22. Harvey, H. J.: Cryosurgery of oral tumors in dogs and cats. Vet. Clin. North Am. 10:821, 1980.
23. Harvey, H. J., et al.: Prognostic criteria for dogs with oral melanoma. J. Am. Vet. Med. Assoc. 178:580, 1981.
24. Helpap, B. and Grouls, V.: Tissue reparation of the liver after thermo- and cryosurgical lesions: Comparative cell analytical investigation. Cryobiology 16:473, 1979.
25. Helpap, B., Sohngen, K., and Breining, H.: Wound healing of the liver after biliary obstruction and cryonecrosis. Res. Exp. Med. 176:143, 1979.
26. Helpap, B., et al.: Wound healing of the kidney after cryonecrosis—autoradiographic investigation with 3H—thymidine on Rats. Virchows Arch. [Pathol. Anat.] 363:123, 1974.
27. Helpap, B., et al.: The proliferative response of the spleen in cryosurgery. Cryobiology 13:54, 1976.
28. Helpap, B., et al.: Wound healing of the brain of rats—autoradiographic investigations with 3H—thymidine. Virchows Arch. [Cell Pathol.] 22:151, 1976.
29. Helpap, B., et al.: Morphological and cell kinetic investigations of the spleen after repeated in situ freezing of liver and kidney. Path. Res. Pract. 164:167, 1979.
30. Holmberg, D. L.: Cryosurgical treatment of canine eyelid tumors. Vet. Clin. North Am. 10:831, 1980.
31. Holmberg, D. L., and Withrow, S. J.: Cryosurgical treatment of palpebral neoplasms: Clinical and experimental results. Vet. Surg. 8:68, 1979.
32. Hoppenbrouwers, R.: An analysis of 400 cases of retinal detachment with the cryoplombage technique. Ophthalmologica 175:52, 1977.
33. Hoyt, R. F., and Seim, H. B.: Veterinary cryosurgery: Mechanism of cell death, cryosurgical instrumentation, and cryogens. Part I. Comp. Cont. Ed. 3:426, 1981.
34. Joyce, J. R.: Cryosurgical treatment of tumors of horses and cattle. J. Am. Vet. Med. Assoc. 168:226, 1976.
35. Karow, A. M., and Pegg, D. E.: *Organ Preservation for Transplantation.* Marcel Dekker, Inc., New York, 1981.
36. Krahwinkel, D. J.: Cryosurgery for the practitioner. Proc. 46th Ann. Mtg. Am. Anim. Hosp. Assoc. 1979, 515.
37. Krahwinkel, D. J.: Cryosurgical treatment of skin diseases. Vet. Clin. North Am. 10:787, 1980.
38. Krahwinkel, D. J., Merkley, D. R., and Howard, D. F.: Cryosurgical treatment of cancerous and noncancerous dis-

eases of dogs, horses, and cats. J. Am. Vet. Med. Assoc. *169*:201, 1976.

39. Lane, J. G.: Practical cryosurgery—an introduction for small animal clinicians. J. Small Anim. Pract. *15*:715, 1974.

40. Lane, J. G., and Burch, D. G. S.: The cryosurgical treatment of canine anal furunculosis. J. Small Anim. Pract. *16*:387, 1975.

41. Liska, W. D.: Anorectal and perianal cryosurgery. Vet. Clin. North Am. *10*:803, 1980.

42. Liska, W. D., Greiner, T. P., and Withrow, S. J.: Cryosurgery in the treatment of perianal fistulae. Vet. Clin. North Am. *5*:449, 1975.

43. Liska, W. D., and Withrow, S. J.: Cryosurgical treatment of perianal gland adenomas in the dog. J. Am. Anim. Hosp. Assoc. *14*:457, 1978.

44. Marcove, R. C., and Miller, T. R.: The treatment of primary and metastatic localized bone tumors by cryosurgery. Surg. Clin. North Am. *49*:421, 1969.

45. Marcove, R. C., et al.: Cryosurgery in the treatment of giant cell tumors of bone: A report of 52 consecutive cases. Clin. Orthop. *134*:275, 1978.

46. Merideth, R. E., and Gelatt, K. N.: Cryotherapy in veterinary ophthalmology. Vet. Clin. North Am. *10*:837, 1980.

47. Neel, H. B.: Immunotherapeutic effect of cryosurgical tumor necrosis. Vet. Clin. North Am. *10*:763, 1980.

48. Norsworthy, G. D., et al.: Cryosurgery in small animal practice. Canine Pract. *4*:18, 1977.

49. Robbins, G. M., and Lane, J. G.: The management of anal furunculosis. J. Small Anim. Pract. *14*:333, 1973.

50. Seim, H. B.: Mechanisms of cold-induced cell death. Vet. Clin. North Am. *10*:755, 1980.

51. Seim, H. B., and Hoyt, R. F.: Veterinary cryosurgery: Part II. Principles of application. Comp. Cont. Ed. *3*:695, 1981.

52. Stoyak, J. M.: Application of cryosurgery in small animals. Proc. 44th Ann. Mtg. Am. Anim. Hosp. Assoc. 1977, pp. 387–389.

53. Torre, D.: Cryosurgical treatment of epitheliomas using the cone-spray technique. J. Dermatol. Surg. Oncol. *3*:432, 1977.

54. Willemse, T.: Cryotherapy in small animal dermatology. *In* Kirk, R. W. (ed.): *Current Veterinary Therapy VII*. W. B. Saunders, Philadelphia, 1980, pp. 495–497.

55. Withrow, S. J.: General principles of cryosurgical technique. Vet. Clin. North Am. *10*:779, 1980.

56. Withrow, S. J.: Application of cryosurgery to primary malignant bone tumors in dogs (Phase I study). J. Am. Anim. Hosp. Assoc. *16*:493, 1980.

57. Withrow, S. J.: Cryosurgical therapy for nasal tumors in the dog. J. Am. Anim. Hosp. Assoc. *18*:585, 1982.

58. Withrow, S. J.: Oncology for the practitioner—cryosurgery. Proc. 49th Ann. Mtg. Am. Anim. Hosp. Assoc. 1982, pp. 243–244.

59. Withrow, S. J., Greiner, T. P., and Liska, W. D.: Cryosurgery: Veterinary considerations. J. Am. Anim. Hosp. Assoc. *11*:271, 1975.

60. Zacarian, S. A.: *Cryosurgical Advances in Dermatology and Tumors of the Head and Neck*. Charles C Thomas, Springfield, IL, 1977.

Chapter **174**

Hyperthermia

Mark W. Dewhirst and William G. Connor

RATIONALE FOR THE USE OF HYPERTHERMIA

Hyperthermia, or heat therapy, is receiving considerable attention as a promising new treatment for neoplasia. It has been the subject of several international congresses[10,69] and symposia.[36,52,54] More recently, several books dealing with hyperthermic biology, clinical treatment,[33,67] and physics and engineering[41,54,67] have been published. Interest in hyperthermia was rekindled after the published reports of its efficacy in murine and pet animal tumors.[9] However, the ancient Greeks observed it to be of value in treating human tumors, and in the late 19th century Busch,[3] Fehleisen,[23] and Coley[8] made similar observations.

The rationale for interest in the development of heat is related to its cytotoxic effects alone and its interactions with both radiation and chemotherapy. In addition, the human and pet animal clinical reports published thus far underscore its relative safety and impressive antitumor effects.

Even though there has been considerable enthusiasm for the use of hyperthermia, several biological and physical problems need to be solved before it can become useful. At the present time it should be considered an experimental modality, and caution should be exercised in its use in private veterinary practice. In this chapter, the use of heat as a single agent and as an adjuvant is reviewed.

BIOLOGICAL EFFECTS OF HEAT

The Cell Survival Curve and the Arrhenius Relationship

Temperatures above 105.8°F (41°C) are cytotoxic, with the degree of cell killing depending on the temperature and duration of heating. *In vitro* the killing effect is described by a survival curve, which measures the ability of treated cells to divide and form a colony. For some cell lines, a small shoulder is present for short heating times. As the heating time is increased, the rate of killing is exponential (Fig. 174–1A).

The inverse of the slope of the exponential portion of the survival curve is described by D_o, which is the time required to reduce survival to 37 per cent of an initial value. Thus, for a given temperature, the D_o describes the heat sensitivity of any cell line. As D_o decreases, the heat sensitivity goes up. For temperatures less than 109.4°F (43°C), a resistant "tail" is

This work was supported in part by grant NIH-NCI CA 17343.

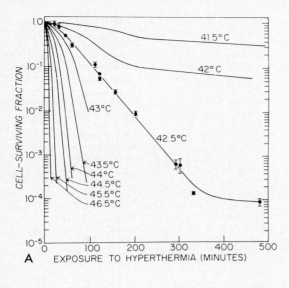

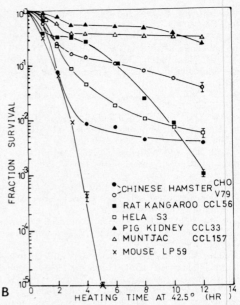

Figure 174–1. *A,* Heat cell survival curves. Temperatures above 41° C are cytotoxic to cells *in vitro*. The degree of cell death achieved by heat depends on the temperature and time, as is demonstrated by an increasing steepness of the survival curves as temperature increases from 41.5 to 46.5° C. The flattening of the survival curves observed for temperatures less than 42.5° C is due to thermotolerance induction. (Reprinted with permission from Dewey, W. C., Hopwood, L. E., Sapareto, S. A., and Gerweck, L. E.: Cellular responses to combinations of hyperthermia and radiation. Radiology *123*:463, 1977.) *B,* Cell survival curves for a variety of cell lines. The heat sensitivity of different cell lines varies considerably in this survival curve for 42.5° C heating. The mouse LP line shows no thermotolerance induction for heating times of up to five hours. (Reprinted with permission from Raaphorst, G. P., Romano, S. L., Mitchell, J. B., Bedford, J. S., and Dewey, W. C.: Intrinsic differences in heat and/or x-ray sensitivity of seven mammalian cell lines cultured and treated under identical conditions. Cancer Res. *39*:396, 1979.)

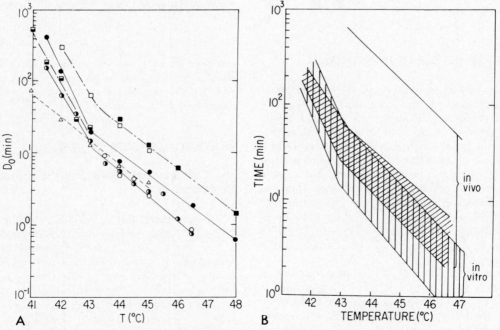

Figure 174–2. *A,* Arrhenius plot for several cell lines *in vitro* displaying the relationship between different time-temperature combinations required to achieve cell killing. The D_0 (time at a given temperature required to reduce survival to 37 per cent of an initial value on the exponential portion of the survival curve) decreases as the temperature increases, indicating a steeper slope on the survival curve for higher temperatures. The break in the plot at roughly 42.5 to 43° C may be related to thermotolerance induction for temperatures of less than 42.5° C. *B,* Comparison of Arrhenius plots for *in vitro* and *in vivo* data. Thermotolerance develops *in vivo* as well as *in vitro* as shown by this comparison of Arrhenius relationships. The relative slopes of the Arrhenius curves are similar, indicating that the mechanisms of *in vitro* and *in vivo* heat killing are probably similar (vertical hatched area = *in vitro*, the diagonally hatched area = *in vivo* data). The brace shows the complete range of reported *in vivo* data. (Reprinted with permission from Henle, K. J.: Arrhenius analysis of thermal responses. *In* Storm, F. K. (ed.): *Hyperthermia in Cancer Therapy.* G. K. Hall Medical Publishers, Boston, 1983.)

often observed for heating times between 1 and 3 hours. The phenomenon is referred to as *thermotolerance*, or induced resistance to further heat killing. Heat sensitivity varies widely between different cell lines, as demonstrated in Figure 174–1B by a range of D_os for a fixed temperature. In addition, the degree of thermotolerance induction varies for those same cell lines.[62] The relationship between different time-temperature combinations required to achieve cell killing is conveniently displayed as *Arrhenius' plot*, where $\ln/D_o$ is plotted as a function of temperature. Using this relationship, one time-temperature combination can be converted to another to achieve the same biological effect. The "break" in the plot at ~108.5°F (~42.5°C) may be related to thermotolerance induction and is observed for most cell lines studied (Fig. 174–2A). The slope of the line gives the inactivation energy of the process involved in cell killing. For most cell lines studied, inactivation energies have been between 100 and 200 kcal/mole. Arrhenius' plots have also been described for *in vivo* systems involving both normal tissue damage and tumor control endpoints. In general, the same type of relationship holds for these studies (Fig. 174–2B).[34]

Clinical Significance

The clinical significance of the preceding discussion relates to the fact that currently available heating techniques most often yield variable tissue temperatures. Consequently, for a given hyperthermic treatment, the degree of cell killing varies widely in different portions of the tumor. In addition, if inactivation energies varied from one tissue to the next, different levels of killing could result from the same time-temperature combination. Therefore, for hyperthermia to be used safely and effectively, the clinician may need working knowledge of these time-temperature relationships for a range of normal and tumor tissues.

Several attempts have been made to make these complex relationships more manageable in a clinical setting. They represent a step toward defining a workable unit for *thermal dose*. The techniques include a simple time-temperature integral,[16] conversion of time-temperature data to equivalent minutes at 109.4°F (43°C),[64] and calculation of thermal dose in standard hyperthermia units.[27] The two latter analyses are based on basic thermodynamic principles and can be adjusted for variations in the heat of inactivation.

THERMOTOLERANCE

Thermotolerance is defined as any heat-induced increase in heat resistance, whether the shoulder or terminal slope of the survival curve is affected.[33] Thermotolerance can be induced in three ways: (1) continuous heating at temperatures less than 109.4°F (43°C) (Fig. 174–1A); (2) heating to temperatures greater than 109.4°F (43°C) followed by cooling to normal body temperature; and (3) the use of some solvents such as ethanol, which can mimic the effect.[43–45]

Clinical Significance

Thermotolerance occurs in human tumors and normal tissues.[33,50] Therefore, it is a clinically relevant phenomenon that can reduce the killing effectiveness of heat. Fortunately, it is not permanent. Thermotolerance decays by 72 hours after induction, regardless of the technique of induction. Clinically, it is advisable to maintain more than a 72-hour interval between heat fractions to maximize cytotoxicity.

PATHOPHYSIOLOGY OF HYPERTHERMIC TUMOR TREATMENT

The vasculature of most tumors is structurally and physiologically abnormal. Tumors have a fixed arteriolar supply, deriving their vasculature from the venular and capillary side of the vascular tree. Because of the exaggerated expansion of the capillary-venous network, tumors are hypotensive and have sluggish and often intermittent blood flow.[61] Many of the vessels are incompletely or abnormally formed, leading to development of large venous sinusoids and spontaneous hemorrhage. This leads to development of regions of tumor that are chronically hypoxic and acidotic.[4,65,73] The acidosis results from anaerobic glycolysis and build-up of lactic acid. This abnormal physiological state makes the tumor especially sensitive to heat for the following reasons:

1. Heat is preferentially cytotoxic to hypoxic-acidotic cells.[29]
2. Heat preferentially destroys tumor microvasculature.[20–23,63,65]
3. Under constant application of heat, tumors are often hotter than adjacent normal tissue because of their impaired ability to carry away the heat via a sluggish vascular network.

Clinical Significance

The clinical significance of tumor microcirculatory pathophysiology is that it does not occur in normal tissues. Hence, it provides a rational basis for expecting heat to have preferentially cytotoxic effects in tumor. Unfortunately, although it is true that selective heating of clinical tumors is often observed, a high response rate does not occur with that modality alone. In fact, response rates and durations of response of tumors treated with heat alone have been relatively poor in tumors in both humans and pet animals.[14,15,40,48–50] The lack of effectiveness may be related to the observation that not all portions of tumor are heated adequately. The implications may be summarized as follows:

1. Not all tumor vasculature is abnormal and is not superheated.

2. Some areas of tumor may be underheated because of poor power distribution from available heating devices.

3. Small nests of tumor cells may reside in or near normal tissue vasculature and may not be adequately heated.

In addition, heat alone may not provide enough cytotoxicity to kill every tumor cell. Clinically, a practical limit to treatment is 30 minutes to 1 hour. From the survival curves in Figure 174–1A, 60 minutes at 111.2°F (44°C) yields about 3 logs of cell kill. By comparison, tumors as small as 1 cm in diameter may have been between 1×10^8 and 1×10^9 cells.

Several laboratories are now investigating a variety of heat-sensitizing agents that effectively lower the D_o and in some cases prevent thermotolerance. Examples of heat-sensitizing agents include ethanol, local anesthetics, polyamines, inhibitors of polyamine synthesis, and steroids.[25,26,28,33,38,76] The highest response rates for heat alone have been in the treatment of bovine ocular squamous cell carcinomas. Four reports have been published, involving a total of several hundred animals. In all reports the complete response rate was near 90 per cent. Local anesthetics, such as lidocaine, were used in most of these animals before heating.[1,18,30,37]

Secondly, it may be possible to enhance preferential tumor heating by manipulating normal tissue blood flow relative to tumor with vasoactive drugs such as hydralazine[51,70,75] or by providing systemic cooling of blood while heating the tumor.[57]

HYPERTHERMIA AS AN ADJUVANT TO RADIATION

Aside from the additive benefits of combined modalities, there are specific biological reasons for interest in heat as an adjuvant to radiation:

1. Heat increases the radiosensitivity of cells and reduces their ability to repair radiation damage.

2. Heat preferentially increases the radiosensitivity of hypoxic-acidotic cells, which are 2.5 to 3.0 times more resistant to radiation than are aerobic cells.

3. Heat is preferentially cytotoxic to radioresistant S-phase cells.[11]

Therefore, in a simplified view, heat would either directly kill or radiosensitize cells in poorly perfused areas, and radiation alone would kill aerobic cells residing near the tumor edge and in adjacent normal tissue where adequate heating may not occur.

Heat radiosensitization is usually described by the *thermal enhancement ratio,* or the ratio of radiation doses for radiation alone compared with heat plus radiation to achieve an isoeffect, such as 50 per cent tumor cure or 50 per cent moist desquamation. Therefore, for an isoeffect, the thermal enhancement ratio is equal to:

$$\frac{\text{radiation alone dose}}{\text{heat} + \text{radiation dose}}$$

For the combined therapy to have an advantageous effect, the thermal enhancement ratio in normal tissue must be less than that in tumor tissue. The *therapeutic gain factor* is defined as the ratio of thermal enhancement ratios for tumor and normal tissue. A thermal gain factor greater than 1 indicates greater effect being achieved in tumor relative to normal tissue.

Both thermal enhancement ratio and therapeutic gain factors are strongly dependent on the *sequence* and time interval between heat and radiation, with the maximum thermal enhancement ratios observed when the two are given simultaneously. Single heat and radiation fraction studies in mice indicated that the largest therapeutic gain factors would be obtained when radiation preceded heat by 2 to 3 hours.[11,59] However, more recent studies with multifractionated heat and radiation do not show such a clear advantage to that sequence.[53]

Clinical Significance

Clinically, the greatest effect in tumor and a minimal effect in normal tissue would be most desirable. Unfortunately, the optimum sequence has yet to be determined. Part of the problem with extrapolation of murine data lies in the fact that for most clinical heating systems the tumor and adjacent normal tissues do not reach the same temperature. In general, tumors have a tendency to superheat compared with adjacent normal tissue. The exact opposite situation occurs in rodent systems, which have typically used water-bath heating. In a water bath, the skin is hotter than the underlying tumor, since heating of the tumor depends on thermal conduction through the skin.

A second problem with murine data is that most of the normal tissue data has been for "early responding" tissues, such as skin, gut epithelium, and so on. Unfortunately, the incidence of these early radiation effects does not reflect the more serious "late" complications such as fibrosis and bone necrosis.[71]

Clinically, simultaneous heat and radiation are technically difficult and economically impossible because this method would occupy a radiotherapy room for hours for one patient.

HEAT COMBINED WITH CHEMOTHERAPY

The biological rationale for the combination of heat and chemotherapy is threefold:

1. Mild hyperthermia (102.2 to 105.8°F, or 39° to 41°C) may increase tumor blood flow, thereby increasing tumor drug concentrations.

2. Hyperthermia may increase cell membrane permeability, thereby allowing for higher intracellular concentrations.

3. Hyperthermia potentiates the cytotoxic effects of a variety of chemotherapeutic drugs, including

adriamycin, bleomycin, cisplatin, alkylating agents, and nitrosureas.

As with heat and radiation, the *in vivo* effects of heat combined with chemotherapy are often synergistic rather than additive. Synergism depends on sequencing, with the best results obtained when the two treatments are given in close proximity.[33] For most drugs studied, the best results are obtained when the temperature is over 109.4°F (43°C).[33]

Clinical Significance

The combination of heat with chemotherapy has some obvious advantages over its combination with radiation. The primary advantage is that such combinations could be used for treatment of systemic disease, whereas radiotherapy can only be used for regional diseases. In addition, some regional diseases could be approached via local perfusion with heated perfusates containing chemotherapeutic agents.[66] The use of chemotherapeutic agents in combination with whole body heating techniques might be of use for disseminated diseases, such as lymphomas or leukemias. However, since neither heating nor chemotherapy could be focused on the tumor, serious normal tissue complications could result.

Methods

Physical Methods—Hyperthermia Production

The available techniques for producing hyperthermia result in three categories of heating: systemic, regional, and localized. The extent and location of disease dictate the type of heating and the method of choice.

Systemic Hyperthermia. Although the procedure is tedious, total body hyperthemia is relatively simple to produce. One technique involves anesthesia followed by administration of intravenous fluids (saline or Ringer's solution) at a rate of 2 to 3 ml/kg/minute. The animal is placed on a heated water blanket, which is used as a heat exchanger. At hourly intervals, atropine is readministered at 0.025 mg/kg. The temperature is maintained by circulating a water and alcohol mixture through the blanket, which is heated by an Aquamatic K-Thermia unit,* which has been modified so that temperatures up to 122°F (50°C) can be achieved. Temperature probes (thermistors or thermocouples) are placed in the rectum and trachea and on the skin. The animal is sealed in a plastic bag and wrapped in the thermal blanket. Inspired air is humidified and warmed to 100.4°F (38°C) to minimize evaporative cooling loss. The blanket temperature is maintained at 116.6°F (47°C) until the desired systemic temperature is attained. Care should be taken to keep skin temperatures below 108.5°F

(42.5°C) to prevent burns, especially at pressure points. Regulation at a given temperature is readily accomplished by regulating the blanket temperature or exposing the animal to ambient temperature. At the completion of the procedure, the blanket temperature is reduced to 59°F (15°C) and the core temperature is reduced below 104°F (40°C). Anesthesia is discontinued and the animal is returned to its cage to allow natural cooling, with periodic observation.

At the beginning of the procedure, dogs generally have core temperatures of between 99.5°F and 101.3°F (37.5° and 38.5°C). Total body heating progresses at a constant rate of approximately 0.4°F (0.2°C) per hour until a temperature 0.9°F (0.5°C) below the desired temperature is attained. Active heating is terminated, and the core temperature will coast to the desired temperature within 15 to 20 minutes.

Alternative methods for induction of systemic hyperthermia include arteriovenous shunts with counter-current heat exchangers,[60] humidified warm-air chambers,[47] and electromagnetic devices, such as the Magnetrode.*[56] The major advantage of these techniques is that the rate of heating is much faster, with steady state being achieved in 30 to 40 minutes instead of the 2 to 3 hours required for the blanket technique. Thermotolerance induction is less of a problem with faster heating techniques. Their major disadvantage relative to blanket heating is the higher cost.

Additional Methods

Regional Hyperthermia

Regional hyperthermia is produced when a major portion of the body is heated. This includes heating total limbs or portions of the thorax, abdomen, or pelvis.

Stehlin and associates[66] and Cavaliere and colleagues[5] have used heated blood for perfusion of extremities to produce regional heating. The technique involves production of an arteriovenous shunt with heating of the shunted blood through a heat exchanger.

Regional heating has been studied[68] using magnetic induction techniques. Successful heating was achieved with a concentric coil operating at 13.56 MHz wrapped around the longitudinal axis of the body. Oleson[55] has described the physical characteristics of this heating technique and concludes that power density distributions that produce direct heating are limited to relatively superficial regions of the human body. Improved depth of heating with magnetic induction has been described using a coaxial coil pair.[58] Improved midplane power deposition is accomplished although the deposition patterns are again quite variable.

Another approach[72] to produce deep heating uses

---

*American Medical Systems, Cincinnati, OH.

*Henry Electric, Los Angeles, CA.

an array of microwave applicators positioned symmetrically around the patient. This approach also produces regional heating. The applicators act as antennae that radiate electromagnetic energy into the patient. The applicators are excited as a phased array such that the incident wave from each applicator interacts with adjacent waves to minimize power distributions at the skin surface. The resultant power distributions are relatively uniform, even at the center of the body.

The critical factor for heating deep-seated tumors to therapeutic temperatures with electromagnetic devices is the difference in perfusion between normal and malignant tissues. Tumors, which have decreased perfusion, may selectively heat because of the decreased capacity to conduct heat away from the tumor mass.

Localized Hyperthermia

The most important application for hyperthermia in veterinary medicine is for the treatment of peripherally accessible lesions. The usual goal of localized hyperthermia is to produce homogeneous tumor temperatures between 107.6°F and 114.8°F (42° and 46°C) in very restricted volumes.

Historically, diathermy or microwaves and ultrasound have been used for many years for physical therapy to relieve a variety of disorders.[46] Currently, microwave frequencies between 500 kHz and 2,450 MHz are used to heat tissue volumes from 1 to 1,000 cm^3 with powers varying from 1 to 200 watts. Recently, Guy[32] has reviewed the biophysics of high-frequency currents and electromagnetic radiation, and Frizzell and Dunn[24] have reviewed the biophysics of ultrasound and the interaction of these energy sources with the biosphere.

Electromagnetic Radiation

Electromagnetic energy is radiated by applicators positioned externally over the surface to be heated. The generators operate at frequencies between 50 and 2,450 MHz and are usually capable of delivering up to 210 watts. The applicators vary in size from a few centimeters in diameter to several centimeters on a side (Fig. 174–3). The depth dose characteristics are such that heating is maximum at the surface, possibly resulting in excessive heating of the skin before an underlying tumor is heated. Since the depth of penetration is small, deep-seated tumors cannot be heated. For example, at 915 MHz the power intensity decreases to 35 per cent of its surface value at a depth of 2.0 cm. The penetration characteristics vary as a function of frequency. At lower frequencies the penetration depth increases. For example, the 35 per cent power intensity depth for 50 MHz increases to 6.0 cm. However, to effectively propagate electromagnetic waves, the applicator must be an appreciable fraction of the wavelength (~60 cm at 10 MHz in tissue). As a consequence, appli-

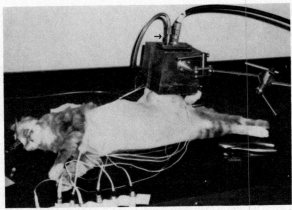

Figure 174–3. Example of a 915-MHz microwave treatment of a large soft tissue sarcoma in the groin of a cat. The thermistor needles used for measurement of tissue temperature are placed at right angles to the electric field of the applicator to minimize disturbance of the field by the thermistors. A vented air port *(arrow)* cools the skin during the treatment.

cators become too large relative to the patient size at low frequencies.

Radiofrequency Current Heating

An alternate approach to radiant techniques for localized heating is to pass an electrical current directly through the tissue to be heated. The tissue acts like an electrical resistor, dissipating power and heating. Frequencies employed vary from 500 kHz to 50 MHz. If the frequency is kept low enough to minimize the capacitive component of current, the power loss in the tissue is simply due to resistance losses, which produce the local heating.

Doss and McCabe[19] have described this low-frequency current field technique for heating using a 500-kHz generator. The current density is deter-

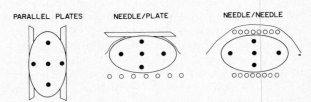

Figure 174–4. Alternative treatment arrangements for 500-kHz radio frequency heating *(LCF).* Two water-cooled copper plates can be placed on either side of the tumor *(parallel plates).* A row of needles, connected in series, can be placed beneath the tumor and a water-cooled copper plate placed on the tumor surface *(needle/plate).* Alternatively, two rows of needles can be placed on either side of the tumor *(needle/needle).* Open circles represent needle placement positions, closed circles represent position of temperature-monitoring thermistors. As in the case of microwave heating, thermistors should be placed at right angles to the electric field to minimize artifacts in temperature measurement. (Reprinted with permission from Dewhirst, M. W., Connor, W. G., and Sim, D. A.: Preliminary results of a phase III trial of spontaneous animal tumors to heat and/or radiation: Early normal tissue response and tumor volume influence on initial response. Int. J. Radiat. Oncol. Biol. Phys. 8:1951, 1982.)

mined by the arrangement of the electrodes used to couple the power generator to the tissue. This in turn determines the heat distributions that result. Figure 174–4 illustrates some of the possibilities for arranging the coupling electrodes. The tissue volume is sandwiched between two parallel plates. Needles implanted into tissue and electrically tied together effectively act as a conducting plate.

A low-frequency current field "heat gun" has been developed that uses the parallel plate concept of heating. The plates are arranged as tweezers, and the tumor volume is pressed between the plates. The tissue acts as a conductive resistor and heats. The power source is small and battery powered so that the unit is portable. This unit is available commercially and has been used for treatment of bovine ocular squamous cell carcinomas, equine tumors, and some small-animal tumors.[1,18,30,31,37]

Ultrasonic Heating

Ultrasound has also been used to produce localized hyperthermia for cancer therapy.[33,42,49] The propagation of ultrasound through tissue is the penetration of oscillating pressure waves into the medium at frequencies ranging from 500 kHz to 10 MHz. These pressure waves cause oscillations of tissue molecules. Damping forces such as viscosity result in an energy transfer from the ultrasound beam to the tissue, causing heating.

A focusing lens on the transducer (applicator) concentrates the energy in the ultrasound beam at the focal depth, thus protecting more superficial structures. A focused beam can be scanned mechanically around the periphery of a tumor to heat the correct volume.[42] Ultrasound beams will not penetrate tissue-bone and tissue-air interfaces and therefore cannot be used to treat tumors behind bone or air.

Frizzell and Dunn[24] have reviewed the biophysics of ultrasound in detail, and Christensen and Durney[7] have published a helpful review of the fundamentals and methods used for localized hyperthermia.

Temperature Measurement

The two primary methods for measuring temperature in tissue are thermistors and thermocouples (Fig. 174–5). A thermistor is an electronic device whose resistance varies as a function of temperature. The relationship between resistance and temperature is complex, requiring conversion tables, but it is very accurate. When properly calibrated, a thermistor is accurate to 0.018°F (0.01°C).

The thermocouple is formed from a junction between two unlike metals (copper and constantan). The junction results in a small voltage differential between the two metals. The voltage difference varies as a function of temperature, thus providing a basis for thermometry. The thermocouple is less accurate than a thermistor but has the advantage that most

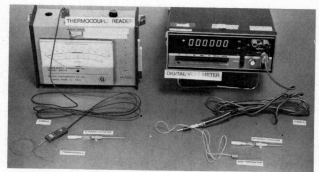

Figure 174–5. Two types of invasive temperature measuring devices. Commercially available thermocouples, a copper constantan device, can be inserted into preplaced 18-gauge catheters for direct measurement of temperature. These devices are accurate to about 0.10° C. Thermistors, also commercially available, can be placed in preplaced 20-gauge catheters for measurement of tissue temperature. The conversion from resistance to temperature is complex, requiring a conversion table. However, the accuracy of this device can be considerably better than that of the thermocouple (± 0.01° C).

commercially available readers are calibrated to give direct measurement of temperature.[6]

CLINICAL RESULTS[13]

Clinical Studies with Heat Alone

Localized Heating

Several studies have been published describing the use of heat alone. In general, the proportion of complete responses has been relatively low and response durations have been short (Table 174–1). The notable exceptions to this trend are the four studies using heat to treat bovine ocular squamous cell carcinomas.[1,18,30,37] In those series the complete response rate was nearly 90 per cent for small tumors requiring one heat treatment. The relatively high response rates observed for those series may have been related to species variation in thermal sensitivity or to the use of local anesthetics, which are potent heat sensitizers.[76] Humans treated with heat alone have had results similar to those in small animals.[40,48,50]

Whole Body Heating

Relatively few studies have investigated whole body heating in animals. We performed a study in dogs with disseminated malignancies (Table 174–2) using the water blanket technique. No concomitant chemotherapy was given.

The most common tumor type treated in this series was the mast cell sarcoma. The overall complete response rate was 33 per cent with only one animal remaining disease free for a significant length of time. The response rate seemed to depend on total tumor burden, in that no animals with tumors achieved complete response, half larger than 100 cm³, in the

TABLE 174–1.   Clinical Effects of Heat Alone—Local Hyperthermia

Author	Method	Species	Number of Tumors	Complete Response Rate	Malignant Histologies* Where Complete Response Obtained	Comments
Dewhirst et al.[15]	500 kHz LCF 111.2°F (44°C), 30 min 1 fx/wk, 4 fx§	Cat, dog	16	25%	SCC, Me, Mast	‡
Marmor et al.[49]	2.97 MHz ultrasound 109.4–113.0°F (43–45°C), 30 min	Cat, dog	22	14%	SCC	——
Grier et al.[31]	2 MHz LCF "heat gun" 122.0°F (50°C), 30 sec	Cat, dog	33	70%	SCC, FSA, Me	——
Doss[18]	2 MHz LCF "heat gun" 122.0°F (50°C), 30 sec	Cattle	200	90%	SCC only	Lidocaine used
Kainer et al.[37]	2 MHz LCF "heat gun" 122.0°F (50°C), 30 sec	Cattle	20	55%†	SCC only	Lidocaine used
Grier et al.[30]	2 MHz LCF "heat gun" 122.0°F (50°C), 30 sec	Cattle	37	67%	SCC only	Lidocaine used
Adams[1]	2 MHz LCF "heat gun" 122.0°F (50°C), 30 sec	Cattle	299	75%†	SCC only	Lidocaine used

*SCC = squamous cell carcinoma, Me = melanoma, Mast = mast cell sarcoma, FSA = fibrosarcoma, LCF = low-frequency current field
†90% complete response rate observed in tumors ≤5 mm
‡Data obtained from a randomized clinical trial. The nonresponse rate was significantly greater than that for radiation alone or heat plus radiation. Response duration was significantly shorter than the other two modalities ($p < .01$ in both cases).
§fx = fractions.

TABLE 174–2.   Clinical Summary of 9 Patients Treated with Whole Body Heat

Case No.	Breed	Histology	Stage	Estimated Tumor Burden	Treatment Summary	Response Type	Complications
49	Australian shepherd female	Mammary adenocarcinoma	$T_4N_0M_2$	>100 cm³	60 min @ 107.6°F (42°C) once weekly × 4	None	Acute liver necrosis. Biliary obstruction. Tumor metastasis to liver present prior to therapy
50	Boxer 6-yr female	Lymphosarcoma	III_a	>100 cm³	60 min @ 107.6°F (42°C) once weekly × 4	None	Pressure burn on point of hip
343	Australian shepherd 8-yr female	Mast cell sarcoma, well differentiated	III_a	10 cm³	60 min @ 107.6°F (42°C) once weekly × 4	None	None. Cimetidine* given during treatment
147	Terrier mix 13-yr female	Mast cell sarcoma	III_a	15 cm³	60 min @ 107.6°F (42°C) once weekly × 4	Partial response	Died of gastric ulceration. No cimetidine therapy given
230	Great Dane 10-yr male	Mast cell sarcoma	III_a	600 cm³	60 min @ 107.6°F (42°C) 1 fraction	No response	Cimetidine therapy given, no gastric ulcer
359	Springer spaniel 10-yr male	Mast cell sarcoma, undifferentiated	III_a	180 cm³	60 min @ 107.6°F (42°C) 2 fractions 2 wk apart	No response	Severe pitting edema in tumor site after heat
170	Cat 10-yr male	Mast cell sarcoma, undifferentiated	III_a	2 cm³	60 min @ 107.6°F (42°C) once weekly × 4 fractions	Complete response 1-mo duration, then regrew	None. Cimetidine not given.
336	Boxer 7-yr female	Mast cell sarcoma, undifferentiated	III_a	2 cm³	60 min @ 107.6°F (42°C) once weekly × 4 fractions	Complete response 7-mo duration then regrew	Pressure burn on chest wall. Was on cimetidine therapy prior to therapy
91	Chihuahua 10-yr female	Mast cell sarcoma	III_a	2 cm³	60 min @ 107.6°F (42°C) once weekly × 4 fractions	Complete response No regrowth at 4-yr post	None. Cimetidine not given.

*Dose of 15 mg/kg three times daily.

range of 10 to 20 cm³, and one-third with tumors of about 2 cm³.

The major toxicities resulting from the therapy included burns at pressure points (i.e., excessive heating at points of contact with the heating blankets) and perforating gastroduodenitis in one animal with a mast cell sarcoma that was not maintained on cimetidine concomitantly with treatment. Transient elevations in blood lactate dehydrogenase, alkaline phosphatase, and creatine phosphokinase were observed. No bone marrow or gut toxicity was seen.

The results of this limited study are somewhat encouraging for treatment of disseminated mast cell disease. The response rate might be improved with the addition of appropriate chemotherapeutic agents, but the risk of serious normal tissue toxicity would also increase with such a combined approach. Without further study it is unclear whether whole body heating is of long-term value in the treatment of either mast cell disease or other malignancies.

In a series of seven dogs with osteosarcoma treated with whole body heating techniques, Kapp and Lord[39] found alterations in normal metastatic behavior. All seven of these animals developed skeletal metastases before pulmonary metastases. A variety of other unusual metastatic sites were also seen at necropsy.

Whole body heating techniques have had very limited success in human patients, even when concomitant chemotherapy has been given. The complete response rates have been less than 5 per cent, with short response durations.[2,35,60]

In general, the use of whole body heating techniques has not been encouraging. For the methods to be efficacious, improvements in complete response rate and duration of response must be attained either via combined therapy with heat sensitizers or with radiation therapy. Trials of this type have yet to be performed in human or veterinary medicine.

In spite of the dismal results obtained for heat alone (either whole body or local), there still may be a role for it in veterinary clinical practice. In contrast to human medicine, radiotherapy facilities are not always available and traditional chemotherapy is either not effective, too toxic, or too expensive. By comparison, interstitial heating devices such as the heat gun are inexpensive and fairly easy to use. It is possible that this method may prove useful as an adjuvant to surgery or heat-sensitizing drugs. For example, adjuvant heat may be an effective treatment for inoperable tumors such as squamous cell carcinomas of the nose and eyelids in cats and as an adjuvant to surgery when incomplete surgical removal is difficult. Alternatively, it is an effective debulking agent and could be used to shrink tumors before surgical resection. Further studies are required to test its effectiveness in these situations.

Clinical Studies with Heat and Radiation

A randomized trial with heat[15] or radiation or both was begun at our institution in 1978, using sponta-

neous pet animal malignancies. In this trial, animals were stratified by histological type and randomized to receive either heat alone (△), radiation alone (XRT), or heat combined with radiation (△ + XRT). The prescription was 111.2 ± 3.6°F (44 ± 2.0°C) for 30 minutes once weekly. The radiation prescription was 460 rads per fraction twice weekly for eight fractions. When heat was given, it preceded radiation by no more than 10 minutes. The heat treatment methods included use of 2,450 MHz microwaves or 500 kHz low-frequency current field heating as described in the methods section of this chapter.

A total of 16 animals were treated by heat alone. That area of study was closed in 1980 because of the early findings that heat alone resulted in a high fraction of nonresponses and significantly shorter response duration than either XRT or △ + XRT.[14,15]

Currently, a total of 130 additional animals have been treated, with 69 receiving XRT and 61 receiving △ + XRT. The population consists of 89 dogs and 41 cats with either mast cell sarcomas (31), mammary adenocarcinomas (15), squamous cell carcinomas (50), melanomas (18), or fibrosarcomas (16).

We have analyzed this population by examining which tumor characteristics and treatment variables are important for prediction of both early and long-term responses. Since the radiation dose was fixed, it was not a variable factor in determination of response. In contrast, tumor temperature distributions were quite variable, depending on the size, location, and type of tumor. Treatment variables included descriptions of thermal gradients and heat treatment methods. The goal of this analysis was to determine which types of tumors could best benefit from adjuvant △ and how best to treat them to ensure that improved response would be obtained.

Prognostic Variables

The complete response rates (complete tumor regression of one month's duration or more) varied between different histological, volume, and site subgroups. The relative improvement in complete response rate with adjuvant heat is described by the *thermal relative risk*, which is the ratio of complete response rates for △ + XRT versus XRT alone.[17] For all subgroups examined, the complete response rates for △ + XRT were greater than those for XRT alone, yielding thermal relative risks greater than one (Table 174–3). Statistically significant improvements in initial complete response rates were observed in melanomas, tumor volumes greater than 50 cm³, oral and subcutaneous sites, and for the overall population of animals.[16]

In some cases the initial response rate differential was not predictive of the differential in response duration. For example, the high initial complete response rate in melanomas treated with △ + XRT of 100 per cent was encouraging, but the response duration of these same tumors was relatively short compared with melanomas treated with XRT alone (Fig. 174–6).[17]

TABLE 174–3. Variation in Complete Response Rates and Relative Responses for Patient Prognostic Variables. Radiation Alone (XRT) vs. Heat Plus Radiation (ΔXRT)

	XRT	Δ XRT	TRR*
Subgroup			
Neoplasm			
Mast cell sarcoma	5/15 (.330)	10/13 (.770)	2.31
Mammary adenocarcinoma	1/8 (.125)	4/7 (.570)	4.57
Melanoma	1/8 (.125)	8/8 (1.00)	8.00†
Squamous cell carcinoma	11/25 (.440)	15/24 (.625)	1.42
Fibrosarcoma	3/9 (.330)	3/7 (.430)	1.29
Volume			
<2cm³	9/14 (.640)	15/19 (.790)	1.23
2–20cm³	10/10 (.500)	12/18 (.670)	1.33
20–50cm³	1/11 (.090)	5/9 (.560)	6.11
50–100cm³	1/11 (.090)	6/7 (.860)	9.43†
>100cm³	0/9 (.000)	2/6 (.330)	0.00†
Site			
Dermal	13/25 (.520)	19/25 (.760)	2.32
Oral	6/19 (.320)	11/15 (.730)	1.46†
Subcutaneous	2/21 (.100)	10/19 (.530)	5.53†
Summary			
All animals	21/65 (.320)	40/59 (.680)	2.10†

*TRR = Thermal relative risk.
†Observed difference in complete response rates statistically significant (p<.01).

Similarly, the response differential steadily increased for increasing tumor volume, with the thermal relative risk varying from 1.23 for small tumors (<2 cm³) to infinity for tumors larger than 100 cm³. In contrast, the response duration differential (described by the relative relapse rate) was greatest for small and large tumors, with no improvement in response for tumors of 20 to 50 cm³.[16]

The type of neoplasm that benefited most from adjuvant heat was the mammary adenocarcinoma, with a thermal relative risk of 4.57 and significantly improved duration of response (Fig. 174–7).[17]

Treatment Variables

Intratumoral thermal gradients varied widely (Fig. 174–8). The gradients were the result of multiple

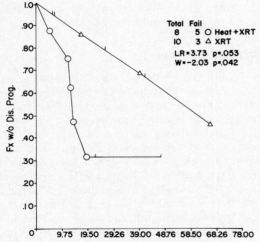

Figure 174–6. Response duration from end of treatment (ENDRX) to last date of contact (LDC) for malignant melanoma. Even though the initial complete response rate for animals receiving the combined therapy was 100 per cent compared with 12 per cent for those receiving radiation alone, the response duration for those animals receiving the combined therapy was significantly shorter than that of those receiving radiation alone. (Reprinted with permission from Dewhirst, M. W., Sim, D. A., Wilson, S., DeYoung, D., and Parsells, J. L.: The correlation between initial and long-term responses of spontaneous pet animal tumors to heat and radiation or radiation alone. Cancer Res. 44:43, 1984.)

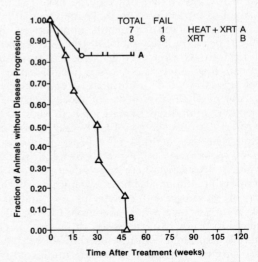

Figure 174–7. Response duration for mammary adenocarcinoma. In contrast to melanomas, the complete response rate for animals in this group receiving heat and radiation was significantly higher than those treated with radiation alone (57 per cent versus 12.5 per cent, respectively). In addition, the response duration of the animals receiving the combined therapy was significantly higher than that of those receiving radiation alone.

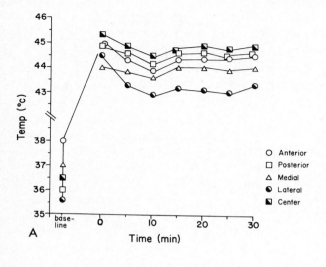

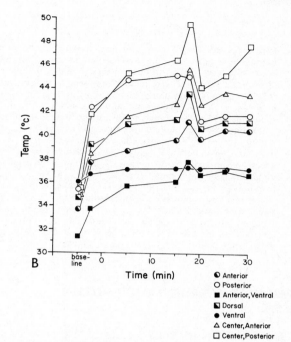

Figure 174–8. Heating curves for two different tumors. *A,* This tumor was a squamous cell carcinoma involving the skin in the groin of a dalmatian. The heating curves represent five different positions within the tumor, which was heated with 2,450-MHz microwaves. Temperature distributions were relatively uniform, the minimum monitored temperature being greater than 43° C.

B, Heating curve for a fibrosarcoma of the oral cavity. In this case, it was not possible to get uniform heating throughout the tumor volume. This tumor was heated with 500-KHz RF heating. The tumor extended onto both sides of the dental arcade. Shielding of parts of the tumor by the intervening teeth prevented adequate heating. (Reprinted with permission from Dewhirst, M. W., Sim, D. A., Wilson, S., De Young, D., and Parsells, J. L.: The correlation between initial and long-term responses of spontaneous pet animal tumors to heat and radiation or radiation alone. Cancer Res. *44:*43, 1984.)

factors including technical difficulties because of tumor location, blood flow, and poor power deposition patterns. We examined the relationship between thermal dose (tumor temperature averages, maxima, minima, and ranges) and clinical outcome, as described by complete response rates and response duration. The time-temperature data were condensed to more usable forms by calculating time-temperature integrals (°-minute),[16] converting to equivalent minutes at 109.4°F (43°C)[64] or standard hyperthermia units.[27] The minimum temperature obtained on the first heat treatment, regardless of how it was con-

verted to thermal dose, was the most important factor for prediction of clinical response (Figs. 174–9 and 174–10).[16]

Effects on Normal Tissue

To achieve a therapeutic gain, the degree of normal tissue damage must be less than the degree of tumor damage. The effects of the combined therapy on normal tissue can be divided into those resulting from heat alone and those resulting from heat enhancement of radiation damage.

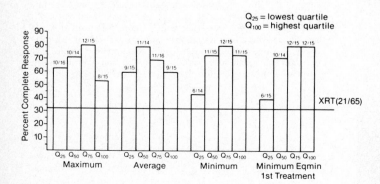

Figure 174–9. Complete response rate as a function of minimum equivalent minutes—quartile variation. A good thermal dose predictor should have an increasing complete response rate as the value of that dose increases. The maximum intratumoral values showed little correlation with complete response rate. The overall average of all tumor temperature-monitored locations shows no such trend. The minimum value obtained on the average and the first treatment indicated an increasing heat complete response rate as a function of increasing value. The horizontal line at 32 per cent represents the complete response rate for radiation alone. The best predictor of initial complete response rate was the minimum temperature achieved on the first heat treatment, described in this case as equivalent minutes at 43° C. (Reprinted with permission from Dewhirst, M. W., Sim, D. A., Sapareto, S., and Connor, W. G.: Importance of minimum tumor temperature in determining early and long-term responses of spontaneous pet animal tumors to heat and radiation. Cancer Res. *44:*43, 1984.)

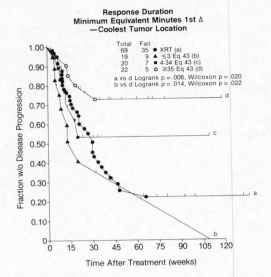

Response Duration
Minimum Equivalent Minutes 1st Δ
—Coolest Tumor Location

Figure 174–10. Response duration as a function of coolest tumor location. A comparison of the response duration curves for radiation alone to animals that were in the lowest, middle, or upper third of the minimum heat dose range demonstrated that for that less than three equivalent minutes at 43° C no significant improvement in response duration is noted. An intermediate duration of response was noted for animals receiving between 4 and 34 equivalent minutes. Those patients receiving greater than 35 equivalent minutes at 43° C had a significant improvement in response duration over radiation alone and animals in the lowest heat dose group. As in complete response rate, the minimum temperature on the first heat treatment was the best predictor of long-term response of tumors treated with combined radiation and heat. (Reprinted with permission from Dewhirst, M. W., Sim, D. A., Sapareto, S., and Connor, W. G.: Importance of minimum tumor temperature in determining early and long-term responses of spontaneous pet animal tumors to heat and radiation. Cancer Res. *44*:43, 1984.)

EFFECTS OF HYPERTHERMIA ON NORMAL TISSUE

Localized hyperthermia can result in four types of normal tissue damage. These side effects can be a significant nursing problem, both for the clinician and the pet owner. With proper care, however, they will heal. The types of complications are edema, skin infarcts, burns, and rapid tumor dissolution.

Tumor bed edema is usually not a clinical problem, lasting from 48 to 72 hours after heating. In some cases, however, edema has been either painful or life-threatening. Examples include chemosis and blepharospasm after treatment of the eyelids,[31] dysphagia or dyspnea after treatment of the base of tongue and pharyngea lesions, and lameness after treatment of large limb lesions.

Skin infarcts occur quite commonly (38.9 per cent incidence), especially when the underlying tumor is closely adherent to or invading skin. These usually become apparent 48 to 72 hours after treatment, although in some cases the latent period has been as

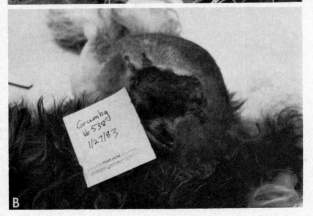

Figure 174–11. A, A 5-MHz plane wave ultrasound transducer positioned over the medial aspect of the right thigh for treatment of a large myxosarcoma. The water bag is coupled to the skin via ultrasound conductive jelly, and the water was maintained at room temperature to prevent surface burning. This patient received one heat treatment. All monitored temperatures within the tumor were between 42 and 46° C. The treatment duration was 30 minutes. *B,* Two weeks after completion of the single heat treatment the patient developed a large skin infarct on the lateral aspect of the thigh. This infarct probably resulted from dissolution of tumor vasculature, which is more sensitive to heat stress than normal tissue. When overlying skin is tightly adherent to tumor, the skin also may lose its blood supply as a result of the tumor infarct. In this case the infarct developed in a site distal from the application site of the ultrasound transducer. Temperatures in this area were not hot enough to have caused direct burning.

long as 2 weeks. By carefully monitoring surface temperatures we have verified that these are not burns. The infarcts slough within 2 weeks of development (Fig. 174–11). Treatment consists of conservative management including debridement of necrotic tissue, twice-daily cleaning with Betadine solution, prophylactic antibiotics to prevent secondary bacterial infection, and epithelialization stimulants. The rate of healing depends on the size of the lesion but usually occurs within 2 months of onset.

Thermal burns are less common (10 per cent incidence) but can happen, since general anesthesia is required for heat treatment. In most cases, the burns are third degree. Clinical management is similar to that for skin infarcts.

Rapid tumor necrosis has been a problem, especially when tumor is closely adherent to underlying bone. Denudation of the mandible, maxilla, and metacarpal bones has occurred, and these lesions have required surgical repair. Heat treatment of tongue lesions has sometimes resulted in severe edema and necrosis in sites distant from the heated volume. In many cases, however, long-term tumor control with good cosmetic results can be achieved (Fig. 174–12).

HEAT ENHANCEMENT OF RADIATION EFFECTS

Little or no enhancement of the incidence or severity of either early or late radiation effects in normal tissue has been observed (Table 174–4). The implications in conjunction with the observed tumor results indicate that a therapeutic gain is possible

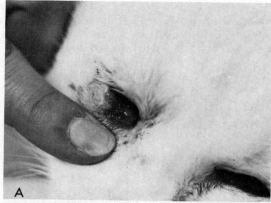
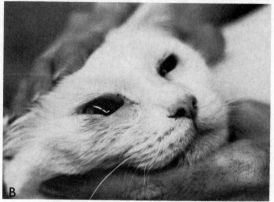

Figure 174–12. A, Appearance of a squamous cell carcinoma of the lower eyelid of a cat prior to receiving a combination of heat and radiation. B, This tumor responded completely and four years have passed with no recurrence. Good cosmetic results were achieved with minimal hair loss.

TABLE 174–4. Comparison of Incidence of Radiation-Induced Normal Tissue Complications of Animals in Table 174–3 Treated with Radiation Alone (XRT) vs. Heat Plus Radiation (Δ + XRT)

Complication	XRT Alone	Δ + XRT
*Early		
Moist desquamation <50% of field	14/65 (21.5%)	4/54 (7.4%)
Moist desquamation >50% of field	10/65 (15.4%)	15/54 (27.8%)
Mucositis <50%	5/27 (18.5%)	3/23 (13.0%)
Mucositis >50%	7/27 (25.9%)	9/23 (39.1%)
*Late		
Periodontal disease	5/7 (71.4%)	0/1 (0.0%)
Fibrosis	8/35 (22.9%)	10/29 (34.5%)
Hair loss	21/35 (60.0%)	18/30 (60.0%)
Bone necrosis	0/21 (0.0%)	3/19 (15.8%)

*Early = Complications occurring during or shortly after treatment
 Late = Complications usually occurring after 4 months after treatment
   Incidence based on at least 6 months follow-up, however

with combined heat and radiation. To achieve a significant gain, however, minimum tumor temperatures must be greater than 35 equivalent minutes at 109.4°F (43°C).

1. Adams, N. J.: Field application of the electrothermal technique for treating cancer eye. Proceedings, Western Section, American Society of Animal Science 30:40, 1979.
2. Bull, J. M., Lees, D. E., Schuette, W. H., et al.: Immunological and physiological responses to whole-body hyperthermia. Nat. Cancer Inst. Monogr. 61:177, 1982.
3. Busch, W.: Über den Einfluss welche heftigere Erysipeln zuwerlig auf organisierte Neubildungen ausüben. Vrh. Naturhist. Preuss Rhein. Westphal. 23:28, 1866.
4. Calderwood, S. K., and Dickson, J. A.: Inhibition of tumor blood flow at high blood sugar levels: Effects on tumor pH and hyperthermia. Nat. Cancer Inst. Monogr. 61:221, 1982.
5. Cavaliere, R., Moricca, G., and Caputo, A.: Regional hyperthermia by perfusion. In Wizenberg, M., and Robinson, J. E. (eds.): Proceedings of the International Symposium on Cancer Therapy by Hyperthermia and Radiation. American College of Radiology Press, Baltimore, 1975.
6. Cetas, T. C.: Invasive thermometry. In Nussbaum, G. H. (ed.): Physical Aspects of Hyperthermia. American Institute of Physics, Inc., New York, 1982.
7. Christensen, D. A., and Durney, C. H.: Hyperthermia production for cancer therapy: A review of fundamentals and methods. J. Microwave Power 16:2, 1981.
8. Coley, W. B.: The treatment of malignant tumors by repeated inoculations of erysipelas with a report of ten original cases. Am. J. Med. Sci. 106:488, 1893.
9. Crile, G.: Heat as an adjunct to the treatment of cancer. Clev. Clin. Q. 28:75, 1961.
10. Dethlefsen, L. A. (ed.): Cancer Therapy by Hyperthermia, Drugs, and Radiation. National Cancer Institute, Washington, D. C., 1982.
11. Dewey, W. C., Freeman, M. L., Raaphorst, G. P., et al.: Cell biology of hyperthermia and radiation. In Meyn, R. E., and Withers, R. (eds.): Radiation Biology in Cancer Research. Raven Press, New York, 1980.
12. Dewey, W. C., Hopwood, L. E., Sapareto, S. A., and Gerweck, L. E.: Cellular responses to combinations of hyperthermia and radiation. Radiology 123:463, 1977.
13. Dewhirst, M. W., and Connor, W. G.: Hyperthermia. In Gourley, I. M., and Vasseur, P. B. (eds.): Textbook of Soft Tissue Surgery. J. B. Lippincott, Philadelphia, 1984.
14. Dewhirst, M. W., Connor, W. G., Moon, T. E., and Roth, H. B.: Response of spontaneous animal tumors to heat and/or radiation: Preliminary results of a phase III trial. Nat. Cancer Inst. Monogr. 61:395, 1982.
15. Dewhirst, M. W., Connor, W. G., and Sim, D. A.: Preliminary results of a phase III trial of spontaneous animal tumors to heat and/or radiation: Early normal tissue response and tumor volume influence on initial response. Int. J. Radiat. Oncol. Biol. Phys. 8:1951, 1982.
16. Dewhirst, M. W., Sim, D. A., Sapareto, S., and Connor, W. G.: The importance of minimum tumor temperature in determining early and long-term responses of spontaneous pet animal tumors to heat and radiation. Cancer Res. 44:43, 1984.
17. Dewhirst, M. W., Sim, D. A., Wilson, S., et al.: The correlation between initial and long-term responses of spontaneous pet animal tumors to heat and radiation or radiation alone. Cancer Res. 43:5735, 1983.
18. Doss, J. D.: Electrothermal treatment of cancer eye. Los Alamos Scientific Laboratory mini-review 77:14, 1977.
19. Doss, J. D., and McCabe, C. W.: A technique for localized heating in tissue: An adjunct to tumor therapy. Med. Instrum. 10:16, 1976.
20. Eddy, A. A., Sutherland, R. M., and Chmielewski, G.: Tumor microvascular response: Hyperthermia and radiation combinations. Nat. Cancer Inst. Monogr. 61:225, 1982.

21. Emami, B., Nussbaum, G. H., Hahn, N., et al.: Histopathological study on the effects of hyperthermia on microvasculature. Int. J. Radiat. Oncol. Biol. Phys. 7:343, 1981.
22. Endrich, B., Zweifach, B. W., Reinhold, H. S., and Intaglietta, M.: Quantitative studies of microcirculator function in malignant tissue: Influence of temperature on microvasculary hemodynamics during the early growth of the BA 1112 rat sarcoma. Int. J. Radiat. Oncol. Biol. Phys. 5:2021, 1979.
23. Fehleisen, R.: In T. Fischer (ed.): Die Atiologie des Erysipels. Verlag, Berlin, 1883.
24. Frizzell, L. A., and Dunn, F.: Biophysics of ultrasound. In Lehmann, J. F. (ed.): Therapeutic Heat and Cold. Williams and Wilkins, Baltimore, 1982.
25. Fuller, D. J. M., and Gerner, E. W.: Delayed sensitization to heat by inhibitors of polyamine-biosynthetic enzymes. Cancer Res. 42:5046, 1982.
26. Fuller, D. J. M., and Gerner, E. W.: Polyamines: A dual role in the modulation of cellular sensitivity to heat. Radiat. Res. 92:439, 1982.
27. Gerner, E. W.: A general concept of thermal dose. Radiat. Res. (submitted), 1983.
28. Gerner, E. W., Stickney, D. G., Herman, T. S., and Fuller, D. J. M.: Polyamines and polyamine biosynthesis in cells exposed to hyperthermia. Radiat. Res. 93:340, 1983.
29. Gerweck, . E., Nygaard, T. G., and Burlett, M.: Response of cells to hyperthermia under acute and chronic hypoxic conditions. Cancer Res. 93:966, 1979.
30. Grier, R. L., Brewer, W. G., Paul, S. R., and Theilen, G. H.: Treatment of bovine and equine ocular squamous cell carcinoma by radiofrequency hyperthermia. J. Am. Vet. Med. Assoc. 177:55, 1980.
31. Grier, R. L., Brewer, W. G., and Theilen, G. H.: Hyperthermic treatment of superficial tumors in cats and dogs. J. Am. Vet. Med. Assoc. 177:227, 1980.
32. Guy, A. W.: Biophysics of high-frequency currents and electromagnetic radiation. In Lehmann, J. F. (ed.): Therapeutic Heat and Cold. Williams and Wilkins, Baltimore, 1982.
33. Hahn, G. M.: Hyperthermia and Cancer. Plenum Press, New York, 1982.
34. Henle, K. J.: Arrhenius analysis of thermal responses. In Storm, F. K. (ed.): Hyperthermia in Cancer Therapy. G. K. Hall Medical Publishers, Boston, 1983.
35. Herman, T. S., Zukoski, C. S., and Anderson, R. M.: Review of the current status of whole-body hyperthermia administered by water circulation techniques. Nat. Cancer Inst. Monogr. 61:365, 1982.
36. Jain, R. K., and Gullino, P. M. (eds.): Thermal characteristics of tumors: Applications in detection and treatment. Ann. N. Y. Acad. Sci. 335, 1980.
37. Kainer, R. A., Stringer, J. M., and Lueker, D. C.: Hyperthermia for treatment of ocular squamous cell tumors in cattle. J. Am. Vet. Med. Assoc. 176:356, 1980.
38. Kapp, D. S.: Thermosensitization and inhibition of thermal tolerance. Abstract from the 29th Annual Meeting of the Radiation Research Society, Minneapolis, May 31–June 4, 1981.
39. Kapp, D. S., and Lord, P. F.: Tolerance of dogs to fractionated systemic hyperthermia. Nat. Cancer Inst. Mongr. 61:391, 1982.
40. Kim, J. H., Hahn, E. W., and Tokita, N.: Combination hyperthermia and radiation therapy for cutaneous malignant melanoma. Cancer 41:2143, 1978.
41. Lehmann, J. F. (ed.): Therapeutic Heat and Cold. Williams and Wilkins, Baltimore, 1982.
42. Lele, P. P.: Local hyperthermia by ultrasound. In Nussbaum, G. H. (ed.): Physical Aspects of Hyperthermia. American Institute of Physics, Inc., New York, 1982.
43. Li, G. C., and Hahn, G. M.: Ethanol-induced tolerance to heat and to adriamycin. Nature 274:699, 1978.
44. Li, G. C., Hahn, G. M., and Shiu, E. C.: Cytotoxicity of commonly used solvents at elevated temperatures. J. Cell. Physiol. 93:331, 1977.

45. Li, G. C., Shiu, E. C., and Hahn, G. M.: Similarities in cellular inactivation by hyperthermia by ethanol. Radiat. Res. 82:257, 1980.

46. Licht, S. (ed.): *Therapeutic Heat and Cold.* Waverly Press, Baltimore, 1965.

47. Macy, D. W., Gillette, E. L., Speer, J. F., et al.: A humidity and temperature-controlled chamber for producing whole body hyperthermia. *Abstract* from the 13th International Cancer Congress, Seattle, September, 1982.

48. Manning, M. R., Cetas, T. C., Miller, R. C., et al.: Results of a phase I trial employing hyperthermia alone or in combination with external beam or interstitial radiotherapy. Cancer 49:205, 1982.

49. Marmor, J. B., Pounds, D., Hahn, N., and Hahn, G. M.: Treating spontaneous tumors in dogs and cats by ultrasound-induced hyperthermia. Int. J. Radiat. Oncol. Biol. Phys. 4:967, 1978.

50. Marmor, J. B., Pounds, D., Postic, T. B., and Hahn, G. M.: Treatment of superficial human neoplasms by local hyperthermia induced by ultrasound. Cancer 43:196, 1979.

51. Mattsson, J., Appelgren, L., Karlsson, L., and Peterson, H. I.: Influence of vasoactive drugs and ischaemia on intratumor blood flow distribution. Eur. J. Cancer 14:761, 1978.

52. Milder, J. W. (ed.): Conference on hyperthermia in cancer treatment. Cancer Res. 39:2232, 1979.

53. Nielsen, O. S., and Overgaard, J.: Importance of preheating temperature and time for the induction of thermotolerance in a solid tumor *in vivo.* Br. J. Cancer 46:894, 1982.

54. Nussbaum, G. H. (ed.): *Physical Aspects of Hyperthermia.* American Institute of Physics, Inc., New York, 1982.

55. Oleson, J. R.: Hyperthermia by magnetic induction: I. Physical characteristics of the technique. Int. J. Radiat. Oncol. Biol. Phys. 8:1747, 1982.

56. Oleson, J. R., Assaad, A., Dewhirst, M. W., et al.: Hyperthermia by magnetic induction methods in a beagle dog model: Analysis of clinical thermometry. Radiat. Res. 98:445, 1984.

57. Oleson, J. R., Babbs, C. F., and Parks, L. C.: Improved preferential tumor hyperthermia with regional heating and systemic blood cooling. *Abstract* From the 31st annual Meeting of the Radiation Research Society. San Antonio, February–March, 1983.

58. Oleson, J. R., Cetas, T. C., and Corry, P. M.: Hyperthermia by magnetic induction: Experimental and theoretical results for coaxial coil pairs. Radiat. Res. 95:175, 1983.

59. Overgaard, J.: Hyperthermic modification of the radiation response in solid tumors. 2nd Rome Interactional Symposium, September, 1980.

60. Parks, L. C.: Clinical evaluation: Induction of systemic hyperthermia by extracorporeal circulation as primary and adjuvant solid tumor malignancies. *In* Nussbaum, G. H. (ed.): *Physical Aspects of Hyperthermia.* American Institute of Physics, New York, 1982.

61. Peterson, H. I. (ed.): *Tumor Blood Circulation.* CRC Press Inc., Boca Raton, 1979.

62. Raaphorst, G. P., Romano, S. L., Mitchell, J. B., et al.: Intrinsic differences in heat and/or x-ray sensitivity of seven mammalian cell lines cultured and treated under identical conditions. Cancer Res. 39:396, 1979.

63. Kang, M., Song, C., and Levitt, S.: Role of vascular function in response of tumors *in vivo* to hyperthermia. Cancer Res. 40:1130, 1980.

64. Sapareto, S. A.: The biology of hyperthermia *in vitro. In* Nussbaum, G. H. (ed.): *Physical Aspects of Hyperthermia.* American Institute of Physics, Inc., New York, 1982.

65. Song, C. W.: Physiologic factors in hyperthermia of tumors. *In* Nussbaum, G. H. (ed.): *Physical Aspects of Hyperthermia.* American Institute of Physics, New York, 1982.

66. Stehlin, J. S., Jr., Giovanella, B. C., delPolyi, P. D., and Anderson, R. F.: Eleven years experience with hyperthermic perfusion for melanoma of the extremities. World J. Surg. 3:305, 1979.

67. Storm, F. K. (ed.): *Hyperthermia in Cancer Therapy.* G. K. Hall, Boston, 1983.

68. Storm, F. K., Harrison, W. H., Elliott, R. S., and Morton, D. L.: Normal tissue and solid tumor effects of hyperthermia in animal models and clinical trials. Cancer Res. 39:2245, 1979.

69. Streffer, C. (ed.): *Cancer Therapy by Hyperthermia and Radiation.* Urban and Schwarzenberg, Baltimore, 1978.

70. Suzuki, M., Hori, K., Abe, I., et al.: A new approach to cancer chemotherapy: Selective enhancement of tumor blood flow with angiotensin II. J. Nat. Cancer Inst. 67:663, 1981.

71. Thames, H. D., Jr., Withers, R. W., Peters, L. J., and Fletcher, G. H.: Changes in early and late radiation responses with altered dose fractionation: Implications for dose-survival relationships. Int. J. Radiat. Oncol. Biol. Phys. 8:219, 1982.

72. Turner, P. F., Paliwal, B., and Gibbs, F.: *A New Technique for Deep Thoracic and Abdominal Hyperthermia.* A manuscript provided by the BSD Corporation, Salt Lake City, 1982.

73. Vaupel, P. W., Frinak, S., and Bicher, H. I.: Heterogeneous oxygen partial pressure and pH distribution in C_3H mouse mammary adenocarcinoma. Cancer Res. 41:2008, 1981.

74. Vaupel, P., Frinak, S., Mueller-Klieser, W., and Bicher, H. I.: Impact of localized hyperthermia on the cellular microenvironment in solid tumors. Nat. Cancer Inst. Monogr. 61:207, 1982.

75. Voorhees, W. G., and Babbs, C. F.: Hydralazine-enhanced selective heating of transmissible venereal tumor implants in dogs. Eur. J. Cancer Clin. Oncol. 18:1027, 1983.

76. Yatvin, M., Clifton, K., and Dennis, W.: Hyperthermia and local anesthetics: Potentiation of survival of tumor-bearing mice. Science 205:195, 1979.

Chapter **175**

Skin

Ralph A. Henderson and Daniel M. Core

The skin is the site of one-third of all canine neoplasms. In the cat, tumors of the skin are more likely to be malignant and account for one-fourth of feline tumors; only lymphohemopoietic tumors are more common. The variety of cutaneous tumors results from the different epithelial and mesenchymal skin components (Fig. 175–1).

ANATOMY OF THE SKIN

The epidermis rests on the basal lamina. The deepest cell layers are composed of basal cells and adjoining prickle cells, called the *stratum germinativum* because they reproduce. The remaining epidermal layers are dying, forming the cornified layer.

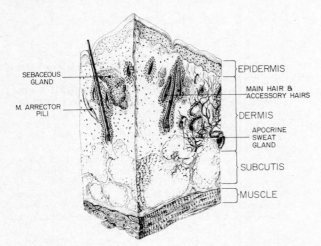

SEBACEOUS GLAND

M. ARRECTOR PILI

EPIDERMIS

MAIN HAIR & ACCESSORY HAIRS

DERMIS

APOCRINE SWEAT GLAND

SUBCUTIS

MUSCLE

Figure 175–1. Cutaneous tumors may arise from the epidermis, hair or glands (appendages), or cells of the dermis or hypodermis. (Reprinted with permission from Swaim, S. F.: *Surgery of Traumatized Skin: Management and Reconstruction in the Dog and Cat.* W. B. Saunders, Philadelphia, 1980.)

They do not undergo neoplastic change. Melanocytes are in the basal layer.

The dermis is situated beneath the basal lamina and is composed of blood vessels, lymphatics, nerves, glands, hair follicles, smooth muscle, adipose tissue, histiocytes, mast cells, connective tissue, and ground substance. The subcutis is a network of connective tissue, nerves, blood vessels, and adipose tissue deep to the dermis. Females have a thicker subcutis than males.[1]

Hair and glands are called *adnexa* and originate from pluripotential cells of the basal layer.[46] In the hair follicle, the inner root sheath is a continuation of the basal layer. Hair matrix cells are differentiated germinative cells, and each hair follicle may have associated sebaceous and apocrine glands and an erector pili muscle.

The cutaneous sebaceous, apocrine sweat, and merocrine glands, singly or in combination, form the specialized glands that have unique locations, such as the caudal tail gland (sebaceous and apocrine sweat), circumanal gland (sebaceous), and anal sac gland (sebaceous and apocrine sweat). Perianal glands are masses of large polygonal cells with no secretory activity and are located deep to the circumanal glands. Sebaceous glands are most numerous in the lips, anus, and dorsum of the body. The large, coiled apocrine sweat glands are usually associated with hair follicles and are especially numerous in the facial and interdigital skin. The smaller coiled merocrine sweat glands are found in the footpads deep in the dermo-hypodermal junction.

MANAGEMENT OF SKIN TUMORS

The client usually presents the pet with a cutaneous lump, ulcer, or discharge. Less frequently, the veterinarian calls the client's attention to these le-

sions. The proper diagnostic protocol includes an assessment of the general health of the patient commensurate with the intended diagnostic or therapeutic risks as well as a progressive inspection of the lesion. The inspection of the lesion should include clinical staging and cytological or histopathological diagnosis.

All canine and feline cutaneous tumors are staged in the same tumor, node, and metastasis (TNM) format (Table 175–1) except mast cell tumor and cutaneous lymphosarcoma. When multiple simultaneous tumors are present, the tumor with the highest T value is identified and the sites of secondary tumors recorded. Successive new tumors are staged independently. A tumor is restaged whenever its stage changes. Once the primary tumor is staged, the regional nodes are evaluated and evidence of distant metastasis is sought through physical, clinical, and radiographic examinations.

Mast cell tumors and lymphosarcomas are staged differently because of their systemic involvement

---

TABLE 175–1. Clinical Stages (TNM) of Canine or Feline Tumors of Epidermal or Dermal Origin (Excluding Lymphosarcoma and Mastocytoma)

T Primary Tumor
Tis Pre-invasive carcinoma (carcinoma *in situ*)
T0 No evidence of tumor
T1 Tumor <2 cm maximum diameter, superficial or exophytic
T2 Tumor 2 to 5 cm maximum diameter, or minimally invasive, irrespective of size
T3 Tumor >5 cm maximum diameter, or invading subcutis, irrespective of size
T4 Tumor invading other structures such as fascia, muscle, bone, or cartilage

N Regional Lymph Nodes (RLN)
N0 No evidence of RLN involvement
N1 Movable ipsilateral nodes
  N1a Nodes not considered to contain growth*
  N1b Nodes considered to contain growth*
N2 Movable contralateral or bilateral nodes
  N2a Nodes not considered to contain growth†
  N2b Nodes considered to contain growth†
N3 Fixed nodes

M Distant Metastasis
M0 No evidence of distant metastasis
M1 Distant metastasis detected† at specified sites

---

*(−) = histologically negative, (+) = histologically positive.

†Including lymph nodes beyond the region in which the primary tumor is situated.

(Reprinted with permission from World Health Organization: *Report of the Second Consultation on the Biological Behavior and Therapy of Tumors of Domestic Animals.* WHO, Geneva, 1978.)

Table 175–2. Clinical Stages of Canine Mastocytoma

Stage I	One tumor confined to the dermis without regional lymph node involvement Ia Without systemic signs Ib With systemic signs
Stage II	One tumor confined to dermis with regional lymph node involvement IIa Without systemic signs IIb With systemic signs
Stage III	Multiple dermal tumors or large infiltrating tumor with or without regional lymph node involvement IIIa Without systemic signs IIIb With systemic signs
Stage IV	Any tumor with distant metastasis or recurrence with metastasis*

*Including blood and/or bone marrow involvement

Note: Multiple tumors occurring simultaneously should have the actual number recorded. The tumor with the highest T category is selected and the number of tumors indicated in parentheses, e.g., T2(5). Successive tumors should be classified independently.

(Tables 175–2 and 175–3). For this reason, cytological assessment should precede clinical staging.

Cytology is valuable because of the rapidity of identification of some tumors and the ability to better direct therapy (Fig. 175–2). Tumors such as malignant melanoma, mast cell tumor, and fibrosarcoma require wide primary excision. Of these tumors, the first two

TABLE 175–3. Clinical Stages of Lymphosarcoma and Lymphoid Leukemia* in Domestic Mammals (Including Lymphosarcoma of Skin)

Anatomical Type
- A. Generalized
- B. Alimentary
- C. Thymic
- D. Skin
- E. Leukemia (true)†
- F. Others (including solitary renal)

Grouping (to include anatomical type)

Stage I	Involvement limited to a single node or lymphoid tissue in a single organ‡
Stage II	Involvement of many lymph nodes in a regional area (± tonsils)
Stage III	Generalized lymph node involvement
Stage IV	Liver and/or spleen involvement (± Stage III)
Stage V	Manifestation in the blood and involvement of bone marrow and/or other organ systems (± Stages I through IV)

*Excluding myeloma.
†Only blood and bone marrow involved.
‡Excluding bone marrow.
Note: each stage is subclassified into: (a) without systemic signs, or (b) with systemic signs.

are relatively easy to diagnose by fine needle aspiration, tissue scrapings, or impression smears. The third does not exfoliate as easily, and excisional (preferred) or incisional biopsies are required for histopathological examination.

EPITHELIAL SKIN TUMORS

Basal Cell and Appendage Tumors

Basal cell and related appendage (adnexal) tumors are common in the dog and cat and originate from the basal cells of the epidermis or hair follicles or in embryonal dermal cells, whereas appendage tumors originate from basal cells of hair follicles, matrices, and cutaneous glands.

Basal Cell Tumors

Incidence. Five to ten per cent of canine and two per cent of feline tumors are basal cell tumors[39,42,48] (also known as basal cell carcinoma, basal cell epithelioma, and basalioma[34]). The mean age of occurrence is six years in the dog and ten years in the cat. Male dogs and cocker spaniels and poodles of both sexes are more commonly affected.[39,42]

Clinical Appearance and Diagnosis. Sessile, firm, solitary, gray, hairless, variably sized tumors on the oral commisures, eyelids, pinna, cheek, jaw, and shoulders are highly suspect. The surface may be ulcerated.

Hypochromatic, palisaded cells with a high mitotic index[48] are arranged in solid, garland, medusoid, adenoid, basosquamous, or combination patterns. A variant morphology has been termed *granular basal cell tumor* because the cytoplasm contains granules thought to be secondary lysozymes. These tumors

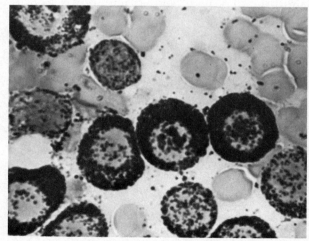

Figure 175–2. Cytological preparation of a well-differentiated mast cell tumor. The diagnostic protocol should be initiated with fine needle aspiration or scraping exfoliation. Melanomas and mast cell tumors are relatively easy to identify, and presurgical diagnosis of some tumors alters the surgical plan.

behave as basal cell tumors.[37] Cystic forms are more common in the cat than the dog.[48]

Treatment and Prognosis. Surgical excision with a 1-cm margin is the treatment of choice. Cryotherapy and radiation are alternatives if excision is impractical. 5-Fluorouracil and cyclophosphamide have been suggested as effective against basal cell tumors.[48]

The recurrence rate is less than 10 per cent.[42] Despite their histological appearance suggesting malignancy, they rarely metastasize, and only the basosquamous variety appears invasive.[50]

Intracutaneous Cornifying Epitheliomas (Keratoacanthoma)

Incidence. The peak occurrence of intracutaneous cornifying epithelioma averages five years of age. These lesions account for 2 to 3 per cent of cutaneous tumors, particularly in the Norwegian elkhound.[40] Males are affected three times more commonly than females.[40] Intracutaneous cornifying epithelioma does not occur in cats.

Clinical Appearance and Diagnosis. Intracutaneous cornifying epitheliomas are solitary or generalized nodules 0.5 to 4.0 cm in diameter with a hard keratinized plug protruding from a pore. The back, neck, thorax, and shoulder are common sites of involvement.[40] When secondarily infected, they mimic draining granulomas. Histopathologically, well-differentiated, stratified squamous cells and connective tissue surround a keratin-filled core.

Treatment and Prognosis. Intracutaneous cornifying epitheliomas are benign. Excision, cryotherapy, or electrocoagulation is usually curative; however, new nodules may appear at different sites. Inflammation results when keratin escapes into the subcutis.

Pilomatrixoma or Calcifying (Mummifying) Epitheliomas

Incidence. Pilomatrixomas originate from differentiated hair matrix[39] and account for 1.6 to 3 per cent of skin tumors in dogs.[48] The highest prevalence seen is between ages five and ten and in Kerry blue terriers and poodles, both of which have a greater number of hairs per follicle.[3] There is no sex predilection, and these tumors are extremely rare in cats.

Clinical Appearance and Diagnosis. Pilomatrixomas are solitary, gray, frequently ulcerated, intradermal tumors of the rump, shoulders, head, and legs. Histopathologically, basophilic cells with ovoid, vesicular nuclei surround "shadow" cells, which have a faintly eosinophilic cytoplasm. Central calcification, melanin deposition, and a foreign body reaction are common.[48]

Treatment and Prognosis. Pilomatrixomas are benign, slow-growing tumors that rarely metastasize and are cured by cryotherapy or excision.

Trichoepitheliomas

Incidence. Trichoepitheliomas originate from primitive hair matrix cells or from the inner hair

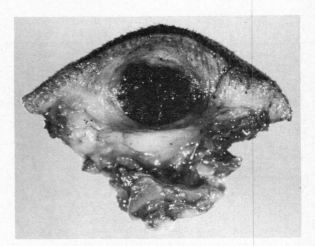

Figure 175–3. Darkly pigmented tumors are not necessarily melanomas. Many tumors may be darkly pigmented, such as this benign tricoepithelioma.

sheath of basal cells and account for 4 per cent of skin tumors of the dog and cat. Animals older than five years are affected more commonly.[39]

Clinical Appearance and Diagnosis. Trichoepitheliomas are round to ovoid, well-circumscribed, gray, ulcerated, solitary tumors of variable size located on the dorsum in the epidermis and subcutis. Morphology varies from undifferentiated to normal hair follicles.[39] Melanin deposition can cause the tumor to appear black (Fig. 175–3).

Treatment and Prognosis. Trichoepitheliomas are benign, and the prognosis is excellent following complete excision or cryotherapy.

Sebaceous Gland Tumors

Incidence. Benign sebaceous gland tumors are very common in the dog but rare in cats.[39] Sebaceous adenomas are more common in cats.[32] Sebaceous gland tumors occur in dogs with a mean age of 9.5 years and in older cats. No breed or sex predilections exist for dogs or cats.[43]

Clinical Appearance and Diagnosis. Sebaceous gland tumors are subdivided into nodular hyperplasia, sebaceous adenoma, sebaceous epithelioma, and adenocarcinoma.[39] In addition, duct obstruction causes sebaceous inclusion cysts.

Sebaceous nodular hyperplasia (discrete nodules covered by hairless epithelium) is yellow and lobulated on the cut surface and is composed of a large gland with fully mature lobules surrounding a central sebaceous duct.[39]

Adenomas are firm, well-circumscribed, freely movable, frequently hairless, and occasionally ulcerated and are less lobulated than sebaceous hyperplasia. Sebaceous adenomas consist of immature lobules of cells with hyperchromatic nuclei and dark cytoplasm peripherally and cells with foamy cytoplasm and pyknotic nuclei located centrally.

Sebaceous epitheliomas are grossly and histopathologically similar to basal cell tumors. Melanin pigmentation is prominent, and sebaceous epitheliomas must be differentiated from melanomas. Infiltrates of inflammatory cells may surround sebaceous epitheliomas.

Sebaceous gland adenocarcinomas are invasive, have ill-defined borders, are often ulcerated, and uncommonly occur on the head.[39,43] These adenocarcinomas are composed of lobules or cords of cells with hyperchromatic nuclei, prominent nucleoli, basophilic cytoplasm, and mitotic figures that invade the adjacent tissues.

Treatment and Prognosis. Sebaceous hyperplasia, adenomas, and epitheliomas are benign, and, when indicated, complete excision or cryotherapy is curative. Chemotherapy (5-fluorouracil) is also reported effective; however, no dosage, route of administration, or reason for suggesting efficacy (remission versus cure) was given.[48]

Since about 20 per cent of sebaceous adenocarcinomas recur, they must be treated by wide excision. About 50 per cent will be 2 cm in diameter or less when first noticed.[43] Metastasis to regional lymph nodes and lungs is late. Radiation should be considered when complete excision is doubtful.[43]

Sweat Gland Tumors

Incidence. Tumors of sweat glands are less common than those of sebaceous glands.[50] Affected animals are usually six to eight years old or older. The prevalence is greater in male dogs and in the cocker spaniel.[10] No sex or breed predispositions have been reported for cats.

Clinical Appearance and Diagnosis. Sweat gland tumors are common on the heads and necks of dogs.[10] Cats have no site predisposition. Adenomas are solitary subcutaneous ulcerations that range from 1 to 4 cm in diameter and are lobulated with a clear, yellowish cut surface. Adenocarcinomas are usually poorly circumscribed.

Adenomas are comprised of a central layer of cuboidal to columnar cells with basal nuclei and a peripheral layer of myoepithelial cells surrounded by inflammatory cells. Although five major classes are distinguished,[50] in general the tumors are characterized by undifferentiated cells with hyperchromatic nuclei, a high mitotic index, and stromal or lymphatic invasion.[39]

Treatment and Prognosis. Excision of adenomas is curative. Adenocarcinomas and involved nodes are excised. Postsurgical irradiation may diminish recurrence of large tumors. Adenocarcinomas are invasive and readily metastasize.[34]

Perianal (Circumanal, Hepatoid) Gland Tumors

Incidence. Perianal gland tumors are the third most common tumor in male dogs and do not occur in cats.[34] Nodular hyperplasia and adenomas (10 per cent of tumors) occur in older dogs and are ten times

more common in males than in females. The high prevalence in intact males, lower prevalence in castrated dogs (male or female), and near absence in intact bitches suggest possible enhancement by testosterone or suppression by estrogen.[51,53]

Adenocarcinomas (2 per cent of tumors) occur with equal frequency in males and females. Tumors in females should be suspected to be malignant. Although no specific breed predisposition has been identified, cocker spaniels, beagles, German shepherds, dachshunds, and fox terriers seem more frequently affected.

Clinical Appearance and Diagnosis. Circumanal glands may be located from the prepuce to the tail and enlarge throughout the lifetime of intact male dogs in response to testosterone.[1] Tumors are solitary or multiple, slow-growing, soft, and often ulcerated (Fig. 175–4), causing bloody discharge, pruritus, tenesmus, and dyschezia. Adenomas are distinguished from adenocarcinomas by microscopic examination. Large polyhedral cells with ovoid nuclei and abundant eosinophilic cytoplasm arranged in lobules that resemble liver, squamous metaplasia, high vascularity, inflammation, and rare mitotic figures are characteristic of adenomas.[34,39]

Adenocarcinomas have a high mitotic index and little cellular differentiation and lack discrete lobules and invasion of stroma and lymphatics by cords of neoplastic cells.[5]

Treatment and Prognosis. The treatment for adenomas is castration and tumor removal. Although castration alone causes regression of adenomas, the possibilities of malignancy, recurrence of a regressed tumor, or the presence of another cell type exist. When multiple tumors are not resectable without causing incontinence, castration and biopsy provide regression and diagnosis. Adenomas are sensitive to radiation and estrogen. The prognosis for adenomas is good; however, histologically "benign" tumors may metastasize.

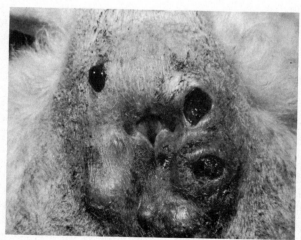

Figure 175–4. Perianal adenomas may be solitary or multiple and must be differentiated from other perianal diseases. The presence of ulceration does not imply malignancy.

Local adenocarcinoma should be treated by castration and excision. Excision may be followed by irradiation. Excision of enlarged lumbar lymph nodes provides long-term remission. Adenocarcinomas are responsive to radiation.[53]

Serum calcium may be elevated secondary to secretion of parathormone-like substance. Hypercalcemia is treated by saline and hypercalcuric diuresis to prevent calcification of soft tissues when the product of serum calcium and phosphorus exceeds 70.

Ceruminous Gland Tumors

Incidence. Tumors from the ceruminous apocrine glands of the external ear canal are more common in the cat than the dog, and most in the cat are malignant.[32] Male cats from 8 to 15 years of age are most commonly affected, but no breed predisposition has been reported.[48]

Clinical Appearance and Diagnosis. Ceruminous gland tumors are nodular and pedunculated or infiltrative.[39] Affected animals are usually presented for chronic nonresponsive otitis externa with a foul odor. Microscopically, ceruminous gland tumors resemble other apocrine gland tumors, except that in ceruminous gland tumors the ducts become cystic, containing papillary projections and pinkish orange secretions.[39] Adenocarcinomas are more anaplastic and invasive than ceruminous gland tumors.

Treatment and Prognosis. Complete excision is difficult because of the location but is curative for adenomas. Because of invasion and metastasis, ablation of the ear or irradiation is recommended for adenocarcinomas.

Squamous Cell Carcinomas

Incidence. Squamous cell carcinomas arise from the stratum spinosum of the epithelium. They are the second most common skin tumor of cats, constituting 9 to 25 per cent of all feline tumors,[32,36] and account for from 3 to 20 per cent of canine skin tumors.[5,44]

Squamous cell carcinomas usually occur in dogs older than six years and cats nine years or older. No breed or sex predilections exist for cats, but Scottish terriers, boxers, Pekingese, and Norwegian elkhounds have a higher incidence than other breeds.[35] Exposure to hydrocarbons of wax or oil, arsenicals, burns, freezing, or solar irradiation (nonpigmented skin only) may be related to the occurrence of the tumor.[25]

Clinical Appearance and Diagnosis. Squamous cell carcinomas are either productive or erosive.[48] Productive carcinomas have an ulcerated, cauliflower appearance with poorly defined borders and are most common in dogs. Ulcerative carcinomas begin as ulcers and develop into crater-like lesions covered by fibronecrotic exudate. Because of their appearance, squamous cell carcinomas may be confused with chronic wounds and be managed by debridement and suture. The limbs of dogs are common sites

of involvement, but the trunk, head, neck, and digits are frequently affected. Digital lesions may be more invasive and may have greater metastatic potential.

Feline squamous cell carcinomas are usually solitary, ulcerated, firm, and broad-based and occur more commonly on the head, especially the ears, lips, nose, and eyelids.

Squamous cell carcinoma invades bone, and metastasis to regional lymph nodes is common. Enlarged lymph nodes or lymph nodes with tumor cells present are excised, en bloc when possible. Metastasis to the lung is usually late.

Histopathologically, squamous cell carcinoma is characterized by large round cells with pyknotic nuclei, mitotic figures, and eosinophilic cytoplasm that form cords, which invade surrounding tissue. Prominent intercellular bridges are present. Well-differentiated tumors produce large amounts of keratin or horn pearls.[5]

Treatment and Prognosis. Early wide excision is optimal. Nail bed squamous cell carcinoma is likely to invade bone, and amputation of the digit or entire limb is necessary when local destruction is extensive.[48] Half of excised squamous cell carcinomas recur within two to four years. Distant metastasis is rare except in long-standing or digital squamous cell carcinoma.

Radiation therapy with 3,500 to 4,500 R delivered in six to ten fractions is an effective primary treatment or adjuvant treatment to prevent recurrence.[11] Localized hyperthermia has also been successful.[23] Chemotherapy with 5-fluorouracil has been suggested for treating primary lesions. Cyclophosphamide is suggested as an adjuvant therapy for systemic involvement.[48]

Lightly pigmented animals should be protected from solar irradiation by sunscreens such as para-aminobenzoic acid, tattooing, or keeping the animal indoors.

Squamous Papillomas

Incidence. Papillomas are benign epidermal tumors and are in some instances caused by species-specific DNA viruses of the Papovaviridae family.[48] Papillomas in older dogs are usually solitary and nonviral, but multiple, virus-induced oral masses are common in young dogs.

Papillomas account for 1 to 2.5 per cent of canine skin neoplasms. No canine or feline breed or sex predispositions exist. Feline papillomas are rare, occur in older cats, and are not induced by viruses.[32]

Clinical Appearance and Diagnosis. Papillomas are usually small (1 cm), friable masses with numerous projections that arise from a flat base, but they can be larger (Fig. 175–5). Pedunculation, ulceration, and secondary infection are common. Canine papillomas usually occur in the oral cavity, head, eyelids, feet, and genitalia. Papillomas are composed of thick layers of epidermal cells with deeply penetrating rete pegs. Papillomas do not invade the dermis.

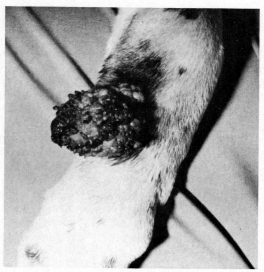

Figure 175–5. Canine papilloma. Although most papillomas are smaller than 1 cm, some become larger and may be pigmented, requiring histopathological examination.

Treatment and Prognosis. Excision, cryotherapy, or electrodesiccation is usually curative. Many papillomas undergo spontaneous regression after one to two months. Removal of several tumors may cause remission of others.[48] Autogenous tumor vaccine is variably successful.[48] Immunodeficiency should be suspected if papillomas recur, which is rare.

Melanocytic Tumors

Incidence. Melanomas constitute 6 to 8 per cent of canine skin tumors and 2 per cent of feline skin tumors.[8,44] Melanocytic tumors are more common in male dogs between 7 and 14 years of age, heavily pigmented breeds, such as Scottish terriers, Boston terriers, Airedale terriers, cocker spaniels, and springer spaniels, are commonly affected.[39] No feline breed or sex predispositions have been reported.

Clinical Appearance and Diagnosis. Melanomas occur in the skin, mucous membranes, and eye. The mucous membrane is the most common site of involvement. Melanomas of the mucous membranes and germinal epithelium of the nail are usually malignant, but the majority of skin melanomas are benign.[21]

Benign melanomas are classified as either dermal or junctional (from the dermoepidermal junction that involves hair follicles) in origin. Junctional melanomas begin as a black macule that progresses to a small, firm, less pigmented nodule. Dermal melanomas are smooth, hairless, dome-shaped, and well-circumscribed and are of variable pigmentation.

Malignant melanomas are usually larger, dark brown to light gray, and ulcerated and are covered by fibronecrotic exudate. Malignant melanomas appear to have a precise margin but deeply invade adjacent tissues and possibly bone. Melanomas may be unpigmented, anaplasia apparently rendering the cell incapable of synthesizing normal quantities of melanin, and special stains may be required for identification.[39]

Although predominantly a round cell tumor, several subclasses of malignant melanoma are distinguished: epithelioid (carcinomatous cells arranged in lobules), spindle cell (an interwoven pattern), epithelioid/spindle cell (varying amounts of both cell types), and dendritic/whorled (heavily pigmented, little anaplasia, and difficult to distinguish from benign melanomas).[21]

Treatment and Prognosis. Cutaneous melanomas are usually benign, but wide excision is recommended for the sake of those that are not. Regional lymph nodes should be removed if they are enlarged. Because of the invasive nature of malignant tumors and the 10 per cent recurrence rate after excision, adjuvant therapy should be considered.[48]

Immunotherapy with bacille Calmette Guérin (BCG) and other agents and combination chemotherapy with adriamycin and imidazole carboxamide (DTIC) have shown minimal reproducible effects.[31] Malignant melanomas are considered radioresistant, but the more anaplastic forms may be palliated by surgery and radiation or radiation alone.

Average survival has been prolonged for humans with melanomas of the extremities by cannulating a major artery and vein of the affected extremity and infusing them with warmed blood (regional hyperthermia) and high-concentration chemotherapy.[41]

Epithelioid malignant melanomas are the most common malignant form and have the worst prognosis. Malignant melanomas metastasize early to the regional lymph nodes and, by blood, eventually to the lungs and elsewhere.[3] Median survival time for individuals with benign melanomas is 110 weeks compared with 30 weeks with malignant melanomas.[8]

Since metastasis and death have been associated with histologically "benign" (according to present criteria) tumors,[8] it has been proposed that melanomas with mitotic indices of two or less (two mitoses/HPF) be classified as benign and those with mitotic indices of three or more be classified as malignant. Under this criteria, benign melanomas would be predicted to have a 90 per cent cure rate two years after excision, and a 70 per cent death rate would be predicted for patients with malignant tumors, 20 per cent dying within six months of surgery.[8]

ROUND CELL TUMORS OF THE SKIN

Round cell tumors have distinct cytological features based on predominant populations of round cells that render exfoliative methods essential, and in some instances superior, to histopathology. Round cell tumors commonly include mast cell tumor, histiocytoma, lymphosarcoma, and transmissible venereal tumor (TVT).

Mast Cell Tumors, Mastocytomas, Mast Cell Sarcomas

Incidence. Mast cells tumors account for 13 and 3 per cent of skin neoplasms in dogs and cats, respectively.[27,39] Mast cell tumors occur in dogs of any age (average 8.5 years) with no sex predisposition. Boxers, Boston terriers, bull terriers, fox terriers, Staffordshire terriers, Labrador retrievers, and English bulldogs have a greater prevalence than others. Older cats are more commonly affected. No feline breed predilection exists, but male cats are affected more often than females.[39]

Clinical Appearance and Diagnosis. Canine mast cell tumors occur in a cutaneous[26,30] and a visceral[17] form. The cutaneous form may be solitary (90 per cent) or multiple (10 per cent)[13,27] and is well-circumscribed, firm, raised, and less than 3 cm in diameter when first seen. Occasional tumors are poorly circumscribed, erythematous, and raised with a soft, mucinous matrix easily mistaken for an inflammatory response.[47] Mast cell tumors may cause pruritus and occur in any cutaneous location. Mast cells contain heparin and histamine. Chronic histamine release may cause hydrochloric acid hypersecretion and gastrointestinal ulceration. Hemorrhage associated with these ulcers may be overt or occult.[15,39]

Feline mast cell tumors may also involve the skin or viscera. Cutaneous tumors may metastasize to the viscera, or visceral tumors may metastasize to the skin.[32] Feline mast cell tumors are hairless, pruritic plaques or nodules and may ulcerate. Common sites on the cat include the head, thigh, and dorsal tail base.

Mast cell tumors should be diagnosed microscopically by cytology. Clinical staging includes buffy coat and bone marrow examination for mast cell leukemia[2] and investigation of pulmonary interstitial densities, splenomegaly, hepatomegaly, lymphadenopathy, and gastrointestinal hemorrhage (See Table 175–2). Microscopically, mast cells possess an eccentrically placed, variably sized nucleus with cytoplasmic granules that stain blue to purple. Eosinophils often accompany mast cell tumors.[39] Mast cell tumors may be histopathologically graded for prognosis.[7,28]

Treatment and Prognosis. The response of mast cell tumors to treatment depends on the clinical stage and histological grade. When clinical staging suggests that the tumor is localized, excision is the treatment of choice. The invasive nature of this tumor dictates a surgical margin around and deep to the tumor that is no less than 3 cm including fascia and muscle. If the margin of the surgical specimen contains tumor, the surgical site should be immediately excised or irradiated. About 25 per cent of tumors recur after surgery alone.[34]

Mast cell tumors are considered to be radiosensitive; 75 per cent undergo remission and about 50 per cent stay in remission for 12 to 48 months (mean 24 months). Radiation of 3,500 to 5,000 R is given in six to ten fractions depending on tumor volume. The response depends on clinical stage and tumor grade, but prospective comparisons have not been reported.[11,20]

Cryotherapy and other necrotizing therapies are able to induce degranulation and release of heparin and vasoactive amines. In practice, the complications of hemorrhage and vasogenic shock are uncommon and do not require pretreatment with antihistamines (H_1 type). However, since the dimensions of the zone of cryonecrosis cannot be critically controlled to adequately circumscribe these tumors, and since margins cannot be examined, it is recommended that cryotherapy not be used on mast cell tumors.

Other forms of therapy are used only for palliation of mast cell tumors. Chemotherapeutic regimens including cyclophosphamide, vincristine, adriamycin,[48] and other drugs have produced inconsistent results. Corticosteroids and their regimens are useful in palliating mast cell tumors. Triamcinolone (3.0 to 6.0 mg) is administered intralesionally at weekly intervals, or prednisone (0.5 to 1.0 mg/kg b.i.d.) is administered by mouth on alternate days.

Cimetidine is a specific antagonist of the gastric H_2 receptors, which are responsible for hyperacidity and ulcers. The recommended dosage is 4 mg/kg q.i.d. per os,[47] and it may be given with other forms of therapy. Cimetidine administration is especially important for patients on chronic steroid therapy.[47]

Animals with grade I (highly undifferentiated) mast cell tumors have a mean survival time of 4½ months following surgery; animals with grade II (moderate differentiation) tumors have a mean survival time of 6 to 7 months following surgery; and animals with grade III (well-differentiated) tumors have a mean survival time of 11 to 12 months following surgery.[7] Half of feline mast cell tumors metastasize.[39]

Canine Cutaneous Histiocytomas

Incidence. Histiocytomas arise from monocyte-macrophage cells and account for about 11 per cent of all canine skin tumors.[21] Half occur in animals younger than two years of age, and the incidence decreases after age two.[29,39] No sex predisposition is reported, but purebred dogs, especially boxers and dachshunds, have a greater prevalence than other breeds.[39]

Clinical Appearance and Diagnosis. Histiocytomas usually are small, erythematous, alopecic, dome-shaped, painless masses less than 2 cm in diameter.[48] The tumor surface may be crusty and may have sparse hair growth. (Fig. 175–6). Common sites of histiocytomas include the pinna of the ear, head, limbs, and trunk.

Fine needle aspirates or tissue scrapings are diagnostic. Histopathologically, histiocytomas consist of sheets of round to oval cells with large nuclei and abundant pale acidophilic cytoplasm. Mitotic figures are quite common and do not indicate malignancy.[39] Four subgroups based on increasing lymphocytic infiltration probably represent a host-mediated response to the tumor.[21]

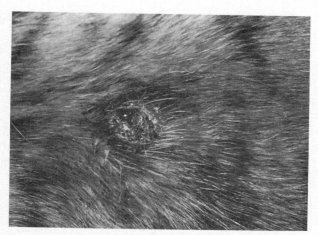

Figure 175–6. Cutaneous histiocytoma may appear as an exudative, crusty lesion rather than a smooth, alopecic, "strawberry" tumor, which is considered characteristic.

Treatment and Prognosis. Histiocytomas are usually excised or frozen at the client's request and for definitive diagnosis, although many are reported to regress spontaneously. About 1 per cent recur aggressively, often as round cell sarcomas.[34]

Cutaneous Lymphosaromas

Incidence. Cutaneous lymphosarcoma may occur as an extension of the three traditional forms of lymphosarcoma (See Table 175–3) or as mycosis fungoides, a rare neoplastic disorder of thymus-derived lymphocytes. Older dogs and perhaps males may be at increased risk.[16,21]

Clinical Appearance and Diagnosis. Cutaneous lymphosarcoma appears as an unresponsive chronic pruritic dermatosis, but the onset may be sudden. Tumors may be solitary or multiple, vary in size, and are often covered by a thick, dry, crust and some degree of alopecia (Fig. 175–7). Lesions begin as

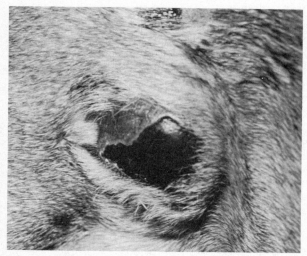

Figure 175–7. Cutaneous lymphosarcoma is often deeply pigmented with epidermal sloughing. Cytologic examination reveals an homogeneous population of lymphocytes.

erythematous macules or nodules and progress at varying rates to tumors and indurated plaques. Occasionally systemic manifestations such as lymphadenopathy, leukemia, or hypergammaglobulinemia may be observed.[16]

Mycosis fungoides is characterized by three clinical stages.[21] Lesions in the premycotic stage present as pruritic erythrodermic patches that may persist for months. In the mycotic stage, the lesions consist of firm, elevated hyperpigmented plaque on a previously unaffected site. The mycotic stage progresses to the third stage of dermal infiltration.

Cutaneous lymphosarcoma consists of a homogeneous population of cells resembling T-lymphocytes.[21] Neoplastic cells have an enlarged convoluted nucleus with densely clumped chromatin and a moderate amount of cytoplasm. Intraepithelial pockets of neoplastic cells are characteristic of mycosis fungoides.[38]

Treatment and Prognosis. Cutaneous lymphosarcoma generally progresses to systemic involvement in dogs, but they have longer survival times than those with other forms of lymphosarcoma. Surgical excision is curative if the lesion is small and solitary. Combination chemotherapy, topical nitrogen mustard, or immunotherapy controls the skin disease for an average of 112 days.[14,16]

CONNECTIVE TISSUE TUMORS OF THE SKIN

Mesenchymal tumors such as fibroma, myxoma, neurofibroma, hemangioma, and their sarcomatous counterparts as well as hemangiopericytoma are characterized by spindled "supporting" cells and account for 25 per cent of cutaneous neoplasms. Because of their pleomorphic capabilities, these tumors are difficult to distinguish clinically, and different histopathological sections from the same tumor may vary.

Fibromas and Myxofibromas

Incidence. Fibromas are benign spindle cell tumors of mesenchymal origin that account for 2.2 and 8.2 per cent of skin tumors in dogs and cats, respectively.[6,48] Myxomas are rare in cats and constitute less than 1 per cent of canine skin tumors. They contain mucin in the intercellular matrix, which distinguishes them from fibromas. Fibromas and myxomas may occur in an animal of any age but usually occur in older animals and demonstrate no sex or breed predisposition.[39]

Clinical Appearance and Diagnosis. Fibromas are well-circumscribed, oval, dermal, or subcutaneous tumors. Fibromas may be pedunculated. They are slow-growing and occur in any location where fibroblasts are found, but appear most commonly on the flank and limbs. Myxomas are soft and mucoid on the cut surface.

Fibromas are composed of fusiform mature fibroblasts combined with collagen fibers. Together they are arranged in whorls and interlacing bundles. Mitotic figures are uncommon. Fibromas are well-differentiated from surrounding tissues. Fibromas must be differentiated from scar tissue.

Treatment and Prognosis. Excision of fibromas or myxomas is usually curative. Neither responds to radiation or chemotherapy.

Fibrosarcomas and Myxosarcomas

Incidence. Fibrosarcomas are made up of malignant fibroblasts and mixed mesenchymal cells capable of collagen production, account for 9 to 14 per cent of canine skin neoplasms, and are the second most common oral tumor in dogs.[6] Myxosarcomas are rare. Fibrosarcomas and myxosarcomas occur in older dogs with no breed or sex predilection.[39]

As the second most common tumor of feline skin, fibrosarcomas account for about 5 per cent of feline tumors occurring naturally or induced by the feline sarcoma and feline leukemia viruses.[48] The sarcoma virus is an incomplete virus and requires the leukemia virus for replication and tumor induction.[32]

Clinical Appearance and Diagnosis. Fibrosarcomas and myxosarcomas are infiltrative, irregularly shaped, and often ulcerated and infected (Fig. 175–8). They may be vascular, firm, or fluctuant, and the center of the tumor may be necrotic. Regional nodes should be palpated, and lungs and nearby bones should be radiographed because 10 per cent metastasize.[9] Feline fibrosarcomas are usually solitary masses of the extremities, body wall, head, or neck. Multiple fibrosarcomas are rare, occur in younger cats, and are often virus-induced.[48]

Histopathological examination is required for diagnosis, since fine needle aspiration often does not dislodge enough tumor cells. Fibrosarcomas are cellular tumors composed of immature fibroblasts, variable amounts of collagen, and common mitotic figures. Myxosarcomas have stellate to fusiform cells with round to ovoid nuclei and multiple nucleoli arranged in whorls, lobules, or sheets distributed in vacuolated basophilic mucinous stroma. Increased numbers of mitotic figures and hyperchromatic nuclei distinguish myxosarcomas from myxomas.

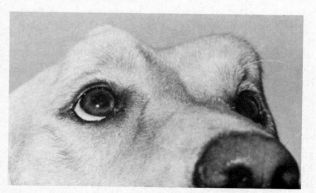

Figure 175–8. A bilaterally symmetrical lesion in a young animal does not rule out neoplasia. The supraorbital nodules in this 18-month-old Labrador retriever are myxofibrosarcomas.

Treatment and Prognosis. Excision with a 4-cm margin is the treatment of choice. Invasive tumors of the extremities should be treated with amputation. The mean survival time of affected animals is 80 weeks, 49 weeks if the mitotic index is nine or more (62 per cent recurrence rate) and 118 weeks if the mitotic index is less than nine (25 per cent recurrence rate).[9] Inoperable or incompletely excised sites should be irradiated. Although fibrosarcomas are considered radioresistant, malignant tumors may be palliated.[11]

Hyperthermia[12] and combination chemotherapy with cyclophosphamide, vincristine, methotrexate or adriamycin, and DTIC[31] have been advocated as adjuvant or palliative therapies.

Feline fibrosarcomas rarely metastasize but have a recurrence rate of 60 to 75 per cent.[31] Cats with fibrosarcomas of the extremities treated by amputation have an excellent long-term survival.[31]

Hemangiopericytomas

Incidence. Hemangiopericytomas stem from adventitial pericytes, which surround small blood vessels,[34] occur in the dermis and subcutis, are malignant, and are unique to dogs. Hemangiopericytomas are more common than fibromas, fibrosarcomas, or hemangiomas.[39] Affected dogs are likely to be female, 6 to 14 years of age, and of the German shepherd, boxer, or spaniel breed.[39]

Clinical Appearance and Diagnosis. Hemangiopericytomas are slow-growing, firm and nodular, average 10 cm in diameter, and involve the lateral surfaces of the elbow, carpus, tarsus, and stifle.[39] Larger masses may be ulcerated and secondarily infected and may cause lameness.

Hemangiopericytomas are infiltrative, surrounding muscle bundles, tendons, and nerves. The cut surface is pink and lobulated and appears well-differentiated from surrounding tissue.[39] Areas of necrosis may be present within the tumor.

Histopathologically, spindle-shaped cells with pink-staining cytoplasmic processes and a single nucleus that contains a prominent nucleolus and marginated chromatin along the nuclear membrane are arranged in whorls around blood vessels in onion skin lamination.[6] The mitotic index varies with the degree of anaplasia. Hemangiopericytomas must be differentiated from fibrosarcomas.

Treatment and Prognosis. Wide excision is optimal but difficult because of infiltration and vascularity. The local recurrence rate is 34 per cent, but only about 1 per cent metastasize.[9] Recurring tumors are more aggressive.[39] Multiple excisions and eventual amputation may be necessary. Irradiation may be used following incomplete excision.[6]

Hemangiomas and Hemangiosarcomas

Incidence. Hemangiomas and hemangiosarcomas are the benign and malignant tumors of vascular endothelium. Both tumors are more common in dogs than cats.[19] The hemangioma is the more common of the two.

Dogs affected with hemangiomas average nine years of age, are of either sex, and are likely to be of Scottish terrier, Airedale, Labrador retriever, or Kerry blue terrier breed.[39] Dogs affected with hemangiosarcoma average ten years of age, are male, and are likely to be of boxer, Boston terrier, or German shepherd breed.[19]

Clinical Appearance and Diagnosis. Dermal hemangiomas are usually less than 1 cm in diameter, sessile or pedunculated, and purple.[39] Subcutaneous hemangiomas are larger, well-circumscribed, and reddish-black on the cut surface. Hemangiomas are composed of well-differentiated endothelial cells that form blood-filled vascular spaces. The leg, flank, face, neck, and eyelid are the most common sites of involvement.[39]

Cutaneous hemangiosarcomas may be primary or metastatic, may occur at any site, and are soft, infiltrative, and reddish-black like a contusion. A contused appearance to the surrounding tissue may indicate neoplastic infiltration. Grossly, cutaneous hemangiosarcomas are difficult to distinguish from hematomas.

Rupture of visceral lesions may cause collapse, shock, and a chronic, although regenerative, anemia. Nonspecific signs such as cachexia, depression, and anorexia may be present. A thorough physical examination, abdominal palpation, thoracic and abdominal radiographs, and paracentesis of body cavities should be performed to stage this tumor.

Hemangiosarcomas are made up of vascular channels formed by elongated spindle-shaped cells with large, round to ovoid hyperchromatic nuclei. Mitotic figures and hemosiderin-filled macrophages are common.[19]

Treatment and Prognosis. Hemangiomas are rarely purposely excised, and they do not recur. Wide excision is the treatment of choice for localized hemangiosarcoma. Radiation is palliative.

Recurrence and metastases are common, occur early, and are widespread. Fewer than 10 per cent of dogs with hemangiosarcoma survive longer than one year,[19] prompting a guarded prognosis.

Lipomas, Infiltrative Lipomas, and Liposarcomas

Incidence. Lipomas are benign tumors of lipocytes and lipoblasts commonly occurring in older purebred bitches.[45] Lipomas constitute 5 to 7 per cent of canine skin tumors[6,45] and 6 per cent of feline skin tumors.[32] Liposarcomas and infiltrative lipomas are much less common, with no age, breed, or sex predispositions.[6,39,48]

Clinical Appearance and Diagnosis. Simple lipomas are slow-growing, smooth, movable, soft, well-encapsulated subcutaneous masses usually of the chest or abdomen. No clinical signs accompany lipo-

mas, and they may be diagnosed by aspirates, but other tumors are often surrounded by or infiltrated with fat. Adipose cells arranged in uniform sheets with fibrous septa distinguish lipomas from normal adipose tissue.[6,48]

Infiltrative lipomas (lipomatosis)[4] are poorly encapsulated and highly invasive. They are often located between planes of tissue or muscle in the perineum, hamstrings, or shoulder. Angiolipoma and parosteal lipoma denote an infiltrative lipoma with high vascularity and a lipoma with osseous attachment, respectively.[18,33,52]

Liposarcomas are highly invasive and poorly circumscribed, adhere to surrounding tissues, and on the cut surface appear cavernous and hemorrhagic.[18] Liposarcomas are more cellular than lipomas, with a finely vacuolated cytoplasm, round nucleus, and one nucleolus. Giant nuclei and multinucleated cells are common, but mitotic figures are rare.[39]

Treatment and Prognosis. Excision, when necessary, is the treatment of choice for lipomas and is usually curative. Lipomas should not be ignored for several reasons: (1) there is the possibility of avascular necrosis, (2) tumors are more difficult to excise when they are larger, and (3) other tumors may mimic a lipoma.[52] Weight reduction in obese dogs may reduce tumor size and allow easier excision.[39]

Infiltrative lipomas and liposarcomas are treated by excision. Recurrence is common owing to their invasiveness. Radical excision including muscle and fascia or amputation is necessary. Adjuvant therapy is not beneficial in the treatment of liposarcomas.[52] Only liposarcomas metastasize.

NONNEOPLASTIC TUMORS OF THE SKIN

A differential diagnosis of cutaneous neoplasia must include nonneoplastic diseases that cause tumors. They are distinguished by cultures and biopsies. Divided here into infectious, nonseptic inflammatory, and cystic groups for convenience, these lists are intended to be representative not exhaustive.

Cutaneous cysts. Epidermal inclusion, dermoid, follicular, and epithelial proliferative cysts.

Infections. Staphlococcal pyogranuloma, *Mycobacterium lepraemurium* (cats,) cutaneous nocardiosis, actinomycosis, pheohyphomycosis, sporotricosis, blastomycosis, histoplasmosis, cryptococcosis, coccidioidomycosis, and zygomycosis.

Nonseptic inflammations. Nodular panniculitis, nodular fasciitis, eosinophilic granuloma, acral lick granuloma, and deep sterile (steroid-responsive) pyogranuloma.

1. Al-Bagdadi, F., and Lovell, J.: The integument. *In* Evans, H. E., and Christensen, G. C. (eds.): *Miller's Anatomy of the Dog.* W.B. Saunders, Philadelphia, 1979, pp. 78–100.
2. Allan, G. S., Watson, A. D. J., Duff, B. C., and Howlett, C. R.: Disseminated mastocytoma and mastocythemia in a dog. J. Am. Vet. Med. Assoc. 165:346, 1974.
3. Alexander, J. W., Dueland, R., and Appel, G. O.: Malignant

melanoma with skeletal metastasis in a dog. J. Am. Vet. Radiol. Soc. 27:7, 1976.

4. Berzon, J. L., and Howard, P. E.: Lipomatosis in dogs. J. Am. Anim. Hosp. Assoc. 16:253, 1980.

5. Bevier, D. F., and Goldschmidt, M. H.: Skin tumors in the dog. Part I. Epithelial tumors and tumorlike lesions. Comp. Cont. Ed. 3:389, 1981.

6. Bevier, D. F., and Goldschmidt, M. H.: Skin tumors in the dog. Part II. Tumors of the soft (mesenchymal) tissues. Comp. Cont. Ed. 3:506, 1981.

7. Bostock, D. E.: The prognosis following surgical removal of mastocytomas in dogs. J. Small Anim. Pract. 14:27, 1973.

8. Bostock, D. E.: Prognosis after surgical excision of canine melanomas. Vet. Pathol. 16:32, 1979.

9. Bostock, D. E., and Dye, M. T.: Prognosis after surgical excision of canine fibrous connective tissue sarcomas. Vet. Pathol. 17:581, 1980.

10. Bostock, D. E., and Owen, L. W.: *Neoplasia in the Cat, Dog and Horse*, 1st ed. Wolfe Medical Publishers, Ltd., London, 1975, pp. 15–53.

11. Brawner, W. R.: Personal communication, 1982.

12. Brewer, W. G., and Turrel, J. M.: Radiotherapy and hyperthermia in the treatment of fibrosarcomas in the dog. J. Am. Vet. Med. Assoc. 181:146, 1982.

13. Brody, R. S.: Canine and feline neoplasia. Adv. Vet. Sci. Comp. Med. 14:309, 1970.

14. Brown, N. O., Nesbit, G. H., Patnaik, A. K., and MacEwen, E. G.: Cutaneous lymphosarcoma in the dog: a disease with variable clinical and histologic manifestations. J. Am. Anim. Hosp. Assoc. 16:565, 1980.

15. Byers, J. C., Fleischman, R. W.: Peptic ulcers associated with a mast cell tumor in a dog. Canine Pract. 8:42, 1981.

16. Conroy, J. D.: Canine cutaneous lymphosarcoma. Vet. Clin. North Am. Small Anim. Pract. 9:141, 1979.

17. Davies, A. P., Hayden, D. W., Klausner, J. S., and Perman, V. S.: Noncutaneous systemic mastocytosis and mast cell leukemia in a dog. A case report and literature review. J. Am. Anim. Hosp. Assoc. 17:361, 1981.

18. Doige, C. ., Farrow, C. S., and Presnell, K. R.: Parosteal lipoma in a dog. J. Am. Anim. Hosp. Assoc. 16:87, 1980.

19. Fees, D. L., and Withrow, S. J.: Canine hemangiosarcoma. Comp. Cont. Ed. 3:1047, 1981.

20. Gilette, E. L.: Radiation therapy of canine and feline tumors. J. Am. Anim. Hosp. Assoc. 12:359, 1976.

21. Goldschmidt, M. H., and Bevier, D. E.: Skin tumors in the dog. Part III. Lymphohistiocytic and melanocytic tumors. Comp. Cont. Ed. 3:588, 1981.

22. Grier, R. L., Brewer, W. G., Paul, S.R., and Theilen, G.H.: Treatment of bovine and equine ocular squamous cell carcinoma by radiofrequency hyperthermia. J. Am. Vet. Med. Assoc. 177:55, 1980.

23. Grier, R. L., Brewer, W. G., and Theilen, G. H.: Hyperthermic treatment of superficial tumors in cats and dogs. J. Am. Vet. Med. Assoc. 177:227, 1980.

24. Grier, R. L., Thoen, C. O., and Harris, D. L.: Regression of cutaneous melanosarcoma following intralesional mycobacterium bovis, BCG, injection: a case report. J. Am. Anim. Hosp. Assoc. 14:76, 1978.

25. Hardy, W. D.: General concepts of canine and feline tumors. J. Am. Anim. Hosp. Assoc. 12:295, 1976.

26. Herman, L. H., Slaughter, L. J., and Martin, D. P.: Malignant mastocytoma in a dog. J. Am. Vet. Med. Assoc. 151:1322, 1967.

27. Hess, P. W.: Canine mast cell tumors. Vet. Clin. North Am. 7:133, 1977.

28. Hottendorf, G. H., and Neilsen, S. W.: Pathologic survey of 300 extirpated canine mastocytomas. Zbl. Veterinar. med. [A] 14:272, 1967.

29. Jeglum, K. A.: Malignant lymphoma in the dog. Comp. Cont. Ed. 1:503, 1979.

30. Lester, S. J., McGonigle, L. F., and McDonald, G. K.: Disseminated anaplastic mastocytoma with terminal mastocythemia in a dog. J. Am. Anim. Hosp. Assoc. 17:355, 1981.

31. MacEwen, E. G.: Melanoma and fibrosarcoma. *In: Surgical Oncology*: Proc. 9th Ann. Vet. Surg. Forum, 1981.

32. Macy, D. W., and Reynolds, H. A.: The incidence, characteristics and clinical management of skin tumors of cats. J. Am. Anim. Hosp. Assoc. 17:1026, 1981.

33. McChesney, A. E.: Infiltrative lipoma in dogs. Vet. Pathol. 17:316, 1980.

34. Nielsen, S. W.: Classification of tumors in dogs and cats J. Am. Anim. Hosp. Assoc. 19:13, 1983.

35. Priester, W. A.: Skin tumors in domestic animals. J. Natl. Cancer Inst. 50:457, 1973.

36. Schmidt, R. E., and Langham, R. F.: A survey of feline neoplasms. J. Am. Vet. Med. Assoc. 151:1325, 1967.

37. Seiler, R. J.: Granular basal cell tumors in the skin of 3 dogs: A distinct histopathologic entity. Vet. Pathol. 18:23, 1981.

38. Shadduck, J. A.: A canine cutaneous lymphoproliferative disorder resembling human mycosis fungoides. Vet. Clin. North Am. Small Anim. Pract. 9:107, 1979.

39. Stannard, A. A., and Pulley, L. T.: Intracutaneous cornifying epithelioma (keratocanthoma) in the dog: a retrospective study of 25 cases. J. Am. Vet. Med. Assoc. 167:385, 1975.

40. Stannard, A. A., and Pulley, L. T.: Tumors of the skin and soft tissues. *In* Moulton, J. E. (ed.): *Tumors in Domestic Animals*. University of California Press, Berkeley, 1978, pp. 16–70.

41. Stehlin, J. S.: Treatment of the primary lesion in melanoma. Surg. Gynecol. Obstet. 125:497, 1981.

42. Strafuss, A. C.: Basal cell tumors in dogs. J. Am. Vet. Med. Assoc. 169:322, 1976.

43. Strafuss, A. C.: Sebaceous gland carcinoma in dogs. J. Am. Vet. Med. Assoc. 169:325, 1976.

44. Strafuss, A. C., Cook, J. E., and Smith, J. E.: Squamous cell carcinoma in dogs. J. Am. Vet. Med. Assoc. 168:425, 1976.

45. Strafuss, A. C., Smith, J. E., Kennedy, G. A., and Dennis, S. M.: Lipomas in dogs. J. Am. Anim. Hosp. Assoc. 9:555, 1973.

46. Swaim, S. F.: *Surgery of Traumatized Skin: Management and Reconstruction in the Dog and Cat*. W. B. Saunders, Philadelphia, 1980.

47. Tams, T. F.: Canine mast cell tumors. Comp. Cont. Ed. 3:869, 1981.

48. Theilen, G. H., and Madewell, B. R. (eds.): Tumors of the skin and subcutaneous tissues. In *Veterinary Cancer Medicine*. Lea & Febiger, Philadelphia, 1979, pp. 123–191.

49. Thrall, D. E.: Radiation therapy in the dog: principles, indications and complications. Comp. Cont. Ed. 4:652, 1982.

50. Weiss, E., and Frese, K.: Tumors of the skin. Bull. W. H. O. 50:79, 1974.

51. Wilson, G. P., and Hayes, H. M.: Castration for treatment of perianal gland neoplasms in the dog. J. Am. Vet. Med. Assoc. 174:1301, 1979.

52. Withrow, S. J.: Lipoma and liposarcoma. *In: Surgical Oncology*. Proc. 9th Ann. Vet. Surg. Forum, 1981.

53. Withrow, S. J.: Perianal adenomas. *In: Surgical Oncology*. Proc. 9th Ann. Vet. Surg. Forum, 1981.

176 Alimentary Tract, Liver, and Pancreas

J. S. Klausner and R. M. Hardy

OROPHARYNGEAL NEOPLASIA

Neoplasia of the oral and pharyngeal cavities is the fourth most frequent canine and feline malignancy. Incidence is reported to be 20/100,000 in the dog and 11/100,000 in the cat.[28] Malignant and benign tumors arising from dental and nondental tissues have been described (Table 176–1).[9,20,27,41,104,108] Squamous cell carcinoma and malignant melanoma are the most frequent malignant oral tumors in dogs, whereas squamous cell carcinoma is the most commonly identified malignant oral tumor in cats.

Most oral tumors arise from the gingiva in the dog and the gingiva or tongue in the cat. Canine lingual tumors are uncommon. Although oral tumors may be encountered in dogs of any age, there is an increased risk in older dogs (Table 176–2). An exception is fibrosarcoma in large dogs, which occurs more frequently in younger dogs than other oral tumors.

Oral tumors occur more frequently in male dogs than female dogs (see Table 176–2). Breeds with a high incidence of oral tumors include cocker spaniel, Weimaraner, German shepherd, German short-haired pointer, golden retriever, and boxer.[27] Small breeds tend to have a higher incidence of malignant melanomas and tonsillar carcinomas, whereas fibrosarcomas and nontonsillar squamous cell carcinomas are more common in large dogs.

The incidence of tonsillar squamous cell carcinomas is higher in urban dogs than in rural dogs, prompting speculation of an environmental cause.[89] Dogs with heavily pigmented oral mucosa are predisposed to malignant melanomas.[26]

Clinical Signs and Diagnosis

Clinically, oral tumors produce proliferative or occasionally ulcerative lesions. Associated clinical signs include decreased appetite, halitosis, and bloody salivation. Dysphagia is common with tonsillar tumors. Histological examination of oral tumors is necessary to differentiate neoplastic from inflammatory lesions and to determine the cell of origin of neoplastic tissue.

Epulides are tumors arising from the periodontal stroma. They are usually located in the gingiva near the tooth and are more common in dogs than cats.[32,57] Three types have been described.[33] The fibromatous and ossifying epulides are benign tumors that form pedunculated nonulcerating, noninvasive masses. The acanthomatous epulides, formally termed *adamantinomas*, are locally invasive, causing bone destruction, but do not metastasize (Fig. 176–1).

Malignant oral tumors are locally invasive, and bone involvement is common (See Table 176–2). Radiographically, involved bones usually appear lytic, but proliferative lesions are occasionally observed. A negative radiograph does not preclude bone involvement. Metastasis to regional lymph nodes may occur,

TABLE 176–1. Canine and Feline Oropharyngeal Tumors

Nonodontogenic Neoplasia
  Benign tumors
    Papilloma, fibroma, lipoma, chondroma, osteoma, hemangioma, histiocytoma, fibromatous epulis, ossifying epulis
  Malignant tumors
    Malignant melanoma, squamous cell carcinoma, fibrosarcoma, acanthomatous epulis, adenocarcinoma, undifferentiated carcinoma, hemangiosarcoma, lymphosarcoma, osteosarcoma, transmissible venereal tumor, mast cell tumor
Odontogenic Neoplasia
  Odontoma
  Ameloblastoma

TABLE 176–2. Epidemiological Features and Biological Behavior of Canine Oropharyngeal Neoplasms*

	Malignant Melanoma	Fibrosarcoma	Tonsillar Squamous Cell Carcinoma	Nontonsillar Squamous Cell Carcinoma
Mean age (yrs)	11	7.6	9.6	8.8
Male: female	4.2:1	1.8:1	1.5:1	1:1
Bone involvement(%)	57	68	ND†	77
Regional lymph node involvement (%)	15	11	35	45
Distant metastases (%)	66	23	41	36

*Data from Todoroff, R. J., and Brody, R. S.: Oral and pharyngeal neoplasia in the dog: a retrospective survey of 361 cases. J. Am. Vet. Med. Assoc. *175*:567, 1979.
†Not determined.

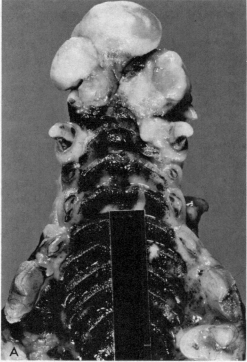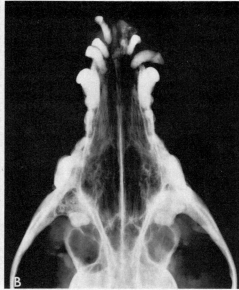

Figure 176–1. A, Upper jaw of a 16-month-old mixed breed dog extensively infiltrated by an acanthomatous epulis. B, Ventrodorsal radiograph of the maxilla. Note the extensive bone lysis surrounding the incisor teeth.

especially with malignant melanoma and squamous cell carcinoma (See Table 176–2). Distant metastasis to pulmonary tissue and other viscera is most often associated with tonsillar squamous cell carcinoma and malignant melanoma (See Table 176–2). Fibrosarcomas are locally invasive but have a relatively low incidence of distant metastasis.

Clinical staging for oral tumors is based on tumor size and the presence of bone invasion, regional lymph node involvement, and distant metastasis (Table 176–3).[109] The clinical stage is determined following careful physical examination of the oral cavity, palpation and biopsy of regional lymph nodes, and thoracic radiology.

Treatment

Dogs without evidence of lymph node or thoracic involvement should receive aggressive local therapy. Short survival times because of tumor recurrence following conventional surgical excision of oral tumors result from failure to completely excise the local tumor and failure to destroy tumor cells that have penetrated bone (Table 176–4). Wide surgical excision can be curative for small tumors that have not invaded underlying bone but is generally only palliative for more aggressive tumors. With bone involvement, tumor and bone excision may be curative. Partial mandibulectomy or maxillectomy and tumor excision have been used successfully for tumors lo-

cated rostral to the canine teeth, whereas hemimandibulectomy has been used for mandibular neoplasms located caudal to the canine teeth. Unfortunately, most oral tumors cannot be totally excised because of their location.

Cryosurgery can be used to treat oral neoplasms. It is especially useful for managing less accessible oral lesions. Other advantages of cryosurgery include its ease of application, low postoperative morbidity, bone-sparing effect, and palliative relief of pain and odor.[44] Postoperative complications, although uncommon, include pharyngeal and lingual edema, air embolism, oronasal fistula, and mandibular fracture. An increased efficacy of cryosurgery compared with convential surgery or radiation therapy has not been established.

Local radiation therapy can be effective in producing remissions and cures of radiosensitive oral tumors.[47,57,102–104] The best responses can be expected with acanthomatous epulides and squamous cell carcinomas (See Table 176–4). The mean survival time in 12 dogs with oral squamous cell carcinomas treated with radiation therapy at the University of Minnesota was 11.8 months (range 1 to 31 months). Results of radiation therapy for oral fibrosarcomas in dogs have generally been poor, although cures are occasionally reported. Increased responsiveness of oral fibrosarcomas has been noted by combining radiation and hyperthermia.[6] Radiation therapy can be used as an adjuvant to surgical excision. By destroying tumor cells remaining in the surgical field and in bone, radiotherapy may decrease the recurrence rate.[39]

TABLE 176–3. Clinical Staging System for Tumors of the Oral Cavity*

T Primary Tumor
  T0 No evidence of tumor
  T1 Tumor < 2 cm maximum diameter
    T1a Without bone invasion
    T1b With bone invasion
  T2 Tumor 2 to 4 cm maximum diameter
    T2a Without bone invasion
    T2b With bone invasion
  T3 Tumor > 4 cm maximum diameter
    T3a Without bone invasion
    T3b With bone invasion
N Regional Lymph Nodes (RLN)
  N0 No evidence of RLN involvement
  N1 Movable ipsilateral nodes
    N1a Nodes histologically negative
    N1b Movable histologically positive
  N2 Movable contralateral or bilateral nodes
    N2a Nodes histologically negative
    N2b Nodes histologically positive
  N3 Fixed nodes
M Distant Metastasis
  M0 No evidence of distant metastasia
  M1 Distant metastasis present

Stage Groupings			
Stage	*T*	*N*	*M*
I	T1	N0, N1a, or N2a	M0
II	T2	N0, N1a, or N2a	M0
III†	T3	N0, N1a, or N2a	M0
IV	Any T		
	Any T	Any N2b or N3	M0
	Any T	Any N	M1

*Reprinted with permission from World Health Organization: *Report of the Second Consultation on the Biological Behavior and Therapy of Tumors of Domestic Animals.* WHO, Geneva, 1978.
†Any bone involvement.

Chemotherapy is used to provide palliative relief in dogs or cats with disseminated oral tumors. Unfortunately, most oral tumors, with the exception of lymphosarcoma and transmissible venereal tumor, are poorly responsive to chemotherapeutic agents.[12]

Prognosis

The prognosis for long-term survival in dogs and cats with most malignant oral tumors is generally guarded to poor because of extensive local involvement at the time of initial diagnosis (See Table 176–4). Tonsillar squamous cell carcinomas and malignant melanomas are locally invasive and rapidly progressive and frequently metastasize to local lymph nodes and distant sites. Nontonsillar squamous cell carcinomas are locally invasive but have a lower incidence of metastatic spread. Fibrosarcomas often do not metastasize but are locally invasive. Acanthomatous epulides have a good prognosis because of their responsiveness to radiation therapy.

ESOPHAGEAL NEOPLASIA

Esophageal neoplasia is rare in the dog and cat except for osteosarcomas and fibrosarcomas associated with *Spirocerca lupi.*[15,58,70,107] A study of 5,854 canine neoplasms observed at necropsy revealed only 19 esophageal tumors.[96] In another report, only two primary esophageal tumors were identified in 49,229 dogs in an 11-year period.[90] Feline esophageal tumors occur more frequently in Great Britain than in the United States. In a report from Great Britain, 13 esophageal carcinomas were identified in a series of 66 feline alimentary tract tumors.[23] In another report by the same author, five esophageal carcinomas were found in a series of 200 feline neoplasms.[25] No esophageal tumors were identified in a series of 46 feline alimentary tract tumors in the United States.[8] Neoplasms that metastasize to the esophagus include thyroid carcinomas, pulmonary neoplasms, and gastric carcinomas.[58,90]

Leiomyoma is the most frequently identified benign esophageal neoplasm.[11,13] Clinical signs result from obstruction of the esophageal lumen. Leiomyomas may be found incidentally at necropsy.

Carcinomas arise from squamous epithelium of the esophagus and infiltrate the lumen, muscularis, and serosa. Annular constriction of the esophagus may result. Metastases to trachea, lung, and mediastinal lymph nodes have been reported.[15,64,90]

Strong evidence exists that *Spirocerca lupi* is an important etiological factor in the development of esophageal osteosarcomas and fibrosarcomas. Esophageal sarcomas are frequent in areas of the world where *S. lupi* is endemic; lesions associated with *S. lupi* (vertebral spondylosis, aortic scarring or aneurysm) are frequent in dogs with esophageal sarcomas;

TABLE 176–4. Response of Canine Oropharyngeal Neoplasms to Surgical Excision or Radiation Therapy*

Neoplasm	Median Survival Time (mo)		
	Untreated	*Surgical Therapy*	*Radiation Therapy*
Malignant melanoma	3	3	4
Fibrosarcoma	3	1	5
Tonsillar squamous cell carcinoma	ND†	2	ND
Nontonsillar squamous cell carcinoma	ND	9	9

*Data from Todoroff, R. J., and Brody, R. S.: Oral and pharyngeal neoplasia in the dog: a retrospective survey of 361 cases. J. Am. Vet. Med. Assoc. *175*:567, 1979.
†Not determined.

and sarcomatous changes have been described in fibroblasts in S. *lupi* granulomas.[4] Esophageal sarcomas frequently metastasize to the lung, and a high incidence of hypertrophic pulmonary osteoarthropathy has been noted.

Clinical Signs

Clinical signs of esophageal neoplasia result from obstruction or altered esophageal motility. Regurgitation, dysphagia, and weight loss are common. Regurgitation may result in aspiration pneumonia and respiratory signs.

Diagnosis

Esophagoscopy, radiographic evaluation, and thoracotomy can be used to establish a diagnosis of esophageal neoplasia. Esophagoscopy may reveal the presence of nodules, ulcerations, mucosal irregularities, lack of distensibility, or stricture. Mucosal lesions can be biopsied through the endoscope with a punch biopsy instrument.

Retention of gas in the esophageal lumen and displacement of mediastinal structures may be noted on survey radiographs.[90] Evaluation of contrast radiographs may reveal an irregular mucosal surface, luminal narrowing, retention of contrast media within the esophagus, or thickening of the esophageal wall. Fluoroscopy may reveal decreased esophageal peristalsis.

Treatment and Prognosis

Neoplasia of the esophagus is associated with a poor prognosis. Small tumors can be surgically removed. Unfortunately, the diagnosis of esophageal neoplasia is often established late in the disease course, thus precluding surgical resection.

GASTRIC NEOPLASIA

Gastric neoplasms are very uncommon in the dog and cat. Adenocarcinoma is the most common canine gastric tumor but accounts for less than 1 per cent of all canine malignancies.[11,60] The incidence of gastric tumor in the cat is less than that in the dog. Lymphosarcoma is the most frequently identified feline gastric neoplasm.[8]

Gastric tumors generally occur in older animals, with vomiting and weight loss the most frequent clinical signs. Signs are usually attributable to gastric outflow obstruction or mucosal ulceration.

Benign Gastric Tumors

Leiomyoma is the most commonly identified benign gastric tumor in dogs.[45,77,92] The average age of

dogs with gastric leiomyomas is 16 years.[77] Leiomyomas originate in the muscle layers of the stomach wall and usually grow into the gastric lumen. They may not cause clinical signs or may be associated with vomiting, especially if outflow obstruction is present. Treatment is by surgical removal.

Adenomatous polyps result from benign gastric mucosal proliferation. Both single and multiple polyps have been reported in the stomach of the dog.[22,29,43,45,73] Grossly, polyps are raised sessile or pedunculated lesions. They may be associated with vomiting, cause pyloric outflow obstruction, or be an incidental finding at necropsy.

Malignant Gastric Tumors

Malignant gastric tumors of dogs and cats include adenocarcinomas, lymphosarcomas, and fibrosarcomas.[8,11,100] Gastric lymphosarcoma may result in nodular, diffusely infiltrative, or ulcerative lesions.[34] The stomach may be the only organ involved, or the disease may be generalized. Therapy includes surgical removal of nodular lesions and chemotherapy.

Adenocarcinomas account for 42 to 72 per cent of all malignant gastric tumors in dogs.[30,49,60,65,74,87] Gastric adenocarcinomas occur in older dogs usually between the ages of 7 and 13 years, with a peak incidence at 8 years. Males are more commonly affected than females. No breed predisposition has been documented. Geographic differences in occurrence similar to those described in man have not been identified in the dog.

Environmental and hereditary factors are thought to increase the risk of gastric cancer in man.[61,91] Substances suspected of being carcinogenic include those associated with pickling or smoking of food for preservation; benzpyrene derived from the cooking process; and nitrosamines derived from high nitrate-containing food.[68] In addition, blood type, atrophic gastritis, and pernicious anemia have been associated with the occurrence of gastric adenocarcinomas in human beings. Canine gastric adenocarcinomas have been induced by the intragastric administration of nitrosamine.[55] The lower frequency of gastric adenocarcinoma in dogs compared with that in man may result from an inherent resistance of the canine stomach to carcinogens or to the shorter life span of the dog.[60]

Gastric adenocarcinomas are usually located in the pyloric antrum or along the lesser curvature of the stomach (Fig. 176–2). Three anatomical types have been described: (1) diffuse infiltration of tumor in the gastric wall resulting in a thickened, nondistensible stomach (linitis plastica); (2) plaque like mucosal lesions usually with large central ulcers; and (3) raised polypoid lesions.[73] The neoplasm originates in the mucosa and spreads laterally, frequently involving all layers of the gastric wall. Histologically, large, pleomorphic tumor cells may be randomly arranged (diffuse type) or may have a distinct glandular structure

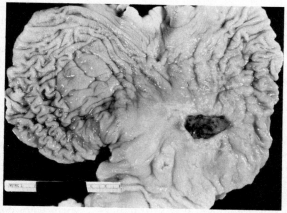

Figure 176–2. Large, nonperforating ulcer on the lesser curvature of the stomach resulting from a gastric adenocarcinoma in an 11-year-old female basset hound.

(intestinal type).[78] Variable amounts of mucin and large central vacuoles may be present within the neoplastic cells. A marked fibrous connective reaction commonly accompanies gastric adenocarcinoma. Early metastasis to regional lymph nodes and liver is common. Other metastatic sites include spleen, omentum, adrenal gland, myocardium, and lung.[45]

Clinical Signs

Chronic vomiting, weight loss, and anorexia are usually noted. In addition, hematemesis, melena, and abdominal pain may be detected. Rarely, an abdominal mass may be palpated. Ascites, icterus, and dyspnea often indicate metastatic spread. The duration of the illness is generally less than three months.[92]

Diagnosis

The presence of chronic vomition and weight loss in an older dog is suggestive of gastric adenocarcinoma. Anemia may be present if mucosal ulceration results in gastric bleeding. A fecal occult blood test may be positive.

Changes detected on abdominal radiographs are usually minimal. An anterior abdominal mass or gastric dilation may be apparent. Contrast radiography, either a barium series or double contrast gastrogram, is usually required to detect gastric lesions (Fig. 176–3). Abnormalities associated with adenocarcinoma include (1) delayed gastric emptying; (2) pyloric or lesser curvature filling defects; (3) thickened gastric wall; (4) mucosal ulceration; and (5) loss of normal rugal pattern.[4,92] Significant abnormalities persist on multiple films. Fluoroscopy is useful in the confirmation of suspicious lesions and the assessment of gastric motility. Diffuse infiltration of the gastric wall results in gastric hypomotility.

Gastric lesions can also be detected with a flexible gastroscope. Gastric neoplasms appear as raised

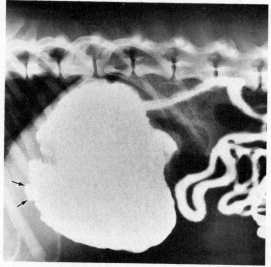

Figure 176–3. Lateral radiograph following stomach tube administration of barium demonstrating multiple filling defects and a large ulcer (arrows) in the anterior margin of the stomach of a 4-year-old male standard poodle. Laparotomy revealed extensive infiltration of lesser curvature of the stomach by adenocarcinoma.

masses that project into the stomach lumen or as thickened rugal folds. Mucosal ulceration or inability to distend the stomach may be apparent. Tumors that diffusely infiltrate the gastric wall are often difficult to see. Directed biopsy of lesions can be achieved with a biopsy forceps passed through the gastroscope.

Surgical exploration is used to confirm a diagnosis of gastric neoplasia, to assess the extent of the tumor in the stomach, and to detect the presence of metastases in regional lymph nodes and the liver. Tissue can be obtained for histopathological evaluation from primary and metastatic lesions.

Treatment

Complete surgical excision is the treatment of choice for gastric adenocarcinomas. Depending on the size and location of the lesion, either segmental resection or partial gastrectomy should be selected. Since the pyloric area of the stomach is often involved, a gastroduodenostomy or gastrojejunostomy may be required. If regional lymph nodes are enlarged, they should be removed. Extensive gastric involvement may preclude complete excision of the primary tumor. Removal of a portion of the neoplasia may provide palliative relief and increased survival time.

Chemotherapy has been used in human beings with extensive metastatic disease and as an adjuvant after complete surgical excision of gastric adenocarcinomas.[21,69] Objective responses in man have been obtained with 5-fluorouracil, mitomycin-C, carmustine (BCNU), and adriamycin. Duration of responses with single agents is generally brief, lasting approximately four months, but combination therapy can extend response time to ten months.[21,62] A beneficial effect of adjuvant chemotherapy has been demonstrated in man.[69] Chemotherapy has not been adequately evaluated in canine gastric adenocarcinoma patients.

Prognosis

Factors that influence prognosis of gastric adenocarcinoma in man include depth of tumor involvement in the gastric wall, involvement of regional lymph nodes, and presence of distant metastases.[61] Most dogs in which gastric adenocarcinoma has been diagnosed have extensive involvement at the time of diagnosis. Survival time in untreated dogs is generally less than three months after the onset of clinical signs. Survival following tumor excision is generally less than six months,[26,60,65] although a five-year survival in one dog has been reported.[29] Earlier gastroscopic diagnosis and adjuvant chemotherapy following surgery may improve the prognosis in the future.

INTESTINAL NEOPLASIA

Intestinal neoplasms are uncommon in the dog and cat. Intestinal adenocarcinoma represents approximately 0.33 per cent of canine malignancies and 0.4 to 2.9 per cent of feline malignancies.[77,86] In dogs, adenocarcinomas are identified more frequently than leiomyosarcomas, lymphosarcomas, or carcinoids.[11,45,46,77] In one report, 53 per cent of canine intestinal tumors were adenocarcinomas.[77] Benign intestinal tumors are recognized less frequently than malignant tumors. In the cat, intestinal lymphosarcoma is identified more frequently than adenocarcinoma.[46] Benign tumors of the feline intestine are very rare.

Intestinal neoplasms usually occur in older animals (Table 176–5), and males are more frequently affected than females. German shepherds and Siamese cats are predisposed to adenocarcinomas,[77,106] and boxers have a high incidence of intestinal lymphosarcoma.[11]

Benign Neoplasms

Leiomyomas occur infrequently in the small and large intestine of dogs and cats.[11,23,24,46,48] They arise from smooth muscle in the intestinal wall and are usually nonulcerated but may obstruct the intestinal lumen. Leiomyomas are occasionally an incidental finding at necropsy.

Adenomatous polyps occur most frequently in the rectum of dogs.[45,46,75] Male and female dogs are equally affected; the mean age of occurrence is 6.9 years, and the collie breed is predisposed.[94] Grossly, rectal polyps vary from a few millimeters to several centimeters in diameter. They are raised, sessile, or pedunculated and may occur in grapelike clusters.[70] Single or multiple polyps may be present. Histolog-

ically, well-differentiated columnar cells cover the surface of the polyp and a fibrous stalk connects the base of the polyp to the mucosa. Polyps generally do not recur following surgical removal.[75] Although carcinomatous change has been described within polyps,[94,95] there is little clinical evidence that adenomatous polyps represent a premalignant lesion in the dog.

Malignant Neoplasms

Adenocarcinomas occur most frequently in the rectum, colon, and jejunum of dogs and in the ileum of cats (See Table 176–5).[10,24,46,53,59,93] Small intestinal adenocarcinomas typically appear as firm, annular, constrictive masses. Neoplastic proliferation begins in the mucosa and spreads throughout the intestinal wall. Extensive stromal fibrosis and muscular hypertrophy contribute to intestinal stenosis. Four histological types of adenocarcinomas have been described: solid, acinar, papillary, and mucinous.[79] The biological behavior of the four types is similar, but each has a predilection for different sites within the intestinal tract.

Intestinal adenocarcinomas frequently metastasize to regional lymph nodes, especially mesenteric and iliac nodes (See Table 176–5). Widespread abdominal lymph node involvement may occur. Diffuse metastasis to peritoneal surfaces (carcinomatosis) results in ascites. Metastasis to abdominal and thoracic viscera including liver, spleen, kidney, myocardium, and lung has been reported.[11,46,79,86]

Lymphosarcoma is most frequently identified in the jejunum of dogs and ileum of cats.[8,24,46] Rectal and colonic involvement occurs less commonly (Fig. 176–4). Multiple sites within the intestinal tract are frequently involved. Grossly, lesions may be fusiform or nodular. Large segments of the intestine may be diffusely thickened. Metastasis to regional lymph nodes, kidney, and liver is common.[46] Affected cats are usually feline leukemia virus–negative.

Leiomyosarcomas have been reported infrequently throughout the intestinal tract of dogs and cats.[14,46,77]

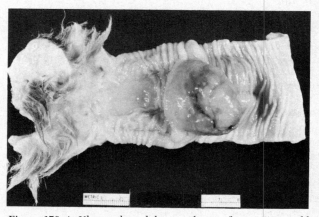

Figure 176–4. Ulcerated, nodular rectal mass from a 5-year-old Shetland sheepdog diagnosed as a lymphosarcoma. There was no evidence of lymphosarcoma in other organs.

TABLE 176–5. Epidemiological Features and Biological Behavior of Canine and Feline Intestinal Neoplasms*

	Mean Age (yrs)	Male:Female	Breed Predisposition	Frequent Sites in Intestine	Frequent Metastatic Sites
CANINE					
Adenocarcinoma	9	1.8:1	German shepherd	Rectum, colon, jejunum	Regional lymph nodes, peritoneum, lung, liver
Leiomyosarcoma	11	1:2	None	Cecum, jejunum	Regional lymph nodes, liver
Lymphosarcoma	6.5	1.6:1	Boxer	Jejunum, ileum	Regional lymph nodes, liver, spleen
FELINE					
Adenocarcinoma	11	2.5:1	Siamese	Ileum	Regional lymph nodes, peritoneum, omentum
Lymphosarcoma	10.5	1.4:1	None	Ileum, duodenum	Regional lymph nodes, peritoneum, omentum, liver

*Data from Brody, R. S., and Cohen, D.: An epizootiologic and clinicopathologic study of 95 cases of gastrointestinal neoplasm in the dog. Sci. Proc. 101st Ann. Mtg. Am. Vet. Med. Assoc., 1964, pp. 167–179; Patnaik, A. K., Hurvitz, A. and Johnson, G. F.: Canine gastrointestinal neoplasms. Vet. Pathol. 14:547, 1977; and Turk, M. A. M., Gallina, A. M., and Russell, T. S.: Nonhematopoietic gastrointestinal neoplasia in cats: a retrospective study of 44 cases. Vet. Pathol. 18:614, 1981.

Cecal and jejunal involvement is most common. Leiomyosarcomas usually arise in the outer muscular layers, are nodular, and may result in intestinal perforation. Metastasis to regional lymph nodes and liver has been reported.[46]

Intestinal carcinoids have been reported in the duodenum, ileum, colon, and rectum of dogs.[18,40,79] An uncommon tumor, carcinoids arise from enterochromaffin cells (Kulchitsky's cells) in the intestinal mucosa. Enterochromaffin cells contain high levels of 5-hydroxytryptamine (serotonin) and are recognized by the presence of intracytoplasmic argyrophilic granules. In man, release of biologically active amines from carcinoid tumors can result in the carcinoid syndrome, which is characterized by cutaneous flushing, abdominal pain, diarrhea, and dyspnea.[3] Canine carcinoid tumors usually metastasize to regional lymph nodes and the liver.[79]

Although uncommon, mast cell tumors may primarily involve the small and large intestine of the cat, resulting in firm, nonulcerated thickenings of the intestinal wall.[1] Metastases to the mesenteric lymph node, liver, and spleen are frequently observed.

Clinical Signs

Clinical signs associated with intestinal neoplasia result from bleeding, intestinal obstruction, peritonitis, or malabsorption. Intermittent vomiting and diarrhea, weight loss, and inappetence are characteristic of small intestinal tumors. Tenesmus, bloody mucoid feces, constipation, rectal prolapse, and increased frequency of defecation are frequent signs with large intestinal tumors.

Intestinal bleeding, which occurs with ulcerative lesions, may result in anemia, thrombocytopenia, and hypoproteinemia. A fecal occult blood test will be positive. Abdominal pain and fever occur with peritonitis resulting from intestinal perforation. Malabsorption occurs when intestinal villi become filled with neoplastic cells, lymphatics become blocked by neoplastic cells, or tumors cause complete or partial intestinal obstruction.

Diagnosis

Intestinal neoplasia should be suspected when an older dog or cat is presented with progressive weight loss and clinical signs referable to the intestinal tract. Unexplained bleeding from the intestinal tract, anemia, ascites, abdominal mass, or peritonitis should also alert one to the possible presence of intestinal cancer.

Intestinal tumors are often identified by abdominal palpation. A nodular mass or diffuse thickening of intestinal loops may be noted. Mesenteric lymph nodes may be enlarged. Diagnosis can sometimes be established by cytological examination of an aspiration biopsy of the abnormal mass.

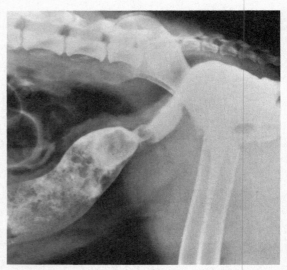

Figure 176–5. Lateral radiograph following administration of a barium enema reveals an annular constriction resulting from an infiltrating adenocarcinoma of the distal colon and rectum in a 7-year-old female German shepherd.

Rectal examination may reveal a polypoid lesion or stricture. Proctoscopic evaluation may reveal a proliferative tumor, ulceration, mucosal irregularity, or stenosis. Lesions can be biopsied with a punch biopsy instrument passed through the proctoscope.

Survey abdominal radiographs and contrast studies (upper GI series, barium enema) are often abnormal (Fig. 176–5). Radiographic abnormalities may include (1) an abdominal mass; (2) intestinal accumulation of fluid, gas, or ingesta; (3) delayed intestinal transit time; (4) mural lesions associated with luminal filling defects; (5) mucosal ulceration; and (6) thickening of the intestinal wall and displacement of adjacent bowel loops.[36] In addition, nodular, patchy, irregular abdominal densities may be noted if diffuse peritoneal metastasis has occurred.[101]

Excisional or incisional biopsy of intestinal tumors can be obtained at laparotomy. In addition, the abdomen can be examined for tumor metastasis.

Treatment

The treatment of intestinal adenocarcinoma is wide surgical excision and intestinal anastomosis. En bloc excision including the tumor, mesentery, and regional lymph nodes may offer the best chance of cure.[101] Tumor removal can provide palliative relief even in the presence of metastatic disease. Chemotherapy has little effect on intestinal adenocarcinomas. In man, treatment of intestinal carcinomas with 5-fluorouracil produces objective responses in only 20 per cent of cases.[19]

Isolated, nodular lymphosarcoma lesions can be surgically excised. Followup combination chemotherapy is indicated. Multiple intestinal lesions or metastatic disease is best treated by chemotherapy alone. Intestinal polyps can be surgically removed through a proctoscope by pedicle ligation or electrocautery or with a tonsil snare.[75] A celiotomy and enterotomy are required to remove polyps in the proximal colon and small intestine.

Prognosis

The prognosis following removal of polyps and other benign tumors is generally good. Recurrences are infrequent.

Malignant intestinal tumors are associated with a guarded to poor long-term prognosis. In man, the absence of lymph node involvement, small tumor size, and lack of penetration into the muscle layers of the intestine are indicators of longer survival times.[7] In cats, survival time varies from two days to two years following surgical resection of intestinal adenocarcinomas.[106] In another report, a cat survived 28 months following surgery and immunotherapy.[83]

HEPATIC NEOPLASIA

Primary Hepatic Tumors

Primary hepatic tumors are uncommon in dogs and cats. They are estimated to constitute from 0.6 to 1.3 per cent of all tumors.[80] Although precise data are not available, several recently published necropsy surveys indicate that primary hepatic tumors are identified in 0.63 to 2.6 per cent of all necropsies performed.[80,99,105] A large veterinary tumor registry estimates the rate of occurrence to be 1.6/100,000 patient years.[63]

Hepatic tumors are of epithelial or mesenchymal origin (Table 176–6). The two most common are hepatocellular carcinoma and cholangiocellular carcinoma. Hepatic neoplasia is most often a disease of aged dogs and cats. The mean age of occurrence is between 10 and 11 years of age, although affected animals as young as 4 years old have been reported.[80, 99] There is no known breed predisposition. Hepatocellular carcinomas and various sarcomas of hepatic origin occur slightly more frequently in male

TABLE 176–6. Classification of Primary Hepatic Neoplasia

Tumors of Epithelial Origin

Hepatocellular adenoma
Cholangiocellular adenoma
Hepatocellular carcinoma (hepatoma)
Cholangiocellular carcinoma (bile duct carcinoma)
Hepatic carcinoids

Tumors of Mesenchymal Origin

Hemangiosarcoma
Fibrosarcoma
Extraskeletal osteosarcoma
Leiomyosarcoma

dogs, whereas cholangiocellular carcinomas are slightly more common in female dogs.[80]

A number of etiological factors have been associated with the development of primary hepatic tumors in man and laboratory animals.[101] Causative factors include (1) chemicals such as azo- compounds, nitrosamines, aflatoxins, methylcholanthrene, acetylaminofluorene, *Senecio* alkaloids, chlorinated hydrocarbons, cycasin, and vinyl chloride, (2) thorotrast, (3) androgens, (4) malnutrition, (5) cirrhosis, (6) hepatitis B virus, and (7) parasites (schistosomiasis, clonorchiasis).[101] Of this list, aflatoxins, polycyclic hydrocarbons, cycasin, and dimethylnitrosamine are well-documented carcinogens. Although the incidence of hepatic neoplasia associated with cirrhosis is high in man, the association in dogs and cats is rare. Only 6 animals out of 110 with primary liver tumors also had histological evidence of cirrhosis; 4 had hepatocellular carcinoma, and two had cholangiocellular carcinoma.[80]

The metastatic potential of primary hepatic tumors is high. The rate of metastasis ranges from 61 per cent for hepatocellular carcinomas to 93 per cent for hepatic carcinoids.[80] Metastasis occurs by direct extension to other parts of the liver or adjacent organs and through blood and lymph to distant sites. The most common sites for metastases of epithelial tumors are regional lymph nodes and lung.[80] Metastatic hepatic sarcomas most often metastasize to the spleen.[80] Additional sites of metastasis for primary hepatic tumors include brain, kidneys, omentum, peritoneum, adrenals, pancreas, gastrointestinal tract, spine, and pituitary gland.[80,101]

Hepatocellular Carcinomas

Hepatocellular carcinomas are the most common hepatic neoplasms. They accounted for 76 of 159 (47.7 per cent) primary hepatic tumors identified in two extensive necropsy studies.[81,105] Clinical signs, although nonspecific, are generally indicative of hepatic failure. Lethargy, weakness, anorexia, weight loss, a pendulous abdomen, and vomiting are commonly present. Less commonly observed signs include ascites, diarrhea, jaundice, and dyspnea. The most significant finding on physical examination is a palpable abdominal mass in as many as 80 per cent of patients with hepatocellular carcinoma.[105] In the majority of cases, the mass is readily localized to the liver.

The ultimate diagnosis of hepatocellular carcinoma requires histological confirmation. However, hematological and biochemical changes are useful for localizing the disease to the liver and for supporting the need for a biopsy. Hematological abnormalities primarily involve varying degrees of anemia (nearly equal to > 50 per cent of patients) and neutrophilia (66 per cent of patients).[81] Significant abnormalities in hepatic biochemical function are very often detected.[81,99,105] Hepatocellular enzyme patterns resemble those seen in a large number of nonneoplastic, inflammatory hepatic diseases. Moderate to marked increases in serum alanine aminotransferase (SGPT) and aspartate aminotransferase (SGOT) frequently occur. Serum alkaline phosphatase concentrations (SAP) are dramatically increased in most cases (82 per cent of patients).[99] Biochemical evidence of functional hepatic failure is less frequently observed. Serum bilirubin concentrations are increased (usually mildly) in 26 per cent of patients, and albumin concentrations are often normal. Increases in serum albumin were reported in 18 per cent of these patients,[80] whereas hypoalbuminemia was found in 16 per cent.[99,105] Blood or serum glucose concentrations were evaluated in 65 animals with hepatocellular carcinoma. Only 4 of 65 (6 per cent) had evidence of hypoglycemia. Hypoglycemia may be so severe that it is the primary reason for presentation to the clinician.[100]

Additional diagnostic tests for evaluation of hepatocellular carcinomas should include radiography, cytology of ascitic fluid, and biopsy. Since an abdominal mass is generally palpable, radiographs localize the lesion to the liver and may determine if extrahepatic, abdominal metastases exist. The presence of ascites may limit the diagnostic usefulness of survey radiographs. Although cytological evaluation of abdominal fluid as an aid in the diagnosis of abdominal neoplasia is commonly practiced, it is not often useful in substantiating a diagnosis of hepatic neoplasia. Biopsy of abdominal masses of undetermined etiology is the diagnostic method of choice. Biopsy techniques include fine needle aspiration, needle core, and incisional and excisional biopsy. Aspiration or needle core biopsies are rapid and technically simple and carry minimal risk for the patient. However, establishing a diagnosis of hepatocellular carcinoma from small biopsy samples may be difficult. Hepatocellular carcinoma cells often retain a normal appearance, mitoses are uncommon, and reasonably normal architecture is maintained.[71]

Exploratory celiotomy is the diagnostic method of choice. Not only does it allow for a visually guided biopsy, but surgical excision may be attempted if no metastases are seen. Hepatocellular carcinomas do not fulfill the usual criteria of malignancy.[71] They are most often found as large, solitary masses with a predisposition for the left lateral hepatic lobe.[80] These cancers are generally well-encapsulated and grow by expansion and compression of adjacent tissue. Their malignant potential is often based on size and degree of local invasion in the absence of detectable metastases.[71] Unfortunately, metastases have been present at the time of diagnosis in 61 per cent of hepatocellular carcinomas.[81] Because these tumors frequently metastasize to the lungs, thoracic radiographs should be included in the presurgical work-up.

Since many hepatocellular carcinomas are single, large masses (Fig. 176–6), surgical excision remains the therapy of choice. Unfortunately, the debilitated state, age, and degree of hepatic or other organ failure in such animals make major surgery risky.

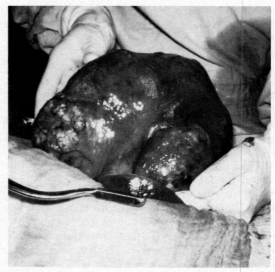

Figure 176–6. Typical large solitary hepatoma at surgery.

Alternatives to surgical excision in man include ligation of either the venous or arterial supply to the affected lobe and chemotherapy. Significant improvement has been noted in human patients with surgically inoperable or metastatic hepatocellular carcinomas by segmental ligation of the portal vein.[48] Tumor vascularity significantly affects whether venous or arterial ligation is selected. Hypovascular neoplasms respond best to segmental portal venous ligation, whereas hypervascular tumors show greater regression if segmental hepatic artery ligation is done. Tumor vascularity is estimated using presurgical radioisotopic scans. Chemotherapy in man has involved the use of systemic or intra-arterial 5-fluorouracil or methotrexate.[101] No controlled clinical trials have been reported using these agents.

The prognosis for patients with hepatocellular carcinoma is usually poor. The high rate of metastasis, size, and degree of invasion of the lesion and the physical status of the patient often preclude corrective surgery. It is hoped that earlier detection and innovative chemotherapeutic approaches will improve this situation in the future.

Cholangiocellular Carcinoma (Bile Duct Carcinoma)

Cholangiocellular carcinomas occur slightly less often than hepatocellular carcinomas. Thirty-nine of 142 (27 per cent) primary hepatic neoplasms have been of this type.[80,105] These tumors arise primarily from intrahepatic bile duct epithelium, although rarely they have arisen from the extrahepatic bile ducts or gallbladder. Several etiologies are known for this tumor in dogs and cats. They include the Chinese liver fluke, *Clonorchis sinensis*, *o*-aminoazotoluene, and the organic sulfite insecticide aramite.[71]

Clinical signs are quite similar to those described for hepatocellular carcinoma. Weight loss, anorexia, depression, vomiting, and an enlarged abdomen are common. Jaundice occurs in 13 to 23 per cent of cases. [82,105] Hepatomegaly is detected by palpation in most cases.

The diagnosis of cholangiocellular carcinoma is ultimately made by microscopic evaluation of the neoplasm. Hematological and biochemical data are similar to those of hepatocellular carcinomas. Increases in SGPT, SGOT, and SAP are common. [82,105] Biochemical data will not differentiate these two primary hepatic neoplasms.

The most important diagnostic and therapeutic procedure is exploratory celiotomy. Cholangiocellular carcinomas are often of the massive type, involving the left lateral lobe primarily. Metastases are even more common than with hepatocellular carcinomas, occurring in roughly 87 per cent of cases. [82] Metastases are most prevalent in the regional lymph nodes, lung, and peritoneum, although widespread metastases are frequent. Cure is not to be expected, because of both dissemination of these cancers prior to diagnosis and their infiltrative nature. The prognosis following diagnosis is obviously poor.

Hepatic Carcinoids

Only two reports mention the occurrence of hepatic carcinoids in the dog. [80,84] The authors concluded that they had observed carcinoids because of the large number of necropsies they performed (12,245) and their awareness of the microscopic features of these tumors. Hepatic carcinoids originate from neuroectodermal tissue scattered throughout the liver. These cells are classified as enterochromaffin or APUD cells. The APUD cell is an acronym for a biochemical characteristic of this group of cells, i.e., they are capable of *a*mine *p*recursor *u*ptake and *d*ecarboxylation. Of the 110 primary hepatic tumors, 15 were of this type. [80] Hepatic carcinoids occur at a slightly younger mean age (eight years) than other hepatic malignancies (ten years). Except for the absence of hepatomegaly, clinical signs, diagnostic criteria, and prognosis for carcinoids are similar to those of the other two primary carcinomas affecting the liver. At necropsy, all 15 tumors were found to be diffuse throughout all liver lobes. Severe hemorrhage and necrosis were present in all dogs. Extrahepatic metastases were identified in 14 of 15 cases.

Nonepithelial Hepatic Neoplasms

Both benign and malignant tumors of mesenchymal origin occur within the liver of dogs and cats. They are much less common than epithelial tumors, however. Tumors involved include hemangiosarcoma, [105] fibrosarcoma, [105] leiomyosarcoma, [80] hepatic mixed sarcoma, [71] and extraskeletal osteosarcomas. [50] Clinical features of hepatic sarcomas are similar to those of other primary tumors; therefore, biopsy is the sole method of differentiation. No effective therapy, short of early surgical excision, is known. The prognosis has been universally poor.

Hepatocellular Adenoma/Nodular Hyperplasia

Nodular hyperplasia is a frequent finding in aged dogs, reportedly occurring in from 15 to 60 per cent of the animals. [72] The differentiation of nodular hyperplasia from hepatocellular adenomas is difficult. [35,80] Nodular hyperplasia occurs most often in dogs over 11 years old and is not thought to be a "precancerous" lesion. [35] These lesions range from 0.1 to 5 cm in diameter and may be single or multiple. They are not associated with clinical signs. They are most often noted during exploratory surgery or at necropsy, and it is important to distinguish them from hepatocellular carcinomas histologically.

Tumors Metastatic to the Liver (Secondary Tumors)

The liver is a major site for metastasis of tumors. The liver, via its portal circulation, serves as a filter between the abdominal organs and the systemic circulation. Thus, it is vulnerable to metastatic cells circulating in the portal system, originating primarily from the gastrointestinal tract. In one series of 1,867 necropsies, 129 cases of metastases to the liver were identified. [105] This amounted to 6.9 per cent of the total cases necropsied, a rate that was 2.6 times the frequency of primary hepatic tumors. Metastases to the liver were identified in 30.6 per cent of all nonhepatic malignancies, exceeding the rate of metastases to the lung (24.2 per cent). [105] The mean age of occurrence for metastatic liver cancer was 7.8 years, whereas that for primary hepatic malignancies was 10 years.

Clinical signs associated with metastatic liver tumors are highly variable. Most often signs relate to the type and location of the primary tumor. The degree of involvement of the liver must be significant before signs of functional failure develop. Hepatomegaly, a common finding in primary hepatic tumors, is uncommon with metastatic tumors. [99,105] Biochemical abnormalities are highly variable. In general, metastatic disease of the liver tends to induce much less dramatic changes in hepatic biochemical profiles than does primary hepatic neoplasia. Mild to moderate increases in SGPT occur in 46[99] to 70 per cent[105] of the cases. The SAP rise may be mild to marked, usually reflecting the degree of major bile duct obstruction, in approximately half the patients. Hyperbilirubinemia occurs 30[105] to 46 per cent[99] of the time.

Tumors metastasizing to the liver arise from three major sources; hematopoietic cells, epithelium, and mesenchyme. [3] Hematopoietic neoplasms, particularly lymphosarcoma (67 cases), accounted for 81 of 129 (63 per cent) secondary liver tumors in one survey. [105] Epithelial tumors, notably pancreatic adenocarcinomas (9 of 27), were the next most common tumors (27 of 129 [21 per cent]). Mesenchymal tumors were the least common type of secondary liver tumor seen, accounting for 21 of 129 (16 per cent) cases.[105] Hemangiosarcoma was the primary tumor diagnosis in 15 of 21 sarcomas. Of these 21 sarcomas, 19 originated in the spleen. Therapy for these tumors is directed at the primary neoplasm, if possible. Since signs and laboratory abnormalities indicative of hepatic disease may dominate the clinical picture, a diagnosis of disseminated cancer may not be made until a liver biopsy is obtained. The prognosis for such cases is generally poor.

PANCREATIC NEOPLASIA

Neoplasms of the pancreas are uncommon in both dogs and cats. Estimates on their frequency of occurrence are from 0.05 to 1.88 per cent of all cancers in dogs[101] and from 1.1 to 2.8 per cent of all cancers in the cat. [71,88] Relative rates for nonendocrine pancreatic tumors are suggested to be 17.8/100,000 patient years in dogs and 12.6/100,000 patient years in cats.[88] This tumor is strongly associated with increasing age. Mean age of occurrence is 10 years in dogs (range 5 to 16 years) and 12 years in cats. Cats over 15 years old have an especially high risk. The only canine breed identified to be at increased risk is the Airedale.

Neoplasms of the pancreas arise primarily from epithelial tissue (Table 176–7). The two most important neoplasms are pancreatic adenocarcinoma and pancreatic islet cell adenocarcinomas.

Pancreatic Adenocarcinomas

Pancreatic adenocarcinomas arise from both ductular and acinar tissue of the exocrine pancreas. Ductular carcinomas are thought to predominate.[52] These tumors metastasize readily, frequently prior to clinical diagnosis. Metastases occur most often in

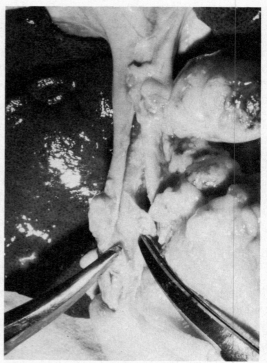

Figure 176–7. Pancreatic adenocarcinoma (at tip of scissors) invading the common bile duct in a 5-year-old Brittany spaniel. Clinical signs were those of extrahepatic bile duct occlusion.

the liver, retroperitoneum, and mesenteric lymph nodes.[71] Less common metastatic sites include the lung, duodenum, adrenal, kidney, heart, and gallbladder.

Clinical signs noted are often nonspecific and frequently relate more to the primary metastatic site (liver) than the organ of origin. Weight loss, anorexia, depression, vomiting, and jaundice are common.[2] Pancreatic adenocarcinomas frequently compress the extrahepatic bile duct, producing jaundice (Fig. 176–7). These tumors are generally small and rarely palpable.

A definitive antemortem diagnosis is rarely made except via exploratory celiotomy. These animals often die or are euthanatized with the diagnosis established at necropsy. Serum amylase and lipase concentrations are usually normal, except in cases where rapidly invading tumors produce mild signs of pancreatitis. Biochemical profiles most often suggest that liver rather than pancreatic disease is present. Mild increases in SGPT, with moderate to marked rises in SAP and serum bilirubin, are typical of metastatic pancreatic adenocarcinoma. Radiographs may detect evidence of mass lesions in the pancreatic region.[2] Abdominocentesis, with or without lavage, may be helpful in establishing a diagnosis. Pancreatic adenocarcinomas exfoliate easily, and cytology of peritoneal fluid may indicate a malignancy. Cytological evaluations rarely establish the site of origin for the exfoliated carcinoma cells, but the prognosis is not altered.

TABLE 176–7. Classification of Pancreatic Tumors Identified in Dogs and Cats*

Epithelial Tumors
Exocrine
Adenoma
Adenocarcinoma
Malignant foregut carcinoid
Undifferentiated carcinomas
Endocrine
Islet cell adenoma
Islet cell adenocarcinoma (insulinoma, gastrinoma)
Non Epithelial Tumors
Unclassified
Metastatic Tumors
Tumorlike Lesions
Nodular hyperplasia
Hyperplasia of pancreatic ducts
Ectopic pancreatic tissue
Cysts

*Data from Kircher, D. H., and Nielsen, S. W.: Tumors of the pancreas. Bull. WHO 53:195, 1976.

The prognosis for animals with pancreatic adeno-carcinoma is invariably poor owing to the tendency for early and widespread metastases. Occasional cases in man have responded to 5-fluorouracil. The therapy for solitary lesions is surgical removal.

Pancreatic Adenoma/Hyperplasia

Pancreatic hyperplasia is considered a frequent finding in aged dogs (7 to 20 years) and does occur in the cat.[71] Pancreatic adenoma is rare, although precise microscopic criteria for separation of these two entities are difficult.[52,71] They occur as small white nodules within the pancreas and have no clinical significance.

Pancreatic Islet Cell Tumors

Two major types of pancreatic islet cell neoplasms are identified in dogs. The most common is the so-called insulinoma or functional tumor of pancreatic beta cells. A much less common neoplasm, the canine gastrinoma, an islet cell tumor of pancreatic G cells that secretes gastrin, has also been identified. Very rare instances of functional beta cell tumors in the cat have occurred.[52]

Insulinomas

So-called insulinomas are much less frequent than pancreatic acinar cell carcinomas. Approximately 70 cases had been reported in dogs up until 1976, with very few cases documented in cats.[52] Between 60 and 70 per cent of these neoplasms were functional. Although the term *insulinoma* is applied to these neoplasms, the vast majority are islet cell carcinomas.[98] Even those that microscopically appear benign often develop recurrent signs at variable intervals postoperatively. The mean age of occurrence is 9 years; however, affected animals range from 3½ to 15 years old.[37,78,97] Reports on breed predispositions are conflicting. Standard poodles, boxers, and fox terriers are considered at increased risk,[88] as are German shepherds, collies, and Irish setters.[54] No sex predilection exists.

Clinical signs are highly variable. All signs may be traced directly to periods of hypoglycemia induced by tumor-produced insulin. Although generalized convulsions occur frequently, they are not always seen.[17,54,97] In addition to convulsions, muscle fasciculations; collapse; weakness, particularly of the rear limb; ataxia; dullness; and disorientation occur. Muscle fasciculations were a frequently observed sign in one recent report.[17] The duration of signs varies from one day to three years prior to diagnosis.[54] Most have had signs for less than six months.[81] Signs are nearly always intermittent, and long periods of time may elapse between clinically evident episodes of hypoglycemia. Generally, signs become more frequent as the disease progresses. In general, a poor correlation exists between the time an animal is fed and the development of clinical signs.

Routine hematological and biochemical screens and urinalysis in animals with functional beta cell tumors are usually normal, except for blood glucose determinations. The first step in diagnosis involves confirming hypoglycemia. Hypoglycemia (blood glucose < 60 mg/dl) is a common finding in most patients, even without fasting.[54] Once hypoglycemia is established, it is important to confirm that the cause is excess insulin production. Multiple etiological possibilities exist for hypoglycemia (Table 176-8). Serum should be analyzed from any hypoglycemic sample for insulin concentrations. Although norms must be established for each individual laboratory, immuno-reactive serum insulin (IRI) concentrations are reported to range from 9.8 to 20 μU/ml.[16] Patients with insulinoma often have IRI values of over 54 μU/ml. In patients with normal IRI values but who also are hypoglycemic, several calculations comparing the ratio of insulin to glucose may be useful in supporting a diagnosis of insulinoma. The insulin/glucose, glucose/insulin, and amended insulin/glucose ratios (AIGR) are all useful in selected instances. It has been suggested that the AIGR may be more reliable than the other ratios for identifying an insulinoma.[54] Abnormal values for insulin/glucose are greater than 0.3, for glucose/insulin less than 2.5, and for AIGR greater than 30.[24] The AIGR is calculated as follows:

$$\text{AIGR } \mu\text{U/mg} = \frac{\text{Serum insulin } (\mu\text{U/ml}) \times 100}{\text{Plasma glucose (mg/dl)} - 30}$$

If hypoglycemia is not detected on random blood samples and insulinoma is still suspected, several provocative tests can be performed to stimulate the neoplastic islet cells to release insulin and induce hypoglycemia. These include "prolonged" fasting and repeated glucose determinations, intravenous and oral glucose tolerance tests, and L-leucine, glucagon, and tolbutamide tolerance tests. Most dogs with insulinomas can be made hypoglycemic by simple fasting.[38,54,97] The other provocative tests are expensive, time-consuming and unreliable and carry a high risk (tolbutamide tolerance) while not improving di-

TABLE 176–8. Differential Diagnosis for Hypoglycemia

Functional islet tumors (insulinomas)
Hepatic failure
   Acquired
   Congenital
Hypoadrenocorticism (Addison's disease)
Large extra pancreatic neoplasms
Hypopituitarism
Hypothyroidism
Sepsis
Iatrogenic (insulin overdosage)
Technical artifacts (sampling/lab errors)

agnostic accuracy. When fasting dogs to induce hypoglycemia, it is best to start the test in the morning so that they may be observed throughout the day. Blood glucose measurements are made every two to three hours until blood glucose concentrations drop below 60 mg/dl.[38] A serum IRI concentration is measured on the first hypoglycemic sample and an AIGR (I/G or G/I ratio) calculated. Most dogs with insulinomas become hypoglycemic within 8 hours, although rare cases may require 24 to 36 hours of fasting to induce hypoglycemia. Patients should be monitored closely throughout this fasting period, particularly if seizures are the primary presenting sign. Once hypoglycemia associated with hyperinsulinism is confirmed, exploratory surgery should be recommended. When serum insulin assays are not available, exploratory surgery should be considered if other known causes for hypoglycemia have been eliminated (See Table 176–8). Routine radiographs of the abdomen are of little value in supporting the diagnosis owing to the small size of these tumors and their location. Thoracic radiographs are also of little value when screening for metastases, as pulmonary metastases of these tumors are quite uncommon.

Preoperative, operative, and postoperative medical management is important for optimum success. Patients are maintained on multiple (3 to 6×/day) feedings of high-protein, low-carbohydrate diets until the evening prior to surgery. Once food is withheld, patients should be started on continuous 5% intravenous dextrose. During surgery, this may be increased to 10% dextrose, as intraoperative hypoglycemia, although rare, does occur.[38] Blood glucose concentrations should be monitored intra- and postoperatively. Dextrose administration is adjusted according to results obtained.

At surgery, the pancreas is gently but thoroughly palpated for evidence of tumor nodules. Most are easily visualized. Islet cell tumors generally range from 1 to 2.5 cm and are round and solitary.[52] Unfortunately, approximately 50 per cent have visible metastases to the regional lymph nodes or liver at surgery (Fig. 176–8).[52,54,97] Tumors are found in the left (splenic) or right (duodenal) limb of the pancreas with approximately equal frequency. Much less often, they are located in the body or angle of the pancreas, and rare, diffuse, nonpalpable tumors have been reported.[54] If no visible or palpable tumors are identified, it has been recommended that the left limb of the pancreas be removed, as it is the most difficult to examine thoroughly.[38]

Postoperatively, dogs with insulinomas may have a highly variable course. Known complications include pancreatitis, diabetes mellitus, acquired epilepsy, and diffuse polyneuropathy.[17,38] Pancreatitis is an infrequent complication in animals, unlike man. Patients should be held off food and water for 36 to 48 hours. Intravenous 5% dextrose is necessary only if evidence of continued postoperative hypoglycemia is detected. Otherwise, balanced fluid and electrolyte solutions and broad spectrum antibiotics are admin-

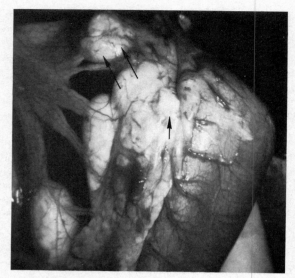

Figure 176–8. Insulinoma (small arrow) with metastasis to the regional lymph node (large arrows).

istered. The development of diabetes mellitus is a unique paradox of this tumor. It is hypothesized that prolonged increases in tumor insulin and subsequent hypoglycemia lead to atrophy of normal islet tissue. Transient diabetes has been reported in approximately 25 per cent of patients.[38] The duration of diabetes may be from a few days to six months. Diabetes may be severe enough to require insulin therapy. Gradual growth of metastases usually corrects the diabetes mellitus. Eventually, signs of hypoglycemia will recur. These patients need careful monitoring because signs of insulin overdosage and tumor recurrence are similar.

Rarer complications of insulinoma are acquired epilepsy and diffuse polyneuropathy.[17,38] Recurrent hypoglycemia was hypothesized to result in organic brain damage in one case of insulinoma. Adult onset seizures persisted despite return of blood glucose concentrations to normal.[17] Two cases of suspected hypoglycemic polyneuropathy have also been reported.[17,38] Neither animal regained normal neurological status despite correction of their hypoglycemic state.

The short-term prognosis for animals with functional islet cell tumors in the absence of visible metastases is good. However, the long-term prognosis is dismal. Surgical cures of insulinomas are not to be expected. When patients are monitored postoperatively for evidence of recurrent hypoglycemia, it invariably develops.[97] The longer the symptom-free duration, the more cause for optimism; however, ultimately the long-term prognosis is poor. Many dogs survive one year or more without signs of hypoglycemia.[16,17,38,54,97] Survival has been reported for one and one-half to two years, even when visible metastases were present at surgery.[17] Combinations of surgical and medical therapy have provided survival for over three and one-half years after diagnosis.[97]

Medical therapy should be reserved for patients with metastatic disease, animals with recurring signs postoperatively, and animals in which surgery is not possible. Medical therapy designed to modify signs of hypoglycemia includes frequent feedings, glucocorticoids, oral hyperglycemic agents, and anticancer drugs. Dietary recommendations include frequent (4 to $6\times$/day) feedings of a high-protein, low-carbohydrate diet. Such diets are thought to induce less stimulation of tumor insulin release. Prednisone or prednisolone may also reduce hypoglycemic attacks through its gluconeogenic effects. Initial dosages of 0.25 to 0.5 mg/kg/day in divided dosages may be used. Dosages should be increased gradually if signs do not abate or if they develop at a later time. The drug diazoxide* has been mentioned as efficacious in the symptomatic control of canine insulinoma for several years. Little published information substantiating these claims has appeared until recently.[37,76] Diazoxide is an oral nondiuretic benzothiadiazine derivative with hyperglycemic effects. Its pharmacological effects include increasing endogenous catecholamine release, inhibiting insulin release, augmenting hepatic glucose release, decreasing peripheral glucose utilization, and increasing free fatty acid mobilization.[38] Side effects include nausea and vomiting. Feeding prior to drug administration reduces gastrointestinal side effects. Diazoxide is available in 50- and 100-mg capsules or a suspension containing 50 mg/ml. Dosages used in the dog are from 10 to 40 mg/kg/day divided into three daily doses. One published report cites successful management of hypoglycemic episodes for 16 months using 15 mg/kg/day of diazoxide plus 5 mg prednisone once daily.[76] Slight increases in dosage were needed over this time interval. A second report indicated clinical success when diazoxide was used at 10 to 20 mg/kg/day for up to one year, at which time the tumor became nonsuppressible.[38]

Streptozotocin is a broad spectrum antibiotic with antineoplastic activity against islet cells. Two case reports on its use in metastatic canine insulinomas indicate that it is highly nephrotoxic in the dog.[66,67] Although the drug is used with some success in man, further investigation is necessary before it can be recommended for use in the dog.

Gastrinomas

Four reports concerning pancreatic islet cell tumors secreting gastrin have appeared.[31,42,51,98] Functional, non-beta islet cell pancreatic tumors have been documented for a number of years in man. This syndrome is characterized by excessive gastric acid production (hyperchlorhydria), peptic esophagitis, and gastric or duodenal ulceration. This complex of signs is produced by a gastrin-secreting tumor of pancreatic islets and is known as the Zollinger-Ellison syndrome. Six dogs have been documented to have

this syndrome. Many more are probably undiagnosed. Clinical signs include chronic vomiting, weight loss, voluminous diarrhea, and melena. Gastric mucosal hypertrophy, diffuse gastritis, and gastric or duodenal ulceration were present in each case. Fasting serum gastrin concentrations were determined in four animals and were found to be markedly increased in each dog. All six dogs had exploratory surgery or were necropsied. Small malignant islet cell tumors that had metastasized were found in every case. The prognosis is obviously poor with gastrinomas. Total gastrectomy is used in man to reduce the severity of clinical signs in cases with identified metastases. Cimetidine, an H_2 receptor antagonist, is also used in man to decrease gastrin-stimulated hydrochloric acid secretion by the stomach. Such therapy is reasonably successful. Cimetidine therapy was attempted in one of six canine cases with a questionable response.[31] Since gastric or duodenal ulcers are uncommon in dogs, except in association with mast cell sarcomas, the pancreas of dogs undergoing surgery for idiopathic upper intestinal ulcers should be carefully examined.

1. Alroy, J., Leav, I., Delellis, R., and Weinstein, R. S.: Distinctive intestinal mast cell neoplasms of domestic cats. Lab Invest. 33:159, 1975.
2. Anderson, N. V., and Johnson, K. H.: Pancreatic carcinoma in the dog. J. Am. Vet. Med. Assoc. 150:286, 1967.
3. Anlyan, W. G.: Carcinoid tumors and the carcinoid syndrome. In Sabiston, D. C. (ed.): Textbook of Surgery. W. B. Saunders, Philadelphia, 1977, pp. 1045–1049.
4. Bailey, W. S.: Spirocerca lupi: a continuing inquiry. J. Parasitol. 58:1, 1972.
5. Berg, P., Rhodes, W. H., and O'Brien, J. B.: Radiographic diagnosis of gastric adenocarcinoma in a dog. J. Am. Vet. Rad. Soc. 5:47, 1964.
6. Brewer, W. G., and Turrel, J. M.: Radiotherapy and hyperthermia treatment of fibrosarcomas in dogs. J. Am. Vet. Med. Assoc. 181:146, 1982.
7. Bridge, M. F., and Perzin, K. H.: Primary adenocarcinoma of the jejunum and ileum. A clinicopathologic study. Cancer 36:1876, 1975.
8. Brody, R. S.: Alimentary tract neoplasia in the cat: a clinicopathologic survey of 46 cases. Am. J. Vet. Res. 27:74, 1966.
9. Brody, R. S.: Biologic behavior of canine oral and pharyngeal neoplasms. J. Small Anim. Pract. 11:45, 1970
10. Brody, R. S.: Canine and feline neoplasia. Adv. Vet. Sci. Comp. Med. 14:309, 1970.
11. Brody, R. S., and Cohen, D.: An epizootiologic and clinicopathologic study of 95 cases of gastrointestinal neoplasm in the dog. Sci. Proc. 101st Ann. Mtg. Am. Vet. Med. Assoc. 1964, pp. 167–179.
12. Buhles, W. C., and Theilen, G. H.: Preliminary evaluation of bleomycin in feline and canine squamous cell carcinoma. Am. J. Vet. Res. 34:289, 1973.
13. Campbell, J. R., and Pirie, H. M.: Leiomyoma of the oesophagus in a dog. Vet. Rec. 77:624, 1965.
14. Carb, A., and Barrett, R. B.: Leiomyosarcoma of the cecum in the dog. J. Am. Anim. Hosp. Assoc. 14:631, 1978.
15. Carb, A. V., and Goodman, D. G.: Oesophageal carcinoma in the dog. J. Small Anim. Pract. 14:91, 1973.
16. Caywood, D. D., Wilson, J. W., Hardy, R. M., and Shull, R. M.: Pancreatic islet cell adenocarcinoma: clinical and diagnostic features of six cases. J. Am. Vet. Med. Assoc. 176:714, 1979.
17. Chrisman, C. L.: Postoperative results and complications of insulinomas in dogs. J. Am. Anim. Hosp. Assoc. 16:677, 1980.

* Proglycem, Schering Corp., Kenilworth, NJ.

18. Christie, G. S., and Jabara, A. G.: Two cases of malignant intestinal neoplasms in dogs. J. Comp. Pathol. 74:90, 1964.

19. Cline, M. J., and Haskell, C. M.: *Cancer Chemotherapy*, W. B. Saunders, Philadelphia, 1980.

20. Cohen, D., Brody, R. S., and Chen, S. M.: Epidemiologic aspects of oral and pharyngeal neoplasms of the dog. Am. J. Vet. Res. 25:1776, 1964.

21. Comis, R. L.: The therapy of stomach cancer. *In* Carter, S. K., Glatstein, E., and Livingston, R. B. (eds.): *Principles of Cancer Treatment*. McGraw-Hill, New York, 1982, pp. 420–425.

22. Conroy, J. D.: Multiple gastric adenomatous polyps in a dog. J. Comp. Pathol. 79:465, 1969.

23. Cotchin, E.: Neoplasms in cats. Proc. R. Soc. Med. 45:671, 1952.

24. Cotchin, E.: Further observations of neoplasms in dogs with particular reference to the site of origin and malignancy. Br. Vet. J. 110:218, 1954.

25. Cotchin, E.: Further examples of spontaneous neoplasms in the domestic cat. Br. Vet. J. 112:263, 1956.

26. Dorn, A. S., Anderson, N. V., Guffy, M. M., Cho, D. Y., and Leipold, H. W.: Gastric carcinoma in a dog. J. Small Anim. Pract. 17:109, 1976.

27. Dorn, C. R., and Priester, W. A.: Epidemiologic analysis of oral and pharyngeal cancer in dogs, cats, horses and cattle. J. Am. Vet. Med. Assoc. 167:1202, 1976.

28. Dorn, C. R., Taylor, D., Schneider, R., Hibbard, M. M., and Klauber, M. R.: Survey of animal neoplasms in Alameda and Contra Costa Counties, California. II. Cancer morbidity in dogs and cats from Alameda County. J. Natl. Cancer Inst. 40:307, 1968.

29. Douglas, S. W., Hall, L. W., and Walker, R. G.: The surgical relief of gastric lesions in the dogs: report of seven cases. Vet. Rec. 86:743, 1970.

30. Drake, J. C., and Hime, J. M.: Gastric carcinoma in the dog: two further cases. J. Small Anim. Pract. 6:131, 1965.

31. Drazner, F. F.: Canine gastrinoma: a condition analogous to the Zollinger-Ellison syndrome in man. Calif. Vet. 35:6, 1981.

32. Dubielzig, R. R.: Proliferative dental and gingival diseases of dog and cats. J. Am. Anim. Hosp. Assoc. 18:577, 1982.

33. Dubielzig, R. R., Goldschmidt, M. H., and Brody, R. S.: The nomenclature of periodontal epulides in dogs. Vet. Pathol. 16:209, 1979.

34. Evans, S. M., and De Frate, L. A.: Gastric lymphosarcoma in a dog: a case report. Am. Coll. Vet. Radiol. 21:55, 1980.

35. Fabry, A., Benjamin, S. A., and Angleton, G. M.: Nodular hyperplasia of the liver in the beagle dog. Vet. Pathol. 19:109, 1982.

36. Feeney, D. A., Klausner, J. S., and Johnston, G. R.: Chronic bowel obstruction caused by primary intestinal neoplasia: a report of five cases. J. Am. Anim. Hosp. Assoc. 18:67, 1982.

37. Feldman, E. C.: Hyperinsulinism in a dog. Mod. Vet. Pract. 60:995, 1979.

38. Feldman, E. C.: Diseases of the endocrine pancreas. *In* Ettinger, S. J. (ed.): *Textbook of Veterinary Internal Medicine, Diseases of the Dog and Cat*, Vol. 1, 2nd ed. W. B. Saunders, Philadelphia, 1983.

39. Fletcher, G. H.: Basic principles of the combination of irradiation and surgery. Radiation oncology. Biol. Phys. 5:2091, 1979.

40. Giles, R. C., Hildebrandt, P. K., and Montgomery, C. A.: Carcinoid tumors in the small intestine of a dog. Vet. Pathol. 11:340, 1974.

41. Gorlin, R. J., Barron, C. N., Chaudhry, A. P., and Clark, J. J.: The oral and pharyngeal pathology of domestic animals. A study of 487 cases. Am. J. Vet. Res. 20:1032, 1959.

42. Happe, R. P., Gaag, V. D., Lemers, C. B. H. W., Toorenburg, J. van, Rehfeld, J. F., and Larsson, L. I.: Zollinger-Ellison syndrome in three dogs. Vet. Pathol. 17:177, 1980.

43. Happe, R. P., Van Der Gaag, I., Wolvekamp, W., and Toorenburg, J. V.: Multiple polyps of the gastric mucosa in two dogs. J. Small Anim. Pract. 18:179, 1977.

44. Harvey, M. J.: Cryosurgery of oral tumors in dogs and cats. Vet. Clin. North Am. Small Anim. Pract. 10:821, 1980.

45. Hayden, D. W., and Nielsen, S. W.: Canine alimentary neoplasia. Zentralbl. Veterinaer Med.[A] 20:1, 1973.

46. Head, K. W., and Else, R. W.: Neoplasia and allied conditions of the canine and feline intestine. Vet. Ann. 21:190, 1981.

47. Hilmes, D. E., and Gillette, E. L.: Radiotherapy of spontaneous fibrous connective-tissue sarcomas in animals. J. Natl. Cancer Inst. 56:365, 1976.

48. Honjo, I., Suzuki, T., Ozawa, K., Takasan, H., Kitamura, O., and Ishikawa, T.: Ligation of a branch of the portal vein for carcinoma of the liver. Am. J. Surg. 30:296, 1975.

49. Howell, J.: Two cases of mucin-secreting carcinoma of the stomach of the dog. J. Comp. Pathol. 74:94, 1964.

50. Jeraj, K., Yano, B., Osborne, C. A., Wallace, L. J., and Stevens, J. B.: Primary hepatic osteosarcoma in a dog. J. Am. Vet. Med. Assoc. 179:1000, 1981.

51. Jones, B. R., Nicholls, M. R., and Badman, R.: Peptic ulceration in a dog associated with an islet cell carcinoma of the pancreas and an elevated plasma gastrin level. J. Small Anim. Pract. 17:593, 1976.

52. Kircher, D. H., and Nielsen, S. W.: Tumors of the pancreas. Bull. WHO 53:195, 1976.

53. Krook, L.: On gastrointestinal carcinoma in the dog. Acta Pathol. Microbiol. Scand. 38:43, 1956.

54. Kruth, S. A., Feldman, E. C., and Kennedy, P. C.: Insulin secreting islet cell tumors: establishing a diagnosis and the clinical course for 25 dogs. J. Am. Vet. Med. Assoc. 181:54, 1982.

55. Kurihara, M., et al.: A new method for producing adenocarcinomas in the stomach of dogs with N-ethyl-N-nitro-N-nitrosoguanidine. Gann 65:168, 1974.

56. Langham, R. F., Mostosky, U. V., and Schirmer, R. G.: X-ray therapy of selected odontogenic neoplasms in the dog. J. Am. Vet. Med. Assoc. 170:820, 1977.

57. Langham, R. F., Keahey, K. K., Mostosky, U. V., and Schirmer, R. G.: Oral adamatinomas in the dog. J. Am. Vet. Med. Assoc. 146:474, 1965.

58. Lawson, D. D., and Pirie, H. M.: Conditions of the canine oesophagus—II. Vascular rings, achalasia, tumors and perioesophageal lesions. J. Small Anim. Pract. 7:117, 1966.

59. Lingeman, C. H., and Garner, F. M.: Comparative study of intestinal adenocarcinomas of animals and man. J. Natl. Cancer Inst. 48:325, 1972.

60. Lingeman, C. H., Garner, F. M., and Taylor, D. D.: Spontaneous gastric adenocarcinomas of dogs: A review. J. Natl. Cancer Inst. 47:137, 1971.

61. Longmire, W. P.: Carcinoma of the stomach. *In* Sabiston, D. C.: *Textbook of Surgery*. W. B. Saunders, Philadelphia, 1977, pp. 983–993.

62. MacDonald, J., Schein, P., Veno, W., and Wooley, P.: 5-FU, mitomycin C and adriamycin: a new combination program for advanced gastrointestinal cancer. Pro. Am. Soc. Clin. Oncol. 176:264, 1976.

63. MacVean, D. W., Monlux, A. W., Anderson, P. S., Jr., Silberg, S. C., and Rozzel, J. F.: Frequency of canine and feline tumors in a defined population. Vet. Pathol. 15:700, 1978.

64. McCaw, D., Pratt, M., and Walshaw, R.: Squamous cell carcinoma of the esophagus in a dog. J. Am. Anim. Hosp. Assoc. 16:561, 1980.

65. McDonald, A.: Primary gastric carcinoma of the dog: review and case report. Vet. Surg. 7:70, 1978.

66. Meyer, D. J.: Pancreatic islet cell carcinoma in a dog treated with streptozotocin. Am. J. Vet. Res. 37:1221, 1976.

67. Meyer, D. J.: Temporary remission of hypoglycemia in a dog with an insulinoma after treatment with streptozotocin. Am. J. Vet. Res. 38:1201, 1977.

68. Miller, A. B.: Epidemiology of gastrointestinal cancer. *In*

Stroehlein, J. R., and Romsdale, M. M. (eds.): *Gastrointestinal Cancer*. Raven Press, New York, 1981, pp. 31–40.

69. Moertel, C. G.: Carcinoma of the stomach: prognostic factors and criteria of response to therapy. *In* Staquet, M. J. (ed.): *Cancer Therapy: Prognostic Factors and Criteria of Response*. Raven Press, New York, 1975, pp. 229–236.

70. Moulton, J. E.: Tumors of the alimentary tract. *In* Moulton, J. E. (ed.): *Tumors in Domestic Animals*, 2nd ed. Univ. of Calif. Press, Berkeley, 1978, pp. 240–272.

71. Moulton, J. E.: Tumors of the pancreas, liver, gall bladder and mesothelium. Univ. of Calif. Press, Berkeley, 1978.

72. Mulligan, R. M.: Neoplasms of the dog. Williams & Wilkins, Baltimore, 1949.

73. Murray, M., McKeating, F. J., and Baker, G. J.: Primary gastric neoplasia in the dog. Vet. Rec. *91*:474, 1972.

74. Nielsen, S. W., and Schroder, J. D.: Gastric carcinoma of dogs: report of three cases. North Am. Vet. *34*:640, 1953.

75. Palminteri, A.: The surgical management of polyps of the rectum and colon of the dog. J. Am. Vet. Med. Assoc. *148*:771, 1966.

76. Parker, A. J., O'Brien, D., and Musselman, E. E.: Diazoxide treatment of metastatic insulinoma in a dog. J. Am. Anim. Hosp. Assoc. *18*:315, 1982.

77. Patnaik, A. K., Hurvitz, A. I., and Johnson, G. F.: Canine gastrointestinal neoplasms. Vet. Pathol. *14*:547, 1977.

78. Patnaik, A. K., Hurvitz, A. I., and Johnson, G. F.: Canine gastric adenocarcinoma. Vet. Pathol. *15*:600, 1978.

79. Patnaik, A. K., Hurvitz, A. I., and Johnson, G. F.: Canine intestinal adenocarcinoma and carcinoid. Vet. Pathol. *17*:149, 1980.

80. Patnaik, A. K., Hurvitz, A. I., and Lieberman, P. H.: Canine hepatic neoplasms: a clinicopathologic study. Vet. Pathol. *17*:553, 1980.

81. Patnaik, A. K., Hurvitz, A. I., Lieberman, P. H., and Johnson, G. F.: Canine hepatocellular carcinoma. Vet. Pathol. *18*:427, 1981.

82. Patnaik, A. K., Hurvitz, A. I., Lieberman, P. H., and Johnson, G. F.: Canine bile duct carcinoma. Vet. Pathol. *18*:439, 1981.

83. Patnaik, A. K., Johnson, G. F., Green, R. W., Hayes, A. A., and MacEwen, E. G.: Surgical resection of intestinal adenocarcinoma, with survival of 28 months. J. Am. Vet. Med. Assoc. *178*:429, 1981.

84. Patnaik, A. K., Lieberman, P. H., Hurvitz, A. I., and Johnston, G. F.: Canine hepatic carcinoids. Vet. Pathol. *18*:445, 1981.

85. Patnaik, A. K., Liu, S. K., Hurvitz, A. I., and McClelland, A. J.: Nonhematopoietic neoplasms in cats. J. Natl. Cancer Inst. *54*:855, 1975.

86. Patnaik, A. K., Liu, S. K., and Johnson, G. F.: Feline intestinal adenocarcinoma. Vet. Pathol. *13*:1, 1976.

87. Pollock, S., and Wagner, B. M.: Gastric adenocarcinoma or linitis plastica in a dog. Vet. Med./Small Anim. Clin. *68*:139, 1973.

88. Priester, W. A.: Data from eleven United States and Canadian colleges of veterinary medicine on pancreatic carcinoma in domestic animals. Cancer Res. *34*:1372, 1974.

89. Reif, J. S., and Cohen, D.: The environmental distribution of canine respiratory tract neoplasms. Arch. Environ. Health *22*:136, 1971.

90. Ridgway, R. C., and Suter, P. F.: Clinical and radiographic signs in primary and metastatic esophageal neoplasms of the dog. J. Am. Vet. Med. Assoc. *174*:700, 1979.

91. Robbins, S. L.: The stomach. *In: Pathologic Basis of Disease*. W. B. Saunders, Philadelphia, 1974, pp. 911–929.

92. Sautter, J. M., and Hanlon, G. F.: Gastric neoplasia in the dog: a report of 20 cases. J. Am. Vet. Med. Assoc. *168*:691, 1976.

93. Schaffer, E., and Schiefer, B.: Incidence and types of canine rectal carcinomas. J. Small Anim. Pract. *9*:491, 1968.

94. Seiler, R. J.: Colorectal polyps of the dog: a clinicopathologic study of 17 cases. J. Am. Vet. Med. Assoc. *174*:72, 1979.

95. Silverman, S. G.: Carcinoma arising in adenomatous polyps. Dis. Col. Rect. *14*:191, 1971.

96. Smith, H. A., and Jones, T. C.: *Veterinary Pathology*. Lea & Febiger, Philadelphia, 1966, pp. 269–274.

97. Steinberg, H. S.: Insulin secreting pancreatic tumors in the dog. J. Am. Anim. Hosp. Assoc. *16*:695, 1980.

98. Strauss, E., Johnson, G. F., and Yalow, R. S.: Canine Zollinger-Ellison syndrome. Gastroenterology *72*:380, 1977.

99. Strombeck, D. R.: Clinicopathologic features of primary and metastatic neoplastic disease of the liver in dogs. J. Am. Vet. Med. Assoc. *173*:267, 1978.

100. Strombeck, D. R., Krum, S., Meyer, D., and Kappesser, R. M.: Hypoglycemia and hypoinsulinemia associated with hepatoma in a dog. J. Am. Vet. Med. Assoc. *169*:811, 1976.

101. Theilen, G. H., and Madewell, B. R.: Tumors of the digestive tract. *In* Theilen, G. H., and Madewell, B. R. (eds.): *Veterinary Cancer Medicine*. Lea & Febiger, Philadelphia, 1979.

102. Thrall, D. E.: Orthovoltage radiotherapy of oral fibrosarcomas in dogs. J. Am. Vet. Med. Assoc. *179*:159, 1981.

103. Thrall, D. E., Goldschmidt, M. H., and Biery, D. N.: Malignant tumor formation at the site of previously irradiated acanthomatous epulides in four dogs. J. Am. Vet. Med. Assoc. *178*:127, 1981.

104. Todoroff, R. J., and Brody, R. S.: Oral and pharyngeal neoplasia in the dog: a retrospective survey of 361 cases. J. Am. Vet. Med. Assoc. *175*:567, 1979.

105. Trigo, F. J., Thompson, H., Breeze, R. G., and Nash, A. S.: The pathology of liver tumors in the dog. J. Comp. Pathol. *92*:21, 1982.

106. Turk, M. A. M., Gallina, A. M., and Russell, T. S.: Nonhematopoietic gastrointestinal neoplasia in cats: a retrospective study of 44 cases. Vet. Pathol. *18*:614, 1981.

107. Vernon, F. F., and Roudebush, P.: Primary esophageal carcinoma in a cat. J. Am. Anim. Hosp. Assoc. *16*:547, 1982.

108. Werner, R. E.: Canine oral neoplasia: a review of 19 cases. J. Am. Anim. Hosp. Assoc. *17*:67, 1981.

109. World Health Organization: *Report of the Second Consultation on the Biological Behavior and Therapy of Tumors of Domestic Animals*. WHO, Geneva, 1978.

Chapter 177

Cardiovascular System

Phillip N. Ogburn

Cardiovascular tumors are now receiving more attention because they are more common than was generally recognized and because improved diagnostic and therapeutic techniques offer increasing chances for clinical improvement and recovery. Cardiovascular tumors may arise from or involve the heart, pericardium, or peripheral vessels. Most reports of cardiac tumors in small animals have dealt mainly with malignancies. Benign tumors are usually undetectable because the clinical features are generally not clinically recognized. Diagnoses of most cardiac tumors have been made at necropsy. Several factors make antemortem diagnosis a clinical challenge: (1) The incidence of cardiovascular tumors is low; (2) clinical signs are variable; and (3) clinical manifestations are nonspecific except with certain tumors like primary hemangiosarcoma of the heart. Recent developments in noninvasive and moderately invasive diagnostic techniques, cardiopulmonary bypass surgery, and chemotherapy have made antemortem diagnosis and treatment of cardiovascular neoplasia possible.

In humans, an antemortem diagnosis was first recorded in 1934,[3] and since that time the diagnosis of heart tumors has become almost routine.[24] There have been many clinical reports of cardiovascular neoplasia in small animals but no accounts of successful corrective surgery or treatment.

TUMORS OF THE HEART

Incidence

Primary tumors of the heart are uncommon. In humans, the reported prevalence of heart neoplasms is between 0.0017 and 0.28 per cent.[38] Epidemiological reports from canine populations suggest a similar rate of occurrence, although a comprehensive study is lacking. In one series of 309 necropsies of dogs with heart disease, only one had a primary cardiac neoplasm, hemangiosarcoma.[15] Two primary neoplasms of the heart were reported in 2,500 necropsied dogs in another series.[35] Of the primary tumors, hemangiosarcoma is the most common.[31,45,50] Several reports describe the occurrence of fibromas of the heart.[15,34,35] Two cardiac tumors, myxoma and rhabdomyoma, named as if they were neoplasms, are thought by Jubb and Kennedy to be developmental anomalies.[30]

Tumors of structures surrounding or adjacent to the heart that influence cardiac function are of considerable importance. Primary tumors of the pericardium, usually mesotheliomas,[28] occur rarely but can significantly affect cardiac activity. Chemodectomas arising from the aortic and carotid bodies are among the most common tumors that affect cardiovascular function. They are not actually derived from cardiac tissue and therefore are not true cardiac neoplasms. Aortic body tumors arise in such close proximity to the heart and in such a well-defined location that their presence is nearly synonymous with cardiac neoplasia. They have been commonly referred to as heart base tumors. Actually, tumors at the base of the heart are relatively common and may be derived from other tissues such as lymph and the thyroid and parathyroid glands.[10,30] Of the metastatic tumors of the heart, hemangiosarcoma, mammary and thyroid gland adenocarcinoma, and melanosarcoma are most common.[1,15,29,30,35,36,45,50,55]

Between January 1962 and June 1976, no primary cardiac tumors were seen in 4,933 necropsied cats.[33,42] Observations of similar cat populations have closely paralleled that data.[6,12,40,49,56] Individual cases of pericardial mesothelioma,[53] fibrosarcoma,[48] chemodectoma,[8] and 18 cases of hemangiosarcoma with metastatic cardiac involvement[42] have been diagnosed in recent reports.

The most common cardiac tumors in cats are metastatic lymphosarcoma, hemangiosarcoma, mammary gland adenocarcinoma, and pulmonary carcinoma.[52] Lymphosarcoma is the most common tumor, comprising one-third of all feline tumors.[21]

Clinical Presentation

Tumors involving the cardiovascular system may cause a broad array of systemic or cardiovascular signs (Table 177–1). Systemic signs such as lethargy, depression, anorexia, and weight loss are commonly

TABLE 177–1. Clinical Signs Associated with Cardiac Tumors

Cardiac	Congestive heart failure (left or right heart)
	Cardiac murmurs
	Muffled cardiac sound (pericardial effusion/tamponade)
	Arrhythmias (ectopic beats/atrioventricular block)
	Bundle branch blocks (intraventricular conduction abnormalities)
	Electrical alternans
Systemic	Fever
	Anorexia/cachexia
	Anemia
	Leukocytosis
	Syncope/seizures

encountered. Along with these general signs, a variety of hematological changes including anemia, thrombocytopenia, leukocytosis, and polycythemia are observed. Because clinical signs differ from animal to animal, it is usually inappropriate to rely on a particular pattern to indicate a specific disease. However, clinical signs produced by cardiovascular tumors are often related to their location within the heart. Therefore, it is usually more helpful to consider the findings typical of tumor location rather than factors that may suggest tumor type.

Myocardial Tumors. Tumors of the heart may cause disturbances in cardiac rhythm or conduction.[23] Tumors involving the right atrium or atrioventricular node can cause sinoatrial or atrioventricular conduction disturbances or ectopic atrial rhythms. Extensive myocardial involvement may give rise to a variety of arrhythmias including atrial fibrillation, paroxysmal atrial tachycardia, atrioventricular nodal rhythm, ventricular tachycardia, and ventricular fibrillation.

Intramural atrial or ventricular masses may cause hemodynamic dysfunction if the tumor is so large that it interferes with cardiac contraction. Impairment of ventricular performance by diffusely infiltrative or multiple disseminated neoplasms such as lymphosarcoma and hemangiosarcoma may simulate heart failure syndromes observed with idiopathic cardiomyopathy, pericarditis, and atrioventricular valve insufficiency.

Intraluminal Tumors. Symptoms associated with intracavity masses depend on the position and size of the tumor.[16,23,34,47,52] Right heart tumors may cause obstruction to right atrial and ventricular filling or to flow of blood to the lung. Prominent clinical features resulting from tumors in the right atrium or ventricle include peripheral edema, hepatomegaly, ascites, dyspnea, pleural effusions, and collapse or syncope.[34,52] Because of elevation in venous pressure, distension and pulsation of the jugular vein may be observed. Systolic murmurs or muffling of the heart sounds may be caused by heart valve dysfunction or fluid accumulation in the pericardial or pleural cavities.[16,48] Pulmonary embolism of tumor particles or from thrombus formation at the tumor site may be suspected in animals with a sudden onset of tachypnea, dyspnea, cyanosis, pale mucous membranes, weakness, collapse, or syncope.

Tumors in the left heart may result in obstruction of atrioventricular or aortic blood flow. Clinical signs produced by these tumors may parallel those of mitral valve disease and include weight loss, cough, dyspnea, paroxysmal nocturnal dyspnea, orthopnea, exertional cyanosis, fatigue, and collapse or syncope. The development of clinical signs may occur suddenly, especially if associated with arrhythmias. Physical examination may disclose heart murmurs or diastolic gallops secondary to valvular regurgitation and ventricular dilatation. In humans, left ventricular tumors may mimic the physical abnormalities found with aortic stenosis, hypertrophic subaortic stenosis,

endocardial fibroelastosis, and coronary artery disease.

Pericardial Tumors. The pericardium may become involved either as a primary site of tumor formation or as a site of metastatic disease. Necropsy observations in small animals have shown that the common neoplasms metastasizing to the heart (hemangiosarcoma, lymphosarcoma and melanoma) frequently involve the pericardium.

Neoplastic pericardial involvement can occur through local extension or via lymphatic or hematogenous spread.

Of the primary tumors that involve the pericardium, mesothelioma, chemodectoma, and sarcoma are common.

Neoplastic pericarditis may ultimately create cardiac dysfunction by compression of the heart or vessels as a consequence of effusion or restrictive changes in the pericardial membrane. Effusions may develop quite rapidly, producing acute cardiac tamponade. Effusions that are largely hemorrhagic are usually associated with sarcomas and may result from erosions on tumor surfaces or from vessel damage.[38]

Pericardial tumors are not usually detected until cardiac compression occurs. Pericardial involvement should be suspected in patients with malignant lesions at other sites. Animals with mammary tumors, lymphosarcoma, melanoma, or hemangiosarcoma that develop cardiac or respiratory-related symptoms should be evaluated for pericardial metastasis. Because the myocardium is often involved in animals with pericardial metastasis, clinical manifestations may result from alteration of both tissues.

Malignant Tumors

A variety of benign and malignant tumors may develop from the hearts of animals (Table 177–2). The incidence of each tumor type cannot be estimated with accuracy because most reported tumors are isolated cases. A high percentage of cardiac tumors exhibit malignant histological characteristics and invasive tendencies. The majority are sarcomas

TABLE 177–2.   Cardiovascular Tumors

Benign	Myxoma
	Fibroma
	Rhabdomyoma
Malignant	Hemangiosarcoma
	Chemodectoma
	Lymphosarcoma
	Mesothelioma
	Fibrosarcoma
	Melanosarcoma
Metastatic	Hemangiosarcoma
	Lymphosarcoma
	Carcinoma
	Sarcoma

that derive from mesenchyme and therefore may display a wide variety of morphological types. They may be classified as hemangiosarcomas, fibrosarcomas, lymphosarcomas, melanosarcomas, and rhabdomyosarcomas. The hemangiosarcoma is the most prevalent. Sarcomas are highly malignant, proliferate rapidly, and generally cause death through widespread involvement of the myocardium (Fig. 177–1), obstruction of blood flow, or metastatic infiltration of other organs.

Clinical signs of cardiac involvement are determined primarily by the location of the tumor and the extent of involvement. Signs include progressive and refractory congestive heart failure (particularly right-sided), pericardial and pleural effusion, arrhythmias, conduction disturbances, obstruction of the vena cava, and sudden death. If tumors involve the left heart, clinical signs may include pulmonary edema, moist rales, dyspnea, and possibly muffling of the heart sounds.[48] Tumors involving only the myocardium without cavity encroachment rarely induce congestive symptoms. If there is extension into the pericardial space, hemorrhagic pericardial effusion and tamponade may occur.

It is often difficult to differentiate benign from malignant tumors prior to surgery or biopsy, although certain characteristics may be helpful. Features suggestive of malignancy include the presence of acute clinical signs, metastatic disease in other organs, rapid growth of the tumor, hemorrhagic pericardial effusion, and local invasion to lymph nodes or other mediastinal structures. Benign tumors are more likely to produce slowly progressive signs of heart failure. The identification of tumor type may occasionally be made from examination of pericardial fluid obtained by pericardiocentesis.

Hemangiosarcomas. Hemangiosarcomas (angiosarcoma, hemangioendothelioma) are highly malignant tumors of endothelial cells and are more commonly found in dogs than cats.[50] There appears to be a predilection toward males in mid to later years.[31] Breeds more notably afflicted are German shepherds,[31] boxers, and Boston terriers.[46] In cats, cardiac

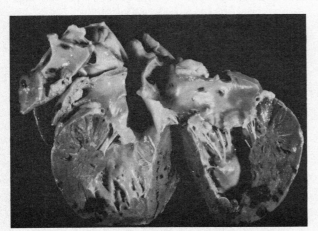

Figure 177–1. Metastases to the left atrium and ventricle from an oral melanosarcoma in a 14-year-old male golden retriever.

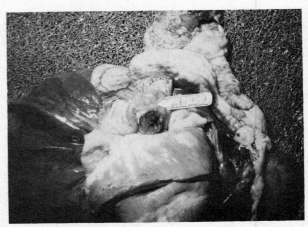

Figure 177–2. A circumscribed primary cardiac hemangiosarcoma, 2.0 cm in diameter, at the junction of the right auricle and atrial body in a nine-year-old male black Labrador retriever.

involvement occurs primarily through metastasis from peripheral tumors.[42] In dogs, a large percentage arise from the heart as primary tumors.[44,45,50] The right heart, specifically the right atrium, is often the site of primary involvement (Fig. 177–2). Hemangiosarcomas frequently originate from the skin in humans;[19] in dogs they occur more commonly from internal sites in the spleen and liver but may arise from any body site. Because the tumor has access to vascular channels, the right heart and lungs are often sites of secondary metastatic spread. The lung usually has diffuse involvement, with spherical nodules scattered throughout the lobes.

Affected animals may have a history of depression, lethargy, anorexia, labored breathing, abdominal fluid accumulation, weakness, collapse, syncope,[26] and central nervous system disorders.[1,31] Examination of affected dogs may reveal pale mucous membranes from anemia or poor perfusion (prolonged capillary refill time), tachycardia, weak femoral pulses, arrhythmias, muffling of cardiac and respiratory sounds, enlarged spleen and liver, ascites, and other general signs of heart failure.

Affected dogs are often anemic. In addition to increased numbers of circulating nucleated erythrocytes resulting from active hematopoiesis and hypoxemia, there may be reticulocytosis, basophilic stippling and leukocytosis with neutrophilia, and left shift.[31] Microangiopathic hemolytic anemia (characterized by moderate numbers of crenated erythrocytes, schistocytes, and poikilocytes), anisocytosis, and polychromasia are often encountered. These changes may result from damage to arteriolar epithelium or from fibrin deposition within vessels triggered by neoplastic cells or secondarily by disseminated intravascular coagulation.[37] Patients with hemangiosarcomas in which large amounts of blood are sequestered are predisposed to disseminated intravascular coagulation. With disseminated intravascular coagulation, the depletion of clotting factors and excessive fibrinolysis causes a paradoxical clotting inadequacy leading to bleeding.[32]

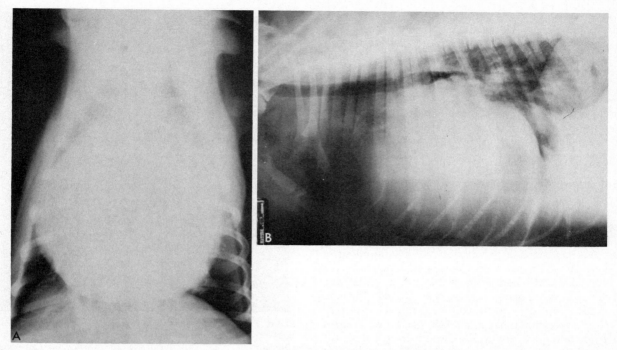

Figure 177–3. Dorsoventral *(A)* and lateral *(B)* thoracic radiographs show cardiomegaly with rounding of the silhouette typical of chronic pericardial fluid accumulation.

Cardiac involvement with hemangiosarcoma often results in effusion or hemorrhage into the pericardial sac. If fluid accumulates slowly there may be gradual distension of the sac, with rounding and enlargement of the cardiac silhouette (Fig. 177–3). Pulmonary congestion and edema accompanied by caudal vena cava enlargement and pleural effusion result as cardiac performance declines. With significant engorgement of the pericardium, the trachea may become dorsally displaced. If pulmonary metastasis occurs, two patterns of radiographic change may develop: (1) a diffuse disseminated interstitial thickening, or more commonly (2) a widely disseminated nodular pattern. Rarely does involvement of the hemangiosarcoma become appreciably nodular or involve the cardiac chambers to the extent that detection by contrast angiocardiography is helpful.

Hemangiosarcomas that originate from the heart are usually located in the right atrium, often at its juncture with the auricle. Myocardial lesions may alter conduction within the heart, giving rise to varying grades of sinoatrial, atrioventricular, or bundle branch block. Certain tumor sites cause local myocardial irritation, triggering arrhythmias such as atrial and ventricular premature beats, paroxysmal atrial and ventricular tachycardia, and atrial fibrillation. With pericardial fluid accumulation, the amplitude of the QRS complexes may become reduced[1] and electrical alternans of the QRS (alternating amplitude changes in the R wave) may occur.[5]

Pericardiocentesis, although of some risk, may occasionally allow the detection of neoplastic cells at cytological examination. The pericardial effusion, which is similar in appearance to venous blood, is distinguished from blood by its inability to clot and the absence of platelets. There is usually close proportionality of packed cell volume and erythroid-myeloid ratio to that in venous blood. Large amounts of fluid creating tamponade can be removed, aiding cardiac compensation. Detection of fluid and estimation of the quantity may be enhanced by echocardiography (Fig. 177–4). The presence of a poorly echogenic fluid between the epicardium and the fibrous pericardium with exaggerated ventricular wall motion is diagnostic of fluid within the pericardial sac.

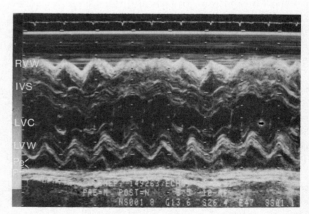

Figure 177–4. An echocardiogram from a dog with pericardial effusion *(Pe)*, which separates the pericardium *(P)* from the left ventricular posterior wall *(LVW)*. Other structures are the left ventricular chamber *(LVC)*, interventricular septum *(IVS)*, and right ventricular wall *(RVW)*.

Chemodectomas. Tumors arising from the non-chromaffin paraganglia of the aortic and carotid bodies, chemodectomas, were first described in dogs in 1936.[29] Although quite common in dogs,[10,30,54] they are rare in cats.[8,54] The majority occur in males 8 years of age and older.[10] Most arise from the aortic body, with ratios of 4.8:1 to 8:1 (aortic to carotid body) being reported.[25,54] Breeds with special predilection are the boxer, Boston terrier, collie, and German shepherd.[16,54] Since the preponderance of tumors occur in brachycephalic breeds, chronic hypoxia has been suggested as a potential cause.[25] Multicentric neoplastic transformation of chemoreceptor tissue occurs frequently in these breeds, as 65 per cent of carotid body tumors also have concurrent aortic body tumors.[14]

Chemodectomas are not secreting tumors. Therefore, clinical signs are related to the development of disease caused by local invasion of adjacent tissue or metastasis. Aortic body tumors may infiltrate the wall of the pulmonary artery and aorta and invade through the wall of the atria, pericardium, and myocardium.[43] Grossly, the tumor has a smooth surface and varies in color and consistency from reddish-brown, hard, and fleshy to gray-white and hard. Aortic body tumors usually grow slowly and may become large, up to 10 cm in diameter, and frequently involve the vagus and phrenic nerves. Clinical signs (e.g., dyspnea, cough, cyanosis, hepatomegaly, venous engorgement, ascites, and subcutaneous edema of the head, neck, and forelimbs) often develop because of serous to bloody pericardial effusion and subsequent cardiac tamponade. If chemodectomas do metastasize, the lung, liver, and bone may be involved.[30,39,41]

Carotid body tumors are more often malignant than are aortic body tumors, with metastasis in 30 per cent of cases evaluated.[14] Metastases to lung, bronchial and mediastinal lymph nodes, liver, pancreas, kidney, and bone have occurred.[17,30] Neoplasms of the carotid body are often rounded, red, and thinly encapsulated, surrounding the bifurcation of the common carotid artery. Carotid body tumors involve the mastoid process and the vagus (X), accessory (XI), and hypoglossal (XII) cranial nerves. Often the cranial sympathetic ganglion and trunk are included in the mass.[14] Pulsation of the mass may be observed in the neck.

Chemodectomas and ectopic thyroid and parathyroid tumors[30] tend to displace the great vessels, heart, and trachea if large. These are often visible as diffuse radiodense masses extending from the dorsal cardiac silhouette or heart base. Angiography may establish the location of these space-occupying masses (Fig. 177–5).[9,16]

Pericardial effusions are almost universally encountered in aortic body tumors and result in reduced amplitude of QRS complexes and often electrical alternans. Effusions are caused by villous proliferation of the pericardium and obstruction of lymph drainage.[10,30] An increase in heart rate secondary to restricted ventricular filling is commonly encoun-

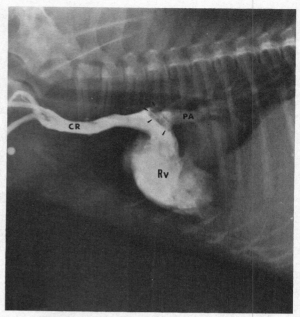

Figure 177–5. A nonselective angiogram shows impaired caudal right atrial filling caused by the presence of a large invasive chemodectoma. Arrows indicate the mass which caused a redirection of blood flow in the right atrium. Other structures include right ventricle *(Rv)*, cranial vena cava *(CR)*, and pulmonary artery *(PA)*.

tered. Echocardiograms may show evidence of pericardial and epicardial separation caused by the pericardial effusion.

The pericardial fluid obtained by pericardiocentesis is classified as a modified transudate and often has reactive mesothelial cell proliferation. It is rare to find neoplastic cells in the fluid, as the tumor does not commonly exfoliate.

Carotid and aortic body tumors are difficult to remove surgically because of local extension involving vessel walls, nerves, and myocardium. Carotid body tumors lend themselves to resection more than aortic body tumors, but the higher degree of malignancy with metastasis must be considered.

Lymphosarcomas. The most common tumor of the cardiovascular system in cats is metastatic lymphosarcoma. Indeed, one-third of all feline tumors are lymphosarcomas. Its cause, an oncogenic RNA virus (oncornavirus) of the family Retroviridae, was first established in 1967.[22] Lymphosarcomas that involve the heart may exhibit two forms or types of distribution. In the nodular form, the neoplasm appears smoothly nodular with masses as large as 5.1 cm (2 in.) in diameter.[30] They resemble fatty accumulations, although they are prone to central necrosis. The majority of foci are found in the right atrium. In the diffusely infiltrative form the myocardium appears irregularly thickened and gray-white, resembling myocardial degeneration and fibrosis (Fig. 177–6). The pericardium, cardiac chambers, and great vessels may be involved.

In cats, the anterior mediastinal form has the highest predilection for developing myocardial involve-

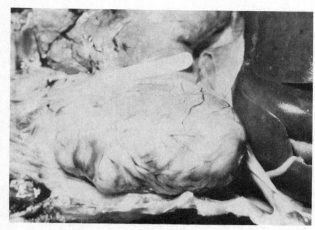

Figure 177–6. Lymphosarcoma with nodular infiltrative characteristics has disrupted the normal surface architecture of a cat's heart.

ment.[52] Involvement of the anterior mediastinum with spread to the heart commonly produces dyspnea, wheezing, coughing, and cyanosis. The anterior mediastinal mass may displace the heart caudally, may result in an incompressible anterior thorax, and may dampen the amplitude of cardiac and respiratory sounds. The electrocardiogram may indicate rhythm and conduction disorders, reduced P-QRS amplitudes, and ST-segment alteration.[52]

Thoracic radiographs may reveal an anterior mediastinal mass with caudal displacement of the heart, dorsal displacement or atelectasis of the cranial lung lobes, tracheal elevation, and frequently pleural effusion.[52]

The hemogram may be normal, but a nonregenerative anemia, lymphocytosis, and abnormal cells ranging from atypical lymphocytes to blast forms are found. Hypercalcemia, secondary to production of parathormone precursor by cancer cells, is occasionally encountered.[11]

The final diagnosis may be clarified by fine-needle biopsy of the mediastinal mass, cytological evaluation of the pleural effusion, or bone marrow examination for blast-transformed lymphocytes. Because cats with anterior mediastinal lymphosarcoma are usually infected with feline leukemia virus,[52] the diagnosis may be further verified by a fluorescent antibody test.[21,52]

Treatment of infected cats is usually not advised because of the infectious nature of the disease. However, treatment programs that have yielded some success include chemotherapy, radiation therapy, and immunotherapy. Surgery is usually not feasible.[13]

Mesothelioma. Mesotheliomas are rare mesodermal neoplasms that arise from the mesothelial cells and supporting tissue covering the pleural, pericardial, and peritoneal cavities. When they arise from the pericardium, they invade the parietal and visceral surface, giving the pericardium a shaggy appearance because of irregular flat to proliferative yellow-brown velvety plaques. Neoplasms may become nodular and invade adjacent fat, myocardium, local lymphatics, and lymph nodes.[28] In humans, metastatic involve-

ment of other organs occurs in 30 per cent to 50 per cent of the cases,[18] but reports on dogs[7,28] and cats[53] do not describe other organ involvement. Most mesotheliomas occur spontaneously and are sometimes found to be congenital in origin.[2,4,20] Asbestosis has been established as a cause of pleural mesothelioma in humans.[51]

There are certain physical features and several diagnostic tests that can be helpful in determining the presence of neoplastic pericardial involvement. Auscultation may reveal the muffling of heart sounds, the arterial pulse may be weak, and jugular vein distension with exaggerated pulsation may be observed. The QRS voltage may be reduced with pericardial fluid accumulation, and electrical alternans may be found. The ST segment may become slurred or deviated. Since pericardial fluid accumulation distends the pericardial sac, the radiographic silhouette of the heart becomes enlarged and rounded, and often pulmonary edema and pleural effusion accumulate. Angiographic evaluation is diagnostically helpful in cases suspected of having some degree of chamber or great vessel compression. In most cases in which pericardial involvement is suspected, pericardiocentesis should be performed not only to provide a cytological diagnosis but also to drain fluid from the sac to relieve the compressed heart. A positive cytological diagnosis is possible in many cases. Pneumopericardiography using carbon dioxide as a contrast agent is helpful in the delineation of pericardial or myocardial involvement in selected cases (Fig. 177–7). More recently, the use of echocardiography has enabled the precise detection of even small amounts of pericardial fluid. In addition to the estimation of effusion volume, this technique may be used to determine the thickness and motion of the epicardium and pericardium in diagnosing constrictive disease.

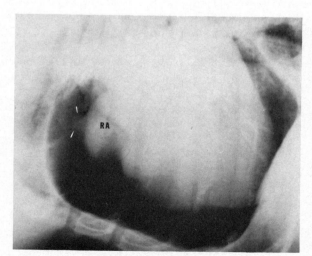

Figure 177–7. A pneumopericardiogram reveals the presence of an enlarged right auricle *(RA)* with nodular masses extending from its surface (arrows). A metastatic squamous cell carcinoma was identified in this eight-year-old female German short-haired pointer.

Treatment for neoplastic pericardial disease depends on the specific tumor involved. Generally, chemotherapy is reserved for those tumors considered most responsive, such as lymphosarcoma. Supportive maneuvers directed at improving cardiac performance are (1) pericardiocentesis with drainage of accumulated fluid and (2) surgical creation of a pericardial window, or pericardiectomy.[53] These forms of treatment combined with specifically directed chemotherapy or radiation therapy may provide added life span in selected cases. With surgical intervention, the clinician must weigh the potential benefit against the risks of high surgical mortality and likely dissemination of tumor cells into the pleural cavity.

Benign Tumors

Some tumors named as though they are neoplasms may actually be developmental anomalies. Myxomas may represent persistence of embryonic myxomatous tissue, of which the endocardial cushions are composed.[30] True myomatous neoplasms do occur in dogs but are exceedingly rare,[47] as are most benign cardiac neoplasms.

Fibromas. Fibromas are benign connective tissue tumors that are possibly congenital in origin.[38] They appear less frequently in the heart than elsewhere in the body. They are usually solitary lesions and may be quite large. If they are located outside the ventricular septum, the usual site of occurrence, they may be amenable to surgical excision (Fig. 177–8). Although fibromas are usually an incidental finding at necropsy, clinical signs associated with mechanical interference with intracardiac flow may occur. They appear to have a predilection for the right heart, and the clinical signs usually mimic tricuspid valve disease and right-sided congestive heart failure.[34]

Myxomas. The occurrence of myxomas in humans contrasts significantly with that observed in dogs. They comprise 30 to 50 per cent of primary tumors

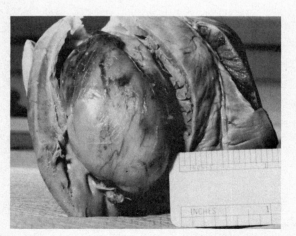

Figure 177–8. Intraluminal mass. A large 2.5 × 4.0 cm smooth-surfaced fibroma located in the right ventricular chamber arose from the moderator brand.

of the heart in humans, occurring most frequently in the left atrium. They are derived from mesenchymal cells of the subendocardial region and they form polypoid, pedunculated masses. They usually arise from the endocardium of the atrial septum and often extend through and sometimes partly occlude the atrioventricular opening.[38] Complete surgical excision along the base of the mass with a rim of unaffected endocardium and myocardium has been the treatment of choice.[38] In dogs they are exceedingly rare and are usually diagnosed at necropsy as an incidental finding.[30,47]

Rhabdomyomas. Rhabdomyomas are rare, benign, striated muscle tumors that sometimes occur in the heart.[27] They represent anomalous formation of myocardial fibers discernible as one or more discrete gray nodules, which may project into the ventricular lumen.[30]

Tumors Of The Peripheral Vessels

Hemangioma. Hemangioma is a benign tumor of endothelial cells that may be confused with vascular malformation, inflamed hematomas, and vascularized neoplasms. Hemangiomas occur mainly in older dogs (> 9 years) with pigmented skin (Scottish terriers, Airedales, Kerry blue terriers, and Labrador retrievers).[50]

The dark red to reddish-black tumors may develop in any location but are usually found in the subcutis or dermis of the leg, flank, neck, face, eyelid, or scrotum.[52] They are usually oval to discoid in shape, 0.5 to 3.0 (0.2 to 1.2 in.) in diameter, and are moderately firm in consistency. Histologically, hemangiomas consist of endothelium-lined spaces, which may contain blood, lymph, or thrombi.[50] If located in scrotal tissue or other sensitive exposed areas of the body, excessive bleeding may result from environmental trauma or self-mutilation. Fatal bleeding has been reported because of disruption of arterial channels supplying the lesion.[52] Tumor recurrence does not appear to be a problem after complete resection of the mass.

Hemangiosarcoma. Hemangiosarcoma is a malignant tumor of endothelial cells originating most frequently from vascular sites in the spleen,[50] liver,[46] heart,[31] bone,[45] muscle, lung, kidney, and skin.[44] The spleen is the most common site of origin in dogs.[30,50] One study of hemangiosarcoma in cats indicated primary involvement of the spleen in a majority of cases.[42] Dog breeds associated with a greater risk than the general population are German shepherds, Labrador retrievers, boxers, Boston terriers, and pointers.[31,44,46] This tumor is more commonly diagnosed in older adult males than in females.[31,46,50]

Hemangiosarcomas are usually nodular, poorly circumscribed, and soft in consistency and may vary in size from 1.0 mm to 20 cm (0.04 to 7.9 in.) or more in diameter. A characteristic physical feature of the tumor is often its hemorrhagic appearance, although its color may vary from mottled reddish-white to reddish-black depending on the degree of cellularity and amount of blood contained in the vascular spaces. In the spleen, it may closely resemble nodular hyperplasia or hematoma.[50] Hemangiosarcomas that occur in the skin are usually found as dark, soft subcutaneous nodules. Ulceration to the surface does occur but is not frequently observed.

Hemangiosarcomas may cause a variety of clinical signs, depending on the location of the primary and metastatic lesions. The differential diagnosis is thus based on history and clinical, radiographic, and laboratory findings. Dogs with primary splenic involvement often have abdominal pain or discomfort in the midventral abdomen. If the spleen is enlarged, the abdomen may appear distended. Splenic rupture is painful and results in blood loss into the abdomen, producing abdominal distension, discomfort, and often a sudden onset of weakness due to blood loss. Signs of hypovolemic shock (collapse, white mucous membranes, tachycardia, weak femoral pulsation, and dyspnea) may occur with major hemorrhage. The character of respiration may become abnormal because of pulmonary metastasis, splenic and hepatic enlargement, blood loss, or because hemothorax restricts ventilatory capacity. Patients with renal hemangiosarcoma may exhibit hematuria and lumbar pain without evident dysuria. Tumor involvement of bone may produce pain in the affected area, lameness, and radiographic evidence of bone lysis.

Hemangiosarcomas are highly malignant neoplasms that metastasize early in the course of their development, often to multiple sites. Complications with blood-loss anemia, disseminated intravascular coagulation, and organ dysfunction as a result of metastatic involvement are often encountered and influence the approach to treatment. Chemotherapy and radiation therapy have not proved to be of major benefit in the treatment of hemangiosarcoma in dogs or cats. Surgical removal of a neoplastic organ or resection of the evident primary mass may be curative in only a small percentage of cases. More commonly, metastatic disease not identified at the time of initial surgery will become a problem within a few weeks to months. The prognosis is justifiably poor.

1. Allan, G.: Hemangioendothelioma in the dog. Aust. Vet. Pract. 10:21, 1980.
2. Andrews, E. J.: Pleural mesothelioma in a cat. J. Comp. Pathol. 83:259, 1973.
3. Barnes, A. R., Beaver, D. C., and Snell, A. M.: Primary sarcoma of the heart: Report of a case with electrocardiographic and pathological studies. Am. Heart J. 9:480, 1934.
4. Baskerwille, A.: Mesothelioma in the calf. Vet. Pathol. 4:149, 1967.
5. Bonagura, J.: Electrical alternans associated with pericardial effusion in the dog. J. Am. Vet. Med. Assoc. 178:574, 1981.
6. Brodey, R. S.: Canine and feline neoplasia. Adv. Vet. Sci. Comp. Med. 14:309, 1970.
7. Brunner, P.: Papillary polypous mesothelioma of the pericardium of a dog. Virchows Arch. (Pathol. Anat.) 357:257, 1972.
8. Buergelt, C. D., and Das, K. M.: Aortic body tumor in a cat: A case report. Vet. Pathol. 5:84, 1968.
9. Cantwell, H. D., Blevins, W. E., and Weirich, W. E.: Angiographic diagnosis of heartbase tumor in the dog. J. Am. Anim. Hosp. Assoc. 18:83, 1982.
10. Capen, C. C.: Tumors of the endocrine glands. In Mouton, J. E.: Tumors in Domestic Animals. 2nd ed., University of California Press, Berkeley, 1978, p. 372.
11. Chew, D. J., Schaer, M., Liu, S.-K., et al.: Pseudohyperparathyroidism in a cat. J. Am. Anim. Hosp. Assoc. 11:46, 1975.
12. Cotchin, E.: Neoplasia in the cat. Vet. Rec. 69:425, 1957.
13. Cotter, S. M.: Feline leukemia virus-associated diseases. In Kirk, R. W. (ed.): Current Veterinary Therapy VI. W. B. Saunders, Philadelphia, 1977. p. 455.
14. Dean, M. J., and Strafuss, A. C.: Carotid body tumors in the dog: A review and report of four cases. J. Am. Vet. Med. Assoc. 166:1003, 1975.
15. Detweiler, D. K.: Wesen und Haufigkeit von Herzkrankheiten bei Hunden. Zentralbl Veterinarmed 9:317, 1962.
16. Edwards, D. F., Bahr, R. J., Suter, P. F., et al.: Portal hypertension secondary to a right atrial tumor in a dog. J. Am. Vet. Med. Assoc. 173:750, 1978.
17. Feher, R. C., and Roullard, P. L.: Aortic body tumor with rare metastasis to the lung in a dog. Vet. Med./Small Anim. Clin. 72:1018, 1977.
18. Fine, G.: Primary tumors of the pericardium and heart. Clin. Cardiol. 5:207, 1973.
19. Glancy, D. L.: Angiosarcoma of the heart. Am. J. Cardiol. 21:413, 1968.
20. Grant, C. A.: Congenital tumors of calves. Report of 2 cases of mesothelioma and a tumor apparently of reticuloendothelial origin. Zentralbl Veterinarmed 5:231, 1958.
21. Hardy, W. D.: Hematopoietic tumors of cats. J. Am. Anim. Hosp. Assoc. 17:921, 1981.
22. Hardy, W. D., and McClelland, A. J.: Feline leukemia virus: Its related diseases and control. Vet. Clin. North Am. 7:93, 1977.
23. Harvey, W.: Clinical aspects of cardiac tumors. Am. J. Cardiol., 21:328, 1968.
24. Hattler, B. G., and Sabiston, D. C.: Tumors of the heart. In Sabiston, D. C., and Spencer, F. C. (eds.): Gibbon's Surgery of the Chest. 3rd ed. W. B. Saunders, Philadelphia, 1976.
25. Hayes, H. M., Jr.: An hypothesis for the aetiology of canine chemoreceptor system neoplasia, based on an epidemiological study of 73 cases among hospital patients. J. Small Anim. Pract. 16:337, 1975.
26. Holmes, J. R., and Welson, M. R.: Cardiac syncope in a dog associated with a hemangiosarcoma. Vet. Rec. 82:474, 1968.
27. Hulland, T. J.: Tumors of muscle. In Moulton, J. E. (ed.): Tumors in Domestic Animals. 2nd ed. University of California Press, Berkeley, 1978. p. 75.
28. Ikede, B. O., Zubaidy, A., and Gill, C. N.: Pericardial mesothelioma with cardiac tamponade in a dog. Vet. Pathol. 17:496, 1980.
29. Jackson, C.: The incidence and pathology of tumors of domesticated animals in South Africa: A study of the Onderstepoort collection of neoplasms with special reference to their histopathology. J. Vet. Sci. Anim. Ind. 6:1, 1936.
30. Jubb, K. V. F., and Kennedy, P. C.: The circulatory system: Neoplasms of the heart. In: Pathology of Domestic Animals. 2nd ed. Academic Press, New York, 1970.
31. Kleine, L. J., Zook, B. C., and Munson, T. D.: Primary cardiac hemangiosarcoma in dogs. J. Am. Vet. Med. Assoc. 157:326, 1970.
32. Legendre, A. M., and Krehbiel, J. D.: Disseminated intravascular coagulation in a dog with hemothorax and hemangiosarcoma. J. Am. Vet. Med. Assoc. 171:1070, 1977.
33. Liu, S. -K.: Pathology of feline heart diseases. Vet. Clin. North Am. 7:323, 1977.
34. Lombard, C. W., and Goldschmidt, M. H.: Primary fibroma in the right atrium of a dog. J. Small Anim. Pract. 21:439, 1980.
35. Loppnow, H., von: Zur Kasuistik primarer Herztumoren beim Hund (2 Falle von Haemangiomen am Rechten Herzohr) Berl. Munch. Tierarztl. Wschr. 74:214, 1961.

36. Luginbuhl, H., and Detweiler, D. K.: Cardiovascular lesions in dogs. Ann. N. Y. Acad. Sci. 127:517, 1965.
37. Madewell, B. R., and Feldman, B. F.: Characterization of anemias associated with neoplasia in small animals. J. Am. Vet. Med. Assoc. 176:419, 1980.
38. McAllister, H. A., Jr.: Primary tumors of the heart and pericardium. In: Sommers, S. C., and Rosen, P. P. (eds.): Pathology Annual: 1979. Part 2. Appleton-Century-Crofts, N. Y., 1979, p. 325.
39. Montgomery, D. L., Bendele, R., and Storts, R. W.: Malignant aortic body tumor with metastasis to bone in a dog. Vet. Pathol. 17:241, 1980.
40. Mulligan, R. M.: Spontaneous cat tumors. Cancer Res. 11:271, 1951.
41. Nilsson, T.: Heart-base tumors in dogs. Acta Pathol. Microbiol. Scand. 37:385, 1955.
42. Patnaik, A. J., and Liu, S. -K.: Angiosarcomas in cats. J. Small Anim. Pract. 18:191, 1977.
43. Patnaik, A. K., Liu, S. -K., Hurvitz, A. I., and McCelland, A. J.: Canine chemodectoma (extra adrenal paragangliomas) a comparative study. J. Small Anim. Pract. 16:785, 1975.
44. Pearson, G. R., and Head, K. W.: Malignant haemangioendothelioma (angiosarcoma) in the dog. J. Small Anim. Pract. 17:737, 1976.
45. Pirie, H. M.: The pathology of heart diseases in the dog. J. Small Anim. Pract. 8:195, 1967.
46. Priester, W. A.: Hepatic angiosarcomas in dogs: An excessive frequency as compared with man. J. Natl. Cancer Inst. 57:451, 1976.
47. Roberts, S. R.: Myxoma of the heart in a dog. J. Am. Vet. Med. Assoc. 134:185, 1959.
48. Ryan, C. P., and Walder, E. J.: Feline fibrosarcoma of the heart. Calif. Vet. 8:12, 1980.
49. Schmidt, R. E., and Langham, R. F.: Survey of feline neoplasms. J. Am. Vet. Med. Assoc. 151:1325, 1967.
50. Stannard, A. A., and Pulley, L. T.: Tumors of the skin and soft tissues. In Moulton, J. E. (ed.): Tumors in Domestic Animals. 2nd ed. University of California Press, Berkeley, 1978, p. 16.
51. Stanton, M. F., and Wrench, C.: Mechanisms of mesothelioma induction with asbestos and fibrous glass. J. Natl. Cancer Inst. 48:797, 1972.
52. Thornburg, L. P., and Breitschwerdt, E. B.: Canine hemangioma of the scrotum with fatal bleeding: A case report. J. Am. Anim. Hosp. Assoc. 12:797, 1976.
53. Tilley, L. R., Bond, B., Patnaik, A. K., Liu, S. -K.: Cardiovascular tumors in the cat. J. Am. Anim. Hosp. Assoc. 17:1009, 1981.
54. Tilley, L. R., Ownes, J. M., Wilkins, R. J., and Patnaik, A. K.: Pericardial mesothelioma with effusions in a cat. J. Am. Anim. Hosp. Assoc. 11:60, 1975.
55. Yates, W. D. G., Lester, S. J., and Mills, J. H. L.: Chemoreceptor tumors diagnosed at the Western College of Veterinary Medicine. 1967–1979. Can. Vet. J. 21:124, 1980.
56. Zook, B. C.: Some spontaneous cardiovascular lesions in dogs and cats. Adv. Cardiol. 13:148, 1974.

Chapter **178** # Hematopoietic System

A. P. Davies, J. S. Klausner, and C. B. Grindem

Hematopoiesis in normal adult animals occurs in the bone marrow and results in the proliferation, differentiation, and release of erythrocytes, granulocytes, monocytes, and platelets into the peripheral circulation. Lymphocytes originate in the bone marrow, but proliferation primarily occurs within the major lymphoid organs.[32,71,111,215] Extramedullary hematopoiesis may occur in multiple organs but is most common in the liver, spleen, and lymph nodes.[111,177]

Experimental evidence strongly supports the concept of a pluripotential stem cell that gives rise to committed stem cells for the lymphoid, erythroid, megakaryocytic, and granulocytic/monocytic series.[158] Under the influence of specific humoral inducers (erythropoietin, granulopoietin, thrombopoietin) and the bone marrow microenvironment, committed stem cells undergo proliferation, differentiation, and maturation.[32,158] In-depth discussion of the factors influencing normal hematopoiesis can be found in recent reviews.[158,215]

Primary hematopoietic neoplasia results from alterations in proliferation, differentiation, or maturation of pluripotent or unipotent stem cells.[32,158] Abnormalities in lymphocytic (both B- and T-cell) and plasma cell development result in lymphoproliferative malignancy. Abnormalities in the erythrocytic, granulocytic, monocytic, megakaryocytic, fibroblast, or osteocyte cells lines result in myeloid neoplasia.

Primary hematopoietic neoplasia is the most common neoplasm in cats, accounting for approximately 35 per cent of all feline cancers.[42,131,156] In dogs, primary hematopoietic neoplasia ranks in frequency behind skin, mammary gland, and digestive tract tumors and accounts for approximately 8 to 10 per cent of all canine neoplasms.[42,131,156]

LYMPHOPROLIFERATIVE DISORDERS

Canine Lymphosarcoma

Lymphosarcoma is the most frequently identified canine hemopoietic neoplasm. The annual reported incidence is approximately 24 to 29 per 100,000 dogs.[41,131] Middle-aged and older dogs are usually affected, with the peak incidence occurring in dogs 5 to 11 years of age.[105] Male and female dogs are affected at approximately the same rate, although a decreased risk in intact females has been noted.[157] Breeds with an increased risk of developing lymphosarcoma include boxers, basset hounds, Saint Bernards, Scottish terriers, Airedale terriers, Labrador retrievers, and bulldogs.[157] Mixed-breed dogs, Pekingese, minature poodles, Chihuahuas, Brittany spaniels, dachshunds, and Pomeranians have a decreased risk.[157]

The cause of canine lymphosarcoma is unknown. Although virus-like particles have been observed in canine lymphosarcoma cells,[22,204] evidence of naturally occurring transmission is lacking. Experimentally, the disease can be induced in neonatal dogs by inoculation with lymphoma cells.[25]

Clinical Findings and Classification

Clinical manifestations of lymphosarcoma are variable, depending primarily on the anatomical location and extent of disease and the presence of paraneoplastic disorders such as hypercalcemia. Five anatomical types have been described (Table 178–1). The multicentric type is identified most frequently.[11,92,198]

Multicentric Lymphosarcoma. Generalized, nonpainful enlargement of lymph nodes characterizes multicentric lymphosarcoma. In addition, tonsilar enlargement, hepatomegaly, splenomegaly, and variable infiltration of other organs including the kidneys, lungs, bone marrow, and heart may occur.[4] At the onset, lymphadenopathy may be the only clinical manifestation. Later, visceral infiltration and organ dysfunction result in a variety of systemic signs including anorexia, fever, weakness, cough, dyspnea, vomiting, diarrhea, and ascites. Obstruction to lymphatics may result in extensive regional edema.

Alimentary Lymphosarcoma. Diffuse or focal involvement of the gastrointestinal tract and mesenteric lymph node enlargement characterize alimentary lymphosarcoma. Gastric lymphosarcoma results in nodular or diffusely infiltrative lesions accompanied by vomiting and weight loss.[51] Lesions associated with intestinal lymphosarcoma may be nodular, annular, or diffusely infiltrative. Malabsorption and intestinal obstruction result in diarrhea, vomiting, and weight loss. An abdominal mass is often palpable.

Thymic Lymphosarcoma. Thymic lymphosarcoma is characterized by an anterior mediastinal mass and pleural effusion resulting in cough and dyspnea. Peribronchial lymph nodes may be enlarged. Dysphagia or regurgitation results if the thoracic esophagus is compressed.

Cutaneous Lymphosarcoma. Cutaneous lymphosarcoma is reported in approximately 6 per cent of cases. Two types of primary skin involvement have

been noted: primary cutaneous lymphosarcoma and mycosis fungoides.[45,98,136,141,185,221] Primary cutaneous lymphosarcoma results in solitary or multiple intradermal nodules, tumors, or plaques, usually on the trunk or upper extremities.[27] Histologically, tumor cells are distributed in the dermis or subcutis. Neoplastic lymphocytes are usually poorly differentiated or histocytic types.[15]

Mycosis fungoides, a T-cell lymphoma, is distinguished from primary cutaneous lymphosarcoma by its protracted clinical course (often months to years) and involvement of the epidermis. Early skin lesions include erythema, scaling, and alopecia.[136] Later, the disease is characterized by the presence of multiple, firm, plaque-like ulcerated tumors.

Cutaneous lymphosarcoma may be localized to the skin, or systemic involvement may occur. In a report of 22 dogs with cutaneous lymphosarcoma, 13 had generalized disease.[15] Lymphadenopathy was the most frequent noncutaneous manifestation. Clinically, cutaneous lymphosarcoma must be differentiated from histiocytoma, mast cell tumor, and transmissible venereal tumor.[185]

Miscellaneous Classification. The miscellaneous classification includes dogs with a variety of clinical manifestations. Lymphosarcoma can originate in any lymphoreticular tissue, remain localized, or disseminate throughout the body. Central nervous system involvement results in spinal cord compression, peripheral nerve damage, or signs of cranial disease.[165] Ocular manifestations include uveitis, glaucoma, exudative retinal detachment, and papillitis.[197] Nasal involvement results in chronic nasal discharge and sneezing.

Hypercalcemia

Ten to 40 per cent of dogs with lymphosarcoma are hypercalcemic (Ca $>$ 11.0 mg/100 ml).[126,148] Hypercalcemia is most often identified in dogs with thymic lymphosarcoma.[126] Clinical manifestations of hypercalcemia frequently overshadow other signs of the neoplasm.

Polyuria and compensatory polydipsia result because of hypercalcemic impairment of renal concentrating mechanisms.[10] Hypercalcemia also induces decreases in renal blood flow and glomerular filtration rate, resulting in azotemia or uremia. Depression, anorexia, and vomiting result from the adverse effects of elevated calcium on the gastrointestinal tract, the nervous system, and renal function.

Prolonged hypercalcemia results in microscopic changes in the kidneys characterized by varying degrees of calcification, degeneration, necrosis, and sloughing of tubular epithelium.[150] Lesions are eventually distributed throughout the renal parenchyma. Reversibility depends on the number of nephrons that are damaged and the extent of the damage.

The pathogenesis of hypercalcemia in lymphosarcoma is incompletely understood.[186] Local bone destruction resulting from tumor infiltration or release

**TABLE 178–1.   Frequency of Types of
Canine Lymphosarcoma**

Anatomical Type	Percentage of Total Cases
Multicentric	84.0
Alimentary	6.9
Cutaneous	6.3
Mediastinal	2.2
Miscellaneous	0.6

of local mediators may increase calcium mobilization from bone. Tumor cells may secrete a substance similar to parathyroid hormone, prostaglandins, an osteoclast activating factor, or other bone-resorbing factor.[83,218]

Diagnosis

In dogs with enlarged peripheral lymph nodes, the diagnosis of lymphosarcoma is made by cytological or histopathological evaluation of lymph nodes. In dogs without peripheral lymphadenopathy, the diagnosis can only be established by initial localization of the disease followed by thorough evaluation of laboratory, radiographic, and biopsy data.

Hematological Findings. Total white blood cell and lymphocyte counts are normal in 80 per cent of dogs with lymphosarcoma.[181] In approximately 50 per cent of dogs, low numbers of lymphoblasts or prolymphocytes are noted in peripheral blood smears.[198] Infrequently, leukemia associated with white blood cell counts in excess of 100,000/μl and immature lymphocytosis are noted.

Normocytic normochromic anemia is present in approximately 30 per cent of animals.[198] Anemia results from replacement of marrow by neoplastic lymphocytes, immune-mediated destruction of red blood cells, shortened red blood cell life span, or blood loss.[198] In one report, 34 per cent of dogs with lymphoid neoplasia were Coombs' positive.[190]

Leukemic dogs are most likely to be thrombocytopenic. Platelet counts are decreased in 20 to 50 per cent of cases, although counts low enough to cause bleeding are unusual.[36,181]

Bone marrow examination reveals increased numbers of immature lymphocytes in approximately 20 per cent of dogs with lymphosarcoma. Rarely, total replacement of normal marrow by neoplastic cells is noted. Occasionally, bone marrow involvement occurs without evidence of neoplastic cells in peripheral blood.

Biochemical Findings. Abnormalities in serum parameters are frequent in dogs with extensive hepatic or renal infiltration and in hypercalcemic dogs. Elevation in serum concentrations of alkaline phosphatase, alanine aminotransferase (SGPT), and bilirubin are noted in most dogs with hepatic lymphosarcoma.[154,195] Elevations in serum urea nitrogen and creatinine concentrations occur in hypercalcemic dogs, in dogs with extensive neoplastic infiltration of both kidneys, and in dehydrated dogs.

Radiographic Findings. Radiography is useful in the detection of occult lymphosarcoma and in determining the extent of disease. Changes identified in thoracic radiographs include sternal and tracheobronchial lymph node enlargement, widening of the anterior mediastinum, pleural effusion, and pulmonary densities. Abdominal radiographs may reveal hepatomegaly, splenomegaly, sublumbar or mesenteric lymph node enlargement, renal enlargement, ileus, and ascites.

Cytological and Histopathological Findings. Cytological evaluation of body fluids and lymph node aspirates frequently is useful in establishing a diagnosis of lymphosarcoma. Increased numbers of lymphocytes or immature lymphocytes may be identified in pleural fluid, ascitic fluid, cerebrospinal fluid, aqueous humor, and pulmonary aspirates. Lymph node aspiration usually reveals large numbers of a monomorphic population of lymphoblasts. Lymphoblasts are large cells with intensely basophilic cytoplasms and a hyperchromatophilic nucleus. One or more nucleoli are usually present. If the results of lymph node aspiration are equivocal, removal and histological examination of an entire lymph node may be necessary to establish a diagnosis. Tissue for histopathological examination can be obtained by either surgical or needle biopsy techniques.[216] Lymph node removal is usually preferable to needle biopsy of the node.

Canine lymphosarcomas have been classified by architectural and cytological characteristics into diffuse or nodular, well-differentiated or poorly differentiated, lymphocytic and histiocytic types.[92,193,209] In the diffuse type, lymph node architecture is completely effaced by neoplastic lymphocytes. Lymphoid nodules predominate in the nodular type. Most canine lymphosarcomas are either diffuse, poorly differentiated lymphocytic or diffuse histiocytic.[92,193,209] In humans, diffuse lymphosarcomas have an unfavorable prognosis.[26] Studies of canine lymphosarcoma patients have not established that histological type affects prognosis.[92,209]

Lymphosarcomas can also be classified by their origin from B- or T-lymphocytes.[2,29] Most multicentric canine lymphosarcomas are derived from B cells, whereas thymic and cutaneous lymphosarcomas are probably derived from T cells.[132,147] In humans, immunological classification of lymphosarcomas and other lymphoproliferative diseases has been useful in predicting response to therapy.[2,29]

Treatment

Therapeutic objectives in lymphosarcoma patients are to produce clinical remission, increase survival time, and improve the animals' well-being. With presently used chemotherapeutic protocols and good supportive care, these goals are often achieved. Mean survival time in untreated dogs is usually less than 2 months, compared with a mean survival time of approximately 7 to 8 months in dogs treated with combination chemotherapy.[116]

Pretreatment Considerations. Before beginning therapy, it is essential to determine the extent of disease and the functional capacity of major body systems and to identify and treat associated metabolic disorders such as hypercalcemia. Classifying dogs according to the World Health Organization (WHO) clinical staging system (Table 178–2) is useful for defining the extent of involvement, formulating a prognosis, and monitoring the response to therapy.

TABLE 178–2.   WHO Clinical Staging for Canine Lymphosarcoma*†

Stage I:	Involvement limited to a single lymph node or lymphoid tissue in a single organ (excluding bone marrow)
Stage II:	Involvement of many lymph nodes in a regional area (± tonsils)
Stage III:	Generalized lymph node involvement
Stage IV:	Liver and/or spleen involvement (± stage III)
Stage V:	Manifestation in the blood and involvement of bone marrow and/or other organ systems (± stages I–IV)

*Reprinted with permission from the internal report of a WHO report of a consultation on the biological behavior and therapy of tumors of domestic animals. WHO, Geneva, 1978 (unpublished WHO document VPH/CMO/78.15).

†Each stage is subclassified as follows: a, without systemic signs; and b, with systemic signs.

Diagnostic tests required to adequately stage canine lymphosarcoma include a complete blood count, platelet count, serum chemistry profile, urinalysis, bone marrow aspiration, and radiographic examination of the chest and abdomen.

Evaluation of kidney and liver function prior to therapy aids selection of chemotherapeutic agents. If hypercalcemia is identified, treatment with parenteral fluids and diuretics should be instituted. Intravenous 0.9 per cent sodium chloride and furosemide (1 to 2 mg/kg) results in rapid lowering of serum calcium concentration. In addition, glucocorticoids are useful in the management of hypercalcemic patients by decreasing intestinal calcium absorption and increasing renal calcium excretion.[23] When possible, administration of glucocorticoids should be delayed until a definitive diagnosis of lymphosarcoma has been established since the drug may alter lymph node morphology, making diagnosis difficult. After induction of tumor remission by chemotherapeutic agents, serum calcium remains within normal limits. Elevation of serum calcium in a patient receiving maintenance chemotherapy suggests relapse of lymphosarcoma.[210]

Chemotherapy. Chemotherapy is the most effective treatment for dogs with multicentric lymphosarcoma. A wide variety of anticancer agents and therapeutic protocols have been used. The decision to use chemotherapy and selection of a specific protocol are based on many factors, including familiarity with specific drugs, ability to monitor laboratory parameters such as complete blood counts and platelet counts, ability to administer blood or platelet transfusions, willingness of the clients to return at scheduled intervals, and monetary constraints imposed by clients.

Anticancer drugs can be administered singly, sequentially, or in combination. Prednisone, cyclophosphamide, vincristine, chlorambucil, and L-asparaginase have been used in single-drug therapy protocols (Table 178–3). Remissions produced usually are of short duration, and mean survival times are generally less than 3 months (Table 178–4). In sequential therapy, a drug is used until a relapse occurs, and then an alternate drug is substituted. One recommended sequence is prednisone followed by cyclophosphamide followed by vincristine.[36] Median survival time with this sequence was reported to be approximately 5 months, with most dogs surviving 4 to 7 months.

Longer remission and survival times can be achieved with combination chemotherapy (Table 178–5). Because the fraction of tumor cells destroyed by each drug is independent of the other drugs used, an increased number of cancer cells can be killed. In addition, rapid destruction of tumor cells by a combination of drugs delays the appearance of resistant cells. Effective combination chemotherapy protocols include drugs that act on different phases of the cell cycle and have different toxic effects on normal tissue.

Combination chemotherapy can be divided into induction and maintenance phases. Aggressive therapy aimed at destroying large numbers of tumor cells is used during the induction phase. Dogs that achieve complete remissions usually survive longer than dogs that have a partial remission.[120] In the maintenance phase, drug dosages are lowered, drug administration intervals are increased, or less toxic drugs are added to allow the bone marrow and immune system time to recover. If the animal relapses, induction therapy is reinstituted or another protocol is substituted.

Immunotherapy. Immunotherapy is beneficial in increasing remission and survival times in dogs with

TABLE 178–3.   Recommended Dosage Schedules for Single-Agent Chemotherapy

Drug	Dosage and Route	Major Adverse Effects
Prednisone	20–50 mg/M² PO every 2 days	Polyuria, polydipsia
Vincristine (Oncovin; Eli Lilly & Co.)	0.5 to 1.0 mg/M² IV, weekly or biweekly	Perivascular irritation, constipation
Cyclophosphamide (Cytoxan; Mead Johnson Pharmaceutical Div.)	50 mg/M² PO once daily for 3 to 4 days per week	Hemorrhagic cystitis, myelosuppression
L-Asparaginase (Elspar; Merck Sharp & Dohme)	10,000 units/M² IP every 7 days	Anaphylaxis
Chlorambucil (Leukeran; Burroughs Wellcome)	2 mg/M² daily for 4 days per week	Myelosuppression

TABLE 178–4. Results of Single-Drug Chemotherapy in Canine Lymphosarcoma*

Drug	No. of Dogs Treated	Mean Objective Remission Time (days)	Mean Survival Time (days)	Reference
Cyclophosphamide	39	NR	57	126
Cyclophosphamide†	8	NR	110	142
Cyclophosphamide	3	NR	137	14
Prednisone	NR	NR	75	14
Prednisone	49	53	NR	193
Chlorambucil	NR	NR	75	14
L-Asparaginase	3	< 30	NR	146

*NR = Not reported.
†Dogs also splenectomized.

small tumor burdens. Mean survival time was approximately 8 months in dogs treated with either Freund's complete adjuvant or autochthonous tumor vaccine after clinical remission was induced with chemotherapy.[211] Survival time in dogs treated only with chemotherapy was approximately 5 months.

Surgical and Radiation Therapy. Regional radiation or lymphadenectomy can be used for dogs with stage I lymphosarcoma.[36] Since occult disease may be present, adjuvant chemotherapy is often indicated.

Solitary lymphosarcomas of the stomach or intestine should be removed surgically. Adjuvant combination chemotherapy has resulted in survival times longer than 18 months in some dogs.[120]

Supportive Therapy and Patient Monitoring. Successful treatment of lymphosarcoma necessitates careful patient monitoring. White blood cell and platelet counts are evaluated every 7 to 21 days. Chemotherapeutic drugs should be temporarily discontinued if the total neutrophil count drops below 3,000/μl or if the platelet count drops below 50,000/ul. Drugs can be reinstituted when counts return to normal.

Defects in humoral and cellular immunity associated with lymphosarcoma and chemotherapy increase susceptibility to viral, fungal, and bacterial infections. In a study of dogs receiving combination chemotherapy, six developed salmonellosis shortly after chemotherapy was initiated.[18] Decreased serum IgG concentrations and altered responsiveness to antigenic stimulation occurred in canine lymphosarcoma patients.[126,212] Cellular immunity as measured by lymphocyte blastogenic response and allogenic skin graft survival may also be abnormal.[17,48,212] Dogs with advanced disease are most immunologically impaired.[17]

All lymphosarcoma patients are monitored closely for infection, but prophylactic use of antibiotics is not always indicated.

Prognosis

Without therapy, most dogs with lymphosarcoma die within 2 months of diagnosis. Although it is usually not curative, chemotherapy can significantly prolong survival times. Factors that influence response to therapy include clinical stage at the time of diagnosis, the presence of systemic signs and hypercalcemia, and body weight. Survival times are shorter in dogs in advanced clinical stages, in hypercalcemic dogs, and in dogs with severe systemic signs.[38,121,193,201,209,210] For unknown reasons, smaller dogs ($\leq$15 kg) survive longer than larger dogs ($\geq$15 kg).[122] Prognosis is not related to age, breed, sex or histological tumor type.[121,193,209]

TABLE 178–5. Results of Combination Chemotherapy in Canine Lymphosarcoma*

Drug Combinations for Induction and Maintenance	No. of Dogs Treated	Percentage of Complete Remission†	Mean Objective Remission Time (Days)	Mean Survival Time (Days)	Reference No.
Vincristine, prednisone, cyclophosphamide, methotrexate, 6-mercaptopurine	20	65	104.8	211.5	116
Vincristine, L-asparaginase, cyclophosphamide, methotrexate	59	89.9	NR	219‡	121
Prednisone, cyclophosphamide	34	38	62	NR	193
Prednisone, cyclophosphamide, vincristine	19	79	184	NR	193
Prednisone, cyclophosphamide, vincristine, 6-mercaptopurine	25	76	136	NR	193
Prednisone, cyclophosphamide, vincristine, cytosine arabinoside	47	67	NR	138	201
Prednisone, cyclophosphamide, vincristine, cytosine arabinoside, L-asparaginase	9	90	101	198	38
Prednisone, chlorambucil	7	NR	NR	69	14

*NR = not reported.
†75% or greater reduction in size of tumor mass.
‡Median survival time.

Canine Lymphocytic Leukemia

In patients with lymphocytic leukemia, neoplastic proliferation of lymphocytes occurs primarily in the bone marrow, resulting in the release of large numbers of malignant cells into the circulation. The spleen, liver, and lymph nodes become infiltrated as the disease progresses. Clinical signs result from the displacement of normal marrow elements by neoplastic cells. Lymphocytic leukemia is found in approximately 10 per cent of dogs with hematopoietic tumors.[126]

Two types of lymphocytic leukemia have been described in dogs.[81,126] Chronic or well-differentiated lymphocytic leukemia (WDLL) is characterized by the presence of large numbers of mature lymphocytes in peripheral blood and bone marrow. This disease is similar to human chronic lymphocytic leukemia. In acute or lymphoblastic leukemia, large numbers of lymphoblasts are present in peripheral blood and bone marrow. This type is similar to human acute lymphoblastic leukemia.

Leukemia may also occur in dogs with advanced lymphosarcoma. This condition, sometimes referred to as lymphosarcoma cell leukemia, should be differentiated from WDLL and lymphoblastic leukemia since the prognosis and treatment of the three conditions may be different.[221]

Well-Differentiated Lymphocytic Leukemia (Chronic Lymphocytic Leukemia)

Thirteen cases of WDLL have been reported in dogs.[13,81,90,124,152,202,213] Average age of affected dogs was 7.3 years (range = 1.5 to 12.0 years). Lethargy, decreased appetite, and weight loss were frequently identified clinical signs. Lymphadenopathy was present in 25 per cent of cases; hepatosplenomegaly was present in 75 per cent of cases. Duration of clinical signs prior to diagnosis varied from 2 weeks to 4 months.

Hematological findings in dogs with WDLL included leukocytosis (25,000 to 478,000/μl and lymphocytosis (18,000 to 468,000/μl). In addition, a nonregenerative anemia was present in most dogs and 20 per cent were thrombocytopenic. Bone marrow examination revealed an increased percentage of lymphocytes. The majority of lymphocytes in peripheral blood and in the bone marrow had the morphological appearance of small lymphocytes, although small numbers of lymphoblasts were occasionally noted.

In humans, chronic lymphocytic leukemia may result from clonal proliferation of B-lymphocytes. Canine WDLL patients had B-cell markers on the surface of their lymphocytes, and some had monoclonal increases in serum immunoglobulins (IgM or IgA) and Bence Jones protein in their urine.[13,124]

In humans, the prognosis for long-term survival is better for WDLL than for other lymphoproliferative disorders. Average survival time is approximately 6 years, and survivals of 35 years have been reported.[166]

The effectiveness of chemotherapy in increasing survival time is controversial.[166] Canine WDLL patients treated with prednisone and chlorambucil typically survived 1.5 to 3.0 years.[90,124,213] One dog survived 23 months without therapy.[81]

Lymphoblastic Leukemia

Lymphoblastic leukemia accounts for 5 to 10 per cent of canine hematopoietic tumors.[126] It occurs most frequently in young dogs less than 4 years of age, but may occur in older dogs. Duration of clinical illness is usually less than 2 weeks, with signs of fever, weight loss, and inappetence. Anemia, splenomegaly, and lymphadenopathy may be present. Large numbers of prolymphocytes and lymphoblasts are identified in peripheral blood and bone marrow. Thrombocytopenia due to myelophthisis is usually noted.

The prognosis for long-term survival in dogs with lymphoblastic leukemia is poor. Clinical remissions were achieved with vincristine and prednisone therapy in six dogs, but average survival time was only 5 months.[126]

Feline Lymphosarcoma and Lymphocytic Leukemia

Lymphosarcoma is the most frequently identified tumor in cats and comprises approximately 75 to 90 per cent of all feline hematopoietic neoplasms.[42,49] The annual reported incidence of feline lymphosarcoma is approximately 200 per 100,000 cats in the population.[198] An increased prevalence in male cats has been noted in some reports[41,95,139] but not in others.[34,181]

Age of affected cats varies with breed, anatomical type of lymphosarcoma, and the presence of a positive test for feline leukemia virus (FeLV). The average age of affected purebred cats is younger (3.7 years) than random-breed domestic cats (6.0 years).[139] Early exposure of purebred cats in catteries to FeLV may account for the difference[71] Cats with alimentary lymphosarcoma and cats that are FeLV negative are often older than cats with other forms of lymphosarcoma and FeLV-positive cats.[71]

Feline Leukemia Virus (FeLV)

Feline lymphosarcoma is caused by a single-stranded RNA virus that is horizontally transmitted between susceptible cats.[73,74,102,104,129] FeLV is classified as a retrovirus because it contains the enzyme reverse transcriptase, which copies RNA into DNA. Three subgroups of FeLV (A, B, and C) have been described.[171]

In addition to causing lymphosarcoma, FeLV has been implicated in the pathogenesis of other malignant and nonmalignant disorders in cats (Table 178–6). The related feline sarcoma virus is a cause of multicentric fibrosarcomas in young cats.[72]

Pathogenesis. FeLV is shed in the saliva and urine of viremic cats.[59] Infection usually occurs via the ocular, oral, or nasal mucous membranes following prolonged contact with infected cats.[70] The virus may also be transmitted by fleas, blood transfusion, and transplacentally.

Viral replication initially occurs in local lymphatic tissue in the head and neck.[163] If the cat mounts an effective immune response, FeLV is eliminated. An ineffective immune response results in FeLV dissemination throughout the body and usually persistent infection. Approximately 30 per cent of exposed susceptible cats become persistently viremic.[74]

Cats become immune to FeLV by producing high titers of serum neutralizing antibody to viral envelope antigens. A titer of 1:10 or greater is protective.[70] Infected cats may also produce antibody to feline oncornavirus-associated cell membrane antigen (FOCMA). FOCMA is induced by FeLV and is expressed on the surface of infected cells. A FOCMA antibody titer of 1:32 or greater protects cats from the development of lymphosarcoma.[70] Antibody to FOCMA does not neutralize virus or protect against nonneoplastic FeLV-related diseases.

Prevalence of FeLV. Persistent FeLV infection is uncommon in the general cat population. In single-cat households with no exposure to FeLV, prevalence of persistent viremia is less than 1 per cent.[74,77] Because of horizontal transmission, prevalence in multiple-cat households after FeLV exposure is 30 to 50 per cent.[32,76,198]

Detection of FeLV. FeLV infection can be detected by an indirect immunofluorescent assay (IFA) or by an immunosorbent assay (ELISA). The IFA test detects FeLV antigens in leukocytes and platelets in peripheral blood.[77] The ELISA test detects soluble FeLV antigens in plasma and serum.[108] The IFA test is both sensitive and specific. Virus can be isolated from 97.5 per cent of cats that test IFA positive and less than 2 per cent of cats that test IFA negative.[75]

Overall agreement between the IFA test and the ELISA test is approximately 80 per cent.[106] When either the IFA or ELISA test is negative, both tests are likely to be negative, but 30 per cent of ELISA-positive cats will be IFA-negative. Virus usually cannot be isolated from the ELISA-positive IFA-negative cats and probably cannot be transmitted to susceptible cats.[106]

FeLV and Lymphosarcoma. Approximately 16 per cent of viremic cats develop lymphosarcoma.[77] The average time between detection of FeLV and the development of lymphosarcoma varies between 5 and 17 months.[57,77] Lymphosarcoma has been noted as early as 1 month following viral detection.[77]

Although FeLV is suspected to be the cause of most feline lymphosarcoma cases, it is identified in the blood in only 66 per cent of cases (Table 178–6). Support for FeLV as the cause of the other 34 per cent of cases comes from laboratory and epidemiological studies.[57,58,75] FOCMA, which is induced by FeLV, has been identified on lymphosarcoma cells from FeLV-negative cats. In addition, the risk of a cat's developing FeLV-negative lymphosarcoma after natural exposure to the virus is similar to the risk of the cat's developing FeLV-positive lymphosarcoma.[75] Epidemiological characteristics of FeLV-positive and FeLV-negative lymphosarcoma cats are similar except that virus-negative cats tend to be older.[57]

Clinical Findings and Classification

Lymphosarcoma can involve any organ in the body, and the clinical manifestations depend on the primary site of involvement. Five anatomical types of feline lymphosarcoma occur: mediastinal, alimentary, multicentric, leukemic, and unclassified.[71] The prevalence of each anatomical type varies in different regions of the world. Leukemia is most frequent in Boston,[32,57] multicentric is most frequent in New York,[71] and alimentary is most frequent in Glasgow.[34,127] The reason for the geographical variation is unknown but may relate to different strains of FeLV in each area.[71]

Mediastinal Lymphosarcoma. Mediastinal (thymic) lymphosarcoma is characterized by tumor infiltration of the thymus, metastasis to mediastinal and sternal lymph nodes, and hydrothorax. Mediastinal lymphosarcoma has been identified in approximately 27 per cent of Boston, 38 per cent of New York, and 10 per cent of Glasgow cats with lymphosarcoma.[4,57,71] Cats with mediastinal lymphosarcoma are younger (average age ⇐ 2.4 years) than cats with other forms of lymphosarcoma and are usually positive for FeLV (Table 178–7). Mediastinal lymphosarcomas are composed of T-lymphocytes.[93]

Acute onset of dyspnea, cyanosis, and cough are often observed. Physical findings usually include muf-

TABLE 178–6.   Feline Leukemia Virus-Associated Diseases*

Disease Diagnosis	Percentage FeLV Positive†
Lymphoid malignancies	66
Myeloproliferative disease	88
Hypoplastic anemia	75
Haemobarteonellosis	41
Feline infectious peritonitis	53
Granulomatous disease	75
Bacterial infections	52
Glomerulonephritis	80
Toxoplasmosis	75
Infertility	91

*Reprinted with permission from Cotter, S. M., Hardy, W. D., Jr., and Essex, M.: Association of feline leukemia virus with lymphosarcoma and other disorders in the cat. J. Am. Vet. Med. Assoc. 166:449, 1975.

†Immunofluorescence test.

TABLE 178–7.   Occurrence of FeLV in Cats with Lymphosarcoma*

Anatomical Type	Percentage FeLV Positive†
Lymphocytic leukemia	69
Mediastinal	68
Multicentric	60
Alimentary	33
Unclassified	66
Total	66

*Reprinted with permission from Cotter, S. M., Hardy, W. D., Jr., and Essex, M.: Association of feline leukemia virus with lymphosarcoma and other disorders in the cat. J. Am. Vet. Med. Assoc., 166:449, 1975.

fled heart sounds, incompressibility of the anterior thorax, and posterior displacement of the apex heartbeat.[95]

Thoracic radiography reveals a widening of the anterior mediastinum, silhouetting of the cranial heart border, elevation of the trachea, displacement of cranial lung lobes, sternal or mediastinal lymphadenopathy, and pleural effusion.[82,95] Fluid removed from the thorax is usually clear or straw-colored, with a specific gravity of 1.020 to 1.040 and a white blood cell count of 5,000 to 295,000/μl.[181] Most of the white blood cells are lymphocytes, prolymphocytes, or lymphoblasts. Similar cells are easily obtained by fine-needle aspiration of the thymic mass.

Alimentary Lymphosarcoma. Alimentary lymphosarcoma is characterized by single or multiple tumors in the stomach, small intestine, colon, or mesenteric lymph nodes. Lesions may be diffusely infiltrative, nodular, or annular. The spleen, liver, and kidneys may also be infiltrated. Alimentary lymphosarcoma has been found in 8 per cent feline lymphosarcoma cases in Boston, 15 per cent in New York, and 50 per cent in Glasgow.[57,71,173] Cats with alimentary lymphosarcoma are older (average age = 8 years) than cats with other anatomical types, and only 33 per cent are FeLV positive (Table 178–7). Alimentary lymphosarcomas are composed of B-lymphocytes.[93]

Chronic weight loss, decreased appetite, diarrhea, and vomiting are characteristic clinical signs.[33,95] Physical findings include emaciation, thickened intestinal loops, palpable abdominal mass, hepatomegaly, and splenomegaly.

Radiographic abnormalities detected on survey radiographs or with contrast studies include (1) an abdominal mass, (2) intestinal accumulation of fluid, gas, or ingesta, (3) delayed intestinal transit time, (4) mural lesions associated with luminal filling defects, (5) mucosal ulcerations, and (6) thickening of the intestinal wall with displacement of adjacent bowl loops.[54] Diagnosis can be established by aspiration or surgical biopsy of gastrointestinal masses or mesenteric lymph nodes.

Multicentric Lymphosarcoma. Multicentric lymphosarcoma is characterized by diffuse involvement of lymphatic tissue throughout the body. Liver, spleen, kidneys, and other visceral organs may be involved. Multicentric lymphosarcoma has been identified in 11 per cent of feline lymphosarcoma cases in Boston, 44 per cent in New York, and 29 per cent in Glasgow.[4,57,71] The average age of affected cats is 4.2 years.[139] Approximately 60 per cent are FeLV positive (Table 178–7). Cells from multicentric lymphosarcomas lack B- and T-cell receptors.[93]

Clinical signs of cats with multicentric lymphosarcoma vary depending on the primary organs involved. Vomiting, decreased appetite, depression, and icterus are noted with hepatic infiltration. Polyuria and polydipsia occur with bilateral renal involvement. Physical findings may include generalized lymph node enlargement, hepatomegaly, splenomegaly, renomegaly, and a palpable abdominal mass. Enlargement of abdominal and thoracic lymph nodes, hepatomegaly, and splenomegaly may be identified on survey radiographs. Diagnosis is usually established by percutaneous or surgical biopsy of affected organs.

Lymphocytic Leukemia. Lymphocytic leukemia is characterized by the presence of neoplastic lymphocytes in blood and bone marrow. Neoplastic cells arise in the bone marrow and are disseminated via the blood throughout the body.[127] In Boston, 50 per cent of cats with lymphosarcoma have lymphocytic leukemia without solid tumor.[31] Much lower prevalences have been reported in California (3.7 per cent)[41] and in Glasgow (3 per cent).[50] The average age of cats with lymphocytic leukemia is 4.2 years, and approximately 70 per cent are FeLV positive (Table 178–7).

Presenting clinical signs are often nonspecific and include lethargy, anorexia, weight loss, and fever. Pallor of mucous membranes is usually noted on physical examination. Splenomegaly and hepatomegaly are sometimes present. Clinical signs result from severe nonregenerative anemia. Packed cell volumes between 8 and 15 per cent are typical. White blood cell counts may be decreased, normal, or increased. Neutropenia is commonly present. Lymphocyte counts are usually elevated (average = 45,178/μl) but may be normal or decreased.[82] Immature or atypical lymphocytes are usually noted in peripheral blood smears.

Diagnosis of lymphocytic leukemia can be confirmed by bone marrow examination. Lymphocytes often comprise 50 to 100 per cent of the nucleated cells in the bone marrow, compared with the normal value of less than 15 per cent.[181] Prolymphocytes and lymphoblasts are often identified.

Unclassified Lymphosarcoma. The least common type of lymphosarcoma, the unclassified or miscellaneous type, includes cats with lymphosarcoma involving a single organ that are not included in other classifications (e.g., lymphosarcomas of the skin, eyes, kidneys, central nervous system, and bone). Six percent of feline lymphosarcoma cases in Boston, 2.9 per cent in New York, and 10 per cent in Glasgow were unclassified.[4,32,71]

Lymphosarcoma involving the central or peripheral nervous system is the most frequent of the unclassified types.[56,71,82] Extradural lymphosarcoma involving the thoracic or lumbar spine results in spinal cord compression and posterior paralysis.[145] Hyperalgesia over the lumbar spine may be an early clinical sign.[31] Most cats with central nervous system involvement are FeLV positive.[71] Analysis of cerebrospinal fluid, myelography, and surgical biopsy of suspected lesions aid in the diagnosis.

Renal lymphosarcoma, which usually involves both kidneys, results in renomegaly and eventual renal failure. Clinical signs include polyuria, polydipsia, depression, anorexia, and weight loss.[95] The easily palpable kidneys are smooth and symmetrically enlarged. Diagnosis is confirmed by aspiration or needle biopsy.

Ocular lymphosarcoma involves the retrobulbar space, third eyelid, iris, or ciliary body.[19,82,95] Examination of aqueous humor obtained by paracentesis may reveal malignant lymphocytes. Cats with ocular lymphosarcoma are usually FeLV positive.[71]

Cutaneous lymphosarcoma is characterized by single or multiple cutaneous nodules or plaques.[82,110] Biopsy is required to differentiate lymphosarcoma from other malignant and nonmalignant skin lesions.

Diagnosis

A presumptive diagnosis of feline lymphosarcoma can often be established following evaluation of clinical, hematological, biochemical, and radiographic information. A definitive diagnosis is established when neoplastic lymphocytes are identified in body tissues or fluids. A positive FeLV test is not equivalent to a diagnosis of lymphosarcoma, and a negative test does not rule out a diagnosis of lymphosarcoma.

Hematological Findings. Anemia is present in approximately 50 per cent of cats with lymphosarcoma.[34,35,198] The average packed cell volume of 49 cats with lymphosarcoma was 27.4, with a range of 4 to 46 per cent. Anemia is identified most frequently in cats with lymphocytic leukemia and least often in cats with alimentary lymphosarcoma.[71]

Total white blood cell count is frequently normal but may be increased or, more commonly, decreased. Leukopenia was present in 21 of 49 cats with lymphosarcoma.[181] Absolute lymphopenia was present in 51 per cent of the cats, whereas only 12 per cent had lymphocytosis. Absolute lymphocyte counts ranged from less than 1500/μl to 693,000/μl. Regardless of the total white blood cell count, 40 per cent of cats had small or large numbers of lymphoblasts or prolymphocytes in peripheral blood smears.

Bone marrow examination may reveal evidence of lymphosarcoma in the absence of abnormalities in the peripheral blood. Abnormal findings include greater than 15 per cent small lymphocytes and the presence of immature or atypical lymphocytes.[181] In a survey of 19 cats with lymphosarcoma, bone marrow examination was suggestive of the diagnosis in 12 of the cats.[181] Only 7 of the 12 cats had abnormalities in peripheral blood.

Biochemical Findings. The anatomical location of lymphosarcoma usually determines which, if any, of the serum biochemical parameters are abnormal. Infiltration of the liver may result in elevation of serum bilirubin, alkaline phosphatase, and alanine aminotransferase (SGPT). Bilateral renal infiltration may result in elevation of serum urea nitrogen, creatinine, and phosphorus.

Hypercalcemia has been reported in only two feline lymphosarcoma cases. An 11-year-old male Siamese cat with cutaneous lymphosarcoma had a serum calcium of 14.6 mg/100 ml, and a 6-year-old female Siamese cat with mediastinal lymphosarcoma had a serum calcium of 16.2 mg/100 ml.[24,47]

Radiographic Findings. Abnormalities on survey radiographs often provide the first clue to lymphosarcoma. Specific changes vary with anatomical type but include a mediastinal mass, pleural effusion, lymphadenopathy, hepatomegaly, splenomegaly, renomegaly, an abdominal mass, ascites, and intestinal ileus.

Cytopathological and Histopathological Findings. A definitive diagnosis of lymphosarcoma is usually made by identifying neoplastic lymphocytes in body fluids or tissues. Depending on location of the disease, aspiration or surgical biopsy is used to collect material for evaluation. Diagnostic criteria of malignancy are similar to those of canine lymphosarcoma.

Treatment

Chemotherapy. The basic principles of chemotherapy discussed in the section on canine lymphosarcoma are generally applicable to cats. Cats tolerate chemotherapy as well as dogs do, although they tend to be in more advanced stages of disease when presented for treatment.[30]

The decision to treat an FeLV-positive lymphosarcoma cat should be made only after a thorough discussion with the client regarding prognosis, cost, potential side effects, potential for infection of other cats, and public health issues. Controversy exists regarding the risk of FeLV to human beings.[70] At present, no danger to humans from exposure to FeLV has been documented. FeLV-positive cats undergoing therapy should be confined to avoid transmission to other noninfected cats.

There is no indication that chemotherapy will benefit an FeLV-positive cat that does not have malignancy. Chemotherapeutic agents should only be administered after a definitive diagnosis of lymphosarcoma has been established.

Prior to treatment, cats should be assessed to rule out concurrent metabolic or infectious diseases. Metabolic abnormalities resulting from lymphosarcoma may regress after effective chemotherapy. Diagnostic tests to document infection such as a chest radiograph, urine culture, and blood culture are advisable in cats that are persistently pyrexic. Bacterial infec-

TABLE 178–8.   Combination Chemotherapy for Feline Lymphosarcoma*

Drugs	No. of Cats Treated	% Complete Remission	Median Objective Remission Duration (Days)	Median Survival Time (Days)	Reference No.
Vincristine, cyclophosphamide, and prednisone	55	64	150	NR	30
Vincristine, L-asparaginase, cyclophosphamide, and methotrexate	26	73	NR	110	125
Prednisone and cyclophosphamide	5	NR	NR	423†	20
Vincristine, cyclophosphamide, cytosine arabinoside, and prednisone	9	NR	NR	102	200

*NR = not reported.

†Average survival time for four of the five cats.

tions should be aggressively treated with antibiotics. In addition, anemia should be corrected with blood transfusion and dehydration corrected with fluid therapy before chemotherapy.

Both single drugs and drug combinations have been successfully used in cats with lymphosarcoma.[14,20,30,125,192,198] Prednisone, cyclophosphamide, vincristine, chlorambucil, doxorubicin, L-asparaginase, methotrexate, and cytosine arabinoside have been used alone or in combination protocols (Table 178–8). Single-drug schedules have fewer side effects than combination therapy, but duration of remission is not as long.[31]

Sixty to 70 per cent of cats treated with combination chemotherapy achieve clinical remission (Table 178–8). In 55 cats treated with vincristine, cyclophosphamide, and prednisone, remission rates were greater in cats with solid tumors (79 per cent) than in cats with leukemia (29 per cent).[30] Median duration of remission was 5 months, with a range of 1 to 42 months. Cats with alimentary lymphosarcoma had the shortest median remission time (4.5 months). Response to treatment was similar for FeLV-positive and FeLV-negative cats.

Complete blood counts and platelet counts should be monitored closely during therapy. Myelosuppressive drugs should be temporarily discontinued if neutrophil counts drop below 3,000/μl or platelet counts drop below 50,000/μl. Supportive therapy including blood transfusions, antibiotics, and fluids is used as needed.

Surgical Therapy. Surgical therapy is usually limited to excision of solitary or localized lesions. Tumors involving the stomach, intestines, mesenteric lymph nodes, skin, eyes, and vertebral canal may be surgically resectable. Since surgery alone is usually not curative, a course of chemotherapy beginning several weeks after surgery is advisable.

Immunotherapy. Complete remission of lymphosarcoma has been reported in cats following administration of whole blood, plasma, serum, or FOCMA antibodies.[71,76] Unfortunately, survival times were less than 6 months. Deaths were attributed to the residual effects of FeLV on the immune system and bone marrow.

Prognosis

Without therapy, approximately 70 per cent of cats with lymphosarcoma die within 8 weeks of diagnosis.[33] Cats that are FeLV negative live longer than those that are FeLV positive.[71]

Overall median survival time of 62 cats treated with a combination drug protocol including vincristine, L-asparaginase, cyclophosphamide, methotrexate, and prednisone was 4 months, and 20 per cent of the cats lived at least 1 year.[71] Survival times longer than 3 years have been reported, and an occasional cat is cured by chemotherapy.[20,31] Cats with lymphocytic leukemia are less likely to respond to therapy than cats with solid tumor.[30] Deaths in treated cats result from relapse of the cancer, myelosuppression, infection, drug toxicity, and anemia.

Multiple Myeloma

Multiple myeloma is a neoplastic disorder resulting from proliferation of mature and immature plasma cells. The clinical manifestations result from neoplastic infiltration of bone marrow and other organs or overproduction of immunoglobulin. Excess immunoglobulin synthesis is typically monoclonal, resulting from a single clone of malignant cells. Protein electrophoresis reveals a spike-like elevation in beta- or gamma-globulins. The increased immunoglobulin, referred to as a paraprotein or M-component, is composed of complete immunoglobulin molecules (usually IgA or IgG) or fragments of immunoglobulin molecules such as light chains. Light chains are small molecules that readily pass through the glomerulus into the urine (Bence Jones proteinuria).

Multiple myeloma is infrequently diagnosed in dogs and cats. Average age of reported canine patients varies from 5.5 to 9.2 years, with a range of 2.5 to 16.0 years.[123,149,202] Average age of feline myeloma patients was 8.3 and 9.7 years in two reports.[43,123] In one canine report, males were affected more frequently than females;[149] but in two other reports, males and females were affected equally often.[123,202] In cats, myeloma has been diagnosed more commonly in males than females.[43,123] Breed predispositions have not been recognized.

The exact cause of multiple myeloma is unknown. Postulated predisposing influences include genetic factors, chronic stimulation of the reticuloendothelial system, and viral infection.[215]

Clinical Findings

Clinical signs result from organ dysfunction caused by proliferation of plasma cells or pathological alterations caused by paraproteins or both. In a review of 22 canine myeloma cases, lameness, pain, and pathological fracture were the most common clinical signs.[149] Less commonly identified findings included anemia, abnormal bleeding tendencies, palpable tumor masses, depression, and weight loss. Depression, anorexia, pallor of mucous membranes, fever, and chronic infection were the most frequent clinical signs in cats.[43]

Skeletal lesions result in bone pain, weakness, and pathological fractures. Radiographic signs include multiple or solitary areas of osteolysis or generalized osteoporosis in the long bones, ribs, vertebrae, skull, or pelvis.[123,149] Neurological abnormalities including paresis, paralysis, and urinary incontinence have been noted as a result of destruction of nervous tissue by neoplastic cells or as a result of pathological fracture of a vertebra.[149]

Infiltration of neoplastic plasma cells into extraosseous tissues may result in splenomegaly, hepatomegaly, or lymphadenopathy. Occasionally, a solitary tumor mass is identified.

Abnormalities caused by the presence of the paraprotein include decreased immune competency, hyperviscosity syndrome, bleeding disorders, and renal dysfunction. Clinical signs vary with the concentration and type of paraprotein.

Decreased resistance to infection is a major cause of death in myeloma patients. Altered immune responses may be related to suppression of normal B-cell function, defective opsonization, and granulocytopenia due to myelophthisis.[215]

Hyperviscosity syndrome results from increased serum concentration of certain immunoglobulins. Molecules with a high molecular weight, such as IgM, or molecules such as IgA that tend to polymerize have the greatest effect on serum viscosity. Clinical manifestations of increased serum viscosity include bleeding abnormalities, circulatory impairment, neurological dysfunction, and retinopathy.[123,214] Bleeding abnormalities may result from complexing of paraproteins with coagulation factors, abnormal platelet function, presence of circulating coagulation inhibitors, and vascular overdistension.[152,187,214] Neurological alterations including dementia, depression,

ataxia, and coma result from vascular occlusion and decreased oxygenation of the brain.[187] Visual dysfunction, retinal vessel dilation, and retinal hemorrhage occur because of circulatory impairment to the eyes.[202,214]

The diagnosis of hyperviscosity syndrome can be confirmed by demonstrating increased serum viscosity with a viscometer or 0.1-ml pipette.[214] Normal serum viscosity in dogs is approximately 1.4 to 1.6 relative to water.[40] Hyperviscosity syndrome was identified in 2 of 22 dogs with myeloma but was absent in 11 cats with myeloma.[43,123]

Clinical manifestations of renal dysfunction include polyuria, polydipsia, azotemia, and uremia. Renal disease may result from a combination of factors including filtration of Bence Jones proteins, tubular obstruction by protein casts, hypercalcemia, amyloidosis, and pyelonephritis.[215]

Diagnosis

Hematological Findings. Normocytic, normochromic anemia is a common finding in myeloma patients. Anemia occurs because of marrow infiltration, decreased red blood cell life span, and chronic renal insufficiency.[149] In addition, elevated serum globulin concentration results in increased rouleaux formation and increased erythrocyte sedimentation rate. Thrombocytopenia and leukopenia occur in approximately 33 per cent of dogs because of myelophthisis.[202] Plasma cell leukemia is unusual, but small numbers of immature plasma cells may be identified in peripheral blood smears.[43]

Bone marrow biopsy usually reveals increased numbers of mature and immature plasma cells. In normal marrow, plasma cells constitute less than 10 per cent of the nucleated cells. An excessive number of plasma cells in bone marrow is not pathognomonic for multiple myeloma since similar findings may occur with other neoplastic, infectious, and immunological diseases. Cats with multiple myeloma are usually negative for FeLV.

Serum Protein Abnormalities. Total serum protein is usually markedly elevated and often provides the first clue to the presence of myeloma. The elevation in protein results from increased serum globulin. Serum albumin is generally normal or decreased. Hypoalbuminemia may result from renal protein loss from glomerulonephritis or amyloidosis.

Plasma electrophoresis generally reveals a monoclonal gammopathy. The paraprotein or M-component appears as a tall, narrow, sharply defined peak with beta or gamma motility. Immunoelectrophoresis can be used to identify the immunoglobulin class of the paraprotein, which is generally IgA or IgG, and the concentration of paraprotein can be determined by radial immunodiffusion.

Urinalysis. The presence of Bence Jones (immunoglobulin light chains) proteins in urine is best determined by urine electrophoresis. Heat precipitation can also be used but is less sensitive. Bence

Jones proteinuria was detected in 7 of 11 dogs and 6 of 11 cats with myeloma.[43,123] Other abnormal findings in urine may include increased albumin concentration, casts, bacteria, and white blood cells.

Biochemical Findings. Serum calcium concentration may be normal, decreased, or increased in myeloma patients. In one report, hypercalcemia was identified in 13 per cent of dogs, but not in cats, with myeloma.[123] Hypercalcemia may result from binding of calcium to the paraprotein or synthesis of an osteoclast activating factor by the tumor.[123]

Differential Diagnosis. Clinical signs of multiple myeloma are often nonspecific, and many disease processes may be considered. None of the clinical findings listed above are pathognomonic. Differentiating myeloma from other plasma cell dyscrasias may be especially difficult. To establish a diagnosis of multiple myeloma at least two of the following should be present: monoclonal gammopathy, increased numbers of plasma cells in bone marrow, Bence Jones proteinuria, and osteolytic bone lesions.[123]

Treatment and Prognosis

Animals with multiple myeloma usually have advanced disease, and survival times are short without therapy. Depending on clinical findings, supportive treatment may include antibiotics to control infection, fluid therapy to correct dehydration, and control of hypercalcemia. In addition, plasmapheresis can be used to rapidly decrease serum viscosity if hyperviscosity syndrome is present.

Combination chemotherapy including melphalan and prednisone has been successfully used in dogs and cats to induce and maintain remission.[43,123] In one report, the therapeutic protocol consisted of melphalan at 0.1 mg/kg body weight once daily, orally for 10 days, then 0.05 mg/kg once daily; and prednisone at a dosage of 0.5 mg/kg body weight once daily, orally.[123] Average survival time in 11 dogs was more than 12 months. Average survival time in five cats treated with melphalan and prednisone was 6.2 months.[43] Remission rates and survival times are generally better for patients with multiple myeloma than for those with other hematopoietic neoplasms.

MYELOPROLIFERATIVE DISEASES

Myeloproliferative disorders are characterized by neoplastic proliferations of erythrocytic, granulocytic, monocytic, thrombocytic, fibroblast, or osteocytic cell lines. Although once considered separate entities, the diseases resulting from myeloproliferative disorders (primary polycythemia, erythemic myelosis, erythroleukemia, granulocytic leukemia, monocytic leukemia, megakaryocytic leukemia, and myelofibrosis) are now considered to represent stages or manifestations of a single, polyphasic proliferative bone marrow disorder. Rationale for this concept includes the following: (1) A pluripotential stem cell gives rise to multiple bone marrow cell lines; (2) although malignant proliferation of one cell type may be predominant, other cell lines are usually concurrently involved; and (3) transitions can occur from one predominant cell type to another during the disease.[32,39,112,158,170,215] William Dameschek introduced the term myeloproliferative disorder to describe this polyphasic disease in 1951, and this term has become widely accepted, although nonlymphocytic[112] and myelomonocytic leukemia[170] are terms sometimes used. Prevalence studies indicate that myeloproliferative disorders account for 5 to 10 per cent of canine and 10 to 25 per cent of feline hematopoietic neoplasms.[42,131,143,184,198]

Etiopathogenesis

Observations in human beings and in experimental animals suggest that myeloproliferative diseases result from the clonal proliferation of a bone marrow pluripotent stem cell.[32,215] Although the exact cause of human myeloproliferative disease remains unknown, studies continue to examine the role of viral infection, environmental factors (chemicals, irradiation), chromosomal aberrations, genetic factors, and immunological dysfunction.[32,215]

In cats, clinical and experimental evidence suggests that FeLV causes myeloproliferative disease. Eighty to 90 per cent of cats with naturally occurring myeloproliferative disease are positive for FeLV, and C-type viral particles have been demonstrated in bone marrow samples from affected cats.[87,89,103,183,198] Myeloproliferative disease has been experimentally induced in cats with FeLV. In one cat, granulocytic leukemia was produced with FeLV isolated from a lymphoid tumor.[103] In another cat, both granulocytic leukemia and thymic lymphosarcoma developed after experimental FeLV infection.[129] In a third cat, reticuloendotheliosis developed following natural exposure to FeLV.[151]

Factors leading to the development of feline myeloproliferative disease after FeLV infection are incompletely understood. It has been suggested that bone marrow cells may have increased susceptibility to malignant clonal proliferation during recovery from bone marrow injury or suppression.[180] In cats, several factors are capable of producing bone marrow injury including infection with panleukopenia virus, *Haemobartonella felis*, and FeLV. Myeloproliferative disease has been reported concurrently with *H. felis* infection in some cats.[37,89,207] In an experimental study, it was noted that reticuloendotheliosis developed during the early phase of bone marrow recovery after FeLV-induced marrow suppression.[151]

Chromosomal aberrations have been described in cats with acute lymphoblastic leukemia[65] and erythroleukemia.[67] The significance of the chromosomal abnormalities and their relationship to FeLV in the pathogenesis of feline myeloproliferative disorders remains to be determined.

The cause of naturally occurring canine myeloproliferative disease is unknown. Granulocytic leukemia has been produced experimentally in dogs by feeding strontium 90, and erythroleukemia has been produced by long-term exposure to cobalt 60.[46,203] The fact that a viral cause has not been identified in dogs may account for the decreased prevalence of myeloproliferative disease in dogs compared with cats.

Preleukemia Syndromes

In humans, a syndrome characterized by chronic anemia, neutropenia, and thrombocytopenia is sometimes recognized prior to the onset of myeloproliferative disease. This hematopoietic abnormality represents hematopoietic dysplasia with ineffective erythropoiesis and granulocytopoiesis. The syndrome has been classified as a preleukemic condition because many patients eventually develop acute blastic nonlymphocytic leukemia.[170] Abnormalities in peripheral blood include marked to moderate anisopoikilocytosis, nucleated red blood cells out of proportion to polychromasia, erythrocyte maturation abnormalities, immature granulocytes, abnormal granulocyte morphology, and abnormally large or small platelets.[32,44,112] Bone marrow is usually hypercellular but may be normal or hypocellular. Erythrocyte hyperplasia and disordered granulocytopoiesis with increased numbers of blasts is common. Megakaryocytes are often increased in numbers and have abnormal morphology (i.e., dwarf megakaryocytes).[32,44,112]

Hematopoietic dysplasia characterized by anemia, leukopenia, lymphopenia, and thrombocytopenia has been recognized in FeLV-positive cats.[32,69,97,128,163] This may represent a preleukemic state, because some cats eventually develop overt myeloproliferative disease.[53,118,134,179]

In addition to hematopoietic dysplasia, a syndrome termed smoldering, or subleukemic, leukemia may occur prior to myeloproliferative disease. This syndrome is characterized by increased numbers of blasts in the bone marrow but not in the peripheral blood.

Diagnosis of Myeloproliferative Disorders

Frequently identified clinical signs in dogs and cats with myeloproliferative disease (excluding primary polycythemia) include weight loss, anorexia, listlessness, pale mucous membranes, and fever.[32,154] Other less commonly identified signs include splenomegaly, hepatomegaly, moderate enlargement of one or more lymph nodes, icterus, recurrent infections, nonhealing wounds, chronic oral disease, and bleeding disorders.[32,155]

Hematological and Bone Marrow Findings

A progressive, nonregenerative anemia is present in most dogs and cats with myeloproliferative disease.[32,155] Increased numbers of nucleated red blood cells, macrocytes, and megaloblastic erythrocytes are commonly noted. Leukocyte numbers may be increased, decreased, or normal. Leukocyte morphology is frequently abnormal. Platelet counts are often reduced in acute myeloproliferative disease and increased in chronic myeloproliferative disease.

Hematological findings in animals with myeloproliferative disorders have to be differentiated from leukoerythroblastic anemias and leukemoid reactions. Leukoerythroblastic anemia is characterized by increased numbers of nucleated red blood cells and low numbers of immature neutrophils in the peripheral blood. Reticulocytosis is slight and is disproportionate to the markedly increased numbers of nucleated red blood cells.[207,215] In humans, leukoerythroblastic anemia is often associated with neoplastic infiltration of the bone marrow but also occurs in nonneoplastic disorders.[209,215] Leukoerythroblastic anemia has been described in FeLV-positive cats with lymphosarcoma and in cats with *H. felis* infection.[62,117,180]

Leukemoid reactions are characterized by leukocytosis, often with a pronounced left shift. Granulocytic, monocytic, and lymphocytic cell lines may be involved. Leukemoid reactions result from infections, intoxications, malignancy, and severe hemorrhage.[215] In dogs, total leukocyte counts of greater than $50,000/\mu l$ with a shift to myelocytes have been noted in pyometra.[181] Cats recovering from panleukopenia virus infection often have pronounced leukemoid reactions.[181]

A diagnosis of myeloproliferative disease is usually established by examination of a blood smear and a bone marrow aspiration sample. The bone marrow is generally hypercellular, with one or more cell lines demonstrating abnormal morphology. Nonaffected cell lines may be hypoplastic.

Miscellaneous Findings

Additional findings in cats with myeloproliferative disease include infection with *H. felis*[37,89,207] or *Toxoplasma gondi*,[208] lupus erythematosus cells in the bone marrow, and hypercalcemia. Hypercalcemia was diagnosed in a cat with subleukemic granulocytic leukemia and myelosclerosis.

Membranous glomerulonephritis was noted in four cats with myeloproliferative disease.[3,64,207] Three of the cats were FeLV positive, and immune complex deposition was demonstrated in two cats.

Necropsy Findings

Generalized splenomegaly and hepatomegaly due to diffuse tumor infiltration are usually noted.[32,155] Lymph nodes are generally less affected than the spleen or liver. Neoplastic infiltration of other organs is not common. In cases of granulocytic leukemia, a greenish hue (chlorma) may be noted in infiltrated organs because of the myeloperoxidase in neoplastic cells.[181]

Classification of Myeloproliferative Disorders

Accurate classification of myeloproliferative disorders is necessary to adequately determine prognosis and to select the optimum therapy.

Classification of myeloproliferative disorders is based on the predominant cell type present in peripheral blood and bone marrow and the degree of cell differentiation (Table 178–9). Classification is often complicated by changes in cell type during the disease course and the simultaneous involvement of more than one cell line. Acute myeloproliferative disorders are characterized by a predominance of undifferentiated blasts, whereas chronic myeloproliferative disorders are characterized by a predominance of more mature types. In general, human patients with acute myeloproliferative disorders have a poorer response to chemotherapy and shorter survival times than those patients with chronic myeloproliferative disorders.[215]

TABLE 178–9.   Classification of Myeloproliferative Disorders*

Neoplastic Syndrome	Cell Type(s)
Acute myeloproliferative disorders	
Acute granulocytic leukemia	Granulocytic
Myelomonocytic leukemia	Granulocytic, monocytic
Monocytic leukemia	Monocytic
Erythroleukemia	Erythroid, granulocytic
Acute erythremic myelosis	Erythroid
Megakaryocytic leukemia	Megakaryocytic
Chronic myeloproliferative disorders	
Chronic granulocytic leukemia	Neutrophilic granulocytes
Eosinophilic leukemia	Eosinophilic granulocytes
Basophilic leukemia	Basophilic granulocytes
Chronic erythremic myelosis	Erythroid
Primary polycythemia	Erythroid
Thrombocythemia	Platelets
Myelofibrosis with myeloid metaplasia	Megakaryocytic, granulocytic, erythroid

*Reprinted with permission from Harvey, J. W.: Myeloproliferative disorders in dogs and cats. Vet. Clin. North Am./Small Anim. Pract. *11*:349, 1981.

Mature cell types can usually be differentiated on Romanovsky's-stained blood or bone marrow smears. Special cytochemical stains may be required to identify immature cell types and to distinguish myeloproliferative from lymphoproliferative disorders (Table 178–10). Considerable overlap often exists between cell types, and cells may be so undifferentiated that they cannot be classified even with special stains.

Acute and Chronic Granulocytic Leukemia. Acute granulocytic leukemia (myelogenous leukemia, neutrophilic leukemia) is characterized by a high proportion of myeloblasts, promyelocytes, and neutrophilic myelocytes in the peripheral blood and bone marrow. Although it is an uncommon disease, acute granulocytic leukemia in dogs and cats has been described in numerous published reports.[7,28,32,52,60,71,85,96,118,137,138, 144,161,164,166,173,174,178,181,182,183,196,199,206,222] Age, breed, and sex predispositions have not been noted.

Hemograms typically reveal nonregenerative anemia and thrombocytopenia. Total leukocyte counts are often increased but may be decreased or normal.[32,63,155] White blood cell counts usually range from 30,000 to 150,000/μl in dogs and 2,700 to 396,000/μl in cats, although counts greater than 400,000/μl have been recorded. Atypical, large neutrophils with abnormally shaped nuclei are commonly noted. Bone marrow examination typically reveals myeloid hyperplasia and maturation arrest at the level of the myeloblast, promyelocyte, or myelocyte.[32,60]

Acute granulocytic leukemia with a predominance of myeloblasts may be difficult to differentiate from lymphoblastic leukemia and myelomonocytic leukemia. Alkaline phosphatase activity is not present in immature lymphocytes (Table 178–10). Monocyte stains (lipase, alpha-naphthyl acetate) are negative in "pure" granulocytic leukemia.

The clinical course in dogs and cats with acute granulocytic leukemia is rapidly progressive. Survival time in untreated animals is usually less than 2 months. Clinical signs can be temporarily improved with blood transfusions, fluids, vitamin-iron supplements, and antibiotics.[60,85]

There are few reports of the use of chemotherapy in dogs and cats with acute granulocytic leukemia. Three cats were treated with different combinations of cytosine arabinoside, cyclophosphamide, vinblastine, and prednisone.[85] Partial remissions were achieved in two of the cats. Average survival time was 41 days after diagnosis.

TABLE 178–10.   Cytochemical Staining Reaction of Normal and Leukemic Cells

Stain	Neutrophil	Monocyte	Lymphocyte	Granulocytic Leukemia	Myelomonocytic Leukemia	Lymphocytic Leukemia
Alkaline phosphatase	−	−	−	+	*	−
Peroxidase	+	*	−	+	*	−
Sudan black	+	*	−	+	*	−
Chloroacetate esterase	+	−	−	+	+	−
Alpha-naphthyl butyrate esterase	−	+	−	−	+	−
Lipase	−	+	−	−	+	−
Alpha-naphthyl acetate esterase	±	+	−	±	+	−

*A few positive granules may be present.

Chronic granulocytic leukemia is characterized by the presence of increased numbers of neutrophils in the peripheral blood and bone marrow, with a relatively orderly maturation sequence.[32] Immature forms generally represent only 3 to 7 per cent of the total leukocyte count. In humans, 90 per cent of patients have the "Philadelphia" chromosome abnormality. Anemia and thrombocytopenia are sometimes present. Human patients with chronic granulocytic leukemia tend to have chronic courses of 3 to 4 years that eventually terminate in an acute "blastic" leukemia.

Chronic granulocytic leukemia has been reported more frequently in dogs than in cats.[32,107,115,144,154,173] Dogs with chronic granulocytic leukemia demonstrate prolonged leukocytosis and neutrophilia. The alkaline phosphatase reaction is helpful in differentiating granulocytic leukemia from an inflammatory response, since alkaline phosphatase activity is absent during reactive leukocytosis.[100] Tissues from affected dogs sometimes have a greenish discoloration due to myeloperoxidase in neutrophils.

Survival times of one to 4 years have been reported in dogs with chronic granulocytic leukemia. Chemotherapy has generally not increased survival time in human patients.[215] The effect of chemotherapy on survival time in canine and feline chronic granulocytic patients is unknown.

Monocytic-Myelomonocytic Leukemia. Monocytic leukemia is characterized by the presence of increased numbers of monocytes or monoblasts in blood and bone marrow. Myelomonocytic leukemia is characterized by blast cells with both myeloid and monocytoid characteristics. Both are considered acute leukemias because response to therapy is poor and survival times are generally short.[78] Abnormal cells frequently stain positive for granulocyte (alkaline phosphatase) and monocyte (alpha-naphthyl acetate esterase, lipase) markers.[101,113] Distinguishing between monocytic and myelomonocytic leukemia is often not possible, and it has been suggested the term myelomonocytic leukemia be used to refer to both entities.[113]

The average age of affected dogs is 5.5 years.[8,66,101,113,130,137,159,162,172] Anorexia, depression, weight loss, and fever are frequently manifestations. Pale mucous membranes, hepatosplenomegaly, and slight to moderate lymphadenopathy are generally present. Neurological signs may occur with central nervous system infiltration.

A complete blood count usually reveals macrocytic normochromic or normocytic normochromic anemia, normoblastosis, and leukocytosis. Total white blood cell count may be in excess of 300,000/μl. Myeloblasts, monocytoid cells, or monocytes predominate in blood and bone marrow.

Survival time in untreated dogs with myelomonocytic leukemia is generally less than 3 weeks. In humans, 6-mercaptopurine, cytosine arabinoside, and daunomycin are used singly or in combination in the treatment of acute myeloid leukemias. Survival times and cure rates are generally less in the treatment of acute lymphocytic leukemia.[215] Three dogs with myelomonocytic leukemia were treated with cytosine arabinoside, 6-thioguanine, and prednisone.[101] Two of the dogs were destroyed because of sepsis within 10 days after the onset of chemotherapy, but the third dog survived 8 months.

Monocytic leukemia has been reported in seven cats[86,96,182,205] and myelomonocytic leukemia in four cats.[80,118,174,194] Clinical findings were similar to those described for dogs except for a lack of peripheral lymph node enlargement in cats. Sixty-three per cent of the cats were FeLV positive. Anemia was generally less severe, and leukocyte counts were generally higher (8,000 to 342,000/μl) than in other feline myeloproliferative disorders. Most cats were thrombocytopenic.

Five cats received antileukemia chemotherapy.[86,118,194,205] Cytosine arabinoside, doxorubicin, cyclophosphamide, 6-mercaptopurine, daunorubicin, prednisolone, and vincristine were used alone or in combination. Clinical responses were transient, and average survival time was only 32 days. Three of the cats bled excessively from venipuncture sites just prior to death.[86,205] Necropsy findings in cats with monocytic and myelomonocytic leukemia included widespread organ infiltration, thrombosis, and infarction.

Basophilic Leukemia. Only two well-documented cases of basophilic leukemia have been reported, one in a dog[122] and one in a cat.[85] Some earlier reports of basophilic leukemia cases were probably mast cell leukemias.[144,181]

In dogs, the white blood cell count was 50,000/μl, with an absolute basophil count of 44,500/μl. The platelet count was greater than 1,000,000/μl. Treatment with hydroxyurea resulted in a remission time in excess of 10 months.

The cat with basophilic leukemia had a white blood cell count of 15,700/μl, with an absolute basophil count of 6,594/μl. Moderate anemia and thrombocytopenia were present, and the cat was FeLV positive. Therapy with cytosine arabinoside, cyclophosphamide, and vinblastine was attempted but the cat died 16 days after diagnosis.

Eosinophilic Leukemia. Chronic eosinophilic leukemia is characterized by persistent eosinophilia, with immature and mature eosinophils in the peripheral blood and bone marrow. Some researchers believe that eosinophilic leukemia in humans is part of a group of diseases associated with eosinophilia and eosinophilic infiltrates.

Eosinophilic leukemia has been reported in cats but not in dogs.[96,181,188,189] Clinical findings included weight loss, lethargy, vomiting, and diarrhea. Hemograms revealed mild anemia and white blood cell counts ranging from 42,645 to 244,000/μl, with absolute eosinophil counts of 29,851 to 203,914/μl. The majority of eosinophils were mature. Cats with eosinophilic leukemia were treated with glucocorticoids alone or in combination with cyclophosphamide. Cats treated with glucocorticoids alone showed no improvement in clinical signs or reduction in eosinophil numbers.[181,158,189] One cat treated with prednisone and cyclophosphamide had a temporary reduction in eosinophil numbers.[181] Survival time in treated cats ranged from 3.5 to 16.0 weeks.

A hypereosinophilic syndrome was diagnosed in six cats and was characterized by a combination of eosinophilic enteritis, disseminated eosinophilic infiltrates, and eosinophilic leukemia.[84] Clinical and laboratory findings were similar to those of feline eosinophilic leukemia. One cat was FeLV positive. All cats were treated with glucocorticoids with poor results. Survival time ranged from 1.5 to 16.0 weeks. The relationship between feline hypereosinophilic syndrome and eosinophilic leukemia remains to be clarified.

Megakaryocytic Leukemia. Megakaryocytic leukemia is characterized by megakaryocytic proliferation in the bone marrow and other reticuloendothelial organs. It may occur alone or in combination with other myeloproliferative disorders. Although the disease is uncommon, several canine and feline cases have been reported.[32,71,79,94,140,167,168,196]

Severe progressive anemia is usually present, but leukocyte and platelet counts are variable.[78] Platelet counts may be decreased, normal, or greater than 1,000,000/μl. Dwarf megakaryocytes and undifferentiated blasts predominate in the blood and bone marrow. Megakaryocytes can be identified by their positive staining reaction with alpha-naphthyl acetate esterase.[94] Splenomegaly is typically present. FeLV has been identified in a cat with megakaryocytic leukemia.[71]

Erythremic Myelosis and Erythroleukemia. Erythremic myelosis and erythroleukemia are myeloproliferative disorders characterized by abnormal proliferation of erythrocytes and their precursors.[32,184,215] Acute erythremic myelosis is characterized by proliferation of immature erythrocyte precursors including blasts and undifferentiated stem cells. Chronic erythremic myelosis is characterized by proliferation of more mature erythrocyte precursors.[32,215] If myeloid precursors are identified, the term erythroleukemia is used.[32,68,215] Since myeloid cells are usually found, hematologists have suggested that the term erythroleukemia (acute and chronic) be used when discussing the various forms of this disease.[78]

In cats, the term reticuloendotheliosis has been used to describe a myeloproliferative disorder in which neoplastic cells were identified in the blood and organs of the reticuloendothelial system.[32,37,61,62,80,99,109,175,176,179,207] Neoplastic cells were large round cells with eccentrically located nuclei, finely dispersed to clumped chromatin, prominent nucleoli, and basophilic cytoplasm. The cytoplasm often contained reddish-brown granules. Recent electron microscopic studies have indicated that these cells are early erythroid precursors, not reticuloendothelial cells. Consequently, it has been suggested the terms

acute erythroleukemia or acute erythemic myelosis be used in place of reticuloendotheliosis.[32,99,133]

Numerous cases of erythroleukemia and erythemic myelosis have been reported in cats,[32,53,80,87,89,133,168,169,175,177,178,179,183,191,207,208,220] but the disease is rare in the dog. Clinical findings include weight loss, anorexia, lethargy, pale mucous membranes, splenomegaly, and less frequently, lymphadenopathy, hepatomegaly, and fever. Male cats are affected more often than females. Most cats are FeLV positive.[37,71]

The progressive anemia that occurs with erythroleukemia is more severe than in other myeloproliferative disorders. Leukocyte counts are variable (average = 22,000/μl) but tend to be lower than counts seen with granulocytic or myelomonocytic leukemias. In one report, 27 of 36 cats with acute and chronic erythroleukemia had left shifts, and in 14 of these cats, shifts were back to the level of myelocytes, promyelocytes, and myeloblasts.[175]

Immature erythrocytes may constitute up to 55 per cent of the total leukocyte count in acute erythroleukemia patients.[61] Increased numbers of macrocytic and megaloblastic nucleated red blood cells, some with bizarre multinucleated forms, predominated in chronic erythremic myelosis and erythroleukemia.[175] Bone marrow aspirates are cellular, with erythroid precursors predominating.

In humans, erythroleukemia may begin with a preleukemic state characterized by chronic cytopenias and refractory anemia. Erythroleukemia, often with megakaryocytic and platelet abnormalities, develops followed by acute (blastic) leukemia or myelofibrosis.[170] In cats, a progression from a preleukemic or erythroleukemic state to a predominately granulocytic leukemia has been noted.[37,62,89,118,176,178,179,207] A progression from erythremic myelosis to acute erythroleukemia (reticuloendotheliosis) has also been observed.[80] Myelofibrosis may be terminal.

With supportive treatment including blood transfusions, fluids, antibiotics, and vitamin-mineral supplements, cats with acute and chronic erythroleukemia survived 2 to 8 weeks. Treatment of four cats with various combinations of cytosine arabinoside, prednisone, cyclophosphamide, and 6-thioguanine resulted in decreased numbers of neoplastic cells in the peripheral blood in three of the cats.[37] Average survival time from diagnosis was 52 days. Death was often attributable to infection, hemorrhage, or organ dysfunction. At necropsy, splenomegaly is a consistent finding, with lymph node and liver enlargements being less common. Histopathology of these organs reveals various degrees of neoplastic infiltration. Other organs are rarely involved.

Primary Polycythemia. Primary polycythemia, or polycythemia vera, is a chronic myeloproliferative disease characterized by an increased hematocrit, red cell mass, and hemoglobin concentration resulting from clonal proliferation of red blood cell precursors. Serum erythropoietin concentration is normal or decreased. Increased red blood cell production results from increased sensitivity of red blood cell precursors to the effects of erythropoietin.[91] The cause of the alteration in sensitivity is unknown.

Primary polycythemia must be differentiated from relative polycythemia and secondary polycythemia. In relative polycythemia, the venous packed cell volume is modestly increased (55 to 65 per cent), but red blood cell mass is normal or decreased.[153] Relative polycythemia usually results from hemoconcentration secondary to intravascular fluid loss. Secondary polycythemia results from excessive erythropoietin produced in response to hypoxia (cardiac or pulmonary disease, hemoglobinopathy, renal cysts, hydronephrosis, polycystic kidneys) or produced by tumors (renal carcinomas, hepatomas, uterine leiomyomas, cerebellar hemangioblastomas). Packed cell volume and red blood cell mass are increased.

Primary polycythemia is rare in dogs and cats. The average age of 11 reported canine cases was 4.3 years (range = 1 to 7 years).[135,153] No predilection for breed or sex was documented. Clinical signs included polyuria and polydipsia (63 per cent), weakness (45 per cent), hemorrhage (45 per cent), seizures (10 per cent), and vomiting or diarrhea (27 per cent). Physical examination revealed hyperemic mucous membranes (100 per cent), splenomegaly (27 per cent), neurological abnormalities (18 per cent), and aortic thrombosis (10 per cent). Thrombotic and neurological complications are thought to result from hyperviscosity, which impairs blood flow.[91]

Hemograms from affected dogs revealed increased hematocrits, red blood cell counts, and hemoglobin concentrations. Hematocrits were usually between 70 and 80 per cent. White blood cell counts and platelet counts were generally normal. In humans, leucocytosis and thrombocytosis are frequent findings.[91]

The only documented feline case of primary polycythemia occurred in a 15-year-old castrated Maltese cat.[160] Dark red-purple mucous membranes was the only abnormal physical finding. Serial hemograms revealed elevations in packed cell volume, hemoglobin concentration, red blood cell count, and white blood cell count.

Red blood cell mass can be calculated following injection of red blood cells labeled with chromium 51.[9] Five polycythemic dogs had red blood cell masses of 70 to 120 ml/kg of body weight (normal = 43.9 ± 5.8 mg/kg of body weight).[135] The single polycythemic cat had a red blood cell mass of 46.3 ml/kg (normal = 19 ml/kg).[160]

Electrocardiography, arterial oxygen tension determination, hemoglobin electrophoresis and intravenous urography performed to rule out causes of secondary polycythemia are all normal.[135,153] In three dogs with primary polycythemia, serum erythropoietin concentration was undetectable.[152]

Primary polythemia has been treated by phlebotomy,[32]P, and administration of cancer chemotherapeutic agents. Reduction in packed cell volume by phlebotomy alleviates many of the acute signs. Removal of 40 ml of blood per kilogram body weight results in a reduction of packed cell volume of approximately 15 per cent.[135] Phlebotomy is repeated as needed to maintain the packed cell volume within the normal range.

The combined use of phlebotomy and ^{32}P or a cancer chemotherapeutic agent can be used for long-term management. Survival times of 1 to 2 years are typical. Radioactive phosphorus is incorporated into the endosteum of bone marrow following oral or intravenous administration. Beta particles released by ^{32}P decrease bone marrow activity. Several months may elapse before the hematocrit returns to normal.[16] An alternative to ^{32}P is the use of chemotherapy. Chlorambucil has been the drug of choice in humans, although a recent report has linked its use to an increased risk of leukemia in primary polycythemia patients.[12] Hydroxyurea has been successfully used to manage primary polycythemia in dogs.[152] Mean remission time was 16.6 months in three dogs treated with hydroxyurea.

1. Ackerman, N., and Madewell, B. R.: Thoracic and abdominal radiographic abnormalities in the multicentric form of lymphosarcoma in dogs. J. Am. Vet. Med. Assoc. 176:36, 1980.
2. Aisenberg, A. C.: Cell surface markers in lymphoproliferative disease. N. Engl. J. Med. 304:331, 1981.
3. Altman, N. H., and Squire, R. A.: Diagnosis of canine lymphoma. J. Am. Vet. Med. Assoc. 157:1676, 1970.
4. Anderson, L. J., and Jarrett, W. F.: Membranous glomerulonephritis associated with leukemia in cats. Res. Vet. Sci. 12:179, 1971.
5. Anderson, L. J., Jarrett, W. F. H., and Crighton, G. W.: A classification of lymphoid neoplasms of domestic animals. Natl. Inst. Cancer. Monogr. 32:343, 1968.
6. Backgren, A. W.: Lymphatic leukosis in dogs. Acta Vet. Scand. 6:(Suppl), 1965.
7. Banyard, M. R., and Taylor, L.: Myeloproliferative disease in a cat. Aust. Vet. Pract. 6:109, 1976.
8. Barthel, C. M.: Acute myelomonocytic leukemia in a dog. Vet. Path. 11:79, 1974.
9. Baum, S. and Bramlet, R.: Basic Nuclear Medicine. Appleton-Century-Crofts, New York, 1975.
10. Benabe, J. E., and Martinez-Maldonado, M.: Hypercalcemic nephropathy. Arch. Intern. Med. 138:777, 1978.
11. Benjamini, E., Theilen, G. H., Torten, M., et al.: Tumor vaccines for immunotherapy of canine lymphosarcoma. Ann. N.Y. Acad; Sci. 277:305, 1976.
12. Berk, P. D., Goldberg, J. D., Silverstein, M. N. et al.: Increased incidence of acute leukemia in polycythemia vera associated with chlorambucil therapy. N. Engl. J. Med. 304:441, 1981.
13. Braund, K. G., Everett, R. M., and Albert, R. A.: Neurologic manifestations of monoclonal IgM gammopathy associated with lymphocytic leukemia in a dog. J. Am. Vet. Med. Assoc. 172:1407, 1978.
14. Brick, J. O., Roenigk, W. J., and Wilson, G. P.: Chemotherapy of malignant lymphoma in dogs and cats. J. Am. Vet. Med. Assoc. 153:47, 1968.
15. Brown, N. O., Nesbitt, G. H., Patnaik, A. K., and MacEwen, E. G.: Cutaneous lymphosarcoma in the dog: A disease with variable clinical and histologic manifestations. J. Am. Anim. Hosp. Assoc. 16:565, 1980.
16. Bush, B. M., and Fankhauser, R.: Polycythemia vera in a bitch. J. Small Anim. Pract. 13:75, 1972;
17. Calvert, C. A., Dawe, D., Leifer, C. E., and Brown, J.: Lymphocyte blastogenesis in dogs with lymphosarcoma. Am. J. Vet. Res. 43:94, 1982

18. Calvert, C. A., and Leifer, C. E.: Salmonellosis in dogs with lymphosarcoma J. Am. Vet. Med. Assoc. 180:56, 1982.

19. Carlton, W. W.: Intraocular lymphosarcoma: Two cases in siamese cats. J. Am. Anim. Hosp. Assoc. 12:83, 1976.

20. Carpenter, J. L., and Holzworth, J.: Treatment of leukemia in the cat. J. Am. Vet. Med. Assoc. 158:1130, 1971.

21. Case, M. T.: A case of myelogenous leukemia in the cat. Zentralbl Veterinarmed 17A:273, 1970.

22. Chapman, A. L., Bopp, W. J., Brightwell, A. S., et al.: Preliminary report on virus-like particles in canine leukemia and derived cell cultures. Cancer Res. 27:18, 1967.

23. Chew, D. J., and Meuten, D. J.: Disorders of calcium and phosphorus metabolism. Vet. Clin. North Amer.: J. Small Anim. Pract. 12:411, 1982.

24. Chew, D. J., Schaer, M., Liu, S., and Owens, J.: Pseudo-hyperparathyroidism in a cat. J. Am. Anim. Hosp. Assoc. 11:46, 1975.

25. Cohen, H., Chapman, A. L., Elbert, J. W., et al.: Cellular transmission of canine lymphoma and leukemia in beagles. J. Natl. Inst. Cancer 45:1013, 1970.

26. Coltman, C. A.: Management of unfavorable histology non-Hodgkin's lymphomas. In Carter, S. K., Glatstein, E., and Livingston, R. B. (eds): Principles of Cancer Treatment, New York, McGraw-Hill Book Company, 1982. pp. 824-331.

27. Conroy, J. D.: Canine skin tumors. J. Am. Anim. Hosp. Assoc. 19:91, 1983.

28. Cooper, B. J., and Watson, A. D. J.: Myeloid neoplasia in a dog. Aust. Vet. J. 5:150, 1975.

29. Cossman, J., and Bernard, C. W.: Malignant lymphomas: The role of immunologic markers in diagnosis, subclassification and management. Hum. Pathol. 11:309, 1980.

30. Cotter, S. M.: Treatment of lymphoma and leukemia with cyclophosphamide, vincristine, and prednisone: II. Treatment of cats. J. Am. Anim. Hosp. Assoc. 19:166, 1983.

31. Cotter, S. M : Feline leukemia virus-associated diseases. In Kirk, R. W. (ed.): Current Veterinary Therapy VI. Philadelphia, W. B., Saunders, 1977, pp. 465–472.

32. Cotter, S. M., Hardy, W. D., Jr., and Essex, M.: Association of feline leukemia virus with lymphosarcoma and other disorders in the cat. J. Am. Vet. Med. Assoc. 166:449, 1975.

33. Crighton, G. W.: Lymphosarcoma in the cat. Vet. Rec. 84:329, 1969.

34. Crighton, G. W.: Clinical aspects of lymphosarcoma in the cat. Vet. Rec. 82:122, 1968.

35. Crighton, G. W.: The hematology of lymphosarcoma in the cat. Vet. Rec. 82:155, 1968.

36. Crow, S. E.: Lymphosarcoma (malignant lymphoma) in the dog: Diagnosis and treatment. J. Cont. Ed. Small Anim. Pract. 4:283, 1982.

37. Crow, S. E., Madewell, B. R., and Henness, A. M.: Feline reticuloendotheliosis: A report of four cases. J. Am. Vet. Med. Assoc. 170:1329, 1977.

38. Crow, S. E., Theilen, G. H., Benjamini, E., et al.: Chemoimmunotherapy for canine lymphosarcoma. Cancer 40:2102, 1977.

39. Dameshek, W.: Some speculations on the myeloproliferative syndromes. Blood 6:372, 1951.

40. Dewhirst, M. W., Stamp, G. L., and Hurvitz, A. I.: Idiopathic monoclonal (IgA) gammopathy in a dog. J. Am. Vet. Med. Assoc. 170:1313, 1977.

41. Dorn, R. C., Taylor, D. N., and Hibbard, H. H.: Epizootiologic characteristics of canine and feline leukemia and lymphoma. Am. J. Vet. Res. 28:993, 1967.

42. Dorn, R. C., Taylor, D. N., Schneider, R., et al.: Survey of animal neoplasms in Alameda and Contra Costa counties, California. II. Cancer morbidity in dogs and cats from Alameda county. J. Natl. Cancer Inst. 40:307, 1968.

43. Drazner, F. H.: Multiple myeloma in the cat. J. Cont. Ed. Vet. Pract. 4:206, 1982.

44. Dreyfus, B.: Preleukemia states: I. Definition and classification, II. Refractory anemia with an excess of myeloblasts in the bone marrow (smoldering acute leukemia). Blood Cells 2:33, 1976.

45. Duncan, J. R., and Prasse, K. W.: Cytology of canine cutaneous round cell tumors. Vet. Pathol. 16:673, 1979.

46. Dungworth, D. L., Goldman, M., Switzer, J. W., and McKenzie, D. H.: Development of a myeloproliferative disorder in beagles continuously exposed to ^{90}Sr. Blood 34:610, 1969.

47. Dust, A. M., and Valli, V. E. O.: Cutaneous lymphosarcoma with IgG monoclonal gammopathy, serum hyperviscosity and hypercalcemia in a cat. Can. Vet. J. 23:235, 1982.

48. Dutta, S. K., Novilla, M. N., Bumgardner, M. K., and Ingling, A.: Lymphocyte responsiveness to mitogens and quantitation to T and B lymphocytes in canine malignant lymphoma. Am. J. Vet. Res. 39:455, 1978.

49. Engle, G. C., and Brody, R. S.: A restrospective study of 395 feline neoplasms. J. Am. Anim. Hosp. Assoc. 5:21, 1969.

50. Essex, M., Cotter, S. M., Hardy, W. D., Jr., et al.: Feline oncornavirus-associated cell membrane antigen. IV. Antibody titers in cats with naturally occurring leukemia, lymphoma, and other diseases. J. Nat. Can. Inst. 55:463, 1975.

51. Evans, S. M., and De Frate, L. A.: Gastric lymphosarcoma in a dog: A case report. Am. Coll. Vet. Radiol. 21:55, 1980.

52. Eyestone, W. H.: Myelogenous leukemia in the cat. J. Natl. Cancer Inst. 12:599, 1951.

53. Falconer, G. J., Irving, A. C., Watson, P. R., and Ludwig J.: A case of erythemic myelosis in a cat. N. Z. Vet. J. 28:83, 1980.

54. Feeney, D. A., Klausner, J. S., and Johnston, G. R.,: Chronic bowel obstruction caused by primary intestinal neoplasia: A report of five cases. J. Am. Anim. Hosp. Assoc. 18:67, 1982.

55. Flecknell, P. A., Gibbs, C., and Kelly D. F.: Myelosclerosis in a cat. J. Comp. Pathol. 88:627, 1978.

56. Fox, J. G., and Gutnick, M. J.: Horner's syndrome and brachial paralysis due to lymphosarcoma in a cat. J. Am. Vet. Med. Assoc. 160:977, 1972.

57. Francis, D. P., Cotter, S. M., Hardy, W. D., Jr., and Essex, M.: Comparison of virus positive and virus negative cases of feline leukemia and lymphoma. Cancer Res. 39:3866, 1979.

58. Francis, D. P., Essex, M., Cotter, S. M., et al.: Epidemiologic association between virus negative feline leukemia and horizontally transmitted feline leukemia virus. Cancer lett. 12:37, 1981.

59. Francis, D. P., Essex, M., and Hardy, W. D., Jr.: Excretion of leukemia virus by naturally injected pet cats. Nature 269:252, 1977.

60. Fraser, C. J., Joiner, G. N., Jardine, J. H., and Gleiser, C. A.: Acute granulocytic leukemia in cats. J. Am. Vet. Med. Assoc. 165:355, 1974.

61. Giles, R. C., Buhles, W. C., and Montgomery, C. A.: Myeloproliferative disorder in a cat. J. Am. Vet. Med. Assoc. 165:456, 1974.

62. Gilmore, C. E., Gilmore, V. H., and Jones, T. C.: Reticuloendotheliosis, a myeloproliferative disorder in cats: A comparison with lymphocytic leukemia. Vet. Pathol. 1:161, 1964.

63. Gilmore, C. E., and Holzworth, J.: Naturally occurring feline leukemia: Clinical, pathologic, and differential diagnostic features. J. Am. Vet. Med. Assoc. 158:1013, 1971.

64. Glick, A. D., Horn, R. G., and Holscher, M.: Characterization of feline glomerulonephritis associated with viral-induced hematopoietic neoplasms. Am. J. Pathol. 92:321, 1978.

65. Goh, K. O., Smith, R. A., and Proper, J. S.: Chromosomal aberrations in leukemic cats. Cornell Vet. 71:43, 1981.

66. Green, R. A., and Barton, C. L.: Acute myelomonocytic leukemia in a dog. J. Am. Anim. Hosp. Assoc. 13:708, 1977.

67. Grindem, C.: Unpublished observations.

68. Gunz, F. W.: Erythroleukemia. In Williams, W. J., Beutter, E., Evslev, A. J., and Rundles, R. W. (eds): Hematology. 2nd ed. New York, McGraw-Hill Book Co., 1977, pp. 802–806.

69. Hardy, W. D., Jr.: Feline leukemia virus non-neoplastic diseases. J. Am. Anim. Hosp. Assoc. 17:941, 1981.

70. Hardy, W. D., Jr.: The feline leukemia virus. J. Am. Anim. Hosp. Assoc. 17:921, 1981.

71. Hardy, W. D., Jr.: Hematopoietic tumors of cats. J. Am. Anim. Hosp. Assoc. 17:921, 1981.

72. Hardy, W. D., Jr.: The feline sarcoma viruses. J. Am. Anim. Hosp. Assoc. 17:981, 1981.

73. Hardy, W. D., Jr.: The virology, immunology and epidemiology of feline leukemia virus In Hardy, W. D., Jr., Essex, M., and McClelland, A. J. (eds.): Feline Leukemia Virus. Elsevier North Holland, New York, 1980.

74. Hardy, W. D., Jr., Hess, P. W., MacEwen, E. G., et al.: Biology of feline leukemia virus in the natural environment. Cancer Res. 36:582, 1976.

75. Hardy, W. D., Jr., McClelland, A. J., Zuckerman, E. E., et al.: Development of virus non-producer lymphosarcomas in pet cats exposed to FeLV. Nature 288:90, 1980.

76. Hardy, W. D., Jr., MacEwen, E. G., Hayes, A. A., and Zuckerman, E. E.: FOCMA antibody as specific immunotherapy for lymphosarcoma of pet cats. In Hardy, W. D., Jr., Essex, M., and McClelland, A. J. (eds.): Feline Leukemia Virus New York, Elsevier North Holland, 1980, pp. 227–233.

77. Hardy, W. D., Jr., Old, L. J., Hess, P. W., et al.: Horizontal transmission of feline leukemia virus. Nature 244:266, 1973.

78. Harvey, J. W.: Myeloproliferative disorders in dogs and cats. Vet. Clin. North Am. Small Anim. Pract. 11:349, 1981.

79. Harvey, J. W., Henderson, C. W., French, T. W., et al.: Myeloproliferative disease with megakaryocytic predominance in a dog with occult dirofilariasis. Vet. Clin. Pathol. 11:5, 1982.

80. Harvey, J. W., Shields, R. P., and Gaskin, J. M.: Feline myeloproliferative disease. Changing manifestations in the peripheral blood. Vet. Pathol. 15:437, 1978.

81. Harvey, J. W., Terrell, T. G., Hyde, D. M., and Jackson, R. I.: Well-differentiated lymphocytic leukemia in a dog: Long-term survival without therapy. Vet. Pathol. 18:37, 1981.

82. Hause, W. R., and Olsen, R. G.: Clinical aspects of feline leukemia diseases. In Olson, R. G. (ed.): Feline Leukemia. CRC Press, Inc., Boca Raton, Florida, 1981, pp. 89–114.

83. Heath, H., Weller, R. E., and Mundy, G. R.: Canine lymphosarcoma: A model for study of the hypercalcemia of cancer. Calcif. Tissue Int. 30:127, 1980.

84. Hendrick, M.: A spectrum of hypereosinophilic syndromes exemplified by six cats with eosinophilic enteritis. Vet. Pathol. 18:188, 1981.

85. Henness, A. M., and Crow, S. E.: Treatment of feline myelogenous leukemia: Four case reports. J. Am. Vet. Med. Assoc. 171:263, 1977.

86. Henness, A. M., Crow, S. E., and Anderson, B. C.: Monocytic leukemia in three cats. J. Am. Vet. Med. Assoc. 170:1325, 1977.

87. Herz, A., Theilen, G. H., Schalm, O. W., and Munn, R. J.: C-type virus in bone marrow cells of cats with myeloproliferative disorders. J. Natl. Cancer Inst. 44:339, 1970.

88. Herz, A., Thelen, G. H., Schalm, O. W., and Munn, R. J.: C-type virus particles demonstrated in bone marrow cells of a cat with myeloproliferative disease. Calif. Vet. 23:16, 1969.

89. Herz, A., Theilen, G. H., Schalm, O. W., and Munn, R. J.: Demonstration of C-type virus particles, Toxoplasma gondii and Hemobartonella felis in a cat with a myeloproliferative disorder. Calif. Vet. 23:18, 1969.

90. Hodgkins, E. M., Zinkl, J. G., and Madewell, B. R.: Chronic lymphatic leukemia in the dog. J. Am. Vet. Med. Assoc. 177:704, 1980.

91. Hoffman, R., and Wasserman, L. R.: Natural history of polycythemia vera. Adv. Intern. Med. 24:255, 1979.

92. Holmberg, C. A., Manning, J. S., and Osburn, B. I.: Canine malignant lymphomas: Comparison of morphologic and immunologic parameters. J. Natl. Inst. Cancer 56:125, 1976.

93. Holmberg, C. A., Manning, J. S., and Osburn, B. I.: Feline malignant lymphomas: Comparison of morphologic and immunologic characteristics. Am. J. Vet. Res. 37:1455, 1976.

94. Holscher, M. A., Collins, R. D., Glick, A. D., and Griffith, B. O.: Megakaryocytic leukemia in a dog. Vet. Pathol. 15:562, 1978.

95. Holzworth, J.: Leukemia and related neoplasms in the cat. J. Am. Vet. Med. Assoc. 136:47, 1960.

96. Holzworth, J.: Leukemia and related neoplasms in the cat. II. Malignancies other than lymphoid. J. Am. Vet. Med. Assoc. 136:107, 1960.

97. Hoover, E. A., and Kociba, G. J.: Bone lesions in cats with anemia induced by feline leukemia virus. J. Natl. Cancer Inst. 53:1277, 1974.

98. Howard, E. B., Nielsen, S. W., and Kenyon, A. J.: Cutaneous lymphomatosis in a boxer dog. Vet. Pathol. 6:76, 1969.

99. Hurvitz, A. I.: Fine structure of cells from a cat with myeloproliferative disorder. Am. J. Vet. Res. 31:747, 1970.

100. Jain, N. C.: Alkaline phosphatase activity in the canine and feline granulocytes. Vet. Rec. 81:266, 1967.

101. Jain, N. C., Madewell, B. R., Weller, R. E., and Grissler, M. C.: Clinical-pathological findings and cytochemical characteristics of myelomonocytic leukemia in five dogs. J. Comp. Pathol. 91:17, 1981.

102. Jarrett, W. F. H.: Cat leukemia. Vet. Rec. 85:553, 1969.

103. Jarrett, W. F., Anderson, L. J., Jarrett, O., et al.: Myeloid leukemia in a cat produced experimentally by feline leukemia virus. Res. Vet. Sci. 12:385, 1971.

104. Jarrett, W. F. H., Crawford, E. M., Martin, W. B., and Davie, F.: Leukemia in the cat. Nature 202:566, 1964.

105. Jarrett, W. F. H., Crighton, G. W., and Dalton, R. G.: Leukemia and lymphosarcoma in animals and man. Vet. Rec. 79:693, 1966.

106. Jarrett, O., Golder, M. C., and Weijer, K.: A comparison of three methods of feline leukemia virus diagnosis. Vet. Rec. 110:325, 1982.

107. Joiner, C. N., Fraser, C. J., Jardine, J. H., and Trujillo, J. M.: A case of chronic granulocytic leukemia in a dog. Can. J. Comp. Med. 40:153, 1976.

108. Kahn, D. E., Mia, A. S., and Tierney, M. M.: Field evaluation of Leukassay *F; an FeLV detection test kit. Feline Pract. 10:41, 1980.

109. Knauer, K. W., and Pierce, K. R.: Feline reticuloendotheliosis. Southwest Vet. 23:53, 1969.

110. Legendre, A. M., and Becker, P. U.: Feline skin lymphoma: Characteristics of tumor and identification of tumor stimulating serum factor(s). Am. J. Vet. Res. 40:1805, 1979.

111. Lewis, H. D., and Rebar, A. H.: Bone Marrow Evaluation in Veterinary Practice. Ralston Purina Company, St. Louis, 1979, p 9.

112. Linman, J. W., and Bagby, G. C.: The preleukemic syndrome: Clinical and laboratory features, natural course, and management. Blood Cells 2:11, 1976.

113. Linnabary, R. D., Holscher, M. A., Glick, A. D., et al.: Acute myelomonocytic leukemia in a dog. J. Am. Anim. Hosp. Assoc. 14:71, 1978.

114. Loeb, W. F.: Blood and blood-forming organs. In Catcott, E. J. (ed.): Feline Medicine and Surgery. 2nd ed. American Veterinary Publications, Inc, Santa Barbara, 1975, pp. 246.

115. Lucke, V. M., and Sumner-Smith, G.: A case of myeloid leukaemia in the dog. J. Small Anim. Pract. 4:23, 1963.

116. Madewell, B. R: Chemotherapy for canine lymphosarcoma. Am. J. Vet. Res. 36:1525, 1975.

117. Madewell, B. R., and Feldman, B. F.: Characterization of anemias associated with neoplasia in small animals. J. Am. Vet. Med. Assoc. 176:419, 1980.

118. Madewell, B. R., Jain, N. C., and Weller, R. E.: Hematologic abnormalities preceding myeloid leukemia in three cats. Vet. Pathol. 16:510, 1979.

119. Madewell, B. R., and Theilen, G. H.: Chemotherapy. In

Theilen, G. H., and Madewell, B. R. (eds): *Veterinary Cancer Medicine*. Lea & Febiger, Philadelphia, 1979, pp. 95–112.

120. MacEwen, E. G.: Canine lymphosarcoma. *In* Kirk, R. W. (ed): *Current Veterinary Therapy VII*, W. B. Saunders, Philadelphia, 1980, pp. 419–422.

121. MacEwen, E. G., Brown, N. O., Patnaik, A. K., et al.: Cyclic combination chemotherapy of canine lymphosarcoma. J. Am. Vet. Med. Assoc. 178:1178, 1981.

122. MacEwen, E. G., Drazner, F. H., McClelland, A. J., and Wilkins, R. J.: Treatment of basophilic leukemia in a dog. J. Am. Vet. Med. Assoc. 106:376, 1975.

123. MacEwen, E. G., and Hurvitz, A. I.: Diagnosis and management of monoclonal gammopathies. Vet. Clin. North. Am. 7:119, 1977.

124. MacEwen, E. G., Hurvitz, A. I., and Hayes, A.: Hyperviscosity syndrome associated with lymphocytic leukemia in three dogs. J. Am. Vet. Med. Assoc. 170:1309, 1977.

125. MacEwen, E. G., Mooney, S., Hayes, A. A., and Harvey, H. J.: Combination chemotherapy of naturally occurring feline lymphosarcoma. Proc. 12th Int. Cancer Res. Cong., Buenos Aires, Argentina. Pergamon Press, New York, 1978.

126. MacEwen, E. G., Patnaik, A. K., and Wilkins, R. J.: Diagnosis and treatment of canine hematopoietic neoplasms. Vet. Clin. North. Am. 7:105, 1977.

127. Mackey, L. J., and Jarrett, W. F.: Pathogenesis of lymphoid neoplasia in cats and its relationship to immunologic cell pathways. I. Morphologic aspects. J. Natl. Cancer Inst. 49:853, 1972.

128. Mackey, L., Jarrett, W., Jarrett, O., and Laird, H. M.: Anemia associated with feline leukemia virus infection in cats. J. Natl. Cancer Inst. 54:209, 1975.

129. Mackey, L. J., Jarrett, W. F. H., Jarrett, O., and Laird, H. M.: An experimental study of virus leukemia in cats. J. Natl. Cancer Inst. 48:1663, 1972.

130. Mackey, L. J., Jarrett, W. F. M., and Lauder, I. M.: Monocytic leukemia in the dog. Vet. Rec. 96:27, 1975.

131. MacVean, D. W., Monlux, A. W., Anderson, P. S., et al.: Frequency of canine and feline tumors in a defined population. Vet. Pathol. 15:700, 1978.

132. Macy, D. W.: Canine malignant lymphoma, Illinois Vet. 16:9, 1973.

133. Maede, Y., and Murata, H.: Erythroleukemia in a cat with special reference to the fine structure of primitive cells in its peripheral blood. Jpn. J. Vet. Sci. 42:531, 1980.

134. Maggio, L., Hoffman, F., Cotter, S. M., et al.: Feline preleukemia: An animal model of human disease. Yale J. Biol. Med. 51:469, 1978.

135. McGrath, C. J.: Polycythemia vera in dogs. J. Am. Vet. Med. Assoc. 164:1117, 1974.

136. McKeever, D. J, Grindem, C. B., Stevens, J. B., and Osborne, CA.: Canine cutaneous lymphoma; J. Am. Vet. Med. Assoc. 180:531, 1982.

137. Meier, H.: Neoplastic diseases of the hematopoietic system in the dog. Zentralbl Veterinarmed 4:633, 1957.

138. Meier, H., and Patterson, D. F.: Myelogenous leukemia in a cat. J. Am. Vet. Med. Assoc. 126:211, 1956.

139. Meincke, J. E., Hobbie, W. V., Jr., and Hardy, W. D., Jr.: Lymphoreticular malignancies in the cat: Clinical findings. J. Am. Vet. Med. Assoc. 160:1093, 1972.

140. Michel, R. L., O'Handley, P., and Dade, A. W.: Megakaryocytic myelosis in a cat. J. Am. Vet. Med. Assoc. 168:1021, 1976.

141. Miller, W. H.: Canine cutaneous lymphomas. *In* Kirk, R. W. (ed.): *Current Veterinary Therapy VII*. W. B. Saunders, Philadelphia, 1980, pp. 493–495.

142. Moldovanu, G., Friedman, M., and Miller, D. G.: Treatment of canine malignant lymphoma with surgery and chemotherapy. J. Am. Vet. Med. Assoc. 148:153, 1966.

143. Nielsen, S. W.: Classification of tumors in dogs and cats. J. Am. Anim. Hosp. Assoc. 19:13, 1983.

144. Neilsen, S. W.: Myeloproliferative disorders in animals. *In* Clark, J. J., Howard, E. G., and Hackett, P. L. (ed.): *Myeloproliferative Disorders in Animals and Man*. Oak Ridge, USAEC Division of Technical Information Extension, 1970.

145. Northington, J. W., and Juliana, M. M.: Extradural lymphosarcoma in six cats. J. Small Anim. Pract. 19:409, 1978.

146. Old, L. J., Boyse, E. A., Campbell, H. A., et al.: Treatment of lymphosarcoma in the dog with l-asparginase. Cancer 20:1066, 1967.

147. Onions, D.: B and T-cell markers on canine lymphosarcoma cells. J. Natl. Cancer Inst. 59:1001, 1977.

148. Osborne, C. A., and Johnston, S. D.: Ectopic hormone production by nonendocrine neoplasmas. *In* Kirk, R. W. (ed.): *Current Veterinary Therapy VI*, W. B. Saunders, Philadelphia, 1977. pp. 1061–1067.

149. Osborne, C. A., Perman, V., Sautter, J. H., et al.: Multiple myeloma in the dog. J. Am. Vet. Med. Assoc. 153:1300, 1968.

150. Osborne, C. A., and Stevens, J. B.: Hypercalcemic nephropathy. *In* Kirk, R. W. (ed.): *Current Veterinary Therapy VI*, W. B. Saunders, Philadelphia, 1977, pp. 1080–1087.

151. Petersen, N. C., Theilen, G., Keane, M. A , et al.: Studies of naturally transmitted feline leukemia virus infection. Am. J. Vet. Res. 38:1523, 1977.

152. Peiffer, R. L., Jeraj, K., Mehlhoff, T., and O'Leary, T. P.: Lymphosarcoma: Small lymphocyte type with ocular manifestations in a dog. Canine Pract. 3:50, 1976.

153. Peterson, M. E., and Randolph, J. F.: Diagnosis of canine polycythemia and management with hydroxyurea. J. Am. Vet. Med. Assoc. 180:415, 1982.

154. Pollet, L., Van Hove, W., and Mattheeuws, D.: Blastic crisis in chronic myelogenous leukaemia in a dog. J. Small Anim. Pract. 19:469, 1978.

155. Prasse, K. W.: White blood cell disorders. *In* Ettinger, S. J. (ed.): *Textbook of Veterinary Internal Medicine*. 2nd ed. W. B. Saunders, Philadelphia, 1983, pp. 2035.

156. Priester, W. A., and Mantel, N.: Occurrence of tumors in domestic animals. Data from 12 United States and Canadian colleges of veterinary medicine. J. Natl. Cancer Inst. 47:1333, 1971.

157. Priester, W. A., and McRay, F. W.: The occurrence of tumors in domestic animals. Bethesda, MD, NCI Monograph #54, NIH Publication #80-2046, 1980.

158. Quesenberry, P., and Levitt, L.: Hematopoietic stem cells. N. Engl. J. Med. 301:755, 1979.

159. Ragan, H. A., Hackett, P. L., and Dagle, G. E.: Acute myelomonocytic leukemia manifested as myelophthisic anemia in a dog. J. Am. Vet. Med. Assoc. 169:421, 1976.

160. Reed, C., Ling, G. V., Gould, D., and Kaneko, J. J.: Polycythemia vera in a cat. J. Am. Vet. Med. Assoc. 157:85, 1970.

161. Reid, J. S., and Marcus, L. C.: Granulocytic leukemia in a cat. J. Small Anim. Pract. 7:421, 1966.

162. Rohrig, K. E.: Acute myelomonocytic leukemia in a dog. J. Am. Vet. Med. Assoc. 182:137, 1983.

163. Rojko, J. L., Hoover, E. A., Matthes, L. E., et al.: Pathogenesis of experimental feline leukemia virus infection. J. Natl. Cancer Inst. 63:759, 1979.

164. Roscher, A. A., Boatwright, R. S., Kupper, H. G., and Egdhal, R. H.: Acute myelogenous leukemia. J. Am. Vet. Med. Assoc. 136:491, 1960.

165. Rosin, A.: Neurologic disease associated with lymphosarcoma in ten dogs. J. Am. Vet. Med. Assoc. 181:50, 1982.

166. Rouse, B. J., Osborne, A. D., and Grunsell, C. S.: Acute granulocytic leukaemia in a bitch. Vet. Rec. 80:408, 1967.

167. Rudolph, R., and Hubner, C.: Megakaryozytenleukase beim hund. Kleintier-Praxis 17:9, 1972.

168. Saar, V. C.: Erythro-megakaryozythamie bei einer Katze. Berl. Munch. Tierarztl. Wochenschr. 83:70, 1970.

169. Saar, V. C.: Erythramie und Erythroleukamie bei der Katze. Berl. Munch. Tierarztl. Wochenschr. 81:423, 1968,

170. Saarni, M. I., and Linman, J. W.: Myelomonocytic leukemia: Disorderly proliferation of all marrow cells. Cancer 27:1221, 1971.

171. Sarma, P. S., and Log, T.: Subgroup classification of feline leukemia and sarcoma viruses by viral interference and neutralization tests. Virology 54:160, 1973.

172. Schalm, O. W.: Acute monocytic leukemia. Canine Pract. 3:19, 1976.

173. Schalm, O. W.: The feline leukemia complex. I. Introduction and leukemic leukemias. Feline Prac. 6:32, 1976.

174. Schalm, O. W : The feline leukemia complex. II. Less common forms of leukemic leukemia. Feline Prac. 6:36, 1976.

175. Schalm, O. W.: Myeloproliferative disorders in the cat. Calif. Vet. 30:32, 1976.

176. Schalm, O. W.: Myeloproliferative disorders in the cats. I. Reticuloendotheliosis. Feline Prac. 5:16, 1975.

177. Schalm, O. W : Myeloproliferative disorders in the cat: II. Erythremic myelosis. Feline Prac. 5:20, 1975.

178. Schalm, O. W.: Myeloproliferative disorders in the cat: IV. Progression from erythroleukemia into granulocytic leukemia. Feline Prac. 5:31, 1975.

179. Schalm, O. W.: Myeloproliferative disorders in a cat with a period of remission followed by a relapse two years later. Calif. Vet. 27:18, 1973.

180. Schalm, O. W.: Comments on feline leukemia: Clinical and pathologic features. Differential diagnosis. J. Am. Vet. Med. Assoc. 158:1025, 1971.

181. Schalm, O. W., Jain, N. C. and Carroll, E. J.: The leukemia complex. In: Veterinary Hematology. Lea & Febiger, Philadelphia, 1975.

182. Schalm, O. W., and Switzer, J. W.: Bone marrow disease in the cat. I. Atypical granulocytic leukemia. Calif. Vet. 22:24, 1968.

183. Schalm, O. W., and Theilen, G. H.: Myeloproliferative disease in the cat, associated with C-type leukovirus particles in bone marrow. J. Am. Vet. Med. Assoc. 157:1686, 1970.

184. Schneider, R.: Comparative epidemiological aspects of naturally occurring malignant lymphoma in domestic cats and rhesus monkeys. In Clemmesen, J., and Yohn, D. S. (eds.): Comparative Leukemia Research, 1975. S. Karger, Basel 1976.

185. Shadduck, J. A., Reedy, L., Lawton, G., and Freeman, R.: A canine cutaneous lymphoproliferative disease resembling mycosis fungoides in man. Vet. Pathol. 15:716, 1978.

186. Sherwood, I. M.: The multiple causes of hypercalcemia in malignant disease. N. Engl. J. Med. 301:1412, 1980.

187. Shull, R. M., Osborne, C. A., Barrett, R. E., et al.: Serum hyperviscosity syndrome associated with IgA multiple myeloma in two dogs. J. Am. Anim. Hosp. Assoc. 14:58, 1978.

188. Silverman, J.: Eosinophilic leukemia in a cat. J. Am. Vet. Med. Assoc. 158:199, 1971.

189. Simar, W., and Holzworth, J.: Eosinophilic leukemia in a cat. Cornell Vet. 57:579, 1967.

190 Slappendel, R. J.: The diagnostic significance of the direct antiglobulin test in anemic dogs. Vet. Immunol. Immunopathol. 1:49, 1979.

191. Sodikoff, C. H., and Schalm, O. W.: Primary bone marrow disease in the cat. II. Erythemic myelosis and myelofibrosis. A myeloproliferative disorder. Calif. Vet. 22:16, 1968.

192. Squire, R. A , and Bush, M.: Comments on treatment of leukemia in the cat. Am. J. Vet. Med. Assoc. 158:1134, 1971.

193. Squire, R. A., Bush, M., Melby, E. C., et al.: Clinical and pathologic study of canine lymphoma: Clinical staging, cell classification and therapy. J. Natl. Cancer Inst. 51:565, 1973.

194. Stann, S. E.: Myelomonocytic leukemia in a cat. J. Am. Vet. Med. Assoc. 174:722, 1979.

195. Strombeck, D. R.: Clinicopathologic features of primary and metastatic neoplastic disease of the liver in dogs. J. Am. Vet. Med. Assoc. 173:267, 1978.

196. Sutton, R. H., McKellow, A. M., and Bottrill, M. B.: Myeloproliferative disease in the cat: A granulocytic and megakaryocytic disorder. N.Z. Vet. J. 26:273, 1978.

197. Szymanski, C,: Intraocular and orbital neoplasia. In Kirk, R. W. (ed.): Current Veterinary Therapy VII. W. B. Saunders, Philadelphia, 1980, pp. 585–587.

198. Theilen, G. H., and Madewell, B. R.: Leukemia—sarcoma disease complex. In Theilen, G. H., and Madewell, B. R. (eds.), Veterinary Cancer Medicine. Lea & Febiger, Philadelphia, 1979.

199. Theilen, G. T., and Schalm, O. W.: Myeloproliferative disease in the dog—A case report of granulocytic leukemia. Calif. Vet. 24:10, 1970.

200. Theilen, G. H., Schalm, O. W., and Pedersen, N. C.: Myeloproliferative disorders and associated leukemias in the cat: Pathogenesis, diagnosis, cytology, therapy and control. Proc. Am. Anim. Hosp. Assoc. 43:171, 1976.

201. Theilen, G. H., Worley, M., and Benjamini, E.: Chemoimmunotherapy for canine lymphosarcoma. J. Am. Vet. Med. Assoc. 170:607, 1977.

202. Thrall, M. A.: Lymphoproliferative disorders. lymphocytic leukemia and plasma cell myeloma. Vet. Clin. North Am. 11:321, 1981.

203. Tolle, D. V., Fritz, T. E., and Norris, W. P.: Radiation-induced erythroleukemia in the beagle dog. Am. J. Pathol. 87:499, 1977.

204. Tomely, F. M., Armstrong, S. J., Nuns De Souza, P. A., et al.: Retrovirus particles associated with canine lymphosarcoma and leukemia. Br. J. Cancer 45:644, 1982.

205. Tsujimoto, H., Shirota, K., Hayashi, T., et al.: Monocytic leukemia in a cat. Jpn. J. Vet. Sci. 43:957, 1981.

206. Wagner, J. E., and Murphy, K.: Granulocytic leukemia in a dog. Illinois Vet. 12:17, 1969.

207. Ward, J. M., Sodikoff, C. H., and Schalm, O. W.: Myeloproliferative disease and abnormal erythrogenesis in the cat. J. Am. Vet. Med. Assoc. 155:879, 1969.

208. Watson, A. D. J., Huxtable, C. R. R., and Hoskins, L. P.: Erythremic myelosis in two cats. Aust. Vet. J. 50:29, 1974.

209. Weiler, R. E., Holmberg, C. A., Theilen, G. H., and Madewell, B. R.: Histologic classification as a prognostic criterion for canine lymphosarcoma. Am. J. Vet. Res. 41:1310, 1980.

210. Weller, R. E., Theilen, G. H., and Madewell, B. R.: Chemotherapy responses in dogs with lymphosarcoma and hypercalcemia. J. Am. Vet. Med. Assoc. 181:891, 1982.

211. Weller, R. E., Theilen, G. H., Madewell, B. R., et al.: Chemoimmunotherapy for canine lymphosarcoma: A prospective evaluation of specific and nonspecific immunomodulation. Am J. Vet. Res. 41:516, 1980.

212. Weiden, P. L., Storb, R., Kolb, H. J., et al.: Immune reactivity in dogs with spontaneous malignancy. J. Natl. Cancer Inst. 53:1049, 1974.

213. Willard, M. D., Krehbiel, J. D., Schmidt, G. M., and Lowrie, P.: Serum and urine protein abnormalities associated with lymphocytic leukemia and glomerulonephritis in a dog. J. Am. Anim. Hosp. Assoc. 17:381, 1981.

214. Williams, D. A : Gammopathies. J. Cont. Ed. Vet. Pract. 4:205, 1982.

215. Wintrobe, M. M., Lee, G. R., Boggs, D. R., et al.: Clinical Hematology. 8th ed. Lea & Febiger, Philadelphia, 1981.

216. Withrow, S. J., and Lowes, N.: Biopsy techniques in small animal oncology. J. Anim. Hosp. Assoc. 17:889, 1981.

217. World Health Organization: Report of a Consultation on the Biological Behavior and Therapy of Tumors of Domestic Animals. WHO, Geneva, 1978.

218. Yarrington, J. T., Hoffman, W. E., Macy, D., and Hawker, C.: Morphologic characteristics of the parathyroid and thyroid glands and serum immunoreactive parathyroid hormone in dogs with pseudohyperparathyroidism. Am. J. Vet. Res. 42:271, 1981.

219. Zacharski, C. R., and Linman, J. W.: Chronic lymphocytic leukemia versus chronic lymphosarcoma cell leukemia. Analysis of 496 cases. Am. J. Med. 47:75, 1969.

220. Zawidzka, Z. Z., Janzen, E., and Grice, H. C.: Erythremic myelosis in a cat: A case resembling DiGuglielmo's syndrome in man. Pathol. Vet. 1:530, 1964.

221. Zenoble, R. D., and George, J. W.: Mycosis fungoides-like disease in a dog. J. Am. Anim. Hosp. Assoc. 16:203, 1980.

222. Zenoble, R. D., and Rowland, G. N.: Hypercalcemia and proliferative, myelosclerotic bone reaction associated with feline leukovirus infection in a cat. J. Am. Vet. Med. Assoc. 175:591, 1979.

INTRACRANIAL NEOPLASMS

Neoplasms of the central nervous system (CNS) occur with greater frequency in the dog than in other domestic species.[52] Neoplasms affecting the CNS may be primary or secondary. Primary tumors arise from cells of neuroectodermal, ectodermal, and mesodermal origin and are normally found within the cranial vault or the spinal column or in the peripheral nerves (Table 179–1). Secondary tumors include those that impinge on the brain from extracranial structures and those that metastasize to the brain from other sites.[21,23,42,73]

The clinical signs associated with these tumors are diverse and vary according to tumor type and location(s). Brain tumors may alter the function of nervous tissue by destruction, compression, impaired circulation, edema, or altered cerebrospinal fluid flow. Other possible effects of brain tumors include

TABLE 179–1. Classification of Central Nervous System Tumors

Neuroectodermal Tumors
  Astrocytoma[6, 49, 50]
  Oligodendroglioma[41, 50, 67]
  Glioblastoma multiforme[61]
  Unclassified glioma[41]
  Ependymoma[47, 50]
  Choroid plexus tumor[22, 35, 39, 55, 80]
  Spongioblastoma[41, 50]
  Medulloblastoma[41, 50]
Mesodermal Tumors
  Meningioma[1, 2, 40, 48, 59]
  Primary reticulosis[2, 16, 32, 62, 69, 70]
  Lipoma[17]
  Chordoma[4]
Ectodermal Tumors
  Craniopharyngioma[63]
  Pituitary adenoma[25, 43, 47]
  Olfactory gland adenocarcinoma[7]
Reported Secondary Tumors[21, 73]
  Mammary gland adenocarcinoma
  Pulmonary carcinoma
  Chemodectoma
  Prostatic carcinoma
  Salivary gland adenocarcinoma
  Hemangiosarcoma
  Fibrosarcoma
  Malignant melanoma
  Lymphosarcoma
Primary Tumors from Surrounding Tissues of the Skull
  Osteoma
  Osteosarcoma
  Fibrosarcoma
  Chondrosarcoma
  Multiple myeloma
  Hemangiosarcoma
  Nasal gland adenocarcinoma
  Chondroma

herniations under the tentorium cerebelli, across the falx cerebri, or through the foramen magnum.

Primary tumors usually grow slowly so that clinical signs progress insidiously. The ability of the nervous system to continue normal function despite these processes makes early diagnosis difficult. Obstruction or erosions of brain vasculature result in infarction or hemorrhage. Consequently, acute presentations of a severe neurological deficit may be seen with primary or secondary tumors.

Secondary tumors, especially those that are highly malignant, have a more rapid progression. In our experience, the rapid deterioration seen with these disorders is often associated with sudden hemorrhage within the brain parenchyma.

Clinical Anatomy of the Brain

The brain is encased and protected by a bony vault. Two principal processes formed by the meningeal layer of the dura mater subdivide and immobilize the brain. The falx cerebri separates the two cerebral hemispheres, and the tentorium cerebelli separates the occipital cortex from the cerebellum. The membranous tentorium attaches to the osseous tentorium cerebelli dorsally and the petrous temporal bones ventrally. Its concave border forms the tentorial notch, which contains the midbrain.

The brain stem and cerebellum, being posterior to the tentorium cerebelli, are regarded as infratentorial or posterior fossa structures. Similarly, the cerebral hemispheres, being anterior to the tentorium cerebelli, are referred to as supratentorial or anterior fossa structures. Finally, the cerebral hemispheres are separated into right and left sides by the falx cerebri.

Knowing these anatomical boundaries is useful in locating a small, single focal lesion to explain the signs exhibited by the patient and makes differential diagnosis easier.

Incidence

Dogs. Although neoplastic disorders of the nervous system may occur at any age, they are most common in dogs over five years of age.[19,53] The reported incidence of primary intracranial tumors in all necropsied dogs varies. A range of from 0.8 to 6.4 per cent is cited in various reports in the veterinary literature.[11,21,64,68] The lower incidence is from unselected necropsies, while the higher incidence is in animals with CNS disease.[11,68] The largest series of primary and secondary CNS tumors was reported by McGrath;[43] in this report of over 6,000 necropsies, the incidence was 2.8 per cent.

Neuroectodermal tumors are the most common

primary intracranial neoplasm in the dog. In fact, neuroectodermal tumors comprise approximately 30 per cent of the total number of nervous system tumors, and all except the choroid plexus papillomas appear more frequently in brachycephalic breeds.[14,41,73]

Astrocytomas are the most common neuroectodermal tumors in dogs at The Animal Medical Center. As noted by other investigators, they occur most frequently in middle-aged boxers and Boston terriers. Cerebral involvement, particularly in the pyriform area of the brain, is common. Other sites of involvement include the thalamus, hypothalamus, midbrain, pons, and rarely the cerebellum.[19,53]

Oligodendrogliomas represent the second most commonly observed neuroectodermal tumor of the central nervous system at The Animal Medical Center. However, oligodendrogliomas are reported more frequently than astrocytomas by other workers. These neoplasms are seen in 5- to 11-year-old dogs and are usually observed in the frontal, olfactory, and temporal lobes.[21,41] Other studies are not in agreement with our findings although all agree that brachycephalic breeds are significantly represented.[20,73]

Ependymal cell tumors of the brain are rare. When observed, however, they are found at the borders of the lateral and fourth ventricles of the brain. Again, brachycephalic breeds are most frequently represented.

Choroid plexus tumors are derived from glial cells which originate from the epithelial cells lining the choroid plexus. Most of the choroid plexus tumors observed at The Animal Medical Center have been in nonbrachycephalic breeds and occurred between the ages of 3 and 10 years. The common location of these usually benign tumors was in the third and fourth ventricles of the brain. These findings are in agreement with earlier reports describing the location of choroid plexus tumors[35] (Fig. 179–1).

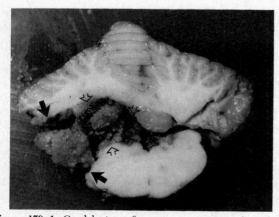

Figure 179–1. Caudal view of a transverse section through the pons, showing the typical appearance of a choroid plexus papilloma (*open arrows*) extending from the fourth ventricle, shifting the brainstem to the right, and overgrowing the cerebellopontine angle (*closed arrows*). The usual clinical presentation of this type of mass reflects vestibular disturbance with or without other cranial nerve involvement, e.g., of nerves five, six, and seven.

Meningiomas are the most common type of central nervous system tumor seen at The Animal Medical Center. They occur most frequently in dolicocephalic breeds. This mesodermal tumor is derived from the meningothelial cells of the meninges of the brain and spinal cord. Common sites include the frontal lobes, the falx cerebri parasagittally, and the cerebellopontine angle (Fig. 179–2). On several occasions, we have observed meningiomas on the floor of the skull. As opposed to the typical irregular, lobulated, well-encapsulated, hard, white bulk meningiomas, these appeared flattened, somewhat roughened, and firmly adherent to the calvarial floor and dura with extension along the base of the brain stem (Fig. 179–3). In each instance, these meningiomas *en plaque* distorted the normal function of peripheral cranial nerves two, three, and six. Furthermore, the compressive and edematous qualities of this tumor cause profound changes in the levels of consciousness owing to involvement of the reticular activating system and hypothalamus. Typical cranial nerve findings include pupillary dilatation, visual deficits, and eye movement and eye position abnormalities. In one predominately retrospective study of meningiomas, a propensity for a ventral location with cranial nerve involvement was noted.[1] In our experience, chiasmic or postchiasmic floor meningiomas, especially with cranial nerve findings, of the bulk type are highly unusual in both the dog and cat.

Another tumor type we have observed on the floor of the cranial vault is extragonadal canine teratocarcinoma. This is a mixed germinal tumor infrequently reported in the veterinary literature. These tumors are composed of recognizable somatic tissue characteristic of fetal or adult stages of development. Histologically, intracranial canine teratocarcinomas are characterized by areas resembling seminoma; acinar-like structures with lipid-containing cells; cystic epithelial structures containing proteinaceous material and cell debris; intercommunicating tubular structures, and well-differentiated glandular elements, containing mucin, that resemble intestinal or bronchial epithelium.[57] These tumors may be benign or malignant and have been classified as teratoma, teratocarcinoma, embryonal carcinoma, or choriocarcinoma.[46,51,54] On gross examination, the neoplasms, found in the hypothalamic area, are flattened, circular masses that infiltrate the thalamus and extend along the border of the brain stem. They adhere to the cranial vault and infiltrate the dura. A potentially important diagnostic feature of this neoplasm is that it has only been reported to occur in young male dogs of mixed breed. However, in one case recently observed here, a 12-year-old male Doberman pinscher was diagnosed as having an extragonadal teratocarcinoma. Additionally, these animals all had an abrupt deterioration of clinical signs following initial presentation. In the four cases observed at The Animal Medical Center, the acute exacerbation of neural signs was related to hypothalamic encroachment and hemorrhage (Fig. 179–4).

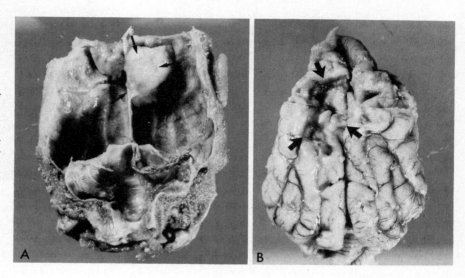

Figure 179–2. A, Ventrodorsal view of anterior and posterior fossas with brain removed. A large meningioma *(arrows)* is shown adhered to the falx cerebri on the left. *B*, Dorsal view of the same brain, depicting cavitation of the frontoparietal areas of the brain *(arrows)* from the falx meningioma.

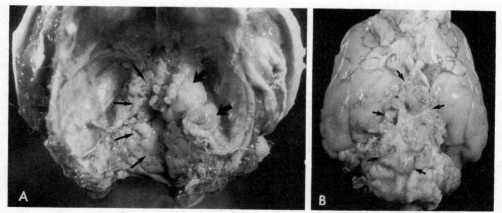

Figure 179–3. A 12-year-old spayed female poodle was presented for lethargy. Neurological examination revealed a bitemporal vision field cut, right medial strabismus, bilaterally fixed dilated pupils, and rotary nystagmus. The dog showed response to glucocorticoid for four months but was euthanized when presented in status epilepticus. *A*, Dorsoventral view of the ventral aspect of the posterior fossa of the cranial cavity at necropsy examination. A meningioma en plaque obliterated much of the posterior fossa *(medium arrows)* and is bulkier on the right *(large arrows)*. *B*, Ventrodorsal view of the brain after removal from the calvarium, showing flattened, moderately irregular, and invasive nature of the meningioma en plaque *(arrows)*.

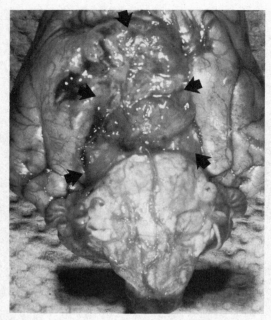

Figure 179–4. A 12-year-old male Doberman pinscher was presented for circling to the right. Left hemiparesis, left hemianopsia, left hemisensory deficits, left lateral ocular deviation, and left pupillary dilatation were found on examination. Dog would lapse and become semicomatose. Sudden death occurred three days after hospital admission. Ventrodorsal view of the brain on postmortem examination shows a large extragonadal teratocarcinoma (*arrows*) extending from the cranial portion of the posterior fossa to the anterior fossa.

The two most common ectodermal tumors involving the brain are pituitary adenomas and olfactory gland adenocarcinomas. Pituitary adenomas, especially pituitary chromophobe adenomas, occur frequently and may approximate the human incidence.[43]

Pituitary tumors develop within the pituitary fossa and are therefore located posterior to the optic chiasm. Despite their localization and usual large size, bitemporal visual difficulties are rarely determined clinically. Additionally, both functional and nonfunctional pituitary tumors have been observed to encroach on the diencephalic zone. Approximately 4 to 5 per cent of over 400 cases of documented canine hyperadrenocorticism were presented with additional signs of hypothalamic dysfunction. Lethargy, irritability, pacing, circling, tetraparesis, sleep disturbance, and nonsustained positional nystagmus were observed in these cases. A slow progression of these signs culminating with a sudden deterioration in all neurological findings was associated with hemorrhage and obstructive hydrocephalus. In general, the masses are observed to adhere to the cranial vault and are regularly raised, reddish in color, and infiltrative (Fig. 179–5).

Olfactory gland adenocarcinomas usually are observed to invade the cribriform plate and compress prefrontal areas of the cerebral hemispheres.[74] Because of their location, the only initial signs of cerebral involvement may be seizures. Their location and propensity to extend ultimately compromise sensory motor function (Fig. 179–6).

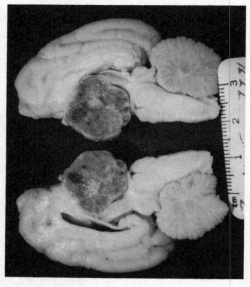

Figure 179–5. A two-year-old male domestic short-hair was presented for lethargy, dullness, and polydipsia. Neurological examination revealed bilaterally fixed dilated pupils with blindness that progressed to right circling and coma. Sagittal section of the brain, on necropsy examination, revealed a pituitary chromophobe adenoma compressing the hypothalamus, thalamus, and brainstem.

The debate about the malignant or inflammatory nature of reticuloendothelial disorders is unresolved. Proliferation of elements within the reticuloendothelial portions of the nervous system are frequently designated by the general term reticulosis. On the basis of cytological features, reticulosis is often classified into inflammatory/granulomatous or neoplastic forms. The exact criteria for this classification vary, since intermediate forms abound. These variations suggest a continuous spectrum of cellular response. The disease is most frequent in young to middle-aged dogs of any breed. In our experience, the inflammatory/neoplastic form of primary reticulosis is most common. The disorder appears as a space-occupying lesion of the cerebral hemispheres or as a multifocal to diffuse process of the cerebral hemi-

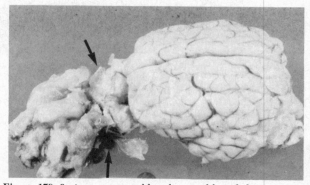

Figure 179–6. A seven-year-old male mixed-breed dog was presented for an uncontrolled seizure disorder that had been controlled with anticonvulsants for one year. Dorsoventral view of the brain at necropsy, revealing a nasal gland adenocarcinoma involving the prefrontal areas of the brain (*arrows*).

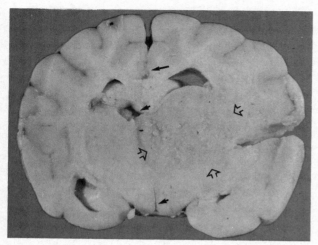

Figure 179–7. Transverse section at the level of the thalamus, showing the inflammatory-neoplastic form of reticulosis. *Open arrows* indicate extent of involvement in the right thalamus. The third ventricle is distorted *(closed arrows)*, the cingulate gyrus is shifted to the left, and the entire right brain is swollen.

spheres, brain stem, cerebellum, and spinal cord (Fig. 179–7). The clinical presentation, therefore, depends on the distribution of inflammatory cells within the brain and meninges.

Reticulosis of the neural tissues of the eye may occur, together with involvement of the central nervous system in dogs. Ocular signs often occur before central nervous system signs, and bilateral involvement is usual. Choroidal invasion with retinal detachment and optic neuritis leads to pupil changes with blindness. Reticulosis should be considered in dogs with ocular findings of this type and neurological signs suggestive of a space-occupying lesion. No breed or sex predilection has been observed by us, although others cite a poodle and terrier breed disposition.[16,32,62,69,74]

Cats. Of 3,915 cats necropsied at The Animal Medical Center during a 12-year period (1962–1974), 87 neoplasms were found in the CNS of 75 cats. There were 52 meningiomas, 28 lymphosarcomas, 1 ependymoma, 1 neurilemoma, 1 astrocytoma, 3 pituitary chromophobe adenomas, and 1 pituitocytoma. Eight of the 75 cats had multiple tumors. Six cats had two meningiomas and two cats had three meningiomas.

Meningiomas were the most frequently encountered intracranial tumor in the cat. This agrees with other reports.[41,73] They occurred as solitary or multiple masses, which were irregularly lobulated, encapsulated, and attached to the dura. Most cats with meningiomas we have encountered are over ten years of age, although we have observed their occurrence in cats as young as one year of age. Male cats appear to have a higher incidence.

In a retrospective study of 36 meningiomas in cats, most cases involved solitary masses which were located supratentorially.[48] Six cats in this study had multiple meningiomas, one of which was located infratentorially. A large percentage (83 per cent) of the solitary meningiomas in this study arose from the supratentorial meninges and were confined to the meninges overlying the cerebral hemisphere. The other solitary meningiomas (17 per cent) were in the following locations: one in the caudal cranial fossa, one arising from the sphenoid bone and compressing the midbrain, one in the third ventricle, and two in either of the lateral ventricles. Our continued experience with this neoplasm, especially from an operative viewpoint, agrees with this retrospective study. Parasagittal, over the frontoparietal lobes, and sphenoid bone origin meningiomas have been the most frequently observed. To date, ten meningiomas have been removed surgically from these areas following selected neurodiagnostic and radiographic criteria (Fig. 179–8).

Meningiomas may have benign or malignant characteristics. In our experience, one cat had an invasive meningioma which eroded the calvarium.[36] The most common pathological change observed at The Animal Medical Center is a hyperostotic reaction of the calvarium adjacent to the tumor. Meningiomas usually compress and distort cerebral tissue. The distorted brain tissue results in appropriate clinical signs compatible with its location and degree of involvement. Distant metastases are very rare in animals and unusual in humans.[31]

In contrast, CNS tumors of neuroectodermal origin are rarely seen in the cat.[41,56,73] However, sporadic reports of ependymomas and gliomas occur in the veterinary literature.[10,15,73]

Pituitary tumors have been considered by some to be nonexistent in the cat.[41] However, tumors of the chromophobe cells of the adenohypophysis[73,75] and of the pituicytes of the adenohypophysis have been described.[72,73]

Lymphosarcoma causes the greatest number of neoplastic changes in the feline CNS.[5,44,65] Most lymphosarcomas, however, are described extracranially (e.g., epidurally in the spinal cord). We have observed one case at The Animal Medical Center oc-

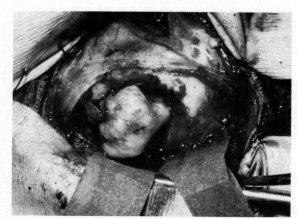

Figure 179–8. A parasagittal frontoparietal meningioma in a 10-year-old male dachshund at surgery. The meningioma is being excised through a craniotomy.

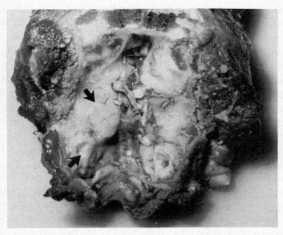

Figure 179–9. A 5-year-old male domestic short-hair presented for a sudden onset of left vestibular signs, left fixed-dilated pupil without visual loss or eye position change, keratitis sicca, facial weakness, and diminished facial sensation. A large kidney was palpable on physical examination. Dorsoventral view of the calvarial floor with brain removed at necropsy, showing lymphosarcoma within the left posterior fossa *(arrows).*

curring within the third ventricle. Another case of lymphosarcoma involved the left fifth, sixth, seventh, and eight cranial nerve roots, a portion of which extended anteroventrally and involved the left semilunar ganglion. The mass compressed the left ventral side of the pons and the anteroventral areas of the medulla (Fig. 179–9). Lymphosarcoma is a relatively infrequent cause of supra- or infratentorial disease.

Secondary Tumors of the Brain

Detailed reports of metastatic brain tumors and their clinical presentation are infrequent. In one study of 48 secondary brain tumors, 38 were metastatic. Primary adenocarcinomas of the mammary gland, thyroid, nasal sinus, and bronchus were the most frequent type seen. Other metastatic tumors included melanomas, hemangiosarcomas, osteosarcomas of mammary origin, and neurogenic sarcomas.[42]

Observations made at our institution suggest the following order of occurrence: in dogs, melanoma, mammary gland adenocarcinoma, hemangiosarcoma, prostatic adenocarcinoma, primary lung tumor (carcinoma nonsmall cell), end-stage lymphocytic leukemia (meningeal infiltration), and hepatic carcinoma. In cats, lymphosarcoma and mammary gland adenocarcinoma.

Clinical Signs

Generalized brain injury associated with space-occupying masses results from hemorrhage, infarction, edema, or herniation. The clinical signs associated with brain tumors may result from compression and infiltration of nervous tissue or obstruction of cerebrospinal fluid flow (Table 179–2). The size,

TABLE 179–2. Common Clinical Signs of Uncomplicated Intracranial Neoplasms*

Supratentorial
Unilateral Intracranial Neoplasms:
  Circling (usually ipsilateral), head pressing, behavior changes, altered mentation, hemianopsia/visual loss (contralateral), hemisensory loss (contralateral), supranuclear (partial) paralysis of cranial nerves 5 and/or 7 (contralateral), hemipostural difficulty (contralateral), hemiparesis (contralateral), seizures
Bilateral Intracranial Cerebral Neoplasms:†
  Circling, head pressing, behavior changes, altered mentation, hyperactivity, hemianopsia (symmetrical or asymmetrical), hemisensory loss, supranuclear paralysis of cranial nerves 5 and/or 7, tetraparesis (symmetrical or asymmetrical), loss of autonomic control, seizures, decerebrate posture
Midline Cerebral Neoplasms:
  Circling, head pressing, behavioral and personality changes, altered mentation, somnolence, hyperactivity, loss of autonomic control, visual loss, hemiparesis/tetraparesis, endocrinopathy, pupil changes, cranial nerve dysfunction (2, 3, and 6), nystagmus
Pituitary Fossa (Diencephalon)
  Visual deficits (cranial nerve 2), hypothalamic signs (abnormal eat/sleep behavior), altered conciousness/awakeness (stupor, coma)
Intratentorial (Mesencephalon)
  Altered conciousness, abnormal pupillary reflexes, eye position and range of motion difficulty, tetraparesis, resting/positional nystagmus, decerebration
Pontomedullary (Metencephalon/Myelencephalon)
  Altered consciousness; facial, trigeminal, abducens, vestibular-cochlear cranial nerve involvement; tetraparesis (asymmetrical/symmetrical); balance disorder/dysequilibrium (head tilt, veering, falling, rolling—ipsilateral); nystagmus (resting or positional); ocular skew deviation, medial or ventrolateral (ipsilateral); temporal/mandibular muscle atrophy

*Modified from Kay, W. J.: Diagnosis of intracranial neoplasms. Vet. Clin. North Am., 7:145, 1977.
†The bilaterality of these signs is often the result of unilateral lesions that herniate, midline neoplasms, or progressive growth of a neoplasm across the midline.

location, extent of invasion, inflammatory qualities, edema, growth rate of the mass, and herniation may influence the severity of clinical signs. For example, rapidly growing tumors generally cause apparent clinical signs. Slow-growing tumors, on the other hand, allow for nervous system compensation and clinical signs are therefore more subtle until tumor growth exceeds this compensation.

Little information on the frequency of brain infarctions or hemorrhage in dogs and cats is available. At The Animal Medical Center, hemorrhagic infarctions due to spontaneous bleeding, infection, vessel erosion, and trauma are commonly observed. The clinical significance of "strokes" is important, since they often occur in conjunction with neoplastic processes. Sudden compromise of neural function complicates this clinical setting by superimposing additional insult to the brain. As a result, even slow-growing tumors of the brain may present with acute clinical signs. A thorough history is essential to establish a time-sign relationship and allow for more reasonable differential considerations. When obtaining a detailed history, the veterinary clinician should inquire about the following areas: (1) personality/behavorial changes, (2) eat/sleep habit changes, (3) overall responsiveness, (4) intellect, (5) restlessness/pacing, (6) gait disturbance, (7) visual difficulty, (8) auditory difficulty, (9) circling, (10) head pressing, (11) balance disorders, (12) muscle atrophy, and (13) seizures. Seizures may be seen with or without any of these signs when associated with intracranial neoplasms. "Silent areas"—e.g., frontal, prefrontal, and subfrontal or temporal lobes—may be compromised by brain tumors yet have little or no other historical or clinical findings. In our experience, meningiomas and nasal gland and olfactory gland tumors involving the prefrontal cortex of dogs frequently present in this manner. In fact, the diagnosis is made following euthanasia, because of the uncontrolled nature of the seizures. Seizures that occur concurrently with other neurological signs generally develop late in the course of the disease process.

Secondary Effects of Intracranial Neoplasia

Brain Edema

Cerebral edema may result from various pathological processes, such as neoplasia, infection, trauma, vascular accidents, metabolic derangements, and malformations. Brain edema is a result of altered blood-brain and blood-CNS barriers. As a consequence, increased amounts of sodium, water, and/or protein accumulate in the substance of the brain. Edema can collect in the extracellular, intracellular, and interstitial spaces. These are commonly referred to as vasogenic, cytotoxic, and interstitial edemas, respectively.[45] Brain tumors generally evoke a vasogenic edema. Vasogenic edema appears to involve the white matter to a greater degree than it does gray matter. The more rapid and extensive the brain edema, the more profound the clinical signs.

Herniation

The cranium houses the cerebrum, cerebellum, brain stem, blood supply, cerebrospinal fluid (CSF), and meninges. Because the skull is an inelastic structure, additional tissue elements—whether they originate from tumors, abscesses, blood, or edema—may cause shifting, or herniation, of neural structures through various anatomical openings.

Four types of pathological herniations occur in domestic animals: (1) cingulate gyrus herniations underneath the falx cerebri to the opposite side, (2) transtentorial herniation in which the occipital or temporal lobes move under the bony tentorium cerebelli, (3) herniations of the medulla or cerebellum or both through the foramen magnum, and (4) rostral cerebellar vermis herniation under the tentorium cerebelli.[34,45] We have not observed rostral cerebellar vermis herniation.

Cingulate gyrus herniations may complicate the clinical assessment of originally lateralizing brain tumors. Clinical signs following this type of herniation mimic bilateral disease. Transtentorial herniations clinically incorporate signs associated with cerebellar or brain stem compression or both. Stupor, coma, changing pupil size, abnormal eye movement, nystagmus, ocular deviations, cardiac arrhythmias, and decerebration may be seen with this process. Herniations through the foramen magnum generally reflect extensive derangement of intracranial contents. A patient with this condition has severe neurologic debilitation which generally results in death.

Differential Diagnosis and Neurodiagnostic Procedures

Focal lateralizing signs of CNS dysfunction may be seen with tumors, vascular insults, and focal inflammatory processes.

Neoplasia often has a progressive but protracted course. Vascular lesions generally are peracute to acute in their onset and have little to no progression. This is true only if the vascular insults are not multiple or if there is an underlying cause, e.g., a primary or secondary brain tumor or systemic infection. Focal inflammatory disease is eliminated as a definitive diagnosis on the basis of selected neurodiagnostics. If focal signs are not present, the differential diagnosis should include degenerative disorders, diffuse inflammatory processes, metabolic disease, toxicities, and midline structural pathology. Routine neurodiagnostic procedures that may be useful in a diagnosis of neoplasia and its location include electroencephalography (EEG), CSF analysis, routine radiographs, various venographic or arterial radiographic studies, and isotope scanning.

The EEG is often useful in the localization of cerebral tumors. Asymmetry, increased amplitudes, and focal slowing will be seen and should coincide with the neurological localization. Deep lesions of the brain may have normal EEGs. Increased intracranial pressure due to cerebral edema or altered CSF flow will dampen the amplitudes of cerebrocortical electrical activity. Generally, a superimposed slow-wave pattern is also seen. Pituitary and small hypothalamic tumors may produce normal EEGs when the animal is alert which become abnormal as the animal relaxes.[8]

Cerebrospinal fluid analysis can further support the suspicion of cerebral neoplasia and is useful in eliminating inflammatory disease as a cause of clinical signs. Despite the usefulness of this procedure, CSF collection is contraindicated when increased intracranial pressure is suspected. Sudden release of this pressure at the time of CSF collection can result in

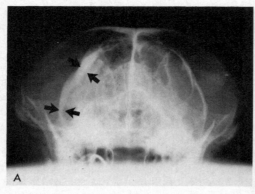

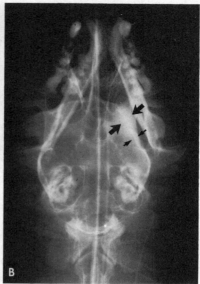

Figure 179–10. A, Modified occipital radiographic view demonstrating hyperostosis *(arrows)* due to a meningioma in a cat. B, Ventrodorsal projection redefining hyperostosis *(arrows)*.

brain herniation and a rapid deterioration of all clinical signs. In instances when CSF collection yields unexpected elevated pressure, precautions should be immediately undertaken to prevent neural shifts. Difficulties in obtaining CSF by cisternal puncture may suggest herniation of the posterior cerebellar vermis and medulla through the foramen magnum. Assuming proper technique when this circumstance occurs, further attempts should be discontinued.[33]

In cerebral tumors (except meningiomas), the CSF pressure (>180 mm CSF) is elevated because of the secondary edema of surrounding nervous tissue. Normal cell counts and increased CSF protein (>30 mg/dl) are usually seen; however, marked pleocytosis may be observed when the tumor causes compression and necrosis that involve the subarachnoid space (ependymomas, choroid plexus papillomas, reticuloses, lymphosarcoma, and meningiomas).

Survey radiography is usually normal unless the mass causes proliferation, hyperostosis, or lysis to the skull (Figs. 179–10 and 179–11). Hyperostotic reactions of the calvarium are frequently associated with meningiomas in cats. Aside from routine positioning for radiography, a modified occipital view is recommended. This position offers an unobstructed view of the foramen magnum and parietal portions of the calvarium. To perform this procedure, the animal is placed in ventrodorsal recumbency. The x-ray tube is positioned at a 30° angle directed caudally. Simultaneously, the head is directed 10° off vertical in the same direction as the tube. The beam is centered just above the orbits. This view has been useful in the diagnosis of 90 per cent of the documented feline cerebral meningiomas observed at The Animal Medical Center. Other radiographic techniques used in diagnosis of intracranial neoplasms include arteriog-

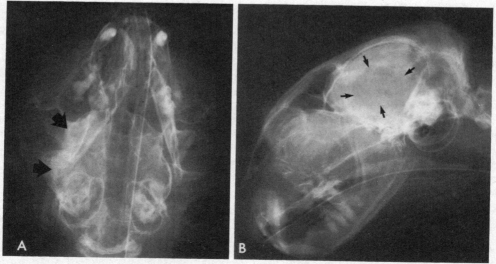

Figure 179–11. A, Ventrodorsal radiograph showing bone destruction *(arrows)* of the right calvarium due to a meningioma in a cat. B, Lateral projection showing calvarial destruction *(arrows)* due to the meningioma.

raphy, ventriculography, and scintography. Their application and usefulness in diagnosing brain tumors have been reported elsewhere.[8,21,26,37] These other radiographic techniques, aside from brain imaging and sinus venography, have been less useful in our experience. Cavernous sinus venography is a safe and easy method for demonstrating lesions on the floor of the cranial vault. We have performed this procedure on a limited number of cases and found the results to be variable.

Treatment of Intracranial Neoplasms

Surgical removal of intracranial neoplasms is the treatment of choice. With the exception of feline cerebral meningiomas, most intracranial neoplasms are intramedullary. Consequently, despite sophisticated localizing techniques, surgery becomes impractical and medical management is often the only alternative.

The objectives of medical management of intracranial neoplasms are the control of brain edema, alleviation of seizures, and the minimizing of herniation tendencies. The degree to which these effects can be managed depends on the tumors' locations, growth rate, and histological type and the metabolic well-being of the patient.[28,45] Glucocorticoids have long been advocated to control and alleviate signs associated with vasogenic brain edema. The administration of glucocorticoids, in cases of suspected intracranial neoplasms, may result in a partial or complete resolution of neurological deficits. This improvement is transient since the growth of the mass will ultimately eliminate the effects of glucocorticoids in limiting edema.

Detailed clinical histories, serial neurological examinations, and other selected neurodiagnostic tests that support a diagnosis of intracranial mass are prerequisites before a glucocorticoid trial is begun. We recommend an initial dose of 0.5 to 1 mg/kg of dexamethasone given intramuscularly or intravenously. This loading dose is followed by a relatively low dose ranging from 0.25 to 1 mg administered three times daily. The animal is carefully assessed within the first 24 to 48 hours for signs of neurological improvement. A schedule of incremental reductions of the individual dosing is prescribed over a two-week period.

Animals with suspected intracranial tumors generally improve clinically during the trial of glucocorticoids. However, when an improvement ceases during the period of reducing the glucocorticoid or after cessation of the drug dosage, the patient is said to have "failed the steroid test." A neoplasm is suspected in this situation, owing to the presumed recurrence of cerebral edema. Animals that are not candidates for further study or surgery may be maintained on the lowest level of glucocorticoids that alleviates the greatest degree of neurological deficits. These animals will ultimately experience a decline in neurological function and will require higher levels of glucocorticoids. Generally, a deterioration occurs over a one- to three-month period, after which glucocorticoids are of little use.

Mannitol can be administered to patients suspected of brain herniations. Precautions should be taken when administering any hypertonic solution. Mannitol can produce sudden elevations in central venous pressure or osmotic fluid shifts, which may complicate congestive heart failure, dehydration, shock, or intracranial bleeding when present. Since hemorrhage and infarction are fairly common with intracranial neoplasms, patients with a sudden exacerbation of a previously slow course are best not treated with mannitol. In addition, a rebound effect may also occur following mannitol administration if the extracellular fluid becomes diluted and the hypertonic fluid penetrates cells, increasing the osmotic concentration intracellularly and drawing water into the cell. These events further exacerbate pre-existing cerebral edema.

NEOPLASIA OF THE SPINE AND SPINAL CORD

Tumors of the spinal column and spinal cord may produce pain and weakness of the neck, shoulders, thorax, abdomen, pelvis, and extremities. These signs can present a most difficult, perplexing, and stimulating clinical problem and are a result of the neoplastic involvement of a very complex system composed of bony elements, multiple joints including the intervertebral disc, ligaments, muscles, and vital vascular and neural structures. Early diagnosis is often difficult, especially when the only sign is intermittent pain that may be projected to a localized region in the thorax, abdomen, or extremity. When pain is associated with paresis or paralysis, however, a spinal cord lesion is immediately suspected.

Because of the prevalence of intervertebral disc disease in the dog, with its associated pain or paresis or both, many other spinal disorders may be overlooked, resulting in ineffective treatment. The presenting signs may be similar, if not identical; in the early development of the pathological processes of spinal meningitis, spinal column osteomyelitis,[24] ankylosing spondylitis, congenital spinal disorders, various traumatically induced diseases, vascular diseases of the spinal cord and meninges,[76-78] intervertebral disc disease, and neoplasia of the vertebral column and spinal cord.[77] Consequently, differential diagnoses in each individual case are essential in strategically launching an immediate as well as long-term diagnostic and therapeutic attack.

Tumor Classification

In this discussion of tumors of the spinal cord, all tumors that exert pressure on the spinal cord and nerve roots are included—the metastatic and primary bone tumors, as well as those tumors affecting the spinal cord, nerve roots, and meninges. Spinal cord tumors are classified according to both their malignancy and their position with respect to the cord and meninges. Therefore, tumors fall into two broad categories: malignant or benign and whether they are extradural, intradural-extramedullary, or intramedullary in location (Table 179–3).

Neural Anatomy

The spinal cord and meninges are contained within the vertebral canal. Dorsal roots entering the spinal cord receive sensory impulses that travel to higher centers in the brain and to the reflex centers of the spinal cord. The ventral roots carry motor impulses

TABLE 179–3.   **Differential Diagnosis of Spinal Cord Tumors**

	Extradural	Intradural-Extramedullary	Intramedullary
*Frequency**	50%	35%	15%
Tumor Types			
Dog	Primary malignant bone tumors	Neurofibromas	Gliomas
	Metastatic tumors to bone and soft tissues	Meningiomas	Ependymomas
	Benign bone tumors		Reticulosis
Cat	Lymphosarcoma: Fibrosarcoma (rare), all others rare	None identified	Rare
Rate of Growth	Rapid	Slow	Most often slow
Location	Equal distribution: C, T, and L	Neurofibroma: Low cervical (C5–C8); less common in other locations in dogs	Gliomas: Equal distribution in C, T, L Reticulosis: Higher frequency in cervical cord
	Meningioma: Equal distribution C,T, and L. Low occurrence rate when compared with neurofibromas	Ependymomas: Lower frequency in any location in dogs	
Clinical Signs			
Pain	Earliest clinical sign: Days to weeks prior to onset of paresis	Earliest clinical sign; months to years prior to onset of paresis	Most often nonexistent If present, observed late when paresis pronounced
	Results from bone and soft tissue disruption as well as nerve root compression	Results from tumors growing from dorsal root (neurofibroma) or adjacent to dorsal root (meningioma)	Hemorrhage of tumor, if it occurs, produces meningeal pain
	Intense, unrelenting; diffuse over several vertebral bodies	Intermittent, focal	
	Increased with activity	Decreased with activity	
	Increased when spine manipulated	Increased when spine manipulated	
	May be referred to extremity resulting in "lameness" ("root signature")	May be referred to extremity resulting in "lameness' ("root signature")	
	May be referred to thoracic or abdominal cavity	May be referred to thoracic or abdominal cavity	
Paresis	Noted within days to weeks of onset of pain	Noted within months to years of onset	Insidious onset Rapid progressive loss of motor function
	Rapid progressive loss of motor function	Insidious onset, very slow progressive loss of motor function	Peracute paresis if intramedullary hemorrhage
Sensory loss	Late clinical sign	Late clinical sign	Late clinical sign
	Observed in nonambulatory state; may be demonstrated prior to nonambulatory state if segments or cord involved (C3–T1, or L4–S4)	Observed in nonambulatory state	Observed in nonambulatory state
		Often demonstrated prior to nonambulatory state if segment of cord involved (C6–T1 or L4–S1)	Often demonstrated prior to nonambulatory state if segment of cord involved (C6–T1 or L4–S1)

Table continued on following page

to the musculature. The meninges are fibrous membranes which envelop and protect the spinal cord, nerve rootlets, and nerve roots and are composed of the dura mater, the arachnoid, and the pia mater. The area between the arachnoid and the pia mater (the subarachnoid space) contains the cerebrospinal fluid (CSF). The space between the dura mater and spinal column is the epidural space and is filled with epidural fat and venous sinuses (Fig. 179–12).

Radiography

Spinal cord tumors are frequently not discernible on plain radiographs unless destructive or proliferative bony changes or both are present. For this reason, myelography is often necessary to localize and identify the neoplastic lesion accurately. The location of the tumor with respect to the dura also permits relatively accurate differential diagnoses of the tumor type and is also of prognostic value.

Positive contrast agents are introduced into the subarachnoid space, by cisternal or lumbar puncture. These agents render the subarachnoid space more radiopaque than the adjacent spinal cord, therefore bringing the spinal cord into relief as a shadow of decreased density (cord shadow).

Extradural Lesions. These are located outside the dura mater and result in attenuation of the dural tube

TABLE 179–3. Differential Diagnosis of Spinal Cord Tumors (*Continued*)

	Extradural	Intradural-Extramedullary	Intramedullary
Sphincter disturbances	Late clinical feature in upper motor neuron lesions; are nonambulatory Early clinical feature in lower motor neuron lesions involving S2–S3 segments or cauda equina	Late clinical feature in upper motor neuron lesions, are nonambulatory Early dysfunction noted in lower motor neuron lesions involving S2–S3 or cauda equina	Early clinical feature in upper motor neuron lesions; however, not with frequency reported in humans Early clinical feature in lower motor neuron lesions involving S2–S3 or cauda equina
Course	Very acute onset with associated rapid neurological deterioration in 2–6 weeks Rapid tumor growth	Very insidious, obscure onset with associated slow progressive deterioration over months to years Slow rate of tumor growth	Insidious onset with rapid progressive deterioration over days to weeks Slow rate of tumor growth; displacement of 50–60% of cord; ischemia and edema result in acute crisis
Diagnostics Cerebrospinal fluid analysis	Elevated protein infrequent	Elevated protein inconsistent	Elevated protein inconsistent RBC, WBC if associated hemorrhage; RBC phagocytized
Radiography	Agressive, lytic, proliferative Subtle lytic lesions Absence of bony lesions	Plain films usually noncontributory; may observe widened intervertebral foramen with neurofibroma	Plain films usually noncontributory
Myelography	Dura displaced from bony canal	"Cup" or "golf tee" configuration	Widened cord shadow on all projections
Therapy Medical	Corticosteroids, muscle relaxants, anti-inflammatory drugs Relieves pain moderately Short-lived response Chemotherapy, immunotherapy, and radiation therapy in selected cases	Corticosteroids, muscle relaxants, anti-inflammatory drugs Relieves pain Pain controlled for months Paresis initially improved, with subsequent progressive deterioration	Corticosteroids, muscle relaxants, anti-inflammatory drugs Improves motor strength Short-lived response and within days progressive deterioration observed
Surgical	Very limited success with malignant tumors Benign tumors, rewarding	Early diagnosis affords rewarding surgical outcome	Very limited success with present state of art

C = Cervical; T = Thoracic; L = Lumbar; S = Sacral.
*Our figures comparable to humans.

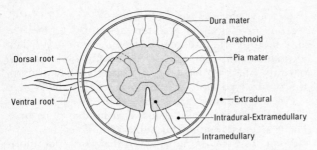

Figure 179–12. Cross-section of spinal cord and meninges. The contrast agent is deposited into the subarachnoid space, between the arachnoid and the pia mater.

and spinal cord (Fig. 179–13). Representative of this type of lesion are extruded disc fragments; bone fragments associated with fractures, vertebral luxations, and subluxations; arachnoiditis with focal constriction of the dural tube; arachnoid cysts; primary and metastatic spinal column tumors; lymphosarcoma of the epidural space; and epidural abscesses.

When performing myelography, if the dye column in any one radiographic view is deflected away from the vertebral canal, resulting in a widened epidural space, the presence of an extradural lesion is confirmed. Rotating the spinal column 90° will result in a widened spinal cord shadow, which alone is not diagnostic since this may be associated with a mass in any one of the three locations (Fig. 179–14).

Intradural-Extramedullary Lesions. These are located in the subarachnoid space which contains the cerebrospinal fluid (Fig. 179–13). The masses most frequently demonstrated are the neurofibroma and the meningioma. A mass in this location acts as a wedge, displacing the dura mater to the bony spinal canal and the spinal cord to the contralateral bony spinal canal. As the contrast material abuts the cranial and caudal margins of the tumor, a "cup" or "golf tee" formation is created, a configuration pathognomonic for an intradural-extramedullary mass. When the spinal column is rotated 90°, a widened cord shadow may be seen (Fig. 179–14).

Intramedullary Lesions. Intramedullary lesions, which include gliomas, ependymomas, reticulosis, hydromyelia, syringomyelia, and vascular disorders, are located within the substance of the spinal cord (Fig. 179–13). These lesions displace the spinal cord substance from within, resulting in a circumferential

enlargement of the spinal cord. The swelling of the spinal cord results in an attenuation of the contrast-filled subarachnoid space as well as expansion of the dura mater. This is generally appreciated in all radiographic projections (ventrodorsal, lateral, and oblique) (Fig. 179–14).

Extradural Tumors

These represent the primary (benign and malignant) and metastatic tumors of the spinal column and epidural space. In humans, extradural tumors represent approximately 50 per cent of all spinal tumors, less than 2 per cent of which are primary bone tumors.[3] There have been few surveys of spinal column tumors in the dog; however, it appears from one study that approximately 50 per cent of the spinal column tumors were extradural.[66] Our experience reflects the same distribution; however, primary bony tumors (osteogenic sarcoma, fibrosarcoma, and chondrosarcoma) far outnumber the metastatic lesions. Osteogenic sarcoma of the spine is the most prevalent tumor identified.

This group of tumors exerts effects on neural tissue by direct extension and compression of the neuraxis from the vertebral structures. As in humans, direct extension of neoplastic tissue through the dura and metastasis to the spinal cord itself are extremely rare in the dog.[60]

Myelographic examination will demonstrate varying degrees of spinal cord attenuation with, at times, such massive shifts of dural tube and spinal cord that the fact of ambulatory status or some neurological function still existing is incomprehensible. It must be appreciated that slow, progressive attenuation of the spinal cord by masses (whether extradural, intradural-extramedullary, or intramedullary) is tolerated rather well when compared with acute, space-occupying lesions of less volume. The spinal cord may be reduced by one-third of its diameter, with minimal neurological deficits. Beyond this state of slow progressive attenuation, neurological signs become evident. Acute paresis may occur subsequent to maximal cord attenuation and is a result of an alteration of blood flow leading to an acute ischemic crisis. In other instances, the dynamics of blood flow are not significantly altered, and progressive paresis ensues.

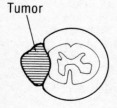
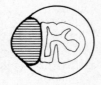

EXTRADURAL

INTRADURAL-EXTRAMEDULLARY

INTRAMEDULLARY

Figure 179–13. Cross-sections depict the relationships of the tumor with respect to the dura mater and the spinal cord.

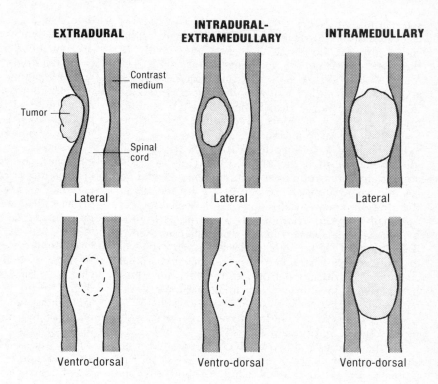

EXTRADURAL

INTRADURAL-EXTRAMEDULLARY

INTRAMEDULLARY

Contrast medium

Tumor

Spinal cord

Lateral

Lateral

Lateral

Ventro-dorsal

Ventro-dorsal

Ventro-dorsal

Figure 179–14. Schematic representations of the myelographic appearance of the three categories of spinal cord tumors.

The earliest sign exhibited in animals with extradural tumors is pain, most often unrelenting and progressive, and usually aggravated by activity. Digital manipulation of the involved area results in exaggerated pain. Unlike other tumors of the spinal cord, extradural tumors generally present with a more diffuse area of exquisite spinal pain upon manipulation. The pain is a consequence of bone destruction or nerve root compression (radiculopathy) or both.

Many dogs and cats with neoplastic disease of the spinal column are treated for weeks for obscure clinical signs, such as shaking, shivering, panting, lethargy, anorexia, abdominal "cramps," constipation, or neck, back, or leg pain. In humans, low thoracic and lumbar lesions resulting in pain radiating to the abdomen have often been mistaken for gallbladder disease, renal disease, appendicitis, cystic ovaries, and other abdominal disorders. Likewise, we have performed abdominal radiographs and, in some instances, have given barium in attempts to identify gastrointestinal pathology or performed intravenous pyelography to define a renal disorder. Prostatic and renal diseases are often diagnosed when pain is referred to the respective sites.

Pathological lesions of the spine attenuating nerve roots frequently result in referred pain to the area enervated by the nerve root; this is termed a "root signature." Compression of the C4–C8, T1–2, L4–L7, or S1 nerve roots often results in referred leg pain. Clinically, the root signature is represented by intermittent or persistent elevation or limping on a leg. These dogs are invariably managed as having a lameness of orthopedic origin. Radiographs of the entire extremity often reveal no pathology, and the dog may be thought to have an obscure musculoskeletal disease. Often, the clinician is lulled into a false sense of security when arthritic changes are radiographically demonstrated, which is quite frequent as most of these animals are elderly.

Interruption of the C8, T1–3 nerve root function may be associated with Horner's syndrome, as the sympathetic pathway to the eye exits from the cord at this level. The miosis may be incomplete, necessitating critical assessment. It is an important localizing feature and a fairly common neurological sign associated with disease of the low cervical and high thoracic spine.

Symptomatic management with corticosteroids and other anti-inflammatory drugs is initially effective but short-lived. Within days to weeks, a refractory state exists.

Generally, within three to five weeks of the onset of pain, paresis is evidenced, at which time the existence of a spinal cord lesion becomes apparent. A state of nonambulatory paresis may occur acutely or within days of the onset of historical pain. The rapid development of neurological weakness with sustained and often excruciating back or neck pain aids in differentiating extradural from intradural-extramedullary tumors. Pain is not generally a feature of intramedullary tumors. The neurological weakness associated with extradural tumors is initially asymmetrical; however, within a matter of days to weeks, symmetrical paresis may be observed. Progressive paresis and paralysis follow rapidly, and corticosteroids, even in large doses, are generally ineffective.

Sensory loss in the extremities is generally a late

sequela to spinal cord compression when the lesion is located in the upper motor neuron segments of the spinal cord (C1–C5 and T2–L3). Pathology involving the lower motor neuron segments (C6–8 to T1, and L4–7, S1–3, and Co1–Co5) and cauda equina may be associated with earlier sensory loss in the corresponding peripheral nerve distribution. Rather profound muscle atrophy is often observed with tumors in the lower motor neuron locations.

Establishing a sensory level is of great value in identifying the site of the lesion. A safety pin is gently applied to the paralumbar skin, moving caudal to rostral. An appropriate response is achieved when the dog responds vocally and/or physically to this minimally noxious stimulus. The transition from a hypalgesic or analgesic zone to a normalgesic zone is thus defined. The lesion is either at the sensory level or immediately rostral by no more than two spinal segments. If critically performed, this test can establish a sensory level even when minimal motor weakness exists. The sensory level is only valuable in assessing thoracic and lumbar disease. Sensory levels of the cervical spine are inconsistent.

The panniculus reflex must be differentiated from the sensory level. A sensory level relies on the animal's ability to perceive and respond to pain whereas a panniculus response is simply a reflex. In addition, because of the variable distribution of the panniculus muscle, we have not found it to be a reliable means of localizing thoracic and lumbar lesions.

Rather consistent localization can be established using hyperpathia (digital manipulation of the spine), the sensory level, and reflex examination of the extremities. The elicitation of a crossed extensor reflex establishes upper motor neuron disease; however, it is not of prognostic value.

Sphincter disturbances resulting in urinary and/or fecal incontinence are late sequelae to spinal cord compression from extradural tumors and develop almost simultaneously with the loss of motor function of the extremities. A paraparetic or tetraparetic non-ambulatory state most often exists prior to the animal's experiencing bowel and bladder dysfunction. Upper motor neuron lesions most often present with late sphincter disturbances. Lower motor neuron lesions involving the S2 and S3 segments or cauda equina more often present with early signs of incontinence and are generally accompanied by extremity weakness. Tumors of the cauda equina may attain massive dimensions prior to altering neurological function of bowel and bladder. These lesions in this location often result in historical and clinical evidence of tail weakness. Urinary bladder dysfunction almost invariably precedes rectal dysfunction. The earliest clinical feature associated with compromise of the S2–S3 segments or their peripheral nerves in the cauda equina may be that of stranguria, which then progress to an overflow, reflex bladder. In the absence of motor deficits, such animals are often treated for urinary tract infection. It is an extreme exception that fecal incontinence precedes urinary incontinence or exists without historical or clinical evidence of urinary incontinence. In such instances, disorders other than those associated with the S2–S3 segments or cauda equina must be investigated.

The radiographic appearance of extradural neoplasia is quite variable, ranging from aggressive, lytic, proliferative lesions to subtle lytic lesions with minimal new bone formation to absence of bony changes.

Primary neoplasia of the spine, as opposed to metastatic disease, is most prevalent in animals. Osteogenic sarcoma is the most frequently defined pathological lesion, followed by fibrosarcoma. Other primary malignant neoplastic lesions, including multiple myeloma, hemangiosarcomas, and chondrosarcomas, are diagnosed with much less frequency. Osteogenic sarcomas are most often aggressive, resulting in readily visible lytic and proliferative bony changes (Fig. 179–15). It is noteworthy that the degree of proliferative changes is not as pronounced as in long bones. Osteogenic sarcomas, as well as many of the metastatic lesions, are often observed to involve the vertebral body or pedicles (lateral bony wall). Therefore, ventrodorsal projections are mandatory to delineate the pathology involving the pedicle (Fig. 179–15B). Fibrosarcomas may be quite elusive as aggressive bone destruction is not always present. Numerous cases have been documented in which the fibrosarcoma originated lateral to the intervertebral foramen. Growth into the spinal canal via the intervertebral foramen was defined. Myelography simply established massive extradural disease.

It is imperative to stress that neoplasia is a disease of the young and the old. Extradural neoplasia of various types, including osteogenic sarcomas, have been diagnosed in dogs as young as six months of age at this institution.

The characteristic multiple, punched out, lytic, minimally proliferative radiographic lesions of multiple myeloma are observed in many bone systems; however, it is our experience that the spinal column is the most common site, followed by the pelvis. Whereas multiple lesions are characteristic, we have demonstrated 14 solitary vertebral body lesions in 9 dogs (Fig. 179–16). Diffuse involvement is characteristic, as defined by bone marrow biopsies, but radiographic lesions were solitary. The diagnosis of multiple myeloma has been made approximately 20 times at this institution, although rarely in cats. Because solitary primary and metastatic neoplasias of the spine are often minimally proliferative and often maximally lytic, the differential diagnosis of myeloma should always be considered. An evaluation of the total protein and albumin/globulin ratio, as well as electrophoresis, is sufficient to make this diagnosis. The presence of Bence Jones protein should be assessed as well. Biopsy of the spinal lesion is contraindicated, as pathological fractures may ensue and diagnosis is most easily established in a totally noninvasive fashion. The importance of considering myeloma as a

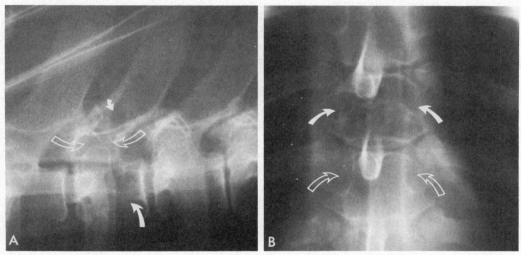

Figure 179–15. An 11-year-old German shepherd was presented for two weeks of back pain and a progressive posterior paresis. *A*, Lateral radiograph of T4 osteogenic sarcoma. Lytic changes are noted in the vertebral body *(large solid arrow)*, dorsal spinous process *(small solid arrow)*, and pedicle *(open arrows)*. Minimal proliferative changes are noted. *B*, Ventrodorsal projection of T4 osteogenic sarcoma. Extensive lysis of the vertebral body is appreciated as well as bilateral destruction of the pedicles *(solid arrows)*. Normal pedicles are depicted by the *open arrows*.

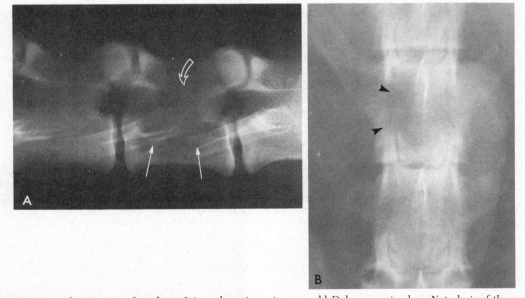

Figure 179–16. *A*, Lateral projection of a solitary L4 myeloma in a nine-year-old Doberman pinscher. Note lysis of the vertebral body *(solid arrows)* and laminar line *(open arrows)*. *B*, Ventrodorsal projection of the L4 myeloma depicts lysis of the right pedicle *(arrow)*. This feature is often more striking than the lucency of the vertebral body on the lateral projections.

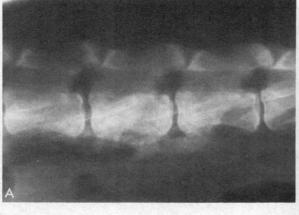

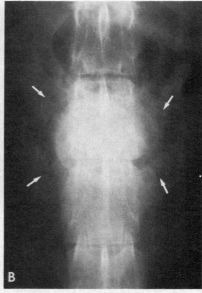

Figure 179–17. *A,* Metastatic prostatic adenocarcinoma of L4, L5, and L6, demonstrating the characteristic aggressive, proliferative, and lytic disease. *B,* The metastatic prostatic adenocarcinoma has actively disrupted the integrity of the transverse processes of L5 and L6 *(arrows).*

differential diagnosis is that it presently is one of the few extradural neoplastic lesions for which therapy is available.

Myelography is indicated to demonstrate and confirm the existence of subtle bony spinal column changes accounting for the neurological deficits demonstrated. It is unnecessary to advise myelography in those animals presenting with readily visible, aggressive, lytic and proliferative lesions of the spine on plain radiographic evaluation.

Metastatic lesions of the spine may be readily apparent on plain radiography or may be extremely obscure, necessitating myelography to demonstrate the lesion(s). The frequency of metastatic disease in the dog and cat is much less than that documented in humans. Metastatic mammary gland neoplasia and prostatic gland neoplasia are the most frequently documented lesions in the dog. These tumors often result in aggressive, proliferative, and lytic bony changes of the spine. Often they are initially diagnosed as active spondylitis or infection of bacterial or fungal origin (Fig. 179–17).

Other sites of origin of tumors that metastasize to the vertebral column have been identified at our institution, but with much less frequency than the mammary or prostatic tumors. These sites include the thyroid, kidney, lungs, uterus, testes, pancreas, and biliary, hepatic, and gastrointestinal tracts. The thyroid and kidney tumors have been documented in greater number than the other tumors. Melanomas and squamous cell carcinomas have been infrequently confirmed as metastatic lesions of the spine. Other tumors arising in the bladder, urethra, and salivary glands and various bone and soft tissue sarcomas have been confirmed occasionally. Splenic hemangiosar-

coma is diagnosed frequently but rarely is metastatic disease to the spine demonstrated. Canine lymphosarcoma, a relatively common entity, is very rarely associated with extradural metastasis or destruction of the spinal column.

Metastatic neoplasia to the spinal column, with subsequent spinal cord attenuation, may present without radiographically visible bony destruction. Metastasis is demonstrated to occur via the venous sinuses on the floor of the canal. Myelography will sometimes demonstrate massive ventral or ventrolateral extradural lesions (Fig. 179–18). Ventral or ventrolateral extradural lesions, unaccompanied by bone destruction and spanning one or more vertebral bodies, is highly suggestive of metastatic disease. Differential considerations, however, must include

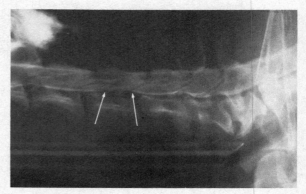

Figure 179–18. A C4 ventral extradural mass documented as a metastatic hepatic adenocarcinoma *(arrows)* to the ventral venous sinuses. The 14-year-old dog had been unsuccessfully treated for pain associated with spondylosis of C5-C6 and C6-C7 for nearly three weeks.

epidural hemorrhage from trauma, laceration of the venous sinus associated with acute disc extrusion, bleeding disorders, and epidural abscess (rare).

As a rule, primary neoplasia of the spine (i.e., osteogenic sarcoma and fibrosarcoma) is most frequently demonstrated in the vertebral body or pedicles or both. On the other hand, lytic aggressive proliferative lesions involving the dorsal elements (lamina and dorsal spinous process) are most frequently associated with metastatic disease (Fig. 179–19).

Rarely will metastatic disease unaccompanied by bone destruction be demonstrated dorsally.

Although uncommon, benign tumors of the spinal column resulting in spinal cord compression do exist and must be recognized in the differential diagnoses. Of primary consideration are the solitary and multiple osteocartilaginous exostoses in dogs and cats.[58] These lesions are quite characteristic radiographically and take on a nonaggressive, expansile, cotton ball–like appearance. Neurological signs generally are noted during the growth phase of the animal. Tumor growth ceases at sexual maturity.

Extradural spinal neoplasia in the cat is reported uncommonly, with the exception of lymphosarcoma. Spinal lymphosarcoma in the cat is an extradural lesion often associated with peracute neural dysfunction (excruciating back pain and paresis), rarely is associated with radiographic bony lesions of the spine, is minimally to not at all responsive to corticosteroid management, and is diagnosed only by myelography. The acute nonambulatory paresis associated with this slowly growing mass lesion reflects upon the ischemic myelopathy demonstrated histopathologically. While feline leukemia virus tests are made routinely, the results are negative in approximately 75 per cent of the cats with spinal lymphosarcoma.

Other primary or metastatic neoplastic lesions are extremely uncommon in the cat. Fibrosarcomas and fibrous histiocytomas have been identified with greater frequency than have osteogenic sarcomas. Multiple myeloma has been documented in our institution in approximately 20 cats.

Infection of the spinal column in the dog or cat must always be considered in the differential diagnosis when radiographs reveal destructive and proliferative changes. However, the clinician must be aware that infection is more likely to involve the disc space than is tumor (very uncommon), and infection is usually confined to the ventral elements of the spine (vertebral body and disc) and transverse spinous processes.

Surgical considerations are quite limited when the characteristic aggressive spinal lesions of extradural neoplasia are radiographically defined. Likewise, solitary or diffuse myelographic signs of extradural metastasis to the venous sinuses or epidural space or both do not reflect an optimistic surgical consideration. Surgical decompressive procedures, with concomitant rhizotomies (cutting the dorsal nerve root to eliminate pain) two levels above and below the lesions bilaterally, have provided relief of pain and significant improvement of motor strength in some instances. This procedure, however, is advisable only when the dorsal elements of the spine (lamina, facets, or pedicles) are involved. Pathological fractures of the vertebral body ensue when laminectomy is performed when a vertebral body tumor is present. Overall, the morbidity is quite high, and any success achieved via surgery is generally short lived.

Chemotherapy, immunotherapy, and radiation therapy may be of value for selected cases. Multiple myelomas have undergone numerous oncological treatment protocols, but rewarding results are quite limited in spinal cases to this date.

Intradural-Extramedullary Tumors

The great majority of tumors in this location in dogs and humans are neurofibromas (also called neurilemomas and schwannomas) and meningiomas. These tumors are very rarely identified in cats. The tumors are benign, well encapsulated, and usually easily separable from the spinal cord.[30] Malignant variants have rarely been reported. Sarcomas, lymphomas, epidermoids, lipomas, melanomas, and neuroblastomas have rarely been reported in this location in humans.[60]

Fifty per cent of all human spinal cord tumors are intradural, and 71 per cent of these are intradural-extramedullary.[60] The meningioma is most commonly reported in the thoracic spine of middle-aged women.[60] The cervical spine and lumbar spine are also represented, albeit in fewer numbers.[12] The neurofibroma is distributed equally in the cervical, thoracic, and lumbar areas with no sex predilection and has a higher incidence than the human meningioma.[12] Neurofibromas may involve a single or multiple nerve roots. Human multiple nerve root neurofibromas exist in a hereditary condition known as neurofibromatosis.[12] Documentation has not been established in the dog or cat. In our experience, the solitary neurofibroma is a fairly common clinical entity in the dog (Fig. 179–20). These tumors have

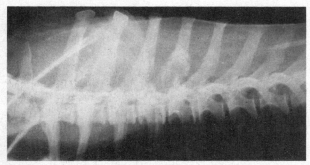

Figure 179–19. Metastatic renal adenocarcinoma of the T4 dorsal spinous process and lamina is demonstrated. The radiographic lesion is aggressive in nature. Although infection is a differential diagnosis, rarely does it involve the dorsal elements of the spine.

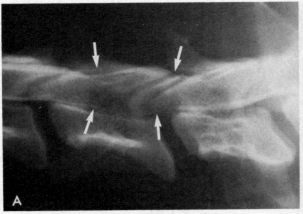

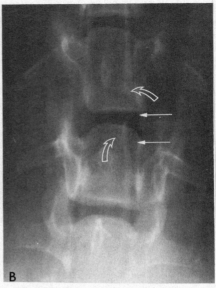

Figure 179–20. A nine-year-old golden retriever was presented with an eight-month course of progressive, left lateralizing tetraparesis. Lameness of the left front leg preceded the paresis by two months. *A*, Widening of the spinal cord shadow and attenuation of the dye column is demonstrated at C5-C6 *(arrows)*. *B*, The left C6 dorsal root neurofibroma is clearly demonstrated by the presence of a myelographic "golf tee" anterior and posterior to the tumor *(open arrows)* characteristic of an intradural-extramedullary mass. An extradural component, also demonstrated *(solid arrows)*, is characteristic of dumbbell-shaped neurofibromas. Spinal meningiomas rarely manifest extradural components. The meningioma was successfully removed surgically.

been identified in the veterinary literature,[66] but because of the limited number of reported cases, statistical data are not available. In our experience of 29 neurofibromas, the most common location was in the mid to low cervical spine with only a few in the thoracic and lumbar spine. Five cases presented with neurofibromas at the C1, C2, C3 root level. One case presented with C1 and C2 root tumors. We have identified and operated on six meningiomas in either the cervical, thoracic, or lumbar spine but in significantly lower numbers than the neurofibroma.

Neurofibromas in dogs and humans characteristically originate intrathecally from the dorsal nerve root.[60] Human and canine meningiomas arise from the meninges, which are typified by arachnoid rest cells that may appear in any location but seem to concentrate at points adjacent to nerve rootlets.[3] In rare instances, this tumor may take on an intramedullary location.[3] Extradural meningiomas of the spine have been identified as well. These extradural tumors may be aggressive and have been associated with destruction of the vertebral body. Meningiomas may be positioned dorsally, ventrally, or laterally. Of interest are the human locations most frequently reported. In one study, 11 of 13 cervical tumors were located ventral to the spinal cord, and both the dorsal tumors were at C1. There were 45 dorsal tumors and 22 ventral tumors in the thoracic and lumbar spine.[38] We have identified and neurosurgically treated six cases. The three cervical tumors were at the C1 level (one dorsal and one ventral) and at the C5 level dorsally. Three thoracolumbar tumors were identified in the dorsolateral position (Fig. 179–21).

Because neurofibromas and meningiomas arise directly from or in close proximity to the dorsal rootlets or roots, radicular discomfort is the earliest clinical feature. Radicular signs frequently precede the signs of spinal cord compression by months or even years, since these tumors characteristically grow very slowly. In humans, radicular signs may be continuous or intermittent and are often most pronounced at rest.[30] Our experience bears out the human clinical features. In contradistinction to extradural tumors, which most often present with excruciating, unrelenting pain generated by activity, intradural-extramedullary tumors may be totally asymptomatic during daily activity.[60] Our observations agree.

The insidious nature of these tumors makes their early diagnosis quite difficult. Radicular pain, the initial sign, may not be recognized as such by the clinician. Just as the nerve roots are compromised by the extension of an extradural tumor, they are likewise functionally altered by this group of benign tumors. Pain associated with the solitary or multiple nerve root tumors is referred to those structures innervated by the involved nerve(s). Depending on the location of the tumor, pain may be referred to the cervical, thoracic, or abdominal musculature, as well as to the muscles of the extremities and tail. The pain is most often not exquisite, as in extradural disease, and the clinician rarely can elicit pain by spinal manipulation.

Some dogs are symptomatically treated for months for intermittent shaking, quivering, lethargy, depression, abdominal tenseness, gastrointestinal disorders, renal disease, prostatitis, and other various disorders

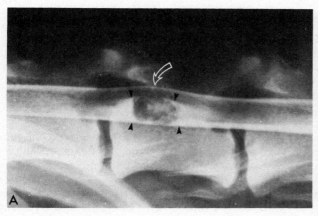
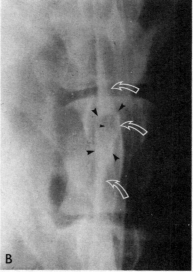

Figure 179–21. A seven-year-old male Collie with progressive right lateralizing posterior paresis of three months' duration. *A,* An intradural-extramedullary mass is documented by the presence of the "golf tee" configuration of the dye column anterior and posterior to the meningioma *(solid arrows).* The spinal cord shadow is widened *(open arrow)* by the presence of the predominantly lateral mass. *B,* The ventrodorsal projection identifies the meningioma *(small arrow)* and a "golf tee" configuration of the dye column anterior and posterior to the mass *(solid arrows).* The spinal cord shadow *(open arrows)* is significantly attenuated by the mass. An extradural component is not demonstrated.

of the thoracic and abdominal cavities. However, the signs more often are obscure and if questioned intensively, the owner often will report the animal's restlessness and inability to sleep in a stationary position, as if agitated. It is common for these dogs to have been repeatedly radiographed for their apparent chronic abdominal distress. Special procedures, including cystograms, pneumocystograms, prostatourethrograms, and gastrointestinal series, have been performed in attempts to identify the disease process. These diagnostic procedures are performed prior to evidence of spinal cord compression and paresis. In some cases, neck or back pain is defined by the clinician, in which case intervertebral disc disease is most frequently diagnosed. Corticosteroids temporarily alleviate the signs; however, exacerbation is inevitable and perplexing.

When the tumor arises from or adjacent to a nerve root that innervates a leg, obscure lameness of an intermittent or progressive nature is a frequent sign. As noted, neurologically related "lamenesses" can be clinically related to pathology of the C4–C8 or T1–2 nerve roots, and likewise to the L4–7 or S1 nerve roots. Intermittent or persistent elevation of the leg is not uncommon. Fasciculations or atrophy is not marked in the early development of the disorder. Corticosteroid administration quite often successfully eliminates the lameness; however, dysfunction recurs when steroids are discontinued. In some instances months may elapse prior to recurrence of signs. The intermittent use of cortisone can maintain a normal state for many months. The lameness is often managed as a musculoskeletal disorder. Older dogs are often radiographed in attempts to establish osteoar-

thritis or other bony lesions that may incidentally be present. In the absence of bony pathology, an obscure lameness is diagnosed.

Tumors involving the C8, T1–3 nerve roots interrupt the sympathetic pathways and therefore create Horner's syndrome. The resultant miotic pupil may be partial, and critical assessment must be applied.

Faced with an animal's progressively less favorable response to corticosteroids, the clinician is drawn to more critical assessment of the dog. Atrophic musculature as well as fasciculations may be observed. Elicitation of neck or back pain (usually minimal) leads the clinician to conduct a thorough neurological examination which is often inconclusive in the earlier stages. Radiographs of the spine, if performed, often demonstrate degenerative disc disease or spondylosis as these dogs are older animals. In some instances, fenestrations have been performed following which progressive deterioration yet occurs.

As the tumor slowly enlarges and more severely attenuates the spinal cord, tetraparesis becomes an important clinical feature. Proprioceptive deficits, which are the initial neurological features, may be quite subtle initially, requiring great patience and serial neurological examinations to confirm. Upper motor or lower motor neuron dysfunction may be present, related to the locations of the tumor. Spinal pain is not likened to the excruciating pain associated with extradural lesions and often is not historically or clinically established. When present, the animal appears more uncomfortable than in pain. Progressive neural dysfunction necessitates myelography to identify the spinal cord attenuation.

While neurofibromas are commonly located in the

low cervical spine and initially produce referred discomfort to a front leg, they have been demonstrated at all cervical levels. Thoracic and lumbar levels have been less commonly identified. The cauda equina is a more frequent site of involvement than the thoracic or lumbar spinal cord. Neurofibromas of the cauda equina frequently involve multiple roots, initially present with referred pain to the leg(s), and characteristically result in low back pain on manipulation, unlike lesions of other spinal locations. Progression results in marked atrophy of the extremities and an increased intensity of back pain. Rectal examination occasionally has defined asymmetrically enlarged sciatic nerves as these tumors extend out from the intervertebral foramina.

Distinction must be made between the neurofibromas originating peripherally (brachial plexus) and those originating from the dorsal rootlet (occasionally, ventral rootlet) zone intradurally. Extension of the intradural neurofibroma to an extradural position may occur and is referred to as a "dumbbell-shaped" neurofibroma (a tumor mass intradurally, narrowing as it grows through the intervertebral foramina and expanding lateral to the foramina).[12] This tumor may continue to extend more peripherally and if in the brachial plexus or pelvic plexus involve multiple peripheral nerves of the extremity. The extension of the tumor along C1–C6 or T3–L4 does not hold the guarded surgical prognosis that is associated with the lesion of C7–T2 and L5–S3. Neurofibromas frequently arise from the brachial plexus, initially induce a lameness that progresses to a palsy, and invariably are associated with considerable pain upon axillary palpation. Often, these nerve tumors are not readily palpable, necessitating surgical exploration. Neurofi-

bromas originating in the brachial plexus rarely if ever ascend through the intervertebral foramina to an intradural-extramedullary position. The growth of the peripheral neurofibromas, on surgical and/or necropsy examination, invariably, terminates at the intervertebral foramina. While intradural-extramedullary neurofibromas are predominantly identified as benign tumors, the purely peripheral tumors are frequently identified as neurofibromas.

In contrast to the extradural tumors, most of which are associated with lytic and proliferative bony changes, the neurofibroma and meningioma are rarely associated with these bony changes. Myelography is necessary to identify the site and space-occupying lesion. In some instances, these slowly expansile tumors induce radiographically visible bony changes via pressure necrosis. Characteristically, this is observed at the intervertebral foramen as a neurofibroma extends from its intradural position laterally. The result is an enlarged foramen. The expansion of the tumor results in pedicle and lamina erosion and vertebral body erosion via pressure necrosis (Fig. 179–22). In rare instances, aggressive lytic and proliferative radiographic changes may be observed. These radiographic features are associated with neurofibrosarcomas and are extremely unusual (Fig. 179–23).

Examination of the cerebrospinal fluid prior to myelography frequently adds little to the diagnosis of these tumors. Spinal fluid protein may be elevated but infrequently in our experience.

Recognition of the neurological features of this class of tumors, followed by myelographic identification, provides the surgeon with a rather favorable prognosis in many instances. Early recognition, level

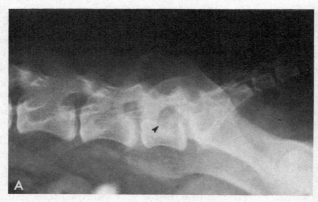
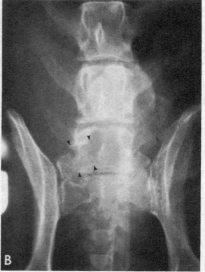

Figure 179–22. A 15-year-old male schnauzer with a two-year history of intermittent and progressive lameness followed by paresis in the sciatic distribution of the right rear leg. *B,* The L7 foramen is enlarged *(arrow)* by a slowly expanding L7 neurofibroma. Note the sclerotic margins of the lamina, pedicle, and vertebral body. This is a classic nonaggressive radiographic picture of a neurofibroma. *B,* A ventrolateral radiograph demonstrating the enlarged and sclerotic foraminal margins of L7 *(arrows).* The radiographic lesion is nonaggressive.

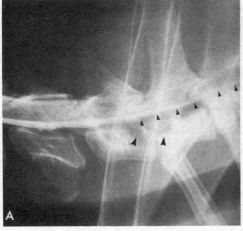
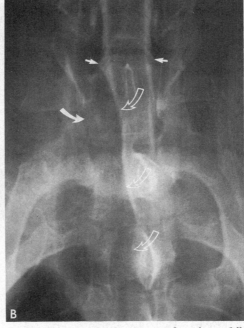

Figure 179–23. A nine-year-old male Airedale with a two-month history of right front leg lameness and weakness followed by a rapid ten-day course of progressive right-lateralizing tetraparesis. *A,* A destructive lesion of C7 and T1 is shown *(large arrows)*. A ventral extradural myelographic defect is present at T1 and T2 *(small arrows)*. Necropsy confirmed a neurofibrosarcoma of the C8 and T1 nerve roots with invasion of the C7 and T1 vertebral bodies and pedicles. *B,* The ventrodorsal projection depicts a massive extradural shift of the dural tube and spinal cord *(open arrows)*. Pedicle erosion is clearly evident *(large solid arrow)* on the right. The C7 nerve rootlets are highlighted by myelography *(small solid arrows)*.

of spinal involvement, presence of a solitary lesion (in the case of neurofibromas), and level of surgical experience all affect the surgical outcome.

Neurofibromas and meningiomas of the feline spinal cord have not been reported in the literature nor documented in our experience.

Intramedullary Tumors

Intramedullary tumors are the least common of the three types of spinal cord tumors. In humans, 50 per cent of all spinal cord tumors are intradural; of these, 20 per cent are intramedullary.[60] Our experience supports this low frequency in the dog. Spinal neoplasia in the cat, other than for extradural lymphosarcoma, is extremely uncommon. Intramedullary tumors in the cat are even more infrequent: only one glioma (C2) was identified in 14 years at this institution.

The majority of these tumors are derived from the glial cells and are therefore collectively called gliomas. The most frequently encountered human types are the astrocytoma and ependymoma.[60] The astrocytoma appears more frequently in the dog.[66] Gliomas may occur in very young dogs—less than one year of age—and should be included in the differential diagnosis of a progressively deteriorating paretic dog. In humans, these tumors make up approximately 20 per cent of all childhood spinal cord tumors. In comparison, they constitute only 12.8 per

cent of adult spinal cord tumors.[3] These tumors progress insidiously and often produce little pain, compared with extradural and intradural-extramedullary tumors. Metastatic tumors to the spinal cord are extremely unusual.[60]

Reticulosis, an often diffuse inflammatory neoplastic disorder of the central nervous system, may present with focal intramedullary spinal cord disease creating a mass effect. It is indistinguishable from other intramedullary disorders. Cerebrospinal fluid analysis may demonstrate a cytological background comparable to that of reticulosis, although this is not consistently demonstrated. While intramedullary in location, reticulosis of the spinal cord often presents with spinal pain, unlike other intramedullary disorders. Reticulosis is most commonly diagnosed in dogs less than 2 years of age, rarely above 5 years of age.

Pain is not generally an early clinical feature of intramedullary neoplasia. When pain is identified, it has been postulated that it is due to compression of the nucleus proprius or crossing fibers of the spinothalamic tract.[3] Others have postulated that pain along the spinal axis is a result of distension of the dural tube which is innervated by the sinu-vertebral nerve.[13] In our experience, the presenting sign of pain is a late sequela and is invariably observed when the animal reaches a nearly nonambulatory or nonambulatory state. Historical investigation, as well as previously conducted neurological examinations, most frequently reveal no evidence of spinal pain.

Unlike intradural-extramedullary tumors, intramedullary tumors often grow rapidly, resulting in rapid and progressive paresis. The onset and course of paresis rarely exceed two to three weeks. Because of the rapid growth of the tumor, spinal cord ischemia and edema or hemorrhage within the tumor mass may occur, resulting in peracute paresis or paralysis. The degree to which motor deficits may lateralize is extreme, resulting in profound deficits in one leg with nearly complete sparing of function in the contralateral leg. Cerebrospinal fluid analysis is most often not rewarding and may be misleading in the event that hemorrhage has occurred.[3] Extradural tumors may also present with rapid deterioration over several weeks; however, historical and clinical evidence of chronic excruciating spinal pain will aid in the differential diagnosis prior to radiographic assessment.

Because of the absence of root or bone pain, referred pain to the thoracic or abdominal areas is infrequent. Tumor growth within the cervical or lumbar intumescence may result in referred pain and subsequent lameness in a leg, and lower motor deficits are demonstrable. In humans, low cervical intramedullary lesions, such as syringomyelia and glioma, have been found to produce upper extremity pain.

Intramedullary tumors at the C8, T1–2–3 spinal cord levels may produce Horner's syndrome in addition to the extremity weakness.

The rapidly progressive asymmetrical motor deficits may initially respond to corticosteroid therapy. However, the positive response is transient, and a refractory state is noted within a matter of days (rarely weeks) of corticosteroid therapy. Progressive paresis ensues and, if undiagnosed, terminates in a nonambulatory paretic or paralytic state.

Characteristically, slowly expanding extradural and intradural-extramedullary lesions of the cervical spinal cord (C1–C8) are initially associated with posterior paresis followed by tetraparesis. This is often observed despite the site of the lesion (upper motor neuron C1–C6 segments or lower motor neuron C7–8 segments). Root signatures may be observed; however, the motor deficits are yet most marked in the rear leg(s). Intramedullary lesions of the cervical spine historically, clinically, and irrespective of the level (C1–C8) present with early front leg weakness, which is then followed by rear leg deficits. This is referred to as a "central cord phenomenon" and relates to the medial anatomical position of the front leg motor pathways with relationship to the rear leg motor pathways within the spinal cord. Central lesions first interrupt the front leg pathway and, based upon the completeness of the lesion, may produce profound front leg deficits with minimal to moderate rear leg weakness. Pathology at C1–C6 produces upper motor neuron dysfunction of the front leg(s) whereas lesions at C7–C8 result in lower motor neuron deficits in the front leg(s). Tetraplegia (complete sensorimotor loss) is but rarely observed in the

dog or cat as most succumb from respiratory failure prior to or soon after hospitalization.

Diminished sensation in the extremities, as with the other tumors, is a late clinical feature and in most instances is established only when ambulation has ceased. Intramedullary tumors at the cervical (C7–T2) or lumbar (L4–S1) intumescence may present with early and distinct sensory loss of an extremity or part of extremity in the face of moderate motor dysfunction of the extremity. Sensory loss of this nature is rarely demonstrated with extradural or intradural-extramedullary tumors.

The sensory level may further enable the clinician to accurately localize the lesion. It is only clinically applicable in the thoracic and lumbar spine, as noted earlier. Animals with intramedullary tumors that involve three or more spinal cord segments (i.e., T12,13–L1), while ambulatory, may present with two distinct sensory levels, or, otherwise stated, a band of hypalgesia over the T12,13–L1 distribution. The sensory status cranial and caudal to the tumor is normal in the early state of the disorder. As the paresis increases, the sensory level is defined at the most cranial level of the tumor.

As a rule, the early onset of urinary and fecal incontinence, preceding major extremity weakness, indicates an intramedullary tumor in humans.[9] This, in our experience, is occasionally documented in the dog or cat. The location of the tumor, however, plays a significant role in the onset of incontinence with respect to extremity weakness. Intramedullary tumors of S2–S3 present with early signs of sphincter dysfunction followed by progressive paresis of the extremities as the mass enlarges. Intramedullary tumors of the cervical, thoracic, and lumbar spinal cord rarely produce incontinence in advance of profound paresis of the extremities in dogs and cats. It is worthy of note that fecal incontinence unaccompanied by urinary incontinence is rarely associated with spinal cord or cauda equina involvement.

Conclusive evidence of intramedullary disease is established following myelography. Cerebrospinal fluid should be routinely submitted for study when performing myelography. In intramedullary lesions in dogs, protein may be elevated although infrequently. Likewise, cytologic study infrequently establishes a firm diagnosis. Spinal cord reticulosis may be diagnosed via cerebrospinal fluid cytology but not consistently.

Myelography will define a swollen cord shadow on all views (Fig. 179–24). Although this myelographic feature represents an intramedullary component, it is not to be concluded that neoplasia is the only differential diagnosis. Spinal cord contusion, fibrocartilaginous embolization of the spinal cord, and syringomyelia are possibilities to consider, although historical assessment more frequently than not will discriminate among them. Intramedullary tumors may present with acute spinal cord dysfunction, as spinal cord ischemia or hemorrhage within the tumor

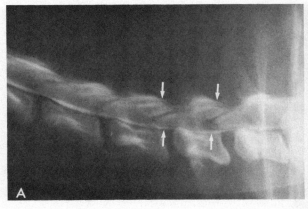

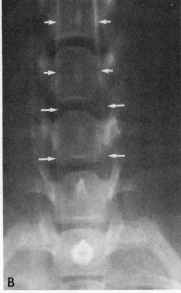

Figure 179–24. A, An intramedullary mass is demonstrated at the C6 spinal level. An enlarged cord shadow and attenuated subarachnoid space are noted *(arrows). B,* The ventrodorsal projection also demonstrates a widened cord shadow and attenuated subarachnoid space at the C6 spinal level *(long arrows).* The subarachnoid space is clearly visible at the C4 and C5 spinal levels *(short arrows).* A glioma was confirmed at necropsy.

may occur.[29] In most instances, this acute paresis is preceded by a progressive paresis that aids in distinguishing neoplasia from the peracute onset of paresis associated with fibrocartilaginous embolization of the spinal cord.

Intramedullary tumors offer a great diagnostic and therapeutic challenge to the surgeon. While many of these tumors are not surgically resectable, some are amenable to surgery as recently reported in the human literature. Successful microsurgical removal of focal and diffuse astrocytomas (often extending from the cervical spinal cord to the conus) has been documented in humans. Surgical removal of intramedullary tumors has not as yet been reported in the veterinary literature, but it is reasonable to expect it with the development of microsurgical skills.

1. Andrews, E. J.: Clinicopathologic characteristics of meningiomas in dogs. J. Am. Vet. Med. Assoc. *163:*151, 1973.
2. Attig, L., and Cusick, P. K.: Osteogenic meningioma in a dog. J. Am. Anim. Hosp. Assoc. *11:*448, 1975.
3. Austin, G.: The Spinal Cord: Basic Aspects and Surgical Considerations. 2nd ed. Charles C Thomas, Springfield, IL., 1972.
4. Ball, V., and Auger, L.: Les chordomas su tumeurs deLahorde dorsale chez l'homme ta les animaux. Rev. Vet. Zootech. *85:*185, 1953.
5. Barker, J., and Greenwood, A. G.: Intracranial lymphoid tumor in a cat. J. Small Anim. Pract. *14:*15, 1973.
6. Berryman, F. C., and deLahunta, A.: Astrocytoma in a dog causing convulsions. Cornell Vet. *65:*212, 1975.
7. Cho, D. Y., Bahr, R. J., and Leipold, H. W.: Adenocarcinoma in the nasal cavity and brain of a dog. J. Am. Vet. Med. Assoc. *165:*350, 1974.
8. Chrisman, C. L.: Behaviour and personality disorders. *In:* Problems in Small Animal Neurology. Lea & Febiger, Philadelphia, 1982. p. 147.
9. Craig, W.: Tumors of the spinal cord. Am. J. Surg. *75:*69, 1948.
10. Cusick, P. K., and Parker, A. J.: Brief communications. Vet. Pathol. *12:*460, 1975.
11. Dahme, E., and Schieter, B.: Intercranielle Geoschwhulste bei Tieren. Zbl. Vet. Med. *7:*341, 1960.
12. Epstein, B. S.: The Spine: A Radiological Text and Atlas. 3rd ed. Lea & Febiger, Philadelphia, 1969.
13. Epstein, F., and Epstein, N.: Surgical treatment of spinal cord astrocytomas of childhood. J. Neurosurg. *57:*685, 1982.
14. Ettinger, S. J. (Ed.): Textbook of Veterinary Internal Medicine: Diseases of the Dog and Cat. 1st ed. Vol. 1. W. B. Saunders, Philadelphia, 1971, Chap. 13.
15. Fox, J. G., Snyder, S. B., Reed, C., and Campbell, L. H.: Malignant ependymoma in a cat. J. Small Anim. Pract. *14:*23, 1973.
16. Frankhauser, R., Fatzer, R., and Luginbuhl, H.: Reticulosis of the central nervous system (CNS) in dogs. J. Vet. Comp. Med. *1:*35, 1972.
17. Funkguist, B.: Hourglass lipoma in a dog. J. Am. Vet. Med. Assoc. *138:*302, 1961.
18. Grant, F. C.: Spinal cord tumors. Am. J. Surg. *23:*89, 1934.
19. Greene, H. J., et al.: Neoplasia in the central nervous system of three canines. J. Am. Anim. Hosp. Assoc. *9:*369, 1973.
20. Hayes, H. M., Priester, W. A., and Pendergrass, T. W.: Occurrence of nervous tissue tumors in cattle, horses, cats, and dogs. Int. J. Cancer *15:*39, 1975.
21. Horlein, B. F. (Ed.): Canine Neurology. 2nd ed. W. B. Saunders, Philadelphia, 1971.
22. Indrieri, R. J., Holliday, T. A., Selcer, R. R., et al.: Choroid plexus papilloma associated with prolonged signs of vestibular dysfunction in a young dog. J. Am. Anim. Hosp. Assoc. *16:*263, 1980.
23. Innes, J. R. M., and Saunders, L. Z.: Comparative Neuropathology. Academic Press, New York, 1962.
24. Johnson, R. G., and Prata, R. G.: Intradiscal osteomyelitis: A conservative approach. J. Am. Anim. Hosp. Assoc., in press.
25. Jubb, R.: The hypophysis in comparative neuropathology. *In:* Innes, I. R. M., and Saunders, L. R. (Eds.): Comparative Neuropathology. Academic Press, New York, 1962.

26. Kallfelz, F. A., deLahunta, A., and Allhands, R. V.: Scintographic diagnosis of brain lesions in the dog and cat. J. Am. Vet. Med. Assoc. *172*:589, 1978.

27. Kay, W. J.: Diagnosis of intracranial neoplasms. Vet. Clin. North Am. 7(1):145, 1977.

28. Kay, W. J.: The use of corticosteroids in neurologic disease. *In*: Proceedings of the Symposium on Effective Use of Corticosteroids in Veterinary Practice. Vet Learning Systems, 1983, p. 43.

29. Kay, W. J., Israel, E., and Prata, R. G.: Cerebrospinal fluid. Vet. Clin. North Am. *4*:419, 1974.

30. Kempe, L. G.: Operative Neurosurgery. Vol. II. Springer-Verlag, New York, 1970.

31. Kernohan, J. W., and Sayre, G. P.: Tumors of the central nervous system. *In*: Atlas of Tumor Pathology. Armed Forces Institute of Pathology, Washington, D. C., 1972.

32. Koestner, A., and Zeman, W.: Primary reticulosis of the central nervous system in dogs. Am. J. Vet. Res. 23:381, 1962.

33. Kornegay, J. N.: Cerebrospinal fluid collection, examination, and interpretation in dogs and cats. Compend. Cont. Ed. *3*:85, 1981.

34. Kornegay, J. N., Oliver, J. E., Jr., and Gorgacz, E. J.: Clinicopathologic features of brain herniation in animals. J. Am. Vet. Med. Assoc. *182*:1111, 1983.

35. Kurtz, H. J., and Hanlon, G. F.: Choroid plexus papillomas in a dog. Vet. Pathol. *8*:91, 1971.

36. Lawson, C., Burk, R., and Prata, R.: Cerebral meningiomas in the cat: Diagnosis and surgical treatment of ten cases. J. Am. Anim. Hosp. Assoc. *20*:333, 1984.

37. Lee, R., and Griffiths, I. R.: A comparison of cerebral arteriography and cavernous sinus venography in the dog. J. Small Anim. Pract. *13*:225, 1972.

38. Levy, W. J., Bay, J., and Dohn, D.: Spinal cord meningioma. J. Neurosurg. *57*:804, 1982.

39. Loomas, L. N.: Choroid plexus papilloma in a dog. Vet. J. *120*:336, 1964.

40. Luginbuhl, H.: Study of meningiomas in cats. Am. J. Vet. Res. *22*:1031, 1961.

41. Luginbuhl, H., Frankhauser, R., and McGrath, J. T.: Spontaneous neoplasm of the nervous system in animals. Prog. Neurol. Surg. *2*:85, 1968.

42. McGrath, J. T.: Neurologic examination of the dog, with clinicopathologic observations. 2nd ed. Lea & Febiger, Philadelphia, 1960.

43. McGrath, J. T.: Intracranial pathology of the dog. *In*: Frauchiger, E., and Seitelberger, F. (Eds.): Symposium über vergleichunde Neuropathologie. Acta Neuropathol. Suppl. *1*:3, 1962.

44. Meincke, J. E., Hobbie, W. V., Jr., and Hardy, W. D., Jr.: Lymphoreticular malignancies in the cat: Clinical findings. J. Am. Vet. Med. Assoc. *160*:1093, 1972.

45. Metz, S. R., Taylor, S. R., and Kay, W. J.: The use of corticosteroids for treatment of neurologic disease. Vet. Clin. North Am. *12*:41, 1982.

46. Mostofi, F. R., and Price, E. B.: Tumors of the male genital system. *In*: Atlas of Tumor Pathology. 2nd series, Fascicle 8. Armed Forces Institute of Pathology, Washington, D. C., 1973. p. 40.

47. Moulton, J. E.: Tumors in Domestic Animals. Univ. of Calif. Press, Berkeley, 1961.

48. Nafe, L. A.: Meningiomas in cats: A retrospective clinical study of 36 cases. J. Am. Vet. Med. Assoc. *174*:1224, 1979.

49. Nelson, R. W., Morrison, W. B., Lurus, A. G., and Miller, J. B.: Diencephalic syndrome secondary to intracranial astrocytoma in a dog. J. Am. Vet. Med. Assoc. *179*:1004, 1981.

50. Nielson, S. W.: Classification of tumors in dogs and cats. J. Am. Anim. Hosp. Assoc. *19*:44, 1983.

51. O'Hare, M. J.: Teratomas, neoplasia, and differentiation: A biological overview. 1. The natural history of teratomas. Invest. Cell Pathol. *1*:39, 1978.

52. Palmer, A. C.: Tumors of the central nervous system. Proc. R. Soc. Med. *69*:49, 1976.

53. Palmer, A. C., Malinowski, W., and Barnett, K. C.: Clinical signs including papilloedema associated with brain tumors in twenty-one dogs. J. Small Anim. Pract. *15*:359, 1974.

54. Patnaik, A. K., et al.: Metastasizing ovarian teratocarcinoma in dogs. A report of 2 cases and review of the literature. J. Small Anim. Pract. *17*:235, 1976.

55. Patnaik, A. K., Erlardson, R. A., Lieberman, P. H., et al.: Choroid plexus carcinoma with meningeal carcinomatosis in a dog. Vet. Pathol. *17*:381, 1980.

56. Patnaik, A. K., Liu, S.-K., Hurvitz, A. I., et al.: Nonhematopoietic neoplasm in cats. J. Natl. Cancer Inst. *54*:855, 1975.

57. Patnaik, A. K., Zaki, F. A., and Herron, A. J.: Extragonadal canine teratocarcinoma. Calif. Vet. *9*:15, 1980.

58. Prata, R. G., Stoll, S. G., and Zaki, F. A.: Spinal cord compression caused by osteocartilaginous exostoses of the spine in two dogs. J. Am. Vet. Med. Assoc. *166*:371, 1975.

59. Riddle, B. L.: Cerebral meningiomas in a cat. Feline Pract. *6*:21, 1976.

60. Rothman, R. H., and Simeone, F. A.: The Spine. Vol. II. W. B. Saunders, Philadelphia, 1975.

61. Russell, D. S., and Rubinstein, L. J.: Pathology of Tumors of the Nervous System. 3rd ed. Williams & Wilkins, Baltimore, 1971.

62. Russo, M. E.: Primary reticulosis of the central nervous system in dogs. J. Am. Vet. Med. Assoc. *174*:492, 1979.

63. Saunders, L. Z., and Richard, C. G.: Craniopharyngioma in a dog with apparent adiposal genital syndrome and diabetes insipidus. Cornell Vet. *42*:490, 1952.

64. Schieter, B., Stavrou, D., Shadduck, J., et al.: Incidence of central nervous system tumors. Tierärztl. Umschau *25*:297, 1970. (Asst. Med.).

65. Shepard, D. E.: Central nervous system in the cat. Comp. Cont. Ed. *11*:306, 1980.

66. Suter, P. F., Morgan, J. P., Holiday, T. A., et al.: Myelography in the dog: Diagnosis of tumors of the spinal cord and vertebrae. J. Am. Vet. Radiol. Soc. *12*:29, 1972.

67. Taylor, F. R., Bucci, T. J., and Garvin, G. T.: Oligodendroglioma in a dog. J. Small Anim. Pract. *13*:41, 1972.

68. Tew, A. B.: The study of the clinical signs and necropsy findings resulting from experimentally produced intracranial lesions in the dog. Thesis, Auburn University, Alabama, 1964.

69. Vandervelde, M., Fatzer, R., and Frankhauser, R.: Immunohistological studies on primary reticulosis of the brain. Vet. Pathol. *18*:577, 1981.

70. Willard, M. D., and deLahunta, A.: Microgliomatosis in a Schnauzer dog. Cornell Vet. *72*:211, 1982.

71. Zaki, F. A.: Spontaneous central nervous system tumors in the dog. Vet. Clin. North Am. *7*:153, 1977.

72. Zaki, F. A., Harris, J., and Budzilovich, G.: Cystic pituicytoma of the neurohypophysis in a Siamese cat. J. Comp. Pathol. *85*:467, 1975.

73. Zaki, F. A., and Hurvitz, A. I.: Spontaneous neoplasms of the central nervous system of the cat. J. Small Anim. Pract. *17*:773, 1975.

74. Zaki, F. A., and Liu, S.-K.: Adenocarcinoma of the olfactory gland in the dog. Vet. Pathol. *11*:138, 1974.

75. Zaki, F. A., and Liu, S.-K.: Pituitary chromophobe adenoma in a cat. Vet. Pathol. *10*:232, 1973.

76. Zaki, F. A., and Prata, R. G.: Necrotizing myelopathy secondary to embolization of herniated intervertebral disk material in the dog. J. Am. Vet. Med. Assoc. *169*:222, 1976.

77. Zaki, F. A., Prata, R. G., Hurvita, A. I., et al.: Primary tumors of the spinal cord and meninges in six dogs. J. Am. Vet. Med. Assoc. *166*:511, 1975.

78. Zaki, F. A., Prata, R. G., and Kay, W. J.: Necrotizing myelopathy in five great Danes. J. Am. Vet. Med. Assoc. *165*:1080, 1974.

79. Zaki, F. A., Prata, R. G., and Werner, L. L.: Necrotizing myelopathy in a cat. J. Am. Vet. Med. Assoc. *169*:228, 1976.

80. Zaki, F. A., and Nafe, L. A.: Choroid plexus tumors in the dog. J. Am. Vet. Med. Assoc. *176*:328, 1980.

81. Zaki, F. A., and Kay, W. J.: Carcinomas of the choroid plexus in a dog. J. Am. Vet. Med. Assoc. *164*:1195, 1974.

LID TUMORS

Tumors of the eyelids may present at any age in dogs and cats but are frequently seen in middle-aged and older dogs (eight to nine years). In the dog, epithelial lid tumors predominate 6 to 1 over mesenchymal tumors, and roughly 75 per cent of the tumors are histologically classified as benign.[19, 20, 23, 62, 63, 79, 100, 102]

Canine Cutaneous Histiocytoma

The tumor is unique to canine skin. Tumor cells arise from the monocyte-macrophage cells of the skin. The incidence has been reported to be 117 per 100,000 dogs and 10.7 per cent of all canine neoplasms reviewed in a three-year period. The tumor is commonly seen in young dogs under two years of age, with a decreasing incidence in older dogs. The tumors are more frequently found in the boxer and possibly Dachshund breeds and especially involve the skin of the head.[18, 43, 61, 71, 102, 111]

The tumors are pink, fleshy, circular, epilated lesions that may involve the lids (Fig. 180–1). The lesions appear erythematous and may become ulcerated. The tumors may range in size from 0.5 to 4.0 cm and involve only the skin. However, if the tumor becomes ulcerated, inflammation may spread into the underlying dermis.

The histological appearance and distribution of infiltrating lymphocytes have been described.[71] There appears to be an immune response to the lesions, and some of them may spontaneously regress or completely disappear. Individual histiocytic cells may have a high mitotic index, but the tumors are benign.

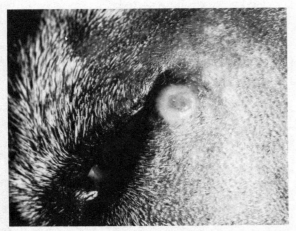

Figure 180–1. A canine histiocytoma of the skin at the lateral canthus. These benign tumors are usually seen in young animals and involve the epidermis and underlying dermis.

Human pathologists may diagnose the tumors as malignant because of their mitotic index.

Because the tumors involve only the skin, they can be removed in a number of ways. Cryosurgery can be done on small lesions. On larger lesions, especially those involving the lid margin, a split thickness lid resection can be performed, the skin and associated tumor removed, and the lid skin closed from side to side. Alternatively, a vertical or horizontal pedicle graft can be created if the lesion involves more than one-fourth of the lid margin.[19, 100] Histiocytomas do not re-occur if completely removed surgically.

Papillomas (Verrucas, Warts)

These benign epithelial tumors are common in dogs, with the incidence reported to range between 1 and 25 per cent of all skin neoplasms.[18, 19, 62, 100, 102]

Cutaneous papillomas involving the lids are most commonly seen in dogs older than eight years.[19] The papillomas may have a broad base or may be on a narrow, pedunculated stalk. The epidermis of the tumor becomes thickened and may appear cauliflowerlike with numerous projections (Fig. 180–2). Frequently as the tumors grow larger they are easily traumatized and their surface ulcerates and they bleed. The tumors do not invade the underlying dermis. Papillomas are frequently found (17 to 20 per cent of lid tumors) in older dogs and may be multiple on one lid.[19, 100]

Because these tumors involve only the epidermis, surgical full thickness wedge resection of the lid is not necessary. These growths can be treated by cryosurgery or split thickness resection of the skin tumor from the lid. If the tumor is completely removed, regrowth will not occur. Cutting the pedunculated stalk of a papilloma may remove the mass of the tumor, but the small remaining stalk may serve as a nidus for regrowth.

Basal Cell Tumors (Basal Cell Carcinoma, Basal Cell Epithelioma)

Basal cell tumors arise from the basal layers of the epidermis or embryonal stratum germinativum or within hair follicles or cells of sebaceous glands.

In terms of the overall incidence of skin tumors in dogs, basal cell tumors are estimated to comprise 10 to 12 per cent, with dogs in the seven- to nine-year-old group having the highest incidence. The incidence of basal cell tumors may be higher in the cat than in the dog, with incidences as high as 26 per cent of all epithelial skin tumors reported.[23, 35, 102]

The tumors may be found on the lids. Size varies from 0.5 to 10 cm, and the skin is elevated, firm,

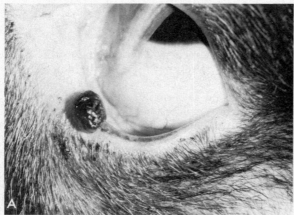

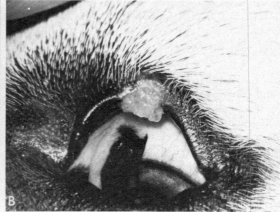

Figure 180–2. A and B, Fibropapillomas of the lid margin. These are commonly seen on the lids of older dogs and may be multiple, with more than one tumor on the lid. They are benign and epithelial in origin.

erythematous, and frequently ulcerated. These tumors do not invade locally but frequently extend into the dermis and are usually well encapsulated. The tumor has been classified on the basis of histological appearance into solid, garland, medusoid, adenoid, cystic, and basosquamous types.[102, 103]

Basal cell tumors are benign, and if the tumor is entirely removed, there is usually no recurrence. If the tumor involves the lid margin and can be palpated over the dermis as well as epidermis, full thickness wedge resection is indicated. Cryotherapy may also be used.

Squamous Cell Carcinoma

These are the most malignant of the epithelial tumors. They originate from the squamous epithelial cells of the epidermis, and the incidence in the dog and cat varies from 3 to 20 per cent of cutaneous tumors. The tumor is more frequently found in animals with lightly pigmented skin following chronic sunlight exposure or long periods of dermatosis. The head, tips of the ears, and eyelids in lightly pigmented or white animals are most frequently affected, e.g., white cats.[18, 35, 73, 102, 106]

The lesion starts as an epitheliomatous "plaque" progressing through stages of *carcinoma in situ* and then invasive carcinoma involving the dermis and subcutaneous tissues. The tumors are frequently rapidly spreading, invasive, and necrotic; are easily traumatized; and tend to bleed. Some tumors consist of cells that are very anaplastic, spread rapidly, and metastasize to regional lymph nodes and lungs. Diagnosis can usually be made based on biopsy of the lesion and histological examination. The tumor should then be staged (Figs. 180–3 through 180–7).[73]

ADNEXAL TUMORS

Tumors of the sebaceous glands of the lids are the most frequently seen adnexal tumors in older dogs

(mean age 9.5 years).[19] These tumors arise from the tarsal (meibomian) glands of the lids and are very common in older dogs. Tumors arising from sebaceous glands can be subdivided into adenomas, adenocarcinomas, and adenomatous hyperplasia.[18, 27, 44, 66, 102]

Tarsal gland adenomas involve the lid margin. As the tumor enlarges, tumor tissue grows through the lid margin. In these cases the overlying skin may be pigmented or the tumor may be easily traumatized and may ulcerate and bleed. Examination of the palpebral conjunctiva reveals that the conjunctiva is elevated because of the tumor growing within the substance of the lid (Figs. 180–8 and 180–9).

These tumors are most easily removed when they are small. A full thickness wedge resection of the lid is performed, and if all tumor tissue is removed, regrowth will not take place. If the tumor is an adenoma, it is benign and noninvasive. If the tumor mass penetrates the margin of the lid and only this extruding tumor tissue is removed, the tumor will regrow until the core of the tumor tissue arising from the gland is surgically resected.[19]

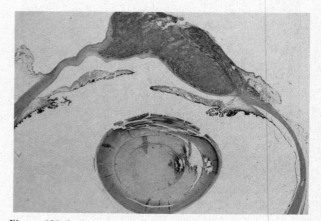

Figure 180–3. Squamous cell carcinoma of the cornea that has grown throughout the corneal stroma but has failed to penetrate Descemet's menbrane and the anterior chamber.

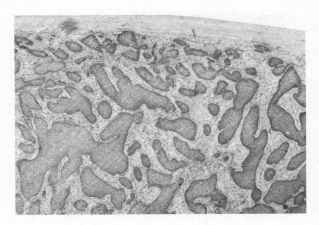

Figure 180–4. Histological section of the squamous cell carcinoma in Figure 180–3 (higher magnification). Nests of squamous tumor cells are present throughout the corneal stroma.

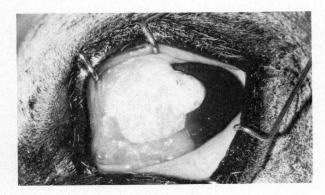

Figure 180–5. A squamous cell carcinoma of the third eyelid as well as the cornea.

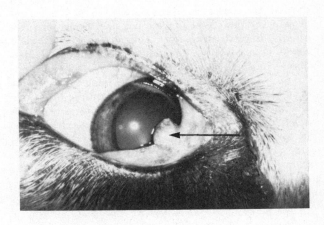

Figure 180–6. Early squamous cell carcinoma on the margin of the third eyelid in a dog. Early surgical removal or cryosurgery is indicated.

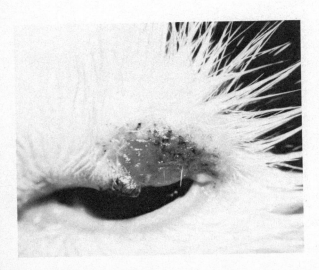

Figure 180–7. Squamous cell carcinoma of the lids of a white cat. Early recognition or wide surgical excision may be curative. Advanced lesions should be staged, and more radical therapy is required.

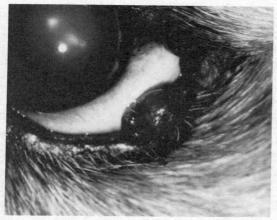

Figure 180–8. A sebaceous gland adenoma of the tarsal glands of the lower lid. This is the most common type of benign growth of the lids in older dogs.

Melanomas

Normal melanocytes are dendritic cells and are located within the epidermis at the epidermal-dermal junction between the cells of the basal layer. Melanoblasts, the precursors of melanocytes, are derived from neuroectodermal tissue.[32]

Melanomas involve the skin of older dogs, with an average age of nine to ten years. The incidence of dermal melanomas is approximately 5 to 7 per cent of skin tumors. Skin melanomas are seen more frequently in Scottish terriers, Boston terriers, Airedale terriers, and springer spaniels. The increased incidence in these breeds may be associated with increased skin pigmentation. The biological behavior of melanomas in dogs varies depending on their location. The tumors arise most frequently from the head, especially the lips and cheeks, the extremities, the prepuce, and mammary area. Those tumors arising at mucocutaneous junctions are malignant, whereas those arising in the skin are usually benign.

An exception is the interdigital area, in which the tumors are usually very malignant.

A classification of skin melanomas in the dog has been established.[32, 102] Benign growths are subdivided according to the presence of abnormal melanocytes at the epidermal-dermal junction. Benign melanocytic growths that show such junctional activity are called *junctional melanocytomas*. Dermal melanocytomas do not have junctional activity and are subdivided into fibrous and cellular tumors. Malignant melanomas invade the dermis and surrounding connective tissue and metastasize.

The more complicated system of dermal melanoma formation used in man referring to nevi formation and junctional and compound nevi cannot be easily applied to the dog.

Melanocytic tumors with junctional activity develop from flat, black maculae into elevated, often pedunculated, lesions that may be from 0.5 to 1.0 cm in diameter. Some junctional nevi regress spontaneously.[32, 102]

Benign dermal melanomas are well-circumscribed elevated masses covered by thin, hairless skin that usually measure 0.5 to 2.0 cm. Malignant melanomas are usually larger than benign dermal melanomas. These tumors are usually rapidly growing and locally invasive, and the overlying skin may be ulcerated. Fortunately, most melanomas of the lids of dogs are either benign junctional or benign dermal (Figs. 180–10 and 180–11).

Bostock has reviewed the prognosis after surgical removal of canine melanomas.[21] Ten per cent of dogs that were diagnosed as having benign dermal melanomas died from the disease. Dogs with malignant melanomas of the skin had a 70-week median survival time, and 45 per cent of the dogs were dead from the tumor in two years. The major histological type found in malignant dermal melanomas was epithelioid; the dogs had a mean survival time of 24 weeks, and 73 per cent died after two years.

Besides the histological type involved in tumor

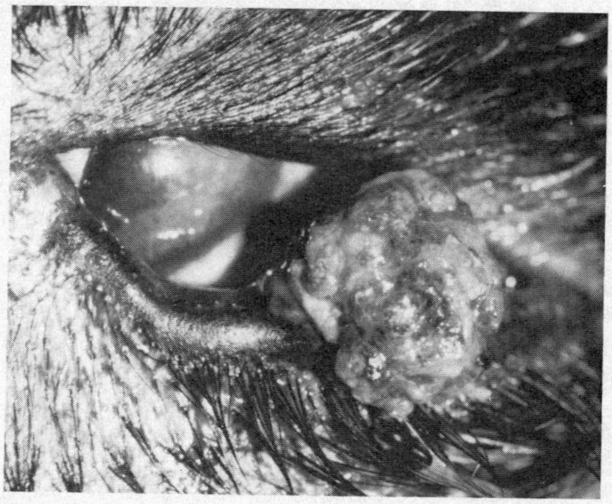

Figure 180–9. A large sebaceous gland adenoma occupying half of the lid margin. Although this tumor is benign, when this large the mass can be easily ulcerated and will bleed.

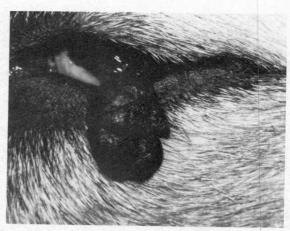

Figure 180–10. A melanoma of the lower lid in a dog. Melanomas of the lid are usually benign compared with those arising from mucous membrane surfaces.

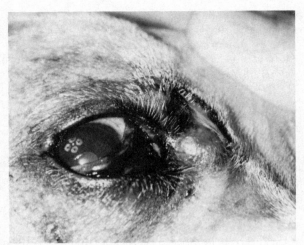

Figure 180–11. A malignant melanoma of the skin and subcutaneous tissue of the medial canthus of a nine-year-old Cairn terrier. The tumor had been surgically removed on three occasions. The time from first surgical removal to metastasis of the melanoma was nine months.

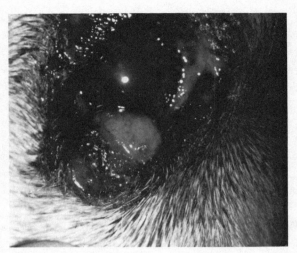

Figure 180–12. A canine mast cell tumor involving half of the lower lid.

formation, the mitotic activity is also of significance in determining prognosis. Dogs with melanomas with two or less mitotic figures per 10 hpf had a median survival time of 104 weeks and a 10 per cent mortality after two years. Dogs with tumors that had three or more mitotic figures per 10 hpf had a 30-week median survival time and a 73 per cent mortality after two years.

Mast Cell Tumors

The mast cell is a normal component of connective tissue. The terms *mast cell tumor, mastocytoma, mast cell sarcoma,* and *mastocytosis* may be used interchangeably. Mast cell tumors in the dog represent 7 to 21 per cent of all skin tumors and 11 to 27 per cent of all malignant skin tumors. The tumor is seen most frequently in dogs eight to ten years of age. There is a breed predilection in the boxer, Boston terrier, English bulldog, and English bull terrier.[18, 40, 53, 66, 102]

The most common tumor sites for those mastocytomas arising from the dermis and subcutaneous tissue are the trunk, perineal region, and head and neck.[18] Lid tumors are elevated, nodular, and firm. Hair is lost from the skin, and the tumors frequently ulcerate on the surface (Fig. 180–12).

Diagnosis of mast cell tumor can be made on impression smears or fine needle aspirates of the tumor. The smears are stained with new methylene blue, a Romanowsky stain, or toluidine blue to demonstrate the metachromatically staining granules of heparin, histamine, serotonin, and eosinophilic chemotactic substance.

Mast cell tumors may be benign or malignant. A histological system has been developed to classify these tumors according to degree of malignancy, and a clinical staging system for these tumors has also been developed.[110] Each patient should be treated based on histological findings and clinical staging.[18] Treatment of lid tumors is by full thickness wedge resection. Additional therapy may involve chemotherapy, radiation therapy, or immunotherapy or any combination thereof.[18, 19]

When a mastocytoma is surgically removed, a wide surgical margin of at least 2 cm should be made. Thus, it is much easier to remove lid tumors cosmetically when they are small. Surgical removal of isolated lid mast cell tumors is most successful when the tumor is confined to stage 1 in which there is no lymph node, peripheral blood, or bone marrow involvement.[110]

Cryosurgery can be used for small mast cell tumors.

TUMORS OF THE CONJUNCTIVA, THIRD EYELID, AND CORNEA

Tumors of the conjunctiva may involve the third eyelid or the bulbar or palpebral conjunctiva. Conjunctival papillomas usually occur on the lid margins or the third eyelid (Fig. 180–13). They may be

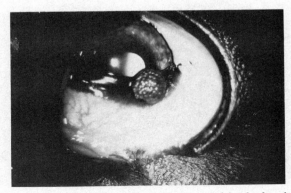

Figure 180–13. A fibropapilloma on the margin of the third eyelid. This fibropapilloma was on a sessile base and could have been removed either surgically or with cryosurgery.

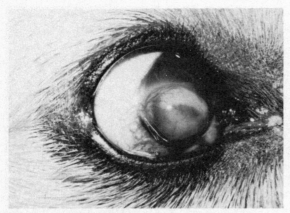

Figure 180–14. A benign fibrous histiocytoma that developed on the conjunctiva and grew to invade the corneal stroma.

pigmented and tend to be pedunculated. Histologically there are usually frond or fingerlike projections covered by acanthotic epithelium and lined by a core of connective tissue.

Carcinoma of the conjunctiva often develops at the perilimbal area or on the third eyelid. The earliest lesion is a leukoplakia or slightly raised fleshy mass (see Figs. 180–5 and 180–6). In these early cases the epithelium is replaced by atypical, pleomorphic epithelial cells, and the epithelium is thickened two to five times normal. The normal polarity of epithelial cells is lost, and mitotic figures are frequently observed in the abnormal cells. The basement membrane of the epithelium is intact, and there is no invasion of the subepithelial tissue.[57, 59, 117] Carcinomas of the conjunctiva spread through the epithelial basement membrane and into the stroma or across the limbus and into the cornea (Fig. 180–14; see also Fig. 180–11).

Dermoids are congenital tumors of the cornea and conjunctiva. A dermoid (dermolipoma) is a choristoma, a congenital tumor composed of elements normally not present in the location under consideration (Fig. 180–15). Dermoids often arise on the

conjunctiva and cross the limbus to involve the cornea. The dermoid is usually composed of epidermis with epidermal appendages (hair follicles, sebaceous glands, keratin). Treatment is by superficial keratectomy. If all the tumor tissue is removed it does not recur.[57, 117]

Intraocular Tumors

Intraocular tumors are not frequently recognized. Reports in the literature cover a total of 24 primary intraocular tumors and 11 secondary intraocular tumors. Undoubtedly more intraocular tumors do occur, but the eye, especially the posterior pole, is seldom examined.[1, 7, 8, 14, 20, 62, 76, 79, 96, 100]

There are a number of clinically significant signs that may indicate the development of an intraocular tumor.

1. The iris may be altered in color, shape, thickness, or mobility. With melanomas, changes in pigmentation and thickess may be diffuse or focal.

2. Keratitis and corneal edema may be associated with neoplastic growth in the iris and invasion of the anterior chamber, damaging the corneal endothelium.

3. Uveitis is commonly seen with lymphosarcomatous infiltration of the anterior uveal tract.

4. Secondary glaucoma may develop when tumor tissue invades the anterior drainage angle.

5. There may be conjunctival and deep scleral vascularization over the area of the tumor cell infiltration in the anterior uveal tract.

6. Additional signs that may be observed with intraocular tumor metastasis include intraocular bleeding, lens luxation, and retinal detachments.

Intraocular tumors can be classified as primary or secondary. Primary tumors arise directly from the neuroepithelium of the retina, ciliary body, or iris; from cells of neural crest origin; from vascular endothelium; or from smooth muscle or neural mesenchymal elements. The most common primary intraocular tumor is the melanoma, which occurs in two forms, localized and diffuse.[1, 2, 77, 112]

Epibulbar Melanomas

Black masses that appear in the sclera, usually near or at the limbus, present a difficult differential diagnosis. The tissue mass may be an epibulbar melanoma arising in the scleral or episcleral tissues and not invading the sclera to involve deeper intraocular tissues. Epibulbar masses may, however, be extensions of intraocular melanomas arising from the ciliary body or iris and growing into the sclera and episcleral tissue. Careful ocular examination usually differentiates the two (Fig. 180–16).

1. Extensions of intraocular melanomas usually have a well-developed vascular supply in the sclera.

2. Gonioscopic examination may show evidence of intraocular spread of melanoma into the sclera.

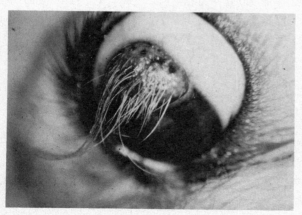

Figure 180–15. A corneal dermoid on the conjunctiva and cornea. Complete surgical removal of the dermoid by a superficial keratectomy will prevent any further growth or irritation.

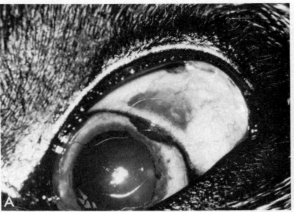
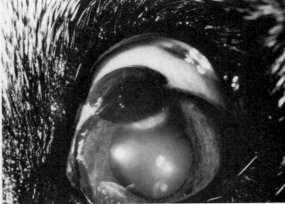

Figure 180–16. *A* and *B,* Episcleral melanomas in the dog. Note that the melanomas are arising on the episcleral tissue and involve the conjunctiva and that there is growth of melanoma into the cornea. Examination of the iris and anterior drainage angle using a gonioscopic lens failed to reveal any spread of the tumor into deeper ocular structures.

3. The iris may show evidence of intraocular involvement with melanoma.

4. Tumor involvement may be seen by dilating the pupil and, using indirect ophthalmoscopy, examining the peripheral retina and pars-plana ciliary body area.

Based on a limited series in dogs, epibulbar melanomas may be more aggressive in their growth patterns in young dogs. In this series tumor growth invaded the cornea from the sclera and grew into the corneal stroma. In older dogs (7 to 11 years) the epibulbar melanomas remained in the sclera and episcleral tissue.[77, 112]

If epibulbar melanomas do not invade and do not grow into the cornea or through the sclera, surgical removal is not recommended. If the tumors begin to grow, either complete enucleation or scleral wall resection with a scleral transplant should be performed.

True melanomas of the posterior choroid are rare in domestic animals.[1, 96] Melanomas usually arise from the pigmented epithelial cells of the ciliary processes, ciliary body, or posterior iridal surface. The growths are not usually recognized until one of the following takes place: (1) a black, elevated mass becomes visible in the well-vascularized sclera adjacent to a thickening of the iris stroma; (2) the surface of the iris assumes a different shape, and iris pigmentation is altered; (3) the anterior chamber is partially filled with pigmented tissue, altering the pupillary space; or (4) hyphema and secondary glaucoma obliterate the anterior ocular segment from view.

The clinical management of intraocular melanomas is being re-evaluated in man as well as in animals.[1, 2, 3, 74, 77, 98, 99, 112, 119] In the dog, melanomas that involve only portions of the iris and small areas of the ciliary body may be treated by surgical sector iridectomy. If postoperative complications are not severe, results have been good, usually without recurrence or metastasis.[1, 29, 77]

The more extensive intraocular melanoma in dogs presents a surgical dilemma. Should the diseased eye

be enucleated? Unfortunately we do not have extensive follow-ups of intraocular melanomas in dogs. There is evidence that intraocular melanomas in dogs grow within the globe but rarely metastasize to regional lymph nodes and lungs.[1, 112] However, my own experience is that if the melanoma is surgically disturbed (i.e., cut during enucleation), rapid spread and dissemination are likely to follow. Another problem encountered with intraocular melanomas in dogs is that, if left alone, the tumor may grow through the scleral wall or cribriform plate and enter the orbit (Figs. 180–17 and 180–18). During the course of enucleation it is usually impossible to avoid disturbing these tumors, and rapid spread over the next two to three months takes place. It is difficult to make concrete recommendations concerning intraocular melanomas in dogs. If the involved eye is not surgically removed, it should be carefully observed for increased tumor size, which is an indication, in my opinion, for careful enucleation.

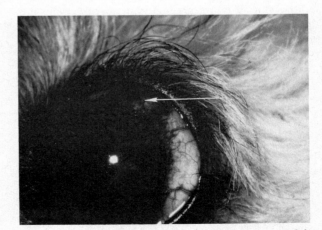

Figure 180–17. A pigmented mass in the superior aspect of the sclera of a dog. The pigmented mass is elevated, and examination of the iris and anterior drainage angle revealed that this is a melanoma arising from the ciliary body that was not grossly visible until the tumor grew into the sclera. In this case, because of the rapid growth of the tumor, the eye was enucleated.

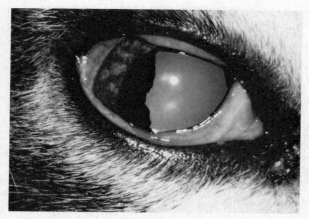

Figure 180–18. A melanoma in a dog arising from the ciliary body and involving the iris and penetrating the sclera. The tumor was not recognized until it grew through the sclera.

Diffuse Feline Melanomas

Another form of melanoma involves the feline eye. In this tumor the melanoma is more diffuse, involves the iris stroma, and results in infiltration of the anterior drainage angle with the development of secondary glaucoma (Fig. 180–19). Neoplastic cells may be seen in the anterior chamber as well as on the anterior lens capsule. The type of tumor cells seen are predominantly anaplastic epithelioid and balloon cells. Although these more diffuse tumor types may spread more rapidly throughout the anterior ocular segment, they do not appear to readily metastasize.[1–3, 33, 86] The treatment of choice is enucleation.

The second most frequently observed intraocular tumors are growths arising from the nonpigmented epithelium of the ciliary body and ciliary processes. These neuroepithelial tumors can be classified morphologically based on whether the tumor is derived from mature neuroepithelium or primitive medullary epithelium. Tumors arising from mature neuroepithelium include adenomas and adenocarcinomas. Tumors arising from more primitive neuroepithelial tissue include medulloepitheliomas and teratoid medulloepitheliomas.[1, 12, 13, 16, 17, 42, 49, 67, 69, 115]

Neuroepithelial Tumors

Neuroepithelial tumors are usually not recognized until they become large enough to be seen through the pupil. More of the tumor mass can be seen if the pupil is dilated. The growth can be deceiving because only a small amount of tumor tissue may be visible in the pupillary space while much more extensive tumor may be present in the vitreous and posterior chamber (Fig. 180–20).

Histologically, the more mature tumors of neuroepithelial tissue—adenomas and adenocarcinomas—are characterized by proliferation of nonpigmented ciliary epithelium. Cells are proliferated in the form of cords, convoluted strands, or pseudorosettes. There may be an eosinophilic staining mucoid material within the center of the rosette, which may be a precursor of vitreous. Although these growths can be locally invasive, they are seldom malignant or metastatic. The more primitive neuroepithelial tumors contain multilayered sheets and tubular structures formed by elongated polarized neuroblastic cells that resemble primitive retina. The teratoid medulloepitheliomas contain structures not normally found as derivatives of the medullary epithelium of the optic cup. These include tissues containing neurons and glia resembling brain, islands of hyaline cartilage, embryonic mesenchyme, and skeletal muscle fibers. These tumors may be locally invasive, but metastasis to other areas is uncommon.[67, 69, 115] Tumors of the nonpigmented epithelium of the ciliary body should be removed by enucleation.

Secondary Intraocular Tumors

The most common secondary intraocular tumor is lymphosarcoma.[31, 72, 84, 93] Immature lymphocytes

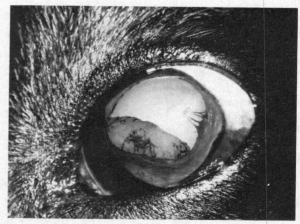

Figure 180–20. The second most common intraocular tumor found in dogs and cats arises from the nonpigmented epithelial tissue of the ciliary body and ciliary processes. These tumors are not usually noticed until the tumor mass is large enough to be seen through the pupil.

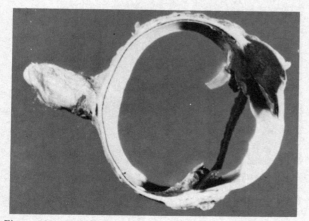

Figure 180–19. Diffuse malignant melanoma arising from the iris and ciliary body of a cat.

commonly infiltrate the third eyelid and anterior uveal tract; infiltration may result in a greatly thickened iris and an irregular, usually miotic pupil. Hypopyon frequently develops, and a severe flare (increased protein) in the anterior chamber obscures the iris and lens from view. There is deep scleral injection and conjunctival chemosis. Thickening of the iris with infiltration of immature lymphocytes can lead to narrowing of the anterior drainage angle and secondary glaucoma.

Lymphocytic infiltration may also involve the posterior choroid. When this occurs there may be an exudative retinal detachment and an outpouring of immature lymphocytes and protein into the vitreous cavity. Retinal hemorrhages and vitreal bleeding may also be observed. The ocular manifestations of lymphosarcoma in the cat are often bilateral, although one eye may show more advanced changes (Figs. 180–21 and 180–22). [1, 31, 84, 96, 100]

Metastatic neoplasms from distant sites most commonly involve the anterior uveal tract. The most frequent tumor type is secondary adenocarcinoma, with metastasis most frequently from the kidney, thyroid, mammary gland, or nasal cavity. Diagnosis of metastatic intraocular tumor involves a careful evaluation of the animal in an attempt to discover the primary tumor. [1, 10, 36, 38, 45, 47, 65, 68, 75, 78, 108, 109] Transmissible venereal tumors may also metastasize to the eye as well as orbital tissue. [1, 17] Hemangiosarcomas may metastasize to the uveal tract and result in intraocular hemorrhage and secondary glaucoma. [108]

ORBITAL TUMORS

Orbital tumors may be primary, arising from one of the many tissues within the orbit, or secondary, spreading by direct extension from the sinuses, nose, and lacrimal gland. In general, orbital tumors in

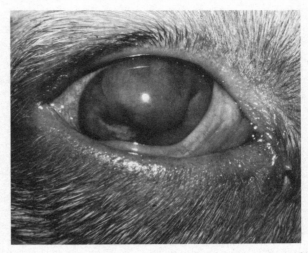

Figure 180–22. Anterior uveal lymphoid infiltration in a dog with lymphosarcoma. The entire uveal tract is filled with immature lymphocytes, and secondary glaucoma, uveitis, and exudative retinal detachments may be observed.

animals are uncommon. [1, 5, 6, 19, 22, 26, 28, 41, 50, 54–56, 64, 82, 87, 89, 96, 97]

Tumors arising primarily from the orbit are sarcomas and meningiomas. Sarcomas are usually very anaplastic, spread diffusely, and may metastasize rapidly to regional lymph nodes and lungs. The tumors often destroy surrounding bone, producing lytic lesions seen on radiographs. These tumors often spread from the orbit into the mouth or nasal cavity.

Meningiomas are usually benign tumors originating from arachnoid cells. [5, 6, 26, 41, 50, 56, 59, 92] Meningiomas may be classified into (1) primary meningiomas that originate from intraorbital optic nerve sheath, or (2) secondary meningiomas that arise within the cranium and extend into the orbit directly through bone or by extension through the optic foramen along sheaths of the optic nerve (Figs. 180–23 and 180–24).

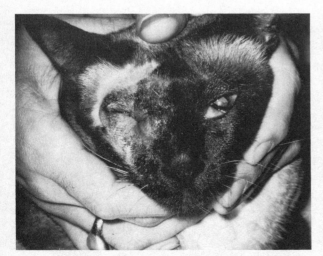

Figure 180–21. Lymphosarcoma in a Siamese cat involving the periorbital tissues of the right eye as well as infiltrating the uvea of the left eye. Deep biopsy of the tissue surrounding the right eye was necessary to confirm the diagnosis of lymphosarcoma.

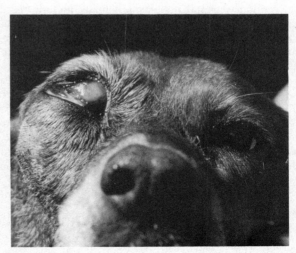

Figure 180–23. Severe exophthalmos in a dog caused by a rapidly growing meningioma of the optic nerve that filled the orbital cavity.

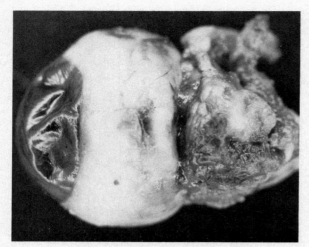

Figure 180–24. Meningioma of the optic nerve as shown in Figure 180–23.

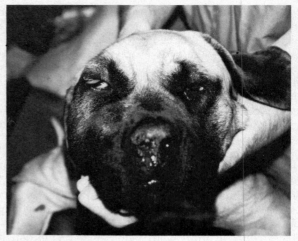

Figure 180–25. A two-year-old dog with a rapidly growing periorbital and orbital mass deforming the right side of the face and compressing the right globe in the orbit. The tumor is typical of the anaplastic sarcomas that involve the periorbital area of young dogs.

Meningiomas have also been classified according to cell type. However, there appears to be some controversy over the naming of these cell types. Basically there are two types: endotheliomatous and fibroblastic. With endotheliomatous meningioma the tumor is composed of polygonal epithelial-like cells with ill-defined cell borders. The cells are diffuse and arranged in elongated sheets or islands separated by scanty vascular connective tissue trabeculae. Cells are almost always present in whorls closely wrapped around one another. The whorls appear fairly frequently with a hyalinized and calcified center and are termed *psammoma bodies*. The word *psammoma* is derived from the Greek *psammos* meaning sand.

The tumor cells of fibroblastic meningiomas are composed of elongated, fusiform cells arranged in wavy, interlacing fascicles. There is a well-developed network of collagen and reticulin fibers between individual cells. Occasional whorls and psammoma bodies may be found.[92] Meningiomas are locally invasive but usually do not metastasize.[5, 6, 26, 56]

Secondary orbital neoplasms usually include nasal carcinoma, anaplastic sarcoma, fibrosarcoma, squamous cell carcinoma, chondrosarcoma, rhadomyosarcoma, osteosarcoma, hemangiosarcoma, chondroma, liposarcoma, and malignant melanoma.

Primary anaplastic sarcomas of the periorbital area have been observed in a series of young dogs one to three years of age. These tumors are small when first recognized but grow rapidly and metastasize early to regional lymph nodes. The cells are very anaplastic, with large numbers of mitotic figures. Bone near these tumors usually undergoes lysis, as seen on radiographic examination (Figs. 180–25 and 180–26).

Orbital and retro-orbital tumors usually present with the following clinical signs[89]:

1. Slowly progressive exophthalmos. Positional deviation of the globe may develop if the tumor is outside the posterior orbital cone of muscles (e.g., tumor of zygomatic salivary gland that causes upward deviation of the globe).

2. Secondary exposure keratitis.

3. Loss of vision; dilated unresponsive pupil.

4. Optic nerve edema, atrophy, retinal detachment.

5. Impaired mobility of the globe.

6. Protrusion of the third eyelid.

Diagnosis of an orbital tumor can be accomplished via a number of techniques (see Chapter 109).

1. Contrast orbital venography may demonstrate a retro-orbital vascular compressive lesion but will not differentiate the type of mass present.

2. Ultrasonography will demonstrate an abnormal mass and its extent but not its type.

3. Radiography of the orbit.

4. Retro-orbital aspiration and cytological examination.

5. Surgical exploration of the orbit. A number of

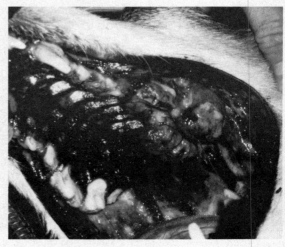

Figure 180–26. The anaplastic sarcoma in Figure 180–25 has grown through the mouth and destroyed large areas of the zygomatic and maxillary bones.

techniques have been described for performing this technique in the dog and cat (see Chapter 109). In many instances, the results of this technique allow a decision to be made about the extent of a retro-orbital mass, i.e., whether it can be surgically removed or if the orbit must be surgically exenterated.[19, 100]

Treatment of orbital neoplasms depends on the extent of the lesion, whether metastasis is present, and the tumor type.[54, 82, 94, 118]

1. Acland, G. M.: Intraocular tumors in dogs and cats. Comp. Cont. Ed. 1:558, 1979.
2. Acland, G. M., McLean, I. W., Aguirre, G., and Trucksa, R.: Diffuse iris melanoma in cats. J. Am. Vet. Med. Assoc. 176:52, 1980.
3. Albert, D. M., Schadduck, J. A., Sang, D. N., and Craft, J.: Feline uveal melanoma model. A.R.V.O. 1977 Supplement to Invest. Ophthalmol. Vis. Sci. April, 1977, p. 35.
4. Albert, D. M., et al.: Retinal neoplasia and dysplasia. Induction by feline leukemia virus. Invest. Ophthalmol. Vis. Sci. 16:325, 1977.
5. Andrews, E. J.: Clinicopathologic characteristics of meningiomas in dogs. J. Am. Vet. Med. Assoc. 163:151, 1973.
6. Barnett, K. C., and Kelly, D. F.: Retrobulbar and chiasmal meningioma in a dog. J. Small Anim. Pract. 8:391, 1967.
7. Barron, C. N., and Saunders, L. Z.: Intraocular tumors in animals. II. Primary nonpigmented intraocular tumors. Cancer Res. 19:1171, 1959.
8. Barron, C. N., Saunders, L. Z., and Jubb, K. V.: Intraocular tumors in animals. III. Secondary intraocular tumors. Am. J. Vet. Res. 24:835, 1963.
9. Barron, C. N., Saunders, L. Z., Seibold, H. R., and Heath, M. K.: Intraocular tumors in animals. V. Transmissible venereal tumors of dogs. Am. J. Vet. Res. 24:1263, 1963.
10. Baskin, G. B., and Depaoli, A.: Primary renal neoplasms of the dog. Vet. Pathol. 14:591, 1977.
11. Belkin, P. V.: Malignant melanoma of the bulbar conjunctiva in a dog. Vet. Med./Sm. Anim. Clin. 70:957, 1975.
12. Bellhorn, R. W.: Ciliary body adenocarcinoma in a dog. J. Am. Vet. Med. Assoc. 159:1124, 1971.
13. Bellhorn, R. W.: Secondary ocular adenocarcinoma in three dogs and a cat. J. Am. Vet. Med. Assoc. 160:302, 1972.
14. Bellhorn, R. W.: Ocular neoplasia. In Kirk, R. W. (ed.): Current Veterinary Therapy VI. W. B. Saunders, Philadelphia, 1977, pp. 652–655.
15. Bellhorn, R. W., and Henkind, P.: Ocular nodular fasciitis in a dog. J. Am. Vet. Med. Assoc. 150:212, 1967.
16. Bellhorn, R. W., and Henkind, P.: Adenocarcinoma of the ciliary body. Pathol. Vet. 5:122, 1968.
17. Bellhorn, R. W., and Vainisis, S. J.: Successful removal of ciliary body adenoma. Mod. Vet. Pract. 50:47, 1969.
18. Bevier, D., and Goldschmidt, M. H.: Skin tumors in the dog: Part I. Epithelial tumors and tumorlike lesions. Part II. Tumors of soft (mesenchymal) tissues. Part III. Lymphohistiocytic and melanocytic tumors. Comp. Cont. Ed. 3:389, 506, 588, 1981.
19. Bistner, S. I., Aguirre, G. D., and Batik, G.: Atlas of Veterinary Ophthalmic Surgery. W. B. Saunders, Philadelphia, 1977.
20. Blodi, F. C., and Ramsey, F. K.: Ocular tumors in domestic animals. Am. J. Ophthalmol. 64:627, 1967.
21. Bostock, D. E.: Prognosis after surgical excision of canine melanomas. Vet. Pathol. 16:32, 1979.
22. Bostock, D. E., and Dye, M. T.: Prognosis after surgical excision of canine fibrous connective tissue sarcomas. Vet. Pathol. 17:581, 1980.
23. Brodey, R. S.: Canine and feline neoplasms. Adv. Vet. Sci. 14:341, 1970.
24. Browne, G., and Mortimer, J. D.: Remission of canine squamous cell carcinoma after nitriloside therapy. Vet. Med./Sm. Anim. Clin. 71:1561, 1976.
25. Bushmann, W., and Hauff, D.: Results of diagnostic ultrasonography in ophthalmology. Am. J. Ophthalmol. 63:926, 1967.
26. Buyukmihci, N.: Orbital meningioma with intraocular invasion in a dog. Proc. Am. Coll. Vet. Ophthalmol. 1976, pp. 1–3.
27. Buyukmihci, N., and Karpinski, L. G.: Cosmetic removal of a sebaceous adenocarcinoma of the eyelid. Vet. Med./Sm. Anim. Clin. 70:1091, 1975.
28. Buyukmihci, N., Rubin, L. F., and Harvey, C. E.: Exophthalmos secondary to zygomatic adenocarcinoma in a dog. J. Am. Vet. Med. Assoc. 167:162, 1975.
29. Carter, J. D.: Extraocular extension of ocular melanoma. Vet. Med./Sm. Anim. Clin. 70:819, 1975.
30. Carter, J. D., and Mausolf, F.: Clinical and histologic features of pigmented ocular cysts. J. Am. Anim. Hosp. Assoc. 6:194, 1970.
31. Cello, R. M., and Hutcherson, B.: Ocular changes in malignant lymphoma of dogs. Cornell Vet. 52:492, 1962.
32. Conroy, J. D.: Melanocytic tumors of domestic animals. Arch. Dermatol. 96:372, 1967.
33. Cordy, R. H.: Primary intraocular melanoma in a Siamese cat. Vet. Pathol. 14:648, 1977.
34. Cotchin, E.: Melanotic tumors of dogs. J. Comp. Pathol. 65:115, 1955.
35. Cotchin, E.: Skin tumors of cats. Res. Vet. Sci. 2:353, 1961.
36. Drazner, F. H.: Multiple myeloma in the cat. Comp. Cont. Ed. 4:206, 1982.
37. Farris, H. E., Fraunfelder, F. T., and Mason, C. T.: Cryotherapy of equine sarcoid and other lesions. Vet. Med./Sm. Anim. Clin. 71:325, 1976.
38. Fischer, C. A., and Liu, S.-K.: Neuro-ophthalmologic manifestations of primary reticulosis of the central nervous system in a dog. J. Am. Vet. Med. Assoc. 158:1240, 1971.
39. Frith, C. H.: Meningioma in a young dog resulting in blindness and retinal degeneration. Vet. Med./Sm. Anim. Clin. 70:307, 1975.
40. Garner, F. M., and Lingeman, C. H.: Mast cell neoplasms of domestic cat. Pathol. Vet. 7:517, 1970.
41. Geib, L. W.: Ossifying meningioma with extracranial metastasis in a dog. Pathol. Vet. 3:247, 1966.
42. Gelatt, K.: Excision of adenocarcinoma of iris and ciliary body. J. Am. Anim. Hosp. Assoc. 6:59, 1970.
43. Gelatt, K. N.: Histiocytoma of the eyelid of a dog. Vet. Med./Sm. Anim. Clin. 70:305, 1975.
44. Gelatt, K. N.: Meibomian adenoma in a dog. Vet. Med./Sm. Anim. Clin. 70:962, 1975.
45. Gelatt, K. N., Guffy, M. M., and Boggess, T. S.: Radiographic contrast techniques for detecting orbital and nasolacrimal tumors in dogs. J. Am. Vet. Med. Assoc. 156:741, 1970.
46. Gelatt, K. N., and Ladds, P. W.: Gonioscopy in dogs and cats with glaucoma and ocular tumors. J. Small Anim. Pract. 12:105, 1971.
47. Gelatt, K. N., Ladds, P. W., and Guffy, M. M.: Nasal adenocarcinoma with orbital extension and ocular metastasis in a dog. J. Am. Anim. Hosp. Assoc. 6:132, 1970.
48. Glick, A. D., Holschner, M., and Campbell, G. R.: Canine cutaneous histiocytoma: Ultrastructural and cytochemical observations. Vet. Pathol. 13:374, 1976.
49. Glickstein, J. M., and Allen, H. L.: Malignant ciliary body adenocarcinoma in a dog. J. Am. Vet. Med. Assoc. 165:455, 1974.
50. Gross, S., Aguirre, G., and Harvey, C.: Tumors involving the orbit of the dog. Proc. 10th Ann. Am. Coll. Vet. Ophthalmol. Mtg, San Francisco, 1979, pp. 229–240.
51. Gwin, R. M., Alsaker, R. D., and Gelatt, K. N.: Melanoma of the lower eyelid of a dog. Vet. Med./Sm. Anim. Clin. 71:929, 1976.
52. Gwin, R. M., Gelatt, K. M., and Peiffer, R. L., Jr.: Ophthalmic nodular fasciitis in the dog. J. Am. Vet. Med. Assoc. 170:611, 1977.
53. Hallstrom, M.: Mastocytoma of the third eyelid of a dog. J. Small Anim. Pract. 11:769, 1970.

54. Hause, W. R.: Treatment of musculoskeletal tumors of the dog and cat, selected cases. Proc. 4th Kal-Kan Symposium, 1980, pp. 45–51.

55. Hayden, D. W.: Squamous cell carcinoma in a cat with intraocular and orbital metastasis. Vet. Pathol. 13:332, 1976.

56. Henderson, J. W.: *Orbital Tumors*, 2nd ed. Brian C. Decker, New York, 1980.

57. Hogan, M. J., and Zimmerman, L. E.: *Ophthalmic Pathology*, 2nd ed. W. B. Saunders, Philadelphia, 1962, pp. 344–466.

58. Howell, R. M., and Alexander, V. G.: Keratoacanthoma on the eyelid of a beagle dog. Vet. Med./Sm. Anim. Clin. 66:1022, 1971.

59. Jakobiec, F. A.: *Ocular and Adnexal Tumors*. Aesculapius Publishing Co., Birmingham, 1978.

60. Jubb, K. V. F., and Kennedy, P. C.: *Pathology of Domestic Animals*, 2nd ed. Vol. 2, Academic Press, New York, 1970, pp. 542–544.

61. Kelly, D. F.: Canine cutaneous histiocytoma: A light and electron microscopic study. Pathol. Vet. 7:12, 1970.

62. Kircher, C. H., Garner, F. M., and Robinson, F. R.: International histologic classificaiton of tumors of domestic animals. Tumors of the eye and adnexa. Bull. WHO 50:135, 1974.

63. Kircher, C. H., Garner, F. M., and Robinson, F. R.: X: Tumors of the eye and adnexia. Bull. Org. Mond. Sante. 50:135, 1974.

64. Koch, S. A.: The differential diagnosis of exophthalmos in the dog. J. Am. Anim. Hosp. Assoc. 5:229, 1969.

65. Koestner, A., and Zeman, W.: Primary reticulosis of the central nervous system in dogs. Am. J. Vet. Res. 23:381, 1962.

66. Krehbiel, J. D., and Langham, R. F.: Eyelid neoplasms of dogs. Am. J. Vet. Res. 36:115, 1975.

67. Langloss, J. M., Zimmerman, L. E., and Krehbiel, J. D.: Malignant intraocular teratoid meduloepithelioma in three dogs. Vet. Pathol. 13:343, 1976.

68. Ladds, P. W., Gelatt, K. N., Strafuss, A. C., and Mosier, J. E.: Canine ocular adenocarcinoma of mammary origin. J. Am. Vet. Med. Assoc. 156:63, 1970.

69. Lahav, M., Albert, D. M., Kircher, C. H., and Percy, D. H.: Malignant teratoid medulloepithelioma in a dog. Vet. Pathol. 13:11, 1976.

70. Lavignette, A. M., and Carlton, W. W.: A case of ocular nodular fasciitis in a dog. J. Am. Anim. Hosp. Assoc. 10:503, 1974.

71. Lockerell, G. L., and Slauson, D. O.: Patterns of lymphoid infiltrate in canine histiocytoma. J. Comp. Pathol. 89:193, 1979.

72. MacEwen, E. G., and Hess, P. W.: Canine lymphosarcoma and leukemia. In Kirk, R. W. (ed.): *Current Veterinary Therapy VI*. W. B. Saunders, 1977, pp. 473–479.

73. Madewell, B. R., Conroy, J. D., and Hodgkins, E. M.: Sunlight-skin cancer association in the dog. J. Cutan. Pathol. 8:434, 1981.

74. McLean, I. W., Foster, W. D., and Zimmerman, L. E.: Prognostic factors in small malignant melanomas of choroid and ciliary body. Arch. Ophthalmol. 95:48, 1977.

75. Magrane, W. G.: Cavernous hemangioma of the iris. North Am. Vet. 35:516, 1954.

76. Magrane, W. G.: Tumors of the eye and orbit in the dog. J. Small Anim. Pract., 6:165, 1965.

77. Martin, C. L.: Canine epibulbar melanomas and their management. Proc. 10th Ann. Am. Coll. Vet. Ophthal. Mtg. San Francisco, 1979, pp. 113–139.

78. Meincke, J. E.: Retinal endothelial malignancies with intraocular involvement in the cat. J. Am. Vet. Med. Assoc. 1966.

79. Morgan, G.: Ocular tumors in animals. J. Small Anim. Pract. 10:563, 1969.

80. Moulton, J. E.: *Tumors in Domestic Animals*, 2nd ed. University of California Press, Berkeley, 1978.

81. Mulligan, R. M.: Melanoblastic tumors in the dog. Am. J. Vet. Res. 22:345, 1961.

82. Owen, L. N.: Biological behavior and therapy of osteosarcoma in the dog. Proc. 4th Kal-Kan Symposium, 1980, pp. 59–62.

83. Peiffer, R. L., Duncan, J., and Terrell, R.: Hemangioma of the nictitating membrane in a dog. J. Am. Vet. Med. Assoc. Submitted for publication, 1983.

84. Peiffer, R. L., Jeraj, K., Mehlhoff, T., and O'Leary, T. P.: Lymphosarcoma, small lymphocyte type, with ocular manifestations in a dog. J. Canine Pract. 3:50, 1976.

85. Peiffer, R. L., and Johnston, S.: Pseudoepitheleomatous hyperplasia of the membrane nictitans of a dog. Vet. Med./Sm. Anim. Clin. 71:635, 1976.

86. Peiffer, R. L., Jr., Seymour, W. G., and Williams, L. W.: Malignant melanoma of the iris and ciliary body in cat. Mod. Vet. Pract. 58:854, 1977.

87. Plitcher, J. M., Koch, S. A., and Stedham, M. A.: Orbital chondroma rodens in a dog. J. Am. Vet. Med. Assoc. 175:187, 1979.

88. Reese, A. B.: *Tumors of the Eye*, 3rd ed. Harper & Row, Hagerstown, 1976.

89. Riis, C. R., and Smith, J.: Diseases of the orbit. In Kirk, R. W. (ed.): *Current Veterinary Therapy VI*. W. B. Saunders, Philadelphia, 1977.

90. Rubin, L. F.: *Atlas of Veterinary Ophthalmoscopy*. Lea & Febiger, Philadelphia, 1974, pp. 210–212.

91. Rubin, L. F., and Koch, S. A.: Ocular diagnostic ultrasonography. J. Am. Vet. Med. Assoc. 153:1706, 1968.

92. Russell, D. S., and Rubinstein, L. J.: Tumors of meninges and related tissues. In *Pathology of Tumors of the Nervous System*, 3rd ed. Williams & Wilkins, Baltimore, 1972, pp. 50–52.

93. Saunders, L. Z., and Barron, C. N.: Intraocular tumours in animals. IV. Lymphosarcoma. Br. Vet. J. 120:25, 1964.

94. Saunders, L. A., and Barron, C. N.: Primary pigmented intraocular tumors in animals. Cancer Res. 18:234, 1958.

95. Saunders, L. Z., Geib, L. W., and Barron, C. N.: Intraocular ganglioma in a dog. Pathol. Vet. 6:525, 1969.

96. Saunders, L. Z., and Rubin, L. F.: *Ophthalmic Pathology of Animals*, 1st ed. S. Karger, New York, 1975, pp. 232–233.

97. Schoster, J. V., and Wyman, M.: Remission of orbital sarcoma in a dog, using doxorubicin therapy. J. Am. Vet. Med. Assoc. 172:1101, 1978.

98. Shammas, H. F., and Blodi, F. C.: Prognostic factors in choroidal and ciliary body melanomas. Arch. Ophthamol. 95:63, 1977.

99. Shields, J. A.: Approaches to the management of choroidal melanoma. In Jakobiec, F. A. (ed.): *Ocular and Adnexal Tumors*. Aesculapius Publishing Co., Birmingham, 1978, pp. 4–12.

100. Slatter, D. H.: *Fundamentals of Veterinary Ophthalmology*. W. B. Saunders, Philadelphia, 1981.

101. Smith, J. S., Bistner, S., and Riis, R.: Infiltrative corneal lesions resembling fibrous histiocytoma: Clinical and pathologic findings in six dogs and one cat. J. Am. Vet. Med. Assoc. 169:722, 1976.

102. Stannard, A. A., and Pulley, T. L.: Tumors of the skin and soft tissues. In Moulton, J. E. (ed.): *Tumors in Domestic Animals*, 2nd ed. University of California Press, Berkley, 1978, pp. 16–74.

103. Strafuss, A. C.: Basal cell tumors in dogs. J. Am. Vet. Med. Assoc. 169:322, 1976.

104. Strafuss, A. C.: Sebaceous gland adenomas in dogs. J. Am. Vet. Med. Assoc. 169:640, 1976.

105. Strafuss, A. C.: Sebaceous gland carcinomas in dogs. J. Am. Vet. Med. Assoc. 169:325, 1976.

106. Strafuss, A. C., Cook, J. E., and Smith, J. E.: Squamous cell carcinomas in dogs. J. Am. Vet. Med. Assoc. 108:425, 1976.

107. Struder, E.: Surgical treatment of cancer of the eye in cattle. Vet. Med./Sm. Anim. Clin. 66:1105, 1971.

108. Szymanski, C. M.: Bilateral metastatic intraocular hemangiosarcoma in a dog. J. Am. Vet. Med. Assoc. 151:803, 1972.

109. Szymanski, C.: Multiple myeloma with hyperviscosity syndrome in a dog. Proc. Am. Coll. Vet. Ophthalmol. 1976, pp. 143–145.

110. Tams, T. R., and Macy, D. W.: Canine mast cell tumors. Comp. Cont. Ed. 3:869, 1981.
111. Taylor, D. O. N., Dorn, C. R., and Luis, O. H.: Morphologic and biologic characteristics of the canine cutaneous histiocytoma. Cancer Res. 29:83, 1969.
112. Trucksa, R., and McLean, I.: Intraocular canine melanomas. Pro. Coll. Vet. Ophthalmol. 12th Ann. Mtg. 1981, pp. 103–114.
113. Van Kampen, K. R., Crisp, W. E., DeMartini, J. C., and Ellsworth, H. S.: The immunologic therapy of squamous cell carcinoma. Am. J. Obstet. Gynecol. 116:569, 1973.
114. Veronesi, U.: A randomized trial of adjuvant chemotherapy and immunotherapy in cutaneous melanoma. N. Engl. J. Med. 307:913, 1982.
115. Verwer, M. A. J., and Thije, P. A. Ten: Tumor of the epithelium of the ciliary body in a dog. J. Small Anim. Pract. 8:627, 1967.
116. Weisse, I., and Stotzer, H.: Intraokulares Melanom bei einem jungen Beagle. Kasuistische Mitteilung. Berl. Munch. Tierarztl. Wschr. 84:328, 1971.
117. Yanoff, M., and Fine, B.: Ocular Pathology. Harper & Row, Hagerstown, 1975, pp. 619–685.
118. Ziegler, J. L. (ed.): Sarcomas of Soft Tissue and Bone in Childhood. National Cancer Institute Monographs, No. 56., NIH Publication 81–2162, Bethesda, 1981.
119. Zimmerman, L. E., McLean, I. W., and Foster, W. D.: Does enucleation of the eye containing a malignant melanoma prevent or accelerate the dissemination of tumor cells? In Jakobiec, F. A. (ed.): Ocular and Adnexal Tumors. Aesculapius Publishing Co., Birmingham, 1978, pp. 31–39.
120. Zimmerman, L. E., and Sobin, L. H.: International Histological Classification of Tumors of Eye and Its Adnexa. World Health Organization, Geneva, 1980.

Chapter 181 Male Reproductive System

Shirley D. Johnston

Reproductive neoplasms in males include those of the testes, prostate, penis and prepuce, and mammary glands. Testicular cancer is the second most common neoplasm in male dogs, and both testicular and prostatic neoplasia occur more often in dogs than in any other domestic animal. Functional testicular tumors may cause a variety of paraneoplastic syndromes (feminization, alopecia, blood dyscrasia), which have been attributed to steroid production by these neoplasms. Tumors of the reproductive organs are very rare in male cats.

World Health Organization (WHO) staging protocols for male reproductive tumors are included in this chapter. These present a uniform system of documenting tumor presence and size (T), involvement of regional lymph nodes (N), and presence of distant metastasis (M). Although stage cannot, at present, be correlated with prognosis or expected survival time, acquisition of such data may permit such correlations in the future.

TESTICULAR NEOPLASIA

Incidence

Testicular neoplasia is more common in dogs than in any other domestic mammal or in humans.[24,35] In male dogs, the testis is the second most common neoplastic organ (after skin).[19,25,35] Testicular tumors constituted 178 of 2,550 (7 per cent), 136 of 2,361 (6 per cent), and 32 of 899 (4 per cent) canine neoplasms and 268 of 299 tumors of the male genitalia.[13,19,20,52] Their incidence has been reported as 33.9 cases per 100,000 male and female dogs.[25]

The Sertoli's cell tumor (SCT), seminoma (SEM), and interstitial cell tumor (ICT) are the most common tumors of the canine testicle. The three tumor types occur with equal frequency.[17,19,35,54,65] Individual cases of testicular fibrosarcoma, hemangioma, granulosa cell tumor, gonadoblastoma, and undifferentiated sarcoma/carcinoma have also been reported in dogs.[17,35,83,93] A 2-cm diameter leiomyoma of the tunica vaginalis of the left testis has been reported as an incidental finding in a 13-year-old miniature poodle at necropsy.[71]

The presence of more than one testicular tumor per dog or per testis is fairly common. Bilateral tumors of the same type were reported in 5 of 46 dogs with SCT (8 scrotal, 2 abdominal), 8 of 47 dogs with SEM (12 scrotal, 4 abdominal), and 21 of 67 dogs with ICT (all scrotal).[50] Thirty-eight of 198 (19.2 per cent) dogs with testicular tumor had more than one type of testicular neoplasm; these included SEM/ICT (16), SCT/ICT (13), SCT/SEM (8), and SEM/ICT/SCT (1) combinations.[50] A survey of testicular tumors in 410 dogs included 46 animals (11.2 per cent) with multiple types (15 SCT/SEM, 15 ICT/SEM, 14 SCT/ICT, 1 SCT/ICT/SEM, and 1 SCT/fibrosarcoma).[35] A survey of 94 male dogs with testicular tumors (from 580 unselected adult dogs submitted for routine necropsy) included 39 (41.5 per cent) with multiple tumor types.[26] Scully and Coffin reported 55 per cent multiplicity, 45 per cent bilaterality, and 35 per cent incidence of two or more tumor types per dog in 86 dogs with 177 testicular tumors.[83]

The incidence of the SCT and SEM is influenced by the presence of cryptorchidism.[35,50,73,77,83] Of 209 canine testicular tumors, 84 (41 per cent) occurred in ectopic testes, with type distribution of 65 SCT, 18 SEM, and 1 ICT.[19] In 410 dogs with testicular neoplasia, cryptorchid animals were determined to have 13.6 times the risk of normal dogs of developing such neoplasms; risk factors by tumor type were 23 times for the SCT, 16 times for the SEM, and 1.6 for the ICT.[35] Cryptorchidism also predisposes to testicular neoplasia in humans; their tumor risk does not decrease if the testis is moved to the scrotum surgically, suggesting that a dysgenetic gonad, rather than abdominal environment, may modulate tumor development.[4,35]

Testicular tumors occur with equal frequency in the right and left scrotal testes.[4,5,19,77] In cryptorchid dogs, testicular tumors occur more frequently in the right testis than the left (R:L = 1.8:1), matching the 1.9:1 right-to-left ratio of cryptorchid testicles in animals without testicular neoplasia.[77] These ratios suggest that tumors arise more often in the right cryptorchid testis because the right testis is retained more often than the left.

Age incidence is influenced by tumor type and location of the affected testis. With advancing age, dogs show increasing risk of developing all testicular tumor types until age 10 to 14 years.[35,78] Mean age of occurrence is 8½ years for the SCT (n = 129), 10 years for the SEM (n = 89) and 11½ years for ICT (n = 45).[19] Mean age incidence of the SCT is 11, 8.8, and 7.8 years in scrotal (n = 50), inguinal (n = 24), and abdominal (n = 34) testes.[77] SEM age incidence by testis location is 10.5, 9.1, and 7.5 years in scrotal (n = 45), inguinal (n = 15), and abdominal (n = 8) testes.[77]

Breed predisposition to testicular neoplasia is reported in the boxer, Chihuahua, Pomeranian, poodle, miniature schnauzer, Shetland sheepdog, Siberian husky, and Yorkshire terrier.[38,91] Breed predisposition to the SCT has only been reported in weimaraners and to the SEM only in German shepherds.[35] Low risk of testicular neoplasia is reported in the mixed-breed dog, dachshund, beagle, and Labrador retriever.[35,91] A syndrome of cryptorchidism, SCT in the abdominal testis, and persistence of the müllerian duct system in individuals that are phenotypically male has been described in miniature schnauzers.[7,63,66]

The incidence of testicular tumors in cats is low; no testicular tumors were present in 56 tumors in 11,909 cats, in 621 feline tumor cases from both sexes, or in surveys of 328 and 571 feline neoplasms.[18,20,24,52] Occasional case reports have documented SCT, undifferentiated carcinomas, and one testicular teratoma in aged male cats.[55,87] One report documents a SCT in the right testis and an adenoma and undifferentiated carcinoma in the left testis of a bilaterally cryptorchid aged domestic short-hair cat.[55]

Diagnosis

Testicular neoplasia is diagnosed by palpation of a testicular mass in the scrotal or ectopic testis, followed by excision biopsy and histopathology.

Paraneoplastic syndromes such as feminization (gynecomastia, pendulous penile sheath, attraction of males), alopecia, or blood dyscrasia (anemia, leukopenia, thrombocytopenia) may cause clinical signs for which the patient is admitted.[2,5,28,48,49,50,54,56,59,84] These are attributed to estrogen production by the neoplastic testis. Other abnormalities associated with testicular neoplasia that may be present in older male dogs are prostatic disease, perineal hernia, perianal gland adenoma, and perianal gland adenocarcinoma. Incidence of these clinical findings in dogs by testicular tumor type is shown in Table 181–1. Paraneoplastic syndromes are present in about half of the dogs with multiple tumor types.[50] Torsion of the scrotal or abdominal neoplastic testis is observed occasionally.[60,72]

Evidence for estrogen production by functional testicular tumors includes (1) in some affected dogs, the presence of clinical findings that are similar to those caused by exogenous estrogen administration,[5,28,50,59,84] (2) the presence of elevated concentrations of urinary estrogens measured by bioassay in some affected dogs,[5] (3) *in vitro* production of labeled estrone and estradiol after addition of tritium or carbon-14 labeled steroid precursors to canine tumor

TABLE 181–1.   Frequency of Clinical Findings in Dogs with Testicular Neoplasia

Finding	Reference	Tumor Type SCT		SEM		ICT	
Feminization (gynecomastia, pendulous prepuce, attraction of males)	5	17/37	(46.0%)				
	19	16/157	(6.4%)	1/107	(0.9%)	4/54	(7.4%)
	50	11/46	(23.9%)	1/47	(2.1%)	0/67	
Alopecia	5	20/37	(54.1%)				
	19	17/157	(10.8%)	2/107	(1.9%)	9/54	(16.7%)
	50	7/46	(15.2%)	2/47	(4.3%)	1/67	(1.5%)
Blood dyscrasia	59	8/60	(13.3%)	1/62	(1.6%)	1/87	(1.1%)
	84	8/76	(10.5%)				
Prostatic disease	5	4/37	(10.8%)				
	50	14/46	(30.4%)	17/47	(36.2%)	20/67	(29.9%)
Perianal gland neoplasia	5	0/37					
	50	5/46	(10.9%)	14/47	(29.8%)	31/67	(46.3%)

TABLE 181–2. Concentrations of Estradiol and Testosterone in Peripheral or Spermatic Vein Plasma from Dogs with Testicular Neoplasia

| Refer-ence | Tumor Type | No. of Cases | Clinical Signs | Plasma Source* | Estradiol (pg/ml) | | Testosterone (ng/ml)† | |
					Tumor Dogs	Normal Range	Tumor Dogs	Normal Range
85	SCT	5	Feminization (5/5)	P	200.0–3,300.0	210.0–750.0	ND–5.0	ND–0.5
				SV	130.0–1,500.0	300.0–600.0	ND–3.6	ND–1.6
	SEM	3	Feminization (2/3)	P	230.0–260.0	210.0–750.0	ND–2.6	ND–0.5
				V	200.0–390.0	300.0–600.0	1.4–2.6	ND–1.6
14	SCT	3	Feminization	P	28.0–31.0	9.5–24.0	0.24–3.16	0.215–2.13
				V	53.0–500.0	15.0–222.0	3.93–13.68	0.364–176.24
	SEM	3	None	P	20.0–121.0	9.5–24.0	0.23–0.86	0.215–2.13
				V	34.0–566.0	15.0–222.0	3.98–4.87	0.364–176.24
2	SEM	1	Alopecia	P			0.063	0.75–2.25
84	SCT	1	Blood dyscrasia	P	342.5	25.0–50.0	0.48	0.75–2.25
59	SCT	6	Blood dyscrasia	P	74.0–486.0	25.0–80.0	0.29–3.5	0.75–2.25
	SEM	1	Blood dyscrasia	P	42.0	25.0–80.0	0.08	0.75–2.25
	ICT	1	Blood dyscrasia	P	51.0	25.0–80.0		

*P = peripheral; SV = spermatic vein.
†ND = nondetectable.

tissue explants,[74] and (4) the presence of increased concentrations of estradiol measured by radioimmunoassay in peripheral or spermatic vein plasma from some affected dogs.[14] Some investigators have been unable to demonstrate elevated plasma or urinary estrogens in some feminized dogs with SCT, and others have been unable to show a correlation between estrogen concentrations and feminizing signs in dogs with testicular tumors.[14,85] Canine estrogen assays are difficult at best, with values from normal dogs varying widely between laboratories.[14,15,36,59,84] In a report of ten dogs with pancytopenia, anemia, or leukopenia and testicular neoplasia (eight SCT), serum estradiol was elevated in only three of the eight dogs in which it was measured (Table 181–2).[59] In a report of bone marrow hypoplasia in eight SCT dogs, plasma estradiol measured in one was elevated.[84] Elevated estradiol was detected in spermatic vein blood from two of three SCT and two of three SEM tumor patients, but there was no correlation between estradiol concentrations and presence or absence of feminizing signs.[14] Peripheral androgen concentrations have been measured in dogs with testicular tumor, both to look for decreased concentrations in feminized patients with hyperestrinism and to look for elevated concentrations in tumor patients (ICT) showing androgen-dependent neoplasia or prostatic disease (Table 181–2). Results have not shown consistent abnormalities in serum testosterone in patients with SCT or SEM.

Diagnosis of testicular tumors in cats has been by histopathology at necropsy. Paraneoplastic syndromes have not been associated with testicular neoplasia in this species.

Metastasis is uncommon, varies with tumor type, and has not been observed in dogs with more than one testicular tumor type.[50] Clinical staging of testicular tumors is by behavior of the primary tumor (T), regional lymph node involvement (N) and the presence of metastasis (M) (Table 181–3).[98] Regional lymph nodes are the sublumbar and inguinal nodes.

Sertoli Cell Tumors. SCTs are among the most easily recognized testicular neoplasms because they are generally the largest of these tumors, are the most common tumor in ectopic testes, and are the most likely to secrete estrogens and therefore cause signs of feminization, alopecia, and blood dyscrasia (Table 181–1).[5,19,50,59] SCTs range in diameter from 1 mm to more than 10 cm.[26] They are homogeneous, pale yellowish-gray or cream-colored masses on cut section.[19,26,83] Classical signs of feminization in dogs with SCT include gynecomastia with or without mammary secretion, pendulous prepuce, attraction of male dogs, and loss of libido. Alopecia involving the ventral thorax and abdomen, posterior lateral aspects of the thighs, neck, and shoulder area are also com-

TABLE 181–3. WHO Clinical Stages of Canine Testicular Tumors*

T: Primary tumor
  T0 No evidence of tumor
  T1 Tumor restricted to testes
  T2 Tumor invading tunica albuginea
  T3 Tumor invading the rete testis and/or the epididymis
  T4 Tumor invading the spermatic cord and/or the scrotum
N: Regional lymph nodes (sublumbar, inguinal)
  N0 No RLN involved
  N1 Ipsilateral RLN involved
  N2 Contralateral or bilateral RLN involved
M: Distant metastasis
  M0 No evidence of metastasis
  M1 Distant metastasis present

*Reprinted with permission from the internal report of a WHO Consultation on the Biological Behaviour and Therapy of Tumours of Domestic Animals, Geneva, 1978 (unpublished WHO document VPH/CMO/78.15).

mon with SCT.[5,83] Estrogen is reported to retard hair growth and cause atrophy of hair follicles and sebaceous glands in affected dogs; large amounts of estrogen also depress testicular and thyroid function by their negative feedback inhibition effect on pituitary gonadotropin releasing hormone and thyroid-stimulating hormone secretion.[5]

Blood dyscrasias that have been described in dogs with SCTs mimic the myelotoxic effects that exogenous estrogens exert on the pluripotential undifferentiated stem cell. These are early anemia, thrombocytopenia, and leukocytosis followed by later decline in the leukocyte count and pancytopenia.[9] Bone marrow aplasia may persist for months after estrogen administration. Sherding and associates described eight dogs with nonregenerative pancytopenia and bone marrow hypoplasia subsequent to SCT; these represented 10.5 per cent of 76 cases of SCT seen over 10 years.[84] The eight cases ranged in age from 2½ to 13 years ($\bar{x}$ = 7 years) and were presented for complaints of anorexia, weakness, acute collapse, hematuria, lameness, or fever. All eight dogs showed one or more feminizing signs. Seven of the eight were treated with castration, antibiotics, fluid therapy, hematinics, androgenic steroids, and blood or platelet-rich plasma transfusions; two of the seven recovered, and five died. One dog was euthanized. In the two dogs that recovered, hemograms showed improvement between 2 and 3 weeks after castration, and by 5 months the hemogram, including platelet count, was normal. Death in the other five was attributed to overwhelming septicemia (3) and profound nonregenerative anemia despite transfusion (2).[84] Morgan also described blood dyscrasias in eight dogs with SCT; these included pancytopenia (6), anemia (1), and leukopenia (1).[59] One of these dogs recovered with treatment. Bone marrow hypoplasia and pancytopenia have been diagnosed in a dog 2 months after castration and removal of a SCT. Original alopecia and feminization were regressing when the dog was returned for hematemesis; the dog died 12 hours after admission.[28]

Testicular torsion is an occasional sequel to testicular neoplasia in dogs; when present, torsion most often occurs in an abdominal testis bearing a SCT.[60,72] Presenting signs include acute anorexia, vomiting, and a painful abdomen; if the affected testis is scrotal or inguinal, marked swelling and pain of the affected gonad are present. Cases have been reported with concurrent alopecia, feminization, and blood dyscrasia.[72] Treatment is immediate castration, with a guarded prognosis until 1 to 2 days postoperatively.

Two cases of SCT in dogs have been described with presenting signs of partially reducible scrotal swelling.[54] In one of these, intravenous tumor extension led to varicosity of the testicular vein; in the other there was hydrocele, varicosity of the testicular vein, and lymphatic spread of the tumor.[54]

Cystic enlargement and squamous metaplasia of the prostate and squamous metaplasia of the renal tubular epithelium have been documented in dogs with metastatic SCT.[11,48,49]

Metastasis occurred in 1 of 46 (2 per cent), 4 of 40 (10 per cent), 2 of 28 (7 per cent), 2 of 138 (1.4 per cent), and 5 of 33 (15 per cent) dogs with SCT.[5,19,26,50,83] When present, metastasis occurs most often to the inguinal and sublumbar lymph nodes; metastasis to the lungs, mediastinal lymph nodes, liver, spleen, kidney, pancreas, mesenteric lymph nodes, and nipple have also been described.[5,11,26,50,83,88]

SCTs have not been associated with paraneoplastic syndromes in cats. These tumors may occur unilaterally or bilaterally and may or may not cause gross gonadal enlargement.[55]

Seminoma. Seminomas are usually round, discrete masses that are pale cream or gray.[26,83] They range in diameter from 1 mm to 10 cm.[26,83] Dow reported that 75 per cent of 41 SEM were less than 2 cm in diameter, whereas Scully and Coffin reported that more than half of 22 SEM they examined were greater than 3 cm in diameter.[26,83] Paraneoplastic syndromes attributable to estrogen production are less common in dogs with SEM than in those with SCT, but feminization and alopecia have been reported in a few SEM patients (Table 181–1). A SEM was present in the scrotal testicle of an 11-year-old toy poodle with progressive nonpruritic alopecia; other endocrine glands were normal, and hair regrowth occurred after castration.[2] Pancytopenia has been reported in an 11½-year-old wire-haired fox terrier presented with weakness, pallor, vomiting, an abdominal mass, and feminization.[59] An abdominal SEM and uterus masculinus were removed at surgery, and the dog recovered. Testicular torsion also has been reported in an abdominal testicle with a SEM.[72]

In one report, incidence of perianal gland neoplasia was nearly 30 per cent in 49 SEM dogs, compared with 10.9 per cent of 46 SCT dogs (Table 181–1).[50]

Metastases of SEMs have been reported in 3 of 47 (6.4 per cent), 0 of 20, 2 of 92 (2 per cent), and 3 of 45 (6.7 per cent) canine patients.[19,26,50,83] Most common sites of metastasis are the sublumbar lymph nodes, followed by the mesenteric lymph nodes, spleen, and lungs.[26,50,86]

Interstitial Cell Tumor. The canine ICT is smaller than other canine testicular neoplasms. Although these tumors range in diameter from 1 mm to 9 cm, 115 of 131 were less than 2 cm, and 50 of 88 were less than 1 cm in diameter.[26,83] They are ochre to yellowish soft friable masses that are sharply demarcated from adjacent seminiferous tubules; they are often incidental findings at necropsy.

As with the SEM, ICT patients occasionally show signs of feminization, alopecia, or blood dyscrasia, which are most typical of the SCT (Table 181–1). The single report of a blood dyscrasia is of pancytopenia in a 15-year-old miniature poodle presented with weakness, pallor, petechiae, and prolonged bleeding time; the dog had an ICT in a scrotal testicle and an adrenocortical adenocarcinoma, either of which may have been responsible for its signs. Intra-abdominal testicular torsion has been described in a 9-year-old unilateral cryptorchid Labrador retriever with a 30 × 10 × 10 cm ICT in the retained right testicle.[60] The patient was presented with a slowly distending abdomen of 6 months duration and vomiting of 2 weeks duration. At laparotomy, 5.2 l of a serosanguinous fluid containing *Pseudomonas aeruginosa* was aspirated from the mass prior to excision; the dog recovered uneventfully.

Lipowitz and colleagues documented prostatic disease in 20 of 67 and perianal gland neoplasia in 31 of 67 cases of ICT.[50] These tumors have not yet, however, been shown to secrete androgens, which might cause such findings.

Metastasis is very rare with the ICT, occurring in only 2 of 332 (0.6 per cent) cases from 4 surveys in the veterinary literature.[19,26,50,83] The 2 cases with metastasis had tumor cells in the sublumbar lymph nodes and lungs; one dog also had inguinal lymph node lesions, and the other had a solitary nodule in the spleen.[19,26]

Treatment and Prognosis

Treatment of canine and feline testicular neoplasia is orchiectomy of the affected testicle(s). Hemicastration may be considered in valuable breeding animals that are not cryptorchid, but bilateral orchiectomy is preferred because of the high incidence of bilateral testicular tumors and because atrophy of the contralateral testis often occurs, reducing fertility.

Prognosis for life of the animal is good in the absence of metastasis and bone marrow suppression. Although incidence of metastasis varies with tumor type, it is generally less than 10 per cent. Dogs with feminizing syndromes may show regression of signs after castration and recurrence of signs if metastasis has occurred.[11,53] Pancytopenia at surgery or as late as 2 months afterward is associated with a poor to grave prognosis, even with aggressive supportive therapy.

PROSTATIC NEOPLASIA

Incidence

Prostatic neoplasia, although not common, occurs more often in dogs than in any other domestic species.[46] Histological types of prostatic neoplasia include adenocarcinoma, poorly differentiated carcinoma, benign mesenchymal neoplasia (leiomyoma, fibroma), sarcoma, and secondary (metastatic) neoplasia to the prostate; most canine prostatic tumors are adenocarcinomas (Table 181–4).[32] A few cases of prostatic adenocarcinoma have been diagnosed in cats.[33,37,69,97]

TABLE 181–4. Clinical Signs and Patterns of Metastasis in Dogs with Prostatic Neoplastia

Parameter	Reference				Total
	46	70	90	95	
No. dogs	20	7	11	15	53
No. intact	16	6		15	
No. M/C	4	1		0	
Age range	6–15 yr	9–12 yr	6–12 yr	6–14 yr	6–15 yr
Age mean	10.1 yr	11.3 yr	8.5 yr	8.8 yr	
No. breeds	13	5	9	9	
Clinical signs (no.)	20	6	8	15	49
Emaciation	14	2	2	4	22
Lameness	10		1	4	15
Tenesmus	9	1	1	8	19
Dysuria	6	1	5	11	23
Polydipsia/polyuria	6			3	9
Lumbar pain	6		1	0	7
Urethral bleeding	5	1	3	2	11
Dyspnea		2			2
Tumor type					
Adenocarcinoma	20	6	9	15	50
Carcinoma			2		2
Transitional cell carcinoma		1			1
Metastasis present (no.)	20/20	5/5	6/7	13/13	44/45
Iliac lymph nodes	15	2	2	13	32
Lung	13	2	3	5	23
Urinary bladder	10	2	2	9	23
Bone	7			3	10
Mesentery	7	1			8
Rectum	6	1		9	16
Pelvic muscles	5	3	1	12	21
Heart	3				3
Adrenal	2			1	3
Kidney	2		3	4	9
Spleen	2				2
Liver	1		1	1	3
Ureter				4	4
Mediastinal lymph node		1			1

Of 4,500 dogs necropsied during 11 years, 430 were identified with prostatic disease and 15 (0.33 per cent) with prostatic adenocarcinoma.[95] Others have estimated that this tumor occurs in 0.29 to 0.6 per cent of all male dogs, and 1.4 to 5.8 per cent of male dogs with carcinomas.[17,45,80] Twenty cases of prostatic adenocarcinoma in dogs were diagnosed over an 11-year period in a veterinary hospital performing 124 necropsies per year; this corresponds to an incidence of 1.5 per cent prostatic tumor cases among all dogs necropsied.[46]

Prostatic neoplasia is age dependent in dogs as it is in humans (Table 181–4); mean age in four studies of 53 dogs was 9.6 years.[46,70,90,95] Mean age of dogs with prostatic adenocarcinoma is not significantly different from that of dogs with other neoplasms.[46] Prostatic adenocarcinoma has occurred in cats 10 and 17 years of age.[33,97]

There is no known hormonal influence on occurrence of prostatic neoplasia in dogs and cats. The canine prostate undergoes androgen-dependent hypertrophy with age, mediated by androgen receptors, which may be induced by estradiol.[23,27,29,39,51] Although castration causes involution of the normal and hyperplastic prostate in dogs, it does not decrease the risk of developing prostatic neoplasia, nor does it alter the course if performed on prostate tumor patients.[46,95] The occurrence of prostatic adenocarcinoma in castrated and intact male dogs and cats and the absence of a correlation between benign prostatic hypertrophy and prostatic adenocarcinoma suggest that the tumor is not hormonally mediated.[33,46] No specific anatomical region of the canine prostate is at increased risk of becoming neoplastic, although different portions vary in their histological response to androgens and estrogens.[46]

Diagnosis

Clinical signs in dogs with prostatic neoplasia are variable and include dysuria, tenesmus, emaciation, rear limb lameness, weakness, and lumbar pain (Table 181–4). Rear limb locomotor disturbance may be the only presenting sign.[46] Duration of clinical signs ranged from 1 to 20 (mean = 3.5) months in a series of 15 dogs with prostatic adenocarcinoma.[95] Clinical signs in cats include hematuria, dysuria, pollakiuria, and outflow obstruction of the urinary tract.[33,69,97]

On rectal palpation, the canine prostate is usually palpably enlarged, firm, and may be cystic or irregularly nodular.[46,95] The median raphe may or may not be palpable.[46] Some glands are painful on digital palpation. Enlarged sublumbar lymph nodes are occasionally palpable.

Metastasis is very common with prostatic adenocarcinoma in dogs and has generally occurred by the time the diagnosis is made. Metastatic lesions are found most often in the iliac lymph nodes, lungs, urinary bladder, pelvic muscles or periprostatic tissue, rectum, bone, mesenteries, and kidneys (Table 181–4).[46,70,90,95] Metastasis also has been reported to the cerebrum in a patient with facial paralysis and loss of balance.[31] Forty-four of 45 cases examined had metastases distant to periprostatic tissue at necropsy.[46,70,90,95] Pulmonary metastases were present in a 10-year-old neutered male cat with prostatic adenocarcinoma; survey radiographs taken prior to euthanasia did not reveal metastatic disease.[33] Metastasis may occur by direct extension or by hematogenous routes via the vena cava and vertebral venous plexus.[46]

Survey radiography generally reveals prostatic enlargement, although the size of the carcinomatous gland varies greatly among dogs and is not different from the size of the hypertrophic gland.[46,95] The largest neoplastic prostate in a series of 15 measured $8 \times 6 \times 5$ cm.[95] Irregularity and filling defects of the prostatic urethra have been detected in both dogs and cats by retrograde urethrography.[33] Thoracic metastases appear as diffuse structured or nonstructured interstitial lung disease. Eight of ten cases with locomotor disturbance had radiographic evidence of metastasis to lower lumbar vertebrae, bones of the pelvis, or long bones of the rear limbs (proximal femur and tibia).[46] Bony lesions were osteolytic, proliferative, or both.[46] One case of hypertrophic osteopathy has been reported in a dog with prostatic adenocarcinoma in the absence of thoracic metastasis; the patient also had a focus of metastatic tumor tissue in the urinary bladder.[79]

Neutrophilia with a slight left shift was present in all of 7 dogs examined in a survey of 20 cases; hematuria and proteinuria were present in 6 of 11.[46] In contrast to some human patients, dogs with prostatic adenocarcinoma have not demonstrated elevations in serum acid phosphatase concentrations.[95]

Definitive diagnosis is achieved by cytological examination of samples collected by ejaculation, prostatic massage, aspiration biopsy, punch biopsy, incision biopsy, or excision biopsy of the prostate gland.[3,47] Ejaculation and prostatic massage are noninvasive and should be attempted initially, although dogs in pain may not achieve erection and ejaculation, and even when samples are obtained they may not be diagnostic. Needle aspiration of the prostate may be performed using a perirectal or transabdominal approach and a long spinal needle. Punch biopsy is performed perirectally, transrectally, or transabdominally after sedation and local anesthesia. Transient (less than 4 days) hematuria and periprostatic hemorrhage are complications of aspiration or punch biopsy.[3] Needle and punch biopsy are contraindicated if abscess is present, because localized peritonitis may follow.[3]

Because many prostates with adenocarcinoma are also hypertrophic and may have prostatic cysts, biopsy specimens must be interpreted with caution. An iliac lymph node should be aspirated at the time of biopsy if possible.[10,46,75,95] Of 15 cases of canine prostatic adenocarcinoma, 6 were diagnosed as prostatic cyst, abscess, or prostatitis after initial biopsy.[95] Prostatic cysts were of variable size and consistency in these patients.

Clinical staging of prostatic tumors is by behavior of the primary tumor (T), regional lymph node involvement (N), and the presence of metastasis (M) (Table 181–5).[98] Regional lymph nodes are the internal and external iliac nodes.

TABLE 181–5. WHO Clinical Stages of Canine Prostatic Tumors*

T: Primary tumor (clinical, radiographic)
  T0 No evidence of tumor
  T1 Intracapsular tumor, surrounded by normal gland
N: Regional lymph nodes (internal and external iliac)
  N0 No RLN involved
  N1 RLN involved
  N2 RLN and juxta RLN (lumbar) involved
M: Distant metastasis (clinical, radiographic)
  M0 No evidence of distant metastasis
  M1 Distant metastasis is present—specify sites

---

*Reprinted with permission from the internal report of the Second WHO Consultation on the Biological Behaviour and Therapy of Tumours of Domestic Animals, Geneva, 1979 (unpublished WHO document VPH/CMO/79.17).

Treatment and Prognosis

Prognosis is grave with all cases of prostatic adenocarcinoma in dogs and cats, because metastasis usually has occurred prior to diagnosis. The only treatment available is prostatectomy. There is no evidence that castration or estrogen therapy alters the course of prostatic neoplasia in dogs. Orthovoltage radiation therapy of these tumors has been used but has not been demonstrated to increase survival time.

Survival time after admission depends on pathological grade and the presence of metastases; 14 dogs with 1 to 6 months duration of signs had postadmission survival times of 1 to 29 ($\bar{x}$ = 2.75) months.[95] A 6-year-old Doberman pinscher with signs for 20 months prior to admission survived for 9 months after diagnosis.[95]

NEOPLASIA OF THE PENIS AND PREPUCE

Incidence

Age-standarized incidence of tumors of the penis and prepuce per 100,000 male dogs per year has been reported as 2.0 cases; these constitute 0.24 per cent of tumors of all sites in male dogs.[82] Penile/preputial tumors diagnosed in dogs include epithelial tumors (papilloma, squamous cell carcinoma) fibropapillomas (fibroma), transmissible venereal tumor (TVT), and other mesenchymal tumors (fibrosarcoma, lymphosarcoma, hemangioma/sarcoma, mast cell sarcoma).[1,21,32] Tumors of the penis and prepuce have not been described in cats.

The median age incidence for all tumors of the reproductive organs of male dogs is between 10 and 11 years, but this is strongly influenced by the large number of testicular tumors that occur in older dogs.[82] The TVT, the most common tumor of the penis and prepuce in dogs, is usually acquired at coitus and therefore occurs in younger dogs. In a series of 78 penile TVTs, 45 were present in dogs younger than 4 years, and 19 were in dogs between 5 and 7.5 years of age.[61] Tumor occurrence in the external genitalia is not influenced by neutering in male dogs.

Diagnosis

Presumptive diagnosis of a tumor of the penis or prepuce is made by inspection at physical examination. Papillomas and TVTs appear as pedunculated or broad-based masses that often ulcerate and bleed. Squamous cell carcinomas may appear wart-like or granular and progress to masses greater than 5 cm in diameter.[43] Final diagnosis is made by cytological examination of aspirated cells or an excision biopsy.

Presenting signs are the presence of a mass or bleeding from the prepuce.[1,61,94] In occasional cases,

TABLE 181–6. WHO Clinical Stages of Canine Tumors of the Penis and Prepuce*

T: Primary tumor
  T0 No evidence of tumor
  T1 Tumor ≤ 1 cm in main dimension, superficial
  T2 Tumor > 1 cm and < 3 cm in its main dimension, with minimal infiltration
  T3 Tumor ≥ 3 cm or every tumor with deep infiltration
  T4 Tumor infiltrating neighboring structures
N: Regional lymph nodes (superficial inguinal)
  N0 No RLN involvement
  N1 Movable unilateral nodes
  N2 Movable bilateral nodes
  N3 Fixed nodes
M: Distant Metastasis
  M0 No evidence of distant metastasis
  M1 Distant metastasis present

*Reprinted with permission from the internal report of the Second WHO Consultation on the Biological Behaviour and Therapy of Tumours of Domestic Animals, Geneva, 1979 (unpublished WHO document VPH/CMO/79.17).

phimosis or lack of libido occurs.[1,61,94] Occasional dogs with genital TVTs also have tumor in the nasal passages and may present with epistaxis.[62]

The TVT is a transmissable tumor that has been maintained in the canine population from a single original neoplasm first identified in 1876 (see chapter 182).[67] Tumor behavior depends on immune competency of the host, with rapid growth, invasion, and metastasis occurring in immune-compromised animals. The tumor may regress spontaneously 2 to 6 months after onset of signs, or it may spread by transplantation to the skin, nasal passages, pharynx, and orbit or by hematogenous or lymphatic spread to the regional lymph nodes, liver, spleen, intestine, lung, or brain.[12,68]

Incidence of metastasis is unknown with spontaneously occurring TVTs; metastases occurred in 5 of 385 (1.3 per cent) dogs in an experimental transplantation project.[44] Extragenital TVT may occur before, or in the absence of, genital lesions.[62]

Tumors of the canine penis and prepuce are clinically staged by behavior of the primary tumor (T), involvement of regional lymph nodes (N), and presence of metastasis (M) (Table 181–6).[98] Regional lymph nodes are the superficial inguinal nodes.

Treatment and Prognosis

Tumors of the penis and prepuce should be removed by wide surgical excision; electrocautery is recommended to minimize bleeding and may be associated with less recurrence of the TVT.[91] Recurrent, invasive, or metastatic TVT should be treated with vincristine* (0.025 mg/kg IV, not to exceed 1

---

*Oncovin[R], Eli Lilly Co., Indianapolis, IN

TABLE 181–7. Reported Cases of Mammary Tumors in the Male Dog

Case No.	Age (yrs)	Breed	Site	Tumor Type	Reference
1	14	German shepherd	5L	Mixed mammary tumor	40*
2	—	Fox terrier	—	Mixed mammary tumor	40*
3	12	—	—	Osteosarcoma	40*
4	—	—	—	Sarcocarcinoma	40*
5	13	Pug	3R	Cystadenochondroma	40*
6	11	Cocker spaniel	2L	Chondroadenocarcinoma	40*
7	12	—	—	Adenocarcinoma	40*
8	—	—	—	Mixed tumor	40*
9	8	Pointer	4	Carcinoma	41*
10	—	—	—	Carcinoma	41*
11	16	Sheepdog cross	1L	Adenocarcinoma	41*
12	14	Bull terrier cross	4R	Papillary cystadenocarcinoma	41*
13	10	Pointer/setter	4,5L 4,5R	Adenocarcinomas (4)	41*
14	12	Gordon setter	2R	Carcinoma	41*
15	6	—	4	Carcinoma	41*
16	10	Cocker spaniel	2R	Cystadenocarcinoma	41*
17	8	Pointer	5L	Adenocarcinoma	41*
18	—	Fox terrier	4R	Fibroadenoma	42*
19	7	Pointer	5R	Fibroadenoma	42*
20	7	Boxer	4,5	Adenomas	42*
21	—	—	—	Mixed tumor	42*
22	Aged	Newfoundland	2	Spindle cell carcinoma	42*
23	15	Cocker spaniel	—	Papillary cystadenocarcinoma	42
24	14	Kelpie cross	4	Benign & malignant mixed tumors	42
25	7	Afghan	1L	Ductal papillary adenoma	76

* = Earlier case cited in reference shown.

TABLE 181–8. Clinical Stages of Canine Mammary Tumors

T Primary Tumor
  T0 No evidence of tumor
  T1 Tumor < 5 cm maximum diameter
  T2 Tumor 5 to 10 cm maximum diameter
  T3 Tumor 11–15 cm maximum diameter; muscle fixation
  T4 Tumor > 15 cm maximum diameter; whole gland involved; infiltration of underlying tissue

N Regional Lymph Nodes (RLN) (axillary, superficial inguinal)
  N0 No RLN involved
  N1 Ipsilateral RLN involved
  N2 Bilateral RLN involved
  N3 Distant LN involved
  NR LN previously removed

M Distant Metastasis
  M0 No evidence of lung metastasis
  M1 Solitary lung metastasis
  M2 Multiple lung metastasis
  M3 Other nonlung sites of metastasis
  M4 Solitary or multiple lung metastasis and other nonlung metastatic sites

mg) once weekly following a hemogram to look for leukopenia until there is no longer evidence of disease.[6,8] Some TVTs refractory to vincristine may respond to doxorubicin* (30 mg/m² IV) administered at three consecutive 7-day intervals.[8]

Orthovoltage radiotherapy using a single dose of 1,000 rads also has been reported effective against TVTs.[92] Radiotherapy (4,000 to 6,000 rads in 500-rad fractions three times weekly) has been recommended following surgical excision of squamous cell carcinomas of the penis and prepuce.[22] When tumor involvement is extensive, the penis may be amputated and a urethrostomy performed.[22,43] Prognosis is good with benign tumors of the penis and prepuce and with TVTs in the absence of central nervous system metastasis; prognosis is guarded to poor with carcinomas and sarcomas.

MAMMARY NEOPLASIA IN MALES

Incidence

Although mammary neoplasia is very common in the bitch and queen (see chapter 182), incidence in male dogs and cats is low. In five reports totaling 1,705 dogs with mammary neoplasms, only 15 affected animals (0.88 per cent) were males.[16,30,42,58,89] Six reports of malignant mammary tumors in cats include 307 females and 4 neutered males (1.3 per cent).[18,34,57,64,81,96]

Twenty-five cases of male canine mammary neoplasia from the literature are listed in Table 181–7. Average age at diagnosis was 10.9 years (n = 18). Nine breeds and four mixed-breed dogs were represented (n = 18). Affected mammary glands were present on both right and left sides (8R:7L), and the fourth and fifth glands were most commonly involved. Two dogs had tumors in more than one gland, and one had bilateral adenocarcinomas in the fourth and fifth glands.

Mammary tumor types in male dogs, in order of decreasing frequency, were the adenocarcinoma (7), malignant mixed mammary tumor (5), carcinoma (4), benign mixed mammary tumor (fibroadenoma) (2), adenoma (2), osteosarcoma (2), cystadenochondroma (1), spindle cell carcinoma (1), and undifferentiated sarcoma/carcinoma (1).[40–42] These total 20 malignant and 5 benign tumors.

The four cases of mammary neoplasia in male cats occurred in castrated males; information on age, tumor type, metastasis, and survival was not presented.[18,57,96]

Diagnosis

Diagnosis is based on palpation of mammary masses and tumor histology. Metastasis of male mammary tumors has been reported, with lesions in the lymph nodes and lungs or axillary lymph nodes only.[40,41] Postmortem information was not provided for most cases in Table 181–7, so frequency of metastasis is unknown. Radiographs of the chest (glands 1 through 3) or abdomen (glands 3 through 5) to look for tumor metastasis are advised prior to surgical excision. No information is available on clinical signs or metastasis in male cats.

Clinical staging of mammary tumors in males is by behavior of the primary tumor (T), regional lymph node involvement (N), and presence of distant metastasis (M) (Table 181–8).[98]

Treatment and Prognosis

Treatment is surgical excision of the affected glands (simple mastectomy). Until more cases are reported, prognosis should be based on histology of the tumor and staging criteria developed for females (see chapter 182).

1. Ball, V., and Rossi, P.: Cancer of the prepuce and glans (round-celled sarcoma) with ganglial metastasis in a dog. Vet. J. 84:530, 1928.
2. Barsanti, J. A., Duncan, J. R., and Nachreiner, R. F.: Alopecia associated with a seminoma. J. Am. Anim. Hosp. Assoc. 15:33, 1979.
3. Barsanti, J. A., Shotts, E. B., Prasse, K., and Crowell, W.: Evaluation of diagnostic techniques for canine prostatic diseases. J. Am. Vet. Med. Assoc. 177:160, 1980.
4. Brodey, R. S.: Canine and feline neoplasia. Adv. Vet. Sci. Comp. Med. 14:309, 1970.
5. Brodey, R. S., and Martin, J. E.: Sertoli cell neoplasms in the dog. The clinicopathologic and endocrinological findings in 37 dogs. J. Am. Vet. Med. Assoc. 133:249, 1958.
6. Brown, N. O., Calvert, C. A., and MacEwen, E. G.: Chemotherapeutic management of transmissible venereal tumor in 30 dogs. J. Am. Vet. Med. Assoc. 176:983, 1980.
7. Brown, T. T., Burek, J. D , and McEntee, K.: Male pseudohermaphroditism, cryptorchidism and Sertoli cell neoplasia in three miniature schnauzers. J. Am. Vet. Med. Assoc. 169:821, 1976.
8. Calvert, C. A., Leifer, C. E., and MacEwen, E. G.: Vincristine for treatment of transmissible venereal tumor in the dog. J. Am. Vet. Med. Assoc. 181:163, 1982.
9. Chiu, T.: Studies of estrogen-induced proliferative disorders of hemopoietic tissues in dogs. Ph.D. thesis, University of Minnesota, 1974.
10. Clark, L., and English, P. B.: Carcinoma of the prostate gland in a dog. Aust. Vet. J. 42:214, 1966.
11. Coffin, D. L., Munson, T. O., and Scully, R. E.: Functional Sertoli cell tumor with metastases in a dog. J. Am. Vet. Med. Assoc. 121:352, 1952.
12. Cohen, D.: The transmissible venereal tumor of the dog—a naturally occurring allograft? Isr. J. Med. Sci. 14:14, 1978.
13. Cohen, D.: Epidemiological analysis of the most prevalent sites and types of canine neoplasia observed in a veterinary hospital. Cancer Res. 34:2859, 1974.
14. Comhaire, F., Mattheeuws, D., and Vermeulen, A.: Testosterone and oestradiol in dogs with testicular tumours. Acta Endocrinol. 77:408, 1974.
15. Concannon, P. W., Hansel, W., and Visek, W. J.: The ovarian cycle of the bitch: Plasma estrogen, LH and progesterone. Biol. Reprod. 13:112, 1975.
16. Cotchin, E.: Neoplasms in small animals. Vet. Rec. 63:67, 1951.
17. Cotchin, E.: Further observations on neoplasms in dogs with

---

*Adriamycin^R, Adria Laboratories, Wilmington, DE.

particular reference to site of origin and malignancy. Part I: Male genital, skeletal, lymphatic and other systems. Br. Vet. J. *110*:274, 1954.

18. Cotchin, E.: Neoplasia in the cat. Vet. Rec. *69*:425, 1957.

19. Cotchin, E.: Testicular neoplasms in dogs. J. Comp. Pathol. *70*:232, 1960.

20. Cotchin, E.: Some tumors in dogs and cats of comparative veterinary and human interest. Vet. Rec. *71*:1040, 1959.

21. Crocker, W. J.: Three thousand autopsies. Cornell Vet. *9*:142, 1919.

22. Crow, S. E.: Neoplasms of the reproductive organs and mammary glands of the dog. *In* Morrow, D. A. (ed.): *Current Therapy in Theriogenology*. W. B. Saunders, Philadelphia, 1980, pp. 640–646.

23. Deklerk, D. P., Coffey, D. S., Ewing, L. L., et al.: Comparison of spontaneous and experimentally induced canine prostatic hyperplasia. J. Clin. Invest. *64*:842, 1979.

24. Dorn, C. R., Taylor, D. O. N., Frye, F. L., and Hubbard, H. H.: Survey of animal neoplasms in Alameda and Contra Costa counties, California. I. Methodology and description of cases. J. Natl. Cancer Inst. *40*:295, 1968.

25. Dorn, C. R., Taylor, D. O. N., Schneider, et al.: Survey of animal neoplasms in Alameda and Contra Costa counties, California. II. Cancer morbidity in dogs and cats from Alameda county. J. Natl. Cancer Inst. *40*:307, 1968.

26. Dow, C.: Testicular tumours in the dog. J. Comp. Pathol. *72*:247, 1962.

27. Dube, J. Y., Frenette, G., and Tremblay, R. R.: Effect of endocrine manipulations on the levels of cytosolic and nuclear receptors for androgens in dog prostate. Invest. Urol. *18*:418, 1981.

28. Edwards, D. F.: Bone marrow hypoplasia in a feminized dog with a Sertoli cell tumor. J. Am. Vet. Assoc. *178*:494, 1981.

29. Ehrlichman, R. J., Isaacs, J. T., and Coffey, D. S.: Differences in the effects of estradiol on dihydrotestosterone-induced prostatic growth of the castrate dog and rat. Invest. Urol. *18*:466, 1981.

30. Frye, F. L., Dorn, C. R., Taylor, D. O. N., et al.: Characteristics of canine mammary gland tumor cases. Anim. Hosp. *3*:1, 1967.

31. Grant, C. A.: Carcinoma of the canine prostate. Acta Pathol. Microbiol. Scand. *40*:197, 1957.

32. Hall, W. C., Nielsen, S. W., and McEntee, K.: Tumors of the prostate and penis. Bull. WHO *53*:247, 1976.

33. Hawe, R. S.: What is your diagnosis? J. Am. Vet. Med. Assoc. *182*:1257, 1983.

34. Hayden, D. W.: Feline mammary tumors. J. Small Anim. Pract. *12*:687, 1971.

35. Hayes, H. M., and Pendergrass, T. W.: Canine testicular tumors: Epidemiologic features of 410 dogs. Int. J. Cancer *16*:482, 1976.

36. Holst, P. A., and Phemister, R. D.: Temporal sequence of events in the estrous cycle of the bitch. Am. J. Vet. Res. *36*:705, 1975.

37. Hornbuckle, W. E., and Kleine, L. J.: Medical management of prostatic disease. *In* Kirk, R. W. (ed.): *Current Veterinary Therapy VII*. W. B. Saunders, Philadelphia, 1980, pp. 1146–1150.

38. Howard, E. B., and Nielsen, S. W.: Neoplasia of the boxer dog. Am. J. Vet. Res. *26*:1121, 1965.

39. Isaacs, J. T., and Coffey, D. S.: Changes in dihydrotestosterone metabolism associated with the development of canine benign prostatic hyperplasia. Endocrinol. *108*:445, 1981.

40. Jabara, A. G.: Canine mixed tumours. Aust. Vet. J. *36*:212, 1960.

41. Jabara, A. G.: Canine mammary carcionomata. Aust. Vet. J. *36*:389, 1960.

42. Jabara, A. G.: Two cases of mammary neoplasms arising in male dogs. Aust. Vet. J. *45*:476, 1969.

43. Johnston, D. E.: Tumors of the prepuce and penis. *In* Catcott, E. J. (ed.): *Canine Surgery*, American Veterinary Publications, Wheaton, IL, 1965.

44. Karlson, A. G., and Mann, F. C.: The transmissible venereal tumor of dogs: Observations on forty generations of experimental transfers. Ann. N.Y. Acad. Sci. *54*:1197, 1952.

45. Krook, L.: A statistical investigation of carcinoma in the dog. Acta Pathol. Microbiol. Scand. *35*:407, 1954.

46. Leav, I., and Ling, G. V.: Adenocarcinoma of the canine prostate gland. Cancer *22*:1329, 1968.

47. Leeds, E. B., and Leav, I.: Perineal punch biopsy of the canine prostate gland. J. Am. Vet. Med. Assoc. *154*:925, 1969.

48. Lindberg, R., Jonsson, O. J., and Kasström, H.: Sertoli cell tumors associated with feminization, prostatitis, and squamous metaplasia of the renal tubular epithelium in a dog. J. Small Anim. Pract. *17*:451, 1976.

49. Lindo, D. E., and Glenn, H. H.: Bilateral Sertoli cell tumor in a canine cryptorchid with accompanying pathologic lesions. Can. Vet. J. *10*:145, 1969.

50. Lipowitz, A. J. Schwartz, A., Wilson, G. P., and Ebert, J. W.: Testicular neoplasms and concomitant clinical changes in the dog. J. Am. Vet. Med. Assoc. *143*:1364, 1973.

51. Lloyd, J. W., Thomas J. A., and Mawhinney, M. G.: Androgens and estrogens in the plasma and prostatic tissue of normal dogs and dogs with benign prostatic hypertrophy. Invest. Urol. *13*:220, 1975.

52. MacVean, D. W., Monlux, A. W., Anderson, P. S., et al.: Frequency of canine and feline tumors in a defined population. Vet. Pathol. *15*:700, 1978.

53. McNeil, P. E., and Weaver, A. D.: Massive scrotal swelling in two unusual cases of canine Sertoli cell tumor. Vet. Rec. *106*:144, 1980.

54. McQueen, S. D., Directo, A. C., and Olson, G.: An unusual case of Sertoli cell neoplasia in a dog. Vet. Med./Small Anim. Clin. *69*:1449, 1974.

55. Meier, H.: Sertoli-cell tumor in the cat: Report of two cases. North Am. Vet. *37*:979, 1956.

56. Michaels, J.: Sertoli cell tumor in a collie dog. Vet. Med./Small Anim. Clin .*69*:192, 1974.

57. Misdorp, W.: Malignant mammary tumors in the dog and cat compared with the same in women. Inaugural Dissertation, Utrecht, 1964.

58. Mitchell, L., de La Iglesia, F. A., Wenkoff, M. S., et al.: Mammary tumors in dogs: Survey of clinical and pathologic characteristics. Can. Vet. J. *15*:131, 1974.

59. Morgan, R. V.: Blood dyscrasias associated with testicular tumors in the dog. J. Am. Anim. Hosp. Assoc. *18*:970, 1982.

60. Naylor, R. W., and Thompson, S. M. R.: Intraabdominal testicular torsion. A report of two cases. J. Am. Anim. Hosp. Assoc. *15*:763, 1979.

61. Ndiritu, C. G.: Lesions of the canine penis and prepuce. Mod. Vet. Pract. *60*:712, 1979.

62. Ndiritu, C. G., Mboguva, S. W., and Sayer, P. D.: Extragenitally located transmissible venereal tumor in dogs. Mod. Vet. Pract. *11*:940, 1977.

63. Neuman, R. H.: Pyometra and a Sertoli cell tumor in a hermaphroditic dog. Vet. Med./Small Anim. Clin. *74*:1757, 1979.

64. Nielsen, S. W.: The malignancy of mammary tumors in cats. North Am. Vet. *33*:245, 1952.

65. Nielsen, S. W., and Lein, D. H.: Tumors of the testis. Bull. WHO *50*:71, 1974.

66. Norrdin, R. W.: A male pseudohermaphrodite dog with a Sertoli cell tumor, mucometra and vaginal glands. J. Am. Vet. Med. Assoc. *156*:204, 1970.

67. Novinsky, M. A.: Zur frage uber die impfung der krebsigen geschwülste. Zentralbl. Med. Wiss. *14*:790, 1876.

68. Oduye, O. O., Ikede, B. O., Esuruoso, G. O., and Apokodje, J. U.: Metastatic transmissible venereal tumor in dogs. J. Small Anim. Pract. *14*:625, 1973.

69. Osborne, C. A.: Personal communication, 1983.

70. O'Shea, J. P.: Studies on the canine prostate gland. II. Prostatic neoplasms. J. Comp. Pathol. *73*:244, 1963.

71. Patnaik, A. K., and Liu, S. K.: Leiomyoma of the tunica vaginalis in a dog. Cornell Vet. *65*:228, 1975.

72. Pearson, H., and Kelly, D. F.: Testicular torsion in the dog: A review of 13 cases. Vet. Rec. 97:200, 1975.
73. Pendergrass, T. W., and Hayes, H. M.: Cryptorchidism and related defects in dogs: Epidemiologic comparisons with man. Teratology 12:51, 1975.
74. Pierrepoint, C. G., Galley, J. M., Griffiths, K., and Grant, J. K.: Steroid metabolism of a Sertoli cell tumor of the testis of a dog with feminization and alopecia and of the normal canine testis. J. Endocrinol. 38:61, 1967.
75. Rabaut, S. M., and Kelch, W. J.: Undifferentiated carcinoma in the canine prostate. Mod. Vet. Pract. 60:401, 1979.
76. Raflo, C. P., and Diamond, S. S.: Neoplasm of the mammary papilla in a male dog. Am. J. Vet. Res. 41:953, 1980.
77. Reif, J. S., and Brodey, R. S.: The relationship between cryptorchidism and canine testicular neoplasia. J. Am. Vet. Med. Assoc. 155:2005, 1969.
78. Reif, J. S., Maguire, T. G., Kenney, R. M., and Brodey, R. S.: A short study of canine testicular neoplasia. J. Am. Vet. Med. Assoc. 175:719, 1979.
79. Rendano, V. T., and Slauson, D. O.: Hypertrophic osteopathy in a dog with prostatic adenocarcinoma and without thoracic metastasis. J. Am. Anim. Assoc. 18:719, 1979.
80. Schlotthauer, C. F., and Millar, J. A. S.: Carcinoma of the prostate gland in dogs—a report of three cases. J. Am. Vet. Med. Assoc. 99:239, 1941.
81. Schmidt, R. E;, and Langham, R. F.: A survey of feline neoplasms. J. Am. Vet Med. Assoc 151:1325, 1967.
82. Schneider, R.: Epidemiological aspects of mammary and genital neoplasia. In Morrow, D. A. (ed.): Current Therapy in Theriogenology. W. B. Saunders, Philadelphia, 1980. pp. 636–639.
83. Scully, R. E., and Coffin, D. L.: Canine testicular tumors. Cancer 5:592, 1952.
84. Sherding, R. G., Wilson, G. P., and Kociba, G. J.: Bone marrow hypoplasia in eight dogs with Sertoli cell tumor. J. Am. Vet. Med. Assoc. 178:497, 1981.
85. Siegel, E. T., Forchielli, E., Dorfman, R. I., et al.: An estrogen study in the feminized dog with testicular neoplasia. Endocrinology 80:272, 1967.
86. Simon, J., and Rubin, S. B.: Metastatic seminoma in a dog. Vet. Med./Small Anim. Clin. 74:941, 1979.
87. Stein, B. S.: Tumors of the feline genital tract. J. Am. Anim. Hosp. Assoc. 17:1022, 1981.
88. Strutt, C. S.: Sertoli cell carcinoma and multiple metastasis in a dog. Cornell Vet. 57:597, 1967.
89. Taylor, G. N., Shabestari, L., and Williams, J.: Mammary neoplasia in a closed beagle colony. Cancer Res. 36:2740, 1976.
90. Taylor, P. A.: Prostatic adenocarcinoma in a dog and a summary of 10 cases. Can. Vet. J. 14:162, 1973.
91. Theilen, G. H., and Madewell, B. R.: Veterinary Cancer Medicine. Lea & Febiger, Philadelphia, 1979.
92. Thrall, D. E.: Orthovoltage radiotherapy of canine transmissible venereal tumors. Vet. Radiol. 23:217, 1982.
93. Turk, J. R., Turk, M. A. M., and Gallina, A. M.: A canine testicular tumor resembling gonadoblastoma. Vet. Pathol. 18:201, 1981.
94. Wasman, S. C.: Cancer of the penis. Vet. Med. 50:31, 1955.
95. Weaver, A. D: Fifteen cases of prostatic carcinoma in the dog. Vet. Rec. 109:71, 1981.
96. Weijer, K., Head, K. W., Misdorp, W., and Hampe, J. F.: Feline malignant mammary tumors. I. Morphology and biology: Some comparisons with human and canine mammary carcinomas. J. Natl. Cancer Inst. 49:1697, 1972.
97. Whitehead, J. E.: Diseases of the male reproductive system. In Catcott, E. J. (ed.): Feline Medicine and Surgery. American Veterinary Publications, Wheaton, IL, 1964.
98. World Health Organization: Report of the Second Consultation on the Biological Behavior and Therapy of Tumours of Domestic Animals. WHO, Geneva, 1979.

Chapter **182**

Female Reproductive System

Shirley D. Johnston

Tumors of the female reproductive organs include those of the ovaries, the tubular tract, and the mammary glands. Tumors of the ovaries and tubular tract are uncommon in companion animals and, when present, are usually benign or can be diagnosed and treated before metastasis occurs. In contrast, mammary tumors are common neoplasms of the bitch and queen. They are malignant in about 50 per cent of dogs and about 90 per cent of cats.

Reproductive neoplasms are not a great diagnostic challenge in companion animals but do present therapeutic challenges when malignant. With the exception of the transmissible venereal tumor, malignant tumors of the ovaries, uterus, and vagina are uncommon enough that good clinical trials to examine their responsiveness to chemo- or immunotherapy have

not been performed. Nor is information on prognostic indicators or post-treatment survival time available. Malignant mammary tumors are a therapeutic challenge because, despite their numbers and the large volume of veterinary literature on them, there is great variation in histological classification schemes (making comparisons difficult) and there are very few randomized prospective clinical trials to document response to the several modes of therapy available.

The World Health Organization (WHO) schema of clinical staging of animal tumors of the reproductive tract based on character of the primary tumor (T), involvement of regional lymph nodes (N), and presence of distant metastasis (M) is recommended to objectively document behavior of these tumors before and after treatment. At present, stages have not been

TABLE 182–1.   Incidence of Ovarian Tumor Types in the Bitch and Queen

Ovarian Tumors Reported in Companion Animals	Tumor Occurrence in the Bitch				Tumor Occurrence in the Queen
	Dow, 1960	Cotchin, 1961	Norris et al., 1970	Total	Nielsen, 1952
Epithelial Origin					
Adenoma/cystadenoma	10	20	20	50 (28%)	1 (10%)
Adenocarcinoma/cystadenocarcinoma	1	7	3	11	1 (10%)
Undifferentiated			10	10	
Gonadal-Stromal Origin					
Granulosa cell tumor	13	30	15	58 (32%)	5 (50%)
Granulosa-theca cell tumor					
Thecoma					
Luteoma		1		1	
Sertoli cell tumor			6	6	
Unspecified			5	5	
Germ Cell Origin					
Dysgerminoma		8	11	19 (10%)	
Teratoma		1	2	3	2 (20%)
Teratocarcinoma					
Mesodermal Origin					
Mixed mesodermal			1	1	
Leiomyoma			1	1	
Fibroma	1			1	
Sarcoma, undifferentiated		2	4	6	
Metastatic Origin					
Lymphosarcoma	2			2	
Uterine adenocarcinoma			1	1	1 (10%)
Mammary adenocarcinoma	1		3	4	
Skin tumor, unspecified			1	1	
Transmissible venereal tumor			1	1	
Totals	28	69	84	181	10

well correlated with prognosis or survival time, but accumulation of standardized data on these tumors will permit such correlations in the future.

OVARIAN NEOPLASIA

Incidence

The incidence of primary ovarian neoplasia in the dog and cat is low. In surveys of 2,917 and 1,150 canine neoplasms, 24 (0.8 per cent) and 14 (1.2 per cent), respectively, were primary ovarian tumors.[23, 38] Surveys of 328, 571, and 254 feline neoplasms revealed the presence of 0.4, 0.3, and 0.2 per cent ovarian tumors, respectively.[40, 42, 114] Tumors in the dog occur with equal frequency in the right and left ovaries and may occasionally occur in both.[43]

Occurrence and behavior of ovarian tumors are influenced by the tissue of origin within the ovary (Table 182–1). The granulosa cell tumor of gonadal-stromal origin is the most common primary ovarian tumor in the dog and cat.

Some granulosa cell tumors produce estrogen, pro-gesterone, or both.[95] These tumors therefore may occur with paraneoplastic syndromes of persistent estrus (vulvar swelling, sanguinous vaginal discharge, attraction of males), estrogen-induced aplastic pancytopenia, or progesterone-induced cystic endometrial hyperplasia and pyometra. Ovarian tumors other than the granulosa cell tumor are often seen in bitches with cystic endometrial hyperplasia or pyometra, and because exogenous progestogens have been demonstrated to cause cystic endometrial hyperplasia, hormonal function has been ascribed to these other tumors.[48] Such uterine change is common in aging bitches, however, and may occur coincidentally with the ovarian tumors, which also occur in the older bitch.[8] In contrast to the bitch, the queen does not routinely exhibit cystic endometrial hyperplasia as a consequence of aging.

Diagnosis

Most ovarian tumors, regardless of histological type, are associated with a palpable mass in the cranial or mid abdomen. Abdominal and thoracic

TABLE 182–2. Clinical Stages of Canine Ovarian Tumors*

T Primary Tumor
 T0 No evidence of tumor
 T1 Tumor limited to one ovary
 T2 Tumors limited to both ovaries
 T3 Tumor extending into ovarian bursa

N Regional Lymph Nodes (sublumbar)
 N0 No regional lymph nodes involved
 N1 Regional lymph nodes involved

M Distant Metastasis
 M0 No evidence of distant metastasis
 M1 Evidence of implantation or other metastases
 M1a   In the peritoneal cavity
 M1b   Beyond the peritoneal cavity
 M1c   Both peritoneal cavity and beyond

*Reprinted with permission from the internal report of the Second WHO Consultation on the Biological Behaviour and Therapy of Tumours of Domestic Animals, Geneva, 1979 (unpublished WHO document VPH/CMO/79.17).

radiographs are indicated in all cases to assess the presence of metastatic lesions, which occur by extension to abdominal surfaces or by lymphatic/hematogenous spread to regional lymph nodes and the thoracic cavity. Radioimmunoassay of plasma estrogen and progesterone are of interest if functional tumors are suspected owing to clinical signs of persistent estrus or pyometra. Reported plasma estrogen concentrations in the cycling bitch vary greatly among laboratories; plasma progesterone concentrations exceeding 2 ng/ml indicate either functional luteal tissue or a functional tumor.

Canine ovarian tumors are clinically staged according to behavior of the primary tumor (T), regional lymph node involvement (N), and presence of distant metastases (M) (Table 182–2).[157] The regional lymph nodes are the sublumbar nodes.

Adenoma/Cystadenoma

Ovarian adenomas are one of the most common primary ovarian tumors of the bitch and have been described in the female cat. Cystadenomas range in diameter from a few millimeters to 7 to 10 cm. Ovarian epithelial proliferation, neoplasia, and metastasis can be induced by prolonged estrogen administration in dogs, but the role of endogenous estrogen in spontaneously occurring tumors is unknown.[120] In 17 spontaneous ovarian adenomas described in the bitch, age at diagnosis ranged from 6 to 14 years, and 8 of 11 patients were nulliparous.[43, 49, 90] Of seven cases, six had abdominal distension, three vomited, and one had abdominal pain on palpation. Because four of these patients had pyometra and two others had cystic endometrial hyperplasia, hormonal function was attributed to the cystadenomas, although these changes are common in all old, intact female dogs.[43] A cystadenoma described in a nine-year-old

cat occurred with a lipoma (from neoplastic transformation of luteinized stromal cells of the ovarian cortex); clinical signs of persistent estrus, virilization, and cystic endometrial hyperplasia were attributed to the lipoma.[15] Diagnois of this tumor is by histopathological examination following surgical excision.

Adenocarcinoma/Cystadenocarcinoma

Ovarian adenocarcinomas usually occur in bitches over nine years of age and are commonly seen in association with cystic endometrial hyperplasia/pyometra. Metastases to omentum, sublumbar lymph nodes, liver, and lungs are described in approximately half the cases in the literature.[43, 49] Clinical signs include an enlarged abdomen associated with a palpable abdominal mass, ascites and hydrothorax when metastatic lesions are present in the liver and lungs, and occasional persistent vaginal hemorrhage. A bilateral ovarian adenocarcinoma with spindle cell transformation has been diagnosed in a five-year-old cat with a palpable abdominal mass, ascites, and hair loss; metastases were present throughout the pelvis and in the peritoneum, liver, and lungs. The endometrium was histologically normal.[115]

Granulosa Cell Tumor

The granulosa cell tumor arises from ovarian sex cords; it is the most common primary ovarian tumor in the dog and cat. Age at diagnosis usually ranges from 4 to 15 years in the bitch, although a granulosa cell tumor with metastasis to the mesentery, omentum, liver, kidneys, and urinary bladder was reported in a 14-month-old golden retriever with a two-day course of lethargy, anorexia, and abdominal distension.[32, 49, 116] The granulosa cell tumor ranges in size from 0.4 to 10 cm in diameter.[49] In one survey, 10 of 13 bitches with this tumor were nulliparous.[49] Clinical signs include abdominal distension and a palpable abdominal mass. The functional granulosa cell tumor may produce estrogens (leading to vulvar enlargement, sanguinous vaginal discharge, persistent estrus, and, occasionally, aplastic pancytopenia), progesterone (leading to cystic endometrial hyperplasia and pyometra), or both.[43, 70, 95, 116] Epidermal and hair follicle atrophy has been described in some dogs with this tumor.[70] Eighty per cent of granulosa cell tumors do not metastasize, so that ovariectomy effects a cure. Metastatic lesions, if present, occur by direct extension to liver, spleen, kidneys, pancreas, adrenals, gastrointestinal tract, and uterus and by lymphatic or hematogenous spread to the mesenteric and bronchial lymph nodes, lungs, meninges, and cerebrum.[6, 32]

Granulosa cell tumors in female cats are usually functional, producing signs of persistent estrus or cystic endometrial hyperplasia, and occur in cats between 3 and 15 years of age.[4, 10, 11, 51] Other reported clinical signs include abdominal enlargement due to a palpable mass, ascites, vomiting and alopecia. Metastases to regional lymph nodes, omentum, liver, spleen, kidneys, and lungs were reported in six of eight cases.[4, 10, 11, 115] One bilateral and one extra ovarian granulosa cell tumor (located at the upper end of the left uterine horn with no connection to the left ovary) have been reported in the cat.[10, 115]

Thecoma

Thecomas originate from ovarian stromal tissue. A thecoma was reported in a ten-year-old toy poodle with a history of depression, vomiting, and anestrus for the previous 18 months.[54] An 8 × 10 cm mass was palpated in the left side of the abdomen and removed surgically from a position caudal to the left kidney. No metastases were present.

Sertoli Cell Tumor

Ovarian tumors arising from sex cord stroma that demonstrate a histological pattern similar to that of Sertoli cell tumors of the testes may occur in the female. Six of these were described in a series of 84 ovarian neoplasms in dogs, and one has been described in the cat.[78, 116] Tumors in the dog occurred in patients 10 to 15 years of age. One bitch had signs of prolonged estrus, two had a purulent vaginal discharge, one had alopecia, and two had mammary carcinomas. In three bitches where the uterus was examined histologically, there was cystic endometrial hyperplasia and pyometra. The feline case occurred in the right ovary of a six-year-old domestic short-haired queen with cystic endometrial hyperplasia. Metastases have not been described with this tumor in the female dog or cat.

Dysgerminoma

Dysgerminomas are malignant tumors arising from undifferentiated germ cells of the ovary; they are comparable to the seminoma of the male. Dysgerminomas constitute about 10 per cent of canine and 15 to 20 per cent of feline ovarian tumors.[43, 45, 116, 140] These tumors are slow-growing and unilateral and may range in diameter from 2 to 30 cm; grossly they appear as nodular masses with bulging, tan, cut surfaces with hemorrhage and necrosis.[45] Dysgerminomas in 18 dogs occurred in 11 breeds in patients ranging from 5 to 20 years of age.[29, 45, 80, 143, 149] Metastases to adjacent peritoneum, adrenals, kidneys, mesenteric lymph nodes, pancreas, liver, and mediastinal lymph nodes occurred in 4 of the 18 cases (22 per cent). Clinical signs included an abdominal mass (16 of 18), sanguinous vaginal discharge (4 of 18), and occasional lethargy and anorexia. Open cervix pyometra was present in the 20-year-old bitch.[143] Five of the 18 cases had other neoplasms in addition to the dysgerminoma, including a papillary cystadenoma of the opposite ovary (one), multiple leiomyomas of the uterus (one), a primary mammary adenocarcinoma

without metastases (one), and an adrenal adenoma (one); one 14-year-old bitch had a metastatic dysgerminoma with a metastatic malignant melanoma, a mixed mammary tumor, and cystic hemangioma of the spleen.[9, 45] Dysgerminomas in cats generally occur in females over six years of age, although bilateral dysgerminomas weighing 40 gm each were reported in a one-year-old domestic short-haired cat presented for routine ovariohysterectomy.[9] Metastasis by extension to adjacent omentum has been reported in a seven-year-old Siamese queen with signs of masculinization.[45]

Teratoma (Dermoid Cyst)

Teratomas are germ cell tumors that show somatic differentiation beyond the primordial germ cell stage into masses with three germ layers (ectoderm, mesoderm, entoderm). They have been called *dermoid cysts*, because the masses typically include cysts lined by hair and keratinized squamous epithelium; they often contain sebaceous fluid, sweat glands, cartilage, fat, muscle fiber, bone, nervous tissue, connective tissue, teeth, and glandular epithelium.

Tumor diameter varies from 2 to 30 cm in dogs[33, 45, 61, 132, 142]; one tumor weighing 3.4 kg was removed from a five-year-old German shepherd bitch.[33] In eight cases reported in dogs, age at diagnosis was 4 to 11 years (mean 6.6 years). Clinical signs include abdominal enlargement with a palpable mass (five of six), weight loss (three of six), anorexia (two of six), vomition (one of six), and polyuria/polydipsia (one of six).[33, 45, 61, 141, 142] Radiographically these tumors are the most likely of all primary ovarian tumors to demonstrate calcific densities. Most bitches with teratomas have normal interestrous intervals; the older ones may have concurrent cystic endometrial hyperplasia.

Teratomas have been reported in cats from two to six years of age.[115] In one case a solid teratoma was present with a unilateral dysgerminoma. In another an extragonadal teratoma was present between the adrenal glands in a domestic short-haired cat from which a dysgerminoma had been removed three months earlier; metastases of the dysgerminoma were present in abdominal and thoracic lymph nodes, lung, liver, adrenals, and kidneys at the time the teratoma was removed. Human teratomas have been described in metastases of dysgerminomas.[61] A two-year-old domestic short-haired cat died suddenly of intra-abdominal hemorrhage from rupture of blood vessels associated with a 1.5-cm diameter teratoma.[45]

Teratocarcinoma

Teratocarcinomas are undifferentiated teratomas containing both mature and embryonal elements.[123] They are much less common than teratomas but have been reported in five bitches ranging from two to ten years of age.[44, 61, 123] Clinical signs included abdominal enlargement, depression, anorexia, and weight loss;

right fore- and hind leg lameness was present in one dog with bony metastases, and dysphagia with neck pain was present in one with cervical metastasis. Metastases may occur to adjacent omentum, regional lymph nodes, pancreas, lung, mediastinum, peripheral lymph nodes, midshaft ulna, olecranon, and tibial crest. Metastases, like the primaries, contain cells originating from two to three germ cell layers. These tumors frequently show radiographic calcific densities and may weigh up to 5 kg each.

Treatment and Prognosis

Excision biopsy is the treatment of choice with all ovarian tumors. Complete ovariohysterectomy is recommended because occasional tumors occur bilaterally, occasional extension to the uterus occurs, and cystic endometrial hyperplasia leading to pyometra is common in the aging bitches in which primary ovarian tumors occur. Care should be taken not to rupture fluid-filled cysts in the tumor, as abdominal implantation of tumor cells from such fluid may occur. Prognosis is good if metastasis has not occurred and poor if it has.

Because of their low incidence, little information is available on the treatment of metastatic ovarian tumors. Cyclophosphamide* (2.2 mg/kg per os once daily while the white blood cell count exceeds 2000/cm³) has been recommended for metastatic cystadenocarcinomas and granulosa cell tumors without case reports of effectiveness.[22] Similarly, intraperitoneal administration of triethylenethiophosphoramide† (0.4 to 0.8 mg/kg body weight) has been recommended after paracentesis to control malignant intraperitoneal effusions.[70] Immunotherapy with intramuscular or intraperitoneal injection of mixed bacterial toxins (*Streptococcus pyogenes, Serratia marcescens*) every

*Cytoxan, Mead Johnson & Co., Evansville, IN.
†Thiotepa, Lederle Laboratories, Pearl River, NY.

four to seven days after surgical excision of the primary tumor reported in one case of metastatic granulosa cell tumor was associated with a two-year period free from tumor recurrence.[70] The authors recommended surgical excision of large tumor masses and paracentesis of ascitic fluid prior to immunotherapy.[70]

UTERINE TUBE (OVIDUCT) NEOPLASIA

Tumors of the uterine tube are extremely rare in the bitch and have not been reported in the queen. Cotchin included 1 papillary cystadenoma of the mesovarium in a list of 266 female genital tumors among 1,150 canine neoplasms[38]; he later listed 2 tumors of the ovarian bursa among 4,187 canine neoplasms.[42] Three cases of uterine tube neoplasia were described in the bitch by McEntee and Nielsen.[96] These were a cauliflower-like adenoma, an adenocarcinoma with implantation to the peritoneal cavity, and a lipoma of the ovarian bursa.

There are no reports of patient signalment, clinical signs, concurrent reproductive disease, if any, or treatment regimens for uterine tube neoplasms in the bitch.

UTERINE NEOPLASIA

Incidence

The occurrence of primary uterine tumors in the dog and cat is shown in Table 182–3. Uterine tumors constitute 0.3 to 0.5 per cent of all canine tumors and 1 to 2 per cent of tumors of the female reproductive organs (including mammary glands). In the cat, uterine neoplasia occurs in 0.2 to 0.4 per cent of all tumor patients and in 1 per cent of patients with tumors of the reproductive organs, including the mammary glands.

TABLE 182–3. Incidence of Uterine Tumors in the Bitch and Queen

No. Tumor Cases	No. Tumors of Reproductive Organs*	No. Primary Uterine Tumors	Reference
Canine			
3,073		11	Brodey and Roszel, 1967
2,923	776	9	Brodey and Roszel, 1967
	266	3	Cotchin, 1954a
2,361	535	9	Cotchin, 1954b
	1,086	11	Cotchin, 1959
1,828		9	Mulligan, 1961
127		1	Thrasher, 1961
Feline			
464		1	Cotchin, 1957
	68	1	Cotchin, 1959
372		1	Engle and Brodey, 1969
256		1	Schmidt and Langham, 1967
165	34	2	Whitehead, 1967

*Including mammae.

Both epithelial (adenoma, adenocarcinoma) and mesenchymal (fibroma, fibrosarcoma, leiomyoma, leiomyosarcoma, lipoma, and lymphosarcoma) tumors have been reported in the uterus of the dog and cat.[26, 38, 42, 60, 86, 96, 108] The most common of these in the bitch is the leiomyoma. In a series of 11 uterine tumors in dogs, 10 were leiomyomas and 1 was a leiomyosarcoma.[26] In a second series of nine canine uterine tumors, seven were leiomyomas, one was a leiomyosarcoma, and one was a lymphosarcoma.[108] There is no relationship between presence of leiomyomas and estrous irregularity or occurrence of signs of false pregnancy; these tumors may, however, occur less frequently in the nulliparous bitch.[26] The most common primary uterine tumor in the cat is the endometrial adenocarcinoma, which may metastasize to the adjacent peritoneum and mesentery, regional lymph nodes, liver, adrenals, ovaries, diaphragm, lung, brain, and eyes.[14, 15, 99, 119, 126] Uterine leiomyomas and leiomyosarcomas have also been reported in cats.[155] A mixed mesodermal tumor, with both carcinomatous and sarcomatous elements, was described in a queen with metastases to the abdominal and thoracic lymph nodes and lungs; mixed histological types occur in 1 per cent of human uterine cancers but have not been otherwise described in companion animals.[53] Primary uterine tumors occur in dogs and cats between 5 and 12 years of age.

Diagnosis

Uterine leiomyomas in dogs are often diagnosed incidentally at ovariohysterectomy or post mortem. These tumors have been diagnosed in bitches with pyometra attributed to obstruction of the uterus by the tumor; pyometra occurs commonly in the aged bitch, however, and may be unrelated to the uterine neoplasm.

TABLE 182–4. WHO Clinical Stages of Uterine and Cervical Tumors*

T Primary Tumor
  T0 No evidence of tumor
  T1 Small noninvasive tumor
  T2 Large or invasive tumor
  T3 Tumor invading neighboring structures

N Regional Lymph Nodes (lumbar, iliacs, sacral)
  N0 No evidence of regional lymph node involvement
  N1 Regional lymph node involved
  N2 Juxtaregional lymph node involved

M Distant Metastasis
  M0 No evidence of distant metastasis
  M1 Evidence of metastasis
    M1a In the peritoneal cavity
    M1b Beyond the peritoneal cavity
    M1c In and beyond the peritoneal cavity

*Reprinted with permission from the internal report of the Second WHO Consultation on the Biological Behaviour and Therapy of Tumours of Domestic Animals, Geneva, 1979 (unpublished WHO document VPH/CMO/79.17).

Clinical signs of uterine adenocarcinomas depend on tumor size and pattern of metastasis. Signs include ascites, anorexia, weight loss, purulent or hemorrhagic vaginal discharge, vomition, constipation, dysuria, and presence of a palpable abdominal mass. Cats with thoracic metastases may have a periodic cough; those with tumor spread to the central nervous system may have blindness or motor incoordination.[14, 119, 126] Diagnosis is based on uterine palpation, abdominal and thoracic radiographs, and surgical exploration. Ultrasonography has been used to detect uterine neoplasia in the diffusely enlarged uterus with pyometra.

Uterine and cervical tumors are clinically staged according to behavior of the primary tumor (T), regional lymph node involvement (N), and presence of metastasis (M) (Table 182–4).[157] Regional lymph nodes are the lumbar, internal iliac, external iliac, and sacral nodes.

Treatment and Prognosis

The recommended treatment for primary uterine neoplasia without metastasis is ovariohysterectomy. Abdominal and thoracic radiographs are indicated prior to surgical exploration to look for metastatic disease. Wide surgical excision without ovariectomy may be considered in the younger purebred bitch with a single leiomyoma if maintenance of her reproductive capacity is essential. Successful treatment regimens for metastatic uterine neoplasia in the dog and cat have not been reported. Prognosis is good for benign tumors (such as leiomyomas) and poor for malignant tumors such as adenocarcinomas when metastases are present.

VAGINAL NEOPLASIA

Incidence

Neoplasms of the vagina and vestibule are the most common of female reproductive tumors in the bitch, excluding those of the mammary gland. In Cotchin's series of 4,187 tumors examined from all tissues of the bitch and dog, 123 vaginal tumors comprised 64 per cent of the 191 genital tumors (excluding those of the mammae).[42] Vaginal tumors are much less common in cats, and reports in this species are of single occasional cases.[87, 155, 156] No vaginal tumors were observed in series of 464, 395, and 256 feline neoplasms from both sexes.[40, 51, 134] Two vaginal leiomyomas were observed in a series of 165 feline tumors (34 of the reproductive organs, including mammary glands) reported by Whitehead.[155]

The leiomyoma and transmissible venereal tumor are the most common vaginal tumors of the bitch.[26, 60] Of 85 canine vaginal tumors, 66 were leiomyomas, 9 were transmissible venereal tumors, 5 were lipomas, 3 were leiomyosarcomas, 1 was a mast cell sarcoma, and 1 was an epidermoid carcinoma. The transmissible venereal tumor may occur with greater frequency in areas with free-roaming populations of dogs.[112, 131] Other reported vaginal tumors of the bitch include the fibroma, fibrosarcoma, neurofibroma, reticulum cell sarcoma, squamous cell carcinoma, and lymphosarcoma.[38, 79, 96, 108, 147] Only benign vaginal tumors (the fibroma and leiomyoma) have been reported in the cat.[87, 96, 155, 156]

Metastases are uncommon in the bitch with a vaginal tumor but may occur with the transmissible venereal tumor, leiomyosarcoma, or the other less common sarcomas. Transmissible venereal tumor metastasis may occur by transplantation of tumor cells to the skin, lip, nasal passage, tongue, pharynx, and tonsils; by direct extension to the cervix, uterus, and uterine tubes; or by hematogenous or lymphatic spread to regional lymph nodes, spleen, liver, intestine, lung, and brain.[1, 3, 13, 36, 93, 98, 112, 118, 125, 129, 133, 139, 154] The frequency of transmissible venereal tumor metastasis is unknown with the spontaneous disease; metastases occurred in 5 of 385 (1.3 per cent) animals in an experimental transplantation study.[88] Leiomyosarcomas of the canine vagina may metastasize to the regional lymph nodes, spleen, lungs, and cervical spinal cord.[26, 72]

Diagnosis

Clinical signs of vaginal tumors include bulging of the perineal region, prolapse of tumor tissue from the vulva, dysuria, and pollakiuria. Intraluminal tumors may become infected and cause sanguinous or purulent vaginal discharge. Initial diagnosis is based on vaginal and rectal palpation and on abdominal and thoracic radiography to look for tumor metastasis. Exfoliative cytology may be diagnostic and should be performed on accessible masses of the vagina and vestibule. Final diagnosis is based on histopathological examination after core or excision biopsy. Vaginal tumors can usually be distinguished clinically from vaginal hyperplasia and prolapse because hyperplasia occurs in young bitches, hyperplastic tissue regresses at the end of estrus, and vaginal hyperplasia most commonly occurs at the ventral midline of the vagina cranial to the urethral orifice, whereas tumors arise from anywhere in the wall of the vagina or vestibule.

Canine tumors of the vulva and vagina are clinically staged according to behavior of the primary tumor (T), regional lymph node involvement (N), and presence of distant metastasis (M) (Table 182–5.)[157] The regional lymph nodes are the inguinal, internal iliac, and sacral nodes.

Leiomyoma

Leiomyomas of the vagina and vestibule occur in bitches from 5 to 16 years of age and occur with greater frequency in the boxer.[26] Tumors are more likely to arise from the vestibule (between the vulva and the urethral orifice) than from the vagina (urethral orifice to cervix). The duration of clinical signs has been reported to depend on whether the tumor is intraluminal (1 day to 2 years; mean 7 weeks) or extraluminal (2 months to 2 years; mean 24 weeks).[26] Intraluminal tumors are firm, white, ovoid masses attached by a thin pedicle to the vestibular wall; extraluminal tumors appear as slowly growing perineal masses. Tenesmus and dysuria may be present with tumors in either location. Leiomyomas occur less frequently in the nulliparous bitch; they are not significantly associated with estrous irregularity or signs of false pregnancy.[26] Two female cats (ages 8 and 14 years) with extraluminal vaginal leiomyomas of 2 × 4 and 7 × 8 cm showed signs of constipation due to compression of the rectum.[156]

Leiomyosarcoma

Vaginal/vestibular leiomyosarcomas are reported in bitches over nine years of age.[26, 72] Clinical signs include perineal swelling, weakness, and dysuria. One tumor was excised and recurred four times in two and one-half years without metastasizing; the patient, a 15-year mixed breed bitch, died of pyometra and nephritis with recurrent tumor still in the vagina.[26] A 3 × 3 × 2 cm vulvar leiomyosarcoma in a 13-year old Standard Poodle was surgically excised one year before the animal presented with a two-month course of progressive bilateral hindlimb weakness; tumor metastasis had occurred to the cervical spinal cord (at C3), the external iliac lymph nodes, and the lungs, and the tumor had recurred adjacent to the surgical site.[72]

Transmissible Venereal Tumor

The transmissible venereal tumor is a naturally occurring neoplasm transmitted by transplantation of

TABLE 182–5. WHO Clinical Stages of Canine Tumors of the Vulva and Vagina*

T Primary Tumor

T0 No evidence of tumor
T1 Tumor ≤ 1 cm in its main dimension, superficial
T2 Tumor > 1 cm and < 3 cm in its main dimension with minimal infiltration
T3 Tumor > 3 cm or deep infiltration present
T4 Tumor infiltrating neighboring structures

N Regional Lymph Nodes (inguinal, iliac, sacral)
N0 No lymph node involvement
N1 Movable, unilateral nodes
N2 Movable, bilateral nodes
N3 Fixed nodes

M Distant Metastasis
M0 No evidence of distant metastasis
M1 Distant metastasis present

*Reprinted with permission from the internal report of the Second WHO Consultation on the Biological Behaviour and Therapy of Tumours of Domestic Animals, Geneva, 1979 (unpublished WHO document VPH/CMO/79.17).

tumor cells to the external genitalia at mating, to scarified skin, or to mucous membranes of the dog.[36] The first successful experimental tumor transmission was reported in 1876 by a Russian veterinarian working with the transmissible venereal tumor.[117] Karyotype, surface antigen, and histocompatibility studies indicate that transmissible venereal tumors have been maintained in the canine population from a single original tumor.[34, 36, 52, 110, 131] Most tumor cells contain 59 chromosomes, of which 17 to 19 are metacentric, in contrast to the normal dog karyotype of 78 acrocentric chromosomes.[2, 110, 151]

The malignancy of spontaneous transmissible venereal tumors is highly variable; tumors may regress spontaneously or may metastasize to the regional lymph nodes, liver, spleen, intestine, lung, and brain. Tumor behavior is associated with immunological response of the host. The tumor shows benign and irregular growth in normal adult dogs and rapid growth with metastasis in neonatal pups and in adults immunosuppressed with whole body x-irradiation prior to tumor transplantation.[35, 158] Both antitumor humoral antibodies and blocking factors that interfere with inhibitory action of these antibodies have been identified in affected dogs; humoral antibodies are present in patients with regressive, progressive, and metastatic disease, whereas blocking factors are present only in patients with locally invasive or metastatic disease.[16, 17, 34, 35, 52] Cell-mediated immunity also influences tumor behavior. In lymphocyte stimulation tests, patients with regressive tumors showed a blastogenic response to transmissible venereal tumor cells, whereas patients with metastatic disease did not.[74]

Because this tumor is generally acquired by coitus, vaginal or vestibular transmissible venereal tumor occurs in younger bitches more frequently than do other vaginal tumors. Case reports describe transmissible venereal tumors in 26 bitches two to six years of age.[26, 27, 112, 118, 130, 131, 148] An intraocular transmissible venereal tumor has been described in a four-month-old mixed breed bitch that did not have a genital tumor.[13] The average duration of clinical signs in 20 bitches was 3.5 months.[26, 27] Vaginal or vestibular transmissible venereal tumors range in size from small nodules to lesions more than 10 cm in diameter.[76, 81, 110, 118] There is no breed predisposition. The transmissible venereal tumor grows from small single or multiple nodules to a pedunculated, cauliflower-like mass, which is friable and may ulcerate. The most common presenting sign of a primary transmissible venereal tumor in the bitch is hemorrhagic vaginal discharge; other signs include the presence of a perineal mass, protrusion of a mass from the vulva, dysuria, and urinary tract infection.[26, 27] The majority of these tumors regress spontaneously two to six months after onset of signs.[131] Local invasion and metastasis of the tumor in other patients may reflect immune suppression of the host. Extragenital transmissible venereal tumor has been reported in 8 of 181 (4.4 per cent) cases of transmissible venereal

tumor.[112] Clinical signs in bitches with extragenital transmissible venereal tumor depend on site of transplantation or metastasis. Common sites of extragenital transmissible venereal tumor due to tumor transplantation include the skin, nasal passages, and orbit, and tumor at these sites may occur in the absence of genital transmissible venereal tumor. Signs of nasal transplantation include epistaxis, dyspnea, and sneezing; severe erosion of the nasal bones may occur.[112] In the skin, tumor nodules are present in the dermis and subcutis and may ulcerate, becoming hemorrhagic and necrotic. Tumor metastasis to the brain has been described in a bitch with vaginal transmissible venereal tumor; clinical signs following surgical removal of the primary tumor included depression and sleepiness.[3] Ocular transmissible venereal tumor has occurred in dogs with and without genital transmissible venereal tumor; the tumor may protrude from the cornea with local invasion, suggesting transplantation, or it may occur internally in the iris or ciliary body.[13] Diagnosis is by vaginal examination and histopathology of exfoliated cells or biopsy samples.

Lipoma

Vaginal or vestibular lipomas ranging in diameter from 5 to 20 cm were reported in five bitches ranging in age from one to eight years.[26] The only clinical sign was presence of a gradually enlarging mass. Lipomas may be intra- or extraluminal and most commonly arise under the mucosa of the vestibule. One lipoma excised from the floor of the vestibule of a seven-year-old German shepherd bitch recurred two years after excision.

Treatment and Prognosis

Vaginal tumors other than the transmissible venereal tumor should be treated by surgical excision following thoracic and abdominal radiography to look for metastatic disease. The need for episiotomy depends on the tumor size and location within the vagina or vestibule. With the exception of the transmissible venereal tumor, no successful treatment of metastatic vaginal neoplasia by chemotherapy or other means has been described in the bitch.

The transmissible venereal tumor responds to surgical excision, chemotherapy, orthovoltage radiotherapy, and immunotherapy.[7, 12, 27, 28, 30, 131, 146] Although the majority regress spontaneously, some are locally invasive, and a small number metastasize widely. Because tumor behavior can be predicted only by immunological methods not widely available (detection of blocking factors, lymphocyte stimulation tests), treatment is recommended.

Advantages of surgical excision include ease of access to most of these tumors and wide availability. A disadvantage is rate of recurrence after surgical excision, which is reported as "common."[7, 26, 88, 125, 146]

Tumors recurred within six months of conventional surgical excision in 4 of 23 (17.4 per cent) dogs with primary tumors only and in 7 of 12 (58.3 per cent) dogs with one primary or metastatic lesion.[7] Five of 18 dogs subsequently treated with radiotherapy and 10 of 41 dogs subsequently treated with chemotherapy were patients with tumor recurrence following surgery.[30, 146] Tumor cell transplantation at the incision site may cause recurrence, and electrosurgery may be associated with less recurrence than conventional surgery.[145] Surgical excision of a large primary tumor has been used with chemo- or radiotherapy, even though these modalities have high success rates with large primary tumors when used alone.[27, 30, 146]

Major advantages of chemotherapy are the high cure rate, ease of administration, and potential usefulness in metastatic or multifocal disease. A disadvantage is the presence of side effects, which include vomiting and transient leukopenia; these occurred in 5 of 41 (13 per cent) patients in one report.[30] Chemotherapy with vincristine* (0.025 mg/kg IV, not to exceed 1 mg) has been demonstrated to be effective against transmissible venereal tumors in one study of 41 dogs.[30] Vincristine is administered once weekly following a hemogram to detect leukopenia. Treatments are given until there is no longer evidence of disease. Of 41 dogs of both sexes with primary or recurrent (but not metastatic) transmissible venereal tumor, 39 experienced complete tumor regression after two to seven weeks of vincristine therapy. One dog failed to respond to vincristine alone and to one week of combination vincristine/cyclophosphamide†/methotrexate‡ therapy (vincristine 0.025 mg/kg IV given once; cyclophosphamide 50 mg/m² per os every other day; methotrexate 2.5 mg/m² per os every other day). Doxorubicin§ (30 mg/m² IV) administered at three consecutive seven-day intervals resulted in complete tumor regression. A second dog that did not undergo complete tumor regression after IV vincristine alone was unresponsive to six weeks of the combination chemotherapy and three weeks of doxorubicin therapy.[30]

Orthovoltage radiotherapy of transmissible venereal tumors in total radiation doses of 1000 to 3000 rads over 1 to 34 days was associated with a tumor-free period of one year after completion of therapy in 18 dogs.[146] Patients were treated one to six times at 2- to 21-day intervals. Tumors in seven of eight dogs were cured with a single dose of 1000 rads, which was the recommended therapy for most dogs.[146] Patients were not treated with other therapy, although three and five had recurrent tumors following previous chemotherapy and surgical excision, respectively. None of the dogs had metastatic disease; one with multicentric tumors (penis, cutaneous flank, cutaneous chest wall, and cutaneous ear) was successfully treated with 1000 rads per site.

Immunotherapy of transmissible venereal tumors has been effective in experimental studies but has not been widely evaluated clinically. Three weekly intralesional injections of Bacillus Calmette Guérin (BCG) were associated with regression of injected and noninjected distant tumors.[74] Another method of immunotherapy, administration of serum from patients in complete remission to dogs with active tumor growth, also may cause tumor remission.[124]

In conclusion, because all modes of therapy reported have been successful, choice of initial mode depends on presence of metastasis, the patient's ability to undergo anesthesia, and availability of orthovoltage x-ray therapy machines. Wide surgical excision using electrocautery is appropriate initial therapy for the single, accessible tumor. Orthovoltage radiotherapy (single dose of 1000 rads), if available, is also appropriate for the single or multicentric accessible tumor and for recurrent or nonresectable tumors. Chemotherapy with vincristine is indicated with metastatic disease, with recurrent invasive tumors when radiotherapy is unavailable, and in patients that are poor anesthetic risks. Treatment failures with vincristine should be treated with doxorubicin. Immunotherapy with intralesional BCG may be considered in chemotherapy treatment failures. Prognosis is good in all patients except those with metastasis to the central nervous system.

MAMMARY NEOPLASIA

Incidence

Patient Signalment

Dog. The mammary gland is the most common site of neoplasia in female dogs.[46] The incidence has been reported at 198.8/100,000 bitches per year and 1,200/100,000 bitches at 10 to 11 years of age.[47] Mammary neoplasms comprised 42 per cent of 2,917 tumors from all sites and 82 per cent of 1,086 tumors of the reproductive organs of the bitch.[23, 42] The bitch has a greater incidence of mammary neoplasia than other female domestic animals or humans.[25] Mammary tumors are rare in bitches under 2 years of age; their frequency increases dramatically after 6 years of age and peaks at 10 to 11 years of age, after which it declines.[37, 47, 107, 109] Median ages of affected bitches in surveys of 318, 201, and 472 bitches with mammary tumors were 9, 10 to 11, and 10.5 years, respectively.[41, 57, 135] Age at peak incidence is the same for neutered and intact females.[25]

Intact females have a three- to sevenfold greater risk of developing mammary cancer than neutered females.[58, 109, 127] Bitches neutered prior to the first estrus were reported to have 0.5 per cent the mammary cancer risk of intact bitches; those neutered after one estrus had 8 per cent risk, and those neutered after two or more estrous cycles had 26 per cent risk; after 2.5 years or four estrous cycles there was no detectable sparing effect of ovariectomy on

---

*Oncovin, Eli Lilly and Co., Indianapolis, IN.
†Cytoxan, Mead Johnson & Co., Evansville, IN.
‡Methotrexate, Lederle Laboratories, Pearl River, NY.
§Adriamycin, Adria Laboratories, Wilmington, DE.

incidence of mammary tumors in the bitch.[136] There is no relationship between presence of mammary tumors and irregular estrus, parity, fecundity, clinical signs of false pregnancy, or serum prolactin concentrations.[24, 64, 135, 136, 150]

Purebred dogs may have increased risk of mammary neoplasia when compared with mixed breed dogs.[47] In a survey of 2,075 mammary neoplasms, 12 breeds (Great Pyrenees, pointer, Samoyed, Airedale terrier, English setter, German short-haired pointer, Irish setter, Brittany spaniel, English springer spaniel, Labrador retriever, miniature/toy poodle, and keeshond) were at significantly higher risk for one or more of the major mammary tumor types.[127] Mixed breeds were at low risk for all tumor types. Others have reported the fox terrier, cocker spaniel, poodle, and Boston terrier at increased risk and the Chihuahua and boxer at reduced risk for mammary neoplasia.[37, 47, 106]

Mammary tumors may occur in any of the five pairs of mammary glands but are present most often in the two caudal pairs.[23, 41, 102, 107, 109, 150] Multiple mammary tumors of the same or different histological type have been reported by many in up to 20 to 66 per cent of affected bitches.[25, 107, 136]

Cat. Mammary tumors are the third most common neoplasm in the cat, following tumors of the skin and lymphoid tissue.[46] The incidence is 25.4/100,000 queens per year. Mammary tumors comprised 56 of 395 (14 per cent) feline tumors and 52 of 68 (76 per cent) tumors of the female reproductive organs of the queen.[23, 40] Age incidence is similar to that of the bitch, increasing most dramatically after 6 years and peaking (at 200/100,000 queens) at 10 to 11 years, after which it declines.[47, 153] Intact female cats, like dogs, have a sevenfold greater risk of mammary cancer when compared with neutered females.[47] In one survey of 136 mammary tumors in 132 cats, Siamese (52) were overrepresented and had twice the risk of developing mammary tumors as the other breeds (domestic, Persian, mixed) combined.[71] All four pairs of mammary glands are equally at risk of developing mammary tumors in the queen.[23, 40, 153]

Incidence of Tumor Type and Patterns of Metastasis

Dog. Many types and histological classification schemes for canine mammary tumors are present in the literature, causing confusion when clinicians attempt to compare therapeutic success and prognosis. Investigators are encouraged to use the WHO histological classification in Table 182–6.[65] Primary carcinomas, sarcomas, carcinosarcomas, and benign tumors may occur in the canine mammary gland. The benign mixed mammary tumor (fibroadenoma) is the most common mammary neoplasm in the dog, comprising nearly half of all mammary tumors, and the adenocarcinoma is the most common malignant neoplasm. Although numbers vary slightly, large surveys of canine mammary tumors from the United States and Europe typically document approximately 50 per cent as benign.[19, 25, 41, 46, 47, 56, 58, 107, 127]

Metastases are common with malignant mammary tumors of all types.[107] Mammary carcinomas in dogs metastasize most commonly to regional lymph nodes and then the lungs. Regional lymph nodes for the three cranial pairs of mammary glands in the bitch are the axillary nodes and for the two caudal pairs the superficial inguinal nodes. There is infrequent anastomosis of lymphatics between the third and fourth pair.[138] Occasionally the third pair of glands may drain solely to the inguinal nodes, but tumors in these glands are reported to spread to the axillary more often than to the inguinal nodes.[56] Lymphatics, like blood vessels, may cross the midline.[138]

Metastases to the liver, kidneys, adrenals, ovaries, heart, bone, brain, urethral and vestibular submucosa, and caudal thigh muscles by retrograde growth through obstructed lymphatics have been reported with mammary adenocarcinomas in the bitch.[25, 107, 145] Primary mammary sarcomas most frequently metastasize to the lungs, suggesting spread of tumor emboli by venous rather than lymphatic drainage.[101, 103–105] Regional lymph nodes, liver, kidney, and bones (femur, humerus, ribs, pelvis, skull, vertebrae, scapula) are also reported sites of metastasis.[25, 101, 102] In one report of 100 necropsies of bitches with malignant mammary tumors (85 adenocarcinomas, 15 sarcomas or carcinosarcomas), 93 per cent had metastatic lesions, with 81 and 65 animals showing metastases to the lungs and lymph nodes, respectively; other sites of metastasis included the kidney (16), liver (14), brain (12 of 54 examined), skeletal muscle (11), adrenals (10), spleen (8), pancreas (5), diaphragm (3), and eyes (2).[56] Absence of bony metastases in necropsy examinations is misleading unless careful radiological and pathological searches are made for these lesions, which are often solitary.[25]

Cat. Feline mammary tumors are usually malignant carcinomas, and the adenocarcinoma is the major type (see Table 182–6).[40, 68, 100] Metastases were detected at necropsy in 120 of 129 cats with malignant mammary tumors and were found in the lungs (83.6 per cent), regional lymph nodes (82.8 per cent), pleura (42.2 per cent), and liver (23.6 per cent).[153] Metastases may also occur in the spleen, omental fat, pancreas, adrenals, kidneys, ovaries, heart, brain, and vertebral column.[31, 40, 68, 100, 113, 153] Lymphatic drainage of the two cranial mammary glands is to the axillary node; the two caudal glands drain to the superficial inguinal lymph node. Lymphatics do not connect anterior and posterior glands or cross the midline in this species.[113] Small veins draining the glands, however, may cross the midline and serve as a metastatic route.[68] In a survey of 132 cats with mammary tumors, 8 had other concurrent neoplasia (lymphosarcoma (2), thyroid carcinoma, squamous cell carcinoma, endometrial adenocarcinoma, cervical leiomyoma, intestinal adenoma, malignant granulosa cell tumor).[71] Mammary tumors have been described in two cats with single thoracic lesions interpreted radiographically as metastases that turned out to be a pulmonary abscess in one and a primary bronchoalveolar adenocarcinoma of the lung in another.[111] Mammary tumors of different histological type (mixed mammary tumor and adenocarcinoma or carcinoma and adenoma) have been reported to occur in the same cat.[21, 71]

Influence of Etiology on Occurrence

Hormones. Reproductive hormones have long been suspected of having a role in the etiology of canine and feline mammary tumors, because (1) the majority of these tumors occur in females, (2) early ovariectomy greatly decreases the risk of acquiring such tumors, and (3) administration of exogenous progestogens causes tumor development and growth in these species.[40, 42, 47, 58, 59, 68, 71, 73, 82, 106, 113, 144, 153] Human mammary cancers may be similarly influenced by sex steroids; between 40 and 50 per cent of these tumors are rich in protein receptors for estradiol and progesterone.[94] Identification of receptor-rich tumors

is clinically important, because these tumors regress after additive (such as antiestrogen) or ablative (ovariectomy, adrenalectomy, hypophysectomy) endocrine therapy.[97] The receptor status of canine and feline mammary tumors has only recently been characterized. When only the estradiol receptor is assayed, mammary adenocarcinomas have been reported estradiol receptor rich in 65 of 129 (50 per cent), 24 of 46 (52 per cent), and 47 of 89 (53 per cent) of canine cases.[63, 92, 122] Estradiol receptor–rich feline mammary tumors have been detected in only 2 of 20 (10 per cent) and 0 of 33 cases examined.[62, 152] Reports of both estradiol and progesterone receptor concentrations in companion animal mammary adenocarcinomas compared with those in humans are listed in Table 182–7. These data indicate that dogs have percentages of receptor-rich tumors similar to those of humans, suggesting that ovariectomy may be of therapeutic value in 44 per cent of those intact bitches with mammary adenocarcinoma. Although the veterinary literature states that ovariectomy at time of mammary tumor excision is not associated with in-

TABLE 182–6. Incidence of Mammary Tumor Types in the Bitch and Queen

	Canine				Feline			
Tumor Type	Cotchin, 1958	Moulton et al., 1970	Bostock, 1977	Total	Cotchin, 1957	Hayden 1971	Hayes et al., 1971	Total
Carcinomas								
Adenocarcinoma, unspecified	14	239			38	27	94	
tubular	19	56	251					
papillary		91	141			19		
papillary-cystic							1	
Solid carcinoma	39	116	276			2		
Spindle cell carcinoma					1			
Anaplastic carcinoma	10		66			2	16	
Squamous cell carcinoma	5	39					2	
Mucinous carcinoma								
Solid adenocarcinoma				1,362 (40%)				202 (86%)
Sarcomas								
Osteosarcoma	23							
Fibrosarcoma		2					1	
Osteochondrosarcoma								
Unspecified	50	7	50				1	
				132 (4%)				2 (0.8%)
Carcinosarcomas (malignant mixed tumors)	27	115	10				4	
				152 (4%)				4 (1.7%)
Benign Tumors								
Adenoma	8	70	82		6	2	11	
Papilloma						1		
Fibroma	2							
Fibroadenoma (benign mixed tumor)	230	616	740			2	4	
Lipoma	9						2	
Myoepithelioma		15						
Benign mesenchymal tumor			9					
				1,781 (52%)				28 (12%)
Total	436	1,366	1,625	3,427	45	55	136	236

TABLE 182–7.   Presence of Estrogen and Progesterone Receptors in Malignant Mammary Tumors

| Species | ER + | | ER − | | Total |
	PR +	PR −	PR +	PR −	
Human[94]	218 (44%)	129 (26%)	27 (5%)	124 (25%)	498
Canine[128]	38 (44%)	8 (9%)	7 (8%)	34 (39%)	87
Feline[84, 85]	0	0	7 (100%)	0	7

Notes: ER = Estrogen receptor.
       PR = Progesterone receptor.

creased survival time, the appropriate study to demonstrate survival after ovariectomy in estradiol and progesterone receptor–rich patients has not been conducted. The presence of progesterone receptors, but not estradiol receptors, in a small number of feline tumors tested is puzzling, as induction of both estradiol and progesterone receptors is dependent on circulating estradiol; the presence of the progesterone receptor, then, in the absence of estradiol receptor is unexplained. A small number of feline patients tested have not shown tumor regression after antiestrogen (tamoxifen) therapy, suggesting that these patients are not really estradiol and progesterone receptor–rich with a masked estradiol receptor undetected by assay.[83]

Conclusions to be drawn from the receptor work of this point, then, are that ovariectomy or instigation of antiestrogen therapy at time of tumor excision may be beneficial in the 44 per cent of canine patients with receptor-rich adenocarcinomas.

Virus. C-type virus particles have been detected in electron microscopic examination of feline but not canine mammary tumors.[50, 71] Their significance is unknown.

Radiation. There is no effect of x-irradiation (100 to 300 R exposure at 10 to 12 months of age, life span studies) on incidence of mammary tumors in the dog.[107]

Diagnosis

Clinical signs of mammary gland neoplasia in the dog and cat are generally restricted to the presence of a mammary mass in the middle-aged to older female. Mammary tumors in both species are firm, well-demarcated nodules that may vary in diameter from several millimeters to 10 to 20 cm. Regional lymph node metastasis may or may not be detected by palpation of increased size or abnormal consistency. Because mixed mammary tumors in dogs are often very large, they may become traumatized, ulcerated, and infected. The wide variety of metastatic patterns with malignant mammary tumors in the bitch and queen leads to a variety of clinical signs. These include dyspnea (pulmonary metastases are the most frequent cause of death), cough, lymphedema of one or more limbs, lameness (if bony metastasis), and hind quarter paresis and emaciation;

locomotor disturbance due to hypertrophic pulmonary osteoarthropathy following thoracic metastasis has also been described.[25, 89, 101, 102] Iridocyclitis and hyphema occur with ocular metastasis.[91] Hypercalcemia, which disappeared following surgical excision of a mammary gland tumor, has also been reported in the dog.[25]

Diagnosis of canine and feline mammary tumors is based on palpation of masses in the glands and tumor histology. Although needle aspiration, scraping of ulcerated lesions, or cytology of fluid expressed from affected glands may yield diagnostic cytological samples with malignant tumors, the absence of neoplastic cells in the sample does not rule out malignancy. Examination of an excision biopsy is often necessary for definitive diagnosis. Several histological grading systems have been proposed that provide prognostic information. In general, the more highly differentiated tumors (with tubule or acinar formation) and those with fewer mitotic figures and more regular nuclear size and shape are associated with a more favorable prognosis.[66, 67, 103, 104] Diagnostic evaluation should include thoracic radiographs to look for metastases; these are usually circular, well-defined radiodensities, although a diffuse interstitial pattern with lymphatic infiltration by tumor cells may occur.[25] Bony metastases are visualized radiographically as irregular osteolytic foci.[25] Radioreceptor assay of estradiol and progesterone receptor in tumor tissue is desirable if available in making decisions on postexcision therapy.

Differential diagnoses include retention cysts in the postlactational gland and mammary hypertrophy lesions (often nodular) in the female treated with progestogens.[5, 69, 77, 137] Mammary hypertrophy (diffuse or nodular) may also be seen in the luteal-phase cat, but these patients are generally younger than those in the mammary tumor population.[5, 69, 77] Occasionally inflammation at the tumor site in a lactating gland may be confused with mastitis, although the former is not usually seen with the fever, leukocytosis, and systemic illness seen in the bitch with bacterial mastitis alone.

Canine and feline mammary tumors are clinically staged according to behavior of the primary tumor (T), regional lymph node involvement (N), and the presence of distant metastasis (M) (Table 182–8).[25] Regional lymph nodes are the axillary and superficial inguinal nodes.

**TABLE 182–8.   Clinical Stages of Canine
Mammary Tumors**

T Primary Tumor
   T0 No evidence of tumor
   T1 Tumor < 5 cm maximum diameter
   T2 Tumor 5 to 10 cm maximum diameter
   T3 Tumor 11–15 cm maximum diameter; muscle fix-
        ation
   T4 Tumor > 15 cm maximum diameter; whole gland
        involved; infiltration of underlying tissue

**N Regional Lymph Nodes (RLN) (axillary, superficial
   inguinal)**
   N0 No RLN involved
   N1 Ipsilateral RLN involved
   N2 Bilateral RLN involved
   N3 Distant LN involved
   NR LN previously removed

M Distant Metastasis
   M0 No evidence of lung metastasis
   M1 Solitary lung metastasis
   M2 Multiple lung metastasis
   M3 Other nonlung sites of metastasis
   M4 Solitary or multiple lung metastasis and other
        nonlung metastatic sites

Treatment and Prognosis

Surgical Excision

Five categories of surgical excision have been used: removal of the tumor alone; removal of the gland bearing the tumor (simple mastectomy, discussed in Chapter 39); removal of the tumor, glands, intervening lymphatics, and regional lymph nodes (en bloc dissection); removal of the gland and adjacent glands if glands 1 and 2 or 4 and 5 are affected (half chain removal); and removal of the entire chain of five mammary glands plus or minus regional lymph nodes (unilateral mastectomy).[25] No clinical trials have adequately demonstrated which of these procedures, if any, are associated with improved survival. Radical surgery in human breast cancer has not been associated with improved patient survival, which leads some investigators to recommend simple mastectomy or en bloc dissection in the dog as well.[25] In one study of canine patients treated by simple mastectomy (211) and en bloc dissection (42), both groups had similar postsurgical survival rates.[105] Nor is the issue of lymph node excision settled. Some argue that regional nodes are a host defense that should not be removed, whereas others argue that they probably contain microscopic tumor foci and should be excised. In a study of canine mammary tumors, the presence or absence of metastases in regional nodes was not associated with prognosis.[103]

Results of surgical treatment that are available are difficult to compare owing to variations in histological diagnosis, staging, surgical procedure used, and patient follow-up. Mean postsurgical survival of bitches with malignant mammary tumors has been reported in several American studies to range from 4 to 10.7 months when treated by mastectomy with or without ovariectomy.[55–57, 136] Duration of clinical signs preoperatively did not have statistical prognostic significance; shorter clinical histories were generally associated with short survival, perhaps owing to more rapidly invasive tumors.[57] In a Dutch report of 253 bitches with malignant mammary neoplasia, 115 (45 per cent) had died or were euthanized because of recurrent or metastatic mammary neoplasia and 63 others (25 per cent) died of other disease within two years of surgical excision.[103] Sarcomas had the worst prognosis (60 per cent of the patients died within one year), and complex carcinomas had the best prognosis.

Postmastectomy survival time of 220 bitches with mammary carcinomas less than 5 cm in diameter has been reported to vary with histological appearance and type of carcinoma.[18] Median survival times of invasive papillary, tubular, solid, and anaplastic carcinomas were 65, 38, 26, and 11 weeks, respectively, and of the well-defined papillary, tubular, and solid tumors were 128, 110, and 82 weeks, respectively.[18, 19]

En bloc dissection has been advocated in the cat, in which frequent lymphatic permeation occurs.[153]

In several studies ovariectomy at time of mastectomy was not associated with improved survival time, although a Russian study of 59 bitches did demonstrate longer mean survival time in the group treated with mastectomy and ovariohysterectomy (18.5 months) than in the group treated with mastectomy alone (6.1 months).[55, 57, 121, 136] The appropriate study examining the effect of ovariectomy plus mastectomy in those bitches with receptor-rich malignant tumors has not been done; if biology of the canine tumors is similar to that of humans, some 44 per cent of mammary adenocarcinoma patients would be expected to benefit from ovariectomy (see Table 182–7).[94, 128] Ovariectomy or ovariohysterectomy should be done prior to mastectomy to avoid seeding the abdomen with exfoliated tumor cells.

Chemotherapy

Chemotherapy following mastectomy is of therapeutic value in human mammary neoplasia but has not been well investigated in the dog or cat. Fifteen bitches with advanced malignant mammary tumors were reported not to respond to combination cytoxin, vincristine, and methotrexate chemotherapy.[91] Antiestrogen (such as tamoxifen) therapy may be of value in intact or neutered bitches with receptor-rich tumors. Tamoxifen was not associated with tumor regression in three cats with advanced mammary adenocarcinoma.[83]

Radiation Therapy

Radiation therapy has not been well evaluated in canine mammary neoplasia, although it is occasionally used.

Immunotherapy

Immunotherapy with intravenous BCG (Bacillus Calmette Guérin), mixed bacterial vaccine (*Streptococcus pyogenes* and *Serratia marcescens*), or levamisol has been used after mammary tumor excision in small numbers of dogs and in some cases was associated with increased survival time or regression of pulmonary metastases.[25] In one report, 34 bitches with invasive mammary carcinoma were randomized into three groups (no treatment, placebo treatment, intravenous BCG); three weeks after mastectomy the bitches were determined to have no palpable local or lymph node metastases or radiological evidence of pulmonary metastasis. Groups 2 and 3 were then treated with intravenous saline or BCG at one-, two-, and four-week intervals and then every eight weeks until one year after surgery. Median survival time for the two control groups was 24 weeks and for the BCG group was greater than 100 weeks, suggesting a BCG-induced delay in pulmonary metastases.[20] Patients with micrometastatic disease and minimal tumor burdens may respond better to this mode of therapy.

Prognosis

In a study of 253 dogs with malignant mammary tumors (211 treated by mastectomy and 42 by en bloc dissection), 75 per cent did not survive more than two years after surgery.[103, 104] Mean survival time after mammary cancer surgery was reported as 8.8 months in 14 animals that died of mammary cancer and 11.3 months in 38 animals that were euthanized owing to mammary neoplasia. Prognosis, defined as two-year survival time, following surgical treatment of canine malignant mammary tumors was shown to be influenced by histological type of tumor, mode of growth, clinical stage of complex carcinomas, and tumor size.[103] Tumor type (with descending malignancy from sarcoma to simple carcinoma to complex carcinoma) and mode of tumor growth (with descending malignancy from highly infiltrating to moderately infiltrating to expansive) were prognostic indicators unaffected by other variables. Clinical stage was associated with two-year survival only with complex carcinomas, where there was a large difference between patients with stage I (tumors less than 5 cm in diameter, skin and underlying tissue not involved) and stage III disease (tumor 11 to 15 cm in diameter, underlying muscle fixation). Tumor location, type of surgery (mastectomy, en bloc dissection), involvement of regional lymph nodes, and duration of signs before treatment were not prognostic indicators.

In the cat, average survival time after tumor detection was reported as 12.3 months in 56 cats; significantly higher one-year survival rates were seen in cats with well-differentiated tumors with low or medium grades of pleomorphism and a low number of mitotic figures.[153] There was also a significant correlation between tumor volume at time of excision and percentage of patients surviving one year; best survival (50 per cent) was seen with tumor volumes less than 8 cm.[19] Time between detection and first surgical excision averaged 7.7 months in 59 cats, suggesting that surgery done this late in the disease is only palliative.

In general, poor prognosis is associated with metastatic lesions, lymphatic infiltration (detected by peripheral lymphedema or satellite nodules between the tumor and regional nodes), widespread cutaneous involvement, infiltration of the thoracic or abdominal wall, infiltration across the midline or along a mammary chain, rapid growth, and recurrence of tumor.

1. Abbott, P. K.: Venereal transmissible tumor on eyelid of dog. Aust. Vet. J. *42*:29, 1966.
2. Adams, E. W., Sapp, W. J., and Carter, L. P.: Cytogenetic observations on the canine venereal tumor in long-term culture. Cornell Vet. *71*:336, 1981.
3. Adams, E. W., and Slaughter, L. J.: A canine venereal tumor with metastasis to the brain. Pathol. Vet. 7:498, 1970.
4. Aliakbrai, S., and Ivoghli, B.: Granulosa cell tumor in a cat. J. Am. Vet. Med. Assoc. *174*:1306, 1978.
5. Allen, H. L.: Feline mammary hypertrophy. Vet. Pathol. *10*:501, 1973.
6. Allen, H. L., and Franklin, G. A.: Malignant granulosa cell tumor in a bitch. J. Am. Vet. Med. Assoc. *166*:447, 1975.
7. Amber, E. I., and Henderson, R. A.: Canine transmissible venereal tumor: evaluation of surgical excision of primary and metastatic lesions in Zaria-Nigeria. J. Am. Anim. Hosp. Assoc. *18*:350, 1982.
8. Andersen, A. C., and Simpson, M. E.: *The Ovary and Reproductive Cycle of the Dog (Beagle)*. Geron-X, Inc., Los Altos, CA, 1973.
9. Andrews, E. J., Stookey, J. L., Helland, D. R., and Slaughter, L. J.: A histopathological study of canine and feline ovarian dysgerminomas. Can. J. Comp. Med. *38*:85, 1974.
10. Arnbjerg, J.: Extra-ovarian granulosa cell tumor in a cat. Feline Pract. *10*:26, 1980.
11. Baker, E.: Malignant granulosa cell tumor in a cat. J. Am. Vet. Med. Assoc. *129*:322, 1956.
12. Banks, W. C.: Results of radiation treatment of naturally occurring animal tumors. J. Am. Vet. Med. Assoc. *166*:1063, 1975.
13. Barron, C. N., Saunders, L. Z., Seibold, H. R., and Heath, M. K.: Intraocular tumors in animals. V. Transmissible venereal tumor of dogs. Am. J. Vet. Res. *24*:1263, 1963.
14. Bellhorn, R.: Secondary ocular adenocarcinoma in three dogs and a cat. J. Am. Vet. Med. Assoc. *160*:302, 1972.
15. Belter, L. F., Crawford, E. M., and Bates, H. R.: Endometrial adenocarcinoma in a cat. Pathol. Vet. 5:429, 1968.
16. Bennett, B. T.: Tumor-blocking and -inhibitory serum factors in the clinical course of canine transmissible venereal tumor. Cancer Res. *35*:2942, 1975.
17. Beschorner, W. E., Hess, A. D., Nerenberg, S. T., and Epstein, R. B.: Isolation and characterization of canine venereal tumor-associated inhibitory and blocking factors. Cancer Res. *39*:3920, 1979.
18. Bostock, D. E.: The prognosis following surgical excision of canine mammary neoplasms. Eur. J. Cancer *11*:389, 1975.
19. Bostock, D. E.: Neoplasia of the skin and mammary glands in dogs and cats. *In* Kirk, R. W. (ed.): *Current Veterinary*

Therapy VI. W. B. Saunders, Philadelphia, 1977, pp. 493–496.

20. Bostock, D. E., and Gorman, N. T.: Intravenous BCG therapy of mammary carcinoma in bitches after surgical excision of the primary tumor. Eur. J. Cancer *14*:879, 1978.

21. Britt, J. O., Howard, E. B., and Ryan, C. P.: Simultaneous mixed mammary tumor and adenocarcinoma in a cat. Feline Pract. *9*:41, 1979.

22. Broadhurst, J. J.: Neoplasms of the reproductive system. *In* Kirk, R. W. (ed.): *Current Veterinary Therapy V.* W. B. Saunders, Philadelphia, 1974, pp. 928–937.

23. Brodey, R. S.: Canine and feline neoplasia. Adv. Vet. Sci. Comp. Med. *14*:309, 1970.

24. Brodey, R. S., Fidler, I. J., and Howson, A. E.: The relationship of estrous irregularity, pseudopregnancy, and pregnancy and the development of K9 mammary neoplasms. J. Am. Vet. Med. Assoc. *149*:1047, 1966.

25. Brodey, R. S., Goldschmidt, M. H., and Roszel, J. R.: Canine mammary gland neoplasms. J. Am. Anim. Hosp. Assoc. *19*:61, 1983.

26. Brodey, R. S., and Roszel, J. F.: Neoplasms of the canine uterus, vagina and vulva. A clinicopathologic survey of 90 cases. J. Am. Vet. Med. Assoc. *151*:1294, 1967.

27. Brown, N. O., Calvery, C., and MacEwen, E. G.: Chemotherapeutic management of transmissible venereal tumor in 30 dogs. J. Am. Vet. Med. Assoc. *176*:983, 1980.

28. Brown, N. O., MacEwen, E. G., and Calvery, C.: Follow-up on chemotherapy of venereal tumors. J. Am. Vet. Med. Assoc. *177*:676, 1980.

29. Buergelt, C. D.: Dysgerminomas in two dogs. J. Am. Vet. Med. Assoc. *153*:553, 1968.

30. Calvert, C. A., Leifer, C. E., and MacEwen, E. G.: Vincristine for treatment of transmissible venereal tumors in the dog. J. Am. Vet. Med. Assoc. 181:163, 1982.

31. Chen, H. C.: A case of feline papilliferous mammary adenocarcinoma with widespread metastases. Can. J. Comp. Med. *32*:465, 1968.

32. Chestnutt, R. K.: Granulosa cell tumor in a Golden Retriever. Vet. Med. Small Anim. Clin. 75:444, 1980.

33. Clayton, H. M.: A canine ovarian teratoma. Vet. Rec. 96:567, 1975.

34. Cohen, D.: Detection of humoral antibody to the transmissible venereal tumor of the dog. Int. J. Cancer *10*:207, 1972.

35. Cohen, D.: The biological behavior of the transmissible venereal tumor in immunosuppressed dogs. Eur. J. Cancer 9:253, 1973.

36. Cohen, D.: The transmissible venereal tumor of the dog—a naturally occurring autograft? Isr. J. Med. Sci. *14*:14, 1978.

37. Cohen, D., Reif, J. S., Brodey, R. S., and Keiser, H.: Epidemiological analysis of the most prevalent sites and types of canine neoplasia observed in a veterinary hospital. Cancer Res. 34:2859, 1974.

38. Cotchin, E.: Further observations on neoplasms in dogs with particular reference to site of origin and malignancy. Br. Vet. J. *110*:218, 1954a.

39. Cotchin, E.: Neoplasia in the dog. Vet. Rec. 66:879, 1954b.

40. Cotchin, E.: Neoplasia in the cat. Vet. Rec. 69:425, 1957.

41. Cotchin, E.: Mammary neoplasms of the bitch. J. Comp. Pathol. 68:1, 1958.

42. Cotchin, E.: Some tumors in dogs and cats of comparative veterinary and human interest. Vet. Rec. 71:1040, 1959.

43. Cotchin, E.: Canine ovarian neoplasms. Res. Vet. Sci. 2:133, 1961.

44. Crane, S. W., Slocum, B., Hoover, E. A., and Wilson, G. P.: Malignant ovarian teratoma in a bitch. J. Am. Vet. Med. Assoc. *167*:72, 1975.

45. Dehner, L. P., Norris, H. J., Garner, F. M., and Taylor, H. B.: Comparative pathology of ovarian neoplasms. 3. Germ cell tumors of canine, bovine, feline, rodent and human species. J. Comp. Pathol. 80:299, 1970.

46. Dorn, C. R., Taylor, D. O. N., Frye, F. L., and Hibbard, H. H.: Survey of animal neoplasms in Alameda and Contra Costa counties, California. I. Methodology and description of cases. J. Natl. Cancer Inst. *40*:295, 1968.

47. Dorn, C. R., Taylor, D. O. N., Schneider, R., Hibbard, H. H., and Klauber, M. R.: Survey of animal neoplasms in Alameda and Contra Costa counties, California. II. Cancer morbidity in dogs and cats from Alameda County. J. Natl. Cancer Inst. *40*:307, 1968.

48. Dow, C.: Experimental production of the cystic-hyperplasia-pyometra complex in the bitch. J. Pathol. Bact. 78:267, 1959.

49. Dow, C.: Ovarian abnormalities in the bitch. J. Comp. Pathol. 70:59, 1960.

50. Else, R. W., and Hannant, D.: Some ultrastructural findings on spontaneous and cultured canine and feline mammary carcinomas. Proc. 6th World Congress WSAVA, 1977, pp. 91–92.

51. Engle, C. G., and Brodey, R. S.: A retrospective study of 395 feline neoplasms. J. Am. Anim. Hosp. Assoc. 5:21, 1969.

52. Epstein, R. B., and Bennett, B. T.: Histocompatibility typing and course of canine venereal tumors transplanted into unmodified random dogs. Cancer Res. *34*:788, 1974.

53. Evans, J. G., and Grant, D. I.: A mixed mesodermal tumor in the uterus of a cat. J. Comp. Pathol. 87:635, 1977.

54. Faulkner, R. T.: Removal of a thecoma in a poodle. Vet. Med./Sm. Anim. Clin. 73:451, 1978.

55. Fidler, I. J., Abt, D. A., and Brodey, R. S.: Biological behavior of canine mammary neoplasms. J. Am. Vet. Med. Assoc. *151*:1311, 1967.

56. Fidler, I. J., and Brodey, R. S.: A necropsy study of canine malignant mammary neoplasms. J. Am. Anim. Hosp. Assoc. *151*:710, 1967.

57. Fowler, E. H., Wilson, G. P., and Koestner, A.: Biologic behavior of canine mammary neoplasms based on a histogenetic classification. Vet. Pathol. 3:197, 1974.

58. Frye, F. L., Dorn, C. R., and Taylor, D. O. N.: Characteristics of canine mammary gland tumor cases. Anim. Hosp. *3*:1, 1967.

59. Giles, R. C., Kwapien, R. P., Geil, R. G., and Casey, H. W.: Mammary nodules in Beagle dogs administered investigational oral contraceptive steroids. J. Natl. Cancer Inst. *60*:1351, 1978.

60. Gilmore, C. E.: Tumors of the female reproductive tract. Mod. Vet. Pract. *45*:38, 1964.

61. Gruys, E., Van Dijk, J. E., Elsinghorst, T. A. M., and van der Gaag, I.: Four canine ovarian teratomas and a non-ovarian feline teratoma. Vet. Pathol. *13*:455, 1976.

62. Hamilton, J. M., Else, R. W., and Forshaw, P.: Oestrogen receptors in feline mammary carcinomas. Vet. Rec. 99:477, 1976.

63. Hamilton, J. M., Else, R. W., and Forshaw, P.: Oestrogen receptors in canine mammary tumors. Vet. Rec. *101*:258, 1977.

64. Hamilton, J. M., Knight, P. J., and Beevers, J.: Serum prolactin concentrations in canine mammary cancer. Vet. Rec. *102*:127, 1978.

65. Hampe, J. F., and Misdorp, W.: Tumors and dysplasias of the mammary gland. Bull. WHO *50*:111, 1974.

66. Harvey, H. J.: General principles of veterinary oncologic surgery. J. Am. Anim. Hosp. Assoc. *12*:335, 1976.

67. Harvey, H. J., and Gilbertson, S. R.: Canine mammary gland tumors. Vet. Clin. North Am. 7:213, 1977.

68. Hayden, D. W.: Feline mammary tumors. J. Small Anim. Pract. *12*:687, 1971.

69. Hayden, D. W., Johnston, S. D., Kiang, D. T., Johnson, K. H., and Barnes, D. M.: Feline mammary hypertrophy/fibroadenoma complex: clinical and hormonal aspects. Am. J. Vet. Res. *42*:1699, 1981.

70. Hayes, A., and Harvey, H. J.: Treatment of metastatic granulosa cell tumor in a dog. J. Am. Vet. Med. Assoc. *174*:1304, 1979.

71. Hayes, H. M., Milne, K. L., and Mandell, C. P.: Epidemiologic features of feline mammary carcinoma. Vet. Rec. *108*:476, 1981.

72. Helphrey, M. L.: Vulvar leiomyosarcoma metastatic to the spinal cord in a dog. J. Am. Vet. Med. Assoc. *172*:583, 1978.

73. Hernandez, F. J., Fernandez, B. B., Chertack, M., and Gage, P. A.: Feline mammary carcinoma and progestagens. Feline Pract. *5*:45, 1975.

74. Hess, A. D., Calchatourian, R., Zander, A. R., and Epstein, R. B.: *In vitro* and *in vivo* response of canine venereal tumors to intralesional BCG therapy. Proc. Am. Soc. Clin. Oncol. *17*:29, 1976.

75. Hess, A., and Cunningham, B.: *In vitro* correlates of the *in vivo* course of the canine transmissible venereal tumor studied by mixed lymphocyte-tumor cultures. Transplant. Proc. *7*:507, 1975.

76. Higgins, D. A.: Observations on the canine transmissible venereal tumor as seen in the Bahamas. Vet. Rec. *79*:67, 1966.

77. Hinton, M., and Gaskell, C. J.: Non-neoplastic mammary hypertrophy in the cat associated either with pregnancy or with oral progestagen therapy. Vet. Rec. *100*:277, 1977.

78. Hofmann, W., Arbiter, D., and Scheele, D.: Sex cord stromal tumor of the cat: so-called androblastoma with Sertoli-Leydig cell pattern. Vet. Pathol. *17*:508, 1980.

79. Howell, J. M. C., Ishmael, J., Tandy, J., and Hughes, I. B.: A 6 year survey of tumors of dogs and cats removed surgically in private practice. J. Small Anim. Pract. *11*:793, 1970.

80. Ishmael, J.: Dysgerminoma of the ovary in a bitch. J. Small Anim. Pract. *11*:697, 1970.

81. Ivoghli, B.: Canine transmissible venereal tumor in Iran. Vet. Pathol. *14*:289, 1977.

82. Jabara, A. G.: Two cases of mammary neoplasms arising in male dogs. Aust. Vet. J. *45*:476, 1969.

83. Johnston, S. D.: Personal observations, 1982.

84. Johnston, S. D., Hayden, D. W., Johnson, K. H., Handschin, B., Theologides, A., and Kiang, D. T.: Progesterone receptors in spontaneously occurring feline mammary adenocarcinomas. Proc. 73rd Ann. Mtg. Amer. Assoc. Cancer Res. 1982, p. 238.

85. Johnston, S. D., Hayden, D. W., Kiang, D. T., Handschin, B., and Johnson, K. H.: Progesterone receptors in feline mammary adenocarcinomas. Am. J. Vet. Res. *45*:379, 1984.

86. Joshi, K. V., Sardeshpande, P. D., Jalnapurkar, B. V., and Ajinkya, S. M.: A case of uterine adenocarcinoma in a dog. Ind. Vet. J. *44*:114, 1967.

87. Joshua, J. O.: *The Clinical Aspects of Some Diseases of Cats.* J. B. Lippincott, Philadelphia, 1965, pp. 119–140.

88. Karlson, A. G., and Mann, F. C.: The transmissible venereal tumor of dogs: observations on forty generations of experimental transfers. Ann. NY Acad. Sci. *54*:1197, 1952.

89. Knight, D., and Hamilton, J. M.: An unusual case of metastatic mammary carcinoma in a bitch. Vet. Rec. *90*:570, 1972.

90. Ladds, P. W.: Ovarian serous cystadenoma in a dog. Cornell Vet. *61*:482, 1971.

91. Ladds, P. W., Gelatt, K. N., Strafuss, A. C., and Mosier, J. E.: Canine ocular adenocarcinoma of mammary origin. J. Am. Vet. Med. Assoc. *156*:63, 1970.

92. MacEwen, E. G., Patnaik, A. K., Harvey, H. J., and Panko, W. B.: Estrogen receptors in canine mammary tumors. Cancer Res. *42*:2255, 1982.

93. Manning, P. J., and Martin, P. D.: Metastasis of canine transmissible venereal tumor to the adenohypophysis. Pathol. Vet. *7*:148, 1970.

94. Martin, P. M., Rolland, P. H., Jacquemier, J., et al.: Multiple steroid receptors in human breast cancer. Cancer Chemother. Pharmacol. *2*:107, 1979.

95. McCandlish, I. A. P., Munro, C. D., Breeze, R. G., and Nash, A. S.: Hormone producing ovarian tumors in the dog. Vet. Rec. *105*:9, 1979.

96. McEntee, K., and Nielsen, S. W.: Tumors of the female genital tract. Bull. WHO *53*:217, 1976.

97. McGuire, W. L.: An update on estrogen and progesterone receptors for primary and advanced breast cancer. *In* Iacobelli, S., King, R. J. B., Lindner, H. R., and Lippman, M. E. (eds.): *Hormones and Cancer.* Raven Press, New York, 1980, pp. 337–344.

98. McLeod, C. G., and Lewis, J. E.: Transmissible venereal tumor with metastasis in 3 dogs. J. Am. Vet. Med. Assoc. *161*:199, 1972.

99. Meier, H.: Carcinoma of the uterus of the cat: Two cases. Cornell Vet. *46*:188, 1956.

100. Misdorp, W.: Malignant mammary tumors in the dog and cat compared with the same in women. Inaugural dissertation, Utrecht, 1964.

101. Misdorp, W., Cotchin, E., Hampe, J. F., Jabara, A. G., and Von Sandersleben, J.: Canine malignant mammary tumors. I. Sarcomas. Vet. Pathol. *8*:99, 1971.

102. Misdorp, W., and den Herder, B. A.: Bone metastasis in mammary cancer. A report of 10 cases in the female dog and some comparisons with human cases. Br. J. Cancer *20*:496, 1966.

103. Misdorp, W., and Hart, A. A. M.: Prognostic factors in canine mammary cancers. J. Natl. Cancer Inst. *56*:779, 1976.

104. Misdorp, W., and Hart, A. A. M.: Canine mammary carcinoma. I. Prognosis. J. Small Anim. Pract. *20*:385, 1979.

105. Misdorp, W., and Hart, A. A. M.: Canine mammary cancer. II. Therapy and causes of death. J. Small Anim. Pract. *20*:395, 1979.

106. Mitchell, L., de la Iglesia, F. A., Wenkoff, M. S., et al.: Mammary tumors in dogs: Survey of clinical and pathological characteristics. Can. Vet. J. *15*:131, 1974.

107. Moulton, J. E., Taylor, D. O. N., Dorn, C. R., and Andersen, A. C.: Canine mammary tumors. Pathol. Vet. *7*:189, 1970.

108. Mulligan, R. M.: Mesenchymal and neurilemmal tumors in the dog. Arch. Pathol. *71*:512, 1961.

109. Mulligan, R. M.: Mammary cancer in the dog: A study of 120 cases. Am. J. Vet. Res. *36*:1391, 1975.

110. Murray, M., James, H., and Martin, W. J.: A study of the cytology and karyotype of the canine transmissible venereal tumor. Res. Vet. Sci. *10*:565, 1969.

111. Nafe, L. A., Hayes, A. A., and Patnaik, A. K.: Mammary tumors and unassociated pulmonary masses in two cats. J. Am. Vet. Med. Assoc. *175*:1194, 1979.

112. Ndiritu, C. G., Mbogura, S. W., and Sayer, P. D.: Extragenitally located transmissible venereal tumor in dogs. Mod. Vet. Pract. *11*:940, 1977.

113. Nielsen, S. W.: The malignancy of mammary tumors in cats. North Am. Vet. *33*:245, 1952.

114. Nielsen, S. W.: Tumors of the genital tract. *In* Catcott, E. J. (ed.): *Feline Medicine and Surgery.* American Veterinary Publications, Wheaton, IL, 1964, pp. 165–168.

115. Norris, H. J., Garner, F. M., and Taylor, H. B.: Pathology of feline ovarian neoplasms. J. Pathol. *97*:138, 1969.

116. Norris, H. J., Garner, F. M., and Taylor, H. B.: Comparative pathology of ovarian neoplasms. IV. Gonadal stromal tumors of canine species. J. Comp. Pathol. *80*:399, 1970.

117. Novinsky, M. A.: Zur frage uber die impfung der krebsigen geschwulste. Zentbl. Med. Wiss. *14*:790, 1876.

118. Oduye, O. O., Ikede, B. O., Esuruoso, G. O., and Akpolodje, J. U.: Metastatic transmissible venereal tumor in dogs. J. Small Anim. Pract. *14*:625, 1973.

119. O'Rourke, M. D., and Geib, L. W.: Endometrial adenocarcinoma in a cat. Cornell Vet. *60*:598, 1970.

120. O'Shea, J. D., and Jabara, A. G.: The histogenesis of canine ovarian tumors induced by stilbestrol administration. Pathol. Vet. *4*:137, 1967.

121. Osipov, N. E., Lagova, N. D., Ponmarkov, V. I.: Spontaneous mammary gland tumors of dogs as a model for experimental tumor therapy. Bull. Exp. Biol. Med. *74*:948, 1972.

122. Panko, W. B., Patnaik, A., and MacEwen, E. G.: Canine mammary adenocarcinoma: biochemical and endocrinologic similarities to human breast cancer. Cancer Treatm. Rep. *63*:1169, 1979.

123. Patnaik, A. K., Schaer, M., Parks, J., and Liu, S. K.:

Metastasizing ovarian teratocarcinoma in dogs. A report of 2 cases and review of the literature. J. Small Anim. Pract. *17*:235, 1976.

124. Powers, R. D.: Immunologic properties of canine transmissible venereal sarcoma. Am. J. Vet. Res. 29:1637, 1968.

125. Prier, J. E., and Johnson, J. H.: Malignancy in a canine transmissible venereal tumor. J. Am. Vet. Med. Assoc. *145*:1092, 1964.

126. Preiser, H: Endometrial adenocarcinoma in a cat. Pathol. Vet. *1*:485, 1964.

127. Priester, W. A.: Occurrence of mammary neoplasms in bitches in relation to breed, age, tumor type, and geographical region from which reported. J. Small Anim. Pract. *20*:1, 1979.

128. Raynaud, J. P., Cotard, M., Andre, F., Mialot, J. P., Rolland, P. H., and Martin, P. M.: Spontaneous canine mammary tumors: A model for human endocrine therapy? J. Ster. Biochem. *15*:201, 1981.

129. Rensburg, I. B.: Extragenital malignant transmissible venereal tumor in a bitch. J. S. Afr. Vet. Assoc. *51*:199, 1980.

130. Rickards, D. A., and Pencis, R. E.: Transmissible venereal tumors. Can. Pract. *3*:23, 1976.

131. Richardson, R. C.: Canine transmissible venereal tumor. Comp. Cont. Ed. *3*:951, 1981.

132. Riser, W. H., Marcus, J. F., Gribor, E. C., and Oldt, C. C.: Dermoid cyst of the canine ovary. J. Am. Vet. Med. Assoc. *134*:27, 1959.

133. Sastry, G. A.: A case of metastatic venereal tumor in a bitch. Ind. Vet. J. *42*:658, 1965.

134. Schmidt, R. E., and Langham, R. F.: A survey of feline neoplasms. J. Am. Vet. Med. Assoc. *151*:1325, 1967.

135. Schneider, R.: Comparison of age, sex and incidence rates in human and canine breast cancer. Cancer *26*:419, 1970.

136. Schneider, R., Dorn, C. R., and Taylor, D. O. N.: Factors influencing canine mammary cancer developments and post surgical survival. J. Natl. Cancer Inst. *43*:1249, 1969.

137. Seiler, R. J., Kelly, W. R., Menrath, V. H., and Barber, R. D.: Total fibroadenomatous change of the mammary glands of two spayed cats. Feline Pract. *9*:25, 1979.

138. Silver, I. A.: Symposium on mammary neoplasia in the dog and cat. I. The anatomy of the mammary gland of the dog and cat. J. Small Anim. Pract. *7*:689, 1966.

139. Spence, J. A., Holt, P. E., Sayer, P. D., Rottcher, D., and Copper, J. E.: Metastasis of a transmissible venereal tumor to the pituitary. J. Small Anim. Pract. *19*:175, 1978.

140. Stein, B. S.: Tumors of the feline genital tract. J. Am. Anim. Hosp. Assoc. *17*:1022, 1981.

141. Stein, B. S., and Velders, R. W.: What is your diagnosis? J. Am. Vet. Med. Assoc. *165*:749, 1974.

142. Storm, R. E.: Dermoid cyst of the ovary. North Am. Vet. *28*:30, 1947.

143. Taylor, D. O. N., and Dorn, C. R.: Dysgerminoma in a 20-year-old female German Shepherd dog. Am. J. Vet. Res. *28*:587, 1967.

144. Taylor, G. N., Shabestari, L., Williams, J., et al.: Mammary neoplasia in a closed Beagle colony. Cancer Res. *36*:2740, 1976.

145. Theilen, G. H., and Madewell, B. R.: *Veterinary Cancer Medicine.* Lea & Febiger, Philadelphia, 1979.

146. Thrall, D. E.: Orthovoltage radiotherapy of canine transmissible venereal tumors. Vet. Radiol. *23*:217, 1982.

147. Thrasher, J. P.: Neoplasms of dogs. J. Am. Vet. Med. Assoc. *138*:27, 1961.

148. Tutt, J. B.: Transmissible venereal tumor in a boxer bitch. Vet. Rec. *84*:13, 1969.

149. Vardija, V. G., and Ajinkya, S. M.: A case of dysgerminoma in a dog. Ind. Vet. J. *46*:475, 1969.

150. Warner, M. R.: Age incidence and distribution of mammary dysplasias in young Beagle bitches. J. Natl. Cancer Inst. *57*:57, 1976.

151. Weber, W. T., Nowell, P. C., and Hare, W. C. D.: Chromosome studies of a transplanted and a primary canine venereal sarcoma. J. Natl. Cancer Inst. *35*:537, 1965.

152. Weijer, K.: Feline malignant mammary tumors. IV. Oestrogen receptors. *In* Weijer, K. (ed.): *Feline Mammary Tumor and Dysplasias.* Drukkerij Van der Molen, 1979, Oosthuizen, The Netherlands, pp. 51–54.

153. Weijer, K., Head, K. W., Misdorp, W., and Hampe, J. F.: Feline malignant mammary tumors. I. Morphology and biology: some comparisons with human and canine mammary carcinomas. J. Natl. Cancer Inst. *49*:1697, 1972.

154. Weir, E. C., and Pond, M. J.: Extragenital occurrence of transmissible venereal tumor in the dog. Literature review and case reports. J. Am. Anim. Hosp. Assoc. *14*:532, 1978.

155. Whitehead, J. E.: Neoplasia in the cat. Vet. Med./Small Anim. Clin. *62*:357, 1967.

156. Wolke, R. E.: Vaginal leiomyoma as a cause of chronic constipation in the cat. J. Am. Vet. Med. Assoc. *143*:1103, 1963.

157. World Health Organization: *Report of the Second Consultation of the Biological Behavior and Therapy of Tumors of Domestic Animals.* WHO, Geneva, 1979, pp. 18–20.

158. Yang, T. J., and Jones, J. B.: Canine transmissible venereal sarcoma: transplantation studies in neonatal and adult dogs. J. Natl. Cancer Inst. *51*:1915, 1973.

Chapter **183**

Urinary System

Dennis D. Caywood and Carl A. Osborne

NEOPLASMS OF THE KIDNEY

Incidence

Benign renal neoplasms are less common than malignant renal tumors in dogs and cats.[3,9,30,43,48,56] They are primarily observed in older animals.[1] The renal hemangioma (Fig. 183–1) is the most commonly encountered benign canine kidney neoplasm (Table 183–1), but it has no breed or sex predilection.

Renal carcinomas (hypernephroma, renal adenocarcinoma, clear cell carcinoma, malignant nephroma) are the most common primary malignant neoplasms of the kidneys of dogs (Fig. 183–2) and cats.[3,9,12,18,30,43,48,53,57] As in humans, there is a higher incidence of these tumors in male dogs. This tumor may be hormonally induced. No sex predisposition has been identified in cats (Table 183–2). The incidence of the tumor increases with age in cats and dogs. Renal carcinomas originate from renal tubular

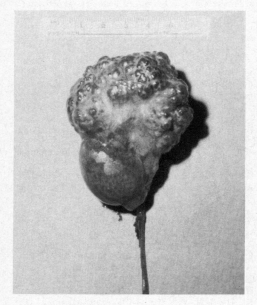

Figure 183–1. Primary renal hemangioma from a ten-year-old female miniature poodle.

TABLE 183–1. Type, Age, and Sex of 176 Dogs with Primary Renal Neoplasms*

Tumor Type	No. of Cases	Male	Female	Not Determined	Mean	Range	Not Determined
Epithelial tissue							
Adenoma	3	1	1	1	8.5	8–9	1
Renal carcinoma	113	57	27	29	8.2	1–15	34
Squamous cell carcinoma	9	6	3	—	8.7	4–14	—
Connective tissue							
Fibroma	2	1	1	—	8.5	5–12	—
Fibrosarcoma	2	1	1	—	6.5	5–8	—
Rhabdomyosarcoma	1	1	0	—	12.0	12	—
Leiomyoma	1	1	0	—	—	—	1
Leiomyosarcoma	1	—	—	1	—	—	1
Lipoma	1	0	1	—	8.0	8	—
Liposarcoma	1	0	1	—	5.0	—	—
Reticulum cell sarcoma	1	1	0	—	3.0	3	—
Unclassified sarcoma	4	1	3	—	7.2	6 mo–12 yr	1
Vascular tissue							
Hemangioma	7	4	3	—	11.3	8–5	—
Hemangiosarcoma	3	3	0	—	10.6	9–12	—
Mixed tissue							
Nephroblastoma	26	11	10	5	4.2	2 mo–11 yr	4
Teratoma	1	0	1	—	2.0	2	—
TOTAL	176	88	52	36	7.4	2 mo–15 yr	42

*Data from the University of Minnesota Veterinary Teaching Hospital, the Veterinary Medical Data Program sponsored by the National Cancer Institute, and the literature.[2,6,8,10,13,16,17,26,27,28,30,32,34,40,42,45,51,54,62,64,70,73,74]

(Reproduced with permission from Caywood, D. D., Osborne, C. A., and Johnston, G. R.: Neoplasms of the canine and feline urinary tracts. *In* Kirk, R. W. (ed.): *Current Veterinary Therapy VII.* W. B. Saunders, Philadelphia, 1980. pp. 1203–1212).

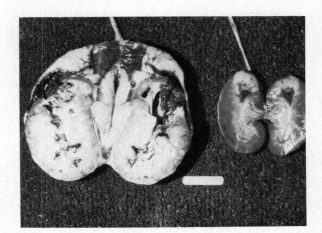

Figure 183–2. Renal adenocarcinoma in an eight-year-old male mixed breed dog. Note the bilateral renal involvement.

TABLE 183–2.   Type, Age, and Sex of 43 Cats with Primary Renal Neoplasms*

Tumor Type	No. of Cases	Sex			Age (Years)		
		Male	Female	Not Determined	Mean	Range	Not Determined
Epithelial tissue							
Adenoma	2	1	1	—	—	—	2
Renal carcinoma	17	3	4	10	9	2–15	6
Transitional cell carcinoma	3	2	1	—	8	6–9	1
Squamous cell carcinoma	2	2	—	—	—	—	2
Connective tissue							
Unclassified sarcoma	8	—	1	7	—	—	8
Muscle tissue							
Leiomyosarcoma	2	—	1	1	—	22	1
Mixed tissue							
Nephroblastoma	9	2	—	7	6	2–8	5
TOTAL	43	10	8	25	7	2–22	25

*Data from the University of Minnesota Veterinary Teaching Hospital, the Veterinary Medical Data Program sponsored by the National Cancer Institute, and the literature.[12,18,37,53,57]

(Reproduced with permission from Caywood, D. D., Osborne, C. A., and Johnston, G. R.: Neoplasms of the canine and feline urinary tracts. *In* Kirk, R. W. (ed.): *Current Veterinary Therapy VII.* W. B. Saunders, Philadelphia, 1980. pp. 1203–1212).

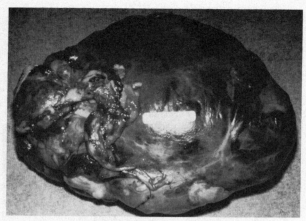

Figure 183–3. Embryonal nephroma in a two-year-old spayed mixed breed dog.

epithelial cells.[60] It has not been resolved whether carcinomas arise directly from renal tubular cells, by evolution through adenomatous hyperplasia, or from renal cortical adenomas.[60]

Embryonal nephroma (Wilms' tumor, nephroblastoma, congenital mixed tumor) is a congenital neoplasm derived from the pluripotential metanephrogenic blastema, which allows production of epithelial and connective tissue elements (Fig. 183–3).[1,44,58] It is regarded as part of the developing kidney and is associated with continued growth but abnormal differentiation.[1,44,58] The neoplasm occurs more often in young dogs and cats, although many cases have been observed in dogs and cats 4 years of age or older (Tables 183–1 and 183–2). No breed or sex predilection is apparent.

Transitional cell and squamous cell carcinomas of the canine renal pelvis are much less common than the same types of tumors in the urinary bladder (Table 183–1) and are rare in cats (Table 183–2). The fact that urothelium maintains the embryonic potential to produce mucus-secreting glandular epithelium and squamous epithelium in addition to transitional epithelium accounts for different morphological varieties of urothelial carcinomas, including transitional cell carcinomas and squamous cell carcinomas.[60] The sequence of events leading to development of transitional cell and squamous cell neoplasms is similar in all species.[9,44,60] Studies of humans, dogs, and laboratory animals have revealed that urothelial cel-

lular hyperplasia precedes formation of many malignant transitional cell neoplasms.[60]

Sarcomas (fibrosarcomas, leiomyosarcomas, rhabdomyosarcomas, undifferentiated sarcomas) of the kidneys of dogs and cats are less common than epithelial neoplasms or nephroblastomas (Tables 183–1 and 183–2).

Metastatic neoplasms are commonly found in the kidneys,[28,43,58,71] possibly because of the large blood volume that the kidneys receive and their abundant supply of capillaries. Renal lymphomas are generally considered metastatic neoplasms of the kidney.[9,47,71] Malignant lymphoma is the most common renal neoplasm of cats but is less frequently encountered in dogs (Tables 183–3 and 183–4).

Clinical Signs

Clinical signs vary with location, size, and duration of neoplasia. Neoplasms of the renal pelvis (Fig. 183–4) are usually associated with local signs (hematuria, hydronephrosis, and others) that precede polysystemic signs.[1,3] This pattern is often opposite to that in patients with renal parenchymal neoplasms.[9,48]

Benign renal neoplasms are rarely of clinical significance and are usually incidental necropsy findings.[9,48] An exception is the renal hemangioma of dogs. This neoplasm is frequently associated with constant or intermittent gross hematuria and varying degrees of enlargement of the affected kidney.[13,17,40,51]

Clinical signs of renal cell carcinomas are nonspecific and may not indicate involvement of the urinary system initially.[8,26,32,42,45,50,73,75] Local signs include persistent or intermittent gross or microscopic hematuria and abdominal distension with an associated palpable mass.[9,42,45,48,50,75] Enlarged kidneys caused by neoplasia must be differentiated from enlarged kidneys caused by hydronephrosis or polycystic disease.[9,48] In addition, neoplastic enlargement of the kidneys must be differentiated from neoplastic enlargement of one or both adrenal glands and the ovaries, spleen, liver, pancreas, and intestine.[9,48] Even though both kidneys are involved, a sufficient quantity of functional renal parenchyma may persist to prevent signs of renal failure.[9,48] Extensive bilateral involvement of the kidneys that destroys 70 to 75 per cent or more of the nephrons is associated with signs of progressive renal insufficiency.[9,48]

TABLE 183–3.   Age and Sex of 40 Cats with Malignant Lymphoma Involving the Kidneys*

Age (Years)			Sex		
Mean	Range	Not Determined	Male	Female	Not Determined
6	1–15	6	20	12	8

*Data from the University of Minnesota Veterinary Teaching Hospital, the Veterinary Medical Data Program sponsored by the National Cancer Institute, and the literature.[47,71]

(Reproduced with permission from Caywood, D. D., Osborne, C. A., and Johnston, G. R.: Neoplasms of the canine and feline urinary tracts. *In* Kirk, R. W. (ed.): *Current Veterinary Therapy VII.* W. B. Saunders, Philadelphia, 1980. pp. 1203–1212).

TABLE 183–4.   Age and Sex of 10 Dogs with Malignant Lymphoma Involving the Kidneys*

Age (Years)			Sex		
Mean	Range	Not Determined	Male	Female	Not Determined
5.5	6 mo–15 yr	1	3	5	2

*Data from the University of Minnesota Veterinary Teaching Hospital, the Veterinary Medical Data Program sponsored by the National Cancer Institute, and the literature.[47]

(Reproduced with permission from Caywood, D. D., Osborne, C. A., and Johnston, G. R.: Neoplasms of the canine and feline urinary tracts. *In* Kirk, R. W. (ed.): *Current Veterinary Therapy VII.* W. B. Saunders, Philadelphia, 1980. pp. 1203–1212).

Polysystemic signs unrelated to the urinary tract are common and may be the first clinical manifestation of renal carcinomas.[9,48] Anemia, pyrexia, anorexia, and weight loss have commonly been reported.[8,9,26,45,48,74] Polysystemic clinical signs may be related to production of excessive quantities of erythrocyte-stimulating factor, renin, parathormone, prostaglandins, and other hormones by these neoplasms.[7,34,64] Polycythemia has been observed in dogs and cats with renal adenomas and adenocarcinomas that elaborated excessive quantities of erythrocyte-stimulating factor.[7,34,64] Clinical signs may be caused by metastatic lesions and on occasion may be the first evidence of their presence.

Renal carcinomas spread by direct extension through the renal capsule or renal pelvis and by invasion of intrarenal veins and lymphatics.[9,34,43,48,60] Invasion and growth of renal carcinomas into renal veins can occur and may account for the high incidence of lung metastases (Fig. 183–5).[9,34,43,48,60] Invasion of the renal vein is less common in dogs than in humans.[9,43,48] The most common sites of metastases in dogs and cats are the lungs, lymph nodes, liver, brain, and bone.[9,43,48] Any tissue may be affected, and metastases to unusual sites are common. Many dogs have metastatic lesions when renal carcinoma is diagnosed.[9,42,43,44,45,48,74] Metastasis may occur prior to the onset of urinary signs.

Clinical signs associated with nephroblastomas are similar to those associated with renal cell carcinomas. Hypertrophic osteoarthropathy has been observed in dogs with renal tumors.[6,10] In one case, characteristic bony lesions of this syndrome developed in the absence of detectable pulmonary metastases.[10]

Embryonal nephromas are usually unilateral; however, bilateral involvement is reported.[9,16] If the tumor penetrates the renal capsule, local invasion of perinephric fat, posterior abdominal muscles, the diaphragm, and neighboring organs may occur.[1,36,37,38] Distant metastases occur via the lymphatics into pararenal and para-aortic lymph nodes or, more commonly, by venous metastasis from the renal vein into the vena cava. The most common site of metastasis is the lung, followed by the liver, mesentery, and lymph nodes.[9,10,15,22,25,33,38,58]

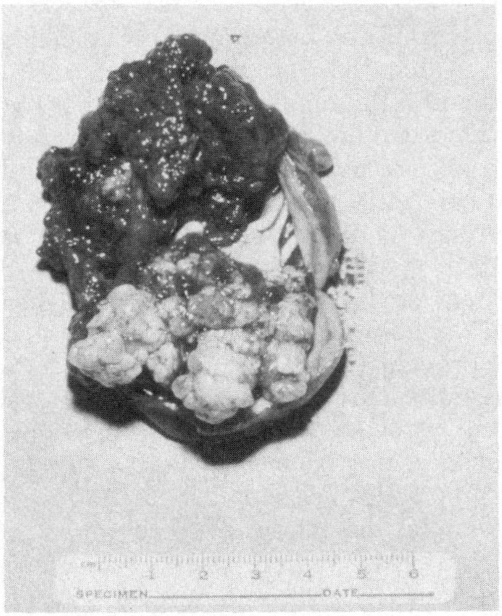

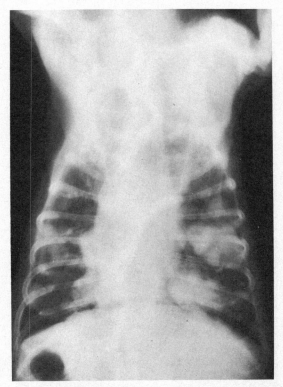

Figure 183–4. Transitional epithelial polyps of the renal pelvis in a nine-year-old male schnauzer.

Figure 183–5. Pulmonary metastases observed on radiographic examination of the dog in Figure 183–2.

In cats, the abdominal form of malignant lymphoma is usually associated with extensive renal involvement. Both kidneys are usually affected and may be palpated as enlarged asymmetrical structures in the abdominal cavity.[9,47,71] Renal failure caused by bilateral renal lymphoma occurs more commonly in cats than in dogs.[47] Nonspecific clinical signs include progressive weight loss, depression, anorexia, vomiting, and diarrhea. Cachexia, fever, anemia, and secondary infections occur during terminal phases.[9,47,71]

Diagnosis

Intravenous urography often helps to localize the site of neoplasia and may permit estimation of the extent of renal parenchymal involvement. Distortion in the shape of the renal pelvis and diverticula and retention of contrast medium are generally seen in the neoplastic kidney (Fig. 183–6).[47] Lack of excretion of detectable quantities of radiopaque contrast material suggests severe hydronephrosis. Selective angiography may also be performed to delineate the precise location and extent of renal destruction (Fig. 183–7). Renal neoplasms associated with enlargement of the kidneys must be differentiated from hydronephrosis and polycystic disease.[9,48]

A definitive antemortem diagnosis may be established by microscopic identification of neoplastic cells. This may be accomplished by biopsy of the kidney or detection of neoplastic cells in urine sediment. Needle biopsy of a unilateral renal neoplasm may be inadvisable if treatment by surgical extirpa-

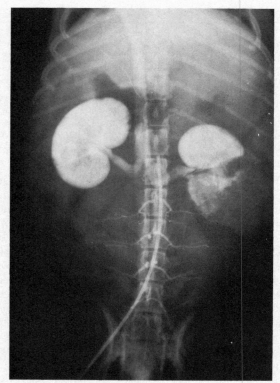

Figure 183–7. Selective angiogram of the kidneys of the dog in Figure 183–1. Note the lack of filling of the distal pole in the left kidney.

tion is contemplated, since the potential for iatrogenic metastasis exists.[9,48] An exploratory celiotomy is advised in such cases because a biopsy may be obtained with less risk of metastasis, the abdomen may be explored for metastases, and nephrectomy can be performed for treatment.

Treatment

Therapy should be based on clinical staging of the neoplasm (Table 183–5).[73] If the tumor has not metastasized and if the opposite kidney is not neoplastic and has adequate function, nephrectomy and partial ureterectomy are indicated. Preoperative abdominal palpation should be restricted to prevent rupture of the tumor and seeding of the abdomen with neoplastic cells.[9,38,58,60] Adequate surgical exposure, careful manipulation of the affected kidney, and ligation of the renal vein are advised prior to mobilizing the tumor to prevent release of neoplastic cells into the blood stream. In addition to complete removal of the tumor, the associated ureter should be removed, since metastasis may occur anywhere along its length. If the lymph nodes are enlarged and appear abnormal, systematic dissection and excision of regional lymph nodes is advised to prevent incomplete removal of tumor cells within lymphatics.[9,38,58,60] There is no information in the veterinary literature on the use of x-ray or chemotherapeutic agents in the treatment of renal cell carcinomas, primary renal tumors

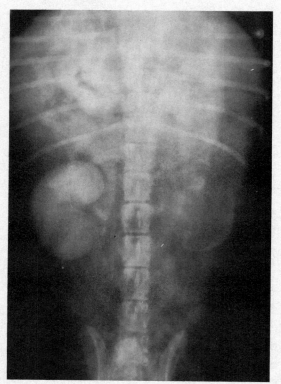

Figure 183–6. Intravenous urogram of the dog in Figure 183–4. Note the thin rim of cortical tissue opacified on the left kidney.

TABLE 183–5. WHO Clinical Stages of Canine Tumors of the Kidney[72]

T: Primary Tumor
T0 No evidence of tumor
T1 Small tumor without deformation of the kidney
T2 Solitary tumor with deformation and/or enlargement of the kidney
T3 Tumor invading perinephric structures (peritoneum) and/or pelvis, ureter, and/or renal blood vessels (renal vein)
T4 Tumor invading neighboring structures

N: Regional Lymph Nodes (RLN) (lumbar LN)
N0 No RLN involved
N1 Ipsilateral RLN involved
N2 Bilateral RLN involved
N3 Other LN involved (abdominal and pelvic LN)

M: Distant Metastasis
M0 No evidence of metastasis
M1 Distant metastasis—specify sites
M1a Single metastasis
M1b Multiple metastases in one organ
M1c Multiple metastases in various organs

arising from the urothelium, or sarcomas. Clinical and experimental studies in humans suggest limited success.[6,59]

Chemotherapy has been very effective in the management of embryonal nephroma in humans. Actinomycin D has prevented metastasis.[20,21,22,24,31,63] In addition to laboratory evidence for direct tumoricidal effect, this drug is also a radiosensitizer that augments the effect of radiation on embryonal nephromas.[31,33,60] The drug acts by binding the guanine moiety of deoxyribonucleic acid, preventing the formation of ribonucleic acid polymerase. As a result of suppressed ribonucleic acid and protein synthesis, cell damage occurs.[24,33] Repeated doses of actinomycin D are much more effective than a single dose in preventing relapse of metastatic disease.[20,21,22,24,31,63] Unfortunately, actinomycin D has many toxic side effects, including depression of immune response and ulceration of the alimentary tract. Serial monitoring of packed cell volume, white blood cell count, and platelet count are recommended during therapy to evaluate toxicity.[24,58,60] Vincristine is a chemotherapeutic agent that has been used with success in the treatment of nephroblastomas in humans. It is much less toxic than actinomycin D and has a synergistic effect when combined with it.[24,33,58,60] Its use in combined therapy may greatly decrease the risks of toxic side effects of actinomycin D.

The use of radiotherapy for nephroblastoma has been limited in veterinary medicine but has significantly improved survival times in humans.[15,58,60] It is probable that cancer cells dislodged during surgery or left behind because of incomplete excision are destroyed by x-ray.[15,58,60] Radiotherapy should be initiated shortly after surgery or administered intraoperatively by single-dose external beam megavoltage or brachytherapy implants.

A unilateral nephroblastoma with metastases was successfully controlled in a 1-year-old female mixed-breed dog by surgical extirpation of the right kidney, local irradiation of tissue adjacent to the right kidney, and periodic administration of actinomycin D (0.015 mg/kg daily for 5 days).[10] Combination therapy, incorporating principles of surgical management, radiotherapy, and chemotherapy, has been extremely effective in management of embryonal nephromas in humans. Cure rates of 70 to 80 per cent have been reported, even in patients with metastatic disease.[21,24,33,58,60]

Prognosis

The prognosis depends on the type, location, and extent of neoplastic involvement, the presence or absence of metastases, and the biological behavior of the neoplasm. A guarded to good prognosis is justified following complete surgical extirpation of a unilateral malignant neoplasm. Unfortunately, early diagnosis is not the rule and metastasis is often present, particularly with parenchymal tumors. In cases in which there is bilateral renal involvement or metastases or in which treatment is not provided, a guarded to poor prognosis should be offered.

NEOPLASMS OF THE URETER

Primary neoplasms of the canine ureter are rare (Table 183-6).[4,9,27,41,48] A good prognosis is associated

TABLE 183–6. Type, Age, and Sex of 5 Dogs with Primary Ureteral Neoplasms*

Tumor Type	No. of Cases	Sex		Age (Years)	
		Male	Female	Mean	Range
Epithelial tissue					
Papilloma	1	1	0	2.0	2
Transitional cell carcinoma	3	0	3	10.6	8–15
Muscle tissue					
Leiomyoma	1	0	1	11.0	11
TOTAL	5	1	4	7.8	2–15

*Data from the University of Minnesota Veterinary Teaching Hospital, the Veterinary Medical Data Program sponsored by the National Cancer Institute, and the literature.[4,41]

(Reproduced with permission from Caywood, D. D., Osborne, C. A., and Johnston, G. R.: Neoplasms of the canine feline urinary tracts. In Kirk, R. W. (ed.): Current Veterinary Therapy VII. W. B. Saunders, Philadelphia, 1980. pp. 1203–1212).

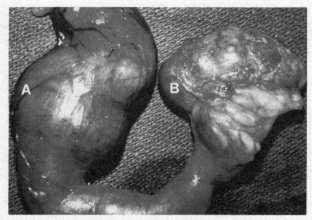

Figure 183–8. Leiomyoma of the ureter of a 11-year-old female mixed breed dog. Note the size of the neoplastic ureter (A) as compared with the kidney (B). (Courtesy of Dr. William Liska.)

with nephroureterectomy of benign and malignant neoplasms confined to the ureter (Fig. 183–8).[4,27,41] Clinical signs are usually associated with hydronephrosis.[4,9,27,41,48] Neoplasms originating from abdominal organs or tissues may encroach on ureters, occlude their lumina, and cause hydronephrosis. Occlusion of the distal ends of ureters by bladder neoplasia invading the trigone is the most common cause of neoplastic involvement of the ureters.[9,48] Primary neoplasms of the ureter have not been reported in cats.

NEOPLASMS OF THE BLADDER

Incidence

Benign and malignant neoplasms of the epithelial lining of the urinary bladder are more common than epithelial neoplasms of the renal pelves, ureters, and urethra.[9,29,46,52,66] The higher incidence of primary epithelial neoplasms in the urinary bladder may be associated with storage of urine, which may enhance the action of carcinogenic agents by allowing increased contact time with tissue.[61] Neoplasms of the urinary bladder are less common in cats than in dogs (Tables 183–7 and 183–8),[9,46] possibly because of a difference in metabolism of potentially carcinogenic agents, including tryptophan.[9,26,46]

Unlike those in humans, canine and feline epithelial neoplasms of the bladder are more common in females.[9,29,46] In all species studied, most epithelial and connective tissue tumors of the bladder were associated with advancing age.[9,29,36,55,65,68] An exception is rhabdomyosarcoma of the urinary bladder. This neoplasm is typically encountered in young dogs and has not been reported in cats.

Papillomas of the canine and feline urinary bladder have been encountered less frequently than carcinomas of the urinary bladder (Fig. 183–9). Although papillomas may occur at any age, they are more common in older dogs.[9,29,46] The biological behavior of naturally occurring papillomas in dogs and cats is

TABLE 183–7. Type, Age, and Sex of 297 Dogs with Primary Neoplasms of Urinary Bladder*

Tumor Type	No. of Cases	Sex Male	Sex Female	Sex Not Determined	Age (years) Mean	Age (years) Range	Age (years) Not Determined
Epithelial tissue							
Papilloma	7	0	3	4	11.1	10–12.5	3
Fibroadenoma	1	0	—	—	10.0	10	—
Adenocarcinoma	15	9	6	—	10.0	2–15	—
Squamous cell carcinoma	19	10	8	1	9.9	5–15	—
Transitional cell carcinoma	143	60	81	2	10.2	2–15	—
Unclassified carcinoma	42	8	13	21	8.9	4–13	15
Muscle tissue							
Leiomyoma	12	1	2	9	12.7	12–13	7
Leiomyosarcoma	12	4	8	—	6.7	2–13	1
Botryoid rhabdomyosarcoma	11	3	5	3	1.7	1–5	4
Connective tissue							
Fibroma	12	0	2	10	7.0	4–11	7
Fibrosarcoma	8	4	3	1	6.3	1–15	1
Unclassified sarcoma	7	3	2	2	3.6	1–5	—
Vascular tissue							
Hemangioma	2	1	0	1	10.0	10	1
Hemangiosarcoma	6	5	1	—	9.3	2–15	—
TOTAL	297	109	134	54	8.3	1–15	40

*Data from the University of Minnesota Veterinary Teaching Hospital, the Veterinary Medical Data Program sponsored by the National Cancer Institute, and the literature.[23,29,36,46,49,52,55,65,66,68]

(Reproduced with permission from Caywood, D. D., Osborne, C. A., and Johnston, G. R.: Neoplasms of the canine and feline urinary tracts. In Kirk, R. W. (ed.): *Current Veterinary Therapy VII.* W. B. Saunders, Philadelphia, 1980. pp. 1203–1212).

TABLE 183–8.   Type, Age, and Sex of 24 Cats with Primary Neoplasms of the Urinary Bladder*

Tumor Type	No. of Cases	Sex			Age (Years)		
		Male	Female	Not Determined	Mean	Range	Not Determined
Epithelial tissue							
Papilloma	2	—	1	1	1.2	0.33–2	—
Cystadenoma	1	—	1	—	12.0	12	—
Transitional cell carcinoma	10	1	6	3	10.6	3–15	1
Squamous cell carcinoma	1	—	—	1	—	—	1
Adenocarcinoma	1	—	—	1	—	—	1
Unclassified carcinoma	5	3	—	2	13.3	13–14	2
Connective tissue							
Myxosarcoma	1	1	—	—	6.0	6	—
Muscular tissue							
Leiomyoma	1	—	1	—	12.0	12	—
Leiomyosarcoma	2	—	2	—	9.8	8.5–11	—
TOTAL	24	5	11	8	9.3	0.33–15	5

*Data from the University of Minnesota Veterinary Teaching Hospital, the Veterinary Medical Data Program sponsored by the National Cancer Institute, and the literature.[12,18,32,46,49,53]

(Reproduced with permission from Caywood, D. D., Osborne, C. A., and Johnston, G. R.: Neoplasms of the canine and feline urinary tracts. *In* Kirk, R. W. (ed.): *Current Veterinary Therapy VII*. W. B. Saunders, Philadelphia, 1980. pp. 1203–1212).

unknown, although they have been removed from patients without recurrence. The size of papillomas is variable (microscopic to several centimeters); they may be single or multiple. As papillomas enlarge they become ulcerated. Ulceration, which frequently is aggravated by bacterial infection, is commonly associated with persistent hematuria.[35]

Fibromas and leiomyomas may be single or multiple. They often grow slowly and therefore are usually asymptomatic.[48] Larger tumors may protrude into the lumen of the urinary bladder but usually do not produce clinical signs until they become large enough to cause mechanical interference with micturition.

Carcinomas are the most common primary malignant tumors of the urinary bladder in dogs and cats. Although transitional cell carcinomas have been observed most frequently, squamous cell carcinomas, adenocarcinomas, and undifferentiated carcinomas may arise from bladder epithelium.[9,29,46,52,66]

Carcinomas may occur as solitary or multiple papillary projections that involve the bladder mucosa or as local or diffuse swellings of the bladder wall, or both. The nonpapillary variety occurs most frequently in dogs (Fig. 183–10).[9,49] Invasion of the bladder wall is common, especially with nonpapillary varieties. The mucosa and underlying muscle layers may be completely destroyed and replaced with neoplastic cells.[9,49] Neoplastic tissue may occlude the urethra or ureters (or both) and cause hydronephrosis.[39] Metastases occur frequently and most commonly involve the lungs and lymph nodes, but other locations are not uncommon.[9,24,48,49]

Sarcomas are much less common than carcinomas, but when present are usually characterized by diffuse

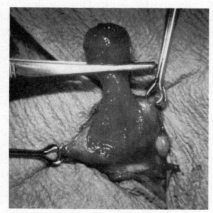

Figure 183–9. Papilloma of the urinary bladder of a ten-year-old female German short-haired pointer with a chronic urinary tract infection.

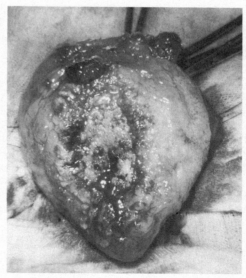

Figure 183–10. Squamous cell carcinoma of the urinary bladder of a six-year-old German shepherd dog. Note the invasive nonpapillary appearance of the neoplasm.

invasive growth into the bladder wall and metastases.[9,48,49]

Metastatic tumors of the urinary bladder are uncommon and are not usually associated with clinical signs.

Clinical Signs

Urinary tract signs of benign or malignant epithelial or connective tissue bladder neoplasms are similar. Intermittent hematuria is frequently observed. Owners often indicate that a wide variety of medications have been used without success to treat hematuria. Increased frequency of urination, a less common complaint, occurs as a result of associated cystitis or reduction in bladder capacity, or both, because of the large size of the neoplasm. Urinary incontinence may be observed and may be caused by partial obstruction of urine outflow (so-called paradoxical incontinence) or destruction of the detrusor muscle. Anorexia and depression are less common complaints.[9,48,49]

Early and potentially curable neoplasms usually do not produce abnormalities detectable by physical examination alone. Later, after tumor growth, clinical signs are similar to those of cystitis. Cystitis is a frequent complication of bladder neoplasia because bacteria readily invade the necrotic and ulcerated surface of neoplasms and stimulate an inflammatory response. Partial or complete obstruction of the urethra may cause dysuria, urinary incontinence, a decrease in the size of the urine stream, overdistension of the bladder with urine, hydronephrosis, signs referable to renal failure, or a combination of these. Obstruction of the ureters at the bladder trigone may also cause signs referable to obstructive uropathy.[9,48,49]

Signs referable to metastatic lesions may occur but are uncommon until advanced stages of neoplasia. Hypertrophic pulmonary osteoarthropathy has been observed in several dogs with malignant bladder neoplasia (Fig. 183–11).[9,36,48,55,65,68]

Diagnosis

Urinalysis may be of value when investigating possible neoplastic diseases of the urinary bladder. Renal function tests are normal unless there is obstruction of urine flow from both kidneys. Urinalysis may indicate cystitis (e.g., proteinuria, hematuria, pyuria, and bacteriuria). In uninfected or treated patients, red blood cells may dominate the microscopic findings in urine sediment. Neoplastic cells may also be found in urine sediment, especially in patients that have carcinoma.[9,48,49]

Evaluation of the morphology of various types of cells (especially transitional epithelial cells) in urine sediment is of proven value in the investigation of neoplastic diseases of the bladder. A diagnosis of

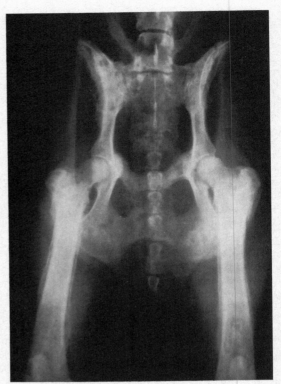

Figure 183–11. Hypertrophic osteopathy of the pelvis and femurs of a two-year-old doberman pinscher with a rhabdomyosarcoma of the urinary bladder.

neoplasia following examination of cytological preparations is based on multiple criteria, including abnormal changes in the nuclei and cytoplasm of individual cells and modification of normal intercellular architecture. Recognition of benign or well-differentiated malignant neoplasms on the basis of cytological preparations may be difficult, since exfoliated cells may differ little from hyperplastic or normal transitional epithelial cells.[9,48,49] Regardless of the type and degree of differentiation of the underlying neoplasm, secondary bacterial infection of neoplastic lesions may result in collection of samples that are composed primarily of inflammatory cells and that contain relatively few neoplastic cells. Thus, a negative result does not rule out neoplasia. Because of difficulties sometimes encountered in evaluating the significance of biopsy findings, results should always be interpreted in association with other clinical, laboratory, and radiographic findings.

Bladder neoplasms are sometimes difficult to demonstrate radiographically, especially if they are diffuse. Radiographic findings are not pathognomonic, as they may be the same as those associated with chronic cystitis. Neoplasms that protrude into the lumen of the bladder may be seen as space-occupying masses. Pneumocystography, positive-contrast cystography, or double-contrast cystography may be used to enhance detection of such masses (Fig. 183–12).[9,48,49]

A definitive diagnosis of bladder neoplasia is based on microscopic detection and evaluation of neoplastic

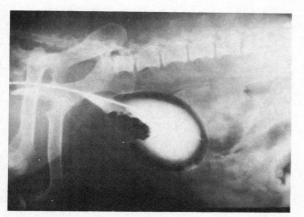

Figure 183–12. Double contrast cystogram of a 12-year-old female beagle with a transitional cell carcinoma of the urinary bladder. Note the papillary mass projecting into the lumen from the ventral wall of the bladder.

TABLE 183–9. WHO Clinical Stages of Canine Tumors of the Urinary Bladder[72]

T: Primary Tumor
  T1s Carcinoma *in situ*
  T0 No evidence of primary tumor
  T1 Superficial papillary tumor
  T2 Tumor invading the bladder wall, with induration
  T3 Tumor invading neighboring organs (prostate, uterus, vagina, anal canal)
The symbol m added to the appropriate T category indicates multiple tumors
N: Regional Lymph Nodes (RLN) (internal and external iliac LN)
  N0 No RLN involved
  N1 RLN involved
  N2 RLN and justa RLN involved
M: Distant Metastasis
  M0 No evidence of metastasis
  M1 Distant metastasis present—specify sites

cells in urine sediment or in biopsy samples obtained via catheter biopsy, cystoscopy, or exploratory celiotomy.[9,48,49] Even when the bladder is examined visually at surgery, differentiation between diffuse neoplasia and cystitis may be difficult because the tissue may be necrotic, inflamed, ulcerated, and thickened in either condition. In such circumstances the lesions should be biopsied, preferably by complete excision, so that a histopathological diagnosis can be established. When excision biopsy is impossible, multiple specimens should be obtained from large solitary lesions, or several lesions should be sampled if many smaller growths are present. The internal iliac and lumbar lymph nodes are examined and, if necessary, biopsied at celiotomy to confirm or rule out metastasis.

Treatment

Therapeutic results are related to the type of tumor, location, and presence of metastasis. Therapy of bladder neoplasms may be curative or palliative and should be based on clinical staging (Table 183–9).[73] Untreated, the majority of animals with malignant bladder neoplasms succumb from the disease. Current methods available to treat bladder neoplasia include surgery, x-ray, and chemotherapy.[9,48,49]

Neoplasms located in accessible areas of the bladder should be removed by partial cystectomy. The neoplastic tissue and a wide zone of healthy tissue, including the entire depth of the bladder wall, are removed. Ureteral transplantation may be necessary. Tumors that occupy the neck of the bladder, the trigone, or a great portion of the bladder surface and wall cannot be removed by partial cystectomy. Several methods of urinary diversion have been used following cystectomy in dogs, including ureteral or trigonal-colonic anastomosis, ureteroileostomy, and gastrocystoplasty.[5,9,14,48,49] Abnormal defecation, azotemia, and pyelonephritis are frequent complications. Gastrocystoplasty involves formation of a substitute bladder from a gastric pouch. The ureters are transplanted into the pouch, and a reversed ileal segment is attached to the pouch and exteriorized in the abdominal flank. The bladder is emptied by catheterization.[14] Postoperative complications and loss of normal function make such approaches impractical for most household pets.

Adjunctive radiotherapy may be of benefit after partial cystectomy of malignant neoplasms of the bladder. X-ray may destroy neoplastic tissue not removed by surgery and may also be of value in cases in which total excision is impossible. External beam megavoltage x-ray is generally not advocated because of excessive scatter radiation. Many veterinary institutions are evaluating intraoperative single-dose x-ray at the surgery site. The initial results are encouraging. Brachytherapy techniques may also be used with surgical excision.[9,14,48]

Apparent growth arrest and partial relief of signs have been obtained by incorporating intravesicular triethylene thiophosphoramide or 5-fluorouracil and systemic administration of doxorubicin, cyclophosphamide, and/or 5-fluorouracil.[14] It is usually necessary to treat the patient for cystitis after surgery. Because of the possibility of postoperative recurrence of the neoplasm, periodic examination of the patient, including radiography and examination of the urine sediment for neoplastic cells, is recommended.

Prognosis

Some indication of prognosis may be given to the owner based on clinical staging of the neoplasm. The location, extent, histological appearance, and depth of penetration are important factors to be considered when establishing a prognosis. The site of the neoplasm is often as closely related to the future course of events as is the histopathological type. In cases in which complete surgical extirpation of solitary non-infiltrating benign tumors has been performed, a fair

TABLE 183–10.   Type, Age, and Sex of 43 Dogs with Primary Neoplasms of the Urethra*

Tumor Type	No. of Cases	Sex			Age (Years)		
		Male	Female	Not Determined	Mean	Range	Not Determined
Epithelial tissue							
Adenoma	4	—	—	4	—	—	4
Adenosarcoma	4	1	2	1	10.6	6–14	1
Squamous cell carcinoma	13	0	13	—	11.0	8–13	—
Transitional cell carcinoma	17	2	15	—	10.5	6 mo–15 yr	1
Unclassified carcinoma	1	0	1	—	15.0	15	—
Connective tissue							
Myxosarcoma	1	0	1	—	9.0	9	—
Muscle tissue							
Rhabdomyosarcoma	1	1	0	—	3.0	3	—
Vascular tissue							
Hemangiosarcoma	2	0	2	—	9.5	9–10	—
TOTAL	43	4	34	5	9.8	6 mo–15 yr	6

*Data from the University of Minnesota Veterinary Teaching Hospital, the Veterinary Medical Data Program sponsored by the National Cancer Institute, and the literature.[32,67,69,72]

(Reproduced with permission from Caywood, D. D., Osborne, C. A., and Johnston, G. R.: Neoplasms of the canine and feline urinary tracts. *In* Kirk, R. W. (ed.): *Current Veterinary Therapy VII.* W. B. Saunders, Philadelphia, 1980. pp. 1203–1212).

to good prognosis is justified. In cases in which malignant neoplasms have been surgically removed, a guarded to fair prognosis should be offered because of the tendency of these tumors to recur and metastasize. In general, tumors that have penetrated the mucosa are more likely to recur and become metastatic than are noninvasive neoplasms. In cases in which no treatment is given or in which the neoplasm has metastasized, a guarded to poor prognosis should be offered. The poor results generally reported in the treatment of urinary bladder neoplasms of dogs and cats are partially related to the fact that the initial diagnosis is usually not established until the condition is inoperable.

NEOPLASMS OF THE URETHRA

Incidence

Primary neoplasms of the urethra are uncommon in dogs and rare in cats.[9,43,72] Canine urethral neoplasms have been observed predominantly in females, and there is increased risk associated with increased age (Table 183–10). Although unproved, it has been suggested that these neoplasms may arise from hyperplastic tissue resulting from irritation associated with chronic urethritis.[9,67,72] Epithelial tumors are the most common and include squamous cell carcinomas (Fig. 183–13), transitional cell carcinomas, and adenocarcinomas.[9,32,72] Other tumor types have rarely been observed. Metastasis to regional lymph nodes has been observed frequently at necropsy. A nonmetastatic transitional cell carcinoma has been reported in the urethra of a 6-year-old male domestic short-hair cat.[71]

Clinical Signs

Dysuria is a constant sign and presumably occurs as a result of obstruction of the urethral lumen and irritation of the urethral mucosa.[2,9,48,67,72] Hematuria is a common but variable sign, and blood may be passed independently of micturition. Urinary incontinence may develop as a result of damage to the urethral sphincter mechanism or partial obstruction of urine outflow (so-called paradoxical incontinence).[9,48] If urethral obstruction is severe or prolonged, varying degrees of postrenal azotemia or hydronephrosis may develop. In the latter instance, a distended, turgid urinary bladder may be detected by abdominal palpation. If the neoplasm is extensive, rectal palpation may reveal thickening and irregularity of the urethra.[9,48]

Diagnosis

Localization of urethral neoplasms may be aided by palpation, catheterization, retrograde contrast ure-

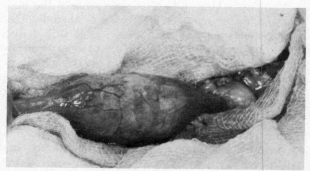

Figure 183–13. Squamous cell carcinoma of the urethra of an 11-year-old female spayed collie mixed breed dog.

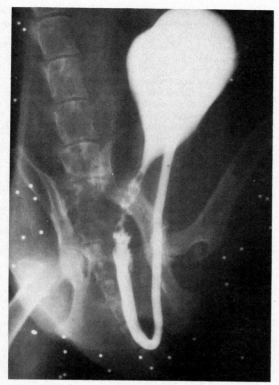

Figure 183–14. Retrograde urethrogram of the dog in Figure 183–13.

thrography, cystoscopy, or exploratory surgery.[9,48,69] Inability to pass the catheter through the urethral lumen or abnormal resistance during insertion of the catheter may be detected. Retrograde catheterization is extremely valuable in tumor localization (Fig. 183–14).[69] Biopsy of mucosal neoplasms may be obtained with a urinary catheter.

Treatment

Therapy is usually limited to excision of operable lesions. Antipubic urethrostomy may be used as a salvage procedure when adequate normal urethra can be maintained proximal to the neoplasm. Trigonal-colonic anastomosis or ureterocolonic anastomosis must be used when the proximal urethra is involved.[5] Single-dose external beam megavoltage x-ray or brachytherapy at surgery may be used in conjunction with surgical excision. Chemotherapeutic measures are unproven in dogs and cats. In humans, systemic administration of doxorubicin, cyclophosphamide, or 5-flurouracil has been used with similar success as in bladder neoplasms.[60]

Prognosis

A fair to guarded prognosis is justified with malignant neoplasms that are localized and surgically removed. Common complications associated with uri-

nary salvage procedures include stricture formation, abnormal defecation, azotemia, and pyelonephritis. In cases in which the neoplasm has metastasized, a guarded to poor prognosis is indicated.

1. Balsaver, A. M., Gibley, C. W., and Tessurer, C. F.: Ultrastructural studies in Wilms' tumors. Cancer 22:417, 1968.
2. Barrett, R. E., and Nobel, A. T.: Transitional cell carcinoma of the urethra in a cat. Cornell Vet. 66:14, 1976.
3. Baskin, G. B., and DePaoli, A.: Primary renal neoplasms of the dog. Vet. Pathol. 14:591, 1977.
4. Berzon, J. L.: Primary leiomyosarcoma of the ureter of a dog. J. Am. Vet. Med. Assoc. 175:374, 1979.
5. Bovee, K. C., Pass, M. A., Wardley, R., et al: Trigonal-colonic anastomosis: A urinary diversion procedure in dogs. J. Am. Vet. Med. Assoc. 174:184, 1979.
6. Brody, R. S., and Craig, P. H.: Hypertrophic osteoarthropathy in a dog with pulmonary metastases arising from a renal adenocarcinoma. J. Am. Vet. Med. Assoc. 132:231, 1958.
7. Brown, N. O.: Paraneoplastic syndromes of humans, dogs, and cats. J. Am. Anim. Hosp. Assoc. 17:911, 1981.
8. Burger, G. T., et al: Renal carcinoma in a dog. J. Am. Vet. Med. Assoc. 171:282, 1977.
9. Caywood, D. D., Osborne, C. A., and Johnston, G. R.: Neoplasms of the canine and feline urinary tract. In Kirk, R. W. (ed.): Current Veterinary Therapy VII. W. B. Saunders, Philadelphia, 1980. pp. 1203–1212.
10. Caywood, D. D., Osborne, C. A., Stevens, J. B., et al.: Hypertrophic osteoarthropathy associated with an atypical nephroblastoma in a dog. J. Am. Anim. Hosp. Assoc. 16:855, 1980.
11. Cope, V., Hackett, M. B., and Raphael, M. J.: Some observations on the value of excretion urography in the detection of renal tumors. Br. J. Urol. 37:691, 1965.
12. Cotchin, E.: Neoplasia in the cat. Vet. Rec. 69:425, 1957.
13. Crow, S. E., Bell, T. G., and Wortman, J. A.: Hematuria associated with renal hemangiosarcoma in a dog. J. Am. Vet. Med. Assoc. 176:531, 1980.
14. Crow, S. E., and Klausner, J. K.: Management of transitional cell carcinomas of the urinary bladder. In Kirk, R. W. (ed.): Current Veterinary Therapy VIII. W. B. Saunders, Philadelphia, 1983.
15. D'Angio, G. J.: Radiation therapy in Wilms' tumor. J. Am. Med. Assoc. 204:124, 1968.
16. Drew, R. A., Done, S. H., and Robins, G. M.: Canine embryonal nephroma: A case report. J. Small Anim. Pract. 13:27, 1972.
17. Dunn, W. H.: Renal neoplasms of dogs. J. Am. Vet. Med. Assoc. 84:119, 1934.
18. Engle, G. C.: A retrospective study of 395 feline neoplasms. J. Am. Anim. Hosp. Assoc. 5:21, 1969.
19. Farah, J., and Lofstrom, J. E.: Angiography of Wilms' tumor. Radiology 90:775, 1968.
20. Farber, S., D'Angio, G., Evans, A., and Metus, A.: Clinical studies of actinomycin D with special reference to Wilms' tumor in children. Ann. N.Y. Acad. Sci. 89:421, 1960.
21. Fernback, D. J., and Martyn, D. T.: Role of dactinomycin in the improved survival of children with Wilms' tumor. J. Am. Med. Assoc. 195:1005, 1966.
22. Garrett, R. A., Donohue, J. I., and Arnold, T. L.: Metastatic renal embryoma: Survival following therapy. J. Urol. 98:444, 1967.
23. Geib, L. W., Billhorn, R. W., and Whitehead, J. E.: Transitional cell carcinoma of the urinary bladder in a dog with unusual clinical signs. J. Am. Anim. Hosp. Assoc. 3:22, 1967.
24. Greene, F. L., and Donaldson, M. H.: Chemotherapy of Wilms' tumor. New Physician 19:598, 1970.
25. Gross, R. E., and Neuhauser, E. B. P.: Treatment of mixed tumors of the kidney in childhood. Pediatrics 6:843, 1950.
26. Habermann, R. T., and Williams, F. P.: Papillary cystic adenocarcinoma of a kidney in a dog. J. Am. Vet. Med. Assoc. 142:1011, 1963.

27. Hanika, C., and Rebar, A. H.: Ureteral transitional cell carcinoma in the dog. Vet. Pathol. 17:643, 1980.

28. Hardy, W. D., Brodey, R. S., and Riser, W. H.: Osteosarcoma of the skull. J. Am. Vet. Rad. Soc. 8:5, 1967.

29. Hayes, H. M.: Canine bladder cancer: Epidemiology features. Am. J. Epidemiol. 104:673, 1976.

30. Hayes, H. M., and Fraumeni, J. F.: Canine renal neoplasm: Epidemiologic features. Cancer Res. 37:2553, 1977.

31. Howard, R.: Actinomycin D in Wilms' tumor: Treatment of lung metastases. Arch. Dis. Child. 40:200, 1965.

32. Jabara, A. G.: Three cases of primary malignant neoplasms arising in the canine urinary system. J. Comp. Pathol. 78:335, 1968.

33. James, D. H., Austu, O., Wren, E. L., and Johnston, W. W.: Childhood malignant tumors—Concurrent chemotherapy with dactinomycin and vincristine sulfate. J. Am. Med. Assoc. 197:1043, 1966.

34. Jay, C. L.: Embryonal nephroma in a dog. Southwestern Vet. 13:234, 1960.

35. Johnston, S. D., Osborne, C. A., and Stevens, J. B.: Canine polypoid cystitis. J. Am. Vet. Med. Assoc. 166:1155, 1975.

36. Kelly, D. F.: Rhabdomyosarcoma of the urinary bladdder in dogs. Vet. Pathol. 10:375, 1973.

37. Kiesel, G. K.: Carcinoma of the kidney of a cat. Cornell Vet. 40:380, 1950.

38. Ladd, W. E.: Embryoma of the kidney (Wilms' tumor). Ann. Surg. 108:885, 1938.

39. Lavingnette, A. M., and Kleine, L. J.: Obstructive uropathy due to a transitional cell carcinoma in a dog. J. Am. Anim. Hosp. Assoc. 3:54, 1967.

40. Lee, R., Weaver, A. D., and Robinson, P. B.: Persistent hematuria in a dog due to a discrete renal hemangioma. J. Small Anim. Pract. 15:621, 1974.

41. Liska, W. D., and Patnaik, A. K.: Leiomyoma of the ureter of a dog. J. Am. Anim. Hosp. Assoc. 13:83, 1977.

42. Lucke, V. M., and Kelley, D. F.: Renal carcinoma in the dog. Vet. Pathol. 13:264, 1976.

43. Moulton, J. R.: Tumors of the urinary system. In Moulton, J. E. (ed.): Tumors in Domestic Animals. 2nd ed. University of California Press Ltd., Berkeley, 1978. pp. 291–295.

44. Mulligan, R. M.: Comparative pathology of human and canine cancer. Ann. N. Y. Acad. Sci. 108:642, 1963.

45. Nielson, S. W., and Archibald, J.: Canine renal disorders. III. Renal carcinoma in three dogs. North Am. Vet. 36:36, 1955.

46. Osborne, C. A., Low, D. G., Perman, V., and Barnes, D. M.: Neoplasms of the canine and feline urinary bladder: Incidence, etiologic factors, occurrence and pathologic features. Am. J. Vet. Res. 29:2041, 1968.

47. Osborne, C. A., Johnson, K. H., Kurtz, H. J., and Hanlon, G. F.: Renal lymphoma in the dog and cat. J. Am. Vet. Med. Assoc. 158:2058, 1971.

48. Osborne, C. A., Low, D. G., and Finco, D. R.: Neoplasms of the kidney. In: Canine and Feline Urology. W. B. Saunders, Philadelphia, 1972. pp. 255–260.

49. Osborne, C. A., Low, D. G., and Perman, V.: Neoplasms of the canine and feline urinary bladder: Clinical findings, diagnosis and treatment. J. Am. Vet. Med. Assoc. 152:247, 1968.

50. Osborne, C. A., Quast, J. F., Barnes, D. M., and Vitz, C. R.: Feline renal pelvic carcinoma. J. Am. Vet. Med. Assoc. 159:1238, 1971.

51. Pamukiu, A. M.: Tumors of the urinary bladder. Bull. WHO 50:43, 1974.

52. Patnaik, A. K., Liu, S. K., Hurvitz, A. I., and McClellund, A. J.: Nonhematopoietic neoplasms in cats. J. Natl. Cancer Inst. 54:855, 1975.

53. Peterson, M. E.: Inappropriate erythropoietin production from a renal carcinoma in a dog with polycythemia. J. Am. Vet. Med. Assoc. 179:995, 1981.

54. Pletchner, J. M., and Dalton, L.: Botryoid rhabdomyosarcoma in the urinary bladder of a dog. Vet. Pathol. 18:695, 1981.

55. Plummer, P. J. G.: A survey of sixty tumours from domesticated animals. Can. J. Comp. Pathol. 15:231, 1951.

56. Puroket, B. L., and Sardeskpande, P. D.: Renal carcinoma in a cat. Indian Vet. J. 41:796, 1964.

57. Richardson, R. C.: Canine transmissible venereal tumor. Compend. Cont. Educ. 3:951, 1981.

58. Rickham, P. P.: Wilms' tumor. In Rob, C., and Smith, R. (eds.): Operative Surgery. 2nd ed. Butterworth and Co., Ltd., London, 1970. pp. 65–66.

59. Rickham, P. P.: Malignant tumors involving the genitourinary system. In Johnston, J. H. and Scholtmeyer, R. J. (eds.): Problems in Pediatric Urology. Excerpta Medica, Amsterdam, 1972. pp. 180–236.

60. Rippe, D. F., Ortiz-Muniz, G., Block, N. L., et al: Urinary bladder carcinogenesis in the dog: Preliminary studies on cellular immunity. Transplant. Proc. 7:495, 1975.

61. Sagartz, J. W., Ayers, K. M., Cushell, I. G., and Robinson, F. R.: Malignant embryonal nephroma in an aged dog. J. Am. Vet. Med. Assoc. 161:1658, 1972.

62. Schweisquth, O., and Schleinger, M. J.: Actinomycin D associated with irradiation in the treatment of Wilms' tumor. Ann. Radiol. 10:657, 1967.

63. Scott, R. C., and Patnaik, A. K.: Renal carcinoma with secondary polycythemia in the dog. J. Am. Anim. Hosp. Assoc. 8:275, 1972.

64. Stamps, P., and Harris, D. L.: Botryoid rhabdomyosarcoma of the urinary bladder of a dog. J. Am. Vet. Med. Assoc. 153:1064, 1968.

65. Strafuss, A. C., and Dean, M. J.: Neoplasms of the urinary bladder. J. Am. Vet. Med. Assoc. 166:1161, 1975.

66. Tarvin, G., Patnaik, A., and Greene, R.: Primary urethral tumors in dogs. J. Am. Vet. Med. Assoc. 172:931, 1978.

67. Teunissen, G. H. B., and Misdorp, W.: Rhabdomyosarcoma of the urinary bladder and fibromatosis of the extremities in a young dog. Zentralbl Veterinarmed 1:81, 1968.

68. Ticer, J. W., Spencer, C. P., and Ackerman, N.: Transitional cell carcinoma of the urethra in four female dogs: Its urethrographic appearance. Vet. Radiol. 21:12, 1980.

69. Weitz, W. L., and McClellan, R. B.: Embryonal nephroma in a dog. J. Am. Vet. Med. Assoc. 97:605, 1940.

70. Willson, J. E., and Gillmore, C. E.: Malignant lymphoma in a cat with involvement of the kidneys demonstrated radiographically. J. Am. Vet. Med. Assoc. 140:1068, 1962.

71. Wilson, G. P., Hayes, H. M., and Casey, H. W.: Canine urethral cancer. J. Am. Anim. Hosp. Assoc. 15:741, 1979.

72. World Health Organization: Internal report of the Second Consultation on the Biological Behaviour and Therapy of Tumours of Domestic Animals, Geneva, 1979 (unpublished WHO document VPH/CMO/79.17).

73. Yang, Y. H.: The multicentric renal adenocarcinomas in situ of a dog. Pathol. Microbiol. 29:181, 1966.

74. Zontinue, W. J.: Renal neoplasia and hematuria. Pulse 8:8, 1966.

184 Musculoskeletal System

J. W. Alexander and Clark S. Patton

INTRODUCTION

William Dock advised medical students that "the most important thing to remember about rare diseases is that they are rare." This statement applies to tumors of the canine musculoskeletal system. Benign and malignant musculoskeletal tumors can arise from each element of muscle and bone and, to varying degrees, recapitulate the histological and biological characteristics of the tissue of origin.[38] Approximately 98 per cent of these neoplasms are malignant,[8] and to arrive at a rapid and accurate diagnosis, the clinician must have a systematic diagnostic plan to follow. The most distressing aspect of musculoskeletal neoplasia is the prognosis. Osteosarcomas in particular have a high rate of metastasis. A dog with a musculoskeletal neoplasm usually has pain, altered function, or a palpable mass. Early diagnosis and treatment are mandatory if the dog is to have any chance for survival. Despite recent advances in chemotherapy and radiotherapy, tumors of the musculoskeletal system are best treated by surgical eradication, using basic principles enunciated many years ago.[29]

Dogs and cats are commonly affected by four primary malignant bone tumors—osteogenic sarcoma, chondrosarcoma, fibrosarcoma, and hemangiosarcoma. Although each of these has a benign counterpart, they are the exception rather than the rule.

TUMORS OF BONE

Osteoma

Biology. Osteomas are characterized by bony excrescences usually arising in intramembranous bones.[22] They are benign lesions in which a major component is mature, lamellar, or woven bone. Osteomas are rare lesions in dogs,[19,25] commonly arising on the inner and outer surfaces of the skull and mandible; however, they have been reported to affect the appendicular skeleton.[19] The lesions are relatively slow growing and are characteristically covered by periosteum.

Clinical Signs. Since osteomas may not be associated with clinical signs, their true prevalence in dogs is unknown. Most affected animals have a painless, slowly enlarging hard mass, which may have been present for a variable period of time. Animals younger than 3 years are most commonly affected. The tumor may be associated with a variety of clinical signs, depending on the location of the mass.

Diagnosis. Radiographic studies of the lesion reveal a solitary dense mass blending into the normal bone and protruding from the surface, while maintaining a distinct and regularly contoured border.[35] Osteomas are initially formed of cancellous bone, which becomes increasingly compact with time.[35] Definitive diagnosis is based on biopsy and histological examination.

Etiology. Long-term multigeneration studies in CF-1 strain of mice revealed the incidence of spontaneous osteomas to be approximately 10 per cent, with the skull being involved in about 90 per cent of the cases.[13] Osteomas in mice have also been induced by injection of the RFB osteoma virus of CF-1 mice.[16]

Treatment and Prognosis. Treatment of osteoma is surgical excision. Complete removal of the mass gives favorable results; however, the location of the lesion may make total excision impossible.

Osteogenic Sarcoma

Biology. Osteogenic sarcoma is a malignant tumor of bone in which the proliferating spindle-cell stroma directly produces osteoid or immature bone.[22] The term "osteogenic" has a double meaning, namely "derived from bone" and "producing bone." Osteogenic sarcomas are the most common tumors of the canine and feline skeleton, accounting for approximately 85 per cent of bone neoplasms.[8]

A number of systems have been proposed to classify these tumors; however, the classification systems are rarely of clinical significance. Osteogenic sarcomas are subclassified into many categories, the most common being sclerosing, osteolytic, subperiosteal, medullary, and telangiectatic.[1]

Incidence. Osteogenic sarcomas generally affect giant and large breeds of dogs, with males being affected slightly more often than females.[8] In the authors' experience the Great Dane, St. Bernard, Irish setter, and German shepherd are the breeds most often affected. The risk of osteogenic sarcoma in giant breeds (over 35 kg) varies from 61 to 185 times the risk in small breeds (under 10 kg).[41] In a study of 194 cases, the average age of affected dogs was 7.74 years, with a range of 1 to 15 years.[8] In this same study, an additional earlier age peak was noted at about 1.5 years of age.

Osteogenic sarcomas most commonly affect the appendicular skeleton, with the forelimbs being involved 1.6 to 1.8 times more often than the hind limbs.[8,44] The most common sites for osteosarcomas in dogs are the (1) distal radius and ulna, (2) proximal humerus, and (3) proximal and distal femur and tibia.

Approximately 24 per cent of canine osteogenic sarcomas are found in the axial skeleton, with about 50 per cent located in the head and 50 per cent in the ribs and vertebrae.[44] The boxer is most commonly affected by osteogenic sarcomas of the skull. Extraskeletal osteogenic sarcomas are rare.[2,5,31] Their biological behavior is similar to osteogenic sarcomas of bone. In cats they are most commonly seen in the metaphysis of the femur and tibia.

Clinical Signs. The earliest clinical sign of osteogenic sarcoma is usually pain. The resulting dysfunction (lameness) is insidious and transitory, eventually becoming persistent and severe. Shortly after the onset of pain, a palpable swelling arises, followed by visible enlargement of the affected site (Fig. 184–1).

Osteogenic sarcomas have a grave prognosis, and an early, correct diagnosis is imperative. This requires close cooperation between the clinician, radiologist, and pathologist.

Diagnosis. The initial identification of this neoplasm is made on the basis of a radiograph. All deep, firm swellings of the extremities should be x-rayed on initial presentation. Park suggests the following four areas be evaluated on radiographs of any suspected bony neoplasm: the bone margins, cortices, neoplastic matrix (new bone production), and the periosteal reaction.[33] The pattern of change on the initial radiographs depends on (1) the cell type, (2) the bone involved, (3) the degree of malignancy, and (4) the biological age of the tumor.[25] In the early stages of an osteogenic sarcoma, the most easily recognized change is cortical destruction, which is subtle at first, beginning with minimal thinning of the cortical shadow; however, as the neoplastic mass enlarges within the medullary cavity, this change progresses to complete cortical destruction (Figs. 184–2 and 184–3). The most suggestive radiographic change noticed in more than 70 per cent of the bone tumors in one series was marked cortical destruction

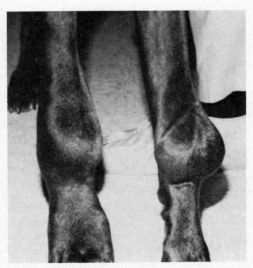

Figure 184–1. Great Dane with bilateral carpal enlargement caused by osteogenic sarcomas.

that progressed to the point of complete disappearance of the cortical shadow.[25]

The periosteal response does not depend on the degree of cortical destruction. In the early stages, an early periosteal response is at times associated with the tumor and resembles a "brush pattern." This early "brush pattern" often progresses to an elevation of the periosteum from the bone. Subperiosteal new bone blends with more normal appearing bone and forms a triangular mass of bone on the periphery of the tumor (Codman's triangle).[25]

The production of neoplastic new bone may be intra- or extramedullary. Neoplastic bone produced within the medullary cavity replaces normal trabecular bone with bone in either amorphous, snowflake-like, or sunburst patterns.[25] Extramedullary neoplastic bone production tends to extend into the soft tissues around the bone. Intra- and extramedullary neoplastic bone production is extremely suggestive of bone neoplasia (Figs. 184–2 and 184–3).[33]

Although the initial identification of a bone tumor is made on a radiograph, the definitive diagnosis is made by the histological examination of a representative excisional biopsy specimen. In selecting a biopsy site, the clinician must avoid collecting only reactive bone. Diagnostic tissue is usually confined to the medullary cavity, and it is important that the biopsy tool completely penetrate the cortex and enter the medullary cavity. The ideal site for biopsy is an area that includes both bone lysis and sclerosis.[25] The biopsy specimen is placed in 10 per cent neutral buffered formalin for fixation.

Typically, osteogenic sarcomas consist of plump, stellate cells producing a hyaline matrix (with hematoxylin and eosin stain) containing collagen fibrils (birefringent with polarized light) and nuclei entrapped in this matrix. The matrix is acidophilic unless mineral makes it basophilic and granular. Matrix can vary in amount from well-formed, wide trabeculae to thin, scalloped wisps between nuclei (Fig. 184–4).

Treatment and Prognosis. Despite recent advances in treatment of osteogenic sarcomas and other malignant bone tumors, these tumors are best managed by surgical excision. Prior to removal of the neoplasm or amputation of the affected limb, a chest x-ray should be obtained. Evidence of pulmonary metastasis has been found on the initial chest radiograph in fewer than 10 per cent of the cases.[25] However, this negative finding in no way rules out the possibility of neoplastic dissemination.

The most common treatment is limb amputation. The majority of affected dogs and cats can still walk satisfactorily, and amputation simply removes a painful and useless extremity. In a series involving 65 dogs with osteogenic sarcoma, there was no statistical correlation between the postsurgical survival time and the age, sex, or breed of the dog, the site of the neoplasm, or the duration of the presurgical clinical signs.[9] In this same study, the median postamputation survival time for dogs with an osteogenic sarcoma

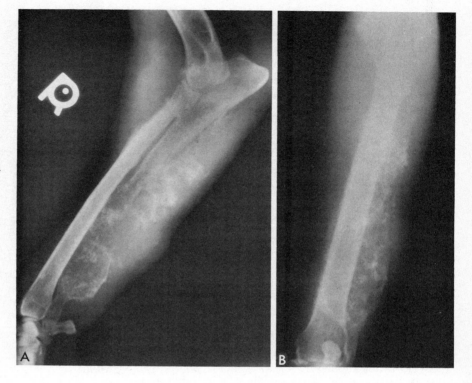

Figure 184–2. Lateral *(A)* and craniocaudal *(B)* radiographs of an adult St. Bernard with an osteogenic sarcoma of the right foreleg. There is complete cortical bone destruction as well as production of extramedullary neoplastic bone in adjacent soft tissues.

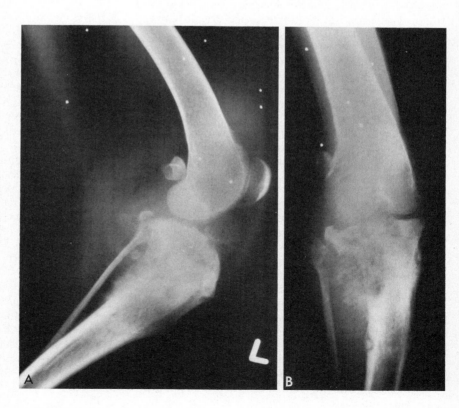

Figure 184–3. Lateral *(A)* and craniocaudal *(B)* radiographs of a dog with an osteogenic sarcoma of the proximal tibia. There is extensive cortical bone destruction, periosteal new bone formation, and extramedullary neoplastic bone in the adjacent soft tissues.

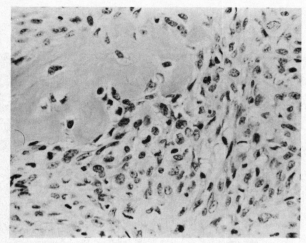

Figure 184–4. A medullary osteogenic sarcoma of the distal radius and ulna of a dog. Elongated and round nuclei separated by small amounts of cytoplasm merge with eosinophilic hyaline material containing single to multiple osteocytes. If calcified, the osteoid stains basophilic and granular. (Hematoxylin-eosin × 230.)

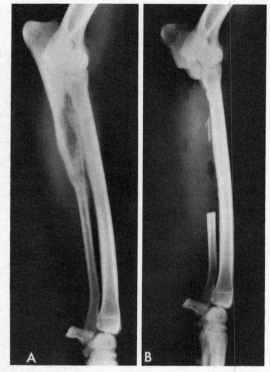

Figure 184–5. A, Lateral radiograph of a dog with an osteogenic sarcoma of the proximal ulna. B, The growth as located in a position on the bone allowing local excision with preservation of the limb.

was 18 weeks, with a range of 3 to 578 weeks. Twenty-six per cent of the dogs were alive 6 months postoperatively, 13.8 per cent were still alive at 9 months, and 10.7 per cent survived more than 1 year. These data indicate that although there is an extremely grave prognosis with this disease, the possibility of recovery is not hopeless.

With such a grave prognosis for a "cure" despite amputation, the alternative of surgical removal of the tumor with limb preservation is especially attractive. Unfortunately, this is possible in selected cases only (Fig. 184–5).

Etiology. One of the most fascinating and intriguing chapters in bone tumor research is the search for etiological factors in the pathogenesis of osteosarcoma. There are several reports of viral-induced tumors.[36] Although several types of RNA and DNA viruses cause bone tumors in experimental animals under specific laboratory conditions, only the FBJ mouse virus has been isolated from a spontaneous sarcoma.[17]

Nearly all radionuclides that localize in bone can produce bone neoplasia in the laboratory, and all mammals thus far tested with appropriate dosages of either internal or external radiation have developed osteogenic sarcomas. Exposure of the distal femur and proximal tibia of mice to 500 rads of x-radiation induces osteogenic sarcoma.[18]

Some authors have postulated a relationship between radiation and virus-induced bone neoplasia. Several reports suggest an interaction between radiation and viruses and that radiation might produce neoplasia by inactivating a viral inhibitor.[36] Some osteogenic sarcomas induced by strontium 90 contain an antigen closely related to the FBJ virus.

Authors of both the human and veterinary literature have attempted to establish a relationship between bone tumors and trauma. Ewing believed that the occurrence of an injury more likely drew a patient's attention to an already existing neoplasm. He referred to this event as "traumatic determinism" and thought that trauma revealed more malignant growths than it produced.[15] In animals, sarcomas have arisen at the sites of fractures and fracture fixation devices.[3,6,20,24,26,28,37,39,42] These sarcomas associated with fractures and fixation devices differ from spontaneous neoplasms in that their location is diaphyseal rather than metaphyseal.[39] Several different fixation devices have been associated with these neoplasms, including bone plates and screws, Steinmann's pins, and Jonas' intramedullary devices. There have been occasional cases in which the fracture-associated sarcomas developed after external fixation or no fixation at all.[39]

Chondrosarcoma

Biology. Chondrosarcoma is a malignant tumor in which the basic neoplastic tissue is fully developed cartilage without tumor osteoid being directly formed by the stroma.[29] Although myxoid changes, calcification, or ossification may be present, the sarcomatous cells do not directly produce neoplastic osteoid or bone, since this is characteristic of osteogenic sarcoma only.[35]

There are two classes of chondrosarcomas—primary and secondary. Primary chondrosarcomas arise in previously normal bone. Secondary chondrosarcomas develop from a preexisting benign cartilaginous mass. In dogs this is an uncommon occurrence and is usually associated with an enchondroma or the cap of a cartilaginous exostosis.

Incidence. Chondrosarcomas are the second most common bone tumor in dogs, constituting about 10 per cent of all canine bone neoplasms.[10] This tumor affects primarily large breeds of dogs but rarely giant breeds, has no sex predilection, and occurs mostly in dogs between 5 and 9 years of age (mean age 5.9 years). Boxers and German shepherds were the most commonly affected breeds in a retrospective study of 35 cases.[10]

The flat bones are more commonly involved than the long bones. In the previously mentioned study, tumors of the ribs, turbinates, and pelvis constituted 60 per cent of the 35 reported chondrosarcomas.[10] Chondrosarcomas of the ribs most commonly arise from the costochondral junction (Figs. 184–6 and 184–7). The intrathoracic portion of the tumor often exceeds the size of the tumor lateral to the rib cage.

Clinical Signs. The clinical signs associated with chondrosarcomas in general depend on the site of skeletal involvement. Tumors of the nasal cavity can cause sneezing, unilateral or bilateral blood-tinged discharges, and nasal obstruction sometimes followed by bone destruction[35] (Fig. 184–8). Rib tumors tend to cause relatively few problems locally, although the intrathoracic portion can lead to varying degrees of pulmonary atelectasis. Pelvic chondrosarcomas can become large enough to cause clinical signs related to compression of the normal structures that pass through the pelvic inlet (e.g., constipation, straining, and so on). Chondrosarcomas of the limbs are very similar to osteogenic sarcomas and cause pain, swelling, and loss of function.

Diagnosis. The radiographic appearance of chondrosarcoma is very similar to osteogenic sarcoma. The tumor is slow-growing and causes an expansion of the medullary canal and eventual erosion of the cortical margins. A soft-tissue mass is often associated with the bony lesions.

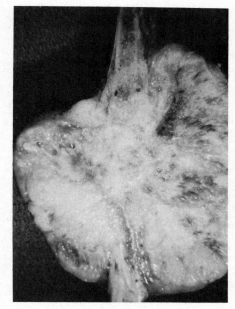

Figure 184–7. Gross specimen of the chondrosarcoma in Figure 184–6. (Courtesy of Dr. C. B. Carrig.)

It is not possible to distinguish chondrosarcoma and other primary malignant bone tumors on clinical signs and radiographic findings. A bone biopsy of any suspected lesion should be obtained before surgical therapy. Histologically, chondrosarcomas consist of spindle to pleomorphic cells, which form a basophilic, hyaline matrix with cells trapped within the matrix. Neoplastic cartilage may undergo ossification (endochondral ossification) and simulate osteogenic sarcoma. Osteogenic sarcomas, on the other hand, often have a cartilaginous component (Fig. 184–9).

Treatment and Prognosis. Chondrosarcomas are slow-growing neoplasms that usually metastasize late

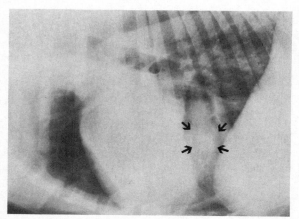

Figure 184–6. Lateral radiograph of a chondrosarcoma of the rib in a ten-year-old mixed breed dog (arrows). (Courtesy of Dr. C. B. Carrig.)

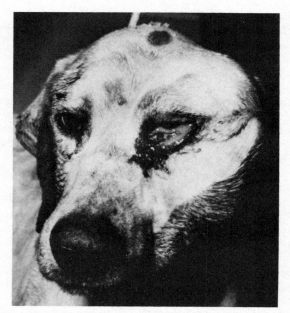

Figure 184–8. Mixed breed dog with a chondrosarcoma of the zygomatic arch and lateral aspect of the skull.

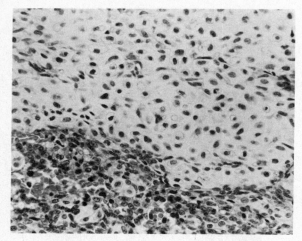

Figure 184–9. A chondrosarcoma of the nasal turbinates of a dog. Hypercellular cartilage consisting of basophilic ground substance with entrapped stellate to oval chondrocytes is bounded by indifferentiated cells. (Hematoxylin-eosin × 230.)

and may be associated with recurrences many years after initial surgical removal.[10] Surgical extirpation of tumor masses located in accessible sites such as the ribs can be curative. Amputation of involved limbs carries a much more favorable prognosis than for osteogenic sarcomas. Chondrosarcomas of the nasal cavity recur locally after surgery and usually demonstrate an increasingly malignant behavior with each clinical recurrence.[35]

Fibrosarcoma

Biology. Fibrosarcoma of bone is a malignant fibroblastic tumor characterized by varying amounts of collagen production and lacking any tendency to form tumor bone, osteoid, or cartilage, either in its primary site or in its metastases.[22]

Incidence. Fibrosarcomas of suspected origin in bone are uncommon, ranging from 0 to 9 per cent in different series of skeletal neoplasms.[25,34,35] Approximately 60 per cent are associated with and have invaded the bones of the maxilla, mandible, and frontal and nasal bones, and approximately 30 per cent are associated with the bones of the extremities.[26,27] Neoplasms arising from the membranous bones of the skull are more malignant than those arising in the long bones.[34]

Diagnosis. Radiographically, fibrosarcomas of bone appear very similar to other previously described primary bone tumors. The primary radiographic lesions are those of cortical destruction and periosteal response similar to that described for osteogenic sarcomas (Fig. 184–10). Histologically, fibrosarcomas consist of spindle to pleomorphic cells separated by variable amounts of collagen fibrils. The cells are poorly organized; mitotic figures and nuclear pleomorphism may be marked (Fig. 184–11).

Treatment and Prognosis. Fibrosarcomas of bone are slower than osteogenic sarcomas both in growth

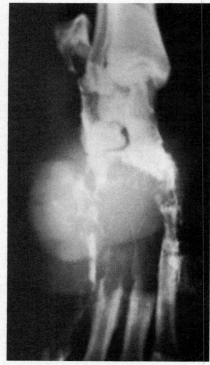

Figure 184–10. Craniocaudal radiograph of the metatarsal bones of a dog with a destructive fibrosarcoma.

at the primary site and in the tendency to metastasize. If the tumor is in an area that allows total resection or if an involved limb can be amputated, the prognosis for a "cure" is much higher than with an osteogenic sarcoma.

Hemangiosarcoma

Biology. Malignant hemangiosarcoma (angiosarcoma) of bone is characterized by the formation of irregular anastomosing vascular channels lined by

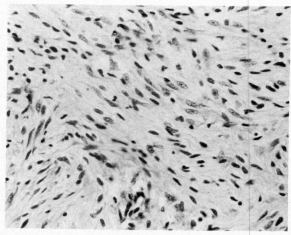

Figure 184–11. A fibrosarcoma of the hard palate of a dog. Poorly organized fusiform cells are separated by small amounts of collagen fibrils (Hematoxylin-eosin × 230.)

one or several layers of atypical endothelial cells having an anaplastic, immature appearance.[22]

Incidence. Primary hemangiosarcoma of bone is an uncommon entity. In a reported series of 152 primary bone tumors, only 4 were hemangiosarcomas.[11] In another retrospective series covering a 20-year period, 22 dogs with hemangiosarcoma of bone were studied.[7] In this latter series, the three most commonly affected breeds were boxers, Great Danes, and German shepherds. The age of affected dogs ranged from 2 to 11 years (median age of 6 years). The proximal humerus and ribs were most often involved.

Clinical Signs and Diagnosis. Hemangiosarcoma of bone causes pain, lameness, loss of function, and bone destruction. Radiographically the lesion is highly lytic with minimal soft-tissue swelling and little periosteal reaction.[14] However, cases have been reported that demonstrated a large soft-tissue element and marked periosteal bone formation,[4] making the tumor very difficult to differentiate radiographically from other primary skeletal neoplasms.

Histologically, hemangiosarcomas are composed of spindle- to pleomorphic-shaped cells giving rise to endothelial lined, irregular vascular channels. Collagen sometimes supports the thin-walled channels (Fig. 184–12).

Treatment and Prognosis. Hemangiosarcomas of bone tend to be well advanced prior to presentation and typically destroy an extensive area of bone before producing clinical signs.[35] By the time clinical signs appear, many tumors have already spread to distant sites. Surgical resection or amputation of an involved limb has not prolonged the animal's life.[7]

Tumors Metastatic to Bone

Biology. Neoplasms arising in the soft tissues or in the skeleton may secondarily involve bone by direct

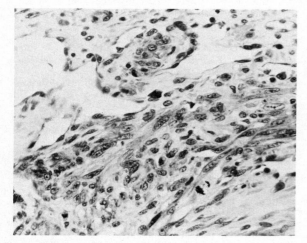

Figure 184–12. An hemangiosarcoma of the humerus of a dog. Fusiform and round undifferentiated cells merge with irregular channels lined by endothelium. Hyaline material adjacent to the endothelium is collagen, which is birefringent under polarized light. (Hematoxylin-eosin × 230.)

extension or by distant metastasis. The routes of metastasis to bone are arterial and venous. The lymphatics are of little importance, as they appear to be absent from bone marrow.[32] Apparently, in humans, metastatic growths in bone are almost always situated initially in the bone marrow.[43] The axial and trunk bones are much more frequently the site of metastatic tumors than peripheral bones of the limbs, and it is significant that in humans these sites still have red marrow even in older individuals. The apparent lack of metastatic tumors in yellow marrow has been attributed to a difference in vascularity. This same phenomenon has been observed in animals when tumor metastases localize in skeletal sites with high vascularity and abundant red marrow.[35]

Local invasion is the most common way in which soft-tissue tumors secondarily involve bone. This is especially true with those growths arising in the oral and nasal cavities.

Incidence. In a study of 24 dogs with metastatic bone disease, the average age was 10 years (range 1 to 15 years), with a peak occurrence at 9 years.[12] In this study, the primary tumor sites were the lung (5 cases), kidney (4 cases), bone (4 cases), spleen (3 cases), skin (3 cases), heart (2 cases), adrenal gland (1 case), urinary bladder (1 case), and tonsil (1 case). The primary neoplasms were sarcomas (11), carcinomas (9), melanomas (2), nephroblastomas (1), and aortic body tumor (1). A total of 39 metastatic tumors were seen in the 24 dogs, 8 of which had 2 or more skeletal lesions. Eleven dogs had tumors in the appendicular skeleton, 8 had tumors in the axial skeleton, and 5 had lesions in both the axial and appendicular skeletons. The 4 most commonly affected sites were the ribs (11 cases), vertebrae (9 cases), humerus (7 cases), and femur (4 cases).

In another study of metastatic bone neoplasm in dogs, the most common sites for the primary growth were the mammary gland, lung, mouth and tonsils, skin, and thyroid gland.[23]

Diagnosis. The radiographic appearance of metastatic bone tumors can be very similar to that of primary bone neoplasms. This, along with the fact that, particularly in the early stages of development, metastatic bone disease can mimic the radiographic appearance of not only primary bone tumors but osteomyelitis and fungal infections of bone makes diagnosis difficult by radiographic examination alone. If the examiner considers the age, breed, and sex of the dog and the tumor's location, multicentric origin, and tendency toward an osteosclerotic appearance, it is possible to suggest whether the lesion is a primary bone tumor or a metastatic one.[30] As a rule, bone biopsy is generally necessary to arrive at a definitive diagnosis.

TUMORS OF SKELETAL MUSCLE

As a general rule, tumors of canine and feline muscle are rare clinical entities. Benign striated muscle tumors are about half as frequent as malignant ones and have been primarily documented in animals other than dogs and cats.[21] The most common tumor of skeletal muscle reported in dogs is rhabdomyosarcoma.

Rhabdomyosarcoma

Clinical Signs. Because of the rare nature of this tumor in dogs and cats, no sex, breed, or regional predisposition has been documented. Congenital rhabdomyosarcomas have been reported in dogs.[40]

Most patients are presented because the owner has observed a mass or swelling under the skin. If a limb is involved, the animal may be lame.

Diagnosis. Because of the diffuse nature of these tumors, incisional biopsies are required for diagnosis. Histologically, rhabdomyosarcomas are characterized by cellular pleomorphism and the presence of striated muscle fibers.[40]

Treatment and Prognosis. Malignant rhabdomyosarcomas are extremely difficult to treat. The tumor is very invasive locally and often is inoperable.[21] In selected cases, early limb amputation may be successful. Metastasis occurs hematogenously to the lungs, liver, spleen, kidneys, lymph nodes, and other structures.[21]

1. Aegerter, E., and Kirkpatrick, J. A.: *Orthopedic Diseases.* 3rd ed. W. B. Saunders, Philadelphia, 1968.
2. Alexander, J. W., Walker, M. A., and Easley, J. R.: Extraskeletal osteosarcoma in the dog. J. Am. Anim. Hosp. Assoc. 15:99, 1979.
3. Banks, W. C., Morris, E., Herron, M. R., et al.: Osteogenic sarcoma associated with internal fracture fixation in two dogs. J. Am. Vet. Med. Assoc. 167:166, 1975.
4. Barber, D. L., Thrall, D. E., Hill, J. R., et al.: Primary osseous hemangiosarcoma in a dog. J. Am. Vet. Rad. 14:17, 1973.
5. Bartels, J. E.: Canine extraskeletal osteosarcoma: A clinical communication. J. Am. Anim. Hosp. Assoc. 11:307, 1975.
6. Bennett, D., Campbell, J. R., and Brown, P.: Osteosarcoma associated with healed fractures. J. Small Anim. Pract. 20:13, 1979.
7. Bingel, S. A., Brodey, R. S., Allen, H. L., et al.: Haemangiosarcoma of bone in the dog. J. Small Anim. Pract. 15:303, 1974.
8. Brodey, R. S., and Riser, W. H.: Canine osteosarcoma, a clinicopathologic study of 194 cases. Clin. Orthop. 62:54, 1969.
9. Brodey, R. S., and Abt, D. A.: Results of surgical treatment in 65 dogs with osteosarcoma. J. Am. Vet. Med. Assoc. 168:1032, 1976.
10. Brodey, R. S., Misdorp, W., Riser, W. H., et al.: Canine skeletal chondrosarcoma: A clinicopathologic study of 35 cases. J. Am. Vet. Med. Assoc. 165:68, 1974.
11. Brodey, R. S., Sauer, R. M., and Medway, W.: Canine bone neoplasms. J. Am. Vet. Med. Assoc. 143:471, 1963.
12. Brodey, R. S., Reid, C. F., and Sauer, R. M.: Metastatic bone neoplasms in the dog. J. Am. Vet. Med. Assoc. 148:29, 1966.
13. Charles, R. T., and Turusov, V. S.: Bone tumors in CF-1 mice. Lab. Anim. 8:137, 1974.
14. Childers, H. Z.: What is your diagnosis: Radiographic diagnosis of a hemangiosarcoma in a dog. J. Am. Vet. Med. Assoc. 157:1379, 1970.
15. Ewing, J.: Bulkey lecture: Modern attitude toward traumatic cancer. Arch. Pathol. Lab. Med. 19:690, 1935.
16. Finkel, M. P., Reilly, C. A., and Biskis, B. O.: Pathogenesis of radiation and virus-induced bone tumors. *In* Grundmann, E. (ed.): *Malignant Bone Tumors.* Springer-Verlag, New York, 1976.
17. Finkel, M. P., Biskis, B. O., and Jinkins, P. B.: Virus induction of osteosarcomas in mice. Science 151:698, 1966.
18. Finkel, M. P., Biskis, B. P., and Farrell, C.: Nonmalignant and malignant changes in hamsters inoculated with extracts of human osteosarcomas. Radiology 92:1546, 1969.
19. Foley, R. H.: Osteoma in two young dogs. J. Am. Anim. Hosp. Assoc. 14:253, 1978.
20. Harrison, J. W., McLain, D. L., Hohn, R. B., et al.: Osteosarcoma associated with metallic implants: Report of two cases in dogs. Clin. Orthop. 116:253, 1976.
21. Hulland, T. J.: Tumors of muscle. *In* Moulton, J. E. (ed.): *Tumors of Domestic Animals.* 2nd ed. University of California Press. Berkeley, 1978.
22. Huvos, H. G.: *Bone Tumors, Diagnosis, Treatment and Prognosis.* W. B. Saunders, Philadelphia, 1979.
23. Kas, N. P., van der Heul, R. O., and Misdorp, W.: Metastatic bone neoplasms in dogs, cats, and a lion (with some comparative remarks on the situation in man). Zentralbl. Veterinarmed. (A) 17:909, 1970.
24. Knecht, C. D., and Priester, W. A.: Osteosarcoma in dogs: A study of previous trauma, fracture, and fracture fixations. J. Am. Anim. Hosp. Assoc. 14:82, 1978.
25. Ling, G. V., Morgan, J. P., and Pool, R. R.: Primary bone tumors in the dog: A combined clinical, radiographic, and histologic approach to early diagnosis. J. Am. Vet. Med. Assoc. 165:55, 1974.
26. Liu, S-K., Dorfman, H. D., Hurvitz, A. I., et al.: Primary and secondary bone tumors in the dog. J. Small Anim. Pract. 18:313, 1977.
27. Liu, S-K.: Tumors of bone and cartilage. *In* Bjorab, M. J. (ed.): *Pathophysiology in Small Animal Surgery.* Lea and Febiger, Philadelphia, 1981.
28. Madewell, B. R., Pool, R. R., and Leighton, R. L.: Osteogenic sarcoma at the site of a chronic nonunion fracture and internal fixation device in a dog. J. Am. Vet. Med. Assoc. 171:187, 1977.
29. Mankin, H. J.: Advances in diagnosis and treatment of bone tumors. N. Engl. J. Med. 300:543, 1979.
30. Morgan, J. P.: *Radiology in Veterinary Orthopedics.* Lea & Febiger, Philadelphia, 1972.
31. Norrdin, R. W., Gobel, J. L., and Chitwood, J. S.: Extraskeletal osteosarcoma in dogs. J. Am. Vet. Med. Assoc. 158:729, 1971.
32. Owen, L. N.: *Bone Tumors in Man and Animals.* Butterworths, London, 1969.
33. Park, R. D.: Radiographic diagnosis of long bone neoplasms in the dog. Comp. Cont. Ed. 3:922, 1981.
34. Peiffer, R. L., Rebar, A., and Burk, R.: Fibrosarcoma involving the skeleton of the dog. Vet. Med. Small Anim. Clin. 4:1143, 1974.
35. Pool, R. R.: Tumors of bone and cartilage. *In* Moulton, J. E. (ed.): *Tumors of Domestic Animals.* 2nd ed. University of California Press, Berkeley, 1978.
36. Pritchard, D. J.: The etiology of osteosarcoma. Clin. Orthop. 111:14, 1975.
37. Sinibaldi, K., Rosen, H., Liu, S-K., et al.: Tumors associated with metallic implants in animals. Clin. Orthop. 118:257, 1976.
38. Spjut, H. J., Dorfman, H. D., Fechner, R. E., et al.: *Introduction, Tumors of Bone and Cartilage.* Armed Forces Institute of Pathology, Washington, D.C., 1971.
39. Stevenson, S., Hohn, R. B., Pohler, O. E. M., et al.: Fracture-associated sarcomas in the dog. J. Am. Vet. Med. Assoc. 180:1189, 1982.

40. Theilen, G. H., and Madewell, B. R.: *Veterinary Cancer Medicine*, Lea & Febiger, Philadelphia, 1979.
41. Tjalma, R. A.: Canine bone sarcoma: Estimates of relative risks as a function of body size. J. Natl. Cancer Inst. 36:1137, 1966.
42. Van Bree, H., Verschooten, F., Hoorens, J., et al.: Internal

43. Willis, R. A.: *The Spread of Tumors in the Human Body*. Butterworths, London, 1952.
44. Wolke, R. E., and Nielsen, S. W.: Site incidence of canine osteosarcoma. J. Small Anim. Pract. 7:489, 1966.

fixation of a fractured humerus in a dog and late osteosarcoma development. Vet. Rec. 107:501, 1980.

======================= Chapter **185**

Respiratory System

Alan M. Norris, Ralph A. Henderson, and Stephen J. Withrow

NEOPLASMS OF THE NASAL AND PARANASAL SINUSES

Incidence

Canine nasal and paranasal sinus tumors are reported as being uncommon,[10,21,62] but in studies involving large numbers of canine neoplasms the incidence of these tumors varied from 1 to 2.5 per cent.[11,24,52,67] Undoubtedly, many nasal and paranasal sinus tumors go undetected because of the difficulty in establishing a diagnosis or the owner's reluctance to subject a pet to the necessary diagnostic procedures. Therefore, the incidence of these tumors is probably higher than reported. Among domestic animals, dogs have the highest occurrence of nasal and paranasal sinus tumors, followed by cats. Dogs frequently have tumor invasion of the paranasal sinuses (Figs. 185–1 and 185–2), whereas cats rarely have sinus involvement (Fig. 185–3).[52]

The Airedale terrier, basset hound, Old English sheepdog, Scottish terrier, collie, Shetland sheepdog, and German short-haired pointer are at increased risk for developing nasal carcinomas.[38] Two breeds, the cocker spaniel and dachshund, have a lower risk

than expected.[38] The reason for these breed variations is not known. The majority of investigators report that nasal tumors are more common in medium to large breeds,[9,11,51,62] although one investigator found no association between body size in mesocephalic breeds and risk of developing nasal carcinoma.[38]

Long-nosed dogs are more frequently affected by nasal tumors.[10,22,68] Of 504 dogs with nasal carcinoma, dolichocephalic breeds had a higher risk, whereas brachycephalic dogs had a reduced risk of developing nasal tumors.[38] The increased surface area and filtering mechanisms of the nasal cavity in long-nosed dogs have been postulated as causative factors,[68] although some dogs with long noses, such as setters, Doberman pinschers and dachshunds, are at a low risk.[38] The observation that brachycephalic dogs commonly mouth-breathe because of upper airway obstruction and stenotic nares and therefore have less exposure to nasal carcinogens may explain the reduced risk in this group. Epidemiological studies have failed to establish a relationship between canine nasal tumors and environmental pollutants.[68] It is evident that a simple relationship between skull type and incidence of nasal tumors does not exist, but complicating factors such as genetics may be involved.[38]

Male dogs have an increased risk of developing nasal carcinoma, as do male cats.[11,38,52,62,67] The tumor

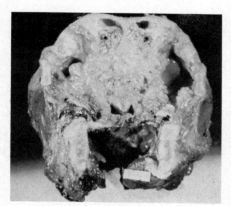

Figure 185–1. Necropsy specimen of the skull of a dog demonstrating an adenocarcinoma of both nasal cavities and the frontal sinus.

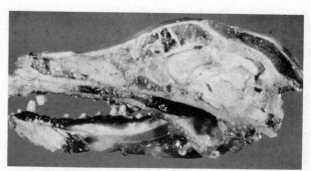

Figure 185–2. Necropsy specimen of a nine-year-old dog with an adenocarcinoma of the nasal cavity.

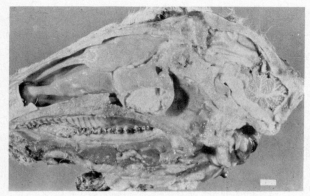

Figure 185–3. Necropsy specimen of a mature cat with an adeno-carcinoma of the nasopharynx.

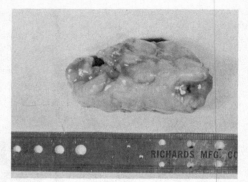

Figure 185–5. Surgical specimen from Figure 185–4 demonstrating the excised tumor.

occurs in older dogs and cats, with a median age of 8 to 10 years.[11,24,51,52,62]

The majority of nasal tumors in both species are malignant, with the percentage of malignant tumors being greater than 90 per cent in dogs and cats.[52,67] The types of tumors found in the nasal cavity are diverse, reflecting the complex structure of this area. Approximately two-thirds of the tumors are carcinomas and one-third sarcomas.[67] Papillomas, adenomas, and fibromas are the most common benign tumors (Figs. 185–4 and 185–5).[67] The biological behavior of nasal tumors is local invasion and destruction, and although metastases do occur, they are seen in the late stages of the disease. Of 504 dogs with nasal carcinoma, only 10 per cent had metastases, with lymph node, brain, and lung being the most common sites of involvement.[67] A difference may exist in the biological behavior of carcinomas and sarcomas, for in one study 5 of 10 carcinomas had evidence of metastatic disease, whereas none of the 12 dogs with nasal sarcomas had metastatic foci.[52]

History

The clinical findings in dogs and cats with tumors of the nasal cavity and paranasal sinuses are nonspecific and must be distinguished from chronic bacterial or fungal rhinitis. The initial sign is often a unilateral nasal discharge that may progress to a bilateral discharge, which may be mucoid or purulent but is most often sanguinous. Severe, periodic epistaxis may be the presenting complaint. A large proportion of affected dogs sneeze, and respiratory stertor is a frequent finding. As the disease progresses, signs develop that are more specific to nasal tumors, including facial deformity (Fig. 185–6), ocular discharge, exophthalmos, oral growths, and neurological signs (Table 185–1). Epiphora results from obstruction of the nasolacrimal duct.

Most animals have received extensive therapy before a definitive diagnosis of neoplasia of the nasal cavity or sinus is established.[52] This is reflected by a 3- to 6-month hiatus between onset of clinical signs and confirmation of the diagnosis.[51,52,62] Prior to radiographic examination of the skull and collection of tissue samples for cytological and histopathological evaluation, the geriatric patient should have a thorough laboratory evaluation. A complete blood count, liver and kidney tests, urinalysis, and thoracic radiographs should be performed to determine if metastatic disease is present. In animals with epistaxis as the sole presenting complaint, von Willebrand's disease, platelet disorders, and other common causes of

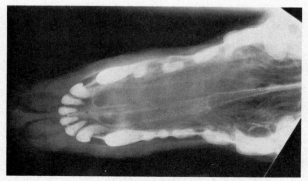

Figure 185–4. Occlusal radiograph of a three-year-old Saluki with a fibroma of the nasal cavity. There is an increased density in the left nasal passage and deviation of the vomer bone.

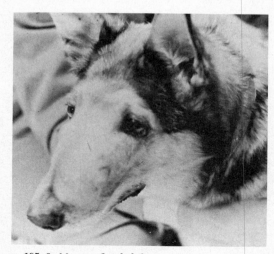

Figure 185–6. Massive facial deformity in a nine-year-old collie cross from an osteosarcoma of the nasal cavity.

TABLE 185–1. Clinical Signs in 120 Dogs with Nasal Tumors[51, 52, 62]

Clinical Sign	Per Cent of Dogs Affected
Nasal discharge:	
Bloody	72
Purulent	29
Mucoid/serous	23
Sneezing	52
Facial deformity	50
Stertorous respiration	39
Ocular discharge	18
Oral/palative disease	12
CNS signs	8

bleeding disorders must be considered. Thoracic radiographs are rarely positive for metastases.[38]

Radiographic Signs

Radiology of the skull is a simple and effective means of determining the presence and extent of a nasal cavity lesion and the site for biopsy. For radiology to be of maximum value, all animals should be anesthetized and properly positioned, and high-quality x-rays should be obtained. Radiology should precede rhinoscopy and biopsy procedures because the hemorrhage from these procedures may result in an increased radiopacity of the nasal cavity and obscure subtle lesions.

A complete radiographic study of the nasal cavity and paranasal sinuses should include the following projections: lateral, intraoral dorsoventral or open-mouth ventrodorsal, and rostrocaudal frontal sinus. Occasionally, oblique views of the skull may be required to see the dental arcade and reduce the superimposition of skull structures that is inherent in a lateral projection.[48]

An occlusal x-ray of the skull or a ventrodorsal projection with the dog in dorsal recumbency and the lower jaw opened widely is most useful (Fig. 185–7).[28,33,56] The use of nonscreen film for intraoral projections results in high-quality radiographs with excellent detail. Lateral views of the skull allow evaluation of cortical bone overlying the sinus and nasal cavity (Fig. 185–8). The rostrocaudal frontal sinus projection or skyline view demonstrates increased opacity of the frontal sinus and erosive lesions (Fig. 185–9). The radiopacity of the frontal sinus in this projection is often the result of mucus accumulation due to obstruction of the frontal sinus ostium. If there is involvement of the sinus with tumor, erosion of the bone is often evident.

The radiographic signs in dogs with chronic nasal disease have been reported.[28,33,52,56,62] Attempts to categorize and diagnose nasal disease based solely on radiographic appearance are difficult and may result in errors. In animals with chronic nasal disease,

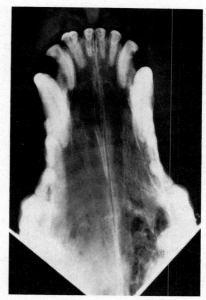

Figure 185–7. Occlusal radiographs of a dog with a squamous cell carcinoma. There is an increased density in the nasal cavity and numerous small lytic areas.

clinical signs have usually been present for months before x-rays are taken, allowing extension of tumors from their origin into adjacent tissue; this further complicates the radiographic appearance.[56] Despite these limitations, certain radiographic features are seen in a high number of cases of neoplasia and aid in diagnosis. Important radiographic findings include an increased density in the frontal sinus, increased opacity of the nasal cavity and the loss of the turbinate trabecular pattern, asymmetry of the nasal cavity, erosion of the vomer bone, destruction of overlying facial bones, and an external mass (Table 185–2).[28,33,34,52,56,69]

Clinically and radiographically, one must differentiate chronic inflammatory lesions and destructive rhinitis from nasal cavity tumors.[28] In inflammatory (hyperplastic) conditions there is an accumulation of mucus and cells, filling the nasal airspaces and causing an increased opacity. Hyperplasia of the mucous

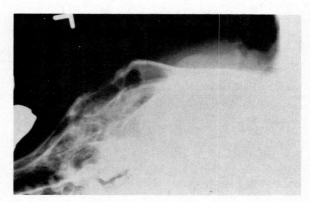

Figure 185–8. Lateral radiograph of a dog with osteolysis of the cortical bone overlying the frontal sinus.

TABLE 185–2. Radiographic Changes in 189 Dogs with Nasal Tumors[28, 33, 52, 56, 69]

Radiographic Sign	Per Cent of Dogs Affected
Increased density of nasal cavity and loss of trabecular turbinates	85
Increased density of frontal sinus	62
Erosion of frontal bone	52
External mass	45
Lysis of vomer bone	40

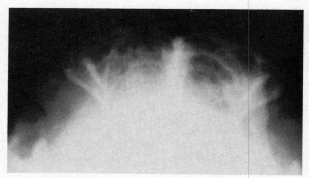

Figure 185–9. Rostrocaudal projection of the frontal sinus of a dog. There is increased density of the right sinus and lysis of the cortical bone.

membranes also contributes to the radiopacity. Destruction of facial bones or erosion of the nasal septum should not occur in inflammatory diseases except in the presence of osteomyelitis, a condition that occurs in chronic rhinitis of cats.

Destructive rhinitis results in erosion of the overlying cortical bone and the nasal septum and may be confused with a nasal tumor.[28,56] Destructive rhinitis is most frequently the result of fungal infections, especially aspergillosis, although other diseases including cryptococcosis, blastomycosis, and penicilliosis have been documented.[13] Destructive rhinitis causes loss of the normal trabecular turbinate pattern and increased lucency of the nasal cavity, which may be observed on x-ray. This radiolucency is typical of destructive rhinitis and is highly suggestive of a fungal cause.[28,33] A comparison of the radiographic appearance of nasal tumors, hyperplastic conditions, and destructive rhinitis is presented in Table 185–3.

Biopsy Techniques

Rhinoscopy using an otoscope speculum introduced via the nares may allow visualization of tumors. The technique is limited to large dogs[22] and only allows examination of the anterior portion of the nasal cavity. Observation of the caudal nasopharynx is possible with a dental mirror and light source.[22] Using a 2.7-mm arthroscope, it is possible to examine the entire nasal cavity from the nares to the cribiform plate. The copious amounts of mucus often present in nasal disease require the use of suction. An 8-French gauge urinary catheter is ideal for suction if the secretions are not too tenacious. Patience and care on the part of the endoscopist are essential, for the nasal cavity in the diseased state may bleed, obscuring the tumor. Polyps, fungal lesions, and tumors may be observed and biopsied.

In most instances diagnostic material can be collected without observation of the tumor. When palpable masses are present, the simplest technique is direct fine-needle aspiration or punch biopsy. For intranasal lesions, two techniques have been described for nasal flushing and collecting tissue samples. With the animal under general anesthesia and in lateral recumbency with the affected side down, a plastic tube is passed through the external nares or nasopharynx. The oropharynx is packed with gauze sponges to prevent fluid and tissue from entering the trachea. Endotracheal intubation with the cuff inflated also reduces the possibility of aspiration pneumonia. Vigorous flushing is performed by injecting 50 to 100 ml of saline through the plastic tube via a 35-ml syringe. Intermittent positive and negative pressure dislodges and flushes material from the nose and into the syringe or onto gauze sponges at the external nares. Tissue is processed for cytological and histological evaluation. A definitive diagnosis can be made in 50 per cent of the cases examined cytologically and 90 per cent of the cases studied histologically.[51]

A nasal flushing technique using a stiff 2- to 5-mm diameter plastic tube beveled at a 45° angle to create a sharp cutting edge has been described.[86] The dis-

TABLE 185–3. Radiographic Changes in 98 Dogs with Intra-nasal Disease

Radiographic Change	Tumors (% of 50 cases)	Hyperplastic Conditions (% of 22 cases)	Destructive Rhinitis (% of 26 cases)
Loss of trabecular pattern	98	0	100
Increased opacity	40	100	0
Mixed density	58	0	11
Increased lucency	0	0	88
Septal destruction	32	0	7
Soft-tissue swelling	40	0	0
Facial bone destruction	42	0	7
Frontal sinus opacification	78	14	11

Modified from Gibbs, C. et al.: Radiological features of intra-nasal lesions in the dog: A review of 100 cases. J. Small Anim. Pract. 20:515, 1979.

tance from the external nares to the medial canthus is measured and an equal length of tubing cut. If the tube extends past the medial canthus, penetration of the cribiform plate is possible. A 35-ml syringe is used to flush saline through the catheter. Positive and negative pressure is applied while the catheter is withdrawn and vigorously inserted to collect core tissue samples.[86] Lowering of the head by tilting the table and placing gauze sponges under the nares enables collection of tissue samples.[86]

Lesions visible on x-ray may be biopsied with a Tru-cut* biopsy needle. The distance and location of the lesion and the area for insertion of the biopsy needle must be determined from radiographs. A good tissue sample may be unobtainable when mucinous carcinomas are biopsied. A Michelle trephine and subsequent curettage often allow an adequate tissue sample to be collected. Once again, the site to be biopsied should be determined from the x-ray films. If these techniques fail to produce tissue samples of diagnostic quality, the nasal cavity should be explored through a dorsal bone flap in the nasal and maxillary bones.[10,49]

Treatment

Since tumors of the nasal cavity and paranasal sinuses are slow growing and locally invasive, with a low incidence of metastasis, management consists of local therapy. Early diagnosis and aggressive therapy may result in improved survival times in the future.

Surgery has been the treatment of choice for nasal tumors, although numerous reports have indicated that survival times are not improved with surgery.[1,18,20] The invasiveness of the tumor usually precludes complete removal from the area of the cribiform plate and orbit. Surgery does not remove the tumor that has invaded bone, and this residual tumor is a cause of treatment failure. Surgery may also result in hypoxic residual tumor that is resistant to radiation therapy. There is an increased morbidity associated with surgery, resulting from blood loss, anesthetic complications, or brain injury. Surgery is rarely palliative, because of secondary rhinitis and extensive turbinate destruction. As a result of these shortcomings, we no longer consider surgery to be the treatment of choice.

Cryosurgery, although not adequately evaluated in the treatment of nasal tumors, does not seem to improve survival times.[57,62,87] A theoretical advantage of cryosurgery is that it can destroy residual neoplastic cells in bone, in areas not accessible to scalpel excision. The dead bone can then serve as a graft, eventually becoming revascularized. Application of the cryogen in the nasal cavity is difficult and if applied haphazardly may result in oronasal fistulas.[87]

Radiation therapy is being evaluated as an adjunct

to surgery and as the primary treatment, resulting in increased survival times. High-energy radiation, supplied by cobalt or megavoltage x-rays, may deliver sufficient radiation to control tumors without prior surgical therapy. When using orthovoltage, volume reduction of the tumor by surgery is probably necessary prior to therapy. A total of 40 gray is delivered to the tumor in 10 to 12 fractions of 4 to 5 gray each. A Monday, Wednesday, Friday regimen is most frequently employed. The sensitivity of the various types of nasal tumors to radiation is not known.

Chemotherapy and immunotherapy have not been adequately evaluated in the management of nasal tumors, but preliminary reports indicate that immunotherapy is of little help.[51]

Prognosis

The prognosis for animals with nasal and paranasal sinus tumors is poor regardless of the method of treatment. Survival times for animals not receiving treatment is about 4 months, based on limited data from a few investigators.[9,5,62] Neither surgery nor cryosurgery has resulted in prolonged survival. In addition, surgery may result in decreased survival times, rendering it an unacceptable method of treatment.

At Colorado State University, 37 dogs with nasal tumors have been irradiated with cobalt therapy or megavoltage x-ray. Results have been encouraging, with mean survival times of 10 months. Carcinomas responded better than sarcomas, and animals managed with surgery and radiation seemed to respond better than those receiving radiation alone. Thirty per cent died with metastases to regional lymph nodes, brain, or lung. Most had recurrence of local disease. In another report of 21 dogs with nasal tumors treated with surgery and orthovoltage x-rays (18 had surgery), the median survival time was 13 months and the mean survival time was 21 months. The 1-year survival rate was 57 per cent.[79]

NEOPLASMS OF THE LARYNX AND TRACHEA

Incidence

Naturally occurring laryngotracheal neoplasms are rare in dogs and cats (Table 185–4). Too few tumors have been reported to establish sex or breed incidence, but most tumors have occurred in older animals. Young dogs are more commonly affected with osteochondromas.

Epidermoid (squamous) cell carcinomas and adenocarcinomas are the most common laryngeal tumors in dogs and cats, respectively. In the trachea, however, mesenchymal tumors are more common in dogs but epithelial tumors are more common in cats.

Experimentally, chemicals such as 9,10-dimethyl-1,2,2-benzanthracene, benzo-α-pyrene,[73] and the by-

---

* Tru-cut disposable biopsy needle. Travenol Laboratories, Inc., Deerfield, IL.

TABLE 185–4. Primary Canine and Feline Laryngeal and Tracheal Tumors Reported to January 1983*

Cell Type	Total Reported	Reference
Canine Laryngeal Tumors		
Epidermoid cell cancer	5	36, 85
Oncytoma	3	64
Mastocytoma	2	5, 36
Reticulum cell sarcoma	1	36
Carcinosarcoma	1	19
Melanoma	1	55
Feline Laryngeal Tumors		
Adenocarcinoma	4	36, 50, 82
Epidermoid cell cancer	1	20
Lymphosarcoma	1	36
Canine Tracheal Tumors		
Osteochondroma	5	26, 31, 43, 80, 88
Leiomyoma	2	8, 17
Osteosarcoma	1	15
Chondrosarcoma	1	1
Mastocytoma	1	37
Adenocarcinoma	1	2
Feline Tracheal Tumors		
Epidermoid cell cancer	4	23, 83
Adenocarcinoma	1	18
Lymphosarcoma	1	70

*Data from Priester, W. A., and McKay, F. W.: The occurrence of tumors in domestic animals (NCI Monograph 54, Bethesda, National Cancer Institute, 1980) are not included because the cases drawn from the Veterinary Medical Data Program (Priester and McKay) may duplicate some of the cases reported.

products of cigarette smoke are carcinogenic in dogs and cats. Inhaled chemical and radioactive carcinogens are concentrated in the mucus of the respiratory tract.[45] Physical and chemical injuries[3,63,73] inhibit mucociliary clearance, further concentrating carcinogens.

Diagnosis

Laryngeal neoplasms cause change of voice, hoarse bark, or dyspnea,[85] whereas tracheal neoplasms cause cough, dyspnea, or noisy respiration. The onset may be acute or slowly progressive. Typically, neoplasia is usually advanced by the time the owner seeks veterinary attention. Transient remission of signs may follow symptomatic therapy with antibiotics and steroids.

The most important diagnostic methods are examination of the upper airway under sedation, endoscopy, and radiography. Intraluminal laryngeal or tracheal masses are easily examined by one of these three methods. Biopsy specimens may be obtained by direct vision, endoscopy, or surgical exploration. An enlarged regional lymph node should be biopsied or aspirated for cell study.

Treatment and Prognosis

Surgical excision is the therapy of choice, and benign tumors such as osteochondromas can be removed, leaving tumor-free margins. Other tumors cannot be resected as cleanly and require excision of a greater quantity of tissue. Chapters 63 and 65 discuss the details of surgical procedures such as laryngectomy and tracheal resection. Although largely untried, preoperative irradiation of susceptible neoplasias may be considered. Irradiation of tracheal anastomoses with greater than 35 gray (3,500 rads) induced stenosis at the anastomotic site in dogs; however, lower quantities of radiation did not affect healing.[81]

Palliative cryonecrosis may be attempted in nonresectable tumors, to enlarge the tracheal lumen. The trachea and bronchi may be frozen three times for 2 to 3 minutes ($-110°C$) with special probes. Mucosal regeneration with squamous-type epithelium occurs in 14 days, and the zone of necrosis is completely replaced by dense, fibrous scar by 180 days.[30,46] The larynx may be frozen twice for 45 seconds, with no loss of mobility if the temperature does not go below -30 to $-40°C$.[42]

Allogenic and xenogenic tracheal prostheses treated with formalin, alcohol, and various agents designed to reduce inflammation were implanted in dogs but resulted in death 7 to 94 days postsurgically.[84] Silicone prostheses may be better tolerated; one human survived 9 months before tumor recurrence (see also Chapter 65).[27]

PRIMARY LUNG TUMORS

Incidence

Primary lung tumors are less common than nasal tumors but are more common than laryngeal and tracheal tumors. Among domestic species, primary lung tumors are most common in dogs, accounting for 0.31[25] to 1.24 per cent[57] of all tumors. The incidence of primary lung tumors in cats at necropsy is 0.38 per cent.[57]

Dogs younger than 7 years are rarely affected, and the average age at diagnosis is 10.5 years.[57] The average age of dogs with small cell anaplastic carcinoma is 7.5 years.[75] No sex or breed predispositions to primary lung tumors have been identified. The right lung lobes, especially the right caudal lobe, are most often affected.[57]

A "natural" cause of primary lung cancer, such as cigarette smoking in humans, has not been established in dogs. Experimentally, however, inhalation of certain agents (e.g., cigarette smoke, asbestos,[44] radioactive plutonium[58,67] and cesium[32]) and instillation of some chemicals (e.g., benzo-α-pyrene,[6,54] 9,10-dimethyl-1,2,2-benzanthracene,[72] and nickel carbonyl[57]) have caused primary lung cancer. Despite these apparent causes, the association of canine lung cancer with industrial or urban areas is disputed, some reports demonstrating no relationship[68] and some demonstrating a positive correlation.[77]

Unlike in humans, in animals primary lung tumors are most likely to originate from the terminal bronchioles and alveoli instead of the primary bronchi.[60] Nearly all lung tumors are malignant. Adenocarcinomas of the papillary or acinar variety are most common in the canine lung (83 per cent).[75] Anaplastic carcinomas of the large or small (oat) cell varieties are less common (8 per cent), as are epidermoid (squamous) cell carcinomas (6 per cent).[75] Other primary neoplasms in the lung include carcinoids, bronchial gland tumors, and mesenchymal tumors, all of which are rare.[29,60] The cell types occurring in cats are similar;[39,74] however, anaplastic carcinomas are not reported in cats.[74] More than one cell type may be found in a single tumor.[4,75]

Diagnosis

As many as one-third of lung tumors are discovered on preanesthetic examination or annual physicians' visits or are detected during radiography for another problem such as intervertebral disc herniation or heartworms. When present, clinical signs range in duration from 1 week to 7 months (mean of 9.6 weeks), and the most common clinical sign is a nonproductive cough.[13] Coughing is the primary owner complaint caused by lung tumors; however, dyspnea, hemoptysis, debilitation, fever, lameness, or general malaise are also seen and may be due to primary tumor, metastasis, or paraneoplastic disease.

Hypertrophic osteopathy is the most common paraneoplastic syndrome caused by lung tumors,[12] but it may occur with other diseases. It usually affects all four limbs, causing a characteristic palisading of the periosteum (Fig. 185–10). The cause is believed to be neurovascular,[41,47] and the lesions may regress when the neoplasm is adequately treated.[16,53] Paraplegia and neuromyopathy have been associated with large cell anaplastic carcinoma.[71] Hypercalcemia has been associated with epidermoid cell carcinoma.[59]

Lung neoplasms metastasize by transairway migration, through blood and lymph, and via direct invasion.[57] Transairway migration by ciliary movement and coughing is the most common route of spread.

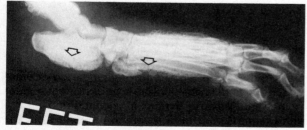

Figure 185–10. Lateral radiograph of the left hind limb. Hypertrophic osteopathy is most commonly seen in association with pulmonary masses. It is characterized by palisading periosteum (arrows), especially of the distal limb bones. The joints are rarely affected. The inciting mass may be extrathoracic.

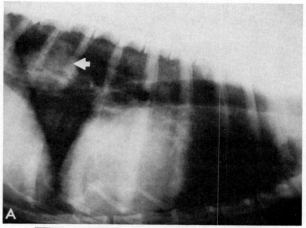

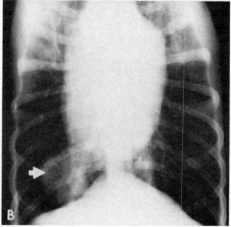

Figure 185–11. *A*, Lateral thoracic radiograph demonstrating a solitary pulmonary nodule (arrow) characteristic of the most common radiographic presentation of primary lung neoplasia. An adenocarcinoma was diagnosed following surgical excision of the left caudal lung lobe. *B*, Ventrodorsal view.

Extrapulmonary metastases may cause myriad clinical signs. Because of their location, blood tumor emboli enter the pulmonary veins and metastasize via the arterial system to the brain, bones, liver, and kidneys. Lymphatic metastases are primarily to the hilar lymph nodes. Invasion of adjacent pericardium or pleura often causes malignant effusions.

Thoracic x-rays are the most valuable diagnostic aid besides biopsy. The lesions seen on radiography can be classified as solitary-nodular (Fig. 185–11), multiple-nodular, or disseminated-infiltrative (Fig. 185–12).[76] A precise nodular density with or without a cavitating center located in a dorsal caudal lung lobe is the most common finding.[7,76] Vessels and adjacent bronchi tend to bend around the neoplasm as it expands.

A thoracotomy is necessary for diagnosis of *solitary* lesions. Punch or needle biopsy is contraindicated in this instance, since finding an abscess, the chief differential, would not alter the treatment plan and increases the risk of implanting the pleural space with tumor cells or bacteria. At thoracotomy each lung lobe is palpated for additional nodules, and the

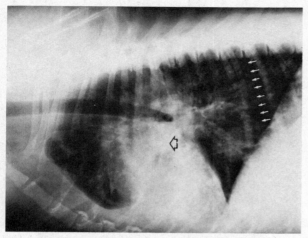

Figure 185–12. Lateral thoracic radiograph demonstrating the diffuse, infiltrative pattern of a primary pulmonary adenocarcinoma. The lesions are most dense at the heart base (black arrow), but the diffuse interstitial pattern may be seen peripherally (white arrows). Pleural effusion is also present. Lung aspiration and pleural cytology were not diagnostic. Biopsy via thoracotomy provided the diagnosis.

primary lesion is completely excised if possible. Secondary lesions and the hilar lymph nodes are biopsied for staging. Lung tumors should be staged according to the TNM system.[14]

Distinguishing diffuse pneumonic diseases is difficult. Endoscopic examination is usually of no value, because most neoplasms arise from the terminal airways. In humans, sputum specimens reveal neoplasia earlier than radiographs, but sputum cannot be collected readily in dogs. Culture and cell or tissue specimens may be obtained from transtracheal washes, lung aspirates, and percutaneous lung biopsy. Despite these diagnostic attempts, open biopsy is often required for diagnosis.

Treatment

When the diagnostic findings indicate that a lung tumor is probably confined to one lobe or one lung, the procedure of choice is lobectomy or pneumonectomy. Intercostal thoracotomy is superior to median sternotomy because it provides adequate exposure for lobectomy and lymph node biopsy. Median sternotomy allows a more thorough exploration and does not preclude lobectomy.

Surgery is valuable for diagnosis only in diffuse disease. Neither primary nor adjuvant regimens of chemotherapy or irradiation have reported efficacy in dogs.

Prognosis

In humans, survival is linked to the presence or absence of respiratory signs at the time of diagnosis.[66] The 5-year survival of humans with respiratory signs is less than 8 per cent compared with those without respiratory signs, of which 80 per cent survive 5 years.[66] Dogs with respiratory signs at the time of diagnosis and surgery have a shorter survival (mean of 10 months) than those without (mean of 18 months).[40]

Necropsy data suggest that nearly 100 per cent of epidermoid carcinomas and 90 per cent of anaplastic carcinomas in dogs metastasize,[13] and only 50 per cent of adenocarcinomas metastasize.[57,78] Treatment is recommended, since clinical data suggest that at least 25 per cent of dogs survive for 18 months to 2 years without recurrence.[40]

1. Aron, D. N., DeVries, R., and Short, C. E.: Primary tracheal chondrosarcoma in a dog: A case report with description of surgical and anesthetic technique. J. Am. Anim. Hosp. Assoc. 16:31, 1980.
2. Ball, V., Douville, M., and Girard, H.: Le cancer de trachea chez l'homme et les animaux. Rev. Vet. 88:447, 1936.
3. Battista, S. P.: Ciliatoxic components of cigarette smoke. Proc. 3rd World Conf. on Smoking & Health. New York. 2–5 Jun 1975 US Dept HEW, NCI, Bethesda Md. Public. No. (NIH) 76–1413, Vol II, 517–534, 1976.
4. Beaumont, P. R.: Intratracheal neoplasia in 2 cats. J. Small Anim. Pract. 23:29, 1982.
5. Beaumont, P. R., O'Brien, J. B., and Allen, H. L.: Mast cell sarcoma of the larynx in a dog: A case report. J. Small Anim. Pract. 20:19, 1979.
6. Benfield, J. R., Shores, E. C., Hammond, W. G., et al.: A clinically relevant canine lung cancer model. Ann. Thorac. Surg. 32:592, 1981.
7. Biery, D. N.: Differentiation of lung diseases of inflammatory or neoplastic origin from lung disease in heart failure. Vet. Clin. North Am. 4:711, 1974.
8. Black, A. P., Liu, S. K., and Randolph, J. F.: Primary tracheal leiomyoma in a dog. J. Am. Vet. Med. Assoc. 179:905, 1981.
9. Bradley, P. A., and Harvey, C. E.: Intra-nasal tumors in the dog: An evaluation of prognosis. J. Small Anim. Pract. 14:459, 1973.
10. Bright, R. M., and Bojrab, M. J.: Intranasal neoplasia in the dog and cat. J. Am. Anim. Hosp. Assoc. 12:806, 1976.
11. Brodey, R. S.: Canine and feline neoplasia. Adv. Vet. Sci. Comp. Med. 14:311, 1970.
12. Brodey, R. S.: Hypertrophic osteoarthropathy in the dog: A clinicopathologic survey of 60 cases. J. Am. Vet. Med. Assoc. 159:1242, 1971.
13. Brodey, R. S., and Craig, P. H.: Primary pulmonary neoplasms in the dog: A review of 29 cases. J. Am. Vet. Med. Assoc. 147:1628, 1965.
14. Brodey, R. S., Gillette, E. L., Milouchine, V. N., et al.: TNM classification in domestic animals. Bull. WHO, 1980. pp. 48–50.
15. Brodey, R. S., O'Brien, J., Berg, P., et al.: Osteosarcoma of the upper airway in the dog. J. Am. Vet. Med. Assoc. 155:1460, 1969.
16. Brodey, R. S., and Wind, A. P.: Surgical management of hypertrophic pulmonary osteoarthropathy in the dog. J. Am. Vet. Med. Assoc. 130:208, 1957.
17. Bryan, R. D., Frame, R. W., and Kier, A. B.: Tracheal leiomyoma in a dog. J. Am. Vet. Med. Assoc. 178:1069, 1981.
18. Cain, G.: Tracheal adenocarcinoma in a cat. J. Am. Vet. Med. Assoc. 182:614, 1983.
19. Cela, M., and Grassi, F.: Tumor of the larynx in a dog. Epithelial neoplasia with sarcomatous features. Ann. Fac. Med. Vet. (Pisa) 27:129, 1975.
20. Collet, P.: Cancer primitif du larynx chez une chatte. Bull. Soc. Sci. Vet. 38:219, 1935.
21. Confer, A. W., and DePaoli, A.: Primary neoplasms of the

nasal cavity, paranasal sinuses, and nasopharynx in the dog. Vet. Pathol. 15:18, 1978.

22. Cook, W. R.: Observations on the upper respiratory tract of the dog and cat. J. Small Anim. Pract. 5:309, 1964.

23. Cotchin, E.: Spontaneous neoplasms of the upper respiratory tract in animals. In: Muir, C. S., and Shanmugaratnam, K. (eds.): Cancer of the Nasopharynx. International Union Against Cancer, monograph Series No 1. Medical Examination Publishing, Flushing, N. Y., 1967. pp. 203–259.

24. Cotchin, E.: Some tumors of dogs and cats of comparative veterinary and human interest. Vet. Rec. 71:1040, 1959.

25. Dorn, C. R., Taylor, D. O. N., Frye, F. L., et al.: Survey of animal neoplasms in Alameda and Contra Costa counties, California. I and II. J. Natl. Cancer Inst. 40:295, 1968.

26. Dubielzig, R. R., and Dickey, D. L.: Tracheal osteochondroma in a young dog. Vet. Med. Small Anim. Clin. 73:1288, 1978.

27. Gamondes, J. P., Boivan, J., Maret, H., et al.: Resection and silicone prosthesis in patients with extensive malignant tumors of the thoracic trachea. Lyon Chir. 77:371, 1981.

28. Gibbs, C., Lane, J. G., and Denny, H. R.: Radiological features of intranasal lesions in the dog: A review of 100 cases. J. Small Anim. Pract. 20:515, 1979.

29. Giesel, O.: Primary lung sarcoma in dogs. Berl. Munch. Tierarzl. Wochenschr. 93:174, 1980.

30. Gorenstein, A., Neel, H. B., and Sanderson, D. R.: Transbronchoscopic cryosurgery: Development of a new technique. Surg. Forum 26:534, 1975.

31. Gourley, T. M., Morgan, J. P., and Gould, D. H.: Tracheal osteochondroma in a dog: A case report. J. Small Anim. Pract. 11:327, 1970.

32. Hahn, F. F., Benjamin, S. A., Bodeker, B. B., et al.: Primary pulmonary neoplasms in dogs exposed to aerosol of 144 CE infused clay particle. J. Natl. Cancer Inst. 50:675, 1973.

33. Harvey, C. E., Biery, D. N., Morello, J., and O'Brien, J.: Chronic nasal disease in the dog: Its radiographic diagnosis. J. Vet. Radiol. Soc. 20:91, 1979.

34. Harvey, C. E.: The nasal septum of the dog: Is it visible radiographically? J. Vet. Radiol. Soc. 20:88, 1980.

35. Harvey, C. E., O'Brien, J. A., Felsburg, P. J., et al.: Nasal penicilliosis in six dogs. J. Am. Vet. Med. Assoc. 10:1084, 1981.

36. Harvey, C. E., and O'Brien, J. A.: Upper airway obstruction surgery: 6. Surgical treatment of miscellaneous laryngeal conditions of dogs and cats. J. Am. Anim. Hosp. Assoc. 18:557, 1982.

37. Harvey, H. J., and Sikes, G.: Tracheal mast cell tumor in a dog. J. Am. Vet. Med. Assoc. 180:1097, 1982.

38. Hayes, H. M., Wilson, G. P., and Fraumeni, J. F.: Carcinoma of the nasal cavity and paranasal sinuses in dogs.: Descriptive epidemiology. Cornell Vet. 72:168, 1982.

39. Head, K. W.: Primary lung tumors in dogs and cats. BTTA Rev. 4:50, 1974.

40. Henderson, R. A., Withrow, S. J., Patnaik, A. K., and MacEwen, E. G.: Survival of dogs following surgical removal of primary lung tumors. (in press).

41. Holling, M. E., Danielson, G. K., Hamilton, R. W., et al.: Hypertrophic pulmonary osteoarthropathy. J. Thorac. Cardiovasc. Surg. 46:310, 1963.

42. Hong, S. W., Silverstein, H., and Sodeghee, S.: The effect of cryosurgery on canine and human larynx. Laryngoscope 87:1079, 1977.

43. Hough, J., Krahwinkel, D. J., Evans, T., et al.: Tracheal osteochondroma in a dog. J. Am. Vet. Med. Assoc. 170:1416, 1977.

44. Humphrey, E. W., Ewing, S. L., Wrigley, J. V., et al.: The production of malignant tumors of the lung and pleura in dogs from intratracheal asbestos instillation and cigarette smoking. Cancer 47:1994, 1981.

45. James, A. C., Greenhalgh, J. R., and Smith, H.: Clearance of lead-212 ions from rabbit bronchial epithelium to the blood. Phys. Med. Biol. 22:932, 1977.

46. Langer, S., and Peters, H.: Endoscopic cryosurgical treatment of inoperable carcinoma of the esophagus and trachea. Therapiewoche 29:4126, 1979.

47. Lavi, Y., Paladugu, R. R., and Benefield, J. R.: Hypertrophic pulmonary osteoarthropathy in experimental canine lung cancer. J. Thorac. Cardiovasc. Surg. 84:373, 1982.

48. Legendre, A. M., Krahwinkel, D. J., and Spaulding, K. A.: Feline nasal and paranasal sinus tumors. J. Am. Anim. Hosp. Assoc. 17:1038, 1981.

49. Legendre, A. M., Spaulding, K., and Krahwinkel, D. J.: Canine nasal and paranasal sinus tumors. J. Am. Anim. Hosp. Assoc. 19:115, 1983.

50. Lieberman, L. L.: Feline adenocarcinoma of the larynx with metastasis to the adrenal gland. J. Am. Vet. Med. Assoc. 125:153, 1954.

51. MacEwen, E. G., Withrow, S. J., and Patnaik, A. K.: Nasal tumors in the dog: Retrospective evaluation of diagnosis, prognosis, and treatment. J. Am. Vet. Med. Assoc. 170:45, 1977.

52. Madewell, B. R., Priester, W. A., Gilette, E. L., and Synder, S. P.: Neoplasms of the nasal passages and paranasal sinuses in domestic animals as reported by 13 veterinary colleges. Am. J. Vet. Res. 37:851, 1976.

53. Madewell, B. R., Nyland, T. G., and Weigel, J. E.: Regression of hypertrophic osteopathy following pneumonectomy in a dog. J. Am. Vet. Med. Assoc. 172:818, 1978.

54. Matsumura, K., Shors, E. C., Fu, P. C., et al.: Sustained release implants of chemical carcinogens in the canine tracheobronchial tree. Ann. Thorac. Surg. 25:112, 1978.

55. McConnell, E. E., Smit, J. D., and Venter, H. J.: Melanoma in the larynx of the dog. J. S. Afr. Vet. Assoc. 42:189, 1971.

56. Morgan, J. P., Suter, P. F., O'Brien, T. R., and Park, R. D.: Tumors in the nasal cavity of the dog: A radiographic study. J. Am. Vet. Radiol. Soc. 13:18, 1972.

57. Moulton, J. E.: Tumors of the respiratory system. In Moulton, J. E. (ed.): Tumors in Domestic Animals. 2nd ed. Univ. of California Press, Berkeley and Los Angeles, 1978. pp. 216–239.

58. Muggenburg, B. A., Guilmette, R. A., Mewhinney, J. A., et al.: P ≠ 114 dose response studies for inhaled plutonium dioxide in beagle dogs (meeting abstract). Health Phys. 43:117, 1982.

59. Nafe, L. A., Patnaik, A. K., and Lyman, R.: Hypercalcemia associated with epidermoid carcinoma in a dog. J. Am. Vet. Med. Assoc. 176:1253, 1980.

60. Nielson, S. W.: Respiratory system: Classification of tumors in dogs and cats. J. Am. Anim. Hosp. Assoc. 19:20, 1983.

61. Nifatov, A. P., Buldakov, L. A., and Kalmykova, Z. I.: Outcome of polymeric plutonium 239 inhalation in dogs. Radiobiologiia 20:140, 1980.

62. Norris, A. M.: Intranasal neoplasms in the dog. J. Am. Anim. Hosp. Assoc. 15:231, 1979.

63. Park, S. S., Kikkawa, Y., Goldring, I. P., et al.: An animal model of cigarette smoking in beagle dogs. Correlative evaluation of effects on pulmonary function, defence and morphology. Am. Rev. Respir. Dis. 115:971, 1977.

64. Pass, D. A., Huxtable, C. R., Cooper, B. J., et al.: Canine laryngeal oncytomas. Vet. Pathol. 17:672, 1980.

65. Patnaik, A. K., Liu, S. K., Hurvitz, A. I., and MacClelland, A. J.: Nonhematopoietic neoplasms in the cat. J. Natl. Cancer Inst. 54:855, 1975.

66. Pool, J.: Primary lung cancer. In Conn, H. F. (ed.): Current Therapy 1981. W. B. Saunders, Philadelphia, 1981. p. 109.

67. Priester, W. A., and McKay, F. W.: The occurrence of tumors in domestic animals. National Cancer Institute Monograph 54. NIH Pub. No 80-2046, National Cancer Institute, Bethesda, 1980.

68. Reif, J. S., and Cohen, D.: The environmental distribution of canine respiratory tract neoplasms. Arch. Environ. Health 21:136, 1971.

69. Sande, R. D., and Alexander, J. E.: Turbinate bone neoplasms in dogs. Mod. Vet. Pract. 51:23, 1970.

70. Schneider, P. R., Smith, C. W., and Feller, D. L.: Histiocytic LSA of the trachea in a cat. J. Am. Anim. Hosp. Assoc. 15:485, 1979.

71. Sorjonen, D. C., Braund, K. G., and Hoff, E. J.: Paraplegia and subclinical neuromyopathy associated with a primary

lung tumor in a dog. J. Am. Vet. Med. Assoc. *180*:1209, 1982.

72. Staub, E. W., Eisenstein, R., Hars, G., et al.: Bronchogenic carcinoma produced experimentally in the normal dog. J. Thorac. Cardiovasc. Surg. *49*:364, 1965.

73. Staub, E. W., Mills, B., Hass, G. M., et al.: Experimental tracheobronchial carcinoma. Proc. Inst. Med. Chic. *24*:298, 1963.

74. Stunzi, H.: Comparative pathology of carcinoma of the lungs in domestic animals. Pathol. Microbiol. *39*:358, 1973.

75. Stunzi, H., Head, K. W., and Nielson, S. W.: Tumors of the lung. Bull. WHO *500*:9, 1974.

76. Suter, P. F., Carrig, C. B., O'Brien, J., et al.: Radiographic recognition of primary and metastatic pulmonary neoplasms of dogs and cats. J. Am. Vet. Radiol. Soc. *15*:3, 1974.

77. Takemoto, K.: Pulmonary cancer and the environment. J. Saitama Med. School *5*:319, 1979.

78. Taylor, G. N., Shabestari, L., Angus, W., et al.: Primary pulmonic tumors in beagles. Am. J. Vet. Res. *40*:1316, 1979.

79. Thrall, D. E.: Radiation therapy in the dog: Principles, indications, and considerations. Comp. Contin. Educ. Pract. Vet. *4*:752, 1982.

80. Troy, G. C.: Surgical removal of a tracheal osteochondroma. Can. Pract. *5*:47, 1978.

81. Tsubota, N., Simpson, W. J., Van-Nostrand, A. W., et al.: The effects of preoperative irradiation on primary tracheal anastomosis. Ann. Thorac. Surg. *20*:152, 1975.

82. Vasseur, P. B., and Patnaik, A. K.: Laryngeal adenocarcinoma in a cat. J. Am. Anim. Hosp. Assoc. *17*:639, 1981.

83. Veith, L. A.: Squamous cell carcinoma of the trachea. Feline Pract. *4*:30, 1974.

84. Wada, G.: Experimental study on tracheal reconstruction utilizing allo- and xenobioprostheses. Nippon Kyobu Geka Gakkai Zasshi *28*:48, 1980.

85. Wheeldon, E. B., Suter, P. F., and Jenkins, T.: Neoplasia of the larynx of the dog. J. Am. Vet. Med. Assoc. *180*:642, 1982.

86. Withrow, S. J.: Diagnostic and therapeutic nasal flush in the dog. J. Am. Anim. Hosp. Assoc. *13*:704, 1977.

87. Withrow, S. J.: Cryosurgical therapy for nasal tumors in the dog. J. Am. Anim. Hosp. Assoc. *18*:585, 1977.

88. Withrow, S. J., Holmberg, D. I., Doige, C. E., et al.: Treatment of a tracheal osteochondroma with an overlapping end to end tracheal anastomosis. J. Am. Anim. Hosp. Assoc. *14*:469, 1978.

Section **XX**

Anesthetic Considerations in Surgery

Donald C. Sawyer
Section Editor

186 Anesthetic Considerations in Surgery

Donald C. Sawyer

Over the past two decades, much change has occurred in veterinary surgery and anesthesia. The transition from intravenous barbiturates for general anesthesia to inhalation anesthesia with halothane, methoxyflurane, or isoflurane with or without nitrous oxide has provided surgeons the opportunity to develop very delicate and complicated surgical maneuvers. Newer and safer anesthetic techniques provide more time to accomplish surgical and diagnostic procedures. The crucial phase of a surgical illness had been thought to be the operation itself, and survival had been thought to depend upon the animal's response to anesthesia. The question whether a patient in poor physical condition could tolerate anesthesia has undergone modification. Anesthesia is still of major importance in surgery, to be given with skill and good judgment, but it is the selection of appropriate anesthetics and techniques and the quality of pre- and postanesthetic care that largely determine a satisfactory outcome. This change in the overall approach to anesthesia has led to a decrease in operative complications and a reduction in postoperative morbidity and mortality in spite of extremes of age and the greater severity of disease in patients who must undergo anesthesia.

PHYSICAL STATUS

It is difficult to define death caused by anesthesia. The effects of the patient's disease, the operation, the species and breed, the inhalant agents, and the lack of a national veterinary record-keeping system make it impossible to indicate the incidence of deaths attributable to anesthesia. Additional risk might involve the technical skills of an anesthetist or surgeon, economic factors in the hospital that limit the availability of monitoring equipment, extremes in atmospheric conditions, or duration of operation. Often a patient is called a poor risk only after a catastrophe has occurred, which may be a means of consciously or unconsciously concealing errors in diagnosis or management. This problem is solved by categorizing the relative physical conditions of all patients. This system provides a common language and a method of examining anesthetic morbidity and mortality. It is also a means of assessing the relative safety of new techniques.

A useful classification for veterinary patients was modified from that adopted by the American Society of Anesthesiologists.[14] The rank is from best to worst: 1—excellent health, 2—minor impairment, 3—major impairment, 4—seriously ill, 5—moribund, E—emergency.

Class 1—Excellent. An animal with no organic disease or systemic disturbance or an animal in excellent health submitted for elective surgery is considered an excellent risk for anesthesia.

Class 2—Good. An animal with slight-to-moderate systemic disturbance is in this group. Patients with minor fractures, slight dehydration, and obesity and some older patients fit into this category.

Class 3—Fair. Animals with moderate-to-major systemic disturbance, such as chronic heart disease, anemia, open or severe fracture subsequent to trauma, and mild pneumothorax are included in this group.

Class 4—Poor. A patient with an extreme systemic disturbance fits this category. Such a disturbance may be severe enough to result in death, for which surgical or medical intervention requiring anesthesia may be needed to change the course. Ruptures of the urinary bladder, internal hemorrhage, and strangulated and diaphragmatic hernias are examples. In some cases, severe airway problems may be part of the clinical picture. This classification should alert the clinician to employ greater safeguards and select anesthetic agents with great care.

Class 5—Critical. Animals in a moribund state are in the worst category because they are close to death or in the process of dying. Patients with gastric dilation of over 1 hour's duration, severe hypotension due to hemorrhage, or comatose conditions from any cause may be categorized as critical. Animals with acute trauma and in severe shock certainly should be placed in this group.

E—Emergency. This is for any patient in one of the previous classes that is operated upon as an emergency.

PATIENT EVALUATION

The health status of patients can be determined by a variety of criteria. A complete history and physical examination can provide valuable information. Too often, problems are created as a result of inadequate physical examination. A physical examination should follow a set format that includes a description for examination of each body system.

Laboratory tests provide useful information not only for the preanesthetic period but also during and following the anesthetic procedure. Table 186–1 lists the criteria for laboratory analysis and radiographic

TABLE 186–1.   Minimum Diagnostic Information for Patients Scheduled for Anesthesia*†

Patient's Physical Status‡	Patient's Age		
	Less Than 5 Years	*5 to 10 Years*	*More Than 10 Years*
Excellent	Packed cell volume (PCV) Total protein (TP)	PCV TP Blood urea nitrogen (BUN) Urinalysis (UA)§	BUN UA Complete blood count (CBC)‖
Good	PCV TP	PCV TP BUN UA	BUN UA CBC
Fair	BUN UA CBC	CBC UA Profile (P)**	CBC UA P
Poor	CBC UA P	CBC UA P	CBC UA P
Critical	CBC UA P	CBC UA P	CBC UA P

*Reprinted with permission from Sawyer, D. C.: *The Practice of Small Animal Anesthesia.* W. B. Saunders, Philadelphia, 1982.

†In all cases, history should be taken and physical examination should be performed.

‡In an emergency: PCV, TP, BUN, UA, others as indicated and as time permits. For trauma: lateral and VD chest radiographs.

§Includes color, turbidity, specific gravity, pH, protein, glucose, ketones, bilirubin, occult blood, urobilinogen, blood cells, casts, bacteria, sperm, and crystals.

‖Includes PCV, TP, hemoglobin, red and white blood cell counts, differential count, and platelet appearance.

**Includes BUN, glucose, SGPT, Na, K, TP, albumin, globulin, and alkaline phosphatase.

examination prior to anesthesia. These provide a minimum data base that may be expanded as individual circumstances dictate.

HOSPITALIZATION

Whenever possible, it is best to hospitalize patients the day before surgery. The extra time allows more opportunity for patient evaluation, laboratory analysis of health status, and adjustment by animals to the hospital environment. Young patients may tolerate hospitalization better than older pets; consequently, in some circumstances it may be best to have older patients spend a restful night in familiar surroundings at home.

The attitude of the patient before anesthesia is a major determinant to the patient's behavior and attitude during recovery. It is important that animals undergo a peaceful anesthetic induction for a smooth recovery to follow. It is important to consider that the first event the animal will recall upon awakening from anesthesia will probably be the last event that occurred before unconsciousness.

Food and Water Fasting

For animals hospitalized the day before surgery, food should be provided at the regular feeding times. Food should be withheld overnight but the animal may have water *ad libitum.* For animals not hospitalized the night before, the same procedure should be followed, but water consumption should be restricted when the patient reaches the hospital. Nervousness may cause excessive water drinking, which may lead to emesis during the anesthetic procedure. Therefore, water may be withheld from patients anesthetized in the morning and restricted for patients operated on in the afternoon. Providing water for geriatric patients is particularly important to maintain normal renal diuresis before anesthesia.

Care should be taken to avoid food being withheld from hospitalized animals. Food intake may have been restricted or limited because of diagnostic procedures or inappetence. Hospitalized animals are usually fed on a regular schedule once per day; if an animal does not reach the hospital before feeding time or if food is withheld for any reason, an evening feeding should be given to the animal if it is willing to eat.

In animals who have been fed in the morning before surgery, emetics may be used to empty the stomach. If the animal is resting quietly, a delay of 2 to 4 hours should provide time for normal emptying. In either case, however, one cannot be assured that the stomach is completely empty, and procedures for induction and intubation of an animal with a full stomach should be followed.[15] Postponing surgery for 18 to 24 hours is an acceptable alternative.

PREANESTHETIC CONSIDERATIONS

The clinician skilled in a variety of anesthetic techniques and well versed in the pharmacology of anesthesia can solve the problem of choice of agent in many ways. However, choice is dictated by several factors: the individual patient (age, breed, condition and complicating disease[s]); the operation to be performed; and the skill and proficiency of the person performing the surgery. Thus, it is unreasonable to state categorically that there is only one agent or technique for a specific situation—recognizing, however, that there are definite contraindications to certain methods of anesthetic management.

Certainly the "emotional" attitude of our patients must be taken into account in planning anesthesia. Fear and apprehension are manifested by many patients and are easily recognized by those experienced in animal behavior. Disciplined animals have learned to control their anxiety, but certain manipulations, tones of voice of hospital personnel, noise, or other influences may cause them to lose control. These emotional states of mind may be seen as cowering, hiding under bedding, snarling, snapping, hissing, shaking, or just casting doubtful or worried looks. For these apprehensive patients, acetylpromazine,* 0.1 mg/kg but not to exceed 3 mg in any patient, results in a remarkable change in attitude with much easier management for everyone concerned. For aggressive dogs, a neuroleptanalgesic such as Innovar-Vet† is recommended, 1 ml/10 to 12 kg subcutaneously, or intramuscularly.

Anticholinergics

In past years, the frequent use of morphine for preanesthetic medication and the copious oral secretions associated with the use of diethyl ether suggested the prophylactic use of a parasympatholytic agent. As a result, atropine was routinely used for this purpose. However, as new, less irritating inhalation anesthetics were introduced, the apparent need for antisialogogues decreased. However, other uses for these drugs, such as prevention or treatment of severe reflex bradycardia, have resulted in continued use by many clinicians. Reflex slowing of the heart may occur following endotracheal intubation, intrathoracic manipulations, traction on abdominal viscera, stimulation of the carotid sinus, or increased intraocular pressure. From an -esthetic standpoint, many practitioners use anticholinergic agents in canine patients to prevent excessive salivation in the postanesthetic period. At times, dogs salivate excessively during recovery, and, since many patients are discharged to the owners on the same day, animals look better dry than wet.

A major side effect is tachycardia, which can usually be avoided if anticholinergics are selectively given to animals with a preanesthetic heart rate of less than 140 beats per minute. Alternatively, they can be given following induction and maintenance during halothane anesthesia. This side effect has been considered so undesirable by some clinicians that its use is recommended only for specific indications.[2,11]

Atropine sulfate can be given 15 to 30 minutes before induction, subcutaneously, intramuscularly, or intravenously. The dose for dogs and cats is 0.04 mg/kg subcutaneously, 0.02 mg/kg intramuscularly, or 0.01 mg/kg intravenously. Anticholinergic agents should be given when narcotics or xylazine is to be used and they are advised for use with other injectable or inhalation agents. Atropine should not be given to patients with heart rates of over 140 beats per minute or to dogs receiving xylazine for urinary cystometry.[13] Although this is not documented, atropine may not be advisable for use in patients with insulinoma.

In spite of its almost universal acceptance, atropine has a relatively short duration (approximately 2 hours), varying effects on pulse rate, and for unexplained reasons it increases recovery time from thiobarbiturate anesthesia in the dog.[9] The quaternary ammonium compound glycopyrrolate (Robinul*) is almost twice as potent as atropine, and the duration of action is at least three times as long. Because it does not cross the blood brain barriers, central stimulation does not occur. At 0.01 mg/kg subcutaneously 10 minutes before induction, Short and Miller demonstrated its safe use in the dog and cat and it was superior to atropine in preventing bradycardia.[17] In earlier studies, Short and colleagues indicated that glycopyrrolate was effective in preventing aspiration of gastric contents not only by producing a higher pH of gastric secretions but also in the reduction of intestinal smooth muscle activity, thus decreasing the possibility of regurgitation.[18] Tachycardia may also be observed with this drug.

Analgesics

Narcotic agents have been used for many decades as premedication for pentobarbital anesthesia. The combination of morphine-atropine has been the most popular in the United States; the main objective has been to minimize the cardiovascular and respiratory effects of barbiturates.

Although narcotics in general have minimal depressant effects on the heart, most depress ventilation, and a high incidence of vomiting is associated with the use of morphine in the dog. As a result, unless there is a specific need for analgesia in the preanesthetic period, narcotics need not be used unless one is prepared to accept the consequences of depressed respiration or to control breathing during the anesthetic procedure.

Three more commonly used analgesics are meper-

---

*Acepromazine, Fort Doge Laboratories, Fort Dodge, IA.
†Pitman-Moore, Inc., Washington Crossing, NJ.

---

*A. H. Robins Co., Richmond, VA.

idine (Demerol*), 1 mg/kg intramuscularly or subcutaneously, oxymorphone (Numorphan†), 0.1 mg/intramuscularly or subcutaneously, or Innovar-Vet,‡ a fixed combination of fentanyl (narcotic) and droperidol (tranquilizer), 1 ml/12 kg subcutaneously or intramuscularly, which may be given to dogs 20 to 30 minutes before induction. Narcotics produce variable effects in cats, but ketamine (Vetelar,§ Ketaset‖), 2 to 4 mg/kg intramuscularly, may be used in feline patients.

Nalbuphine (Nubain†), butorphanol (Stadol), and pentazocine (Talwin) are agonist/antagonist analgesics that produce minimal sedation and little or no respiratory or cardiovascular depression. They can be given subcutaneously or intramuscularly before anesthesia, with sedation provided by diazepam (Valium**), 0.2 mg/kg, or acetylpromazine, 0.05 mg/kg. They are not currently controlled substances under federal drug regulations.

Tranquilizers

The predominant class of tranquilizers used for veterinary patients is the phenothiazines. As indicated, they are excellent for relieving fear and apprehension. An undesirable side effect of arterial hypotension due to central nervous system depression and peripheral alpha-adrenergic receptor blockade must be expected and is usually mild if moderate doses are used. However, in the presence of hypovolemia from any cause, hypotension may be severe and circulatory failure may occur when the drug is used alone or followed by general anesthesia. Intravenous fluids with balanced electrolytes add volume to the dilated vascular bed and increase venous return to allow maintenance of cardiac output.

One of the more commonly used phenothiazine tranquilizers, acetylpromazine, provides a protective effect against epinephrine-induced ventricular arrhythmias.[12] Experience in the use of this drug indicates that a dose of 0.1 mg/kg intramuscularly or subcutaneously is effective and that no more than 3 mg should be given to any patient regardless of size.

The minor tranquilizer diazepam (Valium) is a benzodiazepine derivative that has a negligible effect on respiration and circulation. It produces mild sedation but has analgesic and muscle-relaxant properties. It is commonly used as a component of balanced anesthesia with narcotics or ketamine at a dose of 0.2 to 0.5 mg/kg intravenously or intramuscularly. Its clinical effect is rather short, lasting 15 to 30 minutes under most circumstances. This drug has found widespread use in veterinary anesthesia in recent years, and it is particularly useful in anesthesia in combination with other drugs.

*Winthrop Laboratories, New York, NY.
†Du Pont Pharmaceuticals, Inc., Manati, PR.
‡Pitman-Moore, Inc., Washington Crossing, NJ.
§Parke, Davis & Company, Detroit, MI.
‖Bristol Laboratories, Syracuse, NY.
**Roche Laboratories, Division of Hoffman–La Roche, Inc., Nutley, NJ.

Xylazine (Rompun*), a sedative/hypnotic/analgesic, has been advocated for use either alone or with ketamine in the dog and cat. Klide and colleagues demonstrated depressant properties of xylazine on the cardiovascular system in the dog[8] and more recently other investigators have shown that when it is combined with ketamine severe consequences may result.[1,10] Muir and coworkers found that xylazine, 1.1 mg/kg, lowered the threshold to ventricular dysrhythmias induced by exogenous epinephrine in the dog.[12] In this study, acetylpromazine raised the threshold whereas the threshold of epinephrine-induced dysrhythmias was lower with xylazine than if no drug had been given as premedication. These studies indicate that xylazine, either when used alone or in combination with ketamine, should not be used in aggressive animals, in patients with a history of heart disease, nor in geriatric patients.

GENERAL PRINCIPLES OF ANESTHESIA

Numerous theories propose mechanisms by which certain agents produce general anesthesia. A specific macroscopic site of action has not been identified, but the most likely sites are in the cortical area of brain and in the reticular formation of the medulla or spinal cord. The synapse is most probably the cellular site of action, but it is not known whether the nerve terminal, the synaptic membrane, or another site is primarily affected. It is clearly recognized that the brain is ultimately involved, but the specific mechanism is not completely understood.

Routes of Administration

Drugs for general anesthesia may be given intravenously, intramuscularly, rectally, orally, or by inhalation. They vary in controllability, but the primary objective is to achieve continuous regulation of anesthetic depth. This is accomplished by producing a partial pressure or concentration of anesthetic that can be decreased or increased promptly as the situation demands. Blood levels of intravenous or inhalation agents are achieved by the same manner; with intravenous agents, injection is made directly into the circulation, whereas the inhalation agents gain rapid entry into the circulation through the large pulmonary surface area. Intramuscular, oral, and rectal routes are less predictable, but certain agents have gained popularity because of their rapid uptake from muscle. Although most volatile liquid anesthetics are metabolized, their biotransformation does not greatly influence clinical recovery. However, injectable agents are inactivated in the body to varying degrees by oxidation, reduction, hydrolysis, or conjugation, and the safety (controllability) of these agents depends on the adequacy of their metabolism. They must be carefully titrated to achieve the desired

*Haver-Lockhart Laboratories, Shawnee, KS.

partial pressure, since once these drugs enter the circulation there is no prompt method of removal. With narcotics, the effects can be reversed with a specific receptor site antagonist such as naloxone (Narcan*), but hepatic metabolism and renal excretion, which may be slow and unpredictable, still must be relied upon for removal from the body. Since inhalation agents enter and leave primarily by the lungs, they provide the most controllable method of producing general anesthesia.

The effect of anesthetics varies according to their concentration in the brain. The concentration is the product of the solubility and partial pressure of the agent in that tissue. The solubility if a constant for each tissue, so the levels change according to the partial pressure. Thus, the concentration of a gas in a mixture is proportional to its partial pressure. These two terms are used interchangeably to describe dosages of inhaled anesthetics. The partial pressure divided by the total pressure equals the concentration, usually expressed in volumes per cent. The term "tension" is also used and is synonymous with partial pressure in both gas mixtures and tissues.

Uptake and Distribution

Inspired gases are initially diluted by other gases in the patient's lung. The alveolar exchange of a gas is relatively rapid and depends on ventilation. The faster the alveolar exchange or washing of gases occurs in the alveoli, the faster the uptake of anesthetics by blood. Once the anesthetic reaches the alveoli, uptake of anesthetic by blood occurs, thus slowing the alveolar anesthetic partial pressure rise. Initally the gradient between the alveolar and blood anesthetic partial pressures is high and is also influenced by the inspired anesthetic concentration and minute ventilation. The movement of gas from alveoli is influenced not only by the gradient but also by the solubility of the anesthetic. Cardiac output and alveolar-to-mixed venous partial pressure difference also determine uptake.

SOLUBILITY

The expression of solubility is the blood/gas partition coefficient. It is the ratio of concentrations of a substance in two phases in equilibrium. It describes the relative capacity per unit volume of two solvents, such as blood and gas, for that anesthetic. It is conventional to express this as blood-to-gas rather than the reverse. This expression is applied to any two phases, such as tissue/blood and oil/gas ratios. In common usage, blood solubility is used interchangeably with blood/gas partition coefficient and tissue solubility with tissue/blood partition coefficient.

Agents with relatively low coefficients such as nitrous oxide (0.47), isoflurane (1.4), enflurane (1.8),

*Pitman-Moore, Inc., Washington Crossing, NJ.

and halothane (2.3), are less soluble and have a slower uptake from the alveoli, and thus alveolar concentration rises more rapidly.[3] Conversely, those agents with high coefficients, such as diethyl ether (12.1) and methoxyflurane (12), are highly soluble and have a greater uptake from the alveoli; therefore, alveolar concentration rises more slowly.

Anesthetic induction is much slower for diethyl ether and methoxyflurane than for the others because of their high blood solubility.

CARDIAC OUTPUT

The second factor that determines anesthetic uptake from the alveoli is blood flow. The greater the blood flow past alveoli, the more anesthetic is removed or taken up by blood.

Initially the anesthetic partial pressure in venous blood is almost zero because the tissues remove most of the anesthetic from arterial blood. However, as uptake by the tissues proceeds, the gradient between tissue and blood decreases. As uptake by tissue decreases, anesthetic concentration in venous blood increases. This decreases the alveolar-to-venous blood anesthetic concentration difference and allows the alveolar anesthetic concentration to rise. This is the most important concept to understand in the relationship between alveolar anesthetic concentration, tissue (brain) partial pressures, and anesthetic depth. The mixed venous blood anesthetic concentration reflects the anesthetic concentration in tissues. The higher the concentration in venous blood, the slower the uptake and the faster the rise in alveolar anesthetic concentration. When the anesthetic concentration in *all* tissues is in equilibrium with that of the blood supplying them, uptake from the lung is zero and the anesthetic concentration in alveoli equals that inspired. This condition rarely occurs during clinical anesthesia but is closer with agents of low solubility, such as nitrous oxide. It would take days or weeks for this to occur with more soluble agents.

Uptake by Tissues

The factors of tissue uptake are the same as those for lung, that is, solubility, arterial-to-tissue anesthetic partial pressure difference, and tissue blood flow. To explain how tissue blood flow determines the rate of uptake, body tissues have been assigned to groups defined by blood flow per unit of tissue volume and by solubility characteristics. Eger has designated tissues as the vessel-rich group, the muscle group, the vessel-poor group, and the fat group.[3] The vessel-rich group includes brain, heart, intestines, kidney, liver, spleen, and endocrine glands. Because of the high blood flow per unit of volume, these tissues equilibrate with arterial anesthetic partial pressures in 5 to 15 minutes; thereafter, uptake becomes negligible. The muscle group includes both skin and skeletal muscle, and, although it constitutes more than 50 per cent of the body mass, it receives less than 20 per cent of the cardiac output. This indicates that equilibrium proceeds at a slower rate and uptake continues over a period of hours. The vessel-poor group includes bones, ligaments, cartilage, and tendons but receives less than 2 per cent of the cardiac output. Therefore this has virtually no influence on the effect of anesthetic uptake. The fat group receives about 5 per cent of the blood supply and constitutes about 20 per cent of the body mass. Anesthetics are more soluble in fat than in other tissues, but blood supply to the fat group limits its uptake.

Factors Affecting Induction

Uptake has been discussed to provide a more physiological or pharmacological view of how inhalation anesthetics enter blood, how they are delivered to tissue, and how they enter and leave tissues. From a clinical standpoint, a number of factors affect the rate at which inhalation agents produce anesthesia.

Ventilation is important, since it is the process by which these agents are brought to the pulmonary capillaries. As alveolar ventilation is increased, more anesthetic molecules are presented to blood, resulting in more rapid equilibration of alveolar-to-inspired anesthetic concentration.

By initially increasing inspired concentration to two to three times the maintenance levels, the larger alveolar-to-arterial gradient forces large numbers of anesthetic molecules into blood and then to tissues, resulting in faster induction. Care must be taken not to make this gradient too high to avoid severe depression of cardiac and respiratory function. As a general rule, to prevent an overshoot, inspired levels above three times minimum alveolar concentration should not be used.

The effect of cardiac output is one factor the anesthetist cannot control but also one that must be recognized. The influence of low cardiac output on uptake is important. With highly soluble agents such as methoxyflurane, if blood flows slowly through the lung it equilibrates with the anesthetic and thus delivers high concentrations in a "bolus" to the brain, heart, and other vessel-rich group tissues, resulting in a sudden induction and perhaps depression of vital functions. If hyperventilation occurs, vasoconstriction as a result of hypocapnia may occur. In addition, cardiac output may decrease because of the physical effects induced by controlled breathing.

Ventilation-perfusion abnormalities may be present in disease states or be produced if one bronchus is intubated. When delayed induction is observed with halothane, the endotracheal tube may be beyond the thoracic inlet and into one bronchus. Delayed induction may also occur in patients with diaphragmatic hernias in which abdominal contents compress the lungs.

The most important influence on alveolar rate of rise is the difference between alveolar concentration and anesthetic concentration in venous blood. Early in induction, venous concentration is low and uptake by tissues is high. As tissue uptake decreases, venous concentration rises. Uptake by blood slows, allowing alveolar concentration to approach equilibrium with pulmonary capillary blood. The rate at which this takes place depends on the tissue/blood partition coefficient, tissue mass, and blood flow.

CONCENTRATION EFFECT AND SECOND GAS EFFECT

These two factors also influence the rate of induction of inhalation agents.[5,19] In addition to the mechanical aspects of ventilation, there is another effect on ventilation during induction and recovery. Uptake of anesthetics by blood in high concentration during induction reduces the volume of gas in the alveoli. Before the next breath, gas moves into the alveoli from the bronchioles, which has the effect of augmenting the volume of gas introduced to the alveoli. During recovery, anesthetics move from blood to alveoli, thus increasing the volume of alveolar gas and effectively causing more gas to be expelled from the alveoli during exhalation. This is the concentration effect, which denotes that the higher the inspired concentration, the more rapid the relative rise in alveolar concentration. Thus, the concentration effect results in a more rapid induction of anesthesia and also aids in recovery. This process occurs with diethyl ether and nitrous oxide, which are delivered in significant volumes. However, more potent agents such as halothane, methoxyflurane, enflurane, and isoflurane are used in such low concentrations that the influence on uptake is minimal.

The second gas effect occurs when two anesthetics are given together. Uptake of a large volume of the first gas in the mixture, e.g., nitrous oxide, augments the inspired volume as does the concentration effect, thus increasing delivery of the second gas, e.g., halothane, to the alveoli. In addition, uptake of the first gas, N_2O, has a concentrating effect on the second gas, which results in a more rapid alveolar rate of rise of the second gas in the presence of the first gas than if used alone. Thus, one of the benefits of nitrous oxide is more rapid induction with halothane. Not only is anesthetic induction faster but also the oxygen partial pressure is higher since oxygen is also a second gas.

Significantly, the concentration effect and the second gas effect have their biggest impact during the first 5 to 10 minutes of induction.

Minimum Alveolar Concentration (MAC)

To express something other than a lethal dose midpoint (LD_{50}) for inhalation anesthetics, it was necessary to express potency without its having a close association with death. Obviously, the anesthesia should be reversible. The MAC is defined as the lowest anesthetic concentration in the alveoli at 1 atmosphere that produces immobility in 50 per cent of humans or animals exposed to a noxious stimulus.[4] It is a measure of anesthetic potency, in which the MAC is the level needed to prevent muscular movement in response to a painful stimulus. Experimentally, the stimulus is produced by clamping the tail of an animal with a large hemostat. The response to skin incision also provides a useful stimulus but is limited to only one observation per patient. Movement of the head, torso, or legs may result, but stiffening, coughing, and hyperventilation are not considered movement. MAC is a useful standard by which all anesthetics may be compared and equals the partial pressure in per cent of 1 atmosphere at the anesthetic site of action. To achieve surgical anesthesia, alveolar anesthetic concentration must be equal to or above MAC. A valuable guide in healthy patients is to maintain surgical anesthesia between 1.25 and 1.75 MAC.

Although extremely useful, MAC measures only a single point on a graded dose-response curve for anesthetics. Nevertheless, no alternative method is available, and MAC has been used widely to evaluate factors that influence anesthetic requirements. The variability of MAC in a single species is small and even between species is relatively narrow (Table 186–2). This fact is especially useful when one is required to anesthetize an unusual pet, such as a skunk or raccoon, in which the variability of injectable agents may be quite large.

Factors that have little effect on MAC include duration of anesthesia, circadian rhythms, hyper- or hypothyroidism, arterial P_{CO_2} up to 90 torr, hyperventilation to a P_{CO_2} of 10 torr, severe metabolic acidosis or alkalosis, arterial P_{O_2} from 40 to 500 torr, anemia to a hematocrit of 10 per cent, and phenylephrine-induced hypertension.[3] Reductions in MAC are found if arterial P_{CO_2} is above 90 torr, Pa_{O_2} is less than 40 torr, or hematocrit is less than 10 per cent. Increasing age reduces MAC, as does hypothermia, but elevation in body temperature increases MAC.

Clinically, a puppy or kitten requires a higher MAC than an elderly adult; thus, care must be taken not to overanesthetize geriatric patients. MAC is increased by intravenous administration of amphetamine, a drug that releases catecholamines. In a clinical situation, an aggravated and aroused animal may have high levels of endogenous catecholamines, which require a higher maintenance concentration initially. As catecholamine levels decrease, however, MAC returns to expected levels. Narcotics, tranquilizers, and other depressants reduce MAC, and the interaction between anesthetics is additive. This is a useful concept in understanding the benefits of balanced anesthesia.[16]

DETERMINATION OF ANESTHETIC DEPTH

The four recognizable phases of anesthesia are I, amnesia and analgesia; II, delirium; III, surgical anesthesia; and IV, premortem.[7] For more accurate estimation of depth, stage III is divided into four planes. For the human patient anesthetized with diethyl ether, Guedel described respiratory changes, pupillary alterations, eye movements, and swallowing and vomiting responses.[7] Gillespie added reflex responses: laryngeal and pharyngeal reactivity, lacrimation, and respiratory response to surgical incision.[6] This system applied only to the unpremedicated human patient allowed to breathe spontaneously during ether anesthesia, a situation that does not exist in modern practice. Anesthetists today use a less well-defined system than Guedel's, but one that is more operational. Anesthetics alter the patient's reaction to various stimuli. It is important to evaluate the stimulus and response in terms of the differences among animals, breeds, and species, a problem unique to the veterinary anesthetist.[16]

Stimulus-Response Assessment

Because of the routine use of intravenous "crash" induction techniques, the stages of sedation, analgesia, and delirium usually are not seen. Even during

TABLE 186–2. MAC Values (Per Cent of 1 Atmosphere) for Anesthetics in Various Species and Classes*

Agent	Dog	Cat	Horse	Human	Monkey	Rat or Mouse	Goldfish	Toad
Methoxyflurane	0.23	0.23		0.16		0.27	0.13	0.22
Halothane	0.87	0.82	0.88	0.75	0.89	1.14	0.76	0.67
		1.14						
Isoflurane	1.28	1.63	1.31	1.15		1.38		
Enflurane	2.2	1.2		1.68				
	2.06							
Diethyl ether	3.04	2.1		1.92		3.2	2.2	1.64
	3.29							
N₂O	188			105	200	Mouse 150		82.2
	222	255				Rat 136		

*Reproduced in part with permission from Quasha, A. L., et al.: Determination and applications of MAC. Anesthesiology 53:315, 1980. Reprinted with permission from Sawyer, D. C.: *The Practice of Small Animal Anesthesia.* W. B. Saunders, Philadelphia, 1982.

inhalation induction, Guedel's stages I and II are not easily separated and may be regarded as a single level—presurgical anesthesia. Signs of this change from presurgical to surgical anesthesia are loss of palpebral reflex, onset of muscle relaxation, and onset of rhythmic breathing. If these have not occurred, the patient is still at the presurgical level and stimulation must be avoided. When these signs are present, surgical anesthesia can be evaluated.

Presurgical anesthesia, surgical anesthesia, and anesthetic overdose define the magnitude of anesthetic depression. Surgical anesthesia may be subjectively divided into three planes: too light, adequate, or too deep (Table 186–3). The anesthetist must evaluate the intensity of stimulation to the nervous system, observe the physiological responses, and then interpret the interaction among patient, stimulus, and anesthetic to deduce the level of surgical anesthesia. The difficulty of learning anesthetic assessment is brought into perspective when one compares the signs produced by halothane-nitrous oxide with those produced by ketamine in the cat. With halothane-N_2O, muscle relaxation is present and palpebral responses are absent, whereas the opposite occurs with ketamine.

Stimulus

The intensity of pain stimulation is quite variable. The most intense pain results from skin and joint capsule incision, periosteal stimulation, fracture manipulation, visceral or peritoneal traction, diaphrag-

matic stimulation, manipulation of the cornea, and excessive distension of the urinary bladder. During surgical anesthesia at a level that previously seemed adequate, the patient may show signs of light anesthesia such as tachycardia, tachypnea, or even movement whenever one or more of these events occur. In anticipation, the anesthetist may increase the anesthetic concentration briefly, fully aware of the further depression of cardiopulmonary function, and then return the concentration to the previous level when appropriate. Weak stimulation results from toe pinch, wound debridement, mild distension of the bladder, and manipulation of fascia or muscle without traction. Inflammation of the tissue usually increases the intensity of the stimulus, and careful handling decreases it. Younger animals may show an increased intensity, whereas older animals and animals with a fair, poor, or critical physical status may have a decreased response. For this reason, the high-risk patient is more difficult to monitor.

If the anesthetist is to maintain the appropriate level of anesthesia, surgical activity must be considered along with the patient's responses. Too often anesthesia is maintained unnecessarily deep to prevent any type of movement, instead of being at the appropriate level for the type of surgery being performed.

Response

Evaluation of responses from painful stimulation during anesthesia is difficult for the beginner, but

TABLE 186–3. **Evaluations of Response to Painful Stimulation During Anesthesia***

Level of Anesthesia	Sensory Response	Motor Response	Reflexes		
			Circulatory	*Respiratory*	*Gastrointestinal*
Too light	Breath holding Deep breathing Stiff chest Phonation Laryngospasm Tachycardia Rise or fall in BP Movement with stimulus Coughing	Fine or gross movement Abdominal tightness	Bradycardia and hypotension or Tachycardia and hypertension Arrhythmias	Spasm: laryngeal bronchiolar Salivation Dysrhythmic breathing	Retching Vomiting Swallowing
Adequate	Minimal response to painful stimuli followed by accommodation	Quiet surgical field Relaxation of skeletal muscles	Absence of troublesome CV, respiratory, and GI reflexes		
Too deep	No response	Flaccid muscles Inability to re-establish normal breathing at the end of anesthesia	Bradycardia Tachycardia Hypotension	Arrest (in the absence of hypocapnia)	Intestinal atony Postoperative ileus

*Modified from Dripps, R. D., Eckenhoff, J. E., and Vandam, L. D.: *Introduction to Anesthesia*. 5th ed. W. B. Saunders, Philadelphia, 1977. Reprinted with permission from Sawyer, D. C.: *The Practice of Small Animal Anesthesia*. W. B. Saunders, Philadelphia, 1982.

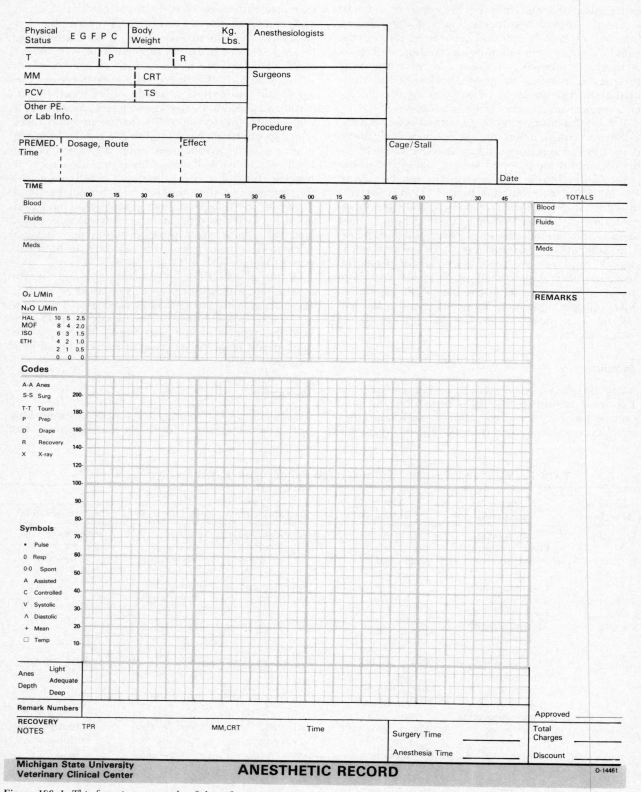

Figure 186–1. This form is an example of the information contained on an anesthetic record. Abbreviations: *E*, excellent; *G*, good; *F*, fair; *P*, poor; *C*, critical; *T*, temperature; *P*, pulse; *R*, respiratory rate; *MM*, mucous membrane color; *CRT*, capillary refill time; *PCV*, packed cell volume; *TS*, total solids; *PE*, physical exam; *Hal*, halothane; *MOF*, methoxyflurane; *Iso*, isoflurane; *ETH*, ethrane. The patient and client information is imprinted in the top right corner.

with experience one finds the combination of signs a useful guide to anesthetic depth. The three components of evaluation are classified as sensory, motor, and reflex functions. Intensity of these responses is separated into three levels: high (light anesthesia), adequate (acceptable anesthesia), and low (deep anesthesia) (Table 186–3). A comparison of strength of the surgical stimulus and observation of intensity of response is what the good anesthetist learns and practices to deliver the appropriate anesthetic level. When the high-risk patient cannot tolerate deeper anesthesia, a neuromuscular blocker may be used to provide the muscle relaxation needed. Also, as uptake of inhaled anesthetic continues and approaches equilibration with levels in body tissues, inspired concentrations are gradually reduced to avoid deeper anesthesia than necessary. Surgical anesthesia usually appears to be deeper than it really is, and one may need to lighten inspired concentrations to determine the appropriate level needed.

THE ANESTHETIC RECORD

The record is an essential part of any anesthetic procedure and is of undeniable value to the patient, surgeon, and anesthetist. An example is presented in Figure 186–1. If pulse rate, respiration, and other variables have been monitored, they should be recorded to better allow continuous assessment of the patient's condition. A good anesthetic record is also helpful if a patient must be anesthetized again, and it is the only means of recording the events occurring from the preanesthetic period through recovery. For medico-legal reasons, it is wise to keep accurate records, because a written review of established events is far better than an account reconstructed from memory. In clinical practice, anesthetic records can be used to better assess procedures and techniques, to establish a good system of disciplined monitoring by technical assistants, and to teach interns and residents. The usefulness of records has been evident at academic institutions for improved patient care, research, and teaching, and the short time spent on making them pays great dividends.

Patient care should never be sacrificed for sake of the record. At times the patient demands the anesthetist's complete attention, and it would be foolish to withdraw attention to maintain the record. However, one can recap the events a short time later, when a reasonably detailed account of the procedure can be made.

Records should also be kept for careful analysis of the circumstances related to the death of every patient who has received an anesthetic. As a general rule, a death that occurs during the interval between induction and recovery is considered an anesthetic death. If anesthetic management in its broadest terms does not appear to have contributed to the death,

then other events may be given as the cause. It is best to be overcritical and not to dismiss anesthesia as the cause. Probably the most common reason for death during anesthesia is the lack of recognition of a cardiac arrest; the most common cause of arrest is cardiovascular depression as a consequence of deeper anesthesia than is needed under the circumstances. Occasionally, an animal may expire during anesthesia and the cause cannot be attributed to anything other than the fact that the patient was anesthetized. This occurrence is relatively rare and may be in the range of 1 in 5,000 to 10,000 procedures.

1. Clark, D. M., Martin, R. A., and Short, C. E.: Cardiopulmonary responses to xylazine/ketamine anesthesia in the dog. J. Am. Anim. Hosp. Assoc. *18*:815, 1982.
2. Dripps, R. D., Eckenhoff, J. E., and Vandam, L. D.: Premedication, transport to the operating room and preparation for anesthesia. *In: Introduction to Anesthesia; The Principles of Safe Practice*. 6th ed. W. B. Saunders, Philadelphia, 1982.
3. Eger, E. I., II: *Anesthetic Uptake and Action*. Williams & Wilkins, Baltimore, 1974.
4. Eger, E. I., II, Saidman, L. J., and Brandstater, B.: Minimum alveolar anesthetic concentration: A standard of anesthetic potency. Anesthesiology *26*:756, 1965.
5. Epstein, R. M., Rachow, H., Salanitre, E., and Wolf, G. L.: Influence of the concentration effect on the uptake of anesthetic mixtures: The second gas effect. Anesthesiology *25*:364, 1964.
6. Gillespie, N. A.: The signs of anesthesia. Anesth. Analg. *22*:275, 1943.
7. Guedel, A. E.: *Inhalation Anesthesia*. 2nd ed. Macmillan, New York, 1971.
8. Klide, A. M., Calderwood, H. W., and Soma, L. R.: Cardiopulmonary effects of xylazine in dogs. Am. J. Vet. Res. *36*:931, 1975.
9. Klide, A. M., Rivas, C., and Peters, J.: Effect of atropine sulfate on thiopental-induced sleeping time in the dog. J. Am. Vet. Med. Assoc. *164*:1029, 1974.
10. Kolata, R. J., and Rawlings, C. A.: Cardiopulmonary effects of intravenous xylazine, ketamine, and atropine in the dog. Am. J. Vet. Res. *43*:2196, 1982.
11. Muir, W. W.: Effects of atropine on cardiac rate and rhythm in dogs. J. Am. Vet. Med. Assoc. *172*:917, 1978.
12. Muir, W. W., Werner, L. L., and Hamlin, R. L.: Effects of xylazine and acetylpromazine upon induced ventricular fibrillation in dogs anesthetized with thiamylal and halothane. Am. J. Vet. Res. *36*:1299, 1975.
13. Oliver, J. E., Jr., and Young, W. O.: Air cystometry in dogs under xylazine-induced restraint. Am. J. Vet. Res. *34*:1433, 1973.
14. Sawyer, D. C.: The preanesthetic period. *In: The Practice of Small Animal Anesthesia*. W. B. Saunders, Philadelphia, 1982.
15. Sawyer, D. C.: The induction period. *In: The Practice of Small Animal Anesthesia*. W. B. Saunders, Philadelphia, 1982.
16. Sawyer, D. C.: The anesthetic period. *In: The Practice of Small Animal Anesthesia*. W. B. Saunders, Philadelphia, 1982.
17. Short, C. E., and Miller, R. L.: Comparative evaluation of the anticholinergic agent glycopyrrolate as a preanesthetic agent. Vet. Med./Small Anim. Clin. *74*:1269, 1978.
18. Short, C. E., Paddleford, R. R., and Cloyd, G. D.: Glycopyrrolate for prevention of pulmonary complications during anesthesia. Mod. Vet. Pract. *55*:194, 1974.
19. Stoelting, R. K., and Eger, E. I., II: An additional explanation for the second gas effect. Anesthesiology *30*:273, 1969.

Chapter 187

Anesthetics and Anesthetic Effects

Donald C. Sawyer

Inhalation anesthesia began in the mid-1800s with the discovery of ether and nitrous oxide as anesthetics, and when cyclopropane was introduced as an anesthetic agent for humans in 1934, true inhalation anesthesia found favor in both England and the United States.[23,26] Precision equipment was developed for delivery of halothane and methoxyflurane. Extensive research has provided improved techniques that allow the opportunity for intricate diagnostic and surgical procedures. Inhalation anesthetics have probably made a larger contribution than injectable agents, but since the development of new narcotic agents, balanced techniques using a combination of agents for anesthesia have been the most significant addition in recent years. Ideally, the use of inhalation agents should permit regulation of partial pressures on a continuous basis to obtain the precise level of anesthesia needed to control response to pain. Although inhalation anesthetics are metabolized to varying degrees, their administration and elimination occur primarily through the alveoli. Inhalation agents provide the most easily controllable method of general anesthesia.

CHARACTERISTICS OF INHALATION ANESTHESIA

Vapor Pressure and Boiling Point

The physical properties of gases and volatile liquids influence their uptake and distribution in the body, determine the way the compounds are provided for use, and dictate the types of vaporizers needed for delivery. General laws of physics govern diffusion, solubility in body fluids, and relationships of pressure, volume, and temperature. The heat of vaporization should be low enough to prevent excessive cooling as the liquid vaporizes, and the vapor pressure must be high enough so that sufficient anesthetic is delivered for the desired effect. The most important function of precision or calibrated vaporizers is to control heat lost from vaporization and to operate efficiently through a wide range of temperatures. If saturation or wick vaporizers are used, attention must be given to the influence of temperature extremes from normal. Table 187–1 lists vapor pressures at 20°C (68°F), but they may be as high as 24°C (75.2°F). When using saturation or wick-type vaporizers, the anesthetist should consult manufacturer's tables if a deviation in ambient temperature greater than 4°C (7.2°F) is anticipated.

Reactivity, Stability, and Flammability

Anesthetics are soluble in rubber and plastic breathing circuits of anesthetic systems.[16] Although the solubility is less in plastic than rubber, plastic circuits are usually not as resistant to deterioration, but either becomes useless with time. Absorption of anesthetics causes deformation, and holes or cracks eventually develop. Absorption of anesthetics in the breathing components may be sufficient (especially with more soluble agents) to affect a second patient given an anesthetic through the same circuit. All volatile liquids are excellent solvents and may corrode brass, solder, and aluminum.

Nitrous oxide supports combustion, but with the exception of diethyl ether, none of the modern agents are flammable in the anesthetic range. Because of its explosive nature, diethyl ether must never be stored in an area where a flame or spark may ignite the vapor. To prevent explosion, it must never be stored in a refrigerator that is not explosion-proof, nor should animals that have been euthanized with the agent be refrigerated.

Part of the emphasis on development of new inhalation agents has been the characteristic of non-flammability. The fluorinated ethers, methoxyflur-

TABLE 187–1.   Some Physical and Chemical Properties of Inhalation Anesthetics

Agent	Formula	Boiling Point (°C)	Vapor Pressure at 20°C (torr)
Nitrous oxide	N_2O	−89	—
Diethyl ether	CH_3-CH_2-O-CH_2-CH_3	35	450
Halothane	$CF_3CHBrCl$	50.2	243
Methoxyflurane	CH_3-O-CF_2-CCl_2H	104.6	23
Enflurane	$CFHCl$-CF_2-O-CHF_2	56.5	180
Isoflurane	CF_3-$CHCl$-O-CHF_2	48.5	250

(From Dripps, R. D., Eckenhoff, J. E., and VanDam, L. D.: *Introduction to Anesthesia.* 5th ed. W. B. Saunders, Philadelphia, 1977.)

ane, isoflurane, enflurane, and the fluorinated hydrocarbon halothane are all nonflammable in clinical concentrations below 25°C (77°F).

Effect of Inhalation Anesthetics on the Heart and Circulation

Cardiac output is controlled primarily by the demand of body tissues for blood. Each area regulates its own vascular supply to provide adequate oxygen and other nutrients and to remove tissue metabolites. In unanesthetized subjects, whatever the demand of tissues for perfusion, the same amount of blood is returned to the heart and ejected. In general, although almost all anesthetics depress cardiovascular function, the heart pumps the blood it receives. Depression of myocardial contractility is one of the fundamental secondary actions of general anesthetics. The effect is dose related and reversible and has been demonstrated both *in vitro* and *in vivo*. The primary effect is inhibition of myocardial contraction, with decreased time of contraction being secondary.

TYPES OF INHALATION AGENTS

Gaseous Anesthetics

Nitrous Oxide. Nitrous oxide was first prepared by Joseph Priestley more than 200 years ago, but Humphrey Davy is credited with describing its anesthetic properties in 1799.[7] Another 50 years passed before its analgesic effects were demonstrated by Horace Wells, when a fellow dentist extracted one of Wells's teeth while Gardner Quincy Colton administered the gas. Since the late 1800s, the popularity of nitrous oxide in human anesthesia has developed to the point that more techniques of general anesthesia are based on its use than on that of any other agent.

The popularity of nitrous oxide in veterinary anesthesia has grown in recent years because of its use at teaching institutions and in practice by clinicians who have learned to appreciate its advantages. Although its maximum allowable concentration (MAC) in dogs is 188 per cent, 66 per cent nitrous oxide reduces halothane MAC 22 ± 8.4 per cent.[5] The lack of potency is obviated by continuous or intermittent intravenous injection of opioids, or inhalation anesthetics. This, combined with the use of a neuromuscular blocker, is especially valuable in high-risk patients. Anesthesia obtained with halothane or methoxyflurane is achieved with lower concentrations when nitrous oxide is used than when either agent is used alone. Spontaneous breathing is enhanced by nitrous oxide; alveolar ventilation is benefited by its sympathomimetic properties. Such a combination provides more satisfactory induction and a better operative and postanesthetic course. Excessive depth of anesthesia may be avoided, and circulatory and respiratory depression of the more potent agents is lessened to some extent by the mild sympathetic-stimulating properties of nitrous oxide, providing a valuable adjunct to general anesthesia.

Precautions. Nitrous oxide must not be used in the presence of pneumothorax or in any situation in which air is trapped in body viscera. Its high partial pressures in blood coupled with its low solubility cause it to diffuse into air-containing body cavities.[10] The relative increase in volume results from the inability of nitrogen to diffuse into blood at the same rate as the influx of nitrous oxide because of the lower solubility of nitrogen in blood. The net result is distension of the intestine or, in the case of pneumothorax, an increase in intrathoracic pressure and a decrease in lung volume. The pressure-volume relationship compromises both ventilation and circulation, and death occurs if the problem is not recognized. Therefore, with intestinal obstruction, air or nitrogen-containing gas is trapped, and nitrous oxide must be avoided. Procedures such as pneumocystography may produce venous emboli. Nitrous oxide dissolved in blood enlarges air emboli, should they occur, and causes death.

Nitrous oxide should not be used in patients with respiratory dysfunction. In these patients, the inspired oxygen tension should be high to avoid hypoxemia. This includes patients with significant space-occupying lesions in the thorax and those with diaphragmatic hernia, pulmonary disease, alveolar-to-arterial diffusion abnormalities, and pulmonary edema.

At the termination of anesthesia with nitrous oxide, the patient must *not* be allowed to breathe room air abruptly. Because of the relative difference in solubility of nitrogen and nitrous oxide, a large volume of nitrous oxide diffuses into the alveoli faster than the uptake of nitrogen by blood. This lowers the alveolar oxygen pressure, producing diffusion hypoxia.[20] This situation can be avoided by administering 100 per cent oxygen 2 to 3 minutes before tracheal extubation, or by mask should the patient be inadvertently extubated while breathing nitrous oxide. The same process occurs during mask induction with nitrous oxide if a patient is allowed to breathe room air for more than 45 seconds while being intubated. Treatment of diffusion hypoxia with oxygen is a simple process, and therefore one need not panic at the sign of cyanosis as long as prompt attention is given to the problem.

Volatile Liquids

Diethyl ether. Diethyl ether (CH_3-CH_2-O-CH_2-CH_3) is an excellent anesthetic and is still used to some extent in veterinary practice. It provides good analgesia and muscle relaxation, but its flammability and explosive properties are its main disadvantages. Its high solubility in blood ($\lambda = 12.1$), high vapor pressure (450 torr at 20°C or 68°F), and high MAC value (3.04 ± 0.53 per cent) all combine to require large amounts of the agent. It is commonly delivered by open drop techniques, although in-the-circle draw-over wick vaporizers are adequate. Because of its flammability, irritating properties, and the advantages of newer and more potent anesthetics, it is seldom used for general anesthesia in clinical practice. It must be stored in sealed metal containers coated with copper or another metal that prevents light oxidation. Diethyl ether should *never* be kept in nonexplosive-proof refrigerators or around any potential source of sparks or flames.

Halothane. This anesthetic, credited with revolutionizing the field of anesthesia, brought with it a more scientific approach to understanding the action and influences of inhalation anesthetics. Halothane has a molecular structure ($CF_3CHBrCl$) that features chemical stability, nonflammability, and good potency. The fluoride group is inert and also provides stability and nonflammability. In 1959, this agent began to gain popularity for human anesthesia, and in the early to mid-1960s veterinarians began to use it. Halothane (Fluothane*, Halothane USP†) has steadily increased in use to become the predominant inhalation agent in veterinary anesthesia. It is relatively inexpensive and provides rapid and smooth induction. Surgical anesthesia is easily maintained, vital functions remain stable, yet anesthetic depth can be quickly adjusted. Because of halothane's relatively low solubility in blood ($\lambda = 2.3$), mask or chamber induction of small patients is easy. Emergence from anesthesia is smooth, and animals usually rest quietly during recovery. With the rapid return of protective airway reflexes and consciousness, most patients become ambulatory within 15 minutes.

Because of its high vapor pressure (243 torr at 20°C or 68°F) and high potency (MAC = 0.90 ± 0.12 per cent), halothane must be delivered from a saturation or precision vaporizer. During clinical anesthesia, equilibration with vessel-rich tissues, which include brain, may be achieved during the first 10 to 15 minutes by keeping inspired concentration between 1.5 and 2.5 per cent. Once surgical anesthesia is reached in healthy patients, the vaporizer setting is maintained between 1.0 and 1.5 per cent until surgery begins. MAC for the dog is 22.2 ± 8.4 per cent lower when combined with 66 per cent nitrous oxide.[5] In general, vaporizer settings can be reduced by 0.5 per cent when halothane is used with 66 per cent nitrous oxide because of the reduction in MAC and the augmented alveolar ventilation by nitrous oxide.

Methoxyflurane. Methoxyflurane (CH_3-O-CF_2-CCl_2H) was introduced as an anesthetic for humans by Artusio in 1959, and by 1963 it gained popularity for use in animals. With the promotion of the anesthetic (Metofane‡) as well as equipment for delivery, inhalation anesthesia began its rise in prominence to replace the use of long-acting barbiturates in clinical veterinary anesthesia. It is the most potent and least

volatile of the liquid anesthetics. Vapor pressure at room temperature ranges between 22 and 25 torr, with the saturated concentration reaching about 3 per cent. Unless the liquid temperature is raised, this is the maximum concentration that can be achieved, which is well below the flammable range. MAC is 0.24 ± 0.03 per cent, and the blood/gas partition coefficient of 12 ranks methoxyflurane with diethyl ether as the most soluble of the inhalation agents. Because of the high solubility coefficient, induction is slow and anesthetic levels change more gradually. Unless vaporizer concentration is reduced early in anticipation of recovery, emergence from anesthesia is delayed. For healthy and spontaneously breathing dogs, the vaporizer in the circle is set at the full open position immediately after thiobarbiturate induction; when anesthetic level is reached, maintenance settings range between 4 and 6. For the vaporizer out of the circle, 2.5 per cent concentration is initially used and then shortly reduced to 1.5 per cent. Maintenance levels range from 0.5 to 1.5 per cent, depending on adequacy of ventilation and duration of the procedure. The high solubility of methoxyflurane in rubber causes loss of large amounts of the drug into the breathing conduits, further slowing induction. However, the absorbed anesthetic can be used to maintain light levels of anesthesia as termination of surgery is approached.

Although it has some limitations because of its high solubility and low vapor pressure, methoxyflurane is still one of the most popular inhalation anesthetics used in small animal practice in the United States.

Enflurane. Chemists have continued to search for better anesthetics that have lower solubility and are more metabolically stable. Interest has been focused on the ethers, and Terrell synthesized enflurane (Ethrane*) ($CFHCl$-CF_2-O-CHF_2) in 1963 and its isomer, isoflurane (Forane, Aerrane),*† in 1965.[8] Enflurane is probably the most popular of the volatile liquids used for anesthesia of humans. It is a stable, nonflammable liquid, slightly less volatile than halothane (Vapor pressure [P_{VAP}] = 180 at 20°C or 68°F); MAC in dogs is 2.2 ± 0.26 per cent, and the blood/gas partition coefficient is 1.78.[8] Enflurane produces rapid induction, easy maintenance when used with thiobarbiturate induction or tranquilizer premedication, and rapid recovery. Cardiac rhythm is stable, and there is only mild sensitization of the heart to epinephrine.

Anesthesia with enflurane alone in dogs is accompanied, in a high percentage of patients, by signs of motor hyperactivity such as muscle twitching and jerks of the head, body, and extremities. These signs are more pronounced at deeper levels of enflurane anesthesia and are accompanied by EEG seizure patterns.

Clinical trials for use in veterinary anesthesia were conducted in late 1979 and early 1980. Because of

---

*Fort Dodge Laboratories, Fort Dodge, IA.
†Halocarbon, Inc., Hackensack, NJ.
‡Pitman-Moore, Inc., Washington Crossing, NJ.

*Anaquest, Madison, WI.
†Forane is human label; Aerrane is veterinary label.

muscle movement that occurs in dogs and the questionable results of its trial use in cats, the popularity of enflurane in veterinary anesthesia will probably not reach the same level as in human anesthesia. Because of the cardiovascular stability associated with its use, this agent could be valuable for high-risk canine patients.

Isoflurane. Isoflurane (Forane, Aerrane)* (CF_3-CHCl-O-CHF_2), an isomer of enflurane, was introduced for clinical trials in human patients in 1969. It was studied extensively but was withdrawn temporarily because of reports of carcinogenic properties in rats.[3] In 1980, isoflurane was approved for use in human anesthesia, and clinical studies for use in veterinary patients were initiated in the same year.

The vapor pressure of isoflurane at 20°C (68°F) is 250 torr, MAC in dogs is 1.28 per cent, and its solubility coefficient is 1.41.[8] It does not produce the central nervous excitation or seizure activity that accompanies enflurane. Arterial pressure is decreased owing to a drop in peripheral vascular resistance, but perfusion in all vascular beds is maintained. Cardiac performance is stable and relaxation is excellent, but isoflurane is a respiratory depressant. With faster induction, metabolic stability, better control of anesthetic levels, and quick recovery, this drug is likely to play a major role in future anesthesia.[9] Its vapor pressure is similar to halothane. Therefore, with certain precautions isoflurane can be used in vaporizers calibrated for halothane.[22]

INJECTABLE ANESTHESIA

Barbiturates and Thiobarbiturates

Ultra-short-acting drugs are commonly used for anesthesia induction. These include thiopental, thiamylal, and methohexital. The principal use of these hypnotics is to quickly achieve anesthesia and unconsciousness, but they can also be used for maintenance. In the absence of inhalation agents, an injectable agent is one alternative for general anesthesia. Pentobarbital, on the other hand, has been used for general anesthesia since the 1930s and still is used to some extent. Because of difficulty in achieving control, prolonged recovery time, and profound respiratory depression associated with the barbituric acid derivatives, their use for general anesthesia has been supplanted by inhalation techniques.

The intravenous barbiturates can produce any degree of central nervous system depression, ranging from mild sedation to deep coma. The individual patient's tolerance, physical condition, and dose administered all determine the total effect. The mode of action is thought to be depression of the short synaptic pathways in the central reticular core of the medulla, with sparing of direct spinolemniscothalamic pathways. Thiobarbiturates are poor analgesics,

and recognition of these differences is essential for the rational use of such agents for general anesthesia. Certain patients may require excessive doses for adequate anesthesia. Often the degree of anesthesia appears adequate, but subsequent to surgical stimulation, movement or struggling may occur, indicating insufficient afferent blockade. The thiobarbiturates also sensitize vagal nerve endings, which may lead to laryngospasm—further evidence that the afferent pathways are not blocked. Under these circumstances, additional anesthetic must be administered carefully.

With thiopental, 22 mg/kg intravenously, or thiamylal, 16 mg/kg intravenously, surgical anesthesia may be provided for 15 minutes. Additional doses may be given to prolong the effect, with the objective of keeping drug levels in plasma and brain sufficient for anesthetic maintenance. The rate of metabolic removal is 10 to 15 per cent per hour; thus the more injected, the longer the recovery.

Complications. Extravascular injection of the alkaline thiobarbiturates may result in vasospasm, with eventual ulceration of the affected area. Careful observation of the site of injection can prevent this unnecessary complication. The best method is to insert an intravascular catheter first and assure proper placement before administering the drug. Either a balanced electrolyte drip is started and the drug given concurrently, or an injection cap is attached to the catheter to permit intermittent injection of the anesthetic.

Ventricular arrhythmias may persist into the anesthetic period with thiobarbiturates. Bigeminal rhythm is most common with thiamylal, and unless pulse rate is below 70, treatment is usually unnecessary in healthy patients. Usually this effect is transient. Muir and others have found that ventricular bigeminy is directly correlated with the increase in tension imposed on the myocardium by increased arterial blood pressure.[17] Transiently decreasing venous return by holding end-inspiratory pressure at 20 to 25 cm H_2O for 15 to 30 seconds may remove the dysrhythmia. Should more frequent and more severe ventricular dysrhythmias occur, appropriate treatment is lidocaine, 0.5 to 3 mg/kg intravenously, in dogs or 0.01 mg/kg acetylpromazine administered intravenously until the problem is resolved. The combined use of thiopental sodium and lidocaine may be indicated for induction of anesthesia in dogs with cardiopulmonary disease.[1]

Dissociative Anesthetics

Ketamine. Ketamine (Ketaset,* Vetalar†), an analogue of phencyclidine, has a shorter duration of action, and its use has become more common in feline anesthesia. The action of this compound is not

---

*Anaquest, Madison, WI; Forane is human label; Aerrane is veterinary label.

*Bristol Laboratories, Syracuse, NY
†Parke, Davis & Company, Detroit, MI

clearly understood, but ketamine seems to interrupt cerebral association pathways while leaving the reticular activating and limbic systems intact and depressing the thalamoneocortical system.[27] The dissociative anesthetic state associated with this drug is characterized by catalepsy, amnesia, profound somatic analgesia, near-normal pharyngeal-laryngeal reflexes, and excessive skeletal muscle tone.

Ketamine has a rapid onset of effect and relatively shorter duration of action than phencyclidine because redistribution from brain to other tissues, metabolism, and excretion are more rapid. Recovery usually occurs in 2 to 6 hours. Prolonged duration of effect may occur in healthy patients, owing probably to abnormal metabolites. Some of the metabolites of ketamine have analgesic effects and contribute to the anesthetic action of the parent compound.[12] The eyes usually remain open, and the cornea must be protected with an ophthalmic solution to prevent drying. Because salivation is common, an anticholinergic may be given as premedication. Circulatory stimulation is evidenced by hypertension and tachycardia, and cerebrospinal fluid pressure is elevated. These adrenergic cardiovascular responses are secondary to vagal inhibition of baroreceptor reflexes. Myocardial oxygen consumption is increased; therefore the use of ketamine in patients with heart disease is inadvisable. Because it is metabolized by the liver and also excreted unchanged by the kidneys, this drug should not be used in animals with hepatic or renal disease. It is currently approved for use only in cats and primates, as clinical evaluation of the drug in the dog was associated with a high incidence of postanesthetic convulsions. Occasionally, tonic-clonic spasms may occur in cats during the recovery phase.

Intramuscular injection of ketamine is usually painful, and restraint is advisable. Dosages range from 10 to 30 mg/kg, which will produce recumbency in 3 to 6 minutes and provide anesthesia for 20 to 60 minutes. In young cats, the higher doses are required and duration may be shorter.

Acetylpromazine, 0.2 to 0.4 mg/kg intramuscularly, can be given with ketamine or, preferably, 10 to 15 minutes before ketamine injection. The dose of intramuscular ketamine should then be kept below 25 mg/kg.

Intravenous administration of 4 to 8 mg/kg of ketamine has a more rapid onset of action, and recovery occurs in 1 to 2 hours. The anesthetic period is shorter, but additional doses of 0.5 to 1 mg/kg may be given as needed. Intubation of the ketamine-anesthetized patient is highly recommended.

Ketamine has been used in mice, rats, dogs, pigeons, and various exotic species. It is used in clinical practice in dogs in combination with acetylpromazine or xylazine for restraint or minor surgery. However, ketamine is not approved by the Food and Drug Administration for use in dogs.

The mixture of diazepam and ketamine is a useful and effective combination. Equal volumes of these two drugs can be placed in the same syringe and given slowly at a dose of 1 ml/5 to 10 kg intravenously. This combination has shown promise for use in human patients,[6] and experience in cats indicates that it is an excellent method for intravenous induction prior to maintenance with inhalation agents. It can also be used alone for minor procedures and may be preferable for balanced techniques in high-risk feline patients.

Indications. Ketamine is useful in cats for short diagnostic procedures and superficial operations such as onychectomy, castration, and minor lacerations. It can also be used intravenously in high-risk patients, but extreme caution must be taken because of the lack of control and the longer recovery periods compared with inhalation agents. The use of nitrous oxide with ketamine is particularly advantageous. Because of its questionable ability to ablate abdominal visceral pain, ketamine should *never* be used alone as an anesthetic for ovariohysterectomy or other abdominal surgical procedures.[11]

Precautions. Because of the simplicity of administration of ketamine, carelessness in its use can occur. Animals given the drug should never be left unattended. Induction should be treated with the same concern as with other drugs. It should not be used in patients with respiratory, hepatic, or kidney disease. In patients with upper airway obstruction such as occurs with sinusitis, 4 to 10 mg/kg may be given intramuscularly for sedation and restraint, and immediately following the onset of action, additional doses may be given intravenously to permit tracheal intubation.

If ketamine or ketamine with diazepam is used as an inducing agent prior to inhalation anesthesia, care must be taken not to produce deep anesthesia with profound respiratory and cardiovascular depression. Concentrations of halothane should be started at 0.2 to 0.5 per cent and then increased as the effects of ketamine dissipate.

Xylazine. Xylazine (Rompun*) is a potent nonnarcotic sedative, analgesic, and muscle relaxant.[4] Sedative and analgesic activity are related to central nervous system depression; the muscle relaxant effect is a result of inhibition of intraneural transmission of impulses in the central nervous system. In the United States, it is currently approved for use in dogs, cats, and horses.

Effects develop in 10 to 15 minutes after intramuscular injection and 3 to 5 minutes after intravenous administration. Emesis occurs in 50 per cent of dogs and 90 per cent of cats. The sleep-like state usually lasts 1 to 2 hours, with analgesia effective for 15 to 30 minutes. Respiratory rate is decreased, as is heart rate and cardiac output. Second-degree atrioventricular block and sinus arrest or sinoatrial block are common. Xylazine may also induce a variety of ventricular dysrhythmias in the presence of epinephrine and halothane.[18] There is a transient increase in arterial blood pressure initially, followed by hypoten-

---

*Haver-Lockhart Laboratories, Shawnee, KS.

sion and bradycardia.[13] Dosage in dogs and cats is 1.0 to 2.0 mg/kg intramuscularly or intravenously. Administration must be preceded by 0.04 mg/kg of atropine to avoid bradycardia.

Xylazine is commonly used with ketamine in veterinary medicine. Recent studies have demonstrated that this combination may produce severe depressant cardiopulmonary changes and should not be used in dogs with diminished cardiopulmonary reserves.[2,14]

Neuroleptanesthesia

Central nervous system depression and analgesia produced without the use of barbiturates or volatile agents is referred to as neuroleptanalgesia. Neuroleptic drugs reduce motor activity, decrease anxiety, and produce a state of indifference. In dogs, this state produces analgesia and sedation to permit surgery, but muscle relaxation is poor and muscle movement may be elicited by auditory stimuli.

Droperidol-Fentanyl. Each milliliter of droperidol-fentanyl (Innovar-Vet*) contains a mixture of 20 mg droperidol and 0.4 mg fentanyl, with 1.8 mg methylparaben and 0.2 mg propylparaben as preservatives. Fentanyl, the narcotic-analgesic, is 70 to 130 times more potent than morphine and has a rapid onset of action, producing analgesia, sedation, and respiratory depression within 3 to 5 minutes. The peak effect occurs in 15 minutes and lasts less than 30 minutes following an intramuscular injection. Panting, adrenergic blockade, hypotension, and bradycardia occur, and defecation is common.[15] Dogs should always receive an anticholinergic to counteract the vagal effects produced by the narcotic unless there is tachycardia before anesthesia.

When 50 to 66 per cent nitrous oxide is added, neuroleptanesthesia is produced. Nitrous oxide usually eliminates auditory responses, defecation, and tachypnea. However, if nitrous oxide is not used, premedication with pentobarbital, 4 to 6 mg/kg intramuscularly, will prevent many undesirable side effects. Innovar-Vet can be given at a dose of 1 ml/9 kg intramuscularly in dogs for minor surgical or diagnostic procedures, and the narcotic component can be reversed with 0.1 to 0.4 mg naloxone intravenously. If used for general anesthesia in high-risk patients, 1 ml/10 to 20 kg of Innovar-Vet is added to 250 ml lactated Ringer's or saline solution and given by intravenous drip over 5 to 10 minutes to effect anesthesia. It may also be given in a 5:1 dilution by syringe. The higher dilution allows better titration to anesthesia in patients with higher risk. The patient gradually becomes sedated and, although appearing to be anesthetized, responds to noise. Therefore, it is helpful to plug the ears with cotton. Oxygen and nitrous oxide should be given by mask at the time of onset of sedative effects. Tracheal intubation can be accomplished within a few minutes as sufficient anesthetic depth is achieved.

The droperidol component of Innovar-Vet causes mild hypotension secondary to alpha-adrenergic blockade and peripheral vasodilation. The threshold to epinephrine-induced arrhythmias is raised, but there is little or no evidence of myocardial depression.[15] Fentanyl also produces mild hypotension and bradycardia, a parasympathomimetic effect that can be blocked by an anticholinergic such as atropine.

Innovar-Vet reduces both respiratory rate and tidal volume, primarily because of the fentanyl. This is a dose-dependent effect and results in an increase in arterial carbon dioxide pressure. The carbon dioxide response curve is shifted to the right, and at high doses the slope is depressed. To avoid this consequence, respiration should be controlled with a rate of 8 to 10 breaths per minute and tidal volume at 20 ml/kg.

Acetylpromazine-Meperidine. This combination of equal volumes can be mixed and given for restraint and minor surgery to provide neuroleptanalgesia similar to that produced with Innovar-Vet. If the combination is given intramuscularly or subcutaneously, 0.5 ml is used for small dogs (7 to 16 kg), and up to 1 ml for larger patients.[25]

Acetylpromazine-Oxymorphone. With the patient sedated with 0.1 mg/kg of acetylpromazine 15 minutes before anesthesia, along with 0.04 mg/kg atropine, 0.1 to 0.3 mg/kg oxymorphone can be given intravenously to effect the desired depth of analgesia. These drugs can be combined and given intramuscularly together, but more control of depth is achieved when they are administered separately as described. In unhealthy dogs, the acetylpromazine dose may be decreased. As with fentanyl, there is mild myocardial depression and hypotension, but because depression to ventilation is greater, control of breathing is advisable. Nitrous oxide is advantageous, as described for the droperidol-fentanyl combination, to provide neuroleptanesthesia.

Diazepam-Oxymorphone. Diazepam, 0.4 mg/kg given intravenously until it becomes effective, is a potent hypnotic, amnesic, and tranquilizer and is advantageous in high-risk patients when used in combination with narcotic-analgesics instead of droperidol or acetylpromazine. It is a mild vasodilator with antiarrhythmic properties, reduces halothane MAC and has minimal depressant effects on myocardial function.[21] The preferred technique is to place the two drugs in separate syringes, and the oxymorphone dose used most commonly for intravenous induction is 0.1 mg/kg. With the drip running, doses of 0.25 to 0.5 ml of each drug are given into the drip at 10- to 15-second intervals. Usually, all of the diazepam is given and thereafter the oxymorphone is given to accomplish endotracheal intubation. Alternatively for sick dogs, diazepam, 0.2 mg/kg, may be given intramuscularly 15 minutes before induction with nitrous oxide, and oxygen may be given by mask prior to intubation; thereafter, halothane or

---

*Pitman-Moore, Inc., Washington Crossing, NJ.

isoflurane may be added at 0.5 per cent increments for the appropriate level of anesthesia. Most often, endotracheal intubation can be accomplished without the appearance of deep anesthesia.

Appraisal of Neuroleptanesthetics

When reversal is needed, profound sedation from the tranquilizer does not mask the sedation of the narcotic. Naloxone is given a few minutes after nitrous oxide is discontinued, at a dose of 0.1 to 0.4 mg intravenously. Alternatively, nalbuphine (Nubain*) may be given at 0.1 mg/kg intravenously. Additional doses of the antagonist can be given as needed, depending on the amount of narcotic given and duration of the procedure. As a general rule, up to 0.4 mg intravenously is sufficient, and no more than 0.8 mg of naloxone should be needed for reversal.

Neuroleptanesthesia is safe and effective, especially for cesarean section, in geriatrics and high-risk patients. The cardiovascular system remains stable as long as adequate fluids are given to prevent hypotension and ventilation is properly controlled. The technique works better in high-risk patients than in normal healthy dogs. That is, it has a more predictable effect in sick patients. In healthy dogs, more sedation is needed with a tranquilizer such as acetylpromazine, and higher doses of the narcotic may be required.

BALANCED ANESTHESIA

The term *anesthesia* denotes loss of sensation to pain with unconsciousness, immobilization, and a certain degree of muscle relaxation. Suppression of muscle tone can be accomplished centrally with intravenous or inhalation anesthetics, with local anesthetics injected into muscle or around nerves supplying muscle, or with drugs that affect transmission of nerve impulses at the neuromuscular junction.

In the resting state, skeletal muscle has a certain amount of tone so that immediate response is made when needed. A voluntary muscle cell acts in an all-or-none response; therefore, muscle cells are not partially activated to produce the resting tone. Motor centers produce a continual random discharge so that only a small fraction of the cells contract at any given time. It is the control of this background activity that provides the degree of muscle relaxation needed during anesthesia.

Muscle relaxation is adequate for most procedures, with halothane or methoxyflurane at 1.2 to 1.5 MAC. When more relaxation is needed, general anesthetics may be used to suppress tone of the motor centers with deep levels. This has the disadvantage of requiring high concentrations, which will compromise the heart, circulation, and respiration and may not be tolerated even in healthy patients. In sick patients, 1.2 MAC may be considered detrimental, and lighter levels would be adequate for analgesia and unconsciousness but not appropriate for muscle relaxation. A second option is to block the nerve signals as they pass through the spinal nerves, as is done with epidural anesthesia. This option is a good one but has certain anatomical limitations for application. Neuromuscular blockade leads to a division of drug effects, such that the anesthetic need not be used to produce unconsciousness and analgesia; therefore, lower and safer doses can be used. Skeletal muscle tone then can be controlled separately with a neuromuscular blocker. *Balanced anesthesia* is the term used to describe this technique. It can be used on any patient but has its best application in high-risk individuals. Since the muscles of breathing are blocked, controlled breathing must be provided.

Any of the narcotic-analgesics, barbiturates, or inhalation agents may be used to block the response to pain. Dosages usually needed for anesthesia and muscle relaxation can be reduced to safer levels. For the inhalation agents, 0.6 to 0.8 MAC may be used as a guide and levels adjusted up or down as needed.

SPECIAL CONSIDERATIONS

Most of the effects of anesthetics on various systems are dealt with in the chapters that follow. However, obese patients present special problems in anesthesia, mostly those associated with ventilation and anesthetic overdose. Because of the increased weight of excess fat and because of the insignificant role of fat in the uptake and distribution of anesthetic agents, a relative overdose of injectable anesthetics may be given unless an allowance is made and the dosage is reduced. In obese patients, increased chest wall mass leads to decreased chest wall compliance. This adds to the work of breathing and may be coupled with a decreased parenchymal compliance secondary to the reduction in lung volume, premature airway closure, and increased pulmonary blood volume. Because of the increases in adipose tissue distributed to the chest wall and abdomen and increases in intra-abdominal pressure, the work of breathing is greater and lung volume is reduced. Depression of alveolar ventilation by anesthetics contributes to this problem; therefore, controlled breathing should be instituted immediately after induction and is continued throughout the procedure. Airway problems may be encountered after induction and extubation. Thus, oxygenation before induction is indicated, and attention must be paid to adequate oxygenation during recovery.

Uptake of the more soluble anesthetics such as methoxyflurane and halothane increases in fat tissue with time. Metabolism of volatile anesthetic agents in markedly obese patients differs quantitatively (methoxyflurane, enflurane) and qualitatively (halothane) from that in nonobese patients. Increased serum ionic

---

*Du Pont Pharmaceuticals, Garden City, NY.

fluoride concentrations have been reported in obese human patients because of increased biotransformation of the inhalation agents, which increases the possibility of postanesthetic renal dysfunction.[19,24]

With prudent management of the anesthetic levels and awareness of the longer duration of action of retained anesthetics, recovery of properly ventilated obese patients is prompt, normal breathing is resumed quickly after anesthesia, and walking is resumed early after operation.

1. Bjorling, D. E., and Rawlings, C. A.: Induction of anesthesia with thiopental-lidocaine combination in dogs with cardiopulmonary disease. J. Am. Anim. Hosp. Assoc. 20:445, 1984.
2. Clark, D. M., Martin, R. A., and Short, C. A.: Cardiopulmonary response to xylazine/ketamine anesthesia in the dog. J. Am. Anim. Hosp. Assoc. 18:815, 1982.
3. Corbett, T. H.: Cancer and congenital anomalies associated with anesthetics. Ann. N.Y. Acad. Sci. 271:58, 1976.
4. Davis, L. E.: Xylazine. J. Am. Vet. Med. Assoc. 176:454, 1980.
5. DeYoung, D. J., and Sawyer, D. C.: Anesthetic potency of nitrous oxide during halothane anesthesia in the dog. J. Am. Anim. Hosp. Assoc. 16:125, 1980.
6. Dhadphale, P. R., Jackson, A. P. F., and Alseri, S.: Comparison of anesthesia with diazepam and ketamine vs. morphine in patients undergoing heart-valve replacement. Anesthesiology 51:200, 1979.
7. Dripps, R. D., Eckenhoff, J. E., and Vandam, L. D.: Introduction to Anesthesia. 5th ed. W.B. Saunders, Philadelphia, 1977. pp. 149.
8. Eger, E. I. II: Anesthetic Uptake and Action. Williams and Wilkins Co., Baltimore, 1974.
9. Eger, E. I., II: Isoflurane: A review. Anesthesiology 55:559, 1981.
10. Eger, E. I., II and Saidman, L. J.: Hazards of nitrous oxide anesthesia in bowel obstruction and pneumothorax. Anesthesiology 26:61, 1965.
11. Haskins, S. C., Peiffer, R. L., and Stowe, C. M.: A clinical comparison of CT 1341, ketamine, and xylazine in cats. Am. J. Vet. Res. 36:1537, 1975.
12. Heavner, J. E., and Bloedow, D. C.: Ketamine pharmacokinetics in domestic cats. Vet. Anesth. 6(2):16, 1979.
13. Klide, A. M., Calderwood, H. W., and Soma, L. R.: Cardiopulmonary effects of xylazine in dogs. Am. J. Vet. Res. 36:931, 1975.
14. Kolata, R. J., and Rawlings, C. A.: Cardiopulmonary effects of intravenous xylazine, ketamine, and atropine in the dog. Am. J. Vet. Res. 43:2196, 1982.
15. Krahwinkel, D. J., Sawyer, D. C., Eyster, G. E., and Bender G.: Cardiopulmonary effects of fentanyl-droperidol, nitrous oxide, and atropine sulfate in dogs. Am. J. Vet. Res. 36:1211, 1975.
16. Lowe, H. J., Titel, J. H., and Hagler, K. J.: Absorption of anesthetic by conductive rubber in breathing circuits. Anesthesiology 34:283, 1971.
17. Muir, W. W., III, Werner, L. L., and Hamilton, R. L.: Arrhythmias in dogs associated with epinephrine and thiamylal anesthesia. Am. J. Vet. Res. 36:1291, 1975.
18. Muir, W. W., III, Werner, L. L., and Hamlin, R. L.: Effects of xylazine and acetylpromazine upon induced ventricular fibrillation in dogs anesthetized with thiamylal and halothane. Am. J. Vet. Res. 36:1299, 1975.
19. Pedersoli W. M.: Blood serum inorganic ionic fluoride, tetracycline, and methoxyflurane anesthesia in dogs. J. Am. Anim. Hosp. Assoc. 13:242, 1977.
20. Roesch, R., and Stoelting, R.: Duration of hypoxemia during nitrous oxide excretion. Anesth. Analg. 51:851, 1972.
21. Sawyer, D. C.: The Practice of Small Animal Anesthesia. W. B. Saunders, Philadelphia, 1982.
22. Steffey, E. P.: Isoflurane concentration delivered by isoflurane and halothane specific vaporizers (abstract). Anesthesiology 53:519, 1980.
23. Stiles, J. A., Neff, W. B., Rosenstine, E. A., and Waters, R. M.: Cyclopropane as an anesthetic agent: A preliminary clinical report. Anesth. Analg. 13:56, 1934.
24. U. S. Dept. of Health, Education and Welfare: Waste Anesthetic Gases and Vapors–Criteria Document. Washington, D. C., Natl. Inst. of Occupational Safety and Health, March, 1977.
25. Warner, H. E.: New drug combination for small animal restraint. Mod. Vet. Pract. 49:20, 1968.
26. Waters, R. M., and Schmidt, E. R.: Cyclopropane anesthesia. JAMA 103:975, 1934.
27. Winters, W. D., Ferrar-Allado, T., Guzman-Flores, C., and Alcaraz, M.: The cataleptic state induced by ketamine: A review of the neuropharmacology of anesthesia. Neuropharmacology 11:303, 1972.

Chapter **188** # Gastrointestinal System—Anesthetic Considerations

Sandee M. Hartsfield

EFFECTS OF ANESTHETICS AND RELATED DRUGS ON GASTROINTESTINAL FUNCTION

Salivary Glands

Glycopyrrolate reduces salivation for approximately two to three times as long as does atropine.[39] Although reducing salivation is not necessary with most currently used anesthetics, some dogs and cats salivate profusely during inhalation by mask.[22] Also, reduced salivation is convenient during oral or pharyngeal surgery. In unintubated anesthetized patients, reducing the volume of saliva may prevent aspiration. Even though most patients maintain laryngeal reflexes during dissociative anesthesia, contrast media placed in the pharynx passed into the trachea of humans anesthetized with ketamine.[5] Finally, during recovery, some patients salivate excessively, making the longer antisialagogue effect from glycopyrrolate desirable.

Gastrointestinal Motility

Anticholinergic drugs reduce gastrointestinal motility, and atropine's duration is shorter than that of glycopyrrolate.[45] Sedatives and tranquilizers may delay gastric emptying.[4,56] Fentanyl and droperidol given together reduce intestinal motility in dogs, a finding based on the transit time of barium sulfate through the stomach and duodenum.[56] In the same study, pentobarbital, halothane, and methoxyflurane profoundly depressed intestinal motility. Acetylpromazine maleate did not change gastrointestinal motility, while triflupromazine hydrochloride reduced motility slightly. Promazine hydrochloride reduced motility more as dosage was increased.[56] Phenothiazine tranquilizers affect intestinal tone and peristalsis less than as the narcotics.[34] Intravenous xylazine markedly prolonged transit time of barium sulfate from the stomach to the duodenojejunal junction in dogs.[23]

In dogs, morphine, oxymorphone, and meperidine initially increase nonpropulsive rhythmic contractions and increase gastrointestinal and sphincter smooth muscle tone and periodic intestinal spasms.[34] Dogs given oxymorphone intravenously often produce flatus or loose stools shortly after administration. The period of small intestinal hypermotility precedes a longer period of relative intestinal atony that results in increased water absorption. This narcotic-induced spasmogenic effect has been related to a central nervous system–mediated increase in parasympathetic tone and possibly to local release of 5-hydroxytryptamine.[34]

Gastric pH and Volume

Several preanesthetic drugs decrease gastric acidity.[10] Since the severity of pulmonary pathology following aspiration of gastric contents is enhanced by low gastric pH,[11] alkalinization of gastric fluid may benefit patients at risk (e.g., in gastric, esophageal, or high intestinal procedures).[45] The degree of alkalinization is limited by time; glycopyrrolate produced greater human alkalinization if the premedication-to-induction period was 60 to 120 minutes.[1] Other anesthetics also affect gastric pH. For example, halothane anesthesia increased gastric pH from 1.8 ± 0.2 to 5.1 ± 0.7 after one hour.[7]

Splanchnic Blood Flow

Anesthetic effects on splanchnic and hepatic blood flow have been studied in humans. All anesthetic techniques decrease hepatic blood flow either by decreasing perfusion pressure or by inducing splanchnic vasoconstriction.[49] Methoxyflurane reduces splanchnic blood flow (SBF) by approximately 50 per cent, and halothane, by about 33 per cent. Nitrous oxide apparently has no effect on SBF or splanchnic vascular resistance. If hypercapnia occurs, splanchnic vasoconstriction ensues. However, SBF depends on systemic blood pressure in the presence of elevated arterial CO_2 tension. By comparison of SBF to splanchnic oxygen consumption during anesthesia in humans, methoxyflurane was shown less desirable than halothane for anesthesia, although direct effects of this concept have not been shown clinically.[2]

Nitrous Oxide Transfer to Closed Gas Spaces

When N_2O is used, its entrance into closed gas spaces within the body causes expansion of volume or increased pressure, depending on the compliance of the walls encompassing the gas. With intestinal gas, N_2O causes expansion of volume. In gastrointestinal obstruction, trapped air is evident in the lumen. Transfer of N_2O into the intestine may cause difficulty with surgical manipulations during abdominal exploratory and surgical closure. Postoperatively, abdominal distension may embarrass ventilation if intraabdominal pressure is increased.[13] In dogs breathing 75 per cent N_2O, intestinal gas volumes increased 1.8 times in two hours and 2.5 times in four hours.[14] Thus, in very short procedures, volume expands very little; therefore, N_2O could be used during induction. Anesthesia for the obstructed patient should not include N_2O.

In laparoscopy, carbon dioxide is infused into the peritoneal space to allow better observation with the laparoscope. If N_2O is used for anesthesia during laparoscopy, abdominal distension may occur, causing reduced ventilatory compliance and reduced blood pressure to complicate anesthetic management.[13] N_2O should not be used for anesthesia during laparoscopy.

ANESTHETIC MANAGEMENT

Preanesthetic Fasting

Withholding food prior to anesthesia reduces vomiting during induction or passive regurgitation during maintenance.[46] Reduced gastric volume limits the amount of material that can be aspirated if vomiting or regurgitation occurs. Generally, small animals are fasted approximately 6 to 12 hours, with water available *ad libitum* prior to anesthesia.[41] Patients weighing less than about 2 kg may be fasted for shorter periods to prevent hypoglycemia, but they should be treated as unfasted animals during anesthesia. Gastric emptying varies from 1.5 to 6 hours in dogs.[46] For emergency surgery or with short periods of fasting prior to anesthesia, rapid intubation and protection of the airway can prevent pulmonary aspiration if vomiting occurs. Gaseous gastric distension may occur in unfasted patients during anesthesia and may affect ventilation and venous return. When recognized, pressure should be relieved by passing a stomach tube to vent gases. Presumably a full stomach may impair venous return in patients positioned in dorsal recumbency. Therefore, emetics such as apomorphine, 0.06 mg/kg subcutaneously in the dog, and xylazine, 0.5 to 1.0 mg/kg intramuscularly in the cat can be useful. However, these drugs produce sedative and tranquilizing effects and may induce cardiopulmonary depression. In addition, their effects are synergistic with anesthetics and anesthetic adjuncts and they should be used judiciously.

Clinical Data Base

The history discloses vomiting or diarrhea, the appetite or period of anorexia, and the attitude and condition of the patient. The physical examination reveals the patient's general condition, such as debilitation versus relatively normal body weight, palpable lesions in the gastrointestinal tract, and concurrent diseases. Finally, blood and urine values can furnish valuable information. With gastrointestinal abnormalities, acid-base and electrolyte imbalances often exist. Therefore, in addition to the usual complete blood count, biochemical profile, and urinalysis, one should determine pH, blood gas, and electrolyte levels in patients with persistent vomiting, diarrhea, or ileus. If hepatic disease is suspected, an extended data base should include a coagulation profile, Bromsulphalein clearance, and protein electrophoresis studies. These data influence selection of drugs, anesthetic dosage, and patient support.

Preanesthetic Selection

No specific guidelines exist for selection of preanesthetic agents for patients scheduled for gastrointestinal surgery. Such drugs must be chosen for the individual patient. Although anticholinergic drugs may affect motility, several indications exist for their use. Endotracheal intubation, surgical manipulation of viscera, and use of certain drugs, including narcotics, neuroleptics, and xylazine, can induce bradycardia. Therefore, anticholinergic premedication seems logical, and glycopyrrolate, because of its longer duration of action and lesser elevation of heart rate, is superior to atropine.[44,45]

Depressant premedication should be based on the needs of each patient. In lethargic patients, preanesthetic depressants are usually unnecessary. In excitable animals, tranquilizers or neuroleptic combinations such as oxymorphone at 0.11 to 0.22 mg/kg and acetylpromazine at 0.11 to 0.22 mg/kg may ease restraint and prevent rough inductions. However, tranquilizers must be used with discretion if hepatic disease is suspected, and the effects of narcotics on gastrointestinal smooth muscle in the dog should be considered in patients with motility abnormalities. Low-dose ketamine (5 to 10 mg/kg intramuscularly)

or acetylpromazine can ease induction in excitable cats.

Maintenance of Anesthesia

Inhalation agents remain the drugs of choice for anesthetic maintenance for gastrointestinal surgery. Based on splanchnic blood flow, controllability, induction, and recovery, halothane is my choice. In patients with dysrhythmias or other pre-existing cardiac disease or in patients requiring complete muscle relaxation, a balanced anesthetic regimen helps avoid complications of deep halothane anesthesia.[41] In some instances, simply providing muscle relaxation with a neuromuscular blocker allows surgical exposure and manipulation with usual or low amounts of halothane and minimal complications. Adequate anesthesia and controlled ventilation must be provided.

Patient Support During Anesthesia

During gastrointestinal surgery, support of vital functions is absolutely essential. Hypothermia caused by tissue exposure, flushing of the abdominal cavity, and cool ambient temperatures is common.[18] Anesthesia and prolonged intestinal exposure and manipulations may cause circulatory shock,[8,9] and fluid loss from hemorrhage, protein depletion, extravasation, and evaporation may contribute to hypovolemia. Cardiac dysrhythmias may occur from visceral manipulations or pre-existing or developing acid-base or electrolyte imbalances.[35] Surgical packing and retraction and patient positioning can impair respiration and venous return. Therefore, cardiac rate and rhythm, pulse quality, blood volume, blood pressure, acid-base balance, electrolytes, respiratory variables, body temperature, and anesthetic depth should be monitored regularly. Deviations from expected values should be corrected. For surgery involving extensive gut manipulation, crystalloid fluids are administered at 20 to 30 ml/kg, and prednisolone sodium succinate, 8 to 10 mg/kg intravenously, is given prior to and during surgery.

Recovery from Anesthesia

Following anesthesia, similar monitoring and support must continue until the patient can maintain homeostasis. After gastrointestinal surgery, fluid volume is a major consideration, and fluid input and output should be monitored for 12 to 24 hours. Postoperative analgesia can be provided as needed.

ANESTHETIC CONSIDERATIONS

Lips, Teeth, Tongue, Pharynx, Soft and Hard Palates, and Related Structures

During surgery in the oral cavity, protection of the airway and control of ventilation are primary considerations. Saliva, blood, clots, tartar, teeth, bone, and other debris may collect and be aspirated if the airway is unprotected. Surgical packing and retraction can also inhibit airway patency. Therefore, endotracheal intubation is highly desirable, if not mandatory, during oral surgery. In many instances, standard endotracheal tube placement through the oral cavity and into the larynx allows surgical exposure and manipulations, but other options include endotracheal intubation by pharyngotomy or by tracheotomy. Endotracheal intubation by external pharyngotomy provides the advantages of routine intubation without interfering with dental occlusion or impairing observation of the operative field, and it avoids tracheotomy and associated postoperative complications.[20]

In patients with space-occupying masses in the oropharynx that interfere with endotracheal intubation, special techniques can be used for endotracheal tube placement. A laryngoscope may allow direct passage of the tube or passage of a canine urinary catheter into the larynx and trachea as a guide over which an endotracheal tube can be advanced. If none of these techniques facilitate intubation, a retrograde guide for intubation can be used.[3]

Some oropharyngeal surgery can be accomplished using analgesics and tranquilizers if the patient maintains protective laryngeal reflexes and adequate ventilation. With concurrent use of nerve blocks or local anesthetic infiltration, even extensive surgical procedures can be performed.[21] Adequate ventilation, oxygenation, and airway patency must be maintained. If normal reflexes do not remain intact, the trachea must be intubated and controlled ventilation and supplemental oxygen used if respiration is depressed.

Following oropharyngeal surgery, the mouth, pharynx, and larynx must be cleared of all debris before the patient is allowed to awaken, regain reflexes, and be extubated. If blood, saliva, or fluids have collected during surgery, removal of the endotracheal tube is done with the head and neck below the median plane of the body and with the endotracheal tube cuff partially inflated. Fluids may collect within the airway between the larynx and the endotracheal tube cuff and are usually removed when this technique is used.

Specific anesthetics for surgery of the oropharynx are more likely to be dictated by the patient's physical status and the function of other body systems than by the oropharyngeal lesion. Anticholinergic premedication should be used to decrease salivation and block vagal-induced bradycardia. Numerous chances for vagal stimulation are possible in salivary gland or oropharyngeal surgery, including carotid sinus and laryngeal and tracheal stimulation.[58] Other preanesthetics should be selected according to the temperament of the patient and the function of the cardiovascular, hepatic, and renal systems. If a lesion impairs the integrity of the airway (e.g., pharyngeal salivary mucocele or pharyngeal tumor), rapid induction with a thiobarbiturate to facilitate immediate intubation of the trachea, or possibly tracheotomy, is a primary consideration. Generally, maintenance of

anesthesia is with inhalation agents. Drugs with relatively low blood solubility (e.g., nitrous oxide and halothane) are preferable if postoperative airway obstruction is a potential complication—e.g., brachycephalic dogs for soft palate resection. Such drugs promote rapid recovery and ventilation. Corticosteroids and diuretics are indicated if edema in the surgical site or surrounding tissues predisposes the patient to airway obstruction following extubation.

Esophagus

Anesthetic requirements for surgery of the esophagus vary with the surgical site, depending on intra- or extrathoracic involvement. The patient's general condition and other affected organ systems dictate anesthetic management, but special considerations exist for certain types of esophageal surgery.

For surgery involving the cervical esophagus (e.g., cricopharyngeal myotomy or esophagotomy), endotracheal tube placement should prevent tracheal collapse resulting from surgical retraction or digital pressure. Positioning of the cuffed end of the tube at the thoracic inlet is appropriate, and the endotracheal tube must be made of material that is not easily collapsed. During anesthesia, monitoring must include periodic assessment of resistance to inspiration so that a patent airway is assured.

In surgery of the thoracic esophagus requiring thoracotomy, one must control ventilation and consider factors required for anesthetic management during thoracic surgery. During surgical correction of vascular rings that cause esophageal pouches, a gastroscope or other rigid instrument may be passed into the esophagus to aid dissection. The trachea may collapse at the thoracic inlet if the endotracheal tube is not of appropriate length or is collapsible. Airway patency and ventilation must be maintained.

Since inability of the patient to swallow and to propel food within the esophagus is present with many esophageal disorders, repeated episodes of food aspiration produce pneumonitis which may complicate anesthetic management. Most aspirated material produces an acute pulmonary inflammatory response. Since patients with esophageal disorders aspirate small amounts of liquid or solid food material that has a pH higher than that of gastric contents, the acute effects of aspirating stomach contents with a pH of less than 2.5 are not usually seen. However, it is possible for solid material to block airways, for liquids to gravitate to alveoli in ventral areas of the lung, and for generalized or localized bacterial pneumonia to develop. In patients with aspiration pneumonia, the condition should be treated medically prior to anesthesia. Before induction, fluid, electrolyte and acid-base balance are evaluated since malnutrition and dehydration are often present. Immediately prior to induction, preoxygenation with 100 per cent oxygen by mask or chamber is appropriate. Otherwise, hypoxemia may predispose the patient to dysrhythmias during induction. Following intubation, anesthetic gases should contain a high fraction of oxygen for the duration of anesthesia, since oxygen administration can reverse hypoxemia due to diffusion impairment and ventilation-perfusion imbalance.[24] If pus or other material collects in the airway during anesthesia, it must be removed by surgical suction. Postoperative management includes maintenance in an oxygen-enriched atmosphere until recovery is complete.

Stomach

Abnormalities Associated with Acute and Chronic Vomiting. Vomiting or sequestration of fluids is common in patients with gastric disease or obstruction of the upper small intestine. Imbalances in fluid volume, electrolytes, and acid-base values are common and may affect patient response to anesthesia. Gastric secretions contain high concentrations of hydrogen, sodium, potassium, and chloride ions, which are lost in vomitus. Therefore, gastric losses promote alkalosis. Alkaline duodenal contents that are expelled along with gastric contents may modify the acid-base imbalance that ensues,[55] and alkalosis may be less marked.

Usually, a metabolic alkalosis occurs after repeated vomiting. Continued vomiting decreases extracellular fluid volume and stimulates renal proximal tubular resorption of bicarbonate. Therefore, metabolic alkalosis is sustained. Hypokalemia, associated with chronic vomiting, also stimulates proximal tubular bicarbonate resorption. However, metabolic alkalosis associated with vomiting is maintained primarily because of decreased extracellular fluid volume, with potassium deficiency probably being of minor importance unless it is severe. When hypokalemia is marked, both volume repletion and potassium administration are necessary to suppress proximal tubular resorption of bicarbonate.[28] Thus, extracellular fluid volume expansion and appropriate use of potassium, based on electrolyte data, are appropriate treatments prior to and during anesthesia in the patient with a history of persistent vomiting.

Alkalotic patients are usually given saline for volume expansion, supplemented with potassium chloride as needed to correct hypokalemia. Potassium chloride is usually added to fluid to yield a concentration not greater than 50 mEq/l, with a maximum infusion rate of 0.5 mEq/kg/hour.[42] Electrocardiographic monitoring is advisable during infusion of fluids containing large amounts of potassium, because of the potential effects on cardiac rate and rhythm.

With chronic vomiting leading to severe nutritional deficiency and emaciation, acidemia instead of alkalemia may be present. Similarly, patients with severe volume depletion are potentially acidotic, arterial acid-base determination and blood-gas analysis are appropriate.

Abnormalities Associated with Gastric Dilation-Torsion Complex. Cardiopulmonary insufficiency complicates anesthetic management of the patient with gastric dilation and volvulus. Gaseous distension of the stomach interferes with diaphragmatic excursions. Tidal volume is decreased, and respiratory rate is increased. Alveolar ventilation becomes inadequate. Ventilation and perfusion balance in pulmonary tissue is altered, and hypoxemia may result. Gastric dilation limits venous return to the heart owing to occlusion or obstruction of the splenic veins, portal vein, and caudal vena cava. Sequestration of blood occurs in the skeletal muscles, portal system, splanchnic organs, and caudal vena cava. Cardiac output is reduced, and arterial hypotension and reduced tissue perfusion occur. Circulatory shock ensues and may be complicated by release of endotoxins from intestinal bacteria and their absorption through lymphatics or through the peritoneum.[55]

Cardiac dysrhythmias occur frequently in dogs with gastric dilation and volvulus and are more likely to be ventricular than supraventricular in origin. Mechanisms for development of abnormal rhythms include low cardiac output reducing coronary blood flow and leading to myocardial ischemia; autonomic imbalance related to sympathetic and parasympathetic hyperactivity; electrolyte, blood gas, and pH abnormalities, including hyperkalemia and hypoxemia; and the reduction of myocardial performance and promotion of electrical instability by low molecular weight proteins (e.g., myocardial depressant factor) from ischemic viscera.[35]

Acid-base and electrolyte disturbances have been examined in dogs with gastric dilation and volvulus.[36] A great variety of pH, blood gas, and electrolyte changes was reported, and metabolic acidosis and hypokalemia were common.

Gastric Surgery

Because of the manipulations required during gastric surgery, preanesthetic fasting is desirable. All fluid and electrolyte abnormalities should be corrected prior to induction, if possible. In patients with uncorrected acid-base, electrolyte, and fluid abnormalities, induction must be done with great care. Preinduction oxygenation is desirable, and glycopyrrolate (0.01 mg/kg) and oxymorphone (0.05 to 0.22 mg/kg intravenously) may be used as preanesthetics. Induction can be performed with halothane in oxygen delivered by mask or by a low dose (1 to 4 mg/kg intravenously) of thiopental. ECG monitoring is desirable during all phases of anesthesia. Since muscle relaxation may facilitate surgical exposure, pancuronium (0.03 to 0.06 mg/kg intravenously) with complete control of ventilation can be recommended, in addition to halothane, for maintenance. Accidental hypothermia is likely because of the large amount of tissue exposure required; therefore, warm fluids and other measures for preserving heat are beneficial.

In patients with gastric dilation-volvulus, preservation of respiratory and cardiovascular function is of primary importance. Prior to induction of general anesthesia, the degree of dilation present should be reduced by means of a stomach tube. Alternatively, a large-needle trocar inserted through the abdominal wall and into the stomach under a local block may be used to evacuate as much gas as possible. In patients with unabated gastric distension, anesthetic induction may be needed prior to relief of cardiopulmonary embarrassment. Control of ventilation must be instituted immediately after induction and intubation; it should be applied with different guidelines than those for manual ventilation in normal patients. A respiratory rate of 12 to 15 breaths per minute, using a tidal volume of about 11 ml/kg, is usually acceptable, with inspiratory pressure reaching levels of 30 cm of H_2O.

Cardiovascular monitoring and support must be extensive. Volume expansion and glucocorticoids in shock doses should begin prior to induction and continue as needed throughout surgery and recovery. Myocardial depression and the high incidence of dysrhythmias demand monitoring of the pulse, heart sounds, arterial blood pressure, and central venous pressure for best evaluation of fluid and drug requirements. Emergency cardiovascular drugs must be readily available, and drugs such as dopamine (Intropin*) or dobutamine (Dobutrex†) may be required in a continuous drip to maintain cardiac output and tissue perfusion in profound myocardial depression.

Intestinal Surgery

Intestinal Obstruction. Obstruction of the intestine produces abnormalities in water, electrolyte, and acid-base balances. If obstruction occurs high in the small intestine, much of the water and electrolyte absorption that occurs in the jejunum from salivary, gastric, and pancreatic secretions is impaired. More distal obstructions have less effect on absorption of normal constituents of intestinal contents.[6] Electrolyte concentrations in dogs change very little, even after five to seven days of complete large intestinal obstruction.[52] Abnormalities caused by intestinal obstruction are related to fluid and electrolyte losses from vomiting, sequestration of fluid in the bowel lumen, and edema of the bowel wall.[6] Because of impaired absorptive functions proximal to an intestinal obstruction, luminal distension and venous congestion can lead to passage of fluid into the peritoneal cavity and to movement of extracellular fluid into the intestinal lumen.[50] Vomiting plays an important role in determining severity of clinical signs. With redistribution of fluid to maintain vascular volume, intracellular fluid depletion becomes significant.[6] Since electrolyte and acid-base changes are common with intestinal obstruction, preanesthetic evaluation and correction of deficits are desirable.

If strangulation and ischemia of the intestine are

associated with obstruction, absorption of products of tissue autolysis and of bacteria and toxins may contribute to the general condition of the patient.[50]

Diarrhea. Diarrhea results in loss of water, sodium, chloride, potassium, and bicarbonate. These losses cause dehydration, hypokalemia, and metabolic acidosis. Decreasing the intracellular-to-extracellular potassium concentration ratio produces clinical signs of muscle weakness, lethargy, and cardiac dysfunction.[31] Cardiac cell membrane changes cause prolonged repolarization. Depression of the ST segment, prominent U waves, and prolonged QT intervals may be seen on an electrocardiogram. Various dysrhythmias may be associated with hypokalemia, including atrioventricular block and ventricular bigeminy, tachycardia, and fibrillation.[42] Thus, to avoid potential dysrhythmias and adverse effects of anesthetics, potassium imbalances should be corrected. Failure to correct abnormalities in water, electrolyte, or acid-base balances can cause devastating effects.

Pancreatic and Hepatic Abnormalities. Pancreatic ischemia may cause release of lysosomal proteases, which can affect the patient systemically. Pancreatic autolysis is associated with increased intestinal damage and formation and release of myocardial depressant factor (MDF).[29] Myocardial depressant factor produces negative inotropic effects on the heart, splanchnic vasoconstriction, and depression of phagocytosis by the reticuloendothelial system. Glucocorticoids prevent formation and effects of MDF by stabilization of lysosomal membranes, if given early in shock or ischemia.[30]

Decreased blood flow to the liver and pancreas may be due to decreased extracellular fluid volume subsequent to intestinal obstruction.[50] Also, if blood flow to these organs is impaired by physical interruption of the blood supply, ischemia can result (see Chapter 11). The anoxic liver releases lysosomal and cytoplasmic enzymes that may have systemic effects, and surgical manipulation of a hypoxic liver (especially following trauma) may release emboli of liver tissue, bile salts, and toxic or vasoactive substances that can promote pulmonary insufficiency.[27]

The physiological functions of the liver and its importance in degradation of anesthetics and anesthetic-related drugs are worthy of consideration. There are various physiological and biochemical effects of liver disease, including portal hypertension and other circulatory changes, impaired protein synthesis, ascites, reduced plasma levels of pseudocholinesterase, impaired detoxification ability, impaired formation of clotting factors, and changes in cerebral function.[16] Portal hypertension and other circulatory changes such as portacaval shunts usually are associated with inadequate blood flow through the liver. In such instances, a patient cannot detoxify anesthetics at the normal rate. If there is evidence of liver dysfunction, it is likely that hepatic ability to degrade drugs is impaired.[16] Protein synthesis, particularly albumin, may be reduced by inhibition of hepatic function. Therefore, protein binding of an-

*Arnar-Stone, Inc., McGraw Park, IL.
†Eli Lilly and Co., Indianapolis, IN.

esthetic drugs may be less, and usual dosages of injectable agents may cause more profound responses than normal. Reduced plasma protein, causing lowered plasma colloid osmotic pressure, may produce ascites, and hypoproteinemia should be considered during fluid replacement. If ascites is extensive, aspiration of some of the fluid prior to or immediately following anesthetic induction may eliminate some of the effects of increased abdominal pressure on pulmonary function. However, rapid aspiration of ascitic fluid can cause hypotension, so this should be done with careful monitoring. When fluids are required, plasma should be considered if total plasma protein is less than 4 gm/dl. Plasma pseudocholinesterase may be reduced in patients with hepatic disease. Therefore, succinylcholine is not the muscle relaxant of choice in these patients. Impaired hepatic synthesis of clotting factors has not been identified as a cause of blood clotting abnormalities in the dog.[48]

Patients with hepatic disease, particularly with portacaval shunts, may show signs of hepatic encephalopathy, including severe depression. Hepatic encephalopathy may occur from an accumulation of toxins and false neurotransmitters in the central nervous system if portal blood has not been detoxified adequately.[51] Hepatic disease and portacaval shuntings are associated with weight loss, which makes these patients particularly susceptible to hypothermia. Finally, since the body's main carbohydrate store is the liver, hypoglycemia may develop in the postoperative period, and glucose administration may be required. Hypoglycemia may exacerbate central nervous system signs.[16]

In liver disease, the choice of anesthetic is not always obvious. The skill with which the drugs are administered is probably more important than the choice. In preanesthetic management, anticholinergic agents can be used. However, depressant premedication should be selected carefully. Phenothiazine tranquilizers are contraindicated because of their high affinity for protein and because hepatic degradation is required for removal. If preanesthetic depressants are required, narcotics are probably best because they can be specifically antagonized. However, hepatic metabolism ultimately will be involved in their degradation and elimination, and narcotic depression may return, requiring repeated reversal. Other premedicants are not recommended, although diazepam has been used in human beings.[16] Induction can be accomplished in various ways, but halothane, N_2O, and O_2 delivered by mask is recommended in depressed, sedated, or small patients. Theoretically, thiobarbiturates in low doses sufficient to facilitate intubation should allow normal clinical recovery. However, high or repeated doses of a thiobarbiturate should not be used with liver impairment.

Maintenance of anesthesia can be facilitated by the inhalation agents. I prefer halothane and oxygen or halothane, N_2O, and O_2. Low concentrations of halothane, usually not greater than 1 per cent, may be used, and also a skeletal muscle relaxant, particularly pancuronium, 0.03 to 0.06 mg/kg intravenously, if required. A second dose at half the original amount should be administered if relaxation becomes inadequate, usually apparent after about 40 minutes. The effects of pancuronium can be reversed by pyridostigmine, 2 to 5 mg, following anticholinergic therapy. Even though up to 30 per cent of injected pancuronium is metabolized by the liver, it is primarily excreted unchanged by the kidney.[33] Therefore, the drug does not totally depend on either organ for termination of its activity. However, it should be used carefully in patients with either renal or hepatic disease.[33] Supportive therapy includes warm fluids for intravenous use and surgical flushing, and monitoring of temperature, pulse quality, electrocardiogram, ventilation, and mucous membrane color is recommended. In surgery of the liver, gallbladder, and bile ducts, surgical retraction can interfere with venous return by impingement on the vena cava. This is usually recognized by an abrupt decrease in pulse quality. With liver disease, treatment of metabolic acidosis should be with bicarbonate instead of lactate because of lactate's requirement for hepatic metabolism.

With regard to the use of halothane in hepatic disease, there is no perfect recommendation. In human anesthesia, the basic contraindication for further use of halothane is unexplained hepatitis following its original use. The presence of hepatic disease does not necessarily result in increased hepatotoxicity following exposure to unpredictable hepatotoxins.[12] Based on the changes in splanchnic blood flow related to halothane and methoxyflurane, on the degree of metabolism of the two drugs, and on clinical impressions following the use of halothane in liver disease, halothane appears to be a reasonable choice for maintenance of anesthesia in patients with liver disease.[19]

Anesthetic and Antibiotic Interactions

Antibiotics are often used in solutions for flushing the peritoneal cavity following potential bacterial contamination. In addition, systemic antibiotics are commonly used. Interactions between antibiotics and anesthetic-related drugs can be important. Some of the drugs that increase the action of nondepolarizing muscle relaxants are neomycin, streptomycin, dihydrostreptomycin, kanamycin, gentamicin, polymyxin A, polymyxin B, colistin, lincomycin, and tetracycline.[26] Penicillin, erythromycin, and chloramphenicol do not have neuromuscular blocking actions.[26] When antibiotics and muscle relaxants interact, neuromuscular blockade is prolonged, and ventilation must be controlled until recovery is complete. In some cases, this potentiated neuromuscular blockade can be reversed by cholinesterase inhibitors. If such reversal is not effective, ventilation must be supported until the block is eliminated by biotransformation and excretion.[26] After initial recovery, neuromuscular blockade may return if antibiotics with neuromuscular effects are given to patients that have received muscle relaxants during anesthesia.[47] Use of a synergistic drug, like an antibiotic, can affect enough other motor units to impair ventilation or produce complete paralysis again.

Perianal Region

The major distinguishing consideration for perianal surgery is 45° tilting of the surgical table.[32,40] Head-down positioning causes the abdominal viscera to rest against the diaphragm, and it prevents epidural analgesia because of migration of the local anesthetic cranially in the epidural space, which impairs ventilation by blocking the nerve supply to the intercostal muscles and the diaphragm.[40] Potentially, respiratory centers in the medullary area of the brain could be blocked. Epidural analgesia can be a definite advantage for perianal surgery in certain high-risk patients, and its use may be limited by positioning.

Based on studies of human Trendelenburg positioning, with a head-down tilt of from 1 to 45°, the effects of head-down positioning are variable, but respiratory and circulatory functions may be altered.[38] The tendency for abdominal viscera to rest against the diaphragm may predispose the patient to pulmonary atelectasis; may decrease pulmonary compliance, total lung volume, and vital capacity; and may increase the work of breathing. Prolonged Trendelenburg positioning may contribute to pulmonary congestion and edema.[37]

Despite these anticipated respiratory changes in the Trendelenburg position, studies in normal dogs and human beings have not shown major abnormalities in blood gases, pH, respiratory rate, or minute volume that can be related to the positioning.[43] However, patients with elevated left atrial blood pressure and obese patients tolerate head-down positioning poorly. Because of increased venous return in the Trendelenburg position, baroreceptor responses can lead to decreased perfusion of vital organs by mediating vasodilation and mild systemic hypotension, even though central blood volume is increased.[38] Carotid blood flow decreases in anesthetized dogs subjected to a 30° tilt.[38] The increase in cranial venous blood pressure may influence intracranial and intraocular pressure, particularly in patients with elevated pressures.[43]

Head-down positioning should be used only if it improves surgical exposure and subsequently shortens operation time. Controlled ventilation should be used to prevent hypoventilation and assure appropriate anesthetic management. Particularly with halothane, controlled ventilation provides a more stable plane of anesthesia.

In patients with hypovolemia, head trauma, thoracic or pulmonary disease, obesity, or cardiac decompensation, head-down positioning is contraindicated and should be selected only after evaluating the potentially harmful physiological changes that may be induced. Because of the influence of the position on central blood volume, blood loss may be underestimated without careful patient monitoring.[38]

Hernias Involving the Gastrointestinal Tract

In patients with herniated gastrointestinal tissues, the degree of physiological disturbance varies with the amount of herniated tissue, the effect on its blood supply and function, and the influence of the herniated tissue on function of other organ systems.

Ischemia of the gastrointestinal tract, liver, or pancreas can produce changes that are important to anesthesia. Strangulation and ischemia of tissues may cause effusion of fluid from the involved organ. Later, organ rupture, toxemia, and septicemia are possible complications. Toxemia is related to bacterial toxins and to autolytic tissue products. Vasoactive amines and polypeptides may be released from ischemic tissues, and bacteria may penetrate walls of strangulated gut.[37] Systemic effects may be marked. Direct myocardial depression, peripheral vasodilation, changes in membrane permeability, variations in pulmonary circulation, and alterations in reticuloendothial function have been associated with ischemia, hypoxemia, and the release of various chemicals into the systemic circulation.

In particular, diaphragmatic hernias may result in serious derangement of both the respiratory and cardiovascular systems. The most common signs in diaphragmatic hernia include dyspnea, hyperpnea, and cyanosis, due to impairment of lung inflation causing reduced tidal volume.[54] Hypoxemia is often present, and hypercapnia may be evident if the patient is unable to compensate for respiratory impairment.

Cardiovascular effects of diaphragmatic hernia may be profound if the incarcerated viscera impinge on the vena cava or impair myocardial contraction. The hernia contents in a pericardioperitoneal defect may restrict cardiac function.[37] In trauma patients with myocardial contusions associated with a diaphragmatic hernia, dysrhythmias may be present although they may not appear until 12 to 24 hours following injury.[25] Hypovolemia may complicate diaphragmatic hernias, and low vascular volume may be associated with fluid loss and decreased fluid intake in depressed patients. In comparison with healthy patients, greater than expected cardiac and central nervous system depression may result during anesthesia.

Acidosis may be present owing to CO_2 retention or poor tissue perfusion. In either instance, certain anesthetic drugs may be less protein bound and have greater activity because of being more undissociated. Both effects may produce greater anesthetic depression of the patient than is usually expected from a "normal" anesthetic dosage.

In trauma-induced hernias, the patient is stabilized prior to anesthesia. Emergency conditions exist if respiratory distress is severe due to the presence of certain viscera in the hernia, e.g., a "trapped" stomach expanding with gas.[25] Rapid control of the airway, ventilation, and oxygenation are major goals of anesthetic management. Avoiding acute cardiovascular depression is an equally important consideration. Preinduction oxygenation by mask or chamber, preanesthetic use of glycopyrrolate, beginning fluid infusion prior to induction through a secure intravenous catheter, and electrocardiographic monitoring during induction are desirable procedures for many high-risk patients, including those with diaphragmatic hernias. In most dogs, intravenous oxymorphone (0.11 to 0.22 mg/kg) followed by a very low intravenous dose of thiopental (2 to 3 mg/kg) facilitates induction, intubation, and maintenance with halothane in oxygen. A similar technique can be used in cats, substituting a low dose of intramuscular ketamine (4 to 6 mg/kg) for the oxymorphone to reduce the thiobarbiturate to a total amount that will be less likely to cause dysrhythmias. In patients without severe respiratory distress, mask or chamber inductions using halothane in oxygen are acceptable. However, pulmonary dysfunction can inhibit anesthetic uptake, prevent adequate depth of anesthesia, and make intubation difficult.

Nitrous oxide should not be used in patients with diaphragmatic hernias because of the potential for expanding gas spaces in incarcerated viscera and because of the pulmonary ventilation and perfusion imbalances that exist in compressed lungs. Controlled ventilation should begin immediately after intubation and should continue throughout the anesthetic period to recovery. While hernia contents remain in the thorax, a high rate (12 to 15 per minute) and a low tidal volume (11 ml/kg) controlled ventilation is recommended. After the hernia is reduced, conventional methods of intermittent positive pressure ventilation can be resumed. Even higher volumes are required to eliminate atelectasis in many patients' lungs. Because of the manipulation of the gastrointestinal tract and liver during reduction of the hernia, glucocorticoids in shock doses (prednisolone, 8 to 10 mg/kg intravenously) at the beginning of surgery may alleviate or reduce the effects of compounds that may be released from ischemic tissues. Monitoring the patient for development of hypotension, dysrhythmias, hypothermia, and acid-base imbalance throughout the anesthetic period is important, and abnormalities should be corrected when recognized. If muscle relaxation is inadequate, pancuronium is probably better than drugs inducing deeper anesthetic levels to facilitate surgery.

Surgery in Patients with Ascites

A broad definition of ascites is collection of serous fluid within the peritoneal cavity. It is a secondary sign of disease and may be associated with abdominal carcinomatosis, congestive heart failure, venous stasis at the level of the liver or within the thoracic cavity, abdominal trauma, hypoproteinemia, hepatic cirrhosis, and peritonitis.[15] All these primary problems influence anesthesia, but this discussion is limited to considerations concerning peritoneal fluid. The effects of abdominal fluid include cranial displacement of the diaphragm, diminishing lung volumes and respiratory gas exchange, and impairment of peripheral arterial blood flow. Many patients with ascites are debilitated, with loss of muscle mass and fat.[15]

In patients with massive ascites, removal of the fluid precedes anesthetic induction to reduce the impairment of respiration and circulation. Protein content and cardiovascular and hepatic function may be less than normal, and appropriate precautions in selection and dosage of drugs must be taken. For abdominal exploration in patients with ascites, fluid is usually removed by suction. Rapid removal of the fluid results in loss of pressure on the blood vessels of the abdominal cavity and the hepatic and splenic blood reservoirs. This may cause a sudden need for increased blood volume to fill the vascular system, and hypovolemic shock may ensue,[17] particularly in anesthetized patients with pharmacologically compromised ability to compensate for changes in blood volume and pressure. Thus, during removal of fluid, close cardiovascular monitoring should be done, and fluid loading should be considered. Fluid selection in patients with ascites must involve evaluation of the patient's total protein and hematocrit levels. Plasma and whole blood should be selected for patients with low plasma protein (especially low albumin) and low packed cell volume, respectively. The presence of respiratory and metabolic acidosis is possible owing to ventilatory and circulatory embarrassment, and appropriate monitoring and treatment (ventilation and bicarbonate) should be a part of the anesthetic regimen.

1. Baraka, A., Saab, M., and Salem, M. R.: Control of gastric acidity by glycopyrrolate premedication in the parturient. Anesth. Analg. 56:642, 1977.
2. Batchelder, B. M., and Cooperman, L. H.: Splanchnic circulation and metabolism. Surg. Clin. North Am. 55:787, 1975.
3. Borland, L. M., Swan, D. M., and Leff, S.: Difficult pediatric endotracheal intubation: A new approach to the retrograde technique. Anesthesiology 55:577, 1981.
4. Carlson, W. D.: Veterinary Radiology. 2nd ed. Lea & Febiger, Philadelphia, 1967, p. 303.
5. Carson, I. W., Moore, J., Palmer, J. P., et al.: Laryngeal competence with ketamine and other drugs. Anesthesiology 38:128, 1973.
6. Chambers, J. N.: Diseases of the intestines. In Bojrab, M. J. (ed.): Pathophysiology in Small Animal Surgery. Lea & Febiger, Philadelphia, 1981, p. 112.
7. Christensen, V., and Skovsted, P.: Effects of general anesthetics on the pH of gastric contents of man during surgery: A survey of halothane, fluroxene and cyclopropane anaesthesia. Acta Anaesth. Scand. 19:49, 1975.
8. Dawidson, I., Applegren, L., Gelin, L. E., et al.: Skeletal muscle microcirculation and oxygenation in experimental intestinal shock: A study on efficacy of different plasma substitutes. Circ. Shock 7:435, 1980.

9. Dawidson, I., Gelin, L. E., and Haglund, E.: Plasma volume, intravascular protein content, hemodynamic and oxygen transport changes during intestinal shock in dogs. Crit. Care Med. 8:73, 1980.

10. Douglas, W. W.: Histamine and 5-hydroxytryptamine (serotonin) and their antagonists. In Gilman, A. G., Goodman, L. S., and Gilman, A. (eds.): The Pharmacological Basis of Therapeutics. 6th ed. New York, MacMillan, 1980, p. 609.

11. Downs, J. B., Chapman, R. L., Modell, J. H., et al.: An evaluation of steroid therapy in aspiration pneumonitis. Anesthesiology 40:129, 1974.

12. Dykes, M. H. M.: Anesthetic hepatotoxicity. In Hershey, S. G. (ed.): Refresher Courses in Anesthesiology. Vol. 10. J. B. Lippincott, Philadelphia, 1982, p. 75.

13. Eger, E. I., II: Anesthetic Uptake and Action. Baltimore, Williams & Wilkins, 1974, p. 171.

14. Eger, E. I., II, and Saidman, L. J.: Hazards of nitrous oxide anesthesia in bowel obstruction and pneumothorax. Anesthesiology 26:61, 1965.

15. Ettinger, S. J.: Ascites, peritonitis, and other causes of abdominal enlargement. In Ettinger, S. J. (ed.): Textbook of Veterinary Internal Medicine. W. B. Saunders, Philadelphia, 1983, p. 121.

16. Farman, J. V.: Anaesthesia in the presence of liver disease and for hepatic transplantation. Br. J. Anaesth. 44:946, 1972.

17. Guyton, A. C.: Circulatory shock and physiology of its treatment. In Textbook of Medical Physiology. 4th ed. W. B. Saunders, Philadelphia, 1971, p. 325.

18. Hartsfield, S. M.: Body temperature variations associated with general anesthesia: A review. Part I: Hypothermia. Southwest. Vet. 32:95, 1979.

19. Hartsfield, S. M.: Anesthesia of the critical patient: General anesthesia for critically ill patients. In Sattler, F. P., Knowles, R. P., and Whittick, W. G. (eds.): Veterinary Critical Care. Lea & Febiger, Philadelphia, 1981, p. 384.

20. Hartsfield, S. M., Gendreau, C. L., Smith, C. W., et al.: Endotracheal intubation by pharyngotomy. J. Am. Anim. Hosp. Assoc. 13:71, 1977.

21. Hartsfield, S. M., and Tholen, M. A.: Dental anesthesia. In Tholen, M. A.: Concepts in Veterinary Dentistry. Veterinary Medicine Publishing Company, Edwardsville, KA, 1983, p. 23.

22. Herzel, W. M.: Use of methoxyflurane in veterinary medicine. Part 3. Pract. Vet. 48:4, 1976.

23. Hsu, W. H., and McNeel, S. V.: Effect of yohimbine on xylazine-induced prolongation of gastrointestinal transit in dogs. J. Am. Vet. Med. Assoc. 183:297, 1983.

24. Hyde, R. W.: Clinical interpretation of arterial oxygen measurements. Med. Clin. North Am. 54:617, 1970.

25. Kagan, K. G.: Thoracic trauma. Vet. Clin. North Am. 10:641, 1980.

26. Katz, R. L.: Drug-relaxant interactions. In Proceedings of the 29th Annual Refresher Course Lectures. No. 217 B. American Society of Anesthesiologists, Chicago, 1978, p. 1.

27. Kolata, R. J., Burrows, C. F., and Soma, L. R.: Shock: Pathophysiology and management. In Kirk, R. W. (ed.): Current Veterinary Therapy 7: Small Animal Practice. W. B. Saunders, Philadelphia, 1980, p. 32.

28. Kurtzman, N. A., White, M. G., and Rodgers, P. W.: Pathophysiology of metabolic alkalosis. Arch. Intern. Med. 131:702, 1973.

29. Lefer, A. M.: Vascular mediators in ischemia and shock. In Cowley, R. A., and Trump, B. F. (eds.): Pathophysiology of Shock, Anoxia and Ischemia. Williams & Wilkins, Baltimore, 1982, p. 165.

30. Lefer, A. M., and Glenn, T. M.: Corticosteroids and the lysosomal protease–MDF system. In Glenn, T. M. (ed.): Corticosteroids in the Therapy of Shock. University Park Press, Baltimore, 1974, p. 233.

31. Lewis, L. D., and Phillips, R. W.: Diarrhea. In Bojrab, M. J. (ed.): Pathophysiology in Small Animal Surgery. Lea & Febiger, Philadelphia, 1981, p. 148.

32. Lowry, E. C.: The perianal and anovaginal regions. In Bojrab, M. J. (ed.): Current Techniques in Small Animal Surgery. Lea & Febiger, Philadelphia, 1975, p. 159.

33. McGrath, C. J., Short, C. E., and Paddleford, R. R.: Pancuronium bromide: An adjunct to anesthetic management of the dog. Vet. Anesth. 2:14, 1975.

34. Muir, W. W.: Drugs used to produce standing chemical restraint in horses. Vet. Clin. North Am. 3:17, 1981.

35. Muir, W. W.: Gastric dilation-volvulus in the dog, with emphasis on cardiac arrhythmias. J. Am. Vet. Med. Assoc. 180:739, 1982.

36. Muir, W. W.: Acid-base and electrolyte disturbances in dogs with gastric dilatation-volvulus. J. Am. Vet. Med. Assoc. 181:229, 1982.

37. Parks, J.: Herniation. In Bojrab, M. J. (ed.): Pathophysiology in Small Animal Surgery. Lea & Febiger, Philadelphia, 1981, p. 420.

38. Prentice, J. A.: Anesthesiologic considerations. In Martin, J. T.: Positioning in Anesthesia and Surgery. W. B. Saunders, Philadelphia, 1978, p. 90.

39. Ramamurthy, S., Ylagan, L. B., and Winnie, A. P.: Glycopyrrolate as a substitute for atropine: A preliminary report. Anesth. Analg. 50:732, 1971.

40. Rawlings, C. A.: Anal sac extraction. In Wingfield, W. E., and Rawlings, C. A.: Small Animal Surgery; An Atlas of Operative Techniques. W. B. Saunders, Philadelphia, 1979, p. 104.

41. Sawyer, D. C.: The Practice of Small Animal Anesthesia. W. B. Saunders, Philadelphia, 1982, p. 4.

42. Schaer, M.: Disorders of potassium metabolism. Vet. Clin. North Am. 12:399, 1982.

43. Schiller, W. R.: The Trendelenburg position; Surgical requirements. In Martin, J. T.: Positioning in Anesthesia and Surgery. W. B. Saunders, Philadelphia, 1978, p. 89.

44. Short, C. E., and Miller, R. L.: Comparative evaluation of the anticholinergic agent glycopyrrolate as a preanesthetic agent. Vet. Med./Small Anim. Clin. 73:1269, 1978.

45. Short, C. E., Paddleford, R. R., and Cloyd, G. D.: Glycopyrrolate for prevention of pulmonary complications during anesthesia. Mod. Vet. Pract. 55:194, 1974.

46. Soma, L. R.: Anesthetic management. In Soma, L. R. (ed.): Textbook of Veterinary Anesthesia. Williams & Wilkins, Baltimore, 1971, p. 287.

47. Standaert, M. D.: Interactions among neuromuscular blocking agents and other drugs. In Refresher Courses in Anesthesiology. Vol. 6. J. B. Lippincott, Philadelphia, 1978, p. 111.

48. Strombeck, D. R., Krum, S., and Rogers, Q.: Coagulopathy and encephalopathy in a dog with acute hepatic necrosis. J. Am. Vet. Med. Assoc. 169:813, 1976.

49. Strunin, L.: The splanchnic, hepatic and portal circulations. In Prys-Roberts, C. (ed.): The Circulation in Anaesthesia. Blackwell Scientific Publications, London, 1980, p. 241.

50. Thurmon, J. C., and Kumar, A.: Physiologic changes affecting anesthetic management in gastrointestinal obstruction. Vet. Clin. North Am. 3:65, 1973.

51. Vulgamott, J. C.: Hepatic encephalopathy associated with acquired portacaval shunt in a dog. J. Am. Vet. Med. Assoc. 175:724, 1979.

52. Weipers, W. L.: Experimental work on intestinal obstruction in the dog. Vet. Rec. 77:581, 1965.

53. White, R. J.: Cardiac arrhythmias during anesthesia. In Soma, L. R. (ed.): Textbook of Veterinary Anesthesia. Williams & Wilkins, Baltimore, 1971, p. 580.

54. Wilson, G. P., Newton, C. D., and Burt, J. K.: A review of 116 diaphragmatic hernias in dogs and cats. J. Am. Vet. Med. Assoc. 159:1142, 1971.

55. Wingfield, W. E.: The stomach. In Bojrab, M. J. (ed.): Pathophysiology in Small Animal Surgery. Lea & Febiger, Philadelphia, 1981, p. 101.

56. Zontine, W. J.: Effects of chemical restraint drugs on the passage of barium sulfate through the stomach and duodenum of dogs. J. Am. Vet. Med. Assoc. 162:878, 1973.

Chapter 189

Anesthesia and the Respiratory System

Jacqueline L. Grandy and Eugene P. Steffy

General anesthesia alters respiratory function in a variety of ways and to varying degrees. The magnitude of the insult depends on the patient's physical status, the drugs employed, techniques of monitoring the patient and supporting the vital functions, and the anesthetist's abilities.

An appreciation of the effects of anesthesia on the respiratory system and an understanding of the anesthetic management of the patient with respiratory disease require as a basis a brief review of respiratory physiology and pathophysiology (see Chapter 62).[12,69,112]

ANESTHESIA AND RESPIRATION

Changes in respiratory function are a common consequence of general anesthesia regardless of the anesthetic technique used. In addition, some drugs used in anesthetic management of small animal patients cause specific respiratory effects. Both nonspecific influences of anesthesia and specific anesthetic-induced respiratory effects are important considerations in devising an appropriate anesthetic plan.

Changes in Functional Residual Capacity

During anesthesia, relaxation of the thoracic and diaphragmatic muscles, forward displacement of the diaphragm by abdominal contents, and recumbent positioning of the patient all decrease intrathoracic volume, tidal volume, and functional residual capacity (FRC).[29,56] As a result of the decrease in FRC, lung compliance is reduced and lung resistance is increased in the anesthetized patient.[18,70] Hypoventilation during general anesthesia is common and results in an increase in Pa_{CO_2} (partial pressure of carbon dioxide) and a decrease in Pa_{O_2} (partial pressure of oxygen) below expected values. Although the respiratory rate may increase in an effort to maintain minute volume, the increase usually is not sufficient to maintain adequate alveolar ventilation owing to an increase in deadspace ventilation.

A reduction in FRC is consistently observed with all types of general anesthesia. It occurs soon after induction but does not necessarily become progressively worse with time.[74] With a decrease in FRC, atelectasis and small airway closure frequently increase. Continued perfusion of these areas results in additional venous admixture and contributes to the increased A-a P_{O_2} difference (the difference between the alveolar (A) and the arterial P_{O_2}).

Changes in Distribution of Ventilation and Perfusion

As a result of the decrease in lung compliance and FRC, ventilation in the anesthetized patient is preferentially distributed to nondependent lung regions[81] (Fig. 189–1). Because hypoxic pulmonary vasoconstriction is also inhibited by many anesthetic agents, perfusion of dependent lung regions continues to be out of proportion to ventilation, resulting in an abnormal distribution of ventilation and perfusion during anesthesia.

An enlargement in respiratory deadspace frequently accompanies general anesthesia.[19] Often this is an increase both in anatomic deadspace subsequent to drug-induced bronchodilation and in alveolar deadspace due to ventilation of unperfused alveoli. Increased deadspace may be further augmented by faulty anesthetic equipment such as an improper sized face mask or endotracheal tube. With anes-

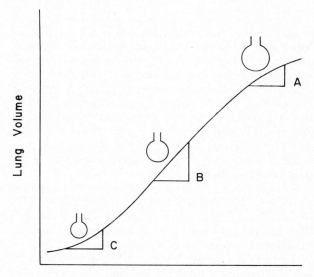

Figure 189–1. Changes in lung volume with varying transpulmonary pressure. With less negative transpulmonary pressure in dependent regions, alveoli are more prone to collapse. In normal awake humans in lateral recumbency the pressure-volume characteristics of the upper lung are represented by A and the lower lung by B. Note the larger change in B (lower lung) for the same change in pressure as in A (i.e., larger volume change of the lower lung). With reductions in functional residual capacity in the anesthetized patient, alveoli in upper lung regions are best represented by B, whereas alveoli in lower regions are represented by C. The change in volume for the same change in pressure is now less in lower lung regions, and ventilation is preferentially distributed to the upper lung.

thetic-induced reductions in tidal volume, this increase in mechanical and physiological deadspace, also referred to as wasted ventilation, further contributes to decreased alveolar ventilation.

Atelectasis During Anesthesia

Production of atelectic areas of lung during general anesthesia is favored by a number of conditions including the absence of spontaneous deep breaths,[3,65] long periods of immobility,[79] increased airway secretions and accumulation of these secretions,[26] low lung volume (decreased FRC), inspiration of high partial pressures of oxygen (O_2), and compression of dependent areas by the mediastinal contents or the pressure of abdominal contents on the diaphragm.

Atelectasis during anesthesia is one of the main causes of an increased A-a P_{O_2} difference. As a result, the venous admixture may increase from less than 5 per cent in the normal awake patient to 22 per cent during uncomplicated anesthesia in humans.[94] In an attempt to minimize the amount of atelectasis, anesthetized patients should be given a large breath (a "sigh") at least twice every five minutes.

Changes in Arterial Oxygen Tensions

Because $P_{I_{O_2}}$ (partial pressure of inspired oxygen) is one of the main determinants of Pa_{O_2}, patients breathing an enriched O_2 mixture should be hyperoxemic. Although the A-a P_{O_2} difference is increased when patients breathe gas mixtures with an elevated $F_{I_{O_2}}$ (fraction of inspired oxygen), a rough estimate of ideal Pa_{O_2} may be obtained by multiplying the $F_{I_{O_2}}$ by 500.[88] When breathing 100 per cent O_2, a Pa_{O_2} of less than 450 mm Hg indicates an increase in venous admixture. Within the time limits of a surgical procedure, inspiration of high partial pressures of O_2 does not produce O_2 toxicity.

If N_2O (nitrous oxide) is being used with O_2 during anesthesia, the $F_{I_{O_2}}$ will vary depending on the ratio of gases in the mixture. It is recommended that not less than 30 per cent O_2 be delivered to the patient to maintain a Pa_{O_2} above 100 mm Hg.

Because of increased hypoventilation, pulmonary vascular shunts, and alveolar ventilation-perfusion ratio (V/Q) mismatch during anesthesia, healthy animals breathing room air may be subjected to varying degrees of hypoxemia. Although this can be tolerated for some time in healthy patients, in older or debilitated animals it may contribute further to morbidity or mortality.

Changes in Control of Ventilation

In the absence of external stimulation, spontaneous ventilation during anesthesia largely depends on

TABLE 189–1.   Causes of Changes in Pa_{O_2} and Pa_{CO_2}

Pa_{O_2}	Pa_{CO_2}
Decreased	
Low $F_{I_{O_2}}$	Hyperventilation
Impaired diffusion	
Hypoventilation	
$\dot{V}/\dot{Q}$ mismatch	
Arterial-to-venous shunting	
Increased	
High inspired $F_{I_{O_2}}$	Hypoventilation
Hyperventilation	Increased inspired CO_2

chemical drive. The responsiveness of both peripheral and central chemoreceptors to changes in Pa_{CO_2} and Pa_{O_2} is reduced by anesthetic agents (Table 189–1). Almost all anesthetic agents depress central control mechanisms in a dose-related fashion. This is manifested by a decreased slope of the CO_2 response curve (Fig. 189–2). Changes in apneic threshold are another index of the way in which ventilatory function is influenced by anesthetic agents. The apneic threshold is the Pa_{CO_2} at which a patient is hyperventilated to the point of apnea.[25,36] Lowering the Pa_{CO_2} below the apneic threshold in the anesthetized patient eliminates spontaneous breathing. The resting Pa_{CO_2} and the apneic threshold generally differ by about 5 mm Hg in human beings.[41] In the presence of respiratory depression and an increase in the Pa_{CO_2}, the apneic threshold is elevated by an equivalent amount.

The response of the patient to hypoxia is mediated solely by the carotid chemoreceptors. Even light levels of barbiturate, halothane, enflurane, or isoflurane anesthesia in dogs markedly depress hypoxic drive,[44] and subanesthetic concentrations of halothane in humans have significantly impaired the

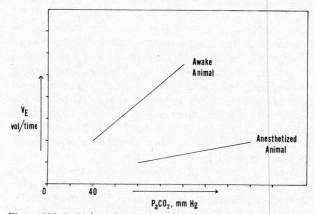

Figure 189–2. Carbon dioxide–ventilation response curve. A moderate increase in Pa_{CO_2} will trigger a marked increase in ventilation in the awake animal. However, the anesthetized animal requires a greater Pa_{CO_2} to initiate a ventilatory response and the magnitude of the response is diminished. (Reprinted with permission from Steffey, E. P., and Gillespie, J. R.: Respiration and general anesthesia. Vet. Clin. North Am 3:45, 1973.)

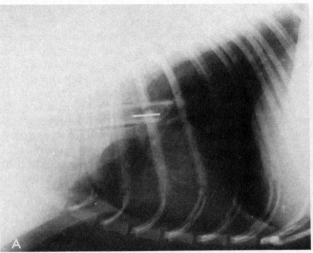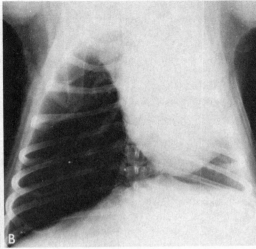

Figure 189–3. *A,* Lateral radiograph of the thorax of a dog. The endotracheal tube has been advanced beyond the carina into a mainstem bronchus. *B,* Ventral-dorsal radiograph of the same dog. Note collapse of left cranial lung lobe as a result of malpositioning of the tube seen in *A.*

response to hypoxia even when the response to increased CO_2 was intact.[53] The reaction to hypoxia is normally augmented by hypercapnia, but this may also be diminished or abolished under anesthesia.[110]

The effects of anesthesia on ventilation may be further modified by premedication, the duration of anesthesia, and surgical stimulation.[86,97] For example, surgical stimulation during light anesthesia may increase minute ventilation and decrease Pa_{CO_2}.[20]

Anesthetic Equipment

Pharyngeal and laryngeal muscle relaxation and suppression of the normal protective airway reflexes predispose the anesthetized patient to airway obstruction. This is an even greater risk in brachiocephalic breeds or in animals with upper airway pathology (e.g., tumor or collapsing trachea). Anesthetic agents also significantly impair tracheal mucociliary flow,[26] and the accumulation of normal respiratory secretions may cause obstruction, laryngospasm,[92] and an increased resistance to breathing.[34]

Endotracheal intubation of the anesthetized patient is an important factor in providing a patent airway and in preventing aspiration, but intubation does not guarantee a patent airway. Endotracheal tubes may become plugged with mucus, or a bronchus may be easily blocked by a tube that has been advanced too far (Fig. 189–3). Once warmed by body heat, endotracheal tubes may become soft and bend easily inside the oral cavity and may therefore be difficult to see. The lumen of the tube may be occluded by excessively high pressure in the endotracheal tube cuff. Herniation of the cuff over the end of the endotracheal tube, resulting in an obstructed airway, may occur if the tube is withdrawn or moved without first deflating the cuff. Choosing the correct length of endotracheal tube is just as important as choosing

the correct diameter. Tubes that are too long add needlessly to the patient's respiratory deadspace, predispose to excessive advancement caudally, or may be easily bent if an excess length of tube lies between the patient and connection to the anesthetic circuit. Surgical drapes covering the endotracheal tube and connections to the anesthetic machine may prevent recognition of a kinked endotracheal tube or disconnection from the anesthetic machine. In a survey of preventable anesthetic mishaps, disconnection of the human patient from the breathing circuit was the most frequent accident.[13] Incorrect fresh gas flow settings and gas supply problems were also common adverse occurrences.

Leaks in the anesthetic circuit (e.g., improper positioning of the soda lime canister or a loose connection between the Y-piece and the endotracheal tube) may result in escape of anesthetic gases and pollution of the environment or dilution of gases in the anesthetic circuit. The latter results in a lower FI_{O_2} and inspired anesthetic gas concentration.

In addition to the increase in respiratory resistance that results from a decrease in FRC, certain equipment-related factors may also increase the work of breathing. Examples include undersized endotracheal tubes, sticky one-way valves on the anesthetic machine, and having small dogs or cats breathe from a circle system rather than from a nonrebreathing system. Although it has been shown that healthy adult cats maintain adequate ventilation on a circle system,[37] this may not be the case in older or debilitated small animal patients.

Surgical Influence

Patient positioning and requirements for surgical exposure, such as severe abdominal retraction, may further decrease lung expansion. Tying the legs tightly across the chest, a surgeon or surgical instruments resting on the chest, or placement of the patient in a head-down position all interfere with ventilation. The changes due to positioning are even more profound in obese patients and those with full stomachs.

Although metabolic demands are reduced under anesthesia, any decrease in hemoglobin (e.g., anemia, hemorrhage), arterial saturation, or cardiac output may result in a deficiency of O_2 delivery to the tissues. Blood for transfusion that has been stored for a period of time will have a decrease in 2,3-diphosphoglycerate (DPG) that will influence the affinity of O_2 for hemoglobin, resulting in a shift in the oxyhemoglobin dissociation curve to the left, thus interfering with O_2 delivery to the tissues.

Lung Defense

Removal of inhaled particles from the lung is a key defense mechanism. The cough reflex is an important means of displacing foreign material from the upper airways, whereas the lower airways depend on functioning of the mucociliary system. By suppressing the cough reflex and decreasing mucociliary clearance, anesthetic agents interfere with lung defense. Additionally, interruption of mucociliary clearance and removal of microbial agents is decreased by accompanying hypoxia, tracheal intubation, hypotension, acidosis, and azotemia.[105] Rapid proliferation of bacteria occurs in the atelectic lung.

Postanesthetic Period

In healthy young persons not undergoing surgery of the thorax or upper abdomen, the deterioration in gas exchange and reduction in lung volume associated with general anesthesia are usually reversed within two to three hours of recovery from anesthesia.[62] Nonetheless, problems with oxygenation and CO_2 retention do not disappear immediately, and ventilation may remain depressed during recovery. Furthermore, hypoventilation slows the removal of volatile anesthetic drugs and may prolong anesthetic recovery.

Because FI_{O_2} is high during inhalation anesthesia, hypoventilation usually does not cause hypoxemia in most patients. However, at the conclusion of anesthesia when the patient is again permitted to breathe room air, hypoventilation and V/Q mismatch may result in a low Pa_{O_2}. Because Pa_{O_2} decreases with age, hypoxemia may more easily occur in older patients.[73] Additionally, the normal ventilatory response to hypoxemia is diminished even by subanesthetic concentrations of many anesthetic agents. Hypoxemia in the postoperative period may delay recovery, exacerbate organ dysfunction, increase central nervous system (CNS) depression, and contribute to mortality.

Pain control during recovery is important not only for the patient's comfort but also because postoperative pain may cause "reluctance" to breathe deeply or to cough, both of which are important in minimizing postanesthetic pulmonary complications. Administration of an analgesic drug is often beneficial to the patient. Narcotics are very effective, but at high doses they may produce severe respiratory depression.[49] Nerve blocks with certain local anesthetics are valuable in controlling pain without retarding postanesthetic return of normal pulmonary function.[93]

Postoperative pain usually decreases with time, the period immediately following surgery being the most painful.[48] Immediate postsurgical reversal of a narcotic analgesic drug with a narcotic antagonist results in a very fast but frequently painful recovery. If possible, at least one to three hours should be allowed to elapse after a painful surgery before a narcotic antagonist is used. Pulmonary function must be closely watched during this time, and arterial blood gases should be measured if possible. Doxapram administered intravenously may be of value in improving ventilation without removing analgesia.

Hypothermia commonly occurs during general anesthesia, especially in small patients[108], and negatively influences respirations and O_2 delivery. Hy-

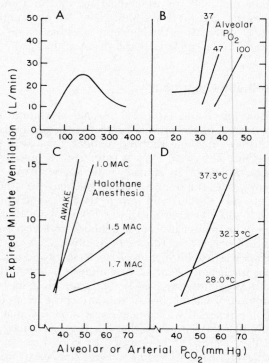

Figure 189–4. A, Effect of Pa_{CO_2} on ventilation in lightly anesthetized (halothane) dogs (from data of Eisele et al., 1967). B, Influence of PA_{CO_2} on CO_2 response curves of conscious human volunteers (from data of Nielsen and Smith, 1951). Influence of increasing dose (MAC) of halothane-O_2 anesthesia (C) and hypothermia (D) on canine CO_2 dose response curves. (From data of Brandstater et al., 1965; and Regan and Eger, 1966, respectively. Reprinted with permission from Ettinger, S. J. (ed.): *Textbook of Veterinary Internal Medicine*, 2nd ed. W. B. Saunders, Philadelphia, 1983, p. 688.)

pothermia increases hemoglobin's affinity for O_2 by displacing the oxyhemoglobin dissociation curve to the left. Hypothermia also causes an increase in anatomic deadspace[87] and, as seen in Figure 189–4D, a reduction in ventilatory responsiveness to increased Pa_{CO2} and decreased Pa_{O2}.[80] Every attempt should be made to maintain normal body temperature during surgery and anesthetic recovery. This is best achieved by using circulating hot water heating pads. Patients may shiver violently during recovery from general anesthesia. In humans, shivering has been found to cause up to a fourfold increase in O_2 consumption.[2] This may place a tremendous burden on the cardiopulmonary system at a time when it may still be compromised by surgery and anesthesia.

Regurgitation, aspiration, and upper airway obstruction are always possible during anesthetic recovery. Premature postanesthetic removal of the endotracheal tube further predisposes the patient to these complications. Patients who do not voluntarily move about during the anesthetic recovery phase should be maintained in a sternal recumbent position or moved from side to side every hour in an attempt to avoid further respiratory depression. If hypoxemia is suspected during recovery, the animal should be allowed to breathe an O_2-enriched gas mixture through either a mask or endotracheal tube until the underlying cause is found and corrected.

CHANGES IN RESPIRATION CAUSED BY DRUGS

Anticholinergic Drugs

Contemporary anticholinergic drugs include atropine, scopolamine, and glycopyrrolate. Atropine is most widely used in veterinary medicine. It inhibits bronchial secretions, increases lung compliance[16] and anatomic deadspace,[87] decreases airway resistance,[32] and may contribute to the reduction in tracheal mucus velocity that accompanies general anesthesia.[1] In the healthy, awake patient the increase in deadspace is usually compensated by a small increase in minute volume so that Pa_{CO2} remains unchanged.[75,91]

Tranquilizers

Probably the most commonly used tranquilizer in small animal practice is acetylpromazine. In general, low doses of acetylpromazine by itself have little effect on respiration but may potentiate the respiratory depression caused by other drugs.[92] Respiratory rate may decrease in the quiet patient, but this decrease is not accompanied by significant changes in Pa_{O2}, Pa_{CO2}, or hemoglobin saturation.[77,107] Large doses of phenothiazine tranquilizers may depress respiration.[47]

The butyrophonone tranquilizer droperidol is widely used in combination with the narcotic fentanyl (Innovar Vet).* Clinically, in low doses droperidol alone appears to have minimal adverse effects on pulmonary function.

Sedatives and Hypnotics

Barbiturates are the most commonly used group of sedative hypnotic drugs employed in small animal anesthesia. These drugs have a dose-related range of effects on the CNS. When used to produce sedation only, respiratory rate alone may be decreased. When used to produce general anesthesia, barbiturates are potent respiratory depressants. Apnea often occurs immediately after injection of an anesthetic induction dose. Alveolar ventilation is decreased and Pa_{CO2} is increased at ordinary surgical levels of barbiturate anesthesia. Patient responsiveness to hypercapnia and hypoxia is also diminished. Generally, protective airway reflexes are maintained in the lighter planes of barbiturate anesthesia. Coughing and laryngospasm can occur; the cough reflex is depressed only with doses that cause respiratory embarrassment. The activity of the cilia lining the respiratory passages is also reduced by barbiturates. Barbiturates do not suppress hypoxic pulmonary vasoconstriction.[4]

Xylazine, at low doses in dogs (1.1 mg/kg intravenously or 2.2 mg/kg intramuscularly) and in cats (4.4 mg/kg intramuscularly), has minimal effects on arterial blood gases.[38,52] Respiratory depression does become significant when xylazine is combined with other drugs. Hypoxemia and hypercapnia have been reported during anesthesia produced by the combination of xylazine and ketamine.[54]

Narcotics and Narcotic Antagonists

Through their effects on the brain stem respiratory center, narcotics cause marked respiratory depression. This depression is drug- and dose-related and is manifested by an increase in Pa_{CO2} and a decrease in Pa_{O2}.[91] Narcotics reduce the responsiveness of the central chemoreceptors to hypoxia and hypercapnia.[109] This is depicted as a shift to the right and a decrease in the slope of the CO_2 response curve (see Fig. 189–2). In most species the cough reflex is suppressed, and bronchoconstriction may also occur.[106] Respiratory rhythm becomes very regular, and there may be an absence of spontaneous deep breaths (sighs). Apnea may occur after intravenous injection of narcotics. In the dog narcotics may also cause panting. Narcotics do not depress hypoxic pulmonary vasoconstriction.[28]

The effects of large doses of narcotics vary among species. In humans and dogs, large doses cause sleep and marked respiratory depression, whereas in cats, excitement or convulsions may result.

Reduced thoracic compliance, or "woody chest" syndrome, is sometimes reported in humans following large doses of intravenous fentanyl. Fentanyl has

---

*Pitman-Moore, Inc., Washington Crossing, NJ.

also been associated with thoracic rigidity in the dog.[64] This stiff chest can be overcome by administration of either a narcotic antagonist or a neuromuscular blocking drug.

Narcotic depression of the CNS can be reversed with narcotic antagonists such as levallorphan, nalorphine, naloxone, and naltrexone. Levallorphan and nalorphine possess both agonist and antagonist properties and may produce respiratory depression. Naloxone and naltrexone are short-acting narcotic antagonists devoid of narcotic agonist properties and are most effective in reversing narcotic-induced respiratory depression.[30]

Dissociative Agents

Ketamine produces a variety of effects on the respiratory system. Although some authors have reported respiratory stimulation with ketamine (5 mg/kg administered intravenously to unmedicated dogs[50]), in general, at clinically used doses ketamine causes dose-dependent respiratory depression, resulting in an increase in Pa_{CO2} and a decrease in Pa_{O2}.[10,38] At higher doses or when combined with other drugs, ketamine causes more profound respiratory depression.[54]

Respiratory control mechanisms are diminished by anesthetizing doses of ketamine, and the slope of the CO_2 response curve is decreased in relation to ketamine dose. However, this depression is not as great as that seen with most other drugs. Unlike many other anesthetic drugs, ketamine alone in dogs causes minimal or no decrease in the ventilatory response to hypoxia and the augmentation of this response by hypercapnia.[43] Hypoxic pulmonary vasoconstriction is not influenced by ketamine.[4]

A change in the pattern of respiration is often seen with ketamine. Apneustic breathing frequently occurs, and with higher doses respiration may become shallow and irregular. An intravenous bolus of ketamine may produce apnea.

Regurgitation and aspiration are possible during ketamine anesthesia. In studies with human patients anesthetized with 2 mg/kg of ketamine, aspiration of a radiopaque contrast material injected over the back of the tongue occurred despite the fact that the material had initiated swallowing in all patients.[103] Aspiration took place without any clinical indication of its occurrence. Tracheal intubation can easily be performed in animals during ketamine anesthesia; therefore, intubation is recommended.

Ketamine usually increases salivation, and anticholinergic premedication is recommended. Bronchoconstriction may be eliminated with ketamine because of its direct relaxation of bronchial smooth muscle.[60]

Inhalation Agents

Halothane, methoxyflurane, enflurane, and isoflurane depress ventilation in a dose-related manner.[9,96]

In dogs, ventilatory depression appears less with halothane or methoxyflurane than with isoflurane.[96] Enflurane is at least as potent a respiratory depressant as is isoflurane.[51] During anesthesia with any of these inhaled agents, Pa_{CO2} and apneic threshold are increased with increasing alveolar dose, the ventilatory responses to increasing CO_2 loads (see Fig. 189–4C) and hypoxia are decreased, and the A-a P_{O2} difference is increased. Bronchodilation,[42] depression of mucociliary flow,[26] and an increase in tracheal compliance[76] have also been reported with halothane.

Volatile anesthetic agents are capable of negatively influencing hypoxic pulmonary vasoconstriction, but results vary among investigators. The widest variation in results has been reported for halothane; some investigators have reported dose-dependent depression,[58,99] whereas others have found no effect on or slight enhancement of hypoxic pulmonary vasoconstriction.[4,23,100] Methoxyflurane has no significant effect on the redistribution of blood flow with hypoxia in the dog lung,[61] but it may cause significant depression of the response in the isolated cat lung.[102] Lack of effect on hypoxic pulmonary vasoconstriction is reported for enflurane,[63] whereas isoflurane shows dose-dependent inhibition of the response.[4]

Except for its influence on Fi_{O2}, the direct effects of nitrous oxide (N_2O) on ventilation are generally minimal. When N_2O is added to other anesthetic agents it may augment respiratory depression. In spontaneously breathing dogs, Pa_{CO2} increased more when halothane and N_2O were administered together than when halothane alone was given.[95] To avoid hypoxemia, N_2O should generally not be administered at a concentration greater than 70 per cent (i.e., 70 per cent N_2O, 30 per cent O_2). Most investigators agree that N_2O inhibits hypoxic pulmonary vasoconstriction.[46,101]

When nitrogen in a closed gas space is replaced by N_2O, the greater solubility of N_2O results in an increase in the volume of gas in the gas space with subsequent expansion of this space. Thus N_2O is contraindicated when air is trapped in any viscus (e.g., intestinal obstruction or pneumothorax). Air injected into the cuff of the endotracheal tube may also be expanded by N_2O. Occasionally this has resulted in overexpansion of the cuff, causing excessive pressure on the tracheal wall or collapse of the endotracheal tube.[71]

Upon discontinuation of N_2O large volumes of the gas are exhaled. If the patient breathes room air as soon as N_2O administration ceases, the large outflow of N_2O into the alveoli decreases alveolar O_2, and hypoxemia may result. This is known as diffusion hypoxia. Diffusion hypoxia may be avoided by administration of O_2 for at least three to five minutes after N_2O has been discontinued.[34]

Respiratory Stimulants

Doxapram is a potent respiratory stimulant that acts on the peripheral chemoreceptors[68] to increase both tidal volume and respiratory rate transiently.[8]

In human patients given doxapram during recovery from anesthesia, Pa_{O_2} remained elevated even after the tidal volume and respiratory rate decreased.[27,57] This may have been due to re-inflation of collapsed or partly collapsed lung by deep breaths. Patients given doxapram following inhalation anesthesia also have shorter anesthetic recovery times.[35,83]

Although doxapram has been used in animals to hasten recovery after anesthesia or heavy sedation, duration of its respiratory effects in cats and dogs is less than five minutes. Doxapram is not necessarily an acceptable treatment for patients in respiratory distress. The underlying cause should be treated and proper support given.

Neuromuscular Blocking Drugs and Cholinesterase Inhibitors

Drugs acting at the neuromuscular junction cause paralysis of all skeletal muscle and should not be used unless ventilatory support is provided. If muscle relaxants have been used during anesthesia, mechanical or manual ventilation should continue throughout recovery until there are signs of adequate neuromuscular function. Although the effects of depolarizing drugs such as succinylcholine disappear relatively quickly, nondepolarizing drugs such as gallamine and pancuronium are more slowly metabolized and require reversal with an anticholinesterase drug such as neostigmine or pyridostigmine to ensure return of adequate respiratory function.

Physostigmine is a cholinesterase inhibitor that, unlike neostigmine, crosses the blood-brain barrier. Physostigmine reverses CNS and respiratory depression of certain drugs such as atropine,[39] scopolamine, phenothiazines,[6] fentanyl-droperidol,[7] and diazepam[55] and has been useful in treating overdoses of these drugs. It transiently antagonizes halothane anesthesia.[45]

ANESTHETIC MANAGEMENT OF THE PATIENT WITH RESPIRATORY SYSTEM DISEASE

Table 189–2 summarizes the anesthetic techniques described in this section.

Preanesthetic Evaluation

Normal pulmonary function is disrupted by general anesthesia. More profound disturbances are anticipated in animals with pre-existing respiratory disease or in animals requiring surgical intervention on some portion of the respiratory system. Abnormalities of the respiratory system may have numerous causes. Regardless of the cause, every effort should be made to have the patient in the best possible physical condition prior to anesthesia. For example, following trauma to the chest that results in lung contusion,

TABLE 189–2. Summary of Anesthetic Techniques for the Patient Undergoing Thoracic Surgery

Premedication:	None
	Atropine (0.02–0.04 mg/kg intramuscularly)
	Meperidine (2–4 mg/kg intramuscularly)
Induction:	Preoxygenate for three to five minutes
	Thiobarbiturate (10 mg/kg intravenously to effect)
	Ketamine (in cats, 2–6 mg/kg intravenously)
	Narcotic ± neuromuscular blocking drug
Maintenance:	Inhalation anesthetic in 100% O_2 ± neuromuscular blocking drug. May supplement with narcotic or ketamine
Support and monitoring:	Electrocardiogram, blood pressure, fluids, arterial blood gases, positive pressure ventilation
Recovery:	Support ventilation Supplement with O_2 Keep patient warm Control pain

pneumothorax, or diaphragmatic hernia, animals should be allowed several days' cage rest if possible. Pneumothorax, hemothorax, and pyothorax all reduce the available lung volume, and removal of the air or liquid significantly improves the animal's ability to ventilate adequately. Dehydration, infection, pulmonary edema, and chronic lung disease should all be treated before anesthesia is induced.

Prior to formulation of an anesthetic plan, every patient should be carefully examined, and all laboratory results should be evaluated. Close attention must always be paid to auscultating the chest and to evaluating the depth of ventilation, the effort involved, and mucous membrane color. Any abnormalities in the pulmonary system should be further investigated with chest radiographs and determination of arterial blood gases. Preanesthetic findings are useful for indicating the extent of pulmonary system disease and the risk of anesthesia. They also serve as baseline measurements against which the patient can be re-evaluated following therapy and during and after anesthesia.

The value of arterial blood gas measurements should not be underestimated. Although the efficiency of gas exchange in the lungs is well evaluated by Pa_{O_2}, Pa_{CO_2} is the clinical measure of ventilation and should always be evaluated along with Pa_{O_2}. In many patients with impaired pulmonary function, Pa_{O_2} is decreased, whereas Pa_{CO_2} may be normal or even lower than normal due to hyperventilation in response to hypoxia. In an unsedated animal the finding of a primary respiratory acidosis, which is always accompanied by a decrease in Pa_{O_2} when the animal is breathing room air, implies the presence of very serious pulmonary disease.

The Anesthetic Period

The patient with reduced pulmonary function is often depressed; further sedation is usually unnecessary and unwarranted. If sedation is needed in dogs, a small dose of narcotic is preferable to a phenothiazine tranquilizer. Meperidine, 2 to 4 mg/kg body weight intramuscularly, usually provides sufficient sedation. At this low dose, meperidine has minimal effects on the respiratory system[107] and is relatively short-acting in the dog, and its actions can be reversed if necessary with a narcotic antagonist. Atropine is usually advisable, except in instances of highly viscous airway secretions, because atropine may further increase the viscosity of these secretions.

Induction of anesthesia should be smooth, and in most cases the time interval between loss of consciousness and endotracheal intubation should be as short as possible. This is especially important in animals prone to upper airway obstruction (e.g., brachiocephalic breeds) or those with little pulmonary reserve (e.g., those with diaphragmatic hernia, lung abscess, or tumor). Administration of O_2 through a face mask for three to five minutes prior to induction (preoxygenation) is encouraged if it can be accomplished with little patient struggling. This minimizes the usual decrease in Pa_{O_2} that occurs after induction and offers some protection to the patient in the event of airway obstruction or apnea (Fig. 189–5). Intravenous catheters should be in place before preoxygenation.

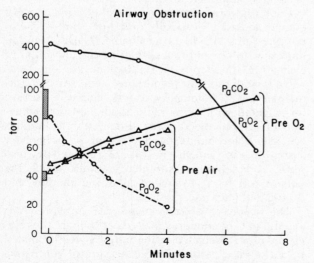

Figure 189–5. Effect of preoxygenation on Pa_{O_2} following airway obstruction. Shaded areas indicate range of Pa_{O_2} and Pa_{CO_2} in normal dogs breathing room air. Note that after four minutes of obstruction Pa_{O_2} is higher in the preoxygenated group (Pre O_2) than in the group breathing room air prior to obstruction (Pre Air).

To preoxygenate an animal, the mask is placed over the animal's muzzle, and O_2 is allowed to flow continuously through the system for three to five minutes. Care must be taken to ensure that the animal's nose is not occluded and that the mask does not traumatize the patient's eyes. Ophthalmic ointment applied to the cornea helps to minimize drying caused by the flow of O_2 over the cornea. Anesthetic induction agents are administered while the animal breathes O_2.

A rapid and smooth induction of anesthesia can usually be accomplished with intravenous thiobarbiturate. A topical anesthetic applied to the vocal cords may aid endotracheal intubation. Induction techniques using intravenous injection of a narcotic or a volatile anesthetic through a mask usually result in a slower onset of anesthesia induction. Consequently, there may be a period during which the animal has lost control of its airway reflexes and may be hypoventilating or even apneic but will not permit tracheal intubation. To achieve a more rapid intubation when using a narcotic for induction of anesthesia, a neuromuscular blocking drug may be administered immediately following intravenous injection of the narcotic drug. When using this technique the patient must be preoxygenated for three to five minutes before the drug is administered. Ketamine injected intravenously has a relatively rapid onset and has sympathomimetic properties that may be desirable in certain patients with poor circulation.

Once intubated, the patient should be immediately connected to the anesthetic machine, and a high concentration of O_2 is established in the circuit. To maintain at least normal patient Pa_{O_2} during anesthesia, N_2O is usually not administered to patients with lung disease or decreased pulmonary reserves. Nitrous oxide should not be used in any patient in whom there is trapped air such as may occur with diaphragmatic hernia, pneumothorax, or pneumomediastinum, because N_2O causes expansion of the gas pocket.

A variety of techniques may be used to maintain anesthesia in the patient with respiratory disease. Requirements differ partly because the degree of pre-existing reduction in pulmonary function varies and partly because surgery of the respiratory tract itself causes further intraoperative considerations. The status of the cardiovascular system and any additional patient disease must also be taken into account. General anesthesia with a volatile anesthetic drug and positive pressure ventilation is usually best for most thoracic procedures. Analgesia may be supplemented by intermittent intravenous administration of narcotics (e.g., oxymorphone, fentanyl). In very depressed, debilitated patients a maintenance technique using only narcotic and neuromuscular blocking drugs (along with O_2 and positive pressure ventilation) may be employed. The actual drugs used may be less important than the skill of the person administering and monitoring the anesthetic.

Monitoring and Support

Monitoring and support of pulmonary function are especially important in the patient with respiratory disease. The measurement of ventilatory rate alone is inadequate; some quantitation of volume is desirable. Ventilatory volume may be crudely assessed by observing chest excursions or movement of the rebreathing bag. It is more accurate and meaningful to measure tidal volume with a ventilometer. The ventilometer should be placed on the expiratory limb of the anesthetic circuit. Because average values for tidal volume or minute volume are quite variable, they should be used only as guidelines. Generally, a minute volume of less than 100 ml/kg/minute in a spontaneously breathing anesthetized dog indicates that mechanical ventilation is required.

Even though a sufficient volume of air may be moving in and out of the lungs, gas exchange may still be inadequate. If possible, arterial blood gases or end-tidal CO_2 should be measured to obtain a more precise measure of pulmonary function. A Pa_{CO_2} of 60 mm Hg or more indicates sufficient hypoventilation to warrant mechanical ventilatory support.

Pre-existing abnormalities in arterial oxygenation frequently become worse under general anesthesia, and, despite a high inspired O_2 concentration, hypoxemia may be a problem. The usual signs of hypoxemia in the awake patient are often masked by anesthetic drugs. If N_2O is used in the anesthetic management of these patients it is desirable to monitor inspired O_2 concentration with an O_2 analyser.

Artificial Ventilation

Mechanical ventilation is required during intrathoracic surgery and is often desirable in patients with pulmonary disease who are undergoing surgery not involving the respiratory system. Patients with a diaphragmatic hernia or other respiratory insult in which lung volume is decreased require mechanical ventilatory support immediately after anesthetic induction. Mechanical ventilation is usually accomplished by raising the ambient gas pressure during inspiration. This causes a pressure gradient between the mouth and the alveoli, resulting in a flow of gas into the lungs. Expiration is usually passive, with the pressure at the mouth and in the alveoli returning to ambient. Artificial ventilation may be accomplished manually by squeezing the inflated rebreathing bag of the anesthetic machine or by replacing the rebreathing bag with a mechanical ventilator. Peak inspiratory pressure achieved, volume of gas delivered, arterial blood gases, and thoracic excursions all serve as guides to the adequacy of positive pressure ventilation. In most patients a Pa_{CO_2} of between 35 and 45 mm Hg should be easily achieved, and with an inspired oxygen concentration of 30 per cent or greater, the Pa_{O_2} should be well in excess of 100 mm Hg.

Peak airway pressure should reach 16 to 20 cm of water in healthy patients, and a rate of eight to ten breaths per minute is sufficient to maintain normal arterial blood gases in most dogs. Faster rates may be needed in small dogs or cats. Expiration should be at least twice as long as inspiration, with inspiratory time set between 1 and 1.5 seconds. If a ventilometer is used, a tidal volume of about 10 to 15 ml/kg is adequate. The volume of air lost through expansion of the tubing in the patient-breathing circuit, which is about 100 to 200 ml in an adult circle system, must also be taken into account.

Positive pressure ventilation may be either assisted or controlled. With a properly adjusted ventilator, assisted ventilation or "patient-triggered" ventilation should produce a Pa_{CO_2} only slightly above the apneic threshold. Mechanically assisted patient ventilation may not ensure normocapnia (normal Pa_{CO_2}) because the apneic threshold may be elevated to varying degrees in the anesthetized patient. Controlled ventilation permits the anesthetist to regulate the patient's Pa_{CO_2} and may be instituted in a number of ways. A neuromuscular blocking agent may be administered, the patient may be hyperventilated to below the apneic threshold, or excessively deep anesthesia may be used. This last method is undesirable because it produces excessive cardiovascular depression. Even with controlled ventilation, on those machines in which it is possible, the ventilator should be adjusted so that the patient can easily trigger a breath, because patient override is usually an indication of inadequate ventilation or insufficient anesthesia.

Mechanical ventilation has certain disadvantages. Ventilation is preferentially distributed to the nondependent areas of lung, resulting in a possible increase in deadspace ventilation.[82] Venous return and pulmonary blood flow may also be diminished, causing concurrent reductions in patient cardiac output and systemic arterial blood pressure. Finally, positive pressure ventilation may rupture airways or alveoli and cause continued leakage of gas. Atelectic areas of lung should be re-inflated during several breaths to avoid rupturing alveoli.

Positive End-Expiratory Pressure

If airway closure is a problem during tidal breathing, as in patients with severe atelectasis or pulmonary edema, hypoxemia may persist despite the administration of 100 per cent O_2. The use of positive end-expiratory pressure (PEEP) elevates end-expired pressure in the airways. As a result, alveoli that have a tendency to close during expiration remain patent throughout the respiratory cycle. By thus increasing the number of alveoli available for gas exchange, the degree of venous admixture is reduced. Usually PEEP of 5 to 10 cm H_2O is sufficient to improve oxygenation and may be used with either spontaneous, assisted, or controlled ventilation. However,

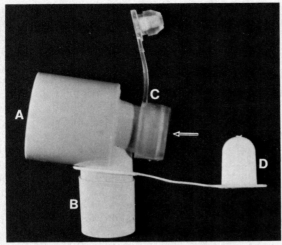

Figure 189–6. Swivel adaptor. The opening *(A)* is connected to the endotracheal tube adaptor with the anesthetic system connected at point *(B)*. The rubber plug *(C)* is then removed, and the endoscope may be inserted through the opening (arrow). If this adaptor is maintained in place for patients on continuous positive pressure ventilation, the entire rubber plug may be removed and replaced by a plastic plug *(D)*, which will not be dislodged by the positive airway pressure, to maintain a tight seal.

it is not desirable to use PEEP in the normal lung because circulatory impairment may occur subsequent to increased intrathoracic pressure.

One-Lung Anesthesia

One-lung anesthesia is indicated to prevent spillage, especially of infected material, from one lung to the other during surgical manipulation of contaminated lung lobes. The mainstem bronchus of the diseased lung may be bypassed by directing the endotracheal tube into the bronchus of the unaffected lung. This is not easily accomplished and almost always needs to be done under bronchoscopy or fluoroscopy. One-lung anesthesia results in a very large A-aP$_{O_2}$ difference due to continued perfusion of the nonventilated lung. Hypoxemia may result. Occluding pulmonary artery blood flow to the nonventilated lung minimizes V/Q imbalance.

Upper Airway Procedures

Upper airway surgery performed through the mouth and oral-tracheal bronchoscopy present a number of unique problems to the anesthesiologist. Special endotracheal tube adaptors* that allow maintenance of the endotracheal tube during bronchoscopy are available (Fig. 189–6). If endotracheal tube positioning cannot be maintained, insufflation with O$_2$ is advisable to minimize the likelihood of hypox-

emia, especially in patients with lung disease. Insufflation may be accomplished through the oral or nasotracheal route. Attention must always be paid to elapsed time to ensure that patients are not attempting to breath through an obstructed airway for too long a period. The amount of time available varies depending on patient status and is shorter in patients with respiratory system disease.

Anesthesia may be maintained using intravenous or inhaled anesthetic agents. Thiobarbiturate anesthesia alone may be unsatisfactory. The amount of thiobarbiturate needed to suppress the cough and swallowing reflexes for relatively long periods of time may result in profound respiratory depression. Narcotic drugs easily abolish upper airway reflexes, but again, respiratory depression may be a problem. Intravenous ketamine (2 to 6 mg/kg) may provide satisfactory conditions in cats provided large doses are not used. The patient must be preoxygenated before bronchoscopy or surgery, especially if O$_2$ supplementation during the procedure is not possible.

Volatile anesthetic agents may also be used for these procedures. Once adequate anesthetic depth has been achieved, the endotracheal tube may be removed, and, especially with methoxyflurane, a relatively long period of anesthesia may be obtained. Inhalation agents may also be supplemented with very small doses of thiobarbiturate, oxymorphone, or ketamine to prolong anesthesia.

Postanesthetic Period

All the considerations mentioned in the previous section for the normal patient are even more important in the patient with poor pulmonary function. Hypoxemia is common following thoracic surgery, and its extent and duration vary in individual cases.[17]

If it is anticipated that positive pressure ventilation or PEEP will be required in the postanesthetic period it is best to perform a tracheostomy at the end of surgery. Positive pressure ventilation should be continued during recovery until it is certain that the patient can maintain adequate alveolar ventilation. The effectiveness of spontaneous ventilation should be judged by determining arterial blood gases. A Pa$_{O_2}$ of less than 60 mm Hg indicates the need for supplemental O$_2$ therapy and possibly PEEP. A Pa$_{CO_2}$ of above 50 mm Hg suggests that positive pressure ventilation is desirable. Administration of O$_2$ to a spontaneously breathing animal with a low Pa$_{O_2}$ and a high Pa$_{CO_2}$ will not improve ventilation or lower Pa$_{CO_2}$; a further increase in Pa$_{CO_2}$ may in fact ensue. Instead, methods of reducing hypoventilation, such as positive pressure ventilation with an enriched O$_2$ mixture, should be employed.

Deliberate hypoventilation, usually achieved by decreasing the patient's respiratory rate, is often used in an effort to raise Pa$_{CO_2}$ and stimulate spontaneous ventilation after a period of controlled ventilation. The time needed for return of spontaneous ventila-

*Olympus Corp. of America, Medical Instrument Div., Strongville, OH.

tion may be prolonged if the apneic threshold is elevated because of anesthetic drugs. Return of spontaneous ventilation may be compounded by a Pa_{CO_2} of below 30 mm Hg. In a patient with impaired oxygenation, a decrease in respiratory rate may easily result in hypoxemia.[98] Rather than hypoventilating such a patient, the delivery of anesthetic gas should be discontinued, the anesthetic circuit flushed several times with O_2, the same rate and depth of ventilation maintained, and the fresh O_2 flow rate increased. This facilitates removal of anesthetic gas from the anesthetic delivery system and the patient. As anesthesia lightens and consciousness returns, spontaneous breathing resumes.

All nondepolarizing neuromuscular blocking drugs should be pharmacologically reversed, and care must be taken to ascertain that the patient has more than adequate muscle function. Thoracic surgery is often painful, and to provide some analgesia during recovery, antagonism of the opiate may be either partially accomplished or not done at all. In these patients the adequacy of ventilation must be assessed, if possible by ventilometry or by determination of arterial blood gases. Hypoventilation due to narcotic depression may be temporarily reversed with doxapram (0.75 to 1.5 mg/kg intravenously in dogs) without removing the analgesia. Pain control is important both to ensure the patient's comfort and to minimize pulmonary complications due to atelectasis by allowing the animal to breathe deeply. With thoracic surgery involving a lateral approach to the chest, a local anesthetic block around the intercostal nerves before surgical closure of the incision provides pain relief. If a long-acting local anesthetic such as bupivacaine (0.5 per cent solution, total dose not to exceed 3 mg/kg) is used, six to eight hours of analgesia usually results.

Brachiocephalic breeds and any animal prone to upper airway obstruction should be observed carefully during the anesthetic recovery period. Halothane or one of the newer volatile anesthetics is preferred over methoxyflurane for anesthetic management of brachiocephalic breeds because anesthetic recovery and return of airway reflexes are faster. Anesthetic recovery should take place in quiet surroundings where the patient will not be stimulated to awaken prematurely. Endotracheal intubation should be maintained as long as possible, and the patient should continue to breathe O_2 until extubation. Higher anesthetic circuit fresh gas flow rates (e.g., 200 to 300 ml/kg/minute) and regular flushing of the circuit with O_2 augment removal of expired anesthetic gases and minimize rebreathing by the patient. It is important to prevent struggling and excitement in patients prone to obstruction. To facilitate quiet anesthetic recovery 2 mg/kg of meperidine intramuscularly 15 to 20 minutes before the end of a painful surgery is sometimes helpful. The body temperature of large heavy breeds prone to airway obstruction, such as English bulldogs, should be monitored closely during recovery. In most cases it is not necessary to place these animals on a circulating hot water heating pad during recovery because their body temperature usually improves quickly without an external heat source. If circulating hot water heating pads are used, hyperthermia may easily occur in these breeds, resulting in fast, shallow breathing that may further increase the chance of airway obstruction. Smaller patients are prone to hypothermia, and a circulating hot water heating pad during recovery hastens rewarming.

Tight bandages or residual intrathoracic air or fluid interfere with postsurgical lung function and delay anesthetic recovery. Chest drains and continuous removal of air and fluid from the thorax may be necessary. Proper monitoring and support are essential during recovery for assessment of the patient's progress and for treatment of complications before they become life-threatening.

1. Annis, P., Landa, J., and Lichtiger, M.: Effects of atropine on velocity of tracheal mucus in anesthetized patients. Anesthesiology 44:74, 1976.
2. Bay, J., Nunn, J. F., and Prys-Roberts, C.: Factors influencing arterial P_{O_2} during recovery from anesthesia. Br. J. Anaesth. 40:398, 1968.
3. Bendixen, H. H., Hedley-White, J., Chir, B., and Laver, M. B.: Impaired oxygenation in surgical patients during general anesthesia with controlled ventilation: A concept of atelectasis. N. Engl. J. Med. 269:992, 1963.
4. Benumof, J. L., and Wahrenbrock, E. A.: Local effects of anesthetics on regional hypoxic pulmonary vasoconstriction. Anesthesiology 43:525, 1975.
5. Berger, A. J., Mitchell, R. A., and Severinghaus, J. W.: Regulation of respiration. N. Engl. J. Med. 297:92, 138, 194, 1977.
6. Bernards, W.: Case history number 74: Reversal of phenothiazine-induced coma with physostigmine. Anesth. Analg. Curr. Res. 52:938, 1973.
7. Bidwai, A. V., Cornelius, L. R., and Stanley, T. H.: Reversal of Innovar-induced postanesthetic somnolence and disorientation with physostigmine. Anesthesiology 44:249, 1976.
8. Bopp, P., Drummond, G., Fisher, J., and Milic-Emili, J.: Effect of doxapram on control of breathing in cats. Can. Anaesth. Soc. J. 26:191, 1979.
9. Brandstater, B., Eger, E. I., and Edelist, G.: Effects of halothane, ether and cyclopropene on respiration. Br. J. Anaesth. 37:890, 1965.
10. Buyniski, J. P., and Christie, G. J.: Ketaset Plus, a new combination anesthetic for cats, 2 pharmacologic aspects. Vet. Med/Sm. Anim. Clin. 72:559, 1977.
11. Clark, J. M.: The toxicity of oxygen. Proceedings of the Conference on the Scientific Bases of Respiratory Therapy. In Am. Rev. Resp. Dis. 110:40, 1974.
12. Comroe, J. H.: Physiology of Respiration. 2nd ed. Year Book Medical Publishers Inc., Chicago, 1979.
13. Cooper, J. B., Newbower, R. S., Long, C. D. and McPeek, B.: Preventable anesthesia mishaps: A study of human factors. Anesthesiology 49:399, 1978.
14. Crosfill, M. L., and Widdicombe, J. G.: Physical characteristics of the chest and lungs and the work of breathing in different mammalian species. J. Physiol. (Lond.) 158:1, 1961.
15. Déry, R., Pelletier, J., Jacques, A., et al.: Alveolar collapse induced by denitrogenation. Can. Anaesth. Soc. J. 12:531, 1965.
16. Don, H. F., and Robson, J. G.: The mechanics of the respiratory system during anesthesia: The effects of atropine and carbon dioxide. Anesthesiology 26:168, 1963.

17. Drummond, G. B., and Milne, A. C.: Oxygen therapy after thoracotomy. Br. J. Anaesth. 49:1093, 1977.

18. Dubin, S.: Lung compliance of normal unanesthetized beagle dogs. Am. J. Vet. Res. 31:895, 1970.

19. Dueck, R., Rathbun, M., and Harrison, W. K.: Canine V̇/Q̇ distribution responses to inhalation anaesthesia and mechanical ventilation. Anesthesiology 55:127, 1981.

20. Eger, E. I., Dolan, W. M., Stevens, W. C., et al.: Surgical stimulation antagonizes the respiratory depression produced by forane. Anesthesiology 36:544, 1972.

21. Eisele, J. H., Eger, E. I., and Muallem, M.: Narcotic properties of carbon dioxide in the dog. Anesthesiology 28:856, 1967.

22. Ettinger, S. F.: *Textbook of Veterinary Internal Medicine, Diseases of the Dog and Cat.* 2nd ed. W. B. Saunders Co., Philadelphia, 1983.

23. Fargas-Babjak, A., and Forrest, J. B.: Effect of halothane on the pulmonary vascular response to hypoxia in dogs. Can. Anaesth. Soc. J. 26:6, 1979.

24. Feigl, E. O., and D'Alecy, L. G.: Normal arterial blood pH, oxygen and carbon dioxide tensions in unanesthetized dogs. J. Appl. Physiol. 32:152, 1972.

25. Fink, B. R., Hanks, E. C., Holaday, D. A., and Ngai, S. H.: Monitoring of ventilation by integrated diaphragmatic electromyogram, determination of carbon dioxide (CO_2) threshold in anesthetized man. J. Am. Med. Ass. 172:367, 1960.

26. Forbes, A. R., and Gamsu, G.: Mucociliary clearance in the canine lung during and after general anesthesia. Anesthesiology 50:26, 1979.

27. Gawley, T. H., Dundee, J. W., Gupta, P. K., and Jones, C. J.: Role of doxapram in reducing pulmonary complications after major surgery. Br. Med. J. 1:122, 1976.

28. Gibbs, J. M., and Johnson, H.: Lack of effect of morphine and buprenorphine on hypoxic pulmonary vasoconstriction in the isolated perfused cat lung and the perfused lobe of the dog lung. Br. J. Anaesth. 50:1197, 1978.

29. Gillespie, D. J., and Hyatt, R. E.: Respiratory mechanics in the unanesthetized dog. J. Appl. Physiol. 36:98, 1974.

30. Gilman, A. G., Goodman, L. S., and Gilman, A.: *The Pharmacological Basis of Therapeutics.* 6th ed. Macmillan Publishing Co., New York, 1980.

31. Glazier, J. B., Hughes, J. M. B., Maloney, J. E., and West, J. B.: Vertical gradient of alveolar size in lungs of dogs frozen intact. J. Appl. Physiol. 23:694, 1967.

32. Goto, H., Whitman, R. A., and Arakawa, K.: Pulmonary mechanics in man after administration of atropine and neostigmine. Anesthesiology 49:91, 1978.

33. Graham, G. R., Hill, D. W., and Nunn, J. F.: Die Wirkung höher CO_2—Konzentrationen auf Kreislauf und Atmung. Anaesthetist 9:70, 1960.

34. Gray, T. C., Nunn, J. F., and Utting, J. E.: *General Anesthesia.* 4th ed. Butterworths, London, 1980.

35. Gupta, P. K., and Dundee, J. W.: Hastening of arousal after general anesthesia with doxapram hydrochloride. Br. J. Anaesth. 45:493, 1973.

36. Hanks, E. C., Ngai, S. H., and Fink, B. R.: The respiratory threshold for carbon dioxide in anesthetized man, determination of carbon dioxide threshold during halothane anesthesia. Anesthesiology 22:393, 1961.

37. Hartsfield, S. M., and Sawyer, D. C.: Cardiopulmonary effects of rebreathing and nonrebreathing systems during halothane anesthesia in the cat. Am. J. Vet. Res. 37:1461, 1976.

38. Haskins, S. C., Peiffer, R. L., and Stowe, C. M.: A clinical comparison of CT1341, ketamine and xylazine in cats. Am. J. Vet. Res. 36:1537, 1975.

39. Heiser, J. F., and Gillin, J. C.: The reversal of anticholinergic drug-induced delirium and coma with physostigmine. Am. J. Psychiat. 127:1050, 1971.

40. Herbert, D. A., and Mitchell, R. A.: Blood gas tensions and acid-base balance in awake cats. J. Appl. Physiol. 30:434, 1971.

41. Hickey, R. F., Fourcade, H. E., Eger, E. I., et al.: The effects of ether, halothane and forane on apneic thresholds in man. Anesthesiology 35:32, 1971.

42. Hickey, R. F., Graf, P. D., Nadel, J. A., and Larson, C. P.: The effects of halothane and cyclopropane on total pulmonary resistance in the dog. Anesthesiology 31:334, 1969.

43. Hirshman, C. A., McCullough, R. E., Cohen, P. J., and Weil, J. V.: Hypoxic ventilatory drive in dogs during thiopental, ketamine, or pentobarbital anesthesia. Anesthesiology 43:628, 1975.

44. Hirshman, C. A., McCullough, R. E., Cohen, P. J., and Weil, J. V.: Depression of hypoxic ventilatory response by halothane, enflurane and isoflurane in dogs. Br. J. Anaesth. 49:957, 1977.

45. Horrigan, R. W.: Physostigmine and anesthetic requirements for halothane in dogs. Anesth. Analg. Curr. Res. 57:180, 1978.

46. Hurtig, J. B., Tait, A. R., Loh, L., and Sykes, M. K.: Reduction of hypoxic pulmonary vasoconstriction by nitrous oxide administration in the isolated perfused cat lung. Can. Anaesth. Soc. J. 24:541, 1977.

47. Jones, L. M., Booth, N. H., and McDonald, L. E.: *Veterinary Pharmacology and Therapeutics.* 4th ed. Iowa State University Press, Ames, Iowa, 1977.

48. Keats, A. S.: Postoperative pain: Research and treatment. J. Chron. Dis. 4:72, 1956.

49. Keats, A. S., and Girgis, K.: Respiratory depression associated with relief of pain by narcotics. Anesthesiology 29:1006, 1968.

50. Kelly, R. W., Wilson, R. D., Traber, D. L., and Priano, L. L.: Effects of two new dissociative anesthetic agents, ketamine and CL-1848C, on the respiratory response to carbon dioxide. Anesth. Analg. Curr. Res. 50:262, 1971.

51. Klide, A. M.: Cardiopulmonary effects of enflurane and isoflurane in the dog. Am. J. Vet. Res. 37:127, 1976.

52. Klide, A. M., Calderwood, H. W., and Soma, L. R.: Cardiopulmonary effects of xylazine in dogs. Am. J. Vet. Res. 36:931, 1975.

53. Knill, R. L., and Gelb, A. W.: Ventilatory responses to hypoxia and hypercapnea during halothane sedation and anesthesia in man. Anesthesiology 49:244, 1978.

54. Kolata, R. J., and Rawlings, C. A.: Cardiopulmonary effects of intravenous xylazine, ketamine, and atropine in the dog. Am. J. Vet. Res. 43:2196, 1982.

55. Larson, G. F., Hurlbert, B. J., and Wingard, D. W.: Physostigmine reversal of diazepam-induced depression. Anesth. Analg. Curr. Res. 56:348, 1977.

56. Laver, M. B., Morgan, J., Bendixen, H. H., and Radford, J. R.: Lung volume, compliance, and arterial oxygen tensions during controlled ventilation. J. Appl. Physiol. 19:725, 1964.

57. Lees, N. W., Howie, H. B., Mellon, A., et al.: The influence of doxapram on postoperative pulmonary function in patients undergoing upper abdominal surgery. Br. J. Anaesth. 48:1197, 1976.

58. Loh, L., Sykes, M. K., and Chakrabarti, M. K.: The effects of halothane and ether on the pulmonary circulation in the innervated perfused cat lung. Br. J. Anaesth. 49:309, 1977.

59. Lumb, W. V., and Jones, E. W.: *Veterinary Anesthesia.* Lea & Febiger, Philadelphia, 1973.

60. Lundy, P. M., Gowdey, C. W., and Colhoun, E. H.: Tracheal smooth muscle relaxant effect of ketamine. Br. J. Anaesth. 46:333, 1974.

61. Marin, J. L. B., Carruthers, B., Chakrabarti, M. K., and Sykes, M. K.: Preservation of the hypoxic pulmonary vasoconstrictor mechanism during methoxyflurane anesthesia in the dog. Br. J. Anaesth. 51:99, 1979.

62. Marshal, B. E., and Wyche, M. Q.: Hypoxemia during and after anesthesia. Anesthesiology 37:178, 1972.

63. Mathers, J., Benumof, J. L., and Wahrenbrock, E. A.: General anesthetics and regional hypoxic pulmonary vasoconstriction. Anesthesiology 46:111, 1977.

64. McLeish, I.: Skeletal muscle rigidity in a dog following fentanyl/droperidol administration: A case report. Vet. Anesth. 4:2, 1977.

65. Mead, J., and Collier, C.: Relation of volume history of lungs to respiratory mechanics in anesthetized dogs. J. Appl. Physiol. 14:669, 1959.

66. Middleton, D. J., Ilkiw, J. E., and Watson, A. D. J.: Arterial and venous blood gas tensions in clinically healthy cats. Am. J. Vet. Res. 42:1609, 1981.

67. Miller, R. D., Fowler, W. S., and Helmholz, H. F.: Changes in relative volume and ventilation of the two lungs with change to the lateral decubitus position. J. Lab. Clin. Med. 47:297, 1956.

68. Mitchell, R. A., and Herbert, D. A.: Potencies of doxapram and hypoxia in stimulating carotid-body chemoreceptors and ventilation in anesthetized cats. Anesthesiology 42:559, 1975.

69. Mountcastle, V. B.: *Medical Physiology*. 14th ed. The C. V. Mosby Co., St. Louis, 1980.

70. Muggenburg, B. A., and Mauderly, J. L.: Cardiopulmonary function of awake, sedated, and anesthetized dogs. J. Appl. Physiol. 37:152, 1974.

71. Munson, E. S., Stevens, D. S., and Redfern, R. E.: Endotracheal tube obstruction by nitrous oxide. Anesthesiology 52:275, 1980.

72. Nielsen, M., and Smith, H.: Studies on the regulation of respiration in acute hypoxia. Acta Physiol. Scand. 24:293, 1951.

73. Nunn, J. F.: Influence of age and other factors on hypoxemia in the postoperative period. Lancet 2:466, 1965.

74. Nunn, J. F.: *Applied Respiratory Physiology*. 2nd ed. Butterworths, London, 1977.

75. Nunn, J. F., and Bergman, N. A.: The effect of atropine on pulmonary gas exchange. Br. J. Anaesth. 36:68, 1964.

76. Palmer, S. K., Zuperku, E. J., Bosnjak, Z., et al.: Halothane, tracheal compliance and upper-airway mechanoreceptors. Anesthesiology 49:260, 1978.

77. Popovic, N. A., Mullane, J. F., and Yhap, E. O.: Effects of acetylpromazine maleate on certain cardiorespiratory responses in dogs. Am. J. Vet. Res. 33:1819, 1972.

78. Rahn, H., and Bahnson, H. T.: Effect of unilateral hypoxia on gas exchange and calculated pulmonary blood flow in each lung. J. Appl. Physiol. 6:105, 1953.

79. Ray, J. F., Yost, L., Moallem, S., et al.: Immobility, hypoxemia and pulmonary arteriovenous shunting. Arch. Surg. 109:537, 1974.

80. Regan, M. J., and Eger, E. I., II: Ventilatory responses to hypercapnea and hypoxia at normothermia and moderate hypothermia during constant depth halothane anesthesia. Anesthesiology 27:624, 1966.

81. Rehder, K., and Sessler, A. D.: Function of each lung in spontaneously breathing man anesthetized with thiopental-meperidine. Anesthesiology 38:320, 1973.

82. Rehder, K., Theye, R. A., and Fowler, W. S.: Function of each lung of dogs during intermittent positive-pressure breathing. Am. J. Physiol. 206:1031, 1964.

83. Riddell, P. L., and Robertson, G. S.: Use of doxapram as an arousal agent in outpatient general anesthesia. Br. J. Anaesth. 50:921, 1978.

84. Robinson, N. E., Gillespie, J. R., Berry, J. D., and Simpson, A.: Lung compliance, lung volumes, and single-breath diffusing capacity in dogs. J. Appl. Physiol. 33:808, 1972.

85. Sackner, M. A., Hirsch, J. A., Epstein, S., and Rywlin, A. M.: Effect of oxygen in graded concentrations upon tracheal mucous velocity, a study in anesthetized dogs. Chest 69:164, 1976.

86. Saidman, L. J., and Eger, E. I.: Effect of nitrous oxide and of narcotic premedication on the alveolar concentration of halothane required for anesthesia. Anesthesiology 25:302, 1964.

87. Severinghaus, J. W., and Stupfel, M.: Respiratory dead space increase following atropine in man and atropine, vagal and ganglionic blockade and hypothermia in dogs. J. Appl. Physiol. 8:81, 1955.

88. Shapiro, B. A., Harrison, R. A., and Walton, J. R.: *Clinical Application of Blood Gases*. 2nd ed. Year Book Medical Publishers Inc., Chicago, 1977.

89. Shappell, S. D., and Lenfant, C. J. M.: Adaptive, genetic, and iatrogenic alterations of the oxyhemoglobin-dissociation curve. Anesthesiology 37:127, 1972.

90. Smith, C. W., Lehan, P. H., and Monks, J. J.: Cardiopulmonary manifestations with high O_2 tensions at atmospheric pressure. J. Appl. Physiol. 18:849, 1963.

91. Smith, T. C., Stephen, G. W., Zeiger, L., and Wollman, H.: Effects of premedicant drugs on respiration and gas exchange in man. Anesthesiology 28:883, 1967.

92. Soma, L. R.: *Textbook of Veterinary Anesthesia*. The Williams & Wilkins Co., Baltimore, 1971.

93. Spence, A. A., and Smith, G.: Postoperative analgesia and lung function: A comparison of morphine with extradural block. Br. J. Anaesth. 43:144, 1971.

94. Stark, D. C. C., and Smith, H.: Pulmonary vascular changes during anesthesia. Br. J. Anaesth. 32:460, 1960.

95. Steffey, E. P., Gillespie, J. R., Berry, J. D., et al.: Circulatory effects of halothane and halothane-nitrous oxide anesthesia in the dog: Spontaneous ventilation. Am. J. Vet. Res. 36:197, 1975.

96. Steffey, E. P., and Howland, D.: Potency of enflurane in dogs: Comparison with halothane and isoflurane. Am. J. Vet. Res. 39:573, 1978.

97. Steffey, E. P., Martucci, R., Howland, D., et al.: Meperidine-halothane interaction in dogs. Can. Anaesth. Soc. J. 21:459, 1977.

98. Sullivan, S. F., and Patterson, R. W.: Posthyperventilation hypoxia. J. Appl. Physiol. 22:431, 1967.

99. Sykes, M. K., Davies, D. M., Chakrabarti, M. K., and Loh, L.: The effects of halothane, trichlorethylene and ether on the hypoxic pressor response and pulmonary vascular resistance in the isolated, perfused cat lung. Br. J. Anaesth. 45:655, 1973.

100. Sykes, M. K., Gibbs, J. M., Loh, L., et al.: Preservation of the pulmonary vasoconstrictor response to alveolar hypoxia during the administration of halothane to dogs. Br. J. Anaesth. 50:1185, 1978.

101. Sykes, M. K., Hurtig, J. B., Tait, A. R., and Chakrabarti, M. K.: Reduction of hypoxic pulmonary vasoconstriction in the dog during administration of nitrous oxide. Br. J. Anaesth. 49:301, 1977.

102. Sykes, M. K., Loh, L., Jastrzebski, J., and Chakrabarti, M. K.: The effect of methoxyflurane on pulmonary vascular resistance and hypoxic pulmonary vasoconstriction in the isolated perfused cat lung. Br. J. Anaesth. 48:191, 1976.

103. Taylor, P. A., and Towey, R. M.: Depression of laryngeal reflexes during ketamine anesthesia. Br. Med. J. 2:688, 1971.

104. Tenney, S. M., and Remmers, J. E.: Comparative quantitative morphology of the mammalian lung: Diffusing area. Nature (Lond.) 197:54, 1963.

105. Tisi, G. M.: Preoperative evaluation of pulmonary function. Am. Rev. Respir. Dis. 119:293, 1979.

106. Toda, N., and Hatano, Y.: Contractile responses of canine tracheal muscle during exposure to fentanyl and morphine. Anesthesiology 53:93, 1980.

107. Turner, D. M., Ilkiw, J. E., Rose, R. J., and Warren, J. M.: Respiratory and cardiovascular effects of five drugs used as sedatives in the dog. Aust. Vet. J. 50:260, 1974.

108. Waterman, A.: Accidental hypothermia during anaesthesia in dogs and cats. Vet. Rec. 96:308, 1975.

109. Weil, J. V., McCullough, R. E., Kline, J. S., and Sodal, I.: Diminished ventilatory response to hypoxia and hypercapnea after morphine in normal man. N. Engl. J. Med. 292:1103, 1976.

110. Weiskopf, R. B., Raymond, L. W., and Severinghaus, J. W.: Effects of halothane on canine respiratory responses to hypoxia with and without hypercarbia. Anesthesiology 41:350, 1974.

111. West, J. B.: Regional differences in gas exchange in the lung of erect man. J. Appl. Physiol. 17:893, 1962.

112. West, J. B.: *Respiratory Physiology—The Essentials*. 2nd ed. The Williams & Wilkins Co., Baltimore, 1979.

113. Wise, W. C.: Normal arterial blood gases and chemical components in the unanesthetized dog. J. Appl. Physiol. 35:427, 1973.

Chapter 190

Anesthesia for Cardiovascular Surgery

Wayne McDonell

The cardiovascular and hemic systems of healthy dogs and cats, or those with minimal disability, can tolerate considerable blood loss, hypoxia, hypercapnia, and drug depression. However, animals with serious cardiac disease invariably have a reduced compensatory "reserve," and relatively minor alterations of oxygen saturation, blood volume, acid-base status, or autonomic nervous function can initiate a lethal sequence of reduced cardiac output, hypotension, myocardial hypoxia, and further reduction in cardiac output.[8,21,30,48] Thus, the operative risk is increased in animals with significant cardiovascular disease, the degree of risk depending on the severity of the disease, the skill with which anesthesia is administered, and the magnitude of the surgical procedure. However, perception of this increased risk is often exaggerated in veterinary medicine, particularly in the geriatric patient with heart disease. In many instances these animals demonstrate little functional reduction in cardiovascular reserve, and anesthesia presents an insignificant risk if done properly with current methods. When surgery is needed, the risk of anesthesia should not dissuade such surgery in most cases, provided all efforts are made to improve the physical status of the animal prior to surgery and appropriate anesthetic techniques are used.

Successful anesthesia of the animal with cardiovascular and hemic dysfunction is based on (1) an understanding of the nature and hemodynamic effect of the dysfunction, (2) logical selection of a technique and drugs to minimize cardiorespiratory depression, (3) adequate monitoring, and (4) meticulous attention to detail in the preoperative, operative, and postoperative periods.[1,3,5,9,29]

In this chapter particular consideration is given to practical anesthetic problems associated with more common surgical procedures on the cardiovascular and hemic systems. For anesthetic considerations during open-heart surgery and cardiopulmonary bypass the reader is referred elsewhere.[7,14,37]

EFFECTS OF ANESTHETIC AND RELATED DRUGS ON THE CARDIOVASCULAR AND HEMIC SYSTEMS

A more detailed description of the pharmacological effects of anesthetic and anesthetic adjuvant drugs is given elsewhere in this section and in standard textbooks.[11,41,53] The following discussion summarizes the more important facts related to the use of these drugs during surgery involving the cardiovascular and hemic systems.

Heart Rate and Rhythm

Apart from serious bradycardia and serious tachycardia, the actual heart rate during anesthesia is not too important in most instances. Serious bradycardia is defined as a heart rate of less than 60 beats per minute (bpm) in the dog and 120 bpm in the cat, and serious tachycardia is a heart rate of more than 160 bpm and 240 in the dog and cat respectively. There is little evidence pointing to an optimum heart rate, although it is rational to suppose that slower heart rates are more mechanically (and energy) efficient than more rapid heart rates.[32] The important thing is not to equate higher heart rates with better cardiac output or blood pressure. Cardiac output is often more dependent on the adequacy of venous return and myocardial contractility than on heart rate. Progressive changes in heart rate during anesthesia are of more significance and warrant careful assessment of the animal.

Although drug selection may modify the propensity to arrhythmias other than bradycardia or tachycardia, many of these arrhythmias are transient and are of little consequence in the majority of animals;[4] they may be of more consequence in patients with cardiac abnormalities. The frequency of arrhythmias is greatest shortly after induction or with prolonged anesthesia, and increases with hypoxia, acidosis, overly deep anesthesia, and electrolyte imbalance regardless of the drugs used.[4,44]

Cardiac Output, Blood Pressure, and Tissue Oxygenation

During general anesthesia, the single most important factor is maintenance of adequate oxygen delivery to body tissues, particularly the brain and myocardium, along with removal of carbon dioxide. This requires effective interaction of the respiratory and cardiovascular systems with adequate hemoglobin levels and oxygen-carrying capacity of blood (Fig. 190–1). Generally, it is possible for the anesthetist to ensure adequate ventilation and an inspired oxygen concentration sufficient to prevent hypoxemia. This may be accomplished through provision of an adequate airway, the use of intermittent positive pressure ventilation (IPPV) when necessary, and enrich-

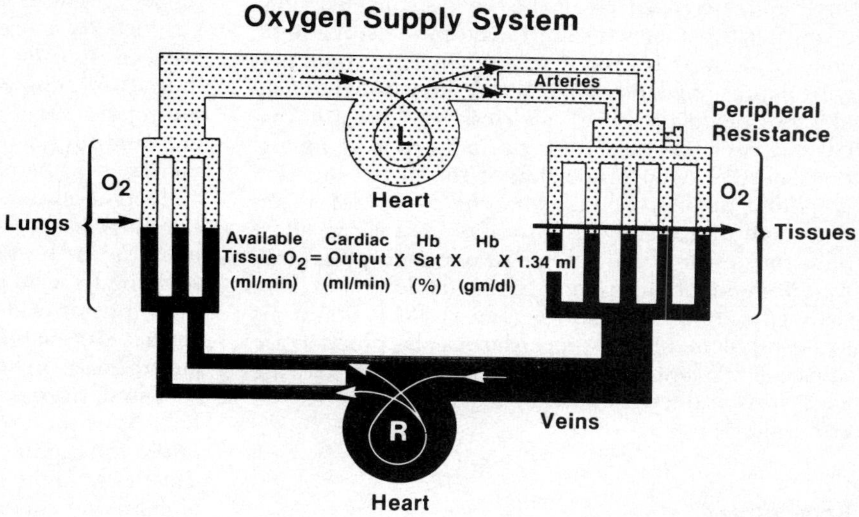

Oxygen Supply System

Figure 190–1. Schematic of the oxygen transport system, showing the interdependency of cardiac output, hemoglobin saturation, and hemoglobin content on available tissue oxygen.

$$\begin{array}{ccccccc}
\text{Available} & & \text{Cardiac} & & \text{Hb} & & \text{Hb} \\
\text{Tissue O}_2 & = & \text{Output} & \times & \text{Sat} & \times & \times\ 1.34\ \text{ml} \\
(\text{ml/min}) & & (\text{ml/min}) & & (\%) & & (\text{gm/dl})
\end{array}$$

ment of the inspired oxygen levels to at least 30 per cent. Higher oxygen levels may be necessary when there is pulmonary disease, a restriction of lung volume (e.g., during a thoracotomy), or right-to-left intracardiac or intrapulmonary shunting of blood flow.

On the circulatory side, the critical factor is the magnitude of blood flow to the various tissues. For the body as a whole, flow can be determined by measurement of cardiac output. Owing to recent advances in catheter technology and the development of thermodilution cardiac output methods, this vital component in circulatory assessment is now being done far more commonly, both in the experimental laboratory and in selected clinical settings.[47] Clinically, during anesthesia information on blood flow to selected accessible vascular fields is obtained by observation of the rate of capillary refill in mucous membranes, determination of urine output, and evaluation of the temperature of the extremities. Maintenance of a "normal" blood pressure is of less importance, particularly in animals in whom coronary insufficiency and myocardial hypoxia from coronary artery atherosclerosis is not a factor. This generality applies within reasonable limits; when diastolic and mean blood pressures fall too low, the myocardium is not adequately perfused and the consequences are grave. Maintenance of a normal blood pressure can be deleterious if it is achieved at the expense of excessive sympathetic stimulation, increased peripheral resistance, and reduced blood flow to vital tissues such as the kidney. Arterial hypertension constitutes an increased afterload on the heart and increased myocardial work.[17]

All of the clinically useful anesthetics, with the possible exception of ketamine, directly impair myocardial function in a dose-dependent, reversible fashion, such that each agent can cause complete cessation of cardiac activity if the dose is high enough. This effect is most obvious in heart-lung preparations or when *in vitro* studies are carried out on cardiac muscle preparations.[38,44] The mechanism of this impairment is poorly understood but seems to involve an interference with myocardial muscle contracture rather than an influence on cellular metabolism.[44] In the intact animal the inotropic myocardial depression may be less obvious, particularly when Pa_{CO_2} levels increase or there is surgical stimulation. In most instances this protective effect seems to be primarily a result of direct or indirect sympathetic stimulation by the anesthetic, often with higher circulating levels of catecholamines.

Inhalation Anesthetics

The contemporary potent inhalation anesthetics all reduce cardiac output and blood pressure in dogs and cats in a dose-related manner.[44,46] At equipotent doses enflurane and methoxyflurane appear to be the most depressive agents, halothane is intermediate, and isoflurane is the least depressive of the four agents.[46] In healthy dogs, maintained eucapneic by IPPV, blood pressure is reduced approximately 20 per cent at 1.5 minimum alveolar concentration (MAC) and 30 to 40 per cent at 2.0 MAC for all four agents. Total peripheral resistance decreases with isoflurane and is minimally affected by the other three drugs. Cardiac output is decreased 15 to 20 per cent at 1.5 MAC and 30 to 40 per cent at 2.0 MAC with methoxyflurane, enflurane, and halothane, whereas isoflurane produces little change in cardiac output.[46] When there is spontaneous ventilation there is less decrease in blood pressure and cardiac output with these agents. This may be due to better venous return during spontaneous ventilation as well as to the sympathetic stimulation that accompanies increased Pa_{CO_2} levels.[45,46]

Nitrous oxide has direct myocardial depressant effects, but these are minimal, and in the intact animal, cardiac output and blood pressure are, if anything, increased by nitrous oxide concentrations of up to 70 per cent owing to the mild sympathetic effect produced by the drug. When it is combined with potent inhalation anesthetics, nitrous oxide may increase blood pressure[44] and lessens the cardiovascular depression caused by the more potent inhalation anesthetics in proportion to the dose reduction in potent agent that may thereby be achieved. In dogs, and presumably also in cats, this sparing effect of nitrous oxide is only about 20 per cent of the dose requirement of the potent agent (at least for halothane),[6] and the resultant beneficial effects of nitrous oxide supplementation on cardiovascular function are minimal.[46] When nitrous oxide is used with narcotic anesthesia, a decrease in ventricular function may be observed.[28]

Barbiturates

At equipotent doses all of the barbiturates produce about the same degree of circulatory depression.[38] During pentobarbital anesthesia cardiac output and stroke volume are decreased by 40 to 45 per cent, mean arterial pressure is increased 8 per cent, and peripheral vascular resistance is increased 86 per cent,[42] and similar effects are produced by thiamylal, thiopental, and methohexital when these are used alone for total anesthesia.[11,40] Thiopental is marginally less depressive and arrhythmogenic than the other barbiturates, however, as with all barbiturates, the degree of myocardial depression is primarily related to the dose administered and the rate of injection. These two factors are the prime determinants of the peak blood concentration attained.[38] In the normal animal, coronary blood flow increases along with myocardial oxygenation, although tachycardia reduces cardiac efficiency.[38] Barbiturate administration produces increased distensibility of the peripheral venous system and leads to pooling of blood in the large veins. Blood pressure is normally well maintained, although serious hypotension may result in hypovolemic animals or in normovolemic animals with cardiovascular disease. These animals are often supported by high levels of endogenous sympathetic activity to maintain ventricular contractility and cardiac output.[38] Sudden loss of part of this support because of venodilation can result in acute cardiac decompensation, hypotension, and cardiac arrest.

Other Injectable Anesthetics

Ketamine exerts little negative inotropic effect on the intact heart at clinical doses.[38,40,44] In cats, 5 mg/kg transiently reduced ventricular contractile force by 20 to 30 per cent, but values returned to normal within five to seven minutes.[38] Generally, when administered to an intact animal that has received no other drug, ketamine enhances cardiac performance in a way that resembles the changes produced by increased activity of the sympathetic system. Arterial

blood pressure, heart rate, and cardiac output are significantly increased, whereas total peripheral resistance remains unchanged.[40] The rise in cardiac output is achieved by a combination of positive inotropic and chronotropic effects on the heart. There are central sympathetic stimulation and consistent increases in the plasma levels of both norepinephrine and epinephrine.[38] Tachycardia and increased contractility lead to increased cardiac work and a large increase in the myocardial oxygen requirement. Interestingly, when ketamine is given during barbiturate, nitrous oxide–narcotic, or halothane anesthesia, cardiac stimulation does not occur unless the level of anesthesia is light.

A new steroid injectable anesthetic, *althesin* (Saffan), has been used extensively in Australia, Canada, United Kingdom, and elsewhere for feline anesthesia. This anesthetic is a mixture of two active drugs, alphaxalone and alphadolone in Cremophor EL. It is not suitable for use in dogs because it causes histamine release and hypotension.[11] Myocardial contractility is not impaired, and cardiac output is well maintained after normal doses in patients with healthy cardiovascular systems.[38] A decrease in peripheral vascular resistance occurs, and there is a dose-dependent decrease in arterial blood pressure in cats, although the degree of hypotension is rarely alarming.[13]

Another new injectable anesthetic, etomidate, shows promise for use in anesthesia induction of cardiac patients because of the relative cardiovascular stability it produces.[35] Etomidate produces negligible effects on cardiac inotropic activity at anesthetic levels, causing a slight decrease in cardiac output, blood pressure, and systemic vascular resistance. Heart rate increases slightly, and arrhythmias are rare.

Narcotic and narcotic-tranquilizer (neuroleptanesthesia) methods of maintaining anesthesia are associated with minimal negative inotropic effects on the heart.[22,38,44] Cardiac output is well maintained, and there is either no decrease in blood pressure (with narcotics alone) or a slight decrease associated with reduction of peripheral vascular resistance when a tranquilizer is incorporated.[22,52]

In summary, all general anesthetics are cardiovascular depressants, the degree of change being dose-related and reversible providing the drug is eliminated by the lungs or hepatic metabolism. It is important to use the lowest dose consistent with the surgical or diagnostic intervention intended. In most instances the dose and manner of administration are more important in the morbidity and mortality associated with anesthesia in the animal with cardiovascular disease than the choice of drugs per se.

EFFECT OF PATHOLOGIC CONDITION ON ANESTHETIC MANAGEMENT

Successful management of a patient with cardiovascular or hemic dysfunction requires an understanding not only of the pharmacology of anesthetics but also of the pathophysiology of the disease entity. From a functional viewpoint, the hemodynamic characteristics of canine and feline cardiovascular disease, whether congenital or acquired, can be ascribed to one or more of the following categories: (1) left-to-right shunting, (2) right-to-left shunting, (3) obstructive lesions, (4) regurgitating lesions, (5) myocardial disease, and (6) noncardiac vascular or hemic disease. It is useful to keep these functional categories in mind when planning an anesthetic regime for an individual animal because they are each associated with specific implications.

Left-to-Right Shunting

Left-to-right shunting of blood occurs in most animals that have a patent ductus arteriosus (PDA) as well as in most of those with atrial and ventricular septal defects. Hemodynamically, a left-to-right shunt produces an increased pulmonary blood flow and filling pressure of the left atrium and ventricle and a reduction in blood flow to the tissues. Arterial oxygenation is generally well maintained. These hemodynamic changes result in left ventricular enlargement and left-sided heart failure,[23] although the right side fails first with ventricular septal defects. The rate at which heart failure develops depends on the magnitude of the shunt, a feature that may not correlate well with the intensity of the murmur. In PDA, pulmonary artery pressures are elevated, producing a gradual increase in pulmonary vascular resistance to a point where the shunt flow may eventually reverse.

Most surgical candidates for ligation of a PDA are reasonable anesthetic subjects if the surgery is not delayed until the animal is too old. These animals tolerate IPPV well and in most instances may be given nitrous oxide as part of the anesthetic regime if desired. Inhalation anesthetic uptake is rapid. Arterial hypoxemia rarely becomes a problem unless myocardial performance is severely compromised owing to secondary cardiac enlargement or unless there is inadequate lung inflation during the thoracotomy. This may happen when the lungs are packed off to provide surgical exposure. Most adverse results in surgery for PDA ligation are associated with the actual exposure and ligature placement around the ductus. If the surgeon accidentally tears the ductus or the dilated thin pulmonary artery, the elastic character of the intrathoracic pulmonary artery and aorta is immediately lost, and the diastolic blood pressure rapidly falls to near zero. This severely curtails coronary blood flow, and the heart arrests, usually in asystole. The rate at which cardiac arrest occurs is out of proportion to the actual amount of blood lost. Unless the major vessel leak can be occluded, it is impossible to start the heart again. When a patent ductus is ligated, there is a sudden change in the proportion of blood remaining in the aorta, and the resulting increase in blood pressure

often produces a reflex bradycardia although this rarely requires treatment even if atropine premedication has not been used.

Right-to-Left-Shunting

A right-to-left shunt flow occurs in patients with tetralogy of Fallot, some early cases of congenital PDA,[36] or when pulmonary artery vascular resistance rises sufficiently to reverse the shunt flow in the more common instances of PDA with initial left-to-right shunting. Animals that have severe pulmonary hypertension or congenital right-to-left PDA are not suitable subjects for surgery,[23,36] but anesthesia may be required for diagnostic procedures. Those animals with tetralogy of Fallot generally require cardiopulmonary bypass for repair, although sometimes an attempt may be made to reduce pulmonic stenosis to increase blood flow through the lungs.

With right-to-left shunts there is a reduced blood flow through the lungs, retarding the uptake of inhalation anesthetics. Cyanosis is common and is often associated with significant polycythemia. With packed cell volumes above 55 to 65 per cent the viscosity of the blood may further impair blood flow to tissues. Anesthetic agents given intravenously reach the brain rapidly because they essentially bypass the lungs. A further deleterious and life-threatening reduction in pulmonary blood flow may be produced by a fall in arterial blood pressure or an increase in pulmonary vascular resistance as may occur with IPPV, additional arterial hypoxemia, or acidosis.[3,29] In these patients induction of anesthesia is particularly hazardous, and the onset of IPPV must be done with great care. High inspired oxygen tensions must be maintained in these animals, and nitrous oxide should not be used in the anesthetic regime unless it is possible to monitor the blood gas status of the animal.

Obstructive Lesions

In dogs, aortic and pulmonic stenoses are the most common congenital defects after PDA; aortic stenosis is also relatively common in cats.[36] All forms of *aortic stenosis* (subvalvular, valvular, and supravalvular) interfere with the ejection of blood from the left ventricle. This limits cardiac output and increases left ventricular pressures; left myocardial hypertrophy and, in severe instances, congestive heart failure follow. Aortic and mitral valve insufficiency may also be present, leading to regurgitant blood flow, atrial distension, and atrial fibrillation.[36] Loss of sinus rhythm with its atrial "kick" can result in a marked drop in cardiac output and blood pressure.[2] On electrocardiographic examination, S-T segment depression, ventricular premature beats, and ventricular tachycardia are seen in severely affected animals. These arrhythmias are related to hypoperfusion of the left ventricular myocardium.

During anesthesia of an animal with aortic stenosis, the animal must be kept in sinus rhythm if at all possible, and all arrhythmias are treated early and vigorously.[2] Bradycardia is prevented with judicious use of anticholinergic agents. Drugs that lower myocardial contractility or systemic arterial blood pressure are to be avoided or used in minimal doses. When the degree of aortic or mitral valve regurgitation is significant, a degree of vasodilation may be desirable to reduce afterload and improve forward flow.[2] However, in veterinary practice, most of these animals are being anesthetized for diagnostic purposes, and it is difficult to estimate the degree of regurgitation present. Corrective surgery requires cardiopulmonary bypass.

Pulmonic stenosis may be subvalvular, valvular, or supravalvular. The severity of the stenosis is variable, and the anesthesic risk varies accordingly. Severe or long-standing pulmonic stenosis is characterized by right-sided cardiac hypertrophy and failure, hepatomegaly, and ascites.[36] Arrhythmias and conduction disturbances are not common, but cardiac output is relatively fixed and depends on a high degree of sympathetic tone and tachycardia. In this regard, the hemodynamic manifestations are similar to those seen with long-standing dirofiloria infestation with secondary pulmonary hypertension. Valvular and subvalvular pulmonic stenoses are now being treated surgically without cardiopulmonary bypass using inflow occlusion techniques and an approach through the pulmonary artery or right ventricular wall.

The restricted blood flow in severe pulmonic stenosis and dirofilaria infestation is vulnerable to the negative influences of alpha-adrenergic drugs, the venodilation produced by barbiturates on induction, right ventricular depression secondary to agents that reduce myocardial contractility, and the mechanical effects of increased pressure in the airway. The induction of anesthesia is best done by a neuroleptanalgesic technique or by careful titration of an inhalation agent, and particular attention must be paid to the adequacy of fluid and blood volume preoperatively and during the procedure.

Animals with constrictive pericardial disease[49] or cardiac tamponade cannot achieve adequate ventricular filling because the effective compliance of the heart is reduced by the pericardium or by fluid in the pericardial sac. Compensatory increased filling pressures and increased heart rate occur in an attempt to maintain the cardiac output, but with acute tamponade or chronic accumulation of large volumes of fluid, cardiac output may be fixed at a life-threatening level. Induction of anesthesia in these animals may be followed by vasodilation and a subsequent profound fall in cardiac output; this effect is exaggerated by IPPV or bradycardia.[2] If at all possible, periocardiocentesis should be performed preoperatively under local anesthesia to improve hemodynamics. When this is not possible, a nonbarbiturate method of induction should be employed, maintaining adequate filling pressures with fluid-volume infusion and judicious use of vasoconstrictor agents.

Vascular ring anomalies such as persistent right aortic arch do not alter cardiovascular hemodynamics directly, and with one or two modifications, anesthesia may be handled the same way as for any thoracotomy. These animals often have varying degrees of aspiration pneumonia and are often moderately dehydrated on presentation. They commonly have semifluid ingesta in the dilated esophagus anterior to the vascular ring anomaly. If precautions are not taken, reflux and aspiration can occur at anesthesic induction. An intravenous method of induction should be used with the animal in a sternal position and the head elevated. The head should be kept elevated until an endotracheal tube is inserted with the cuff inflated to prevent possible aspiration.

Regurgitating Lesions

Hemodynamic regurgitation may occur as a consequence of congenital dysplasias of the semilunar or atrioventricular valves or subsequent to acquired cardiovascular disease—in particular, chronic valvular disease. Atrioventricular regurgitation may also accompany cardiomyopathy if the ventricles dilate sufficiently. Chronic valvular disease is the most common cardiovascular disorder in the dog. The incidence of this acquired disease in aged dogs may approach 50 per cent.[16] Usually the mitral valve is affected, although about 30 per cent of affected dogs have tricuspid valve involvement as well; the pulmonic and aortic valves are rarely affected.[16] During systole, there is regurgitation of blood into the atria with atrioventricular insufficiency, reducing aortic flow. Atrial enlargement and ventricular hypertrophy follow, leading to compensatory sodium and water retention. Sympathetic stimulation augments venous return and increases myocardial contractility, heart rate, and peripheral resistance. Initially, forward stroke volume and arterial blood pressure are supported by these reserve mechanisms, although exercise tolerance may be reduced. However, the disease is progressive, and eventually congestive heart failure occurs with generalized cardiomegaly, pulmonary venous distension, alveolar wall thickening, pulmonary edema, and subnormal gas exchange. When right ventricular failure predominates there is dilation of the caudal vena cava, hepatic congestion, ascites, and pleural effusion.[16] Supraventricular premature complexes are commonly seen; paroxysmal supraventricular tachycardia, atrial tachycardia, and atrial flutter or fibrillation may follow. Ventricular premature complexes are common in advanced chronic valvular disease. Iatrogenic digitalis intoxication is common and produces a variety of arrhythmias, including atrioventricular block, sinus arrest, and premature atrial or ventricular complexes.

Dogs with chronic valvular disease that are free of clinical signs of heart failure (class I) tolerate anesthesia well if reasonable precautions are taken. The same is true of animals that show signs of heart failure only with strenuous exercise (class II). Animals that experience signs of heart failure at night or with routine activity (class III) are significantly greater anesthetic risks, as are class IV dogs, that is, animals showing clinical signs at rest. Whenever possible, the cardiovascular status of class II to class IV dogs should be stabilized (with diuretics, diet and exercise control, and additional drug therapy)[16,18] and improved to an optimal level before they are subjected to anesthesia and surgery.

With regurgitating lesions, changes related to anesthesia are increased blood volume, slower circulation time, increased alveolar-arterial gradient of oxygen tension, and reduced cardiac output and myocardial contractility.[29] Both intravenous and inhalation agents take longer to reach the brain. Myocardial contractility is easily depressed by potent agents, and concentrations must be kept low. Anesthetic requirements are also reduced.[2,3] Inspired oxygen concentrations should be kept at 40 to 50 per cent to ensure adequate arterial oxygenation. With mitral insufficiency, judicious use of vasodilators reduces the ventricular afterload and degree of regurgitation, thereby increasing the forward flow.[27] A moderate degree of tachycardia is also claimed to be beneficial, although excessively high rates are detrimental.[2]

Drug therapy for cardiac failure, such as digitalis and diuretics, tends to deplete body stores of potassium unless the diet is supplemented. Hyperventilation during anesthesia lowers the plasma potassium levels further and may initiate serious arrhythmias. Therefore, preanesthetic examination of plasma potassium levels is always advisable in such cases. Digitalized dogs exhibiting atropine-resistant bradycardia or atrioventricular block should not be subjected to anesthesia and surgery until the digitalis dosage is reduced.

Myocardial Disease

Myocardial disease rarely may result from infectious agents, infiltrative tumors, ischemia, or thyroid dysfunction.[54] Myocardial damage and arrhythmias are also seen as late sequels to chronic valvular disease, after gastric dilation and volvulus or following trauma.[25] Congestive (dilated) and hypertrophic idiopathic cardiomyopathies are common problems in larger young to middle-aged dogs[54] and may be seen in cats as well.[50] With cardiomyopathy, degenerative changes of the myocardium are apparent biochemically, ultrastructurally, microscopically, and grossly. Contractility is greatly reduced, causing a decreased cardiac output and eventually severe congestive heart failure, despite the action of compensatory mechanisms. With congestive cardiomyopathy, eventually the atrial dilation and degenerative lesions become severe enough to cause atrial flutter or fibrillation. This abolishes the atrial "kick" and often leads to a sudden further loss of cardiac output with an acute onset of left or right congestive heart failure in contrast to the gradual onset seen with chronic valvular disease. When congestive heart failure occurs,

there may be atrioventricular regurgitation. Atrial fibrillation is common, as are S-T segment depression, T wave changes, and ventricular premature complexes. With hypertrophic cardiomyopathy, complete heart block is a common electrocardiographic sign.[24]

When the degree of cardiomyopathy is severe and congestive heart failure is present, these animals are poor anesthetic subjects.[24] They are intolerant of even a mild myocardial depressant and are prone to the development of ventricular tachycardia and fibrillation during anesthesia. It is unlikely that animals in failure warrant surgical intervention because of the grave prognosis; however, they may require light anesthesia for diagnostic procedures. More commonly, noncardiovascular surgery is required in dogs that have earlier evidence of cardiomyopathy without signs of overt heart failure; the need is primarily to minimize the anesthetic depression of myocardial contractility and control arrhythmias that develop. Occasionally, atrial fibrillation is precipitated by anesthesia in susceptible dogs. This fibrillation generally reverts to a sinus rhythm spontaneously after recovery from anesthesia.

Noncardiac Vascular or Hemic Disease

Anesthetic considerations for the animal in critical condition, including the traumatized and shocked patient, are discussed elsewhere in this section. Peripheral vascular and lymphatic surgery, surgical biopsy, or excision of lymph glands presents no particular anesthetic problem other than the need to ensure adequate fluid volume replacement if there is significant blood loss. Anesthesia and surgical repair of animals with portosystemic vascular shunts is primarily complicated by the degree of hepatic insufficiency present,[10] and the recommended anesthetic techniques are the same as those used for patients with liver failure. Because the shunt is rarely closed completely at the time of surgery, continued partial bypass of the liver should be anticipated postsurgically, resulting in a prolonged effect of drugs that depend on hepatic metabolism for elimination. Splenectomy may present hemostasis problems, and it is important that a secure, large-bore venous catheter is available. If the spleen is greatly enlarged, the increase in abdominal pressure may interfere with ventilation and necessitate IPPV.

ANESTHETIC TECHNIQUE

Preparation of the Animal and Premedication

Stabilization of the Animal

Whenever possible, cardiac failure should be brought under control prior to surgery. In many instances this may be accomplished with cage rest, diuretic administration, and a low sodium diet as described elsewhere.[17,39] Digitalization may be required, but it is important that this be done carefully over a number of days; prophylactic digitalization is not indicated when heart failure is absent or when cardiac failure can be treated by more conservative methods. Anesthesia and surgery, especially cardiac surgery, can lower the tolerance of an animal to cardiac glycosides. Their action may be greatly increased by a fall in plasma potassium, hypocapnia, catecholamines, or hypoxia.[3] Normally, it is best to discontinue the use of cardiac glycosides 36 hours before anesthesia and surgery, because the reduced blood level at the time of surgery is offset by the animal's increased sensitivity to the drug.[3]

An attempt is made to correct serious arrhythmias such as complete heart block, atrial flutter and fibrillation, ventricular tachycardia, or multiple premature complexes before the animal is subjected to anesthesia. This may require digitalization, propranolol administration, or the use of lidocaine depending on the specific arrhythmia.[19,50] Because lidocaine and propranolol both reduce myocardial contractility, they should not be given prophylactically. When arrhythmias are present, however, this consideration is outweighed by the beneficial effect of an improved cardiac output when arrhythmias are controlled.

Plasma potassium levels should be evaluated and corrected prior to anesthesia, as well as any fluid or blood volume deficits or cardiac effusions. Cardiovascular disease is often accompanied by renal or hepatic insufficiency, and the preoperative evaluation attempts to determine the extent of these problems.

Premedication

When significant tachycardia is already present it is best to avoid preanesthetic use of anticholinergic agents. This is true even when narcotic premedication or neuroleptanesthetic regimes are used. An argument has been made against the routine use of anticholinergic agents in small animal anesthesia[32] on the ground that the tachycardia they produce increases myocardial work and oxygen consumption without a concomitant increase in cardiac output.[32,33] If significant bradycardia develops, it can be readily treated by intravenous administration of atropine or glycopyrrolate, and an appropriate dose should be drawn up and kept at hand.

There may be an increase in heart rate of dogs and cats anesthetized with inhalation agents even if atropine is not used.[46] There is little convincing evidence that atropine premedication at recommended doses produces an additional increase in heart rate during inhalation anesthesia.[41] When preoperative tachycardia is not present, the choice of whether to use an anticholinergic agent is probably a matter of personal preference, which may be influenced by the breed of dog, type of surgery, and subsequent drug selection. In most instances, I prefer to use an anticholinergic, probably because of my preference for using narcotic-based regimes for anesthetic management.

Some type of pre-induction sedation is almost always indicated to reduce the apprehension of the animal and the consequent sympathoadrenal stimulation.[30] High catecholamine levels, struggling, and coughing predispose to the development of arrhythmias on induction and make it more difficult to achieve a smooth, safe transition to a suitable plane of anesthesia with minimal doses of subsequent anesthetic drugs. Preanesthetic sedative or analgesic administration reduces the amount of anesthetic required to abolish response to surgery and greatly facilitates indwelling catheter placement for a secure venous access and preoxygenation by face mask. Phenothiazine tranquilizers, diazepam, narcotics, and the fentanyl-droperidol combination produces little if any reduction of myocardial contractility.[11,21,38,41,44] Because animals with cardiovascular disease often exhibit a reduced requirement for all central nervous system depressants,[21] a low dose of sedative is used initially. If the sedative effect is inadequate, the dose is increased before induction commences.

Xylazine premedication is avoided in all animals with cardiovascular disease because of the degree of cardiovascular depression it produces[20,34] and the fact that it predisposes to development of significant arrhythmias.[20,34] Diazepam (0.2 to 0.6 mg/kg intravenously) is useful if ketamine is to be used for induction, and it can be used to potentiate the sedative effects of narcotic drugs.

In many instances I prefer to use a narcotic alone, usually oxymorphone (0.1 to 0.2 mg/kg intramuscularly or intravenously) or meperidine (2 to 5 mg/kg intramuscularly). Oxymorphone is used when neuroleptanalgesia is to be used; meperidine if induction is to be achieved with a thiobarbiturate. Morphine is best avoided because of the emesis it causes. I prefer to use small doses of acepromazine (0.05 to 0.1 mg/kg intramuscularly or intravenously) if the pathophysiology of the cardiovascular disease indicates that forward flow will be increased by a reduction in afterload. Acepromazine has a useful antiarrhythmic effect.[34] It should not be used if concurrent hypovolemia is present because of the alpha-adrenergic blockade it produces,[52] nor should it be used when peripheral sympathetic tone is important in maintaining venous return or when significant hepatic dysfunction is present.

Induction

A secure venous access should be established before induction is begun using a large-gauge indwelling catheter, depending on the size of the animal. These catheters must be large enough to permit blood, plasma, or rapid fluid administration if necessary. Three to five minutes of oxygen administration by face mask is desirable before induction if the animal tolerates the mask without struggling. To be useful, however, the oxygen administration must be maintained right up to or during anesthesic induction. When the degree of cardiovascular compromise is not great, a thiobarbiturate may be used to induce anesthesia. A low dose of thiopental (8 to 10 mg/kg) should be given slowly after premedication, using a 1 or 2 per cent solution. The arrhythmogenic potential of the thiobarbiturates is directly proportional to the concentration of the drug injected, being greater with higher concentrations[4] or in animals that are not premedicated. Thiopental is considerably less arrhythmogenic than thiamylal.[4]

If a mask induction is indicated, halothane-nitrous oxide is preferred unless there are serious underlying arrhythmic problems. Although isoflurane has a lower solubility coefficient than halothane and should therefore produce a rapid induction, it is more irritating, and animals tend to show greater resistance to face mask induction with it. However, isoflurane is much less arrhythmogenic than halothane,[46] and this feature may be of great benefit when ventricular arrhythmias are a problem.[12]

In seriously compromised dogs, I prefer to sedate the animal with a narcotic or narcotic-tranquilizer mixture and to intubate the animal without using further drugs, using a laryngoscope and topical analgesia of the larynx. This can be accomplished in most ill dogs without difficulty. Unconsciousness may be produced by minimal doses of nitrous oxide and halothane, isoflurane, or methoxyflurane as desired. This method of induction often leads to tachypnea and should be used only if the anesthetist is prepared to institute IPPV. Topical analgesia of the larynx is desirable before endotracheal intubation regardless of the induction regime to prevent coughing and minimize the arrhythmias associated with intubation. In cats, I prefer a mask induction with nitrous oxide and halothane or isoflurane, or the use of althesin (4 to 6 mg/kg intravenously) after premedication with meperidine (5–10 mg/kg IM) or oxymorphone (0.05–0.1 mg/kg IM).

If an animal starts to struggle during induction with any of these regimes, or if intubation is difficult under light levels of anesthesia, pancuronium (0.04 to 0.06 mg/kg) can be given intravenously to achieve muscle relaxation. The onset time is one to two minutes, and the animal is kept on oxygen during this period. Use of a muscle relaxant in this way necessitates the institution of IPPV from the outset, but this is preferable to using unacceptably large doses of induction agents.

Maintenance of Anesthesia

Choice of Agent

It is best to use a drug regime with which you have some familiarity, regardless of the inherent advantages of certain drugs.[2,21] The depth of anesthesia should be adjusted to the degree of surgical stimulation and kept as light as possible.

Diagnostic catheterization and angiocardiography can be carried out under neuroleptanalgesic sedation and nitrous oxide alone if the animal is ill and local anesthesia may be used at the site of catheter insertion. In healthier animals, 0.5 per cent halothane may be administered as well to add to central nervous system depression. If intracardiac blood samples are being obtained for blood gas analysis as part of the diagnostic evaluation, the nitrous oxide-oxygen ratio should temporarily be adjusted to 4:1 at least three minutes before blood collection. This will give an inspired oxygen concentration of 20 per cent to aid in interpretation of the blood gas values. When higher inspired oxygen levels are required to maintain adequate oxygenation of the animal, the concentration should be noted at the time the blood sample is drawn.

For selected minor surgical procedures, it is possible to use neuroleptanalgesia sedation along with local infiltration, epidural, or intravenous administration of a local analgesic agent. Major surgery requires a regime that produces unconsciousness, and generally one of the inhalation anesthetics is preferred. In the most critical patients, the concurrent use of a nondepolarizing muscle relaxant reduces the required dose of inhalation (or injectable) agent and improves cardiovascular stability.[11,14] It is important, however, that the anesthetist be familiar with the use of these agents and methods for their reversal. When good analgesia is a prerequisite for overall patient management, as in orthopedic surgery, I prefer to use methoxyflurane for maintenance of anesthesia; halothane is chosen when rapid induction and recovery are important, as for a thoracotomy or when the patient is a brachycephalic animal. Isoflurane has a number of useful attributes,[46] but it is a comparatively expensive drug at present and is reserved for use in high-risk patients. In the cardiac patient these drugs should all be given with a precision vaporizer at a fresh gas flow rate that is high enough to allow the inspired concentration to be predicted (100 to 200 ml/kg/minute).

Regardless of the drug regime used, it is important to prevent hypothermia and to ensure that no significant hypoxemia or hypercapnia occurs during anesthesia. In many instances this precludes the use of spontaneous ventilation. IPPV should be carried out to maintain eucapnia using a rate of 10 breaths per minute and a tidal volume of 20 ml/kg. Alternatively, a coaxial (Bain) circuit can be used as a partial rebreathing circuit with larger tidal volumes and fresh gas flows equal to 100 ml/kg/minute.[26]

Monitoring

It is important to monitor the cardiopulmonary status of these animals as carefully as possible, based on the availability of equipment. If deleterious changes are detected early, they will be far more amenable to correction. The most useful monitoring aids include electrocardiographic monitoring, use of an esophageal stethoscope for heart and lung auscultation, and determination of the rate of capillary refill, urine output, and central venous pressure. An estimate of arterial blood pressure can be made by palpation of the sublingual and femoral pulses, but measurement by direct or indirect methods is preferred. Serial blood gas and acid-base analyses can be useful, particularly when dealing with pulmonary edema, right-to-left shunts, or low cardiac output.

The preferred treatment for surgical hypotension and low cardiac output depends on the cause and may include any or all of the following: reduction of anesthetic dose, discontinuance or adjustment of the method of IPPV, expansion of blood volume, correction of arrhythmias, and inotropic stimulation of the heart with a dopamine or dolbutamine drip. It is important to estimate the volume of blood loss carefully and to replace this loss accurately and judiciously with whole blood, plasma, or crystalloids. Animals with cardiac disease are less tolerant of both hypo- and hypervolemia. Those animals with left heart failure are more sensitive to the possibility of inducing pulmonary edema owing to the hemodilution produced when crystalloid solutions are used to replace blood loss. Fluid administration should be monitored by serial determinations of packed cell volume and total plasma protein levels.

Intraoperative arrhythmias are treated initially by minimizing the anesthetic dose and ensuring that hypoxia and hypercapnia are corrected. Bradycardia is treated initially with atropine; if refractory, an isoproterenol, dopamine, or dolbutamine drip is given to effect. Atrial arrhythmias are difficult to treat effectively in an acute situation during anesthesia and I prefer to not treat them unless cardiac output is seriously impaired. Lidocaine (1 to 4 mg/kg intravenously) may be tried but is less successful for controlling atrial arrhythmias than arrhythmias of ventricular origin. Lidocaine is the drug of choice for controlling ventricular premature contractions. When these are refractory to lidocaine, a switch to isoflurane may be desirable if available.[12]

Recovery

It is important to maintain oxygen supplementation during the recovery period in animals with cardiovascular disease. Shivering and struggling during recovery may increase oxygen requirements three- to fourfold at a time when the cardiopulmonary system is still depressed with residual drug effects. If a nondepolarizing muscle relaxant has been used, neostigmine (0.01 to 0.02 mg/kg) is administered to ensure complete reversal of the muscle relaxant effect. Although it is possible to reverse any residual narcotic-induced central nervous system depression with naloxone, generally this is not necessary or desirable. Some postsurgical analgesia and sedation is preferred in most animals to keep them quiet and comfortable. Pain relief and a nonexcited, nonapprehensive postanesthetic period are more important considerations than any slight respiratory depression that might accompany continued narcotic sedation.

Continued careful monitoring of vital signs is most important in the recovery period, and most animals with significant cardiovascular disease should be kept under close observation for 12 to 24 hours in an intensive care environment. If shock, cardiac failure, or pulmonary edema develops postsurgically, it must be treated early and vigorously.

1. Bolton, G. R.: Prevention and treatment of cardiovascular emergencies during anesthesia and surgery. Vet. Clin. North Am.—Sm. Anim. Pract. 2:411, 1972.
2. Bull, A. P.: The anesthetic evaluation and management of the surgical patient with heart disease. Surg. Clin. North Am. 63:1035, 1983.
3. Burton, G. W., and Balmer, H. G. R.: Anaesthesia for patients with cardiac disease and hypertension. In Gray, T. C., Nunn, J. F., and Utting, J. E. (eds.): General Anaesthesia. 4th ed., vol. I. Butterworths, Boston, 1980.
4. Cohen, R. B., and Tilley, L. P.: Cardiac arrhythmias in the anaesthetized patient. Vet. Clin. North Am.—Sm. Anim. Pract. 9:155, 1979.
5. Devloo, R. A., Moffitt, E. A., and Sessler, A. D.: Anesthesia for cardiac surgery. Surg. Clin. North Am. 45:871, 1965.
6. DeYoung, D. J., and Sawyer, D. C.: Anesthetic potency of nitrous oxide during halothane anesthesia in the dog. J. Am. Anim. Hosp. Assoc. 16:125, 1980.
7. Eyster, G. E., and Evans, A. T.: Open-heart surgery in the dog. In Kirk, R. W. (ed.): Current Veterinary Therapy: Small Animal Practice. Vol. VI. W. B. Saunders Co., Philadelphia, 1977.
8. Fabian, L. W., and Short, C. E.: Anesthesia for the patient with acquired and congenital heart disease. Vet. Clin. North Am. 3:17, 1973.
9. Gleed, R. D., and Jones, R. S.: Monitoring of cardiac function during anaesthesia. Vet. Rec. 103:428, 1978.
10. Griffiths, G. L., Lumsden, J. H., and Valli, V. E. O.: Hematologic and biochemical changes in dogs with portosystemic shunts. J. Am. Anim. Hosp. Assoc. 17:705, 1981.
11. Hall, L. W., and Clarke, K. W.: Veterinary Anaesthesia. 8th ed. Bailliere Tindall, London, 1983.
12. Harvey, R. C., and Short, C. E.: The use of isoflurane for safe anesthesia in animals with traumatic myocarditis or other myocardial sensitivity. Canine Practice 10:18, 1983.
13. Haskins, S. C., Peiffer, R. L., and Stowe, C. M.: A clinical comparison of CT1341, ketamine and xylazine in cats. Am. J. Vet. Res. 36:1537, 1975.
14. Ionescu, M. E., and Wooler, G. H.: Current Techniques in Extracorporeal Circulation. Buttersworths, Boston, 1976.
15. Kalota, R. J., and Rawlings, C. A.: Cardiopulmonary effects of intravenous xylazine, ketamine, and atropine in the dog. Am. J. Vet. Res. 43:2196, 1982.
16. Keene, B. W., and Bonaguar, J. D.: Valvular heart disease. In Kirk, R. W. (ed.): Current Veterinary Therapy: Small Animal Practice. vol. VIII. W. B. Saunders Co., Philadelphia, 1983.
17. Kittleson, M.: Concepts and therapeutic strategies in the management of heart failure. In Kirk, R. W. (ed.): Current Veterinary Therapy: Small Animal Practice. vol. VIII. W. B. Saunders Co., Philadelphia, 1983.
18. Kittleson, M.: Drugs used in the management of heart failure. In Kirk, R. W. (ed.): Current Veterinary Therapy: Small Animal Practice. vol. VIII. W. B. Saunders Co., Philadelphia, 1983.
19. Kittleson, M.: Drugs used in the therapy of cardiac arrhythmias. In Kirk, R. W. (ed.): Current Veterinary Therapy: Small Animal Practice. vol. VIII. W. B. Saunders Co., Philadelphia, 1983.
20. Klide, A. M., Calderwood, H. W., and Soma, L. R.: Cardiopulmonary effects of xylazine in dogs. Am. J. Vet. Res. 36:931, 1975.
21. Krahwinkel, D. J.: Anesthesia for cardiac surgery. J. Am. Anim. Hosp. Assoc. 8:308, 1972.

22. Krahwinkel, D. J., Jr., Sawyer, D. C., Eyster, G. E., et al.: Cardiopulmonary effects of fentanyl-droperidol, nitrous oxide, and atropine sulfate in dogs. Am. J. Vet. Res. 36:1211, 1975.

23. Liska, W. D., and Tilley, L. P.: Patent ductus arteriosus. Vet. Clin. North Am.—Sm. Anim. Pract. 9:195, 1979.

24. Liu, S. K., Tilley, L. P., and Maron, B. J.: Canine hypertrophic cardiomyopathy. J. Am. Vet. Med. Assoc. 174:708, 1979.

25. Macintire, D. K., and Snider, T. G.: Cardiac arrhythmias associated with multiple trauma in dogs. J. Am. Vet. Med. Assoc. 184:541, 1984.

26. Manley, S. V., and McDonell, W. N.: A new circuit for small animal anesthesia: The Bain coaxial circuit. J. Am. Anim. Hosp. Assoc. 15:61, 1979.

27. McIntosh, J. J.: The use of vasodilators in treatment of congestive heart failure: A review. J. Am. Anim. Hosp. Assoc. 17:255, 1981.

28. Merin, R. G.: The function of the heart: Effects of anesthetics and adjuvant drugs. Am. Soc. Anesth. Refresher Courses in Anesth. 6:81, 1978.

29. Moffitt, E. A., Tarhan, S., and Lundborg, R. O.: Anesthesia for cardiac surgery: Principles and practice. Anesthesiology 29:1181, 1968.

30. Muir, W. W.: Anesthesia for the dog with heart disease. In Kirk, R. W. (ed.): Current Veterinary Therapy: Small Animal Practice vol. VI. W. B. Saunders Co., Philadelphia, 1977.

31. Muir, W. W.: Thiobarbiturate-induced dysrythymias: The role of heart rate and autonomic imbalance. Am. J. Vet. Res. 38:1377, 1977.

32. Muir, W. W.: Anesthesia and the heart. J. Am. Vet. Med. Assoc. 171:92, 1978.

33. Muir, W. W.: Effect of atropine on cardiac rate and rhythm in dogs. J. Am. Vet. Med. Assoc. 172:917, 1978.

34. Muir, W. W., Werner, L. L., and Hamlin, R. L.: Effects of xylazine and acetylpromazine upon induced ventricular fibrillation in dogs anesthetized with thiamylal and halothane. Am. J. Vet. Res. 36:1299, 1975.

35. Nagel, M. L., Muir, W. W., and Nguyen, K.: Comparison of the cardiopulmonary effects of etomidate and thiamylal in dogs. Am. J. Vet. Res. 40:193, 1979.

36. Pyle, R. L.: Congenital heart disease. In Ettinger, S. J. (ed.): Textbook of Veterinary Internal Medicine: Diseases of the Dog and Cat. 2nd ed., vol. I. W. B. Saunders Co., Philadelphia, 1983.

37. Richardson, J. C.: Cardiopulmonary bypass. In Gray, T. C., Nunn, J. F., and Utting, J. E. (eds.): General Anesthesia. 4th ed., vol. 1. Butterworths, Boston, 1980.

38. Roberts, J. G.: Intravenous anesthetic agents. In Prys-Roberts, C. (ed.): The Circulation in Anesthesia: Applied Physiology and Pharmacology. Blackwell Scientific Publications, London, 1980.

39. Ross, J. N.: Heart failure. In Ettinger, S. J. (ed.): Textbook of Veterinary Internal Medicine. 2nd ed., vol. I. W. B. Saunders Co., Philadelphia, 1983.

40. Sawyer, D. C.: Effect of anesthetic agents on cardiovascular function and cardiac rhythm. Vet. Clin. North Am. 3:25, 1973.

41. Sawyer, D. C.: The Practice of Small Animal Anesthesia. W. B. Saunders Co., Philadelphia, 1982.

42. Sawyer, D. C., Lumb, W. V., and Stone, H. L.: Cardiovascular effects of halothane, methoxyflurane, pentobarbital, and thiamylal. J. Appl. Physiol. 30:36, 1971.

43. Short, C. E.: Anesthesia for thoracic surgery. J. Am. Anim. Hosp. Assoc. 8:374, 1972.

44. Smith, N. T.: Myocardial function and anesthesia. In Prys-Roberts, C. (ed.): The Circulation in Anaesthesia: Applied Physiology and Pharmacology. Blackwell Scientific Publications, London, 1980.

45. Smith, T. C.: Carbon dioxide and anesthesia: Respiratory, circulatory, and metabolic effects. Am. Soc. Anesth. Refresher Courses in Anesth. 4:125, 1976.

46. Steffey, E. P.: Circulatory effects of inhalation anesthetics in dogs and horses. Proc. Anesth. Great Britain and Ireland (Suppl. 1st Internat. Congr. Vet. Anesth.) 10:82, 1982.

47. Swan, H. J. C., and Ganz, W.: Use of balloon flotation catheters in critically ill patients. Surg. Clin. North Am. 55:501, 1975.

48. Theye, R. A.: Cardiac performance during anesthesia and operation. Surg. Clin. North Am. 45:841, 1965.

49. Thomas, W. P., Reed, J. R., Bauer, T. G., et al.: Constrictive pericardial disease in the dog. J. Am. Vet. Med. Assoc. 184:546, 1984.

50. Tilley, L. P.: Feline cardiac arrhythmias. Vet. Clin. North Am.—Sm. Anim. Pract. 7:273, 1977.

51. Tilley, L. P., and Weitz, J.: Pharmacologic and other forms of medical therapy in feline cardiac disease. Vet. Clin. North Am.—Sm. Anim. Pract. 7:415, 1977.

52. Turner, D. M., Ilkiw, J. E., Rose, R. J., et al.: Respiratory and cardiovascular effects of five drugs used as sedatives in the dog. Aust. Vet. J. 50:260, 1974.

53. Vickers, M. D., Wood-Smith, F. G., and Stewart, H. C.: Drugs in Anaesthetic Practice. 5th ed. Butterworths, Boston, 1978.

54. Wood, G. L.: Canine myocardial diseases. In Kirk, R. W. (ed.): Current Veterinary Therapy: Small Animal Practice. vol. VIII. W. B. Saunders Co., Philadelphia, 1983.

Chapter **191** # Neuroanesthesiology

Beverly Ann Gilroy

All anesthetic agents and techniques affect the nervous system. Neuroanesthesiology concerns the practice of anesthesiology in patients with neurological diseases, especially those involving the central nervous system (CNS). Patients with acute or chronic CNS disease (e.g., spinal trauma, meningitis, seizure disorders) are not uncommon in veterinary practice and frequently require anesthesia for diagnosis or treatment. Many procedures, such as cerebrospinal fluid (CSF) taps, myelograms, and craniotomies, which can be done on awake humans, require general anesthesia in animals. Moreover, because veterinary patients can only present signs, not verbalize symptoms (e.g., headache, blurred vision), their disease processes may be well advanced when they are first examined. Inappropriate anesthetic techniques can exacerbate pre-existing pathology whereas optimal anesthetic management can contribute to a favorable outcome.

ANATOMICAL, PHYSIOLOGICAL, AND PHARMACOLOGICAL CONSIDERATIONS

Anatomy

The brain and spinal cord, which comprise the CNS, are physically confined within the bony cranium and vertebral column. These bony tissues, as well as meningeal extensions (e.g., tentorium cerebelli, falx cerebri) limit the extent to which the CNS tissues can change in volume without significant changes in pressure. The major components within this confinement, as illustrated in Figure 191–1, are the gray and white matter of the brain and spinal cord, the cerebrospinal fluid, and the blood or intravascular volume flowing through the CNS.

Physiology

The cells of the CNS have unusually high energy requirements. Glucose is the only substrate that can sustain normal function,[8] and oxygen is essential because anaerobic glycolysis cannot provide enough energy for normal cerebral function for more than a few minutes.[8] Increases or decreases in body temperature directly affect CNS metabolic rate and energy requirements. Normally, substrate requirements are met by cerebral blood flow (CBF) and spinal cord blood flow (SBF). Cerebral blood flow is held constant over a range of mean arterial pressures if hypoxia and changes in arterial carbon dioxide

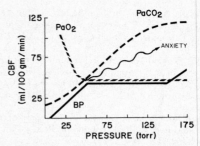

Figure 191–2. Physiological stimuli and cerebral blood flow (CBF). (Reprinted with permission from Shapiro, H. M.: Neuroanesthesia: Physiologic and Pharmacologic Principles. ASA Annual Refresher Course Lectures, 1980.)

(Pa_{CO_2}) are avoided (Fig. 191–2). This phenomenon is referred to as autoregulation. Spinal cord blood flow also varies with Pa_{CO_2}, although sensitivity is less than with CBF, and SBF also autoregulates.[20]

The vasculature of the CNS also differs in that its capillaries are less permeable to many substances than those in other tissues; this is referred to as the blood-brain barrier. This barrier may be diminished or abolished by injury or disease states.

Pharmacology

Many of the drugs used in anesthesia affect CNS metabolism and activity. Some agents are potentially epileptogenic. The CNS seizure threshhold is lowered by phenothiazines.[18] Although most of the clinically used barbiturates are anticonvulsants, methohexital, an ultrashort-acting oxybarbiturate, has convulsant properties and causes seizures in children[17] and myoclonus in dogs.[23] Enflurane, a volatile anesthetic, has been associated with electroencephalographic evidence of epileptic activity,[19] with muscle twitching in dogs[21] and seizures in humans in the postanesthetic period.[14] Studies with ketamine have produced conflicting results; both convulsant and anticonvulsant activity have been seen in various species. However, ketamine should probably be considered potentially epileptogenic in do-

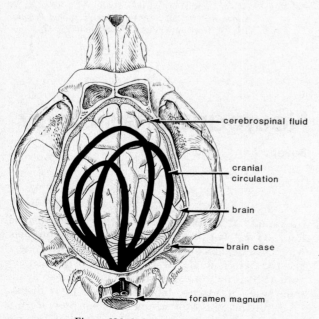

Figure 191–1. Intracranial contents.

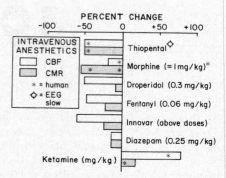

Figure 191–3. Intravenous agents and cerebral blood flow/cerebral metabolic rate (CBF/CMR). (Reprinted with permission from Shapiro, H. M.: Neuroanesthesia: Physiologic and Pharmacologic Principles. ASA Annual Refresher Course Lectures, 1980.)

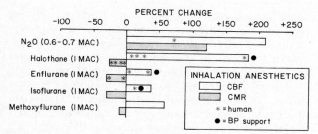

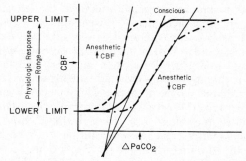

Figure 191–4. Inhalationals and cerebral blood flow/cerebral metabolic rate (CBF/CMR). (Reprinted with permission from Shapiro, H. M.: Neuroanesthesia: Physiologic and Pharmacologic Principles. ASA Annual Refresher Course Lectures, 1980.)

mestic species and should not be used in patients with histories of seizure disorders.[24]

With the exceptions mentioned above, barbiturates and volatile general anesthetics depress electroencephalographic activity and CNS metabolism.

Anesthetic agents can markedly alter CBF and SBF. Ketamine and the inhalation agents increase this flow; thiobarbiturates are cerebral vasoconstrictors and decrease flow. Changes in CBF and cerebral metabolic rate (CMR) produced by anesthetic agents are summarized in Figures 191–3 and 191–4. The effect of volatile anesthetics on autoregulation is dose-dependent (Fig. 191–5). These anesthetic-induced changes in autoregulation can be enhanced or diminished by alterations in Pa_{CO_2} (Fig. 191–6).

Pathophysiology

Injury and other disease states can cause focal or general disruption of CNS autoregulation. Such disruption may cause increases in CBF or SBF, thus increasing the volume of the CNS. Whether such increases produce increases in intracranial pressure (ICP) or intraspinal pressure (ISP) depends on the patient's position on the volume-pressure curve (Fig. 191–7). If the patient already has decreased compliance (e.g., due to a mass lesion such as an abscess or tumor) as designated by positions 3 or 4

Figure 191–6. Cerebral blood flow–carbon dioxide (CBF-CO_2) sensitivity and anesthesia. (Reprinted with permission from Shapiro, H. M.: Neuroanesthesia: Physiologic and Pharmacologic Principles. ASA Annual Refresher Course Lectures, 1980.)

(Fig. 191–7), an increase in CNS blood flow can result in marked elevations in pressure. Such elevations can result in decreases in cerebral (or spinal) perfusion pressure and in brain herniation. Caudal transtentorial, foramen magnum, rostral transtentorial, and cingulate gyrus herniations have been reported in small animals.[13]

Factors that can affect ICP and ISP include patient positioning and venous return, the intravascular volume within the CNS (CBF plus SBF) Pa_{CO_2}, hypoxia, the patient's hydration status, osmolality, the patency of CSF flow and reabsorption, loss of autoregulation secondary to CNS disease, and anesthetic agents.

CLINICAL NEUROANESTHESIA

Relatively few articles[3,11,16] have been published about veterinary neuroanesthesia. Development of specific recommendations has been handicapped by the lack of controlled, prospective clinical trials evaluating anesthetic management and outcome. The following recommendations are based on the previously discussed physiological and pharmacological principles, data from research animals, reports in the human medical literature, and my own experience.

Elective Anesthesia in a Patient with a History of Seizures

The specific technique varies with species, breed, and procedure to be performed. If the etiology of the

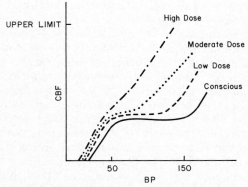

Figure 191–5. Volatile anesthetics and autoregulation. (Reprinted with permission from Shapiro, H. M.: Neuroanesthesia: Physiologic and Pharmacologic Principles. ASA Annual Refresher Course Lectures, 1980).

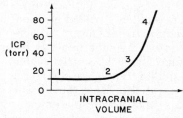

Figure 191–7. Intracranial compliance curve. (Reprinted with permission from Shapiro, H. M.: Neurosurgical anesthesia and intracranial hypertension. *In* Miller, R. D. (ed.): *Anesthesia.* Churchill Livingstone, New York, 1981.)

seizure is known, it may influence the choice of agent. If hypoglycemia is suspected, the patient should receive intravenous dextrose solutions during anesthesia and recovery to prevent potentially devastating neurological damage; general anesthetics prevent hypoglycemia-induced seizures and mask hypoglycemic coma. If hypoglycemia occurs and is not detected, the result can be neurological damage or "failure to awaken" from the anesthetic. If hepatic encephalopathy is suspected, caution must be exercised in administering agents dependent on liver metabolism for inactivation (e.g., morphine). In many cases, however, the etiology of the seizures is unknown.

If the patient is already receiving anticonvulsant therapy, it is important to determine what kind. Chronic administration of barbiturates can produce tolerance to acutely administered barbiturates as well as induction of increased liver enzyme activity.[7] This increased activity can result in increased metabolism of volatile anesthetics and other agents.

The need for premedication in these patients varies with their temperament and degree of CNS depression. Phenothiazines are contraindicated; short-acting narcotics such as meperidine (3 to 4 mg/kg intramuscularly) alone or combined with diazepam (0.4 mg/kg intramuscularly) can be useful. Ketamine and methohexital should be avoided. Acceptable induction techniques include intravenous thiobarbiturates, intravenous Innovar-Vet (unless rapid control of the airway is necessary), and face mask inductions with halothane or isoflurane. These volatile agents are also suitable for maintenance, as is methoxyflurane.

Diagnostic Procedures

Radiological procedures are frequently performed in the diagnosis of neurological disease. General anesthetics (with the probable exception of ketamine) can provide the analgesia and muscle relaxation needed for proper positioning. The choice of anesthetic is generally based on the patient's physical status, breed, and length of the procedure. It is important to ensure that positioning does not compromise the patient's airway. Also, if it is anticipated that the patient will be disconnected from the anesthetic machine or extubated for any reason, nitrous oxide should not be used. Patients receiving nitrous oxide who are suddenly placed on room air exhibit diffusion hypoxia. In prolonged radiographic procedures, inadvertent hypothermia is a common complication, especially in the smaller patient.

Contrast studies can cause significant complications. It is essential to have the patient adequately anesthetized so that needle placement and contrast injection do not produce movement and potential injury. In air-contrast studies (e.g., pneumoencephalograms) nitrous oxide is contraindicated. Subarachnoid injection of radiopaque media such as methiodal and metrizamide can produce significant

alterations in cardiopulmonary parameters.[15] Either apnea or tachypnea may occur. Tachycardia, bradycardia, hypertension, or hypotension may be seen. Convulsions in the postanesthetic recovery period are a significant complication. Premedication may include anticholinergics such as atropine or glycopyrrolate. Phenothiazines are contraindicated. Diazepam (0.4 mg/kg intramuscularly) or phenobarbital (2 to 3 mg/kg intramuscularly) may decrease the incidence of seizures.[16] Thiobarbiturate induction is commonly preferred, although one *in vitro* study has suggested that methiodal, when absorbed into the blood stream, can displace thiopental from serum protein-binding sites and possibly contribute to anesthetic complications.[3] This implication must be weighed against the potential advantages of a rapid, smooth induction and possible anticonvulsant actions. Anesthesia is maintained with halogenated agents (most commonly methoxyflurane or halothane) with or without nitrous oxide. Intravenous fluids such as lactated Ringer's solution aid excretion of contrast agents and help treat hypotension. Some authors recommend maintaining general anesthesia for at least one hour after the myelogram, but this does not always prevent seizures in the recovery period.[5] The head should be kept elevated and fluids continued throughout the procedure and recovery period until the patient has regained full consciousness without evidence of seizures. Twitching or muscle fasciculations during recovery may indicate the onset of seizures, and intravenous diazepam 0.4 mg/kg should be given in such cases. It is better to prevent seizures than to wait until they occur.

Computerized tomography is not yet commonly used in veterinary medicine but has been reported.[12,22] It is noninvasive but does require immobility of the patient. This may be achieved with sedation and restraint or with general anesthesia depending on the patient's overall status.

Cerebrospinal fluid taps are frequently performed in neurological patients. In veterinary patients, the tap is usually done at the cisterna magna. The procedure requires immobility and thus adequate anesthesia. Extreme cervical flexion can result in airway obstruction, so the patient should be intubated with a tube of adequate length.

One of the major factors affecting selection of an anesthetic technique for CSF tap is the effect of the patient's disease on intracranial compliance. Mass lesions (e.g., tumors, abscesses) and meningitis can cause marked decreases in the patient's intracranial compliance. Therefore, anesthetics that increase cerebral blood flow may cause significant increases in intracranial pressure (ICP). Sudden removal of CSF at the cisterna magna may result in herniation of brain through the foramen magnum.[13] Since CSF taps can generally be performed in less than 15 to 20 minutes, thiobarbiturates can be used for anesthesia in most cases. Ketamine should probably be avoided. If CSF taps must be done under inhalation anesthesia, hyperventilation should be instituted before the halogenated agent is administered.

Some clinicians measure the ICP using a three-way stopcock and a plastic manometer such as that used for measuring central venous pressure. The pressure is measured before CSF is withdrawn (opening pressure) and after the sample is collected (closing pressure). Comparison of the two readings can help estimate the patient's, position on the compliance curve (Fig. 191–7). When making comparisons between patients, it is important to know if the same anesthetic technique was used in each case because variations in anesthetics can produce variations in pressure readings.

During and following CSF taps it is advisable to monitor respiration closely. Apnea may result from airway obstruction due to positioning, but this is easily corrected. Persistent apnea not due to airway obstruction may be due to iatrogenic trauma or herniation.

Electroencephalography can be a useful diagnostic tool in neurology. In particular, it may be of potential value in predicting increased ICP prior to performing CSF taps. However, encephalography in veterinary patients can be difficult because of the large bulk of cranial muscles and lack of patient cooperation. Anesthetic agents, as noted previously, have significant and varied effects on the electroencephalogram (EEG). Many clinicians find that they can satisfactorily interpret EEGs in anesthetized patients but others prefer awake patients. Some have chosen to use neuromuscular blocking agents such as succinylcholine to ensure immobility and to minimize artifact. Use of such agents requires positive pressure ventilation until the agents have been metabolized, excreted, or antagonized. Such techniques do not affect the EEG pharmacologically but subject the patient to significant psychological stress if given without unconsciousness-producing drugs. Thus, for humane reasons, neuromuscular blocking agents should not be used alone.

Therapeutic Procedures

Decompressions

Cranial decompressions are occasionally done in veterinary medicine but are much less common than spinal decompressions. Craniotomy may be indicated for treatment or excision of cerebral abscesses or tumors. Hydrocephalus is seen in certain breeds, and surgical procedures for establishing "shunts" have been published. Traumatic injuries may result in the need for cranial decompression, but this is much less common than in human medicine.

Spinal decompression may be indicated in the treatment of vertebral fractures, luxations, and subluxations. One of the most common indications is dorsal rupture of intervertebral disc(s) with protrusion of the disc material into the spinal canal. It is important to differentiate between cervical lesions and lower cord lesions because cervical lesions present more difficult problems with airway management and may present a greater likelihood of arrhythmias and cardiovascular instability.[9]

Anesthetic considerations include not only the location of the lesion, as mentioned above, but also whether the patient has an acute or chronic injury. Acute injuries that require decompression within a few hours to minimize cord injury may be accompanied by other injuries (e.g., pneumothorax) or cardiovascular shock, which greatly increases anesthetic risk. Chronic injuries may have resulted in muscular atrophy or in urinary incontinence, which predisposes the patient to decubital ulcers and renal disease. Human patients who are quadriplegic are extremely sensitive to the effects of depolarizing muscle relaxants such as succinylcholine.[10] Administration of such agents to chronic quadriplegics has resulted in life-threatening hyperkalemia.

Acute cervical injuries in particular require that endotracheal intubation be performed with great care and with minimal flexion or hyperextension of the neck. Use of a laryngoscope and stylet if necessary can be helpful. If a ventral surgical approach is anticipated, a long endotracheal tube extending to the thoracic inlet is needed to prevent airway obstruction during retraction of the trachea. Care must be taken not to use too long a tube, which could result in endobronchial intubation. Auscultation of the cranial portions of both lung fields should be done as soon as the endotracheal tube is tied in place to ensure that bronchial intubation has not occurred.

Positioning of the patient is extremely important not only to ensure a patent airway but also to ensure adequate venous drainage from the affected area. Compression of the jugular veins can result in increases in intracranial pressure.

Fortunately, there are several agents and techniques that can be used to reduce swelling of the brain or spinal cord. One of the most effective techniques is hyperventilation to reduce Pa_{CO_2}, thus reducing cerebral blood flow. Extreme hyperventilation should be avoided; it is generally recommended to keep Pa_{CO_2} just below normal (e.g., approximately 28 to 33 mm Hg). Application of positive end expiratory pressure (PEEP), either intentionally or inadvertently (by failure to open the pop-off or relief valve during expiration), can result in elevations in ICP. Hyperventilation is one of the most rapidly acting and probably one of the safest methods of reducing ICP.

Osmotic agents such as 20 per cent mannitol intravenously have been used to lower ICP. Such agents can markedly increase the patient's intravascular volume, and mannitol has been specifically implicated in cases of acute pulmonary edema in small animals. Mannitol should also be avoided when subdural, intracerebral, or intraspinal hemorrhage is suspected. Hypertonic solutions of glucose and urea are no longer used. Nonosmotic diuretics such as furosemide have also been used to reduce intracranial pressure and may cause fewer acid-base and electrolyte abnormalities.[4]

Pharmacologic doses of corticosteroids have been widely used in the treatment of cerebral and spinal trauma, although their efficacy has not been definitely proved.[19] Corticosteroids are beneficial in reducing cerebral edema surrounding brain tumors and may help to ameliorate clinical signs. Their use in other types of neurological cases is questionable, but they will probably continue to be used owing to their relatively low risk/benefit ratio.

Barbiturates, including the thiobarbiturates, are well documented as effective cerebral vasoconstrictors. These drugs may be of benefit in reducing ICP and intraspinal pressure and in reducing swelling at the site of decompression. However, they have potent cardiopulmonary effects, and the patient must be closely monitored when they are administered.

Because the neuronal tissues have such high oxygen requirements and because injury can result in ischemia of these tissues, efforts have been made to discover methods of pharmacologic protection of these structures. A great deal of research has been done on experimental models of acute, focal and global cerebral and spinal injuries. It is important to consider not only the type of injury created but also the anesthetic technique utilized and the time after injury at which the pharmacologic intervention was made. Thus far, the evidence remains controversial. Corticosteroids have not proved effective. Barbiturates are somewhat effective in focal injuries if they are given within a relatively short period after injury. The nonbarbiturate anticonvulsants such as diphenylhydantoin do not improve the outcome. Two agents that have shown some promise in early studies are naloxone[1] and thyrotropin-releasing hormone (TRH),[6] but it is too early to recommend either for routine clinical use.

A suggested anesthetic protocol for decompression includes stabilization of the patient's cardiopulmonary system and minimal or no premedication. Meperidine in dosages of 3 to 4 mg/kg intramuscularly can be used. If an anticholinergic is desirable, glycopyrrolate may be preferred over atropine. Induction can be performed with intravenous thiobarbiturates unless these are contraindicated by ventricular arrhythmias or other cardiovascular instability. If thiobarbiturates are contraindicated, intravenous Innovar Vet, 1 ml/25 to 30 kg, can be used to accomplish endotracheal intubation. Maintenance is achieved with low levels (less than 1.5 minimum alveolar concentration (MAC) of isoflurane and hyperventilation. If isoflurane is not available, halothane can be used, or methoxyflurane possibly combined with neuromuscular blocking agents. Close monitoring of the patient, including respiratory rate and depth, heart rate and rhythm (ECG), pulse strength, mucous membrane color and capillary refill time, blood pressure, and central venous pressure when possible, should be performed.

Ketamine, high doses of narcotics, and high levels of halogenated agents such as halothane should be avoided, especially when the patient is allowed to breathe spontaneously.

Fracture/Luxation Stabilization

Various surgical techniques have been developed to treat fractures and luxations of the vertebral column. Acute fractures and luxations frequently require decompression of the cord as well as stabilization of the vertebrae. All of the above mentioned factors for decompressive surgery apply in these cases as well.

Abnormalities causing chronic cervical instability (e.g., "wobblers," atlantoaxial subluxation) are now more commonly diagnosed and treated. These cases again require the utmost care in positioning for endotracheal intubation so as not to exacerbate the lesion. Gentle, steady traction on the patient's ears in a rostral direction to keep the neck in mild extension helps minimize movement of the vertebral column. This is most easily done with the patient in a lateral recumbent position. The use of an appropriate laryngoscope blade (e.g., a Michaels and Shapiro blade, or a Miller's blade of adequate length) and an appropriately positioned stylet make intubation much easier.

Although hyperventilation has been recommended to reduce spinal blood flow and to help reduce swelling of the cord, in cervical lesions it may be more beneficial to allow the patient to breathe spontaneously. Close monitoring of the patient then helps to detect possible iatrogenic exacerbation of the lesion interfering with neural control of respiration. In general, the recommendations given for decompressive surgery also apply to stabilization surgery.

Prophylactic Fenestrations

These are commonly performed as part of the management of intervertebral disc disease. Cervical fenestrations require the same attention to airway management as that needed for ventral cervical decompressions. The anesthetic protocol is partly determined by whether or not preoperative radiographs or myelograms are performed. Cervical disc patients frequently have considerable pain and may benefit from premedication with analgesics such as meperidine or oxymorphone.

Thoracolumbar fenestrations can be performed by a number of surgical approaches. One of the techniques used requires a thoracotomy.[2] If such a technique is used, one must be concerned not only with the neurological factors affecting anesthetic choice but also with the effects of thoracotomy on ventilation, oxygenation, and hemodynamics. Controlled ventilation performed either manually or mechanically is required during the thoracotomy. Retraction and packing of the lungs may interfere with oxygenation, and thus it may be wise to avoid the use of nitrous oxide. If nitrous oxide is used, it must be discontinued at least five minutes prior to closure of the chest wall to minimize enlargement of the pneumothorax. Since positive pressure ventilation can interfere with venous return to the heart and cause a decrease in cardiac output, it may be necessary to increase the rate of intravenous fluid administration. Evaporative losses from exposed viscera also increase the fluid requirement as well as the likelihood of inadvertent hypothermia, which is an extremely common complication of this surgical approach. Specific recommendations for anesthesia for thoracotomy are discussed in Chapter 189.

Postanesthestic Considerations

The postanesthetic period is critical for the neurological patient. It is essential to monitor the patient closely to ensure that neither anesthesia nor the diagnostic or therapeutic maneuvers have exacerbated the patient's pre-existing disease. One of the most useful things to monitor is the patient's level of consciousness. Any deterioration in this should be immediately and intensely investigated to determine its cause, which may be progressive neurological injury or a deterioration in the patient's cardiopulmonary status. Other neurological reflexes such as response to deep painful stimulus should also be regularly monitored.

If a myelogram has been performed, the patient should be watched closely for evidence of impending seizures. If seizures should occur, they should be appropriately treated and the patient observed for hyperthermia.

The patient's cardiopulmonary signs should also be followed, as well as body temperature to ensure that any hypothermia that has occurred during anesthesia is abating.

Many neurosurgical patients experience considerable pain during the recovery period, and administration of analgesics such as meperidine, oxymorphone, or nalbuphine may be indicated. Such analgesics may be advisable not only from a humane viewpoint but also to minimize excessive thrashing movements by the patient. These advantages must be weighed against the effect such drug administration will have on the veterinarian's ability to follow the patient's neurological signs.

Perhaps one of the most important factors affecting the outcome of neurological cases is the quality of nursing care provided in the postsurgical period. Such care requires not only the monitoring discussed above but also interventions such as assisting emptying of the bladder in immobile patients to prevent urine burns and rotation of such patients to minimize lung congestion and the incidence of decubitus ulcers. Provision of adequate nutrition to these patients must also be emphasized.

1. Baskin, D. S., and Hosobuchi, Y.: Naloxone reversal of ischaemic neurological deficits in man. Lancet 2:72, 1981.
2. Bojrab, M. J.: Prophylactic thoracolumbar disk fenestration. *In* Bojrab. M. J. (ed.): *Canine Surgery.* Lea & Febiger, Philadelphia, 1975, p. 404.
3. Bonhaus, D. W., Sawyer, D. C., and Hook, J. B.: Displacement of protein-bound thiopental by sodium methiodal may contribute to anesthetic complications during canine myelography. Am. J. Vet. Res. 42:1612, 1981.
4. Cottrell, J. E., Robustelli, A., Post, K., and Turndorf, H.: Furosemide and mannitol induced changes in intracranial pressure and serum osmolality and electrolytes. Anesthesiology 47:28, 1977.
5. Davis, E. M., Glickman, L., Rendano, V. T., and Short, C. E.: Seizures in dogs following metrizamide myelography. J. Am. Anim. Hosp. Assoc. 17:642, 1981.
6. Faden, A. I., Jacobs, T. P., and Holaday, J. W.: Thyrotropin-releasing hormone improves neurologic recovery after spinal trauma in cats. N. Engl. J. Med. 305:1063, 1981.
7. Goodman, L. S., and Gilman, A.: *The Pharmacological Basis of Therapeutics.* Macmillan, New York, 1969, p. 115.
8. Gordon, E. (ed.): *A Basis and Practice of Neuroanaesthesia.* Excerpta Medica, New York, 1981, pp. 51, 100.
9. Greenhoot, J. H., Shiel, F. O., and Mauch, H. P., Jr.: Experimental spinal cord injury: Electrocardiographic abnormalities and fuchsinophilic myocardial degeneration. Arch. Neurol. 26:524, 1972.
10. Gronert, G. A., and Theye, R. A.: Pathophysiology of hyperkalemia induced by succinylcholine. Anesthesiology 43:89, 1975.
11. Hartsfield, S. M., and Thurmon, J. C.: Anesthesia in small animal neurological patients. J. Am. Anim. Hosp. Assoc. 11:396, 1975.
12. Janssen, D. L., Hammock, M. K., Davis, D. O., and Bush, M.: Cranial computed tomography in the evaluation of neurologic disorders in two non human primates. J. Am. Vet. Med. Assoc. 179:1245, 1981.
13. Kornegay, J. N., Oliver, J. E., and Gorgacz, E. J.: Clinicopathologic features of brain herniation in animals. J. Am. Vet. Med. Assoc. 182:1111, 1983.
14. Kruczek, M., Albin, M. S., Wolf, S. and Bertoni, J. M.: Postoperative seizure activity following enflurane anesthesia. Anesthesiology 53:175, 1980.
15. Menhusen, M. J., and Parker, A. J.: Clinical observations of cardiovascular and respiratory changes during contrast myelography with water soluble media. J. Am. Anim. Hosp. Assoc. 11:401, 1975.
16. Riedesel, D. H.: The relationship between premedication and post myelographic seizure activity. Calif. Vet. 34:23, 1980.
17. Rockoff, M. A., and Goudsouzian, N. G.: Seizures induced by methohexital. Anesthesiology 54:333, 1981.
18. Roizen, M. F.: Preoperative evaluation of patients with diseases that require special preoperative evaluation and intraoperative management. *In* Miller, R. D. (ed.): *Anesthesia.* Churchill Livingstone, New York, 1981, pp. 49, 76.
19. Rucker, N. C., Lumb, W. V., and Scott, R. J.: Combined pharmacologic and surgical treatments for acute spinal cord trauma. Am. J. Vet. Med. 42:1138, 1981.
20. Smith, A. L.: Effect of anesthetics and oxygen deprivation on brain blood flow and metabolism. Surg. Clin. North Am. 55:819, 1975.
21. Steffey, E. P., and Howland, D.: Potency of enthrane in dogs: Comparison with halothane and isoflurane. Am. J. Vet. Med. 39:573, 1978.
22. Swengal, J. R.: Computerized tomography for diagnosis of brain tumor in a dog. J. Am. Vet. Med. Assoc. 181:605, 1982.
23. Wauquier, A., Vanden Broeck, W. A., Verheyen, J. L., and Janssen, P. A.: Electroencephalographic study of the short-acting hypnotics etomidate and methohexital in dogs. Eur. J. Pharmacol. 47:367, 1978.
24. Wright, M.: Pharmacologic effects of ketamine and its use in veterinary medicine. J. Am. Vet. Med. Assoc. 180:1462, 1982.

Chapter 192

Male and Female Reproductive Systems

Sandee M. Hartsfield

EFFECTS OF ANESTHETICS AND RELATED DRUGS ON REPRODUCTIVE FUNCTION

The veterinary literature citing the effects of various anesthetics and anesthetic adjuncts on the reproductive system is not extensive, except for the placental transfer of drugs used in cesarean section and the neonatal responses to these drugs. Very little information is derived directly from the dog or the cat.

Anticholinergic Drugs

Atropine in high doses blocks both the uterine response to hypogastric nerve stimulation in rabbits and acetylcholine stimulation of the isolated canine uterus.[12] In normal doses, atropine is likely to produce little effect on the uterus.[12] In very high doses, atropine delays ovulation in cattle.[49] In a study using intravenous glycopyrrolate in women just prior to delivery, no clinically significant changes in uterine activity were noted.[1]

Narcotics

Narcotics and similar analgesics reduce the release of follicle-stimulating hormone, luteinizing hormone, and thyrotropin in women, a fact that may be of significance in breeding animals.[36]

Tranquilizers

The best known effect of phenothiazine tranquilizers on the reproductive systems of animals is the production of paralysis of the retractor penis muscle and penile prolapse in stallions.[36] Significant, permanent effects of a similar nature are not recognized in small animals. Certain phenothiazines in large doses have teratogenic properties in experimental animals, but studies have not shown similar effects in humans. Diazepam has been associated specifically with development of oral clefts in human fetuses.[38]

Xylazine

Because of smooth muscle relaxation, decreased uterine contractions may be expected following xylazine administration, and relaxation and temporary penile prolapse may be seen in horses.[36] However, xylazine has an oxytocinlike effect on the uterus, and it should not be used in late pregnancy because of the possibility of abortion.[27] In evaluation of this contradiction, variation in uterine response may possibly be related to the species, drug dosage, or stage of pregnancy.

Barbiturates

In low doses, barbiturates do not significantly impair uterine contractions during labor. However, doses used to produce general anesthesia decrease the strength and rate of uterine contractions.[23]

Ketamine

Ketamine causes increased arterial blood pressure and heart rate, decreased arterial pH and P_{O_2} and increased arterial P_{CO_2} in pregnant goats near term.[28] This secondary sympathetic response has been associated with decreased uterine blood flow and decreased O_2 delivery to the fetus. However, one study in ewes showed that even though uterine blood flow was reduced dramatically following infusion of vasoactive drugs, fetal blood gases and acid-base variables were not significantly changed.[15]

Ketamine has oxytocic effects on the uterus. It has a dose-related effect in women, and ketamine increases basal uterine tone. By decreasing blood flow to the placenta, such effects could affect the fetus.[14] However, more recent data suggest that low doses of ketamine are not likely to affect the fetus owing to minimal changes in basal uterine tone.[32]

Inhalation Anesthetics

Halothane relaxes uterine smooth muscle, but methoxyflurane has little effect on the uterus.[31]

GENERAL PRINCIPLES OF ANESTHETIC MANAGEMENT

There are several considerations in anesthesia for reproductive system surgery. Elective neutering procedures often involve healthy animals in which anesthetic management requires no special variation. In nonelective procedures involving the male or female reproductive systems, the principles of anes-

---

Parts of this chapter have appeared in, and are reprinted with permission from, Hartsfield, S. M.: Obstetrical anesthesia in small animals. Calif. Vet. 33:18, 1979.

thesia depend on the condition of the patient and the organ systems involved in uptake, distribution, biotransformation, and elimination of anesthetic drugs (e.g., heart, lungs, kidneys, and liver).

At times, pregnant animals must be anesthetized, and the effects of anesthetic drugs and the anesthetic state on the fetus must be considered. The possibility of teratogenic effects of anesthetics also exists.[38] There is no evidence that intrauterine exposure to a properly administered anesthetic results in long-term fetal effects. The most likely time for direct toxic anesthetic effects is early in fetal development.[38] This statement is supported by data collected from pregnant mice.[53] Similarly, the effects of anesthesia on the developing fetus may be related to physiological changes that alter placental blood flow (e.g., if the dam is anesthetized and becomes hypotensive, uterine blood flow is likely to be lowered). Hypovolemia, aortocaval compression causing decreased venous return with the dam in dorsal recumbency, and sympathetic blockade due to regional analgesia are common causes of maternal hypotension.[16] Maternal hypoxia, hypotension, hypocarbia, hypercarbia, electrolyte imbalances, hypertension related to vasoconstrictors, and other alterations in maternal or fetal physiology may be more detrimental than exposure to anesthetic drugs.[38] The following principles may be useful in evaluating and managing an anesthetic regimen for a pregnant animal prior to term:

1. Perform anesthesia only in required cases. Do not expose the fetus to unnecessary drugs.
2. Anesthesia during the first trimester may be more teratogenic.
3. Avoid anesthetics that are highly metabolized because metabolites may affect the fetus.
4. Maintain the physiological status of the dam throughout anesthesia, particularly avoiding hypovolemia, hypotension, hypoxemia, and hypercarbia.
5. Thiopental, morphine, meperidine, succinylcholine, and low concentrations of nitrous oxide have "safe histories" in the first trimester of pregnancy in humans.[38]

FEMALE REPRODUCTIVE SYSTEM

Uterus and Ovaries

Pyometra

This suppurative inflammation of the uterus[5] is associated with progestational and estrogenic factors complicated by bacteria.[19] Renal dysfunction often occurs with pyometra and may be due to prerenal uremia, glomerular disease, tubular abnormalities, or renal pathology not related specifically to the uterine disease. Anemia and azotemia may be present. The anemia may be caused by toxic depression of bone marrow or loss of erythrocytes into the uterus.[5] Dehydration is common, especially if the disease has initiated vomiting, diarrhea, or anorexia. Because surgery is the most likely treatment for pyometra, particularly in animals with a closed cervix, anesthetic management of the sick patient is an important consideration.

Preanesthetic management depends on the specific condition of the patient. The following recommendations assume a toxic, depressed patient with a closed cervix. Blood and urine samples should be taken for baseline data, which should include a complete blood count, a biochemical profile that should report blood urea nitrogen, creatinine, alanine aminotransferase, and alkaline phosphatase, and a urinalysis. Blood gas and acid-base data and electrolyte measurements are useful information as well. The physical examination should include cardiopulmonary function, and a preanesthetic electrocardiogram may be recorded. Rehydration and correction of acid-base and electrolyte derangements should begin prior to induction of anesthesia. A central venous catheter, inserted through the jugular vein with the tip of the catheter near the right atrium, may be placed for fluid infusion and recording of central venous pressure (CVP), and a peripheral catheter (cephalic vein) of relatively large bore is inserted and secured for fluid and drug infusion. The latter catheter is of particular value for rapid fluid administration if circulatory shock occurs. A urinary catheter is beneficial for monitoring urine production, especially if abnormal renal function is evident. However, the patient should not be unduly stressed to accomplish this because the catheter can be placed after anesthetic induction. Because of potential renal dysfunction, dehydration, and septicemia, a large volume of fluid may be required to maintain vascular volume.

Preanesthetic medication is optional, depending on personal preferences and the anesthetic regimen. Glycopyrrolate, 0.011 mg/kg intravenously with an equal dose subcutaneously, may be given immediately prior to induction. Preanesthetic oxygenation by mask helps prevent postinduction hypoxemia. Continuous electrocardiographic (ECG) monitoring should be started prior to induction. Oxymorphone, 0.11 to 0.22 mg/kg given intravenously, can be used for intubation in depressed dogs, or the drug can be used to ease mask induction with halothane in more alert animals. Halothane or halothane and nitrous oxide can be used for induction by mask in premedicated, very depressed, or small patients (e.g., cats). Hypotensive premedicants (e.g., acetylpromazine) should not be used in pyometra patients. Intubation should be done quickly, and maintenance of anesthesia is accomplished with inhalation anesthetics or with a balanced anesthetic protocol. At least 30 per cent oxygen is delivered during anesthesia using an appropriate anesthetic system (e.g., a circle system for a larger patient and a Norman elbow or Bain system for a patient weighing less than 5 kg). Ventilation is assisted or controlled to ensure CO_2 removal. Monitoring and support of vital functions must continue throughout the maintenance and recovery periods until the patient recovers.

Obstetrical Anesthesia

In small animals, anesthesia is needed to facilitate both vaginal and abdominal deliveries. Basic principles of anesthesia and peculiarities of anesthetic management in obstetrical patients are important. Special considerations include maternal and fetal hazards, placental transfer of drugs, and physiologic variations in pregnant and newborn animals. Although information about pregnant and newborn animals may be derived from various species, probably most data come from sheep and humans. Consequently, there are species variations in dogs and cats. However, there are enough similarities to allow this information to be considered and applied logically in anesthetic management.[21]

Maternal and Fetal Hazards in Obstetrical Anesthesia

Anesthesia toward the end of gestation is complicated by the presence of more than one patient. In some cases, efforts may be concentrated on either the dam or the fetuses, depending on the interests of the owner. However, problems consistently arise that can be prevented or treated, resulting in less maternal and fetal mortality. Maternal complications during anesthesia include aspiration of vomitus, hypotension causing circulatory failure, and convulsions.[45] Difficulties arise most often if labor has been prolonged or if the mother has pre-existing physiological abnormalities such as extreme obesity. Fetal complications are related to pharmacologic depression and maternal hypoxemia, acidosis, hyperventilation, or hypothermia.[45]

Aspiration of vomitus can cause maternal mortality. The onset of labor is unpredictable in relation to eating, and gastric emptying slows with the onset of pain or as a result of certain drugs.[16] Displacement of the stomach, increased abdominal pressure, and surgical manipulations increase the tendency toward regurgitation.[16,45] Therefore, a patient receiving drugs that produce general anesthesia or depress laryngeal reflexes should have its airway protected by a properly sized endotracheal tube. Even with regional or local techniques, the patient's head should be positioned below the median plane of the body so that regurgitated material may be easily eliminated from the oropharynx. Aspiration of gastric contents causes hypoxemia due to airway obstruction, bronchospasm, pulmonary vasospasm, and atelectasis. Due to chemical injury, which is most severe if the pH of the aspirated material is less than 2.5, a proteinaceous fluid exudate begins to accumulate. Early deaths are related to hypoxemia, and survivors may succumb to secondary infections and pneumonia.[47] Although mechanical prevention of aspiration is most desirable, use of preanesthetic glycopyrrolate instead of atropine increases gastric pH and may decrease the severity of chemical injury.[44,48] However, time is required for a significant effect on gastric pH, and

more benefit was realized in humans who received the drug 60 to 120 minutes prior to induction.[3]

Hypotension and circulatory failure can be significant reasons for maternal deaths.[45] Causes of hypotension include drug depression, sympathetic blockade, decreased venous return, extracellular fluid volume depletion, and septic or endotoxic shock. Several drugs used in general anesthesia produce arterial hypotension. These include inhalation anesthetics, narcotics, and tranquilizers. They may be peripheral vasodilators or direct myocardial depressants. Spinal or epidural techniques cause sympathetic blockade in the affected posterior area of the body. In the pregnant animal, a likely cause of hypotension is the weight of the gravid uterus on the vena cava when the patient is in dorsal recumbency.[16] In humans, this is alleviated by lateral displacement of the uterus,[45] but this technique may be less useful in animals with two gravid uterine horns. Leaving the patient in lateral recumbency as long as possible may be beneficial. Circulatory shock associated with absorption of bacterial or tissue products of dead, necrotic fetuses may also cause maternal hypotension. Pressures as high as 100 mm Hg (systolic) may be required to maintain uterine perfusion and prevent fetal embarrassment.[45] Repositioning, intravenous fluids, and possibly vasopressors can help to maintain maternal blood pressure.[45] Ephedrine has been useful in humans and sheep for treating epidural or spinal-induced hypotension because it increases maternal blood pressure without reducing uterine blood flow.[41]

Although unusual, convulsions may complicate obstetrical anesthesia. They may be related to hypocalcemia in puerperal tetany, alkalemia subsequent to hyperventilation, or drug toxicity from excessive local anesthetics. Eclampsia with convulsive activity has been reported at calcium blood levels of less than 7 mg/dl.[4,18] Because anesthetics depress seizures, convulsions are most likely to occur in the pre- and postanesthetic periods. Seizure activity is usually controlled by a central nervous system depressant such as thiopental or diazepam.

Fetal hypoxemia may complicate vaginal or abdominal deliveries. Maternal hypotension, increased intramyometrial pressure due to oxytocin or prolonged uterine contractions, and decreased uterine blood flow related to certain drugs contribute to fetal hypoxemia and acidosis.[45] Abnormally low fetal oxygen tension is associated with depressed neonates. Also, drugs that cross the placenta may cause fetal respiratory impairment; barbiturates, narcotics, and inhalation anesthetics may produce prolonged depression in neonates because neonatal hepatic and renal biotransformation and elimination of drugs are usually slow.[33] Also, the lower neonatal blood pH may increase the concentration and activity of the drug.[33]

Traumatic attempts at delivery, insufficient oxygenation of the dam, and diffusion hypoxia after use of nitrous oxide are other possible causes of neonatal hypoxemia. During and after delivery, fetal aspiration of meconium and amniotic fluid may occur, causing asphyxia, particularly if the fetus lodges in the birth canal.[17] In general, neonatal depression and hypoxemia are best prevented by control of maternal blood pressure, adequate ventilation and oxygenation, judicious use of anesthetic and related drugs, and rapid attention to the neonatal airway, ventilation, and oxygenation upon delivery.

Placental Transfer of Drugs

Virtually every anesthetic and anesthetic adjunct commonly administered to pregnant animals has been identified in fetal tissues of at least one species. Most commonly used drugs cross the placenta by simple diffusion according to the Fick equation, the rate of diffusion being primarily determined by the transplacental concentration gradient.[2] The effective blood concentration of a drug injected into the dam is altered by the rate of uptake into the maternal blood (e.g., rate of injection for intravenously administered drugs), degree of protein binding (unbound drug is available to cross the placenta), maternal drug distribution, rate of maternal biotransformation, and rate of maternal excretion of the drug.[2,33] Similar effects on the fetal side of the placenta may also change the concentration gradient.[2] Besides a high concentration gradient, increasing lipid solubility, decreasing the degree of drug ionization, and decreasing molecular size favor drug passage across the placenta.[33] Placental blood flow may affect drug transfer,[2] but the chorioallantoic placentation of domestic animals does not present any major barrier to penetration of drugs.[52] However, a flaccid uterus may have a high blood flow due to decreased resistance, tending to promote drug transfer. In placental disease with increased membrane thickness, drug passage may be impaired.

Inhalation anesthetics traverse the placenta rapidly because of their high lipid solubilities, relatively low molecular weights, and usually undissociated state in maternal blood.[16,46] Neonatal narcosis is proportional to the depth and duration of maternal anesthesia. Minimum alveolar concentration (MAC) of an inhalation anesthetic is decreased during pregnancy, indicating that anesthetic requirements are decreased in the pregnant patient.[37] Methoxyflurane, halothane, and nitrous oxide are the most commonly used inhalation agents. Nitrous oxide allows lower concentrations of the other two more depressant drugs to be used for maintenance. In human infants, neonatal asphyxia becomes apparent if greater than 75 per cent nitrous oxide is administered to the mother.[7] If less than 60 per cent is used, neonatal hypoxemia is not a problem.[7] Presumably, oxygen should be administered for a few minutes upon delivery to prevent diffusion hypoxia.[10] Halothane crosses the placenta readily and is a significant depressant, but like N$_2$O, it is eliminated rapidly from the newborn if respiration begins spontaneously or is controlled. This occurs because of its relatively low blood gas partition coefficient. However, halothane causes profound uterine relaxation, which may increase postsurgical uterine hemorrhage in some species.[8,11] Based on my clinical observations, this effect appears to be significant in dogs. Although methoxyflurane in low concentrations has been used successfully for obstetrical anesthesia in women and in veterinary patients, it has come into disfavor with many veterinary practitioners because neonatal depression is associated with the level of anesthesia required for cesarean section. Like the adult, the neonate probably takes longer to eliminate anesthetics with high partition coefficients.

Barbiturates rapidly cross the placenta because they are lipid soluble and are partially undissociated. Placental transfer is probably higher in the face of maternal acidemia and hypoproteinemia. With thiobarbiturates, equilibrium of placental transfer occurs within three to four minutes, but in humans, doses of less than 8 mg/kg of thiopental produce very little neonatal depression.[46] A short-acting oxybarbiturate like pentobarbital in an anesthetic dose causes extreme neonatal depression and high mortality[16] and should not be used in obstetrical anesthesia as a primary anesthetic. However, pentobarbital may have some value as a preanesthetic in doses of 4.4 to 6.6 mg/kg given intramuscularly 10 to 20 minutes before induction. Although low doses of thiobarbiturates may be useful for induction, they should not be used for maintenance in obstetrical anesthesia.

Local anesthetics given maternally by almost any route can be detected in fetal blood.[46] It has been suggested that local anesthetics are more toxic on a milligram-to-kilogram basis in the fetus or neonate than in adult animals. Neonatal toxicity usually is manifested by cardiovascular depression. Toxicity is most likely to be due to massive overdosage due to a dosage calculation error, inadvertent intravascular injection, or direct fetal injection due to spinal needle misplacement as reported in humans.[45] Spinal or epidural overdosage can cause fetal problems secondary to maternal hypotension and respiratory embarrassment subsequent to elimination of intercostal muscle activity, diaphragmatic activity in the cervical area, and central respiratory drive as the brain stem is blocked. Anterior migration of local anesthetics may be more pronounced than normal due to distended veins within the spinal canal when the patient is in the supine position. The specific choice of a local anesthetic agent is probably immaterial if it is used correctly, and local anesthetics are less likely to cause neonatal depression than other drugs.

Narcotics cross the placenta and may tend to concentrate in fetal blood because of their lower pH.[46] There is generally some neonatal depression even when moderate to low doses are given to the mother. However, moderate doses usually do not produce serious depression in healthy neonatal puppies.[46] In addition, narcotic antagonists will reverse respiratory depression in the neonate. Certain narcotics (e.g., meperidine) have prolonged elimination half-lives in human neonates, and prolonged effects should be expected in the newborn. Patients given narcotic antagonists should be observed carefully, and repeat doses of the antagonist should be used if narcotic depression returns.[29]

Various tranquilizing drugs cross the placenta.[34] Phenothiazine derivatives can be found in fetal blood within two minutes of maternal intravenous injection,[16,46] but they induce very little respiratory depression. Acetylpromazine and droperidol cause alpha blockage and vasodilation and may decrease the dam's ability to respond to cardiovascular insults. Therefore, there may be significant indirect effects on the fetus, causing fetal depression and hypothermia.[7] Phenothiazine tranquilizers are highly protein bound and theoretically should cross the placenta more in the face of maternal hypoproteinemia.[33] Diazepam readily crosses the placenta, and fetal blood levels may exceed maternal blood levels. Significant neonatal depression and hypothermia have been reported.[2,10,29] Xylazine probably crosses the placenta in proportion to maternal dosage, and, based on unpublished observations, neonates from mothers given xylazine are depressed.

Ketamine, although it has been useful in obstetrical anesthesia in dogs, crosses the placenta in dogs, monkeys, goats, and women.[28] Ketamine may increase uterine tone to the point of decreasing uterine blood flow and potentially contributing to neonatal hypoxemia.[15] However, low doses of ketamine did not produce an "unphysiologic" change in uterine tone or activity in pregnant women at term.[32]

Muscle relaxants have been useful adjuncts in obstetrical anesthesia. As a group, they cross the placenta only minimally because of high ionization, low lipid solubility, and large molecular size.[16,46] Gallamine, succinylcholine, and pancuronium have been used in animals. Gallamine crosses the placenta, even in clinical doses, but detrimental effects to the neonate are not apparent.[16] The other relaxants in clinical doses cross the placenta minimally and produce no paralyzing effect on the neonate.[10] Therefore, they may be safely used to facilitate muscle relaxation for surgery, allowing use of lower concentrations of drugs that are depressant to the newborn.

Anticholinergic agents are used to decrease salivary or bronchial secretions and provide vagal blockade during anesthesia. Atropine readily crosses the placenta, increasing fetal heart rate within six minutes of administration to the mother.[55] Elevation of the fetal heart rate above normal values is generally undesirable during cesarean section.[40] In addition, atropine may produce central nervous system effects that are unwanted in human neonates.[40] Glycopyrrolate is an alternative drug that produces similar cardiac and secretory effects without crossing the placenta or blood-brain barrier in significant amounts.[40] Additionally, it has a longer duration than atropine, may be less dysrhythmogenic, and raises gastric pH.[44]

Physiologic Variations in Pregnant and Newborn Patients

Physiologically, several changes occur during pregnancy. Cardiovascular and respiratory changes are of primary concern. As the gestation period progresses, maternal blood volume increases by about 30 per cent, probably because of hormonal influences and placental shunting.[16] Cardiac output increases by 30 to 50 per cent to compensate for this required blood flow through the placenta.[43] Consequently, normal cardiac reserve is decreased, and the patient has less capacity to respond to cardiovascular insults. Such insults occur during obstetrical anesthesia and surgery. They include drug-induced hypotension and cardiac depression. Positional changes, use of retractors and abdominal packs, surgical blood loss, and exteriorization of the gravid uterus may all require increased cardiac performance to maintain cardiovascular homeostasis. Also, oxytocin may be injected to contract the uterus and reduce hemorrhage. Used intravenously, it decreases mean arterial pressure as much as 45 per cent.[51] Although this hypotension is usually transient, it is a hazard that may be intolerable to the marginal patient. Finally, hematocrit in dogs and cats tends to fall by about 20 to 30 per cent toward the termination of pregnancy.[39] This lower red cell concentration should be considered in clinical management of the dam if blood loss is extensive during surgery.

Respiratory system function changes during pregnancy owing to hormonal influences and increased abdominal volume.[43] Many patients, during labor, are panting or are tachypneic. In women with uncomplicated pregnancy, minute volume is increased, and respiratory alkalosis with Pa_{CO_2} as low as 20 torr and pH as high as 7.6 are often present.[16] With expanding abdominal volume, functional residual volume (FRC) decreases progressively because of cranial displacement of the diaphragm.[16,43] Because of decreased FRC, hypoventilation, such as that associated with anesthesia, produces hypoxia and hypercarbia in the gravida more rapidly than in the nonpregnant woman.[43] The decrease in FRC (less volume for dilution of anesthetic gases), the increase in alveolar ventilation (faster alveolar rate of rise of inhalation anesthetic), and lower MAC values during pregnancy may be causes of faster inhalation inductions during pregnancy. Although the above information comes from data collected from women and ewes, similar effects can be presumed in small animal patients.

The physiology of the newborn also varies from that of normal adults. The capacity for drug metabolism is considerably less in the early neonatal period than in later stages of development.[33] Even with a drug that can be effectively metabolized and excreted by the newborn, the drug's half-life may be prolonged due to a greater volume of distribution and greater tissue uptake than occurs in the adult.[14] Therefore, anesthetics and related drugs should be used to encourage minimal transfer to the fetus.

The fetal cardiovascular system functions differently, and these changes persist for a while after birth. Anatomical variations exist because of gas exchange at the placenta. In addition, fetal and neonatal heart rates are greater than those in the adult. A newborn puppy has a heart rate greater than 120, and development of bradycardia leads to decreased cardiac output, acidosis, and depression. In human infants, heart rates of less than 100 are frequently associated with asphyxia and low cardiac output.[17] Bradycardia can be induced by drugs, maternal hypoxemia, and maternal hypotension.

Oxygen-carrying capacity and oxygen exchange vary in the fetus and the newborn.[9] They usually have higher levels of hemoglobin than an adult (e.g., 23 g/dl versus 13.4 g/dl in humans). Also, this hemoglobin has greater affinity for oxygen and is more saturated at any given oxygen tension. The loading tendency assures oxygenation of fetal hemoglobin at the placenta. However, plasma pH of the fetus tends to be lower than adult plasma pH, promoting release of oxygen to fetal tissues. Therefore, alkalinizing agents and excessive ventilation are potentially detrimental to oxygen delivery to tissues in the newborn. Administration of oxygen-enriched gases to a newborn patient may help to decrease hypoxemia caused by ventilation-perfusion imbalances and diffusion impairment. Long-term (greater than a few minutes to a few hours) administration of 100 per cent oxygen is contraindicated, but 40 to 50 per cent oxygen can be used safely.[50]

The newborn animal also has immature thermoregulatory mechanisms that make it vulnerable to cold.[35] Neonates have a large body surface area to body mass ratio, a small amount of subcutaneous fat, and usually a wet body, all of which cause heat loss.[35] Drugs that cross the placenta may have central or peripheral effects that impair retention of body heat (e.g., vasodilation caused by alpha-blockers or halothane.

The Obstetrical Patient

Because anesthetic management of obstetrical patients is difficult to evaluate except on an individual basis, there have been few controlled studies evaluating various anesthetic regimens. There have been neonatal mortality studies at some institutions, but even these are difficult to apply because duration of labor, degree of prematurity, and cardiovascular data during surgery are not readily available.

Four basic approaches to anesthesia for cesarean section are discussed, and these can be modified greatly by the drugs and dosages chosen.[21] Each has advantages and disadvantages. The practicing veterinarian may be unable to apply some procedures due to limitations in equipment and personnel. The technique chosen must be one with which the anesthetist is familiar. Before applying a specific anesthetic technique in a critical obstetrical case, the anesthetist should be experienced with the procedure, having practiced the technique in healthy animals.

The first anesthetic regimen, the one with the least potential detrimental effect on the newborn, is regional anesthesia. In the small animal, an epidural anesthetic, given at the lumbosacral junction, is the usual technique because use of a true spinal is more difficult anatomically.[26] For cesarean section, a dose of approximately 1 ml per 3.5 kg of body weight (nonpregnant weight) using 2 per cent lidocaine provides analgesia caudal to the umbilicus.[26,30,42] This dosage should be reduced in obese or aged animals. To prevent rapid anterior migration of the anesthetic, the patient should not be positioned head-down.

Sedation or tranquilization may be necessary to facilitate restraint. The second regimen includes premedication and regional anesthesia. Acetylpromazine, xylazine, narcotics, dissociatives, and neuroleptics are possible choices. Epidural or infiltration anesthesia (line block) plus fentanyl-droperidol or oxymorphone-acetylpromazine as premedication are acceptable techniques for dogs. Ketamine plus an epidural or local infiltration in the cat is also acceptable. The usual fentanyl-droperidol (fentanyl, 0.4 mg/ml, and droperidol, 20 mg/ml) preparation can be used intramuscularly at the rate of 1 ml for every 9 to 12 kg. Lower doses may be used intravenously. Oxymorphone (0.11 to 0.22 mg per kilogram) and acetylpromazine (0.11 to 0.22 mg per kilogram) can be given intramuscularly or intravenously. I use a maximum dose of 4 mg of each drug for large dogs, and the amount of each drug may be reduced in depressed or high-risk patients. Either drug combination should be preceded by atropine or glycopyrrolate to prevent bradycardia. Ketamine can be used in the cat (less than 11 mg per kilogram) intramuscularly to facilitate restraint during epidural analgesia. All of these drugs can be expected to cause some neonatal depression, to slow the recovery of the mother, and possibly to affect the dam's willingness to accept and care for the newborn animals. If infiltration blocks are employed, the total dose of local anesthetic must be considered. Dilution of procaine or lidocaine to 0.5 to 1 per cent is helpful in small patients.

A third regimen, involving primarily inhalation anesthesia for maintenance, is useful for both cats and dogs. The number of preanesthetic, induction, and maintenance drug combinations is almost infinite. I use halothane in oxygen or halothane in nitrous oxide and oxygen for maintenance. Fifty per cent nitrous oxide and the least possible concentration of halothane are employed. Induction is done with halothane (4 per cent) in oxygen (2 l/min) and nitrous oxide (3 l/min) in patients that are amenable to induction through a mask or that can be placed in an induction chamber.[42] During maintenance, the halothane concentration is kept to a minimum, generally less than 1 per cent, until the fetuses are removed from the uterus. Muscle relaxants may be employed—for example, 0.03 to 0.06 mg per kilogram of pancuronium to provide 20 to 40 minutes of paralysis. When relaxants are employed, intermittent positive pressure breathing is absolutely necessary until the patient regains ability to breathe spontaneously with an adequate tidal volume. Methoxyflurane can be used instead of halothane, but neonatal depression is usually significant. Inhalation agents should be administered with appropriate anesthetic systems based on patient size.

The fourth regimen involves "balanced anesthesia," which employs a combination of drugs to produce narcosis, analgesia, and muscle relaxation.[42] Balanced anesthesia is discussed in Chapter 187.

With any of the regimens discussed, regular patient monitoring, adequate ventilation, supplemental oxygen, maintenance of body temperature, control of fluid balance, and attention to acid-base status are needed for maximal anesthetic management and patient care.

Ovaries

Surgery involving the ovaries alone generally does not require special anesthetic techniques. Manipulation of the ovary and its attachment often causes the patient to respond by increasing respiratory and heart rates, and lightly anesthetized patients may have an even more significant reaction (e.g., raising of the head, limb movements, or vigorous abdominal movements). Therefore, depth of anesthesia should be monitored closely during ovarian manipulations. Because release of catecholamines can induce dysrhythmias, especially during halothane anesthesia, the patient should not be excessively responsive. This is likely to be most important in animals with cardiac disease or a predilection toward dysrhythmias.

MALE REPRODUCTIVE SYSTEM

The major variations in anesthetic management for these surgical procedures are associated with complications during surgery or abnormalities in the patient's physical condition prior to anesthesia.

Penis and Prepuce

Penile surgery can be associated with a significant degree of hemorrhage prior to or during surgery. Blood loss may be the most significant complication of surgery, and this has a direct effect on anesthetic management. Because a tourniquet can be used to control hemorrhage in penile amputations, presurgi-

cal blood loss may be of most consequence. Therefore, fluids to correct and maintain vascular volume, erythrocyte numbers, and total protein should be administered as indicated by volume of blood loss, changes in arterial and central venous pressure, and variations in hematocrit and total protein.

Regional (epidural) analgesia has been recommended for replacement of the glans penis into the prepuce of dogs with paraphimosis.[54] However, except for certain high-risk patients, regional techniques offer no obvious advantages over general anesthesia. Regionally administered, long-acting local anesthetics or repeated injections of shorter-acting local anesthetics have been suggested for postoperative pain relief following penile surgery.

Prostate

Prostatic surgery may involve castration and prostatic drainage, marsupialization, biopsy, or resection. The complications associated with prostatic surgery can be related to prolonged anesthesia and surgery time, hypothermia due to tissue exposure and anesthetic effects, and hypovolemia related to fluid loss and possibly septicemia. Gram-negative (most commonly *E. coli*) and gram-positive bacteria have been isolated from diseased canine prostate glands.[6] Circulatory shock has been related to endotoxins and exotoxins from bacteria in the genitourinary tract, especially during surgical manipulations.[25]

1. Abbound, T. K., Read, J., Miller, F., et al.: Use of glycopyrrolate in the parturient: Effect on maternal and fetal heart rate and uterine activity. Obstet. Gynecol. 57:224, 1981.
2. Alper, M. H.: What drugs cross the placenta and what happens to them in the fetus. *In* Hershey, S. G. (ed.): *Refresher Courses in Anesthesiology*. Vol. 4. J. B. Lippincott Co., Philadelphia, 1976.
3. Baraka, A., Saab, M., and Salem, M. R.: Control of gastric acidity by glycopyrrolate premedication in the parturient. Anesth. Analg. 56:642, 1977.
4. Burke, T. J.: Post-parturient problems in the bitch. Vet. Clin. North Am. 7:693, 1977.
5. Burke, T. J., and Reynolds, H. A.: The female genital system. *In* Bojrab, J. J. (ed.): *Pathophysiology in Small Animal Surgery*. Lea & Febiger, Philadelphia, 1981.
6. Christie, T. R.: The prostate. *In* Bojrab, M. J. (ed.): *Pathophysiology in Small Animal Surgery*. Lea & Febiger, Philadelphia, 1981.
7. Cohen, S. N., and Olson, W. A.: Drugs that depress the newborn. Pediatr. Clin. North Am. 17:835, 1970.
8. Cohen, S. E.: Inhalation analgesia and anesthesia for vaginal delivery. *In* Shnider, S. M., and Levinson, G.: *Anesthesia for Obstetrics*. The Williams & Wilkins Co., Baltimore, 1979.
9. Comroe, J. H.: The transport of oxygen by blood. *In: Physiology of Respiration*. Year Book Medical Publishers, Chicago, 1974.
10. Datta, S., and Alper, M. H.: Anesthesia for cesarean section. Anesthesiology 53:142, 1980.
11. DeVore, J. S.: Effects of anesthesia on uterine activity and labor. *In* Shnider, S. M., and Levinson, G.: *Anesthesia for Obstetrics*. The Williams & Wilkins Co., Baltimore, 1979.
12. Eger, E. I., II: Atropine, scopolamine and related compounds. Anesthesiology 23:365, 1962.

13. Evans, T.: Anesthesia for the geriatric patient. Vet. Clin. North Am. *11*:653, 1981.

14. Finster, M., and Pederson, H.: Perinatal pharmacology. *In* Hershey, S. G. (ed.): *Refresher Courses in Anesthesiology*. Vol. 6. J. B. Lippincott Co., Philadelphia, 1978.

15. Galloon, S.: Ketamine for obstetric delivery. Anesthesiology *44*:522, 1976.

16. Goodger, W. J., and Levy, W.: Anesthetic management of the cesarean section. Vet. Clin. North Am. *3*:85, 1973.

17. Gregory, G. A.: Resuscitation of the newborn: Anesthesiology *43*:225, 1975.

18. Hall, M. A., and Swenberg, L. N.: Genital emergencies. *In* Kirk, R. W. (ed.): *Current Veterinary Therapy VI*. W. B. Saunders Co., Philadelphia, 1977.

19. Hardy, R. M., and Osborne, C. A.: Canine pyometra; pathophysiology, diagnosis and treatment of uterine and extrauterine lesions. J. Am. Anim. Hosp. Assoc. *10*:245, 1974.

20. Hartsfield, S. M.: Body temperature variations associated with general anesthesia: A review. Part I: Hypothermia. Southwest. Vet. *32*:95, 1979.

21. Hartsfield, S. M.: Obstetrical anesthesia in small animals. Calif. Vet. *33*:18, 1979.

22. Harvey, H. J., and Gilbertson, S. R.: Canine mammary gland tumors. Vet. Clin. North Am. 7:213, 1977.

23. Harvey, S. C.: Hypnotics and sedatives. *In* Gilman, A. G., Goodman, L. S., and Gilman, A. (eds.): *The Pharmacological Basis of Therapeutics*. 6th ed. Macmillan Publishing Co., New York, 1980, p. 356.

24. Hayes, A.: Feline mammary gland tumors. Vet. Clin. North Am. 7:205, 1977.

25. Jennings, P. B., Jr., Whitten, N. J., and Sleeman, H. K.: The diagnosis and treatment of shock in the critical care patient. *In* Sattler, F. B., Knowles, R. P., and Whittick, W. G. (eds.): *Veterinary Critical Care*. Lea & Febiger, Philadelphia, 1981.

26. Klide, A. M.: Epidural analgesia. *In* Soma, L. R. (ed.): *Textbook of Veterinary Anesthesia*. The Williams & Wilkins Co., Baltimore, 1971.

27. Knight, A. P.: Xylazine. J. Am. Vet. Med. Assoc. *176*:454, 1980.

28. Kumar, A., Thurman, J. C., Nelson, D. R., et al.: Effects of ketamine hydrochloride or maternal and fetal arterial blood pressure and acid-base status in goats. Vet. Anes. 5:28, 1978.

29. Levinson, G., and Shnider, S. M.: Systemic medication for labor and delivery. *In* Shnider, S. M., and Levinson, G.: *Anesthesia for Obstetrics*. The Williams & Wilkins Co., Baltimore, 1979.

30. Lumb, W. V., and Jones, E. W.: *Veterinary Anesthesia*. Lea & Febiger, Philadelphia, 1973.

31. Marshall, B. E., and Wollman, H.: General anesthetics. *In* Gilman, A. G., Goodman, L. S., and Gilman, A. (eds.): *The Pharmacological Basis of Therapeutics*. 6th ed. Macmillan Publishing Co., Inc., New York, 1980, pp. 281, 287.

32. Marx, G. F., Hwang, H. S., and Chandra, P.: Postpartum uterine pressures with different doses of ketamine. Anesthesiology *50*:163, 1979.

33. Mirkin, B. L.: Perinatal pharmacology: Placental transfer fetal localization and neonatal disposition of drugs. Anesthesiology *43*:156, 1975.

34. Moir, D. D.: *Obstetric Anaesthesia and Analgesia*. The Williams & Wilkins Co., Baltimore, 1976.

35. Moiser, J. E.: The puppy from birth to six weeks. Vet. Clin. North Am. 8:79, 1978.

36. Muir, W. W.: Drugs used to produce standing chemical restraint in horses. Vet. Clin. North Am. Large Anim. Pract. *3*:17, 1981.

37. Palahniuk, R. J., Shnider, S. M., and Eger, II, E. I.: Pregnancy decreases the requirements for inhaled anesthetics. Anesthesiology *41*:82, 1974.

38. Pedersen, H., and Finster, M.: Anesthetic risk in the pregnant surgical patient. Anesthesiology *51*:439, 1979.

39. Perman, V., and Schall, V. D.: Diseases of the red blood cells. *In* Ettinger, S. J.: *Textbook of Veterinary Internal Medicine*. W. B. Saunders Co., Philadelphia, 1983.

40. Proakis, A. G., and Harris, G. B.: Comparative penetration of glycopyrrolate and atropine across the blood-brain and placental barriers in anesthetized dogs. Anesthesiology *48*:339, 1978.

41. Ralston, D. H., Shnider, S. M., and deLorimier, A. A.: Effects of equipotent ephedrine, metaraminol, mephentermine and methoxamine on uterine blood flow in the pregnant ewe. Anesthesiology *40*:354, 1974.

42. Sawyer, D. C.: *The Practice of Small Animal Anesthesia*. W. B. Saunders Co., Philadelphia, 1982, pp. 29–35, 108–109, 114–117, 198–199.

43. Shnider, S. M.: The physiology of pregnancy. Am. Soc. Anesthesiol. Annual Refresher Course Lectures *125*:1, 1978.

44. Short, C. E., Paddleford, R. R., and Cloyd, G. D.: Glycopyrrolate for prevention of pulmonary complications during anesthesia. Mod. Vet. Prac. 55:194, 1974.

45. Smith, B. E.: Maternal and fetal hazards in obstetric anesthesia. *In* Hershey, S. G. (ed.): *Refresher Course in Anesthesiology*. Vol. 2. J. B. Lippincott Co., Philadelphia, 1974.

46. Soma, L. R.: Anesthetic management. *In* Soma, L. R. (ed.): *Textbook of Veterinary Anesthesia*. The Williams & Wilkins Co., Baltimore, 1971.

47. Stewardson, R. H., and Nyhus, L. M.: Pulmonary aspiration. Arch. Surg. *112*:1192, 1977.

48. Stoelting, R. K.: Responses to atropine, glycopyrrolate, riopan of gastric fluid pH and volume in adult patients. Anesthesiology *48*:367, 1978.

49. Stowe, C. M.: Parasympatholytic drugs. *In* Jones, L. M. (ed.): *Veterinary Pharmacology and Therapeutics*. 3rd ed. Iowa State University Press, Ames, Iowa, 1965.

50. Thurmon, J. C.: Oxygen therapy—a review. *In* Proceedings of the Illinois Veterinary Respiratory Symposium, Champaign, Illinois, 1978, pp. 188–202.

51. Weis, F. R., and Peak, J.: Effects of oxytocin on blood pressure during anesthesia. Anesthesiology *40*:189, 1974.

52. Welsch, F.: Placental transfer and fetal uptake of drugs. J. Vet. Pharmacol. Therap. 5:91, 1982.

53. Wharton, R. S., Mazze, R. I., and Wilson, A. I.: Reproduction and fetal development in mice chronically exposed to enflurane. Anesthesiology *54*:505, 1981.

54. Wilson, G. P.: Surgery of the male reproductive tract. Vet. Clin. North Am. 5:537, 1975.

55. Wylie, W. D., and Churchill-Davidson, H. C.: *A Practice of Anaesthesia*. Year Book Medical Publishers, Chicago, 1972.

193 Anesthesia and the Liver

Cynthia M. Trim

Disorders of liver function result in changes in glucose homeostasis, interference with protein synthesis and coagulation, and delayed metabolism of drugs. Anesthesia and surgery can further influence liver function. The object of this discussion is first, to describe the effects of anesthesia and surgery on the function of a normal liver, and second, to enumerate the abnormalities that might be present in an animal with liver disease and suggest appropriate anesthetic management to minimize complications.

EFFECT OF ANESTHESIA AND SURGERY ON LIVER FUNCTION

The hepatic artery supplies the liver with 25 to 35 per cent of its total blood flow and most of its oxygen.[57] The major blood supply is from the portal vein, which drains the stomach, intestines, spleen, and pancreas. The portal vein provides at least one-third of the total hepatic oxygen uptake.

Regulation of Hepatic Blood Flow

Autoregulation has been described in the hepatic circulation of the dog.[36] In the heart, autoregulation maintains constant blood flow despite changes in pressure. In contrast, an increase in pressure in the portal or hepatic vein or hepatic artery initiates vasoconstriction in the hepatic arterioles. This regulation of resistance may be mainly the result of local myogenic activity.[36] However, when portal venous blood flow is decreased, hepatic arterial resistance is decreased, providing some compensation for reduced flow.

The hepatic vessels are also influenced by the sympathetic nervous system. Stimulation of the sympathetic nerves to the liver causes vasoconstriction in the hepatic arterioles and portal venous system.[57] Despite continuous stimulation, vasoconstriction in the hepatic arterioles gradually disappears during a period of minutes, whereas venous constriction persists.[57] Vasoconstriction in the hepatic artery decreases blood flow and the amount of oxygen available for hepatic metabolism. A reduction in hepatic arterial blood flow alone may not be sufficient to cause hepatitis. Hepatic arteries have been ligated without adversely affecting liver function.[54] However, hepatic hypoxia may be an important prerequisite of hepatic injury,[9] and anaerobic conditions may significantly alter anesthetic drug metabolism.

The effect of hypercapnia (increasing the Pa_{CO_2} from 38 to 56 torr) was investigated in humans under thiopental-succinylcholine-nitrous oxide anesthesia using sulfobromophthalein (BSP) clearance.[27] The hepatic blood flow (HBF) and splanchnic vascular resistance did not change significantly with the onset of anesthesia, but HBF decreased 15 per cent with the increase in Pa_{CO_2} in 9 of 13 subjects. Increased heart rate and mean arterial pressure and flushing of the face of human subjects were also observed, indicating both a vasoconstrictor and a vasodilator response. It was suggested that the splanchic vasoconstriction was mediated through the sympathetic nervous system. Increased carbon dioxide in the blood perfusing splanchnic blood vessels causes only vasoconstriction if the splanchnic nerve supply is intact. Increasing the inspired carbon dioxide to 5 per cent in humans anesthetized with halothane resulted in splanchnic vasodilation and a significant increase in HBF.[28] This difference in results may have been due to the addition of halothane. Anesthesia of dogs with halothane at an end-tidal concentration above 0.8 per cent depressed the carotid sinus baroreceptor reflex to hypotension.[7]

Effect of Anesthetic Drugs on Hepatic Blood Flow

Anesthetic drugs influence HBF by decreasing the cardiac output and arterial blood pressure and by affecting the sympathetic nervous system. A decrease in HBF proportional to the decrease in cardiac output and arterial blood pressure has been documented in dogs anesthetized with halothane[73] and with halothane or enflurane.[41] In each study, dogs were anesthetized with a barbiturate for placement of electromagnetic flowmeters before the inhalation anesthetic was tested. In one experiment, the halothane and enflurane concentrations in arterial blood were confirmed using gas-liquid chromatography.[41] This allowed for some comparison between agents (Fig. 193–1). Whereas decreases in hepatic blood flow were similar with halothane and enflurane, 3 per cent enflurane significantly decreased hepatic arterial resistance. Other studies of pentobarbital-halothane anesthesia in dogs have also demonstrated decreases in hepatic blood flow or splanchnic blood flow that are proportional to decreases in cardiac output.[2,10]

The addition of nitrous oxide decreases the requirement for halothane in the dog, producing less cardiovascular depression at equipotent doses.[22,70] Considerable individual variation has been reported. Consequently, less depression of HBF can be expected in some dogs when nitrous oxide is used with halothane. Experiments in swine have demonstrated

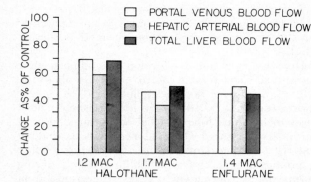

Figure 193–1. Halothane and enflurane decreased hepatic blood flow in pentobarbital-anesthetized greyhounds. MAC, minimum alveolar concentration. (Modified with permission from Hughes, Campbell, D., and Fitch, W.: Effects of enflurane and halothane on liver blood flow and oxygen consumption in the greyhound. Br. J. Anaesth. 52:1079, 1980.)

that the decrease in blood flow to the stomach and intestines was less with halothane and nitrous oxide than with halothane alone.[74]

Results from a study comparing isoflurane with halothane suggested that isoflurane produced a smaller decrease in cardiac output and similar decreases in arterial blood pressure and oxygen consumption at equivalent anesthetic concentrations.[72] Blood flow through the splanchnic region was better maintained with isoflurane than with halothane. In swine, isoflurane anesthesia decreased blood flow to the gastrointestinal tract by about 25 per cent compared with the awake value, but no change was produced in the hepatic arterial blood flow.[52]

Methoxyflurane has been studied in human volunteers. Splanchnic blood flow decreased 46 per cent from awake values.[51] No difference was noted between light and deep anesthesia, or between spontaneous and controlled ventilation. Although some response was undoubtedly due to the decreased arterial pressure, angiography demonstrated specific vasoconstriction of the hepatic artery. Estimations of hepatic blood volume indicated that venoconstriction also occurred. The decrease in splanchnic blood flow was not accompanied by an equal reduction in oxygen consumption. Despite the discrepancy between blood flow and oxygen consumption, no biochemical evidence of splanchnic hypoxia was found from the results of venous lactate and pyruvate determinations.

Narcotic analgesics are used in seriously ill patients because they generally cause less cardiovascular depression than other types of anesthetic. They are also reversible with naloxone. The effect of some narcotics on splanchnic blood flow in the dog has been studied utilizing an electromagnetic flow probe around the cranial mesenteric artery.[61] Morphine (1 mg/kg diluted to 10 ml with saline) infused over five minutes in awake dogs increased heart rate, cardiac output, and mean arterial pressure within the first 2.5 minutes. These changes soon returned to control values. Cranial mesenteric blood flow increased 26 to 55 per cent from control, and mesenteric vascular resistance decreased 22 to 30 per cent. A higher dose of morphine, 3 mg/kg, transiently increased heart rate and cardiac output in the same study. Mean aortic blood pressure did not change significantly. This dose of morphine decreased mesenteric arterial flow by 29 to 44 per cent for most of the 30-minute observation period. Mesenteric vascular resistance was increased throughout. A constricting effect in the splanchnic circulation of high-dose morphine has also been documented in anesthetized dogs.[34] Morphine increases circulating catecholamine levels by stimulating the adrenal medulla,[31,47] and this stimulation may be responsible for the vasoconstriction.

In a similar study, 2 to 6 mg/kg of meperidine was infused over five minutes in awake dogs.[62] The lower dose of meperidine did not significantly alter cranial mesenteric arterial blood flow or resistance. The higher dose initially increased heart rate by 62 per cent and reduced mean aortic blood pressure and peripheral vascular resistance by 28 and 24 per cent, respectively. Cardiac output progressively decreased to 18 per cent at 30 minutes. These systemic effects were accompanied by a severe decrease in mesenteric blood flow and by increased vascular resistance. The cranial mesenteric artery supplies only a proportion of the portal vein blood flow. However, the information indicated that high doses of morphine or meperidine produce adverse effects that may be significant in dogs with compromised liver function.

Reports of the effects of other commonly used narcotics on HBF are not available. Innovar-Vet* (fentanyl and droperidol), 1 ml/12 kg, with atropine had a minimal effect on cardiac output in healthy dogs.[17,48] Another investigation demonstrated that fentanyl, 0.01 or 0.02 mg/kg, or droperidol, 0.5 mg/kg (equivalent to Innovar-Vet 1 ml/20 kg) did not affect left ventricular performance.[59] Nalbuphine† did not change mean arterial pressure, heart rate, or cardiac output in halothane-anesthetized dogs.[66] In contrast, butorphanol,‡ 0.1 and 0.4 mg/kg, produced small but significant decreases in heart rate and mean arterial pressure in awake dogs.[76] Butorphanol, 0.5 mg/kg, infused over five minutes in dogs anesthetized with thiopental, resulted in a 37 per cent decrease in cardiac output.[68] Butorphanol may, therefore, decrease HBF.

Effect of Surgery on Hepatic Blood Flow

HBF is decreased by anesthesia and is further reduced by surgery. Furthermore, the severity of this effect has been demonstrated in humans to be proportional to the proximity of the surgery to the liver.[32] In a clinical study of liver function tests 1

*Pitman-Moore, Inc., Washington Crossing, NJ.
†Nubain, Du Pont Pharmaceuticals, Garden City, NY.
‡Stadol, Torbutrol, Bristol Laboratories, Syracuse, NY.

nour and 24 hours postoperatively, evidence of malfunction was consistently evident at 1 hour in cholecystectomy patients, whereas minimal changes occurred in patients undergoing non–liver-related procedures.[46,77] These patients were healthy and changes were transient, because all variables had returned to normal or near normal values within 24 hours postoperatively. In addition, no significantly different changes were observed between patients receiving different anesthetic techniques, which included narcotics and nitrous oxide, halothane, halothane and nitrous oxide, enflurane, and methoxyflurane.

Effects of Anesthetics on the Biliary System

Abnormalities demonstrated by cholangiography during neuroleptanalgesic sedation in humans led to a study of the effect of anesthetic drugs on the biliary tract. The guinea pig was chosen because of its well-developed bile duct sphincter. Morphine, meperidine, and fentanyl produced significant increases in intrabiliary pressure.[3] Pentazocine produced a slight effect on the sphincter. This increase was reversed by the administration of atropine. Neither halothane nor enflurane produced changes in intrabiliary pressure from control levels.[3]

Postoperative Liver Function

The effect of ketamine anesthesia on serum enzymes has been studied in humans.[23] Serum alkaline phosphatase (SAP), serum aspartate aminotransferase (SAA), and gamma-glutamyl transferase (GGT) were measured on the third to fourth and on the thirteenth to fifteenth days after a minor surgical procedure. Lorazepam and ketamine, with or without nitrous oxide, were compared with thiopental combined with narcotics or halothane. On the third to fourth postoperative days, a significantly greater number of patients who had received ketamine had an enzymatic disturbance that suggested liver disease. Several possible reasons for these changes were proposed, including a hepatotoxic effect, enzyme induction, changes in liver metabolism, or altered HBF.

Serum enzyme levels following methoxyflurane anesthesia have been measured in dogs.[60] The blood urea nitrogen (BUN), SAP, and SAA were measured before anesthesia and one and three days after anesthesia. A BSP clearance test was performed at one and three days after anesthesia, and a phenosulfonphthalein (PSP) clearance test was run at two and five days after anesthesia. The SAP increased significantly after anesthesia, from a baseline of 10.9 King-Armstrong units to 48.5 units at one day and 52.7 units at three days. The other measurements were unchanged, except for one dog who had a 5 per cent BSP retention on the first day after anesthesia. The elevation in SAP may be an indication for cautious use of methoxyflurane in animals with hepatic disease. Hepatic failure has occurred in an apparently healthy dog three days following methoxyflurane anesthesia.[33]

Hepatitis occasionally develops in humans after anesthesia. Considerable controversy exists about the role of halothane in the etiology.[16,26,81] A recent review reported that there are no published clinical cases of hepatitis following halothane anesthesia in veterinary patients.[8] The evidence suggests that, in contrast to organ damage from methoxyflurane that is produced by a toxic metabolite released during normal biotransformation, damage is caused by an increased accumulation of halothane metabolites. The increased level of halothane metabolites occurs when metabolism changes from an oxidative to a reductive pathway. This change may be caused by excessive amounts of halothane to be metabolized or by a decreased hepatic oxygen supply from reduced HBF or hypoxemia. Some patients may have a genetic predilection for the reductive metabolic pathway. The authors concluded that a history of pre-existing liver disease is not necessarily a contraindication to the use of halothane.

Enzyme Induction

Metabolites of inhalation anesthetics, fluoride, bromide, and organic acids, have been implicated in the pathogenesis of organ toxicity.[50] Stimulation of hepatic microsomal activity (enzyme induction) may increase the levels of metabolites and therefore the incidence of hepatic malfunction after anesthesia. Repeated anesthesia with halothane in mink has been associated with abnormal histopathologic changes in the liver and kidney.[35] Methoxyflurane stimulates hepatic enzyme activity in such a way that metabolism is enhanced in subsequent exposures.[15] Hepatic failure has been reported in a dog following multiple prolonged anesthesias with methoxyflurane.[58]

Enzyme induction with phenobarbital has been blamed for hepatic failure in a dog after methoxyflurane anesthesia for ovariohysterectomy[75] and in a human after fluroxene anesthesia for gastrectomy.[64] Rats pretreated with phenobarbital died of massive hepatic necrosis when exposed to fluroxene anesthesia.[39] In a detailed study of postanesthetic hepatic injury in rats, the influences of enzyme induction, HBF alterations, surgery, and anesthesia time were studied.[38] Rats pretreated with phenobarbital and anesthetized with 1 per cent halothane for two hours received surgery to reduce HBF by hepatic artery ligation. These animals demonstrated the greatest degree of microscopic hepatic injury (3.83 on a scale of 0 to 5, in which 5 was equivalent to confluent centrilobular necrosis). Rats that were anesthetized with thiamylal, enflurane, or isoflurane for the same time period and underwent the same procedures had little damage based on a score of less than 0.71.[38] Hepatic injury was less in halothane-anesthetized rats in which the hepatic artery was not ligated, and less when a peripheral incision was substituted for the laparotomy. Hepatic damage was markedly increased when the anesthesia time was increased from two to four hours. Rats that had not received phenobarbital showed no evidence of liver damage following halothane anesthesia or surgery or from reduced HBF.

Multiple administrations of ketamine result in an increase in activity of hepatic drug-metabolizing enzymes, and in this respect ketamine resembles phenobarbital.[53]

ANESTHESIA IN THE PATIENT WITH LIVER DISEASE

Pre-existing hepatic malfunction increases the risk of operative problems and postoperative liver failure. Measurement of hepatic enzymes may detect liver disease.[19] Alanine transaminase (serum glutamic-pyruvic transaminase, SGPT) and sorbitol dehydrogenase (SDH) are essentially liver-specific. In a survey of dogs with metastatic liver disease, SGPT and SAP were elevated in 70 per cent.[55] Ideally, determinations should be made in all patients requiring anesthesia. However, for financial reasons, it is general practice to screen animals five years or older, all sick animals, and all animals requiring major surgery. Certain other dogs should be included. For example, cirrhosis has been ascribed to long-term anticonvulsant drug therapy in dogs.[18] Variable increases in SGPT and SAP have been demonstrated in dogs receiving the anticonvulsant drugs diphenylhydantoin and primidone.[56] Therefore, additional tests of liver function, such as BSP retention, are advisable before a dog receiving anticonvulsants is submitted to general anesthesia.

Drug Binding

Most drugs are bound to some extent with plasma albumin. Decreased production of albumin in patients with liver disease results in a larger unbound fraction and therefore increased activity of the active component. This is of clinical significance when thiopental, thiamylal, or ketamine is used for induction of anesthesia.

Drug Biotransformation

The initial decrease in plasma concentration of thiopental or thiamylal is usually attributed to redistribution of the drug into tissues, primarily skeletal muscle.[67] Analysis of the disposition curve of thiopental in dogs indicated that factors that influence the distribution and redistribution of the drug affect the duration of anesthesia.[13] However, other studies demonstrated that metabolism of thiopental contributed to awakening from anesthesia.[65] Return to nor-

mal is achieved by storage of the drug in fat deposits and subsequent metabolism in the liver. Therefore, animals with little body fat experience a prolonged period of sedation and ataxia after barbiturate anesthesia.[11] For these reasons, a patient with liver disease who is anesthetized with a thiobarbiturate will probably be slow to wake and have a prolonged recovery. Similarly, return to consciousness from ketamine anesthesia is due to redistribution of the drug from the brain to other tissues. An average of 62 per cent of ketamine is biotransformed in the dog, mainly by the liver.[45] Therefore, severe liver malfunction may prolong the duration of activity of ketamine. In humans only a small amount of free ketamine appears in the urine. However, a study in people with evidence of preanesthetic liver insufficiency showed no difference in the rate of metabolism of ketamine when compared with healthy people.[42] Maintenance of anesthesia by halothane slows distribution and redistribution of ketamine and inhibits its hepatic metabolism,[80] thereby prolonging its CNS effects. In cats a large portion of ketamine is excreted unchanged by the kidney, whereas a smaller portion is metabolized,[82] and thus ketamine anesthesia is less likely to be prolonged by liver disease.

In the liver, the inhalation anesthetics are metabolized to varying degrees. Nitrous oxide and isoflurane are essentially not metabolized, and enflurane is metabolized only in small amounts (2.4 per cent).[50] Up to 20 per cent of the inhaled dose of halothane is metabolized, but this is unlikely to cause a prolonged recovery in patients with liver disease. However, as much as 50 per cent of methoxyflurane is metabolized by the liver,[50] and concurrent liver disease results in a poor recovery from anesthesia.

Narcotic analgesics are metabolized by the liver, and prolonged sedation is common in dogs with reduced hepatic function. A large dose may have an unexpectedly long effect in some animals, probably due to severe hemodynamic changes and decreased HBF. In experimentally hepatectomized dogs, prolonged elimination of morphine and fentanyl was documented.[40] The morphine was eventually eliminated by renal excretion of the unchanged drug. The fentanyl was slowly excreted as metabolites and no unchanged fentanyl was detected in the urine. The sites of extrahepatic biotransformation of fentanyl are still to be determined. Reversibility of the action of narcotics with the antagonist naloxone is especially useful with liver disease.

Neuromuscular blocking agents are eliminated from the body in different ways. Succinylcholine is destroyed by plasmacholinesterase produced by the liver. Liver disease is associated with decreased levels of plasmacholinesterase and prolonged activity of succinylcholine.[24] Gallamine is primarily excreted unchanged in the urine; 84 per cent of the drug has been recovered in the urine of dogs within 24 hours.[30] No prolonged duration of action of gallamine was observed in human patients with extrahepatic biliary obstruction.[63] Pancuronium, in contrast, is partly metabolized by the liver, partly eliminated in the bile, and partly excreted unchanged in the urine.[1] Prolonged neuromuscular blockade with pancuronium has been documented in human patients with extrahepatic biliary obstruction,[69] cirrhosis,[25] and fulminant liver failure.[79]

Coagulopathy

The liver is the major site for synthesis of plasma coagulation factors. Considerable liver disease must be present before abnormalities of coagulation occur, and the incidence of clotting disorders is low in clinical practice.[5] Nonetheless, it is important to determine adequacy of clotting before surgery. Coagulopathies associated with hepatic disease in animals have been recently reviewed.[6]

Plasma Glucose

Decreased glucose production in patients with cirrhosis may result in hypoglycemia during general anesthesia. This can be prevented by an infusion of 5 per cent dextrose. An investigation in humans anesthetized for laparotomy and cholecystectomy demonstrated that 5 per cent dextrose infusion at a rate of 6 ml/kg per minute produced a strong hyperglycemic effect.[78] Thiopental-halothane-nitrous oxide anesthesia produced a 40 per cent increase in blood glucose in patients receiving 0.9 per cent sodium chloride solution or Hartmann's solution. In contrast, a 5 per cent dextrose solution produced a 160 per cent increase in blood glucose.

Renal Failure

An increased incidence of renal failure has been described in human patients with jaundice after general anesthesia.[21,83] Similar information for animals is not available, but as a precaution, an intravenous infusion of balanced electrolytes should be started before induction of anesthesia and continued throughout surgery to maintain adequate urine production.

GENERAL CONSIDERATIONS

A list of potential problems associated with liver disease is given in Table 193–1. Management of anesthesia must include methods to circumvent these problems.

The patient must be brought to optimal physiologic status before anesthesia. Antibiotics (cephalosporins, ampicillin) should be administered before anesthesia to diminish intestinal flora and endotoxin production. Parenteral vitamin K may restore prothrombin production.[71]

TABLE 193–1.   Anesthesia of the Dog with Liver Disease

Potential Problems	Management
Decreased hepatic blood flow	Avoid deep anesthesia, maintain blood volume, controlled ventilation.
Drug toxicity	Evaluate liver function with concurrent anticonvulsant therapy.
Prolonged recovery from anesthesia	Use thiobarbiturates cautiously, reverse narcotics; do not use methoxyflurane or succinylcholine; use only low doses of pancuronium.
Hemorrhage	Pretreat with vitamin K, fresh blood transfusion.
Hypoglycemia	Give 5% dextrose.
Renal failure	Infuse fluid to maintain urine output.
Endotoxemia	Pretreat with antibiotics.

Fresh plasma or whole blood infusion is advisable before surgery if clotting time is abnormal. A large-bore, indwelling venous catheter should be installed as a precaution should the need arise for rapid fluid infusion, even when local analgesic techniques are used instead of general anesthesia.

My preference is to use an anticholinergic drug for premedication (atropine, 0.04 mg/kg intramuscularly, or glycopyrrolate,* 0.01 mg/kg intramuscularly). These are not used in the dog with moderate to severe cardiac disease. Drugs that are substantially metabolized by the liver (e.g., thiobarbiturates, ketamine, and methoxyflurane) should be avoided in patients with moderate to severe liver disease. The exception is the narcotic analgesic, because its action can be reversed with naloxone,† 0.01 to 0.02 mg/kg intravenously. Innovar-Vet, up to 1 ml/25 kg, or oxymorphone,‡ up to 0.2 mg/kg, can be injected intravenously over several minutes to achieve sufficient analgesia and depression for endotracheal intubation. A very small dose of acetylpromazine§ (0.03 mg/kg) or diazepam‖ (0.2 to 0.4 mg/kg) may be used with oxymorphone, if necessary. Nalbuphine may be a suitable alternative to Innovar-Vet or oxymorphone. Anesthesia can be maintained with nitrous oxide with halothane, enflurane, or isoflurane. Incorporating a neuromuscular blocking agent such as gallamine (balanced anesthesia) may provide the best conditions for a severely compromised patient who requires major surgery by reducing the need for narcotic or inhalation anesthesia.[37]

---

*Robinul-V, A. H. Robins Company, Inc., Richmond, VA.
†Narcan, Du Pont Pharmaceuticals, Garden City, NY; Naloxone-V, Pitman-Moore, Inc., Washington Crossing, NJ.
‡Numorphan, Du Pont Pharmaceuticals, Garden City, NY.
§Acepromazine, Fort Dodge Laboratories, Fort Dodge, IA.
‖Valium, Roche Laboratories, Nutley, NJ.

Dextrose 5 per cent in water is infused at 5 ml/kg per hour to prevent hypoglycemia. In addition, lactated Ringer's solution (LRS) or other balanced electrolyte solution is given at 5 ml/kg per hour to provide maintenance requirements. Blood loss can be replaced by the addition of LRS at 2.5 times the blood volume lost. Patients with pre-existing low plasma albumin levels will develop severe hypoalbuminemia with this rate of crystalloid infusion. It may be necessary to provide part of the intraoperative fluid requirement as plasma or dextran infusion. The arterial blood pressure and capillary refill time should be monitored to assess tissue perfusion. In the anesthetized dog with severe liver disease it is wise to monitor urine output, and preferably include catheterization of the urinary bladder. Controlled ventilation can be used to ensure normal levels of carbon dioxide. Monitoring should continue into the postoperative period.

LAPAROSCOPY

A liver biopsy can be obtained in dogs without general anesthesia when a laparoscope is used. The laparoscope is inserted through a small incision in the flank.[44] Lidocaine, 2 per cent, is infiltrated in the skin and muscles either at the site of incision or about 2 cm dorsal and cranial to the site (inverted L block). Some sedation and analgesia of the patient may be needed because the abdomen must be distended with nitrous oxide or carbon dioxide to allow a view of the liver. Oxymorphone, 0.2 mg/kg given intravenously, with or without acetylpromazine, has been found useful by the author. The distension of the abdomen impairs ventilation, and oxygen must be supplied by face mask to prevent hypoxemia. Increased intra-abdominal pressure (20 to 40 mm Hg) with either carbon dioxide or nitrous oxide decreases the cardiac output by more than 40 per cent.[43] The results support the view that abdominal pressures of more than 20 mm Hg are potentially dangerous. The blood pressure, heart rate, and capillary refill time must be monitored continuously during laparoscopy to detect unacceptable depression or sudden deterioration. Alternatively, general anesthesia by conventional means may be used in appropriately healthy patients.

PORTOCAVAL SHUNT

Techniques for surgical correction of congenital portocaval shunts in dogs and cats have been reported (Chapter 79).[14,19] Anesthetic management is influenced by the physical status of the patient, and the degree of hepatic impairment depends on the type of anomaly.[20,29] Weight loss decreases the volume of tissue available for anesthetic drug redistribution. Hypoalbuminemia increases the active component of protein-bound drugs. Blood bypassing the liver limits

the amount of anesthetic drug presented to the liver for biotransformation. Hepatic insufficiency results in decreased production of bile salts. In experimental animals, the absence of bile salts in the intestinal tract allows absorption of endotoxin from the intestine.[4] In addition, portal vein hypertension and decreased intestinal blood flow may occur after surgical ligation of the portocaval anastomosis.[20,29] Intestinal ischemia further compromises the intestinal barrier to endotoxin. Flunixin meglumine, 1.1 mg/kg intravenously, improved cardiac output and arterial blood pressure in dogs during experimental endotoxemia.[12] This drug could be used if endotoxemia was suspected in a patient with a portocaval shunt. Systemic arterial blood pressure should be monitored at the time of ligation in case hypotension occurs from decreased venous return to the heart.

1. Agoston, S., Kersten, U. W., and Meijer, D. K. F.: The fate of pancuronium bromide in the cat. Acta Anaesth. Scand. 17:129, 1973.
2. Ahlgren, I., Aronsen, K. F., Ericsson, B., and Fajgelj, A.: Hepatic blood flow during different depths of halothane anaesthesia in the dog. Acta Anaesth. Scand. 11:91, 1967.
3. Arguelles, J. E., Franatovic, Y., Romo-Salas, F., and Aldrete, J. A.: Intrabiliary pressure changes produced by narcotic drugs and inhalation anesthetics in guinea pigs. Anesth. Analg. (Cleve.) 58:120, 1979.
4. Bailey, M. E.: Endotoxin, bile salts and renal function in obstructive jaundice. Br. J. Surg. 63:774, 1976.
5. Badylak, S. F., and Van Vleet, J. F.: Alterations of prothrombin time and activated partial thromboplastin time in dogs with hepatic disease. Am. J. Vet. Res. 42:2053, 1981.
6. Badylak, S. F.: Coagulopathies associated with hepatic disease. Calif. Vet. 36(2):14, 1982.
7. Bagshaw, R. J., and Cox, R. H.: Baroreceptor control of systemic hemodynamics at incremental halothane levels in the dog. Acta Anaesth. Scand. 25:416, 1981.
8. Benson, G. J., and Brock, K. A.: Halothane-associated hepatitis and methoxyflurane-related nephropathy: A review. J. Vet. Pharmacol. Therap. 3:187, 1980.
9. Benumof, J. L., Bookstein, J. J., Saidman, L. J., and Harris, R.: Diminished hepatic arterial flow during halothane administration. Anesthesiology 45:545, 1976.
10. Boettner, R. B., Ankeney, J. L., and Middleton, H.: Effect of halothane on splanchnic and peripheral flow in dogs. Anesth. Analg. (Cleve.) 44:214, 1965.
11. Bogan, J.: Factors affecting duration of thiopentone anaesthesia in dogs, with particular reference to greyhounds. Proc. Ass. Vet. An. G. Br. & Ir 1:18, 1970.
12. Bottoms, G. D., Johnson, M. A., and Roesel, O. F.: Endotoxin-induced hemodynamic changes in dogs: Role of thromboxane and prostaglandin I_2. Am. J. Vet. Res. 44:1497, 1983.
13. Brandon, R. A., and Baggot, J. D.: The pharmacokinetics of thiopentone. J. Vet. Pharmacol. Therap. 4:79, 1981.
14. Breznock, E. M., Berger, B., Pendray, D., et al. Surgical manipulation of intrahepatic portocaval shunts in dogs. J. Am. Vet. Med. Assoc. 182:798, 1983.
15. Brown, B. R.: Hepatic microsomal enzyme induction. Anesthesiology 39:178, 1973.
16. Brown, B. R.: General anesthetic and hepatic toxicity. Ariz. Med. 34:332, 1977.
17. Buckhold, D. K., Erickson, H. H., and Lumb, W. V.: Cardiovascular response to fentanyl-droperidol and atropine in the dog. Am. J. Vet. Res. 38:479, 1977.
18. Bunch, S. E., Castleman, W. L., Hornbuckle, W. E., and Tennant, B. C.: Hepatic cirrhosis associated with long-term anticonvulsant drug therapy in dogs. J. Am. Vet. Med. Assoc. 181:357, 1982.

19. Cornelius, C. E.: Biochemical evaluation of hepatic function in dogs. J. Am. Anim. Hosp. Assoc. 15:259, 1979.

20. Cornelius, L. M., Thrall, D. E., Halliwell, W. H., et al.: Anomalous portosystemic anastomoses associated with chronic hepatic insufficiency in six young dogs. J. Am. Vet. Med. Assoc. 167:220, 1975.

21. Dawson, J. L.: The incidence of postoperative renal failure in obstructive jaundice. Br. J. Surg. 52:663, 1965.

22. DeYoung, D. J., and Sawyer, D. C.: Anesthetic potency of nitrous oxide during halothane anesthesia in the dog. J. Am. Anim. Hosp. Assoc. 16:125, 1980.

23. Dundee, J. W., Fee, J. P. H., Moore, J., et al.: Changes in serum enzyme levels following ketamine infusions. Anaesthesia 35:12, 1980.

24. Durant, N. N., and Katz, R. L.: Suxamethonium. Br. J. Anaesth. 54:195, 1982.

25. Duvaldestin, P., Agoston, S., Henzel, D., et al.: Pancuronium pharmacokinetics in patients with liver cirrhosis. Br. J. Anaesth. 50:1131, 1978.

26. Dykes, M. H. M.: Anaesthesia and the liver: History and epidemiology. Can. Anaesth. Soc. J. 20:34, 1973.

27. Epstein, R. M., Wheeler, H. O., Frumin, M. J., et al.: The effect of hypercapnia on estimated hepatic blood flow, circulating splanchnic blood volume, and hepatic sulfobromophthalein clearance during general anesthesia in man. J. Clin. Invest. 40:592, 1961.

28. Epstein, R. M., Deutsch, S., Cooperman, L. H., et al.: Splanchnic circulation during halothane anesthesia and hypercapnia in normal man. Anesthesiology 27:654, 1966.

29. Ewing, G. O., Suter, P. F., and Bailey, C. S.: Hepatic insufficiency associated with congenital anomalies of the portal vein in dogs. J. Am. Anim. Hosp. Assoc. 10:463, 1974.

30. Feldman, S. A., Cohen, E. N., and Golling, R. C.: The excretion of gallamine in the dog. Anesthesiology 30:593, 1969.

31. Fennessy, M. R., and Ortiz, A.: The behavioural and cardiovascular actions of intravenously administered morphine in the conscious dog. Eur. J. Pharmacol. 3:177, 1968.

32. Gelman, S. I.: Disturbances in hepatic blood flow during anesthesia and surgery. Arch. Surg. 111:881, 1976.

33. Glouten, P.: Personal communication, 1983.

34. Green, J. F., Jackman, A. P., and Parsons, G.: The effects of morphine on the mechanical properties of the systemic circulation in the dog. Circ. Res. 42:474, 1978.

35. Greenham, L. W., and Ware, G. C.: Mustelid anaesthesia and halothane hepatitis. Vet. Rec. 105:104, 1979.

36. Hanson, K. M., and Johnson, P. C.: Local control of hepatic arterial and portal venous flow in the dog. Am. J. Physiol. 211:712, 1966.

37. Hall, L. W., and Clarke, K. W.: Relaxation of the skeletal muscles during anaesthesia. In Hall, L. W., and Clarke, K. W. (eds.): Veterinary Anaesthesia. 8th ed. Balliere Tindall, London, 1983.

38. Harper, M. H., Collins, P., Johnson, B. H., et al.: Postanesthetic hepatic injury in rats: Influence of alterations in hepatic blood flow, surgery, and anesthesia time. Anesth. Analg. (Cleve.) 61:79, 1982.

39. Harrison, G. G., and Smith, J. S.: Massive lethal hepatic necrosis in rats anesthetized with fluoroxene, after microsomal enzyme induction. Anesthesiology 39:619, 1973.

40. Hug, C. C., Murphy, M. R., Sampson, J. F., et al.: Biotransformation of morphine and fentanyl in anhepatic dogs. Anesthesiology 55 (Suppl.): A261, 1981.

41. Hughes, R. L., Campbell, D., and Fitch, W.: Effects of enflurane and halothane on liver blood flow and oxygen consumption in the greyhound. Br. J. Anaesth. 52:1079, 1980.

42. Idvall, J., Ahlgren, I., Aronsen, K. F., and Stenberg, P.: Ketamine infusions: Pharmacokinetics and clinical effects. Br. J. Anaesth. 51:1167, 1979.

43. Ivankovich, A. D., Miletich, D. J., Albrecht, R. F., et al.: Cardiovascular effects of intraperitoneal insufflation with carbon dioxide and nitrous oxide in the dog. Anesthesiology 42:281, 1975.

44. Jones, B. D.: The use of liver function tests: A clinician's perspective. Proc. Am. Anim. Hosp. Assoc. 50:235, 1983.

45. Kaka, J. S., and Hayton, W. L.: Pharmacokinetics of ketamine and two metabolites in the dog. J. Pharmacokin. Biopharm. 8:193, 1980.

46. Kalow, B., Rogoman, E., and Sims, F. H.: A comparison of the effects of halothane and other anaesthetic agents on hepatocellular function in patients submitted to elective operations. Can. Anaesth. Soc. J. 23:71, 1976.

47. Kayaalp, S. O., and Kaymakcalan, S.: Studies on the morphine-induced release of catecholamines from the adrenal glands in the dog. Arch. Int. Pharmacodyn. 172:139, 1968.

48. Krahwinkel, D. J., Sawyer, D. C., Eyster, G. E., and Bender, G.: Cardiopulmonary effects of fentanyl-droperidol, nitrous oxide, and atropine sulfate in dogs. Am. J. Vet. Res. 36:1211, 1975.

49. Levesque, D. C., Oliver, J. E., Cornelius, L. M., et al.: Congenital portacaval shunts in two cats: Diagnosis and surgical correction. J. Am. Vet. Med. Assoc. 181:143, 1982.

50. Levitt, J. D.: The biochemical basis of anesthetic toxicity. Surg. Clin. North Am. 55:801, 1975.

51. Libonati, M., Malsch, E., Price, H. L., et al.: Splanchnic circulation in man during methoxyflurane anesthesia. Anesthesiology 38:466, 1973.

52. Lundeen, G., Manohar, M., and Parks, C.: Systemic distribution of blood flow in swine while awake and during 1.0 and 1.5 MAC isoflurane anesthesia with or without 50% nitrous oxide. Anesth. Analg. (Cleve.) 62:499, 1983.

53. Marietta, M. P., Vore, M. E., and Way, W. L.: Characterization of ketamine induction of hepatic microsomal drug metabolism. Biochem. Pharmacol. 26:2451, 1977.

54. Mays, E. T., and Wheeler, C. S.: Demonstration of collateral arterial flow after interruption of hepatic arteries in man. N. Engl. J. Med. 290:993, 1974.

55. McConnell, M. F., and Lumsden, J. W.: Biochemical evaluation of metastatic liver disease. J. Am. Anim. Hosp. Assoc. 19:173, 1983.

56. Meyer, D. J., and Noonan, N. E.: Liver tests in dogs receiving anticonvulsant drugs (diphenylhydantoin and primidone). J. Am. Anim. Hosp. Assoc. 17:261, 1981.

57. Milnor, W. R.: Regional circulations. In Mountcastle, V. B. (ed.): Medical Physiology. 14th ed. The C. V. Mosby Co., St. Louis, 1980.

58. Ndiritu, C. G., and Weigel, J.: Hepatorenal injury in a dog associated with methoxyflurane (a case report). Vet. Med. Sm. Anim. Clin. 72:545, 1977.

59. Ostheimer, G. W., Shanahan, E. A., Guyton, R. A., et al.: Effects of fentanyl and droperidol on canine left ventricular performance. Anesthesiology 42:288, 1975.

60. Pedersoli, W. M.: Serum fluoride concentration, renal, and hepatic function test results in dogs with methoxyflurane anesthesia. Am. J. Vet. Res. 38:949, 1977.

61. Priano, L. L., and Vatner, S. F.: Morphine effects on cardiac output and regional blood flow distribution in conscious dogs. Anesthesiology 55:236, 1981.

62. Priano, L. L., and Vatner, S. F.: Generalized cardiovascular and regional hemodynamic effects of meperidine in conscious dogs. Anesth. Analg. (Cleve.) 60:649, 1981.

63. Ramzan, I. M., Shanks, C. A., and Triggs, E. J.: Pharmacokinetics and pharmacodynamics of gallamine triethiodide in patients with total biliary obstruction. Anesth. Analg. (Cleve.) 60:289, 1981.

64. Reynolds, E. S., Brown, B. R., and Vandam, L. D.: Massive hepatic necrosis after fluroxene anesthesia—a case of drug interaction? N. Engl. J. Med. 286:530, 1972.

65. Saidman, L. J., and Eger, E. I.: The effect of thiopental metabolism on duration of anesthesia. Anesthesiology 27:118, 1966.

66. Sawyer, D. C., Anderson, D. L., and Scott, J. B.: Cardiovascular effects and clinical use of nalbuphine in the dog. Proc. Ass. Vet. An. G. Br. & Ir. 10 (Suppl.):215, 1982.

67. Sawyer, D. C.: The induction period. In Sawyer, D. C. (ed.): The Practice of Small Animal Anesthesia. W. B. Saunders Co., Philadelphia, 1983.

68. Sederberg, J., Stanley, T. H., Reddy, P., et al.: Hemodynamic

effects of butorphanol-oxygen anesthesia in dogs. Anesth. Analg. (Cleve.) *60*:715, 1981.

69. Somogyi, A. A., Shanks, C. A., and Triggs, E. J.: Disposition kinetics of pancuronium bromide in patients with total biliary obstruction. Br. J. Anaesth. *49*:1103, 1977.

70. Steffey, E. P., Gillespie, J. R., Berry, J. D., et al.: Circulatory effects of halothane and halothane-nitrous oxide anesthesia in the dog: Controlled ventilation. Am. J. Vet. Res. *35*:1289, 1974.

71. Strunin, L.: Preoperative assessment of the patient with liver dysfunction. Br. J. Anaesth. *50*:25, 1978.

72. Theye, R. A., and Michenfelder, J. D.: Individual organ contributions to the decrease in whole-body VO_2 with isoflurane. Anesthesiology *42*:35, 1975.

73. Thulin, L., Andreen, M., and Irestedt, L.: Effect of controlled halothane anaesthesia on splanchnic blood flow and cardiac output in the dog. Acta Anaesth. Scand. *19*:146, 1975.

74. Tranquilli, W. J., Manohar, M., Parks, C. M., et al.: Systemic and regional blood flow distribution in unanesthetized swine and swine anesthetized with halothane and nitrous oxide, halothane, or enflurane. Anesthesiology *56*:369, 1982.

75. Trim, C. M.: Anesthesia and the kidney. Comp. Cont. Educ. *1*:843, 1979.

76. Trim, C. M.: Cardiopulmonary effects of butorphanol tartrate in dogs. Am. J. Vet. Res. *44*:329, 1983.

77. Viegas, O., and Stoelting, R. K.: LDH_5 changes after cholecystectomy or hysterectomy in patients receiving halothane, enflurane, or fentanyl. Anesthesiology *51*:556, 1979.

78. Walsh, E. S., Traynor, C., Paterson, J. L., and Hall, G. M.: Effect of different intraoperative fluid regimens on circulating metabolites and insulin during abdominal surgery. Br. J. Anaesth. *55*:135, 1983.

79. Ward, S., Judge, S., and Corall, I.: Pharmacokinetics of pancuronium bromide in liver failure. Abstract of Proceedings of Anaesthesia Research Society. Br. J Anaesth. 227P, 1982.

80. White, P. F., Marietta, M. P., and Pudwill, C. R.: Effects of halothane anesthesia on the biodisposition of ketamine in rats. J. Pharmacol. Exp. Ther. *196*:545, 1976.

81. Willis, E. J., and Walton, B.: A morphologic study of unexplained hepatitis following halothane anesthesia. Am. J. Pathol. *91*:11, 1978.

82. Wright, M.: Pharmacologic effects of ketamine and its use in veterinary medicine. J. Am. Vet. Med. Assoc. *180*:1462, 1982.

83. Zollinger, R. M., and Williams, R. D.: Appraisal of progress in surgical therapy: Surgical aspects of jaundice. Surgery *39*:1016, 1956.

Chapter **194**

Anesthesia and the Urinary System

Cynthia M. Trim

The kidney is responsible for controlling the volume, tonicity, pH, and electrolyte composition of body fluids. The kidney also influences systemic hemodynamics through the renin-angiotensin system. This chapter includes a discussion of anesthesia and the urinary system from two viewpoints—first, the mechanisms whereby anesthesia and surgery alter renal function and upset homeostasis in the normal animal and second, the ways in which abnormal urinary function can modify the patient's response to anesthesia and surgery.

EFFECTS OF ANESTHESIA AND SURGERY ON RENAL FUNCTION

Anesthesia changes renal function by reduction or redistribution of renal blood flow (RBF), by stimulation of the sympathetic nervous system, by increasing or decreasing levels of aldosterone, antidiuretic hormone (ADH), renin, or prostaglandins, or by exerting a direct toxic effect on the kidney. Anesthetic drugs may act by one or more of these effects, and the final outcome may be modified or emphasized by the combination of two or more drugs. Surgery further modifies renal function through stimulation of the sympathetic nervous system, together with physio-

logic change from fluid loss and tissue trauma. Although urinary function apparently returns after anesthesia in most patients, the ability of the kidney to regulate urine volume and content is impaired for several days.[39]

Because the effects of anesthetic drugs on the function of healthy kidneys have been studied in detail, the most appropriate drugs may be chosen to produce the least adverse effect in a patient with a urinary tract problem.

Renal Blood Flow

Blood flow to the kidney is high when compared with other organs (642 ml/min/100 gm in unanesthetized dogs[89]), and it comprises up to 25 per cent of the cardiac output. Therefore, a change in renal blood flow (RBF) is expected if anesthesia decreases cardiac output.

A decrease in systemic blood pressure does not necessarily result in a decrease in RBF or glomerular filtration rate (GFR). "Autoregulation" occurs in the healthy kidney over a wide range of blood pressures to maintain a constant RBF and GFR (Fig. 194–1). Between mean arterial pressures of 70 and 160 mm Hg, a decrease in arterial pressure is followed within

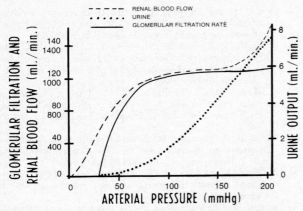

Figure 194–1. Autoregulation of renal blood flow (RBF) and glomerular filtration rate (GFR) and lack of autoregulation of urine flow. (Reprinted with permission from Guyton, A. C.: *Textbook of Medical Physiology.* 6th ed. Philadelphia, W. B. Saunders Company, 1981.)

minutes by dilation of the afferent glomerular arteriole, and glomerular blood flow is maintained. When arterial blood pressure remains depressed for hours, the formation of angiotensin II causes constriction of the efferent arteriole. RBF declines, but GFR is maintained because glomerular hydrostatic pressure is maintained.[30] However, although published information sometimes conflicts because different experimental models and methods have been used, it appears that some anesthetic drugs abolish autoregulation. The final outcome is influenced by the sympathetic, endocrine, and renin-angiotensin systems in the intact animal.

Experiments *in vitro* have demonstrated that the direct effects of halothane on canine kidneys are vasodilation, increased RBF, and increased urine production.[7] Light anesthesia in dogs ventilated with 1 per cent halothane resulted in vasodilation in the kidney with no change in RBF from the awake value,

despite a marked depression of myocardial contractility.[94] Prolonged anesthesia with 2 per cent halothane decreased RBF less than 20 per cent from control values. In dogs anesthetized with atropine, thiopental, and halothane with controlled ventilation, increasing the vaporizer setting to 1.5 per cent (end-tidal halothane, 0.9 per cent) decreased mean arterial pressure but not urine production.[43] Halothane concentrations above this level resulted in a progressive decrease in the volume of urine produced. Enflurane was evaluated in the same study. No decrease in urine production was obtained with a vaporizer setting of up to 3.5 per cent (end-tidal enflurane, 2.1 per cent). Above this concentration the arterial blood pressure fell rapidly and urine production ceased. In another investigation, halothane did not alter the intrarenal distribution of blood flow in normovolemic, normotensive dogs, but when the dogs were made hypotensive with halothane, cortical blood flow (usually 85 per cent of RBF) was decreased more than medullary flow.[5]

Methoxyflurane anesthesia has been reported to decrease RBF in dogs[51] and cats.[44] Autoregulation was impaired because a decrease in mean arterial pressure (to above 70 mm Hg) caused by an increase in methoxyflurane decreased RBF.[51] However, in another investigation of both halothane and methoxyflurane anesthesia during induced diuresis in dogs, RBF was comparable in the two groups.[60] Urine outputs were low relative to the intravenous fluid loads. Less urine was produced with methoxyflurane, but the difference was not statistically significant. Preliminary information indicates that RBF is qualitatively better when it is maintained with isoflurane rather than with halothane at equivalent levels of anesthesia.[54,88]

An increase, no change, and a decrease in RBF have all been described with pentobarbital anesthesia[2,8,13] (Fig. 194–2). Injection of thiopental at a dose rate commonly used to induce anesthesia does

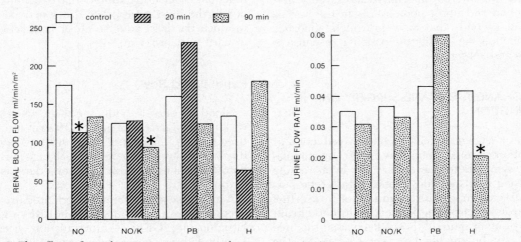

Figure 194–2. The effects of anesthetic agents—nitrous oxide 80 per cent (NO), nitrous oxide 80 per cent and ketamine 5 mg/kg IV (NO/K), pentobarbital 20 mg/kg IV (PB), and halothane 1 to 1.2 per cent (H)—on renal blood flow and urine flow rate in piglets. Measurements were made at 20 minutes and/or 90 minutes after the onset of anesthesia. *Asterisks* refer to statistically significant changes (p<0.05) from control values. (Reprinted with permission from Bailie, M. D., Alward, C. T., Sawyer, D. C., and Hook, J. B.: Effect of anesthesia on cardiovascular and renal function in the newborn piglet. J. Pharmacol. Exp. Therap. 208:298, 1979.)

not decrease RBF in healthy dogs (Fig. 194–3).[81] The reduction in renal vascular resistance that occurred simultaneously with the decrease in aortic pressure may have indicated that autoregulation was not depressed. In a similar experiment, intravenous injections of ketamine, 2.5 or 5.0 mg/kg, increased aortic blood pressure and RBF (Fig. 194–4).[81] Increased arterial blood pressure and cardiac output from ketamine have been previously documented in both dogs and cats.[37,38] Increased urine production has been reported in cats after an intramuscular injection of ketamine, 33 mg/kg.[34]

Use of other anesthetic drugs with ketamine may produce different effects. When ketamine was injected into piglets breathing 80 per cent nitrous oxide, RBF decreased, but no change in urine production occurred (Fig. 194–2).[2] Ketamine injected into dogs anesthetized with nitrous oxide and brevimythal (a barbiturate) resulted in a decrease in cardiac output, RBF, and urinary output.[25] Ketamine is frequently combined with xylazine in clinical practice. Xylazine alone has been reported to increase urine production in several species,[34,90,92] despite a severe decrease in cardiac output. The effect does not appear to be the result of changes in RBF or GFR.[92]

Morphine is known to cause an antidiuresis in humans and animals.[71] Both an increase and a de-

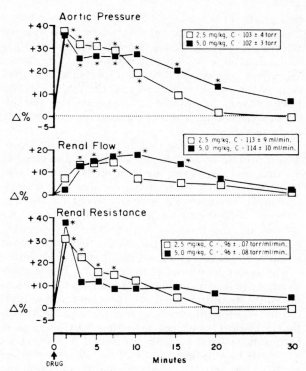

Figure 194–4. Ketamine and renal hemodynamics in dogs. Mean per cent changes in aortic pressure, renal blood flow, and renal vascular resistance after 2.5 mg/kg *(open squares)* and 5.0 mg/kg *(solid squares)* doses of ketamine. *Inset* for each variable indicates mean actual control values ± SEM. Control values are depicted on ordinate as 0. After drug administration (indicated by *arrows*), changes from the control values are expressed as mean per cent change and are followed for 30 minutes. *Asterisks* refer to statistically significant changes (p<0.05) from control values. (Reprinted with permission from Priano, L. L.: Alteration of renal hemodynamics by thiopental, diazepam, and ketamine in conscious dogs. Anesth. Analg. (Cleve.) *61*:853, 1982.)

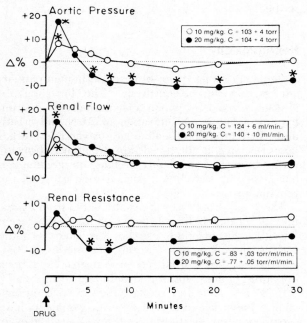

Figure 194–3. Thiopental and renal hemodynamics in dogs. Mean per cent changes in aortic pressure, renal blood flow, and renal vascular resistance after 10-mg/kg *(open circles)* and 20-mg/kg *(solid circles)* doses of thiopental. Inset for each variable indicates actual mean control values ± SEM. Control values are depicted on ordinate as 0. After drug administration (indicated by *arrow*), changes from control values are expressed as mean per cent change and are followed for 30 minutes. *Asterisks* refer to statistically significant changes (p<0.05) from control values. (Reprinted with permission from Priano, L. L.: Alteration of renal hemodynamics by thiopental, diazepam, and ketamine in conscious dogs. Anesth. Analg. (Cleve.) 61:853, 1982.)

crease in RBF and GFR with morphine have been reported.[32,79] Meperidine, 2 mg/kg or 6 mg/kg, infused intravenously over five minutes, produced increases in RBF,[80] whereas pentazocine, 1 mg/kg or 3 mg/kg injected intravenously as a bolus, transiently decreased RBF.[99] These changes appeared to reflect the systemic arterial blood pressure. Early work with Innovar in human patients demonstrated little depression of effective renal plasma flow (ERPF, determined by para-amino hippuric acid clearance) and GFR.[29] Fentanyl given alone, 0.025 mg/kg or 0.05 mg/kg infused over 10 minutes, to conscious dogs caused increased aortic pressure and renal vasoconstriction but no change in RBF.[82] However, fentanyl, 0.025 mg/kg infused intravenously over 10 minutes, administered to dogs anesthetized with atropine, thiopental, and nitrous oxide resulted in a significant fall in ERPF and urine volume.[42]

Renin-Angiotensin-Aldosterone System

The juxtaglomerular apparatus consists of modified muscle cells containing renin-filled granules embedded in the wall of the afferent arteriole.[100] Release of renin into blood and interstitial fluid is initiated through a baroreceptor mechanism by a fall in renal arterial pressure. A change in composition of the fluid in the distal renal tubule also results in renin release. The effect is mediated through a specialized group of cells in the tubule wall known as the macula densa. Furthermore, stimulation of renal nerves and increased circulating levels of catecholamines stimulate renin secretion.

Renin is an enzyme that hydrolyzes a liver-produced protein to angiotensin I. This is converted to a vasoactive substance, angiotensin II, in the lung. In addition to its vasoconstrictive properties, angiotensin II stimulates the adrenal zona glomerulosa to increase aldosterone production. Aldosterone increases tubular reabsorption of sodium, promoting water retention and maintaining the circulating blood volume. In exchange for sodium, potassium is lost.

The systemic arterial blood pressure during anesthesia is partly maintained through the renin-angiotensin system. Increased plasma renin activity (PRA) has been recorded subsequent to pentobarbital anesthesia in dogs[45] but not in piglets.[2] Differences in results have been partially attributed to differences in the dietary sodium intake of the animals. In one study, pentobarbital anesthesia had no effect on the PRA in dogs with normal salt intake but resulted in marked increases in dogs fed a low sodium diet.[27] In another experiment, pentobarbital or thiopental anesthesia produced a severe drop in RBF in dogs on an unrestricted diet but no change in RBF in dogs fed a high sodium diet.[14] The decrease in blood pressure that follows the administration of an angiotensin II inhibitor is used as further evidence of renin activity. Increased activity of the renin-angiotensin system has been documented with halothane[2,63] and enflurane anesthesia[63] but not with ketamine.[2,63] An investigation with human patients demonstrated increased PRA only after surgery began.[64] Surgery stimulates the sympathetic nervous system,[27] and this in turn can initiate renin release. A quiet, smooth induction of anesthesia with minimal effect on systemic hemodynamics is less likely to activate the renin-angiotensin system than an induction in which the patient is anxious or excited. Hypotension caused by hemorrhage increases renin release.[41,45,66]

Antidiuretic Hormone

Antidiuretic hormone (ADH, vasopressin), released from the posterior pituitary, affects the permeability of the renal tubules to water and has a potent vasoconstrictor effect in the splanchnic, renal, and coronary circulations. Increased levels of ADH have been reported with ether, methoxyflurane, halothane, and nitrous oxide-relaxant anesthesia.[19] Other studies with a variety of anesthetic drugs have shown that anesthesia does not result in ADH release but that surgical stress during light anesthesia is a potent stimulus.[76] The level of ADH produced suggests that

ADH contributes significantly to the vasopressor response to surgery. Hypotension due to hemorrhage also causes ADH release through stimulation of the carotid body or aortic arch baroreceptors and decreased blood volume that stimulates atrial stretch receptors. The ADH contributes substantially to the restoration of arterial pressure after hemorrhage.[17]

Controlled ventilation produces no change or a decrease in ADH levels in dogs.[3] Institution of positive end-expiratory pressure (PEEP) with controlled ventilation increases plasma ADH levels and decreases urine production. Current literature on the effect of controlled ventilation on renal function has been reviewed.[9]

Prostaglandins

Prostaglandins synthesized in the kidney are thought to play a part in the autoregulation of RBF and GFR in conditions of reduced renal function. Increased renal secretion of prostaglandins is seen in anesthesia combined with surgical stress[87] and in hypovolemic conditions such as hemorrhagic hypotension.[65] Prostaglandins modulate intrarenal vascular perfusion patterns and preserve inner cortical blood flow.[65] It is assumed that this is a defense mechanism to protect renal function. The influence of prostaglandins on renal circulation has recently been described.[96]

Nephrotoxicity

Renal failure has been reported in human patients after methoxyflurane anesthesia.[56] The clinical picture is characterized by polyuria, hypernatremia, serum hyperosmolality, and elevation of BUN and creatinine. The duration of malfunction is variable but has been responsible for the death of patients. Concurrent administration of tetracycline[50] or gentamicin[4] has been implicated as a participating cause of the renal failure.

The renal tubule damage is attributed to inorganic fluoride, a metabolite of methoxyflurane; the serum fluoride concentrations can be correlated with the severity of malfunction.[56] Serum fluoride levels comparable to those produced in humans have been measured in dogs after methoxyflurane anesthesia[12,74] (Fig. 194–5) and after methoxyflurane with tetracycline.[75] Polyuria and decreased urine osmolality have occurred after anesthesia, but no clinical signs of renal failure have been noted (Fig. 194–6).[12,73,74] However, infusion of sodium fluoride into dogs without methoxyflurane resulted in renal damage.[26] The defect produced is related more to the peak fluoride level than to the duration of exposure to fluoride. Investigation of intrarenal distribution of blood flow during anesthesia indicated that methoxyflurane, but not halothane, reduced outer cortical perfusion and produced a relative increase in inner cortical perfu-

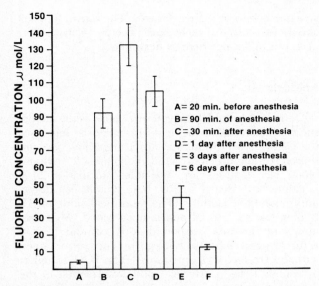

Figure 194–5. Histogram showing effects of three hours of methoxyflurane anesthesia on serum inorganic fluoride in 20 dogs. Values are mean ± SEM. All values B to F are significantly higher than control value *(A)*. (Reprinted with permission from Pedersoli, W. M.: Serum fluoride concentration, renal and hepatic function test results in dogs with methoxyflurane anesthesia. Am. J. Vet. Res. 38:949, 1977.)

sion.[52] This may prolong tubular contact with toxic metabolites.

High levels of fluoride can be achieved by deep methoxyflurane anesthesia or by anesthesia in a patient in which methoxyflurane metabolism is accelerated by enzyme induction. The hepatic microsomal enzyme system for methoxyflurane is induced by exposure to low concentration of methoxyflurane and by pretreatment with phenobarbital.[11] Fatal hepatorenal failure has been reported in a dog that was anesthetized three times in four months with methoxyflurane.[68] Clinical signs of renal failure have also occurred in apparently normal dogs after a single methoxyflurane anesthesia.[91] Renal function was restored in each case by intensive fluid therapy.

The potential for renal failure after methoxyflurane anesthesia clearly exists. Deep anesthesia with methoxyflurane should be avoided, and adequate fluid intake after anesthesia must be ensured. Methoxyflurane cannot be recommended for dogs on anticonvulsant treatment.

Whereas methoxyflurane is highly fat-soluble and up to 50 per cent of the inhaled dose is metabolized, halothane has relatively low solubility, and less than 20 per cent is metabolized.[93] Enflurane is structurally similar to methoxyflurane, but the former undergoes limited biodegradation, and serum fluoride levels after enflurane anesthesia are lower. Some impairment of urine concentrating ability was demonstrated in humans after enflurane, but not halothane, anesthesia.[55] No concentrating defect was discovered in dogs after halothane or enflurane anesthesia.[97] It is unlikely that normal kidneys in small animals are damaged by these anesthetics, but surgical patients

with pre-existing renal disease could be harmed. The rate of increase of serum inorganic fluoride level from the start of enflurane anesthesia is greater in dogs without renal function than in dogs with renal function.[98] Isoflurane is metabolized in minute quantities and increases in fluoride levels are too small to be of concern.[57,95]

ANESTHESIA AND URINARY SYSTEM DISEASE

Case Report

A three-year-old male German Shepherd dog (36 kg) was presented for surgical repair of a ruptured bladder. Preanesthesia examination 17 hours after the accident indicated a heart rate of 160 per minute, respiratory rate 132 per minute, rectal temperature 40°C (104°F), and persistent vomiting. Laboratory values were: packed cell volume (PCV) 65 per cent, total protein (TP) 9.1 gm per cent, blood urea nitrogen (BUN) 181 mg/dl, creatinine 6.1 mg/dl, glucose 181 mg/dl, sodium 158 mEq/l, potassium 6.7 mEq/l, chloride 115 mEq/l, calcium 10 mg/dl, arterial pH 7.24, P_{CO_2} 23 mm Hg, base excess (BE) −14.7 mEq/l. A catheter was inserted into the jugular vein to measure central venous pressure, which was −1.0 cm H_2O. Evidence of pulmonary contusions was observed on the thoracic radiographs.

A large-bore catheter was inserted aseptically into the abdominal cavity for drainage. Lactated Ringer's solution was infused intravenously, and because of metabolic acidosis, sodium bicarbonate was injected in 40 mEq increments at 30-minute intervals for a total of 120 mEq. Two hours later, the PCV was 50 per cent, TP 6.7 gm per cent, sodium 161 mEq/l, potassium 5.1 mEq/l, chloride 119 mEq/l, BUN 115 mg/dl, CVP +1.5 cm H_2O. Treatment was continued for an additional two hours before surgery, and by that time the dog had received 5 liters of lactated Ringer's solution. The CVP was +3.0 cm H_2O, with an arterial pH of 7.34, and BE −4.3 mEq/l.

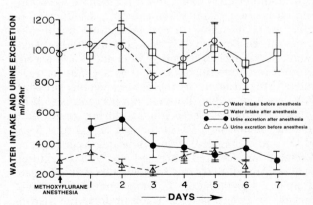

Figure 194–6. Effects of three hours of methoxyflurane anesthesia on 24-hour water intake and urine excretion in 20 dogs before and after anesthesia. Values are mean ± SEM. *Open circles,* water intake before anesthesia; *open squares,* water intake after anesthesia; *open triangles,* urine excretion before anesthesia; *solid circles,* urine excretion after anesthesia. (Reprinted with permission from Pedersoli, W. M.: Serum fluoride concentration, renal and hepatic function test results in dogs with methoxyflurane anesthesia. Am. J. Vet. Res. 38:949, 1977.)

No atropine was administered because the heart rate was 180 beats/min. Anesthesia was induced by slow titration of acepromazine and oxymorphone intravenously over five minutes. A total dose of 1 mg acepromazine and 3.25 mg oxymorphone was required. The trachea was intubated, and the dog was allowed to breathe 100 per cent oxygen spontaneously in a circle CO_2 absorption system. Pancuronium, 0.8 mg, was injected intravenously at the start of surgery to improve muscle relaxation, and controlled ventilation was initiated. Lidocaine, 80 mg, was given five minutes later to control premature ventricular contractions and repeated again at 60 minutes. The oxymorphone was partially reversed at the end of surgery with naloxone, but neostigmine was not needed to antagonize the pancuronium. Total anesthesia time was 1 hour 35 minutes. Recovery from anesthesia was uneventful, with the exception of premature ventricular contractions, which had to be controlled for five days with lidocaine and procaine amide.

This case report illustrates some of the problems encountered during management of traumatic injury to the urinary tract: (1) hypovolemia, (2) acidosis, (3) hyperkalemia, (4) reduced anesthetic requirement (surgery accomplished with a drug dosage that would be insufficient in a healthy dog), (5) reduced renal function (dose of pancuronium used was one-third of that used in animals with normal renal function), and (6) traumatic myocarditis (manifested by premature ventricular contractions). Abnormalities of fluid, electrolyte, and acid-base balance must be corrected before anesthesia to provide the best possible chance of survival. Animals with chronic renal disease may have similar abnormalities, but they often present additional management problems, such as anemia or hepatic malfunction.

Fluid Balance

There is not always sufficient time to correct dehydration before surgery, but it is essential to restore the circulating blood volume before anesthesia because most anesthetic drug combinations further depress the cardiovascular system. During fluid replacement, serial measurements of hematocrit and plasma protein can sometimes be used as a guide to treatment. Measurement of the central venous pressure (CVP), when cardiac disease is not present, is a useful guide to efficacy of treatment during rapid fluid loading. A normal CVP in the dog is +3 to +5 cm H_2O, and a negative value indicates hypovolemia. Lactated or acetated balanced electrolyte solution may be infused to correct hypovolemia and to initiate diuresis. Furosemide, 1 mg/kg injected intravenously, or a continuous infusion of dopamine hydrochloride, 3 μg/kg/per minute, can be used to stimulate urine production. Dopamine increases RBF, GFR, water, and sodium excretion[16] but only if the blood volume is adequate.[69] Forty mg (1 ml) of solution may be added to 500 ml saline or balanced electrolyte solution and administered with a pediatric infusion set. The infusion should be closely monitored to avoid exceeding the recommended dose. Vasocon-

striction occurs at higher dosages. The rate of infusion should be slowed if tachycardia occurs. A urine flow of 1 to 2 ml/kg per hour is desirable.

Acidosis

Dehydration and hypovolemia cause reduced tissue perfusion and lactic acidosis. Acidosis depresses the CNS, myocardium, and other organ function and therefore should be corrected. If facilities for pH and blood gas analyses are available, calculation of a negative base excess ($-BE$, base deficit) can determine metabolic acidosis. The numerical value of BE is identical in arterial and venous blood. Measurements of the total carbon dioxide content (TCO_2) value are less accurate but can be cheaply obtained with the Harleco CO_2 apparatus.* The TCO_2 is higher in venous than in arterial blood. Subtraction of the measured value from the normal value gives an approximate estimate of base deficit. Normal values for BE and TCO_2 differ between species. Values for canine arterial blood have been reported as pH 7.40 ± 0.02, P_{CO_2} 34 ± 3 mm Hg, P_{O_2} 98 ± 6 mm Hg, HCO^-_3 20.5 mEq/l, BE −3 mEq/l, and TCO_2 21.6 mEq/l.[35] The mean TCO_2 for venous blood was 22.7 mEq/l. Other published data place the pH between mean values of 7.39 and 7.44, P_{CO_2} 31 to 33 mm Hg, HCO_3 19.5 to 22.5 mEq/l, and BE −4 to −2 mEq/l.[49,67] The cat is more acidemic, with an arterial pH of 7.34 and P_{CO_2} 34 to 35 mm Hg.[31,61] These values result in a HCO^-_3 of 17.5 ± 3 mEq/l, BE −6.4 ± 5 mEq/l, and T_{CO_2} 18.4 ± 4 mEq/l.[61] The venous TCO_2 was recorded at 20.1 ± 4 mEq/l.

A decrease of 5 mEq/l from the normal value is considered a mild metabolic acidosis, a decrease in 10 mEq/l a moderate acidosis, and a decrease of 15 mEq/l a severe acidosis. Correction of acidosis before anesthesia can be accomplished using the following calculation: The total mEq of bicarbonate required is the deficit (mEq/l) × 0.3 × kg body weight, where 0.3 or 30 per cent of body weight represents the extracellular fluid volume. The total dose is divided, and each half is infused intravenously over five to ten minutes, at least 30 minutes apart. Rapidly infused sodium bicarbonate causes hypotension. If the animal is severely acidotic, the calculated requirement should be infused over a longer period of time to avoid paradoxical cerebral acidosis. This calculation of bicarbonate requirement is inadequate in chronic disease states, and re-evaluation in several hours usually reveals the need for additional bicarbonate. Sodium bicarbonate is available commercially as 5 and 7.5 per cent solutions, which are hypertonic. Correction of a severe metabolic acidosis with these solutions may result in hypernatremia. Dilution with sterile water down to 1.3 per cent (isotonic) before infusion may be necessary. In the absence of any laboratory measurement, a suspected mild deficit can

---

*Division of American Hospital Supply

be corrected fairly safely with 1.5 mEq/kg $NaHCO_3$ intravenously.

Potassium

Patients with oliguria or anuria fail to excrete potassium released from protein catabolism, resulting in elevated levels of potassium in extracellular fluid. The major concern is the effect of potassium on the heart. Signs of disturbed membrane excitability are evident in the ECG when serum potassium reaches 7 mEq/l. Hyperkalemia causes narrow, peaked T waves and shortened Q-T interval. P waves are lost between 8 and 9 mEq/l. The QRS complex becomes widened and merges with the T wave above 10 mEq/l. Cardiac arrest may be initiated by stress or anesthesia in patients with elevated extracellular potassium. Animals with traumatic myocarditis are particularly at risk.

Cats with urethral obstruction have been studied under both clinical and experimental conditions.[23,72] In a report of clinically occurring obstruction, 7 of 15 cats examined had serum potassium levels greater than 9 mEq/l.[72] In a group of 13 cats with experimentally induced urethral obstruction, central nervous system depression and vomiting were observed in 11 cats at 48 hours.[23] At this time the mean serum potassium level of the group was 7.6 mEq/l and the venous TCO_2 was 14.1 mEq/l. The obstruction was removed in a second group of eight cats when severe clinical signs developed. These cats (mean weight 3.5 kg) were treated with a mean volume of 228 ml of balanced electrolyte solution* intravenously followed by 144 ml subcutaneously four hours later. With this treatment, the serum potassium decreased from 9.0 mEq/l at the termination of obstruction to 7.4 mEq/l after one hour and 6.6 mEq/l after four hours.

Three other methods for the treatment of severe hyperkalemia are available. The effect of potassium on the heart can be counteracted by injection of 10 per cent calcium gluconate, up to 10 ml for a large dog, intravenously over several minutes. Correction of the metabolic acidosis drives potassium into the cells. A dose of 1 mEq/kg of sodium bicarbonate should be begun until the results of the laboratory tests are available. Administration of insulin causes glucose to move into cells and promotes simultaneous transfer of potassium. A total dose of 0.5 to 1.0 unit of regular insulin per kg body weight is recommended, with 2 gm dextrose per unit of insulin to prevent hypoglycemia.[84] Balanced electrolyte solution must be used in addition to these treatments to restore blood volume and cardiac output.

Effect on Drug Action

Drugs that have limited lipid solubility or are mainly ionized in the physiologic range of pH are usually eliminated unchanged through the kidneys. This includes quaternary ammonium bases, ganglion blocking drugs, nondepolarizing muscle relaxants, many antibiotics, and digoxin.[78,86] These drugs are passively filtered through the glomeruli, or actively or passively reabsorbed, or actively secreted, by the tubules. Only nonprotein bound drugs can be filtered. Glomerular filtration of the drug is therefore influenced by the degree of protein-binding and by the GFR.

Most of an injected dose of gallamine in dogs is excreted intact in the urine; 84 per cent of the drug was recovered in the urine in 24 hours compared with 3.5 per cent in the bile.[22] In addition, experimentally induced renal failure resulted in elevated blood gallamine levels for 24 hours and prolonged paralysis. Gallamine should therefore be avoided in animals with renal disease. In the cat, pancuronium is partly metabolized in the liver and partly excreted unchanged in bile and urine.[1] Slow elimination of pancuronium has been reported in human patients with chronic renal failure.[58] Antagonism with neostigmine can be satisfactory in patients with renal failure provided that smaller than usual doses of pancuronium are administered.[10] Succinylcholine, a depolarizing muscle relaxant, is entirely dependent on the liver for detoxification. However, injection of succinylcholine causes a transient increase in serum potassium, and, although succinylcholine is not contraindicated in patients in renal failure with normal potassium levels, its use in patients with elevated serum potassium could result in a cardiac arrest.[62]

The antibiotics kanamycin, gentamicin, and cephaloridine rely principally on the kidney for their elimination. Impaired renal function may increase the blood concentration to levels that are toxic or that significantly affect neuromuscular function adversely. A modified dose schedule is recommended for animals with renal disease.[48,83]

The majority of an injected dose of ketamine in cats is excreted unchanged in the urine.[40] Consequently, a lower dose than usual, such as 2 mg/kg intravenously, is advisable to avoid prolonged recovery in cats with urinary tract malfunction. A much greater amount (62 per cent) is metabolized in the dog.[46]

The actions of the commonly used narcotic analgesics are terminated by redistribution or hepatic metabolism. Yet prolonged duration of activity (days) has been reported with narcotics in uremic patients, even in patients with renal disease and no evidence of hepatic malfunction.[20] Consequently, it may be necessary to antagonize narcotic depression with naloxone more than once.

Decreased binding of thiopental to plasma proteins has also been reported in uremic patients—56 per cent compared with 28 per cent in healthy patients.[28] This could not be explained completely by competitive displacement by nitrogenous end-products or by hypoalbuminemia. This is important because the active form of thiobarbiturate is the unbound portion, and this may be the reason why chronic renal failure

---

*Multisol-R, Abbott Laboratories, North Chicago, IL.

patients require up to 50 per cent less barbiturate for anesthesia than healthy patients. Others have determined that the rate and extent of distribution and elimination of thiopental is unchanged in chronic renal failure relative to normal patients.[13] Therefore, a decrease in the rate of administration to accommodate the increase in unbound fraction of thiopental is more important than the total dose.

Chronic Renal Disease

The animal with chronic renal disease usually has other important problems in addition to those relating to the urinary tract. Hepatic function may be decreased, diminishing the ability to metabolize drugs.[18] Prolonged bleeding time, decreased platelet adhesiveness, and abnormal prothrombin consumption occur during uremia and may be the direct effect of urea or one of its metabolites.[21]

Anemia may also be present, either because of deficient erythropoietin production or because of bone marrow suppression by retained metabolites. Physiologic compensation for anemia usually involves increasing the 2,3-diphosphoglycerate (2,3-DPG) in the red cells, shifting the oxygen dissociation curve, and favoring tissue oxygenation. However, the increase in 2,3-DPG is minimal in uremic patients with anemia compared with the increase observed in anemic patients without concurrent renal disease.[6] Halothane anesthesia has been studied in dogs in the presence of anemia.[53] Anemia did not reduce the requirement of halothane for anesthesia, nor were there any differences in cardiac output, blood pressure, or subendocardial-subepicardial blood flow between dogs with a normal level of hemoglobin and anemic dogs. Oxygen delivery to tissues should not be jeopardized until the packed cell volume (PCV) is less than 20 per cent,[59] provided that cardiovascular function is good. However, since cardiac output and blood pressure are depressed by anesthesia, and especially when hemorrhage is expected during surgery, red blood cell replacement to achieve a higher PCV is warranted before induction of anesthesia.

It should be remembered that chronic renal disease may be evident in animals presented for surgery unrelated to the urinary tract (e.g., ovariohysterectomy for pyometra).[33] Therefore, it is very important to include the BUN and creatinine values in the preoperative data base.

Anesthetic Management

A patient with urinary tract disease must be evaluated before anesthesia for the presence of multiple diseases. For example, a high percentage of animals in a survey of urinary bladder neoplasia also had renal, hepatic, or cardiac disease.[15] As indicated before, the patient in renal failure must be treated medically before anesthesia. Hypovolemia and aci-

dosis can be corrected before anesthesia. An obstructed urethra can usually be cleared with a minimum of sedation or anesthesia so that the animal can be treated for several days before a perineal urethrostomy is performed. Ketamine is not contraindicated in cats with urethral obstruction if urine flow can be restored. Highly variable urine output has been reported in cats after relief of urethral obstruction.[23] Small doses of ketamine must be used because pre-existing central nervous system depression reduces the anesthetic requirement. These patients may also have cardiovascular depression from hypovolemia and acidosis and are less able to tolerate anesthetic drug-induced depression. Various combinations are used to anesthetize the cat for urethral catheterization. These include ketamine, 2 mg/kg intravenously, or ketamine, 2 mg/kg intravenously with diazepam, 0.2 mg/kg. A combination that has proved satisfactory in my experience is 0.1 ml ketamine with 0.1 ml atropine and 0.1 ml promazine (or 0.05 ml acepromazine) mixed together in a 1-ml syringe. The combined drugs are slowly injected intravenously until adequate sedation is produced. Xylazine, 0.25 mg/kg, has been used for sedation with ketamine but must be used cautiously because of its severe cardiovascular depressant effect. The obstruction must be removed rapidly because increased urine production occurs within 30 minutes. Induction of anesthesia in an anesthetic chamber with halothane and maintenance of anesthesia with halothane by face mask and a nonrebreathing system provide good anesthesia with a rapid recovery. Halothane should not be used if the serum potassium concentration is elevated.

A lumbosacral epidural nerve block using 1 ml/5 kg of 2 per cent lidocaine is sometimes used instead of sedation or anesthesia.

The choice of anesthetic drugs for the traumatized patient depends on the nature of the damage. Operative fluid infusion should be sufficient to maintain a urine output of 1 to 2 ml/kg per hour. Fluid administration should be continued after anesthesia until oral intake of water is sufficient to maintain urine output. The traumatized patient must also be monitored closely for postoperative renal failure. It has been stated that measuring urine volume alone may not detect failure early enough, and creatinine clearance tests may be warranted.[24,77,85]

Anesthesia for the patient with chronic renal disease must be managed to prevent hypervolemia, hypotension, or hypoxemia. Drugs with marked effects on the kidney should be avoided, and drugs excreted through the kidney should be used in low doses. Low doses of thiopental, thiamylal, or ketamine can be used when some renal function is present. Narcotic or neuroleptanalgesic combinations, with or without halothane, are preferred when renal function is severely compromised.[36] The injectable drugs can be titrated slowly intravenously to effect. Small doses of phenothiazines, butyrophenones, or diazepam should be safe, provided that hypovolemia is corrected. Light surgical anesthesia with halothane or isoflurane has a minimal effect on the kidney. Induction with halothane by face mask without sedation is usually accomplished easily in older patients. Nitrous oxide is a useful adjunct unless the animal has a pneumothorax or severe pulmonary contusions. Hypoventilation does not adversely affect RBF until the arterial P_{CO_2} exceeds 70 mm Hg.[70] However, respiratory acidosis decreases cardiac function; therefore, controlled ventilation is advocated in these patients even when hypoventilation is mild. Epidural analgesia may be a satisfactory alternative for some procedures if the patient has an adequate blood volume and is not unduly anxious.[47]

1. Agoston, S., Kersten, U. W., and Meyer, D. K. F.: The fate of pancuronium bromide in the cat. Acta Anaesth. Scand. 17:129, 1973.
2. Bailie, M. D., Alward, C. T., Sawyer, D. C., and Hook, J. B.: Effect of anesthesia on cardiovascular and renal function in the newborn piglet. J. Pharmacol. Exp. Ther. 208:298, 1979.
3. Baratz, R. A., Philbin, D. M., and Patterson, R. W.: Urinary output and plasma levels of antidiuretic hormone during intermittent positive-pressure breathing in the dog. Anesthesiology 32:17, 1970.
4. Barr, G. A., Mazze, R. I., Cousins, M. J., and Koseh, J. C.: An animal model for combined methoxyflurane and gentamicin nephrotoxicity. Br. J. Anaesth. 45:306, 1973.
5. Bastron, R. D., and Deutsch, S.: Renal effects of anesthesia. In Anesthesia and the Kidney (Scientific Basis of Clinical Anesthesia). Grune & Stratton, New York, 1976.
6. Bastron, R. D., and Deutsch, S.: Anesthesia for the functionally anephric patient. In Anesthesia and the Kidney. Grune & Stratton, New York, 1976.
7. Bastron, R. D., Pyne, J. L., and Inagaki, M.: Halothane-induced renal vasodilation. Anesthesiology 50:126, 1979.
8. Berne, R. M.: Hemodynamics and sodium excretion of denervated kidney in anesthetized and unanesthetized dog. Am. J. Physiol. 171:148, 1952.
9. Berry, A. J.: Respiratory support and renal function. Anesthesiology 55:655, 1981.
10. Bevan, D. R., Archer, D., Donati, F., et al.: Antagonism of pancuronium in renal failure: No recurarization. Br. J. Anaesth. 54:63, 1982.
11. Brown, B. R.: Hepatic microsomal enzyme induction. Anesthesiology 39:178, 1973.
12. Brunson, D. B., Stowe, C. M., and McGrath, C. J.: Serum and urine inorganic fluoride concentrations and urine oxalate concentrations following methoxyflurane anesthesia in the dog. Am. J. Vet. Res. 40:197, 1979.
13. Burch, P. G., and Stanski, D. R.: Pharmacokinetics of thiopental in renal failure. Anesthesiology 55(3A):A176, 1981.
14. Burger, B. M., Hopkins, T., Tulloch, A., and Hollenberg, N. K.: The role of angiotensin in the canine renal vascular respose to barbiturate anesthesia. Circ. Res. 38:196, 1976.
15. Burnie, A. G., and Weaver, A. D.: Urinary bladder neoplasia in the dog; a review of seventy cases. J. Small Anim. Pract. 24:129, 1983.
16. Cadnapaphornchai, P., Taher, S. M., and McDonald, F. D.: Mechanism of dopamine-induced diuresis in the dog. Am. J. Physiol. 232:F524, 1977.
17. Cowley, A. W., Switzer, S. J., and Guinn, M. M.: Evidence and quantification of the vasopressin arterial pressure control system in the dog. Circ. Res. 46:58, 1980.
18. Deutsch, S.: Anesthetic management in acute and chronic renal failure. Vet. Clin. North Am. 3:57, 1973.
19. Deutsch, S.: Effects of anesthetics on the kidney. Surg. Clin. North Am. 55:775, 1975.
20. Don, H. F., Dieppa, R. A., and Taylor, P.: Narcotic analgesics in anuric patients. Anesthesiology 42:745, 1975.
21. Eknoyan, G., Wacksman, S. J., Glueck, H. I., and Will, J. J.: Platelet function in renal failure. N. Engl. J. Med. 280:677, 1969.
22. Feldman, S. A., Cohen, E. N., and Golling, R. C.: The excretion of gallamine in the dog. Anesthesiology 30:593, 1969.
23. Finco, D. R., and Cornelius, L. M.: Characterization and treatment of water, electrolyte, and acid-base imbalances of induced urethral obstruction in the cat. Am. J. Vet. Res. 38:823, 1977.
24. Finco, D. R., Coulter, D. B., and Barsanti, J. A.: Simple, accurate method for clinical estimation of glomerular filtration rate in the dog. Am. J. Vet. Res. 42:1874, 1981.
25. Fischer, D., Omlor, D., and Kreuscher, D.: Influence of ketamine anaesthesia on renal and cardiovascular functions in mongrel dogs. Internat. Urol. Nephrol. 11:271, 1979.
26. Frascino, J. A., O'Flaherty, J., Olmo, C., and Rivera, S.: Effect of inorganic fluoride on the renal concentrating mechanism. Possible nephrotoxicity in man. J. Lab. Clin. Med. 79:192, 1972.
27. Fray, J. C. S., Siwek, L. G., Strull, W. M., et al.: Influence of dietary sodium on renin activity and arterial pressure during anesthesia. Am. J. Physiol. 231:1185, 1976.
28. Ghoneim, M. M., and Pandya, H.: Plasma protein binding of thiopental in patients with impaired renal or hepatic function. Anesthesiology 42:545, 1975.
29. Gorman, H. M., and Craythorne, N. W. B.: The effects of a new neuroleptanalgesic agent (Innovar) on renal function in man. Acta Anaesth. Scand. [Suppl] 24:111, 1966.
30. Guyton, A. C.: Renal mechanisms for concentrating and diluting the urine and for urea, sodium, potassium, and fluid volume excretion. In Guyton, A. C. (ed.): Textbook of Medical Physiology. W. B. Saunders Co., Philadelphia, 1980.
31. Hall, L. W., and Clarke, K. W.: Anaesthesia of the cat. In Hall, L. W., and Clarke, K. W. (eds.): Veterinary Anesthesia. 8th ed. Balliere Tindall, London, 1983.
32. Handley, C. A., and Keller, A. D.: Changes in renal function produced by morphine in normal dogs and dogs with diabetes insipidus. J. Pharmacol. Exp. Ther. 99:33, 1950.
33. Hardy, R. M., and Osborne, C. A.: Canine pyometra: Pathophysiology, diagnosis and treatment of uterine and extra-uterine lesions. J. Am. Anim. Hosp. Assoc. 10:245, 1974.
34. Hartsfield, S. M.: The effects of acetylpromazine, xylazine, and ketamine on urine production in cats. Presented at the American College of Veterinary Anesthesiologists Annual Scientific Meeting, St. Louis, 1980.
35. Haskins, S. C.: Sampling and storage of blood for pH and blood gas analysis. J. Am. Vet. Med. Assoc. 170:429, 1977.
36. Haskins, S. C.: Anesthetic management for the end-stage renal failure patient. Calif. Vet. 33:13, 1979.
37. Haskins, S.: Ketamine and ketamine-sedative combinations in dogs. Presented at the American College of Veterinary Anesthesiologists Annual Scientific Meeting, Las Vegas, 1982.
38. Haskins, S. C., Peiffer, R. L., and Stowe, C. M.: A clinical comparison of CT 1341, ketamine and xylazine in cats. Am. J. Vet. Res. 36:1537, 1975.
39. Hayes, M. A., and Goldenberg, I. S.: Renal effects of anesthesia and operation mediated by endocrines. Anesthesiology 24:487, 1963.
40. Heavner, J. E., and Bloedow, D. C.: Ketamine pharmacokinetics in domestic cats. Vet. Anesth. 6:16, 1979.
41. Hembrough, F. B., Crump, M. H., Wilke, L., and Feher, R. C.: Plasma renin activity during controlled hemorrhage in the dog. Am. J. Vet. Res. 38:245, 1977.
42. Hunter, J. M., Jones, R. S., and Utting, J. E.: Effect of anaesthesia with nitrous oxide in oxygen and fentanyl on renal function in the artificially ventilated dog. Br. J. Anaesth. 52:343, 1980.
43. Hunter, J. M., Jones, R. S., Snowdon, S. L., and Utting, J.

E.: Cardiovascular and renal effects of enflurane and halothane in the dog. Res. Vet. Sci. 31:177, 1981.

44. Irestedt, L., Westermark, L., and Wahlin, A.: Blood circulation in the kidney of the cat under methoxyflurane (Penthrane) anesthesia. Acta Anaesth. Scand. 19:277, 1975.

45. Johnson, M. D., and Malvin, R. L.: Plasma renin activity during pentobarbital anesthesia and graded hemorrhage in dogs. Am. J. Physiol. 229:1098, 1975.

46. Kaka, J. S., and Hayton, W. L.: Pharmacokinetics of ketamine and two metabolites in the dog. J. Pharmacokin. Biopharm. 8:193, 1980.

47. Kanto, J., Vhnamaki, O., Gronroos, M., et al.: Blood glucose, insulin, antidiuretic hormone and renin activity response during caesarian section performed under general anaesthesia or epidural analgesia. Acta Anaesth. Scand. 25:442, 1981.

48. Klausner, J. S., Meunier, P. C., Osborne, C. A., et al.: Half-life of cephaloridine in dogs with reduced renal function. Am. J. Vet. Res. 38:1191, 1977.

49. Kolata, R. J., and Rawlings, C. A.: Cardiopulmonary effects of intravenous xylazine, ketamine, and atropine in the dog. Am. J. Vet. Res. 43:2196, 1982.

50. Kuzucu, E. Y.: Methoxyflurane, tetracycline, and renal failure. J. Am. Med. Assoc. 211:1162, 1970.

51. Leighton, K. M., Koth, B., and Wenkstern, B. M.: Autoregulation of renal blood flow: Alteration by methoxyflurane. Can. Anaesth. Soc. J. 20:173, 1973.

52. Leighton, K., and Bruce, C.: Distribution of kidney blood flow: A comparison of methoxyflurane and halothane effects as measured by heated thermocouple. Can. Anaesth. Soc. J. 22:125, 1975.

53. Loarie, D. J., Wilkinson, P., Tyberg, J., and White, A.: The hemodynamic effects of halothane in anemic dogs. Anesth. Analg. (Cleve.) 58:195, 1979.

54. Lundeen, G., Manohar, M., and Parks, C.: Systemic distribution of blood flow in swine while awake and during 1.0 and 1.5 MAC isoflurane anesthesia with or without 50% nitrous oxide. Anesth. Analg. (Cleve.) 62:499, 1983.

55. Mazze, R. I., Calverley, R. K., and Smith, N. T.: Inorganic fluoride nephrotoxicity: Prolonged enflurane and halothane anesthesia in volunteers. Anesthesiology 46:265, 1977.

56. Mazze, R. I., and Cousins, M. J.: Renal toxicity of anaesthetics: With specific reference to the nephrotoxicity of methoxyflurane. Can. Anaesth. Soc. J. 20:64, 1973.

57. Mazze, R. I., Cousins, M. J., and Barr, G. A.: Renal effects and metabolism of isoflurane in man. Anesthesiology 40:536, 1974.

58. McLeod, K., Watson, M. J., and Rawlins, M. D.: Pharmacokinetics of pancuronium in patients with normal and impaired renal function. Br. J. Anaesth. 48:341, 1976.

59. Messmer, K.: Hemodilution. Surg. Clin. North Am. 55:659, 1975.

60. Messick, J. M., Wilson, D. M., and Theye, R. A.: Canine renal function and VO₂ during methoxyflurane anesthesia. Anesth. Analg. (Cleve.) 51:933, 1972.

61. Middleton, D. J., Ilkin, J. E., and Watson, A. D. J.: Arterial and venous blood gas tensions in clinically healthy cats. Am. J. Vet. Res. 42:1609, 1981.

62. Miller, R. D., Way, W. L., Hamilton, W. K., and Layzer, R. B.: Succinylcholine-induced hyperkalemia in patients with renal failure? Anesthesiology 36:138, 1972.

63. Miller, E. D., Longnecker, D. E., and Peach, M. J.: The regulatory function of the renin-angiotensin system during general anesthesia. Anesthesiology 48:399, 1978.

64. Miller, E. D.: The renin-angiotensin system in anesthesia. In Brown, B. R. (ed.): Anesthesia and the Patient with Endocrine Disease. F. A. Davis Co., Philadelphia, 1980.

65. Montgomery, S. B., Jose, P. A., Slotkoff, L. M., et al.: The regulation of intrarenal blood flow in the dog during ischemia. Circ. Shock 7:71, 1980.

66. Montgomery, S. B., Jose, P. A., and Eisner, G. M.: The role of anesthesia and catecholamines in the renal response to mild hemorrhage. Circ. Shock 9:433, 1982.

67. Nagel, M. L., Muir, W. W., and Nguyen, K.: Comparison of the cardiopulmonary effects of etomidate and thiamylal in dogs. Am. J. Vet. Res. 40:193, 1979.

68. Ndiritu, C. G., and Weigel, J.: Hepatorenal injury in a dog associated with methoxyflurane. Vet. Med./Sm. Anim. Clin. 4:545, 1977.

69. Neiberger, R. E., Levin, J. I., and Passmore, J. C.: Renal effects of dopamine during prolonged hemorrhagic hypotension in the dog. Circ. Shock 7:129, 1980.

70. Norman, J. N., MacIntyre, J., Shearer, J. R., et al.: Effect of carbon dioxide on renal blood flow. Am. J. Physiol. 219:672, 1970.

71. Papper, S., and Papper, E. M.: The effects of preanesthetic, anesthetic, and postoperative drugs on renal function. Clin. Pharmacol. Ther. 5:205, 1964.

72. Parks, J.: Electrocardiographic abnormalities from serum electrolyte imbalance due to feline urethral obstruction. J. Am. Anim. Hosp. Assoc. 11:102, 1975.

73. Pedersoli, W. M., and Jackson, J. A.: Tetracycline, methoxyflurane anesthesia and severe renal failure in dogs. J. Am. Anim. Hosp. Assoc. 9:57, 1973.

74. Pedersoli, W. M.: Serum fluoride concentration, renal, and hepatic function test results in dogs with methoxyflurane anesthesia. Am. J. Vet. Res. 38:949, 1977.

75. Pedersoli, W. M.: Blood serum inorganic ionic fluoride, tetracycline and methoxyflurane anesthesia in dogs. J. Am. Anim. Hosp. Assoc. 13:242, 1977.

76. Philbin, D. M., and Coggins, C. H.: The effects of anesthesia on antidiuretic hormone. In Brown, B. R. (ed.): Anesthesia and the Patient with Endocrine Disease. F. A. Davis Co., Philadelphia, 1980.

77. Polzin, D. J., and Osborne, C. A.: Conservative medical management of canine chronic polyuric renal failure. In Kirk, R. W. (ed.): Current Veterinary Therapy VIII Small Animal Practice. W. B. Saunders Co., Philadelphia, 1983.

78. Prescott, L. F.: Mechanisms of renal excretion of drugs (with special reference to drugs used by anaesthetists). Br. J. Anaesth. 44:246, 1972.

79. Priano, L. L., and Vatner, S. F.: Morphine effects on cardiac output and regional blood flow distribution in conscious dogs. Anesthesiology 55:236, 1981.

80. Priano, L. L., and Vatner, S. F.: Generalized cardiovascular and regional hemodynamic effects of meperidine in conscious dogs. Anesth. Analg. (Cleve.) 60:649, 1981.

81. Priano, L. L.: Alteration of renal hemodynamics by thiopental, diazepam, and ketamine in conscious dogs. Anesth. Analg. (Cleve.) 61:853, 1982.

82. Priano, L. L.: Effects of high-dose fentanyl on renal haemodynamics in conscious dogs. Can. Anaesth. Soc. J. 30:10, 1983.

83. Riviere, J. E.: Checklist of hazardous drugs in patients with renal failure. In Kirk, R. W. (ed.): Current Veterinary Therapy VIII Small Animal Practice. W. B. Saunders Co., Philadelphia, 1983.

84. Schaer, M.: The use of regular insulin in the treatment of hyperkalemia in cats with urethral obstruction. J. Am. Anim. Hosp. Assoc. 11:106, 1975.

85. Shin, B., Isenhower, N. N., McAslan, C., et al.: Early recognition of renal insufficiency in post-anesthetic trauma victims. Anesthesiology 50:262, 1979.

86. Stern, A.: Drug metabolism in renal failure. Comp. Cont. Educ. 5:913, 1983.

87. Terragno, N. A., Terragno, D. A., and McGiff, J. C.: Contribution of prostaglandins to the renal circulation in conscious, anesthetized, and laparotomized dogs. Circ. Res. 40:590, 1977.

88. Theye, R. A., and Michenfelder, J. D.: Individual organ contributions to the decrease in whole body VO₂ with isoflurane. Anesthesiology 42:35, 1975.

89. Thorburn, G. D., Kopald, H. H., Herd, J. A., et al.: Intrarenal distribution of nutrient blood flow determined with krypton[85] in the unanesthetized dog. Circ. Res. 13:290, 1963.

90. Thurmon, J. C., Nelson, D. R., Hartsfield, S. M., and Rumore, C. A.: Effects of xylazine hydrochloride on urine in cattle. Aust. Vet. J. *54*:178, 1978.
91. Trim, C. M.: Anesthesia and the kidney. Comp. Cont. Educ. *1*:843, 1979.
92. Trim, C. M.: The effects of xylazine on renal function and blood glucose of horses. Presented at the American College of Veterinary Anesthesiologists Annual Scientific Meeting, New Orleans, 1981.
93. Tyrrell, M. F.: Metabolism of volatile anesthetic agents. *In* Scurr, C., and Feldman, S. (eds.): *Scientific Foundations of Anesthesia.* Year Book Medical Publishers, Inc., Chicago, 1982.
94. Vatner, S. F., and Smith, N. T.: Effects of halothane on left ventricular function and distribution of regional blood flow in dogs and primates. Circ. Res. *34*:155, 1974.
95. Wade, J. G., and Stevens, W. C.: Isoflurane: An anesthetic for the eighties? Anesth. Analg. (Cleve.) *60*:666, 1981.
96. Weber, P. C., Siess, W., Scherer, B., et al.: Prostaglandins and the renal circulation. *In* Herman, A. G., Vanhoutte, P. M., Denolm, H., and Goossens, A. (eds.): *Cardiovascular Pharmacology of the Prostaglandins.* Raven Press, New York, 1982.
97. Wickström, I., and Stefansson, T.: Effects of prolonged anesthesia with enflurane or halothane on renal function in dogs. Acta Anaesth. Scand. *25*:228, 1981.
98. Wickström, I., Stefansson, T., and Sundström, E.: Effects of renal function on serum fluoride level in dogs during and after enflurane anesthesia. Acta Anaesth. Scand. *25*:258, 1981.
99. Yamashiro, H.: Effect of pentazocine on renal blood flow. Br. J. Anaesth. *50*:133, 1978.
100. Yates, F. E., March, D. J., and Maran, J. W.: The adrenal cortex. *In* Mountcastle, V. B. (ed.): *Medical Physiology.* C. V. Mosby Co., St. Louis, 1980.

Chapter 195 Anesthesia and the Musculoskeletal System

L. Klein and A. M. Klide

PREANESTHETIC DRUGS

Anticholinergic Drugs

Atropine and other anticholinergic drugs have no clinically significant effect on skeletal muscle.[1,4]

Tranquilizers

Phenothiazine Derivatives

All the phenothiazines decrease motor activity; however, occasionally they may increase it. There is some controversy about the neuromuscular effect of the phenothiazine tranquilizers. Two major pharmacology texts[43,108] state exactly opposite effects.

There is conflicting evidence about phenothiazine tranquilizers and central cholinergic mechanisms (i.e., inhibition and potentiation of tranquilization by atropine sulfate). Phenothiazines may inhibit pseudocholinesterase but not true acetylcholinesterase activity.

Studies in chronic cat preparations showed that chlorpromazine modifies descending neural influences at both the spinal and supraspinal levels and diminishes patellar reflexes. It did not act at the neuromuscular junction.[59]

Benzodiazepine Derivatives

The benzodiazepines experimentally produce muscle relaxation. However, in humans in controlled trials they do not have any advantage over either placebos or aspirin.[44,138] These drugs have no presynaptic or postsynaptic action at the neuromuscular junction,[136] nor do they enhance the effects of competitive neuromuscular blocking agents at the neuromuscular junction. Their primary site of action is supraspinal and involves multisynaptic pathways. Specific benzodiazepine receptors are involved.[110] The molecular mechanism of action is enhancement of efficiency of activity of neurons using gamma-aminobutyric acid as a neurotransmitter, but the drugs themselves are not gamma-aminobutyric acid mimetic compounds.[26]

All of the clinically studied compounds in this family have the same pharmacological characteristics in common. The new compound, midazolam, produces muscle relaxation in dogs and cats. This drug does not affect the neuromuscular junction nor does it enhance or inhibit the action of competitive neuromuscular blocking drugs.[6] Zolazepam also has many properties in common with diazepam.[11]

Butyrophenone Tranquilizers

There is no specific information about the effects of these compounds on the musculoskeletal system other than that they are dopamine receptor blocking agents and that this property is the most likely cause for the occasional extrapyramidal reactions (dyskinesia) and parkinsonlike rigidity.

2,6, Substituted Diphenylamino Compounds

The two major drugs in this group are xylazine and clonidine.

Xylazine. This drug produces greater muscle relaxation than mephenesin. The muscle relaxation is not due to effects on the neuromuscular junction.[75] It is produced by inhibition of interneuronal transmission of impulses "at the central level of the central nervous system (CNS)."[17]

Clonidine. This drug is used to treat hypertension in humans and is of interest because it has many properties similar to xylazine.

Narcotics

Narcotics, especially in high dosages given rapidly to humans, may cause skeletal muscle rigidity.[109,122,125] The site of action for this response is not clear, but it does not appear to be at the neuromuscular junction or spinal reflex arc level.[122] Morphine-induced muscle rigidity in rats is due to a functional deficiency of dopamine in nigrostriatal neurons.[135] There are no published reports of narcotic-produced rigidity in dogs. However, this phenomenon occurs with etorphine but not oxymorphone in dogs. Etorphine produces marked muscle rigidity, which is relaxed by small doses of thiopental, in horses, ponies, and zebras. In clinically used doses, narcotics have no effect on neuromuscular transmission.[52,125]

PARENTERAL ANESTHETICS

Barbiturates

There is some controversy about the neuromuscular effects of barbiturates. In toxic dosages, barbiturates increase transmitter release at the neuromuscular junction and reduce the sensitivity of the postsynaptic membrane to the depolarizing effect of acetylcholine and decamethonium. The neuromuscular blocking effects of both a competitive muscle relaxant (*d*-tubocurarine) and a noncompetitive muscle relaxant (decamethonium) are enhanced during barbiturate anesthesia.[56] At the opposite extreme, thiopental and the barbiturates have little effect on the intensity and duration of action of the nondepolarizing relaxants.[41,126]

In general, barbiturates are alkaline, very irritating solutions that may cause inflammation and necrosis when injected perivascularly or subcutaneously. They are sometimes injected intramuscularly but this should be deep into a large muscle.

Saffan

A mixture of two steroid anesthetics, alphaxalone and alphadolone, may be given intramuscularly or intravenously to cats. It does not cause local irritation. Perivascular injection does not cause local irritation, necrosis, or sloughing.[5]

Cyclohexylamines

The drugs in this family, phencyclidine, tiletamine, and ketamine, all produce moderate to severe skeletal muscle rigidity. Ketamine is a relatively potent inhibitor of gamma-aminobutyric acid (GABA) binding.[17] Since benzodiazepine may produce muscle relaxation by enhancing the effect of GABA, it is not unreasonable to suspect that a drug that inhibits GABA binding would produce muscle rigidity. When methiothepin, an antiserotonin neuroleptic agent, is given before ketamine, muscle flaccidity occurs after ketamine administration instead of the expected rigidity.[17] Ketamine does not cause appreciable tissue irritation on intramuscular injection although it causes pain.

Etomidate

When given intravenously etomidate causes a high incidence of pain in humans, especially if injected into a small vein. Necrosis does not usually occur following intra-arterial injection.

INHALATION ANESTHETICS

Nitrous Oxide

Nitrous oxide does not have any effect on sensory receptors and nerve conduction.[102] In general, inhalation anesthetics depress spinal motor neurons so that they fail to respond to afferent stimulation. Areflexia and quiescent motor neurons result in skeletal muscle relaxation. Nitrous oxide may depress spinal reflexes but does not produce muscle relaxation; this difference between it and potent inhalants might be dose-dependent. It is a common clinical observation that during light anesthesia in humans with nitrous oxide and either barbiturates or narcotics that the abdominal muscles are "tight." Electromyography shows increased activity, particularly during the expiratory phase. In decerebrate cats, the segmental spinal reflex may be facilitated or inhibited by electrical stimulation of the brain stem reticular formation. An average of 60 to 65 per cent nitrous oxide completely blocks the reticular inhibition of spinal reflexes (both monosynaptic and multisynaptic). In contrast, the reticular facilitation is not abolished by nitrous oxide concentrations of up to 85 per cent. At the neuromuscular junction, nitrous oxide may increase the twitch response to indirect stimulation.

Volatile Anesthetics

The effects of volatile anesthetics on the neuromuscular junction are succinctly stated by Waud and Waud: "The effects of volatile anesthetics on both indirect and direct twitch responses have been studied for more than 60 years, with considerable variation in the results reported."[134] Volatile anesthetics depress neuromuscular transmission in amphibian and mammalian nerve-muscle preparations studied *in vitro*; the mechanism appears to be desensitization of the postsynaptic membrane.[134] In *in vivo* studies, volatile anesthetics in clinically used concentrations do not usually affect the twitch response to indirect stimulation. Only ethers have some minimal effect when given in high concentrations. Volatile anesthetics do, however, have an action on the neuromuscular junction as demonstrated by the increase in the average neuromuscular refractory period and the occurrence of fade on high-frequency tetanic stimulation.

Volatile anesthetics potentiate the effect of nondepolarizing muscle relaxants, both *in vitro* and *in vivo*. A study in isolated guinea pig nerve-lumbrical muscle preparations showed that the ED_{50} for *d*-tubocurarine was decreased by the following fractional amounts: methoxyflurane, 0.311; halothane, 0.334; isoflurane, 0.335; diethyl ether, 0.462; enflurane, 0.697. Thus, enflurane had the greatest potentiating effect on *d*-tubocurarine. Decreases in dose requirements may be explained by the effects of the anesthetics on chemosensitivity of the end-plate region.[133]

In humans, an increase in anesthetic dose by one minimum alveolar concentration (MAC) of halothane reduces the requirements for relaxants by about 60 per cent.[102] Isoflurane appears at least as potent if not more potent than enflurane in potentiating the action of neuromuscular blocking agents. When compared with halothane at equipotent concentrations (1.25 MAC) in humans, the median effective dose of *d*-tubocurarine during isoflurane anesthesia is 1.7 mg/m²—about one-third of that during halothane anesthesia, which is 5.6 mg/m².[91] Isoflurane is also more potent than halothane in increasing the action of pancuronium, gallamine, and succinylcholine.[92] The median effective dose of pancuronium during halothane anesthesia (1.25 MAC) is 0.49 mg/m² and during isoflurane anesthesia at equipotent concentration, 0.27 mg/m². With gallamine, the respective ED_{50}'s are 22.5 and 9.4 mg/m². As with halothane, increasing alveolar concentration of isoflurane is associated with decreasing median doses of *d*-tubocurarine and pancuronium. In humans, during 0.5, 1.0, and 1.5 per cent isoflurane anesthesia (with 70 per cent N_2O), the ED_{50}'S of *d*-tubocurarine are 2.40, 1.87, and 1.46 mg/m², and those of pancuronium are 0.6, 0.36, and 0.18 mg/m², respectively.[92]

Isoflurane potentiates the action of pancuronium more than it does that of *d*-tubocurarine. Increasing the alveolar concentration of isoflurane by 1.0 per cent reduces the requirement for pancuronium by 70 per cent, but that of *d*-tubocurarine by only 40 per cent.[93] The degree of potentiation of muscle relaxants by volatile anesthetics depends on the particular relaxant, species, and anesthetic used.[102]

NEUROMUSCULAR BLOCKING AGENTS

Neuromuscular blocking agents are valuable adjuncts to veterinary anesthesia, providing physical control of a patient in a number of situations. Examples of cases in which they are particularly useful include intraocular procedures in which eye movement interferes with surgery, animals with sensitive airways that make it difficult to gain ventilatory control, and prevention of movement in hemodynamically and anesthetically unstable animals in which a surgical level of anesthesia is difficult to achieve without significant cardiovascular depression. In the intensive care unit, neuromuscular blockade can aid in the management of severe trauma or animals requiring positive pressure ventilation under sedation.

Mechanisms and Characteristics of Neuromuscular Blockade

An understanding of the physiology and pharmacology of neuromuscular transmission is useful when monitoring clinical blockade. Several excellent review articles are available.[3,78,132] The classic mechanism of nondepolarizing (competitive) blockade is that the agent binds to the acetylcholine (ACh) receptor at the motor end-plate, preventing depolarization and contraction. The degree of weakness of the muscle depends on the number of fibers prevented from depolarizing. Response to a single nerve stimulus is progressively weaker as more fibers are affected by the drug. With rapid repetitive firing of the nerve (tetanic stimulation or voluntary isometric contraction), a large amount of ACh is released, temporarily displacing the blocking agent from the receptor and increasing the force of contraction. However, during this time, the ACh store is depleted, the blocking agent again binds to the receptors, and the muscle fatigues. This is observed or recorded as "fade" or fatigue of the muscle. During and immediately after the period of rapid nerve firing, ACh is mobilized within the motor nerve terminal so that the twitch response immediately after tetanus is enhanced (post-tetanic potentiation [PTP]). During slow repetitive firing (e.g., a train of four pulses at 2 Hz: $[T_4]$), the effects of ACh depletion (resulting in fade) can be observed without the complicating phenomena of increased contractility, drug displacement, and ACh mobilization that occur during tetanic stimulation.

There is some evidence that the nondepolarizing agents, especially gallamine and *d*-tubocurarine, act presynaptically, interfering with ACh mobilization and that they also enter and plug pre- and postsynaptic ion channels.[19,124]

Succinylcholine binds to the ACh receptor initially, causing membrane depolarization and disorganized contractions seen as muscle fasciculations, and remains on the receptor, preventing repolarization.

Weakness is proportional to the number of fibers affected. T_4 and tetanic fade do not occur, nor does PTP because ACh is not competitive with succinylcholine and does not displace it from the receptor. With repeated dosage or prolonged infusion, the character of succinylcholine block changes, and T_4 and tetanic fade occur (phase II block).

Tetanic fade may be due to a combination of pre- and postsynaptic effects. The relationship of twitch depression to fade varies with species, muscle type, specific blocking agent, and the time and type of anesthetic. Fade is more obvious in the limb muscles than on the face during nondepolarizing blockade in the horse and dog,[64] and fade increases with time.[69]

Antagonism of Neuromuscular Blockade

When an incomplete nondepolarizing blockade is present, (<80–90 per cent twitch depression), pharmacologic antagonism of the blockade can be achieved with cholinesterase inhibitors such as neostigmine, edrophonium, or pyridostigmine. These drugs decrease the rate of enzymatic destruction of ACh at the motor end-plate, allowing it to compete more favorably for the receptor, thereby antagonizing the blockade. They may also have presynaptic effects. Antagonism of pancuronium-induced T_4 fade is most pronounced with edrophonium, intermediate with neostigmine, and least rapid with pyridostigmine at equivalent degrees of recovery of the first twitch in the train.[32]

Dosage and Administration of Neuromuscular Blocking Agents

Because of the pronounced individual variation in sensitivity to and duration of action of nondepolarizing agents, it is often desirable to use an incremental method of administration to avoid overdose and subsequent difficulty with reversal. Half the dose expected to produce a 90 per cent twitch depression is a safe first dose, and additional doses based on the response to the first can be given at three- to five-minute intervals while monitoring neuromuscular function until the desired effect is achieved. When spontaneous recovery begins to occur, one-fifth to one-fourth of the total dose initially injected can be given to prolong the blockade. Agents such as pancuronium accumulate if multiple repeated doses are given. The rate of spontaneous recovery decreases with time. The newer drug, vecuronium, is nearly noncumulative with repeated dosage in dogs. In addition, vecuronium is short-acting. In experimental cats, an 80 to 90 per cent block recovered to 90 per cent control in 8 to 13 minutes, and in dogs, vecuronium had a duration of one-third to one-half that of pancuronium. Atracurium, another new nondepolarizer, should also prove to have short duration of action. In eight anesthetized dogs given a 100 per

cent paralyzing dose, twitch strength recovered to 50 per cent control in 9.5 to 29.3 minutes.[66] The nondepolarizing agents currently available have an onset time of two to five minutes, which is not rapid enough for emergency intubation. Significant hypercarbia and hypoxia develop before the jaws are sufficiently relaxed to permit tracheal intubation. Onset time can be shortened by giving very large doses, but recovery from these doses may be excessively prolonged.

Succinylcholine, the only depolarizing agent in clinical use, has a duration short enough that a dose expected to provide 100 per cent twitch depression can be given as an initial bolus. When spontaneous recovery begins, paralysis can be maintained by infusion or repeated injections. With prolonged administration, phase II block develops and may be long-lasting in some individuals. Phase II block is at least partially reversible with cholinesterase inhibitors, but reliable criteria for determining presence and degree of reversibility of phase II block have not been determined in dogs and cats. If a blockade initially established with succinylcholine is to be maintained, a switch should be made to a nondepolarizing agent because the dose of cholinesterase inhibitor providing optimum reversal of a phase II or mixed block is difficult to predict, and overdose can result in an intensification and prolongation of the blockade.

Monitoring During Onset and Maintenance of Blockade

Several hand-held peripheral nerve stimulators* are available. Most have capabilities for single twitch, 2 Hz (train-of-four), and tetanic stimulation. Several peripheral nerves are available for stimulation (Fig. 195–1). The ulnar nerve lies just medial to the elbow joint and can be palpated as it crosses the joint. Stimulation causes flexion of the carpal joint. The peroneal nerve can be palpated as it crosses the shaft of the fibula on the lateral aspect of the hind leg just distal to the stifle. Stimulation causes flexion of the tarsus and extension of digits. The facial nerve can also be used and the lip twitch observed.

It is best to observe responses to stimulation before blockade is established to ensure that electrodes have been placed properly and to allow control responses to be observed for reference during onset and reversal, but this is not always possible. Therefore, one should gain experience observing the responses in anesthetized, nonparalyzed animals prior to relying on them in assessing degree of blockade and reversal.

If a stimulator is not available, weakening of jaw tone or reflexes such as palpebral, knee jerk (and ear flick in the cat), can be used to detect onset of blockade provided they were present prior to admin-

---

*These are available from Dupaco, San Marcos, CA; J. H. Emerson Co., Cambridge, MA; Anesthesia Associates, Inc., San Marcos, CA; and Neuro Technology, Inc., Houston, TX.

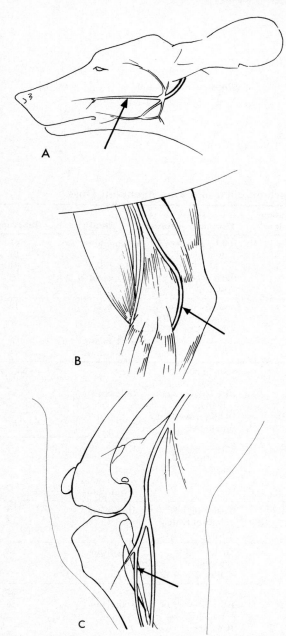

Figure 195–1. Location of peripheral nerves used to monitor neuromuscular blockade. *A,* Facial nerve. *B,* Ulnar nerve (right elbow, medial view). *C,* Peroneal nerve (left stifle, lateral view).

istration of the drug. It is undesirable to use respiratory insufficiency or apnea as an end-point, since hypercarbia, hypoxia, and acidosis develop during the onset of paralysis. Controlled ventilation should be instituted before or during administration of the first dose of the blocking agent. During maintenance of the block, electrical stimulation can be continued. Fade may continue to deepen with time even as twitch strength is recovering.[19,69] With succinylcholine blockade, fade also becomes more prominent with time during infusion or with repeated dosage. Reported dosages for commonly used blocking agents are shown in Tables 195–1 and 195–2.

Pharmacologic Antagonism of Nondepolarizing Blockade

Because depolarization block may occur with excessive administration of cholinesterase inhibitors, it is desirable to titrate reversal of blockade while using a stimulator or observing reflexes. Incremental doses of 10 to 20 µg/kg of neostigmine, or 200 µg/kg of edrophonium, the first increment preceded by 20 to 40 µg/kg of atropine, can be given at five- to seven-minute intervals. The equivalent dosage of pyridostigmine is approximately 40 to 80 µg/kg, but the onset time is somewhat longer. The most sensitive indicator of reversal is a sustained contraction in response to tetanic stimulation. Slight fade during T_4 stimulation is difficult to detect by observation or palpation and thus may not be a safe test for assessing adequate reversal. Most clinical monitors stimulate at frequencies of 50 or 100 Hz. Sustained contraction of limb muscles during five seconds of 50- or 100-Hz stimulation usually parallels adequate respiratory neuromuscular function, but since many other factors may depress respiration in anesthetized animals, respiration should be monitored carefully. A recently established or very deep blockade (>80 or 90 per cent) cannot always be antagonized completely. Residual blockade will wear off in time, during which respiration may have to be controlled. Adequacy of respiratory muscle strength can be assessed by twisting the neck of the rebreathing bag and observing the airway pressure gauge (−10 to 20 cm H_2O is adequate) during an inspiratory effort or by briefly occluding the endotracheal tube and observing the effort needed to overcome the obstruction. Jerky, incomplete, brief, or diaphragmatic efforts indicate a need to continue controlled ventilation or observe spontaneous respiration very closely until residual block has worn off.

Reversal Of Phase II Block

Since tetanic fade may occur after the first succinylcholine dose in some animals, a clear-cut criterion for evidence of phase II block is lacking. In a long-established succinylcholine block that is recovering slowly, a test dose of edrophonium 100 µg/kg preceded by atropine may be given. If improvement is noted, additional increments can be given. Edrophonium is suggested because it is shorter-acting than neostigmine or pyridostigmine and is less likely to cause a prolonged depolarization block.

Factors Affecting Sensitivity to Blocking Agents

Disease States

Any disease causing impaired neuromuscular transmission (myasthenia gravis, botulism) markedly increases sensitivity to nondepolarizing blocking agents.

TABLE 195–1. Potency and Duration of Neuromuscular Blocking Agents in Dogs

Drug	Dose (μg/kg)	Muscle	% Twitch Depression	Duration (Minutes)	Duration Criterion	Anesthetic	Reference
Atracurium	125	Gastrocnemius	97 ± 11.5	22 ± 2.8	100% recovery of twitch	α-Chloralose	61
	80 ± 7	Gastrocnemius	50	—	—	α-Cloralose	61
	200	Ulnar n. carpal flexors	100	24.5	100% recovery of twitch	Thiopental N_2O–O_2	66
d-Tubocurarine	130 ± 19	—	90	100 ± 19	Return to 50% control twitch from 3 × ED 90	Halothane	16
	350	Tibialis	95	—	—	α-Cloralose, morphine	7
Gallamine	500	—	100 (Apnea)	15–20	Spontaneous respiration	—	83, 54
	400	Tibialis	100	26 ± 7*	10% recovery of twitch	Halothane	38
				40 ± 11*	100% recovery of twitch		
Metocurine	63 ± 19	—	90	109 ± 21	Return to 50% control twitch from 3 × ED 90	Halothane	16
	100	—	95	—	—	α-Chloralose, morphine	7
Pancuronium	22 ± 3	—	90	108 ± 10	Return to 50% control twitch from 3 × ED 90	Halothane	16
Vecuronium	14 ± 3	—	90	42 ± 2	Time to 50% recovery of twitch after 3 × ED 90	Halothane	16
Succinylchloride	300	—	100	15–20	—	—	54
	400	Tibialis	100	22 ± 12*	10% recovery of twitch	Halothane	38
				37 ± 19	100% recovery of twitch		
	300	Gastrocnemius	100	25 ± 4†	50% recovery of twitch	Thiopental N_2O–O_2	65
				29 ± 5	100% recovery of twitch		

Mean ± SM except *Mean ± standard deviation or †not stated.

TABLE 195–2. Potency and Duration of Neuromuscular Blocking Agents in Cats

Drug	Dose (μg/kg)	Muscle	% Twitch Depression	Duration (minutes)	Duration Criterion	Anesthetic	Reference
Atracurium	100	—	90	Equal or slightly shorter than pancuronium	—	α-Chloralose	85
	250	Gastrocnemius	99 ± 1.43	29 ± 2.5	100% recovery of twitch	Halothane/α-chloralose/pentobarbital	61
	125	Gastrocnemius	54 ± 12.9	11 ± 2.2	100% recovery of twitch	Halothane/α-chloralose/pentobarbital	61
d-Tubocurarine	350 (100–1020)	Tibialis	95	—	—	α-Chloralose/pentobarbital	113
	200	Gastrocnemius	97 ± 2.7	20 ± 6.2	100% recovery? (not stated)	Halothane/α-chloralose	60
	130 ± 1	—	50	—	—	Halothane/α-chloralose	61
Gallamine	500	—	100 (apnea)	10–20	Spontaneous respiration	—	54, 83
	1200	Gastrocnemius	98 ± 2.6	24 ± 9.4	100% recovery? (not stated)	Halothane/α-chloralose	60
	830 ± 130	Gastrocnemius	50	—	—	Halothane/α-chloralose	61
Metocurine	25 (7–89)	Tibialis	95	—	—	α-Chloralose/pentobarbital	113
	40	Gastrocnemius	98 ± 2.6	42 ± 9.4	100% recovery? (not stated)	Halothane/α-chloralose	60
	20 ± 3	Gastrocnemius	50	—	—	Halothane/α-chloralose	61
Pancuronium	22	—	95	Not stated	—	α-Chloralose	114
	20	Gastrocnemius	80	15 ± 2	100% recovery? (not stated)	Halothane/α-chloralose	60
	22	Tibialis	88 ± 5	14 ± 2	50% recovery of twitch	Pentobarbital	34
	34	Tibialis	50	8.8 ± 2.3	100% recovery? (not stated)	α-Chloralose/pentobarbital	35
Vecuronium	35	Tibialis	88 ± 4†	8.3 ± 1.2	90% recovery of twitch	α-Chloralose/pentobarbital	10
	25–40	Tibialis	81 ± 6	9 ± 1	50% recovery of twitch	Pentobarbital	34
	38	Tibialis	50	3.9 ± 0.5	Not stated	α-Chloralose	35
	24 ± 3	Tibialis	50	5.0 ± 0.5	25% to 75% recovery of twitch	Isoflurane	79
Succinylcholine	75	—	100	—	—	α-Chloralose	85
	50–100	—	—	—	—	—	83
	1500	—	Apnea	4–5	Spontaneous respiration	—	53

Mean ± SEM except †Not stated.

Other disease states causing generalized weakness such as coonhound paralysis or cachexia due to chronic infection or malignancy, although not strictly increasing sensitivity to the agents, may reduce muscle strength so much that residual blockade after antagonism becomes clinically important. If neuromuscular blocking agents are used in these patients, respiration should be monitored carefully in the postanesthetic period.

Patients with severe burns are resistant to nondepolarizing agents.[81,137] The mechanism is not known. Upper motor neuron lesions,[46] denervation, and disuse atrophy[50] also decrease sensitivity to these drugs. Pseudocholinesterase levels may be elevated in hyperthyroidism, resulting in a resistance to succinylcholine.[3] Peripheral nerve injury can result in a spastic muscle response to succinylcholine,[80] as does malignant hyperthermia, which is discussed in Section XVIII.

Myotonic patients have abnormal responses to succinylcholine, manifested as severe, sustained spasms that may interfere with spontaneous and controlled respiration and result in severe postoperative pain. Responses to nondepolarizing agents are normal, but a tonic response to neostigmine may occur.[24,99]

Drug Effects

Antibiotics. Aminoglycoside antibiotics potentiate neuromuscular blocking agents and cause blockade by themselves. The mechanism is prejunctional, where they compete with calcium for binding sites, thereby reducing the quantal content of ACh released during nerve impulse. They may also stabilize postjunctional membranes. The effects may be subclinical in healthy animals but may become clinically important if exhaustion, debilitation, neurologic or muscular disease, electrolyte imbalances, anesthetics, depolarizing or nondepolarizing blocking agents, or cytotoxic drugs are present. Aminoglycoside blockade is poorly antagonized by cholinesterase inhibitors but can be at least partially antagonized with calcium and aminopyridines. Tetracyclines, lincosamides, and polymixin also enhance nondepolarizing blockade. The mechanism is not clear.

Polymyxin blockade is potentiated by neostigmine but can be antagonized by 4-aminopyridine.[74,88,119,121] Clinical situations in which antibiotic blockade is important include animals in which multiple routes of antibiotic administration have been used (e.g., perforated intestinal lesion in which oral and parenteral antibiotic therapy may be given in addition to peritoneal lavage). Neuromuscular and cardiovascular effects of antibiotics can be minimized if these factors are kept in mind and if total dosage, based on body weight, is not excessive. Furosemide potentiates nondepolarizing blockade.[97] Cimetidine in high concentrations potentiates antibiotic blockade.[18] Other conditions potentiating neuromuscular blockade are hypokalemia,[95] hypocalcemia, hypermagnesemia,[120] respiratory acidosis, metabolic alkalosis,[98] severe hypothermia,[94] and hemodilution.[117]

Other Effects

Cardiovascular Effects of Neuromuscular Blocking Agents

Succinylcholine may cause either vagal or sympathetic cardiovascular effects. In humans, profound bradycardia and hypotension can occur when a second dose of succinylcholine is given approximately five minutes after the first. The mechanism may be sensitization of the muscarinic receptor by succinylmonocholine. Atropine may protect against this response.[84,101,116] Succinylcholine produces arrhythmias and hypotension in anesthetized dogs.[127] In burned and severely traumatized patients and in those with denervation and other neurologic disorders including tetanus, succinylcholine administration can cause a massive K^+ release from muscle, resulting in hyperkalemia, cardiac arrhythmias, and cardiac arrest. The mechanism may involve a supersensitivity of the muscle membrane to cholinergic drugs, and the abnormal response can persist for weeks or months following the insult.[51] D-tubocurarine causes histamine release and sympathetic ganglionic blockade. Pronounced hypotension may occur when this agent is given to dogs and cats, and it is not recommended. Gallamine and pancuronium are vagolytic, and pancuronium may release norepinephrine. Dimethylcurarine and the newer agents, vecuronium and atracurium, have little or no autonomic activity at neuromuscular blocking doses.[7,15,22,31,35,60,86] In clinical practice, during potent inhalation anesthesia the results on heart rate and blood pressure are modest with gallamine and pancuronium.[38,111] Dimethylcurarine may cause hypotension in sick dogs.*

Placental Transfer

Although in humans, placental transfer of pancuronium occurs with umbilical cord–maternal blood ratios reaching 0.2 to 0.4 at 20 to 30 minutes after injection, clinical evidence of neuromuscular blockade in the newborn was lacking.[37] In the cat and ferret, fetal twitch depression could not be demonstrated when the mothers were given paralyzing doses of gallamine, succinylcholine, or pancuronium, and in dogs, injection of 30 to 100 times the maternal paralyzing doses of blocking agents caused weakness in some but not all puppies.[105,106] Based on these results, it seems safe to use neuromuscular blocking agents as adjunctive agents for cesarean delivery.

Administration of succinylcholine causes a transient increase in intraocular pressure, while nondepolarizers may cause a slight decrease.[72] Succinylcholine administration with halothane anesthesia has been associated with a high incidence of myoglobinuria in children,[112] and muscle pain is common after succinylcholine administration.

---

*Klide, A.: Unpublished clinical observations.

Excretion

The disposition of nondepolarizing blocking agents may be divided into two phases. The first is the dilutional and distributive phase during which onset of blockade occurs. This phase is usually complete by two to five minutes. During the second phase, plasma levels decrease due to redistribution and excretion. The kidney is virtually the only route of elimination for gallamine in the dog[40] and cat. In patients with marginal renal function, substantial blood levels of gallamine may remain for days, while cholestasis does not affect its duration. Pancuronium elimination occurs by both hepatic and renal excretion, and both cholestasis and renal failure prolongs its half-life.[2,123] Hepatic exclusion prolongs vecuronium blockade, but renal exclusion does not.[36,39]

Atracurium has the unique property of being unstable at physiologic pH and temperature, undergoing "hoffman elimination," thereby requiring neither the kidneys nor the liver for elimination. This drug may be the blocking agent of choice in patients with questionable liver and kidney function.[25]

Much of an injected dose of succinylcholine is inactivated by plasma cholinesterase before reaching the neuromuscular junction. Patients with lower cholinesterase levels have prolonged paralysis from single doses. Conditions that lower cholinesterase levels include administration of organophosphates (anthelmintics, insecticides, cytotoxic drugs, echothiophate eyedrops) and liver disease. In humans, prolonged succinylcholine block occurs in patients with atypical cholinesterase, which does not metabolize succinylcholine. This genetic variant has not been reported in the dog or cat. Succinylcholine blockade is not prolonged in renal failure. Untoward effects of neuromuscular blocking agents in the presence of neuromuscular or muscle disease are described below in the section on muscle disease.

In human anephric patients, neostigmine clearance is reduced and its action prolonged. "Recurarization" after pharmacologic reversal of pancuronium has not been documented.[27]

MUSCLE DISEASES AND THEIR EFFECTS ON RESPONSES TO ANESTHETICS

Myotonia

Myotonia is defined as an abnormal delay in muscle relaxation following active contraction. In *myotonia congenita*, only the skeletal muscles are involved. In *paramyotonia*, signs appear only upon exposure to cold. In *myotonia dystrophia*, skeletal, smooth, and cardiac muscles are involved as well as the central nervous and endocrine systems. Myotonic disorders suggestive of myotonia dystrophica have been described in dogs.[33,48,63,73]

The myotonic response can be triggered by voluntary contraction or electrical or mechanical stimu-lation. The neuromuscular junction responds normally to nondepolarizing blocking agents, but neuromuscular blockade as well as spinal and regional anesthesia does not prevent the myotonic response to direct mechanical stimulation. Succinylcholine is contraindicated in myotonic patients because it may precipitate violent spasms. The jaws and muscles of respiration are involved, and intubation and positive pressure ventilation may be impossible. Cholinesterase inhibitors given for antagonism of nondepolarizing blocking agents may also precipitate myotonic contractures, which can be minimized by titrating the reversal with repeated low doses rather than giving a large bolus.

Shivering in the postoperative period may make myotonia worse, as may agents causing muscle rigidity or twitching, such as ketamine. Patients with myotonic dystrophy are likely to be more at risk than normal patients for severe respiratory and cardiovascular depression during general anesthesia.[28,89,99]

Malignant Hyperthermia

Malignant hyperthermia[49] is a rare pharmacogenetic defect that has been well studied in humans and pigs in which volatile inhalation anesthetics, succinylcholine, and occasionally other stresses may precipitate accelerated muscle metabolism characterized by tachycardia, hypercarbia, hyperpnea, metabolic acidosis, hyperkalemia, hyperphosphatemia, and hyper- or hypocalcemia with or without generalized rigidity. Fatality rates in untreated humans and pigs approach 80 to 100 per cent. In survivors, grossly elevated creatinine kinase and aspartate aminotransferase (AST) (glutamic-oxaloacetic transaminase), as well as myoglobinuria indicate the severe muscle damage that occurs in this syndrome.

Isolated cases suggestive of this syndrome have been reported in the dog[8,9,77,87,115,118] and cat.[30] Definitive diagnosis of susceptibility is made by exposure of live muscle strips to caffeine and halothane. Affected muscle is unusually sensitive to these agents and contracts at lower concentrations than normal muscle.

Three of the five canine case reports suggestive of malignant hyperthermia involve greyhounds, indicating that this breed may be highly susceptible. Some fit coursing and racing greyhounds are affected by an exertional myopathy known as "cramp" or "pinched back" in which affected muscles, usually lumbar and gluteals, become firm and sensitive to palpation. Myoglobinuria may be present, and in some cases muscle damage is severe and the dog is permanently impaired due to the resultant loss of muscle mass. Various factors including spells of hot or cold weather, overexertion, and psychological stresses may predispose to the development of signs in susceptible individuals.[29,45,47,68] The relationship between stress and exertional myopathy to malignant hyperthermia in the greyhound has not been studied.

Successful treatment of malignant hyperthermia depends on early recognition and aggressive action. Early signs usually include tachycardia, hyperpnea, and an apparent lightening of the anesthetic level. Increased metabolism may be evident in a rapid consumption of the CO_2 absorbent in the breathing circuit. These signs are followed by an increase in skin and core temperature with or without muscle rigidity. The patient should be removed from the breathing circuit and given 100 per cent O_2 by positive pressure ventilation from a demand valve or breathing circuit free of contamination by volatile inhalants. Ice packs, surface cooling with cold water or alcohol on the skin over the large blood vessels (neck, groin, axillae), and iced intravenous fluids are helpful. Cold water enemas and gavage should be used if necessary but preclude further temperature monitoring. Sodium bicarbonate (2 to 4 mEq/kg) can be given empirically if acid-base status cannot be evaluated. Cardiac arrhythmias (usually ventricular tachycardia) may be treated with procainamide. The only definitive pharmacologic treatment for malignant hyperthermia is dantrolene. Effective dosage in pigs and humans ranges from 1 to 10 mg/kg. One greyhound was successfully treated with 0.7 mg/kg. Doses of 1 to 2 mg/kg can be given every ten minutes until body temperature begins to decrease and, if rigidity is present, relaxation occurs.

Known or suspected susceptible individuals can be pretreated with dantrolene, 1 to 2 mg/kg intravenously prior to anesthesia. If the parenteral preparation is not available, oral premedication can be given. The effective oral dosage in susceptible small animals is not known, but suggested dosage in humans is 4 to 7 mg/kg per day in divided doses beginning at least 24 hours before anesthesia.[49] Anesthetics and adjuncts considered safe for patients susceptible to malignant hyperthermia include barbiturates, steroid anesthetics, narcotics, nitrous oxide, nondepolarizing relaxants, and ester-linked local anesthetics.

Myasthenia Gravis

Myasthenia gravis is characterized by generalized weakness in which the number of ACh receptors at the motor end-plate is reduced. Studies of congenital myasthenia in dogs suggest that it is inherited as an autosomal recessive trait.[90] In acquired myasthenia gravis antibodies are formed against the cholinergic receptors.[104] Muscle strength can be improved in myasthenia gravis by administration of cholinesterase inhibitors such as neostigmine or, preferably, the longer-acting pyridostigmine. Extreme sensitivity to nondepolarizing relaxants occurs in myasthenia gravis patients, and these drugs should be avoided. Resistance to depolarizing agents may be present. Respiratory muscle weakness results in a tendency toward respiratory insufficiency, and obstruction and endotracheal intubation with assisted or controlled ventilation may have to be maintained well into the recovery period. Antibiotics with neuromuscular depressant effects enhance weakness in myasthenic patients.

Other Muscle Diseases

Thyroid myopathy, steroid myopathy, and glycogen storage disease are associated with cardiomyopathy. Poor ventricular function in these patients may make them poor anesthetic risks. Dogs with chronic polymyositis may have megesophagus and may regurgitate and aspirate during induction of anesthesia. In addition, the mouth may be difficult to open for intubation.

LOCAL ANESTHETICS

Infiltration

Effects on Muscle

Injection of local anesthetics at commonly used concentrations into muscle causes inflammation necrosis and atrophy. Regeneration occurs in two to three weeks.[13,23,55]

Epidural Analgesia

Effects on the Musculoskeletal System

Local anesthetics injected into the epidural space may produce blockade of autonomic nerves, sensory nerves, or motor nerves. In general, the autonomic fibers are the smallest in diameter and are blocked by a low concentration of local anesthetic. Sensory fibers are larger in diameter and require a higher concentration. The motor nerves are the largest in diameter and require the highest concentration of local anesthetic to produce a block. This generalization holds for myelinated fibers but not for unmyelinated C-fibers. These unmyelinated C-fibers may be very resistant to blockade by local anesthesics. When using epidural analgesia for surgery in small animals, it is usually desirable to provide muscle relaxation; therefore, the concentration of local anesthetic used is relatively high (i.e., 1.5 to 2 per cent lidocaine or 0.75 per cent bupivacaine). When these concentrations are used, blockade of autonomic, sensory, and motor nerves is produced in the blocked region. The effect of this block on muscle is profound muscle relaxation within the blocked area, an increase in blood flow, and an increase in the temperature of the overlying skin.

ANESTHETIC TECHNIQUES FOR SURGERY ON THE MUSCULOSKELETAL SYSTEM

Anesthesia and Muscle Surgery

There are not many surgical procedures that are done specifically to muscles except diagnostic muscle biopsy and occasionally, extensor-flexor muscle transposition in dogs in brachial plexus dysfunction and its variants.

Muscle biopsies may be done to aid in diagnosis of several muscle diseases. The anesthetically related problems vary depending on the patient's disease. The most common reason for biopsy is to aid in the diagnosis of the canine polymyositides. The primary anesthetic-related problem is that the animal's mouth can be opened only a small amount even under anesthesia, and therefore oral intubation may be difficult or impossible. One should be prepared to do a rapid tracheotomy if the animal has depressed or absent breathing during or after induction.

A very rare disease for which a muscle biopsy may be desirable is malignant hyperthermia. It is necessary to avoid all of the drugs listed above that are known to trigger the condition (see the above section on Malignant Hyperthermia for suggested management of these cases).

For extensor-flexor muscle transpositions, succinylcholine is avoided.

Anesthesia and Orthopedic Surgery

Relatively healthy patients can be handled for elective procedures in a routine manner with some additional consideration. When maintenance with an inhalation agent is planned, I prefer not to use a phenothiazine tranquilizer or xylazine. Phenothiazine tranquilizers are avoided because they cause a fall in circulating red blood cells and white blood cells and may produce hypotension.[58,76,107,131] Xylazine is avoided in patients who will be receiving an inhalation anesthetic, especially halothane. Xylazine enhances the increased sensitivity of the myocardium that halothane produces to the ventricular arrhythmogenic property of epinephrine.[100] Xylazine also produces a decrease in cardiac output and arterial blood pressure.[70]

Anesthesia may be maintained by injectable or inhalation anesthetics. In general, maintenance with inhalation agents is preferred. Maintenance with barbiturates can lead to prolonged recoveries in any species, especially cats and sighthounds (see below). Methoxyflurane is reported to provide more analgesia than halothane during and after anesthesia and more muscle relaxation than halothane. Experience in our clinic, however, suggests that the muscle relaxation obtained with reasonable levels of halothane anesthesia is satisfactory for most orthopedic procedures. If profound muscle relaxation is required, skeletal neuromuscular blocking agents such as pancuronium, epidural analgesia, or isoflurane may also be used. Halothane produces no clinically significant changes in respiratory rate, heart rate, or blood pressure in dogs or cats. Enflurane does not offer any advantages over the other inhalation anesthetics available and, at present, costs about six times as much as halothane on a kilogram per hour basis.

Isoflurane has some properties that may be useful in small animal orthopedics. Its blood gas solubility coefficient of 1.4 indicates that induction and recovery are faster than with halothane, it seems to provide a great deal of analgesia at relatively light levels of anesthesia, it provides marked muscle relaxation, and it seems to have a lesser depressant effect on the cardiovascular system than halothane. Its major disadvantages are cost and depression of ventilation. This respiratory depression often requires the use of positive pressure ventilation. Isoflurane does not sensitize the myocardium to the arrhythmogenic properties of epinephrine as halothane does.[62]

Special Considerations

Trauma

Traumatized animals can be challenging both anesthetically and orthopedically. As many life-threatening conditions as possible should be treated before the animal is anesthetized for definitive surgery. Some life-threatening conditions require anesthesia for immediate repair. Those areas related to muscle and bone will be discussed here.

An equally high incidence of thoracic trauma accompanies fore and hind limb fractures from motor vehicle injuries in dogs and cats. These injuries include pulmonary contusion, rib fractures, pneumothorax, pleural effusion,[130] hemithorax, and diaphragmatic hernia, all of which may impose limitations on respiratory function. Myocardial contusions can result in conduction disturbances and tachyarrhythmias. Careful physical examination and operative monitoring are necessary to detect these abnormalities so that they can be managed appropriately.

Antibiotics

Effects of antibiotics other than known toxic effects and the susceptibilities of the organism are too often ignored. These effects include increased anesthetic sleeping time, skeletal neuromuscular blockade, hypotension, and hyperkalemia from potassium penicillin.

Chloramphenicol can markedly prolong the sleeping time produced by barbiturates.[17] It can also prolong the sleeping time produced by ketamine in cats as well as that produced by a mixture of tiletamine and zolazepam in cats.[20,21]

Antibiotics in many chemical families, including aminoglycocides, polymixins, tetracyclines, and licosamides, may have a blocking effect on the skeletal neuromuscular junction, producing muscle weakness. Antibiotics may do this by themselves, and they may also have a marked effect when given with neuromuscular blocking agents even after the clinical effect of the neuromuscular blocking agent is gone. Cats are more susceptible than dogs in this respect.

Bleeding

There are many anesthetic techniques for controlling bleeding—some are easy and some are more complicated. Positioning the body so that the surgical site is placed higher than the heart can decrease bleeding significantly; however, careful monitoring to detect venous air embolism is required. Treatment of air embolism involves positioning the patient in left lateral recumbency and aspiration of the air from a right atrial catheter. Inappropriate mechanical ventilation can be used (i.e., increasing inspiratory time). Drug-related methods for decreasing surgical bleeding vary from deepening the level of anesthesia to use of drugs such as sodium nitroprusside, meperidine, or verapamil. Because production of induced hypotension often causes a reflex tachycardia that confounds attempts to produce hypotension a beta-adrenergic blocker such as propranolol is usually given to counteract the reflex tachycardia.

Fat Embolism

Fat embolism occurs relatively frequently in traumatized human patients and in human surgical patients. The most common etiologic factor associated with fat embolism is long bone fracture, especially of the femur and tibia.[12] The incidence after long bone fracture is probably about 5 per cent. In a study of 45 human patients with severe blunt trauma, the incidence of fat embolism syndrome was 13 of 45 (29 per cent).[82] Total hip replacement has been associated with fat embolism,[57,67] severe hypotension, and deep vein thrombosis.[129] The mortality rate in human patients who show signs of this complication has been variously reported as between 10 and 50 per cent.[12] The reason for presenting this subject here, even though the apparent incidence in animals is low,[42] is that the incidence has not been adequately investigated, and a traumatized animal is likely to be anesthetized during the period when signs of fat embolism are most likely to appear (i.e., within five days postinjury). It is unusual for initial symptoms to appear more than a week after injury.[12] A review of 100 human patients with fat embolism showed that 25 per cent showed symptoms within 12 hours of injury, 60 per cent within 24 hours, 75 per cent before 36 hours, and 85 per cent within 48 hours.[12] The signs may include the following: dyspnea, tachypnea, cyanosis, increased central venous pressure, pulmonary edema, decreased arterial oxygen tension, impairment of consciousness including restlessness, delirium, lethargy, stupor or coma, convulsions, hyperpyrexia, tachycardia, petechial hemorrhage, and embolic retinopathy.

The treatment of patients with fat embolism has two parts—treating the complication and treating the underlying disorder. There is only one group of treatments that is unequivocally and significantly effective—the proper management of respiratory failure. All other therapeutic maneuvers are either of much less importance or are of doubtful effectiveness. Supportive therapy of all dysfunctioning systems must be maintained. The various drugs used to treat the underlying condition include ethanol, heparin, adrenal corticosteroids, and dextran.[12]

One report showed that in three dogs insertion of the cement (used for holding artificial hips in place) into the femoral shaft resulted in medullary pressures of between 290 and 900 torr and the appearance of medullary contents in the lungs within 10 to 20 seconds. In five other dogs, pulmonary embolization was not detected when the rise in femoral medullary pressure was prevented by drilling a hole distal to the cemented area.[67] Total arthroplasty produced clearly identifiable lesions in previously healthy veins distant from the surgical site in dogs.[129] Continuous intravenous infusion of lidocaine (loading dose of 1.25 mg/kg followed by continuous infusion of 0.125 mg/kg/min) decreased the incidence of these lesions from 75 per cent to 30 per cent.[128] To avoid complications, epidural analgesia is a good anesthetic technique for total hip replacement.

If severe hypotension occurs during total hip arthroplasty, it must be treated. If the dogs are anesthetized with halogenated anesthetics, especially halothane, adrenergic stimulants may cause various ventricular arrhythmias. We treat hypotension with intravenous ephedrine 0.2 to 0.5 mg/kg or with phenylephrine given by continuous intravenous drip to effect (10 mg diluted in 250 or 500 ml of 5 per cent dextrose solution).

Skeletal Neuromuscular Blocking Agents

Succinylcholine should not be used in animals with burns, trauma, nerve damage, or neuromuscular disease (if used, caution and the capability for determining serial serum potassium levels are needed, as well as the ability to treat acute hyperkalemia).[14,96] (See previous section on Autonomic Effects Of Blocking Agents.) Nondepolarizing blocking agents may be used.

Epidural Analgesia

Epidural analgesia can be a useful technique, especially for the patient with multiple trauma and procedures involving muscle and bone, as long as certain facets of the technique are understood and dealt with. In healthy dogs, epidural analgesia of a level sufficient to perform abdominal surgery does not affect cardiovascular function,[71,103] but if the patient is hypovolemic, severe hypotension may be produced. If the epidural technique is chosen, vascular volume must be vigorously supported before and during the effect of the epidural. If fluid support is not adequate in maintaining blood pressure, a sympathomimetic agent may be needed (e.g., ephedrine 0.1 to 0.25 mg/lb intravenously or intramuscularly).

TABLE 195–3.   List of Drugs and Manufacturers

Generic Name	Brand Name	Manufacturer
Alphadolone	Saffan (a mixture of alphaxalone plus alphadolone)	Glaxo Greenford, Middlesex, England
Alphaxalone	Saffan (a mixture of alphaxalone plus alphadolone)	Glaxo Greenford, Middlesex, England
Atracurium	Tracrium	Burroughs Wellcome Co. Research Triangle Pk, NC 27709
Bretylium	Bretylol	American Critical Care McGaw Pk, IL 60085
Bupivacaine	Marcaine	Breon Laboratories, Inc. Sterling Drug, Inc. New York, NY 10016
Butorphanol	Stadol	Bristol Laboratories Syracuse, NY 13201
d-Tubocurarine	Tubocurarine USP	Eli Lilly & Co. Indianapolis, IN 46285
Dantrolene	Dantrium	Norwich-Eaton Pharmaceuticals Norwich, NY 13815
Diazepam	Valium	Roche Laboratories Nutley, NY 07110
Dimethyltubocurarine	Metubine	Eli Lilly & Co. Indianapolis, IN 46285
Diprenorphine	M50-M50	D-M Pharmaceuticals, Inc. Rockville, MD 20850
Dobutamine	Dobutrex	Eli Lilly & Co. Indianapolis, IN 46285
Dopamine	Intropin	American Critical Care McGaw Park, IL 60085
Droperidol	Innovar-Vet (a mixture of droperidol plus fentanyl)	Pitman-Moore, Inc. Washington Crossing, NJ 08560
Edrophonium	Tensilon	Roche Laboratories Nutley, NH 07110
Enflurane	Ethrane	Ohio Medical Products Madison, WI 53713
Etomidate	Amidate	Abbott Laboratories North Chicago, IL 60064
Etorphine	M99	D-M Pharmaceuticals, Inc. Rockville, MD 20850
Fentanyl	Sublimaze	Janssen Pharmaceuticals, Inc. New Brunswick, NJ 08903
Furosemide	Lasix	Hoechst Corp. Somerville, NJ 08876
Gallamine	Flaxedil	Davis & Geck Pearl River, NY 10965
Glycopyrolate	Robinul-V	A. H. Robins Richmond, VA 23220
Hexafluorenium	Mylaxen	No longer manufactured in U.S.
Hydrolazine	Apresoline	CIBA Summit, NJ 07901
Isoflurane	Forane	Ohio Medical Products Madison, WI 53713
Isoproterenol	Isuprel	Elkins-Sinn, Inc. Cherry Hill, NJ 08034
Ketamine	Vetalar	Parke-Davis Morris Plains, NJ 07950
Levallorphan	Lorfan	Roche Laboratories Nutley, NJ 07110
Lidocaine	Xylocaine	Astra Worcester, MA 01606
Meperidine	Demerol	Winthrop Laboratories New York, NY 10016
Methadone	Dolophine	Eli Lilly & Co. Indianapolis, IN 46285
Methohexital	Brevital	Eli Lilly & Co. Indianapolis, IN 46285
Methoxyflurane	Metofane	Pitman-Moore, Inc. Washington Crossing, NJ 08560
Metocurine	Metubine iodide	Eli Lilly & Co. Indianapolis, IN 46285
Metrizamide	Amipaque	Winthrop Laboratories New York, NY 10016

Table continued on following page

TABLE 195–3.   **List of Drugs and Manufacturers** (*Continued*)

Generic Name	Brand Name	Manufacturer
Nalbuphine	Nubain	Endo Pharmaceuticals, Inc. Manati, Puerto Rico 00701 subsidiary of Dupont Co.
Naloxone	Narcan	Pitman-Moore, Inc. Washington Crossing, NJ 08560
Neostigmine	Prostigmin	Roche Laboratories Nutley, NJ 07110
Oxymorphone	Numorphan	Endo Pharmaceuticals, Inc. Manati, Puerto Rico 00701
Pancuronium	Pavulon	Organon Pharmaceuticals West Orange, NJ 07052
Pentazocine	Talwin V	Winthrop Laboratries New York, NY 10016
Phenylephrine	Neo-synephrine	Winthrop Laboratories New York, NY 10016
Procainamide	Pronestyl	E. R. Squibb & Sons, Inc. Princeton, NJ 08540
Promazine	Sparine	Wyeth Laboratories, Inc. Philadelphia, PA 19101
Propranolol	Inderal	Ayerst New York, NY 10017
Pyridostigmine	Regonol	Organon Pharmaceuticals West Orange, NJ 07052
	Mestinon	Roche Laboratories Nutley, NJ 07110
Quinidine gluconate		Eli Lilly & Co. Indianapolis, IN 46206
Sodium nitroprusside	Nipride	Roche Laboratories Nutley, NJ 07110
Succinylcholine	Anectine	Burroughs Wellcome Co. Research Triangle Pk, NC 27709
Thiamylal	Surital	Parke-Davis Morris Plains, NJ 07950
Thiopental	Pentothal	Abbott Laboratories North Chicago, IL 60064
Tiletamine	Telazol (a mixture of tiletamine plus zolazepam)	Parke-Davis Morris Plains, NJ 07950
Trimethaphan	Arfonad	Roche Laboratories Nutley, NJ 07110
Verapamil	Isoptin	Knoll Pharmaceutical Co. Whippany, NJ 07981
Vecuronium (NC-45)	Norcuron	Organon Pharmaceuticals West Orange, NJ 07052
Xylazine	Rompun	Haver-Lockart Shawnee, KS 66201
Zolazepam	Telazol (a mixture of tiletamine plus zolazepam)	Parke-Davis Morris Plains, NJ 07950

To avoid precipitating a crisis when using an epidural in a severely traumatized patient, an intramuscular injection of ephedrine can be given immediately after the epidural injection. Further treatment of hypotension is given as needed. Local anesthetics most commonly used are lidocaine (2 per cent) and bupivacaine (0.75 per cent). The onset of both is rapid, usually within five minutes. The duration of surgical analgesia expected is: lidocaine 2 per cent without epinephrine, 0.75 to 1 hour; lidocaine 2 per cent with epinephrine, 1.25 to 1.5 hours; bupivacaine 0.75 per cent without epinephrine, 3 hours. In some procedures with unpredictable durations, a continuous epidural may be used. A catheter is placed in the epidural space through which repeated injections of local anesthetic can be made throughout the surgical procedure. The dosage requirements for this technique are: lidocaine (2 per cent with epinephrine), repeat one-half the total initial dose every hour; bupivacaine (0.75 per cent without epinephrine), repeat one-half the original dose every two hours. The initial dosage used is: lidocaine (2 per cent with epinephrine), 1 ml per 5 kg body weight to block the hind limbs or 1 ml per 3.5 kg for an abdominal block; bupivacaine (0.75 per cent without epinephrine), 1 ml per 4 kg, especially in very thin dogs. These dosages may be increased with emaciation or decreased with obesity.

1. Adams, H. R.: Cholinergic pharmacology: Autonomic drugs. *In* Booth, N. H., and McDonald, L. E. (eds.): *Veterinary Pharmacology.* Iowa State University Press, Ames, 1982.

2. Agoston, S., and Kersten, U. W.: The fate of pancuronium bromide in the cat. Acta Anaesth. Scand. *17*:267, 1973.

3. Ali, H. H., and Savarese, J. J.: Monitoring of neuromuscular function. Anesthesiology *45*:216, 1976.

4. Ambache, N.: The use and limitations of atropine for pharmacological studies on autonomic effectors. Pharmacol. Rev. *7*:467, 1955.

5. Anonymous: *A Glaxo Guide To Saffan.* Glaxo, Middlesex, England, 1974, p. 29.

6. Anonymous: *Investigational Drug Brochure.* Hoffman-La Roche, Nutley, N. J., June, 1977.

7. Antonio, R. P., Philbin, D. M., and Savarese, J. J.: Comparative hemodynamic effects of *d*-tubocurarine and metocurine in the dog. Anesthesiology *51*:S281, 1979.

8. Bagshaw, R. J., Cox, R. H., Knight, D. H., and Detweiler, D. K.: Malignant hyperthermia in a greyhound. J. Am. Vet. Med. Assoc. *172*:61, 1978.

9. Bagshaw, R. J., Cox, R. H., and Rosenberg, H.: Dantrolene treatment of malignant hyperthermia. J. Am. Vet. Med. Assoc. *178*:1029, 1981.

10. Baird, W. L. M., Bowman, W. C., and Kerr, W. J.: Some actions of ORG NC45 and of edrophonium in the anaesthetized cat and in man. Br. J. Anaesth. *54*:375, 1982.

11. Baukema, J., Okerholm, R. A., and Glasko, A. J.: The comparative metabolism of zolazepam in rat, dog, and monkey. Res. Commun. Chem. Pathol. Pharmacol. *10*:227, 1975.

12. Beck, J. P., and Collins, J. A.: Theoretical and clinical aspects of post-traumatic fat embolism syndrome. Instr. Course Lect. *22*:38, 1973.

13. Benort, P. W., and Belt, W. D.: Some effects of local anesthetic agents on skeletal muscle. Exp. Neurol. *34*:264, 1972.

14. Birch, A. A., Jr., et al.: Changes in serum potassium response to succinylcholine following trauma. J. Am. Med. Assoc. *210*:490, 1969.

15. Booij, L. H. D. J., Edwards, R. P., Sohn, Y. J., and Miller, R. D.: Cardiovascular and neuromuscular effects of Org NC45, pancuronium, metocurine and d-tubocurarine in dogs. Anesth. Analg. *59*:26, 1980.

16. Booij, L. H. D. J., Edwards, R. P., Sohn, Y. J., and Miller, R. D.: Comparative cardiovascular and neuromuscular effects of ORG NC45, pancuronium, metocurine and *d*-tubocurarine. Anesth. Analg. *19*:26, 1980.

17. Booth, N. H., and McDonald, L. E.: *Veterinary Pharmacology and Therapeutics.* 5th ed., The Iowa State University Press, Ames, Iowa, 1982.

18. Bossa, R., Benvenuti, C., and Galatulas, I.: Cimetidine increases the neuromuscular blocking activity of aminoglycoside antibiotics. Agents Actions *12*:273, 1982.

19. Bowman, W. C.: Prejunctional and postjunctional cholinoceptors at the neuromuscular junction. Anesth. Analg. *59*:935, 1980.

20. Bree, M. M., Park, J. S., and Short, C. E.: Responses of cats to ketamine-antibiotic combinations. Vet. Med./Sm. Anim. Clin. *70*:1309, 1975.

21. Bree, M. M., Park, J. S., Short, C. E., et al.: Effect of chloramphenicol on tilazol (CI-744) anesthesia in cats. Vet. Med./Sm. Anim. Clin. *71*:764, 1976.

22. Brown, B. R., and Crout, J. R.: The sympathomimetic effect of gallamine on the heart. J. Pharmacol. Exp. Ther. *172*:266, 1970.

23. Brun, A.: Effects of procaine, Carbocain, and Xylocaine on cutaneous muscle in rabbits and mice. Acta Anesth. Scand. *3*:59, 1959.

24. Buzello, W., Krieg, N., and Schlickewei, A.: Hazards of neostigmine in patients with neuromuscular disorder. Br. J. Anaesth. *54*:529, 1982.

25. Chapple, D. J., and Clark, J. S.: Pharmacological action of breakdown products of atracurium and related substances. Br. J. Anaesth. *55*:11S, 1983.

26. Costa, E., and Guidotti, A.: Molecular mechanisms in the receptor action of benzodiazepines. Ann. Rev. Pharmacol. Toxicol. *19*:531, 1979.

27. Cronnelly, R., Stanski, D. R., Miller, R. D., et al.: Renal function and the pharmacokinetics of neostigmine in anesthetized man. Anesthesiology *51*:222, 1979.

28. Dalal, F. Y., Bennett, E. J., Raj, P. P., and Lee, D. G.: Dystrophica myotonia: A multisystem disease. Can. Anaesth. Soc. J. *19*:436, 1972.

29. Davis, P. E., and Paris, R.: Azoturia in a greyhound: Clinical pathology aids to diagnosis. J. Small. Anim. Pract. *15*:43, 1974.

30. DeJong, R. H., Heavner, J. E., and Amory, D. W.: Malignant hyperthermia in the cat. Anesthesiology *41*:608, 1974.

31. Domenech, J. S., Garcia, R. C., Sasiain, J. M. R., et al.: Pancuronium bromide: An indirect sympathomimetic agent. Br. J. Anaesth. *48*:1143, 1976.

32. Donati, F., Ferguson, A., and Bevan, D. R.: Twitch depression and train-of-four ratio after antagonism of pancuronium with edrophonium, neostigmine or pyridostigmine. Anesth. Analg. *62*:314, 1983.

33. Duncan, I. D., and Griffiths, I. R.: Myotonia in canine Cushing's disease. Vet. Rec. *100*:30, 1977.

34. Durant, N. N., Houwertjes, M. C., and Crul, J. F.: Comparison of the neuromuscular blocking properties of ORG NC45 and pancuronium in the rat, cat and rhesus monkey. Br. J. Anaesth. *52*:723, 1980.

35. Durant, N. N., Marshall, I. G., Savage, D. S., et al.: The neuromuscular and autonomic blocking activities of pancuronium, Org NC45, and other pancuronium analogues, in the cat. J. Pharm. Pharmacol. *31*:831, 1979.

36. Duvaldestin, P., Berger, J. L., Videcoq, M., and Desmont, J. M.: Pharmacokinetics and pharmacodynamics of Org NC45 in patients with cirrhosis. Anesthesiology *57*:A238, 1982.

37. Duvaldestin, P., Demetriou, M., Henzel, D., et al.: The placental transfer of pancuronium and its pharmacokinetics during caesarean section. Acta Anaesth. Scand. *22*:327, 1978.

38. Evans, A. T., Anderson, L. K., Eyster, G. E., and Sawyen, D. C.: Cardiovascular effects of gallamine triethiodide and succinylcholine chloride during halothane anesthesia in the dog. Am. J. Vet. Res. *38*:329, 1977.

39. Fahey, M. R., Morris, R. B., Miller, R. D., et al.: Pharmacokinetics of Org NC45 (Norcuron) in patients with and without renal failure. Br. J. Anaesth. *53*:1049, 1981.

40. Feldman, S. A., Cohen, E. N., and Golling, B. A.: The excretion of gallamine in the dog. Anesthesiology *30*:593, 1969.

41. Foldes, F. F., Swerdlow, M., and Seker, E. S.: *Narcotics and Narcotic Antagonists.* Charles C Thomas, Springfield, 1964.

42. Furneaux, R. W.: Two cases of fat embolism in the dog. J. Am. Anim. Assoc. *10*:45, 1974.

43. Gershon, S., Neubauer, H., and Sundland, D. M.: Interaction between some anticholinergic agents and phenothiazines. Clin. Pharmacol. Ther. *6*:749, 1965.

44. Gilman, A. G., Goodman, L. S., and Gilman, A.: *The Pharmacological Basis of Therapeutics.* 6th ed. Macmillan Publishing Co., New York, 1980.

45. Gowing, G. M.: "Pinched back," an azoturia-like condition in coursing greyhounds. Southwest. Vet. *28*:183, 1964.

46. Graham, D. H.: Monitoring neuromuscular block may be unreliable in patients with upper-motor-neurom lesions. Anesthesiology *52*:74, 1980.

47. Graham, S., and Lomas, G.: Myoglobinuria in a racing greyhound. Aust. Vet. Pract. *33*:258, 1976.

48. Griffiths, I. R., and Duncan, I. D.: Myotonia in the dog: A report of four cases. Vet. Rec. *93*:184, 1973.

49. Gronert, G. A.: Malignant hyperthermia. Anesthesiology *53*:395, 1980.

50. Gronert, G. A.: Metocurine dose-response in muscle with disuse atrophy. International Symposium on Relaxants, Boston, MA, August 24, 1983.

51. Gronert, G. A., and Theye, R. A.: Pathophysiology of hyperkalemia induced by succinylcholine. Anesthesiology 43:89, 1975.

52. Gudnason, H. V., and Eger, E. E.: Influence of morphine and muscle relaxants in anesthetized dogs. South. Med. J. 62:1394, 1969.

53. Hall, L. W.: Relaxant drugs in small animal anesthesia. Proceedings of 1st International Congress of Veterinary Anaesthesia, Cambridge, England. Assoc. Vet. Anaesth. Great Britain and Ireland 10 (Suppl.): 144, 1982.

54. Hall, L. W., and Clarke, K. W.: Veterinary Anaesthesia 8th ed. Baillière Tindall, London, 1983.

55. Hall-Craggs, E. C. B.: Rapid degeneration and regeneration of a whole skeletal muscle following treatment with bupivacaine (Marcain). Exp. Neurol. 43:349, 1974.

56. Harvey, S. C.: Hypnotics and sedatives. In Gilman, A. G., Goodman, L. S., and Gilman, A. (eds.): The Pharmacological Basis of Therapeutics. 6th ed. Macmillan Publishing Co., New York, 1980.

57. Herndon, J. H., Bechtol, C. O., and Crickenberger, D. P.: Fat embolism during total hip replacement. J. Bone Joint Surg. 56A:1350, 1974.

58. Hoe, C. M., and Wilkinson, J. S.: A diluting effect of chorpromazine hydrochloride on the circulating blood of dogs. Vet. Rec. 69:734, 1957.

59. Hudson, R. D.: Effects of chlorpromazine on motor reflexes of the chronic spinal cat. Arch. Int. Pharmacodyn. 174:442, 1968.

60. Hughes, R., and Chapple, D. J.: Effects of non-depolarizing neuromuscular blocking agents on peripheral autonomic mechanisms in cats. Br. J. Anaesth. 48:59, 1976.

61. Hughes, R., and Chapple, D. J.: The pharmacology of atracurium, A new competitive neuromuscular blocking agent. Br. J. Anesth. 53:31, 1981.

62. Joas, T. A., and Stevens, W. C.: Comparison of the arrhythmic doses of epinephrine during Forane, halothane and fluroxene anesthesia in dogs. Anesthesiology 35:48, 1971.

63. Jones, B. R., Anderson, L. J., Barnes, G. R. G., et al.: Myotonia in related chow chow dogs. N. Z. Vet. J. 25:220, 1977.

64. Jones, R. S.: The experimental investigations of muscle relaxants in small animals. Proceedings of 1st International Congress on Veterinary Anaesthesia, Cambridge, England. Assoc. Vet. Anaesth. Great Britain and Ireland 10 (Suppl.) 156, 1982.

65. Jones, R. S., Heckmann, R., and Wuersch, W.: Observations on the duration of action of suxamethonium in the dog. Br. Vet. J. 134:521, 1978.

66. Jones, R. S., Hunter, J. M., and Utting, J. E.: Neuromuscular blocking action of atracurium in the dog and its reversal by neostigmine. Res. Vet. Sci. 34:173, 1983.

67. Kallos, T., et al.: Intramedullary pressure and pulmonary embolism of femoral medullary contents in dogs during insertion of bone cement and a prosthesis. J. Bone Joint Surg. 56A:1363, 1974.

68. Kirk, H.: "Cramp" in racing greyhounds. Vet. Rec. 54:425, 1942.

69. Klein, L., Hopkins, J., and Rosenberg, H.: Different relationship of train-of-four to twitch and tetanus for vecuronium, pancuronium, and gallamine. Anesthesiology 59:A275, 1983.

70. Klide, A. M., Calderwood, H. W., and Soma, L. R.: Cardiopulmonary effects of xylazine in dogs. Am. J. Vet. Res. 36:931, 1975.

71. Klide, A. M., and Penney, B. E.: Unpublished data, 1978.

72. Konchigeri, H. N., Lee, Y. E., and Venugopal, K.: Effect of pancuronium on intraocular pressure changes induced by succinylcholine. Can. Anaesth. Soc. J. 26:479, 1979.

73. Kramer, J. W., Hegreberg, G. A., Bryan, G. M., et al.: A muscle disorder of labrador retrievers characterized by deficiency of type II muscle fibers. J. Am. Vet. Med. Assoc. 169:817, 1976.

74. Krieg, N., Rutten, M. J., Crul, J. F., and Booij, L. H. D.

75. J.: Preliminary review of the interactions of Org NC45 with anaesthetics and antibiotics in animals. Br. J. Anaesth. 52:33S, 1980.

75. Kroneberg, G., et al.: The pharmacology of 2- (2,6-dimethylphenylamino) -4H -5, 6-dehydro-1, 3-thiazine (BAY 1470). Naunyn-Schmeidebergs Arch. Pharmak. Exp. Pathol. 256:257, 1967.

76. Lang, S. M., Eglen, R. M., and Henry, A. C.: Acetylpromazine administration: Its effect on canine hematology. Vet. Rec. 105:397, 1979.

77. Leary, S. L., Anderson, L. C., Manning, P. J., et al.: Recurrent malignant hyperthermia in a greyhound. J. Am. Vet. Med. Assoc. 182:521, 1983.

78. Lee, C., and Katz, R. L.: Neuromuscular pharmacology: A clinical update and commentary. Br. J. Anaesth. 52:173, 1980.

79. Lee, C., Tran, B. K., Durant, N., and Nguyen, N. B.: Vecuronium, isoflurane and hypotensive anesthesia in the cat. Anesthesiology 59:A271, 1983.

80. Lee, C., Yang, E., and Katz, R. L.: Focal contracture following injection of succinylcholine in patients with peripheral nerve injury. Can. Anaesth. Soc. J. 24:475, 1977.

81. Leibel, W. S., Jeevendramartyn, J. A., Szyfelbein, S. K., et al.: Elevated plasma binding cannot account for the burn-related d-tubocurarine hyposensitivity. Anesthesiology 54:378, 1981.

82. Lepisto, P., et al.: Fat embolism in severely injured patients. Ann. Chir. Gynaecol. Fenniae 64:198, 1975.

83. Lumb, W. V., and Jones, E. W.: Veterinary Anesthesia. Lea & Febiger, Philadelphia, 1973.

84. Magee, D. A., Sweet, P. T., and Holland, A. J. C.: Cardiac effects of self-taming of succinylcholine and repeated succinylcholine administration. Can. Anaesth. Soc. J. 29:577, 1982.

85. Marshall, I. G.: Comparison of atracurium and vecuronium in the cat. Presented at the International Symposium on Relaxants Boston, August 24–25, 1983.

86. Marshall, R. J., McGrath, J. C., Miller, R. D., et al.: Comparison of the cardiovascular actions of Org NC45 with those produced by other non-depolarizing neuromuscular blocking agents in experimental animals. Br. J. Anaesth. 52:21S, 1980.

87. McGrath, C. J., Crimi, A. J., and Ruff, J.: Malignant hyperthermia in dogs. Vet. Med. Small Anim. Clin. 77:218, 1982.

88. McIndewar, E. C., and Marshall, R. J.: Interactions between the neuromuscular blocking drug Org NC45 and some anaesthetic, analgesic and antimicrobial agents. Br. J. Anaesth. 53:785, 1981.

89. Meyers, M. B., and Barash, P. G.: Cardiac decompensation during enflurane anesesthesia in a patient with myotonia atrophics. Anesth. Analg. 55:433, 1976.

90. Miller, L. M., Lennon, V. A., Lambert, E. H., et al.: Congenital myasthenia gravis in 13 smooth fox terriers. J. Am. Vet. Med. Assoc. 182:694, 1983.

91. Miller, R. D., Eger, E. I., Way, W. L., et al.: Comparative neuromuscular effects of forane and halothane alone and in combination with d-tubocurarine in man. Anesthesiology 35:38, 1971.

92. Miller, R. D., et al.: Comparative neuromuscular effects of pancuronium, gallamine and succinylcholine during forane and halothane anesthesia in man. Anesthesiology 35:509, 1971.

93. Miller, R. D., et al.: The dependence of pancuronium and d-tubocurarine induced neuromuscular blockades on alveolar concentrations of halothane and forane. Anesthesiology 37:573, 1972.

94. Miller, R. D., and Roderick, L. L.: Pancuronium-induced neuromuscular blockade, and its antagonism by neostigmine, at 29, 37, and 41°C. Anesthesiology 46:333, 1977.

95. Miller, R. D., and Roderick, L.: The effect of hypokalemia on a pancuronium neuromuscular blockade and its antagonism by neostigmine. Br. J. Anaesth. 50:541, 1978.

96. Miller, R. D., and Savarese, J. J.: Pharmacology of muscle

relaxants, their antagonists, and monitoring of neuromuscular function, *In* Miller, R. D. (ed.): *Anesthesia*. Churchill Livingstone, New York, 1981.

97. Miller, R. D., Sohn, Y. I., and Matteo, R. S.: Enhancement of *d*-tubocurarine neuromuscular blockade by diuretics in man. Anesthesiology 45:442, 1976.

98. Miller, R. D., Van-Nyhuis, L. S., Eger, E. I., et al.: The effect of acid-base balance on neostigmine antagonism of *d*-tubocurarine-induced neuromuscular blockade. Anesthesiology 42:337, 1975.

99. Mitchell, M. M., Ali, H. H., and Savarese, J. J.: Myotonia and neuromuscular blocking agents. Anesthesiology 49:44, 1978.

100. Muir, W. W., III, Werner, L. L., and Hamlin, R. L.: Effects of xylazine and acetylpromazine upon induced ventricular fibrillation in dogs anesthetized with thiamylal and halothane. Am. J. Vet. Res. 36:1299, 1975.

101. Nagee, D. A., Sweet, P. T., and Holland, A. J. C.: Effect of atropine on bradydysrhythmias induced by succinylcholine following pretreatment with *d*-tubocurarine. Can. Anaesth. Soc. J. 29:573, 1982.

102. Ngai, S. H.: Action of general anesthetics in producing muscle relaxation: interaction of anesthetics with relaxants. *In* Katz, R. L.: *Muscle Relaxants*. American Elsevier Publishing Co., New York, 1975.

103. Nolte, I., Watney, G. C. G., and Hall, L. W.: Cardiovascular effects of epidural blocks in dogs. J. Small Anim. Pract. 24:17, 1983.

104. Palmer, A. C., Lennon, V. A., and Beadle, C.: Autoimmune form of myasthenia gravis in a juvenile Yorkshire Terrier and Jack Russell Terrier hybrid contrasted with congenital (non-autoimmune) myasthenia gravis of the Jack Russell. J. Small Anim. Pract. 21:359, 1980.

105. Pittinger, C. B., and Morris, L. E.: Observations of the placental transmission of gallamine triethiodide (Flaxedil), succinylcholine chloride (Anectine), and decamethonium bromide (Syncurine) in dogs. Anesth. Analg. 34:107, 1955.

106. Pittinger, C. B., and Morris, L. E.: Placental transmission of *d*-tubocurarine chloride from maternal to fetal circulation in dogs. Anesthesiology 14:238, 1953.

107. Popovic, N. A., Mullane, J. F., and Yhap, E. O.: Effects of Acetylpromazine on certain cardiorespiratory responses in dogs. Am. J. Vet. Res. 33:1819, 1972.

108. Proctor, C. D., Riolan, S. A., Fudema, J. J., and Prabhu, V. G.: Extension of tranquilizer action by anticholinesterases. Toxicol. Appl. Pharm. 6:1, 1964.

109. Rafferty, T. D.: Respiratory effects of narcotic analgesia, *In* Kitahata, L. M., and Collins, J. G. (eds.): *Narcotic Analgesics in Anesthesiology*. The Williams & Wilkins Co., Baltimore, 1982.

110. Regan, J. W., Roeske, W. R., and Yamamura, H. I.: The benzodiazepine receptor. J. Pharmacol. Exp. Ther. 212:137, 1980.

111. Reitan, J. A., and Warpinski, M. A.: Cardiovascular effects of pancuronium bromide in mongrel dogs. Am. J. Vet. Res. 36:1309, 1975.

112. Ryan, J. F., Kagen, L. J., and Hyman, A. I.: Myoglobinemia after a single dose of succinylcholine. N. Engl. J. Med. 285:824, 1971.

113. Savarese, J. J.: The autonomic margins of safety of metocurine and *d*-tubocurarine in the cat. Anesthesiology 50:40, 1979.

114. Savarese, J. J., and Ali, H. H.: The autonomic margin of safety of alcuronium and pancuronium. Int. Anesth. Res. Soc. Abstracts, Miami, 1977.

115. Sawyer, D. C.: Malignant hyperthermia. J. Am. Vet. Med. Assoc. 179:341, 1981.

116. Schoenstadt, D. A., and Whitcher, C. E.: Observations on the mechanism of succinyldicholine-induced cardiac arrhythmias. Anesthesiology 24:358, 1963.

117. Schuh, F. T.: Influence of haemodilution on the potency of neuromuscular blocking drugs. Br. J. Anaesth. 53:263, 1981.

118. Short, C. E., and Paddleford, R. R.: Malignant hyperthermia in the dog. Anesthesiology 39:462, 1973.

119. Singh, Y. N., Marshall, I. G., and Harvey, A. L.: Pre- and post-junctional blocking effects of aminoglycoside, polymyxin, tetracycline and lincosamine antibiotics. Br. J. Anaesth. 54:1295, 1982.

120. Skaredoff, M. N., Roaf, E. R., and Datta, S.: Hypermagnesemia and anaesthetic management. Can. Anaesth. Soc. J. 29:35, 1982.

121. Sokoll, M. D., and Gergis, S. D.: Antibiotics and neuromuscular function. Anesthesiology 55:148, 1981.

122. Sokoll, M. D., Hoyt, J. L., and Gergis, S. D.: Studies in muscle rigidity, nitrous oxide and narcotic analgesic agents. Anesth. Analg. 55:16, 1972.

123. Somogyi, A. A., Shanks, C. A., and Triggs, E. J.: Disposition kinetics on pancuronium bromide in patients with total biliary obstruction. Br. J. Anaesth. 49:1103, 1977.

124. Standaert, F. G.: Sites of action of muscle relaxants. Am. Soc. Anesthesiol.: Annual Refresher Course Lectures No. 219, 1981.

125. Stanley, T. H.: Pharmacology of intravenous narcotic anesthetics. *In* Miller, R. D. (ed.): *Anesthesia*. Churchill Livingstone, New York, 1981.

126. Stanley, T. H.: Pharmacology of intravenous non-narcotic anesthetics. *In* Miller, R. D. (ed.): *Anesthesia*. Churchill Livingstone, New York, 1981.

127. Stevenson, D. E.: A review of some side effects of muscle relaxants in small animals. J. Small Anim. Pract. 1:77, 1960–61.

128. Stewart, G. J.: Antithrombotic activity of local anesthetics in several canine models. J. Am. Soc. Regional. Anesth. (Suppl.) 7:S89, 1982.

129. Stewart, G. J., Alburger, P. D., Jr., Stone, E. A., and Soszka, T. W.: Total hip replacement induces injury to remote veins in a canine model. J. Bone Joint Surg. In press, 1984.

130. Tamas, R., Paddleford, R. R., and Krahwinkel, D. J.: Incidence of thoracic trauma in conjunction with limb fractures following motor vehicle injuries in dogs and cats. Proc. Sci. Mtg. Am. Coll. Vet. Anesth. Atlanta, 1983, pp. 1–2.

131. Tavernor, W. D.: An assessment of promazine hydrochloride as a sedative in the dog. Vet. Rec. 74:779, 1962.

132. Viby-Mogensen, J.: Clinical assessment of neuromuscular transmission. Br. J. Anaesth. 54:209, 1982.

133. Waud, B. E.: Decrease in dose requirements of *d*-tubocurarine by volatile anesthetics. Anesthesiology 51:298, 1979.

134. Waud, B. E., and Waud, D. R.: Effects of volatile anesthetics in directly and indirectly stimulated skeletal muscle. Anesthesiology 50:103, 1979.

135. Waud, P., Kuschinsky, K., and Sontag, K. H.: Morphine induced muscular rigidity in rats. Eur. J. Pharmacol. 24:189, 1973.

136. Webb, S. N., and Bradshaw, E. G., An investigation, in cats, into the activity of diazepam at the neuromuscular junction. Br. J. Anaesth. 45:313, 1973.

137. Yamashita, M., Shiga, T., Matsuki, A., and Oyama, T.: Unusual resistance to pancuronium in severely burned patients: Case reports. Can. Anaesth. Soc. J. 29:630, 1982.

138. Zbinden, G., and Randall, L. O.: Pharmacology of benzodiazepines. *In* Garattini, S., and Shore, P. A. (eds.): *Advances in Pharmacology*. Vol. 5. Academic Press, New York, 1967.

Chapter 196

Anesthesia and the Endocrine System

Cynthia M. Trim

Considerable endocrine and metabolic changes occur during and after anesthesia and surgery.[52,78] During surgery, cortisol, growth hormone, prolactin, luteinizing hormone, antidiuretic hormone, and catecholamines variably increase, whereas thyrotropin and testosterone values are suppressed.[52,78] Renin may be released and aldosterone synthesized.[86] After surgery, metabolic changes include a negative nitrogen balance, sodium retention and potassium loss, reduced water and glucose tolerance, and increased plasma concentration of free fatty acids.[43,78] A variety of factors initiate these changes: fear and apprehension, some anesthetic agents, consequences of anesthetic technique such as blood pH changes, hypercarbia, hypoxia, or pain, and surgery, including fluid loss, handling of tissues, and sepsis. The responses may be modified by the nutritional and medical state of the patient.

Anesthetic agents influence the endocrine response to anesthesia and surgery, but surgical stress plays the greater part. In humans, halothane anesthesia caused an increase in plasma cortisol, methoxyflurane, no change, and enflurane, a slight decrease in plasma cortisol.[78] The onset of surgery in each case was associated with a large increase in cortisol. In another investigation, serum prolactin, growth hormone, luteinizing hormone, and cortisol were elevated not only in a group of patients for elective surgery under general anesthesia, but also in awake patients after gastroscopy.[101] Attempts at producing stress-free anesthesia have not been completely successful. Anesthesia in human patients with high doses of fentanyl significantly attenuated the hormonal stress response compared with patients anesthetized with halothane without fentanyl.[38,56] When blockade extended to the fourth thoracic vertebra, epidural analgesia prevented increases in blood cortisol and glucose in response to hysterectomy.[28] Our aim should be to minimize the stress response to surgery by maintaining the circulation, by decreasing fear, apprehension, and pain, and by adequate intravenous alimentation.

THE ADRENAL GLANDS

Hyperadrenocorticism

Hyperadrenocorticism is a disorder of excessive production of cortisol from the adrenal cortex. It is caused either by a cortisol-producing adrenocortical adenoma or carcinoma (Cushing's syndrome) or by excessive stimulation of the adrenal glands by hypersecretion of adrenocorticotropic hormone (ACTH) from the pituitary gland (Cushing's disease). In some cases of pituitary-dependent hyperadrenocorticism, a tumor is present in the pituitary. The reason for abnormal function is uncertain in the remainder but may be a defect in neurotransmitter release or function.

Hyperadrenocorticism is usually suspected from the clinical signs of polyuria, polydipsia, polyphagia, pendulous abdomen, alopecia and thin skin, and hyperpigmentation.[60,63,73,81] The diagnosis is confirmed by the ACTH stimulation test and dexamethasone suppression test.[30,81,83] Measurement of the plasma endogenous ACTH concentration and comparison of the results with those of a high-dose dexamethasone suppression test can be used to distinguish between adrenal neoplasia and pituitary-dependent hyperadrenocorticism.[31,63,81]

Before anesthesia is induced in the patient with hyperadrenocorticism a thorough examination of the patient's physical status and clinical laboratory data, with review of any previous anesthetic experience, should be completed. In addition, the metabolic and biochemical changes characteristic of hyperadrenocorticism provide specific management problems. Approximately 10 per cent of dogs with hyperadrenocorticism also have diabetes mellitus,[63,81] which requires special considerations (see later in this chapter). A small number of dogs develop dystrophic calcification of the skin, abdominal organs, and bronchi. Pulmonary insufficiency may accompany the bronchial calcification and fibrosis. Affected patients should be identified by thoracic radiography before anesthesia. If measurement of serum electrolytes confirms hypokalemia, potassium should be given before anesthesia. Hypokalemia can complicate anesthesia with muscle weakness, bradycardia, ventricular dysrhythmias, and hypotension.[65] The potassium deficit can be corrected by oral administration of a commercial potassium-containing preparation, or by intravenous administration of fluids containing up to 20 mEq/l potassium at a rate not exceeding 0.5 mEq/kg per hour.[69] Osteoporosis may have occurred in the animal with hyperadrenocorticism, and this can be confirmed by radiography. Care must be taken to avoid fractures while handling the animal. Obesity and muscle weakness will result in hypoventilation during anesthesia, and controlled ventilation will probably be necessary. However, there appears to be no reason for choosing one anesthetic agent over another based on adrenal disease.[65]

Pituitary-dependent hyperadrenocorticism in animals is usually treated by administering O,P'-DDD (mitotane)* due to the unavailability of facilities for pituitary irradiation and the difficulties involved in

---

*Lysodren, Bristol Laboratories, Syracuse, NY.

hypophysectomy.[82] Adrenal carcinomas are usually aggressive and difficult to resect completely. Chemical adrenalectomy with O,P'-DDD may be more successful. The treatment for an adrenal adenoma is surgical excision.

Massive blood loss may occur during surgery on the adrenals, and therefore one or two venous catheters should be placed in preparation for rapid fluid infusion. The intensity of monitoring of the cardiovascular and respiratory systems during anesthesia depends on the condition of the patient and the equipment available. Heart rate and blood pressure, blood loss, and rate and depth of breathing are assessed frequently. Surgically created pneumothorax is a possible complication because of the proximity of the adrenal glands to the diaphragm.[65] One or both adrenal glands may be removed in treatment for hyperadrenocorticism. Even when the excision is unilateral, treatment with steroids is advisable until the function of the remaining gland increases. The addition of 100 to 200 mg hydrocortisone, 25 to 50 mg prednisolone, or 3 to 5 mg dexamethasone to the fluids infused during surgery is recommended.[81] Cortisone acetate, 2.5 mg/kg twice daily, or prednisone, 0.5 mg/kg twice daily, is given on the first postoperative day. The dosage is decreased over one week to a maintenance level of 0.5 mg/kg of cortisone acetate twice daily or 0.2 mg/kg of prednisone once daily. This is continued until the second adrenal gland is functioning adequately (up to two months).[81]

Hypoadrenocorticism

Adrenocortical insufficiency occurs in dogs[22,98,118,119] and, rarely, in cats.[49] It may be caused by primary adrenocortical insufficiency (Addison's disease) or may arise secondary to a pituitary or hypothalamic lesion, treatment with O,P'-DDD, bilateral adrenalectomy, or long-term administration of glucocorticoids. These patients may be depressed, weak, anorexic, and vomiting. Hyponatremia and hyperkalemia are frequently present due to the mineralocorticoid deficiency, but some patients have normal serum electrolyte values.[92,98] Hypercalcemia was found in 16 of 62 dogs with hypoadrenocorticism.[84]

Decreased aldosterone production by the adrenal cortex results in excessive sodium and water loss by the kidney and potassium retention. Severe hyponatremia affects the central nervous system and may cause seizures or coma. Astroglial cells swell, and neurotransmitter release is impaired.[116] The actions of local and inhalation anesthetics are potentiated, and smaller doses than usual are adequate for anesthesia in these patients.[37,116] Hypovolemia and decreased cardiac output are a consequence of sodium and water depletion. Blood volume must be restored before anesthesia, and anesthetic agents must be administered carefully to minimize cardiovascular depression. Thiopental or thiamylal should either not be used or used with caution.

Skeletal muscle and the heart are significantly affected by hyperkalemia. Muscle weakness combined with respiratory depression from anesthetic drugs cause hypoventilation. Hyperkalemia decreases resting membrane potentials in the heart, slowing heart rate and decreasing conduction velocity, and may result in atrioventricular block. Bradycardia may progress to sinus arrest or fibrillation. Fluid therapy should precede anesthesia to decrease the serum potassium concentration to below 6.5 mEq/l.

The magnitude of hypercalcemia is related to the severity of adrenocortical insufficiency.[84] Hypercalcemia causes muscle weakness, bradycardia, and atrioventricular block. Elevated calcium levels contract smooth muscle, causing vasoconstriction and hypertension. Ultimately, blood volume is reduced. Anesthetic drugs that cause vasodilation then cause unexpected hypotension. Animals with severe biochemical abnormalities should be treated before anesthesia with 0.9 per cent saline infusion and corticosteroids, restoring serum calcium concentration to normal.

A reduction in renal perfusion and urine output occurs when cardiac output is decreased. Prerenal azotemia is present in some dogs with hypoadrenocorticism.[98] An increased intensity of action of anesthetic drugs or a prolonged duration of action may occur in these patients due to altered protein binding from azotemia and acidosis and slowed elimination of the drugs or their metabolites.

Action potentials generated from the neuromuscular junction have had decreased amplitude in experimental animals with adrenal insufficiency.[112,121] Prolonged neuromuscular blockade with pancuronium has been reported in a human patient suspected of having inadequate replacement of adrenocortical hormones.[68]

The preoperative assessment of the patient with hypoadrenocorticism includes measurement of serum electrolytes. Surgery is delayed, if possible, for treatment to correct abnormal electrolyte values and expand blood volume. A venous catheter is inserted and an infusion of saline started before induction of anesthesia. Dextrose, 5 per cent in water, is also given if hypoglycemia is present. Smaller amounts of anesthetic than usual should be used. Controlled ventilation may be necessary during anesthesia. Dosage of neuromuscular blocking agents is reduced because their effect may be prolonged, especially when renal function is decreased.

Acute adrenal insufficiency may occur as sudden hypotension during surgery or as abdominal pain and shock during recovery.[1,94] Acute adrenal insufficiency must be considered in the differential diagnosis of unexpected hypotension during surgery, but other causes are more common, such as hypoxemia, interruption of venous return by the surgeon, low blood volume, or endotoxemia. It is usual to administer an additional dose of corticosteroid before anesthesia to patients that have been on long-term steroid therapy to counteract decreased adrenocortical function. This practice has been rejected by some as unnecessary and possibly deleterious if it creates a false sense of security.[27] A study of 104 glucocorticoid-treated human patients undergoing surgery without supplementary glucocorticoid administration, 74 of which underwent major surgery, indicated that the incidence of acute stress-induced adrenocortical insufficiency is infrequent.[53] Moreover, although eight patients developed unexplained hypotension, only one had low plasma corticosteroid values. A quiet induction of anesthesia, adequate depth of anesthesia, sufficient fluid therapy during surgery, and postoperative pain control minimize but do not abolish "surgical stress."

Pheochromocytoma

Pheochromocytoma is an adrenal medullary tumor that secretes catecholamines. The tumor may produce only norepinephrine or both norepinephrine and epinephrine and, in a few cases, dopamine. The catecholamines are usually released periodically, producing episodes of tachycardia, hypertension, restlessness, panting, and collapse.[113] Large tumors may constantly secrete catecholamines, resulting in persistent hypertension that leads to venous congestion, cardiomyopathy, and congestive heart failure.[7,113] If pheochromocytoma is suspected, the diagnosis may be confirmed by identifying an adrenal tumor by contrast angiography or computerized axial tomography, or by the measurement of abnormally high levels of catecholamines and their metabolites in the urine.[7,55,113] The type and amount of metabolites present may indicate the character, size, and location of the tumor. For example, a pure norepinephrine-secreting tumor produces only normetanephrine in the urine. Preoperative and operative cardiac arrhythmias are less common in pure norepinephrine-secreting tumors.[7]

The danger during anesthesia and surgery is sudden release of catecholamines. This can occur in response to palpation, surgical dissection of the tumor, or some drugs. The resulting tachycardia and hypertension can cause cardiac failure. The current recommendation in anesthesia for human patients with pheochromocytoma is treatment with phenoxybenzamine* orally for several days before surgery.[7,37,114] Phenoxybenzamine is a long-acting, alpha-adrenergic blocking drug that provides cardiovascular stability during surgery by preventing vasoconstriction. The drug causes hypotension in the patient with strong sympathetic tone. Therefore, in animals it might be safer to omit phenoxybenzamine pretreatment and to control hypertension during surgery with phentolamine,† a shorter-acting (20 minutes) alpha-blocker, while the cardiovascular system is being continuously monitored. Continuous tachycardia can be controlled preoperatively by the administration of propranalol.‡

Particular emphasis should be placed on preoperative evaluation of the cardiovascular system, including examination of the electrocardiogram and thoracic radiographs. An elevated packed cell volume may indicate contracted blood volume. Phenothiazine tranquilizers are avoided because hypotension occurs if epinephrine levels increase, the so-called "epinephrine-reversal." The use of droperidol-fentanyl (Innovar) is controversial. Innovar has been used successfully as an induction agent in humans and has been recommended because droperidol reduces the pressor response to epinephrine.[21,37] Other case reports have suggested that droperidol has been associated with release of catecholamines from the tumors.[6,7] Thiopental or thiamylal have been used satisfactorily for induction of anesthesia in both dogs and humans with pheochromocytoma.[7,113,114] The process of endotracheal intubation causes tachycardia and increased blood pressure.[88] In dogs, intravenous administration of lidocaine before intubation reduces this response. A comparison was made of the cardiovascular effects of thiopental, 22 mg/kg, and a combination of thiopental, 11 mg/kg, and lidocaine, 8.8 mg/kg, for induction of anesthesia in healthy, unpremedicated dogs.[90] Smaller increases in heart rate and mean arterial pressure occurred after tracheal intubation in dogs receiving the thiopental and lidocaine combination. The drugs were injected intravenously in alternate per-kilogram boluses of 2.5 mg thiopental, 2.0 mg lidocaine, 1.25 mg thiopental, 2.0 mg lidocaine, 1.25 mg thiopental, and 1.0 mg lidocaine. The catheter must be flushed with saline between injections to prevent the mixing of thiopental, which is alkaline, and lidocaine, which is acid. The total dose administered is adjusted to each individual's requirement. Lidocaine injected intravenously as a bolus exceeding 3 mg/kg decreases the cardiac output and arterial pressure in dogs.[61] However, lidocaine reduces the anesthetic requirement for thiopental such that the combined depressant effect of thiopental and lidocaine on the cardiac output is not greater than the larger dose of thiopental alone.[90] Ketamine should not be used because it increases circulating catecholamine levels, heart rate, and blood pressure when used alone or with xylazine or diazepam.[17,41,42] Halothane may be used to maintain anesthesia. Enflurane or isoflurane causes less myocardial sensitization to catecholamines than halothane,[18,26,109] and either is preferred. More arrhythmogenicity has been demonstrated with halothane-nitrous oxide anesthesia than with halothane alone.[62]

Heart rate, arterial blood pressure, electrocardiogram, and body temperature are monitored closely throughout induction and maintenance of anesthesia. Induction of anesthesia is accomplished quietly, without hypoxemia or hypercapnia. Blood volume should be maintained with a balanced electrolyte solution such as lactated Ringer's. Hypertension resulting from catecholamine release can be treated with phentolamine. An intravenous injection of 1.5 mg phentolamine was reported to satisfactorily decrease arterial pressure in a 12-kg dog during surgery.[113]

---

*Dibenzyline, SmithKline Beckman, Philadelphia, PA.
†Regitine, CIBA Pharmaceutical Company, Summit, NJ.
‡Inderal, Ayerst Laboratories, New York, NY.

Alternatively, phentolamine, 10 mg in 100 ml of 5 per cent dextrose in water, can be infused intravenously until the desired effect is achieved.[7] An increase in heart rate usually occurs as the blood pressure decreases. Arrhythmias may be of various types and may require appropriate treatment. Sinus tachycardia should disappear after the tumor is removed, and treatment may not be needed provided that the arterial pressure and capillary refill time are adequate. Hypotension may occur after the tumor is removed or in the postoperative period due to sudden withdrawal of catecholamine influence. Increased fluid administration or a blood transfusion is the best treatment for hypotension at this point.[21]

THE PANCREAS

Diabetes Mellitus

The most important goal in the anesthetic management of the diabetic animal is to prevent hypoglycemia. Hypoglycemia is almost impossible to diagnose during anesthesia without measurement of blood glucose, and even a short period of hypoglycemia may produce irreversible brain damage. When blood glucose exceeds 200 mg/dl, leukocyte phagocytosis is inhibited.[4] Infection is the leading cause of death in the human diabetic surgical patient, and there is evidence that control of blood glucose to more normal levels is associated with decreased morbidity.[70] A practical approach is to provide moderate hyperglycemia (100 to 250 mg/dl) for a short time, and to anticipate and avoid serious abnormalities of fluid, electrolyte, and glucose balance.

In addition to routine examination before anesthesia, the diabetic patient must be investigated for evidence of other disease, such as hyperadrenocorticism.[14,51] Decreased renal function, although less common in diabetic dogs than in humans, is present in 5 to 10 per cent of diabetic dogs.[59] Peripheral neuropathy may exist without clinical signs of nervous system malfunction. The autonomic nervous system can also be involved, with impaired vascular reflexes resulting in postural hypotension.[50]

No two diabetic patients are alike in their requirement for insulin, and there are many factors that may alter an animal's response to anesthesia and surgery. It is usual to schedule anesthesia early in the morning so that the patient can be monitored for the rest of the day while laboratory facilities are available. If surgery is delayed until late morning or afternoon, hypoglycemia may develop preoperatively. The stressful effect of anxiety, anesthesia, and surgery increases blood levels of catecholamines and glucocorticoids, promoting hyperglycemia. Most anesthetic drugs with the exception of xylazine cause only a minor change in blood glucose. The surgical procedure may cause a greater hyperglycemia by sympathetic stimulation. Xylazine administration causes a decrease in serum insulin and an increase in plasma glucose. In cats, intravenous injection of xylazine, 1 mg/kg, resulted in a 200 to 500 per cent increase in glucose which persisted for three to four hours.[32] Dogs receiving xylazine, 2.2 mg/kg intramuscularly, developed a maximum increase of 69 per cent by 2.5 hours.[5] Blood glucose was above normal for four hours. Xylazine may impose a further stress on the patient by depressing thermoregulation, an effect that continues after the animal has apparently recovered from sedation.[87] In humans, ketamine stimulates the sympathetic nervous system and increases plasma catecholamine levels, producing a mild increase in blood glucose.[102] Halothane, methoxyflurane, or enflurane anesthesia results in a reversible and dose-dependent inhibition of glucose-stimulated insulin release.[8,36,67] Satisfactory drug combinations include premedication with an anticholinergic and a low dose of acepromazine or narcotic analgesic. Anesthesia may be induced with a thiobarbiturate and maintained with an inhalant agent. The exact choice of drugs depends on the physical status of the patient and the requirements of the procedure to be performed. The anesthesia should allow the patient to recover quickly so that the normal routine of feeding and insulin treatment can be instituted as soon as possible.

Several protocols involving the use of dextrose and insulin infusions are used in the anesthetic management of human diabetics.[70,110] In animals, the simplest successful technique for the controlled diabetic is as follows. The patient is fed and treated normally the day before surgery. On the morning of surgery food is withheld, only half the usual dose of insulin is administered. Blood glucose is measured before anesthesia, and if the value is less than 80 mg/dl, syrup or dextrose solution is administered before proceeding. Infusion of 5 per cent dextrose in water at 5 ml/kg per hour during anesthesia maintains adequate blood glucose levels.[117,120] This solution may be given "piggyback" into the infusion line of a non–dextrose-containing fluid, which is also given at 5 ml/kg per hour to achieve a total flow of 10 ml fluid/kg per hour. An alternative solution is 0.45 per cent saline and 2.5 per cent dextrose. Five per cent dextrose, containing 0.5 unit insulin per 100 ml given at 10 ml/kg per hour has also been recommended.[96] Balanced electrolyte solutions are necessary to replace blood loss. For short procedures, adequate surveillance can be provided by measuring blood glucose at the end of anesthesia and again several hours after anesthesia, when the effect of the insulin administered in the morning is increasing. Blood glucose should be measured at least every two hours during long procedures. General anesthesia may result in uneven absorption of insulin from a subcutaneous site by decreasing subcutaneous blood flow. Alternatively, local vasodilation may occur when the animal is placed on a heating pad, and the insulin is absorbed more rapidly. The peak effect of most insulin preparations will occur several hours after surgery is completed, and it is important to ensure that the patient eats its evening meal, if able to do so, or receives additional dextrose.

Insulin requirement increases during pregnancy, but this requirement drops by half when the placenta separates.[103] Therefore, if emergency cesarean section is performed and the animal has already received its regular dose of insulin, it must be monitored closely to prevent hypoglycemia.

A diabetic patient which is poorly regulated is better hospitalized for stabilization for two to three days before anesthesia. Emergency treatment of an uncontrolled diabetic requiring anesthesia and surgery is more complicated. Surgery should be postponed as long as possible to provide time to improve the patient's status. In addition to measurement of blood glucose, preoperative evaluation should include determination of serum potassium and evaluation of the fluid and acid-base status. Management of diabetes mellitus in the dog and cat is discussed in detail elsewhere.[16,29,34,71] It may be necessary to measure blood glucose in these patients every 30 minutes during anesthesia. Insertion of a urinary catheter to monitor urine production and glucose is not routinely done in the diabetic patient because of the increased risk of infection. However, the added information may be valuable in the uncontrolled diabetic. The urine should be allowed to drain continuously through the catheter to sample accurately for glucose determination.

In every case, frequent monitoring of blood glucose in the diabetic patient allows adjustments to be made to avoid hypoglycemia or severe hyperglycemia.

Insulinoma

An insulinoma is a beta islet cell tumor of the pancreas that produces severe hypoglycemia by massive release of endogeous insulin. Our main concern in management of anesthesia is to avoid brain damage from hypoglycemia. Fasting the patient before anesthesia is necessary but can result in potentially dangerously low blood glucose levels. In some dogs, hypoglycemia occurs within four to six hours of beginning a fast.[57] Therefore, monitoring blood glucose levels and infusion of 5 per cent dextrose solution should begin during the preanesthetic preparation time.

In addition to the venous catheter used for fluid infusion, a convenient access for blood sampling should be established before anesthesia. The lingual veins are large enough in most dogs to be used by direct puncture during anesthesia. The puncture site must not be held off by alcohol-drenched material, or the mucous membrane will slough. A theoretical argument can be made for choosing anesthetic drugs that decrease the cerebral metabolic rate and therefore presumably decrease the cerebral metabolism of glucose. Barbiturates, neuroleptic techniques, halothane, methoxyflurane, enflurane, and isoflurane decrease cerebral metabolism.[108,111] Nitrous oxide has variable effects, but increases cerebral metabolic rate in dogs.[93] This increase can be partially counteracted by the prior administration of a thiobarbiturate. Ketamine produces a marked increase in cerebral metabolic rate.[108] However, a variety of anesthetic drug combinations have been used successfully for this surgery: in humans, diazepam-meperidine-thiopental-methoxyflurane-nitrous oxide,[12] meperidine-thiopental-halothane-nitrous oxide,[89] and glycopyrrolate-diazepam - Innovar - thiopental - enflurane - nitrous oxide,[9] and in dogs, atropine-thiamylal-halothane-nitrous oxide, and atropine-diazepam-thiopental-methoxyflurane-nitrous oxide (University of Georgia). A sudden fall in arterial blood pressure was noted after injection of thiopental in two human patients treated with diazoxide.[9] This was explained by two possible mechanisms. First, the thiopental may have displaced the diazoxide from its protein-binding sites, releasing active drug, which would produce vasodilation and a fall in blood pressure. Second, the diazoxide may occupy the protein-binding sites of thiopental, leaving a greater percentage than normal of the thiopental dose unbound and active. However, a significant decrease in blood pressure was also reported after thiopental in one of two patients who had not received diazoxide.[12] In one dog treated with diazoxide, hypotension was not produced, but less than half the calculated dose of thiopental was required for tracheal intubation. These events may suggest that a slower and more cautious administration of thiobarbiturate may be necessary in these patients.

Dogs with insulinoma may be obese, and controlled ventilation during anesthesia may be necessary. Excessive hyperventilation should be avoided because lowered carbon dioxide levels decrease cerebral blood flow and thus glucose delivery to the brain. Hypoglycemia is difficult to recognize during anesthesia. Signs referable to the sympathetic system, such as sweating, tachycardia, hypertension, or hypotension, may occur, but seizures may be masked by anesthetic drugs. Severe hypoglycemia can occur during surgical manipulation of the tumor, whereas a marked increase in blood glucose level may occur after its removal. The latter does not always occur because several tumors may be present that are not apparent during surgery.[57] Consequently, blood glucose should be measured frequently during and after surgery and infusion of 5 per cent dextrose should be adjusted accordingly.

Pancreatitis

Dehydration, azotemia, and decreased renal function are frequently present in patients with pancreatitis.[74,97] Hyperglycemia was present in 88 per cent of a group of animals with pancreatitis, with blood glucose exceeding 200 mg/dl in 67 per cent.[97] Hypocalcemia was identified in 52 per cent of the animals studied.[97] Treatment before anesthesia should at least ensure replacement of blood volume, restored urine production, and correction of hypocalcemia. The animal should also be evaluated for the presence of cardiac or respiratory abnormalities,[58,74] which may alter the management of anesthesia.

Anticholinergic drugs have been recommended in the treatment of pancreatitis because they block vagus-mediated secretion of pancreatic enzymes and prevent increases in flow of secretions and bicarbonate caused by distension of the fundus of the stomach.[39,45] More recently, it has been recommended that anticholinergics be avoided in patients with pancreatitis[74,107] because (1) in an experimental study of acute pancreatitis in dogs, atropine did not alter the course of the disease,[2] and (2) anticholinergics reduce gastric motility, which might result in accumulation of fluid, distension of the antrum of the stomach, and increased pancreatic enzyme secretion. However, general anesthesia produced by a variety of anesthetic agents has been documented to decrease gastric fluid volume, regardless of whether the anticholinergic drugs, atropine or glycopyrrolate, were included.[106] Consequently, use of an anticholinergic during anesthesia to counteract anesthetic drug- or surgically induced bradycardia is not contraindicated.

Dosages of anesthetic drugs should be adjusted for pre-existing central nervous system depression. Anesthesia must be managed to maintain good cardiovascular status. Infusion of dextran 40, 1.5 ml/kg per hour, improves pancreatic blood flow and increases pancreatic oxygen consumption in dogs with experimentally induced pancreatitis.[23,24] The cardiac output and blood pressure were higher in these dogs than in dogs that were not treated. However, the percentage of the cardiac output to the pancreas was increased, suggesting that the regional circulation was also affected.[23] Clinical cases of pancreatitis are currently being treated with dextran 40.[19] Anesthesia and surgery may decrease the cardiac output and blood pressure and decrease splanchnic blood flow by sympathoadrenal activation. Treatment with dextran 40 at this time may partially counter these effects. Arterial blood pressure should be monitored constantly throughout surgery because manipulation of the inflamed pancreas may cause the release of several vasoactive substances that result in vasodilation and hypotension. The reaction can be so severe that the patient may die before treatment with fluids, vasoconstricting drugs, and decreased anesthetic administration can be effectively instituted.

THE THYROID GLAND

Hypothyroidism

Hypothyroidism can be the result of a primary disease of the thyroid or can arise secondary to a pituitary or hypothalamic lesion that interferes with the release of thyrotropin or thyrotropin-releasing hormone.

A major effect of hypothyroidism is to increase the sensitivity of the patient to anesthetic drugs.[54,75] At extremes of thyroid activity, the sensitivity of the central nervous system to anesthetics may be altered.[3] Patients may also be slow to recover from anesthesia and may show prolonged sedation.[20,44] Excessive duration of anesthetic action may result from the decreased hepatic metabolic activity.[75] Normal response to pancuronium and reversal with neostigmine have been reported.[54]

A decrease in cardiac output by up to 40 per cent, due to reductions in heart rate and stroke volume, accompanies hypothyroidism.[75] Structural degeneration of the myocardium and impaired cellular metabolism of the myocardium from decreased thyroid hormone are suggested causes.[75] Hypothyroid patients are usually vasoconstricted and consequently have a low blood volume.[44] Therefore, anesthetic drugs that cause vasodilation may precipitate hypotension. It follows that drugs that maintain peripheral vascular tone, such as ketamine, may be useful for induction of anesthesia. The combination of decreased anesthetic requirements and decreased cardiovascular function may explain why hypotension readily develops in these patients.[54]

Thyroid hormones are necessary to support a normal metabolic rate, and a significant decrease (to 55 or 60 per cent of normal) can occur in patients with overt hypothyroidism.[75] These patients may have a subnormal body temperature and be unable to increase core temperature in response to low temperature stress.[15,76] During anesthesia and the early postoperative period, the hypothyroid patient is particularly susceptible to hypothermia.[75] Hypothermia decreases the patient's requirement for anesthetic drugs. A decrease in anesthetic requirement of 50 per cent has been measured in dogs during a decrease in temperature from 38°C to 28°C.[20] During recovery, shivering increases oxygen demand and stresses the cardiovascular and respiratory systems at a time when they may not be able to respond. Hypoxemia and secondary cardiac dysrhythmias may result.[77]

The hypothyroid animal should be investigated for the presence of diabetes mellitus. In one study of 62 hypothyroid dogs, 11 were diabetic.[40] Otherwise, animals with adequately treated hypothyroidism should not require special treatment. Most patients with mild hypothyroidism tolerate anesthesia and surgery well, but severe hypothyroidism increases the risk of anesthesia and surgery. General anesthesia may also precipitate myxedema coma, which has a high mortality rate.[15,75] Elective procedures should be postponed until the patient is euthyroid. Anesthetic agents are chosen and administered with the knowledge of decreased cardiovascular function in mind. Tranquilizers, sedatives, or narcotics are used only in extremely small doses. Thiobarbiturate should be titrated in small increments rather than administered as a bolus injection. Anesthesia can be maintained with low concentrations of an inhalation agent. Controlled ventilation may be necessary during anesthesia because hypothyroidism decreases respiratory function and the hypoxic ventilatory drive.[44] The patient is evaluated for adequacy of ventilation in the recovery period. Renal blood flow and glomerular filtration rate are generally decreased, and renal function is supported during anesthesia with an intravenous fluid infusion of balanced electrolyte solution.

Hyperthyroidism

Adenomas or carcinomas of the thyroid gland may secrete excessive amounts of thyroxine (T_4) or triiodothyronine (T_3). Symptoms of increased circulating levels of thyroid hormones include weight loss, polyphagia, hyperactivity, polydipsia, polyuria, and vomiting.[13,35,46,47,85] The recommended treatment is surgical excision of the thyroid gland, preferably after localization of the excessively active tissue by a thyroid scan.[35,46,85]

Cardiovascular abnormalities are common in hyperthyroid patients. In a survey of 131 cats with hyperthyroidism, the mean resting heart rate exceeded 240 beats per minute, 16 cats had congestive heart failure, and 40 cats had electrocardiographic changes indicating left ventricular enlargement.[85] Atrial and ventricular dysrhythmias and intraventricular conduction disturbances were also described. Tachycardia and ventricular hypertrophy also occur in humans with hyperthyroidism and have been attributed to a direct effect of excess thyroid hormones on the heart.[33] The ventricular hypertrophy appears to be reversible, disappearing when treatment decreases the levels of T_3 and T_4 to normal[33,100] Treatment with antithyroid drugs to render the patient euthyroid before surgery should decrease the risk of cardiac failure during anesthesia. The dose of propylthiouracil recommended for cats is 50 mg orally three times a day for one to three weeks.[35,80] When surgery cannot wait, the heart rate can be reduced by the administration of propranolol, a beta-adrenergic blocking drug. Propranolol reduces cardiac contractility and heart rate, prolongs atrioventricular conduction, and decreases blood pressure. Propranolol must not be given to patients in congestive heart failure. The suggested dosage for cats is 2.5 mg three times daily. The disadvantages of propranolol treatment in relation to general anesthesia are additional direct myocardial depression and imbalance of the sympathetic nervous system that exist during beta-blockade, when unopposed vasoconstriction from tracheal intubation, surgical stimulation, or blood loss can lead to cardiovascular collapse.[64]

An investigation in dogs pretreated for three weeks with oral propranolol in high dosage (20 mg/kg/day) demonstrated a small degree of additional cardiac depression during halothane anesthesia when compared with a group of untreated dogs.[91] However, the effects were simply additive and did not produce a significant difference in the response of heart rate, cardiac output, and blood pressure to increasing

depths of halothane anesthesia. In a similar study, equipotent concentrations of enflurane depressed the cardiovascular system more than halothane.[48] Propranolol injected intravenously during enflurane anesthesia caused significant myocardial depression and hypotension.

Atropine potentiates the tachycardia and should be avoided. Thiobarbiturates have an antithyroid activity and are the induction agent of choice.[104,117] Ketamine causes sympathetic stimulation and catecholamine release and thus should not be used. Halothane decreases plasma T_4 concentrations[122] and has been used successfully to maintain anesthesia for thyroidectomy.[47] Narcotic drugs may be used as part of the anesthetic technique.

The ECG should be monitored for dysrhythmias during anesthesia. Balanced electrolyte solution should be infused during surgery at the regular rate. Despite polyuria, signs of renal malfunction are usually absent.[85] Large tumors may have a well-developed blood supply, resulting in excessive blood loss during surgery. A thyrotoxic crisis may be manifested by tachycardia, hypertension, hypotension, increased rectal temperature, and cardiac arrest. Differential diagnosis should include malignant hyperthermia and sepsis.[66,79,95,105] Damage to the recurrent laryngeal nerve during surgery can result in laryngeal collapse and airway obstruction after intubation, requiring tracheotomy.

Even when an effort is made to preserve the parathyroid glands, hypocalcemia can occur 24 to 72 hours after surgery owing to damage to the vascular supply of the parathyroids or to decreased function from trauma-induced edema or hemorrhage; this will require treatment with calcium chloride or calcium gluconate.[46,47,80]

THE PARATHYROID GLAND

Hyperparathyroidism

Primary hyperparathyroidism occurs as a result of excess parathyroid hormone (PTH) production by the parathyroid gland. Adenomas are the most frequent cause, but occasionally primary hyperparathyroidism is caused by a carcinoma.[10] The condition has been diagnosed most often in older dogs. The clinical signs include anorexia, depression, weakness, and vomiting.[10] Laboratory tests identify hypercalcemia, with blood calcium values exceeding 11.5 mg/dl, and hypophosphatemia.

Excess PTH production increases mobilization of calcium from bone, ultimately resulting in demineralization of the skeleton. Hypercalcemia adversely affects the function of several systems, with results of significance to anesthesia. The contractility of cardiac and vascular smooth muscle is altered. An increase in blood-ionized calcium concentration to 60 per cent above normal in anesthetized dogs has been documented to cause an increase in mean arterial pressure, a reflex decrease in heart rate, and a nonsignificant decrease in cardiac output.[99] The calcium-induced vasoconstriction results in a decrease in the blood volume. In this situation, decreased peripheral vascular tone during anesthesia may cause hypotension. Hypercalcemia impairs the urine-concentrating ability of renal tubules, reduces glomerular filtration, and causes nephrolithiasis and nephrocalcinosis.[11] Patients with primary hyperparathyroidism have altered renal function varying in degree from polyuria to renal failure with azotemia.[11,115] Therefore, patients requiring anesthesia for parathyroidectomy are examined for hypovolemia and dehydration, remembering that hypertension may mask a contracted blood volume. Laboratory tests should be used to determine the magnitude of the hypercalcemia and the degree of renal malfunction. Blood calcium levels should be lowered before anesthesia by inducing diuresis with 0.9 per cent saline and furosemide.[10,115] The cardiovascular system and serum potassium should be monitored during this time. Hypokalemia should be corrected.

Adenomas are usually sharply demarcated from the thyroid glands by a fibrous capsule, but carcinomas are invasive and infiltrate tissues around the thyroid gland, lymphatics, and veins, requiring extensive dissection. Sometimes the parathyroid glands are normal and surgical exploration of the neck, or the thorax at the base of the heart, is necessary to locate the neoplasm.[10,115] Prolonged surgical time should be anticipated and adequate warmth and fluid administration provided. Surgical exploration at the thoracic inlet may create a pneumothorax. No specific anesthetic drugs have been recommended for surgery of the parathyroid glands, other than precautions related to renal malfunction.

Blood calcium should be monitored for several days after surgery. Until the remaining parathyroid tissue can resume normal function, hypocalcemia is a possibility.[25] Low blood calcium is most likely within 12 to 48 hours[10] but may not occur for three to four days.[11,115] Calcium gluconate is infused to restore the blood calcium to normal.

Anesthesia for patients with pseudohyperparathyroidism, in which hypercalcemia and hypophosphatemia are induced by factor(s) released from nonparathyroid tissue, is performed in a similar fashion. The cause of the disorder is generally a malignant neoplasm, and surgical exploration may be more extensive.[10]

1. Alford, W. C., Meador, C. K., Mihalevich, J., et al.: Acute adrenal insufficiency following cardiac surgical procedures. J. Thorac. Cardiovasc. Surg. 78:489, 1979.
2. Attix, E., Strombeck, D. R., Wheeldan, E. B., and Stern, J. S.: Effects of an anticholinergic and a corticosteroid on acute pancreatitis in experimental dogs. Am. J. Vet. Res. 42:1668, 1981.
3. Babad, A. A., and Eger, E. I., II: The effects of hyperthyroidism and hypothyroidism on halothane and oxygen requirements in dogs. Anesthesiology 29:1087, 1968.
4. Bagdade, J. D., Root, R. K., and Bulger, R. J.: Impaired leukocyte function in patients with poorly controlled diabetes. Diabetes 23:9, 1974.
5. Benson, G. J., Thurmon, J. C., and Tranquilli, W. J.: Effect of xylazine hydrochloride upon plasma glucose and serum insulin in adult Pointer dogs. Proc. Am. Coll. Vet. Anesth. Annual Mtg., Atlanta, 1983, p. 31–32.
6. Blitt, C. D.: Droperidol and pheochromocytoma. Anesth. Analg. (Cleve.) 60:770, 1981.
7. Brown, B. R.: Anesthesia for pheochromocytoma. In Brown, B. R. (ed.): Anesthesia and the Patient with Endocrine Disease. F. A. Davis Co., Philadelphia, 1980.
8. Bradford, M. W., Rusy, B. F., and Ewart, R. L.: Effects of enflurane on rat pancreatic islet metabolism and insulin release. Anesthesiology 55(3A):A184, 1981.
9. Burch, P. G., and McLeskey, C. H.: Anesthesia for patients with insulinoma treatment with oral diazoxide. Anesthesiology 55:472, 1981.
10. Capen, C. C., and Martin, S. L.: Calcium-regulating hormones and diseases of the parathyroid glands. In Ettinger, S. J. (ed.): Textbook of Veterinary Internal Medicine. 2nd ed. W. B. Saunders Co., Philadelphia, 1983.
11. Carillo, J. M., Burk, R. L., and Bode, C.: Primary hyperparathyroidism in a dog. J. Am. Vet. Med. Assoc. 174:67, 1979.
12. Chari, P., Pandit, S. K., Kataria, R. N., et al.: Anaesthetic management of insulinoma. Anaesthesia 32:261, 1977.
13. Chastain, C. B.: Excess triiodothyronine production by a thyroid adenocarcinoma in a dog. J. Am. Vet. Med. Assoc. 177:172, 1980.
14. Chastain, C. B.: Intensive care of dogs and cats with diabetic ketoacidosis. J. Am. Vet. Med. Assoc. 179:972, 1981.
15. Chastain, C. B.: Canine hypothyroidism. J. Am. Vet. Med. Assoc. 181:349, 1982.
16. Chastain, C. B., and Nichols, C. E.: Low-dose intramuscular insulin therapy for diabetic ketoacidosis in dogs. J. Am. Vet. Med. Assoc. 178:561, 1981.
17. Chernow, B., Lake, C. R., Creuss, D., et al.: Plasma, urine, and CSF catecholamine concentrations during and after ketamine anesthesia. Crit. Care. Med. 10:600, 1982.
18. Conner, J. T., Miller, J. D., and Katz, R. L.: Isoflurane anesthesia for pheochromocytoma: A case report. Anesth. Analg. (Cleve.) 54:419, 1975.
19. Cornelius, L. M.: Personal communication.
20. Denlinger, J. K.: Prolonged emergence and failure to regain consciousness. In Orkin, F. K., and Cooperman, L. H. (eds.): Complications in Anesthesiology. J. B. Lippincott Co., Philadelphia, 1983.
21. Desmonts, J. M., Le Houelleur, J., Remond, P., and Duvaldestin, P.: Anaesthetic management of patients with phaeochromocytoma: A review of 102 cases. Br. J. Anaesth. 49:991, 1977.
22. DiBartola, S. P.: Canine hypoadrenocorticism: A brief review. Calif. Vet. 34(4):15, 1980.
23. Donaldson, L. A., Williams, R. W., and Schenk, W. G.: Experimental pancreatitis: Effect of plasma and dextran on pancreatic blood flow. Surgery 84:313, 1978.
24. Donaldson, L. A., and Schenk, W. G.: Experimental acute pancreatitis: The changes in pancreatic oxygen consumption and the effect of dextran 40. Ann. Surg. 190:728, 1979.
25. Edis, A. J.: Prevention and management of complications associated with thyroid and parathyroid surgery. Surg. Clin. North Am. 59:83, 1979.
26. Eger, E. I.: Isoflurane: A review. Anesthesiology 55:559, 1981.
27. Eltherington, L. G.: Complications of prior drug therapy. In Orkin, F. K., and Cooperman, L. H. (eds.): Complications in Anesthesiology. J. B. Lippincott Co., Philadelphia, 1983.
28. Engquist, A., Mogens, R. B., Fernandes, A., and Kehlet, H.: The blocking effect of epidural analgesia on the adrenocortical and hyperglycemic responses to surgery. Acta Anaesth. Scand. 21:330, 1977.
29. Feldman, E. C.: Diabetic ketoacidosis in dogs. Compend. Cont. Educ. Pract. Vet. 2:456, 1980.
30. Feldman, E. C.: Comparison of ACTH response and dexamethasone suppression as screening tests in canine hyperadrenocorticism. J. Am. Vet. Med. Assoc. 182:506, 1983.

31. Feldman, E. C.: Distinguishing dogs with functioning adrenocortical tumors from dogs with pituitary-dependent hyperadrenocorticism. J. Am. Vet. Med. Assoc. *183*:195, 1983.

32. Feldberg, W., and Symonds, H. W.: Hyperglycaemic effect of xylazine. J. Vet. Pharmacol. Ther. *3*:197, 1980.

33. Forfar, J. C., Muir, A. L., Sawers, S. A., and Toft, A. D.: Abnormal left ventricular function in hyperthyroidism. N. Engl. J. Med. *307*:1165, 1982.

34. Foster, D. W., and McGarry, J. D.: The metabolic derangements and treatment of diabetic ketoacidosis. N. Engl. J. Med. *309*:159, 1983.

35. Fox, P. R.: Feline myocardial diseases. *In* Kirk, R. W. (ed.): *Current Veterinary Therapy VIII: Small Animal Practice*. W. B. Saunders Co., Philadelphia, 1983.

36. Gingerich, R., Wright, P. H., and Paradise, R. R.: Effects of halothane on glucose-stimulated insulin secretion and glucose oxidation in isolated rat pancreatic cells. Anesthesiology *53*:219, 1980.

37. Gregory, I. C.: Anaesthesia and the endocrine glands. *In* Churchill-Davidson, H. C. (ed.): *A Practice of Anaesthesia*. 4th ed. W. B. Saunders Co., Philadelphia, 1979.

38. Hall, G. M., Young, C., Holdcroft, A., and Alaghband-Zadeh, J.: Substrate mobilization during surgery: A comparison between halothane and fentanyl anaesthesia. Anaesthesia *33*:924, 1978.

39. Hardy, R. M., and Stevens, J. B.: Exocrine pancreatic diseases. *In* Ettinger, S. J. (ed.): *Textbook of Veterinary Internal Medicine*. W. B. Saunders Co., Philadelphia, 1975.

40. Hargis, A. M., Stephens, L. C., Benjamin, S. A., et al.: Relationship of hypothyroidism to diabetes mellitus, renal amyloidosis, and thrombosis in purebred Beagles. Am. J. Vet. Res. *42*:1077, 1981.

41. Haskins, S. C.: Ketamine and ketamine-sedative combinations in dogs. Presented at the American College of Veterinary Anesthesiologists Annual Scientific Meeting, Las Vegas, 1982.

42. Haskins, S. C., Peiffer, R. L., and Stowe, C. M.: A clinical comparison of CT1341, ketamine, and xylazine in cats. Am. J. Vet. Res. *36*:1537, 1975.

43. Hayes, M. A., and Goldenberg, I. S.: Renal effects of anesthesia and operation mediated by endocrines. Anesthesiology *24*:487, 1963.

44. Hellman, D. E.: The thyroid gland. *In* Brown, B. R. (ed.): *Anesthesia and the Patient with Endocrine Disease*. F. A. Davis Co., Philadelphia, 1980.

45. Hendrix, T. R.: The secretory function of the alimentary canal. *In* Mountcastle, V. B. (ed.): *Medical Physiology*. 14th ed. C. V. Mosby Co., St. Louis, 1980.

46. Hoenig, M., Goldschmidt, M. H., Ferguson, D. C., et al.: Toxic nodular goitre in the cat. J. Small Anim. Pract. *23*:1, 1982.

47. Holzworth, J., Theran, P., Carpenter, J. L., et al.: Hyperthyroidism in the cat: Ten cases. J. Am. Vet. Med. Assoc. *176*:345, 1980.

48. Horan, B. F., Prys-Roberts, C., Hamilton, W. K., and Roberts, J. G.: Haemodynamic responses to enflurane anaesthesia and hypovolaemia in the dog, and their modification by propranolol. Br. J. Anaesth. *49*:1189, 1977.

49. Johnessee, J. S., Peterson, M. E., and Gilbertson, S. R.: Primary hypoadrenocorticism in a cat. J. Am. Vet. Med. Assoc. *183*:881, 1983.

50. Johnson, C. A., Kittleson, M. D., and Indrieri, R. J.: Peripheral neuropathy and hypotension in a diabetic dog. J. Am. Vet. Med. Assoc. *183*:1007, 1983.

51. Katherman, A. E., O'Leary, T. P., Richardson, R. C., et al.: Hyperadrenalcorticism and diabetes mellitus in the dog. J. Am. Anim. Hosp. Assoc. *16*:705, 1980.

52. Kaufman, L.: The endocrine response to surgery and anaesthesia. *In* Scott, C., Feldman, S. (eds.): *Scientific Foundations of Anaesthesia*. William Heinemann Medical Books, London, 1982.

53. Kehlet, H., and Binder, C.: Adrenocortical function and clinical course during and after surgery in unsupplemented glucocorticoid-treated patients. Br. J. Anaesth. *45*:1043, 1973.

54. Kim, J. M., and Hackman, L.: Anesthesia for untreated hypothyroidism: Report of three cases. Anesth. Analg. (Cleve.) *56*:299, 1977.

55. Koizumi, K., and Brooks, C. M.: The autonomic system and its role in controlling body functions. *In* Mountcastle, V. B. (ed.): *Medical Physiology*. 14th ed. C. V. Mosby Co., St. Louis, 1980.

56. Kono, K., Philbin, D. M., Coggins, C. H., et al.: Renal function and stress response during halothane or fentanyl anesthesia. Anesth. Analg. (Cleve.) *60*:552, 1981.

57. Kruth, S. A., Feldman, E. C., and Kennedy, P. C.: Insulin-secreting islet cell tumors: Establishing a diagnosis and the clinical course for 25 dogs. J. Am. Vet. Med. Assoc. *181*:54, 1982.

58. Lees, G. E., Suter, P. F., and Johnson, G. C.: Pulmonary edema in a dog with acute pancreatitis and cardiac disease. J. Am. Vet. Med. Assoc. *172*:690, 1978.

59. Ling, G. V., Lowenstine, L. J., and Pulley, L. T.: Diabetes mellitus in dogs: A review of initial evaluation, immediate and long-term management, and outcome. J. Am. Vet. Med. Assoc. *170*:521, 1977.

60. Ling, G. V., Stabenfeldt, G. H., Comer, K. M., et al.: Canine hyperadrenocorticism: Pretreatment clinical and laboratory evaluation of 117 cases. J. Am. Vet. Med. Assoc. *174*:1211, 1979.

61. Liu, P., Feldman, H. S., Covino, B. M., et al.: Acute cardiovascular toxicity of intravenous amide local anesthetics in anesthetized ventilated dogs. Anesth. Analg. (Cleve.) *61*:317, 1982.

62. Liu, W. S., Wong, K. C., Port, J. D., and Andriano, K. P.: Epinephrine-induced arrhythmias during halothane anesthesia with the addition of nitrous oxide, nitrogen, or helium in dogs. Anesth. Analg. (Cleve.) *61*:414, 1982.

63. Lorenz, M. D.: Diagnosis and medical management of canine Cushing's syndrome: A study of 57 consecutive cases. J. Am. Anim. Hosp. Assoc. *18*:707, 1982.

64. Lowenstein, E.: Beta-adrenergic blockers. *In* Smith, N. T., Miller, R. D., Corbascio, A. N. (eds.): *Drug Interactions in Anesthesia*. Lea & Febiger, Philadelphia, 1981.

65. Maddi, R., and Gabel, R. A.: Anaesthetic considerations for adrenalectomy. *In* Brown, B. R. (ed.): *Anesthesia and the Patient with Endocrine Disease*. F. A. Davis Co., Philadelphia, 1980.

66. McGrath, C. J., Crimi, A. J., and Ruff, J.: Malignant hyperthermia in dogs. Vet. Med./Sm. Anim. Clin. *77*:218, 1982.

67. Merin, R. G., Samuelson, P. N., and Schalch, D. S.: Major inhalation anesthetics and carbohydrate metabolism. Anesth. Analg. (Cleve.) *50*:625, 1971.

68. Meyers, E. F.: Partial recovery from pancuronium neuromuscular blockade following hydrocortisone administration. Anesthesiology *46*:148, 1977.

69. Michell, A. R.: The pathophysiological basis of fluid therapy in small animals. Vet. Rec. *104*:542, 1979.

70. Miller, J., and Walts, L. F.: Perioperative management of diabetes mellitus. *In* Burnell, B. R. (ed.): *Anesthesia and the Patient with Endocrine Disease*. F. A. Davis Co., Philadelphia, 1980.

71. Moise, N. S., and Reimers, T. J.: Insulin therapy in cats with diabetes mellitus. J. Am. Vet. Med. Assoc. *182*:158, 1983.

72. Moore, R. W., and Withrow, S. J.: Gastrointestinal hemorrhage and pancreatitis associated with intervertebral disk disease in the dog. J. Am. Vet. Med. Assoc. *180*:1443, 1982.

73. Mulnix, J. A.: Adrenal cortical disease in dogs. Vet. Scope (Upjohn) *19*:12, 1975.

74. Mulvany, M. H., Feinberg, C. K., and Tilson, D. L.: Clinical characterization of acute necrotizing pancreatitis. Compend. Cont. Educ. Pract. Vet. *4*:394, 1982.

75. Murkin, J. M.: Anesthesia and hypothyroidism: A review of thyroxine physiology, pharmacology, and anesthetic implications. Anesth. Analg. (Cleve.) *61*:371, 1982.

76. Nesbitt, G. H., Izzo, J., Peterson, L., and Wilkins, R. J.: Canine hypothyroidism: A retrospective study of 108 cases. J. Am. Vet. Med. Assoc. *177*:1117, 1980.

77. Orkin, F. K.: Physiologic disturbances associated with induced hypothermia. *In* Orkin, F. K., and Cooperman, L. H. (eds.): *Complications in Anesthesiology.* J. B. Lippincott Co., Philadelphia, 1983.

78. Oyama, T.: Influence of general anesthesia and surgical stress on endocrine function. *In* Brown, B. R. (ed.): *Anesthesia and the Patient with Endocrine Disease.* F. A. Davis Co., Philadelphia, 1980.

79. Peters, K. R., Nance, P., and Wingard, D. W.: Malignant hyperthyroidism or malignant hyperthermia? Anesth. Analg. (Cleve.) *60*:613, 1981.

80. Peterson, M. E.: Diagnosis and treatment of feline hyperthyroidism. Proc. 6th Kal Kan Symposium, 1982, pp.63–66.

81. Peterson, M. E.: Hyperadrenocorticism. *In* Kirk, R. W. (ed.): *Current Veterinary Therapy VIII: Small Animal Practice.* W. B. Saunders Co., Philadelphia, 1983.

82. Peterson, M. E.: O,P'-DDD (mitotane) treatment of canine pituitary-dependent hyperadrenocorticism. J. Am. Vet. Med. Assoc. *182*:527, 1983.

83. Peterson, M. E., Gilbertson, S. R., and Drucker, W. D.: Plasma cortisol response to exogenous ACTH in 22 dogs with hyperadrenocorticism caused by adrenocortical neoplasia. J. Am. Vet. Med. Assoc. *180*:542, 1982.

84. Peterson, M. E., and Feinman, J. M.: Hypercalcemia associated with hypoadrenocorticism in sixteen dogs. J. Am. Vet. Med. Assoc. *181*:802, 1982.

85. Peterson, M. E., Kintzer, P. P., Cavanagh, P. G., et al.: Feline hyperthyroidism: Pretreatment clinical and laboratory evaluation of 131 cases. J. Am. Vet. Med. Assoc. *183*:103, 1983.

86. Pettinger, W. A.: Anesthetics and the renin-angiotensin-aldosterone axis. Anesthesiology *48*:393, 1978.

87. Ponder, S. W., and Clark, W. G.: Prolonged depression of thermoregulation after xylazine administration to cats. J. Vet. Pharmacol. Ther. *3*:203, 1980.

88. Prys-Roberts, C., Greene, L. T., Meloche, R., and Foëx, P.: Studies of anaesthesia in relation to hypertension II: Haemodynamic consequences of induction and endotracheal intubation. Br. J. Anaesth. *43*:531, 1971.

89. Pulver, J. J., Cullen, B. F., Miller, D. R., and Valenta, L. J.: Use of the artificial beta cell during anesthesia for surgical removal of an insulinoma. Anesth. Analg. (Cleve.) *59*:950, 1980.

90. Rawlings, C. A., and Kolata, R. J.: Cardiopulmonary effects of thiopental/lidocaine combination during anesthetic induction in the dog. Am. J. Vet. Res. *44*:144, 1983.

91. Roberts, J. G., Foëx, P., Clarke, T. N. S., and Bennett, M. J.: Haemodynamic interactions of high-dose propranolol pretreatment and anaesthesia in the dog. I. Halothane dose-response studies. Br. J. Anaesth. *48*:315, 1976.

92. Rogers, W., Straus, J., and Chew, D.: Atypical hypoadrenocorticism in three dogs. J. Am. Vet. Med. Assoc. *179*:155, 1981.

93. Sakabe, T., Kuramoto, T., Seiichiro, I., and Takeshita, H.: Cerebral effects of nitrous oxide in the dog. Anesthesiology *48*:195, 1978.

94. Salam, A. A., and Davies, D. M.: Acute adrenal insufficiency during surgery. Br. J. Anaesth. *46*:619, 1974.

95. Sawyer, D. C.: Malignant hyperthermia. J. Am. Vet. Med. Assoc. *179*:341, 1981.

96. Sawyer, D. C.: The anesthetic period: predictable problems. *In* Sawyer, D. C. *The Practice of Small Animal Anesthesia.* W. B. Saunders Co., Philadelphia, 1982.

97. Schaer, M.: A clinicopathologic survey of acute pancreatitis in 30 dogs and 5 cats. J. Am. Anim. Hosp. Assoc. *15*:681, 1979.

98. Schaer, M., and Chen, C. L.: A clinical survey of 48 dogs with adrenocortical hypofunction. J. Am. Anim. Hosp. Assoc. *19*:443, 1983.

99. Scheidegger, D., and Drop, L. J.: The relationship between duration of Q-T interval and plasma ionized calcium concentration: Experiments with acute, steady-state [Ca⁺⁺] changes in the dog. Anesthesiology *51*:143, 1979.

100. Skelton, C. L.: The heart and hyperthyroidism. N. Engl. J. Med. *307*:1206, 1982.

101. Sowers, J. R., Raj, R. P., Hershman, J. M., et al.: The effect of stressful diagnostic studies and surgery on anterior pituitary hormone release in man. Acta Endocrinol. *86*:25, 1977.

102. Stefansson, T., Wickström, I., and Haljamäe, H.: Hemodynamic and metabolic effects of ketamine anesthesia in the geriatric patient. Acta Anaesth. Scand. *26*:371, 1982.

103. Steinke, J.: Management of diabetes mellitus and surgery. N. Engl. J. Med. *282*:1472, 1970.

104. Stehling, L. C.: Anesthetic implications of hyperthyroidism. *In* Brown, B. R. (ed.): *Anesthesia and the Patient with Endocrine Disease.* F. A. Davis Co., Philadelphia, 1980.

105. Stevens, J. J.: A case of thyrotoxic crisis that mimicked malignant hyperthermia. Anesthesiology *59*:263, 1983.

106. Stoelting, R. K.: Gastric fluid volume and pH after fentanyl, enflurane, or halothane-nitrous oxide anesthesia with or without atropine or glycopyrrolate. Anesth. Analg. (Cleve.) *59*:287, 1980.

107. Strombeck, D. R., and Feldman, B. F.: Acute pancreatitis. *In* Kirk, R. W. (ed.): *Current Veterinary Therapy VIII: Small Animal Practice.* W. B. Saunders Co., Philadelphia, 1983.

108. Suffecool, S. L.: Anesthetic management for insulinoma resection. *In* Brown, B. R. (ed.): *Anesthesia and the Patient with Endocrine Disease.* F. A. Davis Co., Philadelphia, 1980.

109. Sumikawa, K., Ishizaka, N., and Suzaki, M.: Arrhythmogenic plasma levels of epinephrine during halothane, enflurane, and pentobarbital anesthesia in the dog. Anesthesiology *58*:322, 1983.

110. Taitelman, U., Reece, E. A., and Bessman, A. N.: Insulin in the management of the diabetic surgical patient. J. Am. Med. Assoc. *237*:658, 1977.

111. Todd, M. M., and Drummond, J. C.: A comparison of the cerebrovascular and metabolic effects of halothane and isoflurane in the cat. Anesthesiology *60*:276, 1984.

112. Torda, C., and Wolff, H. G.: Effect of pituitary hormones, cortisone and adrenalectomy on some aspects of neuromuscular function and acetylcholine synthesis. Am. J. Physiol. *169*:140, 1952.

113. Twedt, D. C., Tilley, L. P., Ryan, W. W., et al.: Pheochromocytoma in the canine. J. Am. Anim. Hosp. Assoc. *11*:491, 1975.

114. Vater, M., Achola, K., and Smith, G.: Catecholamine responses during anaesthesia for phaeochromocytoma. Br. J. Anaesth. *55*:357, 1983.

115. Villar, H. V., and Wangensteen, S. L.: Surgery of the parathyroid glands. *In* Brown, B. R. (ed.): *Anesthesia and the Patient with Endocrine Disease.* F. A. Davis Co., Philadelphia, 1980.

116. Vitez, T. S.: Electrolytes and the anesthesiologist. Am. Soc. Anesth. Annual Refresher Course Lectures, 1983, p. 128.

117. Wase, A. W., and Foster, W. C.: Thiopental and thyroid metabolism. Proc. Soc. Exp. Biol. Med. *91*:89, 1956.

118. Willard, M. D., Schall, W. D., McCaw, D. E., and Nachreiner, R. F.: Canine hypoadrenocorticism: Report of 37 cases and review of 39 previously reported cases. J. Am. Vet. Med. Assoc. *180*:59, 1982.

119. Willard, M. D., Schall, W. D., Nachreiner, R. F., and Shelton, D. G.: Hypoadrenocorticism following therapy with o,p'-DDD for hyperadrenocorticism in four dogs. J. Am. Vet. Med. Assoc. *180*:638, 1982.

120. Woodruff, R. E., Lewis, S. B., McLeskey, C. H., and Graney, W. F.: Avoidance of surgical hyperglycemia in diabetic patients. J. Am. Med. Assoc. *244*:166, 1980.

121. Woodbury, D. M.: Relation between the adrenal cortex and the central nervous system. Pharmacol. Rev. *10*:275, 1958.

122. Wu, W., and Zbuzek, V. K.: Halothane anesthesia and plasma vasopressin concentration in hypo- and hyperthyroid rats. Anesthesiology *55(3)*: A191, 1981.

Chapter 197

Anesthesia and Monitoring for Trauma and Critical Care Patients

T. Evans

Selecting an anesthetic technique for the critical patient includes careful evaluation of the history. Many disease conditions can profoundly affect the course of anesthesia through their actions on dosage, uptake, distribution, and recovery time of anesthetic agents. Trauma, with its inherent physical insult to vital organs, can also influence the choice of anesthetic regimen. The ability to match the safest anesthetic technique with current disease or trauma can only be developed by careful attention to the physical status of the patient combined with knowledge of the effects of anesthetic agents.

THE TRAUMA PATIENT

Premedication

The increasing number of emergency clinics has provided the opportunity to develop improved anesthesia techniques for the trauma patient requiring immediate surgery. The trauma patient presents specialized anesthetic problems that must be resolved quickly, often without benefit of information concerning medical history or previous drug therapy. Thus, the clinician must be able to evaluate and treat airway occlusion, multiple injuries, full stomach, and shock before or concurrent with anesthetic induction. Before anesthesia can proceed, some thought must be given to premedication, which improves chances for a successful recovery. Tranquilizers are used to allay fear and apprehension, but sometimes this aspect of medical management is preempted by the more immediate need for respiratory and circulatory resuscitation of the patient in poor condition. If an analgesic is needed to perform a life-saving palliative maneuver, small incremental doses of a narcotic (oxymorphone,* 0.025 mg/kg) may be given intravenously. Narcotic analgesics should not be used in the disoriented or comatose patient.[34] Barbiturates should not be used in the patient that is excited, delirious, or in pain, because small doses of these agents may augment such symptoms.

Harmful vagal influences and excess secretions can be controlled by atropine† or glycopyrrolate.‡ Unfortunately, gastric secretions already accumulated will not be eliminated, because the drugs prevent further secretion but do not reduce the volume of secretions already present. Because trauma decreases gastric emptying time, one should assume that the stomach contains food or fluid and should be prepared to take appropriate measures to prevent aspiration during anesthetic induction.[34] Glycopyrrolate decreases gastric acidity and may be helpful if aspiration occurs.[66] Aspiration of gastric contents of pH less than 2.5 has almost uniformly resulted in pneumonitis, which is associated with a significant increase in morbidity and mortality.[34] However, anticholinergics may relax the cardiac sphincter, facilitating the movement of stomach contents to the pharynx.[7] In humans, antacids have been recommended as an alternative to raise gastric pH above 2.5. In patients receiving a preinduction antacid, aspiration of gastric contents resulted in a less severe aspiration syndrome.[77] In contrast, Gibbs and colleagues[33] reported contradictory findings in the dog: aspiration of hydrochloric acid at a pH of 1.8 produced effects on PaO_2 and pulmonary shunt fraction similar to those of aspiration of antacid and saline.[33] Although I believe that the mortality rate of dogs and cats is low compared with that in humans, aspiration of stomach contents is still a potential problem that can be diminished by careful attention to positioning, time of last meal, and intelligent use of premedications. Antacids are not recommended because previous studies have shown a questionable effectiveness and because the agents require forced administration to dogs and cats. I recommend the use of either atropine or glycopyrrolate as premedication, positioning to prevent gastric pressure, immediate intubation after loss of consciousness, and the availability of suction equipment to clear the pharynx in the event of regurgitation.

Induction and Intubation

Airway protection of the unconscious traumatized patient is an important first step to successful resuscitation. Intubation is easily accomplished in the comatose patient but may be difficult in the awake patient. Following narcotic-induced analgesia, intravenous succinylcholine may be used to produce sufficient muscle relaxation for intubation. Controlled ventilation must be provided until spontaneous breathing resumes. Intubation without prior analgesics should not be attempted in patients with elevated

---

*E.I Dupont de Nemours and Co., Inc., Wilmington, DE.
†Rugby Laboratories Inc., Rockville Center, NY.
‡A. H. Robins Co., Richmond, VA.

intracranial pressure, penetrating wounds of the eye, or penetrating wounds of the neck. Struggling and increased stress during intubation in the awake patient may further increase intracranial and intraocular pressure and may induce hemorrhage and false airway development in the cervical area. Prior to administration of succinylcholine, the patient should be preoxygenated for three minutes,[75] effectively replacing alveolar nitrogen with oxygen. The patient is then be able to tolerate several minutes of apnea or airway obstruction before the onset of tissue hypoxia. Alternatively, the fiberoptic bronchoscope may be used to simplify intubation in dogs in which conventional methods of intubation are too difficult or dangerous. The fibroscope, after being heated in warm water to prevent fogging, is passed through the endotracheal tube so that the end slightly protrudes beyond the distal endotracheal tube opening. The fibroscope and endotracheal tube are directed through the oropharynx of the dog to the glottis while the operator looks through the fibroscope to observe the glottis and epiglottis. After the combined fibroscope and endotracheal tube are passed through the glottis, the fibroscope is withdrawn, leaving the endotracheal tube in place.

Thoracic Trauma

Considerations for anesthetic management of patients with chest trauma must include a review of the factors affecting delivery of inhalation anesthetics. Pneumothorax causes partial or total collapse of lung lobes. A right-to-left pulmonary shunt results, and uptake of inhalation anesthetics is impaired, especially of relatively insoluble agents such as halothane and enflurane.[19] Accordingly, the depth of anesthesia is difficult to control. Intermittent positive-pressure ventilation may be used to enhance, anesthetic delivery, although it causes an increase in transpulmonary pressure, which may reopen partially healed lung parenchyma, causing the pneumothorax to worsen.

The use of nitrous oxide in the presence of pneumothorax is contraindicated, because nitrous oxide moves from the blood into the air-filled space (pneumothorax) faster than nitrogen (from air) moves from the air-filled space to the blood.[22] The resulting disproportionate movement of gases causes a potentially lethal increase in intrathoracic pressure.

Hemothorax and pulmonary parenchymal hemorrhage also exacerbate right-to-left shunting, thereby contributing to increased difficulty in maintaining a stable anesthetic state, especially with relatively insoluble inhalation agents (Table 197–1).[19] Tachypnea, in the presence of decreased tidal volume, often occurs as a result of pulmonary trauma or secondarily to the effects of inhalation anesthetics on ventilation. Halothane in particular causes a dose-related increase in breathing frequency, especially at higher minimum alveolar concentrations (MAC).[47] The tachypnea has been attributed to increased sensitivity to the Hering-

TABLE 197–1. Partition Coefficients (Solubility) at 37°C

Anesthetic	Blood Gas*
Nitrous oxide	0.47 (20)
Isoflurane	1.4 (15)
Enflurane	1.8 (19)
Halothane	2.3 (20)
Diethyl ether	12 (20)
Methoxyflurane	12 (20)

*Number in parentheses indicates reference for the value.

Breuer inflation reflex.[18] If one considers the effects of pulmonary trauma previously described, one can appreciate the benefits of IPPV, not only in administration of anesthetics but also in the improvement in pulmonary function.

Because of these factors, I prefer a balanced anesthetic technique for the patient with thoracic trauma. The patient should be clipped and scrubbed before anesthesia. Oxygen is given by mask, provided that it is accepted by the patient without struggling. If the patient struggles, the mask is not used. Rapid induction is necessary to allow speedy intubation, especially in animals with fluid or abdominal viscera in the pleural space. An ultra-short-acting barbiturate such as thiamylal sodium or thiopental sodium, given to effect, accomplishes this goal without excessively compromising cardiovascular function. If even less cardiovascular depression is desired for a dog, a low dose of thiamylal (4 mg/kg) is given, and following loss of consciousness, succinylcholine (0.4 mg/kg) is injected intravenously to allow immediate intubation and ventilation. Anesthesia is maintained with small incremental doses of oxymorphone (0.02 to 0.04 mg/kg) intravenously and low concentrations of halothane* (0.5 per cent). Nitrous oxide should not used because of the time that can be saved, with use of 100 per cent oxygen, to apply resuscitation techniques should severe cardiovascular depression occur.

Abdominal Trauma

The incidence of abdominal trauma in the dog and cat is as high as 10 to 13 per cent.[46] Surgery may be required to diagnose abdominal injury to determine its extent, or to repair or remove traumatized organs. Important factors that complicate the administration of anesthetics include: (1) arterial hypotension as a result of blood loss from a ruptured spleen, liver, or blood vessel; (2) metabolic acidosis as a sequel to urinary bladder rupture or shock; (3) gas-filled stomach and intestines, which decrease functional residual capacity and tidal volume with a subsequent delay in the uptake of inhalation anesthetics; and (4) trauma to the liver and kidney, which regulate metabolism

---

*Ft. Dodge Laboratories Inc., Ft. Dodge, IA.

and excretion of anesthetics. The elimination of ketamine, or gallamine, and pancuronium is delayed if abdominal trauma has caused renal failure or urinary bladder rupture.[56,78] If trauma to the liver has been severe enough to interfere with drug metabolism, then narcotics, tranquilizers, and barbiturates, with the exception of the ultra-short-acting thiamylal or thiopental, should not be used because of potential long-lasting effects. Thiopental sodium or thiamylal sodium can be used if dosages are diminished to one-half of the usual general anesthesia dose, because the duration of action of such an agent depends on redistribution rather than on metabolism.

A gas-filled dilated viscus increases in size if nitrous oxide is used.[22] The poorer operating conditions unnecessarily lengthen the time for laparotomy. Methoxyflurane and halothane have been safely used in the presence of abdominal trauma. Halothane, because of its comparatively low tissue solubility, is easier to control and is preferred to methoxyflurane.

Central Nervous System Trauma

Because a blow to the head or a hypoxic episode can result in swelling of the brain and intracranial hypertension, cerebral vasodilation must be avoided. Drugs that produce hypoventilation and hypercapnia are also avoided. Volatile agents, such as halothane, can induce the triad of arterial hypotension, hypercapnia, and intracranial hypertension. These agents can be used if hypotension is prevented, hyperventilation is used, and increased intracranial pressure is prevented with diuretics (e.g., mannitol,* furosemide†).

The administration of large doses of steroids is useful in reducing intracranial pressure due to primary or metastatic brain tumors, but the ability of steroids to reduce cerebral edema due to cerebral ischemia (cardiac arrest) or head injury is questionable.[42] Steroids are often used in the belief that they do not do any harm and may do some good. Continuous use of steroids has produced complications, including hyperglycemia, glucosuria, gastrointestinal bleeding, electrolyte abnormalities, and higher incidence of infection.[12,36] However, for acute brain injury, dexamethasone‡ 1 gm/kg intravenously repeated at eight-hour intervals for the first 24 to 48 hours may be used.

THE CRITICAL CARE PATIENT

Heart Disease

Response to anesthesia in patients with cardiac disease is variable. Young animals with congenital

defects may tolerate anesthesia, whereas older patients with limited cardiac reserve may not tolerate even low doses of anesthetics.

A smooth anesthetic induction is especially important in animals with heart disease. The patient with obstructive cardiac disease such as aortic or pulmonary stenosis cannot respond to the increased need for tissue perfusion because of a relatively fixed cardiac output.[44] The patient with a congenital lesion such as atrial septal defect, ventricular septal defect, or patent ductus arteriosus may have increased pulmonary blood flow, but the higher flow does not affect uptake of anesthetic agents.[19] Increased blood volume allows normal tissue perfusion, and local control of vascular resistance regulates blood flow to satisfy metabolic needs. Tetralogy of Fallot produces a right-to-left shunt and reduced pulmonary blood flow; therefore, in the affected patient, induction time with a relatively insoluble inhalation anesthetic such as halothane is longer than with the more soluble methoxyflurane. An intravenous agent acts rapidly in a patient with right-to-left shunt because the drug goes directly to the brain, a portion of the injected dose being shunted away from the lung. Also, because of the right-to-left shunt, the risk of pulmonary embolization is greater.

If the heart disease has progressed to heart failure, any anesthetic technique is risky, whereas if the patient has some cardiac reserve, almost any anesthetic technique is successful. The patient with cardiac tamponade is one of the most difficult to anesthetize, because the depressant effects of anesthetics cause an immediate reduction in cardiac output, resulting in cardiac failure. Death may occur if cardiac tamponade is not immediately relieved.

A balanced anesthetic technique for the patient with heart disease is recommended. A combination of atropine or glycopyrrolate, tranquilizer (acetylpromazine* or diazepam†), narcotic (oxymorphone), muscle relaxant, and inhalation anesthetic works well for the patient in failure. Less severely affected patients tolerate conventional anesthesia consisting of barbiturate induction followed by halothane for maintenance.

Pulmonary Disease

The patient with pulmonary disease is often presented with a reduced volume between the functional residuals and closing capacities. Conditions such as pulmonary infection, atelectasis, multiple trauma, heart failure (with secondary pulmonary congestion), obesity, and increased age may decrease functional residual capacity.[61] Anesthesia further reduces it and causes a change in the relationship between closing and functional residual capacities, resulting in a grossly low or atelectatic relationship between these

*Travenol Laboratories, Inc., Morton Grove, IL.
†National Laboratories Corp., Sommerville, NJ.
‡Schering Corporation, Kenilworth, NJ.

*Ft. Dodge Laboratories, Inc., Ft. Dodge, IA.
†Roche Laboratories, Nutley, NJ.

parameters.[17] Mucus flow is reduced by anesthesia, especially in the patient with copious amounts of secretions, because of slowing of tracheal ciliary movement.[29] Also, anesthesia inhibits the hypoxic pulmonary vasoconstriction reflex and may increase shunting more in patients with a preexisting reflex than in those without it.[52] Assisted or controlled ventilation, therefore, is very important for the patient with pulmonary disease.

Hepatic Disease

Anesthetics cause changes in hepatic function and hepatic blood flow, whereas inhalation anesthetics depress cellular function.[3] An abnormal Bromsulphalein clearance test result following surgery is probably due to alterations in liver blood flow caused by operative manipulation or preexisting liver disease.[30] Liver function tests also change after use of multiple anesthetics, particularly if one of them is halothane.[8] Hepatic venous pressure may increase with right ventricular failure or as a result of increased intrathoracic pressure secondary to positive-pressure ventilation. Specific anesthetic effects on hepatic blood flow are similar to other changes that cause the sympathetic nervous system to react. In general, splanchnic vascular resistance is regulated primarily by the sympathetic nervous system and reacts similarly to other vascular beds.[38] Direct alpha-receptor stimulation secondary to hypoxia or hypercarbia or relative alpha-receptor stimulation secondary to beta-receptor blockade increases splanchnic vascular resistance and decreases hepatic blood flow. Conversely, decreased splanchnic vascular resistance and increased hepatic blood flow result from beta-receptor stimulation and alpha-receptor blockade and from the direct effect of carbon dioxide on the splanchnic vasculature during halothane anesthesia.[23]

All anesthetic agents and techniques decrease hepatic blood flow, but for different reasons.[3] Halothane decreases flow 29 per cent, probably in relation to decreased perfusion pressure and cardiac output.[23] It can also cause a vascular arteriolar spasm.[5] Methoxyflurane produces a 50 per cent reduction in blood flow owing to decreased perfusion pressure and higher splanchnic vascular resistance.[49] A combination of nitrous oxide and thiopental anesthesia causes little change in resistance.[24] Hypercarbia decreases splanchnic blood flow.[13] Similarly, if carbon dioxide is decreased, blood flow is also reduced because of intermittent positive-pressure ventilation, which causes a reduction in venous return to the heart and cardiac output. Although hepatic blood flow decreases to a greater degree than oxygen consumption, there is little evidence of anaerobic metabolism.[13] Cellular hypoxia apparently does not occur, although the margin of safety for tissue oxygenation is narrowed. Intermittent positive-pressure ventilation, hypocarbia, hypercarbia, and surgical manipulation, particularly during light levels of anesthesia, may play a more important role in decreased hepatic blood flow than the effects of direct agents.[32]

Jaundice in a critical patient causes bradycardia. Tachycardia in a patient with obstructive jaundice may signal ventricular fibrillation and imminent sudden death.[3] The patient with liver disease often has hypoalbuminemia and may have an unusually profound and prolonged response to thiobarbiturates because of decreased protein binding. Also, the diseased liver may not be able to compensate for a decreased clearance of citrate, so blood transfusions using acid-citrate-dextrose as anticoagulant should be given slowly.

Halothane probably does not cause hepatitis in the dog or cat, especially if events common during anesthesia, such as surgical stimulation, intermittent positive-pressure ventilation, and hypocarbia or hypercarbia, which increase splanchnic resistance and decrease splanchnic blood, flow are discounted. Hepatotoxicity after anesthesia is rare and difficult to prove, especially in the dog or cat, in which follow-up is often impossible.

Renal Disease

Anesthesia and the stresses of surgery decrease glomerular filtration rate and renal plasma flow. Halothane produces a 20 to 40 per cent decrease in glomerular filtration rate and a 40 per cent decrease in effective renal plasma flow.[16] The other potent inhalation anesthetics cause dose-dependent changes. Methoxyflurane promotes a reduction in outer cortical perfusion and a relative increase in inner cortical perfusion that may lead to prolonged tubular contact with the toxic products of methoxyflurane.[48] Methoxyflurane is nephrotoxic in humans,[53] but the human syndrome, high-output renal failure, is more difficult to produce in dogs.[9,28,60] Other factors can reduce glomerular filtration rate and renal blood flow. Anxiety, dehydration, stress, drugs used for preanesthetic medication, hypotension, surgical stimulation, and either oliguria or osmotic diuresis can affect renal function.[3] Preoperative hydration prior to halothane anesthesia can nearly eliminate the changes during light anesthesia and lessen the changes seen during deep anesthesia.[2] Ketamine normally decreases renal cortical blood flow and urine output but has no effect on renal blood flow of greyhounds.[6] Also in dogs, fentanyl-droperidol* increases renal cortical blood flow and decreases urine output but does not appreciably alter medullary blood flow.[41] The preanesthetic use of xylazine produces hyperglycemia and diuresis, especially in the cat.[27] In the critical patient requiring continuous positive-pressure ventilation, there is a 29 per cent decrease in cardiac index and a 9 per cent decrease in mean renal arterial pressure.[39] There is also an increase in plasma antidiuretic hormone in dogs ventilated with positive end expiratory pres-

---

*Pitman Moore, Inc., Washington Crossing, NJ

sure.[1] In hypotensive dogs, halothane reduces or abolishes the effects of sympathetic vasoconstriction, allowing renal blood flow to return to normal.[51] Studies using the isolated canine kidney have shown that halothane actually increases renal blood flow, total and fractional sodium excretion, osmolar clearance, and urine flow. Blood is shifted from the outer to the inner cortex.[4] Thus, the changes in renal function observed during anesthesia result primarily from alterations in hemodynamics. In humans during light anesthesia, changes in renal function are minimal and transient as long as hydration is adequately maintained during anesthesia.[2]

Central Nervous System Disease

Anesthetics affect cerebral blood flow, cerebral perfusion pressure, and intracranial pressure. Cerebral blood flow is increased during anesthesia with halothane, nitrous oxide, enflurane, isoflurane, and methoxyflurane, with halothane causing the greatest change (more than 200 per cent).[68] In contrast, injectable drugs, including thiopental, morphine, droperidol, fentanyl, fentanyl-droperidol, and diazepam, decrease cerebral blood flows and ketamine increases it.[68] Increased cerebral blood flow causes a parallel rise in intracranial pressure, especially in animals with central nervous system disease or space-occupying lesions within the cranium. However, there are some species differences. Fentanyl has minimal effects on cerebral metabolic rate for oxygen consumption ($CMRO_2$) in humans but causes a marked transient decrease in both indices in dogs.[55] This effect is reversed by narcotic antagonists. In the dog, nitrous oxide causes cerebral metabolic stimulation, which helps explain the resulting increase in cerebral blood flow and intracranial pressure.[65] Because the effect of barbiturates is to reduce cerebral blood flow, they have been proposed as part of the treatment for ischemic lesions of the brain.[62] Recent evidence has shown that barbiturates do not work in complete ischemia of a dog brain but may still work in partially ischemic lesions.[72] Seizure activity is produced by some anesthetics, particularly the ethers, including enflurane, diethyl ether, forane, and methoxyflurane.[43] Ancillary drugs used during anesthesia, such as succinylcholine, may increase intracranial pressure as much as 25 mm Hg.[40]

Drugs used to treat hypotension—epinephrine, norepinephrine, and isoproterenol—increase cerebral blood flow. Epinephrine does so through a state of CNS arousal; hydralazine also increases intracranial pressure.[59]

In summary, all commonly used inhalation anesthetics produce cerebral vasodilation and decrease brain metabolism. Nitrous oxide can be significantly detrimental to patients with intracranial hypertension. In dogs, methoxyflurane decreases $CMRO_2$ and elevates cerebral blood flow to a lesser extent than other volatile anesthetics. Barbiturates reduce cerebral blood flow and $CMRO_2$, approximately paralleling central nervous system depression.

Acid-Base Disturbances

Acidosis increases the active (non-ionized) fraction of the thiobarbiturate molecule, decreases protein binding, depresses cardiovascular function, increases heart irritability, and shifts the oxyhemoglobin curve to the right.[11,44,64,76] Halothane and xylazine may produce life-threatening changes in cardiac electrical activity during acidosis, because they reduce the threshold to premature ventricular contractions and other dysrhythmias.[57] Alkalosis constricts cerebral vessels, reducing blood flow below metabolic need. It also shifts the oxyhemoglobin dissociation curve to the left, thereby decreasing unloading of oxygen to tissues and promoting local tissue hypoxia.[76] Acidosis should be treated prior to induction of anesthesia, especially if the pH is below 7.2.

Operative Procedure

Operating conditions can be improved by the use of certain anesthetic techniques. Neuromuscular blocking agents reduce patient movement due to electrocautery stimulation or subsequent to manipulation of abdominal viscera. Unfortunately, gallamine is contraindicated in patients with renal disease, because it is eliminated primarily via renal excretion.[74] Succinylcholine should not be used in patients with hepatic disease because serum cholinesterase synthesis by the liver may be decreased.[74] Neither group of relaxants should be used in the patient with muscle weakness, severe tissue damage, or burns. The use of depolarizing muscle relaxants in patients with excessive tissue damage may produce dangerously high serum potassium levels, possibly high enough to cause cardiac arrest.[54]

Postoperative analgesia is not usually required in the dog and cat; however, if after the excitement phase of recovery is over the patient is still in pain, as expressed by whining or restlessness, analgesia is warranted. Pulmonary disease may be a contraindication to the administration of narcotic postoperative analgesics (oxymorphone, merperidine*), because further depression of ventilation may result. The use of phenothiazine tranquilizers in the dog or cat after a painful surgical procedure apparently has good results, but these drugs probably provide little or no analgesia even though clinically the patient seems to rest easier. Arguments against the use of narcotic analgesics include short clinical effect, respiratory depression, and potential abuse by humans. Synthetic agonist-antagonist analgesics show some promise in treating the postoperative patient because they cause little sedation or depression of ventilation.[63]

---

*Winthrop Laboratories, Des Plains, IL.

MONITORING OF THE CRITICAL CARE PATIENT

Factors to consider in the choice of a monitoring system for the critical care patient include the patient's condition, anesthetic agent, operative procedure, equipment available, and the variables requiring monitoring. The patient's condition is determined by the severity of the disease process. A patient that is comatose or has multiple-system trauma may require extensive monitoring, whereas the patient with single organ system disease may require a less sophisticated technique.

The choice of anesthetic agent also influences the choice of monitoring system. Some anesthetic agents produce dysrhythmias with greater frequency than others. Because the halogenated hydrocarbons, particularly halothane, reduce the threshold to dysrhythmias from administration of epinephrine, and monitoring of patients receiving such agents should include an electrocardiogram.[44] Most anesthetic agents, with the exception of ketamine and barbiturates, produce arterial hypotension.[71] The degree of hypotension is dose-dependent. Therefore, monitoring of arterial blood pressure is an excellent means of assessing anesthetic depth.

Consideration of the operative procedure is important not only to determine the need for monitoring but also to predict the problems associated with techniques of monitoring. It is difficult to monitor a patient undergoing head surgery, because most of the important monitoring sites are covered by surgical drapes or are not accessible. Visual assessment of mucous membranes is difficult, evaluation of jaw (muscle) tone is impossible, and palpebral or corneal reflexes are not easily appraised.

Inexpensive monitoring equipment gives the same information as more expensive equipment. For example, an aneroid manometer can be used for mean arterial pressure, an esophageal stethoscope to gauge heart and lung sounds, and a mercury thermometer to determine body temperature. All of these devices can be easily obtained and provide accurate information.

Many criteria are used to assess the critical patient, including depth of anesthesia, functional capacity of the heart and vascular system, packed cell volume, efficiency of the respiratory system, blood pH and gas levels, efficiency of the kidneys, and body temperature.

The depth of anesthesia is monitored both subjectively and objectively. The subjective parameters are: degree of muscle relaxation, strength of peripheral pulse, color of mucous membranes, and vaporizer setting. The objective parameter, end tidal concentration of inhalation anesthetics, can be continuously monitored by means of a breath-by-breath analyzer.*

Monitoring the Cardiovascular System

The cardiovascular system is best monitored by assessing trends. Isolated values provide limited information unless grossly abnormal, and much more can be gained from observing changes and trends. An arterial blood pressure of 100 mm Hg systolic is merely an observation, unless the prior pressure is known. If the pressure has been at 150 mm Hg, a reading of 100 mm Hg becomes highly significant, and its cause demands diagnosis and treatment. Similarly, a pressure of 100 mm Hg may be encouraging during halothane anesthesia because hypotension is usually expected. One of the most effective ways of monitoring the cardiovascular system is by peripheral pulse. Information obtainable via the pulse includes cardiac rate, rhythm, and character of the pulse. If the peripheral pulse is palpable, blood is perfusing coronary and cerebral circulations. If arterial blood is fully oxygenated, metabolic demands of oxygen for those systems will be met. Peripheral pulse can be monitored electronically using a photoplethysmograph.[50]* This type of monitor is usually applied to the tongue or foot of a dog or cat. Such a pulse monitor, however, fails to work when the pulse pressure is low or when there is vasoconstriction at the site of pulse detection. Therefore, it may not work in a patient in which it is potentially most useful. In lengthy operations with the patient breathing spontaneously and the presence of a regular pulse, a photoplethsmograph provides good evidence of adequate peripheral flow.

Arterial pressure is another useful variable to monitor during surgery. Clinically, arterial pressure is a means of assessing tissue blood flow. However, flow is not the only important factor. An adequate head of pressure is important to overcome the critical closing pressures of various organs. Diastolic pressure is particularly important in sustaining coronary artery flow.

Methods of Monitoring

Indirect arterial pressure measurements are obtained by various methods, including oscillotonometry, auscultation of the sounds under a cuff, detection of arterial wall movement under the cuff, and detection of the onset of flow below the cuff. Oscillotonometry was the first indirect method.[50] Recently, a machine has been developed that uses the oscillotonometry principle.† The machine automatically inflates the cuff at set periods from one to 16 minutes and automatically derives the systolic and diastolic pressures as the cuff is deflated. A second method of indirect pressure measurement involves the use of Korotkoff sounds under the cuff. This method correlates well with intravascular measurement,[50] but it is difficult to use in dogs and cats because the small size and conformation of their legs and feet make it difficult to place the cuff properly. A third method involves detection of arterial wall movements and uses the Doppler principle.[31]‡ In the digital method,

---

*LB-2 Infra-red Analyzer, Beckman Instruments, Palo Alto, CA.

*Datascope Corporation, Paramus, NJ.
†Dinamap, Applied Medical Research, Tampa, FL.
‡Arteriosonde, Hoffman–LaRoche, Cranberry, NY.

the cuff is inflated and a finger is used to detect the appearance of a pulse from a peripheral artery. In human medicine, this method is unreliable at pressures below 80 mm Hg, in patients with vasoconstricted arteries, and in small children. In dogs this method is unreliable at femoral artery pressures below 50 mm Hg.

Intra-Arterial Pressure Monitoring

Although indirect monitoring of arterial pressure is probably more practical for veterinarians, the benefits of intra-arterial pressure monitoring sometimes outweigh the risks. Indications for direct monitoring of arterial pressure include the anticipation of an unstable anesthetic state, rapid arterial pressure changes, profound hypotension too low for accurate indirect monitoring (shock), and need for repeated blood gas estimations. During anesthesia, mean arterial pressure should be maintained between 70 and 90 mm Hg in order to provide adequate tissue perfusion to prevent anerobic metabolism. Mean pressure less than 60 mm Hg should be treated with such measures as: (1) decrease in anesthetic level, (2) fluid administration to provide adequate venous return, and (3) pharmacological stimulation of the heart. Direct arterial pressure can be monitored inexpensively with an aneroid manometer, which can be obtained as part of a home blood pressure monitoring kit (Fig. 197–1).[25] In the dog, the technique involves catheterization of the femoral or the cranial tibial artery. After the area is surgically prepared, an "outside the needle" catheter is placed intra-arterially through a pericutaneous puncture and is connected to low-compliance plastic tubing that has been previously filled with fluid. All connections in the system should be tight. The pressure indicated on the aneroid manometer is within 10 per cent of mean arterial pressure.

The catheter is kept patent by periodic flushing with heparinized saline or with a continuous saline flow device.* After the catheter is removed, compression of the puncture site for at least five minutes is needed to prevent hematoma. If the arterial pressure wave form is displayed on an oscilloscope, one can make some assessment of myocardial strength. If the upstroke of the pressure wave decreases in steepness, myocardial depression should be suspected.[50]

Heart Sounds

Heart sounds should be clear, and changes in intensity may be due to changes in myocardial contractility. An esophageal stethoscope is a convenient means of monitoring heart sounds. It is not easily displaced, as is an external stethoscope taped to the animal's chest. Useful information can be obtained

*Statham MFS Microflush System, Statham Instruments, Inc., Oxnard, CA.

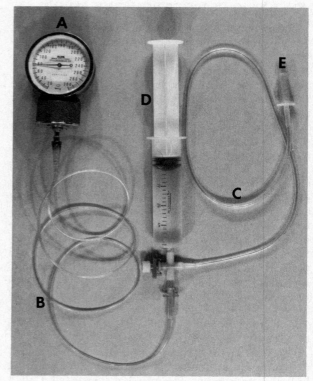

Figure 197–1. Equipment needed to monitor mean arterial pressure. *A,* Aneroid manometer (available from Anesthesia Associates, Inc., P.O. Box 1105, San Marcos, California 92069); *B,* 36-inch transmission set (No. 825–88, available from Cutter Medical, 4th and Parker Streets, Berkeley, California 94710). *C,* Extension tubing and three-way stopcock (available from C. R. Bard, Inc., Murray Hill, New Jersey 07974). *D,* Heparinized saline used to fill tubing and catheter before connection to manometer. *E,* Connection to arterial catheter. (Reprinted with permission from Sawyer, D. C.: *The Practice of Small Animal Anesthesia.* W. B. Saunders, Philadelphia, 1982.)

by listening to the strength, character, and rhythm of the heart sound.

Electrocardiogram

The object of monitoring the electrocardiogram (ECG) is to establish the rate and rhythm of ventricular depolarization. However, during electrical-mechanical dissociation, it is possible to have a normal or near normal ECG with little or no cardiac output. Therefore, the ECG does not substitute for monitoring of peripheral pulse or heart sounds. The ECG is used to determine why, not whether, there is a problem with peripheral pulse. The benefits of using an ECG on a routine basis include determining the frequency of minor or major dysrhythmias, immediate treatment of major dysrhythmias, and availability of equipment in emergencies.

Cardiac Filling Pressure

Central venous pressure is monitored to determine cardiac efficiency and is useful to determine the point at which further transfusion is ineffective. The principal of monitoring central venous pressure is based on the Frank-Starling law, which states that the strength of contraction is related to the myocardial muscle fiber length.[37] An increase in venous return improves cardiac output because strength of contraction of the myocardial muscle is increased. As the myocardial muscle fails, venous pressure increases. Central venous pressure also serves as an early warning of decreased venous return with hypovolemia. An "inside the needle" catheter is placed percutaneously into the jugular vein and advanced to the right atrium.[10] Ideally, the tip of the catheter should be just distal to the entrance of the right atrium. However, if the catheter follows a smaller vein to the thorax, reasonably accurate recordings are obtained.

Monitoring left side ventricular function is done through a Swan-Ganz catheter.[73] A catheter is advanced with ECG monitoring down the right jugular vein, and a small balloon on the end of the catheter is inflated. The balloon floats the catheter via the jugular vein to the vena cava through the right atrium and ventricle and into the pulmonary artery. As the catheter wedges in a peripheral pulmonary artery, the pressure obtained, referred to as wedge pressure, is indicative of left atrial pressure. This method of monitoring cardiac filling pressure is too complicated for routine clinical use in the dog and cat and accordingly is used primarily in research.

Cardiac Output

Cardiac output can be monitored using a thermal dilution computer by injecting room temperature or cold saline as the indicator.[26] The change in temperature is affected by changes in cardiac output. Like pressure monitoring with the Swan-Ganz catheter, thermodilution cardiac output determination is used mostly in the research laboratory.

Peripheral flow of blood is monitored by observing the color and temperature of peripheral limbs. If flow is decreased, the limb becomes pale and cold. As peripheral flow increases, temperature increases and a healthy pink color returns.

Packed Cell Volume

Packed cell volume (PCV) is important to monitor because anesthesia reduces it 15 to 20 per cent.[67] Anesthesia is not advisable if the packed cell volume is below 25 per cent, because oxygen-carrying capacity is decreased. Acute hemorrhage during surgery is not reflected by an immediate drop in packed cell volume unless supplemental fluids are given rapidly.[58]

Respiratory System

The respiratory system can be monitored by observing mucous membrane color, breath sounds, and the force required to inflate the lungs. Oxygen monitors with an alarm system can be used to monitor percentage of oxygen delivered. Expired carbon dioxide concentration can also be monitored continuously. A respirometer is used to monitor volume and derive minute ventilation. Arterial oxygen is usually monitored by intermittent sampling of blood to evaluate PaO_2 and oxygen saturation of hemoglobin. After the use of muscle relaxants, return of spontaneous ventilation is best evaluated by assessment of negative inspiratory force. The procedure involves inserting a 20-gauge needle into the endotracheal tube. An aneroid manometer is connected to the needle via low-compliance tubing. After the endotracheal tube is occluded, inspiratory force can be read on the aneroid manometer. Normal spontaneous inspiratory pressure should be -5 mm Hg.[70]

Body Temperature

The body temperature of small dogs and large dogs with thin hair coats should be monitored by use of an electronic thermometer. Malignant hyperthermia, a rare problem in temperature control characterized by increased levels of carbon dioxide and lactic acid, is triggered by some anesthetics.[35,69] Immediate recognition of this syndrome is necessary if treatment is to be successful.

Anesthetic Recovery

Anesthetic recovery is monitored by noting heart rate, pulse strength, mucous membrane color, capillary refill time, and central venous pressure. Ventilation rate, depth, and character should also be monitored, especially if muscle relaxants have been used. During recovery from anesthesia, a steady progressive improvement in mental alertness should be observed along with improvement in cardiovascular and respiration variables. If recovery is slow, hypothermia, hypotension, or hypoventilation should be suspected, and appropriate therapy instituted.

Summary

Monitoring of the critical care patient requires more intense observation of vital signs than monitoring for elective surgery. In choosing a monitoring system, the veterinarian should consider the patient's condition, the anesthetic agent or technique selected, the operative procedure, the equipment available, and the practicability.

1. Baratz, R. A. and Ingraham, R. C.: Renal hemodynamic and antidiuretic hormone release associated with volume regulation. J. Physiol. *198*:565, 1960.
2. Barry, K. G., Mazze, R. I., and Schwartz, F. D.: Prevention of surgical oligemia and renal-hemodynamic suppression by sustained hydration. N. Engl. J. Med. *270*:1371, 1964.
3. Bastron, R. D.: *In* Miller, R. D. (ed.): *Hepatic and Renal*

Physiology in Anesthesia. Churchill-Livingstone, New York, 1981.

4. Bastron, R. D., Pyne, J. L., and Inagaki, M.: Halothane-induced renal vasodilation. Anesthesiology 50:126, 1979.

5. Benumof, J. L., Brookstein, J. J., Sardman, L. J., and Harris, R.: Diminished hepatic arterial flow during halothane administration. Anesthesiology 45:545, 1976.

6. Bevan, D. R., and Bhudu, R.: The effect of ketamine on renal blood flow in greyhounds. Br. J. Anaesth. 47:634, 1975.

7. Brock-Utne, J. G., Rubin, J., Welman, S., et al.: The effect of glycopyrrolate on the lower esophageal sphincter. Can. Anaesth. Soc. J. 25:144, 1978.

8. Brohult, J.: Liver reaction after halothane and diethyl ether anesthesia. Acta Anaesthesiol. Scand. 11:201, 1967.

9. Brunson, D. B., Stowe, C. M., and McGrath, C. J.: Serum and urine inorganic fluoride concentrations and urine oxalate concentrations following methoxyflurane anesthesia in the dog. Am. J. Vet. Res. 40:197, 1979.

10. Burrows, C. F.: Techniques and complications of intravenous and intraarterial catheterization in dogs and cats. J. Am. Vet. Med. Assoc. 163:1357, 1973.

11. Carson, S., Chorley, G. E., Hamilton, F. N., et al.: Variation in cardiac output with acid-base changes in the anesthetized dog. J. Appl. Physiol. 20:948, 1965.

12. Cooper, P. R., Moody, S., and Clark, W. K.: Dexamethazone and severe head injury: a prospective double-blind study. J. Neurosurg. 51:307, 1979.

13. Cooperman, L. H.: Effects of anaesthetics on the splanchnic circulation. Br. J. Anaesth. 44:967, 1972.

14. Cousins, M. J., and Mazze, R. I.: Anaesthesia, surgery and renal function: immediate and delayed effects. Anaesth. Int. Care. 1:355, 1973.

15. Cromwell, T. H., Eger, E. I., II, Stevens, W. C., and Dolan, W. M.: Forane uptake excretion and blood solubility in man. Anesthesiology 35:365, 1971.

16. Deutsch, S., Goldberg, M., Stephen, G. M., and Wu, W.: Effects of halothane anesthesia on renal function in normal man. Anesthesiology 27:793, 1966.

17. Don, H.: The mechanical properties of the respiratory system during anesthesia. Int. Anesthesiol, Clin. 15:113, 1977.

18. Dundee, J. W., and Drips, R. D.: Effects of diethyl ether, trichlorethylene and trifluoroethylvinyl ether on respiration. Anesthesiology 18:282, 1957.

19. Eger, E. I.: Effect of ventilation perfusion abnormalities. *In* Eger, E. I. (ed.): *Anesthetic Uptake and Action*. Williams & Wilkins, Baltimore, 1974.

20. Eger, E. I.: Uptake of inhaled anesthetics: the alveolar to inspired anesthetic difference. *In* Eger, E. I., (ed.): *Anesthetic Uptake and Action*. Williams & Wilkins, Baltimore, 1974.

21. Eger, E. I., II, and Larson, C. P., Jr.: Anaesthetic solubility in blood and tissues: values and significance. Br. J. Anaesth. 36:140, 1964.

22. Eger, E. I., and Saidman, L. J.: Hazards of nitrous oxide anesthesia in bowel obstruction and pneumothorax. Anesthesiology 26:61, 1965.

23. Epstein, R. M., Deutsch, S., Cooperman, L. H., et al.: Splanchnic circulation during halothane anesthesia and hypercapnea in normal man. Anesthesiology 27:654, 1966.

24. Epstein, R. M., Wheeler, H. O., Furmin, M. J., et al.: The effect of hypercapnia on estimated hepatic blood flow, circulating splanchnic blood volume, and hepatic sulfobromphthalein clearance during general anesthesia in man. J. Clin. Invest. 40:592, 1961.

25. Evans, A. T.: Monitoring the critical patient. *In* Sattler, F. P., Knowles, R. P., and Whittick, W. G. (eds.): *Veterinary Critical Care*. Lea & Febiger, Philadelphia, 1981.

26. Evonuk, E., Imig, C. J., Greenfield, W., and Eckstein, J. W.: Cardiac output measured by thermal dilution of room temperature injectate. J. Appl. Physiol. 16:271, 1961.

27. Feldberg, W., and Symonds, H. W.: Hyperglycemic effect of xylazine. J. Vet. Pharmacol. Ther. 3:197, 1980.

28. Fleming, J. T., and Pedersoli, W. M.: Serum inorganic fluoride and renal function in dogs after methoxyflurane anesthesia, tetracycline treatment, and surgical manipulation. Am. J. Vet. Res. 41:2025, 1980.

29. Forbes, A. R.: Halothane depresses mucociliary flow in the trachea. Anesthesiology 45:59, 1976.

30. French, A. B., Barass, T. P, Fairlie, C. W., et al.: Metabolic effects of anesthesia in man. V: A comparison of the effects of ether and cyclopropane anesthesia on the abnormal liver. Ann. Surg. 135:145, 1952.

31. Garner, H. E., Hahn, A. W., Hartley, J. W., et al.: Indirect blood pressure measurement in the dog. Lab. Anim. Sci. 25:197, 1976.

32. Gelman, S. I.: Disturbances in hepatic blood flow during anesthesia and surgery. Arch. Surg. 111:881, 1976.

33. Gibbs, C. P., Schwartz, D. J., Wynne, J. W., et al.: Antacid pulmonary aspiration in the dog. Anesthesiology 51:380, 1979.

34. Giesecke, A. H., Jr.: Anesthesia for trauma surgery. *In* Miller, R. D. (ed.): *Anesthesia*. Churchill Livingstone, New York, 1981.

35. Gronert, G. A.: Malignant hyperthermia. Anesthesiology 53:395, 1980.

36. Gudeman, S. K., Miller, J. D., and Becker, D. P.: Failure of high dose steroid therapy to influence intracranial pressure in patients with severe head injury. J. Neurosurg. 51:301, 1979.

37. Guyton, A. C.: Heart muscle: the heart as a pump. *In*: *Textbook of Medical Physiology*. W. B. Saunders, Philadelphia, 1976.

38. Guyton, A. C.: Muscle blood flow during exercise; cerebral, splanchnic, and skin blood flows. *In*: *Textbook of Medical Physiology*. W. B, Saunders, Philadelphia, 1976.

39. Hall, S. V., Johnson, E. E., and Hedley-White, J.: Renal hemodynamics and function with continuous positive pressure ventilation in dogs. Anesthesiology 71:452, 1974.

40. Halldin, M., and Wahlin, A.: Effect of succinylcholine on the intraspinal pressure. Acta Anaesthesiol. Scand. 3:155, 1959.

41. Hirasawa, H., and Yonezawa, T.: The effects of ketamine and Innovar on the renal cortical and medullary blood flow in the dog. Anaesthetist 24:349, 1975.

42. Ito, U., Ohno, K., Suganama, Y., et al.: Effect of steroid on ischemic brain edema. Analysis of cytotoxic and vasogenic edema occurring during ischemia and after restoration of blood flow. Stroke 11:166, 1980.

43. Joas, T. A., Stevens, W. C., and Eger, E. I.: Electroencephalographic seizure activity in dogs during anesthesia. Brit. J. Anaesth. 43:739, 1971.

44. Jobes, D. R.: Anesthesia for cardiac surgery. Surg. Clin. North 55:893, 1975.

45. Katz, R. L., and Bigger, J. T., Jr.: Cardiac arrhythmias during anesthesia and operation. Anesthesiology 33:193, 1970.

46. Kolata, R. J., Kraut, N. J., and Johnston, D. E.: Patterns of trauma in urban dogs and cats. A study of 1000 cases. J. Am. Vet. Med. Assoc. 164:499, 1974.

47. Larson, C. P., Eger, E. I., Muallem, M., et al.: The effects of diethyl ether and methoxyflurane on ventilation. Anesthesiology 30:174, 1969.

48. Leighton, K., and Bruce, C.: Distribution of kidney blood flow: a comparison of methoxyflurane and halothane effects as measured by heated thermocouple. Can. Anaesth. Soc. J. 22:125, 1975.

49. Libonati, M., Malsch, E., Price, H. L., et al.: Splanchnic circulation in man during methoxyflurane anesthesia. Anesthesiology 38:466, 1973.

50. Lindop M. J.: Monitoring of the cardiovascular system during anesthesia. Anesth. Clin. 19:1, 1981.

51. MacDonald, A. G.: The effect of halothane on renal cortical blood flow in normotensive and hypotensive dogs. Br. J. Anaesth. 41:644, 1969.

52. Mathers, J. M., Benumof, J. L., and Wahrenbrock, E. A.: General anesthetics and regional hypoxic pulmonary vasoconstriction. Anesthesiology 46:111, 1977.

53. Mazze, R. I., and Cousins, J. M.: Renal toxicity of anesthetics with specific reference to the nephrotoxicity of methoxyflurane. Can. Anaesth. Soc. J. 20:64, 1973.

54. Mazze, R. I., Escue, H. M., and Houston, J. B.: Hyperkalemia and cardiovascular collapse following administration of succinylcholine to the traumatized patient. Anesthesiology *31*:540, 1956.

55. Michenfelter, J. D., and Theye, R. A.: Effects of fentanyl, droperidol and Innovar on canine cerebral metabolism and blood flow. Br. J. Anaesth. *43*:630, 1971.

56. Miller, R. D., and Savarese, J. J.: Pharmacology of muscle relaxants, their antagonists, and monitoring of neuromuscular function. *In* Miller, R. D., (ed.): *Anesthesia.* Churchill Livingstone, New York, 1981.

57. Muir, W. W., Werner, L. L., and Hamlin, R. L.: Effects of xylazine and acetylpromazine upon induced ventricular fibrillation in dogs anesthetized with thiamylal and halothane. Am. J. Vet. Res. *36*:1299, 1975.

58. Nelson, A. W.: The unified concept of shock. Vet. Clin. North Am. *6*:173, 1976.

59. Overgaard, J., and Skinhoj, E.: The effects of hydralazine upon intracranial pressure and cerebral blood flow. *In* Harper, A. M., and Jennett, W. B. (eds.): *Blood Flow and Metabolism in the Brain: Proceedings.* Churchill Livingstone, New York, 1976.

60. Pedersoli, W. M.: Serum fluoride concentration, renal and hepatic function test results in dogs with methoxyflurane anesthesia. Am. J. Vet. Res. *38*:949, 1977.

61. Rehder, K., Marsh, H. M., Rodarti, J. R., and Hyatt, R. E.: Airway closure. Anesthesiology *47*:40, 1977.

62. Rockoff, M. A., and Shapiro, H. M.: Barbiturates following cardiac arrest: possible benefit or Pandora's box? Anesthesiology *49*:385, 1978.

63. Romagnoli, A., and Keats, A. S.: Ceiling effect for respiratory depression by nalbuphine. Clin. Pharmacol. Ther. *27*:478, 1980.

64. Saidman, L. J : Uptake, distribution and elimination of barbiturates. *In* Eger, E. I., II (ed.): *Anesthetic Uptake and Action.* Williams & Wilkins, Baltimore, 1974.

65. Sakabe, T., Kuramoto, T., Inone, S., and Takeshita, H.: Cerebral effects of nitrous oxide in the dog. Anesthesiology *48*:195, 1978.

66. Salem, M. R., Wong, A. Y., Moni, M., et al.: Premedicant drugs and gastric juice pH and volume in pediatric patients. Anesthesiology *44*:216, 1976.

66a. Sawyer, D. C.: The anesthetic period. *In: The Practice of Small Animal Anesthesia.* W. B. Saunders, Philadelphia, 1982.

67. Sawyer, D. C., Lumb, W. V., and Stone, H. L.: Cardiovascular effects of halothane methoxyflurane, pentobarbital and thiamylal. J. Appl. Physiol. *30*:36, 1971.

68. Shapiro, H. M.: Anesthesia effects upon cerebral blood flow, cerebral metabolism, and the electroencephalogram. *In* Miller, R. D. (ed.): *Anesthesia.* Churchill-Livingstone, New York, 1981.

69. Short, C. E., and Paddleford, R. R.: Malignant hyperthermia in a dog (letter). Anesthesiology *39*:462, 1973.

70. Smith, T. C.: Respiratory effects of general anesthesia. *In* Soma, L. R. (ed.): *Textbook of Veterinary Anesthesia.* Williams & Wilkins, Baltimore, 1971.

71. Steffey, E. P., and Howland, D., Jr.: Potency of enflurane in dogs: comparison with halothane and isoflurane. Am. J. Vet. Res. *39*:573, 1978.

72. Steen, P. P., Milde, J. H., and Michenfilder, J. D.: No barbiturate protection in a dog model of complete cerebral ischemia. Ann. Neurol. *5*:343, 1979.

73. Swan, H. J. C., Ganz, W., and Forrester, J. S.: Catherterization of the heart in man with the use of a flow directed balloon tipped catheter. N. Engl. J. Med. *283*:447, 1970.

74. Tavernor, W. D.: Muscle relaxants. *In* Soma, L. R. (ed.): *Textbook of Veterinary Anesthesia.* Williams & Wilkins, Baltimore, 1971.

75. West, J. B.: Diffusion. *In: Respiratory Physiology—The Essentials.* Williams & Wilkins, Baltimore, 1974.

76. West, J. B.: Gas transport to the periphery. *In: Respiratory Physiology—The Essentials.* Williams & Wilkins, Baltimore, 1974.

77. White, F. A., Clark, R. B., and Thompson, D. S.: Preoperative oral antacid therapy for patients requiring emergency surgery. South. Med. J. *71*:177, 1978.

78. Wright, M.: Pharmacologic effects of ketamine and its use in veterinary medicine. J. Am. Vet. Med. Assoc. *180*: 1462, 1982.

Normal Laboratory Values

Jennifer N. Mills

Hematological Values[27]

	Units	Dog	Cat
Hemoglobin (Hb)	g/dl	12–18	8–15
Hematocrit (PCV)*	%	37–55	24–45
Erythrocytes (RBC)	$\times 10^{12}$/L	5.5–8.5	5–10
Mean corpuscular volume (MCV)	fL	60–77	39–55
Mean corpuscular Hb (MCH)	pg	19–25	13–17
Mean corpuscular Hb concentration (MCHC)	%	32–36	30–36
Reticulocyte count	%	0–1.5	0–1
RBC life span	days	120	70
RBC diameter	μ	6.7–7.2	5.5–6.3
Erythrocyte fragility			
% NaCl solution for initial hemolysis	—	0.40–0.50	0.66–0.72
complete hemolysis	—	0.32–0.42	0.46–0.54
Platelet count	$\times 10^9$/L	200–900	300–700
Leukocytes (WBC)	$\times 10^9$/L	6.0–17.0	5.5–19.5
Segmented neutrophils	%	60–77	35–75
	$\times 10^9$	3.0–11.5	2.5–12.5
Band neutrophils	%	0–3	0–3
	$\times 10^9$/L	0–0.3	0–0.3
Lymphocytes	%	12–30	20–55
	$\times 10^9$/L	1.0–4.8	1.5–7.0
Monocytes	%	3–10	1–4
	$\times 10^9$/L	0.15–1.35	0–0.85
Eosinophils	%	2–10	2–12
	$\times 10^9$	0.1–1.25	0–1.5
Basophils	%	rare	rare
	$\times 10^9$	rare	rare
Relative viscosity of whole blood at 38°C[1]	poises	4.7	4.2
Plasma protein (refractometry)*	g/dl	6.0–7.5	6.0–8.0
Plasma fibrinogen (heat precipitation)	mg/dl	150–300	150–300
Total blood volume	ml/kg	80–90	60–66

*Lower in young animals, higher range in greyhounds.

Influence of Age on the Canine Hemogram[27]*

	Units	6–8 Weeks	9–12 Weeks	4–6 Months	1–2 Years
Number of dogs†		24	21	9	13
Hb	g/dl	10.4±0.58	11.8±0.81	14.4±0.82	15.9±1.2
PCV	%	33.1±2.2	37.2±2.9	44±2.4	49.3±3.4
RBC	$\times 10^{12}$/L	4.73±0.38	5.4±0.54	6.56±0.46	6.91±0.60
MCHC	%	31.5±1.4	31.8±1.3	32.7±0.6	32.3±1.2
WBC	$\times 10^9$/L	13.4±2.0	15.0±2.0	13.6±1.7	14.0±2.2
Segmented neutrophils	%	58.8±10.9	56.4±7.8	52.4±5.5	58.1±7.3
Band neutrophils	%	0.65±0.77	0.57±1.1	0.61±0.81	0.27±0.42
Lymphocytes	%	30.1±8	33.5±8.1	36.9±5.5	28.6±7.7
Monocytes	%	6.9±2.6	6.7±2.7	6.0±1.8	5.2±2.1
Eosinophils	%	3.3±1.9	2.3±1.6	4.1±1.9	7.3±3.5
Basophils	%	0.08±0.24	0.07±0.23	0	0.12±0.4
Plasma protein	g/dl	5.33±0.29	5.87±0.46	6.6±0.25	7.03±0.33
Fibrinogen	mg/dl	183±70	200±84	222±66	215±80

*Mean ± standard deviation.
†Basenjis.

Influence of Age on the Feline Hemogram[27]*

	Units	0–6 Hours	1 Week	4 Weeks	8 Weeks	4 Months
Number of Cats		24	21	20	19	21
Hb	g/dl	12.2	10.9	8.4	9.4	10.7
PCV	%	44.7	35.7	29.9	35.6	35.7
RBC	$\times 10^{12}$/L	4.95	5.19	5.84	7.1	8.77
MCV	fl	90.3	68.8	51.2	50.1	40.7
MCH	pg	24.6	21.0	14.4	13.2	12.2
MCHC	%	27.3	30.5	28.1	26.4	29.9
WBC	$\times 10^{9}$/L	7.5	7.8	8.5	8.4	9.3

*Mean.

Bone Marrow Differential Cell Counts*

	Dog[1]	Cat[22]
Number of animals	187	60
Red cell series		
Rubriblasts	0.5	1.71
Prorubricytes and rubricytes	27.2	12.50
Metarubricytes	15.9	11.68
Total erythrocytic cells	43.6	25.88
Granulocytic cell series		
Myeloblasts	1.2	1.74
Promyelocytes	1.4	0.88
Myelocytes—neutrophils	4.8	9.76
Metamyelocytes—neutrophils	7.4	7.32
Band neutrophils	24.6	25.8
Segmented neutrophils	9.6	9.24
Eosinophils—all types	3.1	3.8
Basophils	—	0.002
Total granulocytic cells	52.2	58.53
Other cells		
Lymphocytes	0.9	7.63
Plasma cells	0.3	1.61
Reticulum cells	0.9	0.13
Monocytes	0.2	—
Megakaryocytes	0.4	—
Disintegrated	—	4.6
Unclassified	—	1.62
Mitotic cells	—	0.61
Vacuolated myeloid cells	—	0.21
Myeloid:erythroid ratio[27]	1.2:1	1.6:1.0

*Figures represent mean percentage cellular composition of bone marrow collected from the rib (dogs) and iliac crest (cats) of normal animals.

Blood, Plasma, and Serum Values[17]

	Dog		Cat	
	Traditional units	S.I. Units	Traditional Units	S.I. Units
Acetylcholinesterase-red cells	270 U/L	270 U/L	540 U/L	540 U/L
Ammonia (HP,S)	19–120 μg/dl	10.5–66.8 μmol/L		
Amylase (S,HP)	185–700 U/L	185–700 U/L		
	100–400 Somogyi units	185–740 U/L		
Arginase (S,HP)	0–4.7 U/L	0–4.7 U/L		
Bicarbonate (HCO_3^-) (S,P)	18–24 mEq/L	18–24 mmol/L	17–21 mEq/L	17–21 mmol/L
Bilirubin (S,P,HP)				
Direct	0.06–0.12 mg/dl	1.0–2.0 mmol/L		
Indirect	0.01–0.49 mg/dl	0.2–8.4 mmol/L		
Total[4]	0.07–0.61 mg/dl	1.2–10.4 mmol/L	0.15–0.2 mg/dl	2.5–3.4 mmol/L
Calcium (S,HP)	9.3–11.3 mg/dl	2.32–2.82 mmol/L	6.2–10.2 mg/dl	1.55–2.55 mmol/L
Chloride (S,HP)	105–115 mEq/L	105–115 mmol/L	117–123 mEq/L	117–123 mmol/L
Cholesterol (S,P,HP)				
Total	135–270 mg/dl	3.51–7.02 mmol/L	95–130 mg/dl	2.47–3.38 mmol/L
Free	31–71 mg/dl	0.81–1.85 mmol/L	20–40 mg/dl	0.52–1.04 mmol/L
Ester	40–78 mg/dl	1.04–2.03 mmol/L	40–86 mg/dl	1.04–2.24 mmol/L

Table continued on following page

	Dog		Cat	
	Traditional units	*S.I. Units*	*Traditional Units*	*S.I. Units*
CO_2 total (S,P)	17–24 mEq/L	17–24 mmol/L	17–24 mEq/L	17–24 mmol/L
CO_2 pressure (B)	38 mm Hg	5.05 kPa	36 mm Hg	4.8 kPa
Copper (S)	100–120 µg/dl	15.7–18.8 µmol/L		
Cortisol				
Fluorometric	5–10 µg/dl		1.66 ± 0.12*[24]	
CPB[30]	2–6 µg/dl		2–5 µg/dl	
RIA[23]	1.8–4 µg/dl	49.7–110 nmol/L	1–3 µg/dl	27.6–82.8 nmol/L
Creatine phosphokinase (S)[10]	6–80 U/L	6–80 U/L		
Creatinine (S,P,HP)	0.5–1.5 mg/dl	44–133 µmol/L	0.8–1.8 mg/dl	70–159 mol/L
Fibrinogen (P,HP)	200–400 mg/dl	2–4 g/L	100–400 mg/dl	1–4 g/L
Folate (S)[3]	4.8–13 µg/L (8.9 ± 0.6 (SE) µg/L)	10.8–29.5 nmol/L (20.2 ± 1.3 (SE) nmol/L)		
Folate-red cells[3]	160–350 µg/L (230 ± 13 (SE) µg/L)	363–794 nmol/L (522 ± 29 (SE) nmol/L)		
Glucose (S,P,HP)	65–118 mg/dl	3.57–6.49 mmol/L	70–110 mg/dl	3.85–6.05 mmol/L
δ-Glutamyltransferase (S)	1.2–6.4 U/L	1.2–6.4 U/L	1.3–5.1 U/L	1.3–5.1 U/L
Insulin (S,HP)	5–15 µU/ml	35.9–107 pmol/L		
Iodine total (S)	5–10 µg/dl	0.39–0.79 µmol/L		
Iron (S)	94–122 µg/dl	16.8–21.8 µmol/L	68–215 µg/dl	12–38 µmol/L
Iron-binding capacity—total (S)[5]	280–340 µg/dl	50–60 µmol/L	170–400 µg/dl	30–71 µmol/L
Isocitrate dehydrogenase (S,HP)	0.4–7.3 U/L	0.4–7.3 U/L	2.0–11.7 U/L	2.0–11.7 U/L
Lactic acid (B)	2–13 mg/dl	0.22–1.44 mmol/L		
Lactate dehydrogenase (S,HP)	45–233 U/L	45–233 U/L	63–273 U/L	63–273 U/L
LDH isoenzymes (S,HP)				
LDH-1 (heart, fast)	1.7–30.2% (13.9 ± 9.5%)*		0–8.0% (4.5 ± 2.8%)*	
LDH-2	1.2–11.7% (5.5 ± 4.2%)*		3.3–13.7% (6.1 ± 3.7%)*	
LDH-3	10.9–25.0% (17.1 ± 5.7%)*		10.2–20.4% (13.3 ± 3.4%)*	
LDH-4	11.9–15.4% (13.0 ± 1.2%)*		11.6–35.9% (23.6 ± 8.6%)*	
LDH-5 (liver, slow)	30.0–72.8% (50.5 ± 16.9)*		40.0–66.3% (52.5 ± 9.3%)*	
Lead (B)	0–50 µg/dl	0–2.4 µmol/L		
Lipase (S)	13–200 U/L	13–200 U/L	0–83 U/L	0–83 U/L
Magnesium (S,HP)	1.8–2.4 mg/dl	0.74–0.98 mmol/L	2.2 mg/dl	0.90 mmol/L
Ornithine carbamyltransferase	2.7 ± 0.7 U/L	2.7 ± 0.7 U/L	3.8 ± 1.0 U/L	3.8 ± 1.0 U/L
O_2 pressure (B)	85–100 mm Hg	11.3–13.3 kPa	78–100 mm Hg	10.4–13.3 kPa
pH (b)	7.31–7.42	7.31–7.42	7.24–7.40	7.24–7.40
Phosphatase, acid (S,HP)	5–25 U/L	5–25 U/L	0.5–24 U/L	0.5–24 U/L
Alkaline (S,HP)	20–156 U/L	20–156 U/L	25–93 U/L	25–93 U/L
Potassium (S,HP)	4.37–5.65 mEq/L	4.37–5.65 mmol/L	4.0–4.5 mEq/L	4.0–4.5 mmol/L
Potassium—red cells	9 mEq/L	9 mmol/L	6 mEq/L	6 mmol/L
Protein total (S)	5.4–7.1 g/dl	54–71 g/L	5.4–7.8 g/dl	54–78 g/L
Albumin	2.6–3.3 g/dl	26–33 g/L	2.1–3.3 g/dl	21–33 g/L
Globulin (G)	2.7–4.4 g/dl	27–44 g/L	2.6–5.1 g/dl	26–51 g/L
α_1	0.2–0.5 g/dl	2–5 g/L	0.2–1.1 g/dl	2–11 g/L
α_2	0.3–1.1 g/dl	3–11 g/L	0.4–0.9 g/dl	4–9 g/L
β_1	0.7–1.3 g/dl	7–13 g/L	0.3–0.9 g/dl	3–9 g/L
β_2	0.6–1.4 g/dl	6–14 g/L	0.6–1.0 g/dl	6–10 g/L
δ_1	0.5–1.3 g/dl	5–13 g/L	0.3–2.5 g/dl	3–25 g/L
δ_2	0.4–0.9 g/dl	4–9 g/L	1.4–1.9 g/dl	14–19 g/L
A/G ratio	0.59–1.11		0.45 ± 1.19	
Protoporphyrin—red cells	35 µg/dl	0.63 µmol/L		
Sodium—serum	141.1–152.3 mEq/L	141.1–152.3 mmol/L	147–156 mEq/L	147–156 mmol/L
Red cells	107 mEq/L	107 mmol/L	104 mEq/L	104 mmol/L
Sorbitol dehydrogenase (S,HP)	2.9–8.2 U/L	2.9–8.2 U/L	3.9–7.7 U/L	3.9–7.7 U/L

Table continued on opposite page

Blood, Plasma, and Serum Values[17] (Continued)

	Dog		Cat	
	Traditional units	S.I. Units	Traditional Units	S.I. Units
Thyroxine—RIA (S)	0.6–3.6 µg/dl	7.8–46.8 nmol/L		
CPB (S)	0.3–2.5 µg/dl	3.9–32.5 nmol/L	0.1–2.5 µg/dl	1.3–32.5 nmol/L
Triiodothyronine—RIA (S)	82–138 ng/dl	1.26–2.12 nmol/L		
Transaminase (AST, SGOT) (S,P,HP)	23–66 U/L	23–66 U/L	26–43 U/L	26–43 U/L
(ALT, SGPT) (S,P,HP)	21–102 U/L	21–102 U/L	6–83 U/L	6–83 U/L
Triglycerides (S)[14]	42 ± 19 (SE) mg/dl	4.6 ± 2 mmol/L		
Urea nitrogen (B,P,HP,S)	10–28 mg/dl	3.6–10 mmol/L	20–30 mg/dl	7.1–10.7 mmol/L
Uric acid (S,P,HP)	0–2 mg/dl	0–0.12 mmol/L		
Vitamin B_{12} (S)[3]	200–400 ng/L	148–296 pmol/L		
	(277 ± 14 ng/L)	(205 ± 10.3 pmol/L)		
binding capacity (S)	886 ng/L	655 pmol/L		
Zinc	58–150 µg/dl	9–23 µmol/L		

Notes: B = blood; HP = heparinized plasma; P = plasma; S = serum; CPB = competitive protein binding; RIA = radioimmunoassay; SE = standard error of the mean; * = standard deviation.

Cerebrospinal Fluid Values[8]

	Dog		Cat	
	Traditional Units	S.I. Units	Traditional Units	S.I. Units
Appearance	Clear and colorless		Clear and colorless	
pH	7.4–7.6		7.4–7.6	
Specific gravity[31]	1.004–1.006		1.005–1.007	
Total protein	15.0–34.8 mg/dl	0.15–0.35 g/L	20–27 mg/dl	0.20–0.27 g/L
Albumin	13.9–27.0 mg/dl	0.14–0.27 g/L	19–25 mg/dl	0.19–0.25 g/L
Globulin	5.5–16.5 mg/dl	0.55–0.16 g/L		
Pandy test[32]	Negative		Negative	
Cell count	0–8/µl	0–8 × 10⁶/L	0–5/µl	0–5 × 10⁶/L
Cell type	15–95% small lymphocytes 5–40% large lymphocytes Occasional epithelial cell		Lymphocytes	
Glucose	74–75 mg/dl	4.11–4.17 mmol/L	85 mg/dl	4.72 mmol/L
Calcium	5.6–6.5 mg/dl	1.40–1.62 mmol/L	5.2 mg/dl	1.3 mmol/L
Phosphorus	1.1–3.9 mg/dl	0.27–0.97 mmol/L		
Sodium	151–155 mEq/l	151–155 mmol/L	158 mEq/L	158 mmol/L
Potassium	2.98–3.11 mEq/L	2.98–3.11 mmol/L	3.0–5.9 mEq/L	3.0–5.9 mmol/L
Chloride	131–138 mEq/L	131–138 mmol/L	144 mEq/L	144 mmol/L
Magnesium	2.6–3.8 mg/dl	1.06–1.55 mmol/L	1.33 mg/dl	0.54 mmol/L
Urea nitrogen	10–11 mg/dl	3.57–3.92 mmol/L	10–11 mg/dl	3.57–3.92 mmol/L
Creatinine phosphokinase[16]	3.1 IU/L	3.1 IU/L		
SGOT (AST)	10–20 IU/L	10–20 IU/L		
Pressure	< 170 mm H_2O		< 100 mm H_2O	
Rate of secretion	49 ± 20 µl/min		22.7 ± 3.2 µl/min	

Urine Constituents[5] (per kg body wt per day)

	Dog		Cat	
	Traditional Units	S.I. Units	Traditional Units	S.I. Units
Calcium	1–3 mg	0.025–0.075 mmol	0.2–0.45 mg	0.005–0.01 mmol
Magnesium	1.7–3.0 mg	0.07–0.12 mmol	0.13 mEq	0.065 mmol
Phosphorus	20–30 mg	0.64–0.96 mmol		
Creatine	10–50 mg	0.077–0.38 mmol		
Creatinine	30–80 mg	0.26–0.7 mmol		
Uric acid	0.2–13.0 mg	0.001–0.07 mmol	4.5 mg	0.026 mmol
17-ketosteroids	0.04–0.1 mg	0.14–0.34 µmol		
Chloride	0–10.3 mEq	0–10.3 mmol		
Sodium	0.04–13.0 mEq	0.04–13.0 mmol		

Urine Values[21]

Urine	Dog	Cat
Volume (ml/kg body wt/day)	24–41	22–30
Volume (L per day)	0.5–2	
Specific gravity		
Minimum	1.001	1.001
Maximum	1.060	1.080
Usual range	1.018–1.050	0.018–1.051
	(av 1.025)	(av 1.030)
Osmolality urine (mOsm/kg water)	500–1200	
Maximal limits	2000–2400	
pH	5.5–7.5	5.5–7.5
Effective renal plasma flow	$266 \pm 66^*$ ml/min/m² body surface	
	$13.5 \pm 3.3^*$ ml/min/kg body wt	
Glomerular filtration rate	$84.4 \pm 19^*$ ml/min/m² body wt	
	4 ml/min/kg body wt	
Urinalysis Semiquantitative Values[5]		
Protein	0–trace	0–trace
Glucose	0	0
Ketones	0	0
Bilirubin	0–1 +	0
Urobilinogen (Ehrlich unit)	1	1
(Wallace and Diamond)	< 1:32	< 1:32

Normal Canine Values for Feces[19]

Parameter	Value
Fecal trypsin[19]	Present up to 1:100 or 1:320 dilution[28]
Meat diet	4.96 ± 1.66 mg/kg body wt/day
	450.2 ± 141.6 mg/g feces
Cereal diet	1.11 ± 0.22 mg/kg body wt/day
	56.4 ± 9.6 mg/g feces
Fecal fat	
Meat diet	0.24 ± 0.01 mg/kg/body wt/day
	1.31 ± 0.2 g/day
	3.13 ± 0.53 g/100 g feces
Cereal diet	0.23 ± 0.01 mg/kg body wt/day
	1.64 ± 0.14 g/day
	1.22 ± 0.07 g/100 g feces
Fat assimilation	
Meat diet	96.9 ± 0.8 (SE*) %
Cereal diet	90.0 ± 1.2 (SE) %
Fecal weight	
Meat diet	8.54 ± 0.21 g/kg body wt/day
Cereal diet	19.99 ± 1.61 g/kg body wt/day

*Standard error of the mean.

Canine Synovia*

	Range	Mean
Volume (ml)	0.1–1.00	0.24
pH	7.0–7.8	7.33
Leukocytes (× 10⁹/L)	0–2.9	0.43
Monocytes (%)		39.72
Lymphocytes (%)		44.10
Clasmatocytes (%)		4.20
Neutrophils (%)		1.38
Mucin clot test	Tight ropy clump in clear fluid	

*Carpal, elbow, shoulder, hip, stifle, and hock joints.[26]

Seminal Fluid[25]

	Dog	Cat
Volume	10 ml	0.04 ml
	(1–25 ml)	(0.01–0.12 ml)
Spermatozoan concentration	125 × 10⁹/L	1730 × 10⁹/L
	(20–540 × 10⁹/L)	(96–3740 × 10⁹/L)
pH	6.7	7.4
	(6.0–6.8)	
Approximate total sperm per ejaculation (billions)	1.25	0.057
Glycerophosphorylcholine	180 mg/dl	
	(110–240 mg/dl)	
Sodium	90 mg/dl	
	(50–124 mg/dl)	

Function Tests

Adrenal Gland
ACTH Stimulation Test[13]

Administer | (Dog) 20 Units corticotropin gel intramuscularly
Normal response | After five hours, plasma cortisol increases to 3.0–14.9 μg/dl (av 9.7 μg/dl) measured by fluorimetry or to 0.3–7.3 μg/dl (av 2.6 μg/dl) measured by competitive protein binding

Dexamethasone Suppression Test[13]

Administer | 0.1 mg dexamethasone/kg body wt orally
Normal response | Plasma cortisol drops to 5 g/dl (fluorimetry) or less after 12 hours

Thorn Test[32]

Administer | 20 U ACTH intramuscularly
Normal response | 75 to 99 per cent reduction in eosinophil count seven hours after injection

Intestine
D-*Xylose absorption*[15]

Administer | (Dog) D-Xylose as a 5% solution at 5 g/kg body wt orally (a higher dose appears necessary for the cat)
Normal response | A peak plasma xylose level of at least 675 mmol/L (45 mg/dl) is reached 60 to 90 minutes after oral dosing

Liver
Bromsulfalein (BSP) retention[9]

Administer | (Dog) 5 mg BSP/kg body wt, slowly intravenously over five min
Normal response | Less than 5 per cent BSP retention at 30 minutes[9] (some dogs up to 10 per cent retention); less then 1.5 per cent BSP retention at 45 min

Ammonia Tolerance[20]

Administer | (Dog) 0.1 g NH$_4$Cl/kg body wt orally
Normal Response | Less than 28 μmol/L (< 50 μg/dl) increase in blood ammonia levels at 30 and 60 min

Pancreas
Para-aminobenzoic Acid (PABA)[2, 28]

Administer | (Dog) N-benzoyl PABA by stomach tube at 35 μmol/kg body wt as a 3.5 mmol/L solution.
Normal response | Six-hour urinary excretion of PABA is 63.1% ± 3.5% (SE)
 | Serum values to 20 to 30 μmol/L (0.27–0.41 mg/dl) at 30 and 60 min

IV Glucose Tolerance[7]

Administer | (Dog and cat) 0.5 g glucose/kg body wt as a 50% solution, intravenously, after a 24-hour fast
Normal response | Plasma glucose should return to preinjection levels in one to one and one-half hours

Kidney
Sodium Sulfanilate Clearance

Administer | (Dog and cat) 20 mg sodium sulfanilate/kg body wt intravenously, at 100 mg/ml solution
Normal clearance | (Dog) $t_{1/2}$ 50 to 80 min[17]
 | (Cat $t_{1/2}$ 45.1 ± 7 min[12]

Phenolsulfonphthalein (PSP) Clearance

Administer | (Dog) 5 mg sodium PSP/kg body wt intravenously, at 20 mg/ml solution
Normal clearance | $t_{1/2}$ 18 to 24 min[17]

Endogenous Creatinine Clearance

Normal clearance | (Dog) 20 min—2.8 ± 0.96 ml/min/kg[11]
 | 60 ± 21.9 ml/min/m² body surface
 | range 26 to 70 ml/min/m³
 | 24 hr—3,7 ± 0.77 ml/min/kg[6]
 | 57.6 ± 9.3 ml/min/m² body surface
 | range 32 to 113 ml/minn/m²

Thyroid Gland
TSH Stimulation[17]

Administer | (Dog) 5 units thyrotropin intramuscularly
Response | Minimum response is a doubling of thyroxine (T$_4$) or triiodothyronine (T$_3$), measured by radioimmunoassay, 16 to 24 hours after injection; mean peak response occurs at 16 hours postinjection

1. Albritton, E. C.: *Standard Values in Blood*. W. B. Saunders, Philadelphia, 1952.

2. Batt, R. M., Bush, B. M., and Peters, T. J.: A new test for the diagnosis of exocrine pancreatic insufficiency in the dog. J. Small Anim. Pract. *20*:185, 1979.

3. Batt, R. M., and Morgan, J. O.: Role of serum folate and vitamin B_{12} concentrations in the differentiation of small intestinal abnormalities in the dog. Res. Vet. Sci. *32*:17, 1982.

4. Benjamin, M. M.: *Outline of Veterinary Clinical Pathology*, 3rd ed. Iowa State University Press, Ames, 1978.

5. Bentinck-Smith, J.: A roster of normal values for dogs and cats. *In* Kirk, R. W. (ed.): *Current Veterinary Therapy VII*. W. B. Saunders, Philadelphia, 1981, pp. 1321–1330.

6. Bovee, K. C., and Joyce, T.: Clinical evaluation of glomerular function: 24 hour creatinine clearance in dogs. J. Am. Vet. Med. Assoc. *174*:488, 1979.

7. Coles, E. H.: *Veterinary Clinical Pathology*, 2nd ed. W. B. Saunders, Philadelphia, 1974, p. 277.

8. Coles, E. H.: Cerebrospinal fluid. *In* Kaneko, J. J. (ed.): *Clinical Biochemistry of Domestic Animals*, 3rd ed. Academic Press, New York, 1980, pp. 719–731.

9. Cornelius, C. E.: Liver Function. *In* Kaneko, J. J. (ed.): *Clinical Biochemistry of Domestic Animals*, 3rd ed. Academic Press, New York, 1980, p. 221.

10. Duncan, J. R., and Prasse, K. W.: *Veterinary Laboratory Medicine. Clinical Pathology*. Iowa State University Press, Ames, 1977.

11. Finco, D. R.: Simultaneous determination of phenolsulfonphthalein excretion and endogenous creatinine clearance in the normal dog. J. Am. Vet. Med. Assoc. *159*:336, 1971.

12. Greenwood, L., and Finco, D. R.: Cited in Finco, D. R.: Kidney function. *In* Kaneko, J. J. (ed.): *Clinical Biochemistry of Domestic Animals*, 3rd ed. Academic Press, New York, 1980, p. 388.

13. Halliwell, R. E. W., Schwartzman, R. M., Hopkins, L., and McEvoy, D.: The value of plasma corticosteroid assays in the diagnosis of Cushing's disease in the dog. J. Small Anim. Pract. *12*:453, 1971.

14. Hayden, D. W., and Van Kruiningen, H. J.: Control values for evaluating gastrointestinal function in the dog. J. Am. Anim. Hosp. Assoc. *12*:31, 1976.

15. Hill, F. W. G., Kidder, D. E., and Frew, J.: A xylose absorption test for the dog. Vet. Rec. *87*:250, 1970.

16. Indreri, R. J., Holliday, T. A., and Keen, C. L.: Critical evaluation of creatinine phosphokinase in cerebrospinal fluid of dogs with neurologic disease. Am. J. Vet. Res. *41*:1299, 1980.

17. Kaneko, J. J. (ed.): *Clinical Biochemistry of Domestic Animals*, 3rd ed. Academic Press, New York, 1980, pp. 785–797.

18. Larson, E. J., and Morrill, C. C.: Evaluation of the bromsulfophthalein liver function test in the dog. Am. J. Vet. Res. *21*:949, 1960.

19. Merritt, A. M., Burrows, C. F., Cowgill, L., and Streett, W.: Fecal fat and trypsin in dogs fed a meat-base or cereal-base diet. J. Am. Vet. Med. Assoc. *174*:59, 1979.

20. Meyer, D. J., Strombeck, D. R., Stone, E. A., Zenoble, R. D., and Buss, D. D.: Ammonia tolerance test in clinically normal dogs and in dogs with portosystemic shunts. J. Am. Vet. Med. Assoc. *173*:377, 1978.

21. Osborne, C. A., Low, D. G., and Finco, D. R.: *Canine and Feline Urology*. W. B. Saunders, Philadelphia, 1972, p. 403.

22. Penny, R. H. C., Carlisle, C. H., and Davidson, H.: The blood and marrow picture of the cat. Br. Vet. J. *126*:459, 1970.

23. Reimers, T. J.: Cited in Kirk, R. W. (ed.): *Current Veterinary Therapy VII*. W. B. Saunders, Philadelphia, 1981, p. 1326.

24. Rivas, C., and Borrell, S.: Effects of corticotrophin and dexamethasone on the levels of corticosteroids, adrenaline and noradrenaline in the adrenal glands of cats. J. Endocrinol. *51*:283, 1971.

25. Roberts, S. J.: *Veterinary Obstetrics and Genital Diseases*, 2nd ed. Published by the author, Ithaca, NY, 1971, p. 622.

26. Sawyer, D. C.: Synovial fluid analysis of canine joints. J. Am. Vet. Med. Assoc. *143*:609, 1963.

27. Schalm, O. W., Jain, N. C., and Carroll, E. J.: *Veterinary Hematology*, 3rd ed. Lea & Febiger, Philadelphia, 1975.

28. Strombeck, D. R.: New method for evaluation of chymotrypsin deficiency in dogs. J. Am. Vet. Med. Assoc. *173*:1319, 1978.

29. Thornton, J. R.: Proceedings No. 48 of the University of Sydney Post Graduate Committee in Veterinary Science, 1979, p. 68.

30. Wallace, R.: Cited in Kirk, R. W. (ed.): *Current Veterinary Therapy VII*. W. B. Saunders, Philadelphia, 1981, p. 1326.

31. Wilson, J. W., and Stevens, J. B.: Analysis of cerebrospinal fluid specific gravity. J. Am. Vet. Med. Assoc. *172*:911, 1978.

32. Wright, J. A.: Evaluation of cerebrospinal fluid in the dog. Vet. Rec. *103*:48, 1978.

Index

Note: Page numbers in *italic* type indicate illustrations; page numbers followed by *t* refer to tables.

To avoid qualifying almost every item in the index with the terms *canine* and *feline*, these adjectives are included only where the distinction is required, that is, in discussions pertaining specifically to the dog or the cat.

Adrenal gland(s) *(Continued)*
  cortex of, hormones of, 1853–1854
  cortical tumor of, prognosis for, 1863
  diseases of, 1854–1863
    anesthesia and, 2692–2693
    medullary, 1861–1863
  function tests for, normal values in,
    2718t
  hormone secretion of, 1853–1854
  innervation of, 1852
  left, surgical approach to, 1862, *1862,
    1863*
  right, surgical approach to, 1862, *1862*
  surgical procedures of, 1861–1863
  tumor of, adrenalectomy for, 1861–1863
  vascularization of, 1852
Adrenal medulla, diseases of, 1861
  hormones of, 1854
  sympathetic, in surgical patient, 84–85
Adrenalectomy, 1861–1863
  bilateral, postoperative care for, 1863
    prognosis for, 1863
  feline, 1863
  intraoperative medication for, 1862
  maintenance therapy after, 1863
  postoperative care for, 1863
  preoperative preparation for, 1861–1862
  surgical approach to, 1862, *1862, 1863*
  via retroperitoneal space, in dog, 597,
    598
  vs. medical treatment, for Cushing's dis-
    ease, 1860
Adrenocorticotropic hormone (ACTH),
    82–83, 1843
  basal plasma, measurement of, in Cush-
    ing's disease, 1859
Adrenocorticotropic hormone stimulation
    test, for Cushing's disease, 1858
Adriamycin, toxic effects of, 2393t
Adventitia, esophageal, anatomy of, 653
Afghan hound, cancer types in, 2361t
  high-risk cancer sites in, 2361t
Aftercare, for surgical patient, 373–389.
    See also *Recovery period,* and under
    specific surgical procedures.
Afterload, cardiac, 1041–1042
Agammaglobulinemia, Bruton's, 196
    common variable, 196
Airedale terrier, cancer types in, 2361t
  high-risk cancer sites in, 2361t
Airway(s), functions of, 919
  hydration of, in postoperative care, 1027
  in cardiopulmonary resuscitation, 153
  obstruction of, as operating room emer-
    gency, 392
  patent, in postoperative care, 1023–1024
  resistance of, pulmonary compliance
    and, 921, 921t, *922*
  suctioning of, postoperative, 1024
  upper, obstruction of, as operating room
    emergency, 396
Albumin, plasma, drug binding with, ef-
    fect of anesthetics on, 2661
Alcohol, in scrubbing of surgical patient,
    281
  sterilization with, 268
Aldehydes, sterilization with, 268
Aldosterone, 1854
  adrenal production of, 1853, 1854
  stimuli of, 83, *84*

Aldosterone *(Continued)*
  function of, 1040
Alimentary tract, 605–848. See also *Gas-
    trointestinal tract.*
Alkalemia, preoperative evaluation of, 246
Alkalinizing agents, in shock, 143
Alkalinizing solutions, for fluid therapy,
    100
Alkaloids, chemical burns due to, 530
  plant, in cancer chemotherapy, 2411t,
    2414
Alkalosis, metabolic, 123–124
  compensatory response to, 120t
  etiology of, 121t
  factors in, 376t
  in shock, 143
  treatment of, 129–130
  preoperative evaluation of, 246
  respiratory, 121–122
    compensatory response to, 120t
    etiology of, 121t
    factors in, 376t
    treatment of, 129
Alkylating agents, in cancer chemother-
    apy, 2409, 2410t
Allergy, drug, to antimicrobials, 52,
    54–55t
Allografts, kidney, survival of, *200*
  rejection of, 205–210. See also *Rejec-
    tion.*
Aluminum, as suture material, 339
Alveolar-capillary membrane, structure of,
    925
Alveolar gas exchange, 102
  impaired, in critical care patient, 939
Alveolar ventilation, 923–924, *924*
Amblyopia, and quadriplegia, hereditary,
    features of, 1281t
Ambulation, postoperative, 381
American College of Veterinary Surgeons,
    establishment of, 4
Amino acids, in parenteral nutrition, 229
  metabolic problems of, 237
Aminoglycosides, adverse effects of, 54t
  drugs antagonistic with, 65t
  for urinary tract infections, 1761, 1761t
Ammonia, in hepatic encephalopathy,
    1159
Ammonium acid urate uroliths, in Dalma-
    tians, 1813
  medical dissolution of, 1821–1822
Ammonium compounds, quaternary, steri-
    lization with, 269
Ammonium ion, in renal acid-base regula-
    tion, 117
Amniotic fluid, 1697
  biochemistry of, 1697
  function of, 1697
  origin and fate of, 1697
Amoxicillin, pharmacokinetic data for, 61t
  regimen for, in dog and cat, 62t
Amphibians, regeneration of appendages
    in, 26–27
Amphotericin B, adverse effects of, in
    renal insufficiency, 68t
  regimen for, in dog and cat, 62t
Ampicillin, adverse effects of, 55t
  in renal insufficiency, 68t
  pharmacokinetic data for, 61t
  regimen for, in dog and cat, 62t

Ampicillin *(Continued)*
  time needed for peak concentrations of,
    57t
Amputations, 2276–2286. See also specific
    body parts.
  closure of stump in, 2277
  division of muscles in, 2277
  division of nerves in, 2277
  division of vessels in, 2277
  levels of, 2276–2277
  physiological considerations in, 2277
  techniques of, 2277–2286
  through joint vs. through bone, 2277
Anal canal, hidradenitis of, 778–779, *778,
    779*
Anal sac, diseases of, 775–777
  clinical signs of, 775
  treatment of, 775–777
  excision of, 776–777
  gel and applicator for, 776
  impaction of, 775
  infected, with fistulae, excision of, 777
  noninfected, excision of, 776
  ruptured, 779, *779*
  treatment of, 776, 777
  surgery of, complications in, 777
  infection in, 777
Anal sacculitis, 775
Anal sinuses, fistulae of, 779
Anal sphincter, external, anatomy of, 888
  hypertrophy of, 785–786
    pathogenesis of, 786
    treatment of, 786
  postoperative failure of, 777
Anal sphincter reflex, test of, 1294, *1295*
Anal splitting, in perineal hernia repair,
    896
Analeptics, in cardiopulmonary resuscita-
    tion, 154
Analgesia, epidural, in trauma, 2686
  musculoskeletal effects of, 2684
Analgesics, in shock, 144
  nephropathy due to, 1759
  postoperative, 378t, 379–380
  preanesthetic, 2596
Anamnesis, in cardiovascular disease, 1055
  in neurological disorders, 1287t
Anaphylaxis, passive cutaneous, character-
    istics of, 189t
  reverse passive cutaneous, characteris-
    tics of, 189t
  systemic, characteristics of, 188t
Anastomosis, intestinal, 722–729. See also
    Intestinal anastomosis.
  vascular, technique of, 1149–1151,
    1149–1151
Anconeal process, ununited (elbow dyspla-
    sia), 2322–2323, *2323*
Anemia, and blood loss, in wound healing,
    34–35
  aplastic, examination of bone marrow in,
    1200
  examination of bone marrow in, 1200
  hemolytic, splenectomy for, 1181
    surgical considerations in, 1180
  in systemic lupus erythematosus, 2304
  nonregenerative, surgical considerations
    in, 1181
  of chronic renal failure, 1738
  patients with, preparation for surgery of,
    1181–1182

Bone (*Continued*)
  healing of, in presence of wire implants, 2005–2007, *2006*
    primary, 1943
    secondary, 1943–1944
      fracture impact stage of, 1943
      induction stage of, 1943
      inflammation stage of, 1943
      hard callus stage of, 1944
      remodeling stage of, 1944
      soft callus stage of, 1944
  hyperparathyroid disease of, 2328–2329
  in growth phase, vascular patterns of, 2021, *2021*
  infections of, 2020–2030. See also *Osteomyelitis.*
    exogenous sources of, 2022
    hematogenous spread of, 2020–2022
    routes of contamination in, 2020–2022
  loss of, bone grafting in, 2044–2045
  mechanical properties of, 1939–1941, *1940*
  metabolic diseases of, 2328–2329
    thoracic involvement in, 543
  mineral crystals of, 1935, *1935*
    hormonal control of, 1935
  neonatal development of, *1935*, 1936
  osteolytic erosion of, metal corrosion in, 2025, *2026*
  physiology of, 1933–1937
  radionuclide imaging of, *1326*, 1327–1328
  structural anatomy of, 1933–1937, *1934–1936*
  traumatic injury to, 220
    metabolic response to, *86*
Bone graft(s), creeping substitution in, 2037
  functions of, 2036–2037
  harvesting and handling of, 2045–2047
  incorporation of, 2037–2042
    effect of surgical technique on, 2040
    factors affecting, 2040
    immunogenicity in, 2040
    methods of preservation and, 2040
  mechanical support with, 2037
  osteoconduction in, 2037
  osteogenesis in, 2036–2037
  remodeling in, 2037
  storage of, 2046
Bone grafting, 2035–2048
  allografts in, collection of, 2046
  alloimplants in, collection of, 2046
  autoclaved alloimplants in, 2041
  autografts in, collection of, 2046
  boiled alloimplants in, 2041
  cancellous autografts in, incorporation of, 2037, *2038*
    inflammatory stage of, 2037
    mechanical phase of, 2038
    vascularization and osteoinduction in, 2037
  cortical autografts in, 2038–2039
  decalcified bone in, 2041
  deproteinized alloimplants in, 2041
  freeze-dried alloimplants in, 2041
  fresh cancellous allografts in, 2040
  fresh cortical allografts in, 2040
  frozen alloimplants in, 2041
  immunosuppression in, 2041–2042
  indications for, 2042–2045

Bone grafting (*Continued*)
  merthiolated alloimplants in, 2041
  osteochondral grafts in, 2039–2040
  terminology of, 2036
  vascularized grafts in, 2039
  xenoimplants in, 2041
Bone marrow, 1199–1204
  aspiration of, 1201
    from femur, 1202
    from iliac crest, 1201–1202, *1202*
    needles for, *1201*, 2372, 2373, 2375
  differential cell counts of, 2713t
  examination of, 1200–1203
    evaluation of results in, 1203
    indications for, 1200–1201
    interpretation of samples in, 1200–1201
    preparation of samples for, 1203
    selection of sites for, 1201–1202
    techniques of, 1201–1202
  gross characteristics of, 1199
  organization of, 1199–1200
    microscopic, 1199–1200
  release of blood cells from, 1179
Bone marrow biopsy, 2372–2375
  needles for, 1201, *1201*, 2372, 2373, 2375
  technique of, 1202
    with Jamshidi needle, 2374, 2375
    vs. aspirate, 1201
Bone marrow toxicity, in cancer chemotherapy, 2408
Bone plating, implant removal in, 1971
  interfragmentary compression with, 1965–1966, *1965*
  postoperative management in, 1970–1971
  principles of application of, 1967–1970
  stress protection in, 1971
  theory and technique of, 1964–1971
Bone tumors, 2575–2581
  metastatic, 2581
    diagnosis of, 2581
    incidence of, 2581
Bowel. See *Colon.*
Boxer, cancer types in, 2361t
  high risk cancer sites in, 2361t
Brachial plexus, avulsion of, 1335–1338, *1336*
  diagnosis of, 1336–1337
  salvage procedures for, 1337–1338, *1337, 1338*
  sensory deficits in, *1336*
  functional anatomy of, 1246–1247
  muscles innervated by, 1246t
  nerves of, 1246t
Brachialis tendon, transplantation of, in brachial avulsion, 1337, *1337*
Brachytherapy, interstitial, 2390
Bradycardia, as operating room emergency, 397
  causes of, 397
  high vagal tone in, 397
  prevention of, 397
  treatment of, 397–398
Bradykinin, in shock, 136
Bradypnea, causes of, 394
  in operating room emergencies, 394
Brain, anatomy of, 1247–1250, *1250*, 1266–1268, 2499

Brain (*Continued*)
  arterial supply to, 1253–1254, *1253, 1254*
  biopsy of, 1306–1307
    technique of, 1306–1307
  cerebral blood flow in, chemical regulation of, 1269
    metabolic autoregulation of, 1269
    pressure autoregulation of, 1268, *1268*
  computed tomography of, *1327*, 1328–1329
  concussion of, 1424
  contusion of, 1425, *1425*
  Cushing response in, 1268–1269
  diseases of, categories of, 1269t
    etiology of, 1269t
  edema of, 1273, *1273*
    cytotoxic, 1273
    in intracranial tumors, 2505
    interstitial, 1273, *1273, 1274*
    vasogenic, 1273
  hematomas of, 1425–1426, *1426, 1427*
    treatment of, 1427
  herniation of, 1266, *1267*
  laceration of, 1425
  necrosis of (encephalomalacia), 1269–1271
  nuclear imaging of, 1324–1328
  physiology of, 1268–1269
    changes in, in cardiac bypass, 1140
  radiography of, 1315–1319
    patient positioning in, 1315–1316
    special techniques in, 1318–1319
    technique of, 1315–1316
  radionuclide imaging of, 1325–1327, *1326*
  response to disease of, 1269
  surgery of, 1415–1429
  trauma of, 1424–1427
    malacia in, 1271, *1271, 1272*
  tumors of, 1274–1276, *1274*, 1275t, 1414, 1415–1424, 2499–2507
    clinical signs in, 1415, *1415*
    secondary, 2504
  venous drainage of, 1254–1255, *1254*
  ventricular system of, *1255*
    development of, 1248t
Brain stem, contusion of, 1425, *1425*
Brain stem–evoked responses, 1312, *1312*
Brain stem syndromes, 1262–1265
Breast, anatomy of, 505
  lymphatic drainage of, *505*
  tumors of, 2553–2558. See also *Mammary tumors.*
    in male dog, 2542–2543
      diagnosis of, 2542–2543
      incidence of, 2542, 2542t
      treatment of, 2543
Breathing. See also *Respiration; Ventilation.*
  in cardiopulmonary resuscitation, 153–154
  rapid, as operating room emergency, 392
  work of, 923, *923*
Breathing pattern, changes in, 353
Brodie's abscess, 2023
Brodifacoum (Talon), poisoning with, 1188
Bronchial tree, anatomy of, *912*, 913–916
Bronchiectasis, 1013–1014
Bronchitis, etiologic agents in, 64t

Scapula (*Continued*)
  injury of, radiographic positioning for, 2049, *2049*
  neck of, fractures of, 2052–2056
    stabilization methods for, *2053, 2054, 2055*
Scapulohumeral joint, anatomy of, 2056–2057, *2057*
  luxation of, 2056–2061. See also *Shoulder.*
Scars, constricting, Z-plasty for, 455, *455*
  tension release along, Z-plasty for, 454, *454*
Schiff-Sherrington phenomenon, 1278, 1371
Schroeder-Thomas (traction) splint, 2001–2002, *2001–2003*
Sciatic nerve, evaluation of, 1294
  signs of dysfunction of, 1257t
Sciatic nerve paralysis, in perineal hernia repair, 896
Scissors, surgical, 306–307, *306*
  dissecting, technique for use of, 314–316, *315*
  for blunt dissection, *315*, 316
  hand signal for, at operating table, 297
  Potts, *1103*
  push-cutting with, 316
  technique for use of, 314–316
  types of, 314, *315*
Sclera, anatomy of, 1510, *1511*
  and cornea, 1509–1531
  layers of, 1510, *1511*
  melanoma of, 2528, *2529*
Scleral fixation sutures, 1442
Sclerectomy, with cyclodialysis and iridencleisis, for glaucoma, 1576–1578, *1576, 1577*
Scottish terrier, cancer types in, 2361t
  high-risk cancer sites in, 2361t
Scratching, aural hematoma due to, 1890–1891
Screws, in fixation of fractures, 1965–1966, *1965, 1966*, 1967–1970
Screw tail (ingrown tail), 512–513, *512*
Scrotum, 1649–1650
  ablation of, 1623–1626, *1626*
  anatomy of, *1602,* 1608
  and prepuce, amputation of, incision site for, *1632*
  biopsy of, 1617
  chronic hyperplasia of, 1650
  hernias in, 865–867. See also *Hernias, scrotal.*
  injury to, 1649
  neoplasms of, 1650
  pathophysiology of, 1613
  physiology of, 1611
  skin of, infection of, 1649–1650
  varicosities of, 1650
Scrub, surgical, 272
  sinks for, 289, *289*
Scrub suits, 270–271, *270*
Scrubbing, of skin of surgical patient, 281, 281
Scurvy, canine, 2313–2314, *2313, 2314*
Sebaceous gland tumors, 2444–2445
  of ear, 1898
  of eyelids, 2524, *2526*
Sedatives, effect on respiration of, 2625

Sedatives (*Continued*)
  postoperative, 378t, 379–380
  in excessive anesthesia, 392
Seizures, syndromes associated with, 1265
Self-recognition, and autoimmune diseases, 204
Semen, evaluation of, 1615–1616
  normal values for, 2717t
Seminal fluid, normal values for, 2716t
Seminoma(s), testicular, 2538
Sensitivity, contact, 190
Sensory nerve conduction, 1311
  reference values for, *1311*
Sensory perception, evaluation of, 1296
Sepsis, in chronic catheterization, 235–236
  in loss of skin grafts, 489
Septic arthritis, 2030–2034
  diagnosis of 2032–2033
  exogenous, 2030
  hematogenous, 2030
  pathophysiology of, 2031–2032
  routes of contamination in, 2030–2031, *2031*
  synovial fluid changes in, 2032, 2032t
  treatment of, 2033–2034
Septicemia(s), puppy, etiologic agents in, 64t
  role of spleen in, 1207–1208
Sequestrum, development of, 2023
  radiographic appearance of, *2025*
Seroma, formation of, as complication of wound healing, 440–441
  in loss of skin grafts, 489
Serratus ventralis muscle, rupture of, 2335
Sertoli cell tumor, ovarian, 2548
  testicular, 2537–2538
Serum, normal values for, 2713–2715t
Serum sickness, characteristics of, 189t
Sesamoid fractures, 2137
Sex chromosomes, in dog, 204
Shock, 130–148
  adrenergic drugs for, 142
  analgesics in, 144
  anaphylactic, 132
  anesthetics in, 144
  antiarrhythmic drugs for, 141–143
  anticholinergic drugs for, 142
  arterial venous oxygen difference in, 137
  as surgical complication, 165–166
  basic changes in, 133–134
  body temperature in, 143–144
  burn. See *Burn shock.*
  cardiac drugs for, 141
  cardiogenic, 132–133
    management of, 145
  cell in, 134
  circulatory, types of, 131–133
  classification of, 131t
  clinical indications of, 138
  corticosteroids for, 141
  definition of, 130
  disseminated intravascular coagulation in, 144
  hyperdynamic, 133
  hypodynamic, 133
  hypovolemic, 131
    management of, 144–145
  inciting factors in, 131t
  initial evaluation of, 137–138, 138t
  inotropic drugs for, 142

Shock (*Continued*)
  lactic acid and lactate measurements in, 144
  maldistributive (septic), 133
    management of, 145
  management of, 137–146
  neurogenic, 131. See also *Shock, vasculogenic.*
  organ systems in, 134–137
  oxygen consumption in, 137
  pathophysiology of, 133–137
  postoperative, 374
  recognition of, 137–138, 138t
  reflex mechanisms in, 133–134
  septic, 133
    management of, 145
  spinal, 1277
  traumatic, 133
  treatment of, monitoring patient response to, 138–144
    recent developments in, 145–146
  vasculogenic, 131–132
    management of, 145
  vasodilators for, 141
  ventilation and oxygenation in, 140–141
Shoe covers, surgical, 271
Short bowel syndrome, after intestinal surgery, 734
Shotgun injuries, 222
Shoulder. See also *Scapulohumeral joint.*
  caudal luxation of, 2061
    salvage techniques for, 2061
  cranial luxation of, 2060–2061
    surgical technique for, 2060–2061
  lateral luxation of, 2057–2058
    conservative management of, 2057
    surgical technique for, 2057–2058, *2058*
  medial luxation of, 2058–2060
    conservative management of, 2059
    surgical technique for, 2059–2060, *2059, 2060*
  neurovascular anatomy of, *2063*
  osteochondritis dissecans of, 2317–2319, *2317–2319*
Sialoliths, 649–650, *650*
Siamese cats, peritoneopericardial hernias in, 875t
Siggaard-Andersen nomogram, for blood acid-base alignment, 114, *114*
Sigmoidoscopy, 348
Silica uroliths, 1814–1815
Silicone, in soft tissue implants, 173
Silk, as suture material, 337–338, *338*
Silver, as suture material, 339
Sinus(es). See also *Nasal sinus(es).*
  dermoid, 504, *504*
  frontal, of dog, anatomy of, 905, *906*
  paranasal, functional anatomy of, 905–906, *906*
    orbital walls and, *1555*
Sinus tachycardia, as operating room emergency, 398–400
  consequences of, 398
  treatment of, 398
Sinusitis, chronic, in cats, 970–972
    sinus drainage in, 970
    sinus flushing in, 970, *970*
    surgical approach to, 970–972
  in dogs, sinus drainage in, *971*
    sinus obliteration in, 970, *971*

CARDIOPULMONARY RESUSCITATION [a]

Steve C. Haskins

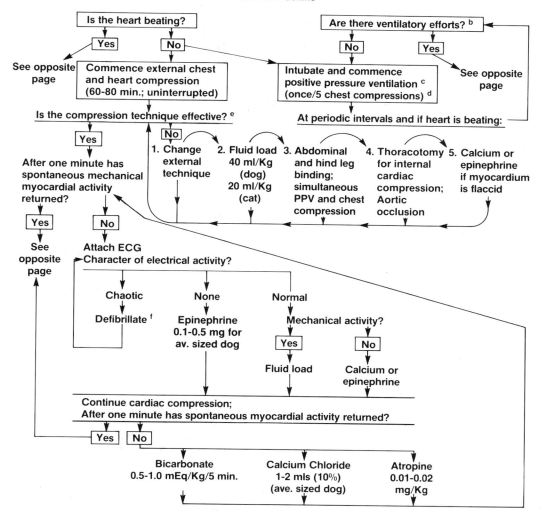

[a] The chart represents diagnostic differentials for the treatment of cardiac and respiratory failure. Emergency support procedures are suggested. The chart is only a guide; specific therapeutic regimens should be tailored to individual patients.

[b] Agonal gaping of the mandible with or without gasps of air constitutes a "No" answer.

[c] Proximal airway pressure 15 cm H_2O; inspiratory time just long enough to achieve a full tidal volume; 10-12 times per minute; and deftly interspersed between continuous chest compressions.

[d] If alone, twice per 15 chest compressions

[e] Peripheral pulse with each compression; mucous membrane color improvement; decreasing pupil size.

[f] Direct current defibrillation   Small patient—internal 10-25 ws; external 100-150 ws
    Large patient—internal 100-150 ws; external 400 ws

    Pharmacologic defibrillation 1) 20-30 mEq K^+ followed by calcium solution
    2) K^+ 1 mEq/Kg plus Acetylcholine 6mg/Kg

[g] Lactated Ringer's solution or equivalent; 20-90 ml/Kg (dog); 10-50 ml/Kg (cat); Whole blood, plasma, or dextran 2-5 ml/Kg/hr up to 20 ml/Kg

[h] Phenylephrine 0.01-0.1 mg/Kg

[i] Dopamine (200 mg in 500 ml D_5W) 2-20 μg/Kg/min; Mephenteramine 0.1-0.75 mg/Kg; Dobutamine 5-10 μg/Kg/min; Isoproterenol 0.01-0.02 μg/Kg/min

[j] Digoxin-Loading 0.1-0.2 mg/Kg divided into 4 doses, Maintenance 0.01-0.02 mg/Kg twice daily

[k] Acepromazine 0.02-0.1 mg/Kg; Hydralazine 0.2-0.5 mg/Kg; Nitroprusside 0.5-10 μg/Kg/min; Phentolamine 5-30 μg/Kg/min; Phenoxybenzamine 0.5-1.0 mg/Kg

[l] Aminophylline 5-20 mg/Kg; Nebulized beta-2 or beta-1 agonists [o]

[m] Glucocorticosteroids; Nebulized alpha-receptor agonists [h]